Robert D. Odze, MD, FRCP(C)
Associate Professor
Department of Pathology
Harvard Medical School
Director, Division of Gastrointestinal Pathology
Brigham and Women's Hospital
Boston, Massachusetts

John R. Goldblum, MD
Professor of Pathology
Cleveland Clinic Lerner College of Medicine
Chairman
Department of Anatomic Pathology
Cleveland Clinic Foundation
Cleveland, Ohio

James M. Crawford, MD, PhD
Professor and Chairman
Department of Pathology, Immunology and
Laboratory Medicine
University of Florida College of Medicine
Gainesville, Florida

Surgical Pathology
of the
GI Tract, Liver, Biliary Tract, and Pancreas

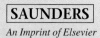
SAUNDERS
An Imprint of Elsevier

SAUNDERS
An Imprint of Elsevier

The Curtis Center
Independence Square West
Philadelphia, Pennsylvania 19106

SURGICAL PATHOLOGY OF THE GI TRACT, LIVER,
BILIARY TRACT, AND PANCREAS   ISBN 0–7216–9318–0

Notice

Pathology is an ever-changing field. Standard safety precautions must be followed but as new research and clinical experience broaden our knowledge, changes in treatment and drug therapy may become necessary or appropriate. Readers are advised to check the most current product information provided by the manufacturer of each drug to be administered to verify the recommended dose, the method and duration of administration, and contraindications. It is the responsibility of the treating physician, relying on experience and knowledge of the patient, to determine dosages and the best treatment for each individual patient. Neither the Publisher nor the author assumes any liability for any injury and/or damage to persons or property arising from this publication.

The Publisher

Library of Congress Cataloging-in-Publication Data

Odze, Robert D.
    Surgical pathology of the GI tract, liver, biliary tract, and pancreas/Robert D. Odze,
John R. Goldblum, James M. Crawford.—1st ed.
        p. cm.
    ISBN 0–7216–9318–0
        1. Pathology, Surgical. 2. Gastrointestinal system—Surgery. 3. Liver—Surgery. 4. Biliary
tract—Surgery. 5. Pancreas—Surgery. I. Goldblum, John R. II. Crawford, James M. III. title.

RD540.O396 2004
617.4′3—dc21   2003054418

Acquisitions Editor: Natasha Andjelkovic
Project Manager: Amy Norwitz

RT/CTP

Printed in China
Last digit is the print number: 9 8 7 6 5 4 3

This book is dedicated, with love, to Tony, Liane,
my dear mother Natasha, and my late father Walter.

ROBERT D. ODZE, MD, FRCP(C)

To those whom I hold most dear: my wife Asmita,
my children Andrew, Ryan, Janavi and Raedan,
my parents Bette and Raymond, and the rest of the
Goldblum and Shirali families whom I also cherish.

JOHN R. GOLDBLUM, MD

To my wife Aleta, my dearest companion in life,
and to my children Bristol and Jenness, parents
Jean and Jim, and parents-in-law Sarah and John.

JAMES M. CRAWFORD, MD, PHD

Contributors

SUSAN C. ABRAHAM, MD
Assistant Professor, Mayo Medical School; Senior
Associate Consultant, Department of Laboratory
Medicine and Pathology, Mayo Clinic, Rochester,
Minnesota
Chapter 15: Polyps of the Large Intestine

N. VOLKAN ADSAY, MD
Associate Professor of Pathology, Wayne State
University School of Medicine;
Harper Hospital, Detroit, Michigan
*Chapter 31: Benign and Malignant Tumors of
the Pancreas*

JORGE ALBORES-SAAVEDRA, MD
Professor of Pathology and Director, Division of
Anatomic Pathology, Louisiana State University, Health
Sciences Center, School of Medicine, Shreveport,
Louisiana
*Chapter 29: Benign and Malignant Tumors of the
Gallbladder and Extrahepatic Biliary Tract*

LILIAN B. ANTONIO, MPH
Laboratory Supervisor, Mount Sinai Hospital, New
York, New York
Chapter 32: Liver Tissue Processing Techniques

DONALD A. ANTONIOLI, MD
Professor of Pathology, Harvard Medical School and
Beth Israel Deaconess Medical Center, Boston,
Massachusetts
Chapter 14: Polyps of the Small Intestine

KAMRAN BADIZADEGAN, MD
Assistant Professor of Pathology, Harvard Medical
School; Assistant Pathologist, Massachusetts General
Hospital, Boston, Massachusetts
Chapter 40: Liver Pathology in Pregnancy

CHARLES BALABAUD, MD
Professor of Medicine, University Bordeaux 2;
Chief, Department of Hepato-Gastroenterology,
Saint André Hospital, University Hospital, Bordeaux,
France
*Chapter 36: Toxic and Drug-Induced Disorders of
the Liver*

KENNETH P. BATTS, MD
Director of Gastrointestinal and Hepatic Pathology,
Hospital Pathology Associates; Department of
Pathology, Abbott Northwestern Hospital,
Minneapolis, Minnesota
*Chapter 35: Autoimmune and Cholestatic Disorders of
the Liver*

PAULETTE BIOULAC-SAGE, MD
Professor of Medicine, University Bordeaux 2; Chief,
Department of Pathology, Pellegrin Hospital,
University Hospital, Bordeaux, France
*Chapter 36: Toxic and Drug-Induced Disorders of
the Liver*

MARY P. BRONNER, MD
Director of GI and Hepatic Pathology Fellowship
Program; Staff Pathologist, Cleveland Clinic
Foundation, Department of Anatomic Pathology,
Cleveland, Ohio
*Chapter 7: Inflammatory Disorders of the
Esophagus*

LAWRENCE J. BURGART, MD
Associate Professor, Mayo Medical School; Chair,
Anatomic Pathology, Mayo Clinic, Rochester,
Minnesota
Chapter 15: Polyps of the Large Intestine

NORMAN J. CARR, FRCPath

Honorary Clinical Lecturer, Southhampton University; Consultant Histopathologist, Department of Cellular Pathology, Southampton General Hospital, Southampton, Hampshire, United Kingdom
Chapter 20: Epithelial Neoplasms of the Appendix

BARBARA A. CENTENO, MD

Associate Professor, University of South Florida School of Medicine; Director of the Cytopathology, H. Lee Moffitt Cancer Center and Research Institute, Tampa, Florida
Chapter 26: Diagnostic Cytology of the Pancreas and Biliary Tract

JAMES M. CRAWFORD, MD, PhD

Professor and Chairman, Department of Pathology, Immunology and Laboratory Medicine, University of Florida College of Medicine, Gainesville, Florida
Chapter 1: Gastrointestinal Tract Endoscopic and Tissue Processing Techniques
Chapter 25: Gallbladder, Extrahepatic Biliary Tract, and Pancreas Tissue Processing Techniques
Chapter 37: Cirrhosis
Chapter 39: Transplantation Pathology of the Liver
Chapter 41: Inherited and Developmental Disorders of the Liver

ANTHONY J. DEMETRIS, MD

Professor of Pathology, University of Pittsburgh, School of Medicine; Professor of Pathology, Director of Transplant Pathology, University of Pittsburgh Medical Center, Pittsburgh, Pennsylvania
Chapter 39: Transplantation Pathology of the Liver

THERESA S. EMORY, MD

Associate Clinical Professor of Pathology, East Tennessee State University, Johnson City, Tennessee; Highlands Pathology Consultants, Kingsport, Tennessee
Chapter 20: Epithelial Neoplasms of the Appendix

FRANCIS A. FARRAYE, MD, MSC

Clinical Director, Section of Gastroenterology; Associate Professor of Medicine and Epidemiology, Boston Medical Center, Boston, Massachusetts
Chapter 1: Gastrointestinal Tract Endoscopic and Tissue Processing Techniques

LINDA D. FERRELL, MD

Professor and Vice Chair of Pathology, University of California, San Francisco, San Francisco, California
Chapter 42: Benign and Malignant Tumors of the Liver

JUDITH A. FERRY, MD

Associate Professor of Pathology, Harvard Medical School; Associate Pathologist and Associate Director of Surgical Pathology, Department of Pathology, Massachusetts General Hospital, Boston, Massachusetts
Chapter 23: Lymphoid Tumors of the GI Tract

ROBERT M. GENTA, MD

Professor and Chief, Division de Pathologie Clinique, Département de Pathologie, Hôpitaux Universitaires de Genève, Geneva, Switzerland; Adjunct Professor of Pathology and Medicine, Baylor College of Medicine, Houston, Texas
Chapter 8: Inflammatory Disorders of the Stomach

JONATHAN N. GLICKMAN, MD, PhD

Assistant Professor of Pathology, Harvard Medical School; Staff Pathologist, Brigham and Women's Hospital, Boston, Massachusetts
Chapter 16: Epithelial Neoplasms of the Esophagus

JOHN R. GOLDBLUM, MD

Professor of Pathology, Cleveland Clinic Lerner College of Medicine; Chairman, Department of Anatomic Pathology, Cleveland Clinic Foundation, Cleveland, Ohio
Chapter 22: Mesenchymal Tumors of the GI Tract

FIONA GRAEME-COOK, FRCP

Assistant Professor, Harvard Medical School; Assistant Pathologist, Massachusetts General Hospital, Boston, Massachusetts
Chapter 21: Neuroendocrine Tumors of the GI Tract and Appendix

JOEL K. GREENSON, MD

Professor of Pathology, Department of Pathology, University of Michigan Health System, Ann Arbor, Michigan
Chapter 10: Inflammatory Diseases of the Large Intestine

CLARA S. HEFFESS, MD

Chief, Endocrine Division, Department of Endocrine and Otorhinolaryngic–Head and Neck Pathology, Armed Forces Institute of Pathology, Washington, DC
Chapter 30: Inflammatory, Infectious, and Other Non-neoplastic Disorders of the Pancreas

CHRISTINE A. IACOBUZIO-DONAHUE, MD, PhD

Instructor, Division of GI/Liver Pathology, Johns Hopkins Medical Institutions, Baltimore Maryland

Chapter 24: Inflammatory and Neoplastic Disorders of the Anal Canal

BRIAN C. JACOBSON, MD, MPH

Assistant Professor of Medicine, Boston University School of Medicine; Associate Director of Endoscopy, Boston University Medical Center, Boston, Massachusetts

Chapter 1: Gastrointestinal Tract Endoscopic and Tissue Processing Techniques

DHANPAT JAIN, MD

Assistant Professor, Department of Pathology, Yale University School of Medicine; Yale-New Haven Hospital, New Haven, Connecticut

Chapter 6: Neuromuscular Disorders of the GI Tract

JOSE JESSURUN, MD

Professor of Pathology, University of Minnesota School of Medicine; Director, Surgical Pathology, Fairview-University Medical Center, Minneapolis, Minnesota

Chapter 28: Infectious and Inflammatory Disorders of the Gallbladder and Extrahepatic Biliary Tract

DAVID S. KLIMSTRA, MD

Associate Professor of Pathology, Weill Medical College of Cornell University; Attending Pathologist, Memorial Sloan-Kettering Cancer Center, New York, New York

Chapter 31: Benign and Malignant Tumors of the Pancreas

A. S. KNISELY, MD

Consultant Histopathologist, Institute of Liver Studies, King's College Hospital, Denmark Hill, London, United Kingdom

Chapter 41: Inherited and Developmental Disorders of the Liver

LAURA W. LAMPS, MD

Associate Professor of Pathology, University of Arkansas for Medical Sciences, Little Rock, Arkansas

Chapter 3: Infectious Diseases of the GI Tract
Chapter 34: Acute and Chronic Hepatitis

GREGORY Y. LAUWERS, MD

Associate Professor of Pathology, Harvard Medical School; Director of Gastrointestinal Pathology Service, Massachusetts General Hospital, Boston, Massachusetts

Chapter 17: Epithelial Neoplasms of the Stomach

AUDREY LAZENBY, MD

Associate Professor of Pathology, University of Alabama School of Medicine, Birmingham, Alabama

Chapter 12: Polyps of the Esophagus

DAVID N. B. LEWIN, MD

Associate Professor, Department of Pathology, Medical University of South Carolina, Charleston, South Carolina

Chapter 5: Systemic Illnesses Involving the GI Tract

MARIDA MINERVINI, MD

Clinical Assistant Professor of Pathology, University of Pittsburgh, School of Medicine, Pittsburgh, Pennsylvania; Chief Pathologist, Instituto Mediterraneo Per Trapianti E Terapie Ad Alta Specializzazione, Palermo, Italy

Chapter 39: Transplantation Pathology of the Liver

ELIZABETH MONTGOMERY, MD

Associate Professor of Pathology, Division of GI/Liver Pathology, Johns Hopkins Medical Institutions, Baltimore, Maryland

Chapter 11: Inflammatory Disorders of the Appendix

LINDA A. MURAKATA, MD

Staff Pathologist, Department of Hepatic and Gastrointestinal Pathology, Armed Forces Institute of Pathology, Washington, DC

Chapter 29: Benign and Malignant Tumors of the Gallbladder and Extrahepatic Biliary Tract

MIKE NALESNIK, MD

Associate Professor of Pathology, University of Pittsburgh, School of Medicine; Associate Professor of Pathology, University of Pittsburgh Medical Center; Staff Pathologist, Presbyterian University Hospital, Pittsburgh, Pennsylvania

Chapter 39: Transplantation Pathology of the Liver

AMY NOFFSINGER, MD

Associate Professor, Department of Pathology and Laboratory Medicine, University of Cincinnati Medical Center, Cincinnati, Ohio

Chapter 18: Epithelial Neoplasms of the Small Intestine

ROBERT D. ODZE, MD, FRCP(C)

Associate Professor, Department of Pathology, Harvard Medical School; Director, Division of Gastrointestinal Pathology, Brigham and Women's Hospital, Boston, Massachusetts

Chapter 10: Inflammatory Diseases of the Large Intestine
Chapter 13: Polyps of the Stomach
Chapter 15: Polyps of the Large Intestine
Chapter 16: Epithelial Neoplasms of the Esophagus

STEFAN PAMBUCCIAN, MD

Assistant Professor, Department of Laboratory Medicine and Pathology, University of Minnesota Medical School; Anatomic Pathologist and Director of Cytopathology, Fairview University Medical Center, Minneapolis, Minnesota

Chapter 28: Infectious and Inflammatory Disorders of the Gallbladder and Extrahepatic Biliary Tract

MARTHA BISHOP PITMAN, MD

Associate Professor of Pathology, Harvard Medical School; Associate Pathologist, Director of the Fine Needle Aspiration Biopsy Service, Massachusetts General Hospital, Boston, Massachusetts

Chapter 33: Diagnostic Cytology of the Liver

PARMJEET RANDHAWA, MD

Associate Professor of Pathology, University of Pittsburgh, School of Medicine; Associate Professor of Pathology, University of Pittsburgh Medical Center; Staff Pathologist, Presbyterian University Hospital, Pittsburgh, Pennsylvania

Chapter 39: Transplantation Pathology of the Liver

MARK REDSTON, MD

Assistant Professor of Pathology, Harvard Medical School; Staff Pathologist, Brigham and Women's Hospital, Boston, Massachusetts

Chapter 19: Epithelial Neoplasms of the Large Intestine

MARIE E. ROBERT, MD

Associate Professor of Pathology, Director, Program in Gastrointestinal Pathology, Yale University School of Medicine; Attending Physician, Yale-New Haven Hospital, New Haven, Connecticut

Chapter 9: Inflammatory Disorders of the Small Intestine

LESLIE H. SOBIN, MD

Professor of Pathology, Uniformed Services University of the Health Sciences; Chief, Division of Gastrointestinal Pathology, Department of Hepatic and Gastrointestinal Pathology, Armed Forces Institute of Pathology, Washington, DC

Chapter 20: Epithelial Neoplasms of the Appendix

ARIEF SURIAWINATA, MD

Assistant Professor of Pathology, Department of Pathology, Dartmouth-Hitchcock Medical Center, Lebanon, Hew Hampshire

Chapter 32: Liver Tissue Processing Techniques

SWAN N. THUNG, MD

Professor of Pathology and Gene Therapy and Molecular Medicine, Mount Sinai School of Medicine; Attending Pathologist, Mount Sinai Hospital, New York, New York

Chapter 32: Liver Tissue Processing Techniques

MICHAEL TORBENSON, MD

Assistant Professor of Pathology, Division of GI/Liver Pathology, Johns Hopkins Medical Institutions, Baltimore, Maryland

Chapter 11: Inflammatory Disorders of the Appendix

JERROLD R. TURNER, MD, PhD

Assistant Professor of Pathology, Department of Pathology, University of Chicago, Chicago, Illinois

Chapter 13: Polyps of the Stomach

HELEN H. WANG, MD, DrPH

Associate Professor of Pathology, Harvard Medical School; Director of Cytopathology, Beth Israel Deaconess Medical Center, Boston, Massachusetts

Chapter 2: Diagnostic Cytology of the GI Tract

IAN R. WANLESS, MD

Professor of Pathology, University of Toronto; Staff Pathologist, Toronto General Hospital, Toronto, Ontario, Canada

Chapter 37: Cirrhosis
Chapter 38: Vascular Disorders of the Liver

KAY WASHINGTON, MD, PhD

Associate Professor of Pathology, Vanderbilt University School of Medicine and Vanderbilt University Medical Center, Nashville, Tennessee

Chapter 4: Immunodeficiency Disorders of the GI Tract
Chapter 34: Acute and Chronic Hepatitis

BRUCE M. WENIG, MD

Professor of Pathology, Albert Einstein College of Medicine, Bronx, New York; Vice Chairman for Anatomic Pathology, Beth Israel Medical Center and St. Luke's-Roosevelt Hospitals, New York, New York

Chapter 30: Inflammatory, Infectious, and Other Non-neoplastic Disorders of the Pancreas

JOSEPH WILLIS, MD

Associate Professor of Pathology, Case Western Reserve University and University Hospitals of Cleveland, Cleveland, Ohio

Chapter 27: Developmental Disorders of the Pancreas, Extrahepatic Biliary Tract, and Gallbladder

JACQUELINE L. WOLF, MD

Associate Professor of Medicine, Harvard Medical School; Staff Physician, Beth Israel Deaconess Medical Center, Boston, Massachusetts

Chapter 40: Liver Pathology in Pregnancy

TONG WU, MD, PhD

Assistant Professor of Pathology, University of Pittsburgh, School of Medicine; Assistant Professor of Pathology, University of Pittsburgh Medical Center; Staff Pathologist, Presbyterian University Hospital, Pittsburgh, Pennsylvania

Chapter 39: Transplantation Pathology of the Liver

RHONDA K. YANTISS, MD

Assistant Professor of Pathology, University of Massachusetts Medical School and University of Massachusetts Memorial Health Care, Worcester, Massachusetts

Chapter 14: Polyps of the Small Intestine

Preface

This book was originally conceptualized on the basis of our perceived need in academic pathology for a book under one cover that includes diseases of all organs (tubular gut, liver, gallbladder, biliary tract, and pancreas) considered part of the field of gastrointestinal pathology. The resulting text, *Surgical Pathology of the GI Tract, Liver, Biliary Tract, and Pancreas,* represents the first complete and comprehensive textbook in gastrointestinal, liver, biliary tract, and pancreatic pathology. The information in this book, and the manner in which it was written, was designed for general pathologists and pathologists in training but particularly for those with a special interest or expertise in gastrointestinal, liver, biliary, or pancreatic disorders. In addition, we have paid special attention to providing only the most relevant, up-to-date clinical, etiologic, and management information necessary for surgical pathologists to make clinically relevant diagnoses. Thus, clinical gastroenterologists, gastroenterologists in training, and surgeons with a special interest in gastrointestinal disorders may also find this book of importance. Wherever possible, we have emphasized relevant clinical-pathologic correlations, with particular focus on management and treatment options, particularly regarding screening and surveillance recommendations for a variety of preneoplastic disorders that occur often in the gastrointestinal tract, liver, biliary tract, and pancreas.

Overall, this is a morphology-based book with particular emphasis on histologic methods that can help differentiate diseases based on evaluation of biopsy and resection specimens. Thus, for each disorder, where applicable, a thorough description of the differential diagnosis is provided, in a predominantly algorithmic manner. We have included many tables or algorithms that provide the key diagnostic tools useful in the pathologic differential diagnosis process. We have included only color photographs that are highly representative of the disorders in question, as well as its common mimickers. The use of recent and new immunohistochemical and other molecular and laboratory techniques is highlighted as well.

One of the other main goals of this book was to organize information in a "user friendly," easily accessible manner, one that would help surgical pathologists gain quick access to diagnostic information regarding particular disease entities without having to spend a lot of time leafing through the index and turning pages. For example, a pathologist who encounters a diagnostically difficult gastric polyp may turn to the chapter on gastric polyps and find differential diagnostic information on these entities in an easy and rapid manner.

The book is organized into parts based on three separate organ systems: the gastrointestinal tract (Part One, Chapters 1 through 24); the gallbladder, extrahepatic biliary tract, and pancreas (Part Two, Chapters 25 through 31); and the liver (Part Three, Chapters 32 through 42). In each part there is an introductory chapter on pertinent tissue processing techniques that provides information on the proper management of tissue specimens related to that particular organ system. In addition, a well-photographed chapter on diagnostic cytology of each of these organ systems is included. We hope that our readers will find this helpful as, in recent years, more and more pathologists are being exposed to cytologic specimens from the gastrointestinal tract and related organs. The section on gastrointestinal pathology (Section I) contains a number of chapters that cover material common to the different components of the gastrointestinal tract, such as infections, immunodeficiency disorders, systemic illnesses, and neuromuscular disorders. This material was organized thus primarily because the pathologic features of these disorders appear similar, regardless of the precise anatomic location of occurrence in the gut. These general chapters are followed by chapters on specific inflammatory lesions (Section II) and neoplastic lesions (Sections IV and V) of each particular anatomic segment of the gastrointestinal tract. A separate section (Section III) on polyps of the esophagus, stomach, small intestine, and large intestine is included, because in clinical practice it is common to receive specimens in which the term "polyp" is perhaps the only or the most significant piece of clinical information available. Neoplasms are separated into epithelial types (Section IV) and nonepithelial types (Section V), similar to the deductive thought process used by pathologists at the time of evaluation of specimens at the microscope.

All chapters in this book were written by pathologists with a special interest or expertise in a particular field. Their contributions emphasize the latest, and sometimes most controversial, aspects of pathology classification systems and diagnostic criteria. In some cases, such as with the inflammatory and neoplastic disorders of the stomach, certain differences between European, Asian, and North American diagnostic philosophies are highlighted where applicable. We took great care to include only the most relevant and up-to-date references and informative review articles.

We are deeply grateful to all of our contributors, not only for writing the chapters but also for being patient and understanding during the laborious editorial process. We believe the result is a comprehensive textbook of gastrointestinal, liver, biliary, and pancreatic pathology that will serve as an excellent foundation for learning the pathologic basis of disorders of the gut and related systems for clinicians and pathologists alike.

ROBERT D. ODZE, MD, FRCP(C)

JOHN R. GOLDBLUM, MD

JAMES M. CRAWFORD, MD, PhD

Acknowledgments

Many people contributed to the conception, writing, editing, and production of this book. On the professional side, I am greatly indebted to my longtime friends and mentors, Dr. Donald Antonioli and Dr. Harvey Goldman, for introducing me to the marvelous world of gastrointestinal pathology, for their guidance, and for teaching me skills that could never be obtained from any other source. Their continuous confidence and support is one of the main reasons why I was capable of conceiving and realizing this work. I also owe a great deal of gratitude to the late Dr. Ramzi Cotran, the former chairman of the Department of Pathology at the Brigham and Women's Hospital, for providing me with all the means for pursuing my academic interests as well as for his wisdom and inspiration. I am also grateful to Dr. Michael Gimbrone, the current chairman; Dr. Fred Schoen, the executive vice-chairman; and Dr. Christopher Fletcher, the director of surgical pathology, as well as to all of my surgical pathology friends and colleagues at the Brigham and Women's Hospital, for providing me with interesting and thought-provoking concepts regarding the art and science of surgical pathology.

Dr. Goldblum would like to acknowledge his mentor in gastrointestinal pathology, Dr. Henry Appelman.

Dr. Crawford gratefully acknowledges his mentors in gastrointestinal and hepatic pathology, Drs. James Madara, John Gollan, and Peter Scheuer.

On a personal level, I cannot emphasize enough the encouragement that I received from my brother Tony and my mother Natasha, who is entirely responsible for making my medical career possible. To my extended family in Boston, Sharon, Mark, John, Eva, and all others close to me, I am blessed for their friendship, advice, and support in all my personal and professional endeavors.

The editors are indebted to all of our technical, administrative, and support staff who were involved in the design and production of this book for their dedicated work, patience, and perseverance. Most notably, we thank our secretaries, Carmen Arjune, Kathleen Ranney, and Nancy Lambka, for their excellent secretarial support.

We would like to thank Natasha Andjelkovic and Michael Houston of Elsevier for providing us with the opportunity to develop this book and for their excellent and creative management skills.

Finally, the editors would like to thank all of the authors for their excellent contributions, and to our gastrointestinal pathology colleagues around the world for providing a fun and exciting academic community that we are a part of.

ROBERT D. ODZE, MD, FRCP(C)

Contents

PART TWO
Gallbladder, Extrahepatic Biliary Tract, and Pancreas

PART THREE
Liver

PART ONE

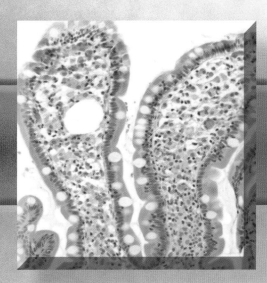

Gastrointestinal Tract

GENERAL PATHOLOGY OF THE GI TRACT

CHAPTER 1

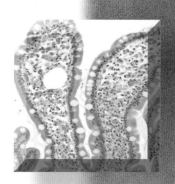

Gastrointestinal Tract Endoscopic and Tissue Processing Techniques

BRIAN C. JACOBSON • JAMES M. CRAWFORD
FRANCIS A. FARRAYE

■ Introduction

Endoscopy provides a unique opportunity for visualization of the mucosal surface of the gastrointestinal tract. When considered within the context of a specific clinical picture, endoscopic images may be all that are needed to make a diagnosis or provide a sound management decision.[1] However, more often than not, an endoscopist will need to sample tissue or remove a lesion to arrive at a diagnosis. Even normal-appearing mucosa may yield underlying histopathologic abnormalities when a biopsy specimen is analyzed by microscopy, such as in mild celiac sprue or microscopic colitis. Estimation of polyp size based on endoscopy is generally inaccurate compared with measurements of gross specimens before fixation.[2,3] Therefore, if the size of a polyp may alter management, as in determination of the need for colonoscopy after screening sigmoidoscopy, polypectomy with ex vivo measurement may be necessary. Tumor stage may be altered by detection of malignancy in a lymph node sampled by endoscopic ultrasound-guided fine-needle aspiration. Hence, histologic examination of specimens obtained at endoscopy by a qualified pathologist is a routine and critical part of managing patients with disorders of the alimentary tract.

■ Bowel Preparation

The effectiveness of endoscopy depends, in part, on the quality of "bowel preparation."[4] Preparation for endoscopy of the upper gastrointestinal tract is typically achieved with a 6-hour fast. Preparation for colonoscopy is achieved by the use of oral purging agents, either with or without enemas. Regimens include the use of a clear liquid diet for 1 to 3 days, cleansing with oral polyethylene glycol (PEG)-electrolyte solution or sodium phosphate lavage solutions, and the use of oral laxatives or prokinetic agents such as magnesium citrate, metoclopramide, cisapride, and senna, as well as rectal enemas (Table 1-1). In general, vomiting is reported more frequently with oral PEG–based high-volume lavage regimens than with oral bowel prokinetics.[5] However, nausea, vomiting, and abdominal cramps are comparable for PEG lavage and oral sodium phosphate regimens.[6] PEG lavage regimens reportedly provide more consistent cleansing.[7,8] Purgative- and laxative-based regimens are more likely to cause flattening of surface epithelial cells, goblet cell depletion, and lamina propria edema; normo-osmotic electrolyte solutions, such as PEG-based solutions, are better agents for preserving mucosal histology.[9] In the most severe form of mucosal damage from purgatives, sloughing of the surface epithelium, neutrophilic infiltration of the lamina propria, and hemorrhage may be encountered and may even resemble pseudomembranous colitis.[10] Chemical-induced colitis from inadequate rinsing of cleansing agents from endoscopic instruments also has been reported. Mucosal changes in this situation may resemble pseudomembranous colitis both endoscopically and microscopically.[11]

■ Methods for Obtaining Tissue Specimens

In general, a limited number of methods are available for obtaining tissue during endoscopy. This section describes several of these methods and the situations in which they are used.

TABLE 1–1. Common Preparation Methods for Colonoscopy

48-hr clear liquid diet, 240-mL magnesium citrate PO, senna derivative laxative (e.g., X-Prep), 12 hr NPO.

48-hr clear liquid diet, senna derivative laxative, rectal enema, 12-hr NPO.

24-hr clear liquid diet, 240 mL magnesium citrate PO, or 4 L PEG-electrolyte lavage,* 12 hr NPO.

24 hr clear liquid diet, 2 L PEG-electrolyte lavage, cascara-based laxative, 12 hr NPO.

24-hr clear liquid diet, oral sodium phosphate,† magnesium citrate PO, 12 hr NPO.

24-hr clear liquid diet, oral sodium phosphate, rectal enema.

*PEG-electrolyte solutions include CoLyte, GoLYTELY, NuLytely, Klean-Prep, and Norgine.

†Oral sodium phosphate solutions include Fleets Phosphosoda, De Witt Phosphosoda.

hr, hours; NPO, nothing per os (mouth); PEG, polyethylene glycol; PO, per os (mouth).

ENDOSCOPIC PINCH BIOPSY

Pinch biopsy performed with the use of a biopsy forceps during endoscopy is the most frequent form of tissue sampling; the biopsy site is usually fully visualized at the time of sampling. Suction capsule biopsy requires fluoroscopic guidance to position a long tube with a biopsy apparatus and is done separately from endoscopy without visualization. Endoscopy without visualization may still be performed in some centers but is less successful than endoscopy-guided biopsies in obtaining tissue and thus has fallen out of favor.[12] Pinch biopsies may be small or large (the latter are sometimes referred to as "jumbo") and can be obtained with or without the use of electrocautery. Electrocautery has value for hemostasis and destruction of residual tissue but may introduce burn artifact into harvested tissue.

All standard biopsy forceps have a similar design (Fig. 1-1). The sampling portion consists of a pair of small cups or a paired set of teeth that are in apposition when closed. In this manner, they can be passed through the 2.8-mm-wide channel of a standard gastroscope or colonoscope. Some biopsy forceps have a spike at the base of the cups or teeth to better seat the forceps against the mucosa and to impale multiple biopsy specimens before the forceps is removed from the endoscope. After emerging from the distal end of an endoscope, the biopsy forceps can be opened to a 4- to 8-mm span that is pressed against a mucosal surface for tissue sampling. (The large cup or jumbo biopsy forceps has jaws that open to a span of 7 to 9 mm.) The biopsy forceps is then closed against the mucosal surface, and the endoscopist simply pulls back the forceps to remove a fragment of tissue. This method often yields a sample that includes the muscularis mucosae, except in regions such as the gastric body, where mucosal folds may be thick.[13] The submucosa is occasionally sampled with either standard or jumbo forceps, but this is not consistently done.[14] Sample size varies according to the amount of pressure the endoscopist applies to the forceps. In addition, application of a fully opened biopsy forceps

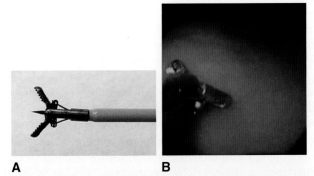

A   **B**

FIGURE 1–1. Endoscopic biopsy forceps. **A,** The biopsy forceps has been opened, revealing two sets of gripping "teeth" and a central spike for impaling the tissue. **B,** The biopsy forceps in use: The biopsy forceps is pressed against the mucosa and subsequently is closed to obtain a tissue sample.

flush against the mucosa before closure usually yields larger pieces of tissue than those obtained by tangential sampling or incomplete opening of the forceps. In general, biopsy specimens are 4 to 8 mm in length.[15,16] The forceps shape does not impart a significant difference in either biopsy specimen size or adequacy of specimens.[15] A new single-use disposable biopsy forceps has also been shown to provide excellent samples.[17] In essence, there is no difference in the quality of tissue samples obtained among the dozen or more biopsy forceps currently available, so the primary consideration in the selection of an endoscopic biopsy forceps is typically one of cost and ease of use.[18]

After obtaining biopsy specimens and removing the forceps from the endoscope, an assistant may dislodge the tissue fragments from the forceps with a toothpick or a similar small, sharp instrument. The tissue is then placed into a container with appropriate fixative, and the container is labeled according to instructions given by the endoscopist.

Specimens obtained with a jumbo forceps often produce tissue samples 6 mm or greater in maximum diameter, but these are not necessarily deeper than standard biopsies. Rather, a jumbo forceps provides more mucosa for analysis. This is particularly useful during surveillance tissue sampling such as in patients with Barrett's esophagus or ulcerative colitis, and a jumbo forceps is as safe as a standard biopsy forceps.[19] However, the use of a jumbo forceps is limited by its size because it cannot fit through a standard endoscope accessory channel. A jumbo forceps requires the 3.6-mm-diameter channel of therapeutic endoscopes, which may be less comfortable for patients. In addition, although jumbo biopsy specimens are larger than standard biopsy specimens, this does not necessarily mean samples are more diagnostic.[20]

The most common indication for mucosal biopsy is the diagnosis of a mucosal abnormality at endoscopy. In addition, it is advantageous to sample normal-appearing mucosa during the evaluation of many conditions to establish "background" features of the mucosa, such as in gastroesophageal reflux disease, nonulcer dyspepsia, diarrhea, and surveillance of premalignant conditions, including Barrett's esophagus and inflammatory bowel disease. The ampulla of Vater may be biopsied during surveillance for adenomatous change in familial adenomatous polyposis because the lifetime incidence of ampullary adenomas in these patients exceeds 50%[21]. Biopsy of biliary or pancreatic strictures may be carried out under fluoroscopic guidance during endoscopic retrograde cholangiopancreatography (ERCP) with the use of either standard or specially designed small biopsy forceps.[22] Even gallbladder lesions noted at ERCP may be amenable to endoscopic biopsy.[23] Endoscopy-directed biopsies are extremely safe. In one study of 50,833 consecutive patients who had an upper endoscopy, none had any biopsy-associated complications.[19]

Occasionally, an endoscopist uses a specialized insulated biopsy forceps to sample a small polyp ("hot biopsy") and then ablates the remaining tissue in situ using electrocautery.[23] Unfortunately, cautery artifact in such small tissue samples often makes the biopsy difficult (or impossible) to interpret histologically.[13,24] In addition, the electrocautery technique carries an excessive risk of perforation secondary to deep tissue burn, particularly in the cecum and ascending colon.[25,26] Finally, destruction of residual dysplastic tissue by electrocautery may be incomplete in as many as 17% of cases.[27]

ENDOSCOPIC SNARE POLYPECTOMY

During endoscopy, a loop of wire may be placed around a polypoid lesion that protrudes into the lumen of the gut for the purpose of removing the polyp (Fig. 1-2). This technique is used primarily for colonic polyps, but polyps throughout the alimentary tract may be excised in this manner. Depending on their size, excised polyps either are retrieved through the suction channel of the endoscope or are held by the snare after resection while the colonoscope is removed. Loss of excised polyps within the recesses of the intestinal lumen is an infrequent occurrence.

Many investigators have reported the successful removal of diminutive polyps (<0.5 cm in diameter) during both "hot" (with electrocautery) and "cold" (without electrocautery) snare polypectomy.[28,29] These techniques use small metal snares called *mini-snares* that open to a size of 1 to 2 cm × 2 to 3 cm. Polyps greater than 0.5 cm in diameter are amenable to snare polypectomy, although the size of the polyp that can be excised may be limited by the size of the loop to be placed around it (and the endoscopist's estimation of perforation risk). Alternatively, large polyps may be removed in a piecemeal fashion and submitted to pathology in several parts. This usually requires multiple transections of the lesion until the entire polyp has been removed.[23] One caveat with this technique is that identifiable tissue margins may be lost, so that the pathologist is

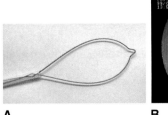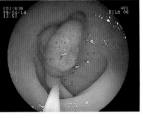

A   **B**

FIGURE 1–2. Endoscopic snare polypectomy. **A,** An open metal snare extends out of a protective plastic sheath. **B,** A polypectomy snare has been placed over a pedunculated polyp and tightened around the polyp stalk. Electrical current is applied through the metal loop of the snare, which helps cut through the stalk and cauterizes blood vessels.

often unable to determine the status of the resection margins.

A hot snare allows the endoscopist to apply current to a metal wire that cuts through the polyp at the base, to assist in both tissue cutting and coagulation. Electrocautery also minimizes bleeding from blood vessels in the stalk of the polyp. Cold polypectomy, without electrical current, avoids the use of cautery, thereby limiting the amount of burn artifact in the specimen and minimizing the risk of perforation. In general, the risk of perforation from either mechanical or electrical injury is minimal but is greater in portions of the colon that have a free serosal surface.

For polyps excised in one piece by either hot or cold polypectomy, the polyp base constitutes the surgical margin of resection. This is true for both pedunculated polyps with a stalk and sessile polyps without a stalk. For polyps removed by hot snare polypectomy, the cauterized portion of the specimen constitutes the surgical margin. An artificial stalk can be created when large sessile lesions are loop-excised. A true pedunculated polyp with a stalk has a narrow base that persists after removal; the base of a sessile polyp is usually as wide as the mucosal surface that is sampled.

Snares are available in a variety of shapes and sizes. Newer snares are also rotatable, which provides the endoscopist with greater control of snare placement. The choice of snare size is typically based on the size of the lesion being removed. The selection of a particular snare shape usually reflects personal choice.

Snare polypectomy is performed in a similar fashion whether colonic, esophageal, gastric, or small bowel lesions are removed. In fact, the ampulla of Vater may be resected by means of standard snare techniques when an ampullary lesion is noted.[30] The risk of perforation during snare polypectomy is less than 0.1%,[31,32] and perforation generally results from transmural burn secondary to cautery. One technique aimed at decreasing the risk of perforation is to pull the snared polyp ("tent") away from the mucosa so that less cautery is applied to the underlying tissue. Another commonly used method is saline-assisted polypectomy.[33,34] A small needle is passed through the endoscope and is inserted into the gut wall adjacent to the polyp. A bolus of normal saline is then injected. Fluid collects within the submucosal plane, thereby "lifting" any mucosal-based polyp away from the muscularis propria. A standard snare polypectomy is then performed, but the cushion of saline insulates the deeper tissue layers from electrical current. Saline-assisted polypectomy is generally reserved for large sessile polyps and, theoretically, results in a decreased rate of polypectomy-associated perforation.

ENDOSCOPIC MUCOSAL RESECTION

The use of a liquid cushion to expand the submucosa and minimize transmural cautery damage is a principal component of endoscopic mucosal resection (EMR). This technique is commonly used to resect premalignant and malignant lesions confined to the mucosa.[35] In general, EMR requires some measure of confidence that a lesion is, in fact, confined to the mucosa or submucosa. Many endoscopists now rely on endoscopic ultrasound (EUS) to determine the depth of a particular lesion. The accuracy of high-frequency EUS (15 or 20 MHz) may be as high as 95% for determining whether a lesion is limited to the lamina propria,[35] but the availability of EUS and variation in operator experience may limit its universal application before EMR.

Several variations of the EMR technique are used. All rely on submucosal injection of a liquid, but there is currently no agreement as to the type or quantity of liquid to be injected.[36] Some endoscopists advocate the use of saline alone. Others add dilute epinephrine to saline in an attempt to constrict small vessels at the base of the lesion. Submucosal fluid collections are eventually absorbed. To lengthen the time that the submucosal cushion lasts, and thus to maximize the time available for performing a safe resection, investigators have used hypertonic solution of 3.5% saline or 50% dextrose. Others advocate the use of sodium hyaluronate instead of saline. The quantity of liquid injected also varies. In general, there is agreement that the target lesion should appear endoscopically to be raised by the cushion of liquid before EMR. In fact, failure to lift the lesion despite the generous use of submucosal saline (the so-called nonlifting sign) may be a sensitive indicator that a lesion has spread into the bowel wall.[37]

Two major types of resection techniques are used—those that do not use suction and those that do. When suction is not used, the endoscopist uses a dual-channel endoscope. A snare, passed through one instrument channel, is opened and placed around the lesion. A biopsy forceps passed through the second channel is used to grab the lesion and pull the mucosa through the snare even farther from the muscularis propria. The snare is then closed around the base of the tented lesion, and electrocautery is applied (Fig. 1-3). This method is referred to as a *lift and cut technique* or a *strip biopsy*.[35,38]

Suction methods of EMR incorporate the use of a cap fitted onto the tip of an endoscope. The cap presents an open surface to the mucosa and creates a short chamber into which the target lesion can be aspirated and held by suction applied through a single-channel endoscope. A specialized snare is opened within the cap before aspiration of the lesion. Once the mucosa has been drawn into the cap, the snare may be closed around the lesion and cautery applied in the usual fashion.[35] This technique, also called *aspiration mucosectomy*, has been widely successful in removing lesions throughout the gastrointestinal tract.[39]

EMR allows the endoscopist to attempt an en bloc resection and thus attempt a potential cure of an early

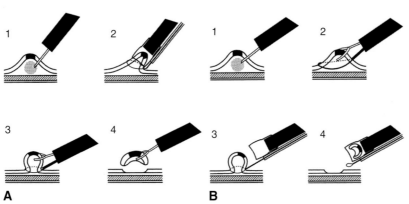

FIGURE 1–3. Endoscopic mucosal resection (EMR). **A,** EMR by strip biopsy: Saline is injected into the submucosal layer, and the area is elevated (1). The top of the mound is pulled upward with forceps, and the snare is placed at the base of the lesion (2 and 3). Electrosurgical current is applied via the snare to resect the mucosa, and the lesion is removed (4). (Reused by permission of the publisher. From Tanabe S, Koizumi W, Kokutou M, et al: Gastrointest Endos 50:819-822, 1999.) **B,** EMR by aspiration: Saline is injected into the submucosa, and the tissue is elevated (1). The lesion is aspirated into a plastic cap at the end of the endoscope, and the snare is closed around the lesion (2). The ensnared lesion is released from the cap (3). Electrosurgical current is applied, and the resected lesion is trapped within the cap by aspiration (4). (Reused by permission of the publisher. From Tanabe S, Koizumi W, Kokutou M, et al: Gastrointest Endos 50:819-822, 1999.)

malignant lesion. En bloc resection is limited, however, to small lesions (1.5 to 2.0 cm in largest diameter).[38] If deep margins are positive for neoplasia, surgical resection of the affected region is advocated.[40] Current indications for EMR include superficial carcinoma of the esophagus and stomach in patients who are nonoperative candidates and large, flat colorectal adenomas with or without high-grade dysplasia (which may require piecemeal resection). EMR as primary therapy for small, superficial cancer has not gained popularity in the United States but is often used in Japan.[35,38,40] EMR may also be indicated as a form of primary therapy for small submucosal lesions, such as rectal carcinoid tumor or leiomyoma. In many cases, the submucosal lesion can be completely resected.[41]

Major complications resulting from EMR include bleeding and perforation. Bleeding is seen in less than 1% to 20% of cases and varies depending on the size of the lesion and its location.[35,38,40] Clinically significant bleeding is rare and is usually amenable to endoscopic hemostatic cauterization. Perforation rates are generally lower than 2%. EMR also provides large specimens for pathologic analysis even in the absence of complete resection. Success rates of en bloc resection of early gastric cancers range from 36% to 74%.[38,40]

Pathologic Features of a Healing Biopsy Site

The complications of gastrointestinal endoscopy are well documented.[42] Although upper endoscopy may involve complications such as bleeding or aspiration in less than 1% of cases,[43] perforation is quite rare. Colonoscopy carries a risk of bleeding or perforation of

about 0.2% for diagnostic procedures without a biopsy, and 1.2% for those with a biopsy or polyp resection.[44] As has been noted earlier, a jumbo biopsy forceps samples a wider region of mucosa but does not necessarily penetrate more deeply; thus, there is no substantive increase in the risk of perforation relative to routine biopsy forceps. Nevertheless, the healing process takes time (Table 1-2). Blood clot and granulation tissue form within several hours following biopsy,[45] as illustrated in Figure 1-4**A** and **B**. Routine superficial biopsies involving only mucosa and submucosa typically reepithelialize within 48 hours after biopsy (Fig. 1-4**C**). Ulcers that penetrate into the muscularis propria often take 3 to 6 days to reepithelialize (Fig. 1-4**D**). Notably, following superficial biopsy, there is no increased risk of perforation during subsequent insufflation (as from repeat endoscopy or from barium enema), even immediately following the biopsy. The risk of perforation following a deep biopsy that involves

TABLE 1-2. Pathologic Features of a Healing Mucosal Biopsy Site

Time	Feature
Immediate	Blood clot with coagulum
Hours	Acute inflammation; granulation tissue reaction
2 days*	Reepithelialization of inflamed biopsy site via ingrowth of epithelial cells from adjacent preserved epithelium; early formation of submucosal scar
1 to 4 weeks	Restoration of mucosa with rudimentary glandular architecture, maturation of submucosal scar
Months	Residual minimal mucosal architectural distortion, submucosal scar

*Longer with deep biopsies involving the muscularis propria.

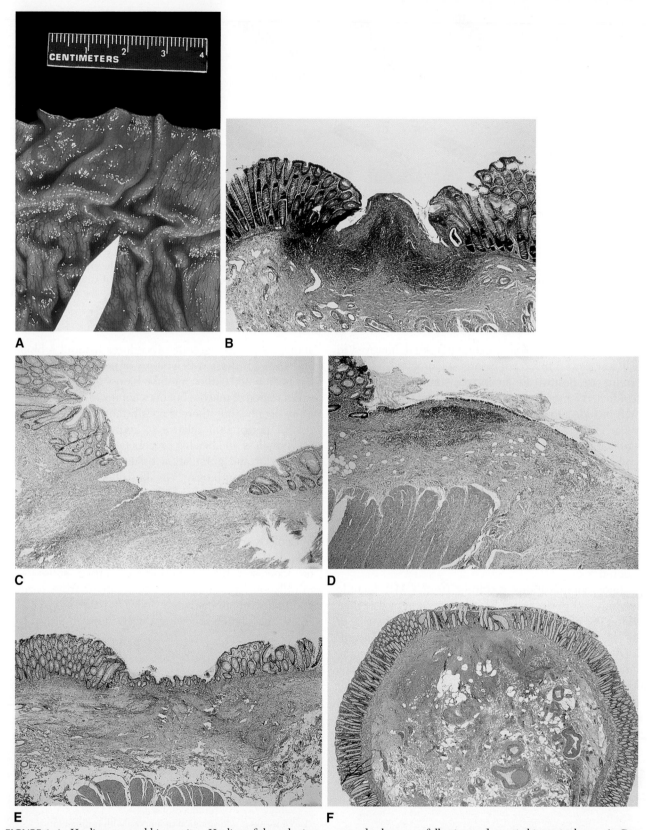

FIGURE 1–4. Healing mucosal biopsy sites. Healing of the colonic mucosa and submucosa following endoscopic biopsy is shown. **A,** Gross photograph of a resected colon specimen 2 days post endoscopic biopsy, with an arrow demonstrating the biopsy site. **B,** Two days after endoscopic polypectomy, the biopsy site shows ulceration, inflammation, and granulation tissue reaction. **C,** Four days after biopsy, the mucosa shows architectural distortion and an attenuated layer of surface epithelium. **D,** Four days after a loop polypectomy, an attenuated layer of epithelium covers portions of the biopsy site, but the ulcer is still present. **E,** Three weeks after biopsy, submucosal scarring and rudimentary crypt restoration are noted. **F,** One month after biopsy of a prominent mucosal fold, the submucosa shows scarring and focal architectural disortion.

the muscularis propria returns to baseline after 3 to 6 days.[45] Regardless of the maximum depth of biopsy penetration (submucosa or muscularis propria; pinch biopsy or loop resection of a polyp), after several weeks a residual submucosal scar may remain, either with (Fig. 1-4**E**) or without (Fig. 1-4**F**) atrophy of the mucosa.

Pathologists should be aware of changes associated with the repair of a biopsy site because these can lead to misinterpretation of architectural distortion as evidence in favor of chronic disease.

◼ Processing of Tissue Specimens for Histologic Analysis

A general framework for processing of bioptic tissue specimens is given in Table 1-3.

FORMALIN

Of the many fixatives used for human tissue, 10% buffered formalin remains the standard and is well suited for mucosal biopsies of the gastrointestinal tract. It is

TABLE 1–3. Techniques of Processing Tissue Specimens Obtained by Endoscopy

Technique	Comment
Formalin fixation	Routine processing of all alimentary tract biopsies; immediate immersion in fixative. Permits immunohistochemistry, molecular analysis.
Flow cytometry	Suspected hematologic malignancy; fresh tissue in sterile culture medium.
Electron microscopy	Suspected poorly differentiated malignancy, infection (e.g., Whipple's disease, microsporidia); immediate immersion in electron microscopy fixative.
Electron microscopy fixative only	Suspected systemic mastocytosis, for which plastic-embedded thick sections with toluidine blue staining are optimal for identifying mast cells.
Microbial culture	Suspected viral, fungal, or parasitic infection; sterile tissue.
Biochemical analysis	Suspected metabolic deficiency (e.g., disaccharidase deficiency); frozen tissue.
Cytogenetics*	Suspected neoplasm (benign or malignant); fresh tissue in sterile culture medium.
Cell culture*	Suspected neoplasm (benign or malignant); fresh tissue in sterile culture medium.

*Usually for investigational purposes only.

inexpensive, the tissue may remain in it for a sustained time, and it is compatible with all of the stains commonly used for morphologic assessment. Hollende's solution, B5, and Bouin's fixative have been used for mucosal biopsies because of better preservation of nuclear morphology compared with formalin. However, the heavy metal content of these fixatives creates biohazard disposal problems that are greater than those of formaldehyde-based fixatives. These fixatives also interfere with isolation of nucleic acid from tissue. On occasion, the formaldehyde of formalin may be an irritant to eyes and the upper respiratory tract, and there is public debate over its potential as a carcinogen.[46] Thus, proper ventilation should be in place to maintain exposure at below 1.0 ppm. This is the lowest concentration that may exert a cytotoxic effect in humans.[46,47] However, typical occupational exposure in the endoscopy suite is exceedingly brief, so that special ventilation is not usually required.

Alimentary tract biopsy specimens should be placed in a volume of formalin fixative that is at least 10 times that of the tissue, and the fixative should surround the specimen on all sides. For routine processing, it is a common mistake to place specimens on saline-soaked gauze for delivery to the pathology suite because severe drying may occur. Fixation of these biopsies should always occur at the bedside. Formaldehyde diffuses into tissue at a rate of approximately 1.0 mm per hour at room temperature.[48] Hence, up to 1 hour is often needed to adequately fix a specimen with a diameter greater than 1.0 mm. More time is needed for larger specimens. Controlled microwave fixation at 63°C to 65°C can greatly speed the process and is useful for rapid processing of specimens.[49]

Orientation of Formalin-Fixed Tissue Obtained at Endoscopy

Esophageal, gastric, and colonic mucosal biopsies do not require precise orientation before tissue processing and embedding. Until the mid-1980s, most peroral small intestinal biopsies were obtained by either a Crosby suction capsule or a Quinton hydraulic assembly.[50,51] These two methods were performed fluoroscopically and thus did not permit direct visualization of the alimentary tract. Biopsies obtained by these methods were carefully oriented under a dissecting microscope before fixation and embedding. Direct endoscopic biopsy of the small intestine replaced the fluoroscopy with suction capsule biopsy procedure by the late 1980s[52,53]; biopsies obtained by this technique are not usually oriented before immersion in fixative, processing, and embedding. Rather, microscopic examination of multiple tissue sections usually permits identification of portions of the small intestinal mucosa that are well oriented and can hence be assessed satisfactorily for tissue architecture.

In contrast, processing of an endoscopic polypectomy specimen in the pathology suite requires diligent effort.[54] The size and surface configuration (bosselated or villiform) of the polyp should be noted, and the base of the polyp should be identified and described as to whether it is sessile or contains a cylindrical stalk. Regardless of the configuration of the stalk, *the base of the polyp should always be inked.* Ink and cautery artifact on a microscopic slide are valuable landmarks for locating the relevant resection margins. Small polyps (<1 cm in diameter) should be bisected along the vertical plane of the stalk so that the surgical margin is included. Both halves of the specimen can then be submitted in one cassette.

Section levels should be numbered consecutively; the first level is the one normally located closest to the middle of the polyp stalk. Large polyps (≥1 cm in diameter) may be sectioned differently if the polyp head is too wide to fit into a single cassette. First, the polyp should be bisected along its long axis and fixed overnight in formalin to allow precise section of the tissue the next day. Once fixed, the sides of the polyp may be trimmed away from the stalk on a vertical axis and submitted in separate cassettes that are labeled accordingly. The middle of the polyp, which contains the base, should be sectioned vertically and submitted in the appropriate number of cassettes.

If the polyp has been excised in a piecemeal fashion, the size, color, surface configuration (bosselated or villiform), and aggregate dimensions of the tissue fragments should be noted. It is important that the number of tissue fragments received be documented because this information is important in determination of whether the surgical margin can be evaluated satisfactorily. Specifically, if a stalk has been identified histologically, the status of the margins should be noted on the surgical pathology report.

FLOW CYTOMETRY

Gastrointestinal lesions suspected of representing a lymphoproliferative process may be processed for flow cytometry.[55] Biopsy specimens intended for flow cytometric analysis, such as gastric biopsies of a mass lesion, should be placed in a sterile culture medium and delivered as rapidly as possible to the flow cytometry laboratory. Ideally, this should occur within several hours, but storage of specimens at 4°C overnight is an acceptable alternative.

Upon receipt in the laboratory, the tissue specimen is disaggregated, and a cell suspension is prepared. Cocktails of fluorescently labeled antibodies appropriate to the diagnostic question are applied to the cell suspension. Current flow cytometry machines can analyze 5000 to 10,000 cells per second, measuring multiple wavelengths of laser-induced fluorescence simultaneously, thus permitting rapid and highly efficient analysis of cell populations. This technique cannot be performed on fixed tissue. It is therefore incumbent on the endoscopist to consider the possibility of a lymphoproliferative disorder at the time of endoscopy to ensure that tissue is preserved in a fresh state.

ELECTRON MICROSCOPY

For those uncommon instances in which electron microscopy of an alimentary tract biopsy is contemplated, tissue samples should be placed directly into an appropriate fixative, which is usually a mixture of paraformaldehyde and glutaraldehyde. Unlike formaldehyde fixatives, the bifunctional glutaraldehyde fixatives penetrate only about 0.5 mm deep into the tissue. Hence, tissue fragments to be placed in fixative for subsequent electron microscopy should ideally be less than $1.0 \times 1.0 \times 1.0$ mm^3 in maximal dimension.

Electron microscopy fixative is also commonly used for processing mucosal biopsy specimens to be analyzed for other conditions, such as systemic mastocytosis or microsporidian infection. Plastic-embedded sections may be stained with toluidine blue to highlight mast cells.

ENDOSCOPY-INDUCED ARTIFACTS

Many types of tissue artifacts may be introduced into tissue as a result of bowel preparation, endoscopic trauma, and/or tissue handling; these are listed in Table 1-4. Histologic features of artifacts are provided in Table 1-5 (see also Chapter 2). The most common type of artifact (or effect) is lamina propria edema and intramucosal hemorrhage ("scope trauma"), as illustrated in Figure 1-5. Other effects include aggregation and clumping of inflammatory cells in the lamina propria, surface flattening, mucin depletion, and even erosion and influx of air into the tissue (pseudolipomatosis).[56-58] The most common histologic artifacts include cautery and crush artifacts (Fig. 1-6). Cautery artifact as a result of hot biopsies is, in fact, a normal and expected component of endoscopic polypectomy with electrocautery. Specifically, the region of cauterization may provide a useful landmark of the surgical margin.

Methods for Obtaining Cytology Specimens

BRUSH CYTOLOGY

Brush cytology is a method used for broad sampling of the mucosal surface.[59,60] Cytology brushes, whether reusable or disposable, have a common design. A cytology brush consists of bristles usually composed of nylon

TABLE 1–4. Endoscopically Related Events That May Affect Tissue Analysis

Artifact	Comment
Trauma	"Scope trauma" (due to mechanical damage from endoscope) or excessive mechanical manipulation for access before biopsy
Cautery artifact	Excessive use of electrical current during "hot" biopsy
Crush artifact	Excessive use of mechanical force during pinch biopsy
Inadequate sampling depth	Absence of submucosa (e.g., evaluate submucosal lesion, rule out amyloid)
Inadequate sampling location	Absence of muscularis propria (for evaluation for Hirschsprung's disease)
	Insufficient regional sampling (e.g., of "normal-appearing" mucosa)
Chemical colitis[56,57]	Inadequate rinsing of cleaning solution from the endoscope
Laxative-induced changes[58]	Edema, damage to surface epithelium from exposure to oral and rectum laxatives
Air-drying	Failure to immerse specimen promptly in fixative
Postbiopsy healing	Sampling of a previous biopsy site during subsequent endoscopy
Wrong fixative	Formalin rather than fixative for electron microscopy; suboptimal but not irretrievable
No fresh tissue	Failure to preserve fresh tissue; precludes flow cytometry, cytogenetics

TABLE 1–5. Histologic Artifacts Related to Endoscopy

Artifact	Feature
"Scope trauma"	Mucosal lamina propria hemorrhage or edema
Bowel prep–related changes	Clumping of inflammatory cells, mucin depletion, epithelial degenerative changes, focal neutrophilic infiltration, hemorrhage, edema, air in mucosa (pseudolipomatosis)
Cautery artifact	Coagulated, eosinophilic tissue without cellular or nuclear detail
Crush artifact	Compressed tissue with markedly elongated, wavy nuclear remnants and no identifiable architecture
Chemical colitis from inadequate cleaning of the endoscope	Degenerative damage to or sloughing of surface epithelium, intraepithelial neutrophils and congestion, focal intramucosal hemorrhage
Laxative-induced changes	Lamina propria edema and neutrophilic infiltration, flattening or sloughing of mucosal surface epithelium, decreased goblet cell numbers
Air-drying	Eosinophilic and compressed tissue and loss of nuclear detail at edge of tissue fragment
Postbiopsy healing	See Table 1–2

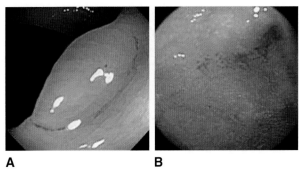

A   **B**

FIGURE 1–5. Endoscopic appearance of "scope trauma." **A,** A duodenal fold is swollen owing to lamina propria edema induced by passage of an endoscope; the region shows a subtle ring of mucosal hemorrhage. **B,** The colonic mucosa demonstrates multifocal areas of mucosal hemorrhage after withdrawal of the colonoscope, these were not present during initial advancement of the colonoscope into the colon. (Photographs courtesy of Dirk Van Leeuwen, Dartmouth Mary Hitchcock Medical Center, Lebanon, NH.)

fibers that branch off a thin metal shaft running within a protective plastic sheath. The various cytology brushes that are currently available do not seem to vary in terms of performance characteristics.[61] The cytology brush is passed through an accessory channel of an endoscope. The end of the sheath is passed out of the tip of the endoscope, and the bristle portion of the brush is then extended from the sheath. The brush is rubbed back and forth several times along the surface of the lesion, or stricture, and is then pulled back into the sheath. The sheath is then withdrawn from the endoscope, and the brush is pushed out of the sheath, thus exposing the bristles. The bristle portion of the brush may be cut off, placed into fixative, and sent in its entirety to the cytopathology laboratory. Alternatively, the bristles can be rolled against glass slides in the endoscopy suite. The slides should be sprayed with fixative immediately, or submerged in it, and subsequently delivered to the cytopathologist. If smears are made in the endoscopy suite, little additional benefit is derived from inclusion of the bristles for cytopathologic analysis.[62]

FINE-NEEDLE ASPIRATION

Fine-needle aspiration (FNA) is another method used for obtaining tissue for cytology.[63-65] FNA needles may be used during standard endoscopy or during EUS. EUS allows an endoscopist to sample tissue from parenchymal lesions and lymph nodes, as well as fluid from cystic lesions. EUS provides real-time imaging to ensure that the intended target is localized and sampled. The needles used for FNA during endoscopy are generally hollow 19- to 25-gauge needles, often fitted with a central stylet to avoid the gathering of intervening tissue. Once the lesion of interest has been

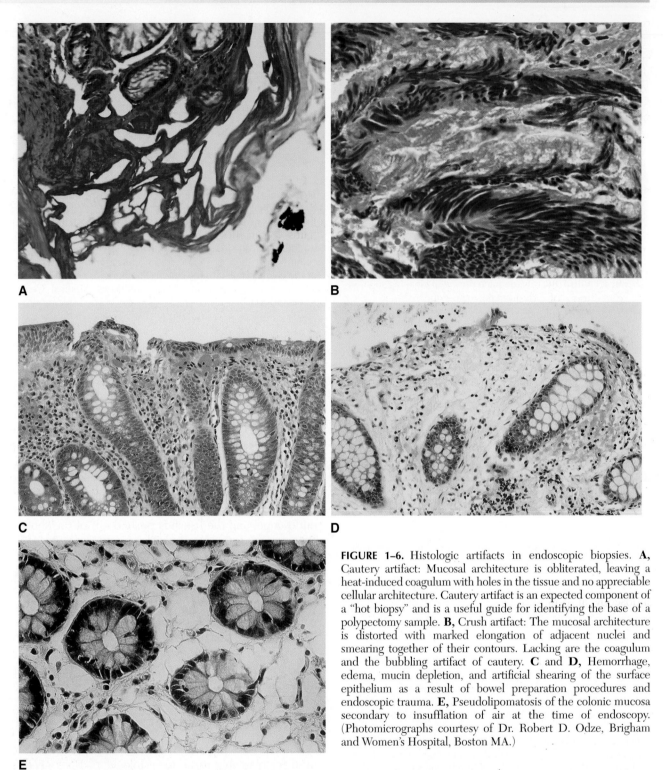

FIGURE 1-6. Histologic artifacts in endoscopic biopsies. **A,** Cautery artifact: Mucosal architecture is obliterated, leaving a heat-induced coagulum with holes in the tissue and no appreciable cellular architecture. Cautery artifact is an expected component of a "hot biopsy" and is a useful guide for identifying the base of a polypectomy sample. **B,** Crush artifact: The mucosal architecture is distorted with marked elongation of adjacent nuclei and smearing together of their contours. Lacking are the coagulum and the bubbling artifact of cautery. **C** and **D,** Hemorrhage, edema, mucin depletion, and artificial shearing of the surface epithelium as a result of bowel preparation procedures and endoscopic trauma. **E,** Pseudolipomatosis of the colonic mucosa secondary to insufflation of air at the time of endoscopy. (Photomicrographs courtesy of Dr. Robert D. Odze, Brigham and Women's Hospital, Boston MA.)

identified, the sheath is pushed out of the endoscope, and the needle is advanced into the target tissue either under fluoroscopic guidance (during ERCP) or under ultrasonographic guidance (during EUS). If a stylet is present, it is then removed, and suction is applied to a syringe at the proximal end of the needle. While suction is applied, the endoscopist moves the needle forward and backward within the lesion, thereby filling the distal needle lumen with tissue. The needle is then withdrawn into the sheath, and the entire apparatus is removed from the endoscope. Complications from FNA biopsy occur in less than 2% of cases and include bleeding and, in the setting of pancreatic mass FNA, acute pancreatitis.

Screening and Surveillance Guidelines in Gastroenterology

This section provides a short review of issues in clinical gastroenterology of interest to pathologists, namely management of Barrett's esophagus, inflammatory bowel disease, and colonic polyps.

SURVEILLANCE IN PATIENTS WITH BARRETT'S ESOPHAGUS

Most authorities recommend that patients with chronic reflux symptoms of longer than 5 years' duration should undergo endoscopy to screen for Barrett's esophagus.[66,67] If Barrett's esophagus is present, it is recommended that the patient enter an endoscopic surveillance program for the detection of dysplasia and adenocarcinoma.[68] Endoscopic surveillance should be undertaken only in patients medically fit to undergo esophagectomy. In the future, nonsurgical ablative endoscopic techniques (e.g., photodynamic therapy, multipolar electrocautery, argon plasma coagulator) may increase the number of possible candidates for surveillance. Aggressive treatment of reflux is warranted before surveillance endoscopy because active inflammation with repair can mimic low-grade dysplasia. Endoscopic surveillance is performed by obtaining four quadrant biopsies at 2-cm intervals with the use of jumbo biopsy forceps. Specific attention is paid to mucosal abnormalities. In the future, complementary techniques may be available to detect high-grade dysplasia, such as laser-induced fluorescence spectroscopy or quasi-elastic light scattering.[69,70]

The appropriate time interval for surveillance of dysplasia in Barrett's esophagus is once every 2 to 3 years. In the presence of biopsy-proven low-grade dysplasia, endoscopy at 6-month to 1-year intervals is recommended. Patients with documented and confirmed high-grade dysplasia should be considered candidates for esophagectomy. "Confirmation" consists of repeat endoscopy, with biopsies, within several weeks after the initial biopsy demonstration of high-grade dysplasia. The prevalence of cancer in resection specimens of patients who have undergone an esophagectomy for high-grade dysplasia ranges from 5% to 41%, and the rate of progression to cancer in patients with high-grade dysplasia approaches 30% at 10 years. If esophagectomy is not performed for high-grade dysplasia, more frequent surveillance (every 3 months) is recommended.

SURVEILLANCE IN INFLAMMATORY BOWEL DISEASE

Although at present no prospective randomized studies are being done to evaluate the efficacy of surveillance for dysplasia in inflammatory bowel disease (IBD), such surveillance has become the standard of care.[71,72] Surveillance colonoscopy should be reserved for patients medically fit to undergo colectomy and, optimally, should be performed at a time of inactive disease, because active inflammation may make challenging the histologic differentiation between dysplasia and reactive epithelial changes. Colonoscopic surveillance should begin after 8 years of disease in patients with pancolitis and after 12 to 15 years in patients with disease confined to the left colon. Patients with ulcerative proctitis or ulcerative proctosigmoiditis are not at increased risk for the development of colorectal cancer and thus should not undergo surveillance. Patients with childhood onset of colitis, or colitis and coexistent primary sclerosing cholangitis, may be at particularly high risk for developing colorectal cancer.[73]

Controversy is ongoing regarding the role of endoscopic surveillance for patients with Crohn's colitis.[74] Crohn's colitis is associated with an increased risk of colorectal carcinoma in patients with long-standing disease, strictures, and fistulas involving the colon.[75] The cumulative probability of detecting dysplasia or cancer in patients with Crohn's colitis after a negative initial screening colonoscopy is 22% by the time of the third follow-up colonoscopy.[74] It is likely that in the near future, pathologists will begin to see an increasing number of patients with Crohn's disease who are undergoing surveillance colonoscopy.

The most appropriate surveillance interval for ulcerative colitis has not been determined, but the current recommendation is once every 1 to 2 years.[75-78] Unfortunately, a recent survey from the United Kingdom demonstrated that a majority of gastroenterologists practice surveillance on a disorganized basis.[79] Thus, there is inconsistency in the management of patients with dysplasia. Furthermore, no standardized protocols are available for obtaining biopsies in patients who undergo surveillance endoscopy. Most endoscopists obtain four-quadrant biopsies at 10-cm intervals, whereas others obtain six specimens from each of the following sections: cecum and ascending colon, transverse colon, descending colon, sigmoid, and rectum. The use of jumbo biopsy forceps is highly recommended.

Additional biopsies should be obtained of any suspicious mucosal lesions. In one study, it was shown that up to 33 specimens are typically needed to detect dysplasia with 90% certainty.[80] The finding of dysplasia of any grade should be confirmed by a pathologist with special expertise in gastrointestinal pathology.[81] For patients with indefinite dysplasia, colonoscopy should be repeated in 4 to 6 months. Most authorities recommend proctocolectomy for patients with long-standing ulcerative colitis or Crohn's colitis and biopsy-proven low-grade dysplasia, particularly if present in multiple biopsies or in successive intervals, because the risk of cancer ranges from 20% to 50%.[82]

The treatment of a dysplastic polyp in ulcerative colitis is complex. The differential diagnosis of a polypoid area of dysplasia is a sporadic adenoma or an ulcerative colitis–associated dysplastic lesion or mass (DALM). If a well-circumscribed adenomatous polyp is found proximal to the extent of histologically demonstrable colitis, it should be managed as a simple adenoma (with the recognition that an adenomatous polyp is, in fact, a dysplastic lesion in its own right). However, when a sessile, plaquelike region of dysplasia is encountered within a region affected by colitis, it should be presumed to be an ulcerative colitis–related lesion and treated accordingly.

More controversial is the management of a small adenomatous polyp within a region of colitis because, in this instance, the polyp may be sporadic (i.e., sporadic adenoma) but may also be an adenoma-like DALM. Two recent studies have shown that ulcerative colitis patients who develop an adenoma-like DALM (i.e., a polyp that histologically resembles a sporadic adenoma), regardless of its location (i.e., whether it is located within or outside of areas of documented colitis), may undergo polypectomy and continued endoscopic surveillance if no other areas of flat dysplasia are detected in the adjacent mucosa or elsewhere in the colon because the risk of adenocarcinoma is negligible.[83,84] In contrast, the finding of flat dysplasia anywhere in the colon would still be regarded as an indication for colectomy. A review of the management of DALMs has been published recently.[85]

SCREENING AND SURVEILLANCE GUIDELINES FOR COLON POLYPS*

The following is a summary of the management of colonic polyps in patients who do not have inflammatory bowel disease. This summary includes postpolypectomy surveillance and the approach to a patient with a malignant polyp.

Definition and Clinical Considerations

Small (<1 cm) tubular adenomas are extremely common and have a low risk of becoming malignant. Only a small proportion of these develop histologic features of high-grade dysplasia and/or cancer. Advanced adenomas are defined as larger lesions (>1 cm in diameter) that contain an appreciable villous component or that contain foci of high-grade dysplasia. Efforts to control colon cancer now focus mainly on strategies to reliably detect and resect advanced adenomas before they become malignant. General guidelines for colonoscopic surveillance of adults with colon polyps who do not have inflammatory bowel disease are provided in Table 1-6. The management of polyps is summarized in Table 1-7.

Initial Management of Polyps

Most patients who have a polyp detected by barium enema or flexible sigmoidoscopy, especially if it is large or if there are multiple polyps, should undergo colonoscopy to excise the lesion or lesions and search for additional neoplasms. The decision as to whether to perform colonoscopy for patients with polyps smaller than 1 cm in diameter must be individualized depending on the patient's age, comorbidity, and past or family history of colorectal neoplasia. Complete colonoscopy should be done at the time of every initial polypectomy to detect and resect all synchronous adenomas. Additional colonoscopic examinations may be required after resection of a large sessile adenoma, if there are multiple adenomas, or if the colonoscopist is not reasonably confident that all adenomas have been found and resected.

TABLE 1–6. Surveillance and Surgical Management of Adults With Colon Polyps Who Do Not Have Inflammatory Bowel Disease

History	Management
1 or 2 colonic adenomas <1 cm in diameter *and* no family history of colorectal cancer	Colonoscopy every 5 years
>2 colonic adenomas, *or* colonic adenoma >1 cm in diameter, *or* colonic adenoma with villous features or with high-grade dysplasia, *or* family history of colorectal cancer	Repeat colonoscopy at 3 years; return to frequency every 5 years after one negative follow-up; remain at every 3 years if additional adenomas are identified
Malignant pedunculated polyp	
All "favorable" features (see Table 1–9)	Follow-up colonoscopy in 3 years
One or more "unfavorable" features (see Table 1–9)	Follow-up colonoscopy within 3 to 6 months, *or* surgical resection of colonic segment*
Malignant sessile polyp	
All "favorable" features (see Table 1–9)	Repeat colonoscopy within 3 to 6 months; return to colonoscopy every 5 years if negative
One or more "unfavorable" features (see Table 1–9)	Surgical resection of colonic segment*

*Surgical resection is recommended *unless* surgical risk is considered unacceptable *and/or* the probability of prolonging the patient's life is considered to be low.

---

*Screening and Surveillance Guidelines for Colon Polyps is reproduced from BondJH: Polyp guideline: Diagnosis, treatment, and surveillance for patients with colorectal polyps. Practice Parameters Committee of the American College of Gastoenterology. Am J Gastroenterology 95: 3053-3063, 2000.

TABLE 1–7. Management of Colonic Adenomas Without Carcinoma

Small adenoma (sessile or pedunculated) (<1 cm in diameter)	Detection by barium enema or flexible sigmoidoscopy: Include age, comorbidity, family history in decision to perform full colonoscopy with resection
	Detection at colonoscopy: Resect
Large pedunculated adenoma (≥1 cm in diameter)	Detection by barium enema or flexible sigmoidoscopy: Perform complete colonoscopy
	Upon performance of colonoscopy: Resect
	If completely resected, no change in surveillance regimen
	If not completely resected, perform follow-up colonoscopy within 3 to 6 months to remove residual adenomatous tissue
Large sessile adenoma (≥1 cm in diameter)	Detection by barium enema or flexible sigmoidoscopy: Perform complete colonoscopy
	Upon performance of colonoscopy: Resect, if possible
	If completely resected, consider follow-up colonoscopy within 3 to 6 months to verify, then return to standard surveillance regimen
	If not completely resected, perform follow-up colonoscopy within 3 to 6 months to remove residual adenomatous tissue; repeat a third time; if adenomatous tissue is still present, recommend surgical resection

Management of Small Polyps

Small polyps (<1 cm and either sessile or pedunculated) are resected with the use of a number of different techniques, both with and without electrocautery. However, a monopolar hot biopsy forceps has limitations and risks that need to be carefully considered, as has been discussed earlier. Considering that a small adenoma left in place is still a premalignant lesion, bioptic resection of any small polyp is justified. A separate question is whether a hyperplastic polyp identified during flexible sigmoidoscopy carries clinical significance. Current evidence supports the recommendation that a hyperplastic polyp found during flexible sigmoidoscopy is not, by itself, an indication for colonoscopy. Although hyperplastic polyps have classically been believed not to be clinically significant, recent discoveries have led to a reappraisal of the significance of large hyperplastic polyps, especially those that occur in the right colon.[86,87] Data are conflicting as to whether small distal adenomas predict the presence of proximal, clinically significant adenomas; therefore, the decision to perform colonoscopy

following identification of an adenoma during flexible sigmoidoscopy must be individualized.

Management of Large Pedunculated Polyps

Large pedunculated polyps (≥1 cm in diameter) resected in one piece should be examined by the pathologist for adequacy of resection; guidelines for polyp specimen processing were given under Orientation of Formalin-Fixed Tissue Obtained at Endoscopy. Piecemeal resection of large pedunculated polyps impedes but does not preclude histopathologic assessment of adequacy of resection. However, in this instance, the pathologist is dependent on the endoscopist to deliver a readily identifiable stalk.

Management of Large Sessile Polyps

Assessment of the adequacy of excision of a large sessile polyp (≥1 cm in diameter) is more problematic and depends on both the endoscopist's assessment of whether a residual lesion is left behind and the pathologist's ability to identify resection margins with confidence (see later). This includes the issue of whether a large sessile polyp is resected intact or piecemeal. Hence, there may be value in tattooing the polypectomy site following endoscopic resection for visualization during a subsequent endoscopic procedure. A patient who has had a successful colonoscopic excision of a large sessile polyp should undergo follow-up colonoscopy in 3 to 6 months so that it can be determined whether the resection was complete. If residual adenomatous mucosa is present, it should be further resected, and the completeness of this resection procedure documented within another 3- to 6-month interval. If complete resection is not possible after two or three examinations, the patient should be considered for a surgical resection.

Postpolypectomy Surveillance

After a complete colonoscopy has been performed following a polypectomy, repeat colonoscopy to evaluate for the presence of metachronous adenomas should be performed after 3 years for patients at high risk of developing metachronous advanced adenomas. This includes patients who at their initial baseline examination have had multiple (more than two) adenomas, a large (≥1 cm) adenoma, an adenoma with villous features, or one with high-grade dysplasia; it also includes patients with a family history of colorectal cancer. Repeat colonoscopy to check for metachronous adenomas should be performed in 5 years for most patients at low risk of developing advanced adenomas. This includes patients who at baseline examination have had only one or two small tubular adenomas (<1 cm) and do not have a family history of colorectal cancer.

After one negative follow-up surveillance colonoscopy, subsequent surveillance may be extended to 5-year intervals. If complete colonoscopy is not feasible, flexible sigmoidoscopy followed by a double-contrast barium enema is an acceptable alternative. Follow-up surveillance should be individualized according to the age and comorbidity of the patient and should be discontinued when it seems unlikely that follow-up can prolong the quality of the patient's life.

Malignant Polyps

Guidelines from the American College of Gastroenterology (ACG) for the management of malignant polyps are provided in Table 1-8.[86] A malignant polyp is defined as an adenomatous polyp with cancer invading the submucosa; favorable and unfavorable histologic features are provided in Table 1-9.

No further treatment is indicated after colonoscopic resection of a malignant polyp if the endoscopic and pathologic criteria listed in Table 1-9 are fulfilled. Patients with a malignant pedunculated polyp with "favorable" criteria may be observed similarly to patients with a history of advanced colonic adenomas. Patients with a malignant sessile polyp that shows favorable prognostic criteria should have follow-up colonoscopy within 3 to 6 months to check for residual neoplastic tissue at the polypectomy site. After one negative follow-up examination, the clinician may revert to a standard surveillance regimen.

TABLE 1–8. Management of Malignant Colonic Polyps

Findings	Management
Pedunculated polyp, all favorable features by histology	No change in surveillance regimen
Sessile polyp, all favorable features by histology	Follow-up colonoscopy within 3 to 6 months; if no evidence of residual adenoma or cancer on follow-up, return to regular surveillance
Pedunculated or sessile polyp, ≥1 unfavorable histologic feature	Consider surgical resection

TABLE 1–9. Favorable and Unfavorable Features in Malignant Colonic Polyps

Favorable	Unfavorable
Cancer is well differentiated to moderately differentiated (grade I or II)	Cancer is poorly differentiated (grade III)
Absence of lymphovascular invasion	Lymphovascular invasion is present
Carcinoma is ≥2 mm from deep margin	Cancer is <2 mm from deep margin

When a patient's malignant polyp has poor ("unfavorable") prognostic features, the relative risk of surgical resection should be weighed against the risk of death from metastatic carcinoma. If a malignant polyp is located in a part of the lower rectum that may require an abdominal-perineal resection, local excision, rather than standard cancer resection, may be justified. In brief, the risk of local recurrence or lymph node metastasis from an invasive carcinoma in a colonoscopically resected malignant adenomatous polyp is considered less than the risk of death from colonic surgery if the following criteria are fulfilled:

1. The polyp is considered to be completely excised by the endoscopist and is submitted in toto for pathologic examination.
2. In the pathology laboratory, the polyp is fixed and sectioned so that it is possible for the pathologist to accurately determine the depth of invasion, grade of differentiation, and completeness of excision of the carcinoma.
3. The cancer is not poorly differentiated (grade III).
4. There is no evidence of vascular or lymphatic involvement.
5. The margin of excision is not involved. Invasion of the stalk of a pedunculated polyp in itself is not an unfavorable prognostic finding as long as the cancer does not extend to within 2 mm of the deep margin of stalk resection.

It should be noted that an adenomatous polyp (with or without malignancy) is not considered adequately resected unless all adenomatous mucosa is removed. Hence, the ultimate goal of any endoscopic resection is to remove all neoplastic mucosa.

References

1. American Society for Gastrointestinal Endoscopy: Tissue sampling and analysis. Gastrointest Endosc 37:663-665, 1991.
2. Fennerty M, Davidson J, Emerson S, et al: Are endoscopic measurements of colonic polyps reliable? Am J Gastroenterol 88:496-500, 1993.
3. Margulies C, Krevsky B, Catalano M: How accurate are endoscopic estimates of size? Gastrointest Endosc 40:174-177, 1994.
4. Tooson JD, Gates LK Jr: Bowel preparation before colonoscopy. Choosing the best lavage regimen. Postgrad Med 100:203-214, 1996.
5. Hangartner PJ, Munch R, Meier J, et al: Comparison of three colon cleansing methods: Evaluation of a randomized clinical trial with 300 ambulatory patients. Endoscopy 21:272-275, 1989.
6. Lee J, McCallion K, Acheson AG, et al: A prospective randomised study comparing polyethylene glycol and sodium phosphate bowel cleansing solutions for colonoscopy. Ulster Med J 68:68-72, 1999.
7. Borkje B, Pedersen R, Lund GM, et al: Effectiveness and acceptability of three bowel cleansing regimens. Scand J Gastroenterol 26:162-166, 1991.
8. Dahshan A, Lin CH, Peters J, et al: A randomized, prospective study to evaluate the efficacy and acceptance of three bowel preparations for colonoscopy in children. Am J Gastroenterol 3497-3501, 1999.
9. Pockros PJ, Foroozan P: Golytely lavage versus a standard colonoscopy preparation. Effect on normal colonic mucosal histology. Gastroenterology 88:545-548, 1985.
10. Meisel JL, Bergman D, Graney D, et al: Human rectal mucosa: Proctoscopic and morphological changes caused by laxatives. Gastroenterology 72:1274-1279, 1977.

11. Jonas G, Mahoney A, Murray J, et al: Chemical colitis due to endoscope cleaning solutions: A mimic of pseudomembranous colitis. Gastroenterology 95:1403-1408, 1988.
12. Achkar E, Carey W, Petras R, et al: Comparison of suction capsule and endoscopic biopsy of small bowel mucosa. Gastrointest Endosc 32:278-281, 1986.
13. Weinstein W: Mucosal biopsy techniques and interaction with the pathologist. Gastrointest Endosc Clin N Am 10:555-572, 2000.
14. Bernstein D, Barkin J, Reiner D, et al: Standard biopsy forceps versus large-capacity forceps with and without needle. Gastrointest Endosc 41:573-576, 1995.
15. Woods K, Anand B, Cole R, et al: Influence of endoscopic biopsy forceps characteristics on tissue specimens: Results of a prospective randomized study. Gastrointest Endosc 49:177-183, 1999.
16. Ladas S, Tsamouri M, Kouvidou C, et al: Effect of forceps size and mode of orientation on endoscopic small bowel biopsy evaluation. Gastrointest Endosc 40:51-55, 1994.
17. Rizzo J, Bernstein D, Gress F: A performance, safety and cost comparison of reusable and disposable endoscopic biopsy forceps: A prospective, randomized trial. Gastrointest Endosc 51:262-265, 2000.
18. Woods KL, Anand BS, Cole RA, et al: Influence of endoscopic biopsy forceps characteristics on tissue specimens: Results of a prospective randomized study. Gastrointest Endosc 49:177-183, 1999.
19. Levine D, Blount P, Rudolph R, et al: Safety of a systemic endoscopic biopsy protocol in patients with Barrett's esophagus. Am J Gastroenterol 95:1152-1157, 2000.
20. Falk G, Rice T, Goldblum J, et al: Jumbo biopsy forceps protocol still misses unsuspected cancer in Barrett's esophagus with high-grade dysplasia. Gastrointest Endosc 49:170-176, 1999.
21. Jailwala J, Fogel E, Sherman S, et al: Triple-tissue sampling at ERCP in malignant biliary obstruction. Gastrointest Endosc 51:383-390, 2000.
22. Watanabe Y, Goto H, Hirooka Y, et al: Transpapillary biopsy in gallbladder disease. Gastrointest Endosc 51:76-79, 2000.
23. Waye J: Techniques of polypectomy: Hot biopsy forceps and snare polypectomy. Am J Gastroenterol 82:615-618, 1987.
24. Kimmey M, Silverstein F, Saunders D, et al: Endoscopic bipolar forceps: A potential treatment for the diminutive polyp. Gastrointest Endosc 34:38-41, 1988.
25. Wadas D, Sanowski R: Complications of the hot biopsy forceps technique. Gastrointest Endosc 33:32-37, 1987.
26. Gilbert D, DiMarino A, Jensen D, et al: Status evaluation: Hot biopsy forceps. American Society for Gastrointestinal Endoscopy Technology Assessment Committee. Gastrointest Endosc 38:753-756, 1992.
27. Peluso F, Goldner F: Follow-up of hot biopsy forceps treatment of diminutive colonic polyps. Gastrointest Endosc 37:604-606, 1991.
28. McAfee J, Katon R: Tiny snares prove safe and effective for removal of diminutive colorectal polyps. Gastrointest Endosc 40:301-303, 1994.
29. Tappero G, Gaia E, De Giuli P, et al: Cold snare excision of small colorectal polyps. Gastrointest Endosc 38:310-313, 1992.
30. Binmoeller K, Boaventura S, Ramsperger K, et al: Endoscopic snare excision of benign adenomas of the papilla of Vater. Gastrointest Endosc 39:205-207, 1993.
31. Lieberman D, Weiss D, Bond J, et al: Use of colonoscopy to screen asymptomatic adults for colorectal cancer. N Engl J Med 343:162-168, 2000.
32. Macrae F, Tan K, Williams C: Towards safer colonoscopy: A report on the complications of 5000 diagnostic or therapeutic colonoscopies. Gut 24:376-383, 1983.
33. Rosenberg N: Submucosal saline wheal as safety factor in fulguration of rectal and sigmoidal polyps. Arch Surg 70:120-123, 1955.
34. Deyhle P, Largiader F, More SJ: A method for endoscopic electroresection of sessile colonic polyps. Endoscopy 5:38, 1973.
35. Soetikno R, Inoue H, Chang K: Endoscopic mucosal resection: Current concepts. Gastrointest Endosc Clin N Am 10:595-617, 2000.
36. Fleischer D: Endoscopic mucosal resection: (Not) made in the USA (so commonly). A dissection of the definition, technique, use, and controversies. Gastrointest Endosc 52:440-444, 2000.
37. Uno Y, Munakata A: The non-lifting sign of invasive colon cancer. Gastrointest Endosc 40:485-489, 1994.
38. Tanabe S, Koizumi W, Kokutou M, et al: Usefulness of endoscopic aspiration mucosectomy as compared with strip biopsy for the treatment of gastric mucosal cancer. Gastrointest Endosc 50:819-822, 1999.
39. Inoue H, Takeshita K, Hori H, et al: Endoscopic mucosal resection with a cap-fitted panendoscope for esophagus, stomach, and colon mucosal lesions. Gastrointest Endosc 39:58-62, 1993.
40. Kojima T, Parra-Blanco A, Takahashi H, et al: Outcome of endoscopic mucosal resection for early gastric cancer: Review of the Japanese literature. Gastrointest Endosc 48:550-554, 1998.
41. Waxman I, Saitoh Y: Clinical outcome of endoscopic mucosal resection for superficial GI lesions and the role of high-frequency ultrasound probe sonography in an American population. Gastrointest Endosc 52:322-327, 2000.
42. Nelson DB: Technical assessment of direct colonoscopy screening: Procedural success, safety, and feasibility. Gastrointest Endosc Clin N Am 12:77-84, 2002.
43. Levine DS, Blount PL, Rudolph RE, et al: Safety of a systematic endoscopic biopsy protocol in patients with Barrett's esophagus. Am J Gastroenterol 95:1152-1157, 2000.
44. Dafnis G, Ekbom A, Pahlman L, et al: Complications of diagnostic and therapeutic colonoscopy within a defined population in Sweden. Gastrointest Endosc 54:302-309, 2001.
45. Maglinte DDT, Strong RC, Strate RW, et al: Barium enema after colorectal biopsies: Experimental data. Am J Roentg 139:693-697, 1982.
46. Bernstein S, Council on Scientific Affairs: Formaldehyde. J Am Med Assoc 261:1183-1187, 1989.
47. Conolly RB, Kimbell JS, Janszen DB, et al: Dose response for formaldehyde-induced cytotoxicity in the human respiratory tract. Regul Toxicol Pharmacol 35:32-43, 2002.
48. Fox CH, Johnson FB, Whiting J, et al: Formaldehyde fixation. J Histochem Cytochem 33:845-853, 1985.
49. Login GR, Dvorak AM: Methods of microwave fixation for microscopy. A review of research and clinical applications: 1970-1992. Prog Histochem Cytochem 27:1-127, 1994.
50. Crosby WH, Kugler HW: Intraluminal biopsy of the small intestine. Am J Dig Dis 2:236-249, 1957.
51. Flick AL, Quinton WE, Rubin CE: A peroral hydraulic biopsy tube for multiple sampling at any level of the gastrointestinal tract. Gastroenterology 40:120-126, 1961.
52. Mee AS, Burke M, Vallon AG, et al: Small bowel biopsy for malabsorption: Comparison of the diagnostic accuracy of endoscopic forceps and capsule biopsy specimens. Br Med J 291:769-774, 1985.
53. Smith JA, Mayberry JF, Ansell ID, et al: Small bowel biopsy for disaccharidase levels: Evidence that endoscopic forceps biopsy can replace the Crosby capsule. Clin Chem Acta 183:317-326, 1989.
54. Lester SC: Manual of Surgical Pathology. New York, Churchill-Livingstone, 2001, p 183.
55. Stetler-Stevenson M, Braylan RC: Flow cytometric analysis of lymphomas and lymphoproliferative disorders. Semin Hematol 38:111-123, 2001.
56. Jonas G, Mahoney A, Murray J, et al: Chemical colitis due to endoscopic cleaning solutions: A mimic of pseudomembranous colitis. Gastroenterology 95:1403-1408, 1988.
57. West AB, Kuan SF, Bennick M, et al: Glutaraldehyde colitis following endoscopy: Clinical and pathological features and investigation of an outbreak. Gastroenterology 108:1250-1255, 1995.
58. Meisel JL, Bergman D, Graney D, et al: Human rectal mucosa: Proctoscopic and morphological changes caused by laxatives. Gastroenterology 72:1274-1279, 1977.
59. Baron T, Lee J, Wax T, et al: An in vitro, randomized, prospective study to maximize cellular yield during bile duct brush cytology. Gastrointest Endosc 40:146-149, 1994.
60. Marshall J, Diaz-Arias A, Barthel J, et al: Prospective evaluation of optimal number of biopsy specimens and brush cytology in the diagnosis of cancer of the colorectum. Am J Gastroenterol 88:1352-1354, 1993.
61. Camp R, Rutkowski M, Atkison K, et al: A prospective, randomized, blinded trial of cytological yield with disposable cytology brushes in upper gastrointestinal tract lesions. Am J Gastroenterol 87:1439-1442, 1992.
62. Ferrari A, Lichtenstein D, Slivka A, et al: Brush cytology during ERCP for the diagnosis of biliary and pancreatic malignancies. Gastrointest Endosc 40:140-145, 1994.
63. Howell D, Beveridge R, Bosco J, et al: Endoscopic needle aspiration biopsy at ERCP in the diagnosis of biliary strictures. Gastrointest Endosc 38:531-535, 1992.

64. Gress F, Hawes R, Savides T, et al: Endoscopic ultrasound-guided fine-needle aspiration biopsy using linear array and radial scanning endosonography. Gastrointest Endosc 45:243-250, 1997.

65. Giovannini M, Seitz J-F, Monges G, et al: Fine-needle aspiration cytology guided by endoscopic ultrasonography: Results in 141 patients. Endoscopy 27:171-177, 1995.

66. Morales TG, Sampliner RE: Barrett's esophagus: Update on screening, surveillance, and treatment. Arch Intern Med 159:1411-1416, 1999.

67. Sampliner RE: Updated guidelines for the diagnosis, surveillance, and therapy of Barrett's esophagus. Am J Gastroenterol 97:1888-1895, 2002.

68. Sonnenberg A, Soni A, Sampliner RE: Medical decision analysis of endoscopic surveillance of Barrett's oesophagus to prevent oesophageal adenocarcinoma. Aliment Pharmacol Ther 16:41-50, 2002.

69. Wallace MB, Perelman LT, Backman V, et al: Endoscopic detection of dysplasia in patients with Barrett's esophagus using light-scattering spectroscopy. Gastroenterology 119:677-682, 2000.

70. Georgakoudi I, Jacobson BC, Van Dam J, et al: Fluorescence, reflectance, and light-scattering spectroscopy for evaluating dysplasia in patients with Barrett's esophagus. Gastroenterology 120:1620-1629, 2001.

71. Eaden JA, Mayberry JF: Guidelines for screening and surveillance of asymptomatic colorectal cancer in patients with inflammatory bowel disease. Gut 51(suppl 5):V10-V12, 2002.

72. Rex DK, Bond JH, Winawer S, et al: Quality in the technical performance of colonoscopy and the continuous quality improvement process for colonoscopy: Recommendations of the U.S. Multi-Society Task Force on Colorectal Cancer. Am J Gastroenterol 97:1296-1308, 2002.

73. Greenson JK: Dysplasia in inflammatory bowel disease. Semin Diagn Pathol 19:31-37, 2002.

74. Friedman S, Rubin PH, Bodian C, et al: Screening and surveillance colonoscopy in chronic Crohn's colitis. Gastroenterology 120:820-826, 2001.

75. Pohl C, Hombach A, Kruis W: Chronic inflammatory bowel disease and cancer. Hepatogastroenterology 47:57-70, 2000.

76. Provenzale D, Wong JB, Onken JE, et al: Performing a cost-effectiveness analysis: Surveillance of patients with ulcerative colitis. Am J Gastroenterol 93:872-880, 1998.

77. Kornbluth A, Sachar DB: Ulcerative colitis practice guidelines in adults. American College of Gastroenterology, Practice Parameters Committee. Am J Gastroenterol 92:204-211, 1997.

78. Hanauer SB, Sandborn W: Management of Crohn's disease in adults. Am J Gastroenterol 96:635-643, 2001.

79. Eaden JA, Ward BA, Mayberry JF: How gastroenterologists screen for colonic cancer in ulcerative colitis: An analysis of performance. Gastrointest Endosc 51:123-128, 2000.

80. Connell WR, Lennard-Jones JE, Williams CB, et al: Factors affecting the outcome of endoscopic surveillance for cancer in ulcerative colitis. Gastroenterology 107:934-944, 1994.

81. Riddell RH, Goldman H, Ransohoff DF, et al: Dysplasia in inflammatory bowel disease: Standardized classification with provisional clinical applications. Hum Pathol 14:931-968, 1983.

82. Bernstein CN, Shanahan F, Weinstein WM: Are we telling patients the truth about surveillance colonoscopy in ulcerative colitis? Lancet 343:71-74, 1994.

83. Engelsgjerd M, Farraye FA, Odze RD: Polypectomy may be adequate treatment for adenoma-like dysplastic lesions in chronic ulcerative colitis. Gastroenterology 117:1288-1294, 1999; discussion 1488-1491.

84. Rubin PH, Friedman S, Harpaz N, et al: Colonoscopic polypectomy in chronic colitis: Conservative management after endoscopic resection of dysplastic polyps. Gastroenterology 117:1295-1300, 1999.

85. Odze RD: Adenomas and adenoma-like DALMs in chronic ulcerative colitis: A clinical, pathological, and molecular review. Am J Gastroenterol 94:1746-1750, 1999.

86. Jass JR, Whitehall VL, Young J, et al: Emerging concepts in colorectal neoplasia. Gastroenterology 123:862-876, 2002.

87. Hawkins NJ, Ward RL: Sporadic colorectal cancers with microsatellite instability and their possible origin in hyperplastic polyps and serrated adenomas. J Natl Cancer Inst 93:1307-1313, 2001.

CHAPTER 2

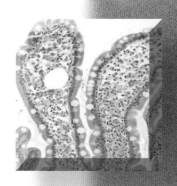

Diagnostic Cytology of the GI Tract

HELEN H. WANG

▌ Introduction

The popularity of gastrointestinal cytology for the diagnosis of infection and malignancy has waxed and waned over the past few decades. The ability to distinguish between a high-grade dysplasia/carcinoma in situ and invasive carcinoma in biopsy specimens and the more prevalent expertise of surgical pathology cause some to consider cytology an unnecessary duplication of gastrointestinal mucosal biopsies.[1,2] However, the combined use of endoscopy, ultrasound guidance, and fine-needle aspiration has expanded the horizons of gastrointestinal cytology.[3-5]

SPECIMEN TYPES

Types of gastrointestinal tract specimens commonly received in the cytology laboratory include endoscopic brushings and ultrasound-guided endoscopic fine-needle aspirations. Endoscopic washing specimens have become unpopular owing to the difficulty involved in handling and processing these specimens, as well as their low yield. Endoscopic fine-needle aspirations have enabled endoscopists to reach farther than they can with biopsy forceps to sample mural lesions, and even lesions adjacent to the gastrointestinal tract. The nonendoscopic specimens obtained with either the balloon- or mesh-type samplers have been evaluated in the research setting to ascertain their utility in the surveillance of high-risk patients.[6-8]

SPECIMEN PREPARATIONS

Direct smears can be made from materials collected on the endoscopic brush, in the needle, or on the balloon and mesh samplers; these can then be either fixed immediately in 95% ethanol and stained with the Papanicolaou method or left to air-dry and stained with Diff-Quik (Dade-Behring, Inc, Deerfield, IL) or Wright-Giemsa stain. Alternatively, the material can be rinsed into a medium, such as CytoLyt (Cytyc Corporation, Boxborough, MA) or 50% ethanol. The specimen can then be processed by means of a concentration method, such as either ThinPrep (Cytyc Corporation, Boxborough, MA) or cytospin, to make slides that are then stained with the Papanicolaou method.

VALUE AND ACCURACY OF SPECIMENS

Cytology specimens have some advantage over specimens obtained by endoscopic biopsy. The brush can sample a wider area and the fine needle can reach deeper lesions than can be reached by biopsy forceps. Also, both the brush and the fine needle are less invasive than biopsy forceps and less likely to cause bleeding. In addition, cytology has shorter turnaround time than histology. Direct smears can be ready for review within minutes with no compromise of the quality of the preparation (unlike frozen sections of biopsy specimens, which compromise the quality of the specimen). However, as was previously mentioned, cytology is limited in its ability to distinguish between high-grade dysplasia/carcinoma in situ and invasive carcinoma.

In spite of the potential duplication of cytology and biopsy, the literature has consistently shown that the highest diagnostic yield is obtained with combined use of these specimens.[9-11] The yield of cytology is significantly higher when the brushing is performed before rather than after the biopsy.[12]

Normal Morphology

ESOPHAGUS

Intermediate-type squamous cells with abundant cytoplasm and vesicular nuclei are seen within the normal esophagus (Fig. 2-1). Superficial-type squamous cells with abundant cytoplasm and small pyknotic nuclei can also be seen in small numbers. Single cells and clusters of ciliated columnar cells from the respiratory tract with no clinical significance may be seen rarely.

STOMACH

Gastric surface foveolar cells can shed as single cells or in sheets. When in sheets, the columnar cells with abundant cytoplasm, regularly spaced nuclei, and open chromatin arrange in a honeycomb or palisaded pattern, depending on the orientation. When they are shed as single cells, they often lose their cytoplasm to become naked nuclei. In endoscopic fine-needle aspiration specimens, the sheets of foveolar cells can mimic cells from a mucinous neoplasm, and the single naked nuclei, because of their small monomorphic appearance, can mimic cells from a pancreatic endocrine tumor.

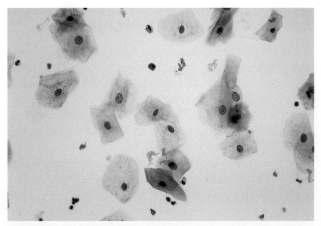

FIGURE 2–1. Brushing specimen from a normal esophagus composed predominantly of intermediate squamous cells. Scattered inflammatory cells are also noted in this field (Papanicolaou).

SMALL INTESTINE

The lining cells from the small intestine can be easily distinguished from gastric foveolar cells by the presence of goblet cells. On low magnification, the specimen typically has a Swiss cheese appearance, with the "holes" representing either goblet cells or gland openings of the crypts. On high magnification, the absorptive cells have either finely granular or vacuolated cytoplasm, and the goblet cells have single large mucin vacuoles and crescent-shaped nuclei with rounded contours. The striated border of the absorptive cells may be seen at the periphery of the sheets.

LARGE INTESTINE

Normal epithelium is characterized on cytology by sheets or strips of tall columnar cells with abundant cytoplasm and basal nuclei. Partial or complete openings of the colonic crypts may be seen.

Infections

Most infections that affect human hosts can infect the gastrointestinal tract. Some infectious agents have a predilection for the gastrointestinal tract. The more common ones are discussed in this section.

CANDIDA

Candida almost exclusively involves the esophagus along the gastrointestinal tract and can occur in both immunocompetent and immunocompromised patients. Brushings are in fact more sensitive than biopsy specimens in the detection of esophageal candidiasis.[9] Contamination by oral *Candida* is usually not a problem because the brush is contained within a sheath when it is passed into and out of the endoscope and is expelled from the sheath only to sample the lesion. The organisms appear as pink to purple pseudohyphae and yeast forms on Papanicolaou stain (Fig. 2-2). Reactive squamous cells as well as inflammatory cells are often noted in the background.

HERPES SIMPLEX VIRUS

Herpes simplex virus infection can theoretically affect epithelial cells anywhere along the gastrointestinal tract, but it is most commonly seen in the esophagus. Multinucleation, nuclear molding, ground-glass chromatin, and eosinophilic intranuclear inclusions are the characteristic features of infected cells (Fig. 2-3).

CYTOMEGALOVIRUS

Cytomegalovirus infection affects epithelial, stromal, and endothelial cells along the gastrointestinal tract and

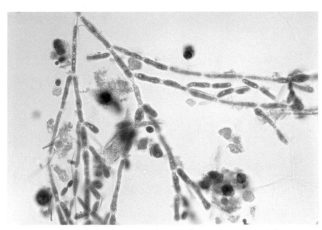

FIGURE 2–2. Pseudohyphae and yeast forms from *Candida* species are seen in this esophageal brushing specimen. Inflammatory cells and debris are in the background (Papanicolaou).

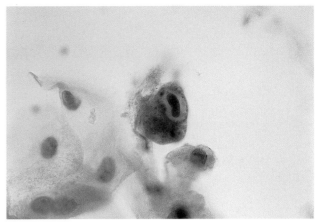

FIGURE 2–4. Both intranuclear and intracytoplasmic inclusions are seen in this cytomegalovirus-infected cell from an esophageal brushing. The intranuclear inclusion is a large amphophilic to basophilic body surrounded by a halo, and the intracytoplasmic inclusion is characterized by small, granular, basophilic to amphophilic bodies (Papanicolaou).

is characterized by large cells with a single large basophilic intranuclear inclusion with a perinuclear halo (Fig. 2-4). Intracytoplasmic textured inclusions can occasionally be seen in the affected cells (see Fig. 2-4).

HELICOBACTER PYLORI

Helicobacter pylori infection occurs exclusively in the stomach and perhaps is the most common infection of the gastrointestinal tract. These organisms can be demonstrated either on imprint smears of gastric biopsies or on brush cytology specimens.[13] Imprint and brushing cytology specimens are comparable in sensitivity (88%) and specificity (61%) with histologic examination of sections stained with hematoxylin and eosin and modified Giemsa.[13] The benefits of imprint and brushing cytology are the rapid results, high specificity, and low cost. However, the efficacy of cytologic detection of these organisms depends on the extent of colonization by the

organism. When present in large quantity, they are evident even at low magnification. They can be difficult to identify when present in small numbers. On Papanicolaou stain, *H. pylori* organisms appear as faintly basophilic, S-shaped rods admixed with mucus in the vicinity of glandular cell clusters (Fig. 2-5). Special stains, such as a triple stain combining silver, hematoxylin and eosin, and Alcian blue at pH 2.5, can enhance their detection by cytology.[14]

GIARDIA

Giardia affects the duodenum of both immunocompetent and immunocompromised hosts. Brush cytology is a useful method for detecting *Giardia* because the organisms are on the luminal surfaces of the intestinal epithelial cells. They are flat, gray, pear-

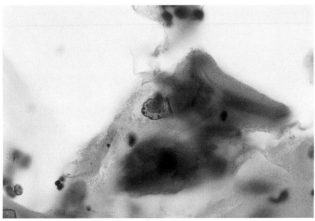

FIGURE 2–3. A Cowdry B inclusion characterized by an eosinophilic intranuclear body surrounded by a halo is seen in the center of the field from an esophageal brushing of herpetic esophagitis (Papanicolaou).

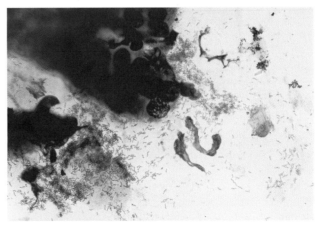

FIGURE 2–5. Numerous S-shaped organisms consistent with *H. pylori* are present in the mucus adjacent to a sheet of epithelial cells on a gastric brushing specimen (Diff-Quik).

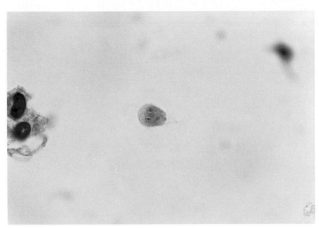

FIGURE 2–6. A pear-shaped, gray, binucleate *Giardia* organism is seen in the center of the field from a duodenal brushing specimen (Papanicolaou).

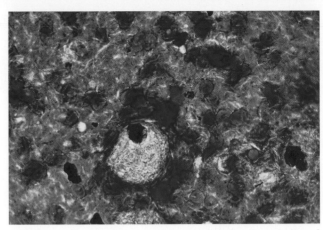

FIGURE 2–8. Numerous negative images of rod-shaped organisms are seen within and outside the histiocyte in the center of the field (from the same case as in Figure 2–7) (Diff-Quik).

shaped, and binucleate with four pairs of flagella (Fig. 2-6).[15]

ATYPICAL MYCOBACTERIA

Because atypical mycobacteria accumulate within macrophages in the lamina propria, very rigorous brushing is required for the infected macrophages to be included in the cytology sample. The presence of isolated foamy histiocytes on the smear should raise the suspicion of an atypical mycobacterial infection (Fig. 2-7). In general, the organisms are present in large numbers. On Diff-Quik–stained smears, the mycobacteria form numerous rod-shaped negative images either within the histiocytes or in the background (Fig. 2-8).[16] Special stains for acid-fast bacilli are necessary to confirm the diagnosis.

CRYPTOSPORIDIA

Cryptosporidia can involve any glandular epithelium of the gastrointestinal tract in human immunodeficiency virus (HIV)–infected patients and can be detected by examination of stool and cytology specimens.[17] Cryptosporidia are 2- to 5-µm round basophilic bodies on the luminal surfaces of the epithelial cells. Therefore, they are seen only when the plane of focus is shifted to the surfaces of the cells where the organisms reside (Fig. 2-9). When in doubt, confirmatory GMS (Gomori's methenamine-silver) stain can be applied.

MICROSPORIDIA

Microsporidia can also be detected on cytologic specimens, such as stool, nasal secretions, duodenal aspirates, and bile, as well as on brushing specimens from the duodenum and biliary tract.[18-20] On Papanicolaou stain, they appear in aggregates as brightly eosinophilic,

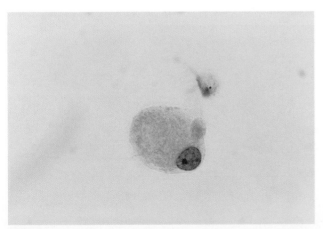

FIGURE 2–7. A histiocyte with abundant granular cytoplasm is present in this duodenal brushing specimen from an HIV-infected man. On special stain, the cell is shown to be filled with acid-fast bacilli, consistent with atypical mycobacteria (Papanicolaou).

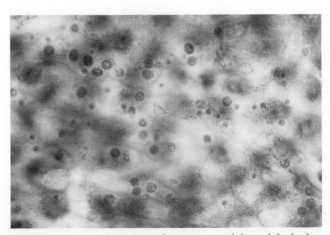

FIGURE 2–9. Many 2- to 5-µm-diameter, round, basophilic bodies are seen on the surface of this sheet of gastric epithelial cells on a brushing specimen (Papanicolaou).

rod-shaped or ovoid organisms, measuring 1 to 3 μm in diameter (Fig. 2-10). They are present in epithelial cells as well as in inflammatory cells. When in the epithelial cells, they are in the supranuclear portion of the cytoplasm and therefore are seen again at a slightly different plane of focus from that of the epithelial nuclei.

Inflammatory/Reactive/Metaplastic Changes

NONSPECIFIC CHANGES

Any injury to the mucosa can evoke a nonspecific inflammatory/reactive epithelial change. When the injury is sufficient to result in ulceration, the change can become so extreme that it may mimic a malignancy and is called *epithelial repair*. It may often be difficult to determine whether the reparative epithelium is of glandular or squamous origin. Although epithelial repair is characterized by prominent eosinophilic nucleoli, they usually are not huge or numerous (more than 3 or 4) (Fig. 2-11). The atypical stromal cells or their stripped nuclei from granulation tissue can also be quite alarming (Fig. 2-12). In spite of striking nuclear enlargement of such cells, hyperchromasia is absent. Instead, they have fine, homogeneous chromatin and a thin, smooth nuclear membrane.

Both cellular arrangements and features of individual cells are useful in the distinction between severe reactive and neoplastic changes. Cells with reactive/reparative changes are usually arranged in flat sheets without three-dimensionality or prominent cell dyshesion. In contrast, dyshesion, presented either as "feathering" (dissociation of cells) at the periphery of cell clusters or as the dispersion of numerous isolated cells, is usually evident with neoplasms, as is three-dimensionality. In

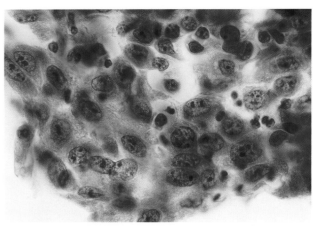

FIGURE 2–11. A loose sheet of reactive epithelial cells with a streaming pattern is seen in an esophageal brushing specimen. The cells are uniformly enlarged with prominent nucleoli. However, irregular nuclear membranes or chromatin aberration is absent. Several inflammatory cells are superimposed on or are infiltrating this sheet. It is difficult to determine whether the cells are squamous or glandular (Papanicolaou).

addition, the enlarged nuclei in reactive/reparative changes usually have uniform size and a similar number of small, prominent nucleoli. These again are in contrast to the variation in nuclear and nucleolar size and shape as well as the chromatin pattern in the neoplastic lesions. Specific types of reactive cells may also be seen, such as those with radiation-induced changes (Fig. 2-13). As in other organs, the cells are proportionally enlarged with metachromatic cytoplasm and nuclear or cytoplasmic vacuoles.

PEMPHIGUS

Rarely, pemphigus vulgaris, an autoimmune disease of the skin and mucous membrane that attacks the intercellular junctions and causes a suprabasilar bleb or

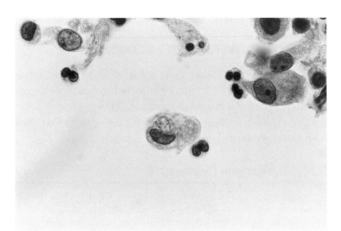

FIGURE 2–10. Several 1- to 3-μm-diameter eosinophilic rods are in the cytoplasm of the cell in the center of this duodenal brushing specimen. They typically are found in the supranuclear portion of the cytoplasm (Papanicolaou).

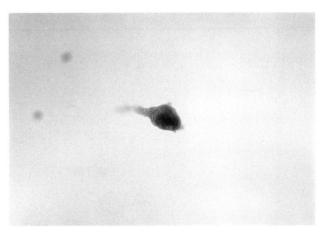

FIGURE 2–12. A single, atypical, ovoid to spindle-shaped cell with enlarged nuclei and prominent nucleoli is seen in a gastric brushing specimen from a patient with resection-proven benign gastric ulcer with abundant granulation at the ulcer bed (Papanicolaou).

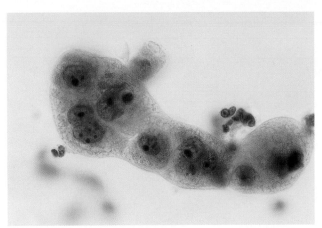

FIGURE 2–13. A group of proportionally enlarged epithelial cells showing prominent nucleoli and finely vacuolated cytoplasm can be seen on this esophageal brushing specimen from a patient with previous radiation therapy for squamous cell carcinoma (Papanicolaou).

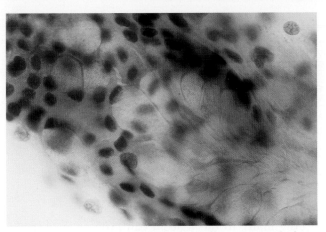

FIGURE 2–15. A sheet of glandular cells, some with large vacuoles expanding the cytoplasm, and crescent-shaped nuclei is seen on a brushing specimen from the esophagogastric junction, consistent with Barrett's esophagus (Papanicolaou).

blister as well as acantholysis, may present with esophageal lesions. Numerous acantholytic cells are usually present. The characteristic cells are round to polygonal, uniform, parabasal-sized isolated cells.[21,22] The cytoplasm is dense and may have perinuclear eosinophilic staining or a clear halo. The cells appear atypical because of the high nucleus-to-cytoplasm ratio, the enlarged nuclei, and the prominent, multiple, even irregular nucleoli (Fig. 2-14). A bar- or bullet-shaped nucleolus is characteristic.[23] However, the cells have smooth nuclear membranes and pale, fine, and even chromatin. Normal mitotic figures can be seen. These atypical cells resemble those in repair except for the increased number of single cells.

BARRETT'S EPITHELIUM

Cytology is not the optimal tool for the diagnosis of Barrett's epithelium. When glandular epithelial cells are seen in a cytology specimen, it is difficult to be certain whether they represent cells from the gastric side of the esophagogastric junction or metaplastic glandular cells from the esophagus. It has also been shown that cytology is neither sensitive nor specific for the detection of goblet cells,[24] a hallmark of Barrett's epithelium, in part because of the absence of a blue hue of acid mucin by the Papanicolaou stain. However, a long segment of Barrett's epithelium is more readily appreciated by cytology owing to the reduced probability of sampling error.[24] Its appearance is similar to that of the lining epithelium of the small intestine, with a Swiss cheese pattern at low magnification and goblet cells with single, large cytoplasmic vacuoles on high magnification (Fig. 2-15). The honeycomb arrangement of the glandular cells in Barrett's epithelium usually tends to be slightly more irregular than that of normal small intestinal epithelium.

■ Neoplastic Lesions

SQUAMOUS DYSPLASIA/CARCINOMA

Squamous dysplastic cells of the esophagus have morphology similar to that of the dysplastic cells on cervicovaginal Papanicolaou smears (Box 2-1).

The cellular features of squamous cell carcinoma vary with the degree of differentiation (Boxes 2-2 and 2-3).

BOX 2–1. **Squamous Dysplasia**

- Some but not all of the malignant features of dysplasia, such as increased nucleus-to-cytoplasm ratio, nuclear enlargement, hyperchromasia, irregular nuclear membrane, and aberrant chromatin pattern
- Fewer atypical cells than carcinoma
- Absent tumor diathesis

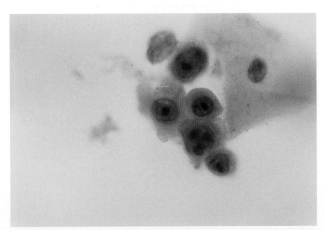

FIGURE 2–14. A loose group of parabasal-sized squamous cells with dense cytoplasm and prominent nucleoli can be seen in this esophageal brushing specimen from a patient known to have pemphigus vulgaris (Papanicolaou).

BOX 2–2. **Well-Differentiated Squamous Cell Carcinoma (Fig. 2-16)**

- Predominantly isolated cells with sharp cytoplasmic borders
- Hyperchromatic/pyknotic nuclei with obscured chromatin
- Variable cell shapes, such as round, oval, or spindle-shaped nuclei
- Keratinized cytoplasm
- Irregular, angulated nuclear contours
- Prominent necrosis/tumor diathesis in the background

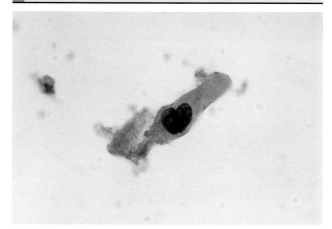

FIGURE 2–16. A keratinized squamous cell with a hyperchromatic nucleus characteristic of well-differentiated squamous cell carcinoma is present in this esophageal brushing specimen (Papanicolaou).

BOX 2–3. **Moderately and Poorly Differentiated Squamous Cell Carcinoma (Fig. 2-17)**

- Less striking keratinization of the cytoplasm
- Tumor cells in crowded, haphazardly arranged cell clusters with indistinct cell borders
- Vesicular chromatin with prominent nucleoli

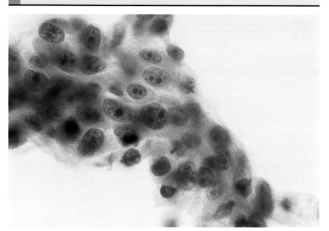

FIGURE 2–17. In contrast to Figure 2–16, a poorly differentiated squamous cell carcinoma has vesicular chromatin and prominent nucleoli and can be difficult to distinguish from a poorly differentiated adenocarcinoma (Papanicolaou).

GLANDULAR DYSPLASIA/CARCINOMA

Glandular dysplasia and carcinoma in the esophagus usually arise in the setting of Barrett's epithelium. The precursor lesions of adenocarcinoma in the stomach and in the intestine can present as either polypoid adenoma or flat dysplastic lesions. Adenoma and dysplasia have a similar appearance on cytology, which varies with the grade of dysplasia. Although the few studies on this topic were based on very small numbers of cases[24-26] and were insufficient to provide definitive conclusions on the utility of cytologic surveillance,[27] the preliminary results appear promising. Low-grade dysplasia may be difficult to distinguish from artifacts, whereas high-grade dysplasia may be confused with either severe reparative change or invasive carcinoma (Boxes 2-4, 2-5, and 2-6).

The amount and characteristics of the cytoplasm of the tumor cells depend on the degree of differentiation. Appearance varies from abundant vacuolated/granular cytoplasm to scant dense cytoplasm that is difficult to distinguish from that of a poorly differentiated squamous cell carcinoma.

Signet ring cell carcinoma, a type of adenocarcinoma that occurs most commonly in the stomach, is worthy of special consideration because it can be difficult to detect on both cytologic and histologic preparations. Because the malignant cells infiltrate predominantly the lamina propria, they are often not included in the brush cytology sample unless mucosal ulceration is present. The reactive/reparative epithelial changes associated

BOX 2–4. **Low-Grade Glandular Dysplasia (Fig. 2-18)**

- Architectural abnormality, i.e., stratification manifested as crowding and overlapping on cytology
- Elongated nuclei with increased nucleus-to-cytoplasm ratio
- Mild hyperchromasia and absent or inconspicuous nucleoli
- Minimal or negligible dyshesion

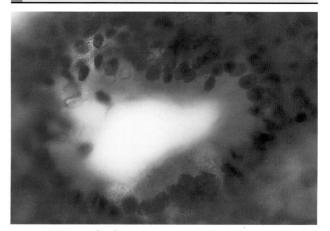

FIGURE 2–18. A gland opening is seen in the center surrounded by stratified, slightly enlarged, and elongated epithelial cells from an esophageal brushing specimen with biopsy-proven Barrett's esophagus and low-grade dysplasia (Papanicolaou).

BOX 2–5. **High-Grade Glandular Dysplasia (Fig. 2-19)**

- Both architectural and cellular abnormalities
- Atypical cells in sheets, crowded haphazardly, arranged in clusters or singly as a result of dyshesion
- Cellular abnormalities similar to those seen in invasive adenocarcinoma but possibly less pronounced

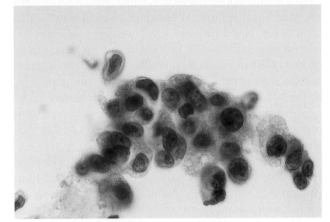

FIGURE 2–19. A loose group of haphazardly arranged, overlapping, atypical glandular cells with nuclear pleomorphism and atypia. The cells do not appear to be definitely malignant, and the background is clean. This is an eosphageal brushing specimen with biopsy-proven high-grade dysplasia in Barrett's esophagus (Papanicolaou).

with an ulcer can distract the attention of the pathologist from the real lesion. In addition, the numerous inflammatory cells from the ulcer can obscure the scattered, isolated tumor cells (Box 2-7).

Even when detected, some signet ring cells have such bland nuclei that they can be mistaken for histiocytes, which themselves have intracytoplasmic phagocytized material and a low nucleus-to-cytoplasm ratio. A high degree of suspicion is the best safeguard against failure to detect a signet ring cell carcinoma by cytology. When in doubt, immunocytochemical studies can be applied to the cytologic material to determine the epithelial versus histiocytic phenotype of the cells of interest. Carcinoma cells should be positive for epithelial markers, such as keratin and epithelial membrane antigen, whereas histiocytes express CD-68 as detected by the KP-1 antibody.

ENDOCRINE TUMORS

Gastrointestinal endocrine tumors are classified into three major categories: (1) well-differentiated endocrine tumors, (2) well-differentiated endocrine carcinoma, and (3) poorly differentiated endocrine (small cell) carcinomas.[28] The distinction of well-differentiated endocrine tumors from well-differentiated endocrine carcinomas is primarily based on features that cannot be evaluated on cytologic preparations, including size, site,

BOX 2–6. **Adenocarcinoma (Fig. 2-20)**

- Increased cellularity
- Abnormal cellular arrangements, such as isolated cells, "feathering" at the edges of cellular groups, and haphazard crowding within the groups
- Variable degree of gland formation by atypical cells
- Atypical cellular features, such as nuclear pleomorphism, high nucleus-to-cytoplasm ratio, nuclear enlargement, chromatin aberration, and irregular nuclear membrane with or without nucleoli
- Possibility of tumor diathesis (old blood and necrotic debris) in the background

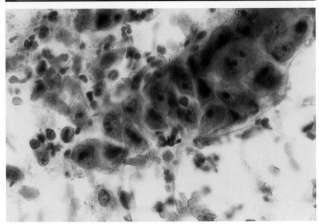

FIGURE 2–20. Compared with the cells in Figure 2–19, the cells in this gastric brushing from an adenocarcinoma have more enlarged nuclei and nucleoli. Inflammatory cells, necrotic debris, and lysed red blood cells are apparent in the background (Papanicolaou).

presence of local invasion, angioinvasion, patterns of hormone production, and metastases. Additional parameters of this classification that can be evaluated to some extent on cytologic preparations include cytologic atypia, mitotic index, and proliferative rate as assessed by MIB-1 staining. Along the gastrointestinal tract, the appendix is the most common site for such tumors, followed by the ileum and rectum,[29] with the stomach a distant fourth. These tumors account for less than 1% of all gastric malignancies.[30] However, cytologic specimens from the appendix, ileum, and rectum are virtually never seen. Our experience with cytology of gastrointestinal endocrine tumors has primarily involved tumors in the stomach and duodenum (Box 2-8).

The term *carcinoid tumor* encompasses all well-differentiated endocrine tumors and carcinomas.[31] The tendency of these tumor cells to lose their cytoplasm causes them to mimic small cell lymphoma owing to their small size and characteristic monomorphism. Such stripped nuclei can be distinguished from low-grade small cell lymphoma by their complete absence of cytoplasm and finely granular ("salt-and-pepper") chromatin pattern. Of course, one should always find

BOX 2–7. **Signet Ring Cell Carcinoma (Fig. 2-21)**

- Prominent inflammation in the background with reactive/reparative epithelial changes
- Isolated cells with moderate to abundant vacuolated cytoplasm and no phagocytic material in cytoplasm
- Variable degree of nuclear atypia

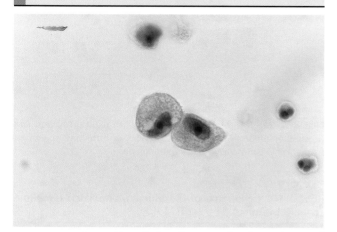

FIGURE 2–21. Two cells with abundant vacuolated cytoplasm and nuclei with slightly irregular nuclear membranes and prominent nucleoli are seen in this gastric brushing specimen of a biopsy-proven signet ring cell carcinoma. No phagocytic material is seen in the vacuolated cytoplasm (Papanicolaou).

BOX 2–8. **Well-Differentiated Endocrine Tumor/Carcinoma (carcinoid tumor) (Fig. 2-22)**

- Dyshesive monomorphic epithelial cells
- Plasmacytoid appearance of the cells with eccentric round to oval nuclei and moderate amount of basophilic dense cytoplasm
- Tendency to lose cytoplasm and to present as stripped nuclei
- "Salt-and-pepper" chromatin pattern

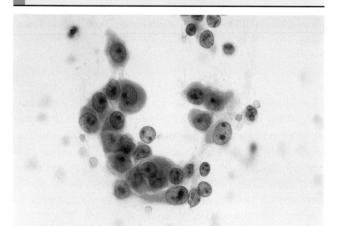

FIGURE 2–22. A loose cluster of epithelial cells and a few single monomorphic epithelial cells are seen in this duodenal brushing specimen from a carcinoid tumor. The eccentric nuclei give the cells a plasmacytoid appearance (Papanicolaou).

intact cells to confirm the diagnosis. Poorly differentiated endocrine carcinomas (small cell carcinoma) of the gastrointestinal tract are similar to those seen elsewhere and are characterized by small cells with scant cytoplasm, showing nuclear molding and a finely dispersed chromatin pattern. Mitoses and necrosis are also prominent features of these tumors.

MESENCHYMAL TUMORS

Mesenchymal tumors common in the gastrointestinal tract include leiomyomas (predominantly of the muscularis mucosae of the esophagus and colorectum), gastrointestinal stromal tumors, and leiomyosarcomas. Owing to their submucosal/mural location, these tumors are not normally accessible by endoscopic brush unless the tumor is ulcerated. Endoscopic fine-needle aspiration with or without ultrasound guidance is the preferred method of sampling. Specimens from leiomyomas usually consist of sparse bland spindle cells. However, specimens from gastrointestinal stromal tumors and leiomyosarcomas are usually cellular with loose and crowded fragments and individual spindle or epithelioid cells (Box 2-9).

The individual cells of gastrointestinal stromal tumors have a tendency to lose their cytoplasm to become stripped spindle-shaped or round to oval nuclei.[32,33] Perinuclear or paranuclear vacuoles are present in some cells. Delicate cytoplasm and prominent nuclear palisading have also been noted.[34] Although leiomyosarcomas tend to show more significant nuclear pleomorphism and atypia as well as a less prominent vascular pattern than gastrointestinal stromal tumors,[35,36] immunocytochemistry and/or polymerase chain reaction analysis of c-*kit* is needed to make the definitive distinction between the two. A majority of gastrointestinal stromal tumors show strong diffuse positivity for CD117 (c-*kit*), whereas leiomyosarcomas are typically positive for desmin and actin[35,37] and negative for CD117.

Although immunocytochemical staining for CD117 is useful in confirming a cytologic diagnosis of gastrointestinal stromal tumor, the diagnosis of malignancy still depends on evaluation of the resected specimen. Most recently, detection of a *kit* mutation on fine-needle aspiration specimen was found to be promising in predicting malignant behavior, although absence of mutation does not preclude malignancy.[38]

LYMPHOID TUMORS

The cytologic appearance of lymphoma of the gastrointestinal tract varies with its subtype. The large cell type usually does not pose any diagnostic difficulty because large malignant lymphoid cells are sufficiently atypical to raise the suspicion of a malignancy (Fig. 2-24). The challenge is to recognize them as being

BOX 2–9. **Gastrointestinal Stromal Tumor (Fig. 2-23)**

- Cellular specimen with fascicles, clusters, and sheets of spindle and/or epithelioid cells
- Cell groups spread out thinly on the slide despite their large size
- Prominent small blood vessels
- Possibility of numerous single cells and naked nuclei
- Delicate fibrillary cytoplasm with wispy cytoplasmic extensions and indistinct cell borders
- Ovoid to spindle-shaped and occasional wavy nuclei
- Uncommon high-grade features, such as marked nuclear atypia, frequent mitoses, and necrosis

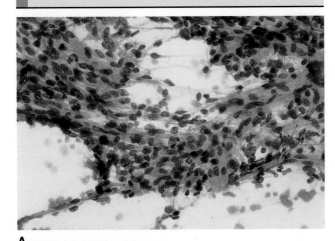

A

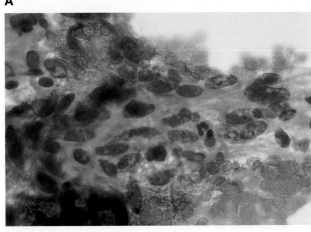

B

FIGURE 2–23. **A,** A hypercellular fascicle of spindle-shaped cells is seen in this endoscopic gastric fine-needle aspiration specimen of a gastrointestinal stromal tumor (Papanicolaou). **B,** On higher magnification, the cells have fibrillary cytoplasm and ovoid to spindle-shaped bland nuclei (Papanicolaou).

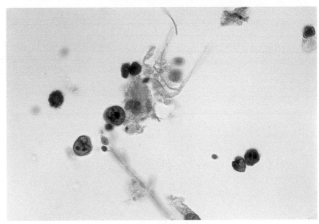

FIGURE 2–24. A few large atypical cells with scant cytoplasm and prominent nucleoli are seen on this gastric brushing specimen from a large cell lymphoma (Papanicolaou).

BOX 2–10. **Lymphoma of the Mucosa-Associated Lymphoid Tissue (MALToma) (Fig. 2-25)**

- Predominance of lymphocytes in an apparent inflammatory specimen
- Monomorphism and subtle atypia in the lymphoid population

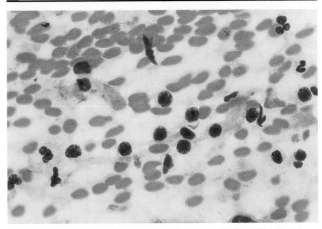

FIGURE 2–25. Several monomorphic small lymphocytes are present in this gastric brushing specimen from a MALToma. These cells can be easily mistaken for reactive lymphocytes. No neutrophils or plasma cells are present (Papanicolaou).

lymphoid and to distinguish them from poorly differentiated epithelial or mesenchymal tumors. Their lymphoid nature may in fact be easier to identify by cytology than from a small biopsy specimen because they shed as isolated, relatively monomorphic, large atypical cells with scant cytoplasm, vesicular nuclei, and a single large nucleolus or multiple prominent nucleoli.[39]

The absence of any true cohesion is the principal diagnostic feature of a lymphoma. Although a poorly differentiated carcinoma may shed predominantly as single cells, cell clusters can usually be found after a careful search. In addition, a poorly differentiated carcinoma often has more abundant cytoplasm, which may or may not be vacuolated, and a greater degree of nuclear pleomorphism than a large cell lymphoma. Immunocytochemical staining may also facilitate the distinction between lymphoma and carcinoma.

A low-grade small cell lymphoma, such as a lymphoma of the mucosa-associated lymphoid tissue (MALToma), can be difficult to diagnose by cytology because it may be mistaken for an inflammatory process (Box 2-10).

A mixed small and large cell lymphoma can pose an even greater challenge. Marker studies are almost always required for a definitive diagnosis of low-grade lymphoma.

References

1. Qizilbash AH, Castelli M, Kowalski MA, et al: Endoscopic brush cytology and biopsy in the diagnosis of cancer of the upper gastrointestinal tract. Acta Cytol 24:313-318, 1980.
2. Cook IJ, de Carle DJ, Haneman B, et al: The role of brushing cytology in the diagnosis of gastric malignancy. Acta Cytol 32:461-464, 1988.
3. Layfield LJ, Reichman A, Weinstein WM: Endoscopically directed fine needle aspiration biopsy of gastric and esophageal lesions. Acta Cytol 36:69-74, 1992.
4. Wiersema MJ, Hawes RH, Tao LC, et al: Endoscopic ultrasonography as an adjunct to fine needle aspiration cytology of the upper and lower gastrointestinal tract. Gastrointest Endosc 38:35-39, 1992.
5. Wiersema MJ, Wiersema LM, Khusro Q, et al: Combined endosonography and fine-needle aspiration cytology in the evaluation of gastrointestinal lesions. Gastrointest Endosc 40:199-206, 1994.
6. Tsang TK, Hidvegi D, Horth K, et al: Reliability of balloon-mesh cytology in detecting esophageal carcinoma in a population of US veterans. Cancer 59:556-559, 1987.
7. Falk GW, Chittajallu R, Goldblum JR, et al: Surveillance of patients with Barrett's esophagus for dysplasia and cancer with balloon cytology. Gastroenterology 112:1787-1797, 1997.
8. Leoni-Parvex S, Mihaescu A, Pellanda A, et al: Esophageal cytology in the follow-up of patients with treated upper aerodigestive tract malignancies. Cancer 90:10-16, 2000.
9. Wang HH, Jonasson JG, Ducatman BS: Brushing cytology of the upper gastrointestinal tract. Obsolete or not? Acta Cytol 35:195-198, 1991.
10. Geisinger KR: Endoscopic biopsies and cytologic brushings of the esophagus are diagnostically complementary. Am J Clin Pathol 103:295-299, 1995.
11. O'Donoghue JM, Horgan PG, O'Donohoe MK, et al: Adjunctive endoscopic brush cytology in the detection of upper gastrointestinal malignancy. Acta Cytol 39:28-34, 1995.
12. Zargar SA, Khuroo MS, Jan GM, et al: Prospective comparison of the value of brushings before and after biopsy in the endoscopic diagnosis of gastroesophageal malignancy. Acta Cytol 35:549-552, 1991.
13. Senturk O, Canturk Z, Ercin C, et al: Comparison of five detection methods for Helicobacter pylori. Acta Cytol 44:1010-1014, 2000.
14. Ghoussoub RA, Lachman MF: A triple stain for the detection of Helicobacter pylori in gastric brushing cytology. Acta Cytol 41:1178-1182, 1997.
15. Marshall JB, Kelley DH, Vogele KA: Giardiasis: Diagnosis by endoscopic brush cytology of the duodenum. Am J Gastroenterol 79:517-519, 1984.
16. Maygarden SJ, Flanders EL: Mycobacteria can be seen as "negative images" in cytology smears from patients with acquired immunodeficiency syndrome. Mod Pathol 2:239-243, 1989.
17. Clayton F, Heller T, Kotler DP: Variation in the enteric distribution of cryptosporidia in acquired immunodeficiency syndrome. Am J Clin Pathol 102:420-425, 1994.
18. Weber R, Bryan RT, Owen RL, et al: Improved light-microscopical detection of microsporidia spores in stool and duodenal aspirates. The Enteric Opportunistic Infections Working Group. N Engl J Med 326:161-166, 1992.
19. Pol S, Romana CA, Richard S, et al: Microsporidia infection in patients with the human immunodeficiency virus and unexplained cholangitis. N Engl J Med 328:95-99, 1993.
20. Chu P, West AB: Encephalitozoon (Septata) intestinalis: Cytologic, histologic, and electron microscopic features of a systemic intestinal pathogen. Am J Clin Pathol 106:606-614, 1996.
21. Kobayashi TK, Ueda M, Nishino T, et al: Scrape cytology of pemphigus vulgaris of the nipple, a mimicker of Paget's disease. Diagn Cytopathol 16:156-159, 1997.
22. Takahashi I, Kobayashi TK, Suzuki H, et al: Coexistence of pemphigus vulgaris and herpes simplex virus infection in oral mucosa diagnosed by cytology, immunohistochemistry, and polymerase chain reaction. Diagn Cytopathol 19:446-450, 1998.
23. DeMay RM: The Art & Science of Cytopathology, vol 1. Chicago, American Society of Clinical Pathologists, 1996.
24. Wang HH, Sovie S, Zeroogian JM, et al: Value of cytology in detecting intestinal metaplasia and associated dysplasia at the gastroesophageal junction. Hum Pathol 28:465-471, 1997.
25. Robey SS, Stanley RH, Gupta PK, et al: Diagnostic value of cytopathology in Barrett esophagus and associated carcinoma. Am J Clin Pathol 89:493-498, 1988.
26. Geisinger KR, Teot LA, Richter JE: A comparative cytopathologic and histologic study of atypia, dysplasia, and adenocarcinoma in Barrett's esophagus. Cancer 69:8-16, 1992.
27. Hughes JH, Cohen MB: Is the cytologic diagnosis of esophageal glandular dysplasia feasible? [see comments]. Diagn Cytopathol 18:312-316, 1998.
28. DeLellis RA: The neuroendocrine system and its tumors. An overview. Am J Clin Pathol 115(suppl 1):S5-S16, 2001.
29. Modlin IM, Sandor A: An analysis of 8305 cases of carcinoid tumors. Cancer 79:813-829, 1997.
30. Thomas RM, Sobin LH: Gastrointestinal cancer. Cancer 75:154-170, 1995.
31. Fenoglio-Preiser CM: Gastrointestinal neuroendocrine/neuroectodermal tumors. Am J Clin Pathol 115(suppl 1):S79-S93, 2001.
32. Dodd LG, Nelson RC, Mooney EE, et al: Fine-needle aspiration of gastrointestinal stromal tumors. Am J Clin Pathol 109:439-443, 1998.
33. Rader AE, Avery A, Wait CL, et al: Fine-needle aspiration biopsy diagnosis of gastrointestinal stromal tumors using morphology, immunocytochemistry, and mutational analysis of c-kit. Cancer 93:269-275, 2001.
34. Boggino HE, Fernandez MP, Logrono R: Cytomorphology of gastrointestinal stromal tumor: Diagnostic role of aspiration cytology, core biopsy, and immunochemistry. Diagn Cytopathol 23:156-160, 2000.
35. Wieczorek TJ, Faquin WC, Rubin BP, et al: Cytologic diagnosis of gastrointestinal stromal tumor with emphasis on the differential diagnosis with leiomyosarcoma. Cancer 93:276-287, 2001.
36. Seidal T, Edvardsson H: Diagnosis of gastrointestinal stromal tumor by fine-needle aspiration biopsy: A cytological and immunocytochemical study. Diagn Cytopathol 23:397-401, 2000.
37. Miettinen M, Sobin LH, Sarlomo-Rikala M: Immunohistochemical spectrum of GISTs at different sites and their differential diagnosis with a reference to CD117 (KIT). Mod Pathol 13:1134-1142, 2000.
38. Li SQ, O'Leary TJ, Sobin LH, et al: Analysis of KIT mutation and protein expression in fine needle aspirates of gastrointestinal stromal/smooth muscle tumors. Acta Cytol 44:981-986, 2000.
39. Sherman ME, Anderson C, Herman LM, et al: Utility of gastric brushing in the diagnosis of malignant lymphoma. Acta Cytol 38:169-174, 1994.

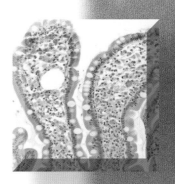

CHAPTER 3

Infectious Diseases of the GI Tract

LAURA W. LAMPS

▒ Introduction

Gastrointestinal (GI) infections are a major cause of morbidity and mortality worldwide. The number of transplant patients and those with other immunocompromising conditions is increasing, and global urbanization and transcontinental travel are becoming more frequent; as a result, the surgical pathologist must now be familiar with infectious diseases that were previously limited to tropical regions of the world, or the realm of esoterica.

The goal of the surgical pathologist in evaluating a GI biopsy for infectious colitis should be twofold. First, acute self-limited and/or infectious processes must be differentiated from chronic idiopathic inflammatory bowel disease (ulcerative colitis or Crohn's disease). Second, dedicated attempts must be made to identify the infecting organism(s).[1] In recent years, the surgical pathologist's ability to diagnose infectious processes in tissue sections has grown exponentially with the advent of new histochemical stains, immunohistochemistry, in situ hybridization, and polymerase chain reaction (PCR) analysis. As these techniques have developed, our knowledge of how histologic patterns of inflammation relate to various organisms has improved.

A majority of enteric infections are self-limited. Those patients who undergo endoscopic biopsy generally have chronic or debilitating diarrhea, systemic symptoms, or a history of immunocompromise or other significant clinical scenarios. A discussion with the gastroenterologist regarding exact symptomatology and colonoscopic findings, as well as facts about travel history, food intake (such as sushi or poorly cooked beef), sexual practices, and immune status, can aid immeasurably in the evaluation of a gut biopsy for infectious diseases.

▒ Viral Infections of the Gastrointestinal Tract

The type of viral infection and the manifestations of disease vary with the site of infection and the immune status of the patient.

Cytomegalovirus. CMV infection may be seen throughout the GI tract from mouth to anus, in both immunocompromised and immunocompetent persons. CMV is best known as an opportunistic pathogen in patients with suppressed immune systems, including those with acquired immunodeficiency syndrome (AIDS) and patients who have had solid organ or bone marrow transplants.[2] Primary infections in healthy persons are generally self-limited. In addition, secondary CMV may be superimposed on chronic GI disease, such as ulcerative colitis and Crohn's disease; in such cases, CMV superinfection is associated with high mortality, toxic megacolon, and exacerbations of the underlying GI disease. Symptoms vary with the immune status of the patient and the site of infection. The most common clinical symptoms are diarrhea (either bloody or watery), abdominal pain, fever, and weight loss.[2] A rare but important entity associated with pediatric CMV infection is hypertrophic gastropathy and protein-losing enteropathy resembling Ménétrier's disease.

CMV causes a remarkable variety of gross lesions. Ulceration is the most common; ulcers may be single or multiple and either superficial or deep. Segmental ulcerative lesions and linear ulcers may mimic Crohn's disease. Other gross lesions include mucosal hemorrhage, pseudomembranes, and obstructive inflammatory masses.

The histologic spectrum of CMV infection is varied; it ranges from minimal inflammation to deep ulcers with prominent granulation tissue and necrosis at the base (Fig. 3-1**A**). The characteristic "owl's eye" inclusions may be seen on routine H&E preparations and can be either intracytoplasmic or intranuclear (Fig. 3-1**B**). Inclusions are preferentially found in endothelial cells and stromal cells, and only rarely in epithelial cells. Unlike adenovirus and herpesvirus, CMV inclusions are often found deep within ulcer bases rather than at the edges of ulcers or in the superficial mucosa. Adjacent nuclei may be enlarged, appear smudged, or have a ground-glass appearance but lack typical inclusions. Associated histologic features include cryptitis, a mixed inflammatory infiltrate that usually includes numerous neutrophils, and mucosal ulceration.[2] Crypt abscesses, crypt atrophy and loss, and numerous apoptotic enterocytes may be seen as well.[3] Characteristic inclusions with virtually no associated inflammatory reaction may occur in immunocompromised patients.

In biopsy specimens, the diagnosis may be easily missed when only rare inclusions are present. Examination of multiple levels and use of immunohistochemistry may be invaluable in the finding of a rare cell containing an inclusion. Other diagnostic aids include viral culture, PCR assays, in situ hybridization, and serologic studies/antigen tests. Isolation of CMV in culture, however, does not imply active infection because virus may be excreted for months to years after a primary infection.[2]

The differential diagnosis is primarily that of other viral infections, particularly adenovirus.[4] Adenovirus inclusions are usually crescent shaped, generally within surface epithelium, and only intranuclear. CMV inclusions have an owl's eye morphology, are generally located within endothelial or stromal cells, and exist within either nucleus or cytoplasm. The ballooning degeneration phase of adenovirus infection, which occurs just before cell lysis, most closely resembles CMV.

The distinction between CMV infection and graft-versus-host disease in bone marrow transplant patients may be particularly difficult in that both clinical and histologic features are similar. Immunohistochemistry or in situ hybridization studies should be employed to rule out CMV infection in this setting; failure to identify CMV infection could result in delay of antiviral therapy.[3]

Herpesvirus. Herpetic infection may be seen throughout the GI tract but is most common in the esophagus and anorectum. Although herpes infections of the gut are often seen in immunocompromised patients, they are not limited to this group.

Patients with herpetic esophagitis present with odynophagia, dysphagia, chest pain, nausea, vomiting, fever, and GI bleeding; many have disseminated herpes infection at the time of diagnosis.[5] Herpetic proctitis is the most common cause of nongonococcal proctitis in homosexual men; it generally presents as severe anorectal pain, tenesmus, constipation, discharge, hematochezia, and fever. Concomitant neurologic symptoms (difficulty in urination and paresthesias of the buttocks and upper thighs) are well described, as is inguinal lymphadenopathy.[6]

Ulcers are the most common gross finding in the esophagus and are generally associated with an exudate. Many patients, however, have a nonspecific erosive

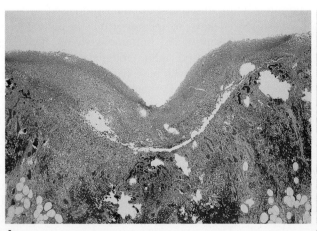

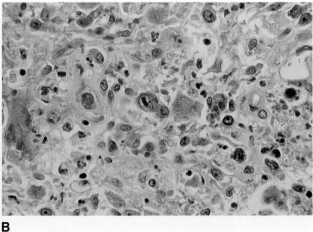

A   B

FIGURE 3–1. A, Colonic ulcer secondary to CMV with granulation tissue and necrosis at the base. **B,** Characteristic "owl's eye" inclusions are seen within endothelial cells in the ulcer base.

esophagitis. In herpetic proctitis, the presence of perianal vesicles is common. Proctoscopic findings include ulceration and mucosal friability, and vesicles are occasionally seen in the rectum or anal canal.[5,6]

Typical histologic findings regardless of site include focal ulceration, neutrophils in the lamina propria, and an inflammatory exudate that often contains sloughed epithelial cells. In the anorectum, perivascular lymphocytic cuffing and crypt abscesses may be seen. Characteristic viral inclusions and multinucleate giant cells are seen in only a minority of biopsy specimens.[6] The best place to search for the atypical cells of herpetic infection is within the squamous mucosa at the edges of ulcers (Fig. 3-2) and in sloughed cells within the exudate. Viral culture is the most valuable diagnostic aid; immunohistochemistry and in situ hybridization are also available.

The differential diagnosis predominantly includes other viral infections such as CMV and varicella-zoster infection. It is important to remember that mixed infections are common in many situations in which herpetic infection is found. In immunocompetent patients, herpetic infection is often self-limited; immunocompromised persons may be at risk for dissemination and life-threatening illness.

Enteric Viruses. Some common enteric viruses known to cause diarrhea include, but are not limited to, adenovirus, rotavirus, coronavirus, echovirus, enterovirus, astrovirus, and Norwalk virus. Many enteric viruses do not cause disease; others seldom if ever are seen by the surgical pathologist because they are detected in stool samples rather than biopsy specimens.

Adenovirus infection is second only to rotavirus as a cause of childhood diarrhea. However, it has gained attention in recent years as a cause of diarrhea in immunocompromised patients, especially those with AIDS. Virtually all patients present with diarrhea, sometimes accompanied by fever, weight loss, and abdominal pain. Characteristic inclusions may be seen, especially in immunocompromised patients, within the nuclei of surface epithelial cells (particularly goblet cells), sometimes accompanied by epithelial degenerative changes.[4] Useful aids in the diagnosis of adenovirus infection include immunohistochemistry, stool examination by electron microscopy, and viral culture. This entity is discussed further and is illustrated in Chapter 4.

Human Papillomaviruses. HPV has been implicated in the pathogenesis of esophageal papillomas, esophageal squamous cell carcinomas, anal condylomas, and anal squamous cell carcinomas. These entities are discussed in detail in Chapters 12, 16, and 24.

Human Immunodeficiency Virus. Histologic abnormalities of the bowel mucosa have been noted in human immunodeficiency virus (HIV)–positive patients, both with and without diarrhea. These features include crypt hypertrophy, increased apoptotic enterocytes, and villous atrophy; the changes resemble those seen in mild graft-versus-host disease and chemotherapy-related mucosal injuries.[7] Many of these patients have chronic diarrhea, but some are asymptomatic. Some workers support the use of the term "AIDS enteropathy" to describe these morphologic findings, provided that the bowel has been adequately sampled and all other entities have been excluded.[7] Others believe that this is a poorly understood term that does not clearly represent a specific disease entity and thus should not be used.

Other Viruses. Other viruses affecting the GI tract include measles (rubeola) and varicella-zoster, which may cause an ulcerative gastroenteritis. In addition, some DNA viruses have been implicated in the pathogenesis of sporadic chronic idiopathic intestinal pseudo-obstruction.

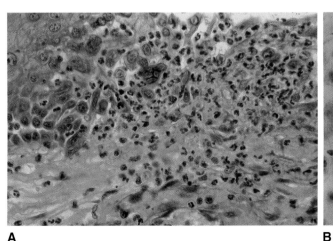
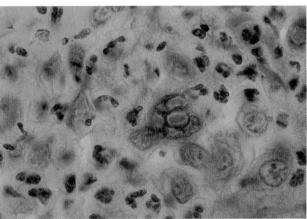

A   B

FIGURE 3–2. A and **B,** Typical herpetic inclusions are seen within the squamous epithelium at the edge of an esophageal ulcer.

Bacterial Infections of the Gastrointestinal Tract

Bacterial diarrhea is a worldwide health problem, with *Escherichia coli* and *Salmonella*, *Shigella*, and *Campylobacter* species the most common pathogens. Many bacterial infections of the gut are related to ingestion of contaminated water or food or to foreign travel. Although these organisms are often recovered by culture, surgical pathologists may play a valuable role in diagnosis (Table 3-1). Despite the dizzying array of bacterial infections that may affect the GI tract, many produce a similar spectrum of histologic features that may be generally categorized as follows:

1. Organisms producing very mild or no histologic changes (such as *Vibrio cholerae* and *Neisseria gonorrhoeae*)
2. Organisms producing the histologic features of acute infectious/self-limited colitis (ASLC) or focal active colitis (FAC), such as *Shigella* and *Campylobacter*
3. Organisms producing suggestive or diagnostic histologic features, such as pseudomembranes, granulomas, or viral inclusions.

The pattern of ASLC is one of the most common in enteric infections. Typical histologic features include neutrophils in the lamina propria, with or without crypt abscesses and cryptitis; preservation of crypt architecture; and lack of basal plasmacytosis.[1,8] The acute inflammatory component may be most prominent in the mid to upper crypts. The lack of both crypt distortion and basal lymphoplasmacytosis helps to distinguish ASLC from early ulcerative colitis. The changes may be focal, as in FAC, or more diffuse. The pathologic details of specific bacterial infections are discussed in the following sections.

MAJOR CAUSES OF BACTERIAL ENTEROCOLITIS

***V. cholerae* and Related Species.** *V. cholerae* is the causative agent of cholera, an important worldwide cause of watery diarrhea and dysentery that may lead to significant dehydration and death. Despite the severity of the illness, *V. cholerae* is a noninvasive, potent toxin producing organisms that cause minimal or no histologic change. Rare nonspecific findings such as small bowel mucin depletion and a mild increase in lamina propria mononuclear cells have been reported.[9] Other species, such as *V. hollisae* and *V. parahaemolyticus*, can also cause severe gastroenteritis.

E. coli. *E. coli* is the most common Gram-negative human pathogen. The diarrheogenic *E. coli* are classified into five groups, based primarily on serotyping; these groups are listed below. If pathogenic *E. coli* is suspected, the clinical laboratory should be notified to search for it specifically because it may be missed on routine culture.

Enterotoxigenic *E. coli* (ETEC) and Enteropathogenic *E. coli* (EPEC). These noninvasive *E. coli* organisms cause nonbloody diarrhea. ETEC is a major cause of traveler's diarrhea, as well as outbreaks within industrialized nations. EPEC is predominantly an infection of infants and neonates. The gross and microscopic pathology of ETEC and EPEC have not been well described in humans.

Enteroinvasive *E. coli*. The pathology of enteroinvasive *E. coli* (EIEC) has not been well described in humans either. These organisms are very similar to *Shigella* genetically and in their clinical presentation and pathogenesis; thus, the pathology could be expected to be similar as well. Symptoms include diarrhea (generally mucoid and watery but nonbloody), tenesmus, fever, malaise, and abdominal cramps. EIEC is transmitted via contaminated cheese, water, and person-to-person contact; it is also a cause of traveler's diarrhea.[10] The

TABLE 3–1. Classification of Bacterial Infections of the Gastrointestinal Tract by Histologic Pattern

Minimal or No Inflammatory Change	Acute Self-Limited Colitis Pattern	Pseudo-membranous Pattern	Predominantly Granulomatous	Diffuse Histiocytic	Predominantly Lymphohistiocytic	Marked Architectural Distortion	Ischemic Pattern
Vibrio cholerae Entero-pathogenic *E. coli* Entero-adherent *E. coli* Spirochetosis *Neisseria* species	*Shigella Campylobacter Aeromonas* Occasionally *Salmonella* (especially nontyphoid) Occasionally *Clostridium difficile* Syphilis (+/– increased plasma cells)	Entero-hemorrhagic *E. coli* *C. difficile* Occasionally *Shigella*	*Yersinia* M. tuberculosis Actinomycosis MAI (immuno-competent patients) Rarely syphilis	*Rhodococcus equi* Whipple's disease MAI (immuno-compro-mised patients)	LGV *Salmonella typhimurium*	*Salmonella typhimurium Shigella*	Enterohemor-rhagic *E. coli*

MAI, *Mycobacterium avium-intracellulare complex;* LGV, lymphogranuloma venereum.

organisms produce a severe dysentery-like illness as well as bacteremia; this can be a particular problem in AIDS patients.

Enteroadherent *E. coli* (EAEC). This noninvasive strain is similar to EPEC. Both have been increasingly recognized as causes of chronic diarrhea and wasting in AIDS patients. Although endoscopic findings are usually unremarkable, right colon biopsies more often yield pathologic findings. Histologic examination shows degenerated surface epithelial cells with associated intraepithelial inflammatory cells. A coating of adherent bacteria at the surface epithelium, which may stain Gram-negative, is the prominent feature (Fig. 3-3).[11]

Enterohemorrhagic *E. coli* (EHEC). The most common strain of enterohemorrhagic *E. coli* is 0157:H7. This pathogen gained national attention in 1993 when a massive outbreak in the western United States was linked to contaminated ground beef. Although contaminated meat is the most frequent mode of transmission, infection may also occur through contaminated water, milk, produce, and person-to-person contact. EHEC produces a cytotoxin similar to that of *Shigella dysenteriae;* however, there is no invasion. Affected persons may develop hemolytic-uremic syndrome or thrombotic thrombocytopenic purpura, and children and the elderly are at particular risk for grave illness.

GI symptoms usually consist of bloody diarrhea with severe abdominal cramps and mild or no fever. Nonbloody, watery diarrhea may occur, however. Only one third of patients have fecal leukocytes. Endoscopically, patients may have colonic edema, erosions, ulcers, and hemorrhage, and the right colon is usually more severely affected. The edema may be so marked as to cause obstruction, and surgical resection may be required to relieve this or to control bleeding. Histopathologic features include marked edema and hemorrhage in the lamina propria and submucosa, with associated mucosal acute inflammation and necrosis (Fig. 3-4). Microthrombi may be seen within small vessels, and pseudomembranes may occasionally be present.[12-13]

Routine stool cultures do not distinguish 0157:H7 from normal intestinal flora; microbiologic diagnosis requires screening on selective agar. An immunohistochemical stain for this organism has recently been described as well.

The differential diagnosis includes *Clostridium difficile*–related colitis, idiopathic inflammatory bowel disease, and especially ischemic colitis, from which EHEC may be histologically indistinguishable.

Salmonella. These Gram-negative bacilli are transmitted through food and water and are prevalent where sanitation is poor. They are an important cause of both food poisoning and traveler's diarrhea.

Typhoid (Enteric) Fever *(Salmonella typhimurium).* Typhoid fever typically presents with abdominal pain, headache, an elevation in fever over several days, and occasionally constipation. An abdominal rash and leukopenia are often seen. Diarrhea, which begins in the second or third week of infection, is initially watery but may progress to severe GI bleeding.[14]

Any level of the alimentary tract may be involved, but the characteristic pathology is most prominent in the ileum, appendix, and colon and is associated with Peyer's patches. Grossly, the bowel wall is thickened, and raised nodules may be seen corresponding to hyperplastic Peyer's patches. Aphthous ulcers overlying Peyer's patches, linear ulcers, discoid ulcers, and full-thickness ulceration and necrosis are common as

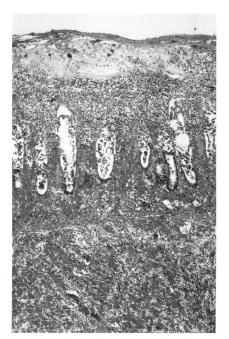

FIGURE 3–4. Enterohemorrhagic *E. coli.* The hemorrhagic necrosis, acute inflammatory exudate, and crypt withering are very similar to the features of ischemic colitis.

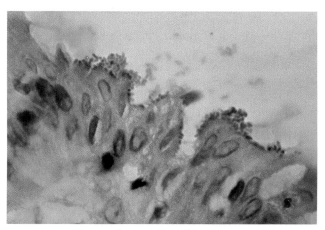

FIGURE 3–3. Enteroadherent *E. coli* in an AIDS patient. A coating of Gram-negative rods with little inflammatory reaction is noted at the surface of the colonic mucosa (Gram stain) (Photograph courtesy of Dr. Mary P. Bronner.)

disease progresses. Associated suppurative mesenteric lymphadenitis may occur. Perforation and toxic megacolon may complicate typhoid fever.[14-16] Occasionally, the mucosa is grossly normal or only mildly inflamed and edematous.[16-17]

The histiocyte is the predominant inflammatory cell. Following hyperplasia of Peyer's patches, acute inflammation of the overlying epithelium develops. Eventually, macrophages, mixed with occasional lymphocytes and plasma cells, infiltrate and obliterate the lymphoid follicles; neutrophils are not prominent.[15] Necrosis then begins in the Peyer's patch and spreads to the surrounding mucosa, which eventually ulcerates. Ulcers are typically very deep. Typhoid fever occasionally shows features more consistent with acute self-limited colitis, including prominent neutrophils, cryptitis, crypt abscesses, and overlying fibrinous exudate.[16-17] Granulomas are occasionally seen.

Nontyphoid _Salmonella_ Species. Nontyphoid _Salmonella_ species (e.g., _S. enterica_ and _S. muenchen_) generally cause self-limited gastroenteritis. Endoscopic findings include mucosal redness, ulceration, and exudates; pathologic features are those of nonspecific acute self-limited colitis. Occasionally, significant crypt distortion may be seen.[17]

The differential diagnosis of typhoid fever includes yersiniosis and other infectious processes, as well as Crohn's disease (Table 3-2), and there may be significant histologic overlap between them.[15,17] Neutrophils and granulomas are often more prominent in Crohn's disease and yersiniosis. The differential diagnosis of nontyphoid _Salmonella_ infection includes other causes of acute self-limited infectious colitis, as well as ulcerative colitis.[17] In addition, _Salmonella_ infection may complicate preexisting idiopathic inflammatory bowel disease. Significant crypt distortion has been reported in some cases of salmonellosis but is generally more pronounced in ulcerative colitis. Clinical presentation and stool cultures may be invaluable to the pathologist in sorting out this differential diagnosis.

TABLE 3–2. Infectious Mimics of Chronic Idiopathic Inflammatory Bowel Disease

I. Mimics of Crohn's Disease
Cytomegalovirus
Salmonella typhimurium
Shigella species
Yersinia species
M. tuberculosis
Lymphogranuloma venereum
Amebiasis

II. Mimics of Ulcerative Colitis
Shigella species
Nontyphoid _Salmonella_ species
Amebiasis

Shigella Species. _Shigella_ organisms are virulent, invasive Gram-negative bacilli that cause severe watery and/or bloody diarrhea and are a major cause of infectious diarrhea worldwide. This infection is transmitted by water contaminated with feces. It has the highest infectivity rate of the enteric Gram-negative bacteria; thus, symptoms may result from ingestion of a very low number of organisms. Infants, young children, and malnourished or debilitated patients are most commonly affected; symptoms include abdominal pain, fever, and diarrhea that is initially watery but turns bloody. Chronic disease is rare.

Grossly, the large bowel is typically affected (the left side usually more severely), but the ileum may be involved. The mucosa is hemorrhagic, with exudates that may form pseudomembranes. Ulcerations are variably present. Histologically, early disease has the features of acute self-limited colitis with cryptitis, crypt abscesses (often superficial), and ulceration. Pseudomembranes similar to _C. difficile_ infection may be seen, as can aphthous ulcers similar to those seen in Crohn's disease. As the disease continues, increased mucosal destruction occurs with many neutrophils and other inflammatory cells in the lamina propria. Marked architectural distortion mimicking idiopathic inflammatory bowel disease is well described.[18]

The differential diagnosis of early shigellosis is primarily that of other infections, particularly enteroinvasive _E. coli_ and _Clostridium difficile_. Shigellosis, especially later in the disease course, may be extremely difficult to distinguish from Crohn's disease or ulcerative colitis, both endoscopically and histologically.[1] Stool cultures and clinical presentation may be helpful in this instance.

Campylobacter Species. These Gram-negative organisms are major causes of diarrhea worldwide and are the most common stool isolate in the United States.[19] This species is found in contaminated meat, water, and milk and is a common animal pathogen. _C. jejuni_ is most commonly associated with gastroenteritis. _C. fetus_ and the other less common species are more often seen in immunosuppressed patients and homosexual men.[19] Patients typically have fever, malaise, abdominal pain (often severe), and watery diarrhea, which may contain blood and leukocytes.[20] Most infections are self-limited, especially in healthy patients. Of note, Guillain-Barré syndrome and reactive arthropathy are associated with _Campylobacter_ infection.[19]

Endoscopic findings include friable colonic mucosa with associated erythema and hemorrhage. Histologic examination shows features of acute self-limited colitis. Mild crypt distortion may occasionally be seen, although architecture overall is preserved.[20]

Yersinia. _Yersinia enterocolitica_ (YE) and _Yersinia pseudotuberculosis_ (YP) are the species that cause human GI disease. _Yersinia_ organisms are among the most common agents of bacterial enteritis in Western and Northern Europe, and the incidence is rising in both Europe and the United States. These Gram-negative coccobacilli may cause appendicitis, ileitis, colitis, and mesenteric lymphadenitis. Although yersiniosis is usually a self-limited process, chronic infections (including chronic colitis) have been well documented. Immunocompromised and debilitated patients, as well as patients on desferrioxamine or with iron overload, are at risk for serious disease.

Yersinia organisms preferentially involve the ileum, right colon, and appendix and may cause a pseudo-appendicular syndrome. In addition, they are responsible for many cases of isolated granulomatous appendicitis.[21] Grossly, involved bowel has a thickened, edematous wall with nodular inflammatory masses centered on Peyer's patches. Aphthous and linear ulcers may be seen. Involved appendices are enlarged and hyperemic, similar to suppurative appendicitis; perforation is often seen. Involved lymph nodes may show gross foci of necrosis.

Both suppurative and granulomatous patterns of inflammation are common, and these are often mixed. *YE* has not typically been associated with discrete granulomas, but it has been characterized by hyperplastic Peyer's patches with overlying ulceration, acute inflammation, hemorrhagic necrosis, and palisading histiocytes.[22] GI infection with *YP* has characteristically been described as a granulomatous process with central microabscesses, almost always accompanied by mesenteric adenopathy (Fig. 3-5).[23] Significant overlap is seen in the histologic features of *YE* and *YP* infection, however, and either species may show epithelioid granulomas with prominent lymphoid cuffing, lymphoid hyperplasia, transmural lymphoid aggregates, mucosal ulceration, and lymph node involvement.[21] Gram's stains are usually not helpful, but cultures, serologic

studies, and PCR assays may be useful in confirming the diagnosis.

The major differential diagnosis includes other infectious processes, particularly *Mycobacterium* and *Salmonella* species. Acid-fast stains and culture results should help to distinguish mycobacterial infection; clinical features and the presence of greater numbers of neutrophils, microabscesses, and granulomas may help to distinguish yersiniosis from salmonellosis.

Crohn's disease and yersiniosis may be difficult to distinguish from one another, and they have a long and complicated relationship. They may show similar histologic features, including transmural lymphoid aggregates, skip lesions, and fissuring ulcers. In fact, isolated granulomatous appendicitis has in the past frequently been interpreted as primary Crohn's disease of the appendix. However, patients with granulomatous inflammation confined to the appendix rarely develop generalized inflammatory bowel disease.[24] Features that may favor a diagnosis of Crohn's disease include cobblestoning of mucosa and creeping fat grossly, as well as microscopic changes of chronicity, including crypt distortion, thickening of the muscularis mucosae, and prominent neural hyperplasia. However, some cases are indistinguishable on histologic grounds alone.

Aeromonas Species. *Aeromonas* species, initially thought to be nonpathogenic Gram-negative bacteria, are increasingly recognized as causes of gastroenteritis in both children and adults. The typical presentation is bloody diarrhea, sometimes chronic, accompanied by nausea, vomiting, and cramping pain. Endoscopically, signs of colitis may be seen; the features are often segmental and may mimic ischemic colitis or Crohn's disease.[25] Histologic features are those of acute self-limited or focal active colitis; organisms are not generally seen on biopsy. Granulomas have been rarely reported.

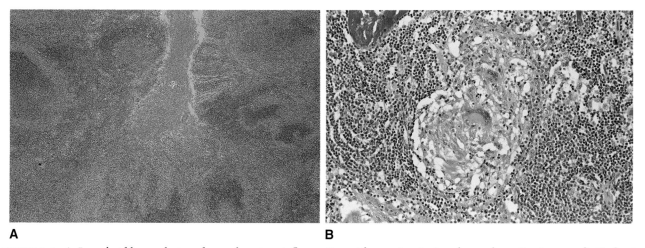

A   **B**

FIGURE 3–5. A, Lymphoid hyperplasia and granulomatous inflammation with prominent microabscess formation in appendicitis due to *Y. pseudotuberculosis*. **B,** Granuloma with lymphoid cuffing in *Y. enterocolitica* infection.

CLOSTRIDIAL DISEASES OF THE GUT

Clostridial organisms are some of the most potent toxigenic bacteria in existence; they are important gut pathogens. Members of this group of bacteria are responsible for pseudomembranous/antibiotic-associated colitis (usually *C. difficile*); necrotizing jejunitis (usually *C. perfringens* [*welchii*]); neutropenic enterocolitis (often *C. septicum*); and botulism (*C. botulinum*).[26]

***C. difficile*–Related Colitis.** *C. difficile* infection is most commonly related to previous antibiotic exposure (especially orally administered); it cannot infect in the presence of normal flora.[26] It is the most common nosocomial GI pathogen. A majority of patients are elderly, although infection is certainly not limited to this group.

The range of disease is variable, from mild diarrhea to fully developed pseudomembranous colitis (PMC) to fulminant disease with perforation or toxic megacolon.[27,28] Watery diarrhea is almost always initially present and may be accompanied by abdominal pain, cramping, fever, and leukocytosis. Bloody diarrhea is sometimes seen. Symptoms can occur up to several weeks after discontinuation of antibiotic therapy.[27]

Endoscopically, classic PMC shows yellow-white pseudomembranes, most commonly in the left colon, that bleed when scraped. The distribution is often patchy, and the rectum may be spared.[27] Atypical findings include mucosal erythema and friability without pseudomembranes. Typical histologic findings may be seen, however, in the absence of gross pseudomembranes. Histologically, classic PMC features "volcano" lesions with intercrypt necrosis and ballooned crypts giving rise

to the laminated pseudomembrane composed of fibrin, mucin, and neutrophils (Fig. 3-6). The ballooned glands are filled with neutrophils and mucin and often lose the superficial epithelial cells.[28] More severe and prolonged PMC may lead to full-thickness mucosal necrosis. Less characteristic lesions, usually focal active colitis with occasional crypt abscesses but lacking pseudomembranes, have been well described in association with a positive *C. difficile* toxin assay.[28]

It is important to remember that the term "pseudomembranous colitis" is a descriptive one, not a specific diagnosis. Although most cases of PMC are related to *C. difficile*, other infectious entities as well as ischemic colitis may have similar appearances. A hyalinized lamina propria favors the diagnosis of ischemia; other features, such as crypt withering, pseudomembranes, and mucosal necrosis, may be seen in either entity.[29] Endoscopically, pseudomembrane formation is more frequent in PMC, although it can be seen in ischemia. A history of antibiotic use and stool assay for *C. difficile* toxin may be invaluable in resolving the differential diagnosis.

***C. perfringens* (*welchii*).** *C. perfringens* causes diarrhea related to food poisoning and is also a cause of antibiotic-associated and nosocomial diarrhea. The notorious pig-bel (segmental necrotizing enterocolitis) is caused by *C. perfringens* type C and usually follows a meal rich in infected meat. It is most common in southeast Asia and New Guinea, where it was initially described following ritual pork feasting. Similar cases have been described after eating binges in Western countries. Symptoms include abdominal pain, bloody diarrhea, and vomiting, often with abdominal distention.

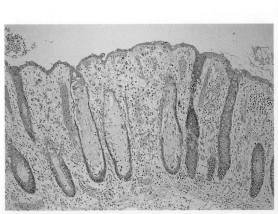 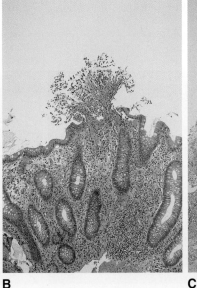 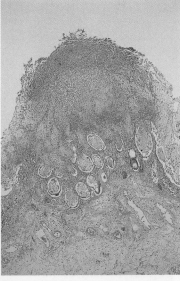

A   **B**   **C**

FIGURE 3–6. A, Early pseudomembranous colitis with ballooned crypts containing neutrophils and intercrypt necrosis, but no pseudomembrane. **B,** Intercrypt necrosis giving rise to early "volcano" lesion. **C,** Classic "volcano" lesion with laminated pseudomembrane composed of fibrin, mucin, and neutrophils.

Complications include perforation, obstruction, bowel gangrene, and septicemia with shock and rapid death. Mild or subacute forms have also been described.[30]

Involvement is predominantly seen in but is not limited to the jejunum. The bowel is often dusky gray-green, as in ischemia. Necrotic areas may be segmental and quite focal, with intervening areas of normal mucosa. The mucosal exudate can be similar to that of PMC, but inflammation and necrosis often become transmural and lead to perforation. Histologically, the mucosa is necrotic and ulcerated, with a heavy acute inflammatory infiltrate at the edges of ulcers. Small vessel vasculitis and microthrombi may be seen.[30] Gram-positive bacilli typical of *Clostridia* can be found in the necrotic exudate.

C. septicum. Neutropenic enterocolitis (typhlitis) is a serious complication of both chemotherapy-related and primary neutropenia. Most patients have received chemotherapy within the previous month. *C. septicum* has been frequently reported as a causative agent, especially in adults; other commonly implicated bacteria include other clostridial species, *E. coli*, *Pseudomonas* species, and enterococci.[31,32] An association with CMV has been noted. Patients usually present with GI hemorrhage, fever, abdominal pain and distention, and diarrhea.[31] Perforation is a well-described complication.

The right colon is preferentially involved, although the ileum and other sites in the colon may be affected. Gross findings include diffuse dilatation and edema of the bowel, with varying severity of ulceration and hemorrhage.[31] Exudates and pseudomembranes resembling *C. difficile* colitis are common. Microscopically, changes range from mild hemorrhage to prominent submucosal edema, ulceration, marked hemorrhage, and focal necrosis, often with a striking absence of inflammatory cells (Fig. 3-7). However, neutrophils may sometimes be found despite peripheral neutropenia.

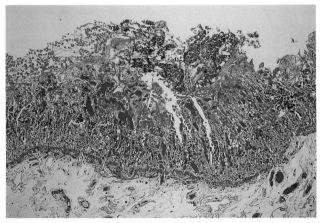

FIGURE 3–7. Typhlitis (neutropenic enterocolitis) in a chemotherapy patient. Ulceration with hemorrhage, prominent submucosal edema, mucosal ulceration and necrosis, and an exudate containing numerous bacteria and yeast are typical features. Neutrophils are scarce.

Sometimes organisms can be detected in the wall of the bowel on Gram's stain.

Differential diagnosis includes ischemic colitis and pseudomembranous colitis. The appropriate clinical setting and dearth of inflammatory cells should favor neutropenic enterocolitis.

MYCOBACTERIAL INFECTIONS OF THE GASTROINTESTINAL TRACT

Mycobacterium tuberculosis. This organism remains common in developing countries and immigrant populations. There has also been a remarkable resurgence of tuberculosis in Western countries, owing in large part to AIDS, but also to institutional overcrowding and immigrant populations. GI (rather than pulmonary) symptoms may be the initial presentation, and primary GI tuberculosis has been well documented. Symptoms and signs are nonspecific and include weight loss, fever, abdominal pain, diarrhea, and palpable abdominal mass.[33-34] Mesenteric adenopathy is common.

Grossly, the ileocecal and jejunoileal areas are most commonly involved, followed by the appendix and ascending colon[33-34]; the ileocecal valve is often deformed and gaping. Rectal, anal, duodenal, and gastroesophageal involvement are much less frequent but are well described.[34] Strictures and ulcers (often occurring together) are the most common endoscopic findings, along with thickened mucosal folds and inflammatory nodules.[33] The ulcers are often circumferential and transverse. Multiple and segmental lesions with skip areas are common. Large inflammatory masses, usually involving the ileocecum, may be seen, and well-described complications include obstruction, perforation, and hemorrhage.

The characteristic histologic lesion is caseating, often confluent granulomas, present at any level of the wall of the gut (Fig. 3-8**A**); a rim of lymphocytes may be present at the periphery. Granulomas may be rare or remote with hyalinization and calcification. Aphthous ulcers, as well as inflammation of submucosal vessels, may be seen. Acid-fast stains sometimes demonstrate organisms within granulomas or necrotic areas (Fig. 3-8**B**), but culture may be required; in addition, PCR assays are available. Purified protein derivative (PPD) tests are unreliable in immunocompromised or debilitated patients.

Differential diagnosis includes other granulomatous infectious processes, especially yersiniosis and fungal disease. The granulomas of yersiniosis are typically noncaseating with striking lymphoid cuffs, but there may be considerable histologic overlap. Crohn's disease may be difficult to distinguish from tuberculosis; features favoring Crohn's disease are linear rather than circumferential ulcers, transmural lymphoid aggregates, and deep fistulas and fissures. Tuberculosis also commonly

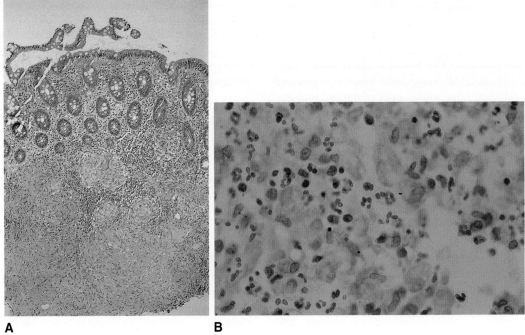

FIGURE 3–8. A, Colonic *M. tuberculosis* with mucosal and submucosal confluent, caseating granulomas. **B,** Rare acid-fast organisms are seen within the necroinflammatory exudate on this Ziehl–Neelsen stain.

lacks mucosal cobblestoning. Atypical mycobacteria such as *Mycobacterium kansasii* and *Mycobacterium bovis* may cause a similar pathologic picture.

Mycobacterium avium-intracellulare **Complex.** This is the most common mycobacterium isolated from the GI tract. Symptoms include diarrhea, abdominal pain, fever, and weight loss and often reflect systemic infection. Endoscopy is usually normal, although white nodules, small ulcers, or hemorrhages may be seen. The small bowel is preferentially involved, but colonic and gastroesophageal involvement may be present, as may mesenteric adenopathy.[35-36]

Immunocompetent patients manifest a granulomatous response, with or without necrosis. Immunocompromised patients generally have villi distended by a diffuse infiltration of histiocytes containing bacilli (Fig. 3-9**A**), with little inflammatory response other than occasional poorly formed granulomas.[35-36] Bacilli stain with acid-fast stains, as well as periodic acid–Schiff (PAS) and Gomori's silver-methenamine (GMS) stains. Culture and PCR assays may also be helpful. Organisms are generally abundant in immunocompromised patients (Fig. 3-9**B**) but may be hard to detect in nonimmunocompromised patients. Differential diagnosis includes Whipple's disease and other infectious processes.

SPIROCHETAL INFECTIONS OF THE GASTROINTESTINAL TRACT

Syphilis *(Treponema pallidum).* GI syphilis predominantly involves the anorectum, although other sites

may be involved, particularly the stomach.[37] Patients are often asymptomatic,[38] but pain, constipation, bleeding, and discharge may be present.

Gross findings in primary syphilis include anal chancres and/or an associated mild proctitis. Signs of secondary syphilis typically present 6 to 8 weeks later and include masses, a mucocutaneous rash, or condyloma lata (raised, moist, smooth warts that secrete mucus and are associated with itching and a foul odor).[36,39] Inguinal adenopathy is typical. Gross signs of primary and secondary infection sometimes coexist.

Gastric involvement may be either an early or a late manifestation of syphilis. The most common presenting sign is upper GI bleeding, and patients typically have antral erosions, ulcers, or features of gastritis endoscopically.[37] Ulcers may have irregular, heaped edges that mimic malignancy.

Histologically, syphilitic chancres typically contain a dense mononuclear cell infiltrate with prominent plasma cells. Syphilitic proctitis is nonspecific, often showing features of acute self-limited or focal active colitis with or without an increase in plasma cells (Fig. 3-10**A**). Syphilitic gastritis often features a dense plasmacytic infiltrate.[37] The glands may be relatively spared by inflammation. Granulomas have been reported, and occasionally prominent, proliferative capillary endothelial cells may be noted.[39,40] Darkfield examination, silver impregnation stains (Fig. 3-10**B**), serologic studies, and immunohistochemistry may be helpful diagnostic aids.

The gross differential diagnosis of chancre includes anal fissures, fistulas, or traumatic lesions; in general,

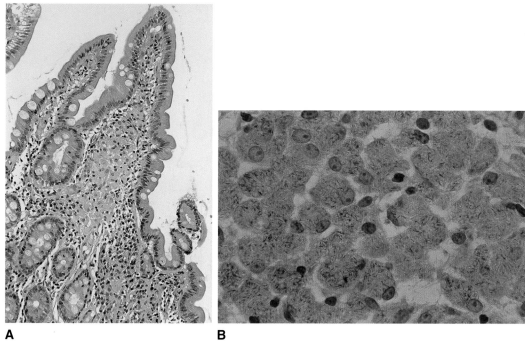

A   B

FIGURE 3–9. A, A villus is distended by a cluster of histiocytes containing *M. avium intracellulare,* with little associated inflammatory response. **B,** The histiocytes are packed with numerous acid-fast organisms typical of MAI, as seen on this Ziehl–Neelsen stain.

condyloma acuminata are more dry and keratinized than condyloma lata. The histologic differential diagnosis primarily includes other infectious processes, such as *Helicobacter pylori* infection in the stomach. If the plasma cell infiltrate is prominent and monomorphic, plasmacytoma should be considered.

Intestinal Spirochetosis. Intestinal spirochetosis is usually seen in homosexual men, although it has been described in a wide variety of other conditions, including diverticular disease, ulcerative colitis, and adenomas. It probably represents infection by a group of related organisms. Although patients with this histologic finding

often have symptoms such as diarrhea or anal pain and discharge, it is not clear that spirochetosis causes these symptoms.[41] Many patients have other infections (especially gonorrhea) complicating the clinical picture. Any level of the colon may be involved, as can the appendix. Typically, endoscopic abnormalities are mild or absent.

On H&E staining, spirochetosis resembles a fuzzy, "fringed" blue line at the luminal border of the colonic mucosa (Fig. 3-11**A**). Invasion is not seen, and the changes can be focal. Most have no associated inflammatory infiltrate, although occasionally, an associated cryptitis is seen. The organisms stain intensely with Warthin-Starry,

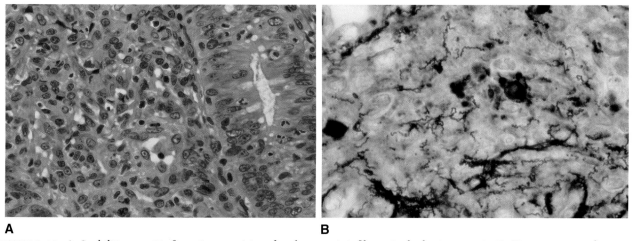

A   B

FIGURE 3–10. A, Syphilitic proctitis featuring cryptitis and a plasmacytic infiltrate in the lamina propria. **B,** Numerous spirochetes are seen on silver impregnation staining (Warthin–Starry). (Photographs courtesy of Drs. Rodger C. Haggitt and Mary P. Bronner.)

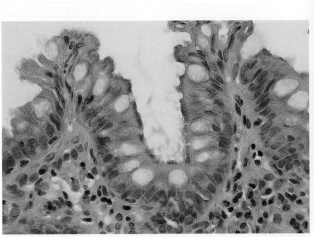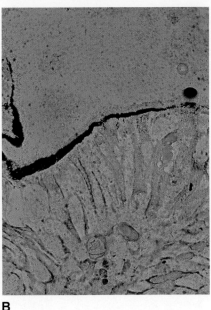

A   **B**

FIGURE 3–11. A, Spirochetosis characterized by a fuzzy, "fringed" blue line at the luminal border of the colonic mucosa. **B,** Organisms stain intensely with silver impregnation stains (Dieterle).

Dieterle, or similar silver stains (Fig. 3-11**B**). They also stain with Alcian blue (pH 2.5) and PAS.[42]

The differential diagnosis primarily consists of a prominent glycocalyx, which should not stain with silver impregnation stains. Occasionally, enteroadherent *E. coli* can give a similar appearance, but *E. coli* should stain strongly Gram-negative and lack spirillar morphology.

OTHER CAUSES OF SEXUALLY TRANSMITTED BACTERIAL PROCTOCOLITIS

Although herpes simplex virus (HSV) is the most common causative agent of infectious proctocolitis among homosexual men, *N. gonorrhoeae*, *T. pallidum*, and *Chlamydia* species are other frequent causes. Patients generally present with anal discharge, pain, diarrhea, constipation, bloody stools, and tenesmus. Proctoscopic findings range from normal to mucosal friability, erosions, and erythema.[38]

Chlamydia trachomatis. Serotypes L1, L2, and L3 cause lymphogranuloma venereum (LGV). Anal pain is usually severe and is accompanied by bloody discharge and tenesmus.[39,43] The anorectum is the most common site, but LGV has been described in the ileum and colon as well.[43] The inflammatory infiltrate is variable; most patients have a lymphoplasmacytic infiltrate in the mucosa and submucosa, but neutrophils may be prominent. Granulomatous inflammation is sometimes present. Histologic features mimicking Crohn's disease have been described.[43,44] In addition, LGV may produce a striking follicular proctitis.[43] Culture, direct immunofluorescence studies, and immunohistochemistry may serve as valuable diagnostic aids.

Granuloma Inguinale *(Calymmatobacterium granulomatis).* Granuloma inguinale causes anal and perianal disease that can be similar to LGV, although extension into the rectum favors LGV.[44] Warthin-Starry or Giemsa stains may aid in visualization of the Donovan bodies typical of granuloma inguinale.

Neisseria gonorrhoeae. Gonorrhea has been reported in up to 20% of homosexual men and is frequently asymptomatic. The anorectum (alone or in combination with pharynx and urethra) is a common site of infection. *N. meningitidis* has also been isolated from the anorectums of homosexual men. Proctoscopic examination is usually unremarkable. Most biopsies in rectal gonorrhea are normal; some reveal a mild increase in neutrophils and mononuclear cells or focal cryptitis.[45] Gram-negative cocci can occasionally be seen on Gram's stain of anal discharge, and culture can be a valuable diagnostic aid.

MISCELLANEOUS BACTERIAL INFECTIONS

Bacterial Esophagitis. Bacterial esophagitis is rare and is usually found in immunocompromised or debilitated patients. Implicated bacteria include *Staphylococcus aureus*, *Lactobacillus acidophilus*, and *Klebsiella pneumoniae*. Endoscopic findings include ulceration, pseudomembrane formation, and hemorrhage. Histologic findings include acute inflammation and necrosis, with bacteria demonstrable within the wall of the esophagus.[46]

Phlegmonous Enteritis, Gastritis, and Esophagitis. Phlegmonous enteritis, gastritis, and esophagitis have all been well documented. They are characterized by a

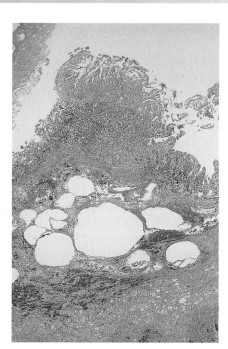

FIGURE 3–12. Emphysematous enteritis due to *C. perfringens*. Note transmural necrosis and mucosal sloughing with associated gas bubbles within the gut wall. (Case courtesy of Dr. David Owen.)

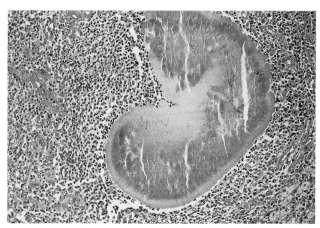

FIGURE 3–13. Actinomycotic ("sulfur") granule consisting of irregularly rounded clusters of bacteria bordered by Splendore-Hoeppli material and an acute inflammatory exudate. (Photograph courtesy of Dr. George F. Gray, Jr.)

suppurative, primarily submucosal inflammatory process, with striking edema. The causative organisms vary and include *E. coli*, clostridial organisms, *Proteus* species, staphylococci, and streptococci group A.[47,48] Most patients are debilitated, and many have cirrhosis or alcoholic liver disease.[48] Patients may have nonspecific GI or systemic symptoms, or phlegmonous disease may be found incidentally at autopsy. Patients typically appear to have an acute abdomen, sometimes complicated by hematemesis or vomiting of purulent material.

Any level of the alimentary tract may be involved. The gut wall is markedly thick and edematous. Sometimes gas-producing organisms such as *C. perfringens* may lead to the formation of gas bubbles in the submucosa (so-called *emphysematous changes*) (Fig. 3-12). Although the mucosa may be red and friable, discrete ulceration is rarely present. Histologically, intense edema and acute inflammation are noted, predominantly in the submucosa, although transmural infiltration may be seen.[48] The mucosa may be spared or sloughed entirely, especially in the stomach. Venous thrombosis may complicate the picture, causing ischemic changes. Gram's stain may show organisms within the bowel wall; in some cases, their identification is required before the diagnosis can be made.

Actinomycosis (*Actinomyces israelii*). This filamentous anaerobic Gram-positive bacterium is a normal inhabitant of the oral cavity and upper GI tract. In rare cases it produces a chronic, nonopportunistic GI infection.[49] Infection usually occurs in a solitary site

and may involve any level of the GI tract. Symptoms include fever, weight loss, abdominal pain, and occasionally a palpable mass. Perianal fistulas and chronic (often granulomatous) appendicitis have been described; sometimes actinomycosis is associated with diverticular disease. Grossly, this organism often produces a large, solitary mass, with or without ulceration, with significant mural infiltration that may extend into surrounding structures.[50]

The organism typically produces actinomycotic ("sulfur") granules consisting of irregularly rounded clusters of bacteria bordered by eosinophilic, clublike projections (Splendore-Hoeppli material). The inflammatory reaction is predominantly neutrophilic, with abscess formation (Fig. 3-13). Palisading histiocytes and giant cells, as well as frank granulomas, often surround the neutrophilic inflammation. A marked associated fibrotic response may be seen. Gram's stains reveal the filamentous, Gram-positive organisms. GMS and Warthin-Starry stains also stain actinomycosis.

The gross differential diagnosis includes peptic ulcer, lymphoma, and carcinoma. The histologic differential primarily includes other infectious processes, particularly *Nocardia* species. Unlike *Nocardia* organisms, actinomycetes are not at all acid-fast. Care should be taken not to confuse actinomycosis with fungi or other bacteria that may form clusters and chains but are not truly filamentous, such as *Pseudomonas* species and *E. coli*.

Whipple's Disease (*Tropheryma whippelii*). Whipple's disease typically presents in middle-aged white men as chronic weight loss, arthritis, malabsorption, and lymphadenopathy. Many patients also have significant neuropsychiatric manifestations.

The small bowel is most often affected, although colonic and appendiceal involvement may be seen. Endoscopically, mucosal folds are thickened and coated with yellow-white plaques, often with surrounding erythema and friability. Histologically, the characteristic lesion is massive infiltration of the lamina propria and submucosa with foamy macrophages (Fig. 3-14**A**); the infiltrate often blunts the distended villi. Involvement may be diffuse or patchy. Typically, no associated mononuclear inflammatory infiltrate is seen, but varying numbers of neutrophils are present. The lamina propria may contain small foci of fat, and there may be overlying vacuolization of enterocytes.[51]

Eighty-four years after Whipple initially reported this disease, Whipple's bacillus was identified as *T. whippelii*, an actinobacterium. This bacillus is strongly PAS-positive (Fig. 3-14**B**); electron microscopy and PCR assays may be useful as well. Differential diagnosis includes predominantly MAI infection, but in rare cases other intracellular organisms such as *Histoplasma* and *Rhodococcus*.

Rhodococcus equi. These Gram-positive coccobacilli occasionally infect humans, particularly those who are immunocompromised. GI infection typically presents as chronic (often bloody) diarrhea and is generally a manifestation of systemic involvement. *R. equi* produces inflammatory polyps, sometimes with associated mesenteric adenitis; histologically, these polyps consist of organism-laden macrophages that pack the mucosa and submucosa, often with an associated granulomatous response. Organisms stain with PAS and Gram's stains and may be partially acid-fast. Histologic

features may mimic infection with MAI or Whipple's disease.[52]

Rocky Mountain Spotted Fever (*Rickettsia rickettsii*). This disease is transmitted by the bite of the common wood or dog tick. Many patients have significant GI findings, including nausea, vomiting, diarrhea, pain, and GI bleeding; these manifestations may precede the rash. Involvement of all levels of the GI tract has been documented.[53] Typical histologic findings include vasculitis at any level of the gut wall, often with accompanying nonocclusive microthrombi and hemorrhage. The inflammatory infiltrate is composed of mononuclear cells with occasional lymphocytes, macrophages, and neutrophils. Immunofluorescence staining demonstrates the organism, and serologic studies may also be of use.

Malakoplakia. This rare disorder, found anywhere in the GI tract, consists of soft, yellow plaques containing a mixture of neutrophils and macrophages; Michaelis-Gutmann bodies are the diagnostic feature. A majority of cases are associated with bacterial infection, particularly *E. coli*, *Klebsiella* species, and mycobacterial organisms; *R. equi* association has also been reported.

Bacillary Angiomatosis. These pyogenic granuloma–like lesions are found in immunocompromised patients and mimic Kaposi's sarcoma. They are usually associated with *Bartonella quintana*.

Helicobacter pylori and ***H. heilmannii.*** These bacteria are discussed in Chapter 8.

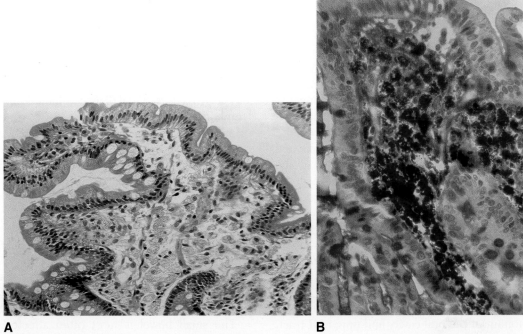

A **B**

FIGURE 3–14. A, Whipple's disease. Villi are distended by an infiltrate of foamy macrophages. **B,** The Whipple bacillus is intensely PAS positive. (Photographs courtesy of Dr. George F. Gray, Jr.)

Fungal Infections of the Gastrointestinal Tract

The importance of fungal infections of the GI tract has increased as numbers of patients with organ transplants, AIDS, and other immunodeficiency states have risen. GI fungal infections are predominantly seen in immunocompromised patients, but virtually all have been described as rare causes of infection in immunocompetent persons. Signs and symptoms of GI fungal infections are in general similar, regardless of fungal agent, and include diarrhea, vomiting, melena, GI bleeding, abdominal pain, and fever. Esophageal fungal infections usually present with odynophagia and dysphagia. It is important to remember that fungal infections of the GI tract are often part of a disseminated disease process, but GI symptoms and signs may well be the presenting manifestations.

Other fungal infections that are occasionally seen in the GI tract but are not discussed here include *Blastomycosis dermatitidis*, *Paracoccidioides brasiliensis* (South American blastomycosis), and *Fusarium*.

Candida Species. *Candida* is the most common source of infection of the esophagus, but it may be seen at any level of the GI tract. The GI tract is a major entryway for disseminated candidiasis because *Candida* species often superinfect ulcers present from other causes. *Candida albicans* is most commonly seen, but *Candida tropicalis* and *Candida (Torulopsis) glabrata* may produce similar manifestations.[54]

Grossly, the esophagus typically contains white plaques that may be scraped away to reveal ulcerated mucosa underneath. Gross features of candidiasis in the remainder of the GI tract are variable and include ulceration, pseudomembrane formation, and inflammatory masses (Fig. 3-15). If vascular invasion is prominent, the gross appearance of infarcted bowel may be seen.[55] Involvement may be diffuse or segmental.

The associated inflammatory response ranges from minimal if any tissue reaction (especially in immunocompromised patients) to prominent neutrophilic infiltrates, abscess formation, erosion/ulceration, and necrosis. Granulomas are occasionally seen. Fungi may invade to any level of the gut wall. Invasion of mucosal and submucosal blood vessels is sometimes a prominent feature of invasive candidal infection.[54,55] *C. albicans* and *tropicalis* produce a mixture of budding yeast forms, hyphae, and pseudohyphae (see Fig. 3-15). *C. (Torulopsis) glabrata* features tiny budding yeast forms similar to *Histoplasma* species and does not produce hyphae or pseudohyphae.[56]

Aspergillus Species. *Aspergillus* infection of the GI tract occurs almost exclusively in immunocompromised patients and is much less frequently seen in the esophagus than is candidiasis. Gross findings are very similar to infection with *Candida* species.[55] A majority of patients with GI aspergillosis have coexistent lung lesions.

The characteristic histologic lesion of aspergillosis is a nodular infarction consisting of a zone of ischemic necrosis centered on a blood vessel containing fungal organisms (Figs. 3-16 and 3-17). The fungal hyphae often extend outward from the infarct in parallel or radial arrays. Inflammatory response ranges from minimal to a marked neutrophilic infiltrate; granulomatous inflammation is occasionally seen.[56] Transmural infarction of the bowel wall is common. The typical hyphae of *Aspergillus* are septate, and they branch at acute angles.

The histologic lesions of mucormycosis and related Zygomycetes are markedly similar to those seen in aspergillosis. In contrast to *Aspergillus* infection, they have broad, ribbonlike, pauciseptate hyphae that branch

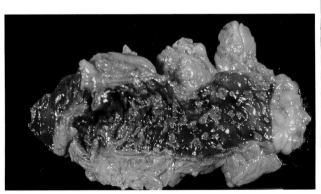

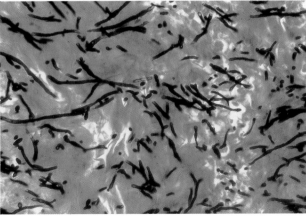

A   B

FIGURE 3–15. A, Colonic candidiasis featuring yellow-white plaques with associated marked mucosal ulceration. **B,** GMS staining shows the mixture of budding yeast forms and pseudohyphae typical of *Candida* species. (Gross photograph courtesy of Dr. Cole Elliott.)

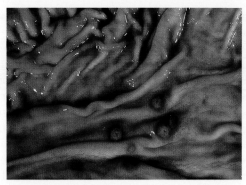

FIGURE 3–16. Typical "target lesion" of aspergillosis, shown in the stomach, consisting of hemorrhagic infarction and necrosis centered on a blood vessel.

randomly at various angles.[56] Ulcers are the most common gross manifestation; they are often large with rolled, irregular edges that may mimic malignancy. These fungi also often superinfect tissues that have been previously ulcerated. Patients with diabetes or other causes of systemic acidosis appear to be at increased risk of developing zygomycosis.[57]

***Histoplasma* Species.** *Histoplasma capsulatum* is endemic to the central United States but has been described in many nonendemic areas as well. GI involvement occurs in more than 80% of patients with disseminated infection. Patients often initially present with signs and symptoms of GI illness and do not always have concomitant pulmonary involvement.[58]

The ileum is the most common site, but any level of the GI tract may be involved. Gross lesions range from normal mucosa to ulcers, nodules, and obstructive masses. Often, a combination of these lesions is seen. Histologic findings include diffuse lymphohistiocytic infiltrates and nodules, usually involving the mucosa and submucosa, with associated ulceration (Fig. 3-18). Often these lesions are present overlying Peyer's patches. Discrete granulomas and giant cells are seen in only a minority of cases. In immunocompromised patients, large numbers of organisms may be seen with virtually no tissue reaction.[58] *Histoplasma* organisms typically are small, ovoid, usually intracellular yeast forms with small buds at the more pointed pole.

Cryptococcus neoformans. This fungus is an unusual but important cause of GI infection. Virtually all patients with GI cryptococcosis have hematogenously disseminated disease with multisystem organ involvement, and most have pulmonary and meningeal disease.[59]

Grossly, cryptococcal infection may be located anywhere in the GI tract. Endoscopic lesions include nodules and ulcers, sometimes associated with a thick white exudate; however, the mucosa is normal in many cases.[59]

Histologic features include typical round to oval yeast forms with narrow-based budding; cryptococci may show considerable variation in size. Occasionally, they produce hyphae and pseudohyphae. Often a "halo" effect can be seen on H&E staining, representing the capsule of the organism. Both superficial and deep

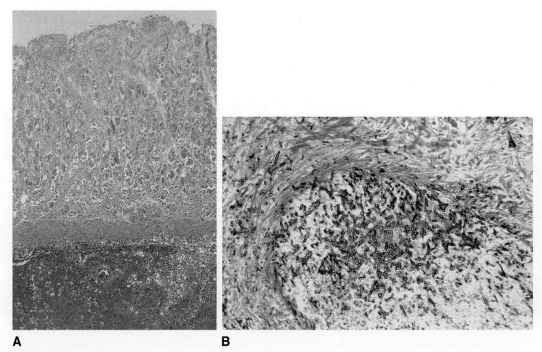

A   B

FIGURE 3–17. **A,** Ischemic necrosis of the mucosa and submucosa in a case of gastric aspergillosis. **B,** *Aspergillus* oganisms fill and penetrate a vessel in the submucosa (GMS).

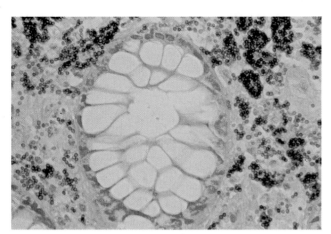

FIGURE 3–18. Numerous *Histoplasma* organisms are seen distending histiocytes within the lamina propria on this GMS stain. (Photograph courtesy of Dr. Patrick J. Dean.)

involvement may occur, and lymphatic involvement is not uncommon. The inflammatory reaction varies according to the immune status of the host, ranging from a suppurative, necrotizing inflammatory reaction, often with granulomatous features (Fig. 3-19**A**), to virtually no reaction at all in anergic hosts.[56,59] The mucopolysaccharide capsule stains with Alcian blue, mucicarmine (Fig. 3-19**B**), and colloidal iron; GMS stains are of course positive as well. Capsule-deficient cryptococci may present a diagnostic challenge, but most have sufficient capsular material left to be seen on mucin stains.[56,59]

Pneumocystis carinii. Although its life cycle more closely resembles that of a protozoan, there is convincing molecular evidence indicating that *P. carinii* has greater homology with fungi. *P. carinii* pneumonia is a major cause of morbidity in the AIDS population, and extrapulmonary (including GI) involvement is occurring more and more frequently.[60]

Endoscopically, *P. carinii* GI infection resembles a nonspecific, often erosive, esophagogastritis or colitis, sometimes with small polypoid nodules. Microscopically, the granular, foamy eosinophilic casts common to pulmonary infection may be seen within mucosal vessels or in the lamina propria.[60] As in the lung, a wide variety of inflammatory responses may occur, including granulomatous inflammation, macrophage infiltrates, and necrosis.

Fungi can often be correctly classified by tissue sections based on morphologic criteria (Table 3-3). Although organisms may be identifiable on H&E sections in heavy infections, GMS and PAS stains remain valuable diagnostic aids. It should be stressed, however, that if there is any doubt as to classification, fungal culture should be relied on as the gold standard of speciation because antifungal therapy may vary according to the type of fungus identified. It is also important to remember that fungi exposed to antifungal therapy or ambient air may produce bizarre and unusual forms. Helpful diagnostic aids, in addition to culture, include serologic assays, antigen tests, and immunohistochemistry.

The differential diagnosis of fungal infections most often includes other infectious processes; occasionally Crohn's disease, ulcerative colitis, sarcoidosis, and ischemic colitis enter the differential as well.

Parasitic Infections of the Gastrointestinal Tract

PROTOZOAN INFECTIONS

Protozoa are prevalent pathogens in tropical and subtropical countries, yet they also cause some of the most common intestinal infections in North America and Europe. Immigration, increasing numbers of

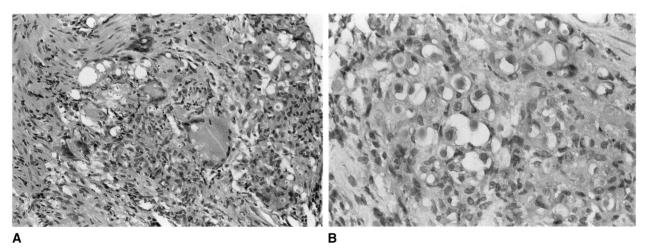

A   **B**

FIGURE 3–19. A, This case of gastric cryptococcosis features a granulomatous reaction with associated giant cells and acute inflammation. A "halo" effect can be seen around the organisms. **B,** The round to oval yeast forms have a mucopolysaccharide capsule that stains with mucicarmine. (Photographs courtesy of Dr. Kay Washington.)

TABLE 3–3. Morphologic Features of Fungi Involving the Gastrointestinal Tract

Organism	Morphologic Features	Host Reaction	Major Differential Diagnoses
Aspergillus species	Hyphae—septate, uniform width Branching—regular, acute angles Conidial head formation in cavitary lesions	Ischemic necrosis with angioinvasion Acute inflammation Occasionally granulomatous	Zygomycetes *Fusarium* *Pseudallescheria boydii*
Zygomycetes	Hyphae—pauciseptate, ribbonlike, thin walls Branching—haphazard	Similar to *Aspergillus*	Similar to *Aspergillus*
Candida albicans; *Candida tropicalis*	Mixture of budding yeast and pseudohyphae; occasional septate hyphae	Usually suppurative May be necrotic and ulcerative Occasionally granulomatous Occasional angioinvasion	*Trichosporon*
Candida glabrata	Budding yeast No hyphae No "halo" effect	Similar to other *Candida* species	*Histoplasma* *Cryptococcus*
Cryptococcus neoformans	Pleomorphic Narrow-based buds Usually mucicarmine-positive	Usually suppurative May have extensive necrosis Sometimes granulomatous	Histoplasmosis Blastomycosis *C. glabrata*
Histoplasma capsulatum	Ovoid, narrow-based buds Intracellular "Halo" effect around organism on H&E	Lymphohistiocytic infiltrate with parasitized histiocytes Occasionally granulomatous	*Cryptococcus* *Penicillium marneffei* *C. glabrata* Intracellular parasites *Pneumocystis carinii*
Pneumocystis carinii	Ovoid Internal enhancing detail Foamy casts	Ranges from suppurative to granulomatous	Histoplasmosis Small parasites

immunocompromised patients, use of institutional child care facilities, and the development of improved diagnostic techniques have impacted our understanding and recognition of these diseases. Many protozoal illnesses are diagnosed by examination of stool samples, but they are also important to the surgical pathologist.

Entamoeba histolytica. Approximately 10% of the world's population is infected with this parasite, predominantly in tropical and subtropical locations. Male homosexuals in Western countries also commonly harbor this pathogen. Although some patients suffer a severe, dysentery-like, fulminant colitis, many others are asymptomatic or have only vague GI symptoms.[61] Complications include serious bleeding and dissemination to other sites, particularly the liver. Rarely, large inflammatory masses (amebomas) may form.

Grossly, small ulcers are initially seen, which may coalesce to form large, irregular ulcers that are often geographic or serpiginous. These ulcers can undermine adjacent mucosa to produce the classic "flask-shaped" lesion; there may be associated inflammation or inflammatory polyps. Intervening mucosa is often normal. The cecum is most commonly involved, but any level of the large bowel or appendix may be infected. Fulminant colitis resembling ulcerative colitis, pseudomembranous colitis resembling that caused by *C. difficile*, and toxic megacolon have been described.[62] Colonoscopy may be normal in asymptomatic patients or those with mild disease.[61]

Histologically, the earliest lesion is a mild neutrophilic infiltrate. In more advanced disease, ulcers are often deep, extending at least into the submucosa, with undermining of adjacent normal mucosa (Fig. 3-20**A**). Necroinflammatory debris is associated; the organisms are generally found within this purulent material. Invasive amebae are occasionally seen within the bowel wall. The adjacent mucosa is usually normal but may show gland distortion and inflammation. The organisms, which may be very few in number, resemble macrophages with foamy cytoplasm and a round, eccentric nucleus; the presence of ingested red blood cells (Fig. 3-20**B**) is pathognomonic of *E. histolytica*.[62] In patients who are asymptomatic or who have mild symptoms, histologic changes may range from normal to a heavy mixed inflammatory infiltrate. Organisms may be particularly difficult (if not impossible) to find in these patients. Invasive amebiasis is not generally seen in patients with mild or absent symptoms.[61]

The differential diagnosis most often is that of amebae versus macrophages within an inflammatory exudate. Amebae are trichrome and PAS positive; in addition, their nuclei are usually more rounded and paler and have a more open nuclear chromatin pattern (see Fig. 3-20**B**). Macrophages also stain with immunostains for alpha-1-antitrypsin and chymotrypsin, whereas amebae do not. The differential diagnosis of amebiasis includes Crohn's disease and ulcerative colitis, as well as other types of infectious colitis. Although some features of amebiasis may mimic idiopathic inflammatory bowel disease, many of the other diagnostic

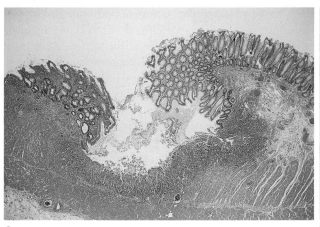
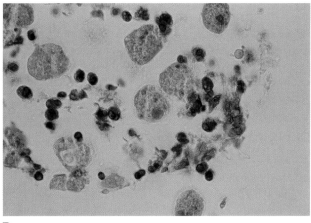

A   **B**

FIGURE 3–20. A, Amoebic ulcer that is deep and flask-shaped, undermining adjacent normal mucosa. **B,** *E. histolytica* within the inflammatory exudate, containing ingested erythrocytes.

features of Crohn's disease (transmural lymphoid aggregates, mural fibrosis, granulomas, and neural hyperplasia) and ulcerative colitis (basal lymphoplasmacytosis, diffuse architectural distortion, pancolitis) are not typically present.

FLAGELLATES

Giardia lamblia. Giardiasis is the leading GI protozoal disease in the United States, reaching a prevalence rate of 2% to 7% overall, and up to 35% in day care centers. Patients present with explosive, foul-smelling, and watery diarrhea; abdominal pain and distention; nausea and vomiting; malabsorption; and weight loss. The infection may resolve spontaneously but often persists for weeks or months if left untreated.[63,64] The cyst (the infective form) is extremely hardy and chlorine resistant and may survive in water for several months. The mechanism by which these organisms cause GI illness is not well understood.

Endoscopic examination is generally unremarkable. Small intestinal biopsies in patients with giardiasis are often normal as well. Biopsies may show mild to moderate villous blunting; increased lamina propria inflammatory cells, including neutrophils, plasma cells, and lymphocytes; and the presence of trophozoites (resembling pears cut lengthwise that contain two ovoid nuclei with a central karyosome) at the luminal surface.[64] Tissue invasion is not seen. Although *Giardia* species are characteristically described as small bowel inhabitants, colonization of the stomach and colon has also been reported.[63] The absence or marked decrease in plasma cells in the lamina propria in a patient with giardiasis should suggest the presence of underlying immunodeficiency (see Chapter 4).

Leishmania donovani **and Related Species.** This disease is endemic in more than 80 countries in Africa,

Asia, South and Central America, and Europe.[65] GI signs and symptoms include fever, abdominal pain, diarrhea, dysphagia, malabsorption, and weight loss; GI involvement is generally part of widely disseminated disease. *Leishmania* species may be found at any level of the alimentary tract, and the spectrum of endoscopic findings includes normal mucosa, focal ulceration, and changes of enteritis.[66]

Histologically, amastigote-containing macrophages are typically present within the lamina propria. In great enough numbers, the laden macrophages distend and blunt small intestinal villi. An associated inflammatory infiltrate is often absent. The amastigotes are round to oval, tiny organisms with a nucleus and a kinetoplast in a "double-knot" configuration. They are highlighted by Giemsa staining. The differential diagnosis is primarily that of other parasitic and fungal infections, and *Leishmania* may be confused with similar organisms such as *Histoplasma* and *Trypanosoma cruzi. Leishmania* organisms are GMS negative and affect the lamina propria rather than the myenteric plexus.[65,66] Serologic studies and immunohistochemistry may aid in diagnosis.

T. cruzi **(Chagas' Disease).** Chagas' disease is one of the most serious public health problems in South America. Parasitic involvement of the enteric nervous system is common in this disease, and an achalasia-like megaesophagus and megacolon are the most frequent manifestations.[67] Histologically, an inflammatory destruction of the myenteric plexus is seen, with loss of up to 95% of neurons. The parasite itself is rarely seen in the myenteric plexuses.[68] Differential diagnosis includes idiopathic primary achalasia and other visceral neuropathies. Many of these latter diseases lack inflammation of the myenteric plexus, but often the differential must be resolved clinically. Unlike primary achalasia, Chagas' disease usually involves other organ systems (especially the heart) or other parts of the GI tract.

CILIATES

Balantidium coli. This ciliate may produce a spectrum of clinical and pathologic changes similar to those of *E. histolytica.* *B. coli* are distinguished from amebae by their larger size, kidney bean–shaped nucleus, and cilia (Fig. 3-21).[69]

COCCIDIANS

Coccidial infection is particularly important when diarrhea is considered in a patient with AIDS, but it is also seen in healthy persons. Transmission is via the fecal-oral route, either directly or via contaminated food and water.[70] All coccidians except microsporidia (which is thought to be limited to the immunocompromised) can cause diarrhea (often prolonged) in healthy patients, especially infants and children, travelers, and the institutionalized. Diarrhea may be accompanied by fever, weight loss, abdominal pain, and malaise. The stool does not usually contain red blood cells or leukocytes. In immunocompetent persons, the infection is usually self-limited, but immunocompromised patients are at risk for chronic, severe diarrhea with malabsorption, dehydration, and death.[70] Many coccidial infections are asymptomatic. Endoscopic findings are usually absent or mild and may include mild erythema, mucosal granularity, mucosal atrophy, and mild erosions.

Although electron microscopy was once considered the gold standard for diagnosis of these organisms, it is expensive and is not widely used. Examination of stool specimens may be helpful in many cases, but mucosal biopsy specimens may actually be more sensitive in others. Enzyme-linked immunosorbent assay (ELISA) techniques, immunohistochemistry, and PCR studies are also available for many of these parasites.

Cryptosporidium parvum. This parasite is most common in the small bowel but can be seen in any segment of the GI tract. Its characteristic appearance is a 2- to 5-μm basophilic spherical body protruding from the apex of the enterocyte (Fig. 3-22).[71] These organisms can be found in the crypts or at the surface. Associated mucosal changes include villous atrophy (occasionally severe), crypt hyperplasia, a mixed inflammatory infiltrate, and crypt abscesses. Giemsa stains may aid in diagnosis, and immunohistochemical antibodies are available. *Cryptosporidia* may be distinguished from most other coccidians by their size and unique apical location; although *Cyclospora* are similar in appearance, they are much larger (8 to 10 μm).

Cyclospora cayetanensis. This is most commonly found in the small bowel. Histologic changes in mucosal biopsy are similar to those of other coccidians.[72] The 8- to 10-μm parasites are usually within enterocytes but can bulge at the surface similar to *Cryptosporidia.* Few detailed light microscopic descriptions are available for this parasite, and there is some disagreement as to their features in tissue sections. They appear to be either crescent shaped or ovoid, and they are sometimes within a parasitiferous vacuole.[73] They are acid-fast with modified Kinyoun or similar stains, and they stain with auramine. They are GMS-negative. The major differential diagnosis involves *Cryptosporidium* species, but *Cyclospora* species are much larger (Fig. 3-23), and they autofluoresce under epifluorescent light.[72] Some crescent-shaped organisms may be confused with *Isospora* species, which are generally larger.

***Isospora belli* and Related Species.** These organisms are most often seen in the small bowel but

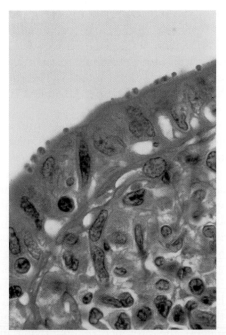

FIGURE 3–22. *Cryptosporidium parvum.* The 2- to 5-μm basophilic spherical bodies protrude from the apex of the enterocytes. (Photograph courtesy of Drs. Rodger C. Haggitt and Mary P. Bronner.)

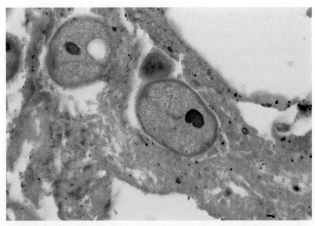

FIGURE 3–21. *B. coli* present within the bowel wall; note large size, kidney bean–shaped nucleus, and cilia. (Case courtesy of Dr. David Owen.)

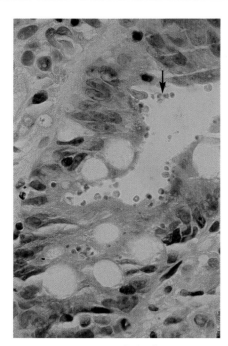

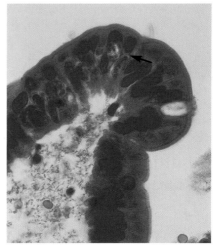

FIGURE 3–24. *Isospora belli.* Banana-shaped intraepithelial inclusions *(arrow)* are seen within apical enterocytes. (Photograph courtesy of Dr. Audrey Lazenby.)

FIGURE 3–23. AIDS patient with both *Cryptosporidium* and *Cyclospora* infections. Cryptosporidia are 2 to 5 μm in size and are located at the apex of the enterocytes *(arrow)*. The round to ovoid *Cyclospora* are similar in appearance but are much larger (8–10 μm).

have also been described in the colon; *Isospora* species may also disseminate. Histologic changes include villous blunting, which may be severe; crypt hyperplasia; a mixed inflammatory infiltrate, often with prominent eosinophils; and fibrosis of the lamina propria in chronic infection. Intraepithelial inclusions, both perinuclear and subnuclear, can be seen in all stages of infection. Rarely, organisms are seen in the lamina propria, often within macrophages.[74,75] The motile parasites are large and banana shaped (Fig. 3-24); trophozoites are round with a prominent nucleus. At some stages, the parasites have a parasitiferous vacuole surrounding them. GMS and Giemsa stains may aid in diagnosis; although the organisms are PAS positive, they may be easily confused with goblet cells. *Isospora* species are differentiated from other coccidia by both their large size and their intracellular location. Patients with isosporiasis are also more likely to have peripheral eosinophilia.

Microsporidia. *Enterocytozoon bieneusi* and *Encephalitozoon intestinalis* are the most commonly seen human pathogens in this group. They are usually seen in the small bowel, but any level of the alimentary tract may be affected. Microsporidia can be difficult to detect in H&E sections. Histologic features include focal villous blunting, a subtle vacuolization of the surface epithelium, and a patchy lymphoplasmacytic infiltrate in the lamina propria.[76,77] A modified trichrome stain can aid greatly in diagnosis (Fig. 3-25); these parasites also stain with Warthin-Starry and Brown-Brenn stains. Sometimes microsporidia polarize within

tissue biopsies because the chitin-rich internal polar filament of the organism is birefringent under polarized light. However, this method of detection is unreliable owing to the unpredictability of spore birefringence, as well as its variability according to the microscope and light source used.

Toxoplasma gondii. GI toxoplasmosis is primarily a disease of the immunocompromised. Ulcers have been described in the bowel, with organisms in the ulcer base. Both crescent-shaped tachyzoites and tissue cysts containing bradyzoites may be seen within tissue sections. Immunohistochemistry and PCR assays, as well as serologic tests, provide useful diagnostic aids.[78]

MISCELLANEOUS PROTOZOAL INFECTIONS

Dientamoeba fragilis is an ameba of low pathogenicity that rarely causes diarrhea. A variety of other amebae are also occasionally associated with mild GI disease,

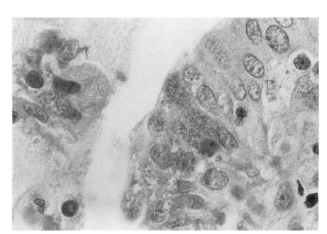

FIGURE 3–25. Tiny microsporidial organisms within enterocytes (modified trichrome).

including *Entamoeba hartmanni, Entamoeba polecki, Iodamoeba buetschlii*, and *Endolimax nana. Blastocystis hominis*, another protozoan of low pathogenicity, may cause enteric disease when present in large numbers. These organisms are rarely seen in tissue sections. When such protozoa of low pathogenicity are identified in tissue sections, symptomatic patients should be evaluated for alternative causes of GI disease.

Helminthic Infections of the Gastrointestinal Tract

Although the most common method of diagnosing GI helminthic infections is examination of stool for ova and parasites, nematodes, trematodes, and cestodes are occasionally seen in biopsy or resection specimens. Hookworms, roundworms (both *Ascaris* and *Enterobius*), and whipworms are the most common helminthic infections in humans.[79] GI helminths have a worldwide distribution, but their clinical importance varies with geographic region. They are more often a cause of serious disease in nations with deficient sanitation systems, poor socioeconomic status, and hot, humid climates. However, helminthic infections are seen in immigrants as well as patients who travel to endemic areas, and they are an increasingly important problem in immunocompromised patients. The nutritional problems caused by helminths can be severe and even life threatening, especially in children.[79] The anatomic site of infection is most often the small bowel, although the stomach and large bowel may certainly be involved.[80]

NEMATODES

Enterobius vermicularis. Pinworms, one of the most common human parasites, have a worldwide distri-

bution but are more common in cold or temperate climates and developed countries. They are extremely common in the United States and northwestern Europe. The infective egg resides in dust and soil, and transmission is believed to be fecal-oral. The worms live and reproduce in the ileum, cecum, proximal colon, and appendix, and the female migrates to the anus to lay her eggs and then die. The eggs and worms produce the typical symptom of pruritus ani. Although many infections are asymptomatic, appendicitis, vulvovaginitis, colitis, and peritoneal involvement have been described,[80-82] and heavy infections may cause abdominal pain, nausea, and vomiting.

The causative role of *E. vermicularis* in appendicitis and colitis is controversial. Although pinworms are found in approximately 0.6% to 13% of resected appendices, their ability to actually cause mucosal damage has been hotly debated.[82] Some believe that the lack of inflammation surrounding even invasive appendiceal pinworms indicates that they invade after the appendix has been surgically removed, to escape decreasing oxygen tension.[81] However, they are capable of mucosal invasion,[81] and they can obstruct the appendiceal lumen and cause inflammation similar to fecaliths.

Grossly, the worms are 2 to 5 mm in length and may be seen with the naked eye (Fig. 3-26). Although the mucosa of the GI tract often appears normal upon examination, hemorrhage and ulceration are occasionally seen with invasion.

Even invasive pinworms usually incite little or no inflammatory reaction, as has been discussed earlier, but an inflammatory infiltrate composed of neutrophils and eosinophils may be seen. Granulomas, sometimes with necrosis, can be seen associated with degenerating worms or eggs. These lesions have been described within the omentum and peritoneum, as well as the appendix, anus, and colon in rare cases.[81] It may be

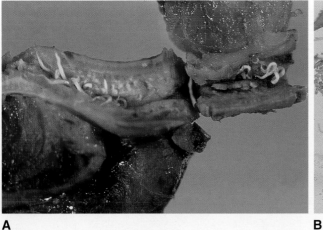

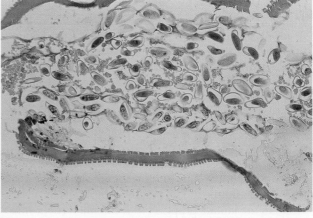

A   **B**

FIGURE 3–26. A, Inflamed appendix containing numerous pinworms (gross photograph). **B,** Section of worm showing cuticle and numerous eggs characteristic of *E. vermicularis*. (Gross photograph courtesy of Dr. George F. Gray, Jr.)

difficult to distinguish between primary *Enterobius* infection and infection complicating a preexisting inflammatory lesion such as an inflamed anal fissure.

***Ascaris lumbricoides* (Roundworms).** *Ascaris* is one of the most frequent parasites in humans. It has a worldwide distribution but is most common in the tropics. These worms are ingested from soil contaminated from feces. Clinical findings are variable and include appendicitis, massive infection with obstruction and perforation, childhood growth retardation, and pancreaticobiliary obstruction. These giant worms (up to 20 cm) may be identified endoscopically, or at resection (Fig. 3-27) if obstruction occurs. Tissue damage occurs primarily at attachment sites.[80]

Ancylostomiasis (Hookworm). Hookworms (*Necator americanus* and *Ancylostoma duodenale*) are a common parasite in virtually all tropical and subtropical countries. The worms attach to the intestinal wall and suck blood from villous capillaries, resulting in anemia. Other clinical symptoms include abdominal pain, diarrhea, hypoproteinemia, and an associated cough with eosinophilia as the worms migrate.[79] Any level of the GI tract may be involved. Endoscopically, the worms (about 1 cm in length) are visible to the naked eye. Histologic changes are often minimal but may include villous blunting and eosinophilic infiltrate.[80] Pieces of worm may occasionally be seen on biopsy.

***Trichuris trichiura* (Whipworms).** Whipworms are a soil helminth with a worldwide distribution. Although many infections are asymptomatic, symptoms and signs of infection include diarrhea, GI bleeding, malabsorption, anemia, and appendicitis. An ulcerative inflammatory process similar to Crohn's disease has been described, as has rectal prolapse.[79,80] The worms live in the small and large intestines, primarily the right colon and ileum. They may cause mucosal hemorrhage and ulceration; the worms are 3 to 5 mm long with a characteristic whiplike tail and may be seen endoscopically. Histologically, the worms thread their anterior ends under the mucosal epithelium, which may

produce enterocyte atrophy and an associated mixed inflammatory infiltrate; crypt abscesses may also be present.[80,83]

Strongyloides stercoralis. *S. stercoralis* is a nematode with a worldwide distribution. In the United States, it is endemic in the southeastern urban areas with large immigrant populations and in mental institutions. This infection occurs primarily in adults, many of whom are hospitalized, suffer from chronic illnesses, or are immunocompromised.[84] Symptoms and signs include diarrhea, abdominal pain and tenderness, nausea, vomiting, weight loss, malabsorption, and GI bleeding. GI manifestations may be accompanied by rash, eosinophilia, urticaria, pruritus, and pulmonary symptoms.[80,84] However, many patients are asymptomatic.

S. stercoralis penetrates the skin, enters the venous system, travels to the lungs, and then migrates up the respiratory tree and down the esophagus to eventually reach the small intestine. The female lives in the small intestine and lays eggs there, thus perpetuating the cycle. This autoinfective capability allows it to reside in the host and produce illness for upward of 30 years. In addition, it may disseminate in immunocompromised patients, causing severe and even fatal illness.[80,84]

Lesions may be seen in the stomach as well as in the small and large intestines. Endoscopically, findings include hypertrophic mucosal folds and ulcers; features typical of pseudomembranous colitis have also been reported. Histologically, both adult worms and larvae may be found in the crypts, but they may be difficult to detect. Adult worms typically have sharply pointed tails that may be curved (Fig. 3-28). Other histologic features include villous blunting, ulcers (which may be fissuring), edema, and a dense eosinophilic and neutrophilic infiltrate. Granulomas are occasionally present.[80,84]

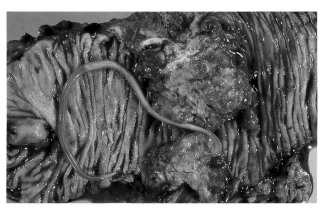

FIGURE 3–27. *Ascaris* atop colon cancer at resection. (Photograph courtesy of Dr. George F. Gray, Jr.)

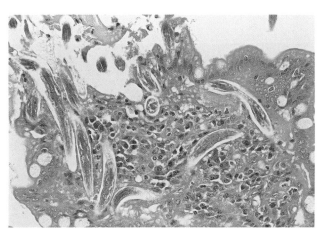

FIGURE 3–28. *S. stercoralis* infection in the small bowel. Typical worms with curved, sharply pointed tails are present within crypts and lamina propria, accompanied by a neutrophilic infiltrate. (Photograph courtesy of Dr. James A. Waldron).

***Anisakis simplex* (Anisakiasis) and Related Species.**
These nematodes parasitize fish and sea mammals, and humans generally ingest them when eating raw and pickled fish. The most common clinical manifestations are those of acute gastric anisakiasis, characterized by epigastric pain, nausea, and vomiting within 12 hours of ingesting parasitized food; the symptoms may mimic peptic ulcer disease.[80,85] The allergenic potential of the *Anisakis* species has also been recognized, and some patients with gastroallergic anisakiasis manifest both GI and hypersensitivity symptoms such as urticaria, angioedema, eosinophilia, and anaphylaxis.[85]

The stomach is the most frequent site of involvement, although small bowel, colon, and appendix may also be involved. Endoscopic findings include mucosal edema, hemorrhage, erosions, ulcers, and thickened mucosal folds. Sometimes larvae may be seen and removed endoscopically. Histologic findings include an inflammatory infiltrate rich in eosinophils that often extends transmurally into serosal and mesenteric tissues (Fig. 3-29). Eosinophilic microabscesses, granulomas, and giant cells may also be seen. Inflammatory changes are often centered around a worm. Larvae (ranging from 0.5 to 3.0 cm in length) are occasionally seen in tissue sections, but *rarely* in stool samples.[86,87]

***Capillaria* Species (Intestinal Capillariasis).**
Capillaria infection is most common in the Philippines, Thailand, and other parts of Asia, although cases have been reported in nonendemic areas. The worms are ingested with infected raw fish. Clinical signs and symptoms include malabsorption accompanied by diarrhea and abdominal pain. The worms measure 2 to 4 cm in length and are most commonly found in the crypts of the small bowel, although they may also invade the lamina propria. Although there is commonly no inflammatory reaction to these parasites upon biopsy, villous blunting, mucosal sloughing, and mild inflammatory changes have been described.[80,88]

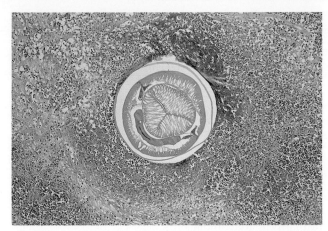

FIGURE 3–29. Gastric anisakiasis. Large worm in the center of a submucosal eosinophilic and neutrophilic abscess. (Photograph courtesy of Dr. David Owen.)

TREMATODES

Schistosomiasis. *Schistosoma* species may cause significant GI disease, and all species have this capability. Patients generally present with diarrhea (often bloody), accompanied by anemia, weight loss, and protein-losing enteropathy. More dramatic GI presentations have been described, including profound dysentery-like illness, obstruction, perforation, intussusception, rectal prolapse, fistulas, and perianal abscesses.[80] Any level of the alimentary tract may be affected. Endoscopically, *Schistosoma* species may cause a striking inflammatory polyposis (particularly in the distal colon) with associated mucosal granularity, friability, and punctate ulcers and hemorrhages. Histologically, inflammatory polyps and mucosal ulcers with associated granulomatous inflammation and an eosinophilic infiltrate are typical. Eggs are occasionally seen in histologic specimens, and sometimes they are calcified.[80,89] Worms are occasionally seen within veins (Fig. 3-30).

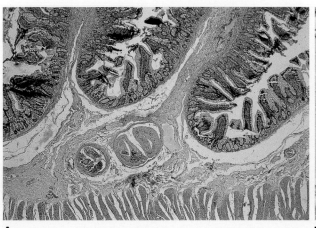

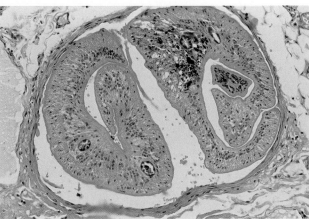

A   **B**

FIGURE 3–30. A and **B,** *Schistosoma* worm within a vein in the submucosa of the small bowel.

Intestinal Flukes (*Fasciolopsis buski* and Related Species). More than 50 species of intestinal flukes have been described in humans, but most clinically significant infections are due to *F. buski*, *Echinostoma* species, and *Heterophyes* species.[90] These flukes are most common in Asia. They are ingested with aquatic plants, and after maturation, the adult worm attaches to the proximal small bowel mucosa.[80,90] A majority of infections are asymptomatic. Symptoms usually occur with heavy infection and include diarrhea, often alternating with constipation; abdominal pain; anorexia; nausea; vomiting; and malabsorption. Ileus, obstruction, and GI bleeding have also been described. The large worms (2 to 7.5 cm) may be seen endoscopically, and mucosal ulceration, inflammation, and abscess formation may occur at attachment sites.

CESTODES

Cestode infections are not usually a problem for the surgical pathologist. *Taenia saginata* (beef tapeworm), *T. solium* (pork tapeworm), and *Hymenolepis nana* (dwarf tapeworm) may occasionally cause GI disease. *Diphyllobothrium lata* (fish tapeworm) is a rare cause of B_{12} deficiency.[80,87]

OTHER HELMINTHIC INFECTIONS

The Central American nematode *Angiostrongylus costaricensis* may cause a dramatic, even fatal ileocecal infection, featuring large obstructive inflammatory masses with perforation and mesenteric vessel thrombosis. *Trichinella spiralis* is a rare cause of diarrhea.[80] Esophagostomiasis, a parasitic disease generally seen in nonhuman primates, may form deep inflammatory masses predominantly in the right colon and appendix.[80]

Differential diagnosis of helminthic infections often involves differentiating between types of worms. Other entities to be considered include causes of ulcerative inflammation, eosinophilic infiltration, and granulomatous inflammation, such as tuberculosis, amebiasis, allergic enteritides, and Crohn's disease.

References

1. Surawicz CM: The role of rectal biopsy in infectious colitis. Am J Surg Pathol 1:82-88, 1988.
2. Chetty R, Roskell DE: Cytomegalovirus infection in the gastrointestinal tract. J Clin Pathol 47:968-972, 1994.
3. Kraus MD, Feran-Doza M, Garcia-Moliner ML, et al: Cytomegalovirus infection in the colon of bone marrow transplant patients. Mod Pathol 11:29-36, 1998.
4. Yan Z, Nguyen S, Poles M, et al: Adenovirus colitis in human immunodeficiency virus infection: An underdiagnosed entity. Am J Surg Pathol 22:1101-1106, 1998.
5. McBane RD, Gross JB: Herpes esophagitis: Clinical syndrome, endoscopic appearance, and diagnosis in 23 patients. Gastrointest Endosc 37:600-603, 1991.
6. Goodell SE, Quinn TC, Mkrtichian E, et al: Herpes simplex virus proctitis in homosexual men: Clinical, sigmoidoscopic, and histopathological features. N Engl J Med 308:868-871, 1983.
7. Bartlett JG, Belitsos PC, Sears CL: AIDS enteropathy. Clin Infect Dis 15:726-735, 1992.
8. Greenson JK, Stern RA, Carpenter SL, et al: The clinical significance of focal active colitis. Hum Pathol 28:729-733, 1997.
9. Pastore G, Schiraldi G, Fera G, et al: A biopsy study of gastrointestinal mucosa in cholera patients during an epidemic in southern Italy. Am J Dig Dis 21:613-617, 1976.
10. Wanger AR, Murray BE, Echeverria P, et al: Enteroinvasive E. coli in travelers with diarrhea. J Infect Dis 158:640-642, 1988.
11. Orenstein JM, Kotler DP: Diarrheogenic bacterial enteritis in acquired immune deficiency syndrome: A light and electron microscopic study of 52 cases. Hum Pathol 26:481-492, 1995.
12. Griffin PM, Olmstead LC, Petras RE: Escherichia coli 0157:H7-associated colitis: A clinical and histologic study of 11 cases. Gastroenterology 99:142-149, 1990.
13. Kelly J, Oryshak A, Wenetsek M, et al: The colonic pathology of E. coli 0157:H7 infection. Am J Surg Pathol 14:87-92, 1990.
14. Kelly JK, Owen DA: Bacterial diarrheas and dysenteries. In Connor DH, Chandler FW, et al (eds): Pathology of Infectious Diseases. Stamford, CT, Appleton and Lange, 1997, pp 421-429.
15. Kraus MD, Amatya B, Kimula Y: Histopathology of typhoid enteritis: Morphologic and immunophenotypic findings. Mod Pathol 12:949-955, 1999.
16. Boyd JF: Pathology of the alimentary tract in Salmonella typhimurium food poisoning. Gut 26:935-944, 1985.
17. McGovern VJ, Slavutin LJ: Pathology of Salmonella colitis. Am J Surg Pathol 3:483-490, 1979.
18. Mathan MM, Mathan VI: Morphology of rectal mucosa of patients with shigellosis. Rev Infect Dis 4:S314-S318, 1991.
19. Fields PI, Swerdlow DL: Campylobacter jejuni. Clin Lab Med 19:489-503, 1999.
20. Blaser JM, Parsons RB, Wang WLL: Acute colitis caused by Campylobacter fetus ss. jejuni. Gastroenterology 78:448-453, 1980.
21. Lamps LW, Madhusudhan KT, Greenson JK, et al: The role of Y. enterocolitica and Y. pseudotuberculosis in granulomatous appendicitis: A histologic and molecular study. Am J Surg Pathol 25:508-515, 2001.
22. Gleason TH, Patterson SD: The pathology of Yersinia enterocolitica ileocolitis. Am J Surg Pathol 6:347-355, 1982.
23. El-Maraghi NRH, Mair N: The histopathology of enteric infection with Yersinia pseudotuberculosis. Am J Clin Pathol 71:631-639, 1979.
24. Dudley TH, Dean PJ: Idiopathic granulomatous appendicitis, or Crohn's disease of the appendix revisited. Hum Pathol 24:595-601, 1993.
25. Deutsch SF, Wedzina W: Aeromonas sobria associated left sided segmental colitis. Am J Gastroenterol 92:2104-2106, 1997.
26. Borriello SP: Clostridial disease of the gut. Clin Infect Dis 2:S242-S250, 1995.
27. Surawicz CM, McFarland LV: Pseudomembranous colitis: Causes and cures. Digestion 60:91-100, 1999.
28. Nash SV, Bourgeault R, Sands M: Colonic disease associated with a positive assay for Clostridium difficile toxin: A retrospective study. J Clin Gastroenterol 25:476-479, 1997.
29. Dignan CR, Greenson JK: Can ischemic colitis be differentiated from C. difficile colitis in biopsy specimens? Am J Surg Pathol 21:706-710, 1997.
30. Murrell TGC, Roth L, Adelaide MB, et al: Pig-bel: Enteritis necroticans. Lancet 1:217-222, 1966.
31. Gomez L, Martino R, Rolston KV: Necrotizing enterocolitis: Spectrum of the disease and comparison of definite and possible cases. Clin Infect Dis 27:695-699, 1998.
32. Lev R, Sweeney KG: Neutropenic enterocolitis: Two unusual cases with review of the literature. Arch Pathol Lab Med 117:524-527, 1993.
33. Horvath KD, Whelan RL: Intestinal tuberculosis: Return of an old disease. Am J Gastroenterol 93:692-696, 1998.
34. Marshall JB: Tuberculosis of the gastrointestinal tract and peritoneum. Am J Gastroenterol 88:989-999, 1993.
35. Roth RI, Owen RL, Keren DF, et al: Intestinal infection with Mycobacterium avium-intracellulare in acquired immune deficiency syndrome (AIDS): Histological and clinical comparison with Whipple's disease. Dig Dis Sci 5:497-504, 1985.
36. Wexner SD: Sexually transmitted diseases of the colon, rectum, and anus. Dis Colon Rectum 33:1048-1059, 1990.

37. Fyfe B, Poppiti RJ, Lubin J, et al: Gastric syphilis: Primary diagnosis by gastric biopsy. Arch Pathol Lab Med 117:820-823, 1993.
38. Quinn TC, Corey L, Chaffee RG, et al: The etiology of anorectal infections in homosexual men. Am J Med 71:395-406, 1981.
39. Rompalo AM: Diagnosis and treatment of sexually acquired proctitis and proctocolitis. Clin Infect Dis 1:S84-S90, 1999.
40. Akdamar K, Martin RJ, Ichinose H: Syphilitic proctitis. Dig Dis Sci 22:701-704, 1977.
41. Surawicz CM: Intestinal spirochetosis in homosexual men. Am J Med 82:587-592, 1988.
42. Rotterdam H: Intestinal spirochetosis. In Connor DH, Chandler FW, et al (eds): Pathology of Infectious Diseases. Stamford, CT, Appleton and Lange, 1997, pp 583-589.
43. de la Monte SM, Hutchins GM: Follicular proctocolitis and neuromatous hyperplasia with lymphogranuloma venereum. Hum Pathol 16:1025-1032, 1985.
44. Geller SA, Zimmerman MJ, Cohen A: Rectal biopsy in early lymphogranuloma venereum proctitis. Am J Gastroenterol 74:433-435, 1980.
45. McMillan A, McNeillage G, Gilmour HM, et al: Histology of rectal gonorrhea in men, with a note on anorectal infection with Neisseria meningitidis. J Clin Pathol 36:511-514, 1983.
46. Walsh TJ, Belitsos NJ, Hamilton SR: Bacterial esophagitis in immunocompromised patients. Arch Intern Med 146:1345-1348, 1986.
47. Schultz MJ, van der Hulst RWM, Tytgat GNJ: Acute phlegmonous gastritis. Gastrointest Endosc 44:80-83, 1996.
48. Rosen Y, Won OH: Phlegmonous enterocolitis. Am J Dig Dis 23:248-256, 1978.
49. Ferrari TC, Couto CA, Murta-Oliveira C, et al: Actinomycosis of the colon: A rare form of presentation. Scand J Gastroenterol 35:108-109, 2000.
50. Skoutelis A, Panagopoulos C, Kalfarentzos F, et al: Intramural gastric actinomycosis. South Med J 88:647-650, 1995.
51. Dobbins WO: Whipple's Disease. Springfield, IL, Charles C Thomas, 1987.
52. Hamrock D, Azmi F, O'Donnell E, et al: Infection by Rhodococcus equi in a patient with AIDS: Histological appearance mimicking Whipple's disease and MAI infection. J Clin Pathol 52:68-71, 1999.
53. Randall MB, Walker DH: Rocky Mountain spotted fever: Gastrointestinal and pancreatic lesions and rickettsial infection. Arch Pathol Lab Med 108:963-967, 1984.
54. Walsh TJ, Merz WG: Pathologic features in the human alimentary tract associated with invasiveness of Candida tropicalis. Am J Clin Pathol 85:498-502, 1986.
55. Prescott RJ, Harris M, Banerjee SS: Fungal infections of the small and large intestine. J Clin Pathol 45:806-811, 1992.
56. Chandler FW, Watts JC: Pathologic Diagnosis of Fungal Infections. Chicago, ASCP Press, 1987.
57. Thomson SR, Bade PG, Taams M, et al: Gastrointestinal mucormycosis. Br J Surg 78:952-954, 1991.
58. Lamps LW, Molina CP, West AB, et al: The pathologic spectrum of gastrointestinal and hepatic histoplasmosis. Am J Clin Pathol 113:64-72, 2000.
59. Washington K, Gottfried MR, Wilson ML: Gastrointestinal cryptococcosis. Mod Pathol 4:707-711, 1991.
60. Dieterich DT, Lew EA, Bacon DJ, et al: Gastrointestinal pneumocystosis in HIV-infected patients on aerosolized pentamidine: Report of five cases and review of the literature. Am J Gastroenterol 87:1763-1770, 1992.
61. Variyam EP, Gogate P, Hassan M, et al: Nondysenteric intestinal amebiasis: Colonic morphology and search for Entamoeba histolytica adherence and invasion. Dig Dis Sci 34:732-740, 1989.
62. Brandt H, Tamayo P: Pathology of human amebiasis. Hum Pathol 1:351-385, 1970.
63. Oberhuber G, Kastner N, Stolte M: Giardiasis: A histologic analysis of 567 cases. Scand J Gastroenterol 32:48-51, 1997.
64. Ortega YR, Adam RD: Giardia: Overview and update. Clin Infect Dis 25:545-550, 1997.
65. Zimmer G, Guillou L, Gauthier T, et al: Digestive leishmaniasis in acquired immunodeficiency syndrome: A light and electron microscopic study of two cases. Mod Pathol 9:966-969, 1996.
66. Hofman V, Marty P, Perrin C, et al: The histological spectrum of visceral leishmaniasis caused by Leishmania infantum MON-1 in acquired immune deficiency syndrome. Hum Pathol 31:75-84, 2000.
67. de Oliveira RB, Troncon LEA, Dantas RO, et al: Gastrointestinal manifestations of Chagas' disease. Am J Gastroenterol 93:884-889, 1998.
68. Krishnamurthy S, Schuffler MD: Pathology of neuromuscular disorders of the colon. Gastroenterology 93:610-639, 1987.
69. Schwartz DA, Mixon JP: Balantidiasis. In Connor DH, Chandler FW et al (eds): Pathology of Infectious Diseases. Stamford, CT, Appleton and Lange, 1997, pp 1141-1145.
70. Goodgame R: Understanding intestinal spore-forming protozoa: Cryptosporidia, Microsporidia, Isospora, and Cyclospora. Ann Intern Med 124:429-441, 1996.
71. Clayton F, Heller T, Kotler DP: Variation in the enteric distribution of Crytosporidia in acquired immunodeficiency syndrome. Am J Clin Pathol 102:420-425, 1994.
72. Curry A, Smith HV: Emerging pathogens: Isospora, Cyclospora, and Microsporidia. Parasitology 117:S143-S159, 1998.
73. Connor BA, Reidy J, Soave R: Cyclosporiasis: Clinical and histopathologic correlates. Clin Infect Dis 28:1216-1221, 1999.
74. Orenstein JM: Isosporiasis. In Connor DH, Chandler FW, et al (eds): Pathology of Infectious Diseases. Stamford, CT, Appleton and Lange, 1997, pp 1185-1190.
75. Brandborg LL, Goldberg B, Breidenbach WC: Human coccidiosis—a possible cause of malabsorption. N Engl J Med 283:1306-1313, 1970.
76. Lamps LW, Bronner MP, Vnencak-Jones CL, et al: Optimal screening and diagnosis of Microsporidia in tissue sections. Am J Clin Pathol 109:404-410, 1998.
77. Kotler DP, Giang TT, Garro ML, et al: Light microscopic diagnosis of microsporidiosis in patients with AIDS. Am J Gastroenterol 89:540-544, 1994.
78. Bertoli F, Espino M, Arosemena JR, et al: A spectrum in the pathology of toxoplasmosis in patients with acquired immunodeficiency syndrome. Arch Pathol Lab Med 119:214-224, 1995.
79. Cooper ES, Whyte-Alleng CAM, Finzi-Smith JS, et al: Intestinal nematode infections in children: The pathophysiological price paid. Parasitology 104:S91-S103, 1992.
80. Cook GC: The clinical significance of gastrointestinal helminths—a review. Trans Roy Soc Trop Med Hyg 80:675-685, 1986.
81. Sinniah B, Leopairut RC, Connor DH: Enterobiasis: A histopathological study of 259 patients. Ann Trop Med Parasitol 85:625-635, 1991.
82. Wiebe BM: Appendicitis and Enterobius vermicularis. Scand J Gastroenterol 26:336-338, 1991.
83. Sinniah B: Trichuriasis. In Connor DH, Chandler FW, et al (eds): Pathology of Infectious Diseases. Stamford, CT, Appleton and Lange, 1997, pp 1585-1588.
84. Milder JE, Walzer PD, Kilgore GK, et al: Clinical features of Strongyloides stercoralis infection in an endemic area of the United States. Gastroenterology 80:1481-1488, 1981.
85. Daschner A, Alonso-Gomez A, Cabanas R, et al: Gastroallergic anisakiasis: Borderline between food allergy and parasitic disease—clinical and allergologic evaluation of 20 patients with confirmed acute parasitism. J Allergy Clin Immunol 105:176-181, 2000.
86. Gomez B, Tabar AI, Tunon T, et al: Eosinophilic gastroenteritis and Anisakis. Allergy 53:1148-1154, 1998.
87. Bruckner DA: Helminthic food-borne infections. Clin Lab Med 19:639-660, 1999.

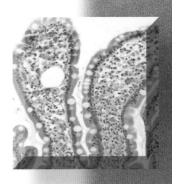

CHAPTER 4

Immunodeficiency Disorders of the GI Tract

KAY WASHINGTON

■ Primary Disorders of Immunodeficiency

Many of the primary disorders of immune deficiency (Table 4-1) are associated with gastrointestinal (GI) lesions. Manifestations of immune deficiency in the GI tract may be broadly divided into the following three categories: (1) increased susceptibility to infection, (2) idiopathic chronic inflammatory conditions, and (3) increased risk of neoplasia. Although many GI lesions are infectious (Table 4-2), chronic inflammatory conditions resembling celiac disease and inflammatory bowel disease (Table 4-3) are seen in many patients with antibody deficiencies and are probably the result of the inability of dysfunctional mononuclear cells to suppress unwanted immune responses. All patients with primary immune deficiencies are at increased risk of neoplasia (Table 4-4), most commonly non-Hodgkin's lymphoma, and the GI tract is often the primary site of involvement. In addition to the risk of lymphoma, some primary immune deficiencies are associated with increased risk for gastric adenocarcinoma[1] and colorectal carcinoma.[2]

HUMORAL IMMUNODEFICIENCIES

Selective IgA Deficiency

This is defined as a serum IgA concentration of less than 50 μg/mL; it is the most common primary immune deficiency, occurring in 1 in 600 persons of northern European ancestry.[3] The disorder is 20 times more common in whites than in blacks.[3] Defects in antibody production in patients with IgA deficiency represent a continuum with those seen in common variable immunodeficiency; 20% to 30% of IgA-deficient patients also have deficits in IgG subclasses. The molecular defect is unknown. Clinical manifestations range from no symptoms to recurrent infections, generally involving mucosal surfaces; autoimmune disorders; allergic diseases; and malignancy. The clinical manifestations of IgA deficiency are typically milder than those seen with common variable immunodeficiency (CVID). Recurrent upper and lower respiratory tract infections are common in both disorders, and both have similar GI manifestations. Infections are less common than might be expected (possibly owing to compensation for lack of mucosal IgA by transport of IgM across the mucosa into the gut lumen). Bacterial enterocolitis causes acute diarrheal illnesses, and persistent *Giardia intestinalis* infection causes chronic diarrhea. Chronic strongyloidiasis has also been reported.[4]

Susceptibility to insulin-dependent diabetes mellitus and celiac disease may be inherited together with IgA deficiency; all three conditions are linked to particular major histocompatibility haplotypes and probably represent genetically linked susceptibilities in certain populations. The prevalence of celiac disease, the most common noninfectious GI complication of IgA deficiency, is 7.7% in IgA-deficient children, compared to 1 in 500 in the general population.[5] Antigliadin IgA and endomysial IgA antibodies cannot be used as screening tools in the IgA-deficient population. A spruelike illness characterized by chronic diarrhea with villous atrophy that does not

TABLE 4–1. Molecular Basis of Primary Immunodeficiency Disorders

Disease	Proposed Cause
IgA deficiency	Impaired IgA synthesis; molecular defect unknown
Common variable immunodeficiency	Impaired B-cell maturation; molecular defect unknown
X-linked agammaglobulinemia	Mutation in *Btk* results in absence of Btk in B cells
Hyper-IgM syndrome	Absence of CD40 ligand on T cells
Hyper-IgE syndrome	Defect on chromosome 4; exact defect unknown
Severe combined immunodeficiency	Multiple defects; most common defect in common γ chain; others include adenosine deaminase deficiency, purine nucleoside deficiency, and T-cell receptor deficiencies
Omenn's syndrome	Missense mutation in *Rag-1*, *Rag-2*
DiGeorge syndrome	Thymic hypoplasia
Chronic mucocutaneous candidiasis	Heterogeneous disorder; mutation in *AIRE* gene in some[94]
Wiskott-Aldrich syndrome	Mutation in *WASP* (gene involved in cell trafficking and motility)
Chronic granulomatous disease	Mutation in gene for component of NADPH oxidase

TABLE 4–2. Gastrointestinal Infections in Primary Immunodeficiency

Disease	Gastrointestinal Infections
IgA deficiency	*Giardia intestinalis*; strongyloidiasis
Common variable immunodeficiency	*Giardia intestinalis*; *Cryptosporidium*; cytomegalovirus
X-linked agammaglobulinemia	*Giardia intestinalis*; *Cryptosporidium*, *Salmonella, Campylobacter*, rotavirus, coxsackievirus, poliovirus
Hyper-IgM syndrome	*Giardia intestinalis, Cryptosporidium, Entamoeba histolytica, Salmonella, Histoplasma capsulatum*
Severe combined immunodeficiency	*Candida; Salmonella* and other bacterial pathogens; cytomegalovirus, rotavirus, Epstein-Barr virus
DiGeorge syndrome	*Candida*
Chronic mucocutaneous candidiasis	*Candida; Histoplasma capsulatum*

TABLE 4–3. Inflammatory Gastrointestinal Lesions in Primary Immunodeficiency

Disease	Manifestation
IgA deficiency	Celiac disease
	Food allergies
	Crohn's disease–like lesion
	Nodular lymphoid hyperplasia
Common variable immunodeficiency	Multifocal atrophic gastritis +/- intestinal metaplasia
	Villous atrophy
	Nodular lymphoid hyperplasia
	Crohn's disease–like lesion
	Granulomatous enteropathy
	Colitis (ulcerative colitis–like; lymphocytic colitis)
X-linked agammaglobulinemia	Crohn's disease–like lesion
	Perianal fistula and perianal abscess
Hyper-IgM syndrome	Nodular lymphoid hyperplasia
	Oral and perianal ulcers
Severe combined immunodeficiency	Graft-versus-host disease–like lesion, small bowel and colon
	Esophageal reflux
Omenn's syndrome	Graft-versus-host disease–like lesion, small bowel and colon
Chronic mucocutaneous candidiasis	Atrophic gastritis
Wiskott-Aldrich syndrome	Crohn's disease–like lesion involving colon
Chronic granulomatous disease	Esophageal and gastric outlet obstruction; Crohn's disease–like lesion in small bowel; colitis (ulcerative colitis–like and Crohn's disease–like)
	Pigmented macrophages

TABLE 4–4. Malignancies Involving the Gastrointestinal Tract in Primary Immunodeficiency

Disease	Gastrointestinal Malignancy
IgA deficiency	Lymphoma
	Gastric adenocarcinoma
Common variable immunodeficiency	Gastric adenocarcinoma
	B-cell lymphoma, involving small bowel
	Colorectal adenocarcinoma, +/- neuroendocrine features
X-linked agammaglobulinemia	Non-Hodgkin's lymphoma
	Gastric adenocarcinoma
	Colorectal adenocarcinoma
Hyper-IgM syndrome	Plasma cell proliferation
	Colorectal adenocarcinoma
Wiskott-Aldrich syndrome	Lymphoma
Ataxia-telangiectasia	Gastric adenocarcinoma

respond to a gluten-free diet may be seen in IgA deficiency, as in CVID. The morphology of celiac disease occurring in the setting of IgA deficiency is similar to that seen in immunocompetent patients. Pernicious anemia complicating chronic atrophic autoimmune gastritis is seen more commonly in IgA deficiency than in CVID. As with other B-cell disorders, the incidence of Crohn's disease and gastric adenocarcinoma appears to be increased in IgA deficiency.[6]

Common Variable Immunodeficiency

Although CVID is not a common disorder, it is probably the most common symptomatic primary immune deficiency. Clinical and immunologic features are heterogeneous, but most patients present with recurrent bacterial infections, usually involving the upper and lower respiratory tracts and leading to chronic lung disease and bronchiectasis. Patients may present with CVID at any age, ranging from infancy to late adult life. Autoimmune manifestations such as thyroid dysfunction, pernicious anemia, autoimmune hemolytic anemia, autoimmune thrombocytopenia, and rheumatoid arthritis are common, and granulomatous involvement of skin and visceral organs mimicking sarcoidosis may be seen.[7] Chronic GI disorders resulting in malabsorption and weight loss occur in about 20% of CVID patients.

CVID is characterized immunologically by hypogammaglobulinemia involving multiple antibody classes. T-cell abnormalities are common; below-normal proliferative responses to mitogens are found in 40% of patients, and 20% have a relative lack of CD4 T cells.[7] The common abnormality shared by IgA deficiency and CVID is failure of terminal maturation of B lymphocytes into plasma cells, which produces various Ig subtypes. A primary B-cell defect is favored in many patients, but in others, defective antigen responsiveness in T-helper cells may be the underlying basis for the disorder.[8]

A genetic basis has long been suspected, based on the observation that familial inheritance of CVID occurs in 20% of cases[9] and that CVID and IgA deficiency tend to occur in the same family; individual family members may gradually switch from one disorder to the other. In multiple-case families, CVID often occurs in parents, with IgA deficiency in the offspring, consistent with the hypothesis that CVID may develop later in life as a more severe manifestation of a common defect involving immunoglobulin class switching. A predisposing locus in the class II or class III major histocompatibility complex (MHC) region has been suggested,[10] although the exact genetic basis has not been identified.

Patients with CVID are at particular risk for chronic inflammatory disorders and malignancies affecting the GI tract. The inflammatory disorders are in some cases a response to acute or chronic infections, but in some

patients, the GI lesions are probably a manifestation of autoimmunity and are associated with other disorders of autoimmunity.[11] In one large clinical study of patients with CVID, 22% had one or more autoimmune diseases, most commonly idiopathic thrombocytopenia purpura (6%) and autoimmune hemolytic anemia (5%).[7]

INFECTIONS IN CVID

Chronic infection with *G. intestinalis* is a common problem in patients with CVID and may or may not cause clinical symptoms. In some cases, malabsorption, steatorrhea, and villous abnormalities can be reversed if *Giardia* organisms are eradicated. Small bowel mucosal abnormalities in giardiasis include villous blunting, increased intraepithelial lymphocytes, and nodular lymphoid hyperplasia. The trophozoite form of the organism can be identified on small bowel biopsy (Fig. 4-1). The prevalence of *Giardia* infections in this population appears to be decreasing, but giardiasis remains a significant cause of chronic diarrhea in CVID.[6]

Other GI infections are less common in CVID. Cryptosporidiosis is occasionally found. The prevalence of common bacterial intestinal infections such as those caused by *Salmonella* species and *Campylobacter* species does not appear to be increased. Although prolonged antibiotic use is common among these patients, an increase in pseudomembranous colitis is not reported.[6] On occasion, viral and fungal organisms infect the GI tract in CVID patients, but such infections are less common in CVID than in acquired immunodeficiency syndrome (AIDS). Cytomegalovirus infection involving the esophagus, stomach, jejunum, and ileocecal area and resulting in multiple ulcers and obstructing strictures has been reported in a patient with CVID.[12]

INFLAMMATORY DISORDERS AND MALIGNANCY IN CVID

Stomach. In some patients with CVID, a nonspecific increase in lamina propria lymphocytes is seen in the

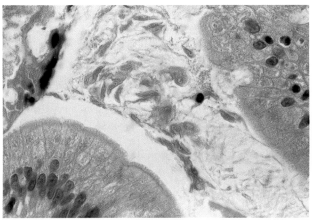

FIGURE 4–1. Giardiasis. Numerous trophozoites in varying orientations are closely associated with the surface of this small-bowel biopsy specimen from a patient with common variable immunodeficiency. The underlying epithelium is normal.

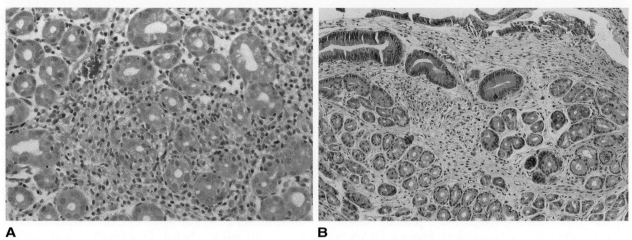

A   **B**

FIGURE 4–2. A, In common variable immunodeficiency, the gastric mucosa often contains a nonspecific mononuclear cell infiltrate. Note the absence of plasma cells. **B,** Loss of gastric glands leads to atrophic gastritis at a young age in patients with CVID. Loss of parietal cells results in pernicious anemia and may occur in the absence of antiparietal cell antibodies.

stomach (Fig. 4-2**A**); increased apoptosis of gastric epithelial cells may be present.[11] In a study of gastric biopsies from 34 patients with CVID and dyspepsia, 41% of patients were infected with *Helicobacter pylori*. All *H. pylori*–positive patients and 20% of *H. pylori*–negative patients had chronic gastritis, and 50% of those infected with *H. pylori* had multifocal atrophic gastritis; 10% of *H. pylori*–negative patients had multifocal atrophic gastritis.[13] Atrophic gastritis resembling autoimmune atrophic gastritis on clinical and morphologic grounds (Fig. 4-2**B**) and resulting in pernicious anemia may occur in the absence of demonstrable anti–parietal cell antibodies in these patients. Atrophic gastritis may develop at a very young age in patients with CVID; it was reported in a 6-year-old who developed multifocal gastric adenocarcinoma at age 11.[14] Adults with CVID are also at increased risk for gastric adenocarcinoma and have a 47-fold increased incidence compared with the general population of Great Britain.[15] Overall, 5% to 10% of CVID patients ultimately develop gastric carcinoma, usually many years after the onset of hypogammaglobulinemia.

Small Bowel. In the small bowel, a spruelike lesion with villous blunting occurs in some patients with CVID and is associated with severe malabsorption, often requiring parenteral nutrition. Villous atrophy associated with CVID generally lacks the degree of crypt hyperplasia seen in celiac disease (Fig. 4-3**A**), but it may be indistinguishable on biopsy. In general, the lamina propria inflammatory infiltrate is not as prominent as in celiac disease, and enterocyte maturation is normal, with preservation of the brush border.[11] Most CVID patients with this small bowel lesion do not respond to a gluten-free diet, although an elemental diet may be beneficial. Plasma cells are absent or are found in only very small numbers in the lamina propria in CVID. Surface intraepithelial lymphocytes are often markedly increased

(Fig. 4-3**B**), even in the absence of villous atrophy. In some cases, an increase in apoptotic bodies is found in crypt epithelial cells (Fig. 4-3**C**).

Granulomatous enteropathy has also been reported in patients with CVID and may be associated with protracted diarrhea unresponsive to antibiotic therapy. Poorly formed non-necrotizing granulomas are found in the lamina propria in multiple sites in the GI tract, including stomach, small intestine, and colon[16]; the diarrhea generally resolves with intravenous immunoglobulin therapy.

Nodular lymphoid hyperplasia (NLH) in the GI tract is characterized by multiple discrete hyperplastic lymphoid nodules in the lamina propria and submucosa of the small intestine (Fig. 4-4), large intestine, or both and is probably a result of chronic antigenic stimulation. The germinal centers of the follicles are composed of proliferating B cells with scattered tingible body macrophages; the mantle zones contain mature and immature B cells; and the extramantle zones contain a mixture of cell types, including B and T cells and macrophages. NLH is found in up to 60% of patients with CVID but may be seen in the setting of giardiasis without antibody deficiency.[17] In contrast to NLH in CVID patients, plasma cells are present in the extramantle zones in non-immunodeficient patients.

NLH is not considered a malignant disorder. However, malignant lymphomas of the GI tract in patients with immunodeficiencies often arise in a background of NLH, and clonal immunoglobulin gene rearrangement has been demonstrated in NLH in the GI tract of a child with CVID.[18] The most common malignancy in CVID is non-Hodgkin's lymphoma, which affects approximately 8% of patients[7]; these lymphomas often originate in extranodal sites, with the small bowel the most common GI site. Most of these lymphomas are of B-cell origin and are classified as diffuse large cell or diffuse mixed small and large cell lymphomas.

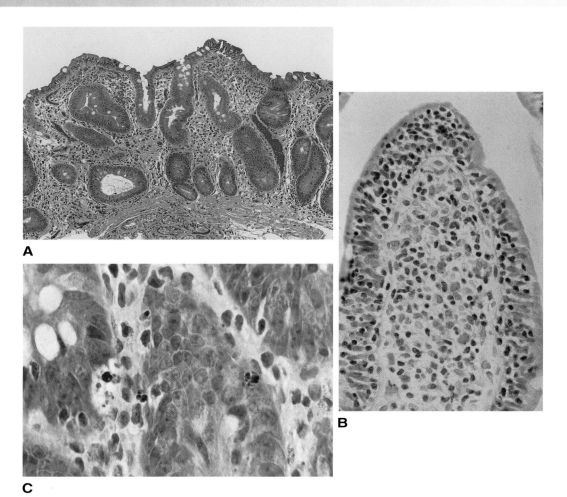

FIGURE 4–3. A, Villous atrophy associated with CVID may be severe and lead to profound malabsorption. Note the relatively sparse inflammatory infiltrate and the lack of crypt hyperplasia. **B,** The surface epithelium of the small intestine often includes a marked increase in the number of intraepithelial lymphocytes in CVID. **C,** An increase in crypt cell apoptosis is often found in small-bowel biopsies with villous atrophy in CVID.

Some patients with CVID develop chronic inflammatory processes involving small or large bowel, clinically similar to inflammatory bowel disease. In the small bowel, the lesions closely resemble Crohn's disease, with transmural inflammation and small bowel obstruction. Granulomas are generally not present in these Crohn's-like disorders.[19]

Large Bowel. The colitis occurring in CVID is variable in morphology. In some patients, the inflammatory process is limited to the colon and clinically mimics ulcerative colitis. Mucosal architectural distortion with crypt destruction is present, although crypt distortion is less pronounced than in most cases of ulcerative colitis, with less crypt branching (Fig. 4-5). Neutrophils are present in the lamina propria and crypt epithelium. In contrast to ulcerative colitis, plasma cells are not present in the lamina propria in CVID-associated colitis. In some cases, the crypt destruction and mucosal distortion are accompanied by increased apoptosis, and the histology is similar to that of colonic graft-versus-host disease.[11] Milder cases of colitis in CVID may resemble lymphocytic colitis, which is characterized by increased intraepithelial lymphocytes and minimal mucosal distortion.[20] The cause and pathogenesis of colitis in these patients remain largely unknown. The association of chronic GI inflammatory and autoimmune disorders in these patients and the resemblance of the lesions to other disorders of immune dysregulation imply that the colitis of CVID may be autoimmune in origin.

Adenocarcinoma of the colon is reported in young patients with CVID. Small cell neuroendocrine carcinoma of the cecum has been reported in a 16-year-old boy, who died of liver metastases 5 months after diagnosis.[21] In another case, nine adenocarcinomas and 20 adenomas were present synchronously in the colon of a 22-year-old man with CVID.[22]

X-Linked Agammaglobulinemia

The typical patient with X-linked agammaglobulinemia (XLAG) is susceptible to bacterial infections resulting from absence of all circulating immunoglobulin subtypes; mature circulating B cells are low to absent. This disorder is characterized by inability to make antibodies

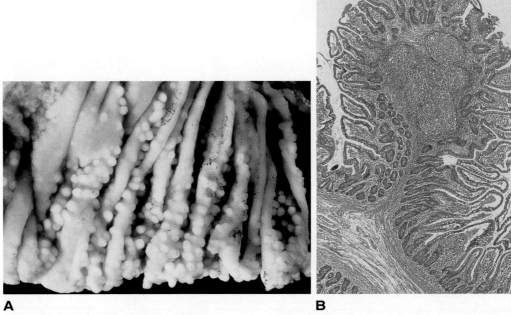

FIGURE 4-4. A, Nodular lymphoid hyperplasia in CVID. Numerous small mucosal and submucosal nodules are present. **B,** Most of the lymphoid nodules contain enlarged germinal centers. Overlying villi are slightly distorted.

to virtually all antigens. The molecular basis of most cases of XLAG was elucidated in 1993, when a defect in the *Btk* (Bruton's tyrosine kinase) gene was found.[23,24] This gene encodes a nonreceptor tyrosine kinase expressed in B-cell and myelomonocytic cell lineages but not in T cells. *Btk* functions in intracellular signaling pathways essential for pre–B-cell maturation, but the exact mechanism by which the defects in *Btk* lead to B-cell maturation arrest remains unclear. XLAG may have greater phenotypic diversity than has previously been recognized; recently, adults with mild or no clinical symptoms but with deficiencies in *Btk* have been described.[25]

GI manifestations are less common in XLAG than in CVID. Age of onset of GI symptoms is younger than in CVID patients, and autoimmune diseases are less common. Small intestinal and colonic mucosal biopsies in the XLAG patient without GI symptoms are notable only for the lack of plasma cells in the lamina propria, resulting in an empty appearance. Mucosal architecture is unremarkable, and villous blunting is not seen. About one third of patients present initially with GI complaints, most commonly diarrhea or perirectal abscess, and in one study, 10% had chronic GI symptoms from persistent infection with *G. intestinalis*, *Salmonella* species, or enteropathic *Escherichia coli*, or secondary to bacterial overgrowth. No cause for chronic diarrhea was found in half of these patients.[26] Chronic infection with rotavirus is also reported in this population.[27] Because biopsies are not routinely performed for chronic rotavirus infection, few descriptions of histopathologic findings are available, but moderate blunting of duodenal villi

with crypt hyperplasia and an increase in lamina propria inflammatory cells are reported in acute infections.[28] Degenerative changes may be noted in epithelial cells on the surface of the villus, but crypt cells are spared and the crypt zone undergoes a compensatory hyperplasia. The histologic changes of acute rotavirus infection are reported to resemble celiac disease but are patchier and quickly revert to normal with resolution of infection.[29]

In addition to GI infections, patients with XLAG may develop a chronic ulcerating inflammatory condition clinically similar to Crohn's disease, manifested by recurrent diarrhea, malabsorption, ulcers, and small bowel strictures (Fig. 4-6). A prominent lymphocytic inflammatory infiltrate without plasma cells or granulomas is seen in the affected areas.[11,30] In one case, enterovirus

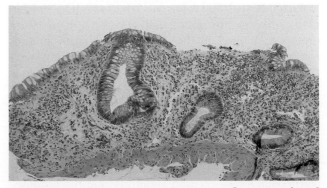

FIGURE 4-5. Colitis in CVID may mimic inflammatory bowel disease, with crypt distortion and loss. The inflammatory infiltrate is relatively sparse, compared with ulcerative colitis, and plasma cells are not present.

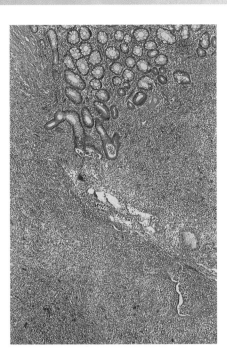

FIGURE 4–6. A chronic inflammatory disorder with fissuring necrosis and small-intestinal ulcers resembling Crohn's disease occurs in some patients with X-linked agammaglobulinemia. Granulomas are typically absent.

was found by polymerase chain reaction (PCR) in inflamed ileum and adjacent mesenteric lymph nodes, suggesting that in some XLAG patients, infection may be responsible for these lesions.[31]

Patients with XLAG are at increased risk for malignancy, even in childhood. The most common malignancy in this group is non-Hodgkin's lymphoma, often involving the GI tract; many of these cases occur in children younger than 10 years of age.[32] Cases of gastric[32] and colorectal adenocarcinoma have been reported rarely.[2] The incidence of colorectal carcinoma for patients with XLAG is calculated as 30-fold, and the mortality as 59-fold, greater than that in the normal European population.[2] In most reported cases, XLAG patients with colorectal carcinoma are young adults in their 20s who present with advanced-stage tumors. In one reported case, both multiple colorectal adenomas and carcinoma were found.[2]

X-Linked Hyper-IgM Syndrome

This syndrome is due to a mutation in the gene for CD40 ligand, resulting in loss of isotype switching. T cells from patients with this disorder lack the CD40 ligand and thus do not interact with CD40 on the B-cell surface, an event necessary for immunoglobulin class switching. These patients have very low levels of IgG and IgA and have normal or elevated IgM levels. They are susceptible to pyogenic infections similar to those encountered in XLAG, as well as to *Pneumocystis carinii* pneumonia. A variety of intracellular pathogens such as

various mycobacterial species, fungi, and viruses (e.g., cytomegalovirus, adenovirus) are implicated in causing disease in these patients. The most common sites of infection are the upper (~88%) and lower respiratory tract (~83%).[33] Disseminated infection[34] and esophageal infection[35] with *Histoplasma capsulatum* may also occur.

Diarrhea occurs in more than half of patients and follows a chronic course in most.[33] Chronic watery diarrhea may be due to *Cryptosporidium* infection; *G. intestinalis*, *Salmonella* species, and *Entamoeba histolytica* have also been implicated. Nodular lymphoid hyperplasia involving the GI tract is reported in approximately 5% of patients.[33] Lymphoid hyperplasia may also result in hepatosplenomegaly, lymphadenopathy, and enlargement of the tonsils.[36] Sclerosing cholangitis is a common (~20% of European patients) and serious complication, often related to chronic infection with *Cryptosporidium*, and may require liver transplantation.[33]

Patients with this disorder are prone to autoimmune hematologic diseases, including cyclic or chronic neutropenia; oral and perianal ulcers are common during neutropenic episodes.[33] Massive proliferation of IgM-producing plasma cells may involve the GI tract, liver, and gallbladder, usually in the second decade of life, and may prove fatal.[37] Small cell carcinoma of the colon has been reported in this disorder,[38] and an increased incidence of liver and biliary tract tumors occurs.[39]

Hyperimmunoglobulin E Syndrome (Job's Syndrome)

This is a rare autosomal dominant multisystem disorder characterized by recurrent staphylococcal skin abscesses, recurrent pneumonia with pneumatocele, elevated serum IgE, eczema, candidiasis, and eosinophilia.[40] The exact genetic defect has not been elucidated, but the disease locus has been mapped to chromosome 4.[41] In addition to findings related to the immune system, characteristic facial features and dental and skeletal abnormalities have been reported in a cohort of 30 patients followed for long periods.[40] GI manifestations appear limited to mucocutaneous candidiasis and tissue-invasive fungal infections with *Cryptococcus* species, reported in the esophagus[42] and colon,[43] and ileocecal histoplasmosis mimicking Crohn's disease.[44] Perforation of the colon, probably related to infection with staphylococcal species, has also been reported.[45] These patients do not appear to be at increased risk for GI malignancy.

COMBINED CELLULAR/HUMORAL IMMUNODEFICIENCIES

Severe Combined Immunodeficiency

Severe combined immunodeficiency (SCID) is a heterogeneous group of congenital disorders characterized by defects in both B- and T-cell function. Children with SCID typically present in the first year of life with severe recurrent bacterial or viral infection. A number of molecular defects may result in SCID. Most are autosomal recessive; these include adenosine deaminase deficiency, accounting for 50% of autosomal recessive SCID; purine nucleoside deficiency; T-cell receptor deficiencies; Zap70 deficiency; JAK3 deficiency; and IL-7 receptor deficiency.[46] X-linked SCID resulting from a defect in the common γ chain is the single most common type of SCID, however.[47] This type of SCID has a characteristic phenotype of absence of T and natural killer (NK) cells but normal B-cell numbers, although the latter cells are dysfunctional.[46]

GI disorders in SCID may be due to a variety of infectious pathogens. Oral, esophageal, and perianal forms of candidiasis are common, and children with SCID may develop profound diarrhea early in life. In general, GI biopsies from these patients show a hypocellular lamina propria without plasma cells or lymphocytes. Because these patients are susceptible to viral infection, examination of stool for viral particles may be indicated. In particular, rotavirus, normally a self-limited infection, may cause chronic diarrhea in these children. Although villous blunting has been described in acute rotavirus infection in normal children[28] and in animal models,[48] the intestinal pathology of chronic rotavirus infection in SCID patients has not been described. Cytopathic viral infections that may be

identified on GI biopsy include cytomegalovirus and adenovirus (Fig. 4-7). *Salmonella* organisms may also cause chronic GI infection in SCID patients. SCID patients receiving nonirradiated blood products and those receiving allogeneic bone marrow transplants are susceptible to graft-versus-host disease (GVHD), although a GVHD-like process affecting the colon and small intestine may occur in those who have not undergone bone marrow transplantation.[49,50] Children with SCID may be at greater risk than the normal population for reflux esophagitis.[51]

Omenn's Syndrome

This syndrome is an autosomal recessive SCID with clinical and pathologic features of GVHD. The immunologic hallmark of the disease is expansion of an oligoclonal population of T cells.[52] Infants with Omenn's syndrome present with diffuse erythroderma, hepatosplenomegaly, and failure to thrive; chronic diarrhea and alopecia are common. Hypereosinophilia and hypogammaglobulinemia are characteristic. Paradoxically, serum IgE levels are increased, although B lymphocytes are not detectable in the circulation, lymph nodes, or skin. Activated circulating T cells are normal to increased in number but constitute an oligoclonal population.

The underlying basis is the impairment but not complete loss of the V(D)J recombination process as a result of mutations in *Rag-1* or *Rag-2*, the recombination-

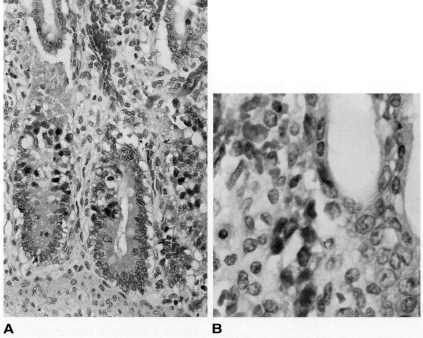

A **B**

FIGURE 4–7. A, Disseminated adenovirus may involve the gastrointestinal tract in patients with SCID. Here, the small bowel crypts are involved; in less severe cases, inclusions may be identified only in surface mucosa. **B,** With adenovirus, infected cells are typically not enlarged. Classic "smudge cells" with homogeneous nuclear staining are shown here.

activation genes.[53] Mutations in these genes were first identified in a subset of SCID patients, those with T-B-SCID; the occurrence of this type of SCID and Omenn's syndrome in the same kindred furnished the clue that Omenn's syndrome was caused by mutations in the same genes. Differences between T-B-SCID and Omenn's syndrome can be explained by the presence of two entirely defective alleles in SCID, as well as the presence of one marginally functional allele that is capable of establishing the oligoclonal T-cell population in Omenn's syndrome patients.[53] Infants with SCID with maternal T-cell engraftment may exhibit GVHD symptoms indistinguishable on clinical grounds from Omenn's syndrome,[54] and a diagnosis of Omenn's syndrome depends on excluding this possibility by appropriate human leukocyte antigen (HLA) typing or molecular analysis. Published accounts of the histopathologic changes in Omenn's syndrome are scant, but skin changes resemble those of GVHD,[55] and numerous apoptotic crypt cells are found in colonic biopsies in a pattern similar to that seen in GVHD. Crypt injury and an increase in lamina propria eosinophils may also be seen (Fig. 4-8).

OTHER PRIMARY IMMUNODEFICIENCIES

DiGeorge Syndrome

This syndrome is due to a congenital malformation of the third and fourth pharyngeal pouches, resulting in thymic and parathyroid hypoplasia. T cells are markedly reduced in number, but B cells are normal in number and functionality. Midline anomalies affecting the GI tract such as esophageal atresia and imperforate anus are seen in some cases; watery diarrhea and malabsorption have been described but are not well characterized.[56] Oral candidiasis is common.

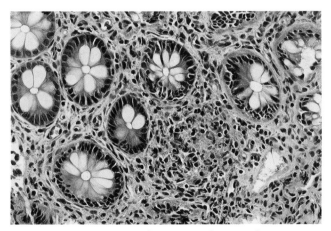

FIGURE 4–8. Omenn's syndrome. Focal crypt destruction is noted, with a localized increase in lamina propria eosinophils.

Chronic Mucocutaneous Candidiasis

This is a heterogeneous group of disorders characterized by persistent *Candida* infection of the skin, nails, and mucous membranes. Autoimmune disorders and a polyglandular endocrinopathy syndrome, including pernicious anemia, occur in more than 50% of patients. Immune defects include disorders of T-cell immunity with variable B-cell involvement. The most common GI manifestation is esophageal candidiasis. Although superficial infection with *Candida* is a defining characteristic, infections with other fungi (such as *H. capsulatum*) and bacteria are common.[57]

Wiskott-Aldrich Syndrome

This syndrome is characterized by early onset of profound thrombocytopenia with small platelets, eczema, and recurrent infections; it is inherited as an X-linked recessive disease. Platelets and T cells are most severely affected. The genetic basis of Wiskott-Aldrich syndrome is mutation of the *WASP* gene, which encodes an intracellular protein expressed exclusively in hematopoietic cells.[58] This protein is involved in transduction of signals from cell surface receptors to the actin cytoskeleton[59] and is important in cytoskeletal architecture and cell trafficking and motility.[60] Diarrhea reported in this disorder has been poorly characterized. Bloody diarrhea may occur and is often attributed to thrombocytopenia[56]; biopsies may not be performed because of the risk of hemorrhage. A Crohn's disease–like inflammatory process with a cobblestone appearance and inflammatory pseudopolyps involving the descending and transverse colon have been reported.[61] Massive hemorrhage from aneurysms involving the liver, small bowel mesentery, and kidney may also occur.[62]

Chronic Granulomatous Disease

Chronic granulomatous disease (CGD) is characterized by phagocytic cells that are unable to reduce molecular oxygen to create the superoxide anion and its metabolites necessary for eradication of certain catalase-positive intracellular microbes. CGD is genetically heterogeneous, resulting from a mutation in any of four components of NADPH oxidase. The most common form of the disease, accounting for 70% of cases, is X-linked recessive; three other forms are autosomal recessive.[63]

As a result of this defect, patients with CGD develop recurrent bacterial and fungal infections; abscesses in a variety of sites and pneumonia are common. Patients are also prone to develop inflammatory and rheumatic diseases, such as an inflammatory bowel disease–like condition and a lupus-like syndrome. GI manifestations are relatively rare in CGD but can be broadly grouped into obstructive and inflammatory categories.

In CGD, obstruction can occur at a number of levels of the GI tract, from esophagus to small bowel. Gastric outlet obstruction is more common in the X-linked form of the disease.[63] In some cases, the obstruction is due to infiltration of the viscus wall by pigment-laden macrophages (the histologic hallmark of CGD) or to granulomatous inflammation. In other cases, the obstruction is reportedly secondary to a functional disturbance in motility. Esophageal obstruction occurs in 1% of CGD patients[63]; biopsies of the esophageal mucosa generally show nonspecific findings or reflux esophagitis,[64] but they may demonstrate pigmented macrophages. Involvement of the gastric antrum and pylorus is somewhat more common, occurring in 16%, and gastric outlet obstruction may be the first manifestation of CGD. Granulomas, giant cells, and macrophages laden with brown-yellow fine pigment are commonly present in gastric biopsies,[65] but in some cases, only nonspecific inflammation is seen.[66] Small bowel obstruction is relatively rare in CGD but is occasionally reported in the context of an inflammatory process.[67]

In a review of small bowel and rectal biopsies from nine patients with CGD, pigment-laden macrophages were found in the lamina propria at both sites. In the small bowel, the macrophages were located deep in the mucosa adjacent to crypts, but when numerous, they also extended up into the villous core (Fig. 4-9). In rectal biopsies, the number of pigmented histiocytes was quite variable, ranging from rare scattered cells to large numbers of histiocytes accumulating between the bases of the crypts and the muscularis mucosae. Granu-

lomas with giant cells were also present in rectal biopsies from some patients. In one of eight cases, distortion of crypt architecture without crypt abscesses was seen.[68]

Chronic inflammatory processes that are indistinguishable from inflammatory bowel disease affecting the small and large bowel may occur in CGD patients[69]; as with obstructive lesions of the GI tract, these lesions are more common in the X-linked form of the disease.[63] Polymorphisms in genes unrelated to NADPH oxidase may modify the clinical phenotype in CGD; certain polymorphisms in the genes for myeloperoxidase and Fcγ receptors are strongly associated with GI complications.[70] Involvement of the small bowel may produce fistulas, longitudinal ulcers, stenosis, and non-necrotizing granulomatous inflammation that are mistaken for Crohn's disease.[71,72] The granulomas seen in intestinal lesions in CGD are often more florid than those usually seen in Crohn's disease,[71] but granulomas are not present in all cases.

In a study of colitis in one CGD patient, the presence of an acute and chronic inflammatory infiltrate confined to the colonic mucosa, the occurrence of crypt abscesses, and the lack of granulomas were more suggestive of ulcerative colitis than Crohn's disease. Mucosal architectural distortion and ulceration were not as prominent as those usually seen in ulcerative colitis, however, and pigmented macrophages were present in the lamina propria.[69]

Other rare disorders of immunity occasionally associated with GI manifestations include leukocyte adhesion deficiency, in which the resulting delayed wound healing and susceptibility to bacterial and fungal infection lead to necrotizing enterocolitis.[73] A chronic inflammatory process with multiple aphthous ulcers involving the gastric antrum, terminal ileum, cecum, and right colon, which resolved with bone marrow transplantation, has also been reported in leukocyte adhesion deficiency.[74] Ataxia-telangiectasia, a chromosomal breakage syndrome, is associated with increased risk of gastric adenocarcinoma; bare lymphocyte syndrome (MHC deficiency) is associated with oral candidiasis and persistent viral infection of the GI tract.

Graft-Versus-Host Disease

Although defined in terms of time of onset following transplantation, acute and chronic forms of GVHD appear to be separate pathogenetic and clinical entities, in that they have different patterns of injury and affect different organ systems.

ACUTE GVHD

Acute GVHD involving the GI tract develops in up to 50% of allogeneic bone marrow transplant recipients[75];

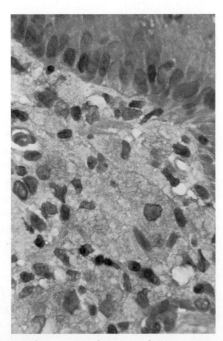

FIGURE 4–9. Chronic granulomatous disease. Accumulation of pigmented macrophages contains light brown dusky material in the small-intestinal mucosa.

skin and liver are also commonly involved. Indeed, the most common cause of persistent nausea and anorexia in patients beyond day 20 after transplant is acute GVHD.[76] Changes identical to those seen in GVHD following allogeneic transplantation may be seen in the GI tract and liver following autologous stem cell transplantation and are considered to be a form of GVHD resulting from a lack of regulation of immune mechanisms by the reconstituting immune system.[77] This syndrome of acute GVHD-like changes in the GI tract following autologous transplantation is rare, occurring in gastric biopsies in only 4% of patients with upper GI symptoms.[78] Rarely, acute GVHD occurs following solid organ transplantation or blood transfusion. Symptoms include profuse diarrhea, crampy abdominal pain, GI hemorrhage, anorexia, nausea and vomiting, and rarely, peritonitis.[75] Involvement of the upper GI tract is slightly more common than that of the large bowel, although simultaneous involvement of both the upper and lower GI tract is common.[79]

On endoscopic examination, the appearance of the mucosa in acute GVHD is variable, ranging from mucosal edema and erythema to more severe changes such as ulcers and mucosal sloughing.[80] The major histologic features of GVHD in the GI tract are epithelial cell apoptosis and a relatively sparse mononuclear inflammatory cell infiltrate (Fig. 4-10**A**). Apoptotic epithelial cells are found primarily in the regenerative compartment of the mucosa, including small intestine and colonic crypts, and the neck area of gastric glands. In the colon, the apoptotic cells are particularly conspicuous and are called *exploding crypt cells;* these cells contain intracytoplasmic vacuoles filled with karyorrhectic nuclear debris (Fig. 4-10**B**).[81] Apoptotic cells are smaller and less conspicuous in the gastric mucosa (Fig. 4-11**A**). In more severe cases of acute GVHD, crypt abscesses as well as crypt dropout may be seen. In the most severe cases, mucosal sloughing and extensive ulceration occur. In the stomach, granular eosinophilic necrotic cellular debris without neutrophils may be present in the lumina of injured gastric glands (Fig. 4-11**B**).[82] Villous blunting is commonly seen in small bowel GVHD. A grading system for acute GVHD affecting the colon has been proposed (Table 4-5)[81]; however, correlation with clinical symptoms and patient outcome is weak.

The changes occurring in the GI tract in acute GVHD are not entirely specific; similar changes are reported in colonic biopsies from patients with severe T-cell deficiencies,[50] malignant thymoma,[83] and common variable immunodeficiency.[11] In the bone marrow transplantation patient, the effects of cytoreductive therapy may resemble the changes of GI GVHD in the early post-transplant period; thus, a diagnosis of GVHD must be made with caution prior to 21 days after transplantation. Recurrence of hematologic malignancies, particularly acute lymphoblastic leukemia, may also mimic acute GVHD.[84] Cytomegalovirus infection may produce mucosal damage characterized by apoptotic epithelial cells, mimicking GVHD[85]; differentiation from GVHD relies on the demonstration of viral inclusions.[86] Furthermore, because GVHD and cytomegalovirus infection may occur simultaneously, it may be difficult to separate the effects of each process on the GI tract. Infection with *Clostridium difficile* has also been reported to be associated with GI GVHD and a high nonrelapse mortality in this group; it is postulated that *C. difficile* toxin may predispose to increased severity of GVHD.[87]

CHRONIC GVHD

The GI tract is less often involved in chronic GVHD, defined as GVHD occurring more than 100 days after

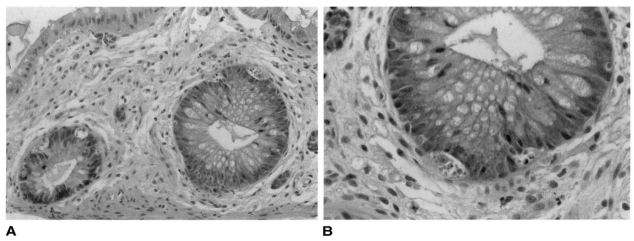

A   **B**

FIGURE 4–10. Acute graft-versus-host disease involving the colon. **A,** The lamina propria inflammatory infiltrate is relatively sparse; no crypt loss is seen in this example, although crypts are slightly distorted and rare apoptotic cells are present. **B,** Large apoptotic bodies known as "exploding crypt cells" are typical of colonic GVHD.

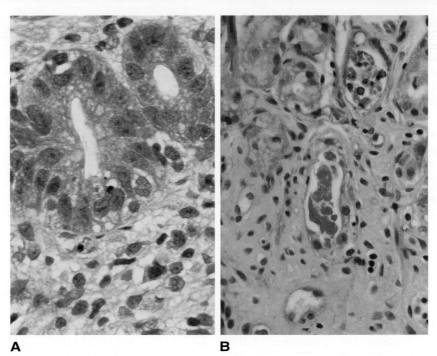

A   **B**

FIGURE 4–11. A, In the stomach, apoptotic bodies in glandular epithelium are small and inconspicuous in acute graft-versus-host disease. **B,** In the gastric fundus, dilated glands containing granular eosinophilic debris are sometimes found in GVHD. As in the colon, the inflammatory infiltrate is relatively sparse.

transplantation. Chronic GVHD is clinically similar in many ways to some of the collagen vascular diseases and has been compared with autoimmune disorders such as scleroderma, Sjögren's syndrome, and primary biliary cirrhosis.[88] Chronic GVHD involves multiple organs, such as salivary gland, mouth, eye, and upper respiratory tract, that are not involved by acute GVHD.

In chronic GVHD, skin changes of dermal fibrosis may resemble scleroderma, and involvement of the oral squamous mucosa leads to painful ulcers and submucosal fibrosis. Involvement of minor salivary glands results in an oral sicca syndrome. In advanced cases, ulcers and submucosal fibrosis occur in the esophagus, the most commonly affected site in the GI tract.[89] Small bowel involvement is less common, and when present it is associated with diarrhea. Focal fibrosis of the lamina propria and segmental submucosal fibrosis, with minimal mucosal changes, have been reported.[89] Mild to moderate crypt distortion in colonic mucosa similar to that seen in

ulcerative colitis has also been reported in allogeneic bone marrow transplant patients, but it is unclear if the mucosal architectural distortion is due to chronic GVHD or other factors.[90]

Neutropenic Enterocolitis

Neutropenic enterocolitis (NEC) is a necrotizing inflammatory process predominantly affecting the cecum, terminal ileum, and ascending colon and occurring most commonly in the setting of neutropenia. Hemorrhagic necrosis of the cecum in this setting has also been called *typhlitis*. Absolute neutrophil counts of less than 1500/mm^3 are typically seen. Historically, most patients with NEC have had acute leukemia, although NEC is now seen in patients undergoing stem cell or autologous bone marrow transplantation for solid malignancies.[91,92] NEC also occurs in patients with aplastic anemia, in renal transplant patients, and in those with other hematologic malignancies. Most patients have received chemotherapy over the previous 30 days.[93] Patients may present with clinical features suggestive of acute appendicitis, such as fever and right lower quadrant pain; one third present with GI hemorrhage,[93] and rarely, a palpable right lower quadrant mass is present. The combination of abdominal pain, diarrhea, and fever is the most common presentation.[92]

TABLE 4–5. Grading of Acute Graft-Versus-Host Disease of the Colon[81]

Grade	Histologic Features
I	Rare apoptotic cells, without crypt loss
II	Loss of individual crypts
III	Loss of two or more contiguous crypts
IV	No identifiable crypts (mucosal ulceration)

On gross examination, the cecum and other affected portions of the GI tract are dilated, edematous, and congested or hemorrhagic. Pneumatosis intestinalis may be seen but is relatively rare. The mucosa is hemorrhagic and is covered with granular necrotic material; no significant inflammatory reaction is present. The pathogenesis of this disorder is initiated with mucosal injury, primarily related to recent administration of chemotherapeutic agents and augmented by neutropenia. Bacterial invasion of the injured mucosa then occurs, with *Clostridium* species implicated as major offenders; fungi such as *Candida* species have also been implicated as causative or contributing agents. Toxins produced by organisms invading the gut wall lead to edema and necrosis. Distention of the bowel wall leads to decreased blood flow, adding an element of ischemic injury. Most patients become septicemic. If untreated, the prognosis is grave, but patients may survive with optimal medical and surgical management; recovery is dependent on the restoration of adequate neutrophil counts.

◾ The GI Tract in HIV Infection

GI illnesses are common in human immunodeficiency virus (HIV)–infected patients, with diarrhea, nausea, vomiting, anorexia, and abdominal pain as presenting symptoms. Prior to the use of new highly effective antiretroviral agents, opportunistic infections with such pathogens as *Isospora, Mycobacterium avium-intracellulare* complex, microsporidia, and *Cryptosporidium* were frequent causes of diarrhea, malabsorption, and wasting. Although the prevalence of intestinal pathogens has decreased in the past decade, from a reported 85% in men with AIDS and diarrhea, to 12% found almost exclusively in homosexual men,[94] current studies continue to show a high prevalence of gastrointestinal dysfunction in HIV-infected patients. Chronic diarrhea is reported in approximately 25% of HIV patients and was not associated with degree of immune suppression in one cohort.[94]

GI dysfunction, as manifested by D-xylose malabsorption, is common, even in early HIV disease, and may be a manifestation of HIV enteropathy, defined as a reduction in small bowel villous surface area associated with chronic diarrhea in the absence of enteric pathogens. In small bowel biopsies, HIV enteropathy is characterized by relatively mild villous blunting without well-developed crypt hyperplasia.[95] The degree of villous atrophy is typically less than that seen in celiac disease. Medications should also be considered as an etiology for diarrhea in these patients and may account for up to 45% of noninfectious cases;[96] commonly implicated medications are nelfinavir, ritonavir, saquinavir, indinavir, and didanosine.

References

1. Filipovich AH, Mathur A, Kersey JH, et al: Lymphoproliferative disorders and other tumors complicating immunodeficiencies. Immunodeficiency 5:91-112, 1994.
2. van der Meer JW, Weening RS, Schellekens PT, et al: Colorectal cancer in patients with X-linked agammaglobulinaemia. Lancet 341:1439-1440, 1993.
3. Burrows PD, Cooper MD: IgA deficiency. Adv Immunol 65:245-276, 1997.
4. Leung VK, Liew CT, Sung JJ: Strongyloidiasis in a patient with IgA deficiency. Trop Gastroenterol 16:27-30, 1995.
5. Meini A, Pillan NM, Villanacci V, et al: Prevalence and diagnosis of celiac disease in IgA deficient children. Ann Allergy Asthma Immunol 7:333-336, 1996.
6. So ALP, Mayer L: Gastrointestinal manifestations of primary immunodeficiency disorders. Semin Gastrointest Dis 8:22-32, 1997.
7. Cunningham-Rundles C, Bodian C: Common variable immunodeficiency: Clinical and immunological features of 248 patients. Clin Immunol 92:34-48, 1999.
8. Conley ME, Cooper MD: Genetic basis of abnormal B cell development. Curr Opin Immunol 10:399-406, 1998.
9. Hammarstrom L, Vorechovsky I, Webster D: Selective IgA deficiency (SIgAD) and common variable immunodeficiency (CVID). Clin Exp Immunol 120:225-231, 2000.
10. Vorechovsky I, Webster ADB, Plebani A, et al: Genetic linkage of IgA deficiency to the major histocompatibility complex: Evidence for allele segregation distortion, parent-of-origin penetrance differences and the role of anti-IgA antibodies in disease predisposition. Am J Hum Genet 64:1096-1109, 1999.
11. Washington K, Stenzel TT, Buckley RH, et al: Gastrointestinal pathology in patients with common variable immunodeficiency and X-linked agammaglobulinemia. Am J Surg Pathol 20:1240-1252, 1996.
12. Tahan V, Dobrucali A, Canbakan B, et al: Cytomegalovirus infection of the gastrointestinal tract with multiple ulcers and strictures, causing obstruction in a patient with common variable immunodeficiency syndrome. Dig Dis Sci 45:1781-1785, 2000.
13. Zullo A, Romiti A, Rinaldi V, et al: Gastric pathology in patients with common variable immunodeficiency. Gut 45:77-81, 1999.
14. Conley ME, Ziegler MM, Borden St, et al: Multifocal adenocarcinoma of the stomach in a child with common variable immunodeficiency. J Pediatr Gastroenterol Nutr 7:456-460, 1988.
15. Cunningham-Rundles C, Siegal FP, Cunningham-Rundles S, et al: Incidence of cancer in 98 patients with common varied immunodeficiency. J Clin Immunol 7:294-299, 1987.
16. Mike N, Hansel TT, Newman J, et al: Granulomatous enteropathy in common variable immunodeficiency: A cause of chronic diarrhoea. Postgrad Med J 67:446-449, 1991.
17. Ward H, Jalan KN, Maitra TK, et al: Small intestinal nodular lymphoid hyperplasia in patients with giardiasis and normal serum immunoglobulins. Gut 24:120-126, 1983.
18. Laszewski MJ, Kemp JD, Goeken JA, et al: Clonal immunoglobulin gene rearrangement in nodular lymphoid hyperplasia of the gastrointestinal tract associated with common variable immunodeficiency. Am J Clin Pathol 94:338-343, 1990.
19. Hermaszewski RA, Webster AD: Primary hypogammaglobulinaemia: A survey of clinical manifestations and complications. Q J Med 86:31-42, 1993.
20. Teahon K, Webster AD, Price AB, et al: Studies on the enteropathy associated with primary hypogammaglobulinemia. Gut 35:1244-1249, 1994.
21. de Bruin NC, de Groot R, den Hollander JC, et al: Small-cell undifferentiated (neuroendocrine) carcinoma of the cecum in a child with common variable immunodeficiency. Am J Pediatr Hematol Oncol 15:258-261, 1993.
22. Adachi Y, Mori M, Kido A, et al: Multiple colorectal neoplasms in a young adult with hypogammaglobulinemia. Report of a case. Dis Colon Rectum 35:197-200, 1992.
23. Tsukada S, Saffran DC, Rawlings DJ, et al: Deficient expression of a B cell cytoplasmic tyrosine kinase in human X-linked agammaglobulinemia. Cell 72:279-290, 1993.
24. Vetrie D, Vorechovsky I, Sideras P, et al: The gene involved in X linked agammaglobulinemia is a member of the src family of protein kinases. Nature 361:226-233, 1993.

25. Hashimoto S, Miyawaki T, Futatani T, et al: Atypical X-linked agammaglobulinemia diagnosed in three adults. Intern Med 38:722-725, 1999.

26. Lederman HM, Winkelstein JA: X-linked agammaglobulinemia: An analysis of 96 patients. Medicine 64:145-156, 1985.

27. Saulsbury FT, Winkelstein JA, Yolken RH: Chronic rotavirus infection in immunodeficiency. J Pediatr 97:61-65, 1980.

28. Davidson GP, Barnes GL: Structural and functional abnormalities of the small intestine in infants and young children with rotavirus enteritis. Acta Paediatr Scand 68:181-186, 1979.

29. Moon HM: Comparative histology of intestinal infections. Adv Exp Med Biol 412:1-19, 1997.

30. Abramowsky CR, Sorensen RU: Regional enteritis-like enteropathy in a patient with agammaglobulinemia: Histologic and immunocytologic studies. Hum Pathol 19:483-486, 1988.

31. Cellier C, Foray S, Hermine O: Regional enteritis associated with enterovirus in a patient with X-linked agammaglobulinemia. N Engl J Med 342:21-22, 2000.

32. Lavillia P, Gil A, Rodriguez MCG, et al: X-linked agammaglobulinemia and gastric adenocarcinoma. Cancer 72:1528-1531, 1993.

33. Levy J, Espanol-Boren T, Thomas C, et al: Clinical spectrum of X-linked hyper-IgM syndrome. J Pediatr 131:47-54, 1997.

34. Hostoffer RW, Berger M, Clark HT, et al: Disseminated *Histoplasma capsulatum* in a patient with hyper IgM immunodeficiency. Pediatrics 94:234-236, 1994.

35. Tu RK, Peters ME, Gourley GR, et al: Esophageal histoplasmosis in a child with immunodeficiency with hyper-IgM. Am J Roentgenol 157:381-382, 1991.

36. Ramesh N, Seki M, Notarangelo LD, et al: The hyper-IgM (HIM) syndrome. Springer Semin Immunopathol 19:383-399, 1998.

37. Rosen FS, Cooper MD, Wedgwood RJ: The primary immunodeficiencies. N Engl J Med 333:431-440, 1995.

38. Hayward AR, Levy J, Facchetti F, et al: Cholangiopathy and tumors of the pancreas, liver, and biliary tree in boys with X-linked immunodeficiency with hyper IgM (X-HIM). J Immunol 158:977, 1997.

39. Zirkin HJ, Levy J, Katchko L: Small cell undifferentiated carcinoma of the colon associated with hepatocellular carcinoma in an immunodeficient patient. Hum Pathol 27:992-996, 1996.

40. Grimbacher B, Holland SJ, Gallin JI, et al: Hyper-IgE syndrome with recurrent infections—an autosomal dominant multisystem disorder. N Engl J Med 340:692-702, 1999.

41. Grimbacher B, Schaffer AA, Holland SM, et al: Genetic linkage of hyper-IgE syndrome to chromosome 4. Am J Hum Genet 65:735-744, 1999.

42. Jacobs DH, Macher AM, Handler R, et al: Esophageal cryptococcosis in a patient with the hyperimmunoglobulin E-recurrent infection (Job's) syndrome. Gastroenterology 87:201-203, 1984.

43. Hutto JO, Bryan CS, Greene FL, et al: Cryptococcosis of the colon resembling Crohn's disease in a patient with the hyperimmunoglobulinemia E-recurrent infection (Job's) syndrome. Gastroenterology 94:808-812, 1988.

44. Alberti-Flor JJ, Granda A: Ileocecal histoplasmosis mimicking Crohn's disease in a patient with Job's syndrome. Digestion 33:176-180, 1986.

45. Hwang EH, Oh J-T, Han SJ, et al: Colon perforation in hyperimmunoglobulin E syndrome. J Pediatr Surg 33:1420-1422, 1998.

46. Jones AM, Gaspar HB: Immunogenetics: Changing the face of immunodeficiency. J Clin Pathol 53:60-65, 2000.

47. Noguchi M, Rosenblatt HM, Filipovich AH, et al: Interleukin-2 receptor gamma chain mutation results in X-linked severe combined immunodeficiency in humans. Cell 73:147-157, 1993.

48. Salim AF, Phillips AD, Walker-Smith JA, et al: Sequential changes in small intestinal structure and function during rotavirus infection in neonatal rats. Gut 36:231-238, 1995.

49. Lee EY, Clouse RE, Aliperti G, et al: Small intestinal lesion resembling graft-vs-host disease. A case report in immunodeficiency and review of the literature. Arch Pathol Lab Med 115:529-532, 1991.

50. Snover DC, Filipovich AH, Ramsay NKC, et al: Graft-versus-host disease-like histopathological findings in pre-bone marrow transplantation biopsies of patients with severe T cell deficiency. Transplantation 39:95-97, 1985.

51. Boeck A, Buckley RH, Schiff RI: Gastroesophageal reflux and severe combined immunodeficiency. J Allergy Clin Immunol 99:420-424, 1997.

52. Brooks EG, Filipovich AH, Padgett JW, et al: T-cell receptor analysis in Omenn's syndrome: Evidence for defects in gene rearrangement and assembly. Blood 93:242-250, 1999.

53. Santagata S, Villa A, Sobacchi C, et al: The genetic and biochemical basis of Omenn's syndrome. Immunol Rev 178:64-74, 2000.

54. Pollock MS, Kapoor N, Dupont B, et al: Identification by HLA typing of intrauterine-derived maternal T cells in four patients with severe combined immunodeficiency. N Engl J Med 307:662-666, 1982.

55. Jouan H, Le Diest F, Nezelof C: Omenn's syndrome—pathologic arguments in favor of a graft versus host pathogenesis: A report of nine cases. Hum Pathol 18:1101-1108, 1987.

56. Ament ME: Immunodeficiency syndromes and the gut. Scand J Gastroenterol Suppl 114:127-135, 1985.

57. Herrod HG: Chronic mucocutaneous candidiasis in childhood and complications of non-*Candida* infection: A report of the Pediatric Immunodeficiency Collaborative Study Group. J Pediatr 116:377-382, 1990.

58. Derry JM, Ochs HD, Francke U: Isolation of a novel gene mutated in Wiskott-Aldrich syndrome. Cell 78:635-644, 1994.

59. Symons M, Derry JM, Karlak B, et al: Wiskott-Aldrich syndrome protein, a novel effector for the GTPase CDC42Hs, is implicated in actin polymerization. Cell 84:723-734, 1996.

60. Zicha D, Allen WE, Brickell PM, et al: Chemotaxis of macrophages is abolished in the Wiskott-Aldrich syndrome. Br J Haematol 101:659-665, 1998.

61. Hsieh K-H, Chang M-H, Lee C-Y, et al: Wiskott-Aldrich syndrome and inflammatory bowel disease. Ann Allergy 60:429-431, 1988.

62. Loan W, McCune K, Kelly B, et al: Wiskott-Aldrich syndrome: Life-threatening haemorrhage from aneurysms within the liver, small bowel mesentery and kidney, requiring both surgical and radiological intervention. J R Coll Surg Edinb 45:326-328, 2000.

63. Winkelstein JA, Marino MC, Johnston RB, et al: Chronic granulomatous disease: Report on a national registry of 368 patients. Medicine 79:155-169, 2000.

64. al-Tawil YS, Abramson SL, Gilger MA, et al: Steroid-responsive esophageal obstruction in a child with chronic granulomatous disease (CGD). J Pediatr Gastroenterol Nutr 23:182-185, 1996.

65. Dickerman JD, Colletti RB, Tampas JP: Gastric outlet obstruction in chronic granulomatous disease of childhood. Am J Dis Child 140:567-570, 1986.

66. Stopyrowa J, Fyderek K, Sikorska B, et al: Chronic granulomatous disease of childhood: Gastric manifestation and response to salazosulfapyridine therapy. Eur J Pediatr 149:28-30, 1989.

67. Lindahl JA, Williams FH, Newman SL: Small bowel obstruction in chronic granulomatous disease. J Pediatr Gastroenterol Nutr 3:637-640, 1984.

68. Ament ME, Ochs HD: Gastrointestinal manifestations of chronic granulomatous disease. N Engl J Med 288:382-387, 1973.

69. Sloan JM, Cameron CH, Maxwell RJ, et al: Colitis complicating chronic granulomatous disease. A clinicopathological case report. Gut 38:619-622, 1996.

70. Foster CB, Lehrnbecher T, Mol F, et al: Host defense molecule polymorphisms influence the risk for immune-mediated complications in chronic granulomatous disease. J Clin Invest 102:2146-2155, 1998.

71. Mitomi H, Mikami T, Takahashi H, et al: Colitis in chronic granulomatous disease resembling Crohn's disease: Comparative analysis of CD68-positive cells between the two disease entities. Dig Dis Sci 44:452-456, 1999.

72. Isaacs D, Wright VM, Shaw DG, et al: Chronic granulomatous disease mimicking Crohn's disease. J Pediatr Gastroenterol Nutr 4:498-501, 1985.

73. D'Agata ID, Paradis K, Chad Z, et al: Leukocyte adhesion deficiency presenting as chronic ileocolitis. Gut 39:605-608, 1996.

74. Hawkins HK, Heffelfinger SC, Anderson DC: Leukocyte adhesion deficiency: Clinical and postmortem observations. Pediatr Pathol 12:119-130, 1992.

75. Chirletti P, Caronna R, Arcese W, et al: Gastrointestinal emergencies in patients with acute intestinal graft-versus-host disease. Leuk Lymphoma 29:129-137, 1998.

76. Wu D, Hockenberry DM, Brentnall TA, et al: Persistent nausea and anorexia after marrow transplantation: A prospective study of 78 patients. Transplantation 66:1319-1324, 1998.

77. Saunders MD, Shulman HM, Murakami CS, et al: Bile duct apoptosis and cholestasis resembling acute graft-versus-host disease after

autologous hematopoietic cell transplantation. Am J Surg Pathol 24:1004-1008, 2000.

78. Tzung SP, Hackman RC, Hockenberry DM, et al: Lymphocytic gastritis resembling graft-vs.-host disease following autologous hematopoietic stem cell transplantation. Biol Blood Marrow Transplant 4:43-48, 1998.

79. Roy J, Snover D, Weisdorf S, et al: Simultaneous upper and lower endoscopic biopsy in the diagnosis of intestinal graft-versus-host disease. Transplantation 51:642-646, 1991.

80. Ponec RJ, Hackman RC, McDonald GB: Endoscopic and histologic diagnosis of intestinal graft-versus-host disease after marrow transplantation. Gastrointest Endosc 49:612-621, 1999.

81. Sale GE, McDonald GB, Shulman HM, et al: Gastrointestinal graft-versus-host disease in man: A clinicopathologic study of the rectal biopsy. Am J Surg Pathol 3:291-299, 1979.

82. Washington K, Bentley RC, Green A, et al: Gastric graft-versus-host disease: A blinded histologic study. Am J Surg Pathol 21:1037-1046, 1997.

83. Wang MH, Wong JM, Wang CY: Graft-versus-host disease-like syndrome in malignant thymoma. Scand J Gastroenterol 35:667-670, 2000.

84. Weisdorf D, Arthur D, Rank J, et al: Gastric recurrence of acute lymphoblastic leukemia mimicking graft-versus-host disease. Br J Haematol 71:559-564, 1989.

85. Snover DC: Mucosal damage simulating acute graft-versus-host reaction in cytomegalovirus colitis. Transplantation 39:669-670, 1985.

86. Kraus MD, Feran-Doza M, Garcia-Moliner ML, et al: Cytomegalovirus infection in the colon of bone marrow transplantation patients. Mod Pathol 11:29-36, 1998.

87. Chakrabarti S, Lees A, Jones SG, et al: *Clostridium difficile* infection in allogeneic stem cell transplant recipients is associated with severe graft-versus-host disease and non-relapse mortality. Bone Marrow Transplant 26:871-876, 2000.

88. Atkinson K: Chronic graft-versus-host disease. Bone Marrow Transplant 5:69-82, 1990.

89. Shulman HM, Sullivan KM, Weiden PL, et al: Chronic graft-versus-host syndrome in man: A long-term clinicopathologic study of 20 Seattle patients. Am J Med 69:204-217, 1980.

90. Asplund S, Gramlich TL: Chronic mucosal changes of the colon in graft-versus-host disease. Mod Pathol 11:513-515, 1998.

91. Song HK, Kreisel D, Canter R, et al: Changing presentation and management of neutropenic enterocolitis. Arch Surg 133:979-982, 1998.

92. Avigan D, Richardson P, Elias A, et al: Neutropenic enterocolitis as a complication of high dose chemotherapy with stem cell rescue in patients with solid tumors: A case series with a review of the literature. Cancer 83:409-414, 1998.

93. Katz JA, Wagner ML Gresik MV, et al: Typhlitis: An 18-year experience and postmortem review. Cancer 65:1041-1047, 1990.

94. Knox TA, Spiegelman D, Skinner SC, Gorbach S: Diarrhea and abnormalities of gastrointestinal function in a cohort of men and women with HIV infection. AM J Gastroenterol 95:3482-3489, 2000.

95. Cummins AG, LaBrooy JT, Stanley DP, et al: Quantitative histologic study of enteropathy associated with HIV infection. Gut 31:317-321, 1990.

96. Call SA, Heudebaert G, Saag M, Wilcox CM: The changing etiology of chronic diarrhea in HIV-infected patients with CD4 cell counts less than 200 cells/mm^3. Am J Gastroenterol 95:3142-3146, 2000.

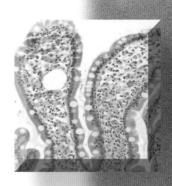

CHAPTER 5

Systemic Illnesses Involving the GI Tract

DAVID N. B. LEWIN

Introduction

Systemic illnesses commonly affect the gastrointestinal (GI) tract. GI symptoms and morphologic changes can result from several different pathogenetic mechanisms, such as nonspecific or constitutional symptoms, pathologic changes common to intestinal and extraintestinal organs, secondary changes such as opportunistic infections or drug reactions, and metastatic disease. This chapter focuses on morphologic alterations in the GI tract due to disorders that primarily affect other organ systems.

Cardiovascular Disorders

CARDIAC SURGERY AND HEART TRANSPLANTATION

GI complications following open heart surgery are uncommon, occurring in approximately 1% of cases; however, the mortality rate is high (approximately 30%).[1,2] Clinical features typically consist of GI hemorrhage secondary to stress ulceration, vascular insufficiency with ischemic necrosis of bowel, and acute diverticulitis. Additional risk factors for ischemia include end-stage renal disease, female sex, non–coronary artery bypass graft, and long pump times.[2]

In contrast to GI complications following open heart surgery, GI complications following cardiac trans-

plantation have been reported in a much greater proportion of patients (up to 20%).[3,4] These complications include the hemorrhagic conditions mentioned previously. Additionally, the use of steroids and immunosuppressive agents increases the risk of intestinal perforation, fistula formation, and infectious GI disease. Finally, these patients are at risk for post-transplant lymphoproliferative disorders.[5]

ISCHEMIC DISEASE

Intestinal ischemic disease can be divided into two major subsets: nonthrombotic (approximately 60% of cases) and thrombotic (approximately 40% of cases).[6] Nonthrombotic causes of ischemic disease include decreased mesenteric blood flow secondary to cardiac failure; shock; atherosclerotic vascular disease; disseminated intravascular coagulation; vasculitis; and fibromuscular dysplasia. Thrombotic causes can be divided into arterial embolism, arterial thrombosis, and venous thrombosis. These diseases are a heterogeneous group of disorders usually seen in elderly individuals.[7] Colonic ischemia, the most common disorder (typically nonthrombotic), has a favorable prognosis. Acute mesenteric ischemia, in contrast, has a poor prognosis, with a survival rate of only 50%.[6] Histologically, resultant lesions range from epithelial and lymphocytic apoptosis[8] to mucosal necrosis and transmural infarction of the bowel (Fig. 5-1). Specifics concerning histology and pathology are discussed in Chapters 9 and 10.

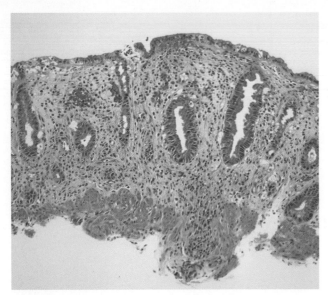

FIGURE 5–1. Early ischemia of the colon. Intermediate magnification reveals atrophy and mucin depletion of the epithelium. A mild acute inflammatory infiltrate is seen. Epithelial apoptosis is present as well. The lamina propria has a characteristic light pink homogeneous appearance.

VASCULAR DISORDERS

Several generalized vascular disorders may involve the GI tract. These also affect a number of other organ systems, most notably the skin. These disorders can be divided into telangiectatic or endothelial proliferative lesions. They typically present with GI hemorrhage and/or vasculitis and may result in infarction.

Hereditary Hemorrhagic Telangiectasia (Rendu-Osler-Weber Disease)

This is an inherited vascular anomaly that shows a widespread distribution of telangiectatic vessels. Approximately 33% of patients with the condition[9] present with repeated bleeding episodes and iron deficiency anemia, typically after the fourth decade of life. The lesions can be identified endoscopically in the GI tract and on the skin. Histologically, they are characterized by tufts of dilated small blood vessels with thinning and ballooning of the wall of the vessels and aneurysmal dilation. The lesions are treated endoscopically with thermal coagulation.

Blue Rubber Bleb Nevus Syndrome (Bean's Syndrome)

This syndrome is characterized by cutaneous and GI cavernous hemangiomas. The lesions can be sporadic or inherited in an autosomal dominant fashion. The syndrome develops in both children and adults. The skin lesions, which occur most commonly on the upper limbs and trunk, consist of blue rubber nipples that are compressible when palpated and then subsequently refill. The GI lesions are similar; thus, patients often present with bleeding or anemia.[10] Histologically, the lesions in both the skin and the GI tract are cavernous hemangiomas. Polypoid lesions include large, dilated vascular spaces in the submucosa. Conservative excision is the treatment of choice.[11]

Kaposi's Sarcoma

Kaposi's sarcoma is a relatively common finding in the GI tract of human immunodeficiency virus (HIV) patients with severe immunologic impairment.[12] Among patients with established skin or lymph node disease, 50% have GI lesions; however, a majority of these (80%) are clinically silent.[13] Patients may present with bleeding, obstruction, and even perforation. Endoscopically, the lesions are relatively distinctive, appearing as red macules or nodules. The diagnostic yield in endoscopic biopsy specimens is low owing to the predominantly submucosal location of the lesions. Because of this, lesions are not typically biopsied. Histologically, one sees a spindle cell proliferation within the submucosa and deep lamina propria with obliteration of the muscularis mucosae (Fig. 5-2). The cells do not show much atypia. Characteristic slitlike spaces containing red blood cells are seen. The endothelial cells are spindled, but plumper (epithelioid) cells often are also present. Eosinophilic periodic acid–Schiff (PAS)-

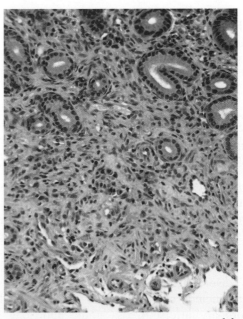

FIGURE 5–2. Kaposi's sarcoma in a gastric mucosal biopsy. A proliferation of spindle cells in seen in the deep lamina propria. Slitlike spaces with red blood cells and extravasated red blood cells are present. A mild chronic gastritis is noted as well.

positive hyaline bodies can also be seen in the endothelial cells.

Vasculitides

In general, the GI tract is usually not the primary organ affected by these diseases. However, it may be affected by systemic inflammatory vasculitides. Solitary GI tract involvement can occur rarely.[14] Classification is based on the size of the involved blood vessels, the anatomic site, and the histologic characteristics of the lesions and clinical manifestations (Table 5-1).[15] Vasculitides can cause local or diffuse pathologic changes that result in nonspecific paralytic ileus, mesenteric ischemia, submucosal edema and hemorrhage, or bowel perforation or stricture.

Takayasu's and Giant Cell Arteritis. These are diseases of medium to large muscular arteries that are characterized by granulomatous inflammation of the vessel wall. Giant cell arteritis, which usually occurs in patients older than 50 years of age, shows granulomatous inflammation in the inner half of the media centered on the internal elastic membrane. Intestinal involvement is unusual, but patients may present with intestinal perforation.[16] Takayasu's arteritis occurs rarely in the GI tract.[17] In contrast to giant cell arteritis, it affects patients younger than 50 years of age. Morphologically, it may be indistinguishable from giant cell arteritis. However, early lesions show an adventitial mononuclear infiltration with perivascular cuffing of the vasa vasorum.

Polyarteritis Nodosa. This is a systemic vasculitis that shows transmural necrotizing inflammation of small and midsized arteries, often in a segmental manner. Acute abdominal syndromes may be seen in 30% of patients.[18] This is a disease of young adults. Lesions have a predilection for branching points and bifurcations of arteries. Aneurysmal dilatation and localized vessel rupture may occur. Histologically, the vasculitis shows a transmural inflammatory infiltrate in the vessel wall with a heavy component of neutrophils, eosinophils, and mononuclear cells. Commonly, fibrinoid necrosis of the wall may be accompanied by thrombosis in the vessel lumen (Fig. 5-3).

Wegener's Granulomatosis. This is a necrotizing granulomatous vascular inflammatory disorder that typically affects the lung and kidney and involves small to medium-sized vessels. Affected patients usually have a positive c-ANCA (antineutrophil cytoplasmic antibody). Rare presentations include abdominal pain that results from GI involvement.[19] The granulomatous inflammation in these cases can be confused with Crohn's disease.[20]

Churg-Strauss Syndrome. This syndrome is characterized by the presence of small vessel vasculitis, extravascular granulomas, asthma, and eosinophilia. GI manifestations occur in at least 30% of patients but are inaugural in only 16%.[21] Typical GI symptoms include abdominal pain, diarrhea, and bleeding. Ulceration and frank perforation can occur.[22] These patients also have a positive c-ANCA. Similar to Wegener's granulomatosis, granulomatous inflammation is seen. However,

Affected Vessel	Disease	Features
Large arteries	Takayasu's arteritis	Under age 50, granulomatous inflammation
	Giant cell arteritis	Over age 50, granulomatous inflammation
Small and medium-sized arteries	Polyarteritis nodosa	Young adults, transmural necrotizing inflammation
	Wegener's granulomatosis	Lung and kidney involvement, granulomatous inflammation, c-ANCA positivity
	Churg-Strauss syndrome	Granulomas, eosinophilia, asthma, c-ANCA positivity
	Thromboangiitis obliterans (Buerger's disease)	Young men, tobacco smokers, acute and chronic inflammation
	Behçet's syndrome	Oral, genital, gastrointestinal ulcers Lymphocytic vasculitis
Small vessels	Microscopic polyangiitis	Necrotizing leukocytoclastic vasculitis, p-ANCA positivity
	Henoch-Schönlein purpura	Children, IgA immune complex vasculitis
	Cryoglobulinemia	IgG-IgM cryoglobulin immune complex vasculitis
	Degos' disease	Endovasculitis and skin lesions
Veins and venules	Diffuse hemorrhagic gastroenteropathy	Stomach and small bowel Neutrophils and endothelial cell swelling
	Enterocolic phlebitis	Small bowel and colon Isolated intestinal vasculitis, lymphocytic phlebitis

TABLE 5–1. Vasculitides of the Gastrointestinal Tract

c-ANCA, cytoplasmic antineutrophil cytoplasmic antibody; p = ANCA, perinuclear antineutrophil cytoplasmic antibody.

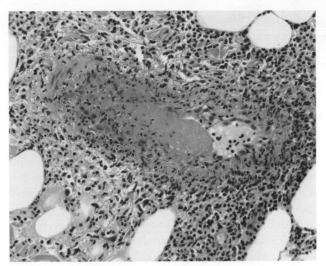

FIGURE 5–3. Polyarteritis nodosa. High-power view of a medium-sized artery containing a heavy infiltrate of neutrophils and lymphocytes. Fibrinoid necrosis of the vessel wall is accompanied by partial thrombosis of the vessel lumen.

eosinophils are usually more numerous, and patients often have associated asthma.

Thromboangiitis Obliterans (Buerger's Disease). This is a nonarteriosclerotic, segmental, inflammatory vaso-occlusive lesion that involves both medium-sized and small arteries. Histologically, one sees a prominent acute and chronic inflammatory infiltrate with thrombosis of the vessels and small microabscesses within the thrombus. The lesion is seen almost exclusively in young men who are habitual tobacco users. Sixteen cases of visceral-intestinal Buerger's disease have been reported.[23]

Behçet's Disease. This is a chronic relapsing vasculitis, characterized by aphthous ulceration of the mouth, inflammatory lesions of the perineal region, and ulcerative lesions of the GI tract. The most frequent sites of GI involvement are the ileocecal region and the colon. Because of the presence of aphthous and ulcerative-type lesions, the disease can mimic Crohn's disease. A lymphocytic inflammatory infiltrate of medium-sized to small arteries and veins is typically present. Occasionally, fibrinoid necrosis is also noted.[24] These features are not characteristic of Crohn's disease. Furthermore, Behçet's disease does not show other typical features of Crohn's disease such as transmural lymphoid aggregates and deep fissuring ulceration.

Microscopic Polyangiitis. These lesions are thought to represent a hypersensitivity reaction and have been given several other names, including *microscopic polyarteritis*, *hypersensitivity vasculitis*, and *leukocytoclastic vasculitis*. This reaction typically affects arterioles, capillaries, and venules. Segmental fibrinoid necrosis of the vessel wall with leukocytoclasia of neutrophils is noted. Usually, no immune deposits are seen in this type

of vasculitis, and most patients are p-ANCA positive. This lesion is usually found in the kidney and lung. However, GI bleeding and involvement may occur.[25]

Henoch-Schönlein Purpura. This is a small vessel vasculitis that primarily affects children. It is believed to be caused by circulating IgA containing immune complexes that deposit in vessel walls. Abdominal pain occurs in 60% of patients; GI bleeding is seen in 33%.[26] Endoscopic and histologic duodenitis have been described.[27]

Cryoglobulinemia. This is another small vessel vasculitis caused by cryoglobulin immune deposits that affect small vessels; it is associated with cryoglobulins in the serum. Immune deposits are IgG-IgM complexes that may be seen secondary to infection with hepatitis C virus.[28] GI involvement often includes the liver and spleen. The intestinal tract is involved less commonly.[29]

Degos' Disease. Malignant atrophic papulosis (Degos' disease) is a rare vascular disorder that is characterized by distinctive skin lesions associated with multiple GI infarctions.[30] Skin lesions typically consist of red papules that become umbilicated in the center.[31] The center eventually becomes porcelain white and atrophic. Lesions in the GI tract begin a few weeks or months after the onset of the cutaneous eruption. Symptoms usually consist of diffuse or localized pain; eventually, intestinal infarction and perforation with peritonitis occur.[32,33] The lesion is often fatal. Histologically, the basic pathologic process is an endovasculitis characterized by endothelial cell swelling and proliferation, sometimes with fibrinoid necrosis within the intima. The intima is the primary site of involvement, and there is an absence of significant inflammation or necrosis in the media or adventitia. Organized thrombi are often present in the vessel lumen. Necrosis of the bowel wall is common.[34]

Diffuse Hemorrhagic Gastroenteropathy. This is an unusual disorder that reveals diffuse hemorrhagic mucosa in the stomach and small bowel. Luminal narrowing of capillaries and postcapillary venules within the lamina propria results from swelling and proliferation of the endothelial cells. Margination and emigration of neutrophils, as well as partial occlusion of some vessels by fibrin thrombi, are always present.[35] This is a localized small vessel vasculopathy of the upper GI tract.

Enterocolic Phlebitis. A number of unusual, isolated intestinal vasculitides have been described; these have been given a variety of descriptive names such as *lymphocytic phlebitis*, *necrotizing and giant cell granulomatous phlebitis*, *idiopathic myointimal hyperplasia of mesenteric veins*, *mesenteric inflammatory veno-occlusive disease*, *intramural mesenteric venulitis*, and *idiopathic colonic phlebitis*.[36] All of these lesions are characterized by the presence of a lymphocyte-rich phlebitis with thrombotic obstruction of the veins (Fig. 5-4). At later stages of the disease, myointimal occlusive proliferation, without the inflammatory component, is typically seen.[37]

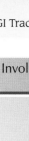

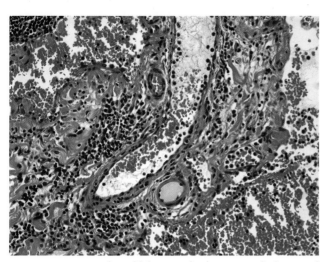

FIGURE 5–4. Enterocolitic phlebitis. High-power view of submucosal vein and artery. A lymphocytic inflammatory infiltrate is seen adjacent to and involving the vein wall. The adjacent artery is uninvolved. Prominent vascular dilatation is noted as well.

Granulomatous and necrotizing inflammation may develop as well. Clinically, the patients seems to have a favorable clinical evolution without either recurrence of intestinal ischemia or development of systemic vasculitis.

Dermatologic Disorders

Both the skin and the GI tract may become involved in a variety of disease processes. These lesions may be divided as follows:

1. Primary dermatologic disorders that also involve the GI tract (Table 5-2). These lesions are discussed in this section.
2. Systemic disorders involving both the skin and the GI tract (Table 5-3). These lesions are discussed in other areas of this chapter.
3. Primary GI disorders with skin manifestations. Only the skin disorders associated with malignancies of the GI tract are discussed in this chapter. The remaining lesions are discussed elsewhere in this textbook.

BULLOUS DISEASES

A majority of primary dermatologic bullous disorders involve the GI tract and typically occur in conjunction with a skin disorder (excluding dermatitis herpetiformis). These typically involve the upper portion of the esophagus. Patients present with symptoms of dysphagia and odynophagia. Histologically, the lesions in esophageal squamous mucosa appear similar to those of the skin. The key distinguishing morphologic features are the level of the plane of separation (vesicle formation), the type of inflammatory infiltrate, and the presence or absence of

TABLE 5–2. Primary Dermatologic Diseases Involving the Gastrointestinal Tract

Bullous diseases
    Epidermolysis bullosa
    Pemphigus vulgaris
    Bullous pemphigoid
    Erythema multiforme
        Stevens-Johnson syndrome
    Dermatitis herpetiformis
Dermatogenic enteropathy
    Eczema
    Psoriasis

acantholysis. Bullae rarely remain intact. Therefore, diagnosis of these lesions on GI biopsy specimen is challenging. The diagnosis is usually made on the basis of appropriate clinical information and biopsy of the skin lesions. In the esophagus, lesions often rupture and produce erosions; occasional fibrosis and stricture formation are also seen.

Epidermolysis Bullosa

Epidermolysis bullosa, a group of more than 12 genetically determined disorders[38] that involve all organs lined by squamous epithelium, is characterized by the formation of vesiculobullous lesions secondary to minor trauma. The site of cleavage can be in the dermis (dermolytic or dystrophic form), at the dermoepidermal junction (junctional form), or in the epidermis (epidermolytic or simplex form). Involvement of the GI tract occurs in 50%

TABLE 5–3. Systemic Diseases Involving the Skin and Gastrointestinal Tract

Vascular disorders
    Hereditary hemorrhagic telangiectasia (Rendu-Osler-Weber disease)
    Kaposi's sarcoma
    Blue rubber bleb nevus syndrome
    Necrotizing angiitis
    Degos' disease (malignant atrophic papulosis)
Metabolic disorders
    Acrodermatitis enteropathica
    Fabry's disease (angiokeratoma corporis diffusum)
    Plummer-Vinson syndrome
Rheumatologic and connective tissue disorders
    Scleroderma
    Dermatomyositis
    Systemic lupus erythematosus
    Polyarteritis nodosa
    Pseudoxanthoma elasticum
    Ehlers-Danlos syndrome
Miscellaneous disorders
    Amyloidosis
    Familial Mediterranean fever
    Mastocytosis

of patients with the dystrophic form and in 33% of patients with the junctional or simplex form.[39] Stricture and esophageal webs occur most frequently in the dystrophic form. However, they can also be seen rarely in the junctional or simplex form.[40] Additionally, anal and perianal disease and perianal blistering is seen in all types. Histologically, this lesion is characterized by separation of the epithelium and formation of bullae, with little or no inflammatory infiltrate.

Pemphigus Vulgaris

Pemphigus vulgaris is a bullous disorder that affects middle-aged and older individuals. The bullae are superficial and flaccid. The lesion is an intraepidermal bulla formed by acantholysis (the loss of intracellular bridges). Histologically, the cells lose their normal angular contours and become rounded. Basal keratinocytes typically remain attached to the epidermal basement membrane. The inflammatory infiltrate is variable; eosinophils and lymphocytes are the most common cells present in the epidermis, both surrounding and within the bullae and within the subjacent lamina propria. Direct immunofluorescence for immunoglobulins is positive in the epidermal intercellular spaces.[41] The incidence of esophageal involvement is unclear. Some studies report endoscopic lesions in up to 80% of patients.[42,43] Additionally, immunofluorescence performed on esophageal mucosa is usually positive in all patients with active disease.[44]

Bullous Pemphigoid

Bullous pemphigoid is a subepidermal bullous disorder characterized by large, tense blisters on the skin. Mucosal involvement of the GI tract is much less common than in pemphigus vulgaris,[45] although one report has described esophageal blisters in 4% of patients with typical bullous pemphigoid.[46] The histology of the bullous lesion has not been described. However, linear deposits of IgG and complement in the basement membrane of the esophagus, and occasionally in the stomach, similar to those found in the skin, have been described.[46] A single case of bullae in the colon has also been reported.[47]

Erythema Multiforme

Erythema multiforme, as the name implies, is a cutaneous reaction pattern characterized by a combination of skin and mucosal lesions. The mucosal lesions usually occur on the lips or in the oral cavity and conjunctiva. However, the esophagus and, rarely, other regions of the GI tract may be involved.[48] Included in this group of disorders is the Stevens-Johnson syndrome (macular trunk lesions with mucosal involvement).[49] Many of these lesions occur secondary to drug reactions or, occasionally, infectious agents such as mycoplasma. In the esophagus, the lesions have been described as small white patches similar to *Candida* species infection. Histologically, superficial ulceration and marked intraepithelial lymphocytosis are noted. Individual squamous cell necrosis most often involves the basal cells but may include the entire thickness of the epithelium. Lesions typically regress; thus, GI complications are uncommon.

Dermatitis Herpetiformis

This is a pruritic vesicular dermatitis with a symmetrical distribution on the skin. Unlike previously discussed bullous disorders of the skin, this disease does not produce bullous lesions in the GI tract. Dermatitis herpetiformis is strongly associated with celiac disease. Approximately 70% of patients with dermatitis herpetiformis have evidence of villous atrophy upon small bowel biopsy.[50] However, most patients are asymptomatic. Of dermatitis herpetiformis patients, 90% are positive for endomysial autoantibodies[51] (typically seen with celiac sprue as well). Human leukocyte antigen (HLA) associations are similar for both dermatitis herpetiformis and celiac sprue. Both the skin disease and the GI symptoms can be controlled by a gluten-free diet.[52]

DERMATOGENIC ENTEROPATHY

Many GI symptoms and histologic findings have been described in patients with active psoriasis and eczema. Steatorrhea and malabsorption are not uncommon, and the terms *dermatogenic enteropathy* and *psoriatic enteropathy* have been applied to these syndromes.[53,54] Histologically, the duodenal mucosa shows an increase in the number of mast cells and eosinophils. A subset of patients have increased numbers of duodenal intraepithelial lymphocytes and antibodies to gliadin (suggestive of latent celiac sprue).[55] Additionally, the colon may show increased lamina propria cellularity, active inflammation, and occasional gland atrophy in the mucosal biopsies of psoriasis patients without bowel symptoms.[56]

DERMATOLOGIC DISORDERS ASSOCIATED WITH MALIGNANCIES OF THE GASTROINTESTINAL TRACT

Acanthosis Nigricans

This disorder consists of numerous brown, hyperpigmented, velvety skin plaques located in the axillae, groin, and flexural areas. The lesion has two major forms—one associated with internal malignancies and the other associated with insulin resistance. Microscopically, dermal lesions are characterized by diffuse hyperkeratosis and papillomatosis. Additionally, epithelial hyperplasia of the esophagus has been described.

When present, this lesion is usually associated with adenocarcinomas of the stomach and colon. At least one report suggests that it is caused by the production of transforming growth factor-α (TGF-α) by tumor cells.[57]

Tylosis

Focal nonepidermolytic palmoplantar keratoderma (tylosis) is a rare autosomal dominant inherited defect of keratinization. It is strongly associated with the development of squamous cell carcinoma of the esophagus, with tumors appearing in 95% of patients.[58] The skin lesion is characterized by thickening of the stratum corneum of the palms and soles. Molecular studies have mapped the defective gene to a small region on chromosome 17q25.[59,60] This same region has been implicated in the development of sporadic squamous cell carcinoma and Barrett's esophagus–associated adenocarcinoma.

Miscellaneous Disorders

Several other nonspecific skin diseases are associated with GI neoplasms.[61] These include generalized dermal pigmentation, migratory thrombophlebitis, and seborrheic keratosis (Leser-Trélat sign).[62]

▇ Endocrine Disorders

Alterations in the secretion of endocrine hormones in endocrine disorders may have a variety of GI effects. Most of these produce functional GI symptoms such as vomiting, diarrhea, constipation, and abdominal pain

secondary to changes in GI motility (Table 5-4). A majority of such diseases do not cause significant morphologic or histologic abnormalities; thus, they are described only briefly here.

ADRENAL GLAND

Addison's disease (primary chronic adrenocortical insufficiency) involves common GI disturbances, including anorexia, nausea, vomiting, and diarrhea.[63] Pheochromocytomas are characterized by hypertension due to high catecholamine levels. Intestinal pseudo-obstruction, megacolon, and even bowel ischemia have also been described and are thought to be secondary to the vasoconstrictive action of excess catecholamine levels.[64]

HYPOTHALAMUS AND PITUITARY

The hypothalamus and the pituitary function as a unit. Disorders of either gland infrequently affect the GI tract. Hypopituitarism affects intestinal motility, as does hypothyroidism. Pituitary adenomas are part of the multiple endocrine neoplasia (MEN) syndrome, discussed later in this chapter. Of the hyperpituitary lesions, acromegaly is of interest with respect to GI neoplasia. Acromegaly is characterized by chronic growth hormone and insulin-like growth factor hypersecretion, usually due to a pituitary adenoma. It is associated with overgrowth of the musculoskeletal system and all organs, including the GI tract. It has been shown to increase epithelial cell proliferation in the colon,[65] and an increased prevalence of colonic adenomas and colonic carcinoma is noted.[66] A less well-established increased risk of gastric carcinoma has also been suggested.[67]

TABLE 5–4. Gastrointestinal Manifestations of Endocrine Disorders

Organ	Endocrine Disorder	Gastrointestinal Manifestation
Adrenal	Addison's disease	Anorexia, weight loss, abdominal pain, diarrhea
	Pheochromocytoma	Watery diarrhea, intestinal ischemia
Hypothalamus and pituitary	Acromegaly	Increased incidence of colonic polyps and neoplasms
Pancreas	Diabetes	Motility disorders, infections, abdominal pain
	Gastrinoma	Peptic ulcers, gastric fundic hyperplasia
	VIPoma	Watery diarrhea
	Somatostatinoma	Diabetes, steatorrhea
	Glucagonoma	Angular stomatitis and glossitis, giant intestinal villi
Parathyroid	Hyperparathyroidism	Nausea, vomiting, abdominal pain
	Hypoparathyroidism	Malabsorption
Thyroid	Hyperthyroidism	Hypermotility: diarrhea or steatorrhea
	Hypothyroidism	Decreased motility: reflux, bezoars, ileus, constipation
	Medullary carcinoma	Watery diarrhea

PANCREAS

Diseases of the exocrine and endocrine pancreas commonly affect the GI tract. These include pancreatic exocrine insufficiency, diabetes, and hormonal effects of functional pancreatic endocrine neoplasms. Pancreatic exocrine insufficiency typically gives rise to steatorrhea and malabsorption and is discussed further in Chapter 30.

Diabetes can involve significant GI symptoms.[68] These appear to result from decreased motility secondary to autonomic nervous system dysfunction. Patients have symptoms such as abdominal pain, bloating, early satiety, nausea, and vomiting. Abdominal bloating appears to correlate best with decreased gastric emptying.[69] The delayed gastric emptying associated with gastric atony and gastric dilatation is called *gastroparesis diabeticorum*, and an increased risk of bezoar formation is apparent. Patients can also experience periodic intractable diarrhea and crampy abdominal pain. Because of hypomotility, these patients are at risk for bacterial infection and malabsorption. Patients are also at increased risk for *Candida* infection of the esophagus.[70] Histologic features are nonspecific. Neuropathic findings with silver stains have been described,[71] as have PAS-positive vascular deposits in the vessels of the submucosa.[72]

Excess hormonal production from the islets of Langerhans of the pancreas can be a result of diffuse hyperplasia (nesidioblastosis) or pancreatic endocrine tumors. Many hormones, such as insulin, glucagon, somatostatin, pancreatic polypeptide, gastrin, ACTH, calcitonin, parathormone, and serotonin, can be produced by these lesions. All GI manifestations reflect altered digestive function and motility.[73]

PARATHYROID

Both hyperparathyroidism and hypoparathyroidism can cause GI symptoms. GI symptoms are common in hyperparathyroidism; they occur in half of patients and may be the presenting symptom in 15% of cases.[74] These patients typically have abdominal pain, nausea, vomiting, and constipation. Many of these symptoms are thought to be due to hypercalcemia, which results from altered neuronal transmission and neuromuscular excitability.[75] Hypoparathyroidism can be associated with malabsorption and steatorrhea. The small intestinal mucosa is typically histologically normal, but rare associations with celiac sprue have been reported.[76]

THYROID

Both hyperthyroidism and hypothyroidism can cause GI symptoms. Hyperparathyroidism produces hypermotility of the gut, and hypoparathyroidism causes hypomotility. Hyperthyroidism can result in rapid gastric emptying, watery diarrhea, and steatorrhea.[77] No constant structural changes in the mucosa or in the wall of the bowel have been consistently reported. Hypothyroidism can be associated with gastric bezoar formation, ileus, volvulus, constipation, and megacolon.[77] In patients with marked myxedema, dilatation, and thickening of the bowel wall with microscopic accumulation of mucopolysaccharide substances within the submucosa, muscularis propria and serosa have been described.[78]

Thyroid neoplasms may also produce GI effects. Medullary carcinoma of the thyroid is a tumor of the calcitonin-producing endocrine C cells of the thyroid. Patients may have prominent "explosive" watery diarrhea as the result of ectopic hormone production.[79] Additionally, papillary carcinoma of the thyroid can be associated with Gardner's syndrome.[80]

MULTIPLE ENDOCRINE NEOPLASIA

The MEN syndromes are a group of autosomal dominant inherited disorders that are associated with hyperplasias and/or neoplasms of several endocrine organs. Three main varieties of this syndrome can occur—MEN I, MEN IIa, and MEN IIb (or III). GI manifestations are caused by the products of the endocrine proliferations.[81,82] Each of these syndromes is associated with a mutant gene locus—MEN I with the *MEN I* gene locus and MEN IIa and IIb with the *RET* gene locus.

■ Hematologic Disorders

HEMORRHAGIC DISORDERS

Patients with bleeding disorders may develop spontaneous hemorrhage in any part of the GI tract. Ten percent to 25% of patients with hemophilia suffer from GI hemorrhage.[83] Von Willebrand's disease,[84] heparin or warfarin overdose, vitamin K deficiencies, platelet deficiency, thrombotic thrombocytopenic purpura, and hemolytic-uremic syndrome can all result in hemorrhage of the GI tract. This is most commonly seen in the upper GI tract and typically is most prominent in the submucosa. It can be severe enough to involve the entire thickness of the bowel wall and give rise to an intramural hematoma.[85] More severe lesions can cause luminal narrowing, rigidity with obstruction, and, rarely, intussusception.[83]

THROMBOTIC DISORDERS

Sickle cell anemia,[86] polycythemia rubra vera,[87] and other thrombotic disorders[88] can produce thrombosis, leading to infarction and hemorrhage of the intestines. Sickle cell anemia causes abnormal sickling and hyperviscosity of the blood and typically produces arterial/capillary obstruction.[86] It involves the watershed areas of the distal transverse colon and splenic flexure, which have the lowest oxygen tension. Sickled red blood cells may be found in the vessels. Polycythemia usually leads to venous obstruction of the portal and mesenteric veins. These lesions involve the deeper parts of the bowel wall, including the muscularis propria. Diagnosis is based on the finding of venous thrombi in the mesenteric and mesocolic tissues not in the field of infarction that occur in conjunction with appropriate clinical history.

MEGALOBLASTIC ANEMIA

Megaloblastic anemias are associated with deficiencies of folic acid and vitamin B_{12}. These anemias are characterized by megaloblastic proliferation of all actively growing cells, as is typically described in bone marrow aspirations but is also seen in the epithelial cells of the GI tract. Owing to impaired DNA synthesis, actively dividing cells in the gastric pits, small bowel, and colonic crypts typically show enlarged, immature-appearing nuclei (Fig. 5-5). The nucleus-to-cytoplasm ratio is decreased. The overall numbers of mitotic figures are also reduced. Additionally, PAS-negative, Alcian blue–negative cytoplasmic vacuoles have been described in duodenal enterocytes.[89] Megaloblastic anemia can be caused by pernicious anemia secondary to autoimmune gastritis; therefore, gastric findings of atrophic autoimmune gastritis may also be present.

LEUKEMIA AND LYMPHOMA

Involvement of the GI tract is often noted in patients with leukemia and lymphoma. This can occur directly by tumor (primary or secondary), secondary to complications of disease, or secondary to therapy.

Autopsy studies have revealed GI involvement in 50% of leukemia patients.[90] In secondary involvement of the GI tract by either leukemia or lymphoma, tumor infiltrates are often multifocal and may be present anywhere from the esophagus to the rectum.[91] These can cause aphthous-type ulcers (typical of leukemic infiltrations) or can result in polypoid, masslike, or large ulcers (typical of lymphomatous involvement).[92] The larger mass lesions can occasionally cause obstruction or intussusception.[93] Histologic features are typical of the particular leukemia or lymphoma. Malignant cells are typically found in the mucosal and submucosal tissue (Fig. 5-6). Tissue should be collected for molecular and cytogenetic analysis because many leukemias and lymphomas include diagnostic and clinically important changes.[94] Primary lymphomas of the GI tract are often solitary lesions, although diffuse forms do occur (typically in the small bowel).

Secondary effects of tumor overgrowth or of chemotherapy resulting in decreased numbers of platelets and inflammatory cells can lead to hemorrhagic lesions of the GI tract and opportunistic infection. Additionally, neutropenic colitis, which is a necrotizing inflammatory disorder of the colon that occurs in neutropenic patients,

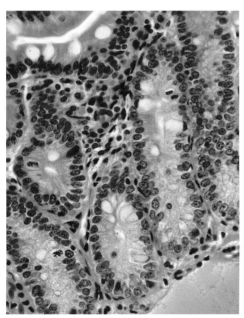

FIGURE 5–5. Nucleomegaly in megaloblastic anemia. High power of actively dividing cells is evident in crypts of the small intestine. Many enlarged immature-appearing nuclei can be seen in the upper third of the crypt.

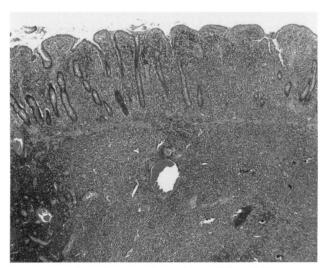

FIGURE 5–6. Lymphoma involving the small bowel. Low-power view of small bowel mucosa and submucosa with massive infiltration by malignant lymphocytes.

can occur with chemotherapy and, rarely, as a complication of acute leukemia.[95] Finally, patients who have received bone marrow transplants may develop graft-versus-host disease, which is characterized by apoptotic destruction of the epithelium throughout the GI tract. It typically presents with diarrhea. Histologically, it is characterized by apoptosis of the epithelial cells, followed by crypt and gland loss and, ultimately, mucosal erosions and ulcerations.[96]

Metabolic Disorders

ACRODERMATITIS ENTEROPATHICA

This systemic disorder occurs secondary to zinc deficiency, which results from a congenital defect in the absorption of dietary zinc. This disorder has recently been localized to a gene (*SLC39A4*) that codes for a transmembrane zinc uptake protein (hZIP4).[97] It typically presents after infancy and weaning (although rare cases have been described in adulthood[98]). It is characterized by chronic diarrhea associated with failure to thrive, periorificial dermatitis, paronychia, nail dystrophy, alopecia, susceptibility to infection, and behavioral change. Serum zinc levels are typically decreased. Treatment is provided in the form of oral zinc. Mucosal biopsy of the small bowel can be normal or can show mild patchy villous lesions. Abnormal inclusion bodies have been described in Paneth cells seen by electron microscopy.[99] Acrodermatitis may also be due to zinc deficiency secondary to Crohn's disease[100] and malnutrition.[101]

PLUMMER-VINSON SYNDROME (PATERSON–BROWN KELLY SYNDROME)

This unusual syndrome has shown a recent decrease in incidence.[102] It is characterized by iron deficiency (its presumed cause), dysphagia, and esophageal webs.[103] Dermatologic findings of angular stomatitis, atrophic tongue, and brittle nails are also seen. Long-standing disease is associated with an increased incidence of postcricoid carcinoma. Iron repletion improves all lesions.

VITAMIN DISORDERS

In general, a majority of vitamin disorders do not involve specific GI symptoms or lesions. Exceptions are brown bowel syndrome, thought to be due to a deficiency of vitamin E (discussed later), and pellagra associated with niacin deficiency. Multiple vitamin deficiencies are often noted in malabsorptive disorders. Vitamins, macronutrients, and minerals are thought to have a protective effect with respect to neoplasia of the

GI tract, especially with esophageal[104,105] and gastric[106] malignancies. Deficiency in vitamin K or anticoagulation therapy leads to a decrease in coagulation factors and can result in hemorrhagic lesions throughout the body.[107] In the GI tract, these range from focal petechial hemorrhage to frank exsanguination. No specific histologic features are associated with these lesions. Similarly, vitamin C deficiency (scurvy) can lead to hemorrhage and delayed wound healing. Deficiencies of folic acid and B$_{12}$ are associated with megaloblastic anemia and megaloblastic changes in the epithelial cells of the stomach and small intestine.[108] Also of interest, Olestra (a nonabsorbed fat replacement) may decrease the absorption of fat-soluble vitamins.[109]

Pellagra

Pellagra is a vitamin deficiency that has major GI effects. It is due to a deficiency of niacin, either dietary (deficiency found in developing countries, alcoholics, and the elderly) or secondary to impaired absorption (such as with Crohn's disease[110] or amyloidosis).[111] It is characterized clinically by diarrhea, dermatitis, and dementia. Diarrhea is often bloody. However, patients can have steatorrhea.[112] The vitamin deficiency causes an interference with the normal renewal of epithelial tissue, hence the effects on the skin and GI tract. Endoscopically, approximately half of patients have lesions. However, all have microscopic inflammation. Endoscopic lesions range from redness and granularity to focal ulceration and more extensive confluent lesions. Microscopically, the inflammatory infiltrate is nonspecific. In the esophagus, mild to severe esophagitis is seen.[113] The small bowel may be normal or may show mild villous blunting and increased inflammatory cells in the lamina propria.[114] In the large bowel, a mild to moderate inflammatory infiltrate with features of colitis cystica superficialis (cystic dilatation of the crypts and crypt abscess formation) has been described. Patients usually respond to niacin replacement therapy.

LIPOPROTEIN DISORDERS

Abetalipoproteinemia

This disease is an autosomal recessive disorder characterized by a defect in the secretion of plasma lipoproteins that contain apolipoprotein B. These patients have steatorrhea, usually in infancy, with central nervous system symptoms of disturbance in gait and balance and fatigue.[115] On peripheral smear, acanthocytes are usually prominent (in 50% of red blood cells). Laboratory findings show an absence of very-low-density lipoproteins (VLDLs), the presence of chylomicrons, and a reduction in triglycerides and other lipids. The defect occurs in a microsomal triglyceride transfer protein that is required for the secretion of plasma lipoproteins containing apolipoprotein B.[116] Normal intraluminal digestion of lipids occurs, along with transport of triglycerides and monoglycerides and their reesterification within enterocytes. However, lipids cannot be excreted on the basal lateral membrane of the enterocytes into blood and lymphatics. Histologically, this translates into prominent accumulation of fine lipid droplets within the basal aspect of the enterocytes (Fig. 5-7). These can be stained with Oil Red O on frozen section tissue or may be seen by electron microscopic examination. The overall architecture of the small bowel is normally well maintained. One pitfall in diagnosis is the similar appearance of lipid droplets identified in normal individuals after a recent lipid-rich meal. Thus, the diagnosis should be made only in fasting patients.

Tangier Disease

Tangier disease is an autosomal recessive disorder characterized by deposition of cholesteryl esters in the reticuloendothelial system, almost complete absence of high-density lipoprotein (HDL) in the plasma, and aberrant cellular lipid trafficking.[117] Clinically, patients present with hepatosplenomegaly, enlarged tonsils, peripheral neuropathy, and, occasionally, diarrhea. Laboratory studies reveal low blood levels of HDL and cholesterol (due to lack of apoprotein A) and high levels of triglycerides. Endoscopically, the lesions are described as tiny yellow nodules or orange-brown spots.[118] Micro-

scopic examination reveals clusters of foamy histiocytes in the lamina propria (Fig. 5-8). Electron microscopic findings include intracytoplasmic vacuoles unbounded by membranes; these are often confluent in appearance.[119]

LYSOSOMAL STORAGE DISORDERS

Lysosomes, which are a major component of the intracellular digestive tract, contain hydrolytic enzymes made in the endoplasmic reticulum. These enzymes break down a variety of complex macromolecules that either are a component of the cell or are taken up by phagocytosis. Lysosomal storage disorders are inherited disorders (usually autosomal recessive) caused by lack of a functional enzyme or defective enzyme lysosome targeting. Substances typically accumulate within cells at the site where most of the material to be degraded is found; degradation typically occurs at this location.

Storage disorders can be divided based on the biochemical nature of the accumulated metabolite into glycogenoses, sphingolipidoses (lipidoses), mucopolysaccharidoses (MPSs), mucolipidoses, and others. Most of these diseases have prominent central or peripheral nervous system effects.[120] In general, except for Fabry's disease, these diseases do not have significant GI effects. Case reports of malabsorption in GM1 gangliosidosis,[121] diarrhea in Niemann-Pick disease,[122] and diarrhea and vomiting in Wolman's disease have been described.[123] The importance of these diseases is that depositions can be identified in a variety of cells in the GI tract

FIGURE 5–7. Abetalipoproteinemia. **A,** High-power view of vacuolated epithelial cells that are clear-staining. **B,** Fat stain highlighting the fat in the surface epithelial cells. (From Lewin D, Lewin KJ: Small intestine. In Weidner N, Cote RJ, Suster S, et al [eds]: Modern Surgical Pathology. Philadelphia, Saunders, 2003, p 742.)

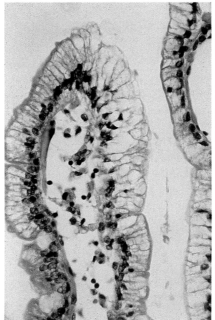

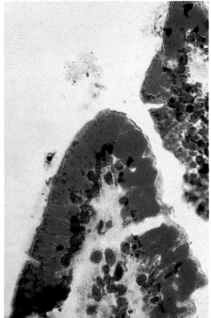

A   B

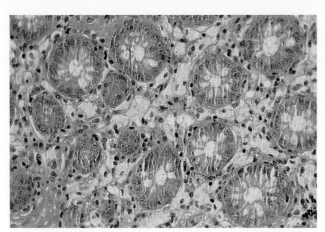

FIGURE 5–8. Tangier disease involving the colon. This condition represents a deposition of cholesterol esters in tissue histiocytes.

(summarized in Table 5-5), typically in the phagocytic cells (macrophages) in the lamina propria. The histologic appearance typically reveals an accumulation of cells with foamy cytoplasm. The material may be positive for fat stains such as Oil Red O or Sudan black on frozen section tissue and/or PAS stain, depending on the particular substance that has accumulated. Electron microscopic examination typically reveals enlarged, unusually shaped lysosomes. Historically, many of these diagnoses have been made on rectal biopsy with histochemical stains and subsequent electron microscopic examination.[124-126] This technique has largely been supplanted by specific enzyme content analysis of circulating lymphocytes or biopsy material. Differentiation among the common mimics of storage disorders is described in the next section.

Fabry's Disease

This rare X chromosome–linked lipid storage disorder, caused by a deficiency of lysosomal a-galactosidase A, results in cellular deposition of glycolipids in many tissues. Clinically, these patients have involvement of multiple organ systems. Symptoms include excruciating pain in the extremities (acroparesthesia), skin vessel ectasia (angiokeratoma), corneal and lenticular opacity, cardiovascular disease, stroke, and renal failure.[127] GI symptoms are seen in 62% of male and 29% of female heterozygotes.[128] Features include vascular ectasia,[129] delayed gastric emptying,[130] diarrhea, and, rarely, ischemic bowel disease with perforation.[131] Histologically, glycolipid deposition is identified in vacuolated ganglion cells in Meissner's plexus and in small blood vessels. By electron microscopy, laminated and amorphous intralysosomal "zebra-like" osmiophilic deposits occur in ganglion cells, smooth muscle fibers, and endothelial cells.[128]

Common Mimickers of Lysosomal Storage Disease

The common mimickers of lysosomal storage disease are often encountered and must be distinguished from them. These can be divided into two general categories—pigmented and nonpigmented. A majority of lesions result from a proliferation of histiocytes with either engulfed infectious organisms or cellular and/or extracellular material. Pigmented lesions, which are in the differential diagnosis of neuronal ceroid lipofuscinosis, include melanosis, pseudomelanosis, brown bowel syndrome, hemosiderosis, and barium granuloma. Nonpigmented lesions are in the differential diagnosis of all the rest of the lysosomal storage diseases and include xanthoma, muciphages, Whipple's disease, *Mycobacterium avium* complex, pseudolipomatosis, malakoplakia, granular cell tumors, signet ring adenocarcinoma, and malignant histiocytosis.

PIGMENTED LESIONS

Melanosis. Melanosis coli is characterized by pigment deposition in macrophages in the lamina propria. Endoscopically, the bowel mucosa can appear normal or brownish in color, depending on the amount of pigment present. Occasionally, the pigment can be so prominent that the mucosa may show multiple foci of tiny white polypoid lesions on a brown background. The white lesions represent normal or hyperplastic lymphoid aggregates that do not contain pigment.[132] Histologically, the pigment in macrophages has a dark brown granular appearance, and these cells may be located anywhere in the lamina propria (Fig. 5-9A). It contains polymerized glycolipids, glycoproteins, and melanin ("melanized ceroid")[2] and is typically associated with anthraquinone laxative use. However, a number of studies have shown an association with increased apoptosis of epithelial cells[133,134] (caused by laxatives as well as chronic colitis,[135] chronic granulomatous disease,[136] bamboo leaf extract,[137] etc.) and suggest that it is a nonspecific marker of increased apoptosis.

Pseudomelanosis. This is a rare benign condition characterized by the presence of discrete, flat, small brown-black spots typically in duodenal mucosa but also reported in gastric mucosa.[138] It occurs in any age group and appears to be associated with upper GI bleeding, chronic renal failure, hypertension, or diabetes mellitus.[139] Unlike melanosis coli, it is not associated with anthraquinone laxatives. Microscopically, the black pigment is located subepithelially in mucosal macrophages, often at the tips of the villi (Fig. 5-9B). Histochemical studies have revealed the pigment to represent a mixture of iron sulfide, hemosiderin, lipomelanin, and ceroid. It is typically negative or only focally positive with iron stains. Electron microscopic studies have revealed the material to be located within lysosomes.

TABLE 5–5. Lysosomal Storage Diseases

Disease	Enzyme Deficiency	Major Accumulating Metabolite	Gastrointestinal Symptoms	Affected Cells	Histologic Features	Electron Microscopic Features
Glycogenoses						
Type 2 Pompe's disease	α-1,4-Glucosidase	Glycogen	None	Hepatocytes, cardiac and skeletal muscle cells	Glycogen within sarcoplasm, PAS-positive	Glycogen
Sphingolipidoses						
GM1 gangliosidosis	GM1 ganglioside β-galactosidase	GM1 ganglioside	Malabsorption	Neurons	Ballooned neurons, fat stain–positive	Whorled configurations
GM2 gangliosidosis						
Tay-Sachs disease	Hexosaminidase-α subunit	GM2 ganglioside	None	Neurons	Ballooned neurons, fat stain–positive	Whorled configurations
Sandhoff's disease	Hexosaminidase-β subunit	GM2 ganglioside	None	Neurons	Ballooned neurons, fat stain–positive	Whorled configurations
Variant AB	Ganglioside activator protein	GM2 ganglioside	None	Neurons	Ballooned neurons, fat stain–positive	Whorled configurations
Sulfatidoses						
Metachromatic leukodystrophy	Arylsulfatase A	Sulfatide	None	Phagocytic cells	Inclusions stain with toluidine blue or other metachromatic stains	Free lipid bodies without cytosomes
Multiple sulfatase deficiency	Arylsulfatases A, B, C	Sulfatide, heparan sulfate, dermatan sulfate	None	Phagocytic cells	Inclusions stain with toluidine blue and other metachromatic stains	Zebra bodies
Krabbe's disease	Galactosylcer-amidase	Galactocere-broside	None	Phagocytic cells	Globoid PAS-positive cells	Curved tubular inclusions
Fabry's disease	α-Galactosidase A	Ceramide trihexoside	Delayed gastric emptying	Phagocytic, ganglion, endothelial cells, smooth muscle fibers	Vacuolization, fat stain–positive	Zebra bodies
Gaucher's disease	Glucocere-brosidase	Glucocere-broside	None	Phagocytic cells	Fibrillary cytoplasm (tissue paper–like), PAS-positive	Elongated lysosomes, stacks of bilayers
Niemann-Pick disease	Sphingomyelinase	Sphingomyelin	Diarrhea	Phagocytic cells, axons, Schwann cells	Innumerable small uniform vacuoles, PAS-positive	Zebra bodies
Mucopolysaccharidoses (MPS)						
Hurler's syndrome (MPS I)	α-L-Iduronidase	Dermatan sulfate, heparan sulfate	None	Phagocytic cells, endothelial cells, intimal cells, fibroblasts	Balloon cells, PAS-positive	Lamellated zebra bodies
Hunter's syndrome (MPS II)	L-Iduronidase sulfatase	Dermatan sulfate, heparan sulfate	None	Phagocytic cells, endothelial cells, intimal cells, fibroblasts	Balloon cells, PAS-positive	Lamellated zebra bodies

Continued

TABLE 5–5. Lysosomal Storage Diseases—**cont'd**

Disease	Enzyme Deficiency	Major Accumulating Metabolite	Gastrointestinal Symptoms	Affected Cells	Histologic Features	Electron Microscopic Features
Mucolipidoses (ML)						
I-cell disease (ML2)	Mannose-6-phospate phosphorylating enzyme	Mucopolysaccharide, glycolipid	None	Gastric chief cells, enterocytes	Vacuolated cells, PAS- and fat stain–positive	Enlarged lysosomes
Other						
Cystinosis	Cystine	Cystine transported	None	Phagocytic cells	Polarizable crystals, unfixed specimen	Membrane-bound crystals
Mannosidosis	Oligosaccharides	Mannosidase	None	Phagocytic cells, nerve, and muscle cells, fibroblasts	Small vacuoles, PAS-positive on frozen section only	Small membrane-bound bodies with fibrillar material
Neuronal ceroid lipofuscinosis (Batten disease and Kufs' disease)	Unknown	Ceroid or lipofuscin-like protein	None	Phagocytic cells, some muscle and Schwann cells, endothelial cells	Large, coarse, granular pigment, positive for Sudan black, PAS, acid-fast, yellow auto-fluorescence	Globules with a granular matrix, "Finnish snowballs"
Wolman's disease	Acid lipase	Cholesterol esters, triglycerides	Diarrhea, vomiting	Phagocytic cells	Large lipid vacuoles, fat stain–positive	Membrane-bound lipid droplets

PAS, periodic acid–Schiff.

Brown Bowel Syndrome. This is a rare acquired disorder associated with malabsorptive states and vitamin E deficiency. It is characterized by accumulation and deposition of lipofuscin pigment predominantly in the smooth muscle of the bowel, which gives a brown color to the bowel. It occurs most often in the small bowel. However, it can involve the colon and/or stomach as well. Vitamin E (α-tocopherol) is an antioxidant that prevents peroxidation of unsaturated fatty acids. It is postulated that a deficiency in this vitamin may result in oxidized lipids, which polymerize with polysaccharides to form the brown pigment. Histologically, the pigment is most prominent in the smooth muscle cells of the muscularis mucosae and propria. Some pigmentation of macrophages, nerves, ganglia, and vascular smooth muscle is usually also noted.[140] The distribution of the pigment in conjunction with an appropriate clinical history often helps in differentiation of this lesion from the others described earlier. The pigment, which stains positive for PAS, acid-fast, and fat stains on unfixed tissues, also shows the typical bright yellow autofluorescence pattern of lipofuscin. Electron microscopic examination usually reveals mitochondrial damage as well as pigment concentrated in the perinuclear Golgi region.[141] Clinically, the pigment does not have any direct effect on the bowel, although defects in contractility,[142] intussusception,[143] and toxic megacolon have been reported.[144]

Hemosiderosis/Hemochromatosis. In advanced iron overload disorders, iron is deposited in parenchymal cells throughout the body. Within the GI tract, these deposits are found most commonly in the parietal cells of the stomach, the Brunner's glands in the duodenum, and the epithelial cells of the gut.[145,146] Some minor amounts of pigment can be seen in macrophages. The pigment appears as finely granular dark brown to black particles. It stains positive with iron stains. The pigment needs to be differentiated from pseudomelanosis duodeni, which is typically larger and is located predominantly in macrophages.

Barium Granuloma. This is a complication of barium examination, typically of the colon. It is secondary to extravasation of barium into the wall of the bowel secondary to mucosal injury, overinflation of the rectal balloon, or intrinsic inflammatory disease.[147] Endoscopically, it may present as a polypoid lesion and may mimic an adenoma or carcinoma. Histologically, one sees a granulomatous reaction surrounding gray, finely granular, refractile, PAS-negative material located in the cytoplasm of histiocytes and in the lamina propria

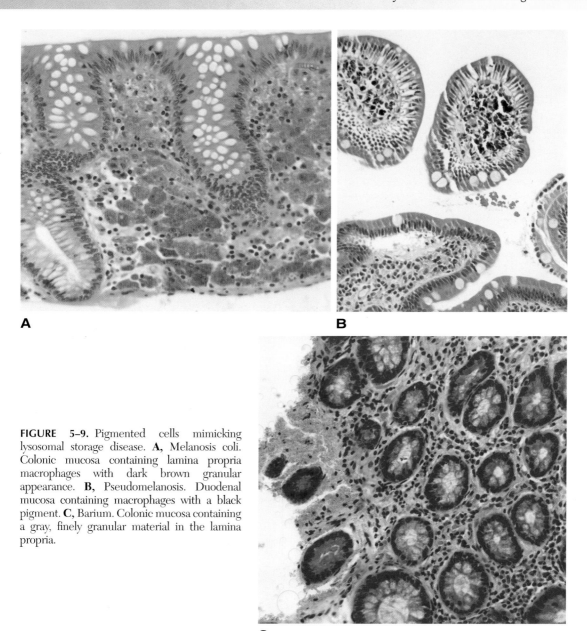

FIGURE 5–9. Pigmented cells mimicking lysosomal storage disease. **A,** Melanosis coli. Colonic mucosa containing lamina propria macrophages with dark brown granular appearance. **B,** Pseudomelanosis. Duodenal mucosa containing macrophages with a black pigment. **C,** Barium. Colonic mucosa containing a gray, finely granular material in the lamina propria.

(Fig. 5-9**C**). The material is not birefringent. X-rays of the paraffin block can help reveal the radiopaque material.[148]

NONPIGMENTED LESIONS

Xanthoma. This is a fairly common lesion of the GI tract that is most commonly found in the stomach. The terms *xanthoma, xanthelasma, lipid island,* and *xanthogranulomatous inflammation* have been used synonymously. Endoscopically, xanthomas appear as small yellow nodules or streaks on the mucosa. They represent an accumulation of lipid and cholesterol within macrophages. Microscopically, one sees a collection of macrophages containing foamy cytoplasm that is positive for fat stains on unfixed tissue (Fig. 5-10**A**). Immunohistochemical stains for alpha-1-antitrypsin and monocyte chemotactic and activating factor are also typically positive,[149] whereas cytokeratin and mucin stains are negative. The lesions are typically associated with chronic inflammatory states[150] but can be seen with malignancies.[149]

Muciphages. These are mucin-rich phagocytes that accumulate as a result of mucosal damage. They are most common in the rectum (up to 40% of all rectal biopsies contain muciphages)[151] and are also commonly found in the lamina propria and in the stalk of adenomatous polyps.[152] Endoscopically, muciphages can present as polyps or nodules. Histologically, foamy histiocytes containing coarse cytoplasmic vacuoles are present in the superficial lamina propria (Fig. 5-10**B**). Mild fibrosis and architectural distortion may occur in cases associated with a previous injury.[153] Histochemical stains for d-PAS (PAS with diastase digesion) and Alcian

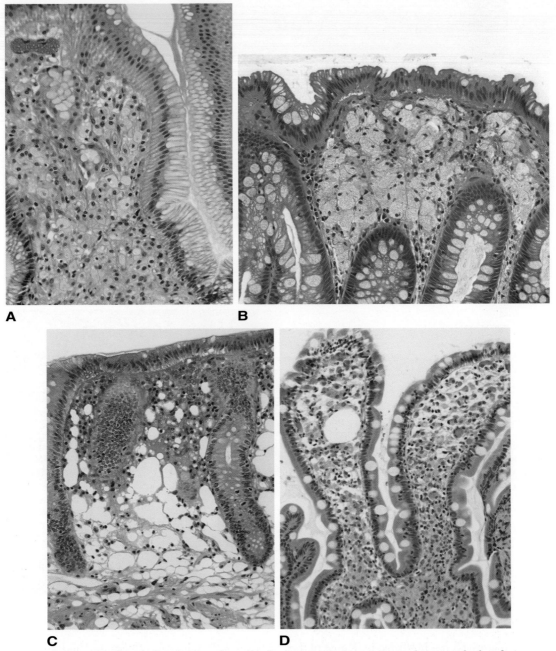

FIGURE 5–10. Nonpigmented cell mimicking lysosomal storage disease. **A,** Xanthoma. Gastric biopsy with abundant macrophages in the lamina propria. The macrophages have a bland central nucleus with foamy cytoplasm. **B,** Muciphages in the rectum. Rectal biopsy containing foamy macrophages with coarse, large cytoplasmic vacuoles in the superficial lamina propria. **C,** Pseudolipomatosis. Colonic biopsy with clear, unlined spaces in the lamina propria. **D,** Whipple's disease. Small bowel biopsy shows expansion of the villus by numerous pink macrophages. A single clear space representing extracellular lipid is present in the tip of one of the villi.

Continued

blue at pH 2.5 and immunohistochemical stains for CD68 and lysozyme are positive in muciphages.

Pseudolipomatosis. This is a common iatrogenic lesion caused by influx of air into the mucosa secondary to endoscopy-related trauma. It is a benign, transient lesion[154] that is characterized histologically by clear open spaces in the lamina propria or submucosa, representing trapped gas, without an epithelial or endothelial cell lining (Fig. 5-10C).[155] These clear spaces do not stain with any immunohistochemical or histochemical reaction.

Whipple's Disease. This is a systemic infection caused by a cultivation-resistant bacterium, *Tropheryma whippelii*. In the GI tract, it is primarily found in the small bowel; however, it can involve the stomach,[156] esophagus, and colon as well.[157] Histologically, one sees characteristic abundant pink-colored foamy macrophages

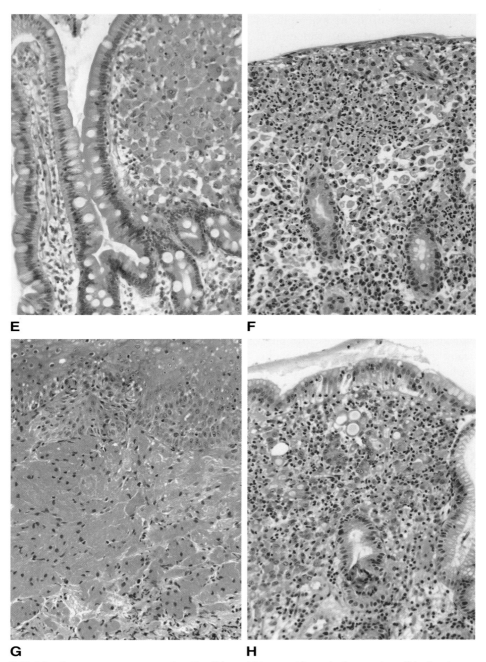

FIGURE 5–10, cont'd E, *Mycobacterium avium* complex. Small bowel biopsy with marked expansion of the lamina propria of the villi by pink homogeneous macrophages. **F,** Malakoplakia. Colonic biopsy with infiltration of the lamina propria with macrophages. A marked acute inflammatory infiltrate is also seen. The macrophages contain small blue inclusions (Michaelis-Gutmann bodies). **G,** Granular cell tumor. Esophageal biopsy with infiltration of large granular cells in the lamina propria below the squamous epithelium. **H,** Signet ring cell adenocarcinoma. Gastric biopsy with infiltration of single cells in the lamina propria. Signet ring cells can be identified in the center of the photograph, just under the surface epithelium. They contain eccentrically located, enlarged atypical nuclei.

filling the lamina propria. These macrophages may contain small granules that are positive for d-PAS. Extracellular lipid is often present as well (Fig. 5-10**D**). Electron microscopic examination reveals intracellular and extracellular bacterial rods in various stages of disintegration. These bacteria are also found within IgA-positive plasma cells.[158] With the use of fluorescence in situ hybridization for rRNA, the active

organism appears to be most prevalent near the tips of intestinal villi in the lamina propria.[159]

Mycobacterium avium **Complex.** This is a common pathogen in acquired immunodeficiency syndrome (AIDS) that may also be seen in other immunocompromised patients.[160] It typically affects the small bowel and colon. Endoscopically, the mucosa can be normal in appearance or coarsely granular.[161] Histologically, abundant variably sized sheets of foamy macrophages are seen in the lamina propria that cause widening of the villi (Fig. 5-10**E**). Diagnosis is made with acid-fast or Fite's stain positivity; numerous elongated organisms are revealed within the macrophages. PAS stain typically reveals a relatively diffuse fibrillary staining pattern in macrophages, as opposed to the granular staining that is characteristic of Whipple's disease. The organisms are typically intact, unlike the various stages of disintegration that are seen in Whipple's disease.

Malakoplakia. This is a rare bacterial infection that affects patients with an underlying macrophage phagolysosome defect (not typically seen in AIDS patients).[162] It is usually caused by *Escherichia coli* or *Klebsiella* species.[163] It is often seen in the urinary tract. However, it can involve any portion of the GI tract. Endoscopically, the mucosa shows numerous soft yellow plaques on the mucosa. Rarely, a mass lesion composed of macrophages may develop as well. Histologically, one sees an infiltration of the lamina propria by neutrophils and abundant macrophages; the latter often contain nuclear grooves (Fig. 5-10**F**). Michaelis-Gutmann bodies, which are small, pale, intracytoplasmic concretions that stain for calcium and iron, are diagnostic. Macrophages also stain for d-PAS. Electron microscopic examination reveals degenerated bacilli in phagolysosomes, similar to those seen in Whipple's disease[164]

Granular Cell Tumor. These tumors are believed to be of neurogenic origin and are typically found in the esophagus, but they can occur anywhere in the GI tract.[165] Rare cases have been described in the small bowel and colon.[166,167] They are mostly benign, but malignant tumors have been described as well. The tumors typically present as nodules in patients with nonspecific GI symptoms. Histologically, these tumors include abundant epithelioid or histiocytic cells with distinct pink granular cytoplasm in the lamina propria or submucosa (Fig. 5-10**G**). The cells are positive for PAS (with diastase) and are strongly S100-positive. Electron microscopic examination reveals cells filled with giant autophagic vacuoles (lysosomes) that contain myelin-like debris of giant lysosomes.

Signet Ring Cell Adenocarcinoma. This tumor (described in detail in Chapters 17 and 19) shows an infiltration of malignant cells with clear cytoplasm and an eccentrically placed hyperchromatic nucleus (Fig. 5-10**H**). It is differentiated from other lesions by the presence of highly atypical nuclear features and by positivity with mucin and cytokeratin stains.[168]

Clear Cell Carcinoid Tumor. A rare case has been reported of a gastric carcinoid composed entirely of clear cells with foamy cytoplasm.[169] Immunopositivity for endocrine markers such as chromogranin A or electron microscopic demonstration of dense core granules helps define the lesion.

Malignant Histiocytosis. Langerhans' cell histiocytosis can involve any portion of the GI tract, either as part of generalized disease or as a separate primary entity. Involved areas may present as a polypoid or mass lesion. Histologically, one sees a mucosal infiltrate composed of Langerhans' cells that have irregular, elongated nuclei and prominent nuclear grooves and folds. The cytoplasm of the tumor cells is abundant and finely granular. These tumors are usually associated with a prominent eosinophilic infiltrate as well. Similar to mucosa-associated lymphoid tissue (MALT) lymphoma, invasion and destruction of the epithelium are common.[170] Immunohistochemical stains for S100 and CD1a are intensely positive in tumor cells. Electron microscopic examination reveals Birbeck granules in the cytoplasm of tumor cells.[171]

AMYLOIDOSIS

Amyloidosis is not a single disease but is the product of a variety of diseases. The common feature of these diseases is the extracellular deposition of amyloid proteins that stain with Congo red and show apple-green birefringence under polarized light. The proteins have a typical fibrillary appearance under electron microscopy. All amyloid fibrils are protein complexes with a common tertiary molecular structure, referred to as a twisted β-pleated sheet pattern.

Classification

Historically, amyloidosis has been classified according to its clinical presentation (localized vs. diffuse) or its underlying cause (primary, secondary, hereditary, or endocrine related); more recently, classification has been determined on the basis of the biochemical composition of the amyloid fibrils (Table 5-6). The most common types that involve the GI tract are AA, AL, and Aβ2M. In addition to the more common proteins listed in the table, a number of other types of amyloid proteins have also been described, such as Aβ (β protein precursor), AapoA1 (apolipoprotein A1), ALys (lysozyme), ACys (cystatin C), and AGel (gelsolin). Finally, a novel and common amyloid protein, called *portal amyloid*, has also been described.[172,173] However, the chemical composition and immunohistochemical staining pattern of this type have not been characterized.

Clinical Features

GI involvement is common in all types of systemic amyloidosis (primary and secondary), ranging from 85% to 100%.[174-176] Additionally, autopsy studies in the elderly (those older than 80 years of age) have identified GI amyloid deposits (portal amyloid) in 35%[172] to 57%[173] of all individuals. This amyloid appears to be a

TABLE 5–6. Amyloidosis

Etiology	Type	Disease	Amyloid Precursor Protein
Primary	AL	Myeloma, Waldenström's, plasma cell dyscrasias, B-cell malignancies	Light chains
	AH	Heavy chain disease	IgG1
Secondary	AA	Chronic inflammatory lesions: Inflammatory bowel disease, rheumatoid arthritis, chronic infections, familial Mediterranean fever Rare malignancies: Gastric and renal carcinoma	Serum amyloid A
	Ab2M	Long-term kidney dialysis	Beta$_2$-microglobulin
Hereditary	ATTR	Familial amyloid polyneuropathy	Transthyretin (prealbumin)
	AFib		Fibrinogen a chain
Endocrine	AIAAP	Endocrine associated	Islet amyloid polypeptide

senile amyloid type without clinical consequence. In most cases associated with systemic amyloidosis, patchy involvement of the GI tract is seen without associated symptoms. However, a variety of GI symptoms, such as bleeding,[177] pseudo-obstruction,[178] decreased motility,[179] and rarely, perforation,[180] may occur on occasion. The greater the number of deposits and the more widespread the involvement, the higher the likelihood of clinical symptoms. Vascular involvement by amyloid produces fragility and rupture of affected vessels, which can lead to the development of petechial hemorrhage of the mucosa and ischemic disease and its manifestations. In fact, ulcerating lesions may mimic inflammatory bowel disease grossly.[181]

Amyloid infiltration within nerve[182] and muscle fibers[183] can cause motility disorders. Malabsorption may result from stasis and bacterial overgrowth. Finally, amyloidosis can occasionally present as a solitary mass lesion or polyp that mimics a malignant tumor.[184]

Endoscopically, the mucosa can appear normal, or it may show a fine granular appearance with erosions, friability, and thickening of the valvulae conniventes.[185,186]

Pathologic Features

Microscopically, amyloid deposits are extracellular and have a classic waxy homogeneous appearance (Fig. 5-11A). Pink hyaline amyloid may contain small slitlike spaces caused by cracking during tissue processing. Histochemical stains for Congo red (the most specific), toluidine blue, crystal violet, fluorochrome, and thioflavine usually stain all types of amyloid (Fig. 5-11B). Amyloid also stains positive with the PAS reaction and negative with lipid and mineral stains. In general, AA amyloid seems to localize to capillaries, small arterioles, and the mucosa. AL amyloid is often found in the muscularis propria and in medium-sized to large vessels. Aβ2M amyloid is found mainly in the muscularis propria

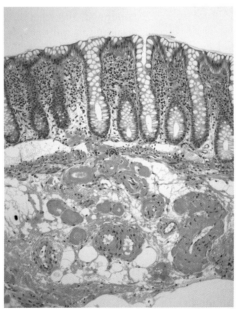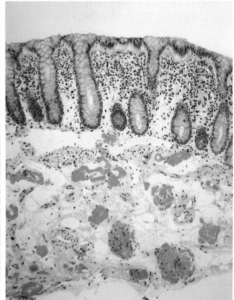

FIGURE 5–11. Amyloidosis. **A,** Intermediate power of a colonic mucosal biopsy. Homogeneous material is present in the vessels in the submucosa and as extracellular deposits. The overlying colonic mucosa is unremarkable. **B,** Same section and microscopic power as used in **A** stained with Congo red. The amyloid deposits have a bright orange-red appearance.

A   **B**

and in small arterioles and venules, forming sub-endothelial nodular lesions.[187] Portal amyloid is usually limited to mesenteric veins as small dotlike or comma-like deposits in close proximity to elastic fibers. Additionally, AL and AA forms can be distinguished by pretreatment with potassium permanganate. This pretreatment abolishes the Congo red affinity of the AA fibrils but not that of the AL fibrils.[188] Immunohistochemical stainings with antibodies to amyloid A, immunoglobulins lambda and kappa light chain amyloid fibril proteins, beta$_2$-microglobulin, and transthyretin characterizes the majority of amyloid deposits (with the exception of portal amyloid). By electron microscopy, one sees an interlocking meshwork of fibrils that measure 7.5 to 10 nm in diameter with variable length.

Amyloidosis should be differentiated from arteriosclerosis in blood vessels and from collagen in the lamina propria, submucosa, and muscularis (in systemic sclerosis). Congo red stains can help with this differential diagnosis in that neither arteriosclerosis nor collagen stains with Congo red. One study suggests that Congo red stain may not be sensitive enough in patients with early amyloidosis in minute amounts.[189]

GI biopsy is a procedure commonly used to diagnosis amyloidosis. Rectal biopsies have a sensitivity of 85% compared with a sensitivity of 54% for fat biopsies.[174] In the rectum, amyloid deposits are most commonly seen in small arterioles and veins within the submucosa; therefore, a deep suction biopsy is usually required for adequate evaluation. Some recent studies suggest that gastric or small bowel biopsies may have a sensitivity as high as 100% in the diagnosis of amyloidosis.[185,190]

FAMILIAL MEDITERRANEAN FEVER (FAMILIAL PAROXYSMAL POLYSEROSITIS, RECURRING POLYSEROSITIS)

Familial Mediterranean fever is an inherited autosomal recessive disorder seen almost exclusively in Sephardic Jews, Arabs, Armenians, and people of Turkish decent. It is characterized by recurring and self-limiting attacks of febrile serosal inflammation involving the peritoneal, synovial, and pleural membranes. This disease typically begins in childhood or adolescence and recurs at irregular intervals throughout life.[191] GI involvement consists of acute inflammation limited to the serosal surfaces of the bowel (peritonitis). Repeated episodes may result in the formation of peritoneal adhesions that may cause obstruction. Systemic amyloidosis may also occur in untreated patients. The amyloid AA type is believed to develop as a consequence of recurrent inflammation. Furthermore, amyloid deposits within the lamina propria and the submucosal vessels may occur without symptoms. The disease is often treated with colchicine.

Pulmonary Disorders

Hypoxia-producing pulmonary disorders can lead to ischemic injury of the GI tract. An increased incidence of peptic ulcer disease has also been described in patients with chronic obstructive pulmonary disease (COPD).[192] This is thought to be due to hypercapnia, which stimulates gastric acid secretion. Pneumonia, bronchitis, asthma, and idiopathic pulmonary fibrosis are all associated with gastroesophageal reflux disease (GERD).[193] It is also believed that GERD may cause or exacerbate several pulmonary diseases.

Reproductive Disorders

EFFECTS OF PREGNANCY AND EXOGENOUS HORMONES

A number of GI problems may develop during pregnancy. Nausea, vomiting, and heartburn are common in the first trimester. Some studies suggest that this is secondary to human chorionic gonadotropin or estrogen secretion,[194] which leads to abnormalities in gastric myoelectrical activity and contractility.[195] Secondary esophagitis may develop as a result of severe vomiting. Reflux, peptic ulcers, *Helicobacter pylori* infection, and cholecystitis are also common during pregnancy. Reflux and cholecystitis appear to be increased in this population. Additionally, constipation is a frequent problem during the late stages of pregnancy. Thrombosed external hemorrhoids, anal fissures, and rectal wall prolapse are all complications that can occur secondary to vaginal delivery.[196] Population studies suggest that maternal inflammatory bowel disease is associated with increased odds of preterm delivery, low birth weight, smallness for gestational age (Crohn's disease), and congenital malformations (ulcerative colitis).[197-199] It is interesting to note that pregnancy does not seem to influence the course of inflammatory bowel disease.[200]

Oral contraceptive pills and exogenous estrogens are associated with nausea and vomiting. Additionally, they are associated with thrombosis and thus an increased risk for ischemia of the small bowel and colon.[201]

ENDOMETRIOSIS

Clinical Features

Endometriosis is a condition characterized by the presence of endometrial glands and/or stroma outside of the uterus. It can involve any portion of the GI tract. The most common sites of involvement are organs in the pelvis such as the rectosigmoid colon, appendix, and small bowel. The GI tract is involved in 12% to 37% of cases.[202] Intestinal endometriosis is usually asymptomatic. However, when symptomatic, it typically presents with obstructive symptoms as a result of adhesions. Complete obstruction of the bowel lumen occurs in less than 1% of cases.[202] Other atypical presentations include diarrhea and GI bleeding. Symptoms are often temporally associated with the onset of menses.

Pathologic Features

Endometriosis may be solitary or multifocal, and it may present as a mass lesion or with volvulus, intussusception, luminal narrowing, or adhesions. Endometrial glands and/or stroma is usually present on the serosal surface but may involve any layer of the bowel wall. On cut surface, the endometriosis often appears sclerotic with punctate hemorrhagic or brown-colored areas. Microscopically, this disorder is characterized by the presence of endometrial-type glands and/or stroma (smaller, slightly elongated cells that are packed together often with intermingled red blood cells) and hemosiderin-laden macrophages (Fig. 5-12). At least two of these three findings must be present for a diagnosis of endometriosis to be established. Additionally, fibrosis and prominent smooth muscle proliferation may surround foci of endometriosis. Fresh hemorrhage may occur. Immunohistochemical staining for estrogen receptors is usually positive in the glands and stromal cells.[203]

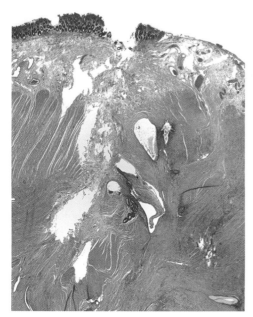

FIGURE 5–12. Endometriosis of the colon. Low-power view of the full thickness of the colon. Glandular epithelium containing blue mucin and dark blue endometrial stroma is identified in the muscularis propria of the colon. Marked muscular hypertrophy is also seen.

Differential Diagnosis

Most importantly, the differential diagnosis includes invasive adenocarcinoma. This may be extremely problematic on fine-needle aspiration specimens. On fine-needle aspiration, the glandular epithelium is preferentially aspirated and may show nuclear atypia, mimicking an adenocarcinoma. The finding of hemorrhage, hemosiderin-laden macrophages, and stromal cells helps to establish a correct diagnosis. On histologic section, this differentiation from adenocarcinoma is dependent on the finding of characteristic stroma and hemosiderin-laden macrophages, in addition to glandular epithelium. Endometriosis may occasionally be present on mucosal biopsy[204] and can resemble colitis cystica profunda. If smooth muscle proliferation is prominent, differentiation from a leiomyoma can be achieved by deeper sectioning of the tissue to look for glandular epithelium. In difficult cases, colonic glands are positive for carcinoembryonic antigen, whereas endometrial glands are negative for this peptide.[205]

◼ Rheumatologic Disorders

Connective tissue disorder may affect the GI tract in a variety of ways. It can cause hypomotility secondary to muscle inflammation and/or atrophy or ischemic disease secondary to vasculitis. A variety of lesions may also develop secondary to pharmacologic therapy of these disorders. Hypomotility is most commonly seen in scleroderma, mixed connective tissue disease, and polymyositis/dermatomyositis. Vasculitis predominates in systemic lupus erythematosus, rheumatoid arthritis, polyarteritis nodosa, and Behçet's syndrome. A majority of these disorders are treated with anti-inflammatory drugs that can have major GI effects. For example, rheumatoid arthritis is typically treated with nonsteroidal anti-inflammatory drugs (NSAIDs), which can cause peptic ulceration and bleeding.

SCLERODERMA

Scleroderma (progressive systemic sclerosis) is a systemic disease of unknown cause characterized by inflammation, fibrosis, upregulated collagen production, and vasculitis. GI involvement is common and is typically characterized by hypomotility. Scleroderma can be part of the CREST syndrome (calcinosis, Raynaud's disease, esophageal involvement, sclerodactyly, and telangiectases). Scleroderma most commonly involves the esophagus; manometric abnormalities are seen in up to 90% of patients.[206] However, abnormalities of the entire GI tract can be noted as well. Colonic dysfunction has been reported in up to 20% of patients.[207]

In the esophagus, lower esophageal sphincter pressure is reduced and gastric emptying of the stomach is delayed.[208] Both of these factors increase the incidence of gastroesophageal reflux disease, erosive esophagitis, and stricture formation. The small and large intestine may also be involved. Typical features include scattered wide-mouthed diverticuli,[209] pseudo-obstruction,[210] and intestinal perforation.[211]

Pathologically, scleroderma is characterized by smooth muscle atrophy and replacement by collagenized fibrous tissue (Fig. 5-13). The lesion most commonly affects the inner circular muscle layer but can involve the entire muscularis propria on occasion. Fibrous tissue can be highlighted by the trichrome stain, which reveals atrophy and loss of muscle tissue. Fibrosis may also involve the submucosa to a variable degree.[212] Muscular atrophy results in atony and dilatation and produces wide-mouthed pseudo-diverticula that can be identified radiographically. In addition, the small vessels of the bowel may show a proliferative endarteritis and mucinous changes of the media.[213] Rarely, ischemic ulcers can occur as a result.

DERMATOMYOSITIS AND POLYMYOSITIS

These are inflammatory myopathies that primarily involve skeletal muscle. However, skin involvement occurs also in dermatomyositis. These disorders may be associated with motor dysfunction of the GI tract.[214] The striated muscle of the cervical esophagus is most frequently affected when delayed esophageal emptying is common.[215] Histologic changes include chronic

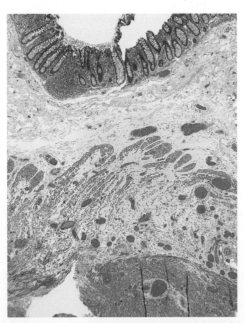

FIGURE 5–13. Scleroderma. Intermediate-power view of the colon stained with trichrome reveals atrophy and increased fibrosis of the inner circular layer of the muscularis propria.

inflammation, edema, and muscle atrophy. Features can mimic scleroderma, but fibrosis is not prominent in these disorders.

SYSTEMIC LUPUS ERYTHEMATOSUS

This systemic multisystem autoimmune disease affects the GI tract in approximately 20% of patients. The development of vasculitis can lead to ischemia[216] and perforation in the GI tract. Additionally, it has been associated with malabsorption, protein-losing enteropathy,[217] and amyloidosis.[218]

MIXED CONNECTIVE TISSUE DISEASE

This is a disease with the features of scleroderma, systemic lupus erythematosus, and polymyositis. GI abnormalities are common.[219] GI features are similar to those of scleroderma, with motility dysfunction[220] and vasculitis being the most common complications.

RHEUMATOID ARTHRITIS

GI involvement occurs in 25% of patients with long-standing rheumatoid arthritis.[221] Notably, this occurs in the form of a necrotizing vasculitis that affects small to medium-sized arteries, similar to polyarteritis nodosa. The condition is usually asymptomatic. However, hemorrhage or even perforation may occur.[222] GI lesions can also be seen in association with long-term use of NSAIDs, and rarely, long-standing inflammation can lead to amyloidosis.

REACTIVE ARTHRITIS

This is a group of inflammatory disorders associated with arthritis (spondyloarthropathy). It includes psoriatic arthritis, Reiter's syndrome, ankylosing spondylitis, and arthritis associated with inflammatory bowel disease. Most affected individuals (70%)[223] have chronic active colitis. Interestingly, clinical remission is always associated with normal gut histology.[224]

SJÖGREN'S SYNDROME

Sjögren's syndrome is a clinicopathologic entity characterized by dry eyes and mouth secondary to immune-mediated destruction of the lacrimal and salivary glands. Patients with Sjögren's syndrome may develop immune-mediated destruction of the pharyngeal and esophageal glands with fissuring and ulceration of the pharynx and esophagus. Esophageal webs have been noted in up to 10% of patients. Atrophic gastritis, atrophy, and chronic inflammation of the esophageal glands have been noted as well.[225] Histologically, the salivary glands of the esophagus show a periductal and perivascular lymphocytic inflammatory infiltrate that can occasionally be quite marked.

HEREDITARY CONNECTIVE TISSUE DISORDERS

Hereditary connective tissue disorders, such as Ehlers-Danlos syndrome and pseudoxanthoma elasticum, result from a defect in collagen synthesis and/or structure. These defects result in thinning of the bowel wall and vascular structures[226]; as a result, these patients are at increased risk for GI hemorrhage and perforation.[227] Ehlers-Danlos patients also have diaphragmatic hernias and GI diverticula. Upper GI tract hemorrhage occurs in 13% of patients with pseudoxanthoma elasticum.[228] In these cases, submucosal yellowish nodular lesions, similar to xanthoma-like skin lesions, may be noted.[229] Histologic examination typically reveals superficial mucosal hemorrhage, erosion, and elastic tissue degeneration of small and medium-sized arteries with calcified plaque formation.

Urologic Disorders

ACUTE RENAL FAILURE

Postsurgical or trauma-associated acute renal failure often results in gastric and/or duodenal erosions, ulceration, and hemorrhage secondary to hypotension, stress, and multiorgan failure.[230]

HEMOLYTIC-UREMIC SYNDROME

Hemolytic-uremic syndrome (HUS) is an acute onset of microangiopathic hemolytic anemia, thrombocytopenia, and renal dysfunction. Cases associated with *E. coli* infection often present with a GI prodrome that is difficult to differentiate histologically from an acute colitis.[231] Presentations mimicking intestinal intussusception[232] and ulcerative colitis have also been described.[233] During HUS, an associated colitis is seen in the majority of patients, and there is a 1% to 2% incidence of colonic perforation.[234] Marked mucosal and submucosal edema and hemorrhage of the colon can occur, but inflammation is not usually significant. Microvascular angiopathy with endothelial cell damage and overt thrombosis may also be noted.[235]

CHRONIC RENAL FAILURE

A variety of GI lesions may develop in patients with chronic renal failure. These are mainly associated with uremia, long-term hemodialysis, or kidney transplantation.

Uremia. GI symptoms that are common among patients with uremia include gastroesophageal reflux,[236] nausea, vomiting, anorexia, epigastric pain, and upper GI hemorrhage. Early studies had suggested that there is an increased incidence of dyspepsia, ulcer disease, and *H. pylori* gastritis. However, recent studies indicate that this is not significantly different from the general population.[237] GI hemorrhage occurs in up to 15% of patients, accounts for 15% to 20% of all deaths in long-term dialysis patients,[238] and is often associated with angiodysplasia. Bleeding abnormalities may also occur as a result of platelet dysfunction. Mucosal abnormalities range from edema to ulceration and occur in 60% of patients who die from uremia.[239] The pathogenesis of uremic syndrome–associated GI tract pathology is unclear. However, many manifestations of uremia are relieved by dialysis, which suggests a role for humoral factors.

Long-term Hemodialysis. Acute fluid loss during the process of dialysis can lead to hypotension and nonocclusive mesenteric ischemia.[240,241] Peritonitis secondary to bacterial infection and acute bowel obstruction secondary to an incarcerated hernia into the catheter tract can also develop in patients on peritoneal dialysis.[242] Dialysis patients are also susceptible to *Salmonella* species enteritis[243] and dialysis-associated beta$_2$-microglobulin amyloidosis.[244]

Kidney Transplantation. GI complications are an important cause of morbidity and mortality in kidney transplant patients.[245] Complications are mainly related to immunosuppression therapy. Patients are at risk for opportunistic infections, including *Candida* species infection, cytomegalovirus, herpesvirus, *Cryptosporidium* species, and *Strongyloides* species. Additionally, these patients are at increased risk for exacerbation of diverticulitis for reasons unknown.[246]

URINARY CONDUITS

Three basic types of urinary diversion have been used for congenital or malignant disorders—ureterosigmoidostomy, ileal neobladder, and antirefluxing colonic conduits.

Ureterosigmoidostomy, whereby the ureter is implanted into the sigmoid colon, is associated with a greatly increased risk for colonic neoplasia at or near the site of anastomosis.[247] Hence, this type of diversion is no longer popular. Adenocarcinomas typically arise 15 to 25 years after surgery and are histologically identical to typical colon adenocarcinomas. Endoscopic surveillance biopsies are recommended to screen for epithelial dysplasia.[248] In addition to dysplasia, one may see inflammatory polyps, edema, crypt branching, and Paneth cell metaplasia.[247,249]

Creation of an ileal neobladder (Kock or Charleston pouch) is now the most common procedure performed in patients who require some form of urinary diversion. These pouches are created from a portion of ileum that is separated from the fecal stream. Thus, risk for malignancy has not been associated with these procedures. However, mucosal biopsy of these pouches may reveal histologic changes over time. Early changes (over the first year) include shortening of villi with loss of microvilli and decreased numbers of goblet cells.[250] Late changes (after 4 years) consist of marked flattening of the epithelium with epithelial stratification, similar to urothelium.[251] Dysplasia has not been described.

Antirefluxing colonic conduits use a segment of colon that is isolated from the fecal stream and appears to be associated with a lower degree of retrograde reflux and thus a decreased incidence of pyelonephritis.

▨ Miscellaneous Disorders

CHRONIC GRANULOMATOUS DISEASE

This is a rare X-linked or autosomal recessive inherited disorder of phagocyte function. It is characterized by recurrent infection in infants and children.[252] Affected children suffer from chronic infections, often with abscess formation, in many organs. The GI system is involved in approximately 25% of patients.[253] Patients may present with B_{12} deficiency and an abnormal Schilling test that is not corrected by the addition of intrinsic factor, steatorrhea, obstruction, or bleeding. The defect lies in the inability of the body to kill catalase-positive bacteria and fungi because of a lack of hydrogen peroxide production by phagocytic leukocytes. This condition may be diagnosed by the finding of a negative nitroblue tetrazolium assay or by other tests that reveal decreased bacteriocidal activity of leukocytes.

The condition is characterized by necrosis, abscess, and sinus tract formation, which may be seen in the form of gastric outlet obstruction,[253,254] perineal abscess, diffuse colitis,[255] or even esophageal narrowing.[256] Histologically, necrotizing lesions often have sparse and poorly formed granulomas, often with marked eosinophilia. Microorganisms are usually not detectable within the lesion. The mucosa of the small and large intestine shows clusters of enlarged macrophages, often located adjacent to the muscularis mucosae in the basal portion of the lamina propria. These macrophages range in size from 50 to 100 mm in diameter and contain a golden brown lipofuscin type of pigment (Fig. 5-14). The pigment stains positively with fat stains and the PAS reaction. The pigment is refractile on standard histologic section as well. Rectal biopsy may show an increase in the number of inflammatory cells (including plasma cells, neutrophils, and eosinophils) in the lamina propria.

The differential diagnosis includes other granulomatous disorders such as mycobacterial and fungal infections, sarcoidosis, and inflammatory bowel disease.

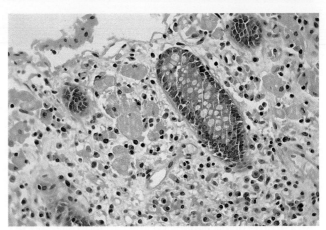

FIGURE 5–14. Chronic granulomatous disease of the colon. Pigmented macrophages are present in the lamina propria and simulate the appearance of melanosis coli.

These lesions can be excluded by stains or cultures and by appropriate clinical history. Pigment-laden macrophages may resemble several storage disorders such as Batten disease and brown bowel syndrome. Other storage disorders typically do not involve PAS-positive pigments. Whipple's disease and *M. avium* complex have PAS-positive material but are not typically refractile. Finally, melanosis coli may have a similar pigment, but macrophages in this condition are usually more prominent in the superficial lamina propria and are not usually present in the small intestine.

SARCOIDOSIS

Sarcoidosis rarely involves the gastrointestinal tract. The stomach is the most common site of sarcoidosis,[257] although involvement of the entire GI tract has been reported. It occurs in middle-aged patients and is usually associated with pulmonary disease, although the GI tract may be the first site of involvement rarely. Sarcoidosis is characterized by an abnormal immune response and the formation of multiple noncaseating granulomas. This condition is also associated with high serum angiotensin-converting enzyme activity. The cause is unknown. In patients with sarcoidosis, a high frequency of humoral autoimmunity (increased incidence of antibodies to H^+,K^+-ATPase, gliadin, and endomysium) is seen.[258] However, there does not appear to be an increased incidence of pernicious anemia or celiac disease.

The pathology of sarcoidosis is variable. The mucosa may show no abnormalities or may be severely involved with a linitis plastica–like appearance of the stomach.[259] Ulceration and bleeding have been reported. Microscopically, the hallmark of sarcoidosis is the presence of noncaseating granulomas. These granulomas are composed of epithelioid histiocytes with or without giant cells and often associated with a rim of lymphocytes at

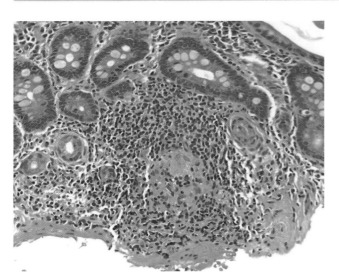

FIGURE 5–15. Sarcoidosis. High-power view of a mucosal granuloma includes epithelioid histiocytes with a rim of lymphocytes. The lesion is present just above the muscularis mucosae in a small bowel biopsy.

the periphery (Fig. 5-15). They may be present in any layer of the bowel wall and may be associated with tissue damage.

The importance of sarcoidosis lies in its differential diagnosis with other causes of granulomas (which are numerous) and with Crohn's disease. Often the cause can be ascertained only with appropriate clinical history. Most sarcoidosis cases are associated with pulmonary pathology, and a high level of serum angiotensin-converting enzyme activity is typical.[260] Sarcoidosis is less common than Crohn's in the GI tract and is more often seen in black patients. Mycobacterial infections (especially in patients with associated pulmonary disease) should also be considered. However, acid-fast stains may be performed on the granulomas in suspected cases. The purified protein derivative (PPD) skin test may also help to differentiate between the two diseases.

Essentially, the diagnosis of sarcoidosis can be established only after other diseases have been excluded.

MASTOCYTOSIS

Both systemic mastocytosis and urticaria pigmentosa (the skin form of mast cell disease) may have GI involvement by disease or by an increase in the number of mast cells. In systemic mastocytosis, 70% to 80% of patients have GI symptoms when a careful history is obtained.[261] Abnormalities include diarrhea, peptic ulcer pain, GI bleeding, nondyspeptic abdominal pain, urgency, and fecal incontinence.[262] A proportion of patients also develop gastric acid hypersecretion caused by hyperhistaminemia. This can lead to ulcer disease and may even mimic the Zollinger-Ellison syndrome. Gastric erosions, duodenal ulceration or varices

secondary to hepatic fibrosis, and portal hypertension can cause GI hemorrhage.[261]

The stomach and duodenum are most commonly involved.[263] A variety of changes can be seen, including focal urticaria–like mucosal lesions, edematous thickening of the mucosal folds, gastric erosions, and peptic-type ulcerations.

Histologically, mastocytosis is characterized by an abnormally increased proliferation of tissue mast cells. The mast cell infiltrate is normally seen throughout the GI tract but predominantly in the mucosa and submucosa. It is often associated with other inflammatory cells such as eosinophils. The infiltrate can be very dense. Associated and mild mucosal villous blunting may be seen. Secondary changes due to gastric acid hypersecretion, such as erosions, may be seen as well. Mast cells can be stained with chloroacetate esterase stains or with the Giemsa stain. Patients with urticaria pigmentosa can also show increased numbers of mast cells in biopsies of the stomach and duodenum, although mast cell numbers do not correlate with elevated skin mast cell counts in this condition.[264]

NEOPLASTIC DISEASE

Neoplastic disease from other sites may involve the GI tract in two ways: (1) by tumor invasion of the GI tract and (2) indirectly via paraneoplastic syndromes.

Tumors can invade the GI tract either by direct extension or via metastasis. Up to 20% of extraintestinal tumors metastasize to the bowel.[265,266] The most common neoplasms that directly involve the small or large intestine are carcinomas from the pancreas, prostate, urinary bladder, and female genital tract or peritoneal seeding from ovarian tumors. Peritoneal seeding typically involves the serosal surface. Tumors that metastasize relatively frequently to the intestines are melanoma and carcinoma of the breast and lung. Primary carcinoma of the digestive tract may also metastasize to other parts of the intestinal tract, particularly the diffuse linitis plastica variant of gastric carcinoma.[267] Metastatic breast carcinoma, particularly the lobular type, can mimic primary signet ring cell carcinoma and may even have a linitis plastica appearance (Fig. 5-16).[268] Immunohistochemical stains for estrogen and progesterone receptors, gross cystic fluid protein, and cytokeratin 5/6 are often positive in breast carcinoma, whereas cytokeratin 20, DAS-1, MUC5AC, and MUC6 are often positive in gastric carcinoma. Epithelial malignancies that metastasize to the GI tract are typically differentiated from primary tumors of the GI tract by the lack of epithelial dysplasia or other (adenoma) precursor lesions adjacent to the tumor and on the finding of prominent lymphatic invasion of metastatic lesions. Metastases are often multicentric as well. Furthermore, colonic tumors are usually cytokeratin 7–negative

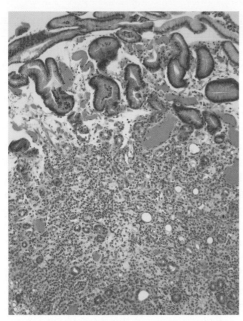

FIGURE 5-16. Metastatic lobular carcinoma of the stomach. Intermediate power of a gastric biopsy shows an infiltrate of numerous small cells in the lamina propria. There is the suggestion of single-cell filing typical of lobular carcinoma of the breast. Signet ring cells are not identified.

and cytokeratin 20–positive, whereas gastric or other foregut tumors are often cytokeratin 7–positive and cytokeratin 20–variable.[269]

Paraneoplastic syndromes may develop secondary to release of hormones or antibodies from tumor cells. Typical examples include the watery diarrhea syndrome seen with bronchial carcinoid tumors and oat cell carcinoma of the lung. The syndrome is caused by the release of serotonin, which causes hypermotility of the gut.[270] Oat cell carcinoma can also lead to gastroparesis secondary to antibody (anti-Hu) production by the tumor.[271] Another example is Zollinger-Ellison syndrome caused by excessive gastrin production from gastrinomas. These patients often present with multiple duodenal ulcers secondary to gastrin-induced acid hypersecretion.[272]

References

1. Aranha GV, Pickleman J, Pifarre R, et al: The reasons for gastrointestinal consultation after cardiac surgery. Am Surg 50:301-304, 1984.
2. Fitzgerald T, Kim D, Karakozis S, et al: Visceral ischemia after cardiopulmonary bypass. Am Surg 66:623-626, 2000.
3. Aleksic I, Czer LS, Admon D, et al: Survival of acute intestinal infarction after cardiac transplantation. Thorac Cardiovasc Surg 43:352-354, 1995.
4. Mueller XM, Tevaearai HT, Stumpe F, et al: Gastrointestinal disease following heart transplantation. World J Surg 23:650-655, 1999.
5. Hsi ED, Singleton TP, Swinnen L, et al: Mucosa-associated lymphoid tissue-type lymphomas occurring in post-transplant patients. Am J Surg Pathol 24:100-106, 2000.
6. Endean ED, Barnes SL, Kwolek CJ, et al: Surgical management of thrombotic acute intestinal ischemia. Ann Surg 233:801-808, 2001.
7. Greenwald DA, Brandt LJ, Reinus JF: Ischemic bowel disease in the elderly. Gastroenterol Clin N Am 30:445-473, 2001.
8. Cobb JP, Karl IE, Buchman TG: Rapid onset of intestinal epithelial and lymphocyte apoptotic cell death in patients with trauma and shock. Crit Care Med 28:3207-3217, 2000.
9. Kjeldsen AD, Kjeldsen J: Gastrointestinal bleeding in patients with hereditary hemorrhagic telangiectasia. Am J Gastroenterol 95:415-418, 2000.
10. Romao Z, Pontes J, Lopes H, et al: Endosonography in the diagnosis of "blue rubber bleb nevus syndrome": An uncommon cause of gastrointestinal tract bleeding. J Clin Gastroenterol 28:262-265, 1999.
11. Domini M, Aquino A, Fakhro A, et al: Blue rubber bleb nevus syndrome and gastrointestinal haemorrhage: Which treatment? Eur J Pediatr Surg 12:129-133, 2002.
12. Ioachim HL, Adsay V, Giancotti FR, et al: Kaposi's sarcoma of internal organs: A multiparameter study of 86 cases. Cancer 75:1376-1385, 1995.
13. Parente F, Cernuschi M, Orlando G, et al: Kaposi's sarcoma and AIDS: Frequency of gastrointestinal involvement and its effect on survival. A prospective study in a heterogeneous population. Scand J Gastroenterol 26:1007-1012, 1991.
14. Burke AP, Sobin LH, Virmani R: Localized vasculitis of the gastrointestinal tract. Am J Surg Pathol 19:338-349, 1995.
15. Jennette JC, Falk RJ, Andrassy K, et al: Nomenclature of systemic vasculitides. Proposal of an international consensus conference. Arthritis Rheum 37:187-192, 1994.
16. Phelan MJ, Kok K, Burrow C, et al: Small bowel infarction in association with giant cell arteritis. Br J Rheumatol 32:63-65, 1993.
17. Usui J, Tekemura H, Yuhara T, et al: Dieulafoy's lesion of the esophagus as a probable complication of Takayasu's arteritis. J Rheumatol 26:454-456, 1999.
18. Levine SM, Hellmann DB, Stone JH: Gastrointestinal involvement in polyarteritis nodosa (1986-2000): Presentation and outcomes in 24 patients. Am J Med 112:386-391, 2002.
19. Storesund B, Gran JT, Koldingsnes W: Severe intestinal involvement in Wegener's granulomatosis: Report of two cases and review of the literature. Br J Rheumatol 37:387-390, 1998.
20. Temmesfeld-Wollbrueck B, Heinrichs C, Szalay A, et al: Granulomatous gastritis in Wegener's disease: Differentiation from Crohn's disease supported by a positive test for antineutrophil antibodies. Gut 40:550-553, 1997.
21. Memain N, De BM, Guillevin L, et al: Delayed relapse of Churg-Strauss syndrome manifesting as colon ulcers with mucosal granulomas: 3 cases. J Rheumatol 29:388-391, 2002.
22. Fraioli P, Barberis M, Rizzato G: Gastrointestinal presentation of Churg Strauss syndrome. Sarcoidosis 11:42-45, 1994.
23. Lie JT: Visceral intestinal Buerger's disease. Int J Cardiol 66:S249-S256, 1998.
24. Lee CR, Kim WH, Cho YS, et al: Colonoscopic findings in intestinal Behcet's disease. Inflamm Bowel Dis 7:243-249, 2001.
25. Ueda S, Matsumoto M, Ahn T, et al: Microscopic polyangiitis complicated with massive intestinal bleeding. J Gastroenterol 36:264-270, 2001.
26. Saulsbury FT: Henoch-Schonlein purpura in children. Report of 100 patients and review of the literature. Medicine 78:395-409, 1999.
27. Gunasekaran TS, Berman J, Gonzalez M: Duodenijejunitis: Is it idiopathic or is it Henoch-Schonlein purpura without the purpura? J Pediatr Gastroenterol Nutr 30:22-28, 2000.
28. Garas G, Morgan CA: Hepatitis C and mixed cryoglobulinaemia: A case of primary gastrointestinal necrotizing vasculitis. Aust N Z J Med 26:110-111, 1996.
29. Jones MP, Pandak WM, Moxley GF: Chronic diarrhea in essential mixed cryoglobulinemia: A manifestation of visceral vasculitis? Am J Gastroenterol 86:522-524, 1991.
30. Fruhwirth J, Mischinger HJ, Werkgartner G, et al: Kohlmeier-Degos's disease with primary intestinal manifestation. Scand J Gastroenterol 32:1066-1070, 1997.
31. Braverman IM: Skin Signs of Systemic Disease, 2nd ed. Philadelphia, WB Saunders, 1981, pp 566-618.
32. Barlow RJ, Heyl T, Simson IW, et al: Malignant atrophic papulosis (Degos' disease)—diffuse involvement of brain and bowel in an African patient. Br J Dermatol 118:117-123, 1988.
33. Rodriguez MA: Ischemic colitis and malignant atrophic papulosis. Am J Gastroenterol 67:163-166, 1977.
34. Owens DW: The skin and the gut. Am J Gastroenterol 55:237-248, 1971.

35. Fishbein VA, Rosen AM, Lack EE, et al: Diffuse hemorrhagic gastroenteropathy: Report of a new entity. Gastroenterology 106:500-505, 1994.
36. Saraga E, Bouzourenne H: Enterocolic (lymphocytic) phlebitis: A rare cause of intestinal ischemic necrosis. A series of six patients and review of the literature. Am J Surg Pathol 24:824-829, 2000.
37. Flaherty MJ, Lie JT, Haggitt RC: Mesenteric inflammatory veno-occlusive disease. A seldom recognized cause of intestinal ischemia. Am J Surg Pathol 18:779-784, 1994.
38. Epstein EH: Molecular genetics of epidermolysis bullosa. Science 256:799-804, 1992.
39. Travis SP, McGrath JA, Turnbull AJ, et al: Oral and gastrointestinal manifestations of epidermolysis bullosa. Lancet 340:1505-1506, 1992.
40. Ergun GA, Lin AN, Dannenberg AJ, et al: Gastrointestinal manifestations of epidermolysis bullosa. A study of 101 patients. Medicine 71:121-127, 1992.
41. Mignogna MD, Lo Muzio L, Galloro G, et al: Oral pemphigus: Clinical significance of esophageal involvement: Report of eight cases. Oral Surg Oral Med Oral Pathol Oral Radiol Endod 84:179-184, 1997.
42. Gomi H, Akiyama M, Yakabi K, et al: Oesophageal involvement in pemphigus vulgaris. Lancet 354:1794, 1999.
43. Trattner A, Lurie R, Leiser A, et al: Esophageal involvement in pemphigus vulgaris: A clinical, histologic, and immunopathologic study. J Am Acad Dermatol 24:223-226, 1991.
44. Torzecka JD, Sysa-Jedrzejowska A, Waszczykowska E, et al: Immunopathological examination of esophagus as a useful criterion of cure in pemphigus vulgaris. J Eur Acad Dermatol Venereol 12:115-118, 1999.
45. Sharon P, Greene ML, Rachmilewitz D: Esophageal involvement in bullous pemphigoid. Gastrointest Endosc 24:122-123, 1978.
46. Bernard P, Souyri N, Pillegand B, et al: Immunofluorescent studies of gastrointestinal tract mucosa in bullous pemphigoid. Arch Dermatol 122:137-138, 1986.
47. Sachsenberg-Studer EM, Runne U, Wehrmann T, et al: Bullous colon lesions in a patient with bullous pemphigoid. Gastrointest Endosc 54:104-108, 2001.
48. Zweiban B, Cohen H, Chandrasoma P: Gastrointestinal involvement complicating Stevens-Johnson syndrome. Gastroenterology 91:469-474, 1986.
49. Mahe A, Keita S, Blanc L, et al: Esophageal necrosis in the Stevens-Johnson syndrome. J Am Acad Dermatol 29:103-104, 1993.
50. Egan CA, O'Loughlin S, Gormally S, et al: Dermatitis herpetiformis: A review of fifty-four patients. Irish J Med Sci 166:241-244, 1997.
51. Koop I, Ilchmann R, Izzi L, et al: Detection of autoantibodies against tissue transglutaminase in patients with celiac disease and dermatitis herpetiformis. Am J Gastroenterol 95:2009-2014, 2000.
52. Hall RP, Owen S, Smith A, et al: TCR Vbeta expression in the small bowel of patients with dermatitis herpetiformis and gluten sensitive enteropathy. Limited expression in dermatitis herpetiformis and treated asymptomatic gluten sensitive enteropathy. Exp Dermatol 9:275-282, 2000.
53. Shuster S, Marks J: Dermatogenic enteropathy: A new cause for steatorrhea. Lancet 1:1367-1368, 1965.
54. O'Laughlin JC, DiGiovanni AM: Psoriatic enteropathy: Report of case and review of literature. J Am Osteopath Assoc 79:107-111, 1979.
55. Michaelsson G, Kraaz W, Hagforsen E, et al: Psoriasis patients have highly increased numbers of tryptase-positive mast cells in the duodenal stroma. Br J Dermatol 136:866-870, 1997.
56. Scarpa R, Manguso F, D'Arienzo A, et al: Microscopic inflammatory changes in colon of patients with both active psoriasis and psoriatic arthritis without bowel symptoms. J Rheumatol 27:1241-1246, 2000.
57. Koyama S, Ikeda K, Sato M, et al: Transforming growth factor-alpha (TGF alpha)-producing gastric carcinoma with acanthosis nigricans: An endocrine effect of TGF alpha in the pathogenesis of cutaneous paraneoplastic syndrome and epithelial hyperplasia of the esophagus. J Gastroenterol 32:71-77, 1997.
58. Harper PS, Harper RMJ, Howel-Evans AW: Carcinoma of the esophagus with tylosis. Q J Med 39:317-333, 1970.
59. Risk JM, Mills HS, Garde J, et al: The tylosis esophageal cancer (TOC) locus: More than just a familial cancer gene. Dis Esophagus 12:173-176, 1999.
60. Iwaya T, Maesawa C, Ogasawara S, et al: Tylosis esophageal cancer locus on chromosome 17q25.1 is commonly deleted in sporadic human esophageal cancer. Gastroenterology 114:1206-1210, 1998.
61. Sher AM: Cutaneous signs of gastrointestinal disease. Compr Ther 12:50-57, 1986.
62. Wagner RF, Wagner KD: Malignant neoplasms and the Leser-Trelat sign. Arch Dermatol 117:598-599, 1981.
63. Tobin MV, Aldridge SA, Morris AI, et al: Gastrointestinal manifestations of Addison disease. Am J Gastroenterol 84:1302-1305, 1989.
64. Salehi A, Legome EL, Eichhorn K, et al: Pheochromocytoma and bowel ischemia. J Emerg Med 15:35-38, 1997.
65. Cats A, Dullaart RP, Kleibeuker JH, et al: Increased epithelial cell proliferation in the colon of patients with acromegaly. Can Res 56:523-526, 1996.
66. Colao A, Balzano A, Ferone D, et al: Increased prevalence of colonic polyps and altered lymphocyte subset pattern in the colonic lamina propria in acromegaly. Clin Endocrinol 47:644-646, 1997.
67. Ladas SD, Thalassinos NC, Ioannides G, et al: Does acromegaly really predispose to an increased prevalence of gastrointestinal tumours? Clin Endocrinol 41:597-601, 1994.
68. Taub S, Mariani A, Barkin JS: Gastrointestinal manifestations of diabetes mellitus. Diabetes Care 2:437-447, 1979.
69. Jones KL, Russo A, Stevens JE, et al: Predictors of delayed gastric emptying in diabetes. Diabetes Care 24:1264-1269, 2001.
70. Kodsi BE, Wickremesinghe C, Kozinn PJ, et al: Candida esophagitis: A prospective study of 27 cases. Gastroenterology 71:715-719, 1976.
71. Hensley GT, Soergel P: Neuropathologic findings in diabetic diarrhea. Arch Pathol Lab Med 85:857-897, 1968.
72. Ivandic A, Bozic D, Dmitrovic B, et al: Gastropathy and diarrhea in diabetic patients: The presence of helicobacteriosis and PAS-positive vascular deposits in the gastric and duodenal mucosa. Wien Klin Wochenschr 113:199-203, 2001.
73. Brentjens R, Saltz L: Islet cell tumors of the pancreas: The medical oncologist's perspective. Surg Clin North Am 81:527-542, 2001.
74. Gardner EC, Hersh T: Primary hyperparathyroidism and the gastrointestinal tract. South Med J 74:197-199, 1981.
75. Eversmann JJ, Farmer RG, Brown CH: Gastrointestinal manifestations of hyperparathyroidism. Arch Intern Med 119:605-609, 1967.
76. Matsueda K, Rosenberg H: Malabsorption with idiopathic hypo-parathyroidism responding to treatment for coincident celiac sprue. Dig Dis Sci 27:269-273, 1982.
77. Miller LJ, Gorman CA, Go VLN: Gut-thyroid interrelationships. Gastroenterology 75:901-911, 1978.
78. Douglas RC, Jacobson SD: Pathologic changes in adult myxedema: Survey of ten necropsies. J Clin Endocrinol Metab 17:1354-1364, 1957.
79. Cox TM, Fagan EA, Hillyard CJ, et al: Role of calcitonin in diarrhea associated with medullary carcinoma of the thyroid. Gut 20:629-633, 1979.
80. Thompson JS, Harned RK, Anderson JC, et al: Papillary carcinoma of the thyroid and familial polyposis coli. Dis Colon Rectum 26:583-585, 1983.
81. Gibril F, Venzon DJ, Ojeaburu JV, et al: Prospective study of the natural history of gastrinoma in patients with MEN1: Definition of an aggressive and a non-aggressive form. J Clin Endocrinol Metabol 86:5282-5293, 2001.
82. Grobmyer SR, Guillem JG, O'Riordain DS, et al: Colonic manifestations of multiple endocrine neoplasia type 2B: Report of four cases. Dis Colon Rect 42:1216-1219, 1999.
83. Pauley MP, Watson-Williams E, Trudeau WL: Intussusception presenting with lower gastrointestinal hemorrhage in a hemophiliac. Gastrointest Endosc 33:115-118, 1987.
84. White LA, Chisholm M: Gastro-intestinal bleeding in acquired von Willebrand's disease: Efficacy of high-dose immunoglobulin where substitution treatments failed. Br J Haematol 84:332-334, 1993.
85. Griffin PH, Schnure FE, Chopra S, et al: Intramural gastrointestinal hemorrhage. J Clin Gastroenterol 88:515-522, 1985.
86. Krauss JS, Freant LJ, Lee JR: Gastrointestinal pathology in sickle cell disease. Ann Clin Lab Sci 28:19-23, 1998.
87. Whelan MA, Kaim P: Mesenteric complications in a patient with polycythemia vera. Am J Gastroenterol 77:526-528, 1982.
88. Gordon MB, Beckman JA: Successful anticoagulation with hirudin in a patient with mesenteric venous thrombosis and multiple coagulation abnormalities. Vasc Med 5:159-162, 2000.
89. Joshi M, Hyams J, Treem W, et al: Cytoplasmic vacuolization of enterocytes: An unusual histopathologic finding in juvenile nutritional megaloblastic anemia. Mod Pathol 4:62-65, 1991.

90. Winton RR, Gwynn AM, Robert JC, et al: Leukemia and the body. Med J Aust 4:89, 1979.
91. Goncalves R, Sousa R, Banhudo A, et al: Endoscopic findings in chronic lymphocytic leukemia. Am J Clin Oncol 23:599-601, 2000.
92. Yoshida Y, Kobayashi M: Endoscopic diagnosis of lower intestinal lesions of leukaemia and malignant lymphoma. J Gastroenterol Hepatol 13:961-967, 1998.
93. Shim CS, Kim JO, Cheon YK, et al: A case of chronic lymphocytic leukemia-complicated colonic intussusception. Gastrointest Endosc 54:77-78, 2001.
94. Barth TF, Bentz M, Dohner H, et al: Molecular aspects of B-cell lymphomas of the gastrointestinal tract. Clin Lymphoma 2:57-64, 2001.
95. Quigley MM, Bethel K, Nowacki M, et al: Neutropenic colitis: A rare presenting complication of acute leukemia. Am J Hematol 66:213-219, 2001.
96. Watanabe N, Okazaki K, Yazumi S, et al: Acute graft-versus-host disease in the small intestine. Gastrointest Endosc 55:716, 2002.
97. Wang K, Zhou B, Kuo YM, et al: A novel member of a zinc transporter family is defective in acrodermatitis enteropathica. Am J Hum Genet 71:66-73, 2002.
98. Bronson DM, Barsky R, Barsky S: Acrodermatitis enteropathica. J Am Acad Dermatol 9:140-144, 1983.
99. Mack D, Koletzko B, Cunnane S, et al: Acrodermatitis enteropathica with normal serum zinc levels: Diagnostic value of small bowel biopsy and essential fatty acid determination. Gut 30:1426-1429, 1989.
100. McClain C, Soutor C, Zieve L: Zinc deficiency: A complication of Crohn's disease. Gastroenterology 78:272-279, 1980.
101. Ecker RI, Schroeter AL: Acrodermatitis and acquired zinc deficiency. Arch Dermatol 114:937-939, 1978.
102. Chen TS, Chen PS: Rise and fall of the Plummer-Vinson syndrome. J Gastroenterol Hepatol 9:654-658, 1994.
103. Hoffman RM, Jaffe PE: Plummer-Vinson syndrome. A case report and literature review. Arch Intern Med 155:2008-2011, 1995.
104. Franceschi S, Bidoli E, Negri E, et al: Role of macronutrients, vitamins and minerals in the aetiology of squamous-cell carcinoma of the oesophagus. Int J Cancer 86:626-631, 2000.
105. Blot WJ, Li JY, Taylor PR, et al: The Linxian trials: Mortality rates by vitamin-mineral intervention group. Am J Clin Nutr 62:1424S-1426S, 1995.
106. Yang CS: Vitamin nutrition and gastroesophageal cancer. J Nutr 130:338S-339S, 2000.
107. Ansell JE, Kumar R, Deykin D, et al: The spectrum of vitamin K deficiency. JAMA 238:545-549, 1979.
108. Hermos JA, Adams WM, Liu YK, et al: Mucosa of the small intestine in folate-deficient alcoholics. Ann Intern Med 76:959-965, 1972.
109. Peters JC, Lawson KD, Middleton SJ, et al: Assessment of the nutritional effects of olestra, a nonabsorbed fat replacement: Introduction and overview. J Nutr 127:1539S-1546S, 1997.
110. Abu-Qurshin R, Naschitz JE, Zuckermann E, et al: Crohn's disease associated with pellagra and increased excretion of 5-hydroxyindoleacetic acid. Am J Med Sci 313:111-113, 1997.
111. Itami A, Ando I, Kukita A, et al: Pellagra associated with amyloidosis secondary to multiple myeloma. Br J Dermatol 137:829, 1997.
112. Spivak JL, Jackson DL: Pellagra: An analysis of 18 patients and review of the literature. Johns Hopkins Med J 140:295-309, 1977.
113. Segal I, Hale M, Demetriou A, et al: Pathological effects of pellagra on the esophagus. Nutr Cancer 14:233-238, 1990.
114. Cook GC: D-xylose absorption and jejunal morphology in African patients with pellagra (niacin tryptophan deficiency). Trans Royal Soc Trop Med Hyg 70:349-351, 1976.
115. Triantafillidis JK, Kottaras G, Sgourous S, et al: A-beta-lipoproteinemia: Clinical and laboratory features, therapeutic manipulations, and follow-up study of three members of a Greek family. J Clin Gastroenterol 26:207-211, 1998.
116. Sharp D, Blinderman L, Combs KA, et al: Cloning and gene defects in microsomal triglyceride transfer protein associated with abetalipoproteinaemia. Nature 365:65-69, 1993.
117. Orso E, Broccardo C, Kaminski WE, et al: Transport of lipids from golgi to plasma membrane is defective in Tangier disease patients and Abc1-deficient mice. Nat Genet 24:192-196, 2000.
118. Barnard GF, Jafri IH, Banner BF, et al: Colonic mucosal appearance of Tangier disease in a new patient. Gastrointest Endosc 40:628-630, 1994.
119. Dechelotte P, Kantelip B, de Laguillaumie BV, et al: Tangier disease. A histological and ultrastructural study. Pathol Res Pract 180:424-430, 1985.
120. Graham DI, Lantos PL: Greenfield's Neuropathology, 6th ed. London, Arnold, 1997, pp 658-718.
121. Kordysz E, Wozniewicz B: Landing disease, GM1 generalized gangliosidosis, and malabsorption syndrome. Pediatr Pathol 9:467-473, 1989.
122. Dinari G, Rosenbach Y, Grunebaum M, et al: Gastrointestinal manifestations of Niemann-Pick disease. Enzyme 25:407-412, 1980.
123. Crocker AC, Vawter GF, Neuhauser EBD, et al: Wolman's disease. Three new patients with a recently described lipidosis. Pediatrics 35:627-640, 1965.
124. Yamano T, Shimada M, Okada S, et al: Ultrastructural study of biopsy specimens of rectal mucosa. Its use in neuronal storage diseases. Arch Pathol Lab Med 106:673-677, 1982.
125. Rapola J, Santavuori P, Savilahti E: Suction biopsy of rectal mucosa in the diagnosis of infantile and juvenile types of neuronal ceroid lipofuscinoses. Hum Pathol 15:352-360, 1984.
126. Ginsel LA, Cambier PH, Daems WTh: Fucosidosis and I-cell disease: A fine structural and silver-staining study of abnormal inclusion bodies in small-intestinal cells. Virchows Arch 27:99-117, 1978.
127. Whybra C, Kampmann C, Willers I, et al: Anderson-Fabry disease: Clinical manifestations of disease in female heterozygotes. J Inherit Metab Dis 24:715-724, 2001.
128. Sheth KJ, Werlin SL, Freeman ME, et al: Gastrointestinal structure and function in Fabry's disease. Am J Gastroenterol 76:246-251, 1981.
129. Okano H, Shiraki K, Tsuneoka K, et al: Esophageal vascular ectasia associated with Fabry's disease. Gastrointest Endosc 53:125-126, 2001.
130. O'Brien BD, Shnitka TK, McDougall R, et al: Pathophysiologic and ultrastructural basis for intestinal symptoms in Fabry's disease. Gastroenterology 82:957-962, 1982.
131. Jardine DL, Fitzpatrick MA, Troughton WD, et al: Small bowel ischaemia in Fabry's disease. J Gastroenterol Hepatol 9:201-204, 1994.
132. Pearce CB, Martin H, Duncan HD, et al: Colonic lymphoid hyperplasia in melanosis coli. Arch Pathol Lab Med 125:1110-1112, 2001.
133. Benavides SH, Morgante PE, Monserrat AJ, et al: The pigment of melanosis coli: A lectin histochemical study. Gastrointest Endosc 46:131-138, 1997.
134. Byers RJ, Marsh P, Parkinson D, et al: Melanosis coli is associated with an increase in colonic epithelial apoptosis and not with laxative use. Histopathology 30:160-164, 1997.
135. Pardi DS, Tremaine WJ, Rothenberg HJ, et al: Melanosis coli in inflammatory bowel disease. J Clin Gastroenterol 26:167-170, 1998.
136. Harris BH, Boles ET: Intestinal lesions in chronic granulomatous disease of childhood. J Pediatr Surg 8:955-956, 1973.
137. Iseki K, Ishikawa H, Suzuki T, et al: Melanosis coli associated with ingestion of bamboo leaf extract. Gastrointest Endosc 47:305-307, 1998.
138. Treeprasertsuk S, Thong-Ngam D, Suwangool P, et al: Pseudo-melanosis duodeni: Association with hypertension and chronic renal failure: Case report. J Med Assoc Thai 83:964-968, 2000.
139. West B: Pseudomelanosis duodeni. J Clin Gastroenterol 10:127-129, 1988.
140. Schnitzer B, Loesel LS: Brown bowel. Am J Clin Pathol 50:433-439, 1968.
141. Horn T, Svendsen LB, Johansen A, et al: Brown bowel syndrome. Ultrastruct Pathol 8:357-361, 1985.
142. Waldron D, Horgan P, Barry K, et al: Anorectal functional deficit in the brown bowel syndrome. Irish J Med Sci 163:404-405, 1994.
143. Drake WM, Winter TA, Price SK, et al: Small bowel intussusception and brown bowel syndrome in association with severe malnutrition. Am J Gastroenterol 91:1450-1452, 1996.
144. Robinson MH, Dowling BL, Clark JV, et al: Brown bowel syndrome: An unusual cause of massive dilatation of the colon. Gut 30:882-884, 1989.
145. Steckman M, Bozymski EM: Hemosiderosis of the duodenum. Gastrointest Endosc 29:326-327, 1983.
146. Conte D, Velio P, Brunelli L, et al: Stainable iron in gastric and duodenal mucosa of primary hemochromatosis patients and alcoholics. Am J Gastroenterol 82:237-240, 1987.

147. Mayorga M, Castro F, Fernandez F, et al: Radiohistology and histochemistry of barium granuloma of the colon and rectum. Histol Histopathol 7:625-628, 1992.

148. Subramanyam K, Rajan RT, Hearn CD: Barium granuloma of the sigmoid colon. J Clin Gastroenterol 10:98-100, 1988.

149. Muraoka A, Suehiro I, Fujii M, et al: Type IIa early gastric cancer with proliferation of xanthoma cells. J Gastroenterol 33:326-329, 1998.

150. Moreto M, Ojembarrena E, Zaballa M, et al: Retrospective endoscopic analysis of gastric xanthelasma in the non-operated stomach. Endoscopy 17:210-211, 1985.

151. Bejarano PA, Aranda-Michel J, Fenoglio-Preiser C: Histochemical and immunohistochemical characterization of foamy histiocytes (muciphages and xanthelasma) of the rectum. Am J Surg Pathol 24:1009-1015, 2000.

152. Rubio CA: Lysozyme-rich muciphages surrounding colorectal adenomas. Anticancer Res 22:879-881, 2002.

153. Shepherd NA: What is the significance of muciphages in colorectal biopsies? Muciphages and other mucosal accumulations in the colorectal mucosa. Histopathology 36:559-562, 2000.

154. Waring JP, Manne RK, Wadas DD, et al: Mucosal pseudolipomatosis: An air pressure-related colonoscopy complication. Gastrointest Endosc 35:581-582, 1989.

155. Snover DC, Sandstad J, Hutton S: Mucosal pseudolipomatosis of the colon. Am J Clin Pathol 84:575-580, 1985.

156. Yanez J, Ulla J, Souto J, et al: Whipple's disease mimicking linitis plastica. Endoscopy 31:S10, 1999.

157. Marcial MA, Villafana M: Whipple's disease with esophageal and colonic involvement: Endoscopic and histopathologic findings. Gastrointest Endosc 46:263-266, 1997.

158. Eck M, Kreipe H, Harmsen D, et al: Invasion and destruction of mucosal plasma cells by *Tropheryma whippelii*. Hum Pathol 28:1424-1428, 1997.

159. Fredricks DN, Relman DA: Localization of *Tropheryma whippelii* rRNA in tissues from patients with Whipple's disease. J Infect Dis 183:1229-1237, 2001.

160. Nguyen HN, Frank D, Handt S, et al: Severe gastrointestinal hemorrhage due to *Mycobacterium avium* complex in a patient receiving immunosuppressive therapy. Am J Gastroenterol 94:232-235, 1999.

161. Cappell MS, Philogene C: The endoscopic appearance of severe intestinal *Mycobacterium avium* complex infection as a coarsely granular mucosa due to massive infiltration and expansion of intestinal villi without mucosal exudation. J Clin Gastroenterol 21:323-326, 1995.

162. Boudny P, Kurrer MO, Stamm B, et al: Malakoplakia of the colon in an infant with severe combined immunodeficiency (SCID) and charge association. Pathol Res Pract 196:577-582, 2000.

163. Lewin KJ, Fair WR, Steilbigel RT, et al: Clinical and laboratory studies into the pathogenesis of malakoplakia. J Clin Pathol 29:354-363, 1976.

164. Lewin KJ, Harrell GS, Lee AS, et al: An electron-microscopic study: Demonstration of bacilliform organisms in malakoplakic macrophages. Gastroenterology 66:28-45, 1974.

165. Voskuil JH, van Dijk MM, Wagenaar SS, et al: Occurrence of esophageal granular cell tumors in The Netherlands between 1988 and 1994. Dig Dis Sci 46:1610-1614, 2001.

166. Thorne MB, Ross BS: Granular cell tumors of the esophagus and colon. J Miss State Med Assoc 43:115-116, 2002.

167. Onoda N, Kobayashi H, Satake K, et al: Granular cell tumor of the duodenum: A case report. Am J Gastroenterol 93:1993-1994, 1998.

168. Ludvikova M, Michal M, Datkova D: Gastric xanthelasma associated with diffuse signet ring carcinoma. A potential diagnostic problem. Histopathology 25:581-582, 1994.

169. Luk IS, Bhuta S, Lewin KJ: Clear cell carcinoid tumor of stomach. A variant mimicking gastric xanthelasma. Arch Pathol Lab Med 121:1100-1103, 1997.

170. Lee RG, Braziel RM, Stenzel P: Gastrointestinal involvement in Langerhans cell histiocytosis (histiocytosis X): Diagnosis by rectal biopsy. Mod Pathol 3:154-157, 1990.

171. Terracciano L, Kocher T, Cathomas G, et al: Langerhans cell histiocytosis of the stomach with atypical morphological features. Pathol Int 49:553-556, 1999.

172. Rocken C, Saeger W, Linke RR: Portal amyloid: Novel amyloid deposits in gastrointestinal veins? Arch Pathol Lab Med 120:1044-1051, 1996.

173. Matsutani H, Hoshii Y, Setoguchi M, et al: Vascular amyloid of unknown origin and senile transthyretin amyloid in the lung and gastrointestinal tract of old age: Histological and immuno-histological studies. Pathol Int 51:326-332, 2001.

174. Breedveld FC, Maarkusse HM, MacFarlane JD: Subcutaneous fat biopsy in the diagnosis of amyloidosis secondary to chronic arthritis. Clin Exp Rheumatol 7:407-410, 1989.

175. Kyle RA, Greipp PR: Amyloidosis (AL): Clinical and laboratory features in 229 cases. Mayo Clin Proc 58:115-119, 1987.

176. Lovat LB, Pepys MB, Hawkins PN: Amyloid and the gut. Dig Dis Sci 15:155-171, 1997.

177. Chang SS, Lu CL, Tsay SH, et al: Amyloidosis-induced gastrointestinal bleeding in a patient with multiple myeloma. J Clin Gastroenterol 32:161-163, 2001.

178. Koppelman RN, Stollman NH, Baigorri F, et al: Acute small bowel pseudo-obstruction due to AL amyloidosis: A case report and literature review. Am J Gastroenterol 95:294-296, 2000.

179. Anan I, El-Salhy M, Ando Y, et al: Colonic enteric nervous system in patients with familial amyloidotic neuropathy. Acta Neuropathol 98:48-54, 1999.

180. Khan GA, Lewis FI, Dasgupta M: Beta 2-microglobulin amyloidosis presenting as esophageal perforation in a hemodialysis patient. Am J Nephrol 17:524-527, 1997.

181. Vernon SE: Amyloid colitis. Dis Colon Rectum 25:728-730, 1982.

182. Yoshimatsu S, Ando Y, Terazaki H, et al: Endoscopic and pathological manifestations of the gastrointestinal tract in familial amyloidotic polyneuropathy type I (Met30). J Int Med 243:65-72, 1998.

183. Tada S, Iida M, Yao T, et al: Intestinal pseudo-obstruction in patients with amyloidosis: Clinicopathologic differences between chemical types of amyloid protein. Gut 34:1412-1417, 1993.

184. Peny MO, Debongnie JC, Haot J, et al: Localized amyloid tumor in small bowel. Dig Dis Sci 45:1850-1853, 2000.

185. Tada S, Iida M, Yao T, et al: Endoscopic features in amyloidosis of the small intestine: Clinical and morphologic differences between chemical types of amyloid protein. Gastrointest Endosc 40:45-50, 1994.

186. Araoz PA, Batts KP, MacCarty RL: Amyloidosis of the alimentary canal: Radiologic-pathologic correlation of CT findings. Abdom Imaging 25:38-44, 2000.

187. Ohashi K, Takagawa R, Hara M: Visceral organ involvement and extracellular matrix changes in beta 2-microglobulin amyloidosis—a comparative study with systemic AA and AL amyloidosis. Virchows Arch 430:479-487, 1997.

188. Wright JR, Calkins E, Humphrey RL: Potassium permanganate reaction in amyloidosis: A histologic method to assist in differentiating forms of the disease. Lab Invest 36:274-279, 1977.

189. Linke RP, Gartner HV, Michels H: High-sensitivity diagnosis of AA amyloidosis using Congo red and immunohistochemistry detects missed amyloid deposits. J Histochem Cytochem 43:863-869, 1995.

190. Yamada M, Hatakeyama S, Tsukagoshi H: Gastrointestinal amyloid deposition in AL (primary or myeloma-associated) and AA (secondary) amyloidosis: Diagnostic value of gastric biopsy. Hum Pathol 16:1206-1211, 1985.

191. Ciftci AO, Tanyel FC, Buyukpamukcu N, et al: Adhesive small bowel obstruction caused by familial Mediterranean fever: The incidence and outcome. J Pediatr Surg 30:577-579, 1995.

192. Glick DL, Kern F Jr: Peptic ulcer in chronic obstructive bronchopulmonary disease. A prospective clinical study of prevalence. Gastroenterology 47:153-160, 1964.

193. Tobin RW, Pope CE, Pellegrini CA, et al: Increased prevalence of gastroesophageal reflux in patients with idiopathic pulmonary fibrosis. Am J Respir Crit Care Med 158:1804-1808, 1998.

194. Goodwin TM: Nausea and vomiting of pregnancy: An obstetric syndrome. Am J Obstet Gynecol 185:S184-S189, 2002.

195. Koch KL: Gastrointestinal factors in nausea and vomiting of pregnancy. Am J Obstet Gynecol 185:S198-S203, 2002.

196. Abramowitz L, Sobhani I, Benifla JL, et al: Anal fissure and thrombosed external hemorrhoids before and after delivery. Dis Colon Rectum 45:650-655, 2002.

197. Friedman S: Management of inflammatory bowel disease during pregnancy and nursing. Semin Gastrointest Dis 12:245-252, 2001.

198. Alstead EM: Inflammatory disease in pregnancy. Postgrad Med J 78:23-26, 2002.

199. Dominitz JA, Young JC, Boyko EJ: Outcome of infants born to mothers with inflammatory bowel disease: A population-based cohort study. Am J Gastroenterol 97:641-648, 2002.

200. Morales M, Berney T, Jenny A, et al: Crohn's disease as a risk factor for the outcome of pregnancy. Hepatogastroenterology 47:1595-1598, 2000.

201. Ghahremani GG, Meyers MA, Farman J, et al: Ischemic disease of the small bowel and colon associated with oral contraceptives. Gastrointest Radiol 2:221-228, 1977.

202. deBree E, Schoretsanitis G, Melissas J, et al: Acute intestinal obstruction caused by endometriosis mimicking sigmoid carcinoma. Acta Gastroenterol Belg 61:376-378, 1998.

203. Bur ME, Greene GL, Press MF: Estrogen receptor localization in formalin-fixed, paraffin-embedded endometrium and endometriotic tissues. Int J Gynecol Pathol 6:140-151, 1987.

204. Bozdech JM: Endoscopic diagnosis of colonic endometriosis. Gastrointest Endosc 38:568-570, 1992.

205. Daya D, O'Connell G, DeNardi F: Rectal endometriosis mimicking solitary rectal ulcer syndrome. Mod Pathol 8:599-602, 1995.

206. Marie I, Levesque H, Ducrotte P, et al: Manometry of the upper intestinal tract in patients with systemic sclerosis: A prospective study. Arthritis Rheum 41:1874-1883, 1998.

207. Trezza M, Krogh K, Egekvist H, et al: Bowel problems in patients with systemic sclerosis. Scand J Gastroenterol 34:409-413, 1999.

208. Bassotti G, Battaglia E, Deernardi V, et al: Esophageal dysfunction in scleroderma: Relationship with disease subsets. Arthritis Rheum 40:2252-2259, 1997.

209. Govoni M, Muccinelli M, Panicali P, et al: Colon involvement in systemic sclerosis: Clinical-radiological correlations. Clin Rheumatol 15:271-276, 1996.

210. Ortiz-Alvarez O, Cabral D, Prendiville JS, et al: Intestinal pseudo-obstruction as an initial presentation of systemic sclerosis in two children. Br J Rheumatol 36:280-284, 1997.

211. Ebert EC, Ruggiero FM, Seibold JR: Intestinal perforation. A common complication of scleroderma. Dig Dis Sci 42:549-553, 1997.

212. D'Angelo WA, Fries JF, Masi AT, et al: Pathologic observations in systemic sclerosis (scleroderma). Am J Med 46:428-440, 1969.

213. Regan PT, Weiland LH, Geall MG: Scleroderma and intestinal perforation. Am J Gastroenterol 68:566-571, 1977.

214. Kleckner FS: Dermatomyositis and its manifestations in the gastrointestinal tract. Am J Gastroenterol 53:141-146, 1970.

215. Horowitz M, McNeil JD, Maddern GJ, et al: Abnormalities of gastric and esophageal emptying in polymyositis and dermatomyositis. Gastroenterology 90:434-439, 1986.

216. Ho MS, The LB, Goh HS: Ischaemic colitis in systemic lupus erythematosus—report of a case and review of the literature. Ann Acad Med Singapore 16:501-503, 1987.

217. Miyata M, Yoshida M, Saka M, et al: Protein-losing gastroenteropathy in system lupus erythematosus: Diagnosis with 99mTc-human serum albumin scintigraphy. Arthritis Rheum 43:1900, 2000.

218. Al-Hoqail I, Naddaf H, Al-Rikabi A, et al: Systemic lupus erythematosus and amyloidosis. Clin Rheum 16:422-424, 1997.

219. Marshall JB, Kretschmar JM, Gerhardt DC, et al: Gastrointestinal manifestations of mixed connective tissue disease. Gastroenterology 98:1232-1238, 1990.

220. Doria A, Bonavina L, Anselmino M, et al: Esophageal involvement in mixed connective tissue disease. J Rheumatol 18:685-690, 1991.

221. Petterson T, Wegelius O, Skrituars B: Gastrointestinal disturbances in patients with severe rheumatoid arthritis. Acta Med Scand 188:139, 1970.

222. McCurley TL, Collins RD: Intestinal infarction in rheumatoid arthritis. Three cases due to unusual obliterative vascular lesion. Arch Pathol Lab Med 108:125-128, 1984.

223. Mielants H, Veys EM, Cuvelier C, et al: The evolution of spondyloarthropathies in relation to gut histology. II. Histological aspects. J Rheumatol 22:2273-2278, 1995.

224. Mielants H, Veys EM, Cuvelier C, et al: The evolution of spondyloarthropathies in relation to gut histology. III. Relation between gut and joint. J Rheumatol 22:2279-2284, 1995.

225. Sheikh SH, Shaw-Stiffel TA: The gastrointestinal manifestations of Sjögren syndrome. Am J Gastroenterol 90:9-14, 1995.

226. Collins MH, Schwarze U, Carpentieri DF, et al: Multiple vascular and bowel ruptures in an adolescent male with sporadic Ehlers-Danlos syndrome type IV. Pediatr Dev Pathol 2:86-93, 1999.

227. Solomon JA, Abrams L, Lichtenstein GR: GI manifestations of Ehlers-Danlos syndrome. Am J Gastroenterol 91:2282-2288, 1996.

228. Fruhwirth H, Rabl H, Hauser H, et al: Endoscopic findings in pseudoxanthoma elasticum. Endoscopy 26:507, 1994.

229. Spinzi G, Strocchi E, Imperiali G, et al: Pseudoxanthoma elasticum: A rare cause of gastrointestinal bleeding. Am J Gastroenterol 91:1631-1634, 1996.

230. Bumaschny E, Doglio G, Pusajo J, et al: Postoperative acute gastrointestinal tract hemorrhage and multiple organ failure. Arch Surg 123:722-726, 1988.

231. Friedland JA, Herman TE, Siegel MJ: Escherichia coli 0157:H7-associated hemolytic uremic syndrome: Value of colonic color Doppler sonography. Pediatr Radiol 25:S65-S67, 1995.

232. Sun Cc, Hill JL, Combs JW: Hemolytic-uremic syndrome: Initial presentation mimicking intestinal intussusception. Pediatr Pathol 1:415-422, 1983.

233. Dillard RP: Hemolytic-uremic syndrome mimicking ulcerative colitis. Lack of early diagnostic laboratory findings. Clin Pediatr 22:66-67, 1983.

234. Saltzman DA, Chavers B, Brennom W, et al: Timing of colonic necrosis in hemolytic uremic syndrome. Pediatr Surg Int 13:268-270, 1998.

235. Richardson SE, Karmali MA, Becker LE, et al: The histopathology of the hemolytic uremic syndrome associated with verocytotoxin-producing Escherichia coli infections. Hum Pathol 19:1102-1108, 1988.

236. Cekin AH, Boyacioglu S, Gursoy M, et al: Gastroesophageal reflux disease in chronic renal failure patients with upper GI symptoms: Multivariate analysis of pathogenetic factors. Am J Gastroenterol 97:1352-1356, 2002.

237. Abou-Saif A, Lewis JH: Gastrointestinal and hepatic disorders in end-stage renal disease and renal transplant recipients. Adv Ren Replace Ther 7:220-230, 2000.

238. Tani N, Harasawa S, Suzuki S, et al: Lesions of the upper gastrointestinal tract in patients with chronic renal failure. Gastroenterol Jpn 15:480-484, 1980.

239. Kang JY: The gastrointestinal tract in uremia. Dig Dis Sci 38:257-268, 1993.

240. Han SY, Kwon YJ, Shin JH, et al: Nonocclusive mesenteric ischemia in a patient on maintenance hemodialysis. Korean J Intern Med 15:81-84, 2000.

241. Flobert C, Cellier C, Berger A, et al: Right colonic involvement is associated with severe forms of ischemic colitis and occurs frequently in patients with chronic renal failure requiring hemodialysis. Am J Gastroenterol 95:195-198, 2000.

242. Rubin J, Rogers WA, Taylor HM, et al: Peritonitis during continuous ambulatory peritoneal dialysis. Ann Intern Med 92:7-13, 1980.

243. Lockyer WA, Feinfeld DA, Cherubin CE, et al: An outbreak of Salmonella enteritis and septicemia in a population of uremic patients: A review of four cases, including infection of an arteriovenous fistula. Arch Intern Med 140:943-945, 1980.

244. Jimenez RE, Price DA, Pinkus GS, et al: Development of gastrointestinal beta$_2$-microglobulin amyloidosis correlates with time on dialysis. Am J Surg Pathol 22:729-735, 1998.

245. Komorowski RA, Cohen EB, Kauffman M, et al: Gastrointestinal complications in renal transplant recipients. Am J Clin Pathol 86:161-167, 1986.

246. Meyers WC, Harris N, Stein S, et al: Alimentary tract complications after renal transplantation. Ann Surg 190:535-542, 1979.

247. Shimamoto C, Hirata I, Takao Y, et al: Alteration of colonic mucin after ureterosigmoidostomy. Dis Colon Rectum 43:526-531, 2000.

248. Sterling JR, Uehling DT, Gilchrist KW: Value of colonoscopy after ureterosigmoidostomy. Surgery 96:784-790, 1984.

249. Tomasino RM, Morello V, Latteri MA, et al: Histological and histochemical changes in the colonic mucosa after ureterosigmoidostomy or colonic conduit. Eur Urol 15:248-251, 1988.

250. Kojima Y, Asaka H, Ando Y, et al: Mucosal morphological changes in ileal neobladder. Br J Urol 82:114-117, 1998.

251. Aragona F, DeCaro R, Parenti A, et al: Structural and ultrastructural changes in ileal neobladder mucosa: A 7 year follow-up. Br J Urol 81:55-61, 1998.

252. Ament ME, Ochs HD: Gastrointestinal manifestations of chronic granulomatous disease. N Engl J Med 288:382-287, 1973.

253. Griscom NT, Kirkpatrick JA, Girdany JA, et al: Gastric antral narrowing in chronic granulomatous disease of childhood. Pediatrics 54:456-460, 1974.

254. Varma VA, Sessions JT, Kahn LB, et al: Chronic granulomatous disease of childhood presenting as gastric outlet obstruction. Am J Surg Pathol 6:673-676, 1982.

255. Mitomi H, Mikami T, Takahashi H, et al: Colitis in chronic granulomatous disease resembling Crohn's disease: Comparative analysis of CD68-positive cells between two disease entities. Dig Dis Sci 44:452-456, 1999.

256. Hiller N, Fisher D, Abrohamov A, et al: Esophageal involvement in chronic granulomatous disease. Case report and review. Pediatr Radiol 25:308-309, 1995.

257. Farman J, Ramirez G, Rybak B, et al: Gastric sarcoidosis. Abdom Imaging 22:248-252, 1997.

258. Papadopoulos KI, Sjoberg K, Lindgren S, et al: Evidence of gastrointestinal immune reactivity in patients with sarcoidosis. J Intern Med 245:525-531, 1999.

259. Hogg SG: Case report: Gastric sarcoid simulating linitis plastica—a 5 year follow-up study. Clin Radiol 44:277-278, 1991.

260. Dumot JA, Adal K, Petras RE, et al: Sarcoidosis presenting as granulomatous colitis. Am J Gastroenterol 93:1949-1951, 1998.

261. Jensen RT: Gastrointestinal abnormalities and involvement in systemic mastocytosis. Hematol Oncol Clin North Am 14:579-623, 2000.

262. Libel R, Biddle WL, Miner PB: Evaluation of anorectal physiology in patients with increased mast cells. Dig Dis Sci 38:877-881, 1993.

263. Scolapio JS, Wolfe J, Malavet P, et al: Endoscopic findings in systemic mastocytosis. Gastrointest Endosc 44:608-610, 1996.

264. Ferguson J, Thompson RP, Greaves MW: Intestinal mucosal mast cells: Enumeration in urticaria pigmentosa and systemic mastocytosis. Br J Dermatol 119:573-578, 1988.

265. Abrams HL, Spiro R, Goldstein N: Metastases in carcinoma: Analysis of 1000 autopsied cases. Cancer 3:74-85, 1950.

266. Washington K, McDonagh D: Secondary tumors of the gastrointestinal tract: Surgical pathologic findings and comparison with autopsy survey. Mod Pathol 8:427-433, 1995.

267. Schuchter LM, Green R, Fraker D: Primary and metastatic diseases in malignant melanoma of the gastrointestinal tract. Curr Opin Oncol 12:181-185, 2000.

268. Ferri LE, Onerheim R, Emond C: Linitis plastica as the first indication of metastatic lobular carcinoma of the breast: Case report and literature review. Can J Surg 42:466-469, 1999.

269. Ramalingam P, Hart WR, Goldblum JR: Cytokeratin subset immunostaining in rectal adenocarcinoma and normal anal glands. Arch Pathol Lab Med 125:1074-1077, 2001.

270. Keren-Rosenberg S, Raats JI, Rapoport BL, et al: Somatostatin in the treatment of paraneoplastic diarrhoea in patients with small cell lung cancer. Ann Oncol 3:409, 1992.

271. Moskovitz DN, Robb KV: Small cell lung cancer with positive anti-Hu antibodies presenting as gastroparesis. Can J Gastroenterol 16:171-174, 2002.

272. Mignon M, Cadiot G: Natural history of gastrinoma: Lessons from the past. Dig Liver Dis 31(suppl 2):S98-S103, 1999.

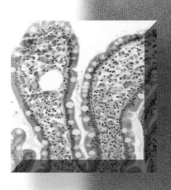

CHAPTER 6

Neuromuscular Disorders of the GI Tract

DHANPAT JAIN

Introduction

Knowledge of the basic organization of the neuromuscular apparatus of the bowel is essential if its motility disorders are to be understood. The neuromuscular organization of the bowel is similar throughout the gastrointestinal (GI) tract, with some minor variations.[1] The smooth muscle forms a superficial thin layer separating mucosa from submucosa (muscularis mucosae) and a thick outer layer (muscularis propria). The muscularis mucosae is organized into inner circular and outer longitudinal layers, except for the esophagus, which has only a single layer of longitudinal muscle coat. Identification of these two distinct layers is often difficult on routine mucosal biopsies. The muscularis propria is organized into inner circular muscle and outer longitudinal muscle layers. The proximal part of the muscularis propria of the esophagus is entirely formed by skeletal muscle that gradually merges with smooth muscle distally. Variable amounts of skeletal muscle may be seen extending into as far as the proximal half of the esophagus. As such, esophageal motility is prone to systemic disorders of both smooth and skeletal muscle.

In the stomach, an additional inner oblique muscle layer is present. The outer longitudinal layer in the colon forms localized thick bands called the *taenia coli*. The muscularis mucosae of the colon continues on into the anal canal. The inner circular layer of the rectum continues distally and becomes thickened to form the internal anal sphincter. The external anal sphincter is formed by striated muscle and is connected to the skeletal muscle of the pelvic floor. The longitudinal muscle of rectum continues between the two anal sphincters to finally break up caudally into multiple septa, which diverge fanwise throughout the subcutaneous part of the external sphincter to reach the skin; these are responsible for the characteristic corrugated appearance of the perianal skin. In addition, the fibers from the longitudinal coat and the internal sphincter extend into the submucosa to form a meshwork around the vascular plexuses (muscularis submucosa ani).

Neural Network of the Bowel

The organization of the neural network in the bowel is complex. The extrinsic nerve supply consists of both sympathetic and parasympathetic nerve fibers that eventually culminate on the intrinsic neural plexuses. The sympathetic fibers originate in the prevertebral ganglia and run along the superior and inferior mesenteric arteries. The parasympathetic fibers run in the posterior branch of the vagus nerve. Generally, the intrinsic neural system is organized into three plexuses: the submucosal plexus (Meissner's plexus), the deep submucosal plexus (Henle's plexus), and the myenteric plexus (Auerbach's plexus) (Fig. 6-1**A**). The most easily

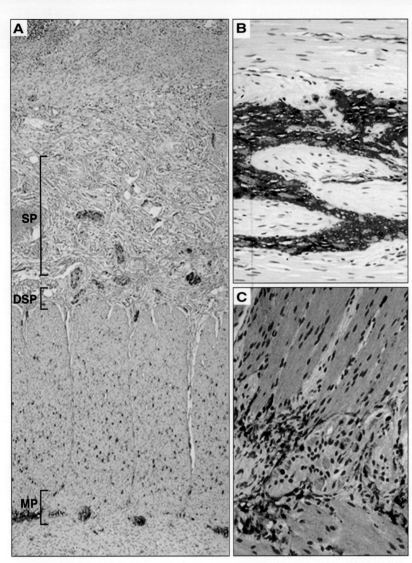

FIGURE 6–1. A, Section of normal colon showing the neural plexuses: submucosal plexus (SP), deep submucosal plexus (DSP), and myenteric plexus (MP) (S100 immunostain). **B,** A tangential section of muscularis propria showing myenteric ganglia in the complex neural network that is not evident in a well-oriented section (S100 immunostain). **C,** A section of small intestine showing interstitial cells of Cajal concentrated around the myenteric plexus and extending into the inner circular and outer longitudinal layers of muscularis propria (c-*kit* immunostain).

identified and prominent is the myenteric plexus, which is composed of clusters of ganglion cells connected by an intricate network of nerves in the space between the circular and longitudinal muscle layers. Although the ganglion cells and nerve bundles are easily identified in these plexuses, their intricate meshwork is not readily appreciated on hematoxylin and eosin–stained sections. Whole mount specimens, silver stains, and/or immuno-histochemical methods are essential for visualization of the overall neural meshwork (Fig. 6-1**B**).[2,3]

In addition to muscle fibers and the neural network, a third population of mesenchymal cells known as the interstitial cells of Cajal (ICCs) is critical for bowel motility. These cells generate a slow wave of depolar-ization and represent the pacemaker cells of bowel peristalsis.[4,5] Their function is in turn modulated by intrinsic and extrinsic neural inputs. These cells cannot be appreciated on routine sections, and most of our knowledge about their morphology and structural organization comes from painstaking ultrastructural

studies.[6-8] Ultrastructurally, these cells show partial basal lamina, many intermediate filaments, darkly staining cytoplasm, abundant rough endoplasmic reticulum, sublamellar caveolae, oval indented nuclei, and lack of myosin filaments. Many of these features overlap with those of smooth muscle cells. It has been shown that these cells express c-*kit*, a tyrosine kinase receptor.[9] Immunohistochemical stains including antibodies against c-*kit* have been used to visualize these cells.[10-12] ICCs have an intricate network and form a close liaison between the smooth muscle cells and the nerve endings. They are most easily identified around the myenteric plexus, especially in the small bowel, from which their network extends into the inner and outer muscular coats (Fig. 6-1**C**). A distinct submucosal ICC plexus has also been recognized. Structural organization of these cells has been described in various segments of the GI tract (from esophagus to anus), and minor differences in regional distribution within each segment have been described.[13]

Normal bowel motility depends on the interplay of smooth muscle, ICCs, the intrinsic and extrinsic nerve supply, and various neuroendocrine peptides. Abnormality in any of these components may result in bowel dysmotility. The clinical manifestations of these disorders vary with the extent and localization of the abnormality. Some of these disorders present with distinctive clinical features (e.g., idiopathic hypertrophic pyloric stenosis, Hirschsprung's disease, achalasia); others have nonspecific manifestations. Diagnostic workup often requires a full-thickness biopsy specimen along with electron microscopy and various special stains. Mucosal biopsies in these conditions often show nonspecific findings and are unrewarding. Pathogenesis of many of these conditions is still poorly understood, and many lack specific diagnostic histomorphology. The diagnosis of bowel motility disorders remains a challenge for both clinicians and pathologists.

Esophagus

PRIMARY ACHALASIA

Achalasia is a motor disorder of the esophagus characterized by failure of the lower esophageal sphincter to relax in response to swallowing.[14,15] It is an uncommon disorder; the overall prevalence has been estimated to be less than 10 cases/10^5 population.[16] Its incidence has been fairly static over the past 50 years. It involves both sexes equally and is primarily a disease of adults, predominantly affecting patients over 60 years of age. It is seen most frequently in North America, northwestern Europe, and Australasia, predominantly among whites.

The main pathologic feature is loss of myenteric ganglion cells. The cause of achalasia is unknown. Current data suggest that myenteric inflammation precedes the loss of ganglion cells, but the inciting events remain unknown.[17] Environmental factors, viral infection, autoimmune mechanisms, and genetic predisposition have all been implicated. There is some suggestion of familial aggregation. Rare familial forms associated with alacrima (absence of tears) and adrenocorticotropic hormone (ACTH) insensitivity are recognized (Allgrove's syndrome, or triple-A syndrome).[18,19] Occasional concordance in monozygotic twins and association with Down syndrome have also been reported. A significant association has been found with class II human leukocyte antigen (HLA) DQw1 in white patients. The alleles identified, HLA DQB1*0602, DQA1*0101, and DRB1*15, are the same alleles that have been found to be associated with a host of other autoimmune disorders, including multiple sclerosis and Goodpasture's syndrome. Further support for an autoimmune mechanism is lent by cases reported in association with

Sjögren's and Sicca syndromes, and the identification of antimyenteric neuronal antibodies in some patients.[20] Varicella-zoster viral DNA has been detected in the myenteric plexus in rare cases by in situ hybridization.[21]

The pathogenesis of this condition is also poorly understood. Progressive inflammatory destruction of myenteric ganglion cells appears to be the critical underlying event, resulting in failure of the lower esophageal sphincter to relax in response to swallowing.[22] Peristalsis in the esophageal body is also decreased or absent. This results in progressive esophageal dilatation with chronic stasis and hypertrophy of the esophageal musculature. Vasoactive intestinal polypeptide (VIP) was initially thought to be the major mediator of relaxation of the lower esophageal sphincter, and studies showed lost or decreased VIP-containing neurons in the distal esophagus.[23,24] Subsequently, it has been established that nitric oxide is the prime esophageal inhibitory neurotransmitter; it colocalizes in the same ganglion cells as VIP. In addition, it has now been shown that intrinsic nitrergic ganglion cells are lost or markedly decreased in achalasia, and that loss of VIP ganglion cells is synonymous with loss of nitrergic ganglion cells.[25,26] Most earlier studies evaluated specimens at the time of autopsy or esophagectomy; thus, the end stage of the disease was reflected. Study of esophagomyomectomy specimens lends some insight into the earlier sequence of events, although very early changes during the asymptomatic stages of the disease are largely unknown.[27] As the disease progresses, however, the inflammatory infiltrate decreases in intensity while ganglionic cell loss and myenteric plexus degeneration become more prominent.

Clinical Features

Young children (<5 years) and infants present with feeding aversion, failure to thrive, choking, recurrent pneumonia, nocturnal cough, aspiration, or nonspecific regurgitation. Older children and adults manifest with vomiting, chest pain, and dysphagia for solids and liquids. Diagnosis is confirmed with imaging studies and manometry. Barium meal typically reveals reduced peristalsis with a characteristic beaklike deformity of the distal esophagus and dilatation of the proximal esophagus. Manometry studies show abnormal peristalsis, increased intraluminal pressure, and incomplete and delayed relaxation of the lower esophageal sphincter. Endoscopy and endoscopic ultrasound are often performed to rule out coexisting mucosal pathology and to exclude secondary causes of achalasia (pseudoachalasia).

Pathologic Features

Grossly, the esophagus is dilated, and the extent of dilatation varies with the severity and the duration of the disease (Fig. 6-2**A**). It often contains stagnant and foul-smelling partially digested food. The distal end is narrowed and strictured.

The main histologic abnormality is seen in the myenteric plexus, although numerous secondary changes are seen throughout the esophageal wall, presumably secondary to prolonged stasis. Widespread near-total to total loss of myenteric ganglion cells is seen. Somewhat better preservation of the ganglion cells may be noted in the most proximal part of the esophagus.[15] Variable amounts of chronic lymphocytic infiltrate admixed with eosinophils, plasma cells, and mast cells are often seen around the myenteric nerves and the residual ganglion cells (Fig. 6-2**B**).[27] Occasionally, lymphocytes may be seen infiltrating the cytoplasm of the ganglion cells (ganglionitis). A majority of chronic inflammatory cells are CD3-positive T cells, most of which are also CD8-positive (Fig. 6-2**C**), although the relative percentage of such cells decreases with disease progression.[22] A large subset of these T cells is resting or activated cytotoxic cells.

Other changes that are frequently seen secondary to distal esophageal obstruction include muscularis propria hypertrophy, muscularis propria eosinophilia, and dystrophic calcification. The hypertrophied muscle may also show degenerative changes, including cytoplasmic vacuolation and liquefactive necrosis. The branches of the vagus nerve in the adventitia appear unremarkable in most cases, although degenerative changes in the vagus nerve and in its dorsal motor nucleus have been described.[14] It has been postulated that these may be due to infection by a neurotrophic virus; however, no specific virus has been identified so far.[28] The mucosa also shows secondary changes such as diffuse squamous hyperplasia, increased intraepithelial lymphocytes (lymphocytic esophagitis), papillomatosis, basal cell hyperplasia, and nonspecific lamina propria inflammation.[29] Some of these changes mimic reflux esophagitis, although sustained lower esophageal pressure does not allow regurgitation of gastric contents in untreated cases.[30] Following esophagomyotomy, gastroesophageal reflux develops in up to 50% of patients and can even lead to Barrett's esophagus in some cases.[31,32]

Prognosis, Treatment, and Follow-up

Achalasia is a chronic disorder, and the treatment is largely palliative. Medications are often tried, but the

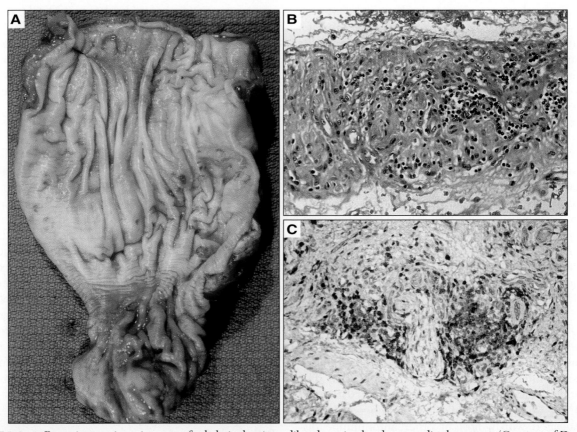

FIGURE 6–2. A, Resection specimen in a case of achalasia showing a dilated proximal and narrow distal segment. (Courtesy of Dr. Henry Appelman.) **B,** Myenteric plexus in a patient with end-stage achalasia. There are no residual ganglion cells, and chronic inflammatory cells are seen in and around a fibrotic nerve. **C,** Strong CD8 staining of lymphocytes within the myenteric plexus of a patient with end-stage achalasia.

best results are obtained with pneumatic dilatation and esophagomyotomy of the lower esophageal sphincter. Resection is reserved for end-stage cases. These patients have a long-term risk for developing squamous cell carcinoma of the esophagus[31,33] (the risk is estimated to be 33-fold higher than that in the general population).[34]

SECONDARY ACHALASIA

Signs and symptoms indistinguishable from primary achalasia may be encountered with other conditions such as Chagas' disease, or in association with a neoplasm that is caused by direct invasion of the myenteric plexus, or that occurs as a paraneoplastic phenomenon.[35,36] The malignancy most commonly associated with paraneoplastic achalasia is small cell carcinoma; however, rare associations with other tumors have also been recognized.

Chagas' disease, which is a rare cause of achalasia, results from infection with the protozoan *Trypanosoma cruzi*.[37,38] This infection is acquired through the bite of blood-sucking reduviid bugs. The geographic distribution of the disease is limited to certain parts of the world such as South or Central America and Africa. Chagas' disease is uncommon in the United States and almost exclusively occurs in immigrants from endemic countries, particularly Brazil. Any part of the GI tract may be affected; the esophagus and the sigmoid colon are the most frequently involved sites, resulting in dysmotility and often massive dilatation (e.g., mega-esophagus, megacolon). In the esophagus, symptoms closely resemble those of achalasia; colonic involvement results in constipation and intestinal pseudo-obstruction. These features are seen in the chronic phase of the disease, and by the time symptoms are noted, the organisms can no longer be demonstrated in the myenteric plexus. Histologically, cases of Chagas' disease cannot be distinguished from other causes of visceral neuropathy.

Stomach

PYLORIC STENOSIS

Infantile and adult forms of this disorder are recognized. Infants present with projectile vomiting, usually within the first 2 to 4 weeks of postnatal life.[39,40] Pyloric stenosis occurs in approximately 1 in 1000 live births, has a high familial incidence and a strong male preponderance, and classically occurs in the first-born of the family. The incidence of this condition seems to be rising in some countries (Britain and Ireland) but decreasing in others (Canada and Denmark).[41] The cause remains unclear.[42] Genetic predisposition and other environmental precipitating factors have been implicated

(e.g., bottle feeding, respiratory distress syndrome). Prenatal use of erythromycin and other macrolide antibiotics has also been implicated as a risk factor; however, the evidence is not conclusive.[43,44]

The pathogenesis of this condition also remains unclear. No evidence of a mechanical obstruction has been found, and the pylorus can be easily intubated.[45] Uncoordinated peristalsis of the stomach and the pyloric musculature (i.e., pylorospasm) has been thought to be the underlying mechanism. Other factors that may play a role include immaturity of the enteric nervous system, hormonal imbalance between gastrin and somatostatin, redundancy of the overlying mucosa, lack of c-*kit*–positive interstitial cells of Cajal, and lack of nitric oxide synthase.[46-51] Homozygous transgenic mice carrying inactivating genes for nitric oxide synthase develop hypertrophy of the pylorus.[52]

Clinical Features

Infants present with progressive nonbilious vomiting, which gradually assumes a more characteristic projectile pattern. The hypertrophied pylorus can be palpated as an olive-sized epigastric mass, and gastric peristalsis may be visible. Some patients also have a congenital diaphragmatic hernia. Idiopathic hypertrophic pyloric stenosis is uncommon in adults; most cases are secondary to scarring caused by juxtapyloric peptic ulceration or tumors.[53] The pathologic features of the adult and pediatric forms are similar.

Pathologic Features

The pylorus is greatly thickened and appears fusiform. The proximal stomach may be dilated depending on the severity and the duration of the obstruction. Microscopically, the inner circular coat of the pylorus is up to 4 times thicker than normal. Muscle fibers are disorganized with increased intercellular collagen, sometimes associated with a mild lymphocytic infiltrate. The longitudinal muscle is frequently attenuated. The enteric nerve plexus is often hypertrophied and shows a relative increase in the number of Schwann cell nuclei. Glial cells show degeneration characterized by pyknosis and vacuolation. ICCs are markedly reduced or absent in the hypertrophied circular muscle, myenteric plexus, and longitudinal muscle, as shown by c-*kit* immunostains and ultrastructure.[46] Only the inner layer of the circular muscle shows somewhat preserved ICCs.

Treatment and Follow-up

Surgical myotomy is the definitive treatment, and pyloric hypertrophy disappears within a few months after the procedure.[54] Pyloric biopsy specimens studied several months after myotomy reveal resolution of the abnormalities of the nerve fibers, glial cells, ICCs, and neuronal nitric oxide synthase[55]; long-term outcome is excellent.[56]

Small and Large Intestine

HIRSCHSPRUNG'S DISEASE

Hirschsprung's disease is a heterogeneous group of disorders characterized by lack of ganglion cells, which results in bowel obstruction.[57,58] The most common form (75% to 80% of cases) involves the distal sigmoid colon and the rectum (short-segment disease, or classic Hirschsprung's disease). In a smaller number of cases (10%), the disease extends proximally beyond the splenic flexure (long-segment disease); rarely (5%), the entire bowel is devoid of ganglion cells (total bowel aganglionosis). Zonal aganglionosis, wherein the absence of ganglion cells is patchy, is extremely rare and may result in failure of surgical correction.

Classic Hirschsprung's disease is a congenital disorder. The estimated incidence is about 1 in 5000 live births, and the disease shows a striking male preponderance (3 to 4.5:1). Rare acquired forms as well as adult cases have also been described. Long-segment disease and total bowel aganglionosis show familial aggregation; however, classic Hirschsprung's disease usually occurs as a sporadic anomaly. A large number of associated conditions have been reported, including Down syndrome, cardiovascular malformations, neurofibromatosis, Waardenburg's syndrome, Laurence-Moon-Bardet-Biedl syndrome, Ondine's curse, multiple endocrine neoplasia, and neuroblastoma; many of these are neural crest disorders (neurocristopathies).

The pathogenesis involves failure of the neural crest–derived ganglion cell precursors to appropriately migrate and colonize the bowel during embryogenesis. Mutations in at least eight different genes, which play a role in various stages of the development and migration of enteric ganglion cells, have been recognized.[57-64] Mutations of the *RET* proto-oncogene, which are the most frequent, have been identified in 20% to 25% of short-segment cases and in 40% to 70% of long-segment cases. Mutations in other genes occur in less than 10% of cases. The mode of inheritance is variable. Familial forms of long- and short-segment disease are autosomal dominant with incomplete penetrance; however, variants associated with other congenital malformations are mostly autosomal recessive. Sporadic cases are thought to have variable patterns of inheritance.

Clinical Features

The earliest and most common presentation is delayed (>48 hours) passage of meconium in the newborn. Infants and older children tend to present with chronic constipation, frequently accompanied by abdominal distention and vomiting. Diagnosis is facilitated with imaging studies and rectal manometry and is established by suction mucosal biopsy. Enterocolitis, which is commonly seen in patients with Down syndrome, is a serious and occasionally life-threatening complication.[65] The etiopathogenesis of this enterocolitis is unknown. Defects in IgA secretion and infection by toxigenic bacteria have been implicated. Histopathology reveals features of acute colitis with cryptitis, crypt abscesses, and sometimes pseudomembrane formation. Severe forms with transmural necrotizing inflammation may progress to perforation.

Pathologic Features

The colon reveals a distal narrow aperistaltic tonic segment, which is aganglionic, and a dilated proximal segment caused by obstruction (Fig. 6-3**A**). The involved segment reveals complete lack of ganglion cells in all the neural plexuses and relative hypertrophy of Schwannian nerve elements (Fig. 6-3**B**). Normally, one to five ganglion cells are found in clusters for every 1 mm of normal rectal mucosa. Ganglion cells are typically large cells with prominent nucleoli and amphophilic to basophilic cytoplasmic Nissl's granules. In newborns, the cells are often smaller, and neither the nucleoli nor the cytoplasmic granules may be prominent, making their identification sometimes difficult. Their arrangement in clusters and association with nerves facilitate recognition. In difficult cases, immunostaining with neuron-specific enolase (NSE), cathepsin D, PGP 9.5, or other neuronal markers may be helpful.[58]

Although a full-thickness transmural biopsy specimen offers better assessment of the neural plexuses because it allows visualization of the more prominent Auerbach's plexus, it requires general anesthesia, risks the development of stricture and perforation, and nowadays is largely restricted to use only in special cases. More commonly, rectal suction mucosal biopsy specimens are obtained to establish the preoperative diagnosis. The biopsy specimen should include submucosa in thickness at least equal to that of the mucosa; however, in practice, this is not always possible. In addition, ganglion cells are scattered and fewer in the submucosa. Therefore, care must be exercised, and proper protocols established at each institution should be followed before the diagnosis is made. Absence of ganglion cells in the submucosa in an adequate biopsy specimen from the rectum farther than 2 cm above the pectinate line is diagnostic of Hirschsprung's disease. Although hypertrophy of nerves by itself should not be considered sufficient evidence to establish the diagnosis, it may represent a useful clue to support this possibility. When ganglion cells are not seen in

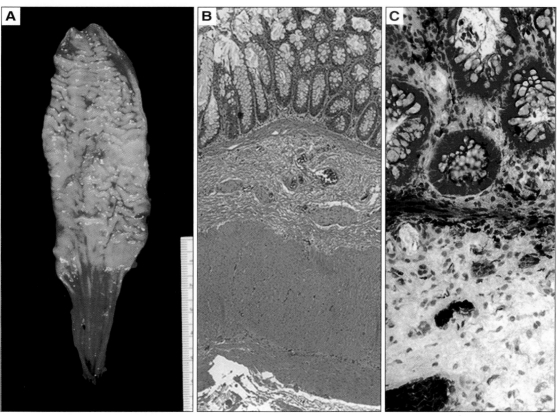

FIGURE 6–3. A, Resection specimen in a case of short-segment (classic) Hirschsprung's disease showing a dilated proximal and narrow aganglionic distal segment. **B,** Section of colon in a case of Hirschsprung's disease showing submucosal neural hyperplasia and lack of ganglion cells. **C,** Acetylcholinesterase stain performed on a frozen section of a mucosal biopsy specimen of the rectum in a case of Hirschsprung's disease showing positively stained fibers in the submucosa, muscularis mucosae, and lamina propria. The presence of acetylcholinesterase-positive fibers in the muscularis mucosae and lamina propria supports the diagnosis of Hirschsprung's disease.

adequately studied serial sections of mucosal biopsies, supportive evidence can be obtained with the use of histochemical stains for acetylcholinesterase.[66] In classic cases, acetylcholinesterase-positive nerve fibers are seen in the muscularis mucosae, as well as in the lamina propria; these are lacking in biopsy specimens from normal individuals (Fig. 6-3**C**). Such fibers are few and difficult to demonstrate in newborns with Hirschsprung's disease and tend to increase with age. Abnormalities of ICCs have also been shown in some studies; however, it appears that this change is secondary to the absence of ganglion cells and is of little diagnostic use.[67,68]

Preoperative biopsies are performed to establish the diagnosis before corrective surgery is planned, and each laboratory should establish a protocol for handling such cases. Ideally, a specimen should be kept frozen and stained for acetylcholinesterase when indicated. Multiple serial sections must be examined before a definitive diagnosis is rendered. The presence of ganglion cells in a colonic biopsy specimen rules out the possibility of conventional Hirschsprung's disease. The 2 cm of rectum immediately above the pectinate line normally has a paucity of ganglion cells with prominent nerve fibers, which may lead to erroneous diagnosis of Hirschsprung's disease. The biopsy specimen in such a situation may reveal a transitional type of epithelium, indicating proximity to the pectinate line; the presence of this epithelium should be specifically mentioned in the report.

Treatment and Follow-up

Treatment involves surgical resection of the involved segment followed by restoration of bowel continuity. This may be performed as a one stage "endorectal pullthrough" procedure, or it may occur in two stages whereby definitive anastomosis is performed following initial colostomy. Biopsy specimens (full-thickness) are often obtained for intraoperative frozen sections to establish the presence of ganglion cells in the segments before completion of the anastomosis, as well as to confirm the lack of ganglion cells in the affected segment. Frozen sections performed for the evaluation of ganglion cells are not without problems and should not replace a preoperative suction mucosal biopsy before the corrective procedure is attempted.[69] At the time of frozen section, toluidine blue, Giemsa, or Diff-Quik stain, in addition to routine stain, may aid in the identification of ganglion cells. The prognosis for surgically treated patients is satisfactory, and most are able to achieve continence.

OTHER DEVELOPMENTAL DISORDERS OF THE ENTERIC NERVOUS SYSTEM

This heterogeneous group includes hypoganglionosis, hyperganglionosis, and abnormal differentiation of ganglion cells. Enteric ganglions may also be involved secondarily by systemic metabolic defects such as lysosomal storage disorders. Neuropathic forms of familial intestinal pseudo-obstruction (discussed later) may be considered another form of developmental abnormality that falls into this category.

Clinically, these disorders resemble Hirschsprung's disease; histology fails to establish aganglionosis, although the acetylcholinesterase stain may mimic the pattern of Hirschsprung's disease. Although diagnostic criteria for aganglionosis (Hirschsprung's disease) are well established, objective criteria needed to define and diagnose other enteric dysganglionoses are poorly defined and often impractical to apply.[70-72] This has resulted in the use of many different terminologies such as "variant Hirschsprung's disease," "pseudo-Hirschsprung's disease," or "Hirschsprung's disease allied disorders."

Hypoganglionosis refers to reduced numbers of ganglia in the neural plexuses, decreased numbers of ganglion cells per ganglion, and ganglia of smaller size.[73] This condition may exist in variable lengths of colon in association with Hirschsprung's disease or as an isolated primary condition that leads to intestinal pseudo-obstruction.

Hyperganglionosis is characterized by increased numbers of ganglion cells or the presence of ectopic ganglia in the lamina propria. Ectopic ganglion cells in the lamina propria are associated with nodular proliferations of ganglion cells (ganglioneuroma), which may occur as a localized lesion or a diffuse condition (ganglioneuromatosis). Diffuse ganglioneuromatosis is almost always associated with multiple endocrine neoplasia (MEN IIB) and mutation in the *RET* proto-oncogene. Intestinal neuronal dysplasia, a controversial entity, shows marked neural hypertrophy and the presence of increased numbers of large ganglion cells in the neural plexuses.[71,74]

It should be recognized that ganglion cell density varies with age, site, and stretching of the tissues during processing. Subtle numeric alterations of ganglion cells are almost impossible to diagnose on routine suction mucosal biopsy. Quantitation of neural plexuses, neural and glial stroma, and ganglion cells is extremely difficult, even on conventionally oriented transmural biopsies. Alterations in specific subtypes of ganglion cells can be resolved only with special staining and electrophysiologic studies.[3] It is likely that underlying the subtle morphologic alteration of ganglion cells may be more marked functional changes that are not evident on routine studies, as was shown in a recent study revealing increased nitric oxide synthase–producing ganglion cells in cases of intestinal neuronal dysplasia.[75] Study of whole-mount sections along with application of special stains has been advocated to better characterize such lesions.

INTESTINAL PSEUDO-OBSTRUCTION

Intestinal pseudo-obstruction is a clinical syndrome caused by inability of the bowel to propel its contents in the absence of a mechanical obstruction. Both acute and chronic forms are recognized.

Acute Intestinal Pseudo-obstruction

PARALYTIC ILEUS

Paralytic ileus is the most common cause of intestinal pseudo-obstruction and generally occurs after abdominal surgery, abdominal trauma, or peritonitis. The entire bowel becomes paralyzed and distended. The diagnosis is made on clinical grounds, and treatment is supportive. No specific histopathologic changes are recognized.

ACUTE IDIOPATHIC INTESTINAL PSEUDO-OBSTRUCTION (OGILVIE'S SYNDROME)

This is a rare and potentially serious development in patients who have just undergone surgery or are ill from other causes.[76] Etiopathogenesis is poorly understood, although temporary autonomic dysfunction is suspected. Patients demonstrate bowel dilatation, most often confined to the right colon, which may lead to transmural ischemia and perforation, most frequently in the cecum. Histopathologic changes are nonspecific and mimic ischemia secondary to increased intramural pressure. The condition in most instances resolves with supportive care.

Chronic Intestinal Pseudo-obstruction

Chronic intestinal pseudo-obstruction is caused by a large number of disorders that may affect various components of the bowel neuromuscular apparatus.[77,78] It most commonly involves the small intestine and/or colon. It may primarily involve the bowel (idiopathic) (Table 6-1)or may be part of a generalized or systemic disorder (secondary) (Table 6-2).

CLINICAL FEATURES

Many of the clinical features of chronic intestinal pseudo-obstruction are common to different subtypes. In most cases, particularly the familial ones, symptoms

TABLE 6–1. Chronic Idiopathic Intestinal Pseudo-obstruction

Myopathic Forms
A. Familial visceral myopathy
  1. Autosomal dominant (type I)
  2. Autosomal recessive (type II)
  3. Autosomal recessive (type III)
  4. Autosomal recessive (type IV)
B. Sporadic visceral myopathy
  1. Degenerative noninflammatory leiomyopathy
    a) Sporadic degenerative noninflammatory leiomyopathy
    b) Nonfamilial South African leiomyopathy
  2. Degenerative inflammatory leiomyopathy
Neuropathic Forms
A. Familial visceral neuropathies
  1. Autosomal recessive
  2. Autosomal recessive with neuronal intranuclear inclusions
  3. Autosomal dominant
  4. X-linked
B. Sporadic visceral neuropathies
  1. Degenerative noninflammatory
  2. Degenerative inflammatory
C. Developmental abnormalities
  1. Hirschsprung's disease
    a) Classic or short-segment disease
    b) Ultra-short-segment disease
    c) Long-segment disease
    d) Total bowel aganglionosis
    e) Zonal aganglionosis
  2. Hirschsprung's disease/allied disorders (pseudo-Hirschsprung's disease)
    a) Hypoganglionosis
    b) Hyperganglionosis
      i) Ganglioneuromatosis
      ii) Intestinal neuronal dysplasia
Disorders of Interstitial Cells of Cajal
  1. With visceral myopathy–type changes
  2. Without other significant pathologic changes
Disorders of Neurohormonal Peptides

TABLE 6–2. Secondary Chronic Intestinal Pseudo-obstruction

A. Systemic disorders
  1. Progressive systemic sclerosis/polymyositis
  2. Systemic lupus erythematosus
  3. Progressive muscular dystrophy
  4. Myotonic dystrophy
  5. Fabry's disease
  6. Parkinson's disease
  7. Multiple sclerosis
B. Endocrine and metabolic disorders
  1. Diabetes mellitus
  2. Hypothyroidism
  3. Hypoparathyroidism
  4. Pheochromocytoma
  5. Acute intermittent porphyria
C. Infiltrative disorders
  1. Amyloidosis
  2. Diffuse lymphoid infiltration
  3. Eosinophilic gastroenteritis
D. Paraneoplastic disorders
  1. Small cell carcinoma
  2. Others
E. Infections
  1. *Trypanosoma cruzi* (Chagas' disease)
  2. Herpesvirus
  3. Cytomegalovirus
  4. Epstein-Barr virus
  5. Lyme disease
F. Miscellaneous conditions
  1. Ceroidosis (brown bowel syndrome)
  2. Small intestinal diverticulosis
  3. Radiation enteritis
  4. Jejunoileal bypass
G. Toxins and pharmacologic agents
  1. Tricyclic antidepressants
  2. Phenothiazines
  3. Ganglionic blockers
  4. Clonidine
  5. Anti-Parkinson's medication
  6. Opiates (narcotic bowel syndrome)
  7. *Amanita phalloides* toxin

begin in childhood. Some patients remain asymptomatic until middle age, and others are entirely asymptomatic. Symptoms are typical of intestinal obstruction with abdominal distention, pain, and vomiting. The distention can be gradual and may become severe, especially when both the small intestine and the colon are involved. Generally, these patients have alternating diarrhea and constipation rather than obstipation. Diarrhea is generally secondary to bacterial overgrowth due to stasis and may result in substantial weight loss. Perforation rarely occurs.

CATEGORIES

PRIMARY (IDIOPATHIC) CHRONIC INTESTINAL PSEUDO-OBSTRUCTION

Among the idiopathic cases, four major categories have been recognized—those with abnormalities of the smooth muscle (myopathic form), those with abnormalities of the neural system (neuropathic form), those with ICC abnormalities, and those with abnormalities of neurohormonal peptides.

Myopathic Forms. Both familial and sporadic myopathic forms are recognized.[77] Care must be exercised before a case is considered to be sporadic because involved family members may be asymptomatic, and a reliable family history may be difficult to elicit. Familial visceral myopathy may also involve other organs (urinary bladder or biliary tract) and has been called "hollow visceral myopathy." Type I is the most common and is characterized by redundant colon, esophageal dilatation, megaduodenum, megacystis, and sometimes uterine inertia. Type II tends to show gastric dilatation, slight small intestinal dilatation often with formation of diverticula, ptosis, and external ophthalmoplegia. In type III, the entire GI tract from esophagus to rectum may be involved and show marked dilatation. Type IV is characterized by gastroparesis, tubular narrow small intestine, normal esophagus, and normal colon.[79] In general, sporadic cases resemble the autosomal recessive familial type III visceral myopathy.

Although smooth muscle degeneration is thought to be responsible for bowel dysmotility, the etiopathogenesis for most of these cases remains obscure. Rare cases with actin or desmin abnormalities have been described.[80,81] In cases of desmin myopathy, systemic skeletal and cardiac muscle involvement is also noted. Rare cases show a T-cell–rich inflammatory leiomyositis and are possibly autoimmune.[82] A distinct type of nonfamilial visceral myopathy has been described in young children from southern, central, and eastern Africa (African visceral leiomyopathy).[83] In some cases, absence of c-*kit*–positive ICC has been thought to be the underlying mechanism[84] (see later). It is likely that this is a heterogeneous group of disorders, and many of the histologic changes likely represent end-stage disease. Many cases probably go unrecognized, and the spectrum of these disorders may be even wider than is now known.

Pathologic Features. The involved segment is often dilated, and the bowel wall may appear thick, normal, or thin, depending on the degree of distention (Fig. 6-4). Although initially no mucosal pathology is noted, inflammation, ulceration, and ischemia may supervene secondary to stasis and extensive dilatation.

Microscopy reveals degeneration and fibrous replacement of the smooth muscle. Degenerative changes are most prominent in the muscularis propria, but they also affect the muscularis mucosae and may be identified in a mucosal biopsy specimen. The longitudinal layer tends to be more severely involved; in some cases, only the circular layer is involved. Muscle degeneration results in fibrosis, cytoplasmic vacuolation, variation in muscle fiber size, and thinning of the bowel wall (Fig. 6-

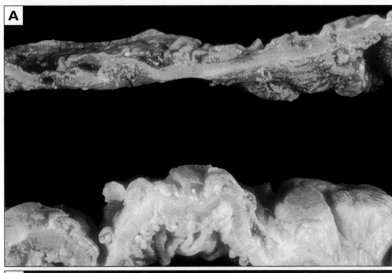

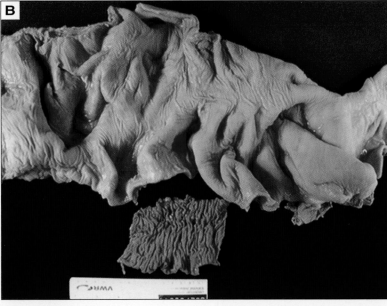

FIGURE 6–4. **A,** Resection specimen of colon in a case of visceral myopathy showing thinning of the wall (*upper segment*) and thickening of the muscle (*lower segment*) in the same case. **B,** Resection specimen of colon in a case of visceral myopathy showing massively dilated colon with flattening of the mucosal folds and a thick wall. A short segment of normal colon has been placed by the side of a dilated colon for comparison.

5**A** and **C**). Fibrosis may be subtle and may require a trichrome stain to be appreciated (Fig. 6-5**B** and **D**). Other changes include nuclear atypia, increased mitotic activity, and periodic acid–Schiff (PAS)-positive intracytoplasmic inclusions. Ultrastructurally, these cytoplasmic inclusions represent aggregates of degenerated myofibrils. However, one must be wary of artifactual changes in the muscle commonly seen in surgical specimens. Rare cases with deficient smooth muscle α-actin show absence of staining with smooth muscle actin antibodies, particularly in the inner circular muscle layer (Fig. 6-6).[51] Electron microscopy shows nonspecific degenerative changes that include mitochondrial vacuolation and may be the only diagnostic evidence of myopathy when light microscopy is normal.

Neuropathic Forms. This group includes patients with abnormalities of the intrinsic or extrinsic neural network of the bowel in both sporadic and familial forms.[77] The mode of inheritance may be autosomal dominant, autosomal recessive, or, rarely, X-linked. Autosomal recessive cases tend to show intranuclear inclusions in ganglion cells; some are characterized by mental retardation and basal ganglia calcification. The autosomal dominant variant does not show any extraintestinal manifestations. The X-linked form is associated with short small intestine, malrotation, and pyloric hypertrophy.[85]

The etiopathogenesis of the neurodegenerative changes remains obscure. Several pathogenetic mechanisms may be involved, including altered calcium signaling, mitochondrial dysfunction, and free radical injury.[86] Rare autosomal recessive cases present with a progressive multisystem neurodegenerative disorder and reveal abnormalities in the mitochondrial DNA.[87] Decreased ganglion cell survival may be a factor in some cases, as is suggested by decreased *BCL2* gene product in the enteric ganglion cells.[88] Some cases reveal inflammatory neuronal degeneration, which suggests an autoimmune or infectious cause[89]; neuronal autoantibodies are found in some patients.[90]

Pathologic Features. Gross findings are similar to those of other forms of intestinal pseudo-obstruction and do not help to differentiate the various subtypes. Examination of routine sections is often unrevealing except in cases in which neurons appear to be markedly decreased in numbers, or when cytomegalovirus-like

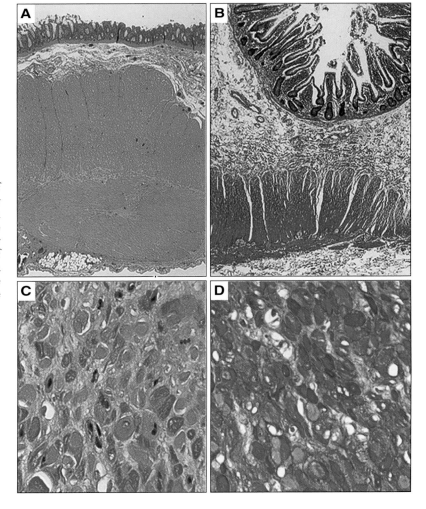

FIGURE 6–5. A, Low-power view of a case of visceral myopathy showing marked hypertrophy of both layers of muscularis propria. **B,** A section of small intestine shows delicate interstitial fibrosis in a case of visceral myopathy (trichrome stain). **C,** Higher magnification of the smooth muscle in the muscularis propria showing degenerative changes. **D,** Same case showing moderate interstitial fibrosis (trichrome stain).

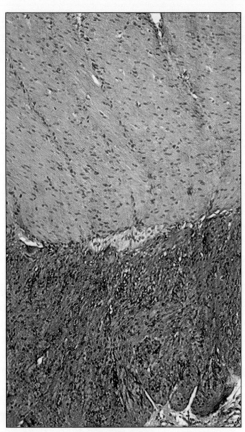

FIGURE 6–6. Immunostain for smooth muscle actin in a case of visceral myopathy showing lack of staining in the inner circular layer; the outer longitudinal layer appears normal.

(CMV-like) intranuclear inclusions can be identified in the neurons.[91] Electron microscopy reveals these inclusions to be proteinic material composed of curving filaments and not viral particles. In addition, subtle degenerative changes in the neurons and abnormal dendritic processes are identified. These changes are best appreciated with silver stains on thick en-face/tangential embedded sections of bowel or whole-mount preparations. Silver stains also help in identification of abnormalities of argyrophobic and argyrophilic ganglion cell populations. However, limited experience with these conditions, the necessity of employing fastidious neuron-counting techniques, and tedious silver stains have limited the study of such cases to a few specialized centers.

ICC Abnormalities. Recent insight into the role of ICCs in bowel motility and their putative role as the pacemaker cells of the bowel has led to speculation that they may play a role in chronic idiopathic intestinal pseudo-obstruction. Steel mutant mice, which lack c-*kit*–positive ICCs, show marked constipation and features suggestive of chronic intestinal pseudo-obstruction.[92,93] Also, blockade of the c-*kit* receptor results in severe disturbance of bowel motility.[94] Piebaldism in humans, a condition associated with inactivation of c-*kit* mutations, is associated with life-

long constipation.[95,96] It has recently been shown that some cases of intestinal pseudo-obstruction show near-total to total loss of c-*kit*–positive ICCs.[84,97-99]

Pathology. Routine stains may show changes typical of visceral myopathy, but some cases do not reveal any obvious histopathologic changes (Fig. 6-7). Immunohistochemistry reveals near-total to total loss of c-*kit*–positive ICCs in the involved segment (small bowel and/or colon).

Neurohormonal Peptide Abnormalities. This ill-defined group includes cases of neuroblastoma and ganglioneuroblastoma associated with chronic intestinal pseudo-obstruction.[100,101] Tumor resection results in resolution of the pseudo-obstruction. VIP produced by the tumors has been implicated as the cause of the intestinal dysmotility.

SECONDARY CHRONIC INTESTINAL PSEUDO-OBSTRUCTION

Systemic Disorders. Patients with scleroderma or progressive systemic sclerosis may have significant involvement of the bowel; the result of this is severe motility problems that often require surgical resection.[102]

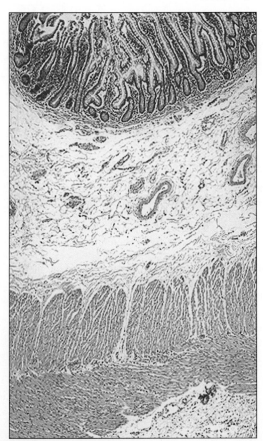

FIGURE 6–7. A case of chronic idiopathic intestinal pseudo-obstruction with no significant histopathologic changes, showing total absence of interstitial cells of Cajal in a section of the small intestine (c-*kit* immunostain).

Clinically, esophageal involvement often predominates. The inner circular layer is often preferentially involved, in contrast to primary visceral myopathy. In scleroderma, collagenous replacement of the muscle layer tends to be nearly complete, unlike the delicate interstitial fibrosis of primary visceral myopathy. Fibrosis may cause wall weakness, resulting in diverticula with squared-mouth ostia. Mucosal changes are nonspecific and are secondary to the underlying motility problem (e.g., reflux esophagitis and villous blunting due to bacterial overgrowth in the small bowel).

Pseudo-obstruction with muscle damage may occur in patients with dermatomyositis/polymyositis, systemic lupus erythematosus, myotonic dystrophy, and progressive muscular dystrophy.[102-105] Amyloid deposition in the muscularis propria (myopathy) or myenteric plexus (neuropathy) may uncommonly present with intestinal pseudo-obstruction. AA-type amyloid is often deposited in the myenteric plexus; AL-type amyloid is more often deposited in the muscularis propria.[106]

Parkinson's disease, familial autonomic dysfunction, and Shy-Drager syndrome may be associated with dysmotility, but no specific pathologic changes are identified. Diffuse polyclonal lymphoid infiltration of the small intestine is another rare condition of uncertain etiopathogenesis.[107] Intestinal pseudo-obstruction may occur with hypoparathyroidism, hypothyroidism, and pheochromocytoma. However, diabetes is by far the most common endocrine disorder associated with bowel dysmotility and may result from autonomic dysfunction, electrolyte abnormalities, and vasculopathy. Eosinophilic gastroenteritis and radiation enteritis may also result in intestinal pseudo-obstruction. Destruction of ganglion cells as a paraneoplastic syndrome has been well described with small cell carcinoma of the lung and rarely with other tumors.[108-110] In such cases, neuronal autoantibodies have been detected, and ganglionic destruction is likely to be immune mediated.

Drugs and Toxins. A variety of pharmacologic agents (e.g., phenothiazines, tricyclic antidepressants, ganglionic blockers, clonidine, and antiparkinsonian medication) have marked effects on bowel motility, and their use (or the presence of naturally occurring toxins such as *Amanita phalloides*) may result in intestinal pseudo-obstruction.

Infections. Viral infection, particularly infection with the herpes group of viruses, has been associated with systemic autoimmune disturbances and bowel dysmotility. Visceral involvement concurrent with varicella-zoster cutaneous involvement has been shown to result in dysmotility of the stomach, small intestine, colon, and anus.[111,112] Bowel dysfunction resolves with improvement in the cutaneous disease. CMV infection has also been implicated in intestinal pseudo-obstruction, especially in immunocompromised individuals.[113,114] In some cases, evidence of Epstein-Barr virus (EBV)

infection has been demonstrated by polymerase chain reaction (PCR) and in situ hybridization studies of the myenteric plexus.[115] Histologically, the only clues may be the presence of inflammatory cells around the ganglia and myenteric plexus, or typical viral inclusions in the ganglion cells. Lyme disease and Chagas' disease may involve the small and/or large intestine, resulting in intestinal pseudo-obstruction.[38,116]

Miscellaneous Conditions

Ceroidosis (Brown Bowel Syndrome). This condition is characterized by deposition of light brown, granular, lipofuscin-like pigment within the smooth muscle cells of the muscularis mucosae and/or the muscularis propria of any bowel segment.[117,118] Ultrastructurally, this granular, electron-dense material contains myelin figures and abnormal distorted mitochondria. Ceroidosis has been seen in many processes associated with malabsorption, including celiac disease, Whipple's disease, and chronic pancreatitis; vitamin E deficiency has been implicated as the underlying factor. It is unclear whether this is a purely nonspecific morphologic marker of a systemic disease or represents a primary smooth muscle disorder.

Irritable Bowel Syndrome. Irritable bowel syndrome is a common disorder of uncertain etiopathogenesis most commonly affecting adult females. Symptoms include any combination of diarrhea, constipation, bloating, and abdominal pain. Disturbance of bowel motility and enhanced visceral sensitivity have been implicated. Colonoscopy is normal, and biopsies do not show any pathologic abnormalities.

Small Bowel Diverticulosis. The most common types of small bowel diverticula are congenital and include Meckel's diverticulum and duodenal diverticulosis. Less commonly, acquired cases of small bowel diverticulosis are encountered secondary to bowel neuromuscular abnormalities.[119] Diverticula result from mucosal outpouchings secondary to fibrosis-induced mural weakness. In cases with scleroderma-like morphologic changes, Raynaud's phenomenon is frequently present, although clinical scleroderma is not evident. Some cases appear to be related to known neurologic disease processes such as Fabry's disease.

Severe Idiopathic Constipation (Slow Transit Constipation, Arbuthnot Lane's Disease). This condition, which is characterized by chronic constipation resulting from reduced colonic propulsive capacity,[120,121] most commonly affects young women. Onset of the disease may be seen in early childhood or late in life. Symptoms persist despite the use of laxatives, and melanosis coli is a common histologic finding. Such cases have often been labeled "cathartic colons"; whether laxative abuse is the underlying cause remains a question. In severe and resistant cases, colectomy may have to be performed. This disorder likely represents a heterogeneous group that comprises myopathic, neuropathic, and ICC abnormalities. Decreased numbers of ganglion cells, intraganglionic neurofilaments, and ICCs have been described.[120,122,123] Amphophilic, hyaline, and round to ovoid (4 to 22 mm) cytoplasmic inclusions of unclear composition may be found in smooth muscle cells.[124] These inclusions appear to be nonspecific and can be identified in normal colon and small bowel, as well as in Chagas' disease.

PROGNOSIS AND THERAPY

Primary intestinal pseudo-obstruction that presents in adulthood usually has a prolonged course of 20 to 30 years; infants and children, however, tend to have a poorer prognosis and die at a young age. Treatment is symptomatic and supportive because no specific and effective therapy is known to date. Surgical resection may be undertaken in resistant cases, and a good outcome is expected in those cases with limited bowel involvement. However, substantial resection of small and/or large bowel may be required, resulting in total parenteral nutrition dependence.

Prognosis and treatment of secondary intestinal pseudo-obstruction vary according to the underlying condition. Patients with progressive systemic sclerosis often die within 5 to 10 years secondary to renal, cardiac, or pulmonary complications. Patients with small cell carcinoma usually die within a year of extraintestinal manifestations. Cases associated with viral infection are generally self-limited; intestinal pseudo-obstruction in cases associated with systemic disease such as systemic lupus erythematosus or amyloidosis generally follows the course of the underlying disease.

References

1. Sternberg SS: Histology for Pathologists, 2nd ed. New York, Lippincott-Raven, 1997, pp 461-571.
2. Nemeth L, Yoneda A, Kader M, et al: Three-dimensional morphology of gut innervation in total intestinal aganglionosis using whole-mount preparation. J Pediatr Surg 36:291-295, 2001.
3. Krisnamurthy S, Heng Y, Schuffler MD: Chronic intestinal pseudo-obstruction in infants and children caused by diverse abnormalities of the myenteric plexus. Gastroenterology 104:1398-1408, 1993.
4. Thuneberg L: Interstitial cells of Cajal: Intestinal pacemaker cells. Adv Anat Embryol Cell Biol 71:1-130, 1982.
5. Rumessen JJ, Thuneberg L: Pacemaker cells in the gastrointestinal tract: Interstitial cells of Cajal. Scand J Gastroenterol 216:82-94, 1996.
6. Faussone-Pellegrini MS, Pantalone D, Cortesini C: Smooth muscle cells, interstitial cells of Cajal and myenteric plexus interrelationship in the human colon. Acta Anat (Basel) 139:31-44, 1990.
7. Rumessen JJ, Mikkelsen B, Qvortrup K, et al: Ultrastructure of interstitial cells of Cajal in circular muscle of human small intestine. Gastroenterology 104:343-350, 1993.
8. Rumessen JJ, Peters S, Thuneberg L: Light- and electron microscopical studies of interstitial cells of Cajal and muscle cells at the submucosal border of human colon. Lab Invest 68:481-495, 1993.
9. Maeda H, Yamagata A, Nishikawa S, et al: Requirement of c-kit for development of intestinal pacemaker system. Development 116:369-375, 1992.
10. Hagger R, Gharaie S, Finlayson C, et al: Distribution of the interstitial cells of Cajal in the human anorectum. J Auton Nerv Syst 73:75-79, 1998.
11. Romert P, Mikkelsen HB: C-kit immunoreactive interstitial cells of Cajal in the human small and large intestine. Histochem Cell Biol 109:195-202, 1998.
12. Wester T, Eriksson L, Olsson Y, et al: Interstitial cells of Cajal in the human fetal small bowel as shown by c-kit immunohistochemistry. Gut 44:65-71, 1999.
13. Vanderwinden JM, Rumessen JJ: Interstitial cells of Cajal in human gut and gastrointestinal disease. Microsc Res Tech 47:344-360, 1999.
14. Casella RR, Brown AL, Sayre GP, et al: Achalasia of the esophagus; pathologic and etiologic considerations. Ann Surg 160:474-486, 1964.
15. Goldblum JR, Whyte RI, Orringer MB, et al: Achalasia: A morphologic study of 42 resected specimens. Am J Surg Pathol 18:327-337, 1994.
16. Mayberry JF: Epidemiology and demographics of achalasia. Gastrointest Endosc Clin N Am 11:235-248, 2001.
17. Paterson WG: Etiology and pathogenesis of achalasia. Gastrointest Endosc Clin N Am 11:249-265, 2001.
18. Allgrove J, Clayden GS, Grant DB, et al: Familial glucocorticoid deficiency with achalasia of the cardia and deficient tear production. Lancet 1:1284-1286, 1978.
19. Dugardeyn C, Anooshiravani M, Christophe C, et al: Achalasia-alacrima-ACTH insensitivity syndrome (triple A-syndrome). J Belge Radiol 76:167-168, 1993.
20. Verne GN, Sallusito JE, Eaker EY: Anti-myenteric neuronal antibodies in patients with achalasia: A prospective study. Dig Dis Sci 42:307-313, 1997.
21. Robertson CS, Martin BAB, Atkinson M: Varicella-zoster virus DNA in the oesophageal myenteric plexus in achalasia. Gut 34:299-302,1993.
22. Clark SB, Rice TW, Tubbs RR, et al: The nature of the myenteric infiltrate in achalasia. An immunohistochemical analysis. Am J Surg Pathol 24:1153-1158, 2000.
23. Uddman R, Alumets J, Edvinsson L, et al: Peptidergic (VIP) innervation of the esophagus. Gastroenterology 75:5-8, 1978.
24. Aggestrup S, Uddman R, Sundler F, et al: Lack of vasoactive intestinal polypeptide nerves in esophageal achalasia. Gastroenterology 84:924-927, 1983.
25. De Giorgio R, Di Simone MP, Stanghellini V, et al: Esophageal and gastric nitric oxide synthesizing innervation in primary achalasia. Am J Gastroenterol 94:2357-2362, 1999.
26. Mearin F, Mourelle M, Guarner F, et al: Patients with achalasia lack nitric oxide synthase in the gastro-oesophageal junction. Eur J Clin Invest 23:724-728, 1993.
27. Goldblum JR, Rice TW, Richter JE: Histopathologic features in esophagomyotomy specimens from patients with achalasia. Gastroenterology 111:648-654, 1996.
28. Birgisson S, Galinski MS, Goldblum JR, et al: Achalasia is not associated with measles or known herpes and human papilloma viruses. Dig Dis Sci 42:300-306, 1997.
29. Lehman MB, Clark SB, Ormsby AH, et al: Squamous mucosal alterations in esophagectomy specimens from patients with end-stage achalasia. Am J Surg Pathol 25:1413-1418, 2001.
30. Csendes A: Results of surgical treatment of achalasia of the esophagus. Hepatogastroenterology 38:474-480, 1991.
31. Peracchia A, Segalin A, Bardini R, et al: Esophageal carcinoma and achalasia. Prevalence, incidence and results of treatment. Hepatogastroenterology 38:514-516, 1991.
32. Jamieson GG: Gastro-esophageal reflux following myotomy for achalasia. Hepatogastroenterology 38:506-509, 1991.
33. Fagge CH: A case of simple stenosis of the esophagus, followed by epithelioma. Guy's Hosp Rep 17:413-415, 1872.
34. Meijssen MA, Tilanus HW, van Vlankenstein M, et al: Achalasia complicated by oesophageal squamous cell carcinoma. A prospective study in 195 patients. Gut 33:155-158, 1992.
35. Kahrilas PJ, Kishk SM, Helm JF, et al: Comparison of pseudo-achalasia and achalasia. Am J Med 82:439-446, 1987.
36. Liu W, Fackler W, Rice TW, et al: The pathogenesis of pseudo-achalasia: A clinicopathologic study of 13 cases of a rare entity. Am J Surg Pathol. 26:784-788, 2002.
37. Koberle F: Chagas' disease and Chagas' syndromes: The pathology of American trypanosomiasis. Adv Parasitol 6:63-116, 1968.
38. Pinotti HW, Felix VN, Zilberstein B, et al: Surgical complications of Chagas' disease: Megaesophagus, achalasia of the pylorus and cholelithiasis. World J Surg 15:198-204, 1991.

39. Rollins MD, Shields MD, Quinn RJ, et al: Pyloric stenosis: Congenital or acquired? Arch Dis Child 64:138-139, 1989.

40. Mitchell LE, Risch N: The genetics of infantile hypertrophic pyloric stenosis. A reanalysis. Am J Dis Child 147:1203-1211, 1993.

41. Nielsen JP, Haahr P, Haahr J: Infantile hypertrophic pyloric stenosis. Decreasing incidence. Dan Med Bull 47:223-225, 2000.

42. Rogers IM: The enigma of pyloric stenosis. Some thoughts on the etiology. Acta Paediatr 86:6-9, 1997.

43. Cooper WO, Ray WA, Griffin MR: Prenatal prescription of macrolide antibiotics and infantile hypertrophic pyloric stenosis. Obstet Gynecol 100:101-106, 2002.

44. Cooper WO, Griffin MR, Arbogast P, et al: Very early exposure of erythromycin and infantile hypertrophic pyloric stenosis. Arch Pediatr Adolesc Med 156:647-650, 2002.

45. Yamashiro Y, Mayama H, Yamamoto K, et al: Conservative management of infantile pyloric stenosis by nasoduodenal feeding. Eur J Pediatr 136:187-192, 1981.

46. Vanderwinden JM, Lui H, De Laet MH, et al: Study of the interstitial cells of Cajal in infantile hypertrophic pyloric stenosis. Gastroenterology 111:279-288, 1996.

47. Guarino N, Shima H, Puri P: Structural immaturity of the pylorus muscle in infantile hypertrophic pyloric stenosis. Pediatr Surg Int 16:282-284, 2000.

48. Hernanz-Schulman M, Lowe LH, Johnson J, et al: In vivo visualization of pyloric mucosal hypertrophy in infants with hypertrophic pyloric stenosis: Is there an etiologic role? Am J Roentgenol 177:843-848, 2001.

49. Dick AC, Ardill J, Potts SR, et al: Gastrin, somatostatin and infantile hypertrophic pyloric stenosis. Acta Paediatr 90:879-882, 2001.

50. Guarino N, Shima H, Oue T, et al: Glial-derived growth factor signaling pathway in infantile hypertrophic pyloric stenosis. J Pediatr Surg 36:1468-1469, 2001.

51. Vanderwinden JM, Mailleux P, Schiffmann SNA, et al: Nitric oxide synthase activity in infantile hypertrophic pyloric stenosis. N Engl J Med 327:511-515, 1992.

52. Huang PL, Dawson TM, Bredt DS, et al: Targeted disruption of the neuronal nitric oxide synthase gene. Cell 75:1273-1286, 1993.

53. Wellman KF, Kagan A, Fang H: Hypertrophic pyloric stenosis in adults. Survey of the literature and report of a case of the localized form. Gastroenterology 46:601-608, 1964.

54. Okorie NM, Dickson JA, Carver RA, et al: What happens to the pylorus after pyloromyotomy? Arch Dis Child 63:1339-1341, 1988.

55. Vanderwinden JM, Liu H, Menu R, et al: The pathology of infantile hypertrophic pyloric stenosis after healing. J Pediatr Surg 31:1530-1534, 1996.

56. Ludtke FE, Bertus M, Voth E, et al: Gasric emptying 16 to 26 years after treatment of infantile hypertrophic pyloric stenosis. J Pediatr Surg 29:523-526, 1994.

57. Kapur RP: Hirschprung disease and other enteric dysganglionoses. Crit Rev Clin Lab Sci 36:225-273, 1999.

58. Reyes-Mugica M: Hirschprung disease. Path Case Rev 5:51-59, 2000.

59. Angirst M, Jing S, Bolk S, et al: Human GFRA1: Cloning, mapping, genomic structure and evaluation as a candidate gene for Hirschprung disease. Genomics 48:354-362, 1998.

60. Doray B, Salmon R, Amiel J, et al: Mutations of the RET ligand, neurturin, supports multigeneic inheritance in Hirschprung disease. Hum Mol Genet 7:1449-1454, 1998.

61. Hofstra RMW, Valenaire O, Arch E, et al: A loss of function mutation in the endothelin converting enzyme 1 (ECE-1) associated with Hirschprung disease. Am J Hum Genet 64:304-308, 1998.

62. Myers SM, Salmon G, Goessling A, et al: Investigation of germline GFR alpha-1 mutations in Hirschprung disease. J Med Genet 36:217-220, 1999.

63. Gath R, Goessling A, Keller KM, et al: Analysis of the Ret, GDNF, EDN3, and EDNRB genes in patients with intestinal neuronal dysplasia and Hirschprung disease. Gut 48:671-675, 2001.

64. Chakravarti A: Endothelin receptor-mediated signaling in Hirschprung disease. Hum Mol Genet 5:503-507, 1996.

65. Teitelbaum DH, Canaiano DA, Qualman SJ: The pathophysiology of Hirschsprung's associated enterocolitis: Importance of histologic correlates. J Pediatr Surg 24:1271-1277, 1989.

66. Nakao M, Suita S, Taguchi T, et al: Fourteen-year experience of acetylcholinesterase staining for rectal mucosal biopsy in neonatal Hirschsprung disease. J Pediatr Surg 36:1357-1363, 2001.

67. Vanderwinden JM, Rumessen JJ, Liu H, et al: Interstitial cells of Cajal in human colon and in Hirschsprung's disease. Gastroenterology 111:901-910, 1996.

68. Horisawa M, Watanabe Y, Torihashi S: Distribution of c-kit immunopositive cells in normal human colon and in Hirschsprung's disease. J Pediatr Surg 33:1209-1214, 1998.

69. Maia DM: The reliability of frozen section diagnosis in the pathologic evaluation of Hirschsprung disease. Am J Surg Pathol 24:1675-1677, 2000.

70. Kapur RP: Developmental disorders of the enteric nervous system. Gut 47(suppl 4):481-483, 2000.

71. Lake B: Intestinal neuronal dysplasia: A little local difficulty? Pediatr Pathol Lab Med 17:687, 1997.

72. Berry CL: Intestinal neuronal dysplasia: Does it exist or has it been invented? Virchows Arch A Pathol Anat Histopathol 422:183-184, 1993.

73. Meier-Ruge WA, Brunner LA, Engert J, et al: A correlative morphometric and clinical investigation of hypoganglionosis of the colon in children. Eur J Pediatr Surg 9:67-74, 1999.

74. Meier-Ruge WA, Longo-Bauer CH: Morphometric determination of the methodological criteria for the diagnosis of intestinal neuronal dysplasia (IND B). Pathol Res Pract 193:465-469, 1997.

75. Bosman C, Devito R, Fusilli S, et al: A new hypothesis on the intestinal pseudo-obstruction by intestinal neuronal dysplasia (IND). Pathol Res Pract 197:789-796, 2001.

76. Vanek VW, Al-Salti M: Acute pseudo-obstruction of the colon (Ogilvie's syndrome): An analysis of 400 cases. Dis Colon Rectum 29:203-210,1986.

77. Krishnamurthy S, Schuffler MD: Pathology of neuromuscular disorder of the small intestine and colon. Gastroenterology 93:610-639, 1987.

78. Coulie B, Camilleri M: Intestinal pseudo-obstruction. Annu Rev Med 50:37-55, 1999.

79. Kansu A, Ensari A, Kalayci AG, et al: A very rare cause of intestinal pseudo-obstruction: Familial visceral myopathy type IV. Acta Pediatr 89:733-736, 2000.

80. Ariza A, Coll J, Fernandez-Figueras MT, et al: Desmin myopathy: A multisystem disorder involving skeletal, cardiac, and smooth muscle. Hum Pathol 26:1032-1037, 1995.

81. Smith VV, Lake BD, Kamm MA, et al: Intestinal pseudo-obstruction with deficient smooth muscle alpha-actin. Histopathology 21:535-542, 1992.

82. Ruuska TH, Karikoski R, Smith VV, et al: Acquired myopathic intestinal pseudo-obstruction may be due to autoimmune enteric leiomyositis. Gastroenterology 122:1133-1139, 2002.

83. Moore SW, Schneider JW, Kaschula RD: Non-familial visceral myopathy: Clinical and pathologic features of degenerative leiomyopathy. Pediatr Surg Int 18:6-12, 2002.

84. Jain D, Moussa K, Tandon M, et al: Role of interstitial cells of Cajal in motility disorders of the bowel. Am J Gastroenterol 98:618-624, 2003.

85. Auricchio A, Brancolini V, Cesari G, et al: The locus of a novel syndromic form of neuronal intestinal pseudoobstruction maps to Xq28. Am J Hum Genet 58:743-748, 1996.

86. Hall KE, Wiley JW: Neural injury, repair and adaptation in the GI tract. I. New insights into neuronal injury: A cautionary tale. Am J Physiol 274:G978-G983, 1998.

87. Haftel LT, Lev D, Barash V, et al: Familial mitochondrial intestinal pseudo-obstruction and neurogenic bladder. J Child Neurol 15:386-389, 2000.

88. De Giorgio R, Santini D, Ceccarelli C, et al: Defective expression of Bcl-2 in the enteric nervous system (ENS): A new potentially useful marker for several functional bowel disorders [abstract]. Ital J Gastroenterol 28(suppl 2):100, 1996.

89. Schobinger-Clement S, Gerber HA, Stallmach T: Autoaggressive inflammation of the myenteric plexus resulting in intestinal pseudoobstruction. Am J Surg Pathol 23:602-606, 1999.

90. Smith VV, Gregson N, Foggensteiner L, et al: Aquired intestinal aganglionosis and circulating autoantibodies without neoplasia or other neural involvement. Gastroenterology 112:1366-1371, 1997.

91. Schuffler MD, Bird TD, Sumi SM, et al: A familial neuronal disease presenting as intestinal pseudo-obstruction. Gastroenterology 75:889-898, 1978.

92. Ward SMA, Burns AJ, Torihashi S, et al: Impaired development of interstitial cells and intestinal electrical rhythmicity in steel mutants. Am J Physiol 269:1577-1585, 1995.

93. Isozaki K, Hirota S, Nakama A, et al: Disturbed intestinal movement, bile reflux to the stomach, and deficiency of c-kit expressing cells in Ws/Ws mutant rats. Gastroenterology 109:456-464, 1995.

94. Torihashi S, Ward SM, Nishikawa S-I, et al: C-kit-dependent development of interstitial cells and electrical activity in the murine gastrointestinal tract. Cell Tissue Res 280:97-111, 1995.

95. Giebel LB, Spritz RA: Mutation of the KIT (mast/stem cell growth factor receptor) protooncogene in human piebaldism. Proc Natl Acad Sci USA 88:8696-8699, 1991.

96. Fleischman RA, Saltman DL, Stastny V, et al: Deletion of the c-kit protooncogene in the human developmental defect piebald trait. Proc Natl Acad Sci USA 88:10885-10889, 1991.

97. Isozaki K, Hirota S, Miyagawa J-I, et al: Deficiency of c-kit(+) cells in patients with a myopathic form of chronic idiopathic intestinal pseudo-obstruction. Am J Gastroenterol 92:332-334, 1997.

98. Yamataka A, Ohshiro K, Kobayashi H, et al: Abnormal distribution of intestinal pacemaker (C-KIT-positive) cells in an infant with chronic idiopathic intestinal pseudoobstruction. J Pediatr Surg 33:859-862, 1998.

99. Kenny SE, Vanderwinden JM, Rintala RJ, et al: Delay of the interstitial cells of Cajal: A new diagnosis for transient neonatal pseudoobstruction. Report of two cases. J Pediatr Surg 33:94-98, 1998.

100. Gohil A, Croffie JM, Fitzgerald JF, et al: Reversible intestinal pseudoobstruction associated with neural crest tumors. J Pediatr Gastroenterol Nutr 33:86-88, 2001.

101. Malik M, Connors R, Schwarz KB, et al: Hormone-producing ganglioneuroblastoma simulating intestinal pseudoobstruction. J Pediatr 116:406-408, 1990.

102. Rohrmann CA Jr, Ricci MT, Krishnamurthy S, et al: Radiologic and histologic differentiation of neuro-muscular disorder of the gastrointestinal tract: Visceral myopathies, visceral neuropathies and progressive systemic sclerosis. Am J Roentgenol 143:933-941, 1984.

103. Nowak TV, Ionasescu V, Anuras S: Gastrointestinal manifestations of the muscular dystrophies. Gastroenterology 82:800-810, 1982.

104. Leon SH, Schuffler MD, Kettler M, et al: Chronic intestinal pseudoobstruction as a complication of Duchenne's muscular dystrophy. Gastroenterology 90:455-459, 1986.

105. Perlemuter G, Chaussade S, Wechsler B, et al: Chronic intestinal pseudo-obstruction in systemic lupus erythematosus. Gut 43:117-122, 1998.

106. Tada S, Iida M, Yao T, et al: Intestinal pseudo-obstruction in patients with amyloidosis: Clinicopathologic differences between chemical types of amyloid protein. Gut 34:1412-1417, 1993.

107. McDonald G, Schuffler M, Kadin M, et al: Intestinal pseudo-obstruction caused by diffuse lymphoid infiltration of the small intestine. Gastroenterology 89:882-889, 1985.

108. Lennon VA, Sas DF, Busk MF, et al: Enteric neuronal autoantibodies in pseudoobstruction with small cell lung carcinoma. Gastroenterology 100:137-142, 1991.

109. Kulling D, Reed CE, Verne GN, et al: Intestinal pseudo-obstruction as a paraneoplastic manifestation of malignant thymoma. Am J Gastroenterol 92:1564-1566, 1997.

110. Lee HR, Lennon VA, Camilleri M, et al: Paraneoplastic gastrointestinal motor dysfunction: Clinical and laboratory characteristics. Am J Gastroenterol 96:373-379, 2001.

111. Kebede D, Barthel JS, Singh A: Transient gastroparesis associated with cutaneous herpes zoster. Dig Dis Sci 32:318-322, 1987.

112. Pai NB, Murthy RS, Kumar HT, et al: Association of acute colonic pseudo-obstruction (Ogilvie's syndrome) with herpes zoster. Am Surg 56:691-694, 1990.

113. Mathias JR, Baskin GS, Reeves-Darby VG, et al: Chronic intestinal pseudoobstruction in a patient with heart-lung transplant. Therapeutic effect of leuprolide acetate. Dig Dis Sci 37:1761-1768, 1992.

114. Sonsino E, Mouy R, Foucaud P, et al: Intestinal pseudoobstruction related to cytomegalovirus infection of myenteric plexus. N Engl J Med 311:196-197, 1984.

115. Debinski HS, Kamm MA, Talbot IC, et al: DNA viruses in the pathogenesis of sporadic chronic idiopathic intestinal pseudo-obstruction. Gut 41:100-106, 1997.

116. Chatila R, Kapadia CR: Intestinal pseudoobstruction in acute Lyme disease: A case report. Am J Gastroenterol 93:1179-1180, 1998.

117. Ruchti C, Eisele S, Kaufmann M: Fatal intestinal pseudo-obstruction in brown bowel syndrome. Arch Pathol Lab Med 114:76-80, 1990.

118. Htizman JL, Weiland LH, Oftedah Gl, et al: Ceroidosis in the "brown bowel syndrome." Mayo Clin Proc 54:251-257, 1979.

119. Krisnamurthy S, Kelly MM, Rohrmann CA, et al: Jejunal diverticulosis: A heterogeneous disorder caused by a variety of abnormalities of smooth muscle or myenteric plexus. Gastroenterology 85:538-547, 1983.

120. Krishnamurthy S, Schuffler MD, Rohrmann CA, et al: Severe idiopathic constipation is associated with a distinctive abnormality of the myenteric plexus. Gastroenterology 88:26-34, 1985.

121. Preston DM, Hawley RR, Lennard-Jones JE, et al: Results of colectomy for severe idiopathic constipation in women (Arbuthnot Lane's disease). Br J Surg 71:547-552, 1984.

122. Wedel T, Spiegler J, Soellner S, et al: Enteric nerves and interstitial cells of Cajal are altered in patients with slow-transit constipation and megacolon. Gastroenterology 123:1459-1467, 2002.

123. He CL, Burgart L, Wang L, et al: Decreased interstitial cell of Cajal volume in patients with slow-transit constipation. Gastroenterology 118:14-21, 2000.

124. Knowles CH, Nickols CD, Sott SM, et al: Smooth muscle inclusion bodies in slow transit constipation. J Pathol 193:390-397, 2001.

INFLAMMATORY DISORDERS OF THE GI TRACT

CHAPTER 7

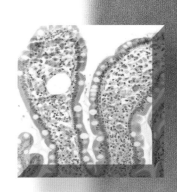

Inflammatory Disorders of the Esophagus

MARY P. BRONNER

▇ Reflux Esophagitis (Gastroesophageal Reflux Disease)

CLINICAL FEATURES

Reflux esophagitis is caused by gastric or duodenal contents entering and injuring the esophagus.[1,2] The cause is multifactorial; hiatal hernia and decreased lower esophageal sphincter pressure appear to play major roles.[3,4] Endoscopic findings include erosions, ulceration, exudates, and stricture formation. However, as many as 50% to 60% of symptomatic patients with objective evidence of reflux disease have normal mucosa or only hyperemia at endoscopy.[5] Furthermore, histologically inflamed esophageal mucosa may appear normal endoscopically, and hyperemia may or may not reflect

histologic esophagitis. Because of these endoscopic/pathologic discrepancies, biopsy is warranted in symptomatic patients both to document tissue injury and to exclude the other important entities in the endoscopic differential, namely, various infections, Barrett's esophagus, and neoplastic change. This is particularly true for those patients who have failed empirical reflux therapy; however, biopsy is undoubtedly warranted in any diagnostic endoscopy.

Biopsy of grossly visible lesions in gastroesophageal reflux disease (GERD) such as erosions, ulcerations, exudates, and strictures characteristically reveals esophagitis, a nonspecific injury pattern resulting from various causes. Pinch biopsies taken through the standard endoscope are generally not adequate for evaluating early changes due to reflux because they often do not include the entire thickness of the mucosa and are difficult to orient properly.[1,5] For this reason, and for patients who have refractory reflux symptoms, an endoscope with a large-caliber biopsy channel and a jumbo biopsy forceps should be used to facilitate a histologic diagnosis. Taking jumbo biopsies does not increase the complication rate,[6] and the greatly improved histologic specimens that result are well worth the effort.

Reflux changes have been shown to be distributed over the distal 8 cm of the esophagus in a patchy fashion, indicating that multiple biopsies are necessary for consistent demonstration of histologic abnormalities.[7] Because occasional single biopsy specimens from the lower 2.5 cm of the esophagus in asymptomatic subjects may reveal microscopic features of GERD,[7] diagnostic biopsy specimens should be taken from more than 2.5 cm above the gastroesophageal junction. The value of these approaches for the diagnosis of reflux esophagitis has been challenged,[8] and as a practical matter, the gastroenterologist who is managing adult patients seldom obtains biopsy specimens from the esophagus for this purpose. Rather, specimens are taken to exclude infection, Barrett's esophagus, and neoplasm. Esophageal biopsies may be more useful for establishing the diagnosis of reflux disease in infants, however.[9]

PATHOLOGIC FEATURES

Reflux esophagitis produces a characteristic, although nonspecific, injury pattern, including squamous hyperplasia and variably present inflammatory components. These are described in turn, followed by the differential diagnosis for reflux esophagitis.

Squamous Hyperplasia

For many years, it was believed that the only diagnostic criterion for esophagitis was inflammation. However, in 1970, Ismail-Beigi and associates found that some patients with clinical symptoms suggesting reflux, but with normal or minimally abnormal endoscopic appearances, had hyperplasia of the esophageal squamous epithelium, a finding they postulated reflected an early histologic manifestation of reflux-induced injury.[10] Hyperplasia was identified when the length of the subepithelial papillae of the lamina propria exceeded two thirds of, and the basal zone occupied more than 15% of, the thickness of the mucosa (Fig. 7-1). Subsequent studies confirmed these observations and demonstrated a significant positive correlation among the severity of reflux as measured by the 24-hour pH score, a composite quantitative evaluation of acid reflux, and the length of the papillae.[11] These correlations are also found in infants and children.[12]

Inflammation

Principal inflammatory cells in reflux esophagitis include the neutrophil, the eosinophil, and the lymphocyte (Fig. 7-2).[13]

NEUTROPHILS

Within the esophageal squamous epithelium, neutrophils are specific for differentiating normal subjects from those with GERD. Unfortunately, intraepithelial neutrophils are an insensitive index of reflux esophagitis in that they are present in less than one third of GERD patients with documented reflux (Fig. 7-2A). On the other hand, their presence can be discerned even in improperly oriented specimens. As an important differential diagnostic consideration, significant numbers of neutrophils, particularly with an erosion, an ulcer, or associated fibrinopurulent exudate, should prompt the pathologist to search for viral or *Candida* infection.

EOSINOPHILS

Increased numbers of eosinophils are likewise present in reflux esophagitis,[14] but because rare eosinophils may

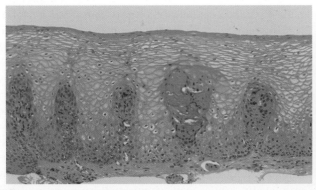
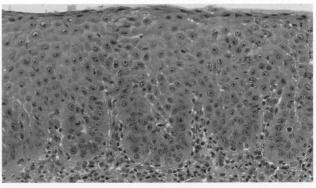

A　　　　　　　　　　　　　　　　　　**B**

FIGURE 7–1. Normal **(A)** and hyperplastic esophageal squamous mucosa **(B).** Normal mucosa shows a basal cell layer that is no more than 15% of the mucosal thickness and lamina propria subepithelial papillae that extend to no more than two thirds of the mucosal thickness.

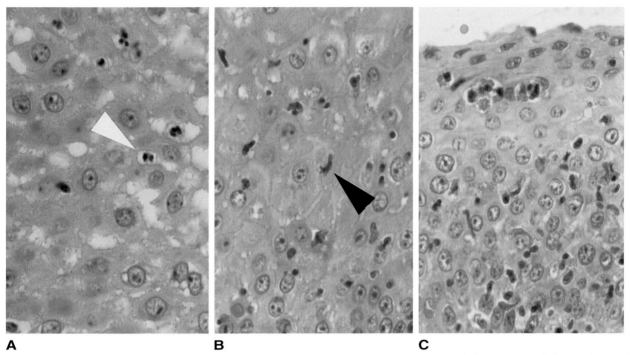

A   **B**   **C**

FIGURE 7–2. The inflammatory cells of GERD include neutrophils (**A**), lymphocytes (**B**), and eosinophils (**C**). Neutrophils are infrequently present and when numerous should prompt a search for fungal or viral pathogens. Lymphocytes, although increased in GERD, are also plentiful in normal esophageal mucosa and therefore assume no practical diagnostic significance. Lymphocytes undergo nuclear deformity (**B**, *black arrowhead*) as they squeeze between squamous cells but should not be mistaken for granulocytes (**A**, *white arrowhead*). Eosinophils may be present in normal esophagi, and in adults they are significant only if numerous (>6 per biopsy).

be found in the mucosa of normal adults, they are not significant unless more than six eosinophils are present in a biopsy section (Fig. 7-2**C**).[13,15] Eosinophilia in esophageal biopsies may be a particularly valuable diagnostic aid in the evaluation of reflux esophagitis in children, however, because eosinophils are not normally present in a child's mucosa.[12,16] Also, the presence of more than one eosinophil in the lamina propria appears to be an even better index of reflux disease in infants.[9] Pediatric patients who demonstrate an allergic history, normal esophageal pH monitoring, and failure to respond to antireflux therapy may have allergic esophagitis.[17] Histologically, these children have marked intraepithelial eosinophilia in the range of 30 eosinophils per high power field, with aggregates of eosinophils usually in the superficial layers of the squamous epithelium.[17] Children who appear to have reflux disease with prominent eosinophilia may improve when given elemental diets, suggesting that certain protein sensitivities may lead to reflux-like symptoms.[17-19]

Occasionally, large numbers of eosinophils are detected in the esophageal biopsies of adult reflux patients.[20] When this is the case, other causes of esophageal eosinophilia, such as eosinophilic gastroenteritis, drug reactions (including Stevens-Johnson syndrome), and pill-induced esophagitis, must be excluded. A more recently described condition called idiopathic eosinophilic esophagitis is discussed later (see under Eosinophilic Esophagitis).

LYMPHOCYTES

Lymphocytes are present in large numbers within the squamous mucosa of GERD patients. Like eosinophils, however, lymphocytes are a normal intraepithelial component of the esophageal squamous mucosa (Fig. 7-2**B**). They are largely T cells that have either round or irregular nuclear contours as they become deformed between squamous epithelial cells. Because of this nuclear deformity, they may bear some resemblance to granulocytes. Although lymphocytes are present in increased numbers in patients with reflux disease,[21] they have no independent diagnostic significance because normal control subjects may have large numbers as well.[22] Lymphocytes within the esophageal mucosa similarly do not correlate with any other parameters of reflux disease in infants.[12]

Inflamed Cardiac and Fundic-Type Mucosae ("Reflux Carditis")

Chronic and active inflammation of cardiac and fundic-type mucosae in the distal esophagus is a common, although nonspecific, feature of GERD. This lesion may be difficult to distinguish from a *Helicobacter pylori*–related chronic active gastritis involving gastric cardiac mucosa. *H. pylori* stains and serologic data, biopsies of the gastric antrum and tubular esophagus, and clinical studies of reflux disease are required for elucidation of the origin of inflamed cardiac or fundic-type mucosae at the gastroesophageal junction. (See Chapter 8 for a detailed discussion.)

Miscellaneous Microscopic Features of GERD

Marked dilatation of capillaries within the mucosa has been described as a characteristic change in reflux esophagitis,[23] but it also occurs frequently in normal controls, probably as a traumatic biopsy artifact.[24] Other features that may be seen in GERD include ballooning degeneration and multinucleation of squamous cells.

Some patients with GERD also have esophageal erosions or ulcers associated with underlying granulation tissue. This granulation tissue may exhibit enlarged and atypical endothelial cells and fibroblasts, resulting in a pseudosarcomatous appearance (Fig. 7-3).[25] These cells are usually distributed as single cells within otherwise typical granulation tissue. Atypical mesenchymal cells in granulation tissue typically do not form solid epithelioid clusters. Furthermore, they have a normal or decreased nucleus-to-cytoplasm ratio. In contrast, carcinoma usually occurs in epithelioid groups or sheets of cohesive cells with overlapping nuclei and increased nucleus-to-cytoplasm ratios. In difficult cases, immunohistochemistry for cytokeratins can be helpful in differentiating carcinoma from these pseudosarcomatous alterations.

Inflammatory exudates from ulcers or erosions within the esophagus characteristically contain many activated and atypical lymphocytes that may simulate lymphoma (Fig. 7-4). As a histologic guideline, these are benign if confined to the surface exudate. They should raise

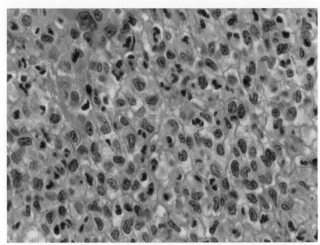

FIGURE 7–4. Benign ulcer exudates in the esophagus and throughout the GI tract characteristically contain cleaved and activated lymphocytes and macrophages that may simulate lymphoma. If limited to the luminal exudate alone, without infiltration of the underlying tissue, they should be considered benign.

concern about potential lymphoma only if they infiltrate the underlying tissue.

DIFFERENTIAL DIAGNOSIS OF GERD

The differential diagnosis of reflux esophagitis includes infectious esophagitis; pill esophagitis; esophagitis caused by the ingestion of corrosive agents such as lye; chemotherapy and radiation-induced esophagitis; squamous dysplasia/carcinoma; eosinophilic esophagitis; a variety of systemic diseases, including collagen vascular disease, Stevens-Johnson syndrome, bullous diseases, and lichen planus; graft-versus-host disease; esophageal stasis syndrome that may develop in esophageal dysmotility states; Crohn's disease; amyloidosis; and trauma-induced injury. Many of these diseases share overlapping morphologic features with reflux esophagitis; thus, it must be emphasized that this diagnosis requires correlation of clinical, endoscopic, and histologic data. No histologic feature or features are entirely specific for reflux esophagitis. The lesions in the differential diagnosis are discussed in greater detail in the following sections.

■ Reactive Hyperplasia and Dysplasia

Occasionally, reactive hyperplasia induced by esophagitis may be pronounced and may resemble squamous dysplasia (Table 7-1; Fig. 7-5). The most helpful differential feature is the cytoarchitectural *uniformity* of squamous hyperplasia in comparison with the cytoarchitectural *pleomorphism* of squamous dysplasia/carcinoma. (See Chapter 16 for a detailed discussion.)

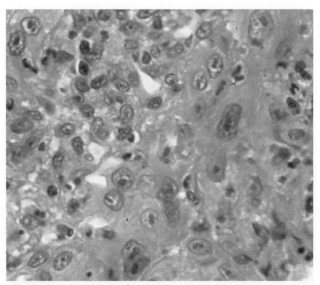

FIGURE 7–3. Benign mesenchymal cells within an esophageal ulcer bed show striking cytologic atypia. These atypical cells can usually be differentiated from carcinoma by their solitary and scattered nature, lack of epithelioid grouping, maintenance of nucleus-to-cytoplasm ratio, and occurrence within otherwise typical granulation tissue.

TABLE 7–1. Differential Diagnosis of Reactive Hyperplasia Versus Dysplasia of Squamous Epithelium

Feature	Hyperplasia	Dysplasia
Papillae	Present, fairly regular	Absent or very irregular
Nuclear enlargement	++	+++
Nuclear pleomorphism	+	+++
Nuclear overlapping	+	+++
Nuclear hyperchromasia	+	+++
Nuclear membrane	Smooth	May be irregular

+, mild degree; ++moderate degree; +++, marked degree.

The mucosal architecture of squamous hyperplasia retains relatively uniform and regular papillae that extend to approximately equal depths within the lamina propria and are also of similar widths. In contrast, dysplastic squamous epithelium typically displays architectural distortion with absent or markedly irregular papillae.

Cytologically, hyperplastic squamous epithelial cells are atypical, but they are characteristically uniformly atypical and quite similar to each other. Specifically, the nuclei are uniformly enlarged with relatively smooth nuclear membranes, generally open chromatin, prominent nucleoli, and limited, if any, nuclear overlapping. Dysplastic squamous epithelial cells on the other hand are characteristically much more pleomorphic in size and shape, are more hyperchromatic, have more irregular nuclear contours, and often overlap one another.

When one is faced with this differential diagnosis, it is also helpful to consider that esophageal squamous dysplasia unassociated with an endoscopically apparent tumor is a rare finding in the United States. Thus, surgical pathologists practicing in the United States see many more examples of esophagitis-induced hyperplasia mimicking dysplasia than a bona fide example of dysplasia.

Infectious Esophagitis

Viruses and fungi cause most forms of acute infectious esophagitis.[26] Bacterial esophagitis occurs in some patients with systemic and upper respiratory infections.

HERPES ESOPHAGITIS

Herpes simplex esophagitis occurs primarily in patients who are immunosuppressed by acquired immunodeficiency syndrome (AIDS), chemotherapy, or transplantation, but it may also occur in otherwise healthy young adults.[27,28] Symptoms of herpetic esophagitis include chest pain, odynophagia, dysphagia, and upper gastrointestinal (GI) bleeding, but it may be asymptomatic.[29] Herpetic ulcers in the esophagus may serve as a portal of entry for other pathogens and are frequently associated with herpetic pneumonitis.[27]

Herpetic ulcers as seen at endoscopy are typically shallow and sharply punched out and are often surrounded by relatively normal appearing mucosa. Microscopic diagnostic criteria include Cowdry type A intranuclear viral inclusion bodies, ground-glass nuclei, nuclear molding, multinucleated giant cells, and ballooning degeneration of infected cells (Fig. 7-6). Inclusion bodies are limited to the squamous epithelial cells at the margin of the ulcer; biopsies taken away from the immediate edge of the lesion may not be diagnostic. Multinucleated giant cell changes in squamous epithelial cells may occur in reflux disease and should not be confused with herpetic cytopathic effects.[30] These cells may have prominent nucleoli, but nuclear inclusion bodies are not present. Large numbers of mononuclear cells, primarily macrophages, in the surface exudate of esophageal ulcers have been described as a characteristic finding in herpetic ulcers[31]; however, similar cells are noted in ulcers throughout the

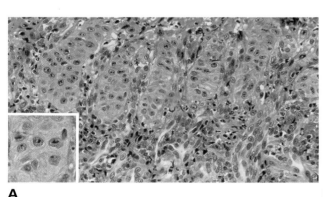

A

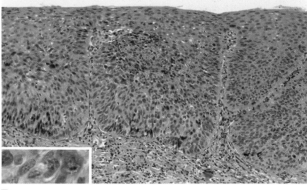

B

FIGURE 7–5. Reactive squamous hyperplasia **(A)** may be difficult to distinguish from squamous dysplasia **(B)** or even carcinoma. The most helpful histologic features are cytoarchitectural uniformity in hyperplasia versus cytoarchitectural pleomorphism in neoplastic squamous proliferations. Note that in squamous hyperplasia **(A)**, the papillae are of uniform length and width, and the nuclei, although atypical, are uniformly atypical and do not overlap one another *(highlighted in inset)*. In high-grade squamous dysplasia **(B)**, the papillae vary greatly in size and shape (or may even be absent), and there is considerable nuclear pleomorphism, hyperchromosia, and overlapping *(highlighted in inset)*.

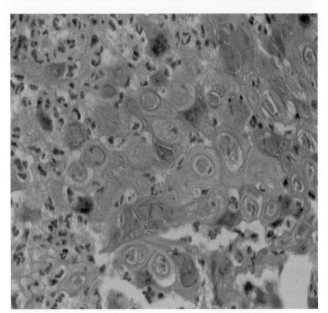

FIGURE 7–6. Herpes esophagitis showing the diagnostic multinucleation, Cowdry type A inclusions, and nuclear molding, involving squamous epithelium at the edge of an ulcer.

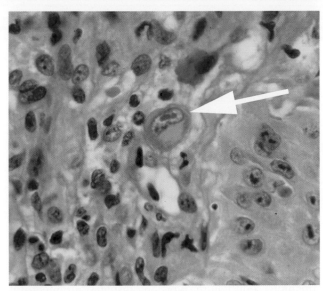

FIGURE 7–7. Cytomegalovirus (CMV) nuclear and cytoplasmic inclusions *(white arrow)* in mesenchymal cells of an esophageal ulcer bed.

GI tract in the absence of herpesvirus infection. Herpes simplex type I is the cause of most herpetic esophagitis, but on morphologic grounds this cannot be distinguished from herpes simplex type II or varicella-zoster. Immunohistochemical staining and in situ hybridization can separate these three viral species, if this becomes important on clinical grounds.

CYTOMEGALOVIRUS ESOPHAGITIS

Cytomegalovirus (CMV) esophagitis is relatively common among AIDS patients; in one study, it was found alone or in combination with *Candida* and herpes in 30% of AIDS patients studied.[32] CMV esophagitis may also occur rarely in immunocompetent individuals.[33] Most patients with CMV esophagitis have multiple, well-circumscribed ulcers.[34] CMV inclusion bodies are found in endothelial cells and fibroblasts within granulation tissue of the esophageal ulcer base (Fig. 7-7) and are not present in the surrounding squamous epithelial cells, in sharp contrast to herpetic inclusions. As in herpetic esophagitis, aggregates of macrophages may also be seen in the luminal exudate of CMV esophagitis,[35] but this finding lacks diagnostic specificity.

Accurate diagnosis of CMV infection is important because effective therapy is available. No single technique for its diagnosis has perfect sensitivity; thus, it has been suggested that a combination of diagnostic modalities be used.[36] For practical purposes, however, if a careful search of a well-prepared H&E section fails to disclose inclusions or even suspicious cells, then additional ancillary immunohistochemical and/or in situ hybridization tests are unlikely to increase the diagnostic yield.

These ancillary techniques have their greatest utility when suspicious but not fully diagnostic cells are identified on routine stained sections.

CANDIDA ESOPHAGITIS

Fungal esophagitis is most commonly caused by *Candida albicans* and *Candida tropicalis* (Fig. 7-8). This infection occurs primarily in patients with some underlying cause, such as AIDS or another immunosuppressive disorder or diabetes, or in patients undergoing antibiotic therapy; it may also be found in otherwise healthy subjects.[37] Because *Candida* organisms are part

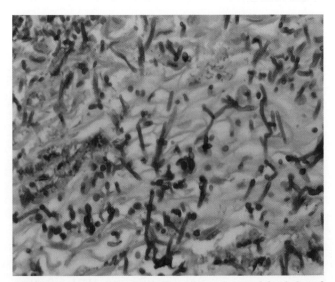

FIGURE 7–8. *Candida* esophagitis showing pseudohyphal and budding yeast forms, as highlighted on this PAS with diastase stain.

of the normal flora of the GI tract, confirmation of this diagnosis requires more than the identification of budding yeast forms; pseudohyphae should be detected within the tissue to document infection.[38] At endoscopy, esophageal candidiasis appears as white plaques of fibrinopurulent exudate in which pseudohyphae and budding yeast forms can be demonstrated. *C. tropicalis* is more virulent than *C. albicans* because of its increased invasiveness.[39] Esophageal candidiasis produces dysphagia and odynophagia but may be asymptomatic and discovered only incidentally at esophagoscopy. The infection generally responds well to antifungal therapy, but in AIDS patients it may be refractory to treatment.[40] All other forms of fungal esophagitis are rare. Esophageal involvement may occur as a complication of mediastinal infection, such as from histoplasmosis.

The endoscopist occasionally identifies small white plaques in the mucosa that resemble *Candida* esophagitis. Often, these plaques represent either glycogenic acanthosis or ectopic sebaceous glands. Glycogenic acanthosis occurs in virtually all esophagi as white mucosal plaques 2 to 5 mm in size.[41] However, it is infrequently recognized endoscopically. Diffuse esophageal glycogenic acanthosis may occur as a rare manifestation of Cowden disease.[42] Biopsy features include distention of squamous epithelial cells with pale-staining material that is periodic acid–Schiff (PAS)-positive and diastase-digestible.[43] Ectopic sebaceous glands, which may also appear as small pale yellow or white punctate elevations of the mucosa, are rare but are easily recognized in biopsy material by their close resemblance to normal dermal sebaceous glands.[44]

OTHER CAUSES OF INFECTIOUS ESOPHAGITIS

Symptoms related to esophageal disease are common in AIDS patients.[32] In most, a specific infectious agent such as *Candida*, herpes, or CMV can be identified.[32,45] Occasionally, one of the less common pathogens, such as *Mycobacterium tuberculosis*, *Mycobacterium avium-intracellulare*, *Histoplasma capsulatum*, or *Toxoplasma gondii*, may be seen.[46,47] In some patients, no apparent cause for the esophagitis or ulcer can be found by the usual techniques; in situ hybridization with the use of specific DNA probes may reveal Epstein-Barr virus in some of these patients.[48] In a study of homosexual men with acute (primary) human immunodeficiency virus (HIV) infection presenting with odynophagia, multiple discrete esophageal ulcers were observed.[49] None of the usual infectious agents could be identified by light microscopy, but electron microscopy revealed viral particles consistent with retrovirus, suggesting that the esophagus may be a target of acute HIV infection. Other AIDS patients develop chronic esophageal ulcers

in which there are no detectable organisms. The term *idiopathic esophageal ulceration* has been used for this condition, and it has been suggested that HIV itself may be causal.[50] However, HIV has been identified with similar frequency in idiopathic esophageal ulcers and in ulcers with detectable infectious agents; thus, it remains unclear whether HIV itself can cause esophageal ulcers.

Pill- and Drug-Induced Esophagitis

Esophageal injury caused by prolonged direct mucosal contact with tablets or capsules taken in therapeutic doses occurs frequently.[51-53] Commonly implicated agents include antibiotics (particularly doxycycline), emepronium bromide, potassium chloride, ferrous sulfate,[54] quinidine, and alendronate.[55] Symptoms include odynophagia, continuous retrosternal pain, and dysphagia. The patient often gives a history of having taken a pill(s) with little or no fluid just before going to bed and being aware that the pill had "stuck in the chest." Most affected individuals do not have any apparent abnormality of esophageal transit[51]; however, several patients with quinidine or potassium chloride injury had preexisting esophageal compression due to either valvular heart disease with left atrial enlargement or esophageal entrapment by fixed mediastinal structures and adhesions following thoracic surgery.[53] The histologic appearance of pill-induced esophagitis, ulceration, and stricture is nonspecific. Prominent eosinophilic infiltration, spongiosis, and necrosis of squamous epithelium should raise the possibility of pill-induced injury. Polarizable crystalline material may be seen in alendronate-induced injury,[55] and crystalline stainable iron can be found in ferrous sulfate–induced disease.[54]

Esophageal erosions and ulcers have been reported in approximately 20% of arthritis patients taking nonsteroidal anti-inflammatory drugs (NSAIDs).[56] NSAID-induced esophageal injury may be caused by both direct and systemic effects, and it may be exacerbated in patients with gastroesophageal reflux disease.[56] Esophageal injury caused by these agents appears to be less common than injury to other parts of the GI tract.[57]

Corrosive or Caustic Esophageal Injuries

Corrosive or caustic esophageal injuries may occur in children or adults and are most commonly the result of alkaline (lye) or acid (nitric) ingestion.[58-60] Gastroduodenal lesions are also common with caustic ingestion. Pathologic features are nonspecific and are related to tissue necrosis and subsequent inflammation. Long-term complications include stricture formation, which may require endoscopic or surgical treatment. Squamous cell carcinoma is a rare complication.[61]

Chemoradiation-Induced Esophagitis

Esophageal injury is a common adverse effect of chemotherapy and radiation therapy.[62,63] The features are similar to those of chemoradiation-induced injury in other portions of the GI tract and consist initially of increased apoptosis within the basal zone. Thereafter, a nonspecific inflammatory reaction with or without erosion/ulceration occurs. Other histologic features include severe or even bizarre epithelial and stromal cells. These atypical cells may be distinguished from neoplastic cells by their low nucleus-to-cytoplasm ratio. Vascular telangiectasia is also a common feature of chemoradiation injury. This reaction often resolves within 4 weeks. Chronic radiation-induced cytologic atypia of stromal cells may persist indefinitely, as may chronic vascular alterations, including sclerosis, dilatation, and intimal foam cell arteriopathy. Finally, mural scarring and strictures may complicate chemoradiation-induced esophageal injury.

Barrett's Esophagus

Barrett's esophagus is an acquired condition in which the stratified squamous epithelium normally lining the esophagus becomes replaced by metaplastic, intestinal-type columnar epithelium, defined by the presence of goblet cells. This condition develops as a result of chronic GERD[64-66] and predisposes to the development of esophageal adenocarcinoma.[64,65] Barrett's esophagus occurs in both adults and children, in whom it has a similar pathogenesis.[67]

There are two main sources of error in the pathologic evaluation of Barrett's esophagus, as outlined in Table 7-2. The first is the overdiagnosis of this serious condition, a problem related to evolving definitions, its histologic mimics, and the vagaries of interpretation of Alcian blue staining at pH 2.5. The second is the problem of overdiagnosing dysplasia in Barrett's esophagus, in particular high-grade dysplasia, given its major clinical consequences. These are explored in detail in the following sections.

DEFINITION

The current definition of Barrett's esophagus requires two components—one endoscopic and one histologic (Fig. 7-9). The diagnosis should not be established unless both are present, as advocated by the American College of Gastroenterology.[68]

TABLE 7–2. Problems in the Pathologic Evaluation of Barrett's Esophagus

1. Overdiagnosis of Barrett's esophagus
   A. Definitional problems
      1. Both endoscopic and histologic components required
      2. Three anatomic landmarks must be separately identified and biopsied
         a. Gastroesophageal junction (GEJ)
         b. Proximally displaced squamocolumnar junction (SCJ) or Z-line
         c. Intervening pink mucosa in tubular esophagus
   B. Pseudogoblet cells
   C. Misinterpretation of Alcian blue staining at pH 2.5
2. Overdiagnosis of high-grade dysplasia in Barrett's esophagus
   A. Atypical cardiac-type mucosa with regenerative changes
   B. Atypia limited to basal glands of Barrett's intestinal metaplasia
   C. Grading accuracy is dependent on both experience and volume
   D. Dysplasia forms a morphologic continuum for which precise boundaries cannot be defined

The endoscopic component requires that columnar mucosa, identified endoscopically by its pink color, must extend proximally from the gastroesophageal junction (GEJ) into the tubular esophagus (see further discussion under Anatomic Landmarks). The histologic component requires that biopsy specimens taken from the endoscopically identified columnar (pink) mucosa must contain metaplastic or intestinalized columnar epithelium with goblet cells.[68] This approach still has its difficulties in that the endoscopic anatomy may be difficult to define, and likewise, the minimum amount of metaplastic epithelium histologically required to confer an increased cancer risk remains unknown.

ANATOMIC LANDMARKS

The following definitions of various endoscopic anatomic landmarks in the distal esophagus have helped to refine the endoscopic identification of Barrett's esophagus (Fig. 7-10). If abnormalities are identified, endoscopists should, at a minimum, identify for the pathologist and separately biopsy these landmarks to enable a correct diagnosis of Barrett's esophagus.[69]

The GEJ in normal individuals is the *anatomic* junction at which the tubular esophagus joins the saccular stomach; it is identified as the proximal margin of the gastric folds. However, the squamocolumnar junction (SCJ), also known as the "Z-line," is a *mucosal* junction that does not always coincide with the anatomic GEJ. Even in patients without Barrett's esophagus, the SCJ may be irregular and, in as many as half of "normal" patients, may lie anywhere within the increased pressure

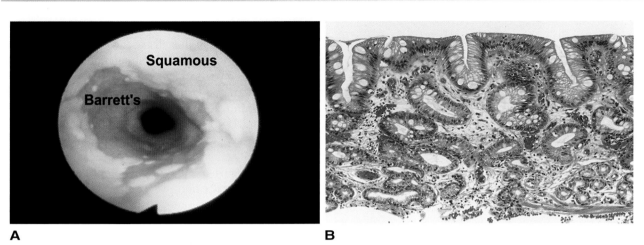

A   **B**

FIGURE 7–9. Barrett's esophagus is defined by both endoscopic (**A**) and histologic (**B**) components. Endoscopically, there must be visible pink columnar epithelium within the tubular esophagus, which on biopsy reveals intestinalized metaplastic columnar epithelium defined by the presence of goblet cells. Barrett's esophagus should not be diagnosed without both components.

region of the lower esophageal sphincter (LES), that is, within the distal 1 cm of the tubular esophagus. Thus, for accurate diagnosis of Barrett's esophagus, separate biopsies should be obtained if endoscopic abnormalities are found; these biopsies should specify (1) the GEJ, (2) the Z-line or the SCJ, and (3) the intervening columnar (pink) mucosa of possible Barrett's esophagus.

Despite these anatomic definitions, endoscopic diagnosis of Barrett's esophagus may be difficult. This is particularly true when the patient has a large hiatal hernia because precise identification of the GEJ is made even more challenging.[70] In normal individuals or in reflux patients without Barrett's esophagus, endoscopically visible columnar or pink epithelium within the distal esophagus/GEJ region is often composed of cardiac or fundic-type mucosa (Fig. 7-11). Thus, cardiac or fundic-type mucosa within the distal 1 to 2 cm of the esophagus may be a variation of normal or may reflect reflux disease that is by definition not diagnostic of Barrett's esophagus.[64,69,71,72] Debate has recently arisen over whether cardiac or cardiofundic-type mucosa in this region is truly "normal" (present congenitally) or represents an acquired alteration caused by reflux disease.[73,74] Recent data favor the concept that most individuals contain less than 0.4 mm of cardiac-type mucosa and that having longer lengths of this type of mucosa is probably a manifestation of reflux disease. This controversy aside, neither cardiac nor fundic-type mucosa in this region is a significant risk factor for malignancy. It cannot be emphasized strongly enough that the histologic component of Barrett's esophagus is limited to intestinal metaplasia with true goblet cells. Lack of understanding of this critical point is one of the major factors generating incorrect diagnoses of Barrett's esophagus, with the attendant and unnecessary risks and consequences these pose for patients.

PATHOLOGIC FEATURES

Epithelial Characteristics

Virtually all columnar epithelium in adults that extends proximal to the LES (i.e., more than 2 to 3 cm above the GEJ) is intestinalized.[71] Occasionally, an individual biopsy specimen may contain only cardiac or fundic-type mucosa when a patient has metaplasia in other specimens. In one report, when the diagnosis of Barrett's esophagus was based on the presence of more than 3 cm of cardiac or fundic-type epithelium, the diagnosis could not be confirmed on second endoscopy in 38% of patients.[75] This observation indicates that endoscopic measurement of columnar epithelium alone is an unreliable determinant. An extremely rare patient, however, may have only cardiac-type mucosa without goblet cells extending well above the LES region. Because of its rarity, the significance of this condition and any potential neoplastic risk it may pose remain unknown. This condition might best be referred to as *columnar-lined esophagus, nonintestinalized,*[76] so that it may be distinguished from classic Barrett's esophagus and its known cancer risk.

Metaplastic epithelium is defined histologically by the presence of acid mucin–containing goblet cells. When it is identified in a biopsy specimen taken from endoscopically visible columnar (pink) epithelium within the tubular esophagus (above the GEJ), it is abnormal, regardless of whether it occupies a 1-cm or a 10-cm segment. Short-segment Barrett's esophagus is defined arbitrarily by the presence of 3 cm or less of metaplastic epithelium within the esophagus.[68,70] When an *endoscopically visible* amount of metaplastic mucosa is present, it is sufficient to confer increased neoplastic risk, regardless of whether it is a short or long segment. However, the minimum *histologic* amount of goblet cell–containing epithelium required to confer an

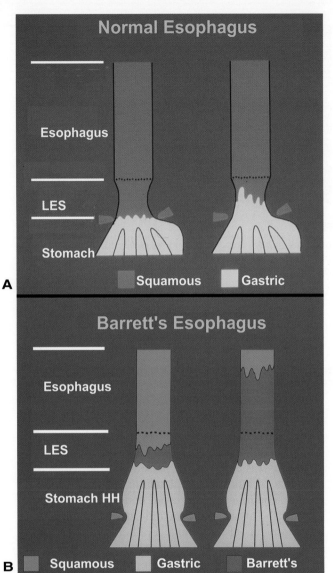

FIGURE 7–10. Anatomic landmarks of the normal lower esophageal sphincter (LES) region **(A)** and of Barrett's esophagus **(B).** Columnar mucosa is common in the normal distal esophagus. In Barrett's esophagus, the squamocolumnar junction is proximally displaced within the tubular esophagus, and the intervening mucosa is composed (at least in part) of intestinalized metaplastic epithelium, noted in red. HH, hiatal hernia.

increased cancer risk remains unknown. Of great importance is that a few metaplastic glands from an endoscopically normal GEJ are quite common and in fact have been found in up to one third of patients undergoing upper endoscopy for reflux symptoms (Fig. 7-12).[77-82]

As has been mentioned earlier, cardiac or fundic-type epithelium may normally reside within the distal 1 to 2 cm of the tubular esophagus. Children with a columnar-lined esophagus have been reported to have fundic or cardiac-type epithelium above the LES region, but the validity of this observation has been challenged.[67] Children with reflux disease who do not initially have

metaplastic epithelium may eventually acquire it.[72] Of the children with reflux disease who had metaplastic epithelium as reported by Qualman and colleagues, the youngest was 5 years of age.[72]

Barrett's metaplastic epithelium is histologically identical to intestinal metaplasia of the incomplete type (type II or III) or, less commonly, the complete type (type I). Subtyping of intestinal metaplasia, however, has no practical clinical significance because neoplastic change may occur in all types. The epithelium covering the mucosal surface and pits, or the villiform projections of Barrett's mucosa, has two major cell types—goblet cells and columnar cells (Fig. 7-13). Paneth cells may also be seen occasionally in complete intestinal metaplasia.

Alcian Blue Stain at pH 2.5

True goblet cells not only have the rounded goblet shape but also contain acidic mucin that stains *intensely* blue with Alcian blue at pH 2.5. Histochemical analyses show that this acidic mucin most often contains a mixture of sialomucins and sulfomucins, but the sialomucins generally predominate. Routine Alcian blue staining at pH 2.5 of potential Barrett's mucosa is not necessary because goblet cells can be readily recognized in most cases on routine staining alone.

Alcian blue staining or the lack thereof can, however, sometimes be helpful in the setting of cardiac-type mucosa with goblet-shaped cells. Distended foveolar cells, which have been called "pseudogoblet" cells (Fig. 7-14), are a potential source of error in the false-positive diagnosis of Barrett's esophagus. Fortunately, these mimickers almost always stain less intensely than true goblet cells with Alcian blue at pH 2.5, if they stain at all. In addition, pseudogoblet cells, unlike true goblet cells, are characteristically arranged in linear continuous stretches without intervening columnar cells.

The columnar cells between goblet cells may resemble normal gastric foveolar cells or intestinal-type absorptive cells, but they do not have all the typical features of either (Fig. 7-15). The brush border, if present, is only partially developed, in contrast to the fully developed, refractile brush border of the mature intestinal absorptive cell.

Distinguishing reactive, inflamed mucosa from dysplastic Barrett's epithelium may be difficult (see Fig. 7-15). In both of these epithelial types, there is a strong tendency toward loss of cytoplasmic mucin, and both show cytologic atypia that may be marked. Clues to distinguishing these epithelia are further discussed in the section to follow on problems in the diagnosis of dysplasia and in Chapter 16.

Alcian blue–positive cells are also found in normal esophageal glands and their corresponding ducts, which may be either mucosal or submucosal in location. As such, they are present within the deeper portions of biopsies and are characteristically intensely Alcian

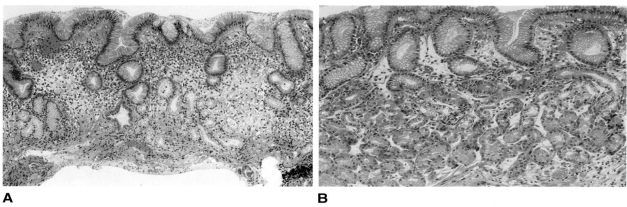

A **B**

FIGURE 7–11. Cardiac (**A**) and fundic (**B**) mucosal type in biopsies from endoscopically visible pink columnar mucosa within the lower esophageal sphincter (LES) region. Note the *absence* of goblet cells, the foveolar surface, and the gastric-type mucinous or oxyntic glands. Gastric epithelium within the LES region occurs in large numbers of normal subjects or GERD patients but is not diagnostic of Barrett's esophagus.

blue–positive. However, they are readily distinguished from Barrett's epithelium by their rounded, grouped or lobular configuration, akin to minor salivary glands, and by their diffuse Alcian blue positivity at pH 2.5 (Fig. 7-16**A**). The ducts draining these glands may have a mucinous or transitional-type epithelium or admixtures of both and may contain Alcian blue–positive cells or surface mucin caps (Fig. 7-16**B** and **C**).

DIFFERENTIAL DIAGNOSIS

Cardia Intestinal Metaplasia

Intestinal metaplasia in biopsy specimens obtained near the GEJ is more common than was previously recognized.[77-82] Given the difficulty in precise localization of the GEJ by means of endoscopic techniques, it may not be clear whether intestinal metaplasia comes from just above or just below the GEJ (see Chapter 8 for details). Although the data are controversial, several studies have found *H. pylori* infection to be a major causative factor for intestinal metaplasia of the cardia.[78-80] In addition, although prospective data are relatively sparse, it has been suggested that the risk of progression to dysplasia and adenocarcinoma for cardia intestinal metaplasia is significantly lower than for short- or long-segment Barrett's esophagus. Immunohistochemical staining for cytokeratins 7 and 20 in this differential diagnosis is controversial (see Chapter 8 for details).[82,83]

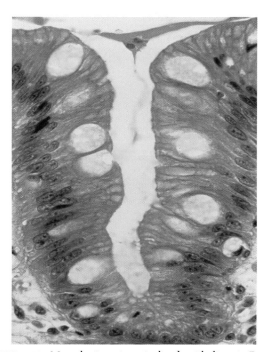

FIGURE 7–12. Rare metaplastic glands at the gastroensophageal junction are insufficient to establish a diagnosis of Barrett's esophagus (Alcian blue at pH 2.5) in the absence of endoscopic confirmation.

FIGURE 7–13. Metaplastic or intestinalized epithelium in Barrett's esophagus with true barrel-shaped goblet cells and intervening columnar cells of either the foveolar cell type or the pseudo-absorptive cell type with an incomplete brush border.

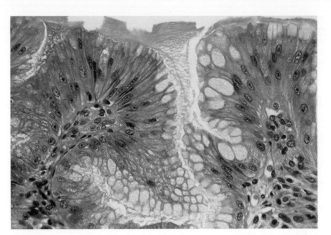

FIGURE 7–14. Pseudogoblet cells are characteristically arranged in a back-to-back continuous linear array and are usually (but not always) negative for Alcian blue staining at pH 2.5 or only faintly positive, as illustrated here. Goblet cells are usually singly dispersed and stain intensely blue with the Alcian blue stain (see also Fig. 7–13 and 7–16**C**).

Pancreatic Acinar Metaplasia

Biopsy specimens obtained from the region of the GEJ not infrequently contain foci of pancreatic acinar metaplasia. This appears to be an incidental finding that has no known clinical importance.[84]

Inlet Patch

Barrett's esophagus should not be confused with congenital islands of ectopic gastric mucosa. These "inlet patches" are found in about 10% of individuals undergoing endoscopy[85]; they occur principally in the cervical esophagus and are separated from the stomach by a large zone of intact squamous epithelium. Inlet patches may have gastric or intestinal-type mucosa, but this should not be confused with Barrett's esophagus that begins in the LES region. Although rare cases of cancer arising in inlet patches have been reported, surveillance is not justified even if there is intestinal metaplasia because of the extremely low neoplastic risk for this prevalent lesion.

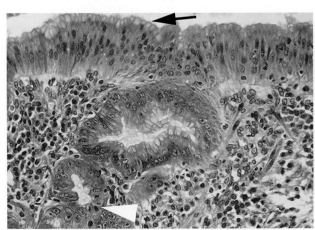

A

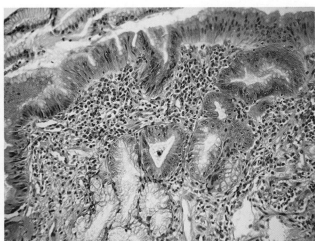

B

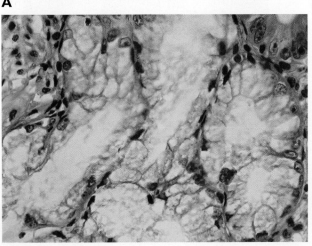

C

FIGURE 7–15. Similarities between reactive cardiac-type mucosa (**A** to **C**) and dysplastic Barrett's mucosa may lead to the overdiagnosis not only of Barrett's esophagus but also of *dysplastic* Barrett's mucosa. Similarities include mucin loss and sometimes marked nuclear atypia, as seen in **A** (at higher magnification) and **B.** Differences include the often more bland mucinous cardiac-type glands (**C**) relative to the more atypical surface (**A**), in comparison with the opposite pattern in Barrett's mucosa, where the atypia is characteristically most severe in the deep glands. Mitotic figures may also be helpful in that the mitotic or regenerative zone of gastric mucosa resides in the central or neck region of the gastric crypt (**A**, *white arrowhead*); in Barrett's epithelium, the regenerative zone emanates from the deepest part of the crypt. Reactive foveolar-type cells commonly retain a linear array of small apical foveolar mucin caps along the mucosal surface (**A**, *black arrow*).

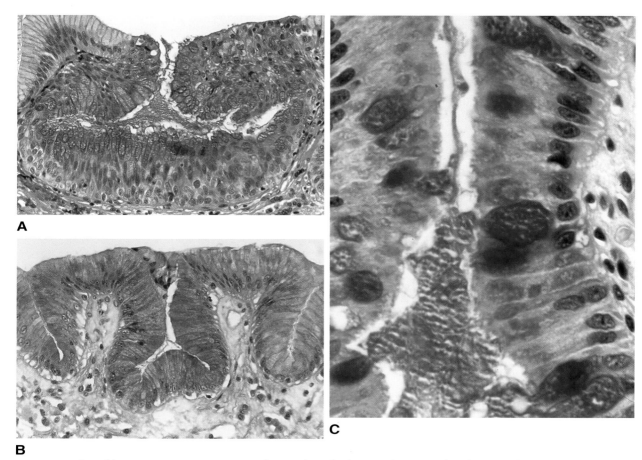

FIGURE 7–16. Alcian blue at pH 2.5 positivity is normal in esophageal submucosal or mucosal cardiac-type glands, the draining ducts of the submucosal glands (**A**), and in reactive cardiac-type mucosa (**B**). This should not be confused with the scattered, intensely blue-staining goblet cells of Barrett's metaplastic epithelium (**C**).

NEOPLASTIC PROGRESSION IN BARRETT'S ESOPHAGUS

General Comments and Definition

Barrett's esophagus predisposes to the development of esophageal adenocarcinoma,[64,66] but the frequency with which it does so is not well established. Part of the difficulty in defining the cancer risk is that the prevalence of Barrett's esophagus itself is not well documented. Barrett's esophagus is present in about 10% to 12% of patients with symptomatic GERD who undergo endoscopy,[64] but an autopsy study has suggested that its true frequency may be as much as 20 times higher.[86] The reported *prevalence* of adenocarcinoma in Barrett's esophagus averages about 10%—that is, about 10% of patients have adenocarcinoma at the time of initial diagnosis of Barrett's esophagus.[64] The estimated *incidence* of adenocarcinoma in Barrett's esophagus ranges from 1 in 52 to 1 in 441 patient-years, representing an increased risk of 30- to 125-fold.[64] Adenocarcinoma of the esophagus appears to be limited to patients who have metaplastic epithelium. Although cancer may arise even in those patients with short segments of Barrett's esophagus, some data support increasing risk with longer lengths of metaplastic epithelium. Cancer arises in Barrett's esophagus through a multistep sequence of events that is initiated by chronic GERD, leading to metaplasia, then dysplasia, and finally adenocarcinoma.

Pathologic Features of Dysplasia

Dysplasia is defined as neoplastic epithelium that remains confined within the basement membrane of the epithelium within which it arises.[87] When the dysplastic epithelium proliferates to form a polyp, the term *polypoid dysplasia*, but not the term *adenoma*, may be applied (see Chapter 16).[88] Dysplasia in Barrett's esophagus is recognized histologically by a combination of architectural and cytologic abnormalities. Dysplastic glands may retain their normal configuration but more often have irregular, crowded, or even grossly distorted architecture. The glands are usually lined by cells with enlarged, irregular, hyperchromatic, crowded, and stratified nuclei. In other examples, the nuclei are large and hyperchromatic, contain large nucleoli, and have lost their polarity, but they lack the crowding and stratification mentioned earlier. In all cases, cytologic features extend from the glands onto the epithelial surface; this is perhaps the single most important criterion in the diagnosis of dysplasia. (See Chapter 16 for further discussion.)

For purposes of clinical utility, dysplasia in Barrett's esophagus has been subdivided into low-grade and high-grade categories. When no features of dysplasia are observed, the diagnosis "negative for dysplasia" is rendered. When the findings are uncertain, the category "indefinite for dysplasia" is assigned. This grading scheme is directly analogous to (and in fact is derived from) that for dysplasia complicating idiopathic inflammatory bowel disease.[87,89] The criteria are as follows:

NEGATIVE FOR DYSPLASIA (Fig. 7-17)

The glandular architecture and cellular morphology are free of neoplastic alterations but may reveal reactive or regenerative change. The glandular architecture is orderly and is not crowded. The regenerative basal glands characteristically display cytologic atypia in Barrett's intestinalized mucosa. This basal atypia includes nuclear enlargement, pleomorphism, outline irregularity, hyperchromasia, and stratification. It may be particularly striking in comparison to frequently admixed nonmetaplastic gastric glands that are usually quite bland. Basal glandular atypia matures completely to the surface in epithelium that is negative for dysplasia. *Surface maturation* refers to the nuclei becoming smaller (less than twice the size of stromal fibroblast nuclei and usually much less), less darkly staining, smoothly contoured, uniform, and largely nonstratified as the cells extend from the basal glands onto the mucosal surface.

Reactive cytologic alterations in the presence of active inflammation are also part of the spectrum of "negative for dysplasia," as long as the cytologic changes still mature to the surface of the biopsy and the glandular architecture is intact. Reactive inflammatory change often produces a more open chromatin pattern and some degree of cytoplasmic mucin depletion.

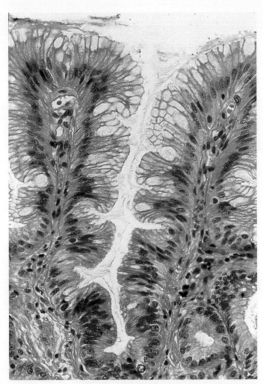

FIGURE 7–17. Baseline glandular atypia in Barrett's metaplasia that is negative for dysplasia. Cells show maturation onto the surface of the mucosa. This baseline glandular atypia is frequently quite marked, especially when viewed in comparison with adjacent nonmetaplastic cardiac or fundic glands.

INDEFINITE FOR DYSPLASIA (Figs. 7-18 and 7-19)

The glandular architecture is intact or may exhibit slight crowding or loss of parallel architecture. The cytologic changes may be mild or focally markedly atypical and lack surface maturation in the presence of pronounced inflammation or erosion/ulceration. Numerous mitotic figures may be present. In *noninflamed*

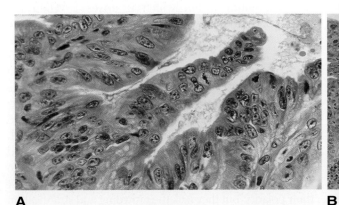
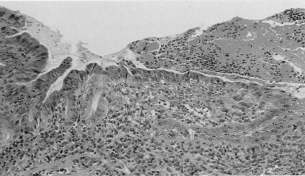

A   **B**

FIGURE 7–18. Indefinite for dysplasia in Barrett's esophagus with severe cytoarchitectural changes (**A**) in the setting of active ulceration (**B**). Changes are concerning not only for dysplasia but also for adenocarcinoma.

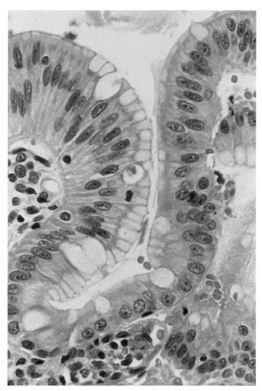

FIGURE 7–19. Indefinite for dysplasia in Barrett's esophagus with cytologic atypia that partially but incompletely matures onto the biopsy surface.

biopsies, marked glandular atypia that matures to the surface and mild atypia that mostly matures to the surface also fall into the indefinite for dysplasia category. Biopsies without intact surface or other obscuring artifacts that limit assessment of maturation may also be categorized as indefinite for dysplasia.

LOW-GRADE DYSPLASIA (Fig. 7-20)

The crypt architecture is relatively preserved, and distortion, if present, is generally mild to moderate. A villiform surface configuration may be present. The nuclei exhibit some combination of stratification, enlargement, hyperchromasia, pleomorphism, and crowding. Abnormal mitotic figures may be present in the upper portion of the crypt. Goblet cell mucin is often diminished and may be absent. "Dystrophic goblet cells" may be seen in which the mucin vacuole is located on the basal rather than the luminal side of the nucleus. Cytologic changes extend from the base of the crypts onto the surface epithelium. Nuclear polarity is preserved, whereby the long axes of the nuclei remain perpendicular to the basement membrane.

HIGH-GRADE DYSPLASIA (Fig. 7-21)

Distortion of crypt architecture is present and may be marked. It consists of some combination of branching and lateral budding of crypts, marked glandular crowding, villiform surface configuration, or intraglandular bridging of epithelium to form cribriform or "back-to-back" gland patterns. Nuclear abnormalities are present as in low-grade dysplasia, but, in addition, more pronounced nuclear enlargement, nuclear membrane irregularity, and hyperchromasia are noted. Loss of nuclear polarity, the most objective criterion for differentiating low- from high-grade dysplasia, refers to cells in which the long axes of the nuclei no longer remain perpendicular to the basement membrane. Nuclei vary markedly in size, shape, and staining characteristics. Cytoplasmic mucin is usually diminished or absent, and dystrophic goblet cells may be present. Cytologic changes extend from the base of the crypts onto the surface epithelium. Because of the major consequences of a diagnosis of high-grade dysplasia, this diagnosis should always be confirmed by at least one experienced GI pathologist.

When high-grade dysplasia is detected for the first time in a patient with Barrett's esophagus, early re-endoscopy with multiple biopsies should be done to rule out a coexisting unsampled carcinoma. Extensive sampling of the mucosa is essential because superficial carcinomas may not be recognizable to the endoscopist.

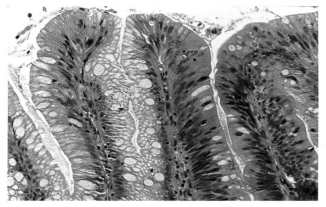

FIGURE 7–20. Low-grade dysplasia (*right*) directly adjacent to mucosa that is negative for dysplasia (*left*) in Barrett's esophagus.

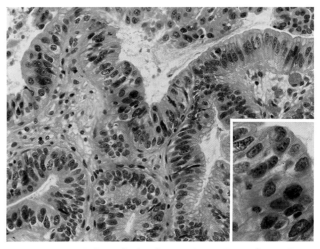

FIGURE 7–21. High-grade dysplasia in Barrett's esophagus. Note the loss of nuclear polarity detailed in the *inset*.

Accordingly, it has been recommended that the sampling be increased to four biopsies every 1 cm throughout the Barrett's segment in patients with high-grade dysplasia. Because high-grade dysplasia is rare in unselected patients with Barrett's esophagus, and because most pathologists therefore do not have the opportunity to study many examples of it, pathologists in this situation would be wise to seek a second opinion regarding the diagnosis of high-grade dysplasia before surgery is undertaken. Patients with superficial carcinoma (either intramucosal or submucosal) who are surgical candidates often undergo esophagectomy; resection of these early carcinomas provides the opportunity for cure.[90,91]

A relatively high prevalence of carcinoma has been found in resected specimens for patients with a pre-operative diagnosis of high-grade dysplasia.[91] This has led to the conclusion that high-grade dysplasia is a marker for coexisting adenocarcinoma, but this conclusion has been based on small numbers of patients, many of whom already had advanced disease because they had symptoms or endoscopic findings suggestive of carcinoma. When thorough endoscopic biopsy sampling is carried out according to the protocols outlined previously, biopsies accurately determine whether a clinically unsuspected carcinoma accompanies the dysplasia.[92,93] Following such a policy has produced a high cure rate for early adenocarcinoma in Barrett's esophagus, but at the same time it has avoided esophagectomy in patients with high-grade dysplasia in whom carcinoma may never develop.[92,93] However, given the intensity of the biopsy protocols mentioned earlier, it is uncertain whether this information can be extrapolated to non-specialized centers.

Problems in the Diagnosis of Dysplasia (see also Chapter 16)

SAMPLING

Mapping studies of esophagectomy specimens containing adenocarcinoma have shown that dysplasia often is not detectable grossly and involves a highly variable amount of esophageal mucosa surrounding the invasive carcinoma.[92] Dysplastic mucosa may occupy most of or the entire esophagus, or it may be limited in extent.[94] Thus, the endoscopist must thoroughly sample the mucosa to avoid missing small areas of dysplasia or carcinoma. Four-quadrant, well-oriented jumbo biopsies obtained every 2 cm or at shorter intervals throughout the length of the Barrett's segment are recommended, combined with additional biopsies of any endoscopic lesions.[95] Shortening of the interval to every 1 cm is recommended for patients with high-grade dysplasia who are maintained under endoscopic surveillance.[96] Adherence to this or similar protocols produces excellent correlation between the preoperative endoscopic

diagnosis and the final diagnosis rendered in resection specimens.[92-95]

BASELINE GLANDULAR ATYPIA OF BARRETT'S METAPLASTIC EPITHELIUM

Metaplastic Barrett's epithelium that is negative for dysplasia consistently shows nuclear atypism, especially when viewed in contrast to gastric epithelium. This is particularly true of the deepest metaplastic glands closest to the muscularis mucosae (see Fig. 7-17). However, they are usually separable from dysplasia because they are confined to the deep glands, while the upper portions show less abnormality or are normal (surface maturation); this feature is best recognized in well-oriented biopsy specimens. Thus, the diagnosis of dysplasia should be made with great caution, if ever, when the changes do not involve the mucosal surface.

INTEROBSERVER VARIATION

The distinction of Barrett's dysplasia from reactive or regenerative changes caused by inflammation is difficult and at times impossible. Reactive changes in biopsies from the edges of ulcers may be indistinguishable from dysplasia. In cases with marked inflammation or ulceration, the atypia may be so severe that even carcinoma may be suspected (see Fig. 7-18). If inflammation or ulceration is present, repeat biopsies after intensive medical antireflux therapy often show resolution of the abnormalities. Problematic cases also include those with cytoarchitectural abnormalities in noninflamed Barrett's epithelium, with cytologic alterations that mature partially but incompletely onto the surface epithelium (see Fig. 7-19).

Because the epithelial abnormalities in dysplasia form a continuous morphologic spectrum, the boundaries between the grades of dysplasia cannot be sharply defined. Thus, observer variation exists in the diagnosis and grading of dysplasia, particularly at the indefinite/low-grade interface.[89] For this reason, the categories of indefinite for dysplasia and low-grade dysplasia are combined in most endoscopic protocols for practical clinical management purposes. Fortunately, at the high end of the spectrum, namely high-grade dysplasia and intramucosal carcinoma, wherein the diagnosis may lead to invasive therapy, excellent agreement has been reached among GI pathologists.[89,96] Thus, histopathologic diagnosis can be highly reliable and accurate, especially at the lowest and highest ends of the spectrum, at which diagnostic management decisions are most important.

OVERDIAGNOSIS OF HIGH-GRADE DYSPLASIA IN BARRETT'S ESOPHAGUS

A significant tendency exists for pathologists to overdiagnose high-grade dysplasia in Barrett's esophagus. One of the more frequent errors is the misinterpretation of severe reactive change as high-grade dysplasia (see

Fig. 7-15). However, the deeper glands in reactive cardiac-type mucosa tend to retain most or all of their mucin. Reactive mucosa may also retain some surface mucin in the form of markedly shortened but back-to-back foveolar mucin caps over the surface. These features, in combination with bland, mitotically inactive mucinous glands, are good criteria for distinguishing reactive epithelium from dysplastic Barrett's epithelium.

HIGH-GRADE DYSPLASIA VERSUS CARCINOMA

When high-grade dysplasia develops, architectural distortion may reach a point at which the diagnosis of carcinoma is impossible to exclude with certainty on the basis of superficial biopsy samples. This occurs when glands grow in a cribriform or dense back-to-back pattern, when ill-defined abortive glands are present in the lamina propria, or when dilated glands are present with luminal necrotic debris. High-grade dysplasia in the setting of an ulcer is another significant risk factor for carcinoma. In such cases, a diagnosis such as "high-grade dysplasia with marked distortion of glandular architecture, invasive adenocarcinoma cannot be excluded" is appropriate (Fig. 7-22). When numerous individual invasive cells or sheets of malignant cells or angulated infiltrative and abortive glands infiltrate the lamina propria, or a well-defined desmoplastic stroma can be identified separate from inflammatory stromal change, the diagnosis of invasive adenocarcinoma can usually be made (Fig. 7-23).

In practice, these two diagnostic categories (high-grade dysplasia and intramucosal adenocarcinoma) may be difficult to separate, especially with endoscopic biopsies.[97] Nevertheless, because a few groups have published natural history data on dysplasia in Barrett's esophagus and have shown that continued endoscopic surveillance may be a safe option for patients with high-grade dysplasia (see later), the precise distinction between high-grade

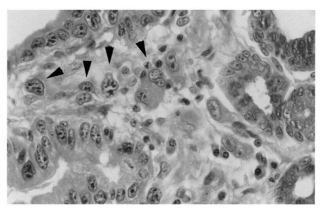

FIGURE 7–23. Intramucosal adnocarcinoma in Barrett's esophagus showing numerous isolated malignant cells invading the lamina propria *(black arrowheads).*

dysplasia and intramucosal carcinoma is becoming more important. This is an area ripe for more study.

Adjunctive Techniques in Evaluating Neoplastic Progression

Brush cytology is not as sensitive or specific as histology in detecting Barrett's metaplastic epithelium.[98] Although it was thought to be useful in detecting dysplasia in one study,[98] another found that its addition to histology increased the cost but not the diagnostic yield for dysplasia and cancer.[99]

DNA content flow cytometry has been extensively evaluated in the study of neoplastic progression in patients with Barrett's esophagus. The prevalence of DNA aneuploidy and/or greater 4N (G2/tetraploid) and S-phase fractions increases with increasing histologic grade.[96] DNA aneuploidy can be detected in paraffin-embedded mucosal biopsy specimens, which may help the clinician to determine the significance of epithelial alterations in negative, indefinite, and even possibly low-grade dysplastic biopsy categories.[95,96] It appears to be adjunctive; experts in this field do not recommend that it replace histology.[96] Once the histologic diagnosis of high-grade dysplasia and probably unequivocal low-grade dysplasia has been made, DNA flow cytometry adds no additional prognostic information.[64]

Molecular Genetic Alterations

Many genetic abnormalities that tend to correlate with advancing histologic grades of neoplastic progression have been documented in Barrett's esophagus. However, to date, long-term prospective studies for determining the potential clinical utility of these markers are virtually nonexistent. No genetic marker has ever been shown to be a better predictor of cancer than histologic neoplastic progression, and in particular, high-grade dysplasia.[64] Reproducibility studies regarding

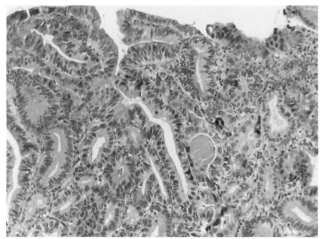

FIGURE 7–22. High-grade dysplasia with marked distortion of glandular architecture; invasive adenocarcinoma cannot be excluded. Note the severe crowding and the presence of dilated glands with necrotic debris.

genetic biomarkers of cancer risk are also limited, and ease of extrapolation of these methods to routine use remains unknown.

NATURAL HISTORY AND MANAGEMENT OF DYSPLASIA (see also Chapter 16)

Management of the patient with dysplasia complicating Barrett's esophagus presents a difficult task. Until recently, insufficient numbers of patients with dysplasia had been followed for a long enough period using adequate numbers of biopsies for the natural history of dysplasia in Barrett's esophagus to be determined precisely. Two large cohorts of patients with Barrett's esophagus have been followed extensively by means of similar rigorous high-density surveillance biopsy protocols. One program is at the Hines VA Hospital in Chicago[93]; the other is at the University of Washington in Seattle.[96]

At the Hines VA program,[93] a total of 1099 patients with Barrett's esophagus were followed over a 20-year period. Of these, 79 (7.2%) patients had high-grade dysplasia, of which 34 had prevalent high-grade dysplasia (present at the first endoscopy) and 45 had incident high-grade dysplasia (detected during surveillance and therefore probably earlier in its natural history). Of the 75 who remained without detectable cancer during the first year of intensive biopsy surveillance, only 12 patients (16%) developed cancer over a mean of 7.3 years of surveillance. Further, 11 of the 12 who were compliant with the surveillance protocol were considered cured of their early cancers by surgical or ablative therapy. These findings support that high-grade dysplasia does not inexorably and rapidly progress to cancer, as was previously feared.

In the 15-year prospective longitudinal study at the University of Washington,[96] a total of 327 patients were evaluated by rigorous surveillance endoscopy for progression from their baseline alterations. Median surveillance intervals were 24.4 months for baseline negative histology, 18.2 months for indefinite histology, 15.7 months for low-grade dysplasia, and 4.6 months for high-grade dysplasia. Mean and median follow-up periods were 3.9 and 2.4 years, respectively. Overall, a total of 42 patients developed cancer; 35 developed cancer within 5 years of their first endoscopy. No patient with negative, indefinite, or low-grade dysplasia with normal flow cytometric studies developed cancer within 5 years. This indicates that surveillance intervals could be lengthened to 5 years for this majority subset, with the use of the intensive Seattle surveillance protocol, including baseline intensive biopsies and flow cytometry with expert preparation and interpretation.

Squamous Overgrowth

Successful antireflux therapy can eliminate or reduce the intensity of reactive changes secondary to inflammation that may be misinterpreted as dysplasia. Successful medical or surgical antireflux therapy may also be associated with some downward migration of the SCJ and with the development of squamous "islands" within the Barrett's segment; however, complete regression of all Barrett's epithelium rarely occurs. Prior biopsy sites, proton pump inhibitor therapy, and ablative therapies are associated with the development of squamous islands. Such squamous overgrowth may cause an underestimation of the endoscopic extent of Barrett's mucosa because metaplastic epithelium, dysplastic epithelium, or both may persist beneath squamous reepithelialized areas in Barrett's esophagus.[100,101] The magnitude of this problem remains unknown.

Endoscopic Ablative Therapy in Barrett's Esophagus

Nonsurgical methods for the treatment of patients with high-grade dysplasia are being explored with promising results. These include photodynamic therapy, multipolar electrocoagulation, heater probe, and argon plasma coagulation.[102-108] Study of photodynamic therapy (PDT) is now nearing the stage of completion of a phase III FDA-controlled trial of more than 200 patients for the treatment of Barrett's esophagus with high-grade dysplasia.[102,106,107] Interim results demonstrate that after a mean follow-up of 1 year (of a total follow-up plan of 5 years), 80% had complete ablation of all Barrett's epithelium, including high-grade dysplasia. Further, compared with controls with high-grade dysplasia on proton pump inhibitor therapy alone, without PDT but under identical surveillance and selection conditions, the PDT patients have a greater than twofold reduction in cancer development.[106,107] The durability of this response is now under study.

Eosinophilic Esophagitis

The esophagus is one of the sites of involvement of eosinophilic gastroenteritis.[109] (See Chapter 9 for details.) Esophageal pathology in this condition, however, is nonspecific in that eosinophilic inflammation is common to all forms of esophagitis. As in all other sites of GI involvement, including gastric and intestinal sites, eosinophilic gastroenteritis involving the esophagus is a diagnosis of exclusion. Peripheral blood eosinophilia is required for the diagnosis. Disorders to be excluded include gastroesophageal reflux disease, idiopathic eosinophilic esophagitis (which may be part of the spectrum of systemic eosinophilic gastroenteritis), fungal and parasitic infection, and allergic and collagen vascular diseases.

Esophageal Involvement in Collagen Vascular Disorders

Collagen vascular disorders, including progressive systemic sclerosis (scleroderma),[110] systemic lupus erythematosus,[111] rheumatoid arthritis,[112] mixed connective tissue disorders, polymyositis, dermatomyositis,[113] and Sjögren's syndrome,[114] may involve the esophagus (see also Chapter 5).[115] Esophageal manifestations range from myoneurenteric dysmotility disorders to esophagitis secondary to reflux, drug-induced esophagitis, or opportunistic infection. Esophageal pathology may relate to the underlying collagen vascular disease or to the adverse effects of NSAID therapy or immunosuppressive or other therapies. Increased rates of Barrett's esophagus and its neoplastic complications have been reported in association with scleroderma.[116]

Esophageal Manifestations of Dermatologic Diseases

The esophagus may be involved in numerous dermatologic conditions, including drug-induced disease such as Stevens-Johnson syndrome[117] and bullous disease such as bullous pemphigoid, benign mucous membrane pemphigoid, epidermolysis bullosa acquisita, pemphigus vulgaris,[118,119] and lichen planus (see also Chapter 5).[120] The esophagus may be involved primarily with these disorders or in conjunction with dermatologic involvement. Esophageal histology mimics that in the skin. Erosions and ulcers with subsequent webs and strictures may develop.

Graft-Versus-Host Disease

Esophageal graft-versus-host disease (GVHD) may manifest as acute GVHD, bullous disease, and complete sloughing of the esophageal mucosa, with formation of an esophageal cast.[121-124] The features of esophageal GVHD are the same as those of GVHD in the remainder of the GI tract, namely, increased intraepithelial lymphocytosis, cell damage manifested in squamous mucosa as dyskeratotic keratinocytes, and increased apoptosis in the regenerative or basal squamous cell layers (see Chapter 5).

Achalasia

Esophageal achalasia is a dysmotility disorder characterized by failure of the LES to relax. Esophageal mucosal and mural histologic involvement may be related to chronic stasis of luminal contents and includes diffuse

squamous hyperplasia, lymphocytic squamous mucosal esophagitis, lymphocytic inflammation of the lamina propria and submucosa with germinal center formation, and submucosal periductal and glandular inflammation and atrophy. Resection specimens demonstrate inflammation and fibrosis of myenteric nerves with markedly diminished numbers of myenteric ganglion cells. Hypertrophy or degeneration and fibrosis and eosinophilia of the muscularis propria are also common manifestations.[125,126]

Esophageal Involvement in Crohn's Disease

Although Crohn's disease may involve the esophagus, this is a rare occurrence with a prevalence of 0.2% in one series.[127] The diagnosis is one of exclusion, as it is throughout the GI tract. Because the histopathologic features are those of nonspecific esophagitis, the diagnosis of esophageal Crohn's disease cannot be established outside of the presence of extraesophageal involvement by gastric, small bowel, or colonic disease.

Esophageal Amyloidosis

The esophagus may be involved in systemic amyloidosis, which, in addition to the amyloid deposition, may result in nonspecific, secondary esophagitis. The frequency of esophageal amyloidosis in one series of GI amyloidosis was 72%[128] (see Chapter 5).

Mallory-Weiss Tears and Other Traumatic Esophageal Diseases

Full-thickness (Boerhaave's syndrome) or partial-thickness (Mallory-Weiss tears) esophageal perforations and hematomas are manifestations of spontaneous and iatrogenic traumatic esophageal disease.[129] In general, these disorders are diagnosed clinically or radiologically. Thus, resection specimens are rarely obtained.

References

1. Frierson HF: Histology in the diagnosis of reflux esophagitis. Gastroenterol Clin N Am 19:631-644, 1990.
2. Vaezi MF, Richter JR: Role of acid and duodenogastroesophageal reflux in gastroesophageal reflux disease. Gastroenterology 111:1192-1199, 1996.
3. Pope CE: Acid-reflux disorders. N Engl J Med 331:656-660, 1994.
4. Mittal RK, Balaban DH: The esophagogastric junction. N Engl J Med 336:924-932, 1997.
5. Knuff TE, Benjamin SB, Worsham GF, et al: Histologic evaluation of chronic gastroesophageal reflux: An evaluation of biopsy methods and diagnostic criteria. Dig Dis Sci 29:194-201, 1984.

6. Levine DS, Blount PL, Rudolph RE, et al: Safety of a systematic endoscopic biopsy protocol in patients with Barrett's esophagus. Am J Gastroenterol 95:1152-1157, 2000.

7. Weinstein WM, Bogoch ER, Bowes KL: The normal human esophageal mucosa: A histological reappraisal. Gastroenterology 68:40-44, 1975.

8. Schindlbeck NE, Wiebecke B, Klauser AG, et al: Diagnostic value of histology in non-erosive gastro-esophageal reflux disease. Gut 39:151-154, 1996.

9. Orenstein SR: Gastroesophageal reflux. Curr Probl Pediatr 21:193-241, 1991.

10. Ismail-Beigi F, Horton PF, Pope CE: Histological consequences of gastroesophageal reflux in man. Gastroenterology 58:163-174, 1970.

11. Johnson LF, DeMeester TR, Haggitt RC: Esophageal epithelial response to gastroesophageal reflux: A quantitative study. Am J Dig Dis 23:498-509, 1978.

12. Black DD, Haggitt RC, Orenstein SR, et al: Esophagitis in infants: Morphometric histological diagnosis and correlation with measures of gastroesophageal reflux. Gastroenterology 98:1408-1414, 1990.

13. Haggitt RC: Histopathology of reflux induced esophageal and supraesophageal injuries. Am J Med 6(suppl 4a):109S-111S, 2000.

14. Brown LF, Goldman H, Antonioli DA: Intraepithelial eosinophils in endoscopic biopsies of adults with reflux esophagitis. Am J Surg Pathol 8:899-905, 1984.

15. Tummala V, Barwick KW, Sontag SJ, et al: The significance of intraepithelial eosinophils in the histologic diagnosis of gastroesophageal reflux. Am J Clin Pathol 87:43-48, 1987.

16. Winter HS, Madara JL, Stafford RJ, et al: Intraepithelial eosinophils: A new diagnostic criterion for reflux esophagitis. Gastroenterology 83:818-823, 1982.

17. Walsh SV, Antonioli DA, Goldman H, et al: Allergic esophagitis in children: A clinicopathologic entity. Am J Surg Pathol 23:390-396, 1999.

18. Kelly KJ, Lazenby AJ, Rowe PC, et al: Eosinophilic esophagitis attributed to gastroesophageal reflux: Improvement with an amino acid-based formula. Gastroenterology 109:1503-1512, 1995.

19. Attwood SEA, Smyrk, TC, DeMeester TR, et al: Esophageal eosinophilia with dysphagia: A distinct clinicopathologic syndrome. Dig Dis Sci 38:109-116, 1993.

20. Lee RG: Marked eosinophilia in esophageal biopsies. Am J Surg Pathol 9:475-479, 1985.

21. Mangano MM, Antonioli DA, Schnitt SJ, et al: Nature and significance of cells with irregular nuclear contours in esophageal mucosal biopsies. Mod Pathol 5:191-196, 1992.

22. Wang HH, Mangano MM, Antonioli DA: Evaluation of T-lymphocytes in esophageal mucosal biopsies. Mod Pathol 7:55-58, 1994.

23. Geboes K, Desmet V, Vantrappen G, et al: Vascular changes in the esophageal mucosa. An early histologic sign of esophagitis. Gastrointest Endosc 26:29-32, 1980.

24. Collins BJ, Elliott H, Cloan JM, et al: Oesophageal histology in reflux esophagitis. J Clin Pathol 38:1265-1272, 1985.

25. Shekitka KM, Helwig EB: Deceptive bizarre stromal cells in polyps and ulcers of the gastrointestinal tract. Cancer 67:2111-2117, 1991.

26. Baehr PH, McDonald GB: Esophageal infections: Risk factors, presentation, diagnosis, and treatment. Gastroenterology 106:509-532, 1994.

27. Buss DH, Scharyj M: Herpes virus infection of the esophagus and other visceral organs in adults: Incidence and clinical significance. Am J Med 66:457-462, 1979.

28. McDonald GB, Sharma P, Hackman RC, et al: Esophageal infections in immunosuppressed patients after marrow transplantation. Gastroenterology 88:111-1117, 1985.

29. McBane RD, Gross JB: Herpes esophagitis: Clinical syndrome, endoscopic appearance, and diagnosis in 23 patients. Gastrointest Endosc 37:600-603, 1991.

30. Singh SP, Odze RD: Multinucleated epithelial giant cell changes in esophagitis: A clinicopathologic study of 14 cases. Am J Surg Pathol 22:93-99, 1998.

31. Greenson JK, Beschorner WE, Boitnott JK, et al: Prominent mononuclear cell infiltrate is characteristic of herpes esophagitis. Hum Pathol 22:541-549, 1991.

32. Bonacini M, Young T, Laine L: The causes of esophageal symptoms in human immunodeficiency virus infection. Arch Intern Med 151:1567-1572, 1991.

33. Chetty R, Roskell DE: Cytomegalovirus infection in the gastrointestinal tract. J Clin Pathol 47:968-972, 1994.

34. Wilcox CM, Straub RF, Schwartz DA: Prospective endoscopic characterization of cytomegalovirus esophagitis in AIDS. Gastrointest Endosc 40:481-484, 1994.

35. Greenson JK: Macrophage aggregates in cytomegalovirus esophagitis. Hum Pathol 28:375-378, 1997.

36. Hackman RC, Wolford JL, Cleaves CA, et al: Recognition and rapid diagnosis of upper gastrointestinal cytomegalovirus infection in marrow transplant recipients. Transplantation 57:231-237, 1994.

37. Kodsi BE, Wickremeisinghe PC, Kozinn PJ, et al: *Candida* esophagitis: A prospective study of 27 cases. Gastroenterology 71:715-719, 1976.

38. Mathieson R, Dutta SK: Candida esophagitis. Dig Dis Sci 28:365-370, 1983.

39. Walsh TJ, Merz WG: Pathologic features in the human alimentary tract associated with invasiveness of *Candida* tropicalis. Am J Clin Pathol 85:498-502, 1986.

40. Tavitian A, Raufman JP, Rosenthal LE, et al: Ketoconazole-resistant *Candida* esophagitis in patients with acquired immunodeficiency syndrome. Gastroenterology 90:443-445, 1986.

41. Rywlin AM, Ortega R: Glycogenic acanthosis of the esophagus. Arch Pathol 90:439-443, 1970.

42. Kay PS, Soetikno RM, Mindelzun R, et al: Diffuse esophageal glycogenic acanthosis: An endoscopic marker of Cowden's disease. Am J Gastroenterol 92:1038-1040, 1997.

43. Bender MD, Allison J, Cuartas R, et al: Glycogenic acanthosis of the esophagus: A form of benign epithelial hyperplasia. Gastroenterology 65:373-380, 1973.

44. Bertoni G, Sassatelli R, Nigrisoli E, et al: Ectopic sebaceous glands in the esophagus: Report of three new cases and review of the literature. Am J Gastroenterol 89:1884-1887, 1994.

45. Connolly GM, Hawkins D, Harcourt-Webster JN, et al: Oesophageal symptoms, their causes, treatment, and prognosis in patients with the acquired immunodeficiency syndrome. Gut 30:1033-1039, 1989.

46. Eng J, Sabanathan S: Tuberculosis of the esophagus. Dig Dis Sci 36:536-540, 1991.

47. Forsmark CE, Wilcox CM, Darragh TM, et al: Disseminated histoplasmosis in AIDS: An unusual case of esophageal involvement and gastrointestinal bleeding. Gastrointest Endosc 36:604-605, 1990.

48. Kitchen VS, Helbert M, Francis ND, et al: Epstein-Barr virus associated esophageal ulcers in AIDS. Gut 31:1223-1225, 1990.

49. Rabeneck L, Popovic M, Gartner S, et al: Acute HIV infection presenting with painful swallowing and esophageal ulcers. JAMA 263:2318-2322, 1990.

50. Wilcox CM, Zaki SR, Coffield LM, et al: Evaluation of idiopathic esophageal ulceration for human immunodeficiency virus. Mod Pathol 8:568-572, 1995.

51. Kikendall JW, Friedman AC, Oyewole MA, et al: Pill-induced esophageal injury. Case reports and review of the medical literature. Dig Dis Sci 28:174-182, 1983.

52. Bott S, Prakash C, McCallum RW: Medication-induced esophageal injury: Survey of the literature. Am J Gastroenterol 82:758-763, 1987.

53. Boyce HW: Drug-induced esophageal damage: Diseases of medical progress. Gastrointest Endosc 47:547-550, 1998.

54. Abraham SC, Jardley JH, Wu T-T: Erosive injury to the upper gastrointestinal tract in patients receiving iron medication: An unrecognized entity. Am J Surg Pathol 23:1241-1247, 1999.

55. Abraham SC, Cruz-Correa M, Lee LA, et al: Alendronate-associated esophageal injury: Pathologic and endoscopic features. Mod Pathol 12:1152-1157, 1999.

56. Semble EL, Wu WC, Castell DO: Nonsteroidal anti-inflammatory drugs and esophageal injury. Semin Arthritis Rheum 19:99-109, 1989.

57. Taha AS, Dahill S, Nakshabendi I, et al: Oesophageal histology in long term users of non-steroidal anti-inflammatory drugs. J Clin Pathol 47:705-708, 1994.

58. Isolauri J, Markkula H: Lye ingestion and carcinoma of the esophagus. Acta Chir Scand 155:269-271, 1989.

59. de Jong AL, Macdonald R, Ein S, et al: Corrosive esophagitis in children: A 30-year review. Int J Pediatr Otorhinolaryngol 57:203-211, 2001.

60. Garcia Diaz E, Castro Fernandez M, Romero Gomez M, et al: Upper gastrointestinal tract injury caused by ingestion of caustic substances. Gastroenterol Hepatol 24:191-195, 2001.
61. Appelqvist P, Salmo M: Lye corrosion carcinoma of the esophagus: A review of 63 cases. Cancer 45:2655-2658, 1980.
62. Novak JM, Collins JT, Donowitz M, et al: Effects of radiation on the human gastrointestinal tract. J Clin Gastroenterol 1:9-39, 1979.
63. Slavin RE, Dias MA, Sarai R: Cytosine arabinoside induced gastrointestinal toxic alterations in sequential chemotherapeutic protocols. A clinico-pathologic study of 33 patients. Cancer 42:1747-1759, 1978.
64. Haggitt RC: Barrett's esophagus, dysplasia and adenocarcinoma. Hum Pathol 25:982-993, 1994.
65. Riddell RH: The biopsy diagnosis of gastroesophageal reflux disease, "carditis," and Barrett's esophagus, and sequelae of therapy. Am J Surg Pathol 20(suppl 1):S31-S50, 1996.
66. Antonioli DA, Wang HH: Morphology of Barrett's esophagus and Barrett's-associated dysplasia and adenocarcinoma. Gastroenterol Clin North Am 26:495-506, 1997.
67. Hassal E: Barrett's esophagus: New definitions and approaches in children. J Pediatr Gastroenterol 15:345-364, 1993.
68. Sampliner RE, Practice Parameters Committee of the American College of Gastroenterology: Updated guidelines for the diagnosis, surveillance, and therapy of Barrett's esophagus. Am J Gastroenterol 97:1888-1895, 2002.
69. Ofman JJ, Shaheen NJ, Desai AA, et al: The quality of care in Barrett's esophagus: Endoscopist and pathologist practices. Am J Gastroenterol 96:876-881, 2001.
70. Sharma P, Morales TG, Sampliner RE: Short segment Barrett's esophagus—the need for standardization of the definition and of endoscopic criteria. Am J Gastroenterol 93:1033-1036, 1998.
71. Weinstein WM, Ippoliti AF: The diagnosis of Barrett's esophagus: Goblets, goblets, goblets. Gastrointest Endosc 44:91-95, 1996.
72. Qualman SJ, Murray RD, McClung J, et al: Intestinal metaplasia is age related in Barrett's esophagus. Arch Pathol Lab Med 114:1236-1240, 1990.
73. Chandrasoma PT, Der R, Ma Y, et al: Histology of the gastroesophageal junction: An autopsy study. Am J Surg Pathol 24:402-409, 2000.
74. Kilgore SP, Ormsby AH, Gramlich TL, et al: The gastric cardia: Fact or fiction? Am J Gastroenterol 95:921-924, 2000.
75. Kim SL, Waring P, Spechler SJ, et al: Diagnostic inconsistencies in Barrett's esophagus. Gastroenterology 107:945-949, 1994.
76. Spechler SJ, Goyal RK: The columnar-lined esophagus, intestinal metaplasia, and Norman Barrett. Gastroenterology 110:614-621, 1996.
77. El-Serag HB, Sonnenberg A, Jamal MM, et al: Characteristics of intestinal metaplasia in the gastric cardia. Am J Gastroenterol 94:622-627, 1999.
78. Hirota WK, Loughney TM, Lazas DJ, et al: Specialized intestinal metaplasia, dysplasia, and cancer of the esophagogastric junction: Prevalence and clinical data. Gastroenterology 116:277-285, 1999.
79. Hackelsberger A, Gunther T, Schultze V, et al: Intestinal metaplasia at the gastro-oesophageal junction: *Helicobacter pylori* or gastro-oesophageal reflux disease? Gut 43:17-21, 1998.
80. Goldblum JR, Vicari JJ, Falk GW, et al: Inflammation and intestinal metaplasia of the gastric cardia: The role of gastroesophageal reflux and *H. pylori* infection. Gastroenterology 114:633-639, 1998.
81. Oberg S, Peters JH, DeMeester TR, et al: Inflammation and specialized intestinal metaplasia of cardiac mucosa is a manifestation of gastroesophageal reflux disease. Ann Surg 226:522-532, 1997.
82. Voutilainen M, Färkkilä M, Juhola M, et al: Complete and incomplete intestinal metaplasia at the esophagogastric junction: Prevalences and associations with endoscopic erosive esophagitis and gastritis. Gut 45:644-648, 1999.
83. Ormsby AH, Goldblum JR, Rice TW, et al: Cytokeratin subsets can reliably distinguish Barrett's esophagus from intestinal metaplasia of the stomach. Hum Pathol 30:288-294, 1999.
84. Wang HH, Zeroogian JM, Spechler SJ, et al: Prevalence and significance of pancreatic acinar metaplasia at the gastroesophageal junction. Am J Surg Pathol 20:1507-1510, 1996.
85. Borhan-Manesh F, Farnum JB: Incidence of heterotopic gastric mucosa in the upper oesophagus. Gut 32:968-972, 1991.
86. Cameron AJ, Zinsmeister AR, Ballard DJ, et al: Prevalence of columnar-lined (Barrett's) esophagus: Comparison of population-based and autopsy findings. Gastroenterology 99:918-922, 1990.
87. Riddell RH, Goldman H, Ransohoff DF, et al: Dysplasia in inflammatory bowel disease: Standardized classification with provisional clinical applications. Hum Pathol 14:931-968, 1983.
88. Lee RG: Adenomas arising in Barrett's esophagus. Am J Clin Pathol 85:629-632, 1986.
89. Montgomery E, Bronner MP, Goldblum JR, et al: Reproducibility of the diagnosis of dysplasia in Barrett esophagus (BE): A reaffirmation. Hum Pathol 32:368-378, 2001.
90. Rusch VW, Levine DS, Haggitt RC, et al: The management of high-grade dysplasia and early cancer in Barrett's esophagus. Cancer 74:1225-1229, 1994.
91. Rice TW, Falk GW, Achkar E, et al: Surgical management of high-grade dysplasia in Barrett's esophagus. Am J Gastroenterol 88:1832-1836, 1993.
92. Levine DS, Haggitt RC, Blount PL, et al: A systematic endoscopic biopsy protocol can differentiate high-grade dysplasia from early adenocarcinoma in Barrett's esophagus. Gastroenterology 105:40-50, 1993.
93. Schnell TG, Sontag SJ, Chejfec G, et al: Long-term nonsurgical management of Barrett's esophagus with high-grade dysplasia. Gastroenterology 120:1607-1619, 2001.
94. Cameron AJ, Carpenter HA: Barrett's esophagus, high-grade dysplasia, and early adenocarcinoma: A pathological study. Am J Gastroenterol 92:586-591, 1997.
95. Reid BJ, Blount PL, Rubin CE, et al: Predictors of progression to malignancy in Barrett's esophagus: Endoscopic, histologic and flow cytometric follow-up of a cohort. Gastroenterology 102:1212-1219, 1992.
96. Reid BJ, Levine DS, Longton G, et al: Predictors of progression to cancer in Barrett's esophagus: Baseline histology and flow cytometry identify low- and high-risk patient subsets. Am J Gastroenterol 95:1669-1676, 2000.
97. Ormsby AH, Petras RE, Henricks WH, et al: Observer variation in the diagnosis of superficial esophageal adenocarcinoma. Gut 51:671-676, 2002.
98. Wang HH, Sovie S, Zeroogian JM, et al: Value of cytology in detecting intestinal metaplasia and associated dysplasia at the gastroesophageal junction. Hum Pathol 28:465-471, 1997.
99. Alexander JA, Jones SM, Smith CJ, et al: Usefulness of cytopathology and histology in the evaluation of Barrett's esophagus in a community hospital. Gastrointest Endosc 46:318-320, 1997.
100. Sharma P, Morales TG, Bhattacharyya A, et al: Squamous islands in Barrett's esophagus: What lies underneath? Am J Gastroenterol 93:332-335, 1998.
101. Biddlestone LR, Barham CP, Wilkinson SP, et al: The histopathology of treated Barrett's esophagus. Am J Surg Pathol 22:239-245, 1998.
102. Overholt BF: Evaluating treatments of Barrett's esophagus that shows high-grade dysplasia [review]. Am J Manag Care 6(16 suppl):S903-S908, 2000.
103. Sampliner RE, Faigel D, Fennerty MR, et al: Effective and safe endoscopic reversal of nondysplastic Barrett's esophagus with thermal electrocoagulation combined with high-dose acid inhibition: A multicenter study. Gastrointest Endosc 53:554-558, 2001.
104. Van Laethem JL, Cremer M, Peny MO, et al: Eradication of Barrett's mucosa with argon plasma coagulation and acid suppression: Immediate and mid term results. Gut 43:747-751, 1998.
105. Michopoulos S, Tsibouris P, Bouzakis H, et al: Complete regression of Barrett's esophagus with heat probe thermocoagulation: Mid-term results. Gastrointest Endosc 50:165-172, 1999.
106. Overholt BF, Panjehpour M, Haydek JM: Photodynamic therapy for Barrett's esophagus: Follow-up in 100 patients. Gastrointest Endosc 49:1-7, 1999.
107. Overholt BF, Haggitt RC, Bronner MP, et al: A multicenter, partially blinded, randomized study of the efficacy of photodynamic therapy (PDT) using porfimer sodium (PDR) for the ablation of high-grade dysplasia (HGD) in Barrett's esophagus (BE): Results of 6-month follow-up. Gastroenterology 120:A79, 2001.
108. Lightdale CJ: Ablation therapy for Barrett's esophagus: Is it time to choose our weapons? Gastrointest Endosc 49:122-125, 1999.
109. Matsushita M, Hajiro K, Morita Y, et al: Eosinophilic gastroenteritis involving the entire digestive tract. Am J Gastroenterol 90:1868-1870, 1995.
110. Rose S, Young MA, Reynolds JC: Gastrointestinal manifestations of scleroderma. Gastroenterol Clin North Am 27:563-594, 1998.

111. Chua S, Dodd H, Saeed IT, et al: Dysphagia in a patient with lupus and review of the literature. Lupus 11:322-324, 2002.

112. Lopez-Cepero Andrada JM, Jimenez Arjona J, Amaya Vidal A, et al: Pseudoachalasia and secondary amyloidosis in a patient with rheumatoid arthritis. Gastroenterol Hepatol 25:398-400, 2002.

113. de Merieux P, Verity MA, Clements PJ, et al: Esophageal abnormalities and dysphagia in polymyositis and dermatomyositis. Arthritis Rheum 26:961-968, 1983.

114. Palma R, Freire A, Freitas J, et al: Esophageal motility disorders in patients with Sjogren's syndrome. Dig Dis Sci 39:758-761, 1994.

115. Fitzgerald RC, Triadafilopoulos G: Esophageal manifestations of rheumatic disorders. Semin Arthritis Rheum 26:641-666, 1997.

116. Katzka DA, Reynolds JC, Saul SH, et al: Barrett's metaplasia and adenocarcinoma of the esophagus in scleroderma. Am J Med 82:46-52, 1987.

117. Lamireau T, Leaute-Labreze C, LeBail B, et al: Esophageal involvement in Stevens-Johnson syndrome. Endoscopy 33:550-553, 2001.

118. Wise JL, Murray JA: Esophageal manifestations of dermatologic disease. Curr Gastroenterol Rep 4:205-212, 2002.

119. Stewart MI, Woodley DT, Briggaman RA: Epidermolysis bullosa acquisita and associated symptomatic esophageal webs. Arch Dermatol 127:373-377, 1991.

120. Abraham SC, Ravich WJ, Anhalt GJ, et al: Esophageal lichen planus: Case report and review of the literature. Am J Surg Pathol 24:1678-1682, 2000.

121. Sodhi SS, Srinivasan R, Thomas RM: Esophageal graft versus host disease. Gastrointest Endosc 52:235, 2000.

122. Otero Lopez-Cubero S, Sale GE, McDonald GB: Acute graft-versus-host disease of the esophagus. Endoscopy 29:S35-S36, 1997.

123. Minocha A, Mandanas RA, Kida M, et al: Bullous esophagitis due to chronic graft-versus-host disease. Am J Gastroenterol 92:529-530, 1997.

124. Nakshabendi IM, Maldonado ME, Coppola D, et al: Esophageal cast: A manifestation of graft-versus-host disease. Dig Dis 18:103-105, 2000.

125. Goldblum JR, Whyte RI, Orringer MB, et al: Achalasia. A morphologic study of 42 resected specimens. Am J Surg Pathol 18:327-337, 1994.

126. Lehman MB, Clark SB, Ormsby AH, et al: Squamous mucosal alterations in esophagectomy specimens from patients with end-stage achalasia. Am J Surg Pathol 25:1413-1418, 2001.

127. Decker GA, Loftus EV Jr, Pasha TM, et al: Crohn's disease of the esophagus: Clinical features and outcomes. Inflamm Bowel Dis 7:113-119, 2001.

128. Tada S, Iida M, Iwashita A, et al: Endoscopic and biopsy findings of the upper digestive tract in patients with amyloidosis. Gastrointest Endosc 36:10-14, 1990.

129. Younes Z, Johnson DA: The spectrum of spontaneous and iatrogenic esophageal injury: Perforations, Mallory-Weiss tears, and hematomas. J Clin Gastroenterol 29:306-317, 1999.

CHAPTER 8

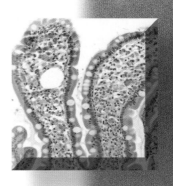

Inflammatory Disorders of the Stomach

ROBERT M. GENTA

▓ Introduction

In 1947, at the dawn of gastroscopy, Rudolf Schindler deemed gastritis "one of the most debated diseases of the human body" and predicted that its significance would be discussed "for some time to come."[1] Indeed, from the mid-1800s, when Cruveiller exposed the inaccuracies of Broussais's first descriptions of gastritis in autopsy material,[2] to the early 20th century, the concept of gastritis as a disease had been virtually abandoned. When gastritis was finally acknowledged to be a distinct entity, the search for its cause began. Since 1870, tiny curved bacteria in the gastric mucosa had been described by both human and veterinary pathologists but were dismissed as irrelevant contaminants.[3,4] Schindler himself claimed that the "bacteriologic etiology of chronic gastritis has not been proven convincingly in a single case."[1] Instead, a wide range of etiologic theories sprang up, including improper mastication, a "coarse" or "miserable" diet, alcohol, caffeine, nicotine, condiments and spices, drugs, heavy metals, thermal injury, chronic infections of tonsils and sinuses, circulatory disturbances, and psychogenic factors. Not surprisingly, many researchers were quite successful at debunking their colleagues' theories but unsuccessful at proving their own.

Meanwhile, increasingly accurate morphologic information was being gathered through the histopathologic examination of properly fixed autopsy material[5] and later of endoscopic biopsy specimens. With better morphology and reliable topographic information, distinct types and distribution patterns of gastritis were recognized, and innumerable classifications were conceived, presented, dismissed, and replaced. Some rested on solid morphologic grounds and proposed valid clinico-pathologic associations (e.g., with peptic ulcer and gastric cancer), but the lack of any therapeutic implications reduced all these classifications to little more than academic exercises.

Therefore, it is hardly surprising that when Warren and Marshall proposed in 1984 that chronic "idiopathic" gastritis had a bacterial cause (i.e., *Helicobacter pylori*),[6] their hypothesis was met with a small wave of skepticism. Yet, within a few years, the association between *H. pylori* gastritis, peptic ulcer, and gastric cancer became recognized and accepted, albeit with different degrees of enthusiasm and with a wide range of opinions regarding the clinical implications.[7] Furthermore, investigations of gastritis prompted by the discovery of *H. pylori* led to the recognition of other distinctive forms such as lymphocytic and chemical gastritis.

To acknowledge these developments and to try to remove diagnostic confusion, a working group of gastro-enterologists met in Sydney, Australia, in 1990, to establish guidelines for the classification and grading of gastritis. The resulting Sydney System had both endoscopic[8] and histologic[9] components. Although the endoscopic component never gained significant acceptance, the histologic component did by combining topographic, morphologic, and etiologic information into a schema that would help generate reproducible and clinically useful diagnoses. Four years after its introduc-

143

tion, the Sydney System was reappraised by an international group of pathologists. This group established a consensus terminology of gastritis and resolved some of the problems associated with the original Sydney System. Their work resulted in the updated Sydney System, currently the most widely used and cited system for the classification of gastritis.[10]

Subsequent long-term studies of the effects of *H. pylori* infection on the oxyntic component of the gastric mucosa helped highlight some limitations of the updated Sydney System, especially with regard to its definitions and criteria of atrophy and atrophic gastritis. To address these shortcomings, a working group of gastrointestinal (GI) pathologists was established in 1998; over the next 3 years, this group proposed a number of modifications.[11,12] In this chapter, the terminology and combined diagnostic approaches of the updated Sydney System and its subsequent modifications are used and advocated.

■ Classification and Grading of Gastritis: The Updated Sydney System

The updated Sydney System (Table 8-1)[10] classifies chronic gastritis on the basis of topography, morphology, and etiology into three broad categories—acute, chronic, and special (or distinctive). The last category includes gastropathies. This system also further separates chronic gastritis into atrophic and nonatrophic forms, representing the extremes of the spectrum of gastritis (Fig. 8-1). Thus, the system can account for nonatrophic antrum-predominant gastritis, or pangastritis, that is initially caused by *H. pylori* but that in conjunction with other yet unknown environmental, bacterial, and host factors may become atrophic multifocal gastritis. Atrophic gastritis restricted to the corpus, which is virtually always autoimmune, is considered to be a distinct atrophic form.

TABLE 8–1. Classification of Chronic Gastritis Based on Topography, Morphology, and Etiology

Type of Gastritis	Etiologic Factors	Gastritis Synonyms
Nonatrophic	*Helicobacter pylori* ?Other factors	Superficial Diffuse antral gastritis (DAG) Chronic antral gastritis (CAG) Interstitial–follicular Hypersecretory Type B
Atrophic Autoimmune	Autoimmunity ?*H. pylori*	Type A Diffuse corporal
Multifocal atrophic (MAG)	*H. pylori* Environmental factors	Pernicious anemia–associated Type B, type AB Environmental Metaplastic Atrophic pangastritis Progressive intestinalizing pangastritis
Special Forms Chemical	Chemical irritation Bile NSAIDs ?Other agents	Reactive Reflux
Radiation	Radiation injury	
Lymphocytic	?Idiopathic ?Autoimmune mechanisms ?Gluten Drugs (ticlopidine) ?*H. pylori*	Varioliform Celiac disease–associated
Noninfectious granulomatous	Crohn's disease Sarcoidosis Wegener's granulomatosis Foreign substances ?Idiopathic	Isolated granulomatous
Eosinophilic	Food sensitivity ?Other allergies	Allergic
Other infectious gastritides	Bacteria (other than *H. pylori*) Viruses Fungi Parasites	Phlegmonous, syphilitic, etc. Cytomegalovirus Anisakiasis

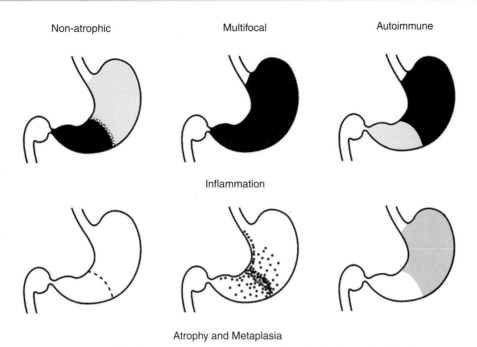

FIGURE 8–1. Schematic representation of the three main types of gastritis as classified in the updated Sydney System. This classification is founded on the distinction between atrophic and nonatrophic gastritis and on the topographic distribution of atrophy.

Acute gastritis is a clinicopathologic term that refers exclusively to the earliest stages of *H. pylori*, to the extremely rare suppurative infections of the gastric mucosa, and to gastric changes that occur as part of acute systemic viral infections. Because biopsy specimens are only rarely obtained from patients with these disorders, the morphologic features of these unusual types of gastritis are poorly described. The Sydney System does not provide a systematic classification of acute gastritis. The term *acute* is also used in conjunction with various types of vascular injury that may occur in patients who ingest nonsteroidal anti-inflammatory drugs (NSAIDs). In this instance (see later in this chapter), the term *acute hemorrhagic gastritis* has been retained in deference to tradition, but *acute hemorrhagic gastropathy* is considered more appropriate.

Under the "special" category of gastritis, the updated Sydney System enumerates several well-characterized gastritides and cites possible causes for them. However, some causative agents may play a role in more than one type of gastritis, and a subject may have histopathologic evidence of more than one type of gastritis as a result of exposure to multiple etiologic agents. A common example is the simultaneous presence of gastritis due to chronic ingestion of NSAIDs and *H. pylori* in the same patient.[13-15] The cause of gastritis can be established in most patients, but in some cases, only nonspecific types and patterns of change may be identified. In these cases, patients should be categorized as "unclassifiable" or "type-indeterminate."

Histopathologic Features of Gastritis

The different types of gastritides and gastropathies are characterized by overlapping histologic changes, which often result from a generalized inflammatory response. However, the presence or absence and relative intensity of the inflammatory response may provide important etiologic clues. Therefore, to facilitate the pathologist's assessment of the various features, it is helpful to describe each of them separately.

EPITHELIAL DEGENERATION

Surface epithelial degeneration is a nonspecific response to injury seen, to a variable degree, in all forms of gastritis, but it is most conspicuous in two conditions—chemical gastritis (resulting from bile reflux or NSAID use) and *H. pylori* gastritis.[16]

The intimate contact of *H. pylori* with the surface cell membrane makes epithelial degeneration particularly prominent in this condition (Fig. 8-2).[17] Several bacterial products, such as the toxins Vac A and cag A, urease, ammonia, acetaldehyde, and phospholipases, have a direct effect on epithelial cells.[18-21] Furthermore, *H. pylori* causes mast cells to release a platelet-activating factor, which leads to platelet activation and thrombosis. This results in disturbances of the local microcirculation and loss of epithelial integrity caused by ischemic damage.[17-23]

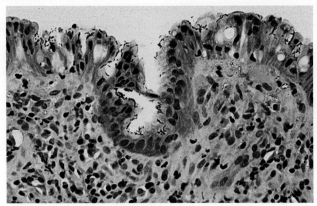

FIGURE 8–2. Architectural disarray and mucin depletion of the gastric surface epithelium associated with adhesion of *H. pylori*. Bacteria, stained with a modified triple stain that includes silver, are visible as dark, slightly curved rods.

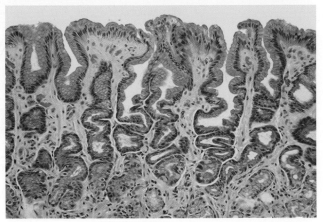

FIGURE 8–3. Foveolar hyperplasia in the antral mucosa. The lack of significant inflammation suggests chemical gastropathy.

In duodenogastric bile reflux, mucosal damage is caused by a direct effect of alkaline pancreatico-duodenal secretions, acids, bile salts, and lysolecithin on the gastric epithelium.[24] NSAID-induced chemical gastritis is due to the decreased synthesis of cytoprotective prostaglandin induced by most first-generation NSAIDs.[25] Injury caused by the use of NSAIDs can be partly prevented by the simultaneous administration of prostaglandin analogues[26] or by reduction of gastric acidity by means of proton pump inhibitors.[27] New NSAIDs specifically designed to selectively inhibit cyclooxygenase-2 (i.e., COX-2 inhibitors) and to minimize gastric damage[28] are now available.

Regardless of the cause, cell injury and necrosis can lead to the development of erosions. Erosions are seen endoscopically either as flat superficial lesions (often due to acute damage caused by drugs, bile reflux, or ischemia) or as elevated lesions whose chronic nature is suggested by the presence of polypoid regenerative mucosa at the margins of the erosion. The latter types of erosions are usually associated with *H. pylori* gastritis. Lesser degrees of surface epithelial degeneration (epithelial cells that are cuboidal rather than columnar in shape with mucin depletion) are common but are not usually visible macroscopically. Such changes are typically found in *H. pylori*–infected stomachs, even in areas where bacteria are rare and difficult to detect. In some areas, focal loss of cells (microerosion) may occur. Regenerative activity in the epithelium is often seen as "buds" made up of multiple cells at the surface, also a feature of *H. pylori* gastritis (see Fig. 8-2).[29]

FOVEOLAR HYPERPLASIA

Foveolar hyperplasia, which is a compensatory response to increased surface epithelial exfoliation, can be viewed as a visual surrogate for increased epithelial cell turnover (Fig. 8-3). Whereas marked hyperplastic foveolae are easily recognized, lesser degrees of foveolar elongation and tortuosity may not be apparent. As an empirical tool, it has been suggested that if more than four cross sections of the same pit are seen in a well-oriented gastric biopsy specimen, one can confidently diagnose the presence of foveolar hyperplasia.[30] The diagnosis of hyperplasia is also facilitated by the finding of hyperchromatic nuclei, by the presence of mitotic activity that reaches higher levels of the pit epithelium, and by signs of cellular immaturity such as mucin depletion, a cuboidal shape of the cells, and a high nucleus-to-cytoplasm ratio.

Foveolar hyperplasia has long been recognized as a prominent feature of bile reflux gastritis.[31] Hyperplasia is also a key feature of gastropathy associated with long-term NSAID treatment.[30] In addition, lesser degrees of hyperplasia are seen in *H. pylori* gastritis; marked hyperplasia suggests coexistent chemical injury (Fig. 8-4).[13]

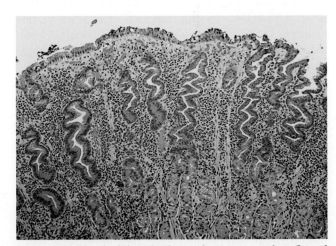

FIGURE 8–4. Marked foveolar hyperplasia in severely inflamed oxyntic mucosa in a patient positive for *H. pylori*. Although the cause of foveolar hyperplasia may be *H. pylori* infection, a superimposed contribution of chemical injury cannot be excluded.

HYPEREMIA AND EDEMA OF THE LAMINA PROPRIA

Mucosal hyperemia is considered to be an indicator of bile reflux gastritis, and a significant correlation has been found between the degree of hyperemia and the concentration of bilirubin in gastric juice.[31] Histologically, marked edema of the lamina propria associated with a lack of inflammation is a characteristic finding in bile gastritis.[31] However, edema and congestion can also be prominent in *H. pylori* gastritis because of an increase in the number of mast cells (Fig. 8-5) and degranulation induced by the infection.[32,33]

NEUTROPHIL INFILTRATION

The presence of neutrophils characterizes the *active* component of chronic gastritis. The term is used to indicate that there is a sustained release of inflammatory mediators and, presumably, an active cause for this release. The cause is *H. pylori* in most cases, but other infectious and inflammatory conditions (e.g., syphilis[34] and Crohn's disease[35]) may be responsible for the presence of neutrophils.

If sufficient numbers of biopsy specimens are examined, neutrophils are found in virtually every subject with *H. pylori* infection.[36,37] The intensity of neutrophil infiltration may help differentiate the acute phase of an infectious gastritis (e.g., phlegmonous gastritis), a particularly active *Helicobacter*-induced

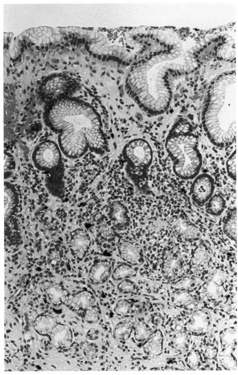

FIGURE 8–5. Increased numbers of mast cells in the lamina propria in chronic *H. pylori* gastritis (anti–human mast cell tryptase).

gastritis (due to *H. pylori* or *Helicobacter heilmannii*), and an acute hemorrhagic gastritis secondary to NSAID- or alcohol-induced chemical injury in which neutrophil infiltration is usually minor.

In *H. pylori* gastritis, neutrophil chemotaxis is stimulated by low-molecular-weight peptide moieties (*porins*) released by the bacteria,[38] by complement activation,[39] and by the release of a variety of chemokines (mostly interleukin-8 [IL-8], IL-10, and IL-12).[40,41] Neutrophils are seen both in the lamina propria and within the epithelium of the foveolae and surface epithelium (Fig. 8-6). Neutrophils may fill the pit lumen, forming so-called pit abscesses (Fig. 8-7), or they may produce a surface exudate (Fig. 8-8). In *H. pylori* infection, active inflammation is seen only in gastric-type mucosa; it is almost never found in areas of intestinal metaplasia. Neutrophils disappear rapidly after successful eradication therapy; thus, their persistence is a good indicator that therapy has failed.[36]

EOSINOPHIL INFILTRATION

Rare, scattered eosinophils may be seen in the gastric lamina propria of normal subjects, particularly in populations who live in suboptimal public health conditions. However, a prominent eosinophilic infiltration in the gastric wall may represent a manifestation of either eosinophilic gastritis or gastroenteritis.[42,43] In either case, the cause, although believed to have an allergic basis, is essentially unknown. Eosinophils are also a prominent component of the inflammatory response in gastric anisakiasis and may be a constituent of granulomas that may form around fragments of helminths in the gastric wall.[44]

In adults with *H. pylori* gastritis, variable but usually small numbers of eosinophils occur (Fig. 8-9). In contrast, children have been reported to have a greater eosinophilic component in *H. pylori*–infected gastric mucosa.[45] After eradication, eosinophils may increase for some time, then decline in parallel with mononuclear cells.[36]

MONONUCLEAR CELL INFLAMMATION

Although normal antral mucosa may contain few chronic inflammatory cells, and the oxyntic mucosa contains includes virtually none, the density of mononuclear cells in the lamina propria of normal subjects varies considerably according to geographic location and ethnicity.[46] Thus, pathologists ought to set a standard for normal that is relevant to the population from which gastric specimens are obtained. The presence of lymphocytes and plasma cells in the superficial portions of the mucosa is a nonspecific response to a variety of agents; their density and distribution provide categoric or etiologic clues in only a minority of instances.

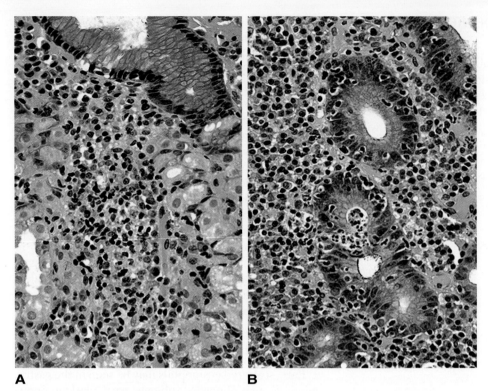

FIGURE 8–6. In *H. pylori* infection, neutrophils typically infiltrate the lamina propria (**A**) as well as the surface and foveolar and glandular epithelium (**B**).

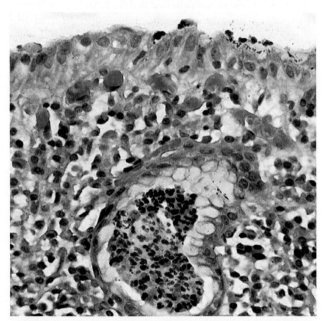

FIGURE 8–7. Pit (foveolae) abscess. *H. pylori* organisms are visible on the upper right portion of the superficial epithelium.

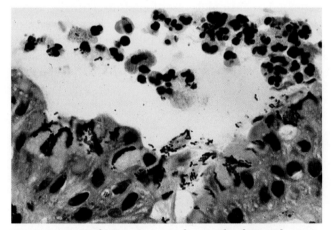

FIGURE 8–8. High-power view of severely damaged gastric surface epithelium with innumerable *H. pylori* infiltrating into intercellular spaces and into gaps created by the dropout of cells (microerosion). Neutrophilic exudate is present on the surface.

Infiltration by lymphocytes, plasma cells, and small numbers of eosinophils and mast cells in the mucosa is a prominent feature of chronic *H. pylori* gastritis, except in areas of severe atrophy and metaplasia, in which the infiltrate may be sparser. In *H. pylori* gastritis, mononuclear cells are found mostly in the lamina propria (Fig. 8-10); only exceptionally do they infiltrate the glandular or superficial epithelium. When this is a prominent feature, even if *H. pylori* and its other accompanying features are present, the possibility of lymphocytic gastritis (see later in this chapter) should be considered.[47] In autoimmune gastritis (also discussed later in this chapter), a diffuse infiltrate of mucosal plasma cells and lymphocytes,[48] which may also extend to deeper portions of the oxyntic mucosa, is usually noted.

In some cases, the only detectable histologic abnormality is a mild to moderate mononuclear infiltrate in the lamina propria. If an exhaustive search for *Helicobacter* (*pylori* or *heilmannii*) or other known

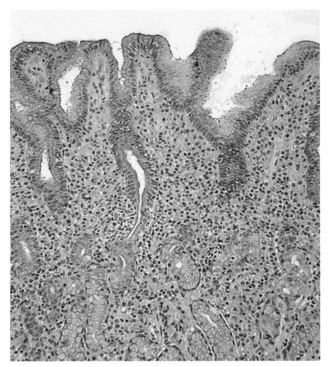

FIGURE 8–9. A case of *H. pylori* gastritis in which eosinophils are more prominent than usual.

causes of gastric inflammation produces a negative result, a diagnosis of chronic inactive gastritis can be made. The word *inactive*, by convention, indicates a lack of neutrophils. This diagnosis is best accompanied by a description of the histologic findings, emphasizing the absence of other abnormalities. It may represent a variation of normal or an immune response to as yet unidentified antigens.

LYMPHOID FOLLICLES

The gastric mucosa, and particularly the corpus, may contain occasional small lymphoid aggregates often located close to the muscularis mucosae. However, lymphoid aggregates with germinal centers are exceedingly rare in the stomach of normal, *H. pylori*–negative adults. When an extensive standardized biopsy protocol is used, lymphoid follicles or aggregates are found in virtually all subjects with *H. pylori* gastritis (Fig. 8-11).[49] In infected children and young adults, lymphoid follicles may be sufficiently prominent to produce a distinctive nodularity of the gastric antrum, endoscopically referred to as *follicular gastritis*.[50]

The presence of lymphoid follicles in the gastric mucosa is virtually restricted to *H. pylori*–associated gastritis. Therefore, *H. pylori* infection is the major cause of acquired mucosa-associated lymphoid tissue (MALT) in the stomach and is a crucial factor in the etiology of primary gastric B-cell lymphoma (MALT lymphoma).[51,52]

Rarely, the lymphoid infiltrate may show an expanded lymphoid population containing large follicles and lymphoepithelial lesions that raise a suspicion of gastric lymphoma. In these circumstances, the biopsy may be tentatively diagnosed as containing an atypical lymphoid proliferation.[53] Further investigation by immunocytochemical and molecular techniques often resolves the diagnostic problem.

ATROPHY

Gastric atrophy is defined as a loss of gastric glands.[11] Recently, however, the narrower definition of "loss of specialized cells" has been proposed.[54] Whenever the gastric mucosa is damaged, irrespective of the mechanism or cause, it may either regenerate and return to normal (*restitutio ad integrum*) or undergo an adaptive reparative change that leads to the replacement of the native glands with other types of tissue (Fig. 8-12).[55] In the event that injured glands fail to regenerate, the space that they previously occupied in the lamina propria may be replaced by fibroblasts and extracellular matrix. The end result of this process is the loss of

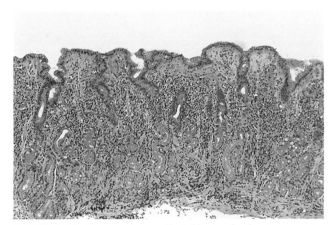

FIGURE 8–10. Mononuclear cells infiltrate the lamina propria, but not the epithelium, in *H. pylori* gastritis.

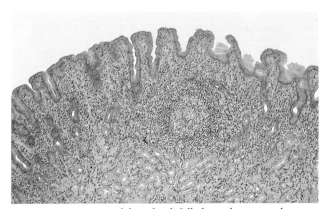

FIGURE 8–11. Mucosal lymphoid follicle with germinal center formation is characteristic of *H. pylori* gastritis.

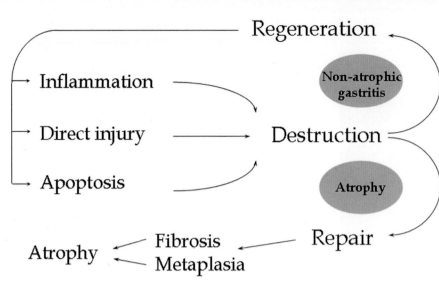

FIGURE 8–12. Mechanisms of atrophy and repair—pathways to atrophic and nonatrophic gastritis.

functional epithelium (i.e., atrophy). In other, often coexisting pathways, the native glands may be replaced by those with a pyloric appearance ("pseudopyloric metaplasia") or by intestinal-type epithelium containing goblet cells—intermediate, so-called absorptive cells, either with or without a brush border (intestinal metaplasia). In chronic *H. pylori* infection, all types of gland repair occur.[46] Widespread atrophy also occurs in autoimmune gastritis as a consequence of immune-mediated epithelial destruction of the oxyntic mucosa (Fig. 8-13). Less severe atrophic changes may also occur in reactive (reflux-type) gastritis. Atrophy may develop focally in reactive gastritis secondary to long-term NSAID use.[30]

Although any of these repair processes may prevent the gastric mucosa from functioning normally (e.g., by secreting acid), pathologists should not let functional considerations influence their assessment of atrophy. For example, because atrophy can be patchy, oxyntic glands may be completely absent from a single biopsy

specimen in a patient who has normal gastric function. Conversely, a dense chronic inflammatory infiltrate may cause severe hypochlorhydria in patients who have no apparent gland loss.

INTESTINAL METAPLASIA

Intestinal metaplasia is defined as the replacement of gastric mucous cells with an epithelium similar to that of the small intestine (Fig. 8-14). Several variations of intestinal metaplasia may occur. Metaplastic epithelium

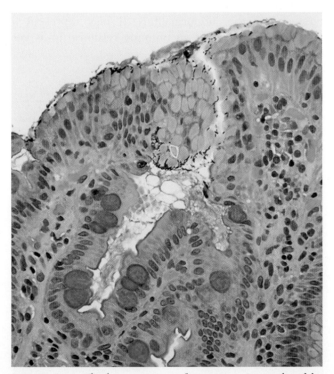

FIGURE 8–13. Complete atrophy of oxyntic mucosa in a patient with end-stage autoimmune gastritis. The oxyntic glands are replaced by pyloric-type glands and fibrosis. At this stage, the inflammatory component is mild.

FIGURE 8–14. The lower portion of a gastric pit is replaced by intestinal metaplasia with goblet cells in a case of active *H. pylori* gastritis. Organisms adhere to nonmetaplastic epithelium.

may resemble normal small intestinal epithelium, showing the presence of acidic mucin–producing goblet cells and absorptive enterocytes with a brush border (complete). Various types of incomplete metaplasia may show a disorderly mixture of irregularly shaped goblet cells and immature "intermediate" mucous cells that contain a wide range of acidic sialomucins (example, type 2a or II) and sulfomucins (incomplete type 2b or III) (Fig. 8-15). The different types of intestinal metaplasia have been classified as complete (type 1) or incomplete (type 2a or 2b; type II or III).[56] Although this classification of intestinal metaplasia is widely accepted, its application is limited owing to the fact that it is common to find a mixture of types in any one individual. Type I intestinal metaplasia poses no increased risk of carcinoma,[57] whereas type III is considered by some to represent an early dysplastic lesion.[58] This notion, however, is disputed by many. In general, the degree of type III (incomplete) metaplasia parallels the proportion of metaplasia itself. Because cancer risk is related to the extent of intestinal metaplasia, there is also a correlation with the extent of the incomplete type.[59]

Intestinal metaplasia is almost always present as a component of atrophic gastritis. Despite some degree of interobserver variability, pathologists can recognize its presence and extent with the use of special mucin histochemical stains. The Alcian blue/periodic acid–Schiff (PAS) technique at pH 2.5 is an excellent stain to demonstrate the type and extent of intestinal metaplasia. A high iron diamine stain can help distinguish type III (positive) from type II (negative) intestinal metaplasia. Because data regarding cancer risk for each type of intestinal metaplasia are equivocal, histochemical subtyping should be reserved for research.

Several studies have shown that intestinal metaplasia occurs more frequently in subjects with *H. pylori*

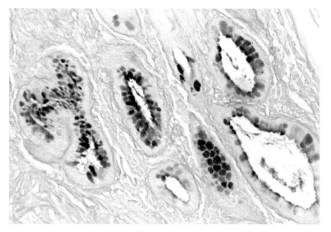

FIGURE 8–15. A high-iron diamine stain is useful for determining the type of intestinal metaplasia. Sulfated mucins, characteristic of type III intestinal metaplasia, stain brown, and nonsulfated acidic mucins stain blue when combined with an Alcian blue stain at pH 2.5.

gastritis.[60,61] Because *H. pylori* does not usually adhere to intestinal-type epithelium (see Fig. 8-14) and because it usually disappears from stomachs with extensive metaplastic atrophy, one could view intestinal metaplasia as a type of host defense response against *H. pylori* infection. Furthermore, the changes in mucus composition may provide an additional defense against *H. pylori*, or they may represent an adaptation to altered bacterial flora. In fact, bacterial overgrowth may underlie the development of intestinal metaplasia in the late stages of autoimmune gastritis. Sulfomucins are more resistant than other types of mucins to bacterial enzyme–related degradation and in this manner may provide an effective means of protection from the effects of bacterial overgrowth. Small foci of intestinal metaplasia are also frequently found in bile reflux gastropathy.[31,62]

ENDOCRINE CELL HYPERPLASIA

Endocrine cell hyperplasia develops as a consequence of functional changes in chronic gastritis. It is most prominent in autoimmune atrophic gastritis. In this condition, hypochlorhydria or achlorhydria often leads to antral G-cell hyperplasia and an accompanying elevation in serum gastrin.[63,64] Hypergastrinemia in turn causes histamine-producing enterochromaffin-like (ECL) cells in the oxyntic glands to undergo hyperplasia.[65]

On hematoxylin and eosin (H&E)–stained section of gastric mucosa, endocrine cells are difficult to detect and impossible to assess qualitatively or quantitatively. To evaluate their number and distribution, it is necessary to perform immunostains, which have now largely replaced the use of classic argentaffin and argyrophil–based histochemical stains (Fig. 8-16). The most widely used criteria for the diagnosis and classification of gastric endocrine cell proliferations are those proposed by Solcia.[66] This classification distinguishes among hyperplasia, adenomatoid hyperplasia, dysplasia, and neoplasia. For instance, hyperplasia is defined as micronodular clusters of five or more cells, not exceeding the diameter of gastric glands, present either within the glands or in the lamina propria. Endocrine cell dysplasia is defined as enlargement and fusion of at least five micronodules (between 150 and 500 mm in diameter) with loss of intervening basement membrane and possible microinvasion. Cells that form dysplastic proliferations may show atypia, irregular shape, and reduced numbers of cytoplasmic endocrine granules.

Mild degrees of neuroendocrine proliferation may be seen in routine gastric biopsies as a result of the widespread use of proton pump inhibitors.[65,67] Hypertrophy occurs almost exclusively in ECL cells, the most common type of endocrine cell in the oxyntic mucosa, and is likely dependent on the trophic effect of hypergastrinemia.[68] Carcinoid tumors have not been reported to develop from hyperplasia in humans.

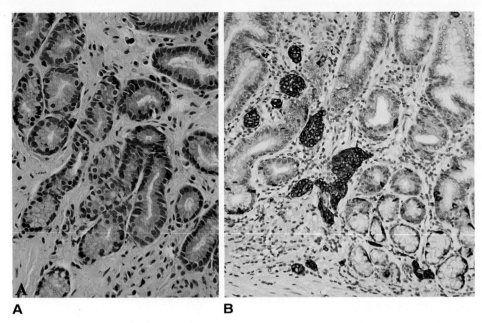

FIGURE 8–16. Endocrine cell hyperplasia. Crowding of G cells, characterized by a centrally located round nucleus and clear cytoplasm, is detectable in sections from the antrum stained with hematoxylin and eosin or the triple stain (**A**). For a semiquantitative evaluation of endocrine cell hyperplasia and for the detection of microcarcinoids, silver-based stains or immunostains (such as chromogranin) are necessary (**B**).

PARIETAL CELL ALTERATIONS

Parietal cell pseudohypertrophy of oxyntic cells is a characteristic yet reversible response to the long-term administration of proton pump inhibitors (Fig. 8-17). This change has also been described in patients with gastric ulcer disease, although the pathogenetic mechanism remains unclear.[68-72]

Helicobacter pylori Gastritis

Chronic *H. pylori* gastritis is one of the most common chronic conditions of humans and one that affects an estimated two thirds of the world's population.[6,73] It is associated with most duodenal and gastric ulcers that are unrelated to NSAIDs and with most gastric MALT

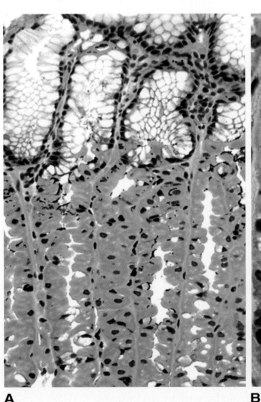
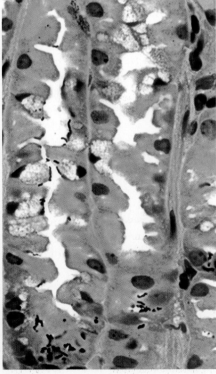

FIGURE 8–17. Long-term treatment with proton pump inhibitors may induce characteristic changes in the oxyntic glands. Their lumina, normally vertical in biopsy specimens, may become dilated, and individual hyperplastic oxyntic cells may protrude into the lumina, creating a jagged appearance (**A**). In some patients, *H. pylori* can be seen in the deeper portions of the oxyntic glands, as well as within the canaliculi of individual parietal cells (**B**). (See also Figure 8-33.)

lymphomas. In certain regions of the world, a considerable proportion of infected subjects develop atrophic gastritis, which is a known precursor of gastric carcinoma.

CLINICAL FEATURES

The initial phase of *H. pylori* infection elicits an acute inflammatory response referred to as *acute gastritis*. At this stage, significant clinical manifestations are uncommon and usually short lived. Therefore, patients rarely undergo endoscopy, and information regarding the clinical aspects of acute *H. pylori* infection is limited to a few well-documented case reports.[74-76] Iatrogenic *H. pylori* infection may also result from the use of inadequately disinfected endoscopes.[77]

Endoscopically, acute *H. pylori* gastritis shows hemorrhagic lesions and multiple antral erosions or ulcers. Both the endoscopic and histopathologic appearances of the gastric mucosa in these patients are virtually identical to those reported in subjects from human ingestion studies[78] and in patients with epidemic gastritis and achlorhydria, a condition described before the discovery of *H. pylori* as a cause of gastritis.[79,80]

Because chronic *H. pylori* gastritis is usually asymptomatic, it is often viewed as a "condition" rather than a "disease." The prevalence of nonulcer dyspepsia is similar among *H. pylori*–infected and noninfected subjects,[81,82] and the eradication of *H. pylori* in patients with nonulcer dyspepsia has not been shown conclusively to improve patients' symptoms, further suggesting the absence of a clear relationship between gastritis and GI symptoms.[83] However, even in the absence of hard data linking chronic gastritis and dyspepsia, the immense impact of *H. pylori* infection on human health cannot be overemphasized: *H. pylori* infection is estimated to be directly responsible for approximately 5% of GI ailments in the community,[84] and patients with *H. pylori* gastritis are at increased risk for duodenal and gastric ulcers, gastric cancer, and lymphoma.

EPIDEMIOLOGY

The prevalence of *H. pylori* is essentially identical to that of gastritis reported in previous studies,[85,86] and the association between chronic gastritis and low socioeconomic class, age, peptic ulcer disease, and gastric carcinoma, demonstrated in regions as diverse as Central and South America, Finland, and China, holds true for *H. pylori* infection as well.[77,87-90] The prevalence of *H. pylori* in adults reaches 90% in many developing tropical countries. In fact, cross-sectional studies have revealed a high prevalence rate of infection in children, indicating that exposure to the bacterium probably occurs early in life. In industrialized parts of the world (western Europe, United States, Canada, and Australia), exposure occurs later in life, which results in a lower percentage of infected adults (approximately 30% by age 50). In the stronger economies of eastern Asia (e.g., Japan and South Korea), where the recent introduction of widespread sanitation measures has paralleled the change from "third world" to "first world" status, a clear trend has been seen toward lower rates of *H. pylori* infection. Furthermore, the prevalence of *H. pylori* is declining in industrialized countries, which is probably a reflection of improved sanitary conditions, as well as the widespread use of antibiotics in both children and adults. Nevertheless, *H. pylori* infection is so common, even in areas of low risk, that it should always be sought in any gastric biopsy specimen examined, regardless of the patient's age or provenance.

PATHOLOGIC FEATURES

Gross Pathology

No distinct endoscopic pattern of chronic *H. pylori* gastritis has been observed. Depending on the stage and type of gastritis, hyperemia, erosions, hypertrophy, and atrophy may coexist in various combinations in the same patient. None of these features has proved useful for predicting the presence or absence of chronic *H. pylori* gastritis. Therefore, the diagnosis of *H. pylori* gastritis rests entirely on histopathologic evaluation of gastric biopsies.

Microscopic Pathology

The gastric mucosa is normally covered by a thick mucous gel layer that is believed to play a protective role. This mucous layer, best visualized in Carnoy's-fixed tissues, is an indispensable site of *H. pylori* colonization and as such often contains large numbers of bacteria.[91] *H. pylori* organisms characteristically attach to surface mucous cells. In rare instances, however, intercellular invasion by *H. pylori* has been observed in surface mucous cells, chief cells, and rarely in parietal cells, particularly in patients who have received proton pump inhibitors (Fig. 8-18; see also Fig. 8-17).

Initially, *H. pylori* was believed to preferentially colonize antral mucosa. However, it has now been shown that oxyntic mucosa and cardiac mucosa are colonized as frequently as the antrum.[37,92] In patients with extensive intestinal metaplasia of the antrum, infection is usually confined to the nonmetaplastic areas of the corpus.[93] This is also the case in patients who use proton pump inhibitors.

Gastric mucosa infected by *H. pylori* shows all the inflammatory changes detailed previously. In the acute stage, endoscopically visible pseudomembranes and pus adherent to inflamed mucosa have been described in severe cases of *H. pylori* infection (Fig. 8-19). In chronic active *H. pylori* gastritis, neutrophils are the

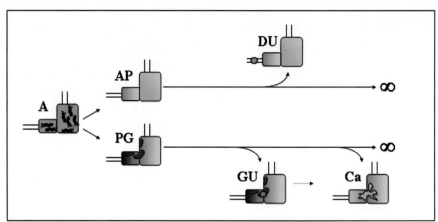

FIGURE 8–18. Pathways of gastritis: From the initial acute infection (A), presumed to be pangastritis, two main courses may develop. The gastritis may become predominantly antral (AP), leaving the corpus, and its ability to produce acid may be relatively unaffected. These patients are at increased risk of developing duodenal ulcers (DUs). In another pathway, pangastritis (PG) may proceed to atrophy and metaplasia. These patients, who become hypochlorhydric in the more advanced stages of the disease, may develop gastric ulcers (GUs) and may have a higher risk of intestinal-type adenocarcinoma (Ca). In the majority of infected individuals with either type of gastritis, the infection may last indefinitely without clinically detectable consequences.

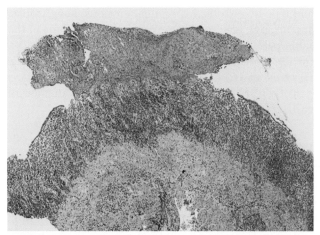

FIGURE 8–19. Acute severe *H. pylori* infection: Fibrinopurulent material is present over a superficial erosion. In addition, the mucosa is extensively infiltrated by neutrophils.

most frequent characteristic feature and are generally more abundant in the antrum and cardia than in the corpus, where they may be completely absent in spite of the presence of visible organisms. This observation may have been the basis for the fallacious concept of "inactive *H. pylori* gastritis." In the lamina propria, neutrophils are always mixed with mononuclear cells and variable numbers of eosinophils. However, neutrophils are typically the only inflammatory cells to infiltrate the gastric epithelium in *H. pylori* infection (see Fig. 8-17).

Lymphoid follicles are virtually always found in infected patients.[94,95] Their density is usually greatest in the region of the angulus and lowest in the proximal greater curvature. These anatomic sites correspond, respectively, to the most and least common origins of gastric lymphomas.[49]

In areas without atrophy or intestinal metaplasia, inflammation tends to be most intense in the superficial portions of the lamina propria (Fig. 8-20) (hence the now abandoned term *superficial gastritis*, which is still occasionally used as a synonym for nonatrophic gastritis). Atrophy, characterized by the decrease or absence of glands, is usually accompanied by fibrosis or intestinal metaplasia (Fig. 8-21).

STAINING OF *H. PYLORI*

In 70% to 80% of gastric biopsy specimens from infected subjects, *H. pylori* organisms are easily visualized by H&E staining. In another 10% to 15%, a careful search is often needed to detect bacteria. In the remaining 10% to 20% of cases, a special stain is needed. Common inexpensive stains, such as Giemsa and Diff-Quik, are usually adequate.[96] Another option is

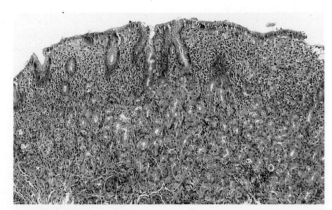

FIGURE 8–20. Superficial gastritis. Although the term is not used in the Sydney System, it describes the bandlike distribution of inflammation in nonatrophic oxyntic mucosa.

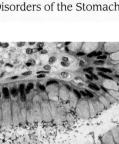

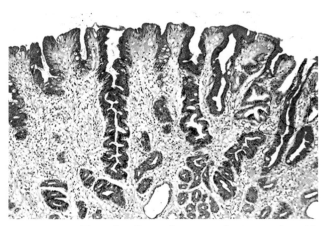

FIGURE 8–21. Example of complete metaplastic atrophy with fibrosis of the lamina propria.

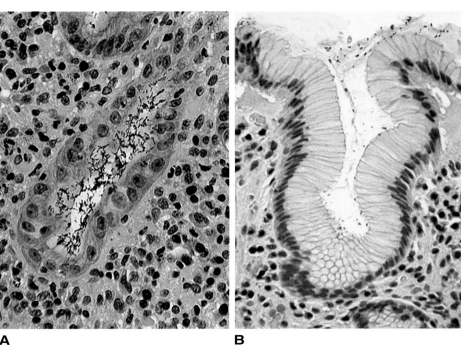

FIGURE 8–22. Triple stain for the simultaneous visualization of *H. pylori* and the features of gastritis. Innumerable organisms are adherent to the epithelium within the lumen of the pit.

silver-based triple stain that simultaneously allows visualization of *H. pylori* and the morphologic changes in the mucosa (Fig. 8-22; see also Figs. 8-2, 8-6, 8-8, and 8-14).[97] Because this stain includes Alcian blue at pH 2.5, it makes detection of small foci of intestinal metaplasia easier (see Fig. 8-14). Immunohistochemical stains for the demonstration of *H. pylori* are also available and may be particularly useful for detecting coccoid forms of the organism (Fig. 8-23).[98,99]

HELICOBACTER HEILMANNII INFECTION

More than 35 species of *Helicobacter* have been described, but only a few have been shown to cause gastritis in humans. These include *Helicobacter felis, H. fennelliae, H. cinaedi,* and *H. heilmannii.* Among these,

H. heilmannii (formerly known as *Gastrospirillum hominis*) is the most common,[100,101] with an estimated prevalence of approximately 1% of all human *Helicobacter* infections.[101,102] In some rural areas in eastern Europe, it is more common, leading to the hypothesis that it is acquired by zoonotic transmission.[101-103] The organisms measure 5 to 9 μm in length (twice as long as *H. pylori*) and have five to seven spirals that are easily visible with the use of a silver stain (Fig. 8-24).

Gastritis caused by *H. heilmannii* is often milder and more patchy than *H. pylori* gastritis. The inflammation tends to be more circumscribed and affects mostly the antrum, although cases with severe corpus active inflammation may be seen as well. Erosions and ulcers are less common than in *H. pylori* gastritis.

FIGURE 8–23. A, Innumerable *H. pylori* (stained with the triple stain) within the lumen of a pit and in the intercellular spaces of foveolar cells. **B,** A gastric pit stained with anti-*H. pylori* immunostains. This is particularly useful to specifically stain the coccoid forms of *H. pylori*, many of which are visible as small dots adherent to the right side of the foveola.

A   **B**

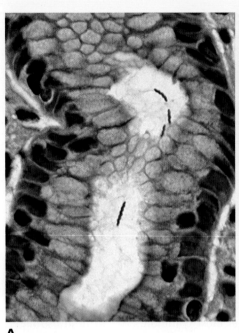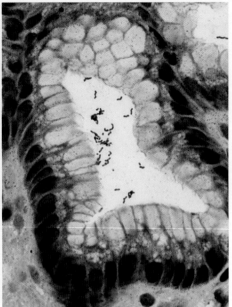

A   **B**

FIGURE 8–24. A, *Helicobacter heilmannii.* The organisms are at least twice as long and are considerably thicker than *H. pylori* **(B).** Their spiral shape is clearly visible at high power.

Diagnosis rests on the morphologic recognition of the bacterial organisms, although the distinction between *H. heilmannii* and *H. felis* is not possible by light microscopy.

EVOLUTION AND COMPLICATIONS OF *H. PYLORI* GASTRITIS

H. pylori gastritis is a lifelong infection that, depending on its phenotype (atrophic vs. nonatrophic), carries an increased risk of duodenal ulcer, gastric ulcer, gastric adenocarcinoma, and primary MALT lymphoma.[104] The relative risk for each of these conditions varies greatly in different populations and is related to bacterial, environmental, and genetic factors. The specific features of each of these major complications are detailed in Chapters 9, 17, 21, and 23.

▮ Autoimmune Gastritis

Autoimmune gastritis is defined as a corpus-restricted chronic atrophic gastritis associated with the presence of serum anti–parietal cell and anti–intrinsic factor antibodies and an intrinsic factor deficiency, with or without pernicious anemia.[48]

CLINICAL FEATURES

Pernicious anemia is a relatively rare disease with a prevalence rate of less than 1%, even among subjects older than 65 years of age and in high-incidence countries.[105-107] Most clinical manifestations of autoimmune gastritis become apparent when the decrease

in parietal cell mass reaches a critical point. These manifestations include hypochlorhydria and achlorhydria, hypergastrinemia, loss of pepsin and pepsinogens, iron deficiency with microcytic anemia, vitamin B_{12} deficiency with megaloblastic anemia, and a moderately increased risk of gastric neoplasms.

Achlorhydria, which is the most direct result of the destruction of acid-producing oxyntic cells, typically occurs in the most advanced stage of the disease. However, hypochlorhydria may occur in patients with large numbers of preserved parietal cells, suggesting a possible role for anti–proton pump antibodies or inhibitory lymphokines released by inflammatory cells. Patients with corpus atrophy and achlorhydria have hypergastrinemia that tends to correlate with disease severity.[108] Damage to chief cells leads to a reduction in pepsin activity in gastric juice and in pepsinogens in blood. The finding of a low pepsinogen I level (<20 ng/mL) is sensitive and specific for the presence of corpus atrophy.[108,109]

A considerable proportion of patients with autoimmune gastritis develop either iron deficiency anemia or pernicious anemia. Hypochromic anemia is associated with corpus-restricted chronic atrophic gastritis in approximately 15% of patients.[48] Occult bleeding from gastric mucosa may account for some of these cases, but achlorhydria seems to be the major contributor to the pathogenesis of anemia. Gastric acid is important in the absorption of nonheme iron, which supplies at least two thirds of nutritional iron needs in most Western diets.[110] Pernicious anemia is usually preceded by corpus-restricted chronic atrophic gastritis and reduced or absent acid secretion for at least 10 years; it is generally associated with end-stage atrophic gastritis.[111]

Autoimmune gastritis is a risk factor for hyperplastic and adenomatous polyps, carcinomas, and endocrine tumors. Polyps, which are found in 20% to 40% of patients with pernicious anemia, are mostly sessile, less than 2 cm in diameter, and often multiple. Most are hyperplastic, but up to 10% contain dysplastic foci.[112] Gastric cancers associated with pernicious anemia are mostly of the intestinal type and arise from intestinal metaplasia, suggesting that the pathogenesis of carcinoma in this disease likely progresses through a metaplasia-dysplasia-carcinoma pathway.[113]

PATHOGENESIS

Recently, the hypothesis that autoimmune gastritis may be initiated by *H. pylori* infection has received considerable attention. However, studies that have investigated the prevalence of *H. pylori* infection among patients with autoimmune gastritis and/or pernicious anemia have yielded a wide range of results.[114] A high prevalence of antibodies with specificity for gastric mucosal antigens has been reported among patients with *H. pylori*–associated gastritis.[115] Furthermore, 20% of subjects have autoantibodies that react with the canaliculi of parietal cells, one of the main targets in autoimmune gastritis. In other studies, *H. pylori*–positive patients with anti-canalicular antibodies had a 30% prevalence of anti-H$^+$,K$^+$-ATPase antibodies.[116] *H. pylori* lipopolysaccharides have been shown to express Lewis x and y blood group antigens, which are also expressed by either H$^+$,K$^+$-ATPase or gastric epithelial cells.[117,118] These studies provide support for the concept that a cross-mimicking mechanism between *H. pylori* and gastric epithelial antigens may be responsible for, or at least participate in, the pathogenesis of autoimmune gastritis.

PATHOLOGIC FEATURES

Gross Pathology

In the corpus, the mucosa is usually thinner than normal; thus, fine submucosal vessels are easily recognizable on endoscopic examination in advanced disease. Hyperplastic polyps are common in advanced stages of disease.

Microscopic Pathology

The main pathologic features of autoimmune gastritis include diffuse corpus-restricted chronic atrophic gastritis with mild to moderate intestinal metaplasia. In the absence of concurrent *H. pylori* infection, the antrum is normal. This pattern of involvement is characteristic of advanced disease and is found in patients with pernicious anemia. Patients without pernicious anemia

but with parietal cell antibodies show a broad spectrum of atrophic changes, from minimal oxyntic gland loss to severe and diffuse atrophy of the oxyntic mucosa. Solcia's group has identified three phases in the development of autoimmune gastritis in the oxyntic mucosa: early, florid, and end stage.[48]

The *early* phase is characterized by diffuse or multifocal dense mononuclear cell infiltration of the entire thickness of the lamina propria, often mixed with eosinophils and mast cells. Patchy destruction of individual oxyntic glands by lymphocytes may be seen (Fig. 8-25), as may patchy pseudopyloric metaplasia and hypertrophic changes of the remaining parietal cells. Similar changes, indicative of a high level of functional stimulation and possibly related to hypergastrinemia, are found in the parietal cells of patients who have received proton pump inhibitor therapy.[119,120] Intestinal metaplasia occurs rarely and only focally in the early phase of pure autoimmune gastritis. At this stage, diagnosis requires demonstration of circulating parietal cell autoantibodies—a test rarely performed in clinical practice.

The *florid* phase reveals marked atrophy of the oxyntic glands, diffuse mononuclear cell infiltration of the lamina propria, and normal or reduced thickness of the mucosa with a relative increase in the foveolar component. Pyloric metaplasia is often extensive, and intestinal metaplasia tends to be focal. At this stage, the pathologic features of autoimmune atrophic gastritis are sufficiently distinctive. However, the demonstration of parietal cell and intrinsic factor antibodies remains necessary for confirmation.

The *end stage* is characterized by a marked reduction in oxyntic glands, foveolar hyperplasia with elongation and microcystic change, hyperplastic polyp formation, and various degrees of pyloric, pseudopyloric, pancreatic acinar, or intestinal metaplasia. At this stage, parietal cells are difficult to detect. Inflammation is

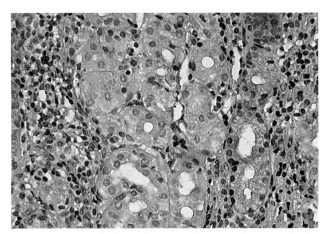

FIGURE 8–25. Marked lymphocytic infiltration of oxyntic glands. This feature can be seen in autoimmune gastritis and in *H. pylori* infection; it usually precedes the development of atrophic gastritis.

usually minimal or absent, although scattered lymphoid aggregates and follicles may still be present. The muscularis mucosae may be thickened three- to fourfold.

In the majority of patients, the antral mucosa either is normal or shows only focal areas of mild chronic inflammation with intestinal metaplasia, similar in degree to that observed in the general asymptomatic population. Hyperplasia of gastrin cells, secondary to achlorhydria, is often seen. Although ECL-cell carcinoids may arise during the florid phase, they are found more commonly in association with end-stage disease.[113]

Lymphocytic Gastritis

CLINICAL FEATURES

As the name implies, lymphocytic gastritis is characterized by the presence of large numbers of mature lymphocytes infiltrating the surface and foveolar epithelium.[47] Initially, lymphocytic gastritis was believed to correspond to an entity described by François Moutier in 1945 as *varioliform gastritis*.[121-123] However, the histologic features of lymphocytic gastritis may also be found in subjects with an endoscopically normal appearance and in patients with celiac disease. Lymphocytic gastritis is relatively rare, found in 1% to 4% of the endoscoped population.[124,125] It is most commonly diagnosed in the sixth decade and affects men and women equally.

In contrast to subjects with uncomplicated chronic active gastritis, patients with the varioliform type of lymphocytic gastritis are often symptomatic. Presenting symptoms include rapid weight loss and anorexia in about half of affected patients. Hypoproteinemia, hypoalbuminemia, and peripheral edema suggesting the presence of a protein-losing gastroenteropathy have been documented in approximately 20% of patients.[47] Lymphocytic gastritis is a chronic disease. Few cases of spontaneous resolution have been reported. No specific therapy is available, but proton pump inhibitors are often used to treat ulcers. If concurrent *H. pylori* infection is present, its eradication is advisable.[126]

Virtually all intraepithelial lymphocytes in lymphocytic gastritis are CD8+ suppressor T cells, similar to those in celiac disease (Fig. 8-26). Thus, an allergic or autoimmune pathogenesis has been proposed. This hypothesis is further supported by the increasingly apparent association between lymphocytic gastritis and celiac disease.[125,127,128]

PATHOLOGIC FEATURES

Gross Pathology

About 80% of patients have endoscopic lesions described as varioliform, aphthous, verrucous, or erosive.[47,129] A complex pattern of enlarged folds covered by a thick layer of mucus may be seen in the corpus. Elevated aphthous nodules may be present at the tops of gastric folds. Flat erosions may be found in the antrum. The remaining 20% of patients (including those with celiac disease) have less dramatic lesions characterized by scattered superficial erosions in the corpus or antrum. Some patients have a normal-appearing mucosa. Some authors have postulated a relationship between lymphocytic gastritis and Ménétrier's disease.[130]

Microscopic Pathology

The increase in severity of intraepithelial lymphocytes ranges from mild to severe. In mild cases, there is

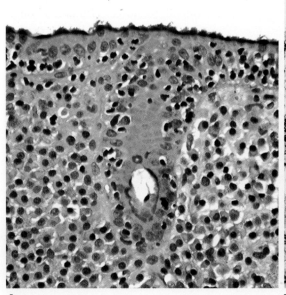

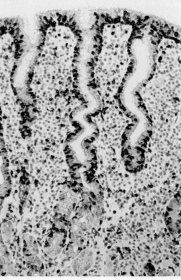

FIGURE 8–26. Lymphocytic gastritis with large numbers of T lymphocytes infiltrating the gastric epithelium (triple stain, **A**). Although not necessary for the diagnosis, the T-cell nature of the infiltrate can be demonstrated with an anti-CD8 immunostain **(B)**. These lymphocytes are mostly T suppressor cells that stain with anti-CD3.

A   **B**

only a minor increase in chronic inflammation with no activity. At the other extreme, marked chronic inflammation may be seen in the lamina propria and is associated with erosions. The histologic features are readily distinguishable from *H. pylori* gastritis (see Fig. 8-24). In *H. pylori* gastritis, few intraepithelial lymphocytes may be present (rarely more that 5 or 6 per 100 epithelial cells). However, in lymphocytic gastritis, more than 25 intraepithelial lymphocytes per 100 epithelial cells is typical.[131] The degree of intraepithelial lymphocytosis is more prominent in the corpus than in the antrum.

Granulomatous Gastritis

Granulomatous gastritis is an entity characterized by the presence of granulomas as the main pathologic feature. It often develops secondary to other disorders but rarely may be primary. In most cases, the morphologic appearance of the granulomas does not provide useful clues as to their cause, except when foreign material, acid-fast bacilli, or fungal forms are identified. Thus, a specific diagnosis can be made only by integrating pathologic data with appropriate clinical and laboratory information. Granulomas may be found in the gastric mucosa of patients with infectious, inflammatory, and neoplastic diseases, as well as in otherwise healthy individuals. Therefore, the endoscopic appearance of the stomach may be normal, or it may exhibit characteristics of the associated diseases. A list of possible causes of granulomas in the gastric mucosa is provided in Table 8-2; these are discussed further in the following sections.

MYCOBACTERIUM TUBERCULOSIS AND HISTOPLASMA CAPSULATUM INFECTIONS

Tuberculosis is the most common cause worldwide of granulomatous disease of the GI tract, but the stomach is rarely affected. Primary gastric tuberculosis has been reported mostly from developing countries with a high prevalence of *Mycobacterium tuberculosis* infection.[132,133] In almost all cases, gastric tuberculosis presents with a large nonhealing ulcer. A few cases of primary infection of the stomach by the dimorphic fungus *Histoplasma capsulatum* have also been reported. Similar to patients with gastric tuberculosis, these patients often present with signs and symptoms of a large gastric ulcer.[134,135]

H. PYLORI INFECTION

Unexplained granulomas may be found in patients with *H. pylori* gastritis, but this is rare. In a historic series of more than 30,000 gastric biopsy specimens examined over

TABLE 8–2. Possible Causes of Gastric Mucosal Granulomas
Infections
Bacterial
Tuberculosis
Syphilis
Whipple's disease
Helicobacter (?)
Fungal
Histoplasmosis
Parasitic
Anisakiasis
Strongyloidosis (?)
Foreign bodies
Sutures
Food
Xanthogranuloma
Tumors
Carcinoma
Lymphoma
Plasma cell granuloma
Granulomatous diseases of unknown cause
Immune-mediated vasculitis
Wegener's granulomatosis
Crohn's disease
Sarcoidosis
Isolated granulomatous gastritis

the course of several years, granulomas were found in 23 subjects, 11 of whom had *H. pylori* infection (Genta et al, unpublished data). In infected subjects, granulomas were few in number and small in size. *H. pylori* was seen only on the luminal surface and not within granulomas (Fig. 8-27). Neither my personal experience nor data from the literature support a causative role for *H. pylori* in the pathogenesis of granulomatous gastritis.[136,137]

ANISAKIASIS

Gastric anisakiasis is discussed in greater detail in Chapter 3. The early lesions of anisakiasis range from interstitial edema accompanied by a loose, predominantly eosinophilic inflammatory infiltrate to overt eosinophilic abscesses. Well-preserved larvae are often detected. In later lesions, the most common finding is the presence of foreign body granulomas, sometimes associated with fragments of helminthic cuticles.[138,139]

FOREIGN BODIES

A common cause of gastric foreign body granulomas is suture material in patients who have undergone a partial gastrectomy. These granulomas are usually found in the vicinity of the anastomotic site. In patients with gastric ulcer, food particles may become engulfed in the ulcer crater, where they may cause a foreign body reaction. When such granulomas are found in biopsy specimens obtained from active ulcers, their origin is

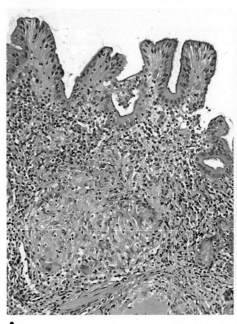
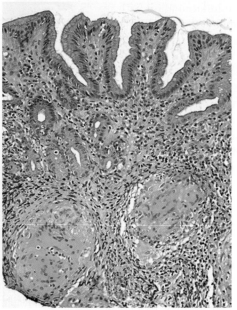

A   **B**

FIGURE 8–27. Multiple non-necrotizing granulomas of undetermined etiology in the gastric mucosa of a 65-year old asymptomatic volunteer. There may be considerable histologic differences among granulomas, with looser giant cells and abundant inflammatory cells (**A**) or more compact structures with less inflammation (**B**). Rarely, however, can the etiology be determined on morphologic grounds. When the cause for granulomas is not evident, clinicians should be alerted to the possibility of Crohn's disease or sarcoidosis.

readily apparent. However, diagnostic difficulties may arise when granulomas are found in specimens from healed ulcers and the pathologist lacks the appropriate clinical information.

TUMORS

Rarely, adenocarcinomas (particularly those that produce mucin) may induce the formation of mucin granulomas in the gastric mucosa or gastric lymph nodes. Granulomas have also been noted in patients with gastric non-MALT lymphoma.[140]

OTHER UNUSUAL CAUSES

In rare instances, granulomatous gastritis may be part of an immune-mediated vasculitis syndrome, or Wegener's granulomatosis. Sometimes, it may assume a form akin to xanthogranulomatous cholecystitis.[141]

GASTRIC INVOLVEMENT IN SYSTEMIC GRANULOMATOUS DISEASE

Granulomas may be detected in the gastric mucosa of patients with established sarcoidosis or Crohn's disease, and in this setting they may be assumed to be part of the systemic process with no further investigation required. However, the finding of granulomas in the stomach may precede the discovery of disease in other organs. In these cases, careful interpretation of gastric biopsy findings, together with evaluation of other clinical and laboratory tests, may lead to the prompt diagnosis of a condition that might otherwise remain obscure for a long time.[136]

In sarcoidosis, involvement of the GI tract is occasionally discovered at autopsy, but it rarely has clinical importance. However, severe disease can produce gastric outlet obstruction or bleeding. Endoscopic findings may include nodularity, polypoid changes, erosions, ulcers, and segmental, usually distal, rigidity resembling linitis plastica.[142,143]

Recent studies have challenged the perception that gastric involvement is rare in Crohn's disease and have found a prevalence of gastric granulomas between 10% and 15%. Focally enhanced *H. pylori*–negative active gastritis may be present in 30% to 70% of patients.[35,144,145] In these patients, focal gastritis was almost twice as frequent in the corpus as in the antrum, and epithelioid granulomas were twice as prevalent in the antrum.

ISOLATED (PRIMARY) GRANULOMATOUS GASTRITIS

The diagnosis of idiopathic granulomatous gastritis should be made only after all of the numerous alternatives previously discussed have been ruled out and appropriate additional tests have been performed. Isolated granulomatous gastritis should not be considered a separate nosologic entity but rather a "holding category," applied as a temporary diagnostic term to cases of granulomatous gastric inflammation for which the cause has yet to be determined. Support for this approach is derived from a number of studies showing that a majority of gastric granulomas are an expression of either concurrent or incipient Crohn's disease or systemic sarcoidosis.[136,146-148] Even after careful evaluation, a proportion of cases of gastric granulomas often remain unexplained. These patients are usually asymptomatic. Thus, a descriptive diagnosis such as *nonnecrotizing granuloma in the gastric mucosa* may be preferable to the use of a name (e.g., *idiopathic granulomatous gastritis*) that may perpetuate the impression that it represents a specific disease.

■ Chemical (or Reactive) Gastropathy

CLINICAL FEATURES

Although an association between the presence of bile in the stomach and mucosal damage was first postulated by William Beaumont in 1859, Dewar and associates were the first to comprehensively describe the pathologic changes found in association with bile reflux in patients who have had a partial gastrectomy, as well as in patients with duodenal or gastric ulcers.[62] Initially, they proposed the term *bile reflux gastritis* to describe a distinct clinicopathologic entity.[31,62,149-151] Subsequently, it was determined that NSAID-induced changes may be similar to those induced by bile reflux, and the term *chemical gastritis* was introduced. The terms *reactive gastritis*, *type C gastritis*, and *chemical gastropathy* have also been used in this setting. Chemical gastropathy, the currently preferred term, is defined as the constellation of endoscopic and histologic changes caused by chemical injury to the gastric mucosa. This tautologic definition reflects the lack of independent specificity of the endoscopic or histologic features seen in subjects with a history of endogenous or exogenous chemical damage to the stomach.

PATHOGENESIS

The pathologic changes referred to as chemical gastropathy (Table 8-3) are not directly associated with any characteristic signs or symptoms. Three categories of patients may exhibit the endoscopic and histologic changes of chemical gastropathy—those who have alkaline reflux after a partial gastrectomy, those who have duodenogastric bile reflux as part of a poorly understood dysmotility syndrome, and those who ingest NSAIDs.

Patients with postgastrectomy alkaline reflux may present with a syndrome characterized by burning midepigastric pain unresponsive to antacids and aggravated by eating and recumbency.[152,153] Bilious vomiting, anemia, and weight loss may occur. Endoscopic confirmation of bile reflux and documentation of the characteristic pathologic findings support the diagnosis, and corrective surgery (e.g., creation of a 40- to 50-cm Roux-en-Y gastrojejunostomy) is successful in about half of cases.[154] No relationship has been demonstrated between symptoms and the gross or microscopic appearance of the gastric mucosa.

Duodenogastric bile reflux secondary to gastroduodenal dysmotility is rare in nonoperated patients.[24] This controversial condition is rarely considered in the differential diagnosis of dyspepsia. Thus, the frequency of histologic changes of chemical gastropathy in these patients is unknown.

As a consequence of frequent NSAID use, patients may experience gastric pain; approximately 10% per year develop erosions or ulcers, and 1% to 2% per year have a major gastric bleeding episode.[155,156] Reactive gastropathy has been documented in 10% to 45% of long-term users of NSAIDs, but no relationship

TABLE 8–3. Endoscopic and Histopathologic Features of *Helicobacter pylori* Gastritis and Chemical Gastropathy

Feature	*H. pylori* Gastritis	Chemical or Reactive Gastritis	Predictive Value in Establishing Diagnosis
Endoscopic			
Mucosal congestion	Frequent	Frequent	Minimal
Edema	Variable	Variable	Minimal
Superficial erosions	Uncommon	Frequent	High
Proximal ulcer	Uncommon	Occasional	Moderate/High
Distal ulcer	Common	Occasional	Low
Polypoid appearance of gastric stump	Virtually never	Frequent post gastrectomy (Billroth II)	High
Histologic			
Active inflammation	Virtually always	Rare in the absence of ulcer	High
Chronic inflammation	Virtually always	Minimal	Moderate
Eosinophils	Common	Uncommon	Low
Atrophy	Variable, may be extensive	Absent or focal	Low
Intestinal metaplasia	Variable, may be extensive	Absent, minimal, or focal	Low
Foveolar hyperplasia	Rare	Frequent	Moderate/High
Regenerative changes	Infrequent	Frequent	Moderate/High
Superficial smooth muscle fibers	Rare	Frequent	Moderate
Ulcer or erosion with normal surrounding mucosa	Virtually never	Frequent	Very high

between the appearance of the mucosa and dyspeptic symptoms has been documented.

MECHANISM OF INJURY

Duodenogastric reflux (with alkaline pancreatico-duodenal secretions, as well as acids, bile salts, and lysolecithin) results in disruption of the mucous barrier and direct damage by chemicals to the surface epithelium. Loss of the mucous barrier allows back-diffusion of hydrogen ions and secondary injurious effects.[25] The combined injury leads to accelerated exfoliation of surface epithelial cells and a histamine-mediated vascular response that manifests as edema and hyperemia. Repetitive injury may lead to the release of other proinflammatory agents such as platelet-derived growth factor, which, among its many actions, stimulates smooth muscle and fibroblastic proliferation.[16]

Epithelial injury following exposure to NSAIDs appears to be mediated by reduced prostaglandin synthesis. Prostaglandins are important cytoprotective agents in the gastric mucosa and exert their effects by maintaining mucosal blood flow, by increasing the secretion of mucus and bicarbonate ions, and by augmenting epithelial defenses against cytotoxic injury. Thus, NSAID-induced injury can be partially prevented by simultaneous administration of prostaglandin analogues such as misoprostol[157] and by suppression of gastric acid production with proton pump inhibitors.[158] New selective COX-2 inhibitors (second-generation NSAIDs or selective NSAIDs) are reportedly much better tolerated by the gastric mucosa.[159]

Although not strictly caused by chemical injury, mucosal lesions may also develop secondary to irradiation of the epigastric region or to intra-arterial chemotherapy in areas of gastric perfusion. Early changes consist of necrosis of fundal glands, edema, and mononuclear cell infiltration. Although reversal of mucosal damage occurs upon cessation of treatment, disruption of the mucosal architecture, fibrosis, and vascular abnormalities may persist indefinitely.[160-162]

PATHOLOGIC FEATURES

Gross Pathology

In postgastrectomy patients with alkaline reflux, the mucosa at the anastomotic site may have a polypoid appearance in association with congestion, edema, and friability.[163,164] Superficial erosions may occur in more proximal areas of the gastric stump, but these are not specific because they can be caused by a variety of injuries. In patients with nonoperated stomachs and possible duodenogastric bile reflux, the mucosa may exhibit congestion, edema, and surface erosions. In

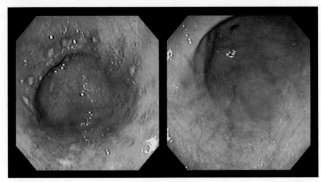

FIGURE 8–28. Endoscopic appearance of acute hemorrhagic gastritis.

long-term NSAID users, the mucosa may be normal or may show congestion, erosions, or ulcers (Fig. 8-28).

Microscopic Pathology

If a set of easily applicable criteria were available, and if the sensitivity, specificity, prevalence, and reliability of the histologic features of chemical gastritis were known, pathologists could provide important diagnostic clues as to the causes of gastric ulcers and erosions and could help identify patients who might benefit from discontinuation of NSAID treatment. Unfortunately, although some features are noted more frequently in long-term NSAID users, the pathologic diagnosis of chemical gastropathy remains a challenging problem.

The specificity and predictive value of the features outlined here are low because of several potential confounding factors, including surreptitious use of NSAIDs, the presence of other substances in the diet (e.g., alcohol, spices, salt) that may cause similar mucosal changes in some individuals, and clinically silent bile reflux.[24,151] Also, *H. pylori* infection may induce some of the features traditionally considered characteristic of chemical gastropathy such as mucosal hyperemia and edema (Fig. 8-29), superficial erosions (Fig. 8-30), foveolar hyperplasia (Fig. 8-31; see also Figs. 8-3 and 8-4), and regenerative changes. Therefore, the pathologist can suspect chemical gastropathy and can communicate this suspicion to the clinician, but a firm histopathologic diagnosis can be made only when supportive clinical data are available and *H. pylori* infection is absent.[13]

Hemorrhagic Gastritis and Vascular Gastropathies

Hemorrhagic gastritis and vascular gastropathies are part of a heterogeneous group of conditions characterized by vascular changes and their effects. *Acute hemorrhagic gastritis* is characterized by diffuse

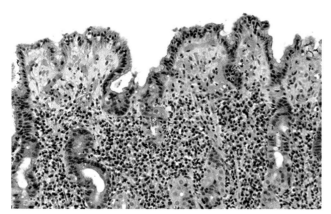

FIGURE 8–29. Subepithelial edema, congestion of the superficial lamina propria, and a paucity of neutrophils are characteristic features of acute hemorrhagic gastritis. In this case, however, *H. pylori* organisms are present (on the surface epithelium at both extremities of the photomicrograph, and within the central foveola), emphasizing the difficulties of the distinction between chemical gastropathy and *H. pylori* gastritis.

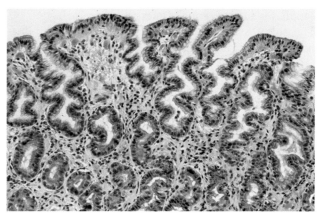

FIGURE 8–31. Moderate foveolar hyperplasia with minimal inflammation. Although this feature is suggestive of chronic chemical injury, it is a nonspecific finding that can be seen in a variety of disorders.

ACUTE HEMORRHAGIC GASTRITIS

Clinical Features

Acute hemorrhagic gastritis has been a recognized nosologic entity for at least a century; Curling documented the association between severe burns and duodenal ulceration—so-called Curling's ulcer.[165] However, the prevalence and importance of stress-induced gastric mucosal breakdowns have been fully appreciated only recently. Most patients admitted to an intensive care unit have mucosal lesions, approximately 20% of them develop overt bleeding, and 2% to 5% die from life-threatening hemorrhage.[166] Ingestion of large doses of aspirin or other NSAIDs may induce acute mucosal injury ranging from edema and hyperemia to erosions and ulcerations. Such lesions may occur suddenly, without previous pain or discomfort, in first-time NSAID users and in patients who have taken NSAIDs regularly for years. Similar but usually less severe changes can be caused by ingestion of large quantities of alcohol. Because alcohol and aspirin may act synergistically to break down mucosal defenses, one wonders how many hemorrhagic gastritides have been caused by attempts to prevent hangovers by taking two aspirin tablets after an alcoholic binge.[167]

The pathogenesis of stress-induced hemorrhagic gastritis is unknown, but luminal acid seems to be essential. Acid exerts its noxious effects when mucosal defense mechanisms (e.g., the mucus-bicarbonate barrier and the epithelial layer) lose their integrity.[166] Vascular disturbances—in association with stasis, vasoconstriction, and increased vascular permeability—may further contribute to mucosal vulnerability. Aspirin and NSAIDs act by interfering with prostaglandin synthesis, as noted earlier. Alcohol causes direct damage to the gastric mucosa. At a concentration of 12.5%, it induces hyperemia and petechiae. At concentrations above 40%, it causes necrosis of the surface epithelium and

mucosal hyperemia associated with bleeding, erosions, and ulcers precipitated by a sudden stress-induced imbalance between aggressive and protective factors involved in the maintenance of mucosal integrity. *Vascular gastropathies* are defined endoscopically as distinct alterations in the gastric mucosal vessels accompanied by little or no inflammation. The most important vascular gastropathies are the watermelon stomach syndrome and portal hypertensive gastropathy.

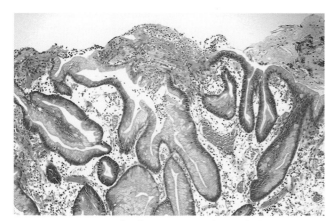

FIGURE 8–30. Superficial erosion with underlying altered foveolar architecture and a small aggregate of fibrinopurulent material in direct continuity with the lamina propria in the area of the eroded epithelium. This latter feature helps distinguish a true erosion from an artifactual detachment of epithelium, which is never accompanied by inflammation or fibrin deposition. Such erosions are typically found in chemical erosive gastropathy, in some patients with *H. pylori* gastritis, and on the surface of inflammatory polyps.

capillaries and subsequent interstitial hemorrhage.[168,169] The suppression of acid with proton pump inhibitors helps reduce the severity of mucosal damage and facilitates healing.

Pathologic Features

GROSS PATHOLOGY

Acute hemorrhagic gastritis is characterized by a hyperemic edematous mucosa with erosions and various degrees of active bleeding (see Fig. 8-28). The clinical history (e.g., shock, burns, ingestion of large doses of aspirin) rather than the pathologic features helps the endoscopist in determining the precipitating factors.

MICROSCOPIC PATHOLOGY

Acute hemorrhagic gastritis, regardless of its cause, is characterized by dilatation and congestion of mucosal capillaries, edema, and various degrees of interstitial hemorrhage in the lamina propria. Epithelial erosions are generally small. Aggregates of fibrin and polymorphonuclear cells replace the eroded epithelium and may project above the surface to form small, elevated clumps of necrotic debris (see Fig. 8-30). The epithelium of gastric pits underlying the erosions, as well as the edges of erosions and ulcers, shows pronounced regenerative atypia that should not be misinterpreted as dysplasia. In the absence of concurrent *H. pylori* infection, neither significant chronic inflammation nor activity in the unaffected areas of the stomach occurs. Therefore, a diagnosis of erosive hemorrhagic gastritis can be made, and possible etiologic agents (e.g., alcohol or NSAID ingestion) may be suggested in the pathology report. If *H. pylori* gastritis occurs, widespread active inflammation often obscures or worsens the changes caused by other agents.

VASCULAR GASTROPATHIES

Watermelon Stomach

CLINICAL FEATURES

Watermelon stomach, or gastric antral vascular ectasia (GAVE) syndrome, is a rare condition of unknown cause frequently associated with gastric atrophy and autoimmune and connective tissue disorders.[170-172] More than 70% of cases occur in women older than 65 years of age. Occult bleeding is seen at presentation in up to 90% of cases, melena or hematemesis in 60%. In most patients, chronic blood loss causes iron deficiency anemia. Treatment is empirical; iron supplements are sufficient in patients with limited bleeding, but therapeutic endoscopy with obliteration of the dilated vessels or antrectomy may be necessary in severe cases.

PATHOLOGIC FEATURES

GROSS PATHOLOGY

Watermelon stomach was so named[173] because of the "longitudinal antral folds seen converging on the pylorus, containing visible and ectatic vessels resembling the stripes on a watermelon" (Fig. 8-32). In other metaphors, the prominent dilated vessels have been compared with "a large flat mushroom" or a "honeycomb." In addition to these picturesquely described vascular ectasias, various amounts of bleeding and blood clotting may be seen.[170,171]

MICROSCOPIC PATHOLOGY

Watermelon stomach has a characteristic pathologic appearance, particularly in the antrum. The lamina propria, which is usually devoid of inflammation, appears expanded owing to smooth muscle proliferation and mild fibrosis; it also contains markedly dilated mucosal capillaries, which are not increased in number but show a significant increase in cross-sectional area.[173,177] In most cases, fibrin thrombi are found within the dilated capillaries (see Fig. 8-32). The presence of thrombi is particularly important for ruling out other causes of mucosal congestion and, although not pathognomonic, is highly suggestive of this disorder.

Portal Hypertensive Gastropathy

CLINICAL FEATURES

Portal hypertensive gastropathy is defined as a dilatation of the mucosal vessels, more prominent in the proximal stomach, that occurs in a high proportion of patients with portal hypertension.[172] Patients with severe portal hypertension usually have diffuse lesions and a high rate of gastric bleeding. Portal decompression surgery is the only measure that may help reduce the risk of hemorrhage.

PATHOLOGIC FEATURES

GROSS PATHOLOGY

The endoscopic appearance of portal hypertensive gastropathy is nonspecific and does not correlate well with the degree of portal hypertension.[174] Endoscopic patterns have been variously described as snake skin, scarlatina rash, cherry-red spots, and mosaic.[175] The mosaic pattern was found by a consensus conference[176] to be the most reliable indicator of mild portal hypertensive gastropathy (low risk of hemorrhage). Red marks suggest a more severe degree of hypertension and a greater risk of hemorrhage.

MICROSCOPIC PATHOLOGY

The pathologic changes of portal hypertensive gastropathy consist of dilatation and tortuosity of small

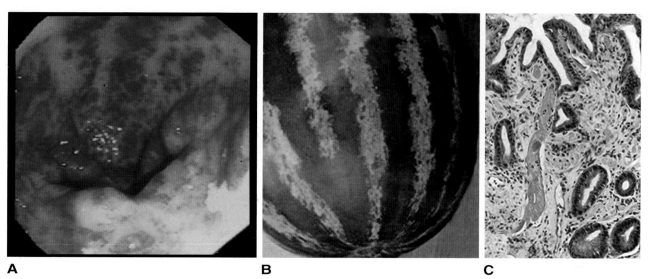

A   **B**   **C**

FIGURE 8–32. Watermelon stomach (gastric antral vascular ectasia). Erythematous lines appear to converge at the pyloric region of the stomach (**A**). The appearance resembles the stripes of a watermelon (**B**). Histologically, dilated mucosal vessels containing thrombus material (**C**) are characteristic of this rare entity.

arteries and veins, with occasional thickening of the walls of the vessels. Changes are more prominent in the corpus and are more likely to be detected in submucosal vessels than in mucosal capillaries. Because of the location of these changes and the reluctance of most gastroenterologists to obtain large and deep biopsy samples from patients who may have an increased risk of bleeding, the diagnosis of portal hypertensive gastropathy is not often made by evaluation of mucosal biopsy specimens. In patients with concurrent *H. pylori* gastritis, it is difficult if not impossible to separate the respective contribution of infection and congestion in the resulting complex of changes observed in the mucosa.[178,179]

Special Problems in the Diagnosis of Gastric Biopsies

NON–*H. PYLORI* CHRONIC ACTIVE GASTRITIS

In most cases, the findings of a mixed inflammatory infiltrate in the lamina propria and a neutrophilic infiltrate in the epithelium associated with degeneration (i.e., mucin loss, cuboidal flattening of the cells, cell dropout) are associated with *H. pylori* infection. Occasionally, bacteria may not be identified in a single biopsy specimen but will be visible after careful examination of multiple specimens (the recommended number of specimens to examine is five, as is discussed in the next section). However, there are still circumstances when, after all appropriate histologic measures have been taken (i.e., deeper cuts, specimen reorientation, special stains, and immunostains), organisms remain undetected.

In such cases, the pathology report should provide a diagnosis based on the features observed (e.g., chronic active gastritis) and should indicate that, in spite of the pathologic characteristics usually associated with *H. pylori* infection, an exhaustive search for bacteria failed to reveal *Helicobacter*-like organisms. This broader wording is suggested because it includes other *Helicobacter* species, such as *H. heilmannii*. A comment regarding possible explanations for this finding, as well as management suggestions, should also be included. For example, if specimens were obtained after antibiotic treatment for *H. pylori*, the persistence of active inflammation would almost certainly indicate that eradication was unsuccessful.[36] If another test (urea breath test or serology) is known to have yielded a positive result, this might represent one of the atypical cases in which bacteria are so rare that customary sampling is insufficient to reveal them. Another uncommon but important possibility is Crohn's disease. Patchy *H. pylori*–negative chronic active gastritis (focally enhanced gastritis) has been shown to be a manifestation of gastric Crohn's disease, even when signs or symptoms of intestinal involvement are not evident.[35]

PROTON PUMP INHIBITOR THERAPY

In addition to changes in the oxyntic mucosa as described earlier in the chapter (i.e., oxyntic cell hyperplasia and oxyntic gland dilatation), prolonged use of proton pump inhibitors can induce the formation of multiple fundic polyps.[72,180] Because these lesions have no known association with neoplastic progression and are reversible upon discontinuation of therapy, no action is considered necessary. Patients with *H. pylori*

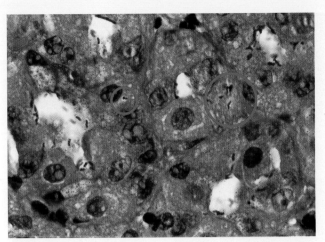

FIGURE 8–33. *H. pylori* is present in the deep portion of the oxyntic glands and within the canaliculi of oxyntic cells *(red circles)*. This feature is seen virtually only in patients receiving long-term proton pump inhibitor therapy.

gastritis who receive proton pump inhibitors for prolonged periods may experience significant changes in the intensity and distribution of inflammation. Most patients who require proton pump inhibitors for treatment of chronic gastroesophageal reflux produce either normal or excessive amounts of acid; therefore, they are likely to have antral-predominant gastritis with only mild inflammatory changes in the corpus. Acid suppression causes a shift in the bacterial and inflammatory burden; after months of therapy, inflammation is often reduced in the antrum and increased in the corpus.[181] At this stage, *H. pylori* organisms are often easier to detect in the corpus, sometimes deep in the oxyntic glands, and even within canaliculi of oxyntic cells (Fig. 8-33). The significance of these changes is uncertain, although it has been suggested that an increased severity of corpus gastritis can accelerate the development of atrophy and might eventually increase the risk of gastric cancer.[182] Current evidence does not indicate that this effect results in an increased incidence of gastric cancer. However, from a pathologic viewpoint, it seems reasonable to avoid increasing inflammation (a potentially destructive phenomenon) in the corpus. Therefore, the guidelines of the Maastricht Consensus of the European *H. pylori* Group recommend detection and treatment of *H. pylori* before initiation of long-term proton pump inhibitor therapy.[183] No consensus in this regard has been reached in the United States.

THE GASTRIC CARDIA AND CARDITIS

Until a few years ago, a commonly accepted definition of the cardia was "the segment of mucosa that extends for about 2 cm distal to the Z-line and consists of mucous-type glands similar to those of the antrum and prepyloric region."[184] Because no particularly interesting pathologic processes were thought to affect this minuscule territory of mucosa connecting two well-characterized segments of the digestive system, the gastric cardia was virtually ignored by gastroenterologists, pathologists, and physiologists alike. However, over the previous several decades, there has been a dramatic rise in the incidence of adenocarcinoma of the cardia in the same populations in which the incidence of gastric cancer has been decreasing. Thus, there has been a recent explosion of interest in exploring the pathology of this ill-defined area of the stomach. Recently, the gastric cardia has been defined as the most proximal portion of the stomach, albeit an extremely small zone that is identifiable only by histologic analysis.[185] Cardiac-type mucosa, characterized by unequivocal PAS-positive mucous glands (either with or without admixed oxyntic glands) arranged in a lobular configuration, has a mean length of only 1.8 mm, with a range of 1.0 to 4.0 mm. This area is susceptible to inflammation (carditis) as a result of at least two (and perhaps more) common forms of injury—gastroesophageal reflux disease (GERD) and *H. pylori* infection.[186] Both of these conditions may lead to the development of carditis and eventually to intestinal metaplasia, if the injurious insult is long-standing (see Figs. 8-34 through 8-36).

Reflux-induced carditis is probably the earliest and most common manifestation of GERD.[187-189] In fact, reflux-induced inflammation of the cardia often coexists with reflux esophagitis; thus, over time, the distal esophagus may undergo columnar metaplasia with the development of mucous glands.[186] This results in an apparent lengthening of the cardia (defined histologically as an area of mucosa occupied predominantly by mucous glands), which in reality represents ultra-short Barrett's esophagus[186] contiguous to the original gastric cardia. In contrast, *H. pylori* carditis usually is not associated with reflux esophagitis but is more commonly associated with corpus and antral gastritis.[186]

In 1994, it was shown that virtually all patients who have *H. pylori* gastritis in the antrum and/or corpus also have bacteria and inflammation in the cardia.[92] Subsequently, it was confirmed that *H. pylori* infection of the cardia represents not a distinct entity but rather an extension of one condition—*H. pylori* chronic active gastritis.[190-195] A variety of clinical, endoscopic, pathologic, and immunohistochemical methods can be used to help distinguish reflux carditis from *H. pylori* carditis in biopsies from the gastroesophageal junction (GEJ) region; these are summarized in Table 8-4.

Intestinal Metaplasia of the Gastroesophageal Junction

Recent reports indicate that intestinal metaplasia in the cardia may be found in up to 20% of patients, even in the absence of *H. pylori* infection, and in apparently

TABLE 8–4. Reflux Carditis Versus *Helicobacter pylori* Carditis

Feature	Reflux Carditis	*H. pylori* Carditis
GERD clinical profile	+	–
Irregular Z-line	+	–
Esophagitis (histologic)	+	–
Gastritis (histologic)	–	+
H. pylori	–	+
Eosinophils	++	+
Neutrophils	+/–	++
Lymphocytes, plasma cells	+	++
Multilayered epithelium	+	–
BE CK7/20 pattern		
(if IM present)	+	+/–
Complete > incomplete IM	–	+

BE, Barrett's esophagus; GERD, gastroesophageal reflux disease; IM, intestinal metaplasia.

normal subjects as well.[196,197] This finding has prompted investigations regarding the possible relationship between intestinal metaplasia of the cardia, intestinal metaplasia of the distal esophagus (Barrett's esophagus), and the development of adenocarcinoma.[190-192] In fact, several studies have shown a different natural history and risk of dysplasia and carcinoma in cases of intestinal metaplasia of the distal esophagus (Barrett's esophagus) versus those with intestinal metaplasia of the proximal stomach (carditis).[198-201] For this reason, it has become important for clinicians to try to differentiate intestinal metaplasia of the cardia from an ultra-short segment of Barrett's esophagus (see Table 8-4).

Some studies have suggested that cytokeratin 7 and 20 (CK7/20) immunoreactive patterns may help to distinguish long-segment Barrett's esophagus from gastric intestinal metaplasia, but their utility in distinguishing short-segment Barrett's esophagus from carditis with intestinal metaplasia is unreliable.[197] For instance, Ormsby and colleagues[202] have shown that a unique pattern of immunoreactivity, designated the "Barrett's CK7/20 pattern" (superficial CK20 staining and strong CK7 staining of superficial and deep glands), is present in 94% of esophageal resection specimens and 100% of biopsy specimens from patients with long-segment Barrett's esophagus. A Barrett's CK7/20 pattern was not observed either in gastric cardia biopsy specimens or in gastric resection specimens of patients with histologic evidence of intestinal metaplasia. The sensitivity, specificity, and positive predictive value of a Barrett's CK7/20 pattern for the diagnosis of long-segment Barrett's esophagus were found to be 97%, 100%, and 100%, respectively. However, other investigators have not been able to confirm these findings.[198,199] Recently, a hybrid "multilayered" type of epithelium, which combines features of squamous and columnar epithelia, has been noted in up to 35% of cases of Barrett's esophagus and also in cases of carditis related to GERD but not *H. pylori* infection.[203] This type of epithelium

has been shown to be highly associated with intestinal metaplasia of the esophagus, and thus its presence is a strong indicator of GERD and incipient Barrett's esophagus (Fig. 8-34).

In fact, some cases of short-segment Barrett's esophagus may be difficult or impossible to separate from intestinal metaplasia in the cardia[199,203] by histologic or histochemical means, even with the use of information outlined in Table 8-4, if appropriate clinical and endoscopic information is not available. In clinical practice, endoscopic information regarding the precise anatomic location of the biopsy and the appearance of the GEJ region (i.e., the presence or absence of tongues of gastric-appearing mucosa protruding into the esophagus) is most helpful in facilitating determination of the location of intestinal metaplasia (i.e., whether it is esophageal or gastric in origin).

In addition, the following heuristic approach may be helpful:

1. If only scattered goblet cells are present within cardia-type mucosa in the absence of complete intestinal metaplasia, then the pathology report should be descriptive and should suggest that correlation with the biopsy site is necessary to determine its origin. Further sampling should be considered from above (i.e., proximal to) the anatomic GEJ if Barrett's esophagus is suspected endoscopically.
2. If complete intestinal metaplasia is noted adjacent to or within oxyntic-type mucosa (in the absence of endoscopic evidence of short-segment Barrett's esophagus), then the pathology report should state that this is more likely an expression of metaplastic atrophic gastritis, particularly if the patient has *H. pylori* infection.
3. Further, if complete or incomplete intestinal metaplasia is detected within cardia-type mucosa in a specimen designated as originating from the distal esophagus, the favored diagnosis should be Barrett's epithelium, an interpretation that is further strengthened if the patient has a normal stomach, both endoscopically and histologically.

Reporting of a Biopsy From the Gastroesophageal Junction

Even if the issues regarding the prevalence and significance of carditis and intestinal metaplasia at the GEJ remain unresolved,[204] endoscopists continue to sample the gastric cardia and the GEJ with increasing frequency. Thus, pathologists should be able to recognize and report the histologic changes that occur in this region. Virtually all subjects infected with *H. pylori* have chronic active gastritis and organisms within the cardia. This finding should be reported as part of the presence

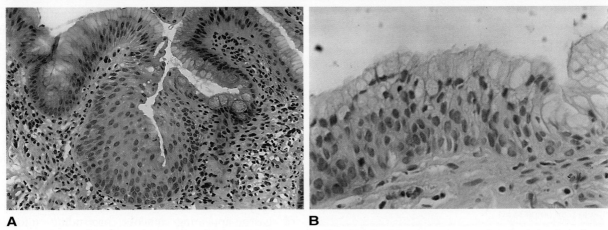

A   **B**

FIGURE 8–34. **A,** High-power section of the squamocolumnar junction from the distal esophagus/proximal stomach (cardia) of a patient with gastroesophageal reflux and no evidence of *H. pylori* infection. In patients without *H. pylori,* mixed inflammation, often with goblet cells, is usually limited to the cardiac region, while the remainder of the stomach is normal. A focus of multilayered epithelium is present in the center. **B,** High-power section of multilayered epithelium showing "squamoid" cells at the base and "columnar" mucous cells at the surface. This epithelium is highly associated with GERD and Barrett's esophagus.

of gastritis elsewhere in the stomach. However, many patients either with or without clinical GERD with an absence of *H. pylori* infection present with significant inflammation in the cardia. It is likely that most of these patients have nonclinically detectable GERD, but this has yet to be proven. Thus, in this setting, the term *carditis* (chronic or chronic active) should be reported only if the biopsies are known to be from the cardia; otherwise a descriptive term indicating the type of mucosa (cardiac, oxyntic, or mixed), the type (neutrophilic, eosinophilic, or mononuclear) and intensity of inflammation (mild, moderate, or severe), the location of inflammation (lamina propria or epithelium), and the occurrence of erosions, if present, is probably best.

A tissue section stained with Alcian blue at pH 2.5 may be helpful for facilitating the detection of intestinal metaplasia, but this is usually not necessary because goblet cells are normally easily identifiable on routine H&E staining. Unfortunately, this stain cannot help distinguish pseudogoblet "blue cells" commonly found in this region from true goblet cells because both types of cells are often Alcian blue–positive.[205-207] Thus, the distinction should be made on a histologic basis (Fig. 8-35). If a biopsy specimen that contains inflamed cardia-type mucosa, either with or without intestinal metaplasia, has been obtained from the GEJ region, and it is unclear to the pathologist if the tissue represents distal esophagus or proximal stomach, then a generic diagnosis is recommended (e.g., squamo-columnar junctional mucosa with mild chronic active inflammation of the columnar component [cardia type]).

A comment on the presence or absence of intestinal metaplasia is also warranted. If squamous epithelium is included in the specimen, the presence or absence of active esophagitis, based on degree of inflammation, basal cell hyperplasia, papillary length, and integrity of

the epithelium, should also be included in the description. In about 1% to 5% of biopsy specimens from the cardia, a small aggregate of pancreatic-type glands may be present, usually in deeper portions of the mucosa (Fig. 8-36). This finding is usually reported as pancreatic acinar metaplasia, although neither its origin (metaplasia or heterotopia) nor its significance is known with absolute certainty. Thus, reporting its presence should be considered optional. Dysplasia may rarely develop in the cardia, as well as in Barrett's esophagus, so one should also report this finding when noted.

Finally, a pathologic diagnosis of Barrett's esophagus should not be established on the basis of a biopsy from the distal esophagus/GEJ region unless intestinal metaplasia is present *and* there is endoscopic evidence that the tissue was obtained from above the anatomic GEJ.

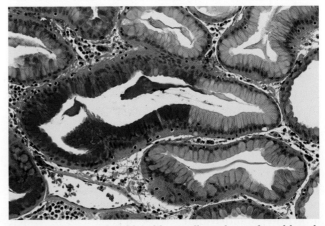

FIGURE 8–35. Pseudogoblet "blue" cells in the cardia. Although the mucus in these cells stains blue with Alcian blue at pH 2.5, the cells appear columnar in shape. The significance of these cells is unclear, although a hypothesis that these cells represent an early form of metaplasia has been proposed.

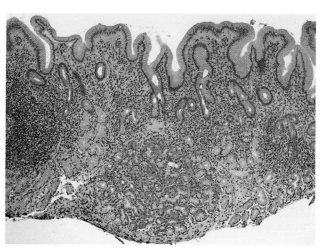

FIGURE 8–36. A well-defined nodule of pancreatic metaplasia is present in the cardia.

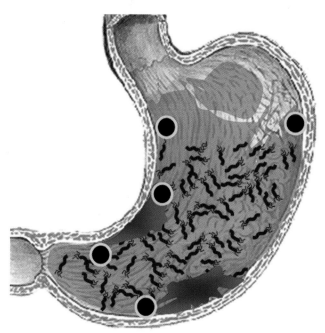

FIGURE 8–37. Mapping protocol of the updated Sydney System. The locations recommended for biopsies have been chosen in an attempt to provide the best sampling for the detection of infection, atrophy, and metaplasia (represented as blue patches in the red, inflamed mucosa).

Diagnosis of Gastritis: Approach to Pathologic Evaluation of Gastric Biopsy Specimens

One advantage of the updated Sydney System is that it provides the pathologist with guidelines for generating a systematic, uniform diagnostic report. The ultimate goal of the guidelines is to make gastric biopsy pathology reporting homogeneous in format and content so that clinical studies may be evaluated meaningfully. To create the report suggested by the updated Sydney System, five recommended biopsy specimens should be methodically evaluated and the findings synthesized (Fig. 8-37).

Unfortunately, endoscopists do not always provide the recommended number of biopsies. To account for this, two types of guidelines are described here—one that uses the updated Sydney System and one that uses an empirical approach in the event that fewer than the recommended number of biopsy specimens are available for review.

Using the Updated Sydney System

BIOPSY

To obtain enough samples for proper classification of gastritis, the biopsy protocol depicted in Figure 8-37 is recommended. Biopsy specimens from three compartments (i.e., antrum, incisura angularis, and corpus) should be separately identified when submitted to the pathology laboratory. Proper orientation is indispensable for optimal histologic evaluation and may be accomplished either in the endoscopy suite or in the histopathology laboratory at the time of tissue embedding.

THE FOUR A'S: ASSESSMENT, ANALOGUE SCALE, ASSIGNMENT, AND AVERAGING

Assessment. Each biopsy specimen must be assessed for its suitability for histopathologic examination. An acceptable slide should show several well-oriented cuts that leave both the mucosal surface and the muscularis mucosae visible. Examples of acceptable sections are depicted in Figures 8-10, 8-11, 8-19, 8-20, 8-34 and 8-36. Unacceptable sections may still be useful for evaluating certain aspects of the gastric mucosa, but clinicians and pathologists should be aware of the pitfalls of this approach. Among errors that result most commonly from examination of inadequate specimens are misinterpretation of cancer in poorly oriented mucosal biopsies (e.g., tangential cuts can give the mistaken impression of invasiveness) and missed visualization of a change present only on some levels of an insufficiently sectioned specimen (the "dark side" effect).[208]

Analogue Scale. For translating pathologic observations into well-defined topographic patterns, or for purposes of comparison, it is desirable that each relevant feature be graded on a standardized reproducible scale. To this end, the Houston consensus working group uses a visual analogue scale originally devised by Karttunen (Karttunen T, unpublished data)[10] that contains several

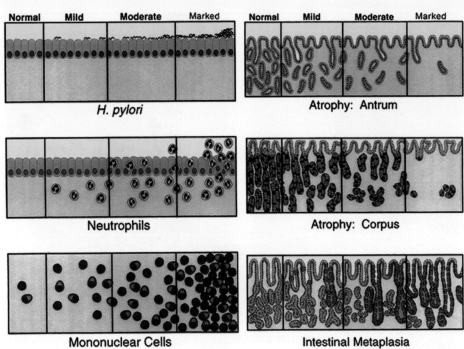

FIGURE 8–38. Visual analogue scale of the updated Sydney System for assistance in the semiquantitative evaluation of the pathologic variables (density of *H. pylori*, intensity of neutrophilic and mononuclear inflammation, atrophy, and metaplasia).

graded variables (density of *H. pylori*, intensity of neutrophilic and mononuclear inflammation, atrophy in the antrum and corpus, and intestinal metaplasia) (Fig. 8-38). Each section deemed suitable for evaluation is examined, and each variable is graded with the use of the analogue scale.

Assignment and Averaging. Each feature is assigned a numeric or descriptive value: 0 for absent, 1 for mild, 2 for moderate, and 3 for marked (or severe). The values of each specimen are averaged separately for each compartment—two specimens from the antrum, one from the incisura angularis, and two from the corpus. Thus, two averaged values are generated—one that represents the severity of a feature in the antrum and one that stands for the corpus.

INFLAMMATION GRADIENT

Once the four A's have been completed, the next step is to compare the relative degree of inflammation in the two main compartments (antrum and corpus), then determine whether the inflammation is similar (i.e., pangastritis) or more severe in the antrum (antrum-predominant gastritis) or the corpus (corpus-predominant gastritis). For the inflammation in one compartment to be characterized as predominant with respect to the other, the difference should be of at least two grades. This helps minimize the effects of interobserver variability. The degree of atrophy and metaplasia can also be assessed according to the recently developed classification of atrophy. Finally, a decision should be made as to whether "focal atrophy—metaplastic or not" or diffuse "atrophic gastritis" is present.

FINAL DIAGNOSIS

The final diagnosis should represent a synthesis of the observations outlined previously—for example, "*H. pylori* antrum-predominant gastritis" or "corpus-restricted atrophic gastritis without *H. pylori* infection, suggestive of autoimmune gastritis."

EVALUATION OF SPECIAL TYPES OF GASTRITIS AND GASTROPATHY

The updated Sydney System is also suitable for evaluating special types of gastritis. A sample diagnosis might read "lymphocytic gastritis, corpus predominant, with *H. pylori* infection." For gastropathies, the updated Sydney System is helpful for assessing the pathologic features of the mucosa, but grading each specimen is not necessary.

EVALUATION OF ATROPHY

The updated Sydney System has incorporated the concept of multifocal atrophic gastritis (MAG) as a distinct nosologic entity separate from nonatrophic gastritis.[207] However, the updated system does not adequately define the range of atrophy, nor does it define the boundary at which gastritis with focal atrophy ends and atrophic gastritis begins. This is a relevant issue because a few scattered foci of intestinal metaplasia can be found in the antrum of most subjects with *H. pylori* and in a small percentage of noninfected adults. Clearly, it would not be appropriate to classify these individuals as having atrophic gastritis, a diagnosis

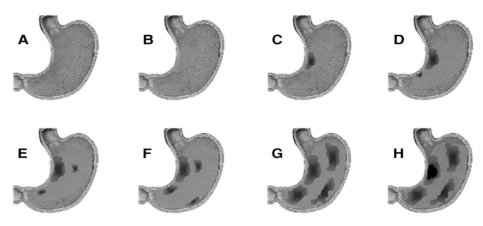

FIGURE 8–39. Spectrum of atrophy (represented by pale-pink discoloration) and metaplasia (represented by blue areas). Although it is obvious that stomach A has nonatrophic gastritis and that stomachs F, G, and H have atrophic metaplastic gastritis, stomachs B through E are difficult to assign to a specific category, particularly if the extent of biopsy sampling was limited.

that would imply altered gastric function and an increased risk of gastric cancer. The inability to clarify the boundary between nonatrophic and atrophic gastritis reflects the difficulty of classifying a disease that evolves on a continuous scale into discrete categories (Fig. 8-39).

The recognition of atrophy in mucosal biopsies is the first step toward understanding the nature of atrophic gastritis. Recent workshops devoted to this issue have formulated methods for grading atrophy.[11,12] Briefly, to reach a satisfactory level of interobserver agreement, the algorithm represented in Figure 8-40 is used. First, the observer must decide whether atrophy is absent, unequivocally present, or impossible to assess because of interference due to inflammation ("indefinite for atrophy"). If present, atrophy is then evaluated according to its two subtypes—nonmetaplastic and metaplastic. Nonmetaplastic atrophy is defined by the presence of an area of lamina propria, normally occupied by glands native to the region from which the biopsy is obtained, that is collapsed to form thin, gland-depleted mucosa with or without fibrosis. Conversely, metaplastic atrophy is defined by the replacement of native glands by intestinal-type (in the corpus) or pyloric (or pseudo-

pyloric) glands. In both cases, the degree of gland loss is graded from mild to severe on a scale of 1 to 3. This algorithm has been helpful in guiding a diverse group of pathologists to an acceptable level of agreement, and efforts are being made to disseminate it to a wider audience.

INCOMPLETE BIOPSY SET

The recommendation made by the updated Sydney System to obtain a five-biopsy set is precisely that—a recommendation. Realistically, most gastroenterologists do not follow this recommendation either because they do not know about it or because they do not believe it is helpful. Some simply fail to see any benefit to the patient of obtaining five biopsy specimens from a normal-appearing stomach. Still others, who work in a highly regulated health care system, simply would not be allowed to do it.

What should a pathologist who would like to use the updated Sydney System do when only a portion of the recommended biopsy specimen set is available? The answer depends on the number of specimens available.

FIGURE 8–40. Algorithm for the evaluation of atrophy proposed at the Atrophy 2000 Consensus Workshop. The semi-quantitative scale of atrophy and metaplasia in each biopsy specimen is recommended only for use in clinical study protocols. However, the concept that atrophy and metaplasia represent an expression of a single phenomenon is helpful in the distinction between atrophic and nonatrophic gastritis.

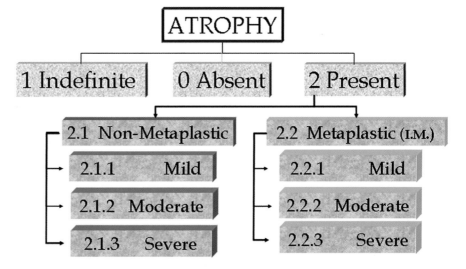

A four-specimen set (two from the antrum and two from the corpus) is suboptimal but acceptable. A three-specimen set (one from the antrum and two from the corpus) is marginally useful for diagnosing *H. pylori* gastritis and for evaluating atrophy in the corpus, where it is more likely to be clinically significant. Although examination of one- or two-specimen sets may still be enhanced by use of the updated Sydney System's step-by-step approach, no attempt should be made to reach topographic conclusions.

It should be noted that even a full five-biopsy protocol provides no more than a glimpse of the morphology of the entire stomach. Although biopsy specimens from the antrum and corpus are adequate for establishing both the *H. pylori* status and the background level and distribution of gastritis, additional biopsy specimens are required from any lesions that may occur for mapping the distribution and extent of intestinal metaplasia and dysplasia. Furthermore, the patchy nature of many pathologic processes, particularly atrophy and metaplasia, makes it difficult to determine their true extent with a sampling procedure that represents less than one thousandth of the gastric mucosal surface area. Although it is generally true that maximal degrees of atrophy and intestinal metaplasia are found in the region of the incisura angularis,[59] and that this is the site most likely to harbor dysplasia,[209-212] it is also true that more extensive biopsy protocols have some advantages over less extensive ones in detecting these types of lesions.[213]

COMMUNICATION BETWEEN THE ENDOSCOPIST AND THE PATHOLOGIST

An accurate clinicopathologic correlation (as in most other conditions) is ultimately achievable only when the pathologist is aware of the locations of biopsy specimens and of relevant endoscopic and clinical information. Thus, endoscopists should as a rule furnish pathologists with narrative and diagrammatic summaries of the patient's findings. In many centers, a set of endoscopic photographs that contain indicators of the locations of biopsy samples, as well as other key features, is routinely forwarded to the pathologist. Conscientious pathologists should initiate and stimulate the development of these and other communication channels that will ultimately benefit the patient, the clinician, and the pathologist alike.

References

1. Schindler R: Gastritis. London, William Heinmann (Medical Books), 1947.
2. Broussais FJ: Histoire des phlegmasies ou inflammations croniques. In Gabor, Crochard (eds): Nouvelles Observations de Clinique et d'Anatomie Pathologique, vol 2, 2nd ed. Paris, 1816.
3. Figura N, Oderda G: Reflections on the first description of the presence of *Helicobacter* species in the stomach of mammals. Helicobacter 1:4-5, 1996.
4. Kidd M, Modlin IM: A century of *Helicobacter pylori*: Paradigms lost-paradigms regained. Digestion 59:1-15, 1998.
5. Faber K: Gastritis and Its Consequences. London, Humphrey Milford, Oxford University Press, 1935.
6. Marshall BJ, Warren JR: Unidentified curved bacilli in the stomach of patients with gastritis and peptic ulceration. Lancet 1:1311-1315, 1984.
7. Genta RM: A year in the life of the gastric mucosa. Gastroenterology 119:252-254, 2000.
8. Tytgat GN: The Sydney System: Endoscopic division. Endoscopic appearances in gastritis/duodenitis. J Gastroenterol Hepatol 6:223-234, 1991.
9. Price AB: The Sydney System: Histological division. J Gastroenterol Hepatol 6:209-222, 1991.
10. Dixon MF, Genta RM, Yardley JH, et al: Classification and grading of gastritis. The updated Sydney System. International Workshop on the Histopathology of Gastritis, Houston 1994. Am J Surg Pathol 20:1161-1181, 1996.
11. Genta RM, Rugge M: Gastric precancerous lesions: Heading for an international consensus. Gut 45(suppl 1):I5-I8, 1999.
12. Ruiz C: Morphometry of atrophy (Orlando 2000). Histopathology 99:1-10, 2001.
13. El Zimaity HM, Genta RM, Graham DY: Histological features do not define NSAID-induced gastritis. Hum Pathol 27:1348-1354, 1996.
14. Barkin J: The relation between *Helicobacter pylori* and non-steroidal anti-inflammatory drugs. Am J Med105:22S-27S, 1998.
15. Atherton JC, Wight NJ: *H. pylori* and risk of ulcer bleeding among users of NSAIDS. Gastroenterology 118:451-452, 2000.
16. Dixon MF: The components of gastritis: Histology and pathogenesis. In Graham DY, Genta RM, Dixon MF (eds): Gastritis. Philadelphia, Lippincott Williams & Wilkins, 1999, pp 51-66.
17. Dixon MF: Pathophysiology of *Helicobacter pylori* infection. Scand J Gastroenterol Suppl 201:7-10, 1994.
18. Crabtree JE, Farmery SM, Lindley IJ, et al: CagA/cytotoxic strains of *Helicobacter pylori* and interleukin-8 in gastric epithelial cell lines. J Clin Pathol 47:945-950, 1994.
19. Shimoyama T, Crabtree JE: Bacterial factors and immune pathogenesis in *Helicobacter pylori* infection. Gut 43(suppl 1):S2-S5, 1998.
20. Dunn BE: Pathogenic mechanisms of *Helicobacter pylori*. Gastroenterol Clin North Am 22:43-57, 1993.
21. Megraud F: Toxic factors of *Helicobacter pylori*. Eur J Gastroenterol Hepatol 6(suppl 1):S5-S10, 1994.
22. Sommi P, Ricci V, Fiocca R, et al: Significance of ammonia in the genesis of gastric epithelial lesions induced by *Helicobacter pylori*: An in vitro study with different bacterial strains and urea concentrations. Digestion 57:299-304, 1996.
23. Denizot Y, Sobhani I, Rambaud JC, et al: Paf-acether synthesis by *Helicobacter pylori*. Gut 31:1242-1245, 1990.
24. Sobala GM, King RF, Axon AT, et al: Reflux gastritis in the intact stomach. J Clin Pathol 43:303-306, 1990.
25. Hawkey CJ: Nonsteroidal anti-inflammatory drug gastropathy. Gastroenterology 119:521-535, 2000.
26. Hawkey CJ: Management of gastroduodenal ulcers caused by nonsteroidal anti-inflammatory drugs. Baillieres Best Pract Res Clin Gastroenterol 14:173-192, 2000.
27. Richardson P, Hawkey CJ, Stack WA: Proton pump inhibitors. Pharmacology and rationale for use in gastrointestinal disorders. Drugs 56:307-335, 1998.
28. Wight NJ, Gottesdiener K, Garlick NM, et al: Rofecoxib, a COX-2 inhibitor, does not inhibit human gastric mucosal prostaglandin production. Gastroenterology 120:867-873, 2001.
29. Genta RM. *Helicobacter pylori*, inflammation, mucosal damage, and apoptosis: Pathogenesis and definition of gastric atrophy. Gastroenterology 113:S51-S55, 1997.
30. Quinn CM, Bjarnason I, Price AB: Gastritis in patients on nonsteroidal anti-inflammatory drugs. Histopathology 23:341-348, 1993.
31. Dixon MF, O'Connor HJ, Axon AT, et al: Reflux gastritis: Distinct histopathological entity? J Clin Pathol 39:524-530, 1986.
32. Plebani M, Basso D, Vianello F, et al: *Helicobacter pylori* activates gastric mucosal mast cells. Dig Dis Sci 39:1592-1593, 1994.
33. Nakajima S, Krishnan B, Ota H, et al: Mast cell involvement in gastritis with or without *Helicobacter pylori* infection. Gastroenterology 113:746-754, 1997.

34. Greenstein DB, Wilcox CM, Schwartz DA: Gastric syphilis. Report of seven cases and review of the literature. J Clin Gastroenterol 18:4-9, 1994.

35. Oberhuber G, Puspok A, Oesterreicher C, et al: Focally enhanced gastritis: A frequent type of gastritis in patients with Crohn's disease. Gastroenterology 112:698-706, 1997.

36. Genta RM, Lew GM, Graham DY: Changes in the gastric mucosa following eradication of *Helicobacter pylori*. Mod Pathol 6:281-289, 1993.

37. Genta RM, Graham DY: Comparison of biopsy sites for the histopathologic diagnosis of *Helicobacter pylori*: A topographic study of *H. pylori* density and distribution. Gastrointest Endosc 40:342-345, 1994.

38. Mai UE, Perez-Perez GI, Allen JB, et al: Surface proteins from *Helicobacter pylori* exhibit chemotactic activity for human leukocytes and are present in gastric mucosa. J Exp Med 175:517-525, 1992.

39. Rautelin H, Blomberg B, Fredlund H, et al: Incidence of *Helicobacter pylori* strains activating neutrophils in patients with peptic ulcer disease. Gut 34:599-603, 1993.

40. Crabtree JE, Lindley IJ: Mucosal interleukin-8 and *Helicobacter pylori*-associated gastroduodenal disease. Eur J Gastroenterol Hepatol 6(suppl 1):S33-S38, 1994.

41. Hida N, Shimoyama T Jr, Neville P, et al: Increased expression of IL-10 and IL-12 (p40) mRNA in *Helicobacter pylori* infected gastric mucosa: Relation to bacterial cag status and peptic ulceration. J Clin Pathol52:658-664, 1999.

42. Wehut WD, Olmsted WW, Neiman HL, et al: Eosinophilic gastritis. Radiologic-pathologic correlation (RPC) from the Armed Forces Institute of Pathology (AFIP). Radiology 120:85-89, 1976.

43. Milman PJ, Sidhu GS: Case report: Eosinophilic gastritis simulating a neoplasm. Am J Med Sci276:227-230, 1978.

44. Ikeda K, Kumashiro R, Kifune T: Nine cases of acute gastric anisakiasis. Gastrointest Endosc 35:304-308, 1989.

45. Whitney AE, Guarner J, Hutwagner L, et al: *Helicobacter pylori* gastritis in children and adults: Comparative histopathologic study. Ann Diagn Pathol 4:279-285, 2000.

46. Genta RM, Gurer IE, Graham DY: Geographical pathology of *Helicobacter pylori* infection: Is there more than one gastritis? Ann Med 27:595-599, 1999.

47. Haot J, Jouret A, Mainguet P: Lymphocytic gastritis. In Graham DY, Genta RM, Dixon MF (eds): Gastritis. Philadelphia, Lippincott Williams & Wilkins, 1999, pp 109-118.

48. Capella C, Fiocca R, Cornaggia M, et al: Autoimmune gastritis. In Graham DY, Genta RM, Dixon MF (eds): Gastritis. Philadelphia, Lippincott Williams & Wilkins, 1999, pp 79-96.

49. Genta RM, Hamner HW, Graham DY: Gastric lymphoid follicles in *Helicobacter pylori* infection: Frequency, distribution, and response to triple therapy. Hum Pathol 24:577-583, 1993.

50. Dohil R, Hassall E, Jevon G, et al: Gastritis and gastropathy of childhood. J Pediatr Gastroenterol Nutr 29:378-394, 1999.

51. Isaacson PG: Gastric lymphoma and *Helicobacter pylori*. N Engl J Med 330:1310-1311, 1994.

52. Isaacson PG: Gastric MALT lymphoma: From concept to cure. Ann Oncol 10:637-645, 1999.

53. Isaacson PG: Gastrointestinal lymphoma. Hum Pathol 25:1020-1029, 1994.

54. Dixon MF: Prospects for intervention in gastric carcinogenesis: Reversibility of gastric atrophy and intestinal metaplasia. Gut 49:2-4, 2001.

55. Genta RM: Review article: Gastric atrophy and atrophic gastritis—nebulous concepts in search of a definition. Aliment Pharmacol Ther 12(suppl 1):17-23, 1998.

56. Jass JR, Filipe MI: Sulphomucins and precancerous lesions of the human stomach. Histopathology 4:271-279, 1980.

57. Ectors N, Dixon MF: The prognostic value of sulphomucin positive intestinal metaplasia in the development of gastric cancer. Histopathology 10:1271-1277, 1986.

58. Tosi P, Filipe MI, Luzi P, et al: Gastric intestinal metaplasia type III cases are classified as low-grade dysplasia on the basis of morphometry. J Pathol 169:73-78, 1993.

59. Cassaro M, Rugge M, Gutierrez O, et al: Topographic patterns of intestinal metaplasia and gastric cancer. Am J Gastroenterol 95:1431-1438, 2000.

60. Stemmermann GN: Intestinal metaplasia of the stomach. A status report. Cancer 74:556-564, 1994.

61. Sugimura T, Sugano H, Terada M, et al: First International Workshop of the Princess Takamatsu Cancer Research Fund: Intestinal metaplasia and gastric cancer. Mol Carcinog 11:1-7, 1994.

62. Dewar EP, Dixon MF, Johnston D: Bile reflux and degree of gastritis after highly selective vagotomy, truncal vagotomy, and partial gastrectomy for duodenal ulcer. World J Surg 7:743-750, 1983.

63. Solcia E, Vassallo G, Sampietro R: Endocrine cells in the antropyloric mucosa of the stomach. Z Zellforsch Mikrosk Anat 81:474-486, 1967.

64. Solcia E, Capella C, Vassallo G, et al: Endocrine cells of the gastric mucosa. Int Rev Cytol 42:223-286, 1975.

65. Solcia E, Fiocca R, Villani L, et al: Morphology and pathogenesis of endocrine hyperplasias, precarcinoid lesions, and carcinoids arising in chronic atrophic gastritis. Scand J Gastroenterol Suppl 180:146-159, 1991.

66. Solcia E, Bordi C, Creutzfeldt W, et al: Histopathological classification of nonantral gastric endocrine growths in man. Digestion 41:185-200, 1988.

67. Lamberts R, Creutzfeldt W, Struber HG, et al: Long-term omeprazole therapy in peptic ulcer disease: Gastrin, endocrine cell growth, and gastritis [see comments]. Gastroenterology 104:1356-1370, 1993.

68. Bordi C, D'Adda T, Azzoni C, et al: Neuroendocrine proliferation in the gastric mucosa: Biological behaviour and management. Verh Dtsch Ges Pathol 81:103-110, 1997.

69. Cats A, Schenk BE, Bloemena E, et al: Parietal cell protrusions and fundic gland cysts during omeprazole maintenance treatment. Hum Pathol 31:684-690, 2000.

70. Krishnamurthy S, Dayal Y: Parietal cell protrusions in gastric ulcer disease. Hum Pathol 28:1126-1130, 1997.

71. Lubensky IA, Schiffmann R, Goldin E, et al: Lysosomal inclusions in gastric parietal cells in mucolipidosis type IV: A novel cause of achlorhydria and hypergastrinemia. Am J Surg Pathol 23:1527-1531, 1999.

72. Stolte M, Bethke B, Seifert E, et al: Observation of gastric glandular cysts in the corpus mucosa of the stomach under omeprazole treatment. Z Gastroenterol 33:146-149, 1995.

73. Marshall BJ: The *Campylobacter pylori* story. Scand J Gastroenterol Suppl 146:58-66, 1988.

74. Caletti G, Fusaroli P, Tucci A, et al: Severe acute gastritis associated with *Helicobacter pylori* infection. Dig Liver Dis 32:34-38, 2000.

75. Sobala GM, Crabtree JE, Dixon MF, et al: Acute *Helicobacter pylori* infection: Clinical features, local and systemic immune response, gastric mucosal histology, and gastric juice ascorbic acid concentrations. Gut 32:1415-1418, 1991.

76. Sugiyama T, Naka H, Yachi A, et al: Direct evidence by DNA fingerprinting that endoscopic cross-infection of *Helicobacter pylori* is a cause of postendoscopic acute gastritis. J Clin Microbiol 38:2381-2382, 2000.

77. Kosunen TU, Aromaa A, Knekt P, et al: *Helicobacter* antibodies in 1973 and 1994 in the adult population of Vammala, Finland. Epidemiol Infect 119:29-34, 1997.

78. Marshall BJ, Armstrong JA, McGechie DB, et al: Attempt to fulfil Koch's postulates for pyloric *Campylobacter*. Med J Aust 142:436-439, 1985.

79. Sonnenberg A, Bartmess J, Kern L, et al: [Achlorhydria in acute gastritis.] Z Gastroenterol 17:776-777, 1979.

80. Thompson CE, Ashurst PM, Butler TJ: Survey of haemorrhagic erosive gastritis. Br Med J 3:283-285, 1968.

81. Talley NJ, Stanghellini V, Heading RC, et al: Functional gastroduodenal disorders. Gut 45(suppl 2):II37-II42, 1999.

82. Malfertheiner P: The Maastricht recommendations and their impact on general practice. Eur J Gastroenterol Hepatol 11(suppl 2):S63-S67, 1999.

83. Talley NJ, Vakil N, Ballard ED, et al: Absence of benefit of eradicating *Helicobacter pylori* in patients with nonulcer dyspepsia. N Engl J Med 341:1106-1111, 1999.

84. Moayyedi P, Forman D, Braunholtz D, et al: The proportion of upper gastrointestinal symptoms in the community associated with *Helicobacter pylori*, lifestyle factors, and nonsteroidal anti-inflammatory drugs. Leeds HELP Study Group. Am J Gastroenterol 95:1448-1455, 2000.

85. Danesh J: *Helicobacter pylori* infection and gastric cancer: Systematic review of the epidemiological studies. Aliment Pharmacol Ther 13:851-856, 1999.

86. Fukao A, Hisamichi S, Ohsato N, et al: Correlation between the prevalence of gastritis and gastric cancer in Japan. Cancer Causes Control 4:17-20, 1993.

87. Correa P, Haenszel W, Tannenbaum S: Epidemiology of gastric carcinoma: Review and future prospects. Natl Cancer Inst Monogr 62:129-134, 1982.

88. Chang-Claude J, Raedsch R, Waldherr R, et al: Prevalence of *Helicobacter pylori* infection and gastritis among young adults in China. Eur J Cancer Prev 4:73-79, 1995.

89. Perez-Perez GI, Bhat N, Gaensbauer J, et al: Country-specific constancy by age in cagA+ proportion of *Helicobacter pylori* infections. Int J Cancer 72:453-456, 1997.

90. Wong BC, Lam SK, Ching CK, et al: Differential *Helicobacter pylori* infection rates in two contrasting gastric cancer risk regions of South China. China Gastric Cancer Study Group. J Gastroenterol Hepatol 14:120-125, 1999.

91. Shimizu T, Akamatsu T, Ota H, et al: Immunohistochemical detection of *Helicobacter pylori* in the surface mucous gel layer and its clinicopathological significance. Helicobacter 1:197-206, 1996.

92. Genta RM, Huberman RM, Graham DY: The gastric cardia in *Helicobacter pylori* infection. Hum Pathol 25:915-919, 1994.

93. Genta RM, Gurer IE, Graham DY, et al: Adherence of *Helicobacter pylori* to areas of incomplete intestinal metaplasia in the gastric mucosa. Gastroenterology 111:1206-1211, 1996.

94. Eidt S, Stolte M: Prevalence of lymphoid follicles and aggregates in *Helicobacter pylori* gastritis in antral and body mucosa. J Clin Pathol 46:832-835, 1993.

95. Wyatt JI, Rathbone BJ: Immune response of the gastric mucosa to *Campylobacter pylori*. Scand J Gastroenterol Suppl 142:44-49, 1988.

96. Rotimi O, Cairns A, Gray S, et al: Histological identification of *Helicobacter pylori*: Comparison of staining methods. J Clin Pathol 53:756-759, 2000.

97. Genta RM, Robason GO, Graham DY: Simultaneous visualization of *Helicobacter pylori* and gastric morphology: A new stain. Hum Pathol 25:221-226, 1994.

98. Cartun RW, Kryzmowski GA, Pedersen CA, et al: Immunocytochemical identification of *Helicobacter pylori* in formalin-fixed gastric biopsies. Mod Pathol 4:498-502, 1991.

99. Jonkers D, Stobberingh E, DeBruine A, et al: Evaluation of immunohistochemistry for the detection of *Helicobacter pylori* in gastric mucosal biopsies. J Infect 35:149-154, 1997.

100. Heilmann KL, Borchard F: Gastritis due to spiral shaped bacteria other than *Helicobacter pylori*: Clinical, histological, and ultrastructural findings. Gut 32:137-140, 1991.

101. Lopez JA, Tamayo MC, Mejia GI, et al: *Gastrospirillum hominis* in a child with chronic gastritis. Pediatr Infect Dis J 12:701-702, 1993.

102. Debongnie JC: *Gastrospirillum hominis* prevalence. Dig Dis Sci 39:1618, 1994.

103. Svec A, Kordas P, Pavlis Z, et al: High prevalence of *Helicobacter heilmannii*-associated gastritis in a small, predominantly rural area: Further evidence in support of a zoonosis? Scand J Gastroenterol 35:925-928, 2000.

104. Go MF, Smoot DT: *Helicobacter pylori*, gastric MALT lymphoma, and adenocarcinoma of the stomach. Semin Gastrointest Dis 11:134-141, 2000.

105. Akinyanju OO, Okany CC: Pernicious anaemia in Africans. Clin Lab Haematol 14:33-40, 1992.

106. Harakati MS: Pernicious anemia in Arabs. Blood Cells Mol Dis 22:98-103, 1996.

107. Jacobson DL, Gange SJ, Rose NR, et al: Epidemiology and estimated population burden of selected autoimmune diseases in the United States. Clin Immunol Immunopathol 84:223-243, 1997.

108. Varis K, Ihamaki T, Harkonen M, et al: Gastric morphology, function, and immunology in first-degree relatives of probands with pernicious anemia and controls. Scand J Gastroenterol 14:129-139, 1979.

109. Kekki M, Samloff IM, Varis K, et al: Serum pepsinogen I and serum gastrin in the screening of severe atrophic corpus gastritis. Scand J Gastroenterol Suppl 186:109-116, 1991.

110. Skikne BS, Lynch SR, Cook JD: Role of gastric acid in food iron absorption. Gastroenterology 81:1068-1071, 1981.

111. Strickland RG, Mackay IR: Letter: Natural history of atrophic gastritis. Lancet 2:777-778, 1974.

112. Abraham SC, Singh VK, Yardley JH, et al: Hyperplastic polyps of the stomach: Associations with histologic patterns of gastritis and gastric atrophy. Am J Surg Pathol 25:500-507, 2001.

113. Solcia E, Rindi G, Fiocca R, et al: Distinct patterns of chronic gastritis associated with carcinoid and cancer and their role in tumorigenesis. Yale J Biol Med 65:793-804, 1992.

114. Franceschi F, Genta RM: Autoimmune gastritis and antigenic mimicking. In Hunt RH, Tytgat GN (eds): *Helicobacter pylori*—Basic Mechanisms to Clinical Cure 2000. Dordrecht, Kluwer Academic Publishers, 2000, pp 289-294.

115. Negrini R, Savio A, Poiesi C, et al: Antigenic mimicry between *Helicobacter pylori* and gastric mucosa in the pathogenesis of body atrophic gastritis. Gastroenterology 111:655-665, 1996.

116. Claeys D, Faller G, Appelmelk BJ, et al: The gastric H+,K+-ATPase is a major autoantigen in chronic *Helicobacter pylori* gastritis with body mucosa atrophy. Gastroenterology 115:340-347, 1998.

117. Appelmelk BJ, Negrini R, Moran AP, et al: Molecular mimicry between *Helicobacter pylori* and the host. Trends Microbiol 5:70-73, 1997.

118. Appelmelk BJ, Martino MC, Veenhof E, et al: Phase variation in H type I and Lewis a epitopes of *Helicobacter pylori* lipopolysaccharide. Infect Immun 68:5928-5932, 2000.

119. Krishnamurthy S, Dayal Y: Parietal cell protrusions in gastric ulcer disease [see comments]. Hum Pathol 28:1126-1130, 1997.

120. Stolte M, Bethke B, Ruhl G, et al: Omeprazole-induced pseudo-hypertrophy of gastric parietal cells. Z Gastroenterol 30:134-138, 1992.

121. Haot J, Hamichi L, Wallez L, et al: Lymphocytic gastritis: A newly described entity: A retrospective endoscopic and histological study. Gut 29:1258-1264, 1988.

122. Haot J, Berger F, Andre C, et al: Lymphocytic gastritis versus varioliform gastritis. A historical series revisited. J Pathol 158:19-22, 1989.

123. Haot J, Jouret A, Willette M, et al: Lymphocytic gastritis—prospective study of its relationship with varioliform gastritis. Gut 31:282-285, 1990.

124. Dixon MF, Wyatt JI, Burke DA, et al: Lymphocytic gastritis—relationship to *Campylobacter pylori* infection. J Pathol 154:125-132, 1988.

125. Hayat M, Arora DS, Wyatt JI, et al: The pattern of involvement of the gastric mucosa in lymphocytic gastritis is predictive of the presence of duodenal pathology. J Clin Pathol 52:815-819, 1999.

126. Hayat M, Arora DS, Dixon MF, et al: Effects of *Helicobacter pylori* eradication on the natural history of lymphocytic gastritis. Gut 45:495-498, 1999.

127. Karttunen T, Niemela S: Lymphocytic gastritis and coeliac disease. J Clin Pathol 43:436-437, 1990.

128. Wu TT, Hamilton SR: Lymphocytic gastritis: Association with etiology and topology. Am J Surg Pathol 23:153-158, 1999.

129. Haot J, Weynand B, Jouret-Mourin A: Chronic lymphocytic gastritis. Gut 31:840, 1990.

130. Wolfsen HC, Carpenter HA, Talley NJ: Menetrier's disease: A form of hypertrophic gastropathy or gastritis? Gastroenterology 104:1310-1319, 1993.

131. Lynch DA, Dixon MF, Axon AT: Diagnostic criteria in lymphocytic gastritis. Gastroenterology 112:1426-1427, 1997.

132. Misra RC, Agarwal SK, Prakash P, et al: Gastric tuberculosis. Endoscopy 14:235-237, 1982.

133. Tromba JL, Inglese R, Rieders B, et al: Primary gastric tuberculosis presenting as pyloric outlet obstruction. Am J Gastroenterol 86:1820-1822, 1991.

134. Hartmann F. [Diseases resulting from a failure of self-recognition and self-induced decay of tissues.] Klin Wochenschr 47:581-593, 1969.

135. Sanguino JC, Rodrigues B, Baptista A, et al: Focal lesion of African histoplasmosis presenting as a malignant gastric ulcer. Hepato-gastroenterology 43:771-775, 1996.

136. Ectors NL, Dixon MF, Geboes KJ, et al: Granulomatous gastritis: A morphological and diagnostic approach. Histopathology 23:55-61, 1993.

137. Shapiro JL, Goldblum JR, Petras RE: A clinicopathologic study of 42 patients with granulomatous gastritis. Is there really an "idiopathic" granulomatous gastritis? Am J Surg Pathol 20:462-470, 1996.

138. Bouree P, Paugam A, Petithory JC: Anisakidosis: Report of 25 cases and review of the literature. Comp Immunol Microbiol Infect Dis 18:75-84, 1995.

139. Kato T, Saito Y, Niwa M, et al: *Helicobacter pylori* infection in gastric carcinoma. Eur J Gastroenterol Hepatol 6(suppl 1):S93-S96, 1994.
140. Leach IH, Maclennan KA: Gastric lymphoma associated with mucosal and nodal granulomas: A new differential diagnosis in granulomatous gastritis. Histopathology 17:87-89, 1990.
141. Talseth T: Isolated gastric involvement in Crohn's disease. Report of a case simulating scirrhus carcinoma. Acta Chir Scand 142:611-613, 1976.
142. Tukiainen H, Vaara J, Syrjanen K, et al: Granulomatous gastritis as a diagnostic problem between sarcoidosis and other granulomatous disorders. Sarcoidosis 5:66-67, 1988.
143. Fireman Z, Sternberg A, Yarchovsky Y, et al: Multiple antral ulcers in gastric sarcoid. J Clin Gastroenterol 24:97-99, 1997.
144. Halme L, Karkkainen P, Rautelin H, et al: High frequency of *Helicobacter* negative gastritis in patients with Crohn's disease. Gut 38:379-383, 1996.
145. Oberhuber G, Hirsch M, Stolte M: High incidence of upper gastrointestinal tract involvement in Crohn's disease. Virchows Arch 432:49-52, 1998.
146. Shapiro JL, Goldblum JR, Petras RE: A clinicopathologic study of 42 patients with granulomatous gastritis. Is there really an "idiopathic" granulomatous gastritis? Am J Surg Pathol 20:462-470, 1996.
147. Laine L, Johnson E, Suchower L, et al: US double-blind, controlled trials of omeprazole and amoxycillin for treatment of *Helicobacter pylori*. Aliment Pharmacol Ther 12:377-382, 1998.
148. Kuipers EJ: *Helicobacter pylori* and the risk and management of associated diseases: Gastritis, ulcer disease, atrophic gastritis and gastric cancer. Aliment Pharmacol Ther 11(suppl 1):71-88, 1997.
149. Dewar P, Dixon MF, Johnston D: Bile reflux and degree of gastritis in patients with gastric ulcer: Before and after operation. J Surg Res 37:277-284, 1984.
150. Dixon MF: Reflux gastritis. Acta Gastroenterol Belg 52:292-296, 1989.
151. Sobala GM, O'Connor HJ, Dewar EP, et al: Bile reflux and intestinal metaplasia in gastric mucosa. J Clin Pathol 46:235-240, 1993.
152. Adson MA, Akwari OE: Management of gastrointestinal dysfunction after gastric surgery. Surg Clin North Am 51:915-926, 1971.
153. Cooperman AM: Postgastrectomy syndromes. Surg Annu 13:139-161, 1981.
154. Ritchie WP Jr: Alkaline reflux gastritis. Late results on a controlled trial of diagnosis and treatment. Ann Surg 203:537-544, 1986.
155. Graham DY, Smith JL: Gastroduodenal complications of chronic NSAID therapy. Am J Gastroenterol 83:1081-1084, 1988.
156. Schoenfeld P, Kimmey MB, Scheiman J, et al: Review article: Nonsteroidal anti-inflammatory drug-associated gastrointestinal complications—guidelines for prevention and treatment. Aliment Pharmacol Ther 13:1273-1285, 1999.
157. Sung J, Russell RI, Nyeomans Chan FK, et al: Non-steroidal anti-inflammatory drug toxicity in the upper gastrointestinal tract. J Gastroenterol Hepatol 15(suppl):G58-G68, 2000.
158. Weilert F, Smith AC, Stokes PL: Therapies for ulcers associated with nonsteroidal antiinflammatory drugs. N Engl J Med 339:349-351, 1998.
159. Everts B, Wahrborg P, Hedner T: COX-2-specific inhibitors—the emergence of a new class of analgesic and anti-inflammatory drugs. Clin Rheumatol 19:331-343, 2000.
160. Berthrong M, Fajardo LF: Radiation injury in surgical pathology. Part II. Alimentary tract. Am J Surg Pathol 5:153-178, 1981.
161. De Sagher LI, Van den HB, Van Houtte P, et al: Endoscopic appearance of irradiated gastric mucosa. Endoscopy 11:163-165, 1979.
162. Roswit B: Complications of radiation therapy: The alimentary tract. Semin Roentgenol 9:51-63, 1974.
163. Cox AG, Cullen JB: Polyps after gastrectomy. Proc R Soc Med 62:1039-1040, 1969.
164. Pickford IR, Craven JL, Hall R, et al: Endoscopic examination of the gastric remnant 31-39 years after subtotal gastrectomy for peptic ulcer. Gut 25:393-397, 1984.
165. Dixon MF: Acute hemorrhagic gastritis. In Graham DY, Genta RM, Dixon MF (eds): Gastritis. Philadelphia, Lippincott Williams & Wilkins, 1999, pp 147-156.
166. Chamberlain CE: Acute hemorrhagic gastritis. Gastroenterol Clin North Am 22:843-873, 1993.
167. Kaufman DW, Kelly JP, Wiholm BE, et al: The risk of acute major upper gastrointestinal bleeding among users of aspirin and ibuprofen at various levels of alcohol consumption. Am J Gastroenterol 94:3189-3196, 1999.
168. Laine L, Weinstein WM: Histology of alcoholic hemorrhagic "gastritis": A prospective evaluation. Gastroenterology 94:1254-1262, 1988.
169. Laine L, Weinstein WM: Subepithelial hemorrhages and erosions of human stomach. Dig Dis Sci 33:490-503, 1988.
170. Gostout CJ, Viggiano TR, Ahlquist DA, et al: The clinical and endoscopic spectrum of the watermelon stomach. J Clin Gastroenterol 15:256-263, 1992.
171. Viggiano TR, Batts KP: Vascular gastropathies. In Graham DY, Genta RM, Dixon MF (eds): Gastritis. Philadelphia, Lippincott Williams & Wilkins, 1999, pp 157-168.
172. Bernstein DE, Phillips RS: Portal hypertensive gastropathy. Gastrointest Endosc Clin N Am 6:697-708, 1996.
173. Jabbari M, Cherry R, Lough JO, et al: Gastric antral vascular ectasia: The watermelon stomach. Gastroenterology 87:1165-1170, 1984.
174. Misra SP, Dwivedi M, Misra V, et al: Endoscopic and histologic appearance of the gastric mucosa in patients with portal hypertension. Gastrointest Endosc 36:575-579, 1990.
175. Lin WJ, Lee FY, Lin HC, et al: Snake skin pattern gastropathy in cirrhotic patients. J Gastroenterol Hepatol 6:145-149, 1991.
176. Spina GP, Arcidiacono R, Bosch J, et al: Gastric endoscopic features in portal hypertension: Final report of a consensus conference, Milan, Italy, September 19, 1992. J Hepatol 21:461-467, 1994.
177. Gilliam JH III, Geisinger KR, Wu WC, et al: Endoscopic biopsy is diagnostic in gastric antral vascular ectasia. The "watermelon stomach." Dig Dis Sci 34:885-888, 1989.
178. Foster PN, Wyatt JI, Bullimore DW, et al: Gastric mucosa in patients with portal hypertension: Prevalence of capillary dilatation and *Campylobacter pylori*. J Clin Pathol 42:919-921, 1989.
179. McCormack TT, Sims J, Eyre-Brook I, et al: Gastric lesions in portal hypertension: Inflammatory gastritis or congestive gastropathy? Gut 26:1226-1232, 1985.
180. Choudhry U, Boyce HW Jr, Coppola D: Proton pump inhibitor-associated gastric polyps: A retrospective analysis of their frequency, and endoscopic, histologic, and ultrastructural characteristics [see comments]. Am J Clin Pathol 110:615-621, 1998.
181. Graham DY, Genta R, Evans DG, et al: *Helicobacter pylori* does not migrate from the antrum to the corpus in response to omeprazole [see comments]. Am J Gastroenterol 91:2120-2124, 1996.
182. Kuipers EJ, Lundell L, Klinkenberg-Knol EC, et al: Atrophic gastritis and *Helicobacter pylori* infection in patients with reflux esophagitis treated with omeprazole or fundoplication. N Engl J Med 334:1018-1022, 1996.
183. Malfertheiner P, Megraud F, O'Morain C, et al: Current European concepts in the management of *Helicobacter pylori* infection—the Maastricht Consensus Report. The European *Helicobacter Pylori* Study Group (EHPSG). Eur J Gastroenterol Hepatol 9:1-2, 1997.
184. Owen DA: Stomach. In Sternberg SS (ed): Histology for Pathologists. New York, Raven Press, 1992, chapter 27, pp 533-545.
185. Kilgore SP, Ormsby AH, Gramlich TL, et al: The gastric cardia: Fact or fiction? Am J Gastroenterol 95:921-924, 2000.
186. Wieczorek TJ, Wang HH, Antonioli DA, et al: Pathologic features of reflux and *Helicobacter pylori*-associated carditis; a comparative study. Am J Surg Pathol (in press).
187. Chandrasoma PT, Lokuhetty DM, Demeester TR, et al: Definition of histopathologic changes in gastroesophageal reflux disease. Am J Surg Pathol 24:344-351, 2000.
188. Oberg S, Peters JH, Demeester TR, et al: Inflammation and specialized intestinal metaplasia of cardiac mucosa is a manifestation of gastroesophageal reflux disease. Ann Surg 226:522-532, 1997.
189. Chandrasoma PT, Der R, Ma Y, et al: Histology of the gastroesophageal junction: An autopsy study. Am J Surg Pathol 24:402-409, 2000.
190. Riddell RH: The biopsy diagnosis of gastroesophageal reflux disease, "carditis," and Barrett's esophagus, and sequelae of therapy. Am J Surg Pathol 20(suppl 1):S31-S50, 1996.
191. Chen YY, Antonioli DA, Spechler SJ, et al: Gastroesophageal reflux disease versus *Helicobacter pylori* infection as the cause of gastric carditis. Mod Pathol 11:950-956, 1998.

192. Goldblum JR: Inflammation and intestinal metaplasia of the gastric cardia: *Helicobacter pylori*, gastroesophageal reflux disease, or both. Dig Dis 18:14-19, 2000.

193. Hackelsberger A, Gunther T, Schultze V, et al: Prevalence and pattern of *Helicobacter pylori* gastritis in the gastric cardia. Am J Gastroenterol 92:2220-2224, 1997.

194. Voutilainen M, Farkkila M, Mecklin JP, et al: Chronic inflammation at the gastroesophageal junction (carditis) appears to be a specific finding related to *Helicobacter pylori* infection and gastroesophageal reflux disease. The Central Finland Endoscopy Study Group. Am J Gastroenterol 94:3175-3180, 1999.

195. Goldblum JR, Vicari JJ, Falk GW, et al: Inflammation and intestinal metaplasia of the gastric cardia: The role of gastroesophageal reflux and *H. pylori* infection. Gastroenterology 114:633-639, 1998.

196. Ormsby AH, Kilgore SP, Goldblum JR, et al: The location and frequency of intestinal metaplasia at the esophagogastric junction in 223 consecutive autopsies: Implications for patient treatment and preventive strategies in Barrett's esophagus. Mod Pathol 13:614-620, 2000.

197. Voutilainen M, Farkkila M, Juhola M, et al: Specialized columnar epithelium of the esophagogastric junction: Prevalence and associations. The Central Finland Endoscopy Study Group. Am J Gastroenterol 94:913-918, 1999.

198. Odze RD: Cytokeratin 7/20 immunostaining: Barrett's oesophagus or gastric intestinal metaplasia. Lancet 359:1711-1713, 2000.

199. Glickman JN, Wang HH, Das KM, et al: Phenotype of Barrett's esophagus and intestinal metaplasia of the distal esophagus and gastroesophageal junction. An immunohistochemical study of Cytokeratins 7 and 20, Das-1 and 45MI. Am J Surg Pathol 25:87-94, 2001.

200. Morales TG, Camargo E, Bhattacharyya A, et al: Long-term follow-up of intestinal metaplasia of the gastric cardia. Am J Gastroenterol 95:1677-1680, 2000.

201. Spechler SJ: The role of gastric carditis in metaplasia and neoplasia at the gastroesophageal junction. Gastroenterology 117:218-228, 1999.

202. Ormsby AH, Goldblum JR, Rice TW, et al: Cytokeratin subsets can reliably distinguish Barrett's esophagus from intestinal metaplasia of the stomach. Hum Pathol 30:288-294, 1999.

203. Glickman JN, Chen YY, Wang HH, et al: Phenotypic characteristics of a distinctive multilayered epithelium suggests that it is a precursor in the development of Barrett's esophagus. Am J Surg Pathol 25:569-578, 2001.

204. Richter JE: Intestinal metaplasia and the squamocolumnar junction: What does it all mean? Gut 42:604-605, 1998.

205. Chen YY, Wang HH, Antonioli DA, et al: Significance of acid-mucin-positive nongoblet columnar cells in the distal esophagus and gastroesophageal junction. Hum Pathol 30:1488-1495, 1999.

206. Lembo T, Ippoliti AF, Ramers C, et al: Inflammation of the gastro-oesophageal junction (carditis) in patients with symptomatic gastro-oesophageal reflux disease: A prospective study. Gut 45:484-488, 1999.

207. Offner FA, Lewin KJ, Weinstein WM: Metaplastic columnar cells in Barrett's esophagus: A common and neglected cell type. Hum Pathol 27:885-889, 1996.

208. Cassaro M, Di Mario F, Leandro G, et al: The dark side of the gastric biopsy. Hum Pathol 30:741-744, 1999.

209. Correa P: Chronic gastritis: A clinico-pathological classification. Am J Gastroenterol 83:504-509, 1988.

210. Correa P, Haenszel W, Cuello C, et al: Gastric precancerous process in a high risk population: Cohort follow-up. Cancer Res 50:4737-4740, 1990.

211. Antonioli DA: Precursors of gastric carcinoma: A critical review with a brief description of early (curable) gastric cancer. Hum Pathol 25:994-1005, 1994.

212. Rugge M, Farinati F, Baffa R, et al: Gastric epithelial dysplasia in the natural history of gastric cancer: A multicenter prospective follow-up study. Interdisciplinary Group on Gastric Epithelial Dysplasia. Gastroenterology 107:1288-1296, 1994.

213. El Zimaity HM, Graham DY: Evaluation of gastric mucosal biopsy site and number for identification of *Helicobacter pylori* or intestinal metaplasia: Role of the Sydney System. Hum Pathol 30:72-77, 1999.

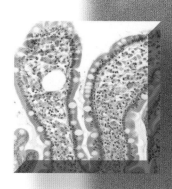

CHAPTER 9

Inflammatory Disorders of the Small Intestine

MARIE E. ROBERT

■ Congenital Anomalies Associated With Inflammation

Numerous developmental abnormalities may involve the small intestine. Some of these include atresia, stenosis, abnormal fixation and malrotation, duplications, cysts, and fistulas. Several medical diseases, such as cystic fibrosis, also affect the small intestine. Some of the more common disorders that may be associated with inflammation are described here.

MECKEL'S DIVERTICULUM

Meckel's diverticulum is the most common congenital abnormality of the gastrointestinal tract, occurring in 1% to 3% of the population.[1-3] It results from persistence of the proximal portion of the vitelline (or omphalomesenteric) duct, which normally undergoes obliteration during the fifth to seventh weeks of embryogenesis. The vitelline duct attaches the yolk sac to the primitive gastrointestinal tract until the time at which the placenta replaces the yolk sac as the primary source of nutrition. Persistence of the intestinal end of the duct results in a diverticulum, which is located almost invariably on the antimesenteric aspect of the ileum, within 1 meter of the ileocecal valve.

The clinical importance of Meckel's diverticulum lies in its association with symptomatic complications, the

most common of which is gastrointestinal hemorrhage.[3] It is estimated that the total lifetime complication rate of Meckel's diverticulum is only 4%. However, more than 40% of complications occur in children younger than age 10.[2] Bleeding accounts for 25% to 50% of complications and is usually due to ileal or diverticular ulceration near a focus of heterotopic gastric oxyntic mucosa within the diverticulum.[2-4] Ulcers are believed to be caused by acid secretion from the oxyntic glands.

Other complications include obstruction (25%), diverticulitis (20%), calculi, and rarely, neoplasms. Obstruction is due either to ileoileal or to ileocolic intussusception. In these instances, the partially inverted diverticulum serves as the leading edge of the intussusception. Volvulus around a diverticulum may also occur rarely.[5] Tumors are a rare but well-documented complication of Meckel's diverticulum, with a reported overall incidence of 0.5% to 4.9%.[2,3] A variety of benign and malignant tumors have been reported, including carcinoid tumor, adenocarcinoma, leiomyoma, leiomyosarcoma, lymphoma, and melanoma.[6-11]

Pathologic Features

Meckel's diverticula are typically present on the antimesenteric border of the ileum (Fig. 9-1). The external shape can vary from an elongated tubular structure to a sacculated outpouching. The site of attachment to the ileum may be narrow (less than 1 cm) or up to 3 cm.[2,3]

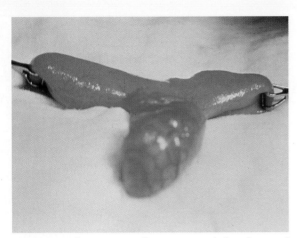

FIGURE 9–1. This image shows a Meckel's diverticulum extending from the antimesenteric border of the ileum.

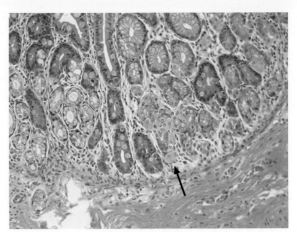

FIGURE 9–2. Meckel's diverticulum. This image shows a focus of heterotopic gastric mucosa consisting of oxyntic and mucinous glands *(arrow)*.

As is the case for all "true" diverticula, all layers of the bowel wall are present in the outpouching.

Microscopically, up to 50% of diverticula contain heterotopic epithelium. Of these, a majority contain gastric oxyntic mucosa (64%), although pancreatic metaplasia is present in 4% to 16%, and "colonic" mucosa in 6% of cases (Fig. 9-2).[12,13] Gastric metaplasia can be recognized grossly as thickened, heaped-up regions of mucosa.[2,3] In areas of gastric metaplasia, "gastritis" and *Helicobacter pylori* organisms may be detected.[14,15]

NON-MECKEL'S DIVERTICULOSIS OF THE SMALL INTESTINE

Diverticulosis of the small intestine is exceedingly rare. The vast majority are acquired and consist of outpouchings of mucosa and muscularis mucosae in areas of muscle weakness, such as the site of perforation of the muscle by vessels.[16-18] The duodenum is the most common site of diverticulosis, with an incidence of 1.7% in radiologic studies.[17] Duodenal diverticula are usually an incidental finding; they frequently occur in the second portion of the duodenum near the ampulla of Vater.[17] Jejunal diverticula are more likely to be multiple, forming numerous sacculated, thin outpouchings on the mesenteric aspect of the bowel wall (Fig. 9-3).[16] The ileum has the lowest incidence of acquired diverticula in the small intestine. Complications are rare and include perforation, hemorrhage, diverticulitis, obstruction, pseudo-obstruction (secondary to a background of visceral myopathy), bacterial overgrowth, and steatorrhea.[16-18]

MECONIUM ILEUS

Approximately 15% of infants with cystic fibrosis develop intestinal obstruction due to accumulation of meconium in the terminal ileum.[19-21] Ileal resections

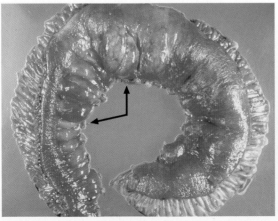

A

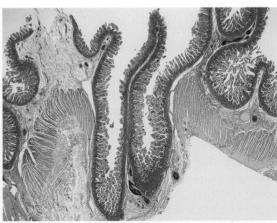

B

FIGURE 9–3. Jejunal diverticulosis. **A,** The serosal surface of this specimen reveals numerous saccular outpouchings on the mesenteric aspect of the intestine *(arrows)*. **B,** Jejunal diverticulosis showing pseudodiverticuli, consisting of mucosa and muscularis mucosae, invaginating through the muscularis propria.

may show marked distention as a result of accumulation of thick plugs of tenacious, brown, mucoid material. Histologic sections usually reveal only minimal changes in mucosal architecture, and variable but mild inflammation. However, a thick layer of periodic acid–Schiff (PAS)-positive mucin can be demonstrated overlying the microvillous brush border and filling crypt lumina (Fig. 9-4). Goblet cells are distended and may be increased in number. The diagnosis is confirmed by a sweat test and/or by genetic phenotyping.[22,23]

Older children and young adults with cystic fibrosis may also become obstructed with secretions by a "meconium ileus equivalent" condition.[20,24] Duodenal biopsies obtained from older patients may reveal distended goblet cells, prominent Brunner's glands, and a prominent layer of mucin overlying surface enterocytes and within crypt lumina.

Ischemic Disorders of the Small Intestine

The intestines are supported by a rich, anastomosing network of blood vessels that originate from three main vessels—the celiac artery, the superior mesenteric artery (SMA), and the inferior mesenteric artery.[25] The small intestine derives its blood supply almost exclusively from the SMA and its branches, although the first portion of the duodenum is also frequently supplied by a branch of the hepatic artery. Because of the extensive network of communicating vessels, vascular insufficiency of the small intestine does not usually occur until there has been a severe compromise in blood flow.

The injury in intestinal ischemia occurs via two mechanisms. The first is the deprivation of oxygen that is needed for normal cellular metabolism.[26] The second is reperfusion injury that occurs when blood flow is reestablished to a previously anoxic region.[27] This process results in the generation of superoxide radicals that increase the permeability of capillaries and other cell membranes. Implicit in reperfusion injury is a transient loss of blood flow. Hence, reperfusion injury does not account for the changes seen in bowel infarcts following acute vascular occlusion.

Ischemic injury may occur as the result of a vast array of conditions (Table 9-1). Furthermore, the outcome following an ischemic episode is variable and depends on its severity, the abruptness of onset of oxygen deprivation, the length of bowel involved, and the length of time of the disruption.[26-31] Most of the entities listed in Table 9-1 are described in other chapters. In this chapter, ischemia due to acute mesenteric insufficiency, focal segmental ischemia, and neonatal necrotizing enterocolitis is discussed.

ACUTE MESENTERIC INSUFFICIENCY

Acute disruption of mesenteric blood flow is a catastrophic condition associated with a high mortality rate secondary to infarction and perforation of the intestines.

Causes

The four main causes of mesenteric insufficiency are embolism, arterial thrombosis, nonocclusive (low-flow) ischemia, and mesenteric vein thrombosis.[26,28,30,31]

TABLE 9–1. Causes of Vascular Insufficiency of the Small Intestine
Occlusive
Embolic
Superior mesenteric artery
Thrombotic
Superior mesenteric artery
Mesenteric vein
Low flow
Low cardiac output
Hypotension/shock
Mechanical
Hernia
Volvulus (including Meckel's diverticulum)
Trauma
Hypercoagulable states
Disseminated intravascular coagulation
Clotting disorders
Infections
Neonatal necrotizing enterocolitis
Bacterial infections (clostridial)
Collagen vascular diseases
Vasculitis
Radiation injury
Drugs
Potassium chloride
Digitalis
Vasopressor agents
Oral contraceptives

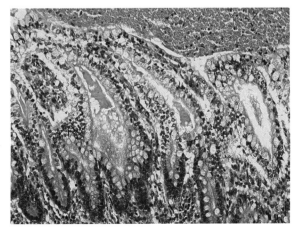

FIGURE 9–4. Cystic fibrosis. Several crypts are plugged with densely eosinophilic acellular material. The goblet cells are also distended with mucin.

Embolism accounts for 25% to 30% of acute intestinal ischemia.[28,30,31] A vast majority of emboli arise from the heart in the setting of atrial fibrillation. Other sources of emboli include left ventricular thrombi, valve vegetations, and atheromatous plaques in the aorta. The clinical presentation is that of acute abdominal pain, usually in a patient with a history of a cardiac abnormality. Vomiting and bloody diarrhea ensue as the tissue injury progresses from reversible ischemia to frank infarction. Peritoneal signs and shock indicate transmural necrosis. Treatment usually consists of emergency embolectomy and resection of the infarcted bowel segment.

Arterial thrombosis accounts for 10% to 15% of cases of acute mesenteric ischemia.[28,30,31] This syndrome occurs in the setting of severe atherosclerosis of the superior mesenteric artery at its origin and may be temporally related to episodes of low flow. The clinical presentation is often milder than that of embolism, with intermittent, mild to moderate abdominal pain or an absence of symptoms until frank infarction sets in.

Nonocclusive mesenteric ischemia also occurs in the setting of low cardiac output and low mesenteric blood flow.[28,30,31] Predisposing factors are congestive heart failure and, potentially, the use of cardiac glycosides, such as digitalis (because of their vasoconstrictive action). Again, the severity of symptoms is variable. However, once significant tissue ischemia occurs, the syndrome is identical to that of mesenteric artery occlusion.

Mesenteric vein thrombosis causes less than 10% of cases of acute intestinal ischemia.[28,30,31] This condition occurs in a variety of clinical settings, including trauma, hypercoagulable states, portal vein thrombosis, low-flow states, intra-abdominal sepsis, neoplasms, and mechanical bowel obstruction. Symptoms are often subtle and of long duration before frank infarction occurs.

Pathologic Features

GROSS PATHOLOGY

The length of the small intestine affected in acute mesenteric ischemia depends primarily on the point of occlusion of the affected vessel or the severity of loss of cardiac output, and the length of time before embolectomy/thrombectomy is performed.[26,32,33] For instance, an embolus lodged at the origin of the SMA will result in infarction of the entire small bowel from the ligament of Treitz to the splenic flexure of the colon.

Evidence of ischemia/infarction may be diffuse and confluent, or patchy and multifocal. The serosal aspect often appears congested and blue/black (Fig. 9-5). Perforations may be present but may not be accompanied by a well-developed fibrinous exudate if the resection occurred within a short period of time after presentation. In arterial occlusions, the mesentery is usually pale, whereas in venous thrombosis, the mesentery is usually congested and hemorrhagic. There is usually an abrupt demarcation between normal and involved segments of bowel.[28,31] The intestinal lumen is invariably filled with blood. The mucosal surface may appear beefy red, boggy, and ulcerated and may contain irregularly protruding mucosal islands. This mucosal appearance gives rise to the "thumbprinting" sign commonly seen on abdominal radiographs of patients with this condition. Pseudo-membranes may also be present. Transmural hemorrhage may be seen, and the wall may be friable and thin. In mesenteric vein thrombosis, thrombi may be seen in mesenteric veins on gross examination.[32]

MICROSCOPIC PATHOLOGY

Microscopically, the features of arterial ischemia are similar throughout the gastrointestinal tract.[34] The earliest changes may occur in the mucosa, but occasionally, the

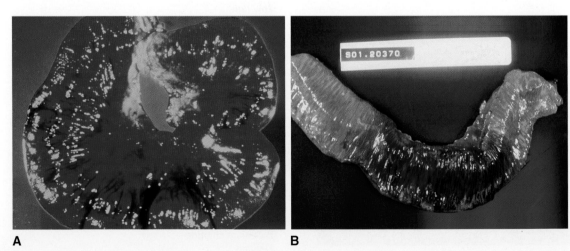

A   **B**

FIGURE 9–5.   Ischemia. **A,** In this example of superior mesenteric artery embolism, a large segment of jejunum is infarcted. The serosal surface is intensely congested and hemorrhagic. (Image courtesy of Dr. Brian West). **B,** This specimen illustrates focal, segmental infarction as might occur with an incarcerated hernia.

submucosa is affected first, with initial sparing of the mucosa.[34,35] Early histologic changes consist of hemorrhage, congestion, and edema of the submucosa, sometimes associated with preservation of the overlying mucosa. Submucosal changes may then lead to various degrees of mucosal necrosis with or without ulceration, luminal hemorrhage, and pseudomembrane deposition (Fig. 9-6).[33] In the acute setting, there is typically an absence of a chronic inflammatory response, although neutrophils may be seen if enough time has elapsed since the onset of the occlusion.

Characteristically, the mucosa shows loss of epithelium, which occurs progressively from the tips of the villi to the base of the crypts and is associated with various degrees of edema and congestion. Within hours of the injury, neutrophils influx into the damaged area. Depending on the extent and severity of injury, the mucosal changes may reverse to normal if the ischemic insult is stopped. However, if ischemia is persistent or severe, tissue healing may result in fibrosis and stricture formation.

Examination of mesenteric vessels may be confusing in that thrombi may form acutely as a response to stasis and congestion. Clinically significant thrombi show evidence of organization, implying their presence over a significant period. Fibrin thrombi may be present in small arterioles in areas of necrosis and do not, by themselves, indicate vasculitis or a hypercoagulable state.

FOCAL SEGMENTAL ISCHEMIA

Vascular compromise that involves short segments of intestine is clinically less severe than the more global insults discussed above. Focal segmental ischemia may be due to atheroemboli, trauma, or mechanical abnormalities, such as bands and adhesions, incarcerated hernias, volvulus, intussusception, neoplasms, and con-genital anomalies.[36,37] The gross and microscopic findings of focal segmental ischemia are similar to those seen in acute mesenteric insufficiency. The main difference is that in focal segmental ischemia, smaller lengths of intestine are involved and a spectrum of changes may occur, ranging from mild reversible disease to chronic irreversible injury.

NEONATAL NECROTIZING ENTEROCOLITIS

This disorder occurs in premature infants during the first week of life and affects the colon and terminal ileum. The pathogenesis is related to ischemia and subsequent infection of the bowel. The hallmark radiologic and pathologic findings include pneumatosis intestinalis and ischemic necrosis of the bowel wall. This disorder is discussed in greater detail in Chapter 10.

■ Disorders of Malabsorption

(Table 9-2)

GLUTEN-SENSITIVE ENTEROPATHY (CELIAC DISEASE)

Epidemiology and Clinical Features

Gluten-sensitive enteropathy (GSE), or celiac disease, is an immune-mediated disorder that results in damage to the small intestinal mucosa and leads to malabsorption of nutrients. Although this disease was described more than a century ago,[38,39] it is only over the past 50 years that the role of dietary gluten in the pathogenesis of this disorder has been recognized.[40] GSE has a worldwide distribution, although it is rare among Asians and blacks. Prevalence rates of 0.05% to 0.2% have been estimated in European countries.[41,42]

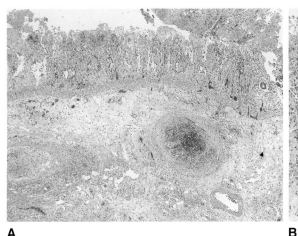
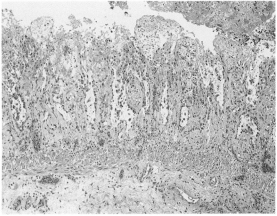

FIGURE 9–6. Ischemia. **A,** Transmural infarction due to ischemia. **B,** High-power view revealing surface epithelial necrosis with focal crypt preservation. There is a fibrinous neutrophilic exudate on the surface.

TABLE 9–2. Classification of Intestinal Malabsorptive Disorders by Category of Disease

Autoimmune
Gluten-sensitive enteropathy
Autoimmune enteropathy
Hypersensitivity
Protein allergy (milk, soy)
Eosinophilic gastroenteritis
Infection
Tropical sprue
Bacterial overgrowth/blind loop
Other infections
Nutritional Deficiencies
B$_{12}$/folate deficiency
Protein-calorie deficiency
Zinc deficiency
Iron deficiency
Inherited/Metabolic/Malformation
Microvillous inclusion disease
Abetalipoproteinemia
Primary intestinal lymphangiectasia
Chronic granulomatous disease
Disaccharide deficiencies
Neoplastic/Infiltrative Disorders
Waldenström's macroglobulinemia
Amyloidosis
Lymphoma
Immune Disorders
Graft-versus-host disease
Radiation/chemotherapy
AIDS enteropathy
Systemic Diseases
Lipid storage diseases
Histiocytosis X
Other
Nonintestinal Diseases
Pancreatic insufficiency
Bile salt insufficiency
Short gut syndrome

Pathogenesis

GSE is an immunologic disorder that occurs in genetically susceptible hosts. Environmental influences are important as well. The familial nature of the disease was originally established in a study of 17 probands and their families who underwent small bowel biopsies.[43] This study found an increased incidence of GSE in first-degree relatives of symptomatic patients. Genetic studies have shown that at least two separate genes are involved in GSE—major histocompatibility complex class I HLA B8, and class II HLA DR3 and DQw2 (the latter two are present in 80% of white patients).[51,52] Up to 95% of patients carry two specific HLA-DQ alleles—DQA1*0501 and DQB1*0201.[53-55] In addition, a group of GSE-associated B-cell alloantigens have been identified. However, these genetic phenotypes do not explain the pathogenesis entirely in that 20% of the normal population is HLA DR3- and DQw2-positive, and not all GSE patients carry this specific phenotype.[51,52]

In the proper genetic environment, exposure to gliadin or the prolamin fraction of gluten found in wheat, rye, and barley results in a local immune response.[44,56] An additional environmental component may be related to previous infection with adenovirus 12.[57] The E1b protein of this virus has been shown to have amino acid sequence homology with alpha gliadin, such that antibodies and T cells that recognize these viral proteins may cross-react with gliadin.

The immune response to dietary gluten involves both antibody- and cell-mediated injury. Antibody-induced injury may occur via antigen-antibody complex deposition with complement activation, and also by the induction of cell-mediated cytotoxicity. Activated mucosal T cells have been shown to cause epithelial injury, probably through the release of cytokines.[57]

The clinical diagnosis of GSE usually depends on the finding of the appropriate combination of symptoms, combined with laboratory evidence of malabsorption and the presence of serum autoantibodies. The findings of serum antigliadin and antiendomysial (smooth muscle) antibodies are fairly specific when used together.[44,58] Testing for antiendomysial antibodies has a sensitivity and specificity of 90% in untreated GSE.[59,60] Recently, a specific endomysial autoantigen, tissue transglutaminase (TTG), has been discovered.[61,62] In fact, testing for serum antibodies to TTG has now largely replaced testing for antiendomysial antibodies in the diagnosis of GSE.

Studies have documented that 10% to 20% of asymptomatic first-degree relatives have mild histologic changes such as increased intraepithelial lymphocytes in the absence of villous blunting, or mild mucosal lesions.[43,63,64] In this setting, a diagnosis of GSE should not be made unless there is other clinical evidence of disease such as malabsorption.

GSE may present at any time in life from early childhood to late adulthood. Classic symptoms include abdominal discomfort, diarrhea, and steatorrhea.[43,44] However, some patients do not develop diarrhea but instead exhibit other signs and symptoms, including short stature, infertility, recurrent aphthous stomatitis, or dermatitis herpetiformis.[42,43,45-47] In adults with occult GSE, complaints of fatigue often lead to a discovery of iron deficiency anemia, which ultimately leads to the correct diagnosis.[48] In fact, some patients are entirely asymptomatic and present initially only with histologic changes on biopsy analysis. The term *latent celiac disease* has been used to describe patients with this presentation.[49,50] Factors governing the type of clinical presentation and the expression of symptoms are poorly understood. It is likely that the development and severity of symptoms are related to the length of intestine involved more than to the severity of mucosal pathology.[49] It is presumed that patients who present in adulthood have had a mild form of disease for a long time.

Pathologic Features

GROSS PATHOLOGY

Endoscopic findings in patients with GSE are often subtle and unreliable. However, a flat, scalloped appearance of the duodenal mucosa, likely reflecting the loss of villi, may be seen.[65] In a landmark study, Rubin and associates described the appearance of normal duodenal mucosa with the use of a hand lens and showed that the mucosa is characterized by numerous slender villi with a delicate capillary network that floats in formalin, similar to "the tentacles of a sea anemone."[66] In contrast, biopsies from patients with GSE have a barren, stubby surface, without normal villi, and contain widely spaced irregular capillaries (Fig. 9-7).

MICROSCOPIC PATHOLOGY

Accurate evaluation of small bowel biopsies in suspected cases of GSE depends on two important prerequisites. Biopsies should be well oriented and obtained from areas distal to the duodenal bulb. Proper orientation allows the best opportunity for evaluating the true mucosal architecture while avoiding the overinterpretation of short villi, invariably seen in poorly oriented sections, as abnormal. Similarly, the duodenal bulb is an area susceptible to peptic injury and to prominent mucosal Brunner's glands, both of which may lead to the presence of short and broad-appearing villi. However, one must keep in mind that GSE does involve the duodenal bulb and that it may be diagnosed in biopsies from that location in the appropriate clinical setting.

Biopsies from GSE are characteristically most severe proximally, and they decrease in severity distally. In untreated disease, the duodenum is always involved, often with severe lesions. The proximal jejunum is usually involved, and in very ill patients, the histologic changes may extend to the terminal ileum, but they are generally less severe at that site.[67]

Histology of Untreated Disease

The normal small bowel mucosa shows a villous height–to–crypt depth ratio of 3 to 5:1, depending on the anatomic location. Villus epithelial cells contain basally located nuclei with abundant mature cytoplasm and a preponderance of absorptive cells admixed with goblet cells. A faint density, representing the microvillous brush border, can be appreciated on H&E-stained tissue sections. Intraepithelial lymphocytes number approximately 1 per 5 to 10 epithelial cells. The lamina propria normally contains a mixture of plasma cells, lymphocytes, and occasional eosinophils (Fig. 9-8). Each of these three mucosal components (architecture, epithelium, and lamina propria) should be carefully examined in cases of suspected GSE.

In untreated GSE, biopsies from the duodenum reveal a loss of normal architecture caused by a decrease in the height of villi. In many cases, the mucosa appears completely flat with no appreciable villi. In others, the villi may be broad and only mildly to moderately shortened, and they may show irregularity (Fig. 9-9). Loss of villous height is matched by crypt elongation or hyperplasia, such that the overall width of the mucosa usually remains intact.[66] The degree of flattening is used to grade the severity of disease as mild, moderate, or severe. The phrase "crypt hyperplastic villous atrophy," although used extensively in the past, is no longer appropriate and should be replaced by the descriptive terms *mild*, *moderate*, and *severe*.[68]

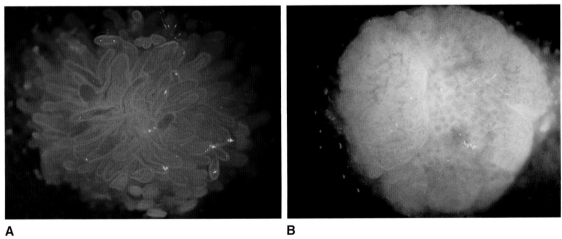

A   **B**

FIGURE 9–7. A, Normal small bowel mucosa viewed with a dissecting microscope (zirconium arc lighting). The villi are slender and translucent, allowing visualization of the underlying delicate capillary network (unstained). **B,** Small bowel mucosa from a patient with celiac disease. The surface is irregular and devoid of villi (unstained). (From Rubin CE, Brandborg LL, Phelps PC, et al: Studies of celiac disease. I. The apparent identical and specific nature of the duodenal and proximal jejunal lesion in celiac disease and idiopathic sprue. Gastroenterology 38:28-49, 1960.)

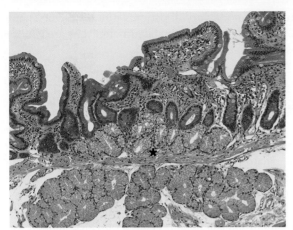

FIGURE 9–8. Normal duodenal bulb. The duodenal bulb is a transition zone that is normally subjected to physiologic peptic injury. Brunner's glands (★) and increased mononuclear inflammation are frequently present in the mucosa, resulting in broader and shorter villi.

The degree of abnormality seen in the surface and crypt epithelium can vary widely and does not always reflect the degree of villous flattening or the severity of symptoms.[66] When severely affected, the surface epithelium shows loss of its normal columnar shape, mucin depletion, vacuolization, and enlargement of cell nuclei (see Fig. 9-9**A**). Cells may show loss of nuclear basal polarity, with stratification, pyknosis, and fragmentation of nuclei. An increase in the number of intraepithelial lymphocytes is characteristic. One study using morphometric analysis found an average of 3 lymphocytes per 10 epithelial cells.[49] Phenotypic analyses from several studies have shown that intraepithelial lymphocytes in GSE are predominantly gamma/delta T cells.[69-71] It is interesting to note that the epithelium on the sides of blunted villi may appear entirely normal, despite its proximity to severely affected cells at the surface of the mucosa. Epithelium lining hyperplastic crypts shows a variable degree of nuclear enlargement and mitosis, likely a reflection of an increase in proliferative activity.

The lamina propria in GSE typically shows an increase in the number of plasma cells, the degree of which may vary widely. Neutrophils and crypt abscesses are uncommon in GSE but may occasionally be present. However, the finding of diffuse or marked acute inflammation should prompt consideration of another diagnosis such as peptic duodenitis, Crohn's disease, or refractory sprue.

Some patients with genetic, serologic, and clinical evidence of GSE show only mild or near-normal pathologic changes.[49,50,72] Marsh and associates have demon-

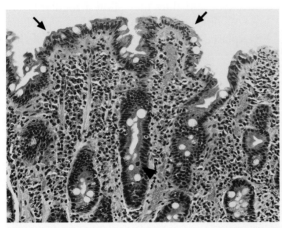

A

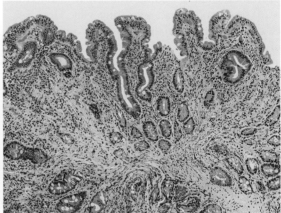

B

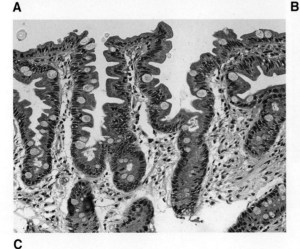

C

FIGURE 9–9. Celiac disease. **A,** Severe lesion. The surface epithelium shows loss of its columnar shape and mucin depletion. A marked increase in intraepithelial lymphocytes is revealed (*arrows*). The elongated crypts show increased mitotic activity and enlarged nuclei. The lamina propria is expanded by plasma cells and lymphocytes. (*Arrowhead* shows a mitotic figure.) **B,** Moderate lesion. In many cases of untreated celiac disease, only mild to moderate villous blunting may be present. In this duodenal biopsy with moderate villous blunting, all the other hallmarks of the disease, including increased intraepithelial lymphocytes and crypt hyperplasia, are present. **C,** Treated celiac disease. Duodenal biopsies obtained on a gluten-free diet may reveal persistent mild abnormalities. In this example, the villous architecture is normal, but there is a slight increase in intraepithelial lymphocytes and mild reactive changes.

strated that some GSE patients show increased intraepithelial lymphocytes with normal architecture (infiltrative type) (Fig. 9-10), whereas others show completely flat mucosa (flat, destructive type) (see Fig. 9-9A).[49,72] Thus, Marsh redefined the histologic diagnosis of GSE to include the entire spectrum of abnormalities. Patients whose only abnormality is increased intraepithelial lymphocytes should have this finding correlated with serologic markers and clinical symptoms before a diagnosis of GSE is established. The proportion of patients with minimal histologic changes who will eventually develop severe histologic lesions and symptoms is unknown.[49,50,73] In a small study, 4 of 12 GSE patients with "mild" lesions had developed flat mucosa at follow-up.[73]

The pathologic features of GSE are entirely nonspecific and may be seen in a variety of diseases, such as tropical sprue,[74] bacterial overgrowth,[75,76] unclassified sprue,[77] specific food allergies,[78] and occasionally in common variable immune deficiency (Table 9-3).[79] Thus, a definite diagnosis of GSE should be made in conjunction with the appropriate clinical information.

Histology of Treated Disease (Response to Gluten-Free Diet)

Small bowel biopsies obtained 1 week to several months after exclusion of dietary gluten may show only a modest improvement in villous architecture and persistently elevated numbers of intraepithelial lymphocytes, despite an excellent clinical response.[67] However, biopsies taken several months after a gluten-free diet return to normal or near normal ("mild" mucosal lesion) in most cases (see Fig. 9-9C). Nevertheless, some patients show a persistence of moderate or even severe lesions in the setting of marked clinical improvement. It should

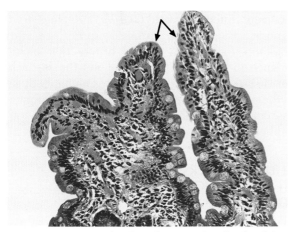

FIGURE 9–10. Untreated celiac disease. This duodenal biopsy was taken from an asymptomatic patient who was discovered to have anti–tissue transglutaminase antibodies. Normal villi are present, but there is a marked increase in the number of intraepithelial lymphocytes *(arrows)*.

TABLE 9–3. Conditions Associated With Flat Mucosal Biopsy Appearance

Gluten-sensitive enteropathy
Refractory sprue
Autoimmune enteropathy
Microvillous inclusion disease
Protein intolerance
Common variable immune deficiency
Tropical sprue
Bacterial overgrowth
Nutritional deficiency
Eosinophilic gastroenteritis

be noted that repeat biopsies are not required when the clinical response to a gluten-free diet is positive. Repeat biopsies are usually indicated only when the clinical response is poor so that other disorders, such as refractory sprue, lymphoma, or infection, can be excluded.

Refractory (Unclassified) Sprue

Refractory, or "unclassified," sprue is defined as an absent or incomplete clinical response to a gluten-free diet.[80,81] Inadvertent gluten ingestion must be ruled out in addition to other potential causes of diarrhea or malabsorption, such as pancreatic insufficiency, concomitant collagenous colitis, lymphoma, or other rare entities, such as adult-onset autoimmune enteropathy.[82-84] Thus, idiopathic refractory sprue remains a diagnosis of exclusion.

Many patients with refractory sprue show abnormalities in their intraepithelial T lymphocytes, such as an abnormal phenotype and monoclonality.[85-88] Cellier, Bagdi, and others have demonstrated that intraepithelial T lymphocytes in refractory sprue show a loss of surface CD4, CD8, and T-cell receptors and contain CD3e and monoclonal rearrangements of the TCRγ gene.[85-88] These findings have led to the theory that a significant proportion of refractory sprue cases represent a form of in situ, or cryptic, T-cell lymphoma. Furthermore, the risk of progression to overt T-cell lymphoma is increased in refractory sprue patients with abnormal intraepithelial lymphocytes.[81,86,88] Some authors have suggested that chemotherapy may be appropriate treatment for such patients.[87,88]

In clinical practice, immunostains for CD3 and CD8 may help distinguish between responsive celiac disease (CD3+ and CD8+) and refractory sprue (CD3+, CD8–). Polymerase chain reaction (PCR) to detect T-cell receptor gene rearrangements can also be performed on paraffin-embedded tissue.[88a]

From a histologic (not causative) standpoint, small bowel biopsies in refractory sprue show moderate to severe villous flattening despite adherence to a gluten-free diet. The lesions are typically patchy and variable in distribution. In some cases, similarity is noted between the histologic appearance of untreated but responsive GSE and refractory sprue. However, in a longitudinal study of 10 refractory sprue patients, several histologic features were strongly associated with a refractory course.[77] In that study, collagenous sprue developed in 5 patients. In addition, basal plasmacytosis and mucosal thinning (atrophy) were found almost exclusively in biopsies from refractory patients.

Collagenous sprue, similar to its counterpart in the colon, is characterized by increased deposition of collagen beneath the surface epithelium basement membrane and is associated with a poor prognosis.[89] Rigorous diagnostic criteria that include the entrapment of small capillaries and fibroblasts within the collagen layer should be applied when the diagnosis is made (Fig. 9-11). A trichrome stain to highlight the collagen is often helpful. Collagen deposition may be patchy and may appear late in the course of illness.

Malignancy in GSE

The association of intestinal lymphoma with GSE was first documented in 1937[90] and occurs in 5% to 10% of patients in some series.[91-93] Lymphomas that arise in this setting were originally classified as reticulum cell sarcomas[94] and/or malignant histiocytosis.[95] In some reports, the term *ulcerative jejunitis* (now understood to be synonymous with lymphoma) was used to describe similar-appearing tumors that develop in the setting of malabsorption.[96] In addition, the term *enteropathy-associated T-cell lymphoma* has been applied to these cases.[97] In 1985, Isaacson characterized these tumors as T-cell lymphomas.[98] However, rarely, B-cell lymphomas arise in association with refractory sprue.[77]

Lymphoma may present as solitary or multiple tumors and may involve any portion of the small bowel, with or without involvement of the mesenteric lymph nodes.[91-93] Clinically, the onset of lymphoma is frequently associated with a relapse of malabsorption in a previously gluten-responsive patient. Although this is controversial, some studies suggest that the risk of lymphoma is increased in patients who fail to adhere to a strict gluten-free diet.[99,100]

In addition to lymphoma, carcinomas, especially those arising in the gastrointestinal tract, occur more frequently in patients with GSE.[91-93,101] In many studies, the most common site of carcinoma is the esophagus, with a fairly equal incidence of occurrence in the stomach and large and small intestines.[91-93] Carcinomas of the oropharynx, bladder, ovary, lung, and breast have also been reported in this setting.

Other Complications in GSE

A variety of intestinal and extraintestinal pathologic conditions occur in GSE. These include lymphocytic[102] and collagenous gastritis,[103] lymphocytic[104] and collagenous colitis,[83,105,106] dermatitis herpetiformis,[45,107] and nonspecific intestinal ulceration,[108,109] as well as a variety of other associations.[110,111]

Differential Diagnosis (see Tables 9-2 and 9-3)

Flattening of small intestinal villi can be seen in several conditions, such as tropical sprue, common variable hypogammaglobulinemia, and bacterial overgrowth; it is also noted in infants and young children with viral gastroenteritis or cow's milk intolerance. Small bowel Crohn's disease and eosinophilic gastroenteritis may also, rarely, result in villous blunting.[112,113] The distinction of these entities from GSE rests primarily on clinical, not pathologic, data. However, in the rare instance of a flat mucosal biopsy in common variable hypogammaglobulinemia, a lack of lamina propria plasma cells and concurrent infection with *Giardia* are clues to the diagnosis. Biopsies in tropical sprue are rarely completely flat, and a clinical history that includes residence in a tropical climate allows the distinction from GSE to be made. Above all, serum antibody tests and the response to a gluten-free diet are of paramount importance in distinguishing GSE from all other conditions.

OTHER DISORDERS OF PROTEIN INTOLERANCE (COW'S MILK AND SOY PROTEIN)

The syndromes of cow's or breast milk and soy protein intolerance in infancy and childhood are well documented.[78,114-118] Other types of food hypersensitivities in children and adults are not as well understood. This section is limited to a discussion of milk and soy allergy

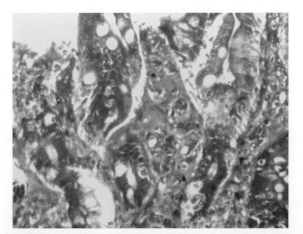

FIGURE 9–11. Collagenous sprue. Cellular elements, including blood vessels and fibroblast, are entrapped within a thickened collagen layer (trichrome).

because these disorders are associated with reproducible histologic patterns of injury to the gastrointestinal tract. Clinically, affected infants introduced to either cow's milk or soy-based formulas develop acute, frequently bloody diarrhea or vomiting, abdominal pain, and weight loss. Symptoms usually improve rapidly following removal of the inciting agent. However, in some, the symptoms may be prolonged, and steroids may be required.

Prospective studies have documented that early histologic injury in soy protein intolerance develops within 12 hours of ingestion and may resolve within 4 days after dietary exclusion.[78] In some patients, an overlap is seen between milk protein intolerance and the more generalized condition of eosinophilic gastroenteritis. Both disorders may be associated with peripheral eosinophilia. Patients with eosinophilic gastroenteritis may initially present with symptoms apparently related to milk protein intolerance. However, their clinical course is more refractory, and they are more likely to have an atopic phenotype.[115]

Histologic abnormalities in soy and milk protein intolerance occur most frequently in the colorectum but can be found throughout the gastrointestinal tract. They consist of mild to severe lamina propria eosinophils, intraepithelial eosinophils associated with epithelial injury, and edema.[115] In the small bowel, varying degrees of villous blunting may be seen with mucosal edema, mucin depletion, and increased intraepithelial lymphocytes and eosinophils. When severe, the histologic features may resemble untreated GSE. However, the finding of increased eosinophils can help distinguish these two entities. Eosinophils are not always significantly increased in protein intolerance. In such cases, clinical correlation is required to make the appropriate diagnosis. Colorectal changes in allergic disease are discussed in Chapter 10.

◾ Autoimmune Enteropathy

CLINICAL FEATURES

Autoimmune enteropathy is a condition characterized by protracted, watery diarrhea and malabsorption associated with variably severe small bowel mucosal lesions in infants. Rarely, adults may be affected by a similar process.[84] The disease was first described by Unsworth and Walker-Smith,[119] who defined the condition using the following four criteria: (1) presentation with protracted diarrhea and severe enteropathy; (2) no response to an exclusion diet or total parenteral nutrition (TPN); (3) evidence of a predisposition to autoimmune disease (presence of circulating autoantibodies and/or associated autoimmune diseases); and (4) absence of severe immune deficiency.[119] Although autoimmune enteropathy was initially described as a disorder of the small bowel, it is clear that the colon may be involved as

well.[120] Also, cases associated with immune deficiency have now been described.[121]

Antienterocyte antibodies are present in approximately 50% of cases and are a fairly specific marker of the disease.[119,120,122,123] Anti–goblet cell antibodies have also been reported in some patients.[124] Concomitant autoimmune diseases of other organs, such as diabetes, nephropathy, thyroiditis, and autoimmune hepatitis, are frequently found in patients and their families.[120,122] Children with this condition are often severely ill, requiring elemental diets and TPN to survive. In the past, many patients died in infancy, although treatment with immunosuppressive regimens, such as steroids, cyclosporine, and tacrolimus, now results in prolonged survival.[125]

PATHOGENESIS

The pathogenesis of autoimmune enteropathy has been studied extensively. Although it is associated with enterocyte autoantibodies, the mechanism of injury is more likely related to abnormalities in T- and B-cell regulation.[123] Upregulation and abnormal expression of HLA class II MHC (HLA-DR) antigens have been shown to be present on crypt epithelial cells.[122] Recently, a 75-kilodalton antigen present on the surface and crypt epithelium in the small and large intestines that reacts with the serum of patients with autoimmune enteropathy has been identified.[126] This antigen may be the target of antienterocyte antibodies, but this has yet to be proved.

PATHOLOGIC FEATURES

Pathologic features of small bowel biopsies include variable flattening of the villi with an increase in the number of lamina propria plasma cells and no increase in the number of intraepithelial lymphocytes (a feature that may help in the distinction from GSE). Crypt hyperplasia is usually but not always present, and neutrophils may be noted in the lamina propria. The severity of the lesion has been shown to correlate with the level of circulating antienterocyte antibodies.[122] Biopsies from the colon in patients with autoimmune enteropathy may reveal variable histology, from normal to severe inflammation.[120]

DIFFERENTIAL DIAGNOSIS

The features of autoimmune enteropathy are entirely nonspecific. Thus, the diagnosis can be made only in conjunction with the appropriate clinical data. Other entities that may have a similar morphologic pattern include GSE, bacterial overgrowth, and immune deficiencies, but these conditions can usually be distinguished by the appropriate clinical information.

■ Tropical Sprue

EPIDEMIOLOGY AND CLINICAL FEATURES

Tropical sprue is defined as a chronic malabsorptive syndrome, often associated with folate and B_{12} deficiency, that occurs in residents of or visitors to the Indian subcontinent and parts of Southeast Asia, Central America, and the Caribbean Islands.[127-130] Notable exceptions are Jamaica and sub-Saharan Africa. Patients may present with chronic diarrhea and a variety of nutritional disorders. In tropical populations, adults are more severely affected than children. The disease occurs in both endemic and epidemic forms.

The cause of tropical sprue remains unknown, although the preponderance of evidence supports an infectious origin.[131-134] The illness probably begins with an acute infection of the small or large intestine that may be bacterial, viral, or parasitic in origin.[133] Subsequently, a chronic infection, with colonization of the small bowel by enterotoxigenic bacteria, is believed to occur, which probably results in ongoing injury to enterocytes. Bacteria isolated from patients with tropical sprue include *Klebsiella pneumoniae*, *Escherichia coli*, and *Enterobacter cloacae*.[133] An environment conducive to bacterial overgrowth may result from the release of enteroglucagon, a potent inhibitor of peristalsis, during the acute infectious phase of the disease.[133] The theory of bacterial overgrowth is strongly supported by the response of some patients to broad-spectrum antibiotics, such as tetracycline, along with folic acid. The entire small bowel is usually affected in tropical sprue, including the ileum,[129,135] leading to vitamin B_{12} and folate deficiency in most symptomatic patients. Vitamin deficiencies may lead to proliferative injury of the intestinal crypts and other epithelia, such as megaloblastic change.[136] Megaloblastic change, or macrocytosis, refers to the nuclear and cytoplasmic enlargement of epithelial cells that occurs in the setting of interrupted DNA synthesis and cell division (see Chapter 5).

PATHOLOGIC FEATURES

Asymptomatic native populations susceptible to tropical sprue usually reveal pathologic changes that include villous shortening and increased inflammation. The degree of abnormality in asymptomatic people is generally minor but occasionally may be pronounced.[128,129] Evidence of malabsorption is also frequently found in asymptomatic native residents.

The entire small bowel, including the ileum, is usually affected in tropical sprue.[129,135] This is in contrast to GSE, in which pathologic lesions are present in the duodenum and jejunum and only rarely extend into the ileum. The patterns of distribution of these two diseases are consistent with their pathogenesis. Tropical sprue is caused by colonization of the bowel by bacteria, whereas GSE is a response to a dietary antigen that is present in highest concentrations in the proximal gut.

Gross Pathology

Early studies of small bowel mucosa with the use of a dissecting microscope revealed that biopsies from symptomatic patients and from some asymptomatic patients in endemic areas show an abnormal villous pattern characterized by fusing and broadening of the villi.[129,135,136] The jejunum is usually more greatly affected than the ileum, which may appear normal under the dissecting microscope despite being abnormal histologically.[135]

Microscopic Pathology

Small bowel biopsies in tropical sprue reveal varying degrees of villous blunting, crypt hyperplasia, and increased mitotic activity (Fig. 9-12).[136,137] An increase in lamina propria lymphocytes, plasma cells, and eosinophils, as well as intraepithelial lymphocytes, is seen. The intraepithelial lymphocytes in tropical sprue are more numerous in the crypts than the surface cells, unlike GSE, in which the reverse situation occurs.[138] In severe cases, decreased mitotic activity is combined with a lack of surface epithelial cell maturation. The cells acquire a cuboidal shape, become mucin depleted, and accumulate fat droplets within their cytoplasm.[128,129,135,136] Concomitant folate and B_{12} deficiency may lead to mucosal atrophy, manifested by crypts lined by cells with markedly enlarged (megaloblastic) nuclei. Completely flat mucosa, common in GSE, is almost never seen in tropical sprue.

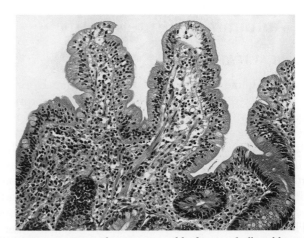

FIGURE 9–12. Tropical sprue. A variable degree of villous blunting is seen in tropical sprue. In this duodenal biopsy, only mild villous blunting is present. A marked increase in intraepithelial lymphocytes can be seen, which is more prevalent in the crypts than in the surface epithelium. The lamina propria is expanded with mononclear cells. (Image courtesy of Raymond Yesner).

Electron microscopic studies of small bowel biopsies in tropical sprue have revealed irregularities of the microvilli, increased lysosomes, accumulation of fat within surface epithelium, and the presence of dense material beneath the basal lamina of the epithelium.[128]

DIFFERENTIAL DIAGNOSIS

The histologic changes in tropical sprue are nonspecific and can be seen in a variety of conditions (see Table 9-3). Thus, a clinical history of residence in or prolonged visits to endemic areas is critical in establishing a correct diagnosis. Parasitic and other specific infections must be excluded before a diagnosis of tropical sprue can be made confidently. Biopsies that show completely flat mucosa should arouse suspicion for other diseases, such as GSE. However, mild to moderate mucosal lesions can be seen in both GSE and tropical sprue. Clinical improvement following treatment with broad-spectrum antibiotics further supports the diagnosis.

▪ Bacterial Overgrowth Syndrome (Blind Loop Syndrome, Stasis Syndrome)

PATHOGENESIS

Bacterial overgrowth by coliform bacteria in the small intestine occurs in a variety of conditions, all of which predispose the individual to decreased motility and stasis.[76,139,140] These include motor/neural disorders such as scleroderma, diabetes mellitus, pseudo-obstruction, and amyloidosis; structural defects such as diverticulosis and strictures; and surgical manipulations that lead to isolated bowel segments, such as Billroth II gastrojejunal anastomosis.[141-149] Immune deficiency states, such as acquired immunodeficiency syndrome (AIDS) and common variable immune deficiency, may also result in bacterial overgrowth and may contribute to the diarrheal illness that frequently occurs in these conditions.[76,140]

CLINICAL FEATURES

Regardless of the underlying cause, bacterial overgrowth by anaerobic bacteria that are normally confined to the colon develops in the small intestine.[76,139,140] Patients with this condition typically have diarrhea and steatorrhea, although malabsorption of vitamin B_{12}, carbohydrates, and other nutrients can occur as well. Proposed theories of pathogenesis are as follows. First, anaerobic bacteria deconjugate bile salts, which leads to fat malaborption.[76] Certain nutrients, such as vitamin B_{12}, may be depleted by luminal bacteria. In addition,

ultrastructural studies in this condition have revealed damage to surface epithelium and the brush border, with some evidence of defective fat transport and absorption.[150]

When bacterial overgrowth is suspected or proven (by breath tests, cultures, or other techniques), antibiotic therapy results in marked improvement.[76,151-153]

PATHOLOGIC FEATURES

Small bowel biopsies from patients with bacterial overgrowth may be histologically normal, despite clinical evidence of malabsorption. When abnormal, biopsies typically reveal mild to moderate villous blunting with increased chronic inflammation in the lamina propria and epithelium, as well as crypt hyperplasia.[76,150,154] Vacuolated epithelial cells, probably containing lipid, may also be seen. When present, the changes are patchy and vary from segment to segment, such that different biopsies taken during the same procedure may show different degrees of abnormality. This pattern of involvement helps to distinguish bacterial overgrowth from GSE.

As in other conditions characterized by villous blunting, the histologic features are entirely nonspecific and do not correlate with the severity of clinical symptoms.[150]

▪ Microvillous Inclusion Disease

Microvillous inclusion disease (MID), also known as congenital or familial microvillous atrophy, is a rare, inherited, autosomal recessive condition that results in severe refractory diarrhea and steatorrhea, as well as carbohydrate malabsorption, in newborns.[155] Severe, life-threatening symptoms usually begin during the first few days of life. Few infants survive beyond infancy, although with the use of TPN, life can be sustained for several years.[156-158] Small bowel and liver transplantation is the only potentially curative therapy.

The light and electron microscopic findings are pathognomonic. At endoscopy, the mucosa in MID appears scalloped or atrophic. Duodenal biopsies typically reveal moderate to severe villous blunting, usually with complete loss of villous architecture. No increase is seen in either lamina propria inflammation or intra-epithelial lymphocytes, unlike in GSE. Careful examination of H&E-stained sections reveals characteristic loss of the microvillous brush border, which can be highlighted with a PAS stain.[156,158] Instead of the normal brush border staining, strong staining with PAS, alkaline phosphatase (normally present in the brush border), and carcinoembryonic antigen is present in the apical cytoplasm of enterocytes in this disease.[157,159] Recently, the immunostain for CD10 has also been shown to have a characteristic staining pattern in the cytoplasm of enterocytes in MID.[160] Normally, CD10 staining reveals a linear brush border staining pattern (similar to that in PAS) in the small intestine. In MID, prominent cytoplasmic CD10 staining is noted within enterocytes.[160] Early observers noted a relative lack of "crypt hyperplasia," noting instead the presence of a thin mucosa and a relative lack of mitotic activity, especially when compared with untreated GSE.[156] However, a recent study has documented both increased proliferation and increased apoptosis in MID.[161]

Electron microscopic findings in MID are pathognomonic and reveal characteristic changes within surface enterocytes (Fig. 9-13).[155] Surface microvilli are markedly decreased in number and shortened and disorganized in appearance. In addition, intracytoplasmic vesicles or inclusions lined by microvilli are present in the apical cytoplasm of many enterocytes. These structures appear to be fragments of the brush border. Also seen is an increase in the number of lysosomes and secretory granules within enterocytes.

Studies of the pathogenesis of MID point to a failure of cytoskeletal and microfilament proteins to bind properly with other cellular elements.[162,163] Cutz and colleagues[155] have proposed that defects in subcellular protein trafficking may lead to assembly of microvilli within intracytoplasmic vesicles instead of at the cell surface. In addition to the small intestine, microvillous inclusions are found in the stomach, large intestine, gallbladder, and kidney.[155,156,164,165]

Abetalipoproteinemia

Abetalipoproteinemia and hypobetalipoproteinemia are rare inherited autosomal codominant disorders that result from mutations in the apolipoprotein B gene.[166-168] In these disorders, plasma concentrations of apolipoprotein B, cholesterol, triglycerides, very low density lipoprotein (VLDL), and low density lipoprotein (LDL) are very low or absent. Clinical manifestations of abetalipoproteinemia are systemic and include acanthocytosis, steatorrhea, severe hypolipidemia, retinitis pigmentosa, cerebellar ataxia, and mental retardation. Since its original description in 1950,[169] numerous studies have confirmed that the major defect in this disease is an inability to synthesize certain apoproteins. In particular, the intestinal manifestations are secondary to a lack of apo-B48 synthesis in intestinal absorptive cells,[166,167,170] although other defects of chylomicron retention have been described as well.[171]

Normal fat absorption from the intestinal lumen occurs via passive diffusion of fatty acids across the absorptive cell membrane. These molecules are then transported to the endoplasmic reticulum where triglyceride resynthesis takes place and chylomicron formation is initiated.[171,172] The assembly of triglycerides into chylomicrons requires phospholipids, cholesterol, and apolipoproteins B, A-I, and A-II. Finally, chylomicrons accumulate in the Golgi apparatus, where glycosylation and final assembly take place. Chylomicrons are then ejected by exocytosis into the intercellular spaces where they enter the mucosal lymphatics. In patients with abetalipoproteinemia, dietary fat diffuses normally into intestinal cells. However, a lack of effective formation of chylomicrons and VLDL occurs in the endoplasmic reticulum and the Golgi apparatus, which leads to accumulation of lipid within absorptive cells.

Patients with abetalipoproteinemia usually present in infancy or early childhood. Intestinal symptoms are frequently the earliest manifestation of disease. Patients have diarrhea, steatorrhea, and failure to thrive, all of which are accentuated after a high-fat meal. Patients often are suspected of having GSE but do not improve on a gluten-free diet.

Small intestinal biopsies show characteristic findings on light and electron microscopy (Fig. 9-14). The cardinal finding is the accumulation of fat vacuoles in the basal portion of the cytoplasm of absorptive cells

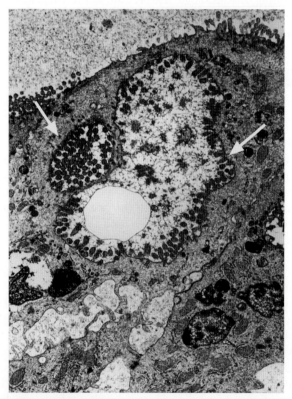

FIGURE 9–13. Microvillous inclusion disease. The diagnosis is usually established by electron microscopy. The surface microvilli are decreased in number, shortened, and disorganized in appearance. Inclusions lined by microvilli are present in the cytoplasm (*arrows*), giving the appearance of an intracellular lumen (transmission electron microscopy). (From Groisman GM, Amar M, Livne E: CD10: A valuable tool for the light microscopic diagnosis of microvillous inclusion disease [familial microvillous atrophy]. Am J Surg Pathol 26:902-907, 2002.)

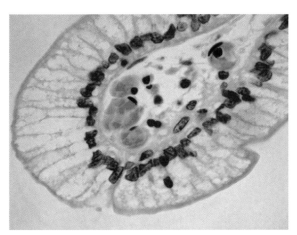

FIGURE 9–14. Abetalipoproteinemia. In this duodenal biopsy, the enterocytes appear vacuolated and have a tall columnar shape. This is due to the accumulation of fat within the cytoplasm and is most pronounced at the tips of the villi. (Image courtesy of Dr. Mary P. Bronner.)

along small bowel villi.[173,174] Vacuolated cells have a tall columnar shape with basally located nuclei. This finding is most marked in the villous tips and decreases progressively along the sides and at the bases of villi. In contrast, goblet cells appear normal. The villous architecture is intact, and there is no increase in inflammation. However, abundant lipid-laden macrophages may be present in the lamina propria. Frozen tissue stained with Oil Red O shows strong positivity in vacuolated epithelial cells. On electron microscopy, normal organelles and a normal brush border are present, but one sees numerous lysosomes filled with lipid and containing membrane-bound structures such as myelin. Characteristically, a lack of lipid within Golgi vacuoles and an absence of chylomicrons are seen.[173]

The differential diagnosis of biopsies that show epithelial cells with marked vacuolization includes normal tissue from a patient who had a recent fatty meal before undergoing endoscopy. Rare cases of severe malnutrition in GSE can have a similar histologic picture. In the latter case, the presence of a severe mucosal lesion characteristic of GSE easily prevents confusion with abetalipoproteinemia.

Eosinophilic Gastroenteritis

Eosinophilic gastroenteritis (EG) includes a spectrum of diseases characterized by eosinophilic infiltration of one or more segments of the gastrointestinal tract, peripheral eosinophilia in some patients, and the frequent occurrence of a previous history of allergy or asthma.[112,175-177] This condition typically presents in children or young adults with symptoms related to the particular segment of bowel that is involved with disease. The stomach is the most common site of involvement,

followed by the duodenum, esophagus, jejunum, and ileum, which are involved in roughly equal numbers. Small bowel and gastric disease often occur together.[112] Following earlier descriptions, Klein categorized EG into three anatomic patterns based on the primary layer of the bowel wall that is infiltrated by eosinophils. These are the mucosal, mural, and serosal types (Table 9-4).[176]

CLINICAL FEATURES

Symptoms associated with mucosal involvement include gastrointestinal hemorrhage, nausea, vomiting, and diarrhea. Protein-losing enteropathy and other forms of malabsorption may occur as well in this type. Patients with primarily mural disease usually present with abdominal pain and symptoms of small bowel obstruction, such as nausea and vomiting. The serosal form often presents with ascites, as well as abdominal pain, nausea, and vomiting.

Once the condition has been accurately diagnosed, treatment consists of steroids. Surgical resection of obstructed segments of small bowel is frequently performed before diagnosis because it is often difficult to make a diagnosis by biopsy analysis if the mucosa is not involved or cannot be sampled. Although some diagnostic importance is given to the finding of peripheral eosinophilia, this may be absent in up to 25% of patients.[112]

PATHOGENESIS

The pathogenesis of EG remains unknown but may be different for the three types. Familial cases do occur,[178] but no specific genetic abnormalities or inheritance patterns have been identified. In some patients with mucosal disease, EG appears to be due to food allergy.[177,179] IgE is elevated in some as well. On the other hand, several studies have shown that the degree of

TABLE 9–4. Eosinophilic Gastroenteritis

Type	Clinical Characteristics	Pathology
Mucosal	Diarrhea, hemorrhage, protein-losing enteropathy	Mucosal eosinophils with degranulation, crypt abscesses, variable villous blunting
Mural	Abdominal pain, obstruction, nausea, and vomiting	Thickened wall, mural and subserosal eosinophilic infiltrates, edema; mucosa may be normal
Serosal	Abdominal pain, obstruction, ascites, nausea, and vomiting	Eosinophils and edema limited to serosa and subserosa, ascitic fluid with abundant eosinophils

From Klein NC, Hargrove RL, Sleisenger MH, et al: Eosinophilic gastroenteritis. Medicine 49:299-319, 1970.

tissue injury and the severity of symptoms are related to the degree of eosinophilic infiltration and to eosinophilic activation and degranulation.[178,180,181]

PATHOLOGIC FEATURES

Pathologic changes in EG depend on the anatomic location of disease.[176,180] Mucosal biopsies are frequently normal in the mural and serosal forms of disease; thus, the finding of normal mucosa in biopsies from patients suspected of having EG does not exclude a diagnosis of EG. In the mucosal type, an increase is seen in intact and degranulated eosinophils both in the lamina propria and infiltrating the epithelium (Fig. 9-15). Some biopsies may show eosinophilic crypt abscesses, surface erosion, or ulceration. The infiltrate can be severe and diffuse, or mild and patchy. Thus, biopsies from multiple sites are needed to detect the presence of mucosal disease.[112,177,178,180,182] In the small intestine, the mucosal architecture is usually normal, or it may show mild villous blunting. However, severe mucosal lesions (flat mucosa) have also rarely been reported.[177] In addition to the lamina propria, eosinophils may accumulate in the muscularis mucosae and the superficial submucosa. The density of eosinophils is often greatest in the deepest portion of the mucosa.

The pathology of the mural form of EG is characteristic. Resection specimens show thickening and induration of the intestinal wall on gross examination. Ulceration may be present.[112,183] Microscopically, prominent edema and a marked eosinophilic infiltrate are the hallmarks of mural EG. Submucosal edema is frequently prominent and may also extend into the muscle layer. As in mucosal biopsies, eosinophilic infiltration is usually of a severe degree but can be patchy. Dense eosinophilic infiltrates may extend into the subserosa (Fig. 9-16).[112,180,183,184] In some cases, edema

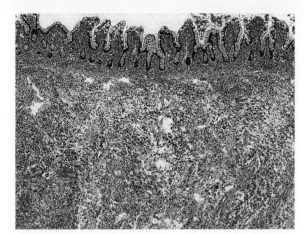

FIGURE 9–16. Eosinophilic gastroenteritis. In the mural form, edema and eosinophils extend into the submucosa and muscularis propria.

and eosinophils are limited to the subserosal layers; this is referred to as the "serosal" type. In this setting, the diagnosis can usually be made by ascitic fluid cytology.

DIFFERENTIAL DIAGNOSIS

The diagnosis of EG in resection specimens is usually straightforward. The differential diagnosis includes many other conditions that can lead to elevated tissue eosinophil levels, such as parasitic infections, vasculitis, and Crohn's disease. Parasites must be excluded by careful examination of tissue sections and by stool examination. In vasculitis, the inflammation tends to be centered within and around blood vessels, and ischemic changes may be present as well. Although clinical and radiologic confusion with Crohn's disease often occurs, the distinction from Crohn's disease is relatively simple in histologic sections. The differential diagnosis in mucosal biopsies is more difficult, especially if the stomach is not involved and the degree of eosinophilic infiltrate is patchy. However, certain features of Crohn's disease, such as focally enhanced neutrophilic exudates and granulomas, are never seen in EG. Occasionally, cases of GSE can be associated with increased mucosal eosinophils.[180] However, clinical correlation with serum autoantibodies and attention to the other characteristic features of GSE usually make distinction from EG straightforward. Of interest, the concurrent or subsequent development of GSE and dermatitis herpetiformis has been reported in patients with EG.[185]

◼ Nutritional Deficiencies

A variety of nutritional deficiencies may lead to characteristic morphologic abnormalities in the small intestine. Changes related to vitamin B_{12}, protein, zinc, and iron deficiencies are described here.

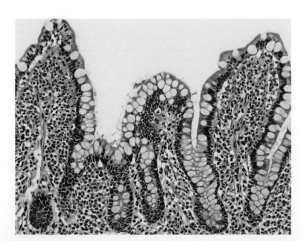

FIGURE 9–15. Eosinophilic gastroenteritis. The epithelium may not show significant injury. In other cases, the epithelium may be infiltrated by eosinophils, with the formation of crypt abscesses and ulceration.

VITAMIN B$_{12}$ DEFICIENCY

Vitamin B$_{12}$ deficiency, such as that due to pernicious anemia, is characterized by macrocytosis, a decrease in the number of mitoses, and villous blunting.[186,187] These changes, which are similar to those seen in folate deficiency, chemotherapy, and radiation, are reversed by B$_{12}$ administration. Tropical sprue may also result in B$_{12}$ deficiency and may show identical small intestinal pathology. After treatment, the mitotic rate has been shown to return to normal within several days, whereas the macrocytic and architectural changes take longer (approximately 2 months) to normalize. Vitamin B$_{12}$ is necessary for normal DNA synthesis. The mechanism by which B$_{12}$ deficiency leads to macrocytosis is thought to be impaired DNA synthesis and inhibition of cell division.[186] Of note, B$_{12}$ deficiency secondary to pernicious anemia rarely, if ever, is associated with evidence of malabsorption.

PROTEIN DEFICIENCY

Protein malnutrition, although rare in Western societies, remains an important cause of infant and child death in African and Asian countries. Kwashiorkor is a syndrome associated with low protein intake but normal or high caloric intake, and marasmus is a condition of both low protein and low caloric intake. Most patients also show concurrent parasitic infection or tropical sprue, which complicates the histologic picture.[188-190]

Pathologic features of untreated patients with kwashiorkor typically include mild to moderate villous blunting, increased mononuclear lymphocytes in the lamina propria, normal or mildly decreased mucosal width, cuboidalization of epithelial cells, and a decrease in the number of mitotic figures.[188-190] In some studies, Paneth cells are also decreased in number, and cytoplasmic lipid droplets are present in epithelial cells.[191] Interestingly, macrocytosis may be present and may reflect dietary folate deficiency. The overall appearance is similar to that of GSE. Changes vary from minimal to severe and correlate with the degree of protein malnutrition, but severe changes are uncommon.

Electron microscopic studies in malnutrition reveal abnormalities in the microvillous brush border, decreased endoplasmic reticulum, dilated cytoplasmic vesicles, and phagocytic vacuoles.[192] Functional studies have revealed a decrease in mucosal disaccharidase, as well as other enzyme activity that may contribute to nutrient malaborption.[188,189] The biopsy appearance in marasmus is less pronounced than that in kwashiorkor, despite a higher degree of caloric depletion. The mucosa is normally slightly thin with a marked decrease in mitotic rate. However, a near-normal crypt-to-villus ratio is usually seen.[190]

After therapy, one long-term study found a return to normal histology only after 4 to 10 years of protein supplementation.[189]

ACRODERMATITIS ENTEROPATHICA (ZINC DEFICIENCY)

Acrodermatitis enteropathica (AE) is a rare autosomal recessive syndrome characterized by the presence of dermatitis, alopecia, diarrhea, growth retardation, and depressed mental function in early childhood.[193] It occurs in all races and affects men and women equally. The discovery in 1973 that AE is caused by zinc deficiency has allowed for successful treatment of this once fatal condition by dietary supplementation with zinc sulfate.[194] It has since been determined that the basic defect in AE may be an abnormality in an intestinal oligopeptidase that cleaves zinc from an oligopeptide carrier. Thus, in AE, zinc remains bound to this peptide and is unavailable for absorption.[195]

Small bowel mucosal biopsies in patients with AE may be entirely normal. However, a number of studies have reported varying degrees of villous blunting, lamina propria inflammation, and edema.[193,196,197] In rare cases, flat lesions similar to those seen in GSE have been documented.[197] The degree of abnormality may reflect the severity of zinc deficiency at the time of biopsy. In any case, the histologic features are nonspecific. Several electron microscopic studies have revealed peculiar rhomboid and ovoid lysosomes within Paneth cells in AE.[196,198] These changes may be related to zinc deficiency; at least one study reported their disappearance following zinc replacement.[198]

IRON DEFICIENCY

Iron deficiency is a well-known result of malabsorption, such as that seen in GSE. However, iron deficiency itself may lead to mucosal injury and subsequent steatorrhea and malabsorption. In a study of 14 infants and children with iron deficiency anemia, in whom GSE had been excluded, duodenal biopsies revealed mild to moderate villous blunting and increased lamina propria inflammation in approximately 50% of patients.[199] The mechanism of injury is unknown but may be related to the role of iron in the normal metabolism of epithelial cells.[200]

◼ Intestinal Lymphangiectasia

Lymphangiectasia can be primary or secondary, the latter of which is common.

PRIMARY LYMPHANGIECTASIA

Clinical Features

Primary intestinal lymphangiectasia (PIL) is a rare congenital disorder characterized by severe protein loss (protein-losing enteropathy), peripheral edema, steatorrhea, chylous effusion, and lymphocytopenia.[201-203] Patients with this condition usually present in childhood or young adulthood. They require a specially formulated diet and occasionally steroids and/or TPN to control the amount of protein loss. Recently, octreotide has been used successfully to treat protein loss associated with PIL.[204]

The basis for this disease is a profound structural abnormality of the lymphatic system consisting of dilation and tortuosity of lymphatic channels that results in lymph stasis within the intestinal tract. These abnormalities may also occur in other sites, most notably the extremities. In addition to hypoalbuminemia, immunoglobulins and certain T-cell populations are selectively decreased, such that immune deficiency may occur.[205,206] For example, a susceptibility to cutaneous viral warts and lymphoma is associated with PIL.[207]

Pathologic Features

The endoscopic appearance has been well described.[201-203,208] At endoscopy, the length of small bowel involvement is variable, with both duodenal and jejunal disease common. A spectrum of visible lesions may be seen. Numerous minute white dots scattered throughout the mucosa ("white-tipped villi") are a common finding.[209] This appearance has been shown by electron microscopy to be due to chylomicron accumulation within surface enterocytes and in the lamina propria.[209] Larger white nodules, often measuring between 1 and 8 mm in size, may be scattered throughout the mucosa as well. Finally, larger, plaquelike, cystic or mass lesions may be present. On biopsy, chylous material may be noted to leak from open lesions. Lymphangiectasia is often patchy in distribution, so that multiple samples should be obtained to ensure adequate tissue for diagnosis.

Microscopic features of PIL include cystically dilated lacteals with minimal to moderate villous blunting, and edema of the lamina propria. Inflammation is not increased. In fact, there may be a decrease in the number of intraepithelial lymphocytes compared with the normal number.[205] Dilated lymphatic channels may extend into the deep mucosa and submucosa, and these can be seen throughout the bowel wall and serosa and in mesenteric lymph nodes (Fig. 9-17).[201,210] The lymphatic channels are lined by endothelium, and the spaces may appear optically clear or may contain foamy proteinaceous material and macrophages.[201-203] Electron microscopic studies have shown increased basal lamina, collagen, and supporting cells in the vicinity of dilated lymphatics.[211]

Differential Diagnosis

The differential diagnosis of PIL includes macroglobulinemia, Whipple's disease, and pneumatosis intestinalis. Immunoglobulin deposits in macroglobulinemia are densely eosinophilic, unlike the proteinaceous material seen in the dilated lymphatics of PIL. Immunohistochemical stains for IgM can also help in differentiating between these two entities. Whipple's disease results in more extensive macrophage infiltrates than are seen in PIL, and these are intensely PAS postive. The cysts in pneumatosis intestinalis lack a clearly defined endothelial lining and instead are usually lined by foreign body giant cells.

In addition to differentiating PIL from other specific diseases, care should be taken not to overinterpret the finding of focally dilated lymphatics, which often occur in mucosal biopsies in the normal population. In addition, tissue artifact may lead to the creation of a space (likely representing trapped air) immediately beneath the epithelial basement membrane of small bowel villi that can be mistaken for a dilated lymphatic. False spaces can be distinguished from true lymphatic vessels by the lack of a lining endothelium in the former.

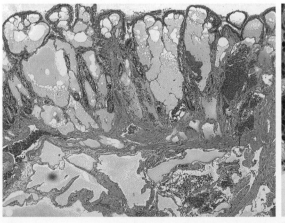
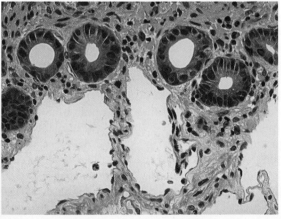

A **B**

FIGURE 9–17. Primary intestinal lymphangiectasia. **A,** Dilated lymphatic channels are present in the mucosa and throughout the bowel wall, including the serosa and draining lymph nodes. **B,** The dilated spaces are lined by endothelial cells.

SECONDARY LYMPHANGIECTASIA

Secondary lymphangiectasia refers to dilated lymphatics not associated with protein-losing enteropathy but instead related to either a local inflammatory or neoplastic process. These include lymphoma, carcinoma, Crohn's disease, systemic lupus erythematosus, Behçet's syndrome, and radiation therapy.[212-214] Clinical correlation with symptoms allows for the distinction between primary and secondary forms, and all secondary causes should be excluded before a consideration of PIL is made.

Waldenström's Macroglobulinemia

Waldenström's macroglobulinemia is an indolent lymphoproliferative disorder of B cells characterized by cells with plasma cell differentiation and the production and deposition of monoclonal IgM throughout the body (hyperviscosity syndrome).[215] Patients develop diarrhea and malabsorption secondary to IgM deposits within mucosal lymphatics.[216,217] Symptoms of intestinal involvement vary from mild to severe and can sometimes be the presenting complaint that ultimately leads to the correct diagnosis.

The endoscopic appearance of the small intestine is that of numerous gray/white granular mucosal nodules. On microscopy, a variable degree of "clubbing" and blunting of villi is seen, combined with a mildly increased lymphoplasmacellular infiltrate. The most striking histologic finding is the deposition of acellular, eosinophilic material within lymphatic channels in the tips of villi and in the base of the mucosa (Fig. 9-18). Foamy macrophages are also frequently present within the lamina propria. Occasional atypical lymphocytes may be seen as well.[216,217] Macroglobulinemia may be associated with diffuse lymphangiectasia, which in turn may cause malabsorption and protein-losing enteropathy. The

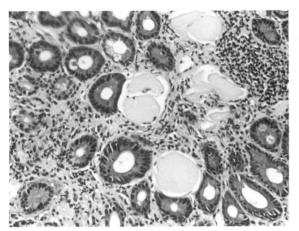

FIGURE 9–18. Waldenström's macroglobulinemia. Acellular monoclonal IgM deposits fill lymphatic channels.

amorphous deposits are PAS positive, diastase resistant, and Congo red negative and may be focally positive with Oil Red O. Immunohistochemical stains reveal strong diffuse positivity for IgM, with light chain restriction.[217] Deposits show a mixture of granular electron-dense material and lipid droplets on electron microscopy.[217] Amyloid and collagen fibrils are not normally present.

The differential diagnosis of Waldenström's macroglobulinemia in mucosal biopsies includes amyloidosis (which tends to accumulate around vessels and can be distinguished by Congo red stains), lymphangiectasia (which lacks the densely eosinophilic material within the lymphatic spaces), Whipple's disease and *Mycobacterium avium-intracellulare* infection (both of which can be distinguished by stains for organisms, electron microscopy, and PCR), and any other disorder that leads to macrophage accumulation.

Inflammatory Bowel Disease

CROHN'S DISEASE (see also Chapter 10)

Crohn's disease is an idiopathic chronic inflammatory condition that is distinguished from other inflammatory bowel diseases by the fact that it can involve any segment of the gastrointestinal tract and is characterized by transmural inflammation with frequent stricture and fistula formation, as well as the presence of noncaseating granulomas in approximately 50% of biopsy and resection specimens.

Epidemiology

Although much has been learned recently about the epidemiology and genetic associations of Crohn's disease, the underlying cause is still unknown and is beyond the scope of this textbook.[218] However, one significant recent discovery is the association between frameshift mutations in the *NOD2* gene, on chromosome 16, and increased susceptibility to Crohn's disease.[219,220]

Crohn's disease has a worldwide distribution but is more prevalent in Western countries. The annual incidence in northern Europe and North America has risen sharply in recent years and is now roughly 8 per 100,000 population. Genetic susceptibility has been demonstrated in both family and population studies, with a higher incidence in relatives of patients with Crohn's disease and in certain ethnic populations, such as Jews.[221] Most patients present in the second decade of life. However, a smaller, second peak also occurs in the eighth decade of life.[222] In this chapter, involvement of the small intestine is considered, with emphasis on the terminal ileum, the most common site of involvement, and the duodenum. A discussion of Crohn's colitis and its distinction from ulcerative colitis can be found in Chapter 10.

TABLE 9–5. Differential Diagnosis of Crohn's Disease in Small Intestine Biopsies

Terminal Ileum	Duodenum
NSAID injury	NSAID injury
Backwash ileitis	Peptic duodenitis
Yersinia infection	Eosinophilic gastroenteritis
Behçet's disease	Involvement by ulcerative colitis (rare)
Vasculitis/Ischemia	Infection
	Gluten-sensitive enteropathy

NSAID, nonsteroidal anti-inflammatory drug.

Pathologic Features

GROSS PATHOLOGY (Table 9-5)

Grossly, Crohn's disease of the small intestine is characterized by thickening of the bowel wall, strictures, fistula formation, and fat wrapping (Fig. 9-19).[223-226] The bowel wall is usually firm and stiff, owing to a combination of fat wrapping, submucosal fibrosis, and hypertrophy of the muscularis propria.[227,228] *Fat wrapping*, or "creeping fat," is the term used to describe adherence of mesenteric adipose tissue to the intestinal wall, in part or in whole. This finding is usually associated with transmural inflammation in the underlying bowel segment, and there is evidence to suggest a role of adipocytes in the secretion of inflammatory mediators.[229,230] Fat wrapping is frequently found in association with stiff, "hose pipe" strictures of the involved segment of bowel. Bowel loops frequently adhere to one another via mesenteric fat. When this occurs, fistula tracts can extend from one segment to another or to other abdominal organs. It is especially common to find a diseased segment adherent to a normal segment of bowel. Enlarged mesenteric lymph nodes are usually noted as well.

The mucosal surface in Crohn's disease shows a variety of changes that may be seen radiologically, endoscopically, or surgically.[223-226] The earliest change consists of aphthous lesions, which are tiny erosions that develop over lymphoid aggregates and are frequently seen in the ileum but can occur anywhere in the gut.[231] As the inflammatory process worsens, aphthous lesions tend to coalesce and deepen, forming bearclaw-shaped ulcers. With progression of disease, longitudinal ulcerations and crevices often develop, which tend to outline areas of uninvolved mucosa and give rise to a "cobblestone" appearance of the mucosa, as well as inflammatory "pseudopolyps" (see Fig. 9-19**C**). Knifelike fissures that penetrate into or through the muscularis propria often develop with time.[228] Intramural and mesenteric abscess cavities and sinus tracts may also

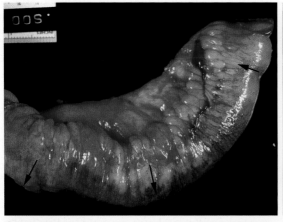

A

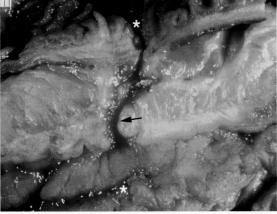

B

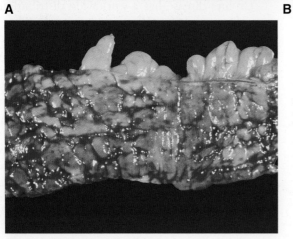

C

FIGURE 9–19. Crohn's disease. **A,** Fat wrapping *(arrows)* is prominent in this case. **B,** In this example, two segments of intestine (*★*) are connected by a fistula tract *(arrow).* **C,** The mucosal surface may exhibit a cobblestone appearance, characterized by the presence of serpiginous, anastomosing ulcers outlining islands of residual intact mucosa.

develop in advanced cases. Skip areas of involvement are characteristic of Crohn's disease. One often sees an abrupt transition between grossly involved and uninvolved segments. The presence of mucosal ulceration at surgical margins should be noted in pathology reports because this finding may portend a high risk of recurrence at the surgical anastomosis.[229]

MICROSCOPIC PATHOLOGY

Varying degrees of active (neutrophilic) inflammation and chronic inflammatory changes (architectural distortion, chronic inflammation, fibrosis, stromal hypertrophy) are usually present in some, or all, layers of the bowel wall (Table 9-6).

Aphthous lesions in the mucosa consist of a small surface erosion associated with a neutrophilic infiltrate (Fig. 9-20**A**).[232,233] They frequently occur in epithelium overlying lymphoid aggregates and are often surrounded by normal mucosa. In the earliest stage, neutrophils infiltrate the base of a single crypt and protrude into the lumen. Fissuring ulceration, which develops in more advanced cases, begins at the base of aphthous ulcers and extends into the deeper layers of the bowel wall (Fig. 9-20**B** and **C**). In addition to aphthous lesions, the mucosa in Crohn's disease shows other chronic and active changes, such as increased lymphocytes, plasma cells, crypt architectural irregularity, and neutrophilic infiltrates. Of note, cryptitis and increased neutrophils within the lamina propria are more common than are true crypt abscesses. Hyperplasia of Paneth cells and pseudopyloric metaplasia (mucous gland metaplasia) within the deep mucosa are also frequently present.[234]

TABLE 9–6. Characteristic Pathologic Features of Crohn's Disease*

Gross Pathology	Microscopic Pathology
Serosal	Aphthous lesions
Fat wrapping	Crypt architectural irregularity
Wall stiffness	Increased lymphocytes and plasma cells
Adhesions to other structures	Neutrophilic cryptitis, crypt abscesses
	Pseudopyloric metaplasia
Fistulas	Submucosal fibrosis
Strictures	Neuronal and muscular hypertrophy
Mucosal	Noncaseating granulomas
Aphthous lesions	Fissuring ulcers, sinus tracts
Cobblestone appearance	Transmural lymphoid aggregates
Serpiginous and "bearclaw" ulcers	Vasculitis

*Segmental involvement is characteristic.

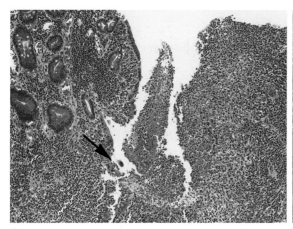

A

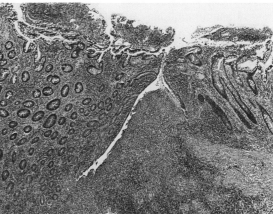

B

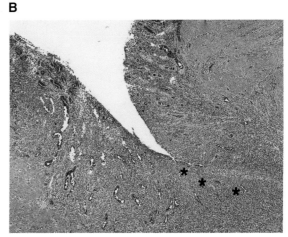

C

FIGURE 9–20. Crohn's disease–aphthous ulcer. **A,** Aphthous ulcers are small erosions associated with a neutrophilic infiltrate *(arrow).* They frequently occur on the surfaces of lymphoglandular complexes. **B,** Early fissures often develop, initially from the base of an aphthous ulcer. **C,** An early fissuring ulcer extends into the submucosa (⋆).

The latter refers to a proliferation of small glands lined by cells that contain clear mucin, similar to those seen in the gastric antrum. A marked variation in the degree of morphologic changes, even within one involved segment of bowel, is a hallmark of Crohn's disease. When present in resection specimens, the mucosal changes described here are typically patchy.

Mural changes in Crohn's disease, loosely called *transmural inflammation*, consist of a myriad of findings. Deep, flask-shaped or knifelike (fissure) ulcers may extend into the submucosa or muscularis propria in a haphazard, irregular fashion and are associated with acute and chronic inflammation, granulation tissue, edema, and fibrosis. Neuronal and smooth muscle hypertrophy within the submucosa and muscularis propria are common. Deep fissuring ulcers are often lined by abundant histiocytes and/or foreign body giant cells, which should not be mistaken for granulomas. One feature that is characteristic of Crohn's disease is the presence of transmural lymphoid aggregates, with or without germinal centers that may be present anywhere in the bowel wall, from the mucosa to the subserosa. A frequent observation in resection specimens is referred to as "the string of beads" (or "rosary" sign) of Crohn's disease. This refers to a linear distribution of lymphoid aggregates in the submucosa and subserosa commonly seen in this disease (Fig. 9-21).[223-226]

Non-necrotizing granulomas are also a characteristic finding in Crohn's disease. However, some granulomas may show a small amount of central necrosis. Granulomas are found in 50% to 60% of resection specimens[223,235,236] and in approximately 35% of biopsy specimens (Fig. 9-22).[223,236,237] They may be found in any segment of the intestine, including uninvolved areas, and may be located throughout the bowel wall, from mucosa to serosa. Regional lymph nodes contain granulomas in up to 40% of cases.[223,235] Granulomas may vary in size and shape, ranging from small, loose collections of epithelioid cells to large, well-formed granulomas with giant cells. The latter frequently are surrounded by a rim of lymphocytes. Special stains to exclude infection should be used in cases that show unusual clinical or histologic features, or in cases in which the granulomas are necrotic.

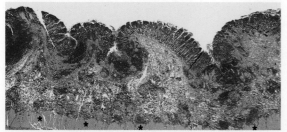

FIGURE 9–21. Crohn's disease. Transmural lymphoid aggregates are a hallmark of Crohn's disease (*). They frequently form a string-of-beads appearance at the junction of the muscularis propria and the subserosa.

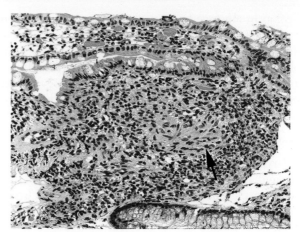

FIGURE 9–22. Crohn's disease. A small collection of epithelioid histiocytes is seen in this mucosal biopsy *(arrow)*.

Vascular changes are common in Crohn's disease as well. The changes observed in mural vessels include endothelial injury, intimal proliferation, thrombosis, and rarely, granulomatous or fibrinoid vasculitis.[238,239] Most of these changes have been observed in arterioles that are located adjacent to or underneath areas of ulceration. Granulomas may also occur in a perivascular distribution. These findings have led some authors to suggest that vasculitis may be an important mechanism of injury in Crohn's disease.[238,239]

Features in Biopsy Specimens

Although a diagnosis of Crohn's disease can usually be made in resection specimens, evaluation of biopsy specimens from the small intestine may be difficult owing to the lack of specificity of the inflammatory changes (see Table 9-5). The histologic features of Crohn's disease in terminal ileal biopsies vary with the severity of disease and the site of biopsy (Fig. 9-23). Characteristic features include increased acute and chronic inflammation in the lamina propria, neutrophilic cryptitis and crypt abscesses, and surface erosion or ulceration, as well as features of chronic injury, such as pseudopyloric metaplasia, crypt and villous architectural changes (atrophy, branching, cystic change), fibrosis, and granulomas. These changes often occur in a patchy or segmental fashion. Severe inflammation, ulceration, and features of chronicity serve to differentiate Crohn's disease of the ileum from "backwash" ileitis associated with severe fulminant ulcerative colitis (see Chapter 10 for further discussion).

Duodenal Crohn's Disease

Duodenal involvement in Crohn's disease is rare (noted in 1% to 7% of cases).[240,241] However, the incidence of involvement is on the rise, which is probably related to the growing use of upper endoscopy as a diagnostic tool. Most patients with involvement of the

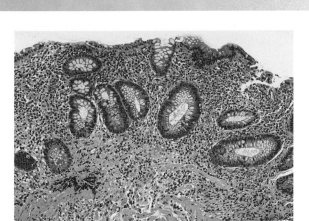

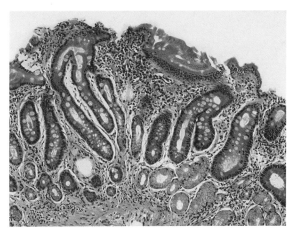

FIGURE 9–23. Crohn's disease. Inflammatory changes in the terminal ileum of a patient with Crohn's disease. Findings include architectural distortion, villous blunting, and increased plasmacellular inflammation. Granulomas are found in only a minority of biopsies.

FIGURE 9–24. Crohn's disease. Duodenal involvement by Crohn's disease may be difficult to distinguish from peptic or NSAID injury. In this patient with both ileal and gastroduodenal Crohn's disease, mild architectural distortion and increased lamina propria inflammation can be seen.

duodenal bulb also have involvement of the gastric antrum. However, distal duodenal involvement is not always associated with gastric involvement.[239-244] The vast majority of patients with duodenal involvement have distal ileal or colonic disease. Rarely, the duodenum is the only site involved by Crohn's disease.[240-242,245]

The clinical manifestations of proximal small bowel Crohn's disease are similar to those of distal disease. Symptoms are usually related to ulceration and stricture formation and include epigastric pain, hemorrhage, nausea, and vomiting. Of note, many Crohn's patients without upper gastrointestinal tract symptoms show endoscopic and histologic evidence of involvement. In two studies, histologic involvement of the duodenum or stomach was found in 24% and 64% of patients without symptoms.[241,244]

The endoscopic findings of proximal Crohn's disease are variable. Asymptomatic patients frequently have small aphthous lesions, whereas symptomatic patients may show granularity, a cobblestone mucosal pattern, linear ulcerations, and stricture formation.[241-243]

Histologic findings in the proximal intestine are similar to those in distal disease. Noncaseating granulomas have been reported in only 7% to 15% of duodenal biopsies[241-243,246] but in up to 75% of resection specimens from this area.[240] Granulomas may be found in endoscopically normal mucosa as well. Because granulomas are relatively uncommon in proximal small bowel biopsies, the diagnosis frequently relies on the presence of other chronic inflammatory changes (Fig. 9-24). These include increased lymphocytes, plasma cells, and eosinophils; basal plasmacytosis; crypt architectural irregularity; and cryptitis and crypt abscesses with or without surface erosions or ulceration. Severe villous blunting is rare, but patchy architectural distortion may be present.[240-244] One study of 49 patients reported that

acute inflammation within otherwise normal small bowel mucosa was seen only in Crohn's disease, not in *H. pylori*–related gastritis.[246] Thus, a diagnosis of duodenal involvement by Crohn's disease relies heavily on the finding of patchy or segmental inflammatory changes, with or without granulomas, in patients without another obvious cause of inflammation (such as peptic injury). Most patients have concomitant distal disease.

Differential Diagnosis

In the ileum, Behçet's disease and vasculitis may in rare cases resemble Crohn's disease. Behçet's disease of the gastrointestinal tract is rare in Western countries, occurs primarily in Asians, and is frequently associated with generalized thrombosis and large genital ulcers. This condition can be difficult to distinguish from Crohn's disease based on histologic analysis because small erosions and superficial ulcers of the terminal ileum may occur in both diseases. However, strictures and sinus tracts do not occur in Behçet's disease, and clinical information often helps in separating these two entities. Other forms of vasculitis can be distinguished from Crohn's disease by the predominant vascular and perivascular location of the inflammatory response, the presence of ischemic changes, and the clinical history of a generalized vasculitic syndrome.

Backwash ileitis in ulcerative pancolitis is uncommon and can be distinguished from Crohn's disease primarily by the lack of severe activity or chronic inflammatory changes in the former (Fig. 9-25). *Yersinia* infection may cause appendicitis and ileocolitis that may also resemble Crohn's disease histologically (see Chapter 3).[247] In biopsy specimens, nonsteroidal anti-inflammatory drug (NSAID)-induced injury may resemble Crohn's disease. However, once again, chronic pathologic changes

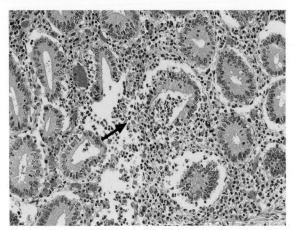

FIGURE 9–25. Backwash ileitis. As shown in this resection, backwash ileitis consists of a mild influx of neutrophils within the lamina propria and/or epithelium *(arrow)*. The villous architecture is normal.

such as crypt irregularity and lymphoplasmacytic infiltrates are less common in NSAID injury. However, because aphthous lesions may occur with NSAID injury, it is prudent to recommend a trial of NSAID removal before making a definitive diagnosis of Crohn's disease in equivocal cases (see Table 9-5).

In the proximal small intestine, other less common mimickers of Crohn's disease include peptic duodenitis, eosinophilic gastroenteritis, GSE, and infectious enteritis (see Table 9-5).

DUODENAL INVOLVEMENT BY ULCERATIVE COLITIS

Several recent studies have reported the presence of chronic active inflammation in the duodenum and/or stomach in patients with ulcerative colitis.[248-252] However, this is controversial because long-term follow-up is ultimately needed if Crohn's disease is to be definitively ruled out in these patients. Nevertheless, pathologically, these cases have been reported to show mild to moderate chronic inflammation, with or without neutrophils, in the lamina propria in biopsies obtained from the first and second portions of the duodenum.[248,252] Others may show diffuse inflammation with crypt and villous architectural distortion, basal plasmacytosis, and crypt abscesses involving the duodenum and, occasionally, the ileum and jejunum (see also Chapter 10).[250]

PNEUMATOSIS CYSTOIDES INTESTINALIS

Pneumatosis cystoides intestinalis refers to the accumulation of gas-filled cysts within the wall of the intestine and may occur at any site in the gastrointestinal tract. It frequently occurs in the setting of an underlying intestinal disease, such as inflammatory bowel disease, neonatal necrotizing enterocolitis, infectious

colitis or enteritis, or diverticulosis. It also occurs in association with a variety of pulmonary diseases, such as cystic fibrosis and chronic obstructive lung disease. Pathologically, the entity is characterized by the presence of empty cysts, lined by macrophages and giant cells within the submucosa and subserosa. This disorder is discussed in greater detail in Chapter 10.

PEPTIC DUODENITIS–DUODENAL ULCER

Peptic duodenitis and duodenal ulcer, once considered separate disease entities, are now recognized to represent two ends of the spectrum of peptic injury.[253,254] In fact, the proximal duodenum may be viewed as an extension of the gastric antrum but without the protective coating of mucus and bicarbonate-secreting surface cells. The duodenal bulb, in particular, is physiologically exposed to a higher acid content than is the rest of the small intestine. In the setting of increased gastric acid secretion, such as occurs in antral predominant *H. pylori* gastritis, duodenal inflammation and ulceration may occur. An extreme version of peptic injury is seen in Zollinger-Ellison syndrome, in which ulceration and diffuse Brunner's gland hyperplasia also involve the distal duodenum and jejunum.[255]

The current understanding of the pathophysiology of peptic duodenitis is that chronic exposure to acid induces both gastric surface metaplasia and hyperplasia of Brunner's glands in the duodenal bulb.[254,256-261] In patients with *H. pylori* gastritis, foci of gastric surface metaplasia may become colonized with bacteria and incite an inflammatory response that can lead to ulceration.[254,260-262] This hypothesis is strongly supported by the fact that a vast majority (95% to 100%) of duodenal ulcers occur in patients with *H. pylori* gastritis, and by the finding that duodenal ulcers heal faster and recur less frequently following eradication of the *H. pylori* organism.[260,263,264]

Studies by Kreuning and coworkers were among the first to document the presence of duodenitis in asymptomatic volunteers.[253,256] Patients with dyspepsia are more likely to have moderate to severe duodenitis or duodenal ulcer.[253] In addition, a high proportion of asymptomatic (64%) and symptomatic (94%) patients have foci of gastric surface metaplasia and prominent mucosal Brunner's glands in duodenal bulb biopsies.[253,256] Rarely, fundic gland heterotopia, found less frequently than gastric surface metaplasia in duodenal biopsies, may also be associated with the development of duodenitis and duodenal ulcer.[254,260,265]

Pathologic Features

Peptic duodenitis is characterized by three features, all of which may vary in severity—increased plasma cell infiltration, neutrophils in the lamina propria and/or epithelium, and reactive epithelial changes, including villous blunting.[253,254,256,259] Gastric surface metaplasia is not always used as an absolute criterion for peptic duodenitis because it may be found in cases without inflammation and thus may simply represent an adaptive response to chronic acid exposure.[254] However, most cases of peptic duodenitis show extensive gastric surface metaplasia, which can be highlighted with a PAS stain (Fig. 9-26). The distribution of changes is often extremely patchy and thus can be missed as a result of sampling error.

In mild cases, one may see nearly normal mucosa with a borderline increase in plasma cells and subtle reactive epithelial changes. These changes are not usually associated with symptoms and thus may be "physiologic."[253,254,256] In moderately active peptic duodenitis, the epithelium is infiltrated by neutrophils and shows mucin depletion, a syncytial growth pattern, and more marked reactive epithelial changes such as nuclear hyperchromasia and increased mitoses. Surface cells containing abundant PAS-positive mucin (gastric surface metaplasia) are usually easily identifiable. Brunner's glands are hyperplastic and, as a result, may be present above the level of the muscularis mucosae. Severe cases show erosion or ulceration. If the ulcer is indeed due to peptic injury, concomitant *H. pylori* gastritis is frequently present.[260,262]

Differential Diagnosis

The pathologic changes in peptic duodenitis are nonspecific. NSAID injury, Crohn's disease, celiac disease, and many infections may have a similar histologic appearance. Clinical correlation and stains for organisms (including *H. pylori*) should be performed to help differentiate these conditions. However, the degree of gastric surface metaplasia combined with prominent Brunner's glands, especially in a patient with documented *H. pylori*

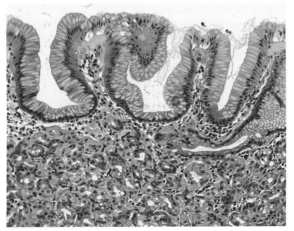

FIGURE 9–26. Peptic duodenitis secondary to heterotopia. This case includes both gastric mucuous cells and oxyntic glands.

gastritis, often helps in establishing a diagnosis of peptic duodenitis.

▮ Radiation- and Drug-Induced Enteritis

RADIATION INJURY

The gastrointestinal tract is exquisitely sensitive to radiation. In fact, the small intestine is the most sensitive portion of the gut, followed by the stomach, colon, and esophagus.[266-269] Radiation injury related to therapeutic use can be subdivided into acute and chronic forms.

Acute Radiation Injury

In the acute stage, the clinical symptoms related to small intestinal involvement include diarrhea, abdominal pain, and bloating. This syndrome, frequently called *radiation enteritis*, occurs in 20% to 70% of exposed patients[270] and can appear within hours after exposure. However, biopsies are not usually obtained at this stage unless the clinical features suggest that other conditions such as opportunistic infections may be involved. The earliest histologic changes occur in the surface and crypt epithelium, which show mitotic arrest, nuclear enlargement, and hyperchromasia, as well as flattening and separation of cells.[271] Increased numbers of apoptotic bodies in the crypts are typical.[272,273] Ultrastructurally, loss of microvilli, vacuolization of endoplasmic reticulum, and other changes have been noted.[274]

After 7 to 14 days of therapy, the epithelial surface is reduced in area by approximately 40%,[271,275] and one sees villous blunting, crypt hypoplasia, and a marked decrease in the number of lymphocytes in the lamina propria. Ulceration can occur at this stage and may be widespread if exposure is continued. In addition to the epithelial changes, endothelial cells are similarly damaged, which results in increased permeability and submucosal edema.[268,269] The acute syndrome is transient; symptoms and histologic changes usually resolve within several weeks after cessation of radiation.

The most important differential diagnosis in the setting of acute radiation therapy is opportunistic infection. Special stains and cultures should be used to exclude infections in these as in all other immunocompromised patients. In addition, the degree of epithelial atypia often present in acute radiation injury may occasionally be mistaken for dysplasia if the clinical history is unknown.

Chronic Radiation Injury

Chronic radiation injury develops years after radiation exposure, regardless of the presence and severity of previous acute radiation injury. The incidence of chronic radiation injury is approximately 5%.[268,269] Some studies cite an incidence rate as high as 36%.[276,277] Clinical symptoms are variable but usually consist of chronic ulceration, stricture formation, or perforation. The symptoms are related to long-term, irreversible pathologic changes within mesenchymal tissue combined with the subsequent development of vascular insufficiency. Epithelial and villous architectural changes usually return to normal after acute radiation injury, whereas stromal cells, especially fibroblasts, and endothelial cells undergo a variety of persistent changes. Enlargement of fibroblasts with expansion and vacuolization of their cytoplasm, as well as an increase in nuclear size, and hyperchromasia are common. Although the cells increase in size, typically the nucleus-to-cytoplasm ratio stays within the normal range.[278,279] Submucosal fibrosis and, occasionally, fibrosis of the muscularis propria may be present as well (Fig. 9-27**A** and **B**). Intimal proliferation of small and medium-sized arteries, with partial or total occlusion of the vascular lumen, is a frequent finding in

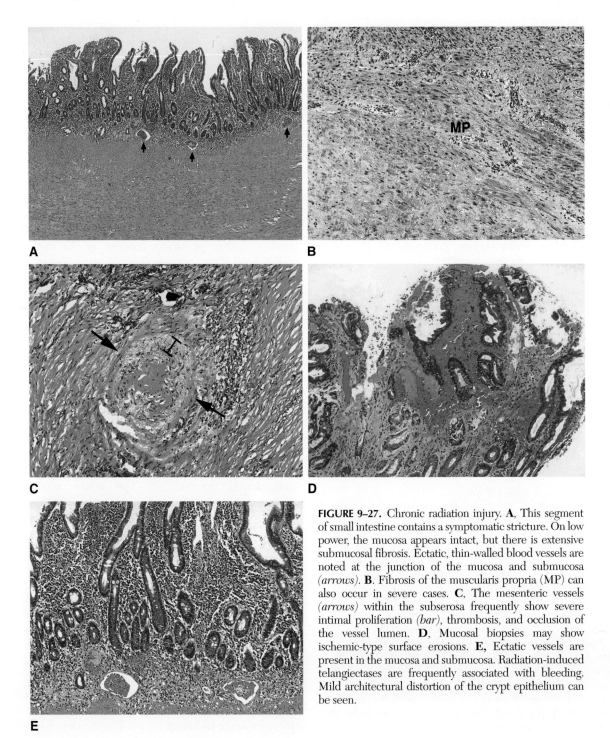

FIGURE 9–27. Chronic radiation injury. **A,** This segment of small intestine contains a symptomatic stricture. On low power, the mucosa appears intact, but there is extensive submucosal fibrosis. Ectatic, thin-walled blood vessels are noted at the junction of the mucosa and submucosa (*arrows*). **B.** Fibrosis of the muscularis propria (MP) can also occur in severe cases. **C,** The mesenteric vessels (*arrows*) within the subserosa frequently show severe intimal proliferation (*bar*), thrombosis, and occlusion of the vessel lumen. **D,** Mucosal biopsies may show ischemic-type surface erosions. **E,** Ectatic vessels are present in the mucosa and submucosa. Radiation-induced telangiectases are frequently associated with bleeding. Mild architectural distortion of the crypt epithelium can be seen.

surgical specimens removed secondary to stricture formation; it often leads to ischemic changes in the overlying mucosa (Fig. 9-27**C**).[278,280] Mucosal biopsies taken from strictured segments may show ulceration, mucosal fibrosis, crypt branching, and inflammation (Fig. 9-27**D**). Although these findings are nonspecific, they are compatible with chronic radiation injury in the proper clinical setting.

Mucosal telangiectases can also develop as a long-term sequela of radiation therapy (Fig. 9-27**E**).[279,281] They may be missed on histologic examination because these thin-walled vessels frequently collapse following biopsy.

CHEMOTHERAPY INJURY

Chemotherapy agents can cause acute enteritis.[282,283] The histologic changes seen in small intestinal biopsies after chemotherapy are similar to those seen in acute radiation injury. Biopsies taken shortly after chemotherapy show reactive nuclear and cytologic atypia and macrocytosis (Fig. 9-28). These changes reflect an arrest of maturation, which occurs within hours following administration of the drug.[284,285] Mitotic figures are usually decreased, and an increase in apoptotic bodies is noted in epithelial crypts, along with villous blunting, which may be severe. Necrosis of crypt epithelium may follow, with the development of surface erosions. These changes are transient, and the mucosa usually returns to normal within a few weeks after cessation of treatment.

Graft-Versus-Host Disease

Acute and chronic graft-versus-host disease (GVHD) occurs in the setting of bone marrow transplantation and, rarely, in heart transplant patients. In this disorder, donor cytotoxic T lymphocytes incite an immunologic reaction to certain host cells. The gastrointestinal tract is a common site of injury; epithelial apoptosis, gland destruction and loss, and surface erosions develop and are associated with gastrointestinal symptoms (Fig. 9-29). Acute and chronic forms of GVHD likely occur via different mechanisms. This disorder is discussed in detail in Chapters 4 and 10.

Nonsteroidal Anti-inflammatory Drug–Induced Enteropathy

CLINICAL FEATURES

Gastrointestinal toxicity as a result of the use of NSAIDs is an increasingly common occurrence, causing up to 20,000 hospital admissions per annum in the United States.[286,287] Ulceration of the stomach and proximal duodenum due to NSAIDs has long been recognized.[288] However, it has only recently been recognized that the distal small bowel and colon may also ulcerate as a result of NSAID use.[289-291] The term *NSAID enteropathy* has been used to describe this condition. Patients may present with persistent iron deficiency anemia despite the absence of gastroduodenal involvement.[289,290] The incidence of small bowel inflammation and ulceration has been reported to be as high as 46% to 70% in long-term NSAID users.[291] A more modest increase was found in an autopsy series wherein 8.4% of patients previously taking NSAIDs had jejunal or ileal ulcers, compared with 0.6% among controls.[289]

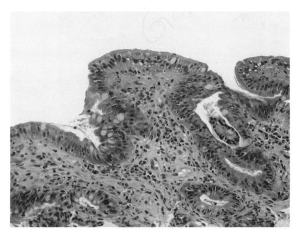

FIGURE 9–28. Chemotherapy injury. Small bowel biopsies obtained shortly after chemotherapy often reveal villous blunting, nuclear enlargement, and cytoplasmic basophilia. A decrease in mitotic activity is seen, caused by an arrest of cell proliferation. No significant inflammation is noted.

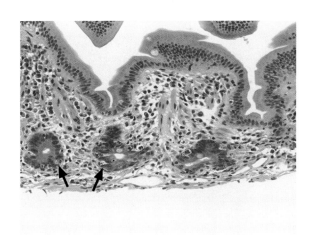

FIGURE 9–29. Graft-versus-host disease. This biopsy shows mild GVHD characterized by an increased number of apoptotic epithelial cells within the crypts (*arrows*). No increase is seen in the amount of inflammation, architectural distortion, or villous blunting.

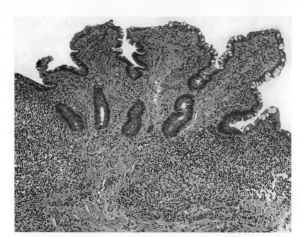

FIGURE 9–30. NSAID injury. In this terminal ileum biopsy, marked expansion of the lamina propria is noted, with occasional crypts containing neutrophils.

PATHOGENESIS

The cause of NSAID enteropathy is poorly understood. However, patients on NSAIDs show increased mucosal permeability secondary to cellular injury and loss of tight junction function.[290,292,293] This may allow for infiltration of luminal antigens, bile, and bacterial products, which in turn may be followed by an inflammatory response.

PATHOLOGIC FEATURES

A spectrum of histologic changes may occur in the small bowel as a result of NSAID injury. Mild lesions consist of superficial erosions with nonspecific neutrophilic and plasmacytic infiltrates (Fig. 9-30).[294-296] Erosions are frequently multiple and can progress to form deep ulcers, which may cause severe hemorrhage.[297] In one surgical study of 11 patients who underwent emergent small bowel resection for NSAID-induced ulceration, ulcers were confined to the ileum in 8 and the jejunum in 11 and were multiple in 50% of cases.[297] The ability to obtain jejunal biopsies during push enteroscopy has led to the documentation of more subtle changes, including mild villous blunting in some cases.[298] However, severe, diffuse villous blunting has not been reported in NSAID injury.

A rare but more distinctive form of NSAID enteropathy is referred to as "diaphragm" disease (Fig. 9-31).[299,300] This condition involves numerous thin, weblike mucosal septa that project into the lumen and cause significant narrowing and obstruction. The mid small intestine and the ileum are the preferred sites of involvement. Mucosal diaphragms consist of mucosa with reactive epithelial changes, with or without surface erosions, and prominent submucosal fibrosis. The bands of fibrous tissue are characteristically oriented perpendicular to the surface of the mucosa. Mild chronic inflammation is usually present. The fibrosis is thought to be due to recurrent

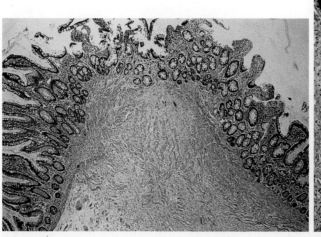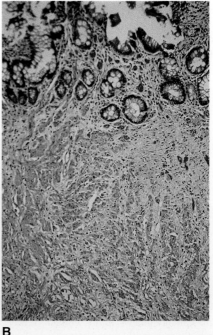

A   **B**

FIGURE 9–31. NSAID injury. **A**, Low-power view of NSAID-induced "diaphragm" disease. This is a cross section through one of the thin fibrous septa that form the luminal diaphragm. Submucosal fibrosis is prominent. **B**, High-power view shows a slightly disorganized mucosa, with reactive changes and submucosal fibrosis.

ulceration and scarring. These "diaphragms" are fairly specific for NSAID injury. However, other conditions such as radiation/chemotherapy, chronic ischemia, and Crohn's disease should be considered in the differential diagnosis.

DIFFERENTIAL DIAGNOSIS

The differential diagnosis of NSAID injury includes peptic and *H. pylori*–induced duodenitis, Crohn's disease, and, rarely, infections such as *Giardia*. The lack of specificity of the histologic changes seen in some of the previously discussed entities can cause diagnostic dilemmas, especially in biopsies of the terminal ileum, wherein the distinction between NSAID injury and Crohn's disease has significant clinical implications. Aphthous lesions may occur in both diseases, but significant plasma cell infiltrates, crypt distortion, and pseudopyloric metaplasia are much less commonly seen in NSAID injury. In the upper gastrointestinal tract, gastric biopsies help to distinguish between *H. pylori* and NSAID injury. In addition, peptic duodenitis, which is frequently associated with marked gastric surface metaplasia in the duodenum, is not specifically associated with NSAID injury. It must be emphasized that appropriate clinical information is important in helping to differentiate these other disorders.

▆ Ileal-Anal Pouch Inflammation (Pouchitis)

CLINICAL FEATURES

Pouchitis is a syndrome defined by the presence of inflammation in the pouch mucosa associated with clinical signs and symptoms and with endoscopic abnormalities. Many clinicians diagnose pouchitis exclusively on the basis of clinical criteria, reserving endoscopic examination, with biopsy, for patients with chronic refractory pouchitis or for those with possible Crohn's disease involving the pouch.

Pouchitis is the most common complication of ileal pouch anal anastomosis (IPAA), the procedure of choice for the surgical management of patients with chronic ulcerative colitis (CUC)[301-304] Pouchitis has also been reported in Kock's continent ileostomies, but this is a poorly understood entity. Pouchitis occurs almost exclusively in patients with CUC.[303] It is uncommon in patients who have had an IPAA procedure for familial adenomatous polyposis.[303,304]

The incidence of pouchitis varies significantly. However, it is well known that the incidence of pouchitis increases proportionally to the length of follow-up. Approximately 50% of patients who have had an IPAA procedure experience at least one episode of pouchitis. In one study, the risk of pouchitis was 80% 1 year after surgery and 48% 10 years after surgery.[302] Interestingly, the incidence of pouchitis decreases dramatically after the first 6 months after surgery. Nevertheless, despite the overall incidence of pouchitis, pouch excision is necessary in less than 1% of patients.[301]

Patients with pouchitis usually present with an increased frequency of bowel movements, with or without bloodly diarrhea, tenesmus, low-grade fever, malaise, and anorexia. Occasionally, patients develop anal fissures, perianal abscesses, strictures, and fistulas, all of which should raise a strong suspicion of an alternative diagnosis such as Crohn's disease involving the pouch.

PATHOGENESIS

A variety of risk factors have been associated with the development of pouchitis.[305,306] Some of these include the extent of inflammation, the presence of extraintestinal manifestations, tobacco smoking, serum positivity for antineutrophil cytoplasmic antibodies (p-ANCA), and the presence of primary sclerosing cholangitis. Recent studies also suggest that severe panulcerative colitis and the presence of ulcerating appendicitis associated with CUC may also increase the risk of development of pouchitis after surgery.[306]

The etiology of pouchitis is essentially unknown.[301,307] Some support the theory that pouchitis represents a form of CUC that has developed (or recurred) within pouch mucosa. Others suggest that various immunologic alterations, combined with stasis of luminal contents, represents the initial inciting events that may, in turn, affect the balance of the bacterial flora and the metabolism of the ileal reservoir. Finally, a deficiency of epithelial nutrients, such as a lower concentration of various short-chain fatty acids, has been documented in patients with pouchitis. It has been proposed that a lack of mucosal nutrients caused by an increase in pouch output and a subsequent dilution of intraluminal sugars can lead to a reduction in the availability of various short-chain fatty acids (butyrate, glutamine) that are necessary for cell metabolism.

PATHOLOGIC FEATURES

Grossly, the most frequent findings in pouchitis are erythema, edema, granularity and friability, loss of vascular pattern, hemorrhage, and superficial erosions and ulcerations. Rarely, pseudomembranes may develop as well. The presence of fissures, fistulas, sinus tracts and/or deep bearclaw ulcers, or fissuring ulcers should raise a strong suspicion that the pouchitis is due to recurrent Crohn's disease.

Microscopically, pouchitis may be classified as active, chronic, or chronic-active. Typical findings include a mixed neutrophilic and lymphocytic infiltrate in the lamina propria and epithelium, either with or without

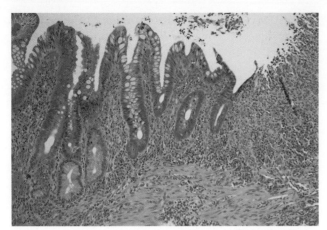

FIGURE 9–32. Example of chronic idiopathic pouchitis in a patient who had an IPAA procedure for severe panulcerative colitis. The biopsy shows acute and chronic inflammation, villous atrophy, ulceration, and a focus of pseudo-pyloric metaplasia.

erosions or ulcerations.[301,308,309] Mild to moderate villous atrophy is common. However, severe cases may show complete villous atrophy. Chronic changes, such as crypt and villous distortion; pseudo-pyloric metaplasia; crypt hyperplasia; expansion of the lamina propria by a mixed inflammatory infiltrate composed of lymphocytes, eosinophils, plasma cells, and histiocytes; and Paneth cell hyperplasia are common in severe cases and, particularly, in recurrent cases (Fig. 9-32). Granulomas, either necrotizing or, more commonly, non-necrotizing, may be present and do not necessarily indicate a definite diagnosis of Crohn's disease, because granulomas may be related to mucin, foreign material (e.g., sutures), and infectious agents as well. Rarely, dysplasia and even adenocarcinoma may develop in pouch mucosa.[310] In 1994, Sandborn and colleagues developed a pouchitis disease activity index (PDAI), which combines information from clinical, endoscopic, and histologic findings, but it is not widely used in clinical practice.[311] Most ileal pouches undergo an early adaptive response to the new luminal environment, characterized by a mild neutrophilic and eosinophilic inflammatory infiltrate in the lamina propria, partial villous atrophy, Paneth cell hyperplasia, and a partial transition to a colonic mucin phenotype characterized by an increase in sulfomucins.[312] These changes should not be misinterpreted as indicative of pouchitis in the absence of appropriate clinical symptoms and/or signs.

DIFFERENTIAL DIAGNOSIS

The differential diagnosis of pouchitis includes ischemia, infection, and recurrent Crohn's disease.[301] The features of ischemia in pouch mocusa are similar to those observed in other portions of the GI tract (see Chapters 9 and 10) and usually develop within a short period of time after surgery. Infections, such as with

Shigella, E. coli, Salmonella, or *Clostridium,* can induce histologic features similar to those of chronic idiopathic pouchitis, but these causes can usually be identified by stool cultures. Crohn's disease involving the pouch should be considered in cases that contain non-necrotizing granulomas of undetermined etiology, deep and/or fissuring type ulcers, sinus tracts, fistulas, or fissures. In these cases, examination of the patients' prior colectomy specimen is essential because it may reveal subtle changes of Crohn's disease. Other less frequent causes of pouch dysfunction should also be considered prior to definitive treatment. These include pelvic sepsis, inflammation of the retained cuff of rectal mucosa (referred to as "cuffitis"), and anastomotic strictures with obstruction. Finally, because virtually all ileal pouches develop early and persistent morphologic, inflammatory, phenotypic, mucin histochemical, and kinetic changes characteristic of colonic metaplasia, a diagnosis of pouchitis should not be made in the absence of appropriate clinical and endoscopic findings.

TREATMENT

The first line of treatment of pouchitis is antibiotics. Anti-inflammatory agents and steroids are typically used for antibiotic-resistant cases. Immunosuppressive agents, such as azathioprine, may be used for long-term maintenance therapy. Replacement therapy with short-chain fatty acids, such as butyrate or glutamine, has met with variable success but has been used when other forms of treatment have failed.[307] Finally, surgical excision of the pouch should be considered when all available drugs have failed.

References

1. Soderlund S: Meckel's diverticulum: A clinical and histologic study. Acta Chir Scand 248:13-233, 1959.
2. Turgeon DK, Barnett JL: Meckel's diverticulum. Am J Gastroenterol 85:777-781, 1990.
3. Cullen JJ, Kelly KA: Current management of Meckel's diverticulum. Adv Surg 29:207-214, 1996.
4. Brown RL, Azizkhan RG: Gastrointestinal bleeding in infants and children: Meckel's diverticulum and intestinal duplication. Semin Pediatr Surg 8:202-209, 1999.
5. Moore GP, Burkle FM Jr: Isolated axial volvulus of a Meckel's diverticulum. Am J Emerg Med 6:137-142, 1988.
6. Al-Dabbagh AI, Salih SA: Primary lymphoma of Meckel's diverticulum: A case report. J Surg Oncol 28:19-20, 1985.
7. Blamey SL, Woods SD: Leiomyoma of Meckel's diverticulum. Med J Aust 145:232-234, 1986.
8. Bloch T, Tejada E, Brodhecker C: Malignant melanoma in Meckel's diverticulum. Am J Clin Pathol 86:231-234, 1986.
9. Adams HW, Rehak EM: Carcinoma in a Meckel's diverticulum: Case report and literature review. J Miss State Med Assoc 28:59-61, 1987.
10. Dixon AY, McAnaw M, McGregor DH, et al: Dual carcinoid tumors of Meckel's diverticulum presenting as metastasis in an inguinal hernia sac: Case report with literature review. Am J Gastroenterol 83:1283-1288, 1988.
11. Shimizu N, Kuramoto S, Mimura T, et al: Leiomyosarcoma originating in Meckel's diverticulum: Report of a case and a review of 59 cases in the English literature. Surg Today Jpn J Surg 27:546-549, 1997.

12. Seagram CGF, Lough RE, Stephen CA, et al: Meckel's diverticulum: A 10 year review of 218 cases. Can J Surg 11:369-373, 1968.

13. Yamaguchi M, Takeuchi S, Awazu S: Meckel's diverticulum: Investigation of 600 patients in the Japanese literature. Am J Surg 136:247-249, 1978.

14. Dye KR, Marshall BJ, Frierson HF, et al: *Campylobacter pylori* colonizing heterotopic gastric tissue in the rectum. Am J Clin Pathol 93:144-147, 1990.

15. Cserni G: Gastric pathology in Meckel's diverticulum: Review of cases resected between 1965 and 1995. Am J Clin Pathol 106:782-785, 1966.

16. Christensen N: Jejunal diverticulosis. Am J Surg 118:612-618, 1969.

17. Brian JE Jr, Stair JM: Noncolonic diverticular disease. Surg Gyn Obstet 161:189-195, 1985.

18. Maglinte DDT, Chernish SM, DeWeese R, et al: Acquired jejunoileal diverticular disease: Subject review. Radiology 158:577-580, 1986.

19. Donnison AB, Shwachman H, Gross RE: A review of 164 children with meconium ileus seen at the Children's Hospital Medical Center, Boston. Pediatrics 37:833-850, 1966.

20. Oppenheimer EH, Esterly JR: Pathology of cystic fibrosis: Review of the literature and comparison with 146 autopsied cases. Perspect Pediatr Pathol 2:241-278, 1975.

21. Rosenstein BJ, Langbaum TS: Incidence of meconium abnormalities in newborn infants with cystic fibrosis. Am J Dis Child 134:72-73, 1980.

22. Eggermont E: The role of the small intestine in cystic fibrosis patients. Acta Paediatr Scand (Suppl) 317:16-21, 1985.

23. Eggermont E: Gastrointestinal manifestations in cystic fibrosis. Eur J Gastroenterol Hepatol 8:731-738, 1996.

24. Jeffrey I, Durrans D, Wells M, et al: The pathology of meconium ileus equivalent. J Clin Pathol 36:1292-1297, 1983.

25. Marston A: Applied anatomy of the intestinal circulation. In Marston A (ed): Vascular Disease of the Gastrointestinal Tract: Pathophysiology, Recognition and Management. Baltimore, Williams and Wilkins, 1986, pp 1-15.

26. Marston A, Clarke JMF, Garcia JG, et al: Intestinal function and intestinal blood supply: A 20 year surgical study. Gut 26:656-666, 1985.

27. McCord JM: Oxygen-derived free radicals in postischemic tissue injury. N Engl J Med 312:159-163, 1985.

28. Boley SJ, Brandt LJ, Veith FJ: Ischemic disorders of the intestines. Curr Probl Surg 15:1-85, 1978.

29. Brandt LJ, Boley SJ: Ischemic intestinal syndromes. Adv Surg 15:1-45, 1981.

30. Ottinger LW: Acute mesenteric ischemia. N Engl J Med 307:535-537, 1982.

31. Moossa AR, Shackford S, Sise MJ: Acute intestinal ischaemia. In Marston A (ed): Vascular Disease of the Gastrointestinal Tract: Pathophysiology, Recognition and Management. Baltimore, Williams and Wilkins, 1986, pp 64-85.

32. Grendell JH, Ockner RK: Mesenteric venous thrombosis. Gastroenterology 82:358-372, 1982.

33. Ming S-C: Hemorrhagic necrosis of the gastrointestinal tract and its relation to cardiovascular status. Circulation 32:332-341, 1965.

34. Boley SJ, Allen AC, Schultz L, et al: Experimental aspects of peripheral vascular occlusion of the intestine. Surg Gynecol Obstet 121:789, 1965.

35. Allen AC: The vascular pathogenesis of enterocolitis of varied etiology. In Boley SJ, Schwartz SS, Williams LF Jr (eds): Vascular Disorders of the Intestine. New York, Appleton-Century-Crofts, 1971, pp 57-102.

36. McIver MA: Acute intestinal obstruction. I. The disease. Am J Surg 19:163-206, 1933.

37. Marston A: Focal ischemia of the small intestine. In Marston A (ed): Vascular Disease of the Gastrointestinal Tract: Pathophysiology, Recognition and Management. Baltimore, Williams and Wilkins, 1986, pp 143-151.

38. Gee S: On the coeliac affection. St. Bartholomew's Hosp Rep 24: 17-20, 1888.

39. Thaysen TEH: Non-Tropical Sprue. Copenhagen, Levin & Munksgaard, 1932.

40. Dicke WK: Coeliac Disease: Investigation of Harmful Effects of Certain Types of Cereal on Patients With Coeliac Disease [doctoral thesis]. The Netherlands, University of Utrecht, 1950.

41. Logan RFA: Descriptive epidemiology of celiac disease. In Branski D, Rozen P, Kagnoff MF (eds): Gluten-Sensitive Enteropathy. Basel, Karger, 1992, pp 1-14.

42. Fasano A, Catassi C: Current approaches to diagnosis and treatment of celiac disease: An evolving spectrum. Gastroenterology 120: 636-651, 2001.

43. MacDonald WC, Dobbins WO III, Rubin CE: Studies of the familial nature of celiac sprue using biopsy of the small intestine. N Engl J Med 272:448-456, 1965.

44. Trier JS: Celiac sprue and refractory sprue. In Feldman M, Scharschmidt BF, Sleisenger MH (eds): Sleisenger & Fordtran's Gastrointestinal and Liver Disease, 6th ed. Philadelphia, WB Saunders, 1998, pp 1557-1573.

45. Weinstein WM: Latent celiac sprue. Gastroenterology 66:489-493, 1974.

46. Shanahan F, Weinstein WM: Extending the scope in celiac disease. N Engl J Med 319:782-783, 1988.

47. Farrell RJ, Kelly CP: Celiac sprue. N Engl J Med 346:180-188, 2002.

48. Croese J, Harris O, Bain B: Celiac disease: Hematologic features and delay in diagnosis. Med J Aust 2:335-338, 1979.

49. Marsh MN, Crowe PT: Morphology of the mucosal lesion in gluten sensitivity. Baillieres Clin Gastroenterol 9:273-293, 1995.

50. Corazza GR, Andreani ML, Biagi F, et al: Clinical, pathological, and antibody pattern of latent celiac disease: Report of three adult cases. Am J Gastroenterol 91:2203-2207, 1996.

51. Kagnoff MF: Immunopathogenesis of celiac disease. Immunol Invest 18:499-508, 1989.

52. Pena AS, Mann DL, Hague NE, et al: Genetic basis of gluten-sensitive enteropathy. Gastroenterology 75:230-235, 1978.

53. Mearin ML, Biemond I, Pena AS, et al: HLA-DR phenotypes in Spanish coeliac children: Their contribution to the understanding of the genetics of the disease. Gut 24:532-537, 1983.

54. Sollid LM, Markussen G, Ek J, et al: Evidence for a primary association of celiac disease to a particular HLA-DQ α/β heterodimer. J Exp Med 169:345-350, 1989.

55. Sollid LM, Thorsby E: HLA susceptibility genes in celiac disease: Genetic mapping and role in pathogenesis. Gastroenterology 105:910-922, 1993.

56. Schuppan D: Current concepts of celiac disease pathogenesis. Gastroenterology 119:234-242, 2000.

57. Kagnoff MF, Paterson YJ, Kumar PJ, et al: Evidence for the role of a human intestinal adenovirus in the pathogenesis of coeliac disease. Gut 28:995-1001, 1987.

58. Chorzelski TP, Beutner EH, Sulej J, et al: IgA anti-endomysium antibody: A new immunological marker of dermatitis herpetiformis and coeliac disease. Br J Dermatol 3:395-402, 1984.

59. Ferreira M, Davies SL, Butler M, et al: Endomysial antibody: Is it the best screening test for coeliac disease? Gut 33:1633-1637, 1992.

60. Corrao G, Corazza GR, Andreani ML, et al: Serological screening of coeliac disease: Choosing the optimal procedure according to various prevalence values. Gut 35:771-775, 1994.

61. Dieterich W, Laag E, Schöpper H, et al: Autoantibodies to tissue transglutaminase as predictors of celiac disease. Gastroenterology 115:1317-1321, 1998.

62. Anderson RP, Degano P, Godkin AJ, et al: In vivo antigen challenge in celiac disease identifies a single transglutaminase-modified peptide as the dominant A-gliadin T-cell epitope. Nature Med 6:337-342, 2000.

63. Stenhammar L, Brandt A, Wagermark J: A family study of coeliac disease. Acta Paediatr Scand 71:625-628, 1982.

64. Rostami K, Mulder CJJ, van Overbeek FM, et al: Should relatives of coeliacs with mild clinical complaints undergo a small-bowel biopsy despite negative serology? Eur J Gastroenterol Hepatol 12:51-55, 2000.

65. Brocchi E, Corazza GR, Caletti G, et al: Endoscopic demonstration of loss of duodenal folds in the diagnosis of celiac disease. N Engl J Med 319:741-744, 1988.

66. Rubin CE, Brandborg LL, Phelps PC, et al: Studies of celiac disease. I. The apparent identical and specific nature of the duodenal and proximal jejunal lesion in celiac disease and idiopathic sprue. Gastroenterology 38:28-49, 1960.

67. MacDonald WC, Brandborg LL, Flick AL, et al: Studies of celiac sprue. IV. The response of the whole length of the small bowel to a gluten-free diet. Gastroenterology 47:573-589, 1964.

68. Lewin KJ, Riddell RH, Weinstein WM: Small bowel mucosal disease. In Lewin KJ, Riddell RH, Weinstein WM (eds): Gastrointestinal Pathology and Its Clinical Implications. New York, Igaku-Shoin Medical Publishers, 1992, pp 750-811.

69. Halstensen TS, Scott H, Brantzaeg P: Intraepithelial T-cells of the TCRγ/δ⁺CD8⁻ and Vδ1/Jδ1⁺ phenotypes are increased in celiac disease. Scand J Immunol 30:665-672, 1989.

70. Savilahti E, Arato A, Verkasalo M: Intestinal, gamma/delta bearing T lymphocytes in celiac disease and inflammatory bowel diseases in children: Constant increase in celiac disease. Pediatr Res 28:579-581, 1990.

71. Kutlu T, Brousse N, Rambaud C, et al: Numbers of T-cell receptor (TCR) α/β⁺ but not of TCR γ/δ⁺ intraepithelial lymphocytes correlate with the grade of villous atrophy in coeliac patients on a long term normal diet. Gut 34:208-214, 1993.

72. Marsh MN: Gluten sensitivity and latency: The histological background. Dyn Nutr Res 2:142-150, 1992.

73. Goldstein NS, Underhill J: Morphologic features suggestive of gluten sensitivity in architecturally normal duodenal biopsy specimens. Am J Clin Pathol 116:63-71, 2001.

74. Swanson VL, Thomassen RW: Pathology of the jejunal mucosa in tropical sprue. Am J Pathol 46:511-551, 1965.

75. Perera DR, Weinstein WM, Rubin CE: Small intestinal biopsy. Hum Pathol 6:157-217, 1975.

76. King CE, Toskes PP: Small intestine bacterial overgrowth. Gastroenterology 76:1035-1055, 1979.

77. Robert ME, Ament ME, Weinstein WM: The histologic spectrum and clinical outcome of refractory and unclassified sprue. Am J Surg Pathol 24:676-687, 2000.

78. Ament ME, Rubin CE: Soy protein: Another cause of the flat intestinal lesion. Gastroenterology 62:227-234, 1972.

79. Ross IN: Primary immunodeficiency and the small intestine. In Marsh MN (ed): Immunopathology of the Small Intestine. New York, Wiley, 1987, pp 283-332.

80. Trier JS, Falchuk ZM, Carey MC, et al: Celiac sprue and refractory sprue. Gastroenterology 75:307-316, 1978.

81. Ryan BM, Kelleher D: Refractory celiac disease. Gastroenterology 119:243-251, 2000.

82. Weinstein WM: Intractable celiac sprue: Management, maintenance, and maladies. In Barkin J, Rogers A (eds): Difficult Decisions in Digestive Diseases. St. Louis, MO, Mosby, 1994, pp 257-263.

83. Fine KD, Meyer RL, Lee EL: The prevalence and causes of chronic diarrhea in patients with celiac sprue treated with a gluten-free diet. Gastroenterology 112:1830-1838, 1998.

84. Corazza GR, Biagi F, Volta U, et al: Autoimmune enteropathy and villous atrophy in adults. Lancet 350:106-109, 1997.

85. Murray A, Cuevas EC, Jones DB, et al: Study of the immuno-histochemistry and T-cell clonality of enteropathy-associated T-cell lymphoma. Am J Pathol 146:509-519, 1995.

86. Carbonnel F, Grollet-Bioul L, Brouet JC, et al: Are complicated forms of celiac disease cryptic T-cell lymphomas? Blood 92:3879-3886, 1998.

87. Cellier C, Patey N, Mauvieux L, et al: Abnormal intestinal intra-epithelial lymphocytes in refractory sprue. Gastroenterology 114:471-481, 1998.

88. Bagdi E, Diss TC, Munson P, et al: Mucosal intra-epithelial lymphocytes in enteropathy-associated T-cell lymphoma, ulcerative jejunitis, and refractory celiac disease constitute a neoplastic population. Blood 94:260-264, 1999.

88a. Patey-Mariaud de Serre N, Cellier C, Jabri B, et al: Distinction between coeliac disease and refractory sprue: A simple immuno-histochemical method. Histopathology 37:70-77, 2000.

89. Weinstein WM, Saunders DR, Tytgat GN, et al: Collagenous sprue: An unrecognized type of malabsorption. N Engl J Med 283:1297-1301, 1970.

90. Fairley NH, Mackie FP: The clinical and biochemical syndrome in lymphadenoma and allied diseases involving the mesenteric lymph glands. Br Med J 1:375-380, 1937.

91. Harris OD, Cooke WT, Thompson H, et al: Malignancy in adult coeliac disease and idiopathic steatorrhoea. Am J Med 42:899-912, 1967.

92. Holmes GKT, Stokes PL, Sorahan TM, et al: Coeliac disease, gluten-free diet, and malignancy. Gut 17:612-619, 1976.

93. Cooper BT, Holmes GKT, Ferguson R, et al: Celiac disease and malignancy. Medicine 59:249-261, 1980.

94. Gough KR, Read AE, Naish JM: Intestinal reticulosis as a complica-tion of idiopathic steatorrhoea. Gut 3:232-239, 1962.

95. Isaacson P, Wright DH: Malignant histiocytosis of the intestine: Its relationship to malabsorption and ulcerative jejunitis. Hum Pathol 9:661-677, 1978.

96. Jeffries GH, Steinberg H, Sleisenger MH: Chronic ulcerative (nongranulomatous) jejunitis. Am J Med 44:47-59, 1968.

97. O'Farrelly C, Feighery C, O'Brian DS, et al: Humoral response to wheat protein in patients with coeliac disease and enteropathy associated T-cell lymphoma. Br Med J 293:908-910, 1986.

98. Isaacson PG, Spencer J, Connolly CE, et al: Malignant histiocytosis of the intestine: A T-cell lymphoma. Lancet September 28:688-691, 1985.

99. Holmes GKT, Prior P, Lane MR, et al: Malignancy in coeliac disease—effect of a gluten free diet. Gut 30:333-338, 1989.

100. Corrao G, Corazza, GR, Bagnardi V, et al: Mortality in patients with coeliac disease and their relatives: A cohort study. Lancet 358:356-361, 2001.

101. Selby WS, Gallagher ND: Malignancy in a 19-year experience of adult celiac disease. Dig Dis Sci 24:684-688, 1979.

102. Wolber R, Owen D, Del Buono L, et al: Lymphocytic gastritis in patients with celiac sprue or sprue-like intestinal disease. Gastroenterology 98:310-315, 1990.

103. Lagorce-Pages C, Fabiani B, Bouvier R, et al: Collagenous gastritis: A report of six cases. Am J Surg Pathol 25:1174-1179, 2001.

104. Wolber R, Owen D, Freeman H: Colonic lymphocytosis in patients with celiac sprue. Hum Pathol 21:1092-1096, 1990.

105. Breen EG, Farren C, Connolly CE, et al: Collagenous colitis and coeliac disease. Gut 28:364, 1987.

106. Zins BJ, Tremaine WJ, Carpenter AH: Collagenous colitis: Mucosal biopsies and association with fecal leukocytes. Mayo Clin Proc 70:430-433, 1995.

107. Brow JR, Parker F, Weinstein WM, et al: The small intestinal mucosa in dermatitis herpetiformis. I. Severity and distribution of the small intestinal lesion and associated malabsorption. Gastroenterology 60:355-361, 1971.

108. Baer AN, Bayless TM, Yardley JH: Intestinal ulceration and malab-sorption syndromes. Gastroenterology 79:754-765, 1980.

109. Weiss AA, Yoshida EM, Poulin M, et al: Massive bleeding from multiple gastric ulcerations in a patient with lymphocytic gastritis and celiac sprue. J Clin Gastroenterol 5:354-357, 1997.

110. Maclaurin BP, Matthews N, Kilpatrick JA: Coeliac disease associated with auto-immune thyroiditis, Sjogren's syndrome, and a lympho-cytotoxic serum factor. Aust N Z J Med 4:405-411, 1972.

111. Regan PT, DiMagno EP: Exocrine pancreatic insufficiency in celiac sprue: A cause of treatment failure. Gastroenterology 78:484-487, 1980.

112. Johnstone JM, Morson BC: Eosinophilic gastroenteritis. Histo-pathology 2:335-348, 1978.

113. Schuffler MD, Chaffee RG: Small intestinal biopsy in a patient with Crohn's disease of the duodenum: The spectrum of abnormal findings in the absence of granulomas. Gastroenterology 76:1009-1014, 1979.

114. Iyngkaran N, Robinson MJ, Prathap K, et al: Cows' milk protein-sensitive enteropathy: Combined clinical and histological criteria for diagnosis. Arch Dis Child 53:20-26, 1978.

115. Goldman H, Proujansky R: Allergic proctitis and gastroenteritis in children: Clinical and mucosal biopsy features in 53 cases. Am J Surg Pathol 10:75-86, 1986.

116. Phillips AD, Rice SJ, France NE, et al: Small intestinal intraepithelial lymphocyte levels in cow's milk protein intolerance. Gut 20:509-512, 1979.

117. Rosekrans PCM, Meijer CJLM, Cornelisse CJ, et al: Use of morphometry and immunohistochemistry of small intestinal biopsy specimens in the diagnosis of food allergy. J Clin Pathol 33:125-130, 1980.

118. Maluenda C, Phillips AD, Briddon A, et al: Quantitative analysis of small intestinal mucosa in cow's milk-sensitive enteropathy. J Pediatr Gastroenterol Nutr 3:349-356, 1984.

119. Unsworth DJ, Walker-Smith JA: Autoimmunity in diarrheal disease. J Pediatr Gastroenterol Nutr 4:375-380, 1985.

120. Hill SM, Milla PJ, Bottazzo GF, et al: Autoimmune enteropathy and colitis: Is there a generalized autoimmune gut disorder? Gut 32:36-42, 1991.

121. Alarcón B, Regueiro JR, Arnaiz-Villena A, et al: Familial defect in the surface expression of the T-cell receptor-CD3 complex. N Engl J Med 319:1203-1208, 1988.

122. Mirakian R, Richardson A, Milla PJ, et al: Protracted diarrhea of infancy: Evidence in support of an autoimmune variant. Br Med J 293:1132-1136, 1986.

123. Murch SH: The molecular basis of intractable diarrhea of infancy. Baillieres Clin Gastroenterol 11:413-438, 1997.

124. Moore L, Xu X, Davidson G, et al: Autoimmune enteropathy with anti-goblet cell antibodies. Hum Pathol 26:1162-1168, 1995.
125. Bousvaros A, Leichtner AM, Book L, et al: Treatment of pediatric autoimmune enteropathy with tacrolimus (FK506). Gastroenterology 111:237-243, 1996.
126. Kobayashi I, Imamura K, Kubota M, et al: Identification of an autoimmune enteropathy-related 75-kilodalton antigen. Gastroenterology 117:823-830, 1999.
127. Baker SJ, Mathan VI: Syndrome of tropical sprue in South India. Am J Clin Nutr 21:984-993, 1968.
128. Brunser O, Eidelman S, Klipstein FA: Intestinal morphology of rural Haitians: A comparison between overt tropical sprue and asymptomatic subjects. Gastroenterology 58:655-668, 1970.
129. Baker SJ, Mathan VI: Tropical enteropathy and tropical sprue. Am J Clin Nutr 25:1047-1055, 1972.
130. Mathan VI: Tropical sprue. Springer Semin Immunopathol 12:231-237, 1990.
131. Gorbach SL, Mitra R, Jacobs B, et al: Bacterial contamination of the upper small bowel in tropical sprue. Lancet 1:74-77, 1969.
132. Klipstein FA, Schenk EA: Enterotoxigenic intestinal bacteria in tropical sprue. II. Effect of the bacteria and their enterotoxins on intestinal structure. Gastroenterology 68:642-655, 1975.
133. Cook GC: Etiology and pathogenesis of postinfective tropical malabsorption (tropical sprue). Lancet March 31:721-723, 1984.
134. Ramakrishna BS, Mathan VI: Role of bacterial toxins, bile acids, and free fatty acids in colonic water malabsorption in tropical sprue. Dig Dis Sci 32:500-505, 1987.
135. Wheby MS, Swanson VL, Bayless TM: Comparison of ileal and jejunal biopsies in tropical sprue. Am J Clin Nutr 24:117-123, 1971.
136. Swanson VL, Wheby MS, Bayless T: Morphologic effects of folic acid and vitamin B_{12} on the jejunal lesions of tropical sprue. Am J Pathol 49:167-191, 1966.
137. Mathan MM, Ponniah J, Mathan VI: Epithelial cell renewal and turnover and relationship to morphologic abnormalities in jejunal mucosa in tropical sprue. Dig Dis Sci 31:586-592, 1986.
138. Marsh MN, Mathan M, Mathan VI: Studies of intestinal lymphoid tissue. VII. The secondary nature of lymphoid cell "activation" in the jejunal lesion of tropical sprue. Am J Pathol 112:302-312, 1983.
139. Bjørneklett A, Høverstad BA, Hovig T: Bacterial overgrowth. Scand J Gastroenterol 20(suppl 109):123-132, 1985.
140. Sherman P, Lichtman S: Small bowel bacterial overgrowth syndrome. Dig Dis Sci 5:157-171, 1987.
141. Bishop RF, Anderson CM: The bacterial flora of the stomach and small intestine in children with intestinal obstruction. Arch Dis Child 487-491, 1960.
142. Wirts CW, Goldstein F: Studies of the mechanism of postgastrectomy steatorrhea. Ann Intern Med 58:25-35, 1963.
143. Kahn IJ, Jeffries GH, Sleisenger MH: Malabsorption in intestinal scleroderma: Correction by antibiotics. N Engl J Med 274:1339-1344, 1966.
144. Pearson AJ, Brzechwa-Ajdukiewicz A, McCarthy CF: Intestinal pseudo-obstruction with bacterial overgrowth in the small intestine. Am J Dig Dis 14:200-205, 1969.
145. Goldstein F, Wirts CW, Kowlessar OD: Diabetic diarrhea and steatorrhea: Microbiologic and clinical observations. Ann Intern Med 72:215-218, 1970.
146. Giannella RA, Rout WR, Toskes PP: Jejunal brush border injury and impaired sugar and amino acid uptake in the blind loop syndrome. Gastroenterology 67:965-974, 1974.
147. Simon GL, Gorbach SL: Intestinal microflora. Med Clin North Am 66:557-574, 1982.
148. Denison H, Wallerstedt S: Bacterial overgrowth after high-dose corticosteroid treatment. Scand J Gastroenterol 24:561-564, 1989.
149. Johnston KL: Small intestinal bacterial overgrowth. Vet Clin North Am Small Anim Pract 29:523-550, 1999.
150. Ament ME, Shimoda SS, Saunders DR, et al: Pathogenesis of steatorrhea in three cases of small intestinal stasis syndrome. Gastroenterology 63:728-747, 1972.
151. Fromm H, Hofmann AF: Breath test for altered bile-acid metabolism. Lancet September 18:621-625, 1971.
152. Hoverstad T, Bjørneklett A, Fausa O, et al: Short-chain fatty acids in the small-bowel bacterial overgrowth syndrome. Scand J Gastroenterol 20:492-499, 1985.
153. Masclee A, Tangerman A, Van Schaik A, et al: Unconjugated serum bile acids as a marker of small intestinal bacterial overgrowth. Eur J Clin Invest 19:384-389, 1989.
154. Toskes PP: Gut damage in the human blind loop syndrome. Gastroenterology 66:1345-1346, 1980.
155. Cutz E, Rhoads JM, Drumm B, et al: Microvillus inclusion disease: An inherited defect of brush-border assembly and differentiation. N Engl J Med 320:646-651, 1989.
156. Phillips AD, Schmitz J: Familial microvillous atrophy: A clinicopathological survey of 23 cases. J Pediatr Gastroenterol Nutr 14:380-396, 1992.
157. Groisman GM, Ben-Izhak O, Schwersenz A, et al: The value of polyclonal carcinoembryonic antigen in the diagnosis of microvillous inclusion disease. Hum Pathol 24:1232-1237, 1993.
158. Phillips AD, Szafranski M, Man L-Y, et al: Periodic acid–Schiff staining abnormality in microvillous atrophy: Photometric and ultrastructural studies. J Pediatr Gastroenterol Nutr 30:34-42, 2000.
159. Lake BD: Microvillous inclusion disease: Specific diagnostic features shown by alkaline phosphatase histochemistry. J Clin Pathol 41:880-882, 1988.
160. Groisman GM, Amar M, Livne E: CD10: A valuable tool for the light microscopic diagnosis of microvillous inclusion disease (familial microvillous atrophy). Am J Surg Pathol 26:902-907, 2002.
161. Groisman GM, Sabo E, Meir A, et al: Enterocyte apoptosis and proliferation are increased in microvillous inclusion disease (familial microvillous atrophy). Hum Pathol 31:1404-1410, 2000.
162. Carruthers L, Phillips AD, Dourmashkin R, et al: Biochemical abnormality in brush border membrane protein of a patient with congenital microvillus atrophy. J Pediatr Gastroenterol Nutr 4:902-907, 1985.
163. Fish EM, Molitoris BA: Alterations in epithelial polarity and the pathogenesis of disease states. N Engl J Med 330:1580-1588, 1994.
164. Cutz E, Sherman PM, Davidson GP: Enteropathies associated with protracted diarrhea of infancy: Clinicopathological features, cellular and molecular mechanisms. Pediatr Pathol Lab Med 17:335-367, 1997.
165. Schofield DE, Agostini RM, Yunis EJ: Gastrointestinal microvillous inclusion disease. Am J Clin Pathol 98:119-124, 1992.
166. Gotto AM, Levy RI, John K, et al: On the protein defect in abetalipoproteinemia. N Engl J Med 284:813-818, 1971.
167. Young SG, Hubl ST, Chappell DA, et al: Familial hypobetalipoproteinemia associated with a mutant species of apolipoprotein B (B-46). N Engl J Med 320:1604-1610, 1989.
168. Narcisi TME, Shoulders CC, Chester SA, et al: Mutations of the microsomal triglyceride-transfer-protein gene in abetalipoproteinemia. Am J Hum Genet 57:1298-1310, 1995.
169. Bassen FA, Kornzweig AL: Malformation of the erythrocytes in a case of atypical retinitis pigmentosa. Blood 5:381-387, 1950.
170. Levy E, Marcel YL, Milne RW, et al: Absence of intestinal synthesis of apolipoprotein B-48 in two cases of abetalipoproteinemia. Gastroenterology 93:1119-1126, 1987.
171. Roy CC, Levy E, Green PHR, et al: Malabsorption, hypocholesterolemia, and fat-filled enterocytes with increased intestinal apoprotein B: Chylomicron retention disease. Gastroenterology 92:390-399, 1987.
172. Kane JP, Havel RJ: Disorders of the biogenesis and secretion of lipoproteins containing the B apolipoproteins. In The Metabolic Basis of Inherited Diseases, 6th ed. New York, McGraw-Hill,1989, pp 1139-1164.
173. Dobbins WO III: An ultrastructural study of the intestinal mucosa in congenital β-lipoprotein deficiency with particular emphasis upon the intestinal absorptive cell. Gastroenterology 50:195-210, 1966.
174. Greenwood N: The jejunal mucosa in two cases of A-beta-lipoproteinemia. Am J Gastroenterol 65:160-162, 1976.
175. Ureles AL, Alschibaja T, Lodico D, et al: Idiopathic eosinophilic infiltration of the gastrointestinal tract, diffuse and circumscribed: A proposed classification and review of the literature, with two additional cases. Am J Med June:899-909, 1961.
176. Klein NC, Hargrove RL, Sleisenger MH, et al: Eosinophilic gastroenteritis. Medicine 49:299-319, 1970.
177. Leinbach GE, Rubin CE: Eosinophilic gastroenteritis: A simple reaction to food allergens? Gastroenterology 59:874-889, 1970.
178. Keshavarzian A, Saverymuttu SH, Tai P-C, et al: Activated eosinophils in familial eosinophilic gastroenteritis. Gastroenterology 88:1041-1049, 1985.

179. Caldwell JH, Tennenbaum JI, Bronstein HA: Serum IgE in eosinophilic gastroenteritis: Response to intestinal challenge in two cases. N Engl J Med 292:1388-1390, 1975.

180. Talley NJ, Kephart GM, McGovern TW, et al: Deposition of eosinophil granule major basic protein in eosinophilic gastroenteritis and celiac disease. Gastroenterology 103:137-145, 1992.

181. Desreumaux P, Bloget F, Seguy D, et al: Interleukin 3, granulocyte-macrophage colony-stimulating factor, and interleukin 5 in eosinophilic gastroenteritis. Gastroenterology 110:768-774, 1996.

182. Talley NJ, Shorter RG, Phillips SF, et al: Eosinophilic gastroenteritis: A clinicopathological study of patients with disease of the mucosa, muscle layer, and subserosal tissues. Gut 31:54-58, 1990.

183. Suen KC, Burton JD: The spectrum of eosinophilic infiltration of the gastrointestinal tract and its relationship to other disorders of angiitis and granulomatosis. Hum Pathol 10:31-43, 1979.

184. McNabb PC, Fleming CR, Higgins JA, et al: Transmural eosinophilic gastroenteritis with ascites. Mayo Clin Proc 54:119-122, 1979.

185. Bennett RA, Whitelock T III, Kelley JL Jr: Eosinophilic gastroenteritis, gluten enteropathy, and dermatitis herpetiformis. Dig Dis Sci 19:1154-1161, 1974.

186. Foroozan P, Trier JS: Mucosa of the small intestine in pernicious anemia. N Engl J Med 277:553-559, 1967.

187. Bianchi A, Chipman DW, Dreskin A, et al: Nutritional folic acid deficiency with megaloblastic changes in the small-bowel epithelium. N Engl J Med 282:859-861, 1970.

188. Stanfield JP, Hutt MSR, Tunnicliffe R: Intestinal biopsy in kwashiorkor. Lancet September 11:519-523, 1965.

189. Cook GC, Lee FD: The jejunum after kwashiorkor. Lancet December 10:1263-1267, 1966.

190. Brunser O, Reid A, Monckeberg F, et al: Jejunal mucosa in infant malnutrition. Am J Clin Nutr 21:976-983, 1968.

191. Theron JJ, Wittmann W, Prinsloo JG: The fine structure of the jejunum in kwashiorkor. Exp Mol Pathol 14:184-199, 1971.

192. Shiner M, Redmond AOB, Hansen JDL: The jejunal mucosa in protein-energy malnutrition: A clinical, histological, and ultrastructural study. Exp Mol Pathol 19:61-78, 1973.

193. Braun OH, Heilmann K, Pauli W, et al: Acrodermatitis enteropathica: Recent findings concerning clinical features, pathogenesis, diagnosis and therapy. Eur J Pediatr 121:247-261, 1976.

194. Moynahan EJ, Barnes PM: Zinc deficiency and a synthetic diet for lactose intolerance. Lancet 1:676, 1973.

195. Walling A, Householder M, Walling A: Acrodermatitis enteropathica. Am Fam Physician 39:151-154, 1989.

196. Lombeck I, von Bassewitz DB, Becker K, et al: Ultrastructural findings in acrodermatitis enteropathica. Pediatr Res 8:82-88, 1974.

197. Kelly R, Davidson GP, Townley RW, et al: Reversible intestinal mucosal abnormality in acrodermatitis enteropathica. Arch Dis Child 51:219-222, 1976.

198. Braun OH, Heilmann K, Rossner JA, et al: Acrodermatitis enteropathica. II. Zinc deficiency and ultrastructural findings. Eur J Pediatr 125:153-162, 1977.

199. Naiman JL, Oski FA, Diamond LK, et al: The gastrointestinal effects of iron-deficiency anemia. Pediatrics 83-99, 1964.

200. Jacobs A: Iron-containing enzymes in the buccal epithelium. Lancet 2:1331, 1961.

201. Waldmann TA, Steinfeld JL, Dutcher TF, et al: The role of the gastrointestinal system in "idiopathic hypoproteinemia." Gastroenterology 41:197-207, 1961.

202. Waldmann TA: Protein-losing enteropathy. Gastroenterology 50:422-443, 1966.

203. Abramowsky C, Hupertz V, Kilbridge P, et al: Intestinal lymphangiectasia in children: A study of upper gastrointestinal endoscopic biopsies. Pediatr Pathol 9:289-297, 1989.

204. Kuroiwa G, Takayama T, Sato Y, et al: Primary intestinal lymphangiectasia successfully treated with octreotide. J Gastroenterol 36:129-132, 2001.

205. Heresbach D, Raoul J-L, Genetet N, et al: Immunological study in primary intestinal lymphangiectasia. Digestion 55:59-64, 1994.

206. Fuss IJ, Strober W, Cuccherini BA, et al: Intestinal lymphangiectasia, a disease characterized by selective loss of naïve CD45RA lymphocytes into the gastrointestinal tract. Eur J Immunol 28:4275-4285, 1998.

207. Bouhnik Y, Etienney I, Nemeth J, et al: Very late onset small intestinal B-cell lymphoma associated with primary intestinal lymphangiectasia and diffuse cutaneous warts. Gut 47:296-300, 2000.

208. Aoyagi K, Iida M, Yao T, et al: Characteristic endoscopic features of intestinal lymphangiectasia: Correlation with histological findings. Hepatogastroenterology 44:133-138, 1997.

209. Riemann JF, Schmidt H: Synopsis of endoscopic and other morphological findings in intestinal lymphangiectasia. Endoscopy 13:60-63, 1981.

210. Persic M, Browse NL, Prpic I: Intestinal lymphangiectasia and protein losing enteropathy responding to small bowel resection. Arch Dis Child 78:194-196, 1998.

211. Dobbins WO III: Electron microscopic study of the intestinal mucosa in intestinal lymphangiectasia. Gastroenterology 51:1004-1017, 1966.

212. Rao SS, Dundas S, Holdsworth CD: Intestinal lymphangiectasia secondary to radiotherapy and chemotherapy. Dig Dis Sci 32:939-942, 1987.

213. Van Tilburg AJ, van Blankenstein M, Verschoor L: Intestinal lymphangiectasia in systemic sclerosis. Am J Gastroenterol 83:1417-1419, 1988.

214. Mak K-L, Hui P-K, Chan W-Y, et al: Mucosal lymphangiectasia in gastric adenocarcinoma. Arch Pathol Lab Med 120:78-80, 1996.

215. Waldenström J: Incipient myelomatosis or "essential" hyperglobulinemia with fibrinogenopenia: A new syndrome? Acta Med Scand 117:216-247, 1944.

216. Bedine MS, Yardley JH, Elliott HL, et al: Intestinal involvement in Waldenström's macroglobulinemia. Gastroenterology 65:308-315, 1973.

217. Pruzanski W, Warren RE, Goldie JH, et al: Malabsorption syndrome with infiltration of the intestinal wall by extracellular monoclonal macroglobulin. Am J Med 54:811-818, 1973.

218. Kornbluth A, Sachar D, Salomon P: Crohn's disease. In Feldman M, Scharschmidt BF, Sleisenger MH (eds): Sleisenger & Fordtran's Gastrointestinal and Liver Disease: Pathophysiology, Diagnosis, Management, 6th ed Philadelphia, WB Saunders, 1998, pp 1708-1734.

219. Hugot J-P, Chamaillard MC, Zouali H, et al: Association of NOD2 leucine-rich repeat variants with susceptibility to Crohn's disease. Nature 41:599-603, 2001.

220. Ogura Y, Bonen D, Inohara N, et al: A frameshift mutation in NOD2 associated with susceptibility to Crohn's disease. Nature 41:603-606, 2001.

221. Roth MP, Peterson GM, McElree C, et al: Geographic origins of Jewish patients with inflammatory bowel disease. Gastroenterology 97:900, 1989.

222. Whelan G: Epidemiology of inflammatory bowel disease. Gastroenterol Clin North Am 19:1, 1990.

223. Price AB, Morson BC: Inflammatory bowel disease: The surgical pathology of Crohn's disease and ulcerative colitis. Hum Pathol 6:7-29, 1975.

224. Warren S, Sommers SC: Cicatrizing enteritis (regional ileitis) as a pathologic entity: Analysis of 120 cases. Am J Pathol 24:475-501, 1948.

225. Rappaport H, Burgoyne FH, Smetana HP: Pathology of regional enteritis. Milit Surg 109:463-502, 1951.

226. Geboes K: Morphological aspects of Crohn's disease. Maldegem, Druk Van Hoetenberghe, 1984.

227. Greenstein AJ, Mann DA, Sachar DB, et al: Free perforation in Crohn's disease. I. A survey of 99 cases. Am J Gastroenterol 80:682-689, 1985.

228. Kelly JK, Siu TO: The strictures, sinus, and fissures of Crohn's disease. J Clin Gastroenterol 8:594-598, 1986.

229. Sheehan AL, Warren BF, Gear MWL, et al: Fat-wrapping in Crohn's disease: Pathological basis and relevance to surgical practice. Br J Surg 79:955-958, 1992.

230. Desreumaux P, Ernst O, Geboes K, et al: Inflammatory alterations in mesenteric adipose tissue in Crohn's disease. Gastroenterology 117:73-81, 1999.

231. Watier A, Devroede G, Perey B, et al: Small erythematous mucosal plaques: An endoscopic sign of Crohn's disease. Gut 21:835-839, 1980.

232. Dourmashkin RR, Davies H, Wells C, et al: Epithelial patchy necrosis in Crohn's disease. Hum Pathol 14:643-648, 1983.

233. Rickert RR, Carter HW: The "early" ulcerative lesion of Crohn's disease: Correlative light and scanning electron microscopic studies. J Clin Gastroenterol 2:11-19, 1980.

234. Ming SC, Simon M, Tandar BN: Gross gastric metaplasia of ileum after regional enteritis. Gastroenterology 44:63-68, 1963.

235. Cook MG: The size and histological appearances of mesenteric lymph nodes in Crohn's disease. Gut 13:970-972, 1972.

236. Surawicz CM, Meisel JL, Ylvisaker T, et al: Rectal biopsy in the diagnosis of Crohn's disease: Value of multiple biopsies and serial sectioning. Gastroenterology 81:66-71, 1981.

237. Chong SKF, Blackshaw AJ, Boyle S, et al: Histological diagnosis of chronic inflammatory bowel disease in childhood. Gut 26:55-59, 1985.

238. Geller SA, Cohen A: Arterial inflammatory cell infiltrate in Crohn's disease. Arch Pathol Lab Med 107:473-475, 1983.

239. Wakefield AJ, Dhillon AP, Rowels PM, et al: Pathogenesis of Crohn's disease: Multifocal gastrointestinal infarction. Lancet 2:1057-1062, 1989.

240. Nugent FW, Roy MA: Duodenal Crohn's disease: An analysis of 89 cases. Am J Gastroenterol 84:249-254, 1989.

241. Weterman IT: Oral, oesophageal and gastro-duodenal Crohn's disease. In Allen RN (eds): Inflammatory Bowel Diseases. New York, Churchill Livingstone, 1983, pp 299-306.

242. Nugent FW, Richmond M, Park SK: Crohn's disease of the duodenum. Gut 18:115-120, 1977.

243. Ariyama J, Wehlin L, Lindstrom CG, et al: Gastroduodenal erosions in Crohn's disease. Gastrointest Radiol 5:121-125, 1980.

244. Korelitz BI, Waye JD, Kreuning J, et al: Crohn's disease in endoscopic biopsies of the gastric antrum and duodenum. Am J Gastroenterol 76:103-109, 1981.

245. Wilder WM, Davis WD Jr: Duodenal enteritis. South Med J 59:884-888, 1966.

246. Wright CL, Riddell RH: Histology of the stomach and duodenum in Crohn's disease. Am J Surg Pathol 22:383-390, 1998.

247. Gleason TH, Patterson SD: The pathology of *Yersinia enterocolitica* ileocolitis. Am J Surg Pathol 6:347-355, 1982.

248. Ruuska T, Vaajalahti P, Arajärvi P, et al: Prospective evaluation of upper gastrointestinal mucosal lesions in children with ulcerative colitis and Crohn's disease. J Pediatr Gastroenterol Nutr 19:181-186, 1994.

249. Kaufman SS, Vanderhoof JA, Young R, et al: Gastroenteric inflammation in children with ulcerative colitis. Am J Gastroenterol 92:1209-1212, 1996.

250. Valdez R, Appelman HD, Bronner MP, et al: Diffuse duodenitis associated with ulcerative colitis. Am J Surg Pathol 24:1407-1413, 2000.

251. Terashima S, Hoshino Y, Kanzaki N, et al: Ulcerative duodenitis accompanying ulcerative colitis. J Clin Gastroenterol 32:172-175, 2001.

252. Tobin JM, Sinha B, Ramani P, et al: Upper gastrointestinal mucosal disease in pediatric Crohn disease and ulcerative colitis: A blinded, controlled study. J Pediatr Gastroenterol Nutr 32:443-448, 2001.

253. Kreuning J, Wal AM, Kuiper G, et al: Chronic nonspecific duodenitis: A multiple biopsy study of the duodenal bulb in health and disease. Scand J Gastroenterol 24:16-20, 1989.

254. Yardley JH: Pathology of chronic gastritis and duodenitis. In Goldman H, Appelman HD, Kaufman N, et al (eds): Gastrointestinal Pathology. Baltimore, William and Wilkins, 1990, pp 69-143.

255. Ellison EH, Wilson SD: The Zollinger-Ellison syndrome: Reappraisal and evaluation of 260 registered cases. Ann Surg 160:512-530, 1964.

256. Kreuning J, Bosman FT, Kuiper G, et al: Gastric and duodenal mucosa in "healthy" individuals: An endoscopic and histopathological study of 50 volunteers. J Clin Pathol 31:69-77, 1978.

257. Hasan M, Sircus W, Ferguson A: Duodenal mucosal architecture in non-specific and ulcer-associated duodenitis. Gut 22:637-641, 1981.

258. Shousha S, Spiller RC, Parkins RA: The endoscopically abnormal duodenum in patients with dyspepsia: Biopsy findings in 60 cases. Histopathology 7:23-34, 1983.

259. Jenkins D, Goodall A, Gillet FR, et al: Defining duodenitis: Quantitative histological study of mucosal responses and their correlations. J Clin Pathol 38:1119-1126, 1985.

260. Wyatt JI, Rathbone BJ, Dixon MF, et al: *Campylobacter pyloridis* and acid induced gastric metaplasia in the pathogenesis of duodenitis. J Clin Pathol 40:841-848, 1987.

261. Khulusi S, Badve S, Patel P, et al: Pathogenesis of gastric metaplasia of the human duodenum: Role of *Helicobacter pylori*, gastric acid, and ulceration. Gastroenterology 110:452-458, 1996.

262. Steer HW: Surface morphology of the gastroduodenal mucosa in duodenal ulceration. Gut 25:1203-1210, 1984.

263. Coghlan JG, Gilligan D, Humphries H, et al: *Campylobacter pylori* and recurrence of duodenal ulcers: A 12-month follow-up study. Lancet 2:1109-1110, 1987.

264. Marshall BJ, Goodwin CS, Warren JR, et al: Prospective double-blind trial of duodenal ulcer relapse after eradication of *Campylobacter pylori*. Lancet 2:1438-1442, 1988.

265. Johansen AA, Hansen OH: Heterotopic gastric epithelium in the duodenum and its correlation to gastric disease and acid level. Acta Pathol Microbiol Scand (A) 81:676-680, 1973.

266. Bloomer WD, Hellman S: Normal tissue responses to radiation therapy. N Engl J Med 293:80-83, 1975.

267. Novak JM, Collins JT, Donowitz M, et al: Effects of radiation on the human gastrointestinal tract. J Clin Gastroenterol March:9-39, 1979.

268. Berthrong M, Fajardo LF: Radiation injury in surgical pathology. II. Alimentary tract. Am J Surg Pathol 5:153-178, 1981.

269. Carr KE: Effects of radiation damage on intestinal morphology. Int Rev Cytol 208:1-118, 2001.

270. Classen J, Belka C, Paulsen F, et al: Radiation-induced gastrointestinal toxicity: Pathophysiology, approaches to treatment and prophylaxis. Strahlenther Onkol 174:82-84, 1998.

271. Touboul E, Balosso J, Schlienger M, et al: Small bowel radiation injury: Radiobiological and radiopathological aspects, risk factors and prevention. Ann Chir 50:58-71, 1996.

272. Wiernik G: Changes in the villous pattern of the human jejunum associated with heavy radiation damage. Gut 7:149-153, 1966.

273. Hugon J, Borgers M: Fine structure of the nuclei of the duodenal crypt cells after x-irradiation. Am J Pathol 52:701-723, 1968.

274. Wartiovaara J, Tarpila S: Cell contacts and polysomes in irradiated human jejunal mucosa at onset of epithelial repair. Lab Invest 36:660-665, 1977.

275. Trier JS, Browning TH: Morphologic response of the mucosa of human small intestine to x-ray exposure. J Clin Invest 45:194-204, 1966.

276. Sher ME, Bauer J: Radiation-induced enteropathy. Am J Gastroenterol 85:121-128, 1990.

277. Donaldson SS, Jundt S, Ricour C, et al: Radiation enteritis in children: A retrospective, review, clinicopathologic correlation, and dietary management. Cancer 35:1167-1178, 1975.

278. Hasleton PS, Carr N, Schofield PF: Vascular changes in radiation bowel disease. Histopathology 9:517-534, 1985.

279. Coia LR, Myerson RJ, Tepper JE: Late effects of radiation therapy on the intestinal tract. Int J Radiat Oncol Biol Phys 31:1213-1236, 1995.

280. Kirkpatrick JB: Pathogenesis of foam cell lesions in irradiated arteries. Am J Pathol 50:291-309, 1967.

281. Hirschowitz L, Rode J: Changes in neurons, neuroendocrine cells and nerve fibers in the lamina propria of irradiated bowel. Virchows Arch A Pathol Anat Histopathol 418:163-168, 1991.

282. Weston JT, Guin GH: Epithelial atypias with chemotherapy in 100 acute childhood leukemias. Cancer 8:179-186, 1955.

283. Slavin RE, Dias MA, Saral R: Cytosine arabinoside induced gastrointestinal toxic alterations in sequential chemotherapeutic protocols: A clinical-pathologic study of 33 patients. Cancer 42:1747-1759, 1978.

284. Trier JS: Morphologic alterations induced by methotrexate in the mucosa of human proximal intestine. II. Electron microscopic observation. Gastroenterology 43:407-424, 1962.

285. Lubitz L, Ekert H: Reversible changes in duodenal mucosa associated with intensive chemotherapy followed by autologous marrow rescue. Lancet September 8:532-533, 1979.

286. Beardon PM, Brown SV, McDevitt DG: Gastrointestinal events in patients prescribed non-steroidal anti-inflammatory drugs: A controlled study using record linkage. Q J Med 266:497-505, 1989.

287. Fries JF, Miller SR, Spitz W, et al: Towards an epidemiology of gastropathy associated with non-steroidal anti-inflammatory drug use. Gastroenterology 96:645-647, 1989.

288. Silvoso G, Ivey KJ, Butt J: Incidence of gastric lesions in patients with rheumatic disease on chronic aspirin therapy. Ann Intern Med 91:517-520, 1979.

289. Allison MC, Howatson AG, Torrance CJ, et al: Gastrointestinal damage associated with the use of nonsteroidal anti-inflammatory drugs. N Engl J Med 327:749-754, 1992.

290. Bjarnason I, Hayllar J, MacPherson AJ, et al: Side effects of non-steroidal anti-inflammatory drugs on the small and large intestine in humans. Gastroenterology 104:1832-1847, 1993.

291. Davies NM, Saleh JY: Detection and prevention of NSAID-induced enteropathy. J Pharm Pharmaceut Sci 3:137-155, 2000.

292. Bjarnason I, Williams P, So A, et al: Intestinal permeability and inflammation in rheumatoid arthritis: Effects of non-steroidal anti-inflammatory drugs. Lancet 2:1171-1174, 1984.

293. Smith MD, Gibson RA, Brooks PM: Abnormal bowel permeability in ankylosing spondylitis and rheumatoid arthritis. J Rheumatol 12:299-305, 1985.

294. Bjarnason I, Zanelli G, Smith T, et al: Nonsteroidal anti-inflammatory drug-induced intestinal inflammation in humans. Gastroenterology 93:480-489, 1987.

295. Bjarnason I, Prouse P, Smith T, et al: Blood and protein loss via small intestinal inflammation induced by non-steroidal anti-inflammatory drugs. Lancet 2:711-714, 1987.

296. Bjarnason I, Zanelli G, Smith T, et al: The pathogenesis and consequence of non-steroidal anti-inflammatory drug induced small intestinal inflammation. Scand J Rheumatol 64:55-62, 1987.

297. Kessler WF, Shires GT III, Fahey TJ III: Surgical complications of nonsteroidal anti-inflammatory drug induced small bowel ulceration. J Am Coll Surg 185:250-254, 1997.

298. Morris AJ, Lee FD, MacKenzie JF: Small bowel enteroscopy: Should jejunal biopsy be routine? Gastroenterology 108:A880, 1995.

299. Lang J, Price AB, Levi AJ, et al: Diaphragm disease: Pathology of disease of the small intestine induced by non-steroidal anti-inflammatory drugs. J Clin Pathol 41:516-526, 1988.

300. Fellows IW, Clarke JMF, Roberts PF: Non-steroidal anti-inflammatory drug-induced jejunal and colonic diaphragm disease: A report of two cases. Gut 33:1424-1426, 1992.

301. Stocchi L, Pemberton JH. Pouch and pouchitis. Gastroenterol Clin North America 30:223-241, 2001.

302. Meagher AP, Farouk R, Dozois RR, et al: J ileal pouch-anal anastomosis for chronic ulcerative colitis: Complications and long-term outcome in 1310 patients. Br J Surg 85:800, 1998.

303. Dozois RR, Kelly KA, Welling DR, et al: Ileal pouch-anal anastomosis: Comparison of results in familial adenomatous polyposis and chronic ulcerative colitis. Ann Surg 210:268, 1989.

304. Stahlberg D, Gullberg K, Liljeqvist L, et al: Pouchitis following pelvic pouch operation for ulcerative colitis: Incidence, cumulative risk, and risk factors. Dis Colon Rectum 39:1012, 1996.

305. MacRae HM, McLeod RS, Cohen Z, et al: Risk factors for pelvic pouch failure. Dis Colon Rectum 40:257, 1997.

306. Sapp H, Farraye F, El-Zammar O, et al: Severe pancolitis, early fissuring ulceration, and severe involvement of the appendix are associated with the development of pouchitis after colectomy for chronic ulcerative colitis. Modern Pathol 15:143A, 2002.

307. Wischmeyer P, Pemberton JH, Phillips SF: Chronic pouchitis after ileal pouch-anal anastomosis: Response to butyrate and glutamine suppositories in a pilot study. Mayo Clin Proc 68:978, 1993.

308. Shepherd NA, Hulten L, Tytgat GN, et al: Pouchitis. Int J Colorectal Dis 4:205, 1989.

309. Moskowitz RL, Shepherd NA, Nicholls RJ: An assessment of inflammation in the reservoir after restorative proctocolectomy with ileonal ileal reservoir. Int J Colorectal Dis 1:167, 1986.

310. Sarigol S, Wyllie R, Gramlich T, et al: Incidence of dysplasia in pelvic pouches in pediatric patients after ileal pouch-anal anastomosis for ulcerative colitis. J Pediatr Gastroenterol Nutr 28:429, 1999.

311. Sandborn WJ, Tremaine WJ, Batts KP, et al: Pouchitis after ileal pouch-anal anastomosis: A pouchitis disease activity index. Mayo Clin Proc 69:409, 1994.

312. Apel R, Cohen Z, Andrews CW, et al: Prospective evaluation of early morphological changes in pelvic ileal pouches. Gastroenterology 107:435-443, 1994.

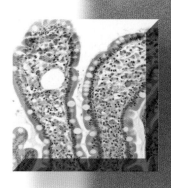

CHAPTER 10

Inflammatory Diseases of the Large Intestine

JOEL K. GREENSON • ROBERT D. ODZE

▉ Introduction

Pathologists are asked to evaluate colorectal biopsy specimens for a variety of reasons, but one of the more common reasons is to identify a pattern of injury with the hope that a specific diagnosis can be rendered. Some forms of colitis, including lymphocytic colitis, collagenous colitis, and ischemic colitis, have specific histologic features. In addition, a host of features are fairly specific for chronic inflammatory bowel disease, although it is often difficult or impossible to distinguish between ulcerative colitis (UC) and Crohn's disease (CD) on the basis of colorectal biopsy specimens.

Perhaps the most important aspect of evaluating colorectal biopsy specimens is having a keen sense of the normal colon. Often, it is difficult to decide whether a biopsy specimen is at the upper limit of normal or the lower limit of abnormal, and in many respects, this is a subjective evaluation. However, the most common diagnosis rendered is "normal colon," and often this is the diagnosis the gastroenterologist is seeking. Thus, the pathologist should not be afraid to make a diagnosis of normal colon; terms such as *nonspecific chronic inflammation, nonspecific colitis*, and *acute and chronic inflammation* are inappropriate pathologic diagnoses that will render the treating gastroenterologist helpless.

The clinician must be aware of several important caveats when evaluating colorectal biopsy specimens in terms of what constitutes normal colon. For example, plasma cells are always present in the lamina propria of the colorectal mucosa, regardless of where the biopsy specimen is taken. However, lamina propria cellularity varies among sites in the colon. In general, the cecum/right colon is more cellular than other portions of the colon, and a progressive decrease in lamina propria cellularity is noted as one moves from right to left colon. In addition, although the crypts throughout the colon are generally straight and evenly distributed and extend to touch the superficial aspect of the muscularis mucosae, there is a bit more crypt irregularity in the distal rectum compared with other portions of the colon. Finally, lymphocytes are normally found in the surface epithelium of the colorectal mucosa. Approximately 5 lymphocytes per 100 epithelial cells are found in the colon.[1] However, more surface epithelial lymphocytes are generally found in the cecum/right colon than in the remainder of the colon, although this is not well known. In addition, one must be careful in counting surface epithelial lymphocytes in epithelium overlying lymphoid follicles, given the increased numbers of intraepithelial lymphocytes normally found in this location.[2,3] Given all of these caveats, it is important for the clinician to know the precise site of the colorectal biopsy specimen so that determination can be made about whether the changes present are normal or pathologic. This has become increasingly difficult because gastroenterologists have tended to group biopsy specimens from different sites in the colon into one specimen container.

Evaluation of patterns of injury in colorectal biopsy specimens is best performed at low magnification. In fact, virtually all of the important information that one can gather from such specimens can be obtained from low magnification. For example, lamina propria cellularity and crypt architecture are easier to evaluate at low magnification than at higher magnifications. In addition, it is easier to compare changes among different fragments within the same specimen container with this mode of evaluation.

The first distinction that the pathologist must make is to determine whether colitis is present, and if it is, whether the colitis is acute or chronic. The most reliable markers of chronic colitis are crypt architectural distortion and basal plasmacytosis. Many colitides, including acute colitides, result in an expanded lamina propria by plasma cells; however, it has been shown that basal plasmacytosis filling the space between the base of the crypts and the superficial aspect of the muscularis mucosae is probably the single best marker of chronic colitis.[4] This has also been found to be true in differentiating acute colitis from acute-onset inflammatory bowel disease in that these features of chronicity are virtually always present, even in the initial biopsy specimen from such patients.[5] Paneth cells are also a useful marker of chronic colitis, although it must be kept in mind that Paneth cells are normally present in the proximal transverse cecum/right colon.

The term *activity* refers to active epithelial injury mediated by either neutrophils or eosinophils. By definition, activity is always present in acute colitis; activity may or may not be present in chronic colitis. When activity is not present in a biopsy specimen showing features of chronic colitis, the colitis can be called *quiescent*.

Ulcerative Colitis

CLINICAL FEATURES

UC is a chronic, episodic disease that has a propensity to arise in adolescents and young adults, although there is a second incidence peak among middle-aged men. Estimates of the annual incidence of UC in North America and Europe range from 4 to 20 per 100,000 individuals.[6] The incidence of UC appears to have equilibrated over the past two decades and is no longer increasing, unlike that of CD, which seems to continue to be increasing in incidence. In fact, it has been estimated that approximately 1% of the U.S. and European population may develop UC during their lifetime.

The etiology and pathogenesis of UC have yet to be fully elucidated. A variety of factors appear to be important, including both environmental and genetic factors. For example, smoking has been found to be protective against the development of UC.[7] Similarly, appendectomy is associated with a significantly lower risk for sub-

sequent development of UC.[8] Other potentially relevant environmental factors include childhood infection, exposure to a variety of microbial agents, diet, occupation, climate, and physical activity.[6] In addition, genetic factors appear to be of significance. For example, the incidence of inflammatory bowel disease (IBD) is twofold to ninefold higher among Ashkenazi Jews compared with the general population, although genetic influence is lower in UC than in CD. Multiple susceptibility genes are likely involved for both UC and CD. A significantly increased frequency of HLA-A11 and HLA-A7 has been noted to occur in UC[9]; among Japanese patients, HLA-DR2 is closely associated with the development of UC.[10] In contrast, this HLA haplotype has not been observed in Western patients with IBD, although an association with DRB*103 and DRB*12 has been found in Western UC patients.[11,12]

PATHOLOGIC FEATURES

Grossly, UC classically involves the rectum with continuous involvement of the colon proximally. Although some cases involve only the rectum (proctitis), others involve the entire colon (pancolitis). The mucosa often has a hemorrhagic or granular appearance, and gross appearance depends in part on the activity of the disease.

Histologically, UC diffusely involves a region of the colon, usually starting at the anal verge and extending proximally in a contiguous fashion. All biopsy specimens from the same region of the colon have a similar appearance, and each biopsy fragment shows a homogeneous pattern of injury across its breadth.

Inflammation

UC is a lymphoplasmacytic predominant process. Dense, homogeneous lymphoplasmacytic inflammation expands and thickens the lamina propria and produces an irregular (luminal) surface[13-15] (Fig. 10-1). All biopsy specimens procured from the same region of the colorectum usually have a similar, uniform density of lymphoplasmacytic inflammation. The density of plasma cells is greatest in the basilar region of the lamina propria (basal plasmacytosis).

Neutrophils may be scattered in the lamina propria or may cause active crypt injury (cryptitis) or form crypt abscesses. The density of neutrophils in untreated UC is also usually similar across each biopsy fragment and between biopsy fragments from the same region of the colon (Fig. 10-2), resulting in a similar degree of mucin depletion in crypt epithelial cells. Crypt rupture can produce histiocytic aggregates and occasional giant cells around the focus (Figs. 10-3 and 10-4), resulting in mucin granulomas. These should not be interpreted as granulomas of CD (see under Crohn's Colitis).

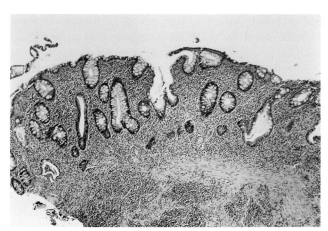

FIGURE 10–1. Active ulcerative colitis, distal rectum. Dense lymphoplasmacytic inflammation involves the entire biopsy. Some crypts are branched (architectural distortion), indicating previous injury and regeneration.

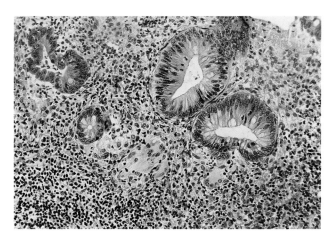

FIGURE 10–4. Active ulcerative colitis. Several foreign body giant cells are surrounded by neutrophils adjcent to ruptured crypts (not shown). Alone, they should not be construed as supportive features of Crohn's disease.

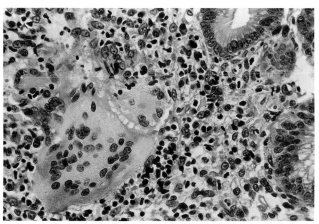

FIGURE 10–2. Moderately active ulcerative colitis. Neutrophils perforate the crypt epithelium and form a crypt abscess.

Crypt Injury and Architectural Distortion

The hallmark morphologic feature of UC is crypt architectural distortion, characterized by irregularly arranged, branched crypts and focal crypt shortening[16] (Fig. 10-5). Crypt injury in UC is usually similar both within and between biopsy fragments procured from the same region of the colon. Crypt branching and shortened crypts are morphologic manifestations of crypt regeneration. Most UC patients have several weeks of subclinical or minimal symptoms during which the lamina propria is inflamed, numerous plasma cells congregate in the basilar region of the lamina propria, and significant crypt injury with regeneration occurs. Crypt architectural distortion is generally considered to be the requisite criterion of chronic colitis; any disease that can produce sufficient persistent crypt injury can result in crypt architectural distortion. In addition to UC, CD, chronic ischemia (usually from radiation therapy),

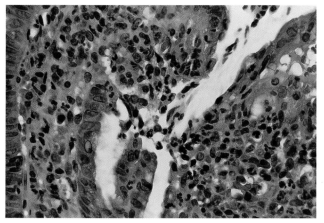

FIGURE 10–3. Active ulcerative colitis. Several foreign body giant cells are located adjacent to crypts. The crypt in the left upper corner has a crypt abscess and is perforated by neutrophils (mucin granuloma).

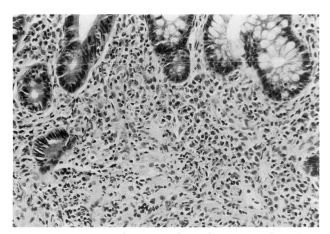

FIGURE 10–5. Active ulcerative colitis. The crypt on the right is branched and short. It does not extend down to the muscularis mucosae (compare with length of crypt to the left).

and persistent or recurrent *Clostridium difficile* infection are the most common causes of architectural distortion in colorectal biopsy specimens procured from patients in the United States.

DISEASE DISTRIBUTION

Occasionally, the rectum can endoscopically appear to be free of active disease or to have less activity than the more proximal colon, suggesting rectal or relative rectal sparing. Histologically, the rectum is abnormal in most of these cases with crypt architectural distortion and mild activity.[17] UC that is limited to the rectum has been referred to as ulcerative proctitis. This disease is thought to be less severe and to have a lower rate of dysplasia and adenocarcinoma than cases of ulcerative pancolitis.[18,19] Histologically, ulcerative proctitis is identical to typical UC. Biopsies from approximately 10 cm above the endoscopic end of active disease must be normal; otherwise, the patient should be classified as having left-sided UC.

Endoscopically normal colonic mucosa proximal to the region of active colitis can display a spectrum of abnormalities. Most commonly, lymphoplasmacytic inflammation fills but does not expand the lamina propria. Crypts are usually evenly arranged (Fig. 10-6). A few neutrophils may be present in the lamina propria and occasionally within a crypt, but no crypt abscesses are found. Eosinophils may also be increased and may produce small crypt abscesses. In the context of classic UC in more distal colon, we consider these changes in proximal bowel to be caused by the colitic process.

RESOLUTION PHASE

Most UC patients enter into a resolution phase of decreasing activity and symptomatology following an active colitis episode; this phase is morphologically characterized by decreasing activity and crypt injury with crypt regeneration followed by crypt remodeling. Neutrophils and the accompanying crypt injury decrease first, which can produce a patchy appearance (Fig. 10-7). Lymphocytes and plasma cells persist and are the last cells to vacate the mucosa. The decreased lympho-plasmacytic inflammation can also result in a patchy process, producing mucosa with no or mild lympho-plasmacytic inflammation interspersed with mucosa with moderate to markedly dense lymphoplasmacytic inflammation.

Healing of ulcers occurs by surface epithelial regrowth that secondarily develops downgrowth of crypt buds. Injured crypts heal from the base toward the surface. Initially, the regenerative cells are cuboidal to columnar with slightly basophilic cytoplasm. Mucin slowly re-appears, first in cuboidal cells and later in goblet cells. Over time, goblet cells can become numerous. Crypt branching and focal shortening are usually prominent during the early resolution phase. Metaplastic Paneth cells appear within regenerative crypt bases in mucosa distal to the hepatic flexure. Together with crypt architectural distortion and basal plasmacytosis, Paneth cell metaplasia can be used as a morphologic marker of previous significant crypt injury (chronic colitis).

Some patients develop prominent lymphoid follicles that are most numerous in the distal colon and rectum (follicular proctitis)[20,21] (Fig. 10-8). Follicular proctitis appears to identify a subgroup of patients who have a less favorable response to medical therapy.[20] Follicular proctitis should be diagnosed only in patients with no more than minimal activity.

CHRONIC ULCERATIVE COLITIS

The resolution period of decreasing activity lasts for several months in most patients and shifts imperceptibly

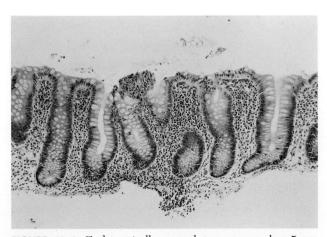

FIGURE 10–6. Endoscopically normal transverse colon 5 cm proximal to the segment of left-sided colitis. Mild lympho-plasmacytic inflammation is seen within the lamina propria.

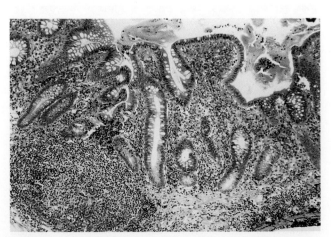

FIGURE 10–7. Resolving ulcerative colitis. Crypt distortion, a prominent lymphoid follicle, and patchy lymphoplasmacytic inflammation are noted, but no crypt abscesses.

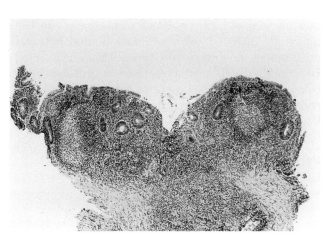

FIGURE 10–8. Follicular proctitis. Prominent lymphoid follicles expand the lamina propria and produce an irregular, bumpy surface. Crypt architectural distortion is seen, but no active colitis.

into the phase of chronic ulcerative colitis (CUC). Between episodic active episodes, most CUC is either inactive or minimally active.

Architecturally distorted crypts remain the telltale sign of previous active colitis. The speed at which this occurs is variable. Patients with only mildly active colitis of short duration can have restitution of architecturally normal mucosa several months after the episode. The pace of crypt remodeling is slow in most patients; such remodeling occurs over many years, if not several decades (Fig. 10-9). Most patients also have additional active colitis episodes or persistent, minimal active colitis that can hamper the remodeling process. Some patients do not achieve complete remission of activity and have persistent chronic minimally active colitis. Many of these patients are receiving medical therapy. The morphology is usually of a patchy colitis with regions of activity separated by inactive areas.

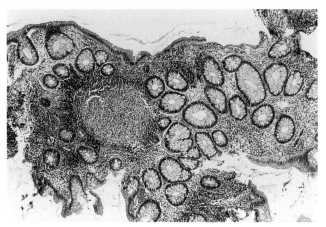

FIGURE 10–9. Chronic ulcerative colitis. Slight crypt disarray and architectural distortion, patchy lymphoplasmacytic inflammation, and a prominent germinal center are evident.

UNUSUAL MORPHOLOGIC VARIANTS OF ULCERATIVE COLITIS

Numerous exceptions to the classic principles of IBD pathology may lead to diagnostic confusion. A summary of the causes of unusual morphologic patterns of disease in UC is provided in Table 10-1. It is important that pathologists recognize these variants so they may avoid falling into diagnostic traps.

EFFECTS OF ORAL AND TOPICAL THERAPY

Classic teaching emphasizes that CUC is characterized morphologically by the presence of diffuse fixed architectural and/or cellular mucosal changes that categorize the process as chronic. However, in 1993, Odze and associates prospectively evaluated 123 rectal mucosal biopsy specimens from 14 patients with pathologically confirmed UC treated with either 5-ASA (5-aminosalicylic acid) or placebo enemas.[22] Overall, over the course of treatment, 29% of rectal biopsies from 64% of patients were histologically normal, showing no evidence of chronic or active disease. In fact, patients treated with 5-ASA showed a significantly higher percentage of normal biopsy specimens (obtained from areas of mucosa previously shown to be involved with chronic active disease) in comparison with the placebo group. This was the first report to demonstrate that "fixed" chronic features in UC may revert to normal in the natural course of the patient's illness and that this phenomenon may be enhanced by topical therapy. Subsequent studies by Kleer and colleagues,[23] Bernstein and coworkers,[24] and Kim and associates,[25] all of whom evaluated patchiness of disease and patterns of involvement in UC colorectal biopsy specimens over time, confirmed and expanded the initial findings of Odze.

In these studies, 30% to 59% of patients, some of whom were treated with oral sulfasalazine and/or steroids, showed either patchiness of disease or rectal sparing on follow-up biopsies. Awareness of these data should prevent misinterpretation of the finding of a normal rectal biopsy specimen or patchiness of disease in treated UC patients as evidence against this diagnosis or as representing skip areas characteristic of CD. In addition, patients with low-grade indolent disease, particularly

TABLE 10–1. Summary of Causes of Unusual Patterns of Disease in Ulcerative Colitis
Treatment effect
Low-grade disease in remission
Appendiceal involvement as a skip lesion
Cecum/ascending colon inflammation in left-sided colitis
Pediatric UC (initial presentation)
"Backwash" ileitis
Rare upper gastrointestinal tract involvement (e.g., duodenitis)
Fulminant colitis

those in clinical and pathologic remission, may show minimal architectural features of chronicity, or perhaps even a completely normal biopsy specimen appearance, during the natural waxing and waning course of their illness. However, it must be emphasized that that these data relate primarily to biopsy material from treated patients. They do not apply to patients who present initially before treatment, or in whom a diagnosis is being considered on the basis of evaluation of a resection specimen. Large portions of mucosa from a resection specimen with a normal histologic appearance are an indication of true segmental disease and normally provide reliable evidence in support of an alternative diagnosis such as CD.

ASCENDING COLON, CECUM, AND APPENDICEAL INVOLVEMENT AS "SKIP" LESIONS IN ULCERATIVE COLITIS

Some patients with either subtotal or left-sided colitis may show patchy, mild, cecal, and/or ascending colon chronic active inflammation that may be falsely interpreted as CD because of the impression of segmental involvement.[26-28] In fact, up to 65% of UC patients present initially with limited left-sided involvement, which may spread to involve more proximal portions of the colon in 29% to 58% of cases.[26,29,30] In one study by D'Haens and colleagues of 20 patients with established left-sided UC, 6 showed a sharp demarcation between affected and unaffected portions of colon, whereas 14 showed a more gradual transition.[26] The area of transition may appear somewhat patchy and may give the false impression of skip lesions. Furthermore, 75% of the latter group of patients showed an area of inflammation in the cecum, primarily in the periappendiceal mucosa, that was separate from the distal inflamed segment. In a previous study by Mutinga and coworkers, 14 patients with both left-sided UC and pathologically confirmed patchy right-sided chronic inflammation were compared with 35 control patients with limited left-sided UC only.[31] These two groups of patients showed similar demographic features, extraintestinal manifestations, severity of disease, prevalence of extension to pancolitis, and natural history, which suggests that patchy right-sided inflammation in patients with left-sided colitis has little clinical significance and should be recognized by pathologists so that a false diagnosis of CD can be prevented.

Similarly, since the original description by Davison and associates in 1990 of discontinuous involvement of the appendix in 21% of 62 cases of UC,[32] several other studies have shown that the appendix may be involved as a skip lesion in this disease,[33,34] although at least one other study failed to confirm this finding.[35] In another study, by Groisman and colleagues, ulcerative appendicitis was present in 86% and 87% of patients with nonuniversal and universal UC, respectively.[33] In fact, this study included two cases with limited left-sided involvement combined with appendiceal involvement. In summary, both appendiceal and/or cecal/ascending colon involvement may occur in patients with subtotal colitis and should be recognized as a potential skip lesion in UC.

INITIAL PRESENTATION OF ULCERATIVE COLITIS IN PEDIATRIC PATIENTS

Several recent studies have shown that pediatric patients who present initially with untreated UC may show evidence of relative, or complete, rectal sparing or patchy disease.[36-41] For instance, in one study by Markowitz and coworkers of 12 pediatric patients with untreated UC, 5 (42%) showed patchy, mild active inflammation and mild crypt changes in the rectum in comparison with more proximal colonic biopsy specimens.[36] In fact, one patient had a completely normal rectal biopsy specimen. More recently, a study by Glickman and associates compared the rectal mucosal biopsy appearance of 70 pediatric UC patients with that of 44 adult patients, all at initial presentation.[37] Compared with adults, the pediatric group showed significantly fewer cases of chronic active disease and a greater number of patients with microscopic skip areas and relative rectal sparing. Two of the 70 pediatric patients showed completely normal rectal biopsy specimens at initial presentation in contrast to none of the adult patients. Thus, the absence of features of chronicity, and/or the presence of mild active disease, and microscopic skip areas at initial presentation in pediatric patients does not exclude the possibility of UC.

BACKWASH ILEITIS

It is commonly recognized that patients with severe pancolitis may show a mild degree of active inflammation in the distal few centimeters of terminal ileum that is presumably related to reflux of colonic contents[42,43] and is called *backwash ileitis*. This condition should not be confused with CD of the terminal ileum, which typically shows longer lengths of involvement and is normally associated with chronic active inflammation; nor should it be confused with other features of CD such as fissuring ulceration, granulomas, and transmural lymphoid aggregates.[43] Unfortunately, strict histopathologic criteria for backwash ileitis have not been defined. In fact, studies regarding the morphology of backwash ileitis date back to the 1960s. Although backwash ileitis has not been shown to be a significant risk factor for the development of pouchitis, rarely, premalignant dysplastic changes and even adenocarcinoma have been shown to develop in this setting.[44,45] In fact, one recent study by Heuschen and colleagues showed a strong association of backwash ileitis with the development of colorectal cancer in patients with UC who had undergone proctocolectomy.[46] However, even in that study, discrete pathologic criteria for backwash ileitis were not defined.

As a general rule, a mild degree of neutrophilic inflammation in the epithelium and/or lamina propria of the distal 1 to 2 cm of ileum, without features of chronicity such as pyloric metaplasia, granulomas, or architectural distortion, may be considered backwash ileitis if the patient has severe pancolitis (Fig. 10-10). However, inflammation that extends for more than 3 to 5 cm or is associated with features of chronicity, ulceration, or submucosal inflammation should be considered suspicious for involvement with Crohn's disease, particularly if the patient has only subtotal colitis or does not have severe disease up to and including the proximal cecum.

UPPER GASTROINTESTINAL INVOLVEMENT IN ULCERATIVE COLITIS

Rarely, gastric and/or duodenal involvement has been reported in association with clinically and pathologically confirmed UC.[47-50] A recent study by Valdez and coworkers described four patients with chronic active inflammation in the duodenum similar in appearance to the patients' colonic disease.[47] Until these cases are followed for longer intervals, it is difficult to know if the upper GI involvement represents truly a manifestation of UC or simply an as-yet-unidentified associated disorder. Precise characterization of these cases with

long-term follow-up is needed to help establish specific criteria for upper gastrointestinal involvement in patients with UC.

Crohn's Colitis

CLINICAL FEATURES

Although CD was originally described more than three centuries ago, Crohn, Ginzberg, and Oppenheimer are credited with the first modern description of CD in 1932.[51] This disease may involve any portion of the upper or lower gastrointestinal tract. Approximately 30% to 40% of patients have small bowel involvement only; 30% to 40% have ileocolonic involvement; and only 10% to 20% have exclusive involvement of the colon (Crohn's colitis [CC]). CD can be categorized by its clinical behavior/pattern of disease, including inflammatory, fistulizing, or fibrostenotic disease. The pattern of disease determines the signs, symptoms, and complications. For example, in inflammatory CD, patients usually present with abdominal pain, diarrhea, weight loss, fever, and sometimes lower gastrointestinal bleeding. In contrast, patients with fibrostenotic disease present with intestinal obstruction and/or jaundice.[52]

Most patients with CD present during their second to fourth decades of life, although there is a smaller peak between the fifth and seventh decades of life. Although all ethnic groups may be affected, CD is clearly more prevalent among white North Americans, Northern Europeans, Ashkenazi Jews, Scandinavians, and the Welsh.

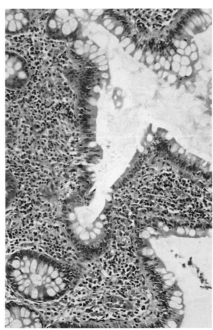

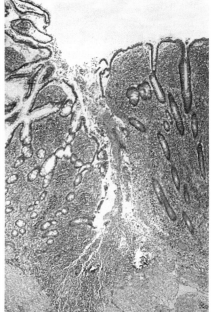

FIGURE 10–10. Backwash ileitis versus Crohn's ileitis. **A,** High-power view of backwash ileitis in a patient with severe pancolitis. A mild degree of neutrophilic inflammation in the superficial lamina propria and epithelium is associated with mild regenerative changes. No features of chronicity or ulceration are noted. **B,** In contrast, this photograph of Crohn's ileitis shows an aphthous-type ulcer with a superficial necroinflammatory infiltrate surrounded by villi that are slightly broad and shortened and show increased inflammation in the lamina propria.

A   **B**

The cause of CD is unknown but likely involves a combination of environmental factors (e.g., luminal bacteria/infectious agents), abnormalities in immune regulation, and a genetic predisposition. For example, unlike in patients with UC, smoking is an independent risk factor for clinical, surgical, and endoscopic recurrence in CD; it also influences disease activity after surgery.[6,53] Dietary factors may also play an important role; zinc deficiencies are associated with immunologic dysfunction in patients with CD,[54] and some data suggest that an elemental diet may improve CD by reducing intestinal permeability.[55]

An infectious cause has been proposed for CD as well, and although traditional methods have failed to detect a specific pathogen, molecular techniques have detected *Mycobacterium paratuberculosis* in the tissues of some patients with CD.[56]

Genetic factors are clearly important in predisposing individuals to CD. Studies have found a familiar risk as well as a higher rate of concordance for monozygotic twins with CD compared with dizygotic twins.[57,58] Although results are inconsistent and vary with the population being studied, numerous studies have found both positive and negative associations between HLA antigens and the development of CD.[59,60] More recently, polymorphisms in *NOD2 (CARD15)*, a gene mapping to the chromosome 16 IBD1 susceptibility locus, have been associated with susceptibility to CD,[61-63] particularly in those with early-onset and severe disease.[64]

PATHOLOGIC FEATURES

On gross examination, colectomy specimens for CC typically show complete or relative rectal sparing with segmental disease involving variable extents of the colonic mucosa and wall. Bearclaw-type ulcers are often present, and areas of edematous but histologically normal mucosa are found between these ulcers, resulting in a cobblestone appearance. Fissures, fistulous tracts, and mural or pericolonic abscesses may be seen. As with small bowel disease, fat wrapping is often present in involved segments.

Histologically, as can be appreciated grossly, CC shows areas of segmental colitis separated by areas of uninvolved colon (skip areas). The diagnosis of CC based on biopsy specimens can be problematic because many of the characteristic features of CC are located beyond the reach of the biopsy forceps. Most of the mucosal abnormalities found in CC are nonspecific if they are interpreted in isolation, and this diagnosis is based on the appreciation of heterogeneity of abnormalities, their patchy distribution between biopsy specimens procured from the same region of the colon, and their patchy distribution across the breadth of each tissue fragment.[65,66] Biopsy specimens from the same region usually have different appearances; normal, inflamed, and ulcerated fragments can be admixed. Often,

numerous tissue fragments from separately identified regions of the colon in conjunction with clinical and endoscopic information are necessary to make a diagnosis of CC (Figs. 10-11 to 10-14). It is usually not possible for the clinician to make a definitive diagnosis of CC without clinical and endoscopic information because treated UC can be morphologically identical to untreated CC.

Inflammation

Inflammatory foci in CC can be an even admixture, or they may be predominantly composed of lymphocytes and plasma cells, neutrophils, or granulomas. Differences in the predominant cell type between foci of mucosal involvement are a major component of the heterogeneity characteristic of CC.

LYMPHOCYTES AND PLASMA CELLS

Heterogeneity in the density and distribution of lymphoplasmacytic inflammation is a morphologic hallmark of CC. Normal mucosa can be situated immediately adjacent to segments with dense lymphoplasmacytic inflammation. Small patches of lymphoplasmacytic inflammation are frequently separated by regions of paucicellular-appearing edematous mucosa. Well-circumscribed, focal collections of lymphocytes that surround several crypts (lymphoid aggregates) simulate normal lymphoid follicles. However, lymphoid aggregates in CC have crypts within their centers; these are pushed to the periphery in normal lymphoid follicles.

NEUTROPHILS

Neutrophils in CC are also focal and patchy. They can be admixed with lymphoplasmacytic inflammation or can be the predominant cell in otherwise normal mucosa. In the latter case, they usually are located in the basal lamina propria and congregate around or minimally infiltrate crypt bases that appear to contain increased amounts of karyorrhectic debris.

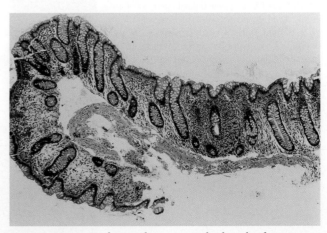

FIGURE 10–11. Crohn's colitis. A single lymphoid aggregate surrounds a crypt.

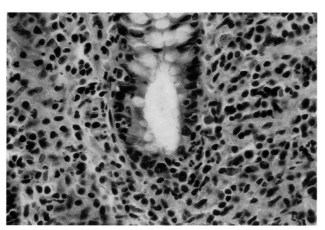

FIGURE 10–12. Crohn's colitis. High-power view of Figure 10-18. Neutrophils focally infiltrate the crypt, which is surrounded by lymphocytes. This is the early lesion that precedes an aphthous ulcer.

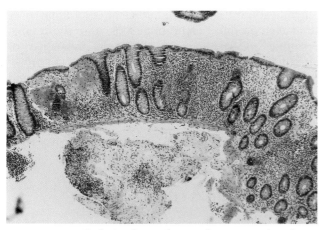

FIGURE 10–13. Crohn's colitis with crypt disarray, patchy edema, and a focal lymphoid aggregate. The crypts are haphazardly arranged.

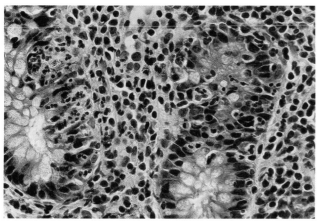

FIGURE 10–14. Crohn's colitis with focal crypt injury.

GRANULOMAS

Two types of granulomas are found in CC. Small pericryptal collections of closely arranged histiocytes have been called *pericryptal microgranulomas*[67] (Fig. 10-15). Segmental injury to crypts from pericryptal microgranulomas is suggestive of CC but occasionally can be seen in UC and other colitides.[68-70] This should not be used as the sole criterion in making this diagnosis. In typical CC, pericryptal microgranulomas are admixed with patchy lymphoplasmacytic inflammation and rare neutrophils. Serial step sections can greatly enhance the likelihood that pericryptal microgranulomas will be found.[71-73] Pericryptal microgranulomas should be distinguished from *mucin granulomas* that form around ruptured crypts. Mucin granulomas have no diagnostic significance because they may be found in UC, CC, and other colitides. CD-associated granulomas are smaller and have more sharply defined edges than mucin granulomas. The macrophages within mucin granulomas usually have greater amounts of bubbly or clear cytoplasm caused by phagocytosis of mucin and crypt contents. Foreign body giant cells are usually not a component of CD granulomas but can be found in mucin granulomas. Mucin stains are not useful in this distinction because in our experience, small amounts of mucin can be found in the cytoplasm of macrophages constituting CD granulomas.

Well-formed, non-necrotizing granulomas are usually located in the submucosa but occasionally can be found in the mucosa (Fig. 10-16). They are diagnostic of CC if found in endoscopically normal mucosa. Thick-walled capillaries, the pericryptal fibroblastic sheath, and tangential sections of germinal centers can mimic the well-formed granulomas of CC.

Crypt Injury and Ulcers

Crypt injury in active CC is usually not a homogeneous, cryptocentric process that produces extensive

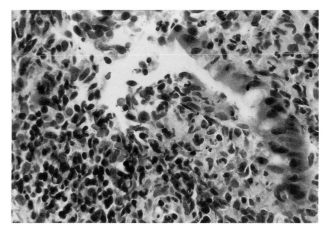

FIGURE 10–15. Crohn's colitis. A pericryptal microgranuloma has perforated the superficial crypt region and produced a superficial erosion.

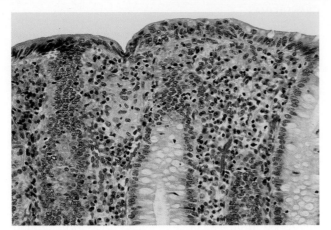

FIGURE 10–16. Crohn's colitis with a small, well-formed granuloma in the lamina propria.

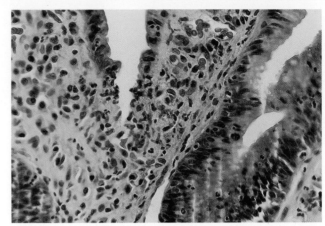

FIGURE 10–17. Crohn's colitis. Base of jagged aphthous ulcer. Neutrophilis infiltrate the epithelium and cause epithelial injury.

crypt destruction and abnormally shaped regenerative crypts, as seen in UC. Typically, one or several injured and inflamed crypts with focal mucin depletion are situated adjacent to normal crypts. The injured crypts are focally infiltrated by neutrophils, and mucin depletion is limited to the epithelial cells immediately around the focus of crypt injury.

Ulcers develop with increasing activity and crypt and surface epithelial injury. Two types of ulcers are morphologically characteristic of CC—aphthous ulcers and fissuring ulcers. Aphthous ulcers arise in focal, mildly active CC. They are well delineated, small, and superficial and are usually limited to two to four crypts; they arise from lymphoid aggregates. The earliest stage is a mild neutrophilic infiltrate in the superficial half of the lymphoid aggregate.[74] Neutrophils infiltrate the crypt(s) and form a small basilar crypt abscess, producing epithelial necrosis and intraluminal exudate. Concomitant neutrophil infiltration and erosion of the superficial epithelium eventuate into a small microabscess that covers the lymphoid aggregate as the ulcer expands. Irregularly shaped crypts with regenerative epithelial changes are found at the edges of older healing ulcers (Fig. 10-17). Aphthous ulcers can continue to expand and connect to form serpiginous or longitudinally predominant ulcers.

Fissuring-type ulcers can extend through the bowel wall. Biopsy specimens from the luminal edge or wall are usually composed of nonspecific granulation tissue and fibrinopurulent debris. Numerous histiocytes may be loosely clustered, suggesting the earliest stages of a granuloma. Their diagnostic importance lies predominantly in the evaluation of resection specimens in that they are a useful feature in distinguishing CC from UC.

Crypt Architectural Disarray and Distortion

Foci of lamina propria inflammation, edema, aphthous ulcers, and focal crypt injury together produce an irregular distribution of crypts in the lamina propria.

Variation in crypt size can also be seen if crypt injury has resulted in patchy crypt architectural disarray, a feature most easily appreciated at medium or low magnification (Fig. 10-18). Sufficient crypt injury over time can produce crypt branching and shortening, resulting in architectural distortion indicative of chronicity (Fig. 10-19). Crypt disarray is a feature of mucosal involvement in Crohn's disease and should not be considered sufficient morphologic evidence of chronicity because it can be found in any phase of CC. Similar to UC, chronic CC should be diagnosed only when metaplastic elements or architectural distortion is seen.

CHRONIC CROHN'S COLITIS

Morphologic features of chronicity are important in the diagnosis of Crohn's disease because other types of colitides may cause a similar-appearing active colitis.

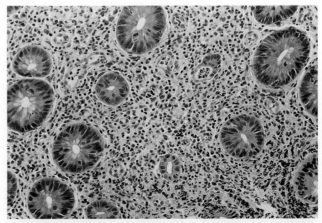

FIGURE 10–18. Crohn's colitis. Cross section of mucosa showing crypt disarray. The crypts are irregularly arranged and vary in size and shape. A small crypt in the center has sustained more serious injury than the adjacent crypts.

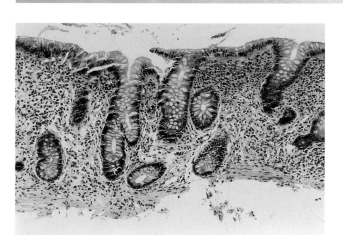

FIGURE 10–19. Chronic Crohn's colitis. The branched crypt is a feature of chronicity.

However, establishing chronicity in CC may be difficult because crypt branching or shortening is usually focal, and isolated branched crypts can be interspersed between regions of normal colon. Paneth cell and mucous gland metaplasia, both markers of chronicity, are found more often in CC than in UC.[75] Paneth cells are not normally found distal to the hepatic flexure and should be considered metaplastic if they are identified beyond this point. Mucous gland (pyloric gland) metaplasia is most commonly found in the cecum and the right colon (Fig. 10-20).

SUPERFICIAL CROHN'S COLITIS

Occasionally, the inflammation in CC is limited to the mucosa, closely mimicking UC.[76] The diagnosis of CC is established in these cases by observation of typical CC in other regions of the colon, or small bowel disease. Superficial CC is rare in our experience. More often, inadequate sampling produces a pattern simulating superficial CC.

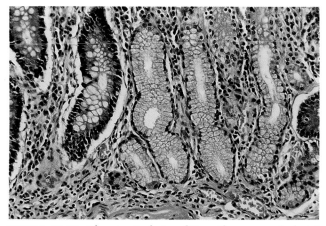

FIGURE 10–20. Chronic Crohn's colitis with mucous (pyloric) metaplasia.

■ Chronic Inflammatory Bowel Disease, Type Unknown (Indeterminate Colitis)

GENERAL COMMENTS

In approximately 5% of IBD cases, a definite diagnosis of UC or CD cannot be established, most commonly owing to insufficient clinical, radiologic, endoscopic, or pathologic data or to prominent overlapping features between these two disorders.[77-81] In these circumstances, the term *indeterminate colitis (IC)* has been used. However, this is a grossly overused term in IBD diagnostic pathology. It must be emphasized that IC is not a specific disease entity; it has no diagnostic criteria. Rather, it represents a provisional descriptive term to be used by pathologists only when a definite diagnosis of UC, CD, or another cause of chronic colitis cannot be established with the information available at the time of surgical signout. In fact, in up to 80% of cases, the true nature of the patient's underlying IBD usually becomes apparent during the ensuing few years of follow-up, or when all of the patient's clinical, endoscopic, and previous pathology material has been obtained and reviewed in detail.[82]

The most common reasons for a diagnosis of IC are listed in Table 10-2. In addition to those reasons outlined in Table 10-2, pathologists often fall back on a diagnosis of IC when a definite diagnosis of UC or CD cannot be made on the basis of biopsy specimen analysis; this practice is highly discouraged. In other instances, the diagnosis is used because of a lack of awareness

TABLE 10–2. Common Reasons for Making a Diagnosis of Indeterminate Colitis

Fulminant colitis (fissures, transmural inflammation, rectal sparing in UC)
Insufficient clinical, radiologic, and/or pathologic information
Interpretation of mucosal biopsy specimens
Failure to recognize unusual variants of UC and CD
- UC with
  - Relative rectal sparing
  - Superficial fissures
  - Granulomas related to ruptured cysts
  - Right-sided involvement in left-sided colitis
  - Appendiceal involvement as a skip lesion
  - "Backwash" ileitis
  - Therapy effect
- CD with diffuse mucosal involvement
Failure to use hard criteria for CD
- Transmural inflammation
- Granulomas
- Deep fissuring ulceration
- Ileal involvement
- Segmental disease
Presence of secondary disease (e.g., pseudomembranous colitis, ischemic colitis, infection)

regarding unusual variants of UC that can lead to apparent skip lesions in UC (previously described), or because of the unwillingness of pathologists to accept a particular finding, such as segmental disease, granulomatous inflammation, transmural lymphoid aggregates, or deep fissuring ulceration, as the solitary criterion for CD.

PATHOLOGIC FEATURES

Historically, the term *indeterminate colitis* was applied to cases of fulminant pancolitis (i.e., severe colitis with systemic toxicity often associated with colonic dilatation), a disease in which the classic features of UC may be obscured by severe ulceration with early superficial fissuring ulceration, transmural lymphoid aggregates, and relative rectal sparing (features normally associated with CD)[83] (Fig. 10-21). However, recently, the term has been broadened to describe any IBD case in which a definite diagnosis

cannot be established. Naturally, the prevalence of establishing a "diagnosis" of IC is highly dependent on the level of awareness of the pathologist regarding the wide range of morphologic features seen in IBD. For instance, in a recent study by Farmer and associates, 84 IBD colectomy specimens were reviewed by 24 university pathologists, whose diagnostic accuracy was compared with that of a single gastrointestinal pathologist with a particular interest in IBD.[80] Not unexpectedly, the gastrointestinal pathologist rendered a diagnosis that was different from that of the others in 45% of specimens; in most cases, this resulted in a change of diagnosis from UC to CD.

In most instances, cases diagnosed as IC are really UC, but a variable proportion (10% to 40%) turn out to be CD. Rarely, other pathologic mimics of IBD such as nonsteroidal anti-inflammatory drug (NSAID) colitis, diverticular disease–associated colitis, radiation or ischemic colitis, or infectious colitis may be interpreted as IC.[78] Unfortunately, there is a strong clinical need for

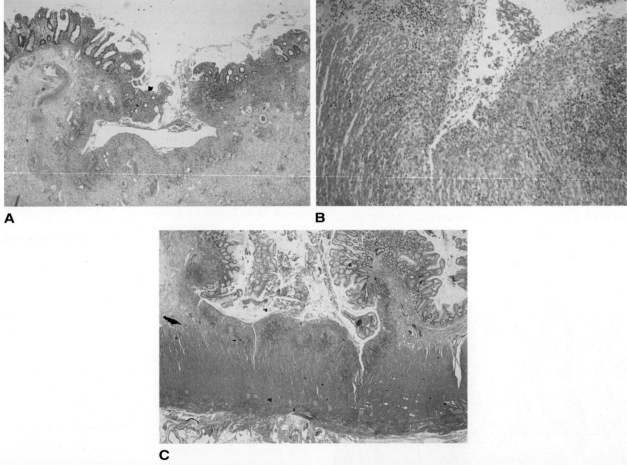

A   **B**   **C**

FIGURE 10–21. Fulminant ulcerative colitis. **A,** In cases of acute severe (fulminant) ulcerative colitis, one may see deep, flask-shaped ulcerations. Note that the surrounding mucosa shows diffuse severe chronic active disease characteristic of ulcerative colitis. **B,** Occasionally, in cases of fulminant ulcerative colitis, superficial "early" fissuring-type ulcers may be identified. However, in contrast to the true fissures seen in Crohn's disease, these fissures are only superficial and appear more like cracks in the wall of the bowel. **C,** Crohn's disease of the colon shows true deep fissuring ulceration extending into the middle portion of the muscularis propria. In addition, the adjacent colonic mucosa shows patchy disease with areas of ulceration altering with areas of uninvolved mucosa.

definitive classification of IBD patients as having CD or UC (or other); an ileal pouch–anal anastomosis (IPAA) ("pouch") procedure is generally contraindicated in CD owing to a high risk of morbidity related to pouchitis, fistulas, incontinence, or anastomotic leaks.[84,85] In 1998, Swan and colleagues evaluated 95 cases of "fulminant colitis" (IC) with the aim of identifying features that could separate UC from CD.[83] After all pathologic material and clinical follow-up information had been reviewed, microscopic examination correctly diagnosed UC or CD in 91% of cases. It is interesting to note that granulomas and transmural lymphoid aggregates away from areas of ulceration were the most specific indicators of CD.

NATURAL HISTORY AND TREATMENT

Many studies have evaluated the pathologic features, natural history, and outcomes of ileoanal pouches in patients with IC.[79-82,86-90] Results vary considerably owing to the fact that most of these studies are retrospective, use varying and undefined criteria for IC, and lack sufficient follow-up information. Nevertheless, in general, approximately 20% of IC patients experience severe pouch complications, which is intermediate in frequency between that seen in UC (8% to 10%) and CD (30% to 40%).[81,84,86,88] This is to be expected, given that in most studies, the IC study group is composed of a mixture of true UC and CD patients. In a recent study by Yu and coworkers of 82 cases of IC and 1437 cases of UC, all of which involved an IPAA operation, patients with IC had higher incidences of pelvic sepsis, pouch fistulas, and pouch failure compared with UC patients.[79] However, ultimately, 15% of IC patients had their diagnosis changed to CD, and when CD patients were removed from the analysis, the rates of pouch complications in IC and UC patients were similar.

Similarly, in another study by McIntyre and associates in 1995, 71 patients with IC and 1232 UC patients were compared for frequency of bowel movements, incontinence, and prevalence of pouchitis and pouch failure.[86] Although the failure rate in IC was higher than that in UC (19 vs. 8%), overall, IC and UC patients had similar outcomes, suggesting again that most patients with IC probably have UC. It is interesting to note that although a substantial proportion of CD patients who receive an IPAA operation experience pouch failure (30% to 45%), some recent studies suggest that CD patients whose pouches can be retained in situ have acceptable pouch function.[84,91]

ANCILLARY DIAGNOSTIC TESTS

In certain circumstances, serologic testing for antineutrophil cytoplasmic antibodies (ANCAs) and anti–*Saccharomyces cerevisiae* antibodies (ASCAs) may be helpful in classification of IC cases into UC or CD.[92]

For instance, ANCAs are detected in the serum of 60% to 70% of UC patients but in only 10% to 40% of CD patients. Of those CD patients who are ANCA-positive, most have left-sided colitis with clinical, endoscopic, and/or histologic features of UC. ASCAs are present in 50% to 60% of CD patients; ASCA has a sensitivity of 67% and a specificity of 92% as a serum marker for CD. Unfortunately, the use of ANCA and ASCA in IC has not been extensively studied, and further investigation is needed.

▮ Differential Diagnostic Considerations

DIFFERENTIAL DIAGNOSIS OF ULCERATIVE COLITIS VERSUS CROHN'S DISEASE

A summary of the classic microscopic features of UC and CD is given in Table 10–3. Important features of untreated UC in biopsy specimens include diffuse involvement of the colorectum without skip lesions, lack of submucosal involvement, lack of granulomas (except those related to mucin or foreign bodies), and lack of terminal ileum involvement (with the exception of a minor degree of inflammation associated with backwash ileitis). In resection specimens, diffuse continuous mucosal disease (including the rectum) in the absence of deep fissuring ulceration, sinus tract formation, transmural lymphoid aggregates (away from areas of ulceration), small intestinal involvement (except in backwash ileitis), or granulomas, and in appropriate clinical, radiologic, and endoscopic settings, is a finding normally considered consistent with UC.

Typical features of CD include segmental involvement, less severe disease in the distal colon compared with the proximal colon, rectal sparing, submucosal inflammation, patchiness of inflammation, granulomas unrelated to mucin or foreign bodies, terminal ileum involvement, upper gastrointestinal involvement, and a less pronounced degree of mucosal architectural changes and mucin depletion compared with UC. Under normal circumstances, any of these features should be considered

TABLE 10–3. Classic Microscopic Features of Untreated Ulcerative Colitis and Crohn's Disease

Ulcerative Colitis	Crohn's Disease
Diffuse, continuous disease	Segmental disease
Rectal involvement	Variable rectal involvement
Disease worse distally	Variable disease severity
No fissures	Fissures, sinuses, fistulous tracts
No transmural aggregates	Transmural aggregates
No ileal involvement (exception: "backwash")	Upper gastrointestinal tract involvement
No granulomas	Granulomas

sufficient for a diagnosis of CD. However, in some cases, as in fulminant colitis, a definite diagnosis of UC or CD cannot be made owing to the presence of overlapping features. Furthermore, several exceptions to the classic pathologic features outlined here have been noted (see under Unusual Morphologic Variants of Ulcerative Colitis), and these may contribute to diagnostic confusion.

DIFFERENTIAL DIAGNOSIS OF INFECTIOUS-TYPE COLITIS VERSUS INFLAMMATORY BOWEL DISEASE

Diffuse, regional, or focal active colitis without crypt architectural distortion and prominent cryptitis without crypt abscesses favor the diagnosis of infectious colitis. Crypt architectural distortion, crypt dropout, basal plasmacytosis with lymphoid aggregates, and giant cells in the lower region of the lamina propria usually indicate a diagnosis of IBD[93-95] (Figs. 10-22 and 10-23). Giant cells are also seen in infectious-type colitis, but in this instance most are found around the upper regions of crypts.

◼ Dysplasia in Inflammatory Bowel Disease

DYSPLASIA IN CROHN'S DISEASE

General Comments and Pathology

Several studies suggest that given a similar duration and extent of disease, the risk of neoplasia is similar in CD and UC.[96-99] In CD, there is also an increased risk of dysplasia and adenocarcinoma in excluded segments of bowel and in the small intestine.[100] In one study by

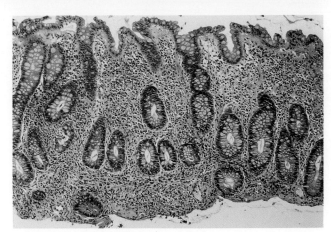

FIGURE 10–23. Ulcerative colitis seven days after onset of first episode of symptoms. Crypt branching is focally present in the left portion of the slide.

Bernstein and colleagues, the relative risk of colon cancer in CD and UC was 2.6 and 2.7, respectively.[101]

Most studies also support a dysplasia/carcinoma sequence in CD similar to that which occurs in UC.[102] For instance, in a study by Friedman and coworkers, a screening and surveillance program detected dysplasia or cancer in 16% of 259 patients who had follow-up for a mean of 24 months.[102] The reported frequency of dysplasia in CD patients with colorectal carcinoma ranges from 40% to 100%.[103,104] Dysplasia in CD occurs more often in areas close to, rather than distant from, the primary tumor. In fact, in 2% to 16% of CD patients, dysplasia is detected during the course of their illness. Regardless of the location of the primary tumor, neoplasia always develops in areas of chronic inflammation in CD, as it does in UC. In a study by Sigel and associates, dysplasia was found adjacent to carcinoma in 87% of cases and distant from carcinoma in 41% of cases.[100] In this study of 30 cases of CD-related adenocarcinoma, 27% occurred in the small intestine and 73% occurred in the colon. In a population-based study from Sweden, the relative risk of colon cancer was 2.5 in patients with CD and 5.6 in CD patients with disease restricted to the colon.[96] The relative risk was even greater in patients who were younger than 30 years of age at the time of diagnosis.

The pathologic features of dysplasia in CD are also similar to those of UC (see under Dysplasia in Ulcerative Colitis); dysplasia is classified in a similar manner (negative, indefinite, positive [low or high grade]). Some authors have also described unusual hyperplastic changes in the mucosa adjacent to carcinoma in CD, which may represent a form of low-grade dysplasia.

Treatment

Overall, the survival benefit of endoscopic surveillance in CD is controversial, primarily because of the

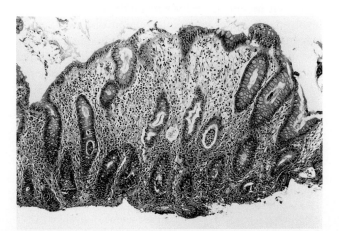

FIGURE 10–22. Ulcerative colitis three days after onset of first episode of symptoms. No crypt architectural distortion is seen. This biopsy specimen reveals the architectural and inflammatory changes of infectious-type colitis rather than ulcerative colitis.

lack of prospective studies.[96,102,105] However, there is a growing trend toward endoscopic surveillance in patients with long-standing CD.[105] Unfortunately, surveillance is often difficult to perform owing to the frequent presence of strictures that often require the use of a pediatric endoscope. In fact, up to 12% of CD-related strictures are malignant from the onset.[106] However, at present, both the American Gastroenterological Association (AGA) and the American College of Gastroenterology (ACG) recommend a surveillance strategy in CD similar to that used in UC.

DYSPLASIA IN ULCERATIVE COLITIS

General Comments

Dysplasia in UC, as elsewhere in the gastrointestinal tract, is defined as unequivocal neoplastic epithelium confined to the basement membrane; at present, it is the best and most reproducible marker of malignancy risk in patients with this condition.[16] It is present in 90% of UC patients with carcinoma, both adjacent to and distant from the primary tumor. Dysplasia may occur in any portion of the colon but often parallels the location of cancer; it may occur as an isolated focus but is more often multiple and rarely diffuse. Dysplasia may be grossly classified as either flat or elevated (dysplasia-associated lesion or mass [DALM]). This classification is important because the treatments for these various gross types of dysplasia are different, as is discussed in the following sections.[107-110]

The strongest risk factors for the development of dysplasia/carcinoma in UC are the extent and duration of disease.[111-115] Some studies also suggest that sclerosing cholangitis is a significant risk factor.[116,117] Controversial risk factors include early age of onset, family history of colon cancer, and folate deficiency.[118-120] It is generally accepted that patients with UC for at least 8 years are at risk for developing dysplasia/carcinoma and thus should be entered into a colonoscopic surveillance program.[121,122]

The incidence of dysplasia in UC is difficult to estimate; studies suggest a 5% incidence of dysplasia after 10 years and a 25% incidence after 20 years.[122-126] The overall incidence of colorectal cancer after 25 to 35 years of UC ranges from 3% to 43%. A reasonable rule is that the risk of carcinoma increases by approximately 1% to 2% per year after the first 10 years of disease. The annual incidence rate of cancer in UC patients with disease for longer than 20 years ranges from 0.5% to 3%.[125,126]

Pathologic Features

Grossly, two general patterns of dysplasia occur in UC—flat (endoscopically undetectable) and raised (endoscopically detectable).[107,127] Raised lesions, other-

wise known as DALMs, are graded morphologically, similarly to flat dysplasia, but are treated differently, as is discussed here. Microscopically, atypical changes in UC are separated into three distinct categories—negative for dysplasia, indefinite for dysplasia, and positive for dysplasia (low and high grade).[16] Dysplastic epithelium shows cells with nuclear hyperchromatism and enlargement (often pencil-shaped), a clumped chromatin pattern often with multiple nucleoli, and hypereosinophilic mucin-depleted cytoplasm (Fig. 10-24). Cells are often arranged in a pseudostratified or stratified manner. Most importantly, dysplastic epithelium does not show maturation to the surface of the mucosa. Mitotic figures are often plentiful, and atypical mitotic figures are not uncommon. Architectural aberration is common as well. Dysplastic crypts tend to have more of a "back-to-back" configuration with little intervening lamina propria, which is sometimes associated with irregular crypt budding, cystic change, villiform surface change, or cribriforming of the crypt lumen. With progression from low- to high-grade dysplasia, the cells acquire a more oval/round nuclear contour and show a greater nucleus-to-cytoplasm ratio and a more distinct loss of nuclear polarity. Mitotic figures are numerous and typically abnormal in quality. In addition, architecturally, a more complex crypt pattern is seen, with greater back-to-back gland formation.

Cases are best considered indefinite for dysplasia when the cytologic and architectural features approach those of low-grade dysplasia, but there is abundant inflammation and perhaps ulceration in the area, which may make interpretation of the atypical changes difficult (i.e., reactive vs. neoplastic). In general, surface maturation is usually indicative of a regenerative process and should always evoke caution in the interpretation of dysplasia. A negative for dysplasia finding is reserved for non-neoplastic crypt regeneration, which can be extreme in cases with fresh erosions or ulcerations.

Sampling error and interobserver variability continue to be common problems encountered in the interpretation of dysplasia in UC.[16] Since Riddell's study in 1983, several interobserver studies have shown only moderate levels of interobserver agreement.[16,128-130] In general, levels of agreement between pathologists are highest for high-grade dysplasia and for biopsy specimens that are negative for dysplasia; they are lowest for biopsy specimens with low-grade dysplasia or that are indefinite for dysplasia. Thus, recent studies have focused on finding other, more reproducible adjunctive methods of assessing malignancy risk in UC. These include a variety of histochemical markers (e.g., mucins, sialosyl-TN) and immunohistochemical (e.g., proliferation markers, *TP53*) and molecular (*APC*, *p27*, *p16*, aneuploidy) methods.[131-136] However, at present, none of these methods has been shown to be more effective than histologic evaluation for dysplasia.

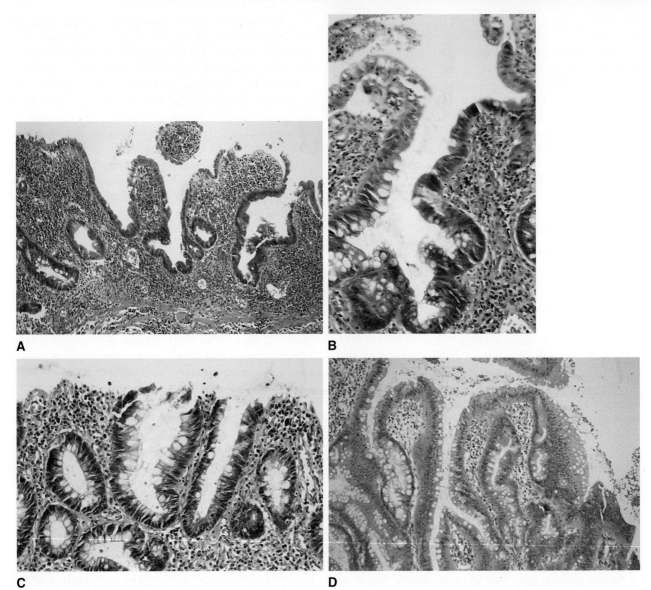

FIGURE 10–24. Dysplasia in ulcerative colitis. **A** and **B,** Low- and high-power view of marked regenerative changes in ulcerative colitis considered negative for dysplasia. In **A,** areas of superficial erosion and severe chronic active inflammation of the lamina propria are seen. The crypts show cells with marked hyperchromaticity, pseudostratification, mucin depletion, and increased mitosis. However, there is a slight degree of surface maturation, and it appears that cells are trying to reepithelialize a previously eroded mucosa. **C,** Atypia considered indefinite for dysplasia. Although the cytologic features are suggestive of low-grade dysplasia, the surface of the mucosa has separated from the specimen; therefore, it is difficult for the clinician to assess the presence or absence of surface maturation. In addition, marked active inflammation is noted in the lamina propria and in the crypts, which makes interpretation of the dysplasia difficult. **D,** Low-grade dysplasia in ulcerative colitis. This slightly villiform mucosa shows a slightly irregular proliferation of long crypts lined by cells that are hyperchromatic and pseudostratified and that show increased mitosis and a distinct lack of surface maturation. Inflammation of the lamina propria and in the epithelium is minimal.

Continued

Natural History, Treatment, and Surveillance

The initial subdivision of dysplasia into flat and raised categories is important for management purposes and relies heavily on endoscopic findings. In summary, many studies have shown that flat low-grade dysplasia has a low incidence of associated carcinoma in patients who have had a colectomy (<20%). Furthermore, the natural history of low-grade dysplasia is not fully understood, and given that there is significant interobserver variability in interpretation of biopsy specimens with low-grade dysplasia, most patients with this finding are treated with increased colonoscopic surveillance.[137,138] However, recent reports suggest that the 5-year predictive value of low-grade dysplasia for the development of either high-grade dysplasia or carcinoma may be as high as 54%.[126] Thus, many institutions now recommend colectomy for patients with flat low-grade dysplasia, particularly if it is found on initial colonoscopy, is multi-

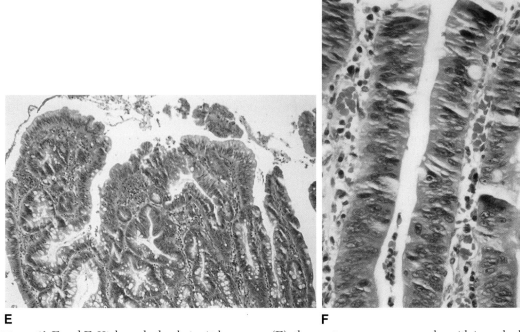

E   F

FIGURE 10–24, cont'd E and **F,** High-grade dysplasia. At low power **(E),** the crypts appear more complex with irregular budding and a more prominent back-to-back glandular arrangement. In **F,** the cytologic features of high-grade dysplasia are evident; a greater degree of atypia is characterized by marked hyperchromaticity, full-thickness pseudostratification, stratification of the nuclei, an increased degree of pleomorphism, and a distinct loss of cell polarity. Once again, no evidence of surface maturation is noted.

focal, or appears in a metachronous fashion.[126,137] In contrast, flat high-grade dysplasia involves a high probability both of cancer at colectomy (40% to 67%) and of progression to carcinoma (40% to 90% 5-year predictive value).[126,138] For these reasons, flat high-grade dysplasia is generally treated with colectomy in medically fit patients. Patients with biopsy specimens considered indefinite for dysplasia should be treated for their inflammation and should have a repeat endoscopy in 6 months to 1 year, preferably after the inflammation has subsided.[137] In all cases of dysplasia assessment, it is important and highly recommended by the AGA and the ACG that the presence or absence of dysplasia be confirmed by at least two pathologists who are skilled in gastrointestinal pathology or who have broad experience with dysplasia in UC.

The optimal surveillance strategy for patients with UC remains controversial.[139] Much debate revolves around the sensitivity of the detection system, the predictive value of dysplasia for assessing the risk of colorectal cancer, and the cost.[140-142] Data supporting the effectiveness of surveillance in patients with UC are not uniform but do suggest a reduction in mortality from carcinoma in patients who undergo surveillance and are willing to undergo prophylactic colectomy should dysplasia be detected. As a result, the overall balance of evidence supports surveillance for dysplasia in UC.

Unfortunately, widespread agreement on appropriate surveillance strategies in patients with UC has not been established.[138,143] The AGA recommends that surveillance should begin after 8 years of disease in patients with pancolitis and after 15 years in patients with colitis involving the left colon only. Colonoscopy should be repeated every 1 to 2 years. Four-quadrant biopsy specimens should be obtained from every 10 cm of mucosa from the cecum to the sigmoid colon and from every 5 cm thereafter. In addition, any suspicious lesions or masses should be biopsied. The finding of dysplasia, when confirmed by an expert pathologist, is usually an indication for colectomy. For patients in whom a colectomy is not feasible or is unacceptable, frequent surveillance (e.g., every 3 to 6 months) is considered an acceptable alternative. At present, surveillance is not indicated in patients with ulcerative proctitis.

ELEVATED (RAISED) DYSPLASIA

. Recent evidence suggests that, in fact, several different subtypes of raised dysplastic lesions (DALMs) occur in UC.[108-110] These are separated grossly into "adenoma-like" and "nonadenoma-like" lesions based on their endoscopic appearance (see Chapter 15). Nonadenoma-like lesions are large, sessile, irregular masses, strictures, or ill-defined nodules with a broad base. Any of these types of lesions should lead one to strongly consider colectomy because of their high association with adenocarcinoma. Biopsy specimens from these lesions often show only dysplastic epithelium, which usually represents only the surface of the underlying carcinoma. More commonly, raised dysplastic lesions in UC appear as well-circumscribed, isolated polypoid lesions that are endoscopically similar to a sporadic adenoma (adenoma-like).[110] In this instance, the clinical differential diagnosis includes adenoma-like DALM in UC versus a sporadic adenoma that has occurred coincidentally in a patient with underlying UC. This distinction is important because the former is generally treated with a colectomy, whereas the latter is treated more appropriately by polypectomy.[107]

Until recently, few data have helped to separate a sporadic adenoma from an adenoma-like DALM. A detailed summary of the pathologic, immunohistochemical, and molecular features that can help distinguish these two types of lesions is provided in Chapter 15. For instance, compared with sporadic adenomas, adenoma-like DALMs show a higher degree of inflammation within the lamina propria, show a mixture of normal and dysplastic crypts at the surface of the polyp, often reveal stalk dysplasia, and demonstrate a significantly higher degree of *TP53* and a lower degree of nuclear beta-catenin immunostaining.[107-110] Adenoma-like DALMs also show a higher prevalence of *3p* and *p16* mutations on polymerase chain reaction (PCR).[144] Unfortunately, although several histologic, immunohistochemical, and molecular parameters can help distinguish these two groups of lesions, in individual cases, clinicians are usually forced to use their clinical judgment in making a treatment decision.

The treatment of adenoma-like lesions in UC is summarized in Chapter 15. Compelling recent data suggest that UC patients with an adenoma-like lesion may be treated adequately by polypectomy and continued surveillance, regardless of the pathogenesis of the lesion.[110,145] It must be emphasized that the most important element in the management decision process is the endoscopic appearance of the lesion (i.e.,

adenoma-like vs. irregular, sessile, nonadenoma-like) (Fig. 10-25).

NONINFLAMMATORY BOWEL DISEASE–RELATED DYSPLASIA

Aside from a common sporadic adenoma, which is by definition a "polypoid area of dysplasia," dysplasia may rarely arise in polyps associated with polyposis syndromes such as juvenile polyposis coli and Peutz-Jeghers syndrome and in inflammatory polyps associated with IBD.

Contrary to common practice, the grading by pathologists of dysplasia in sporadic adenomas is usually not necessary because lesions with high-grade dysplasia do not have significant ramifications with regard to treatment of the particular polyp. In both cases, the adenoma should be excised in total with negative margins. However, recent data suggest that patients with "advanced" adenomas (i.e., those that are large [>1 to 2 cm] or that have a significant villous component or areas of high-grade dysplasia) may have a significantly increased risk of developing additional, more proximally located, advanced adenomas and perhaps should be surveyed more frequently.

Dysplasia in juvenile polyps occurs almost exclusively in patients with the autosomal dominant condition, juvenile polyposis coli (JPC); in this instance, the dysplastic epithelium usually appears morphologically similar to that in common sporadic adenomas[146-148] (see Chapter 15). Patients with JPC who have dysplastic juvenile polyps are considered strong candidates for colectomy.[149] Similarly, dysplasia may develop in isolated Peutz-Jeghers polyps in the colon of patients with Peutz-Jeghers syndrome, although this is extremely rare.[149] Treatment for patients with dysplastic Peutz-Jeghers polyps is controversial, but at minimum, a complete polypectomy with negative margins should be performed, in addition to removal of any other possible dysplastic lesions.[149] Finally, rarely, dysplasia may develop in otherwise typical inflammatory polyps associated with IBD. In these cases, the dysplasia is usually similar to that which occurs in the flat mucosa, and it should be treated in a similar manner.

◼ Other Colitides

ACUTE INFECTIOUS-TYPE COLITIS OR ACUTE SELF-LIMITED COLITIS

Clinical Features

Acute infectious-type colitis is a transient, presumably infectious colonic inflammation that presents with acute-onset bloody diarrhea.[4] This process resolves (usually within 2 to 4 weeks) without residual inflammation or recurrent symptoms. A variety of infectious

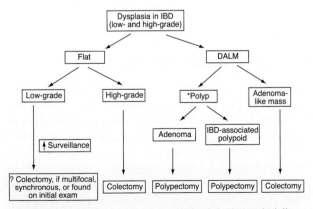

FIGURE 10–25. Algorithmic approach to treatment of dysplasia in IBD.

agents may give rise to acute self-limited colitis (ASLC). In some instances, the infection may not be self-limited, leading many pathologists and clinicians to prefer the term *acute infectious-type colitis*. Bacterial pathogens such as *Campylobacter, Salmonella,* and *Shigella* species are most often to blame; however, viral and parasitic infections may also cause acute infectious colitis.[5] In many instances, the exact cause of ASLC is not determined (see Chapter 3).

Patients with acute infectious-type colitis may present with the same symptoms as those with acute-onset ulcerative colitis; hence, colon biopsy specimens may be required to distinguish between infectious colitis and chronic IBD. Several studies have confirmed that histopathology can differentiate these two processes.[4,5,95]

Pathologic Features

The hallmark of acute infectious-type colitis is an intact crypt architecture with neutrophilic infiltrates in the crypt epithelium (Figs. 10-26 to 10-28). Although the lamina propria may be hypercellular, the cells present are generally lymphocytes, histiocytes, and neutrophils, rather than plasma cells. Basal plasma cells should not be seen in acute colitis because these are a marker of a chronic process. Crypt abscesses and crypt rupture granulomas may be seen in infectious-type colitis. Damage to the surface epithelium is also seen, with erosions and flattening of surface epithelial cells. The full-blown histologic picture of acute infectious-type colitis is increasingly uncommon in the current managed care environment because it may take a patient 2 to 3 weeks to be seen by a gastroenterologist and undergo endoscopy with biopsy, by which time the lesions may have healed. The resolving phase of infectious colitis is more challenging to diagnose because one may find only occasional foci of cryptitis (focal active colitis) with a patchy increase in lamina propria inflammation. This

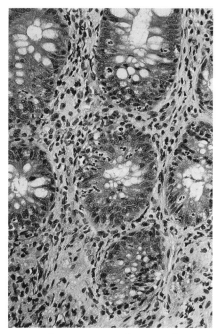

FIGURE 10–27. High-power view of acute infectious-type colitis showing foci of cryptitis.

pattern of inflammation can also be seen in smoldering Crohn's disease. Some cases of resolving infection may have residual surface epithelial damage with increased intraepithelial lymphocytes reminiscent of lymphocytic colitis.

FOCAL ACTIVE COLITIS

Focal active colitis (FAC) is the term used to describe the isolated finding of focal neutrophilic crypt injury. This term may encompass a spectrum of histologic changes from a single crypt abscess or a single focus of cryptitis to multiple discrete foci of cryptitis or crypt abscesses within a series of colorectal biopsy specimens (Figs. 10-29 and 10-30).

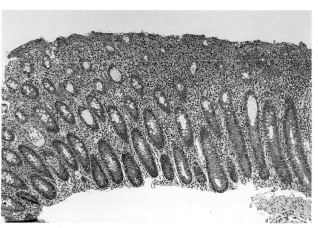

FIGURE 10–26. Low-power view of acute infectious-type colitis showing intact crypt architecture, one of the key diagnostic features of this entity.

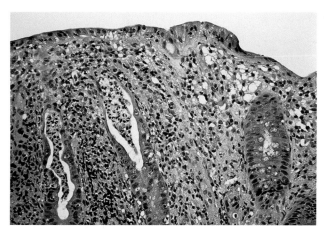

FIGURE 10–28. Acute infectious-type colitis showing several crypt abscesses and damage to the surface epithelium. Surface damage is another common finding in acute colitis.

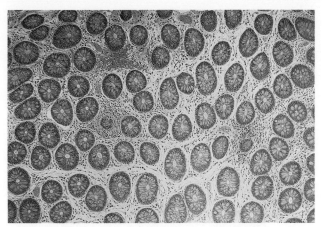

FIGURE 10–29. Low-power view of a tangential section of colon showing foci of cryptitis (focal active colitis). The two damaged crypts have a smaller diameter than the adjacent normal crypts, as well as a cuff of mononuclear cells.

Two studies of FAC have found that the most common cause of this pattern of inflammation is resolving infectious colitis.[150,151] Oral sodium phosphate bowel preparations are another important cause of this pattern of injury.[152] These preparations appear to cause cryptitis that is often centered on lymphoid follicles, identical to the small aphthous lesions that may be seen in infectious colitis and Crohn's disease. An increase in apoptosis that can mimic mild graft-versus-host disease can also be found. Other causes of FAC are shown in Table 10-4.

ISCHEMIC COLITIS

Clinical Features

Ischemia can give rise to a wide range of clinical presentations and pathologic changes. Although many cases of ischemia occur in older patients with known cardiovascular disease, ischemic colitis can also be seen

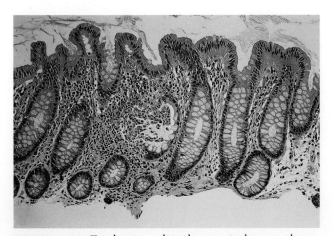

FIGURE 10–30. Focal active colitis shows a single crypt abscess with adjacent lamina propria inflammation composed of neutrophils, lymphocytes, and macrophages.

TABLE 10–4. Prevalence of Conditions Associated With a Focal Active Colitis Pattern of Injury

Type of Colitis	Number of Cases (%)
Acute infectious-type colitis	38/73 (52.1)
Incidental*	26/73 (35.6)
Ischemia	5/73 (6.8)
Crohn's disease	4/73 (5.5)

*Incidental colitis refers to cryptitis found in biopsy specimens taken from patients undergoing endoscopy for colon polyps in whom no symptoms of IBD ever developed.
Combined data on focal active colitis from Volk EE, Shapiro BD, Easley KA, et al: The clinical significance of a biopsy-based diagnosis of focal active colitis: A clinicopathologic study of 31 cases. Mod Pathol 11:789-794, 1998 and Greenson JK, Stern RA, Carpenter SL, et al: The clinical significance of focal active colitis. Hum Pathol 28:729-733, 1997.

in younger people such as long-distance runners and women taking oral contraceptives. Histologic changes can range from focal areas of acute mucosal necrosis that may be transient and require only supportive care to full-blown gangrene of the gut that may be fatal despite emergency surgery.

Although lack of blood flow to the mucosa is the underlying mechanism of disease, there is a long list of possible causes. Anything from occlusion of a major blood vessel to low-flow states secondary to hypovolemia may cause colonic necrosis[153] (Table 10-5). In addition, many drugs have been associated with an ischemic pattern of injury. In some instances, the drug may induce vasospasm (e.g., cocaine); in other cases, the medication may cause thrombosis.[154] Enterohemorrhagic strains of *Escherichia coli* (such as *E. coli* O157:H7) also cause an ischemic-type colitis, presumably because of the numerous fibrin thrombi that develop during this toxin-mediated infection. Mechanical obstruction may also lead to ischemia secondary to compression/obstruction of blood vessels. Vasculitis due to collagen vascular disease or cytomegalovirus (CMV) may cause ischemia as well.

Pathologic Features

Grossly, ischemia often shows geographic areas of ulceration with pseudomembranes. This is typically accompanied by marked submucosal edema, a finding that gives rise to the "thumbprinting" pattern seen on barium enemas.[153] Endoscopically, submucosal edema can be prominent enough to appear masslike. Watershed areas around the splenic flexure are the most common sites for ischemic lesions of the colon; however, nearly any site can be ischemic, even the proximal rectum.[155] Healed ischemic lesions may form strictures that mimic Crohn's disease.[155]

Histologically, acute ischemic lesions of the colon show necrosis of the superficial portion of the mucosa that often spares the deeper portion of the colonic

TABLE 10–5. Colonic Ischemia: Etiologic Factors

Idiopathic (spontaneous)
Major vascular occlusion
 Trauma
 Thrombosis, embolization of
  mesenteric arteries
 Arterial embolus
 Cholesterol embolus
 Aortography
 Colectomy with inferior
  mesenteric artery ligation
 Midgut ischemia
 Post abdominal aortic
  reconstruction
 Mesenteric venous thrombosis
 Hypercoagulable states
 Portal hypertension
 Pancreatitis
Small vessel disease
 Diabetes mellitus
 Rheumatoid arthritis
 Amyloidosis
 Radiation injury
 Systemic vasculitis disorders
  Systemic lupus erythematosus
  Polyarteritis nodosa
  Allergic granulomatosis
  Scleroderma
  Behçet's syndrome
  Takayasu's arteritis
  Thromboangiitis obliterans
  Buerger's disease
Shock
 Cardiac failure
 Hypovolemia
 Sepsis
 Neurogenic insult
 Anaphylaxia

Medications
 Digitalis preparations
 Diuretics
 Catecholamines
 Estrogens
 Danazol
 Gold
 NSAIDs
 Neuroleptics
Colonic obstruction
 Colon carcinoma
 Adhesions
 Stricture
 Diverticular disease
 Rectal prolapse
 Fecal impaction
 Volvulus
 Strangulated hernia
 Pseudo-obstruction
Hematologic disorders
 Sickle cell disease
 Protein C deficiency
 Protein S deficiency
 Antithrombin III
  deficiency
Cocaine abuse
Long-distance running

From Gandhi SK, Hanson MM, Vernava AM, et al: Ischemic
colitis. Dis Colon Rectum 39:88-100, 1996.

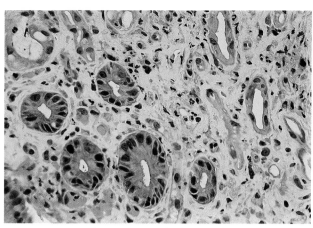

FIGURE 10–32. High-power view of ischemic colonic mucosa shows small withered or atrophic crypts with marked regenerative atypia. These changes should not be misinterpreted as dysplasia.

crypts[155,156] (Fig. 10-31). Remaining crypts usually have an atrophic or withered appearance that reveals striking cytologic atypia, which can be mistaken for dysplasia (Fig. 10-32). Other findings include pseudomembranes, hemorrhage into the lamina propria, and hyalinization of the lamina propria, which can be highlighted by trichrome stain[156] (Figs. 10-33 and 10-34). Cryptitis and crypt abscesses can be seen, but these are usually not prominent. These lesions may regress on their own, or perforation and/or stricture formation can occur. The chronic phase of ischemia may be much more difficult to diagnose because the only histologic findings may be areas of submucosal fibrosis and stricture that are rather nonspecific.

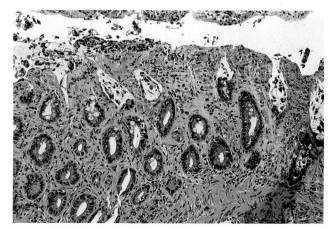

FIGURE 10–31. Ischemic colitis shows superficial mucosal necrosis with regenerative-appearing crypts in the deeper portions of the mucosa and a smudgy hyalinized appearance of the lamina propria, a specific finding in ischemic colitis.

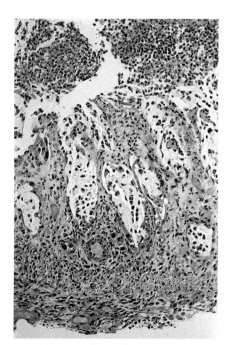

FIGURE 10–33. Pseudomembrane in ischemic colitis.

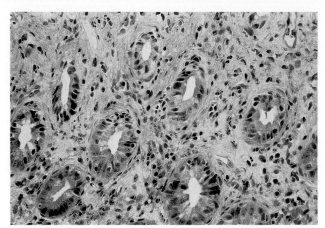

FIGURE 10–34. Trichrome-stained section shows blue staining of lamina propria in hyalinized areas, allowing distinction of ischemia from *Clostridium difficile* colitis in cases of pseudomembranous colitis.

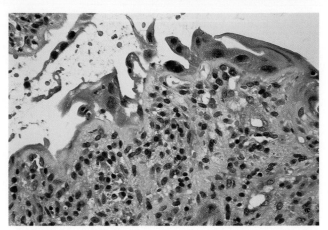

FIGURE 10–35. High-power view of acute radiation colitis shows marked cytologic atypia in the surface epithelium. Care must be taken to avoid overcalling these changes as dysplastic. (Photo courtesy of Henry D. Appelman, MD.)

Differentiating ischemia from *C. difficile* colitis can be difficult in that both may present with pseudo-membranous colitis. A hyalinized lamina propria and atrophic crypts are specific findings in ischemia that are not seen in *C. difficile* colitis[156] (see Figs. 10-32 and 10-33). In addition, pseudomembranes tend to be diffuse in *C. difficile* and patchy in ischemia. An ischemic-appearing lesion with pseudomembranes in the right colon should also make one consider enterohem-orrhagic *E. coli*, especially if fibrin thrombi are present. Pseudomembranous colitis is discussed in detail in Chapter 3.

RADIATION COLITIS

Damage to the colon caused by radiation can be either acute or chronic. The incidence of radiation colitis increases with the dose given. A dose of 4500 rads is usually required to cause clinically significant com-plications; a dose of 5000 to 6000 rads causes lesions in 25% to 50% of patients.[157] Acute radiation damage is often subclinical, and chronic radiation damage has been reported in 5% to 15% of patients receiving radiation to the pelvis.[158] Patients receiving radiation therapy for cervical and prostate cancer have the highest risk, which is no surprise, given the proximity of these organs to the gut.

Acute radiation injury occurs within hours to days of radiation exposure and is caused by damage to the epithelium. This damage usually heals within 8 weeks. Endoscopically, edema and a dusky mucosal appearance may be noted. Histologically, apoptosis with epithelial flattening, loss of mucin content, and decreased mitoses may be seen. Erosions may develop, and eosinophils are typically prominent in the lamina propria and epithelium. As the mucosa recovers from this insult, marked regenerative atypia can be seen, which should not be

misinterpreted as dysplasia (Fig. 10-35). Chronic radiation colitis occurs secondary to damage to the mesenchymal tissues of the gut. These changes may remain clinically silent for long periods, with an average range of 6 to 24 months.[158] Unfortunately, once symptomatic, these lesions can remain problematic for the lifetime of the patient.

Many of the changes seen in chronic radiation damage are due to ischemia; radiation induces occlusive damage to vessels in the submucosa and mesentery. Strictures, fistulas, ulcers, and serosal adhesions may be seen. Endoscopically, patchy erythema often correlates with telangiectasia of the mucosal capillaries—a histologic hallmark of chronic radiation damage. In addition, areas of hyalinization are often found around these dilated mucosal vessels (Fig. 10-36). Atypical "radiation fibroblasts" are

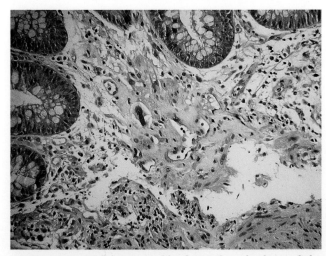

FIGURE 10–36. Telangiectatic blood vessel at the base of the lamina propria in chronic radiation colitis. Note the hyalinized area surrounding the blood vessel and the adjacent atypical-appearing radiation fibroblast.

seen in areas of hyalinized connective tissue, as occurs with radiation damage seen elsewhere in the body.

Key to making a diagnosis of radiation colitis is knowledge of the clinical history. Acute radiation damage, although not often biopsied, can mimic allergic/eosinophilic gastroenteritis. Chronic radiation damage can be subtle in biopsy specimens because vascular changes in the capillaries are easily overlooked. Occasionally, hyalinized changes in the lamina propria can mimic collagenous colitis; however, these hyalinized areas do not stain as intensely on trichrome stain.[159] In addition, the characteristic inflammatory changes of collagenous colitis are absent. Distinguishing ischemic injury due to radiation therapy from primary ischemia is often impossible on histologic grounds alone.

NEONATAL NECROTIZING ENTEROCOLITIS

Neonatal necrotizing enterocolitis (NEC) is largely a disease of premature infants that develops within the first week of life. These babies present with vomiting and abdominal distention; abdominal x-rays may show gas within the intestinal wall, peritoneal cavity, and/or portal vein branches.[160] The overall mortality rate ranges from 20% to 30% and is even higher in lower-birth-weight infants.[160,161]

The exact cause of NEC remains elusive; however, it is clear that hypoperfusion of an immature gastrointestinal tract plays a role.[161] It has also been shown that a delay in oral feeding or a switch from formula to breast milk can greatly reduce the incidence of NEC.[160,161] The role of both pathogenic and commensal bacteria is also under investigation.

The pathology of NEC is essentially that of ischemic colitis.[162,163] The most commonly involved segments of the gut are the ileum and the right colon. In addition to typical ischemic changes, the pathologist may identify intramural gas bubbles corresponding to those seen radiographically. Portions of the gut that are injured but are not surgically removed may develop strictures and become atretic.[163]

ALLERGIC PROCTOCOLITIS

Allergic proctocolitis is a disease of infants in the first year of life who develop an allergy to formula or breast milk.[164] These children present with bloody diarrhea or rectal bleeding, which often needs to be distinguished from infectious colitis, NEC, and the colitis associated with Hirschsprung's disease.[165]

Mild and nonspecific endoscopic findings of focal erythema and friability have been reported in allergic proctocolitis.[164] Ulcers or erosions have been reported rarely. The histologic features of allergic proctitis can be focal and quite subtle. The major finding is that of increased eosinophils both in the lamina propria and

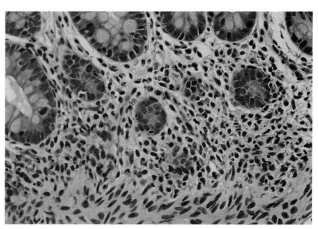

FIGURE 10–37. Allergic colitis in a young infant with bloody stools. Note the increased eosinophils in the deep aspects of the lamina propria, some of which are infiltrating the crypt epithelium. (Photo courtesy of Henry D. Appelman, MD.)

within the epithelium and muscularis mucosae[164-166] (Fig. 10-37). Several studies have found that the presence of more than 60 eosinophils per 10 high-power fields in the lamina propria correlates with allergic proctocolitis.[164,165] Because the normal number of eosinophils in the lamina propria of the colon varies by geographic region, this number may not be appropriate in more southern climates, where eosinophil counts tend to be higher.[167] The distribution of eosinophils is also important because their presence in the epithelium or muscularis mucosae and at the periphery of lymphoid aggregates also correlates with allergy. One may also find foci of neutrophilic cryptitis in allergic proctocolitis. Because of the focal nature of the histologic changes, multiple biopsy specimens from multiple sites in the colon may be required for diagnosis.[164]

The pathologic differential diagnosis of allergic proctitis is similar to the clinical one. Differentiation of allergy from infection and ischemia rests largely on the finding of abnormal numbers and distributions of eosinophils because all may show cryptitis.

Treatment of allergic proctocolitis generally involves dietary manipulation to eliminate the offending agent.

MICROSCOPIC COLITIS

The term *microscopic colitis* was first coined by Read and colleagues in 1980 to describe a group of patients with chronic diarrhea, normal colonoscopy, and a normal barium enema, who had evidence of mucosal inflammation in their colonic biopsy specimens.[168] From this subset of colitides, at least two well-defined clinicopathologic conditions have been described: collagenous and lymphocytic colitis. In addition, other less well-described lesions that cause chronic diarrhea may fall into this category.[169]

Collagenous Colitis

CLINICAL FEATURES

In 1976, Lindstrom published the first report of chronic watery diarrhea in a patient with deposition of collagen underneath the colonic mucosa and coined the term *collagenous colitis*.[170] Patients with collagenous colitis have a history of chronic watery diarrhea with a normal or near-normal colonoscopic examination. Although mild erythema may be seen, friable mucosa with exudates and/or ulcers is generally not seen in collagenous colitis unless a superimposed infectious or ischemic process is present. Women patients outnumber men by 8:1, and most patients are middle-aged or older.

NSAIDs have been implicated as a possible cause of collagenous colitis.[171] In addition, there is a well-known association between collagenous colitis and celiac disease.[172] Jarnerot and colleagues found that diversion of the fecal stream caused the histologic changes to regress, and reestablishing the fecal stream induced a relapse of the colitis.[173] These seemingly disparate findings all point to some form of luminal antigen as central to the pathogenesis of collagenous colitis.

PATHOLOGIC FEATURES

Histologically, biopsy specimens of collagenous colitis show remarkably intact crypt architecture with an increase in superficial lamina propria mononuclear cells (Figs. 10-38 and 10-39). In many cases, a pink subepithelial "stripe" may be evident, even at low magnification. At higher power, the superficial lamina propria reveals increased plasma cells and eosinophils (see Fig. 10-39). The surface epithelium shows patchy infiltration by lymphocytes with damage to the epithelium. The surface may also be stripped of the thickened collagen table (presumably an artifact of brittle collagenous

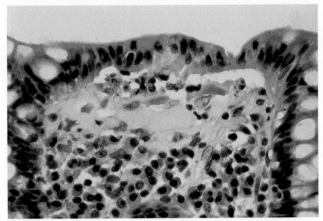

FIGURE 10–39. High-power view of collagenous colitis shows the characteristic subepithelial collagen table that is entrapping small capillaries. Also, increased numbers of plasma cells and eosinophils are noted in the superficial lamina propria, as is damage to the surface epithelium with intraepithelial lymphocytes.

tissue sectioning). The collagenous thickening typically blends imperceptibly with the basement membrane to form a hypocellular pink fibrous band that often entraps small capillaries (see Fig. 10-39). Eosinophils are often closely associated with this band.

Collagen thickness may vary dramatically from site to site in individual patients and should be evaluated only in well-oriented sections. The normal basement membrane of the colon measures 2 to 3 μm; thickness ranges from 10 to 30 μm in collagenous colitis.[174] Distal biopsies, particularly those from the rectum and sigmoid, may show less thickening that may be in the normal range. A trichrome stain highlights the collagenous band and shows the irregular nature of its lower border (Fig. 10-40). Care should be taken to avoid misinterpreting a thickened basement membrane as evidence of collagenous colitis.

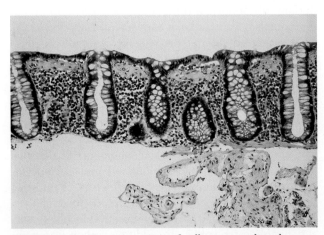

FIGURE 10–38. Low-power view of collagenous colitis shows an intact crypt architecture and a visible pink stripe across the superficial aspect of the lamina propria.

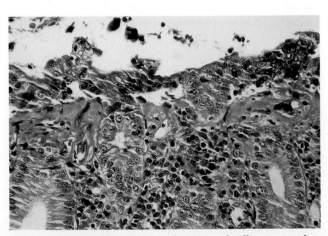

FIGURE 10–40. Trichrome-stained section of collagenous colitis highlights the subepithelial collagenous band that surrounds capillaries. Note the irregular, jagged appearance of the lower border of the collagen. (Photo courtesy of Henry D. Appelman, MD.)

Surface epithelial damage with increased intraepithelial lymphocytes should always be present in cases of collagenous colitis. Cryptitis and intraepithelial neutrophils may be seen, but these are usually much less prominent than the intraepithelial lymphocytes. Although one may rarely encounter a crypt abscess, large numbers of crypt abscesses probably indicate either superimposed infection or a separate diagnosis such as ulcerative colitis. Paneth cell metaplasia may also be seen in collagenous colitis, and this may be a marker of disease that is refractory to therapy.[175]

DIFFERENTIAL DIAGNOSIS

Several lesions, including lymphocytic colitis, chronic IBD, solitary rectal ulcer/mucosal prolapse, enema effect, ischemia, and radiation colitis, may mimic some of the histologic changes of collagenous colitis.[159] Lymphocytic colitis appears identical to collagenous colitis except for the absence of the subepithelial collagen table. Compared with collagenous colitis, chronic IBD typically shows greater architectural distortion, and the fibrosis involves deeper aspects of the lamina propria. However, some cases of collagenous colitis reveal chronic features closely simulating IBD.[176] Mucosal prolapse also shows fibrosis in deeper portions of the lamina propria, as well as muscular proliferation and crypt distortion. Enema effect may mimic some of the surface epithelial damage seen in collagenous colitis and may make it difficult for clinicians to evaluate the surface epithelium in general. Ischemia often involves fibrosis and hyalinization of the lamina propria that may be misdiagnosed as collagenous colitis; however, the other inflammatory changes of collagenous colitis are absent. Radiation colitis also shows hyalinization of the lamina propria, often with telangiectatic blood vessels, and atypical endothelial cells and fibroblasts. The hyaline material in radiation colitis does not stain as intensely on the trichrome stain as the collagen in collagenous colitis.

Lymphocytic Colitis

CLINICAL FEATURES

In 1989, Lazenby and coworkers described a subset of patients with microscopic colitis that had increased intraepithelial lymphocytes as a prominent histologic feature.[1] Lymphocytic colitis shares many of the clinical and pathologic features of collagenous colitis. Patients typically have chronic watery diarrhea with normal endoscopic findings. There tends to be a more even sex distribution in lymphocytic colitis than in collagenous colitis.

Lymphocytic colitis has also been associated with the use of medications such as ranitidine and Cyclo 3 Fort; both have been reported to cause colitis that recurred

with rechallenge.[177] An even stronger association has been found between lymphocytic colitis and celiac disease than between collagenous colitis and celiac disease.[178-180] In addition, an increased incidence of HLA-A1 haplotype and other autoimmune processes has been noted in lymphocytic colitis patients.[181]

PATHOLOGIC FEATURES

Surface epithelial damage with increased intraepithelial lymphocytes is the hallmark of lymphocytic colitis[1] (Figs. 10-41 and 10-42). In addition, a superficial plasmacytosis is generally seen without crypt distortion. The lamina propria often has fewer eosinophils than are seen in collagenous colitis, and the surface epithelium may have a greater number of lymphocytes. Surface damage and lymphocytosis are often patchy, and plasmacytosis tends to be diffuse. Care must be taken to avoid evaluating intraepithelial lymphocytes overlying a lymphoid follicle, because these are usually increased in number in this location. It should also be recognized that in normal individuals, a greater number of intraepithelial lymphocytes are generally found in the right colon than in the left colon.[1] As in collagenous colitis, a few foci of cryptitis or a rare crypt abscess may be seen, but more activity than this suggests another diagnosis.

DIFFERENTIAL DIAGNOSIS

The differential diagnosis of lymphocytic colitis includes the resolving phase of infectious colitis. In a study of epidemic chronic diarrhea linked to the water supply of a cruise ship, Bryant and associates described a colonic epithelial lymphocytosis that was similar to lymphocytic colitis (so-called Brainerd diarrhea).[182] The authors noted that surface damage was less than in lymphocytic colitis. The pathologist must ensure that the clinical history is consistent with lymphocytic colitis before making this diagnosis. Wang and colleagues reported lymphocytic colitis–like histology in patients

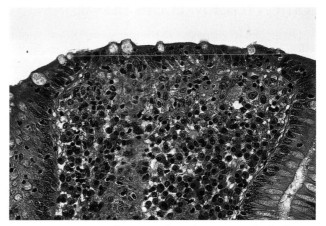

FIGURE 10–41. Lymphocytic colitis shows superficial plasmacytosis of the lamina propria and increased numbers of surface lymphocytes.

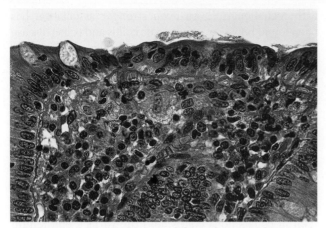

FIGURE 10–42. High-power view of lymphocytic colitis reveals damaged surface epithelium with increased intraepithelial lymphocytes. No thickening of the subepithelial collagen table is seen.

with constipation, as well as in patients with endoscopic abnormalities.[183] In addition, reported cases of Crohn's disease with patchy areas show a lymphocytic colitis–like pattern.[184] Some cases of collagenous colitis may be confused with lymphocytic colitis, particularly when only rectal biopsies are obtained or when the subepithelial collagen table in collagenous colitis is patchy.

Other Microscopic Colitides

Several other variants of microscopic colitis have been described. Bo-Linn and coworkers described a group of patients with chronic watery diarrhea and a nondistorting colitis with focal neutrophilic infiltrates.[185] McKenna and associates described a group of patients with watery diarrhea, normal endoscopic findings, and a marked increase in apoptosis (so-called apoptotic colopathy); the cause remains unknown.[186]

DIVERTICULAR DISEASE–ASSOCIATED COLITIS: ULCERATIVE COLITIS–LIKE VARIANT

Diverticular disease, particularly in the sigmoid colon, is common among patients over the age of 60. Recently, several reports of diverticular disease–associated colitis have been published that describe a chronic segmental colitis that is present in the distribution of the diverticula.[187-190] This colitis is restricted to the mucosa and is not related to diverticulitis. Patients typically present with hematochezia.

The pathogenesis of this condition is uncertain, but its clinical course and histologic features resemble those of mild ulcerative colitis. Endoscopically, changes range from patchy areas of hemorrhage and exudate to diffuse granularity. These changes are confined to the distribution of the diverticula; hence, rectal sparing often occurs.

Histologically, a range of chronic changes occur in the lamina propria, from mild plasmacytosis and mild crypt distortion to a full-blown ulcerative colitis–like appearance. Cryptitis and crypt abscesses are also seen. Classification of this colitis is difficult if the pathologist is not informed of the presence of diverticula. Key to making the correct diagnosis is the recognition that the colitis is present only in the distribution of the diverticula.

Treatment of diverticular disease–associated colitis varies from therapies aimed at diverticulitis (dietary fiber and antibiotics) to anti-inflammatory therapies similar to those used for ulcerative colitis.[188] Some patients are refractory to medical management and require surgical resection; others have developed classic ulcerative colitis.[188]

DIVERTICULAR DISEASE–ASSOCIATED COLITIS: CROHN'S DISEASE–LIKE VARIANT

Another form of diverticular disease-associated colitis mimics Crohn's disease. This form occurs in patients with diverticulitis who do not have evidence of Crohn's disease elsewhere in the gastrointestinal tract. Resection specimens demonstrate a Crohn's-like reaction to the diverticulitis.[191-193]

Grossly, segmental thickening of the bowel wall is seen with fat wrapping, a cobblestone pattern of the mucosa, and bearclaw-like ulcers. Serosal exudates and transmural sinuses are usually noted.[191]

Microscopically, nearly all of the histologic features of Crohn's disease may be present (Fig. 10-43). Of note, in one study, absence of neural hyperplasia, gastric antral gland–type metaplasia, and villiform mucosal surface changes was recorded.[191]

The cause of this reaction pattern is unknown, but follow-up studies have found that a vast majority of patients do not develop Crohn's disease (much like patients with isolated granulomatous appendicitis do not develop Crohn's disease). Pathologists must recognize this reaction pattern and must not rush to make the diagnosis of Crohn's disease in a patient with no other history or risk factors for the disease.

DIVERSION COLITIS

Clinical Features

Diversion colitis is an inflammatory process that occurs in segments of the colon excluded from the fecal stream. Although this is often an incidental finding in asymptomatic patients, some may present with mucoid or bloody discharge and/or abdominal pain.[194,195] The condition occurs 3 to 36 months following colonic exclusion and completely regresses within 3 months of reestablishment of the fecal stream.[195]

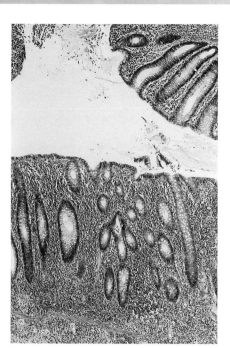

FIGURE 10–43. Low-power view of Crohn's-like diverticulitis reveals chronic inflammation of the lamina propria with crypt distortion, mimicking chronic inflammatory bowel disease.

The cause of diversion colitis is thought to be a deficiency of short chain fatty acids, which are usually derived from fermentation of dietary starches by normal colonic bacterial flora.[196] Short chain fatty acids are the main source of energy for colonocytes. Once the fecal stream has been diverted, dietary starches are no longer present. Somehow, this lack of colonocyte nutrition leads to an inflammatory disorder. Inflammation can be reversed by short chain fatty acids given via enemas several times a week.[196]

Pathologic Features

Gross and endoscopic features of diversion colitis include erythema, friability, edema, and nodularity with aphthous ulcers.[194] Histologically, the nodularity corresponds with large lymphoid aggregates with prominent germinal centers[197] (Fig. 10-44). The remaining features of diversion colitis are variable. In some instances, inflammation may mimic severe ulcerative colitis, complete with crypt distortion and marked chronic inflammation of the lamina propria. In other cases, patchy cryptitis and aphthous lesions may mimic Crohn's disease[194,195,197] (Fig. 10-45).

Because the histology is so variable, the key to making this diagnosis rests in the knowledge that the biopsy specimens come from a diverted segment of colon. Pathologists should remember that Hartmann's pouch is a diverted segment of colon that virtually always shows some element of diversion colitis (not pouchitis). Even in patients with Crohn's disease, an

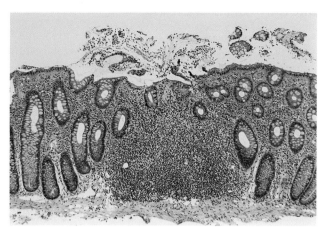

FIGURE 10–44. Low-power view of diversion colitis shows characteristic enlarged lymphoid aggregates with a small aphthous erosion.

FAC with aphthous ulcers in a diverted segment of colon should be regarded as diversion colitis because previous studies have shown that these changes quickly regress once the fecal stream has been reestablished.[198]

Biopsy specimens of a diverted segment are often taken before the fecal stream has been reestablished; once this occurs, it is critical that the pathologist make the correct diagnosis. Some form of chronic IBD will probably be diagnosed if the pathologist is not told that the biopsy specimens in question have been taken from a diverted segment of colon. This errant diagnosis will likely delay surgery and lead to unnecessary anti-inflammatory therapy.

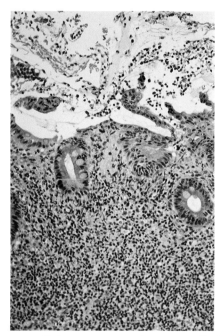

FIGURE 10–45. High-power view shows superficial erosion overlying a lymphoid follicle. These aphthous lesions can be seen in Crohn's disease and infectious colitis, as well as in diversion colitis.

DRUG-INDUCED COLITIS

Drug-induced colitis can present with a wide variety of clinical symptoms and histologic changes. Chemotherapeutic agents are often associated with ulcerative lesions of the entire gastrointestinal tract, and antibiotics are well known for causing pseudomembranous colitis secondary to *C. difficile*.[199] Other drugs are associated with less specific reaction patterns that make difficult the diagnosis of a drug-induced colitis. Perhaps the most ubiquitous agents associated with colitis are NSAIDs. These have been linked to a number of inflammatory lesions in the colon, including FAC, chronic nonspecific ulcers, ischemic-type lesions, collagenous colitis, and increased apoptosis.[200-204] Estrogen compounds have also been associated with colonic lesions. Both oral contraceptives and hormone replacement therapies have been associated with ischemic-type ulcers in the colon.[205,206]

Fibrosing colonopathy is an inflammatory lesion of the colon that was first described in pediatric patients taking high-strength replacement pancreatic enzymes.[207,208] Children with this lesion present with bloody diarrhea and typically have strictures in the right colon. The distal ileum may also be involved, but the sigmoid colon and rectum are usually spared. Grossly, the mucosal surface has a cobblestone appearance with thickening of the colonic wall. Microscopically, dense fibrosis of the submucosa and lamina propria is noted, as is thickening of the muscularis propria. Cryptitis with a hypercellular lamina propria is usually seen in the mucosa.[207] Eosinophils are prominent in the mucosa and may be present within the muscularis propria.[207] Mast cells are also increased throughout all layers of the colonic wall. Granulomas, crypt distortion, and transmural inflammation of the type seen in Crohn's disease are not seen in this disorder.[208]

▉ Preparation Artifacts

To accurately assess colorectal biopsy specimens, the pathologist must always be aware of what type of bowel preparation is used before endoscopy. Sodium phosphate enema preparations are hyperosmolar solutions that can cause damage to the rectal mucosa. Endoscopically, the rectal mucosa may appear erythematous and friable with abundant mucus, mimicking IBD and prompting biopsy.[209,210]

Histologically, enema effect is typified by flattening of the surface epithelium with edema of the lamina propria. In some cases, the surface epithelium may be completely stripped away. This can be particularly frustrating when one is attempting to evaluate the surface epithelium for changes of lymphocytic or collagenous colitis. Extravasated red blood cells, some of which may be lysed, are also found in the lamina

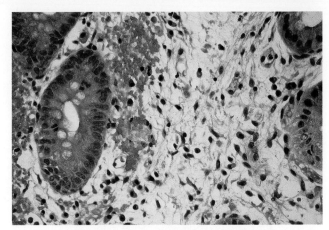

FIGURE 10–46. Enema effect indicates edema of the lamina propria with extravasated red blood cells, many of which are lysed.

propria (Fig. 10-46). In addition, mucin is often extruded onto the surface of the epithelium, and mucin depletion is seen in the crypts. The longer the time interval is between the enema and the endoscopy, the more pronounced these changes can become. If the patient has an enema the night before a procedure, one may even find neutrophils in the epithelium, mimicking acute colitis. More intense mucosal damage and inflammation can be seen if enemas containing soap or hydrogen peroxide are used.[211] Occasionally, some of the changes of enema effect are seen in patients who have not had an enema but instead have had some endoscopic trauma. This can occur in patients undergoing colonoscopy when the entire colon is visually inspected first and rectal biopsies are subsequently obtained. At academic centers, this phenomenon may be more common during the summer months when the gastrointestinal fellows are new to the endoscopy service.

Oral sodium phosphate solutions have also been associated with histologic changes in the colon. Small aphthous lesions have been seen endoscopically; histologically, these show foci of cryptitis and apoptosis centered around lymphoid aggregates.[152,211] These changes can easily be misinterpreted as smoldering Crohn's disease, infectious colitis, or graft-versus-host disease.[152]

▉ Solitary Rectal Ulcer/Mucosal Prolapse Syndrome

CLINICAL FEATURES

The solitary rectal ulcer syndrome is a bit of a misnomer in that this lesion is not always ulcerated, nor is it always solitary. It is found in the rectum, mostly along the anterior rectal wall between 4 and 10 cm from the anal verge.[212] Most patients with this condition are relatively young, otherwise healthy people who complain of blood in their stools, pain or discomfort with defecation, and alternating diarrhea or constipation.

The process is thought to be caused by malfunction of the puborectalis muscle such that excessive straining upon defecation results.[212] This straining leads to mucosal prolapse that ultimately may ulcerate and form polypoid masses. Endoscopically, these lesions can appear threatening in that the mass lesions mimic carcinoma and the ulcerative lesions mimic CD.[212-214] When this process occurs at the anal verge and a polyp is formed, it is known as an inflammatory cloacogenic polyp.[215] Similar polypoid lesions are seen in the sigmoid colon in patients with diverticular disease.[216] Small polyps develop on the mucosal folds at the mouths of diverticula, referred to as polypoid prolapsing mucosal folds. Ileostomy and colostomy stomas may also show mucosal prolapse.

PATHOLOGIC FEATURES

The characteristic finding in mucosal prolapse at any site is fibromuscular hyperplasia of the lamina propria (Figs. 10-47 and 10-48). Strands of smooth muscle growing perpendicular to colonic crypts are diagnostic of prolapse (see Fig. 10-48). Occasionally, the amount of fibrosis can overshadow the smooth muscle proliferation. The epithelium is often inflamed and ulcerated, and in some cases, an ischemic appearance may be noted, complete with small pseudomembranes. In

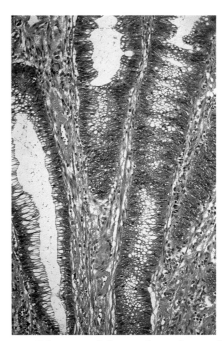

FIGURE 10–48. Solitary rectal ulcer syndrome (mucosal prolapse) reveals the characteristic smooth muscle proliferation between the crypts.

polypoid cases, the mucosa often takes on a villiform configuration that can mimic a villous adenoma. One must study the mucosa carefully to determine whether the cytologic changes are reactive or dysplastic, because the treatment for solitary rectal ulcer syndrome is different from that for a sessile adenoma. In some cases, glands may become trapped in the submucosa (colitis cystica profunda).[217] Care should be taken to avoid diagnosing this process as a neoplasm; the epithelium lining the cysts in colitis cystica profunda is cytologically bland. The smooth muscle proliferation may mimic a Peutz-Jeghers polyp; however, the branching or arborizing architecture of these lesions is absent. Because prolapsed lesions contain distorted and inflamed mucosa, it is also possible for these findings to be misinterpreted as representing IBD, especially when ulcers dominate the picture. Smooth muscle growing between the crypts is the best hint that one is dealing with mucosal prolapse rather than chronic IBD.

Solitary rectal ulcer syndrome tends to be a chronic condition, and treatment options vary considerably from increased dietary fiber to local excision of ulcerated mass lesions.[212]

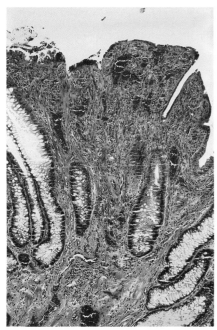

FIGURE 10–47. Solitary rectal ulcer syndrome (mucosal prolapse) shows an ulcerated mass with a villiform architecture. Care must be taken not to interpret these changes as neoplastic.

■ Behçet's Syndrome

Behçet's syndrome is a rare condition typified by oral and genital ulcers and iritis.[218,219] Systemic involvement, including gastrointestinal tract disease, may be seen. Ulcerative lesions of the colon, anus, and ileum have been described.[218] Overall distribution of disease is similar to that in Crohn's disease in that the right colon is more often involved and rectal sparing may be seen. The ulcers have a punched-out appearance that may be transmural. Transmural lymphoid aggregates and submucosal fibrosis are absent in Behçet's syndrome.[218] In addition, in most cases of colitis in Behçet's syndrome, evidence of vasculitis is noted. It has been postulated that much of the gastrointestinal tract damage that occurs in this disease is due to vasculitis-induced ischemia.

References

1. Lazenby AJ, Yardley JH, Giardiello FM: Lymphocytic ("microscopic") colitis: A comparative histopathologic study with particular reference to collagenous colitis. Hum Pathol 20:18-28, 1989.
2. Goldman H, Antonioli DA: Mucosal biopsy of the rectum, colon and distal ileum. Hum Pathol 13:981-1012, 1982.
3. Levine DS, Haggitt RC: The colon. In Sternberg SS (ed): Histology for Pathologists. New York, Raven Press, 1992, pp 573-591.
4. Nostrant TT, Kumar NB, Appelman HD: Histopathology differentiates acute self-limited colitis from ulcerative colitis. Gastroenterology 92:318-328, 1987.
5. Surawicz CM, Belic L: Rectal biopsy helps to distinguish acute self-limited colitis from idiopathic inflammatory bowel disease. Gastroenterology 86:104-113, 1984.
6. Fiocchi C: Inflammatory bowel disease: Etiology and pathogenesis. Gastroenterology 115:182-205, 1998.
7. Bridger S, Lee JC, Bjarnason I, et al: In siblings with similar genetic susceptibility for inflammatory bowel disease, smokers tend to develop Crohn's disease and non-smokers develop ulcerative colitis. Gut 51:21-25, 2002.
8. Russel MG, Dorant E, Brummer RJ, et al: Appendectomy and the risk of developing ulcerative colitis or Crohn's disease: Results of a large case-control study. Gastroenterology 113:337-382, 1997.
9. Asquith P, Stokes PL, Mackintosh P, et al: Histocompatibility antigens in patients with inflammatory bowel disease. Lancet 1:113-115, 1974.
10. Asakura H, Tsuchiya N, Aiso S, et al: Association of the human lymphocyte-DR2 antigen with Japanese ulcerative colitis. Gastroenterology 82:413-418, 1982.
11. Satsangi J, Welsh KI, Bunce M, et al: Contribution of genes of the major histocompatibility complex to susceptibility and disease phenotype in inflammatory bowel disease. Lancet 347:1212-1217, 1996.
12. Roussomoustakaki M, Satsangi J, Welsh K, et al: Genetic markers may predict disease behavior in patients with ulcerative colitis. Gastroenterology 112:1845-1853, 1997.
13. Le Berre N, Heresbach D, Kerbaol M, et al: Histological discrimination of idiopathic inflammatory bowel disease from other types of colitis. J Clin Pathol 548:749-753, 1998.
14. Schumacher G: First attack of inflammatory bowel disease and infectious colitis. A clinical, histological and microbiological study with special reference to early diagnosis. Scand J Gastroenterol Suppl 198:1-24, 1993.
15. Price AB, Morson BC: Inflammatory bowel disease: The surgical pathology of Crohn's disease and ulcerative colitis. Hum Pathol 6:7-29, 1975.
16. Riddell RH, Goldman H, Ransohoff DF, et al: Dysplasia in inflammatory bowel disease: Standardized classification with provisional clinical applications. Hum Pathol 14:931-968, 1983.
17. Markowitz J, Kahn E, Grancher K, et al: Atypical rectosigmoid histology in children with newly diagnosed ulcerative colitis. Am J Gastroenterol 88:2034-2037, 1993.
18. Meucci G, Vecchi M, Astegiano M, et al: The natural history of ulcerative proctitis: A multicenter, retrospective study. Gruppo di Studio per le Malattie Infiammatorie Intestinali (GSMII). Am J Gastroenterol 95:469-473, 2000.
19. Toyoda H, Yamaguchi M, Uemura Y, et al: Successful treatment of lymphoid follicular proctitis with sulfasalazine suppositories. Am J Gastroenterol 95:2403-2404, 2000.
20. Flejou JF, Potet F, Bogomoletz WV, et al: Lymphoid follicular proctitis. A condition different from ulcerative proctitis? Dig Dis Sci 33:314-320, 1988.
21. Bogomoletz WV, Flejou JF: Newly recognized forms of colitis: Collagenous colitis, microscopic (lymphocytic) colitis, and lymphoid follicular proctitis. Semin Diagn Pathol 8:178-189, 1991.
22. Odze R, Antonioli D, Peppercorn M, et al: Effect of topical 5-aminosalicylic acid (5-ASA) therapy on rectal mucosal biopsy morphology in chronic ulcerative colitis. Am J Surg Pathol 17:869-875, 1993.
23. Kleer CG, Appelman HD: Ulcerative colitis: Patterns of involvement in colorectal biopsies and changes with time. Am J Surg Pathol 22:983-989, 1998.
24. Bernstein CN, Shanahan F, Anton PA, et al: Patchiness of mucosal inflammation in treated ulcerative colitis: A prospective study. Gastrointest Endosc 42:232-237, 1995.
25. Kim B, Barnett JL, Kleer CG, et al: Endoscopic and histological patchiness in treated ulcerative colitis. Am J Gastroenterol 94:3259-3262, 1999.
26. D'Haens G, Geboes K, Peeters M, et al: Patchy cecal inflammation associated with distal ulcerative colitis: A prospective endoscopic study. Am J Gastroenterol 92:1275-1279, 1997.
27. Okawa K, Aoki T, Sano K, et al: Ulcerative colitis with skip lesions at the mouth of the appendix: A clinical study. Am J Gastroenterol 93:2405-2410, 1998.
28. Yang SK, Jung HY, Kang GH, et al: Appendiceal orifice inflammation as a skip lesion in ulcerative colitis: An analysis in relation to medical therapy and disease extent. Gastrointest Endosc 49:743-747, 1999.
29. Ekbom A, Helmick C, Zack M, et al: The epidemiology of inflammatory bowel disease: A large, population-based study in Sweden. Gastroenterology 100:350-358, 1991.
30. Pena AS, Meuwissen SGM: Evidence for clinical subgroups in inflammatory bowel disease. In Targan S, Shanahan D (eds): Inflammatory Bowel Disease, From Bed to Bedside. Baltimore, Williams and Wilkins, 1994, pp 272-278.
31. Mutinga M, Farraye F, Wang H, et al: Clinical significance of right colonic inflammation in patients with left sided chronic ulcerative colitis: A study of 34 patients. Gastroenterology 120:A450, 2001.
32. Davison AM, Dixon MF: The appendix as a 'skip lesion' in ulcerative colitis. Histopathology 16;93-95, 1990.
33. Groisman GM, George J, Harpaz N: Ulcerative appendicitis in universal and nonuniversal ulcerative colitis. Mod Pathol 7:322-325, 1994.
34. Kroft SH, Stryker SJ, Rao MS: Appendiceal involvement as a skip lesion in ulcerative colitis. Mod Pathol 7:912-914, 1994.
35. Goldblum JR, Appelman HD: Appendiceal involvement in ulcerative colitis. Mod Pathol 5:607-610, 1992.
36. Markowitz J, Kahn E, Grancher K, et al: Atypical rectosigmoid histology in children with newly diagnosed ulcerative colitis. Am J Gastroenterol 88:2034-2037, 1993.
37. Glickman J, Bousvaros A, Farraye F: Relative rectal sparing and skip lesions are not uncommon at initial presentation in pediatric patients with chronic ulcerative colitis. Mod Pathol 15:127A, 2002.
38. Washington K, Greenson JK, Montgomery E, et al: Histopathology of ulcerative colitis in initial rectal biopsy in children. Am J Surg Pathol 26:1441-1449, 2002.
39. Robert ME, Skacel M, Ullman T, et al: Histologic rectal sparing (RS) at initial presentation of ulcerative colitis (UC). Mod Pathol 13:87A, 2000.
40. Tang LH, Reyes-Mugica M, Hao L, et al: Histologic differences between children and adults presenting with ulcerative colitis. Mod Pathol 14:96A, 2000.
41. Schumacher G, Kollberg B, Sandstedt B: A prospective study of first attacks of inflammatory bowel disease and infectious colitis. Histologic course during the 1st year after presentation. Scand J Gastroenterol 29:318-332, 1994.
42. McCready FJ, Bargen A, Dockerty MB, et al: Involvement of the ileum in chronic ulcerative colitis. N Engl J Med 240:119-127, 1949.
43. Saltzstein SL, Rosenberg BF: Ulcerative colitis of the ileum and regional enteritis of the colon: A comparative histopathologic study. Am J Clin Pathol 40:610-623, 1963.
44. Schlippert W, Mitros F, Schulze K: Multiple adenocarcinomas and premalignant changes in "backwash" ileitis. Am J Med 66:879-882, 1979.

45. Gustavsson S, Weiland LH, Kelly KA: Relationship of backwash ileitis to ileal pouchitis after ileal pouch-anal anastomosis. Dis Colon Rectum 30:25-28, 1987.
46. Heuschen UA, Hinz U, Allemeyer EH, et al: Backwash ileitis is strongly associated with colorectal carcinoma in ulcerative colitis. Gastroenterology 120:841-847, 2001.
47. Valdez R, Appelman HD, Bronner MP, et al: Diffuse duodenitis associated with ulcerative colitis. Am J Surg Pathol 24:1407-1413, 2000.
48. Igarashi M, Hirokado K, Suziki Y, et al: A case report of ulcerative colitis complicated with ulcerative duodenitis. J Soc Coloproct Col 37:255-260, 1984.
49. Sasaki M, Okada K, Koyama S, et al: Ulcerative colitis complicated by gastroduodenal lesions. J Gastroenterol 31:585-589, 1996.
50. Mitomi H, Atari E, Eusugi H, et al: Distinctive diffuse duodenitis associated with ulcerative colitis. Dig Dis Sci 42:684-693, 1997.
51. Crohn BB, Ginzburg L, Oppenheimer GD: Regional ileitis. A pathological and clinical entity. October 15, 1932.
52. Lopez I, Sellin JH: Crohn's disease: Clinical challenges. Clin Perspect Gastroenterol 5:137-146, 2001.
53. Somerville KW, Logan RFA, Edmond M, et al: Smoking and Crohn's disease. BMJ 289:954-956, 1984.
54. Ainly C, Cason J, Slavin BM, et al: The influence of zinc status and malnutrition on immunological function in Crohn's disease. Gastroenterology 100:1616-1625, 1991.
55. Teahon K, Smethurst P, Pearson M, et al: The effect of elemental diet on intestinal permeability and inflammation in Crohn's disease. Gastroenterology 101:84-89, 1991.
56. Lamps LW, Madhusudhan KT, Havens JN, et al: Pathogenic *Yersinia* DNA is detected in bowel and mesenteric lymph nodes from patients with Crohn's disease. Am J Surg Pathol 27:220-227, 2003.
57. Orholm M, Munkholm P, Langholz E, et al: Familial occurrence of inflammatory bowel disease. N Engl J Med 324:84-88, 1991.
58. Tysk C, Lindberg E, Jarnerot G, et al: Ulcerative colitis and Crohn's disease in unselected population of monozygotic and dizygotic twins: A study of heritability and the influence of smoking. Gut 29:990-996, 1988.
59. Toyoda H, Wang S-J, Yang H-J, et al: Distinct associations of HLA class II genes with inflammatory bowel disease. Gastroenterology 104:741-748, 1993.
60. Nakajima A, Matsuhashi N, Kodama T, et al: HLA-linked susceptibility and resistance genes in Crohn's disease. Gastroenterology 109:1462-1467, 1995.
61. Hugot JP, Laurent-Puig P, Gower-Rousseau C, et al: Mapping of a susceptibility locus for Crohn's disease on chromosome 16. Nature 379:821-823, 1996.
62. Ohmen JD, Yang HY, Yamamoto KK, et al: Susceptibility locus for inflammatory bowel disease on chromosome 16 has a role in Crohn's disease, but not in ulcerative colitis. Hum Mol Genet 5:1679-1684, 1996.
63. Brant SR, Fu Y, Fields C, et al: American families with Crohn's disease have strong evidence for linkage to chromosome 16 but not chromosome 12. Gastroenterology 115:1056-1061, 1998.
64. Brant SR, Panhuysen CIM, Bailey-Wilson JE, et al: Linkage heterogeneity for the IBD 1 locus in Crohn's disease pedigrees by disease onset and severity. Gastroenterology 119:1483-1490, 2000.
65. Farmer RG, Hawk WA, Turnbull RB Jr: Regional enteritis of the colon: A clinical and pathologic comparison with ulcerative colitis. Am J Dig Dis 13:501-514, 1968.
66. Kleer CG, Appelman HD: Surgical pathology of Crohn's disease. Surg Clin North Am 81:13-30, 2001.
67. Rotterdam H, Korelitz BI, Sommers SC: Microgranulomas in grossly normal rectal mucosa in Crohn's disease. Am J Clin Pathol 67:550-554, 1977.
68. Dundas SA, Mansour P: Defining epithelioid cell granulomas. J Clin Pathol 50:880, 1997.
69. Lee FD, Maguire C, Obeidat W, et al: Importance of cryptolytic lesions and pericryptal granulomas in inflammatory bowel disease. J Clin Pathol 50:148-152, 1997.
70. Warren BF, Shepherd NA, Price AB, et al: Importance of cryptolytic lesions and pericryptal granulomas in inflammatory bowel disease. J Clin Pathol 50:880-881, 1997.
71. Surawicz CM, Meisel JL, Ylvisaker T, et al: Rectal biopsy in the diagnosis of Crohn's disease: Value of multiple biopsies and serial sectioning. Gastroenterology 80:66-71, 1981.
72. Kuramoto S, Oohara T, Ihara O, et al: Granulomas of the gut in Crohn's disease. A step sectioning study. Dis Colon Rectum 30:6-11, 1987.
73. Petri M, Poulsen SS, Christensen K, et al: The incidence of granulomas in serial sections of rectal biopsies from patients with Crohn's disease. Acta Pathol Microbiol Immunol Scand [A] 90:145-147, 1982.
74. Rickert RR, Carter HW: The "early" ulcerative lesion of Crohn's disease: Correlative light- and scanning electron-microscopic studies. J Clin Gastroenterol 2:11-19, 1980.
75. Dundas SA, Dutton J, Skipworth P: Reliability of rectal biopsy in distinguishing between chronic inflammatory bowel disease and acute self-limiting colitis. Histopathology 31:60-66, 1997.
76. McQuillan A, Appelman HD: Superficial Crohn's disease: A study of 10 patients. Surg Pathol 2:3-10, 1989.
77. Geboes K: Crohn's disease, ulcerative colitis or indeterminate colitis—how important is it to differentiate? Acta Gastroenterol Belg 64:197-200, 2001.
78. Nicholls RJ, Wells AD: Indeterminate colitis. Baillieres Clin Gastroenterol 6:105-112, 1992.
79. Yu CS, Pemberton JH, Larson D: Ileal pouch-anal anastomosis in patients with indeterminate colitis. Dis Colon Rectum 43:1487-1496, 2000.
80. Farmer M, Petras RE, Hunt LE, et al: The importance of diagnostic accuracy in colonic inflammatory bowel disease. Am J Gastroenterol 95:3184-3188, 2000.
81. Marcello PW, Schoetz DJ, Roberts PL, et al: Evolutionary changes in the pathologic diagnosis after the ileoanal pouch procedure. Dis Colon Rectum 40:263-269, 1997.
82. Meucci G, Bortoli A, Riccioli FA, et al: Frequency and clinical evolution of indeterminate colitis: A retrospective multi-centre study in northern Italy. Eur J Gastroenterol Hepatol 11:909-913, 1999.
83. Swan NC, Goeghan JG, O'Donoghue DP, et al: Fulminant colitis in inflammatory bowel disease. Dis Colon Rectum 41:1511-1515, 1998.
84. Sagar PM, Dozois RR, Wolff BG: Long-term results of ileal pouch-anal anastomosis in patients with Crohn's disease. Dis Colon Rectum 39:893-898, 1996.
85. Grobler SP, Hosie KB, Affie E, et al: Outcome of restorative proctocolectomy when the diagnosis is suggestive of Crohn's disease. Gut 34:1384-1388, 1993.
86. McIntyre PB, Pemberton JH, Wolff BG, et al: Indeterminate colitis: Long term outcome in patients after ileal pouch-anal anastomosis. Dis Colon Rectum 38:51-54, 1995.
87. Pezim ME, Pemberton JH, Beart RW Jr, et al: Outcome of "indeterminate" colitis following ileal pouch-anal anastomosis. Dis Colon Rectum 32:653-658, 1989.
88. Koltun WA, Schoetz DJ, Roberts PL, et al: Indeterminate colitis predisposes to perineal complications after ileal pouch-anal anastomosis. Dis Colon Rectum 34:857-860, 1991.
89. Riegler G, Arimoli A, Esposito P, et al: Clinical evolution in an outpatient series with indeterminate colitis. Dis Colon Rectum 40:437-439, 1997.
90. Kangas E, Matikainen M, Mattila J: Is "indeterminate colitis" Crohn's disease in the long-term follow-up? Int Surg 79:120-123, 1994.
91. Wells AD, McMillan I, Price AB, et al: Natural history of indeterminate colitis. Br J Surg 78:179-181, 1991.
92. Papadakis KA, Targan SR: Serologic testing in inflammatory bowel disease: Its value in indeterminate colitis. Curr Gastroenterol Rep 1:482-485, 1999.
93. Anand BS, Malhotra V, Bhattacharya SK, et al: Rectal histology in acute bacillary dysentery. Gastroenterology 90:654-660, 1986.
94. Tsang P, Rotterdam H: Biopsy diagnosis of colitis: Possibilities and pitfalls. Am J Surg Pathol 23:423-430, 1999.
95. Kumar NB, Nostrant TT, Appelman HD: The histopathologic spectrum of acute self-limited colitis (acute infectious-type colitis). Am J Surg Pathol 6:523-529, 1982.
96. Ekbom A, Helmick C, Zack M, et al: Increased risk of large-bowel cancer in Crohn's disease with colonic involvement. Lancet 336:357-359, 1990.
97. Rubio CA, Befrits R: Colorectal adenocarcinoma in Crohn's disease: A retrospective histologic study. Dis Colon Rectum 40:1072-1078, 1997.
98. Greenstein AJ, Sachar DB, Smith H, et al: Comparison of cancer risk in Crohn's disease and ulcerative colitis. Cancer 48:2742-2745, 1981.

99. Gyde SN, Prior P, Macartney JC, et al: Malignancy in Crohn's disease. Gut 21:1024-1029, 1980.

100. Sigel JE, Petras RE, Lashner BA, et al: Intestinal adenocarcinoma in Crohn's disease: Report of 30 cases with a focus on coexisting dysplasia. Am J Surg Pathol 23:651-655, 1999.

101. Bernstein CN, Blanchard JF, Kliewer E, et al: Cancer risk in patients with inflammatory bowel disease: A population-based study. Cancer 91:854-862, 2001.

102. Friedman S, Rubin PH, Bodian C, et al: Screening and surveillance colonoscopy in chronic Crohn's colitis. Gastroenterology 120:820-826, 2001.

103. Connell WR, Sheffield JP, Kamm MA, et al: Lower gastrointestinal malignancy in Crohn's disease. Gut 35:347-352, 1994.

104. Hamilton SR: Colorectal carcinoma in patients with Crohn's disease. Gastroenterology 89:398-407, 1985.

105. Hanauer SB, Meyers S: Practice guidelines. Management of Crohn's disease in adults. Am J Gastroenterol 92:559-566, 1997.

106. Yamazaki Y, Ribeiro MB, Sachar DB, et al: Malignant colorectal strictures in Crohn's disease. Am J Gastroenterol 86:882-885, 1991.

107. Torres C, Antonioli D, Odze RD: Polypoid dysplasia and adenomas in inflammatory bowel disease. Am J Surg Pathol 22:275-284, 1998.

108. Odze RD: Adenomas and adenoma-like DALMs in chronic ulcerative colitis: A clinical, pathologic, and molecular review. Am J Gastroenterol 94:1746-1750, 1999.

109. Odze R, Brown CA, Noffsinger AE, et al: Genetic alterations in chronic ulcerative colitis associated adenoma-like DALMs are similar to non-colitic sporadic adenomas. Am J Surg Pathol 24:1209-1216, 2000.

110. Engelsgjerd M, Farraye F, Odze RD: Polypectomy may be adequate treatment for adenoma-like dysplastic lesions in chronic ulcerative colitis. Gastroenterology 117:1288-1294, 1999.

111. Bernstein CN: Cancer surveillance in inflammatory bowel disease. Curr Gastroenterol Rep 1:496-504, 1999.

112. Ekbom A, Helmick C, Zack M, et al: Ulcerative colitis and colorectal cancer: A population-based study. N Engl J Med 323:128-133, 1990.

113. Lennard-Jones JE, Melvill DM, Morson BC, et al: Precancer and cancer in extensive ulcerative colitis: Findings among 401 patients over 22. Gut 31:800-806, 1990.

114. Greenstein AJ, Sachar DB, Smith H, et al: Cancer in universal and left-sided ulcerative colitis: Factors determining risk. Gastroenterology 77:290-294, 1979.

115. Collins JH, Feldman M, Fordtran JS: Colon cancer, dysplasia and influence of surveillance in patients with ulcerative colitis. N Engl J Med 316:1654-1658, 1987.

116. Brentnall TA, Haggitt RC, Rabinovitch PS, et al: Risk and natural history of colonic neoplasia in patients with primary sclerosing cholangitis and ulcerative colitis. Gastroenterology 110:331-338, 1996.

117. Shetty K, Rybicki L, Brzezinski A, et al: The risk of cancer or dysplasia in ulcerative colitis patients with primary sclerosing cholangitis. Am J Gastroenterol 94:1643-1649, 1999.

118. Sugita A, Sachar DB, Bodian C, et al: Colorectal cancer in ulcerative colitis: Influence of anatomical extent and age at onset on colitis-cancer interval. Gut 32:167-169, 1991.

119. Nuako KW, Ahlquist DA, Mahoney DW, et al: Familial predisposition for colorectal cancer in chronic ulcerative colitis: A case-control study. Gastroenterology 115:1079-1082, 1998.

120. Lashner BA, Silverstein MD, Hanauer SB: Hazard rates for dysplasia and cancer in ulcerative colitis: Result from a surveillance program. Dig Dis Sci 34:1536-1541, 1989.

121. Nugent FW, Haggitt RC, Gilpin PA: Cancer surveillance in ulcerative colitis. Gastroenterology 100:1241-1248, 1991.

122. Woolrich AJ, DaSilva MD, Korelitz BI: Surveillance in the routine management of ulcerative colitis: The prediction value of low-grade dysplasia. Gastroenterology 103:431-438, 1992.

123. Rozen P, Baratz M, Fefer F, et al: Low incidence of significant dysplasia in a successful endoscopic surveillance program of patients with ulcerative colitis. Gastroenterology 108:1361-1370, 1995.

124. Kewenter J, Ahiman H, Hulten L: Cancer risk in extensive ulcerative colitis. Ann Surg 188:824-828, 1987.

125. Langholz E, Munkholm P, Davidsen M, et al: Colorectal cancer risk and mortality in patients with ulcerative colitis. Gastroenterology 103:1444-1451, 1992.

126. Connell WR, Lennard-Jones JE, Williams CB, et al: Factors affecting the outcome of endoscopic surveillance for cancer in ulcerative colitis. Gastroenterology 107:934-944, 1994.

127. Blackstone MO, Riddell RH, Rogers BHG, et al: Dysplasia-associated lesion or mass (DALM) detected by colonoscopy in long-standing ulcerative colitis: An indication for colectomy. Gastroenterology 8:366-374, 1981.

128. Odze RD, Goldblum JR, Noffsinger A: Interobserver variability in the diagnosis of ulcerative colitis-associated dysplasia by telepathology. Mod Pathol 15:379-386, 2000.

129. Dixon MF, Brown LJR, Gilmour HM, et al: Observer variation in the assessment of dysplasia in ulcerative colitis. Histopathology 13:385-397, 1988.

130. Melville DM, Jass JR, Morson BC, et al: Observer study on the grading of dysplasia in ulcerative colitis: Comparison with clinical outcome. Hum Pathol 20:1008-1014, 1990.

131. Burmer GC, Rabinovitch, PS, Haggitt RC, et al: Neoplastic progression in ulcerative colitis: Histology, DNA content, and loss of a p53 allele. Gastroenterology 103:1602-1610, 1992.

132. Lofberg R, Brostom O, Karlen P, et al: DNA aneuploidy in ulcerative colitis: Reproducibility, topographic distribution, and relation to dysplasia. Gastroenterology 102:1149-1154, 1992.

133. Itzkowitz SH, Young E, Dubois D, et al: Sialosyl-Tn antigen is prevalent and precedes dysplasia in ulcerative colitis: A retrospective case-control study. Gastroenterology 110;694-704, 1996.

134. Itzkowitz SH, Greenwald B, Meltzer SJ: Colon carcinogenesis in inflammatory bowel disease. Inflamm Bowel Dis 1:142, 1995.

135. Greenwald BD, Harpaz N, Yin J, et al: Loss of heterozygosity affecting the p53, Rb, and mcc/apc tumor suppressor gene loci in dysplastic and cancerous ulcerative colitis. Cancer Res 52:741-745, 1992.

136. Rubin CE, Haggitt RC, Burmer GC, et al: DNA aneuploidy in colonic biopsies predicts future development of dysplasia in ulcerative colitis. Gastroenterology 103:1611-1620, 1992.

137. Itzkowitz SH: Inflammatory bowel disease and cancer. Gastroenterol Clin North Am 26:129-139, 1997.

138. Bernstein CN, Shanahan F, Weinstein WM: Are we telling patients the truth about surveillance colonoscopy in ulcerative colitis? Lancet 343:71-74, 1994.

139. Provenzale D, Wong JB, Onken JE, et al: Performing a cost-effectiveness analysis: Surveillance of patients with ulcerative colitis. Am J Gastroenterol 93:872-880, 1998.

140. Lennard-Jones JE: Cancer risk in ulcerative colitis: Surveillance or surgery. Br J Surg 72(suppl):S84, 1985.

141. Collins RH, Feldman M, Fordtran JS: Colon cancer, dysplasia, and surveillance in patients with ulcerative colitis. A critical review. N Engl J Med 316:1654-1658, 1987.

142. Axon AT: Cancer surveillance in ulcerative colitis. A time for reappraisal. Gut 35:587-589, 1994.

143. Karlen P, Kornfeld D, Bromstrom O, et al: Is colonoscopic surveillance reducing colorectal cancer mortality in ulcerative colitis? A population based case control study. Gut 42:711-714, 1998.

144. Walsh SV, Loda M, Torres CM, et al: P53 and beta catenin expression in chronic ulcerative colitis–associated polypoid dysplasia and sporadic adenomas: An immunohistochemical study. Am J Surg Pathol 23:963-969, 1999.

145. Rubin PH, Friedman S, Harpaz N, et al: Colonoscopic polypectomy in chronic colitis: Conservative management after endoscopic resection of dysplastic polyps. Gastroenterology 117:1295-1300, 1999.

146. Desai DC, Neale KF, Talbot IC, et al: Juvenile polyposis. Br J Surg 82:14-17, 1995.

147. Jass JR, Williams CB, Bussay HJR, et al: Juvenile polyposis—a precancerous condition. Histopathology 13:619-630, 1988.

148. Coburn MC, Pricolo VE, DeLuca FG, et al: Malignant potential in intestinal juvenile polyposis syndromes. Ann Surg Oncol 2:386-391, 1995.

149. Wirtzfeld DA, Petrelli NJ, Rodriguez-Bigas MA: Hamartomatous polyposis syndromes: Molecular genetics, neoplastic risk, and surveillance recommendations. Ann Surg Oncol 8:319-327, 2001.

150. Volk EE, Shapiro BD, Easley KA, et al: The clinical significance of a biopsy-based diagnosis of focal active colitis: A clinicopathologic study of 31 cases. Mod Pathol 11:789-794, 1998.

151. Greenson JK, Stern RA, Carpenter SL, et al: The clinical significance of focal active colitis. Hum Pathol 28:729-733, 1997.

152. Driman DK, Preiksaitis HG: Colorectal inflammation and increased cell proliferation associated with oral sodium phosphate bowel preparation solution. Hum Pathol 29:972-978, 1998.

153. Gandhi SK, Hanson MM, Vernava AM, et al: Ischemic colitis. Dis Colon Rectum 39:88-100, 1996.

154. Deana DG, Dean PJ: Reversible ischemic colitis in young women. Association with oral contraceptive use. Am J Surg Pathol 19:454-462, 1995.

155. Haggitt RC: Differential diagnosis of colitis. In Goldman H, Appelman HD, Kaufman N (eds): Gastrointestinal Pathology, 1st ed. Baltimore, Williams and Wilkins, 1990, pp 342-348.

156. Dignan CR, Greenson JK: Can ischemic colitis be differentiated from *Clostridium difficile* colitis in biopsy specimens? Am J Surg Pathol 21:706-710, 1997.

157. Berthrong M, Fajardo LF: Radiation injury in surgical pathology. II. Alimentary tract. Am J Surg Pathol 5:153-176, 1981.

158. Oya M, Yao T, Tsuneyoshi M: Chronic irradiation enteritis: Its correlation with the elapsed time interval and morphological changes. Hum Pathol 27:774-781, 1996.

159. Lazenby AJ, Yardley JH, Giardiello FM, et al: Pitfalls in the diagnosis of collagenous colitis: Experience with 75 cases from a registry of collagenous colitis at the Johns Hopkins Hospital. Hum Pathol 21:905-910, 1990.

160. Caplan MS, Jilling T: Neonatal necrotizing enterocolitis: Possible role of probiotic supplementation. J Pediatr Gastroenterol Nutr 30:S18-S22, 2000.

161. Coit AK: Necrotizing enterocolitis. J Perinat Neonatal Nurs 12:53-66, 1999.

162. Stevenson JK, Graham CB, Oliver TK Jr, et al: Neonatal necrotizing enterocolitis. Am J Surg 118:260-272, 1969.

163. Beardnore HE, Rodgers BM, Outerbridge E: Necrotizing enterocolitis (ischemic enteropathy) with the sequel of colonic atresia. Gastroenterology 74:914-917, 1978.

164. Odze RD, Bines J, Leichtner AM, et al: Allergic proctocolitis in infants: A prospective clinicopathologic biopsy study. Hum Pathol 24:668-674, 1993.

165. Winter HS, Antonioli DA, Fukagawa N, et al: Allergy-related proctocolitis in infants: Diagnostic usefulness of rectal biopsy. Mod Pathol 3:5-10, 1990.

166. Goldman H, Proujansky R: Allergic proctocolitis and gastroenteritis in children: Clinical and mucosal biopsy features in 53 cases. Am J Surg Pathol 10:75-86, 1986.

167. Pascal RR, Gramlich TL, Parker KM, et al: Geographic variations in eosinophil concentration in normal colonic mucosa. Mod Pathol 10:363-365, 1997.

168. Read NW, Krejs GJ, Read MG, et al: Chronic diarrhea of unknown origin. Gastroenterology 78:264-271, 1980.

169. Kingham JG, Levison DA, Ball JA, et al: Microscopic colitis—a cause of chronic watery diarrhoea. Br Med J Clin Res Ed 285:1601-1604, 1982.

170. Lindstrom CG: "Collagenous colitis" with watery diarrhea. A new entity? Pathol Eur 11:87-89, 1976.

171. Riddell RH, Tanaka M, Mazzoleni G: Non-steroidal anti-inflammatory drugs as a possible cause of collagenous colitis: A case-control study. Gut 33:683-686, 1992.

172. Breen E, Rarren C, Connolly C, et al: Collagenous colitis and celiac disease. Gut 28:364, 1987.

173. Jarnerot G, Tysk C, Bohr J, et al: Collagenous colitis and fecal stream diversion. Gastroenterology 109:449-455, 1995.

174. Jessurun J, Yardley JH, Giardiello GM, et al: Chronic colitis with thickening of the subepithelial collagen layer (collagenous colitis). Hum Pathol 18:839-848, 1987.

175. Goff JS, Barnett JL, Pelke T, et al: Collagenous colitis: Histopathology and clinical course. Am J Gastroenterol 92:57-60, 1997.

176. Ayata G, Ithamukkala S, Sapp H, et al: Prevalence and significance of inflammatory bowel disease-like morphologic features in collagenous and lymphocytic colitis. Am J Surg Pathol 26:1414-1423, 2002.

177. Beaugerie L, Luboinski J, Brousse N, et al: Drug induced lymphocytic colitis. Gut 35:426-428, 1994.

178. Beaugerie L, Patey N, Brousse N: Ranitidine, diarrhea, and lymphocytic colitis. Gut 37:708-711, 1995.

179. Wolber R, Owen D, Freeman H: Colonic lymphocytosis in patients with celiac sprue. Hum Pathol 21:1092-1096, 1990.

180. DuBois RN, Lazenby AJ, Yardley JH, et al: Lymphocytic enterocolitis in patients with 'refractory sprue.' JAMA 262:935-937, 1989.

181. Giardiello FM, Lazenby AJ, Yardley JH, et al: Increased HLA A1 and diminished HLA A3 in lymphocytic colitis compared to controls and patients with collagenous colitis. Dig Dis Sci 37:496-499, 1992.

182. Bryant DA, Mintz ED, Puhr ND, et al: Colonic epithelial lymphocytosis associated with an epidemic of chronic diarrhea. Am J Surg Pathol 20:1102-1109, 1996.

183. Wang N, Dumot JA, Achkar E, et al: Colonic epithelial lymphocytosis without a thickened subepithelial collagen table: A clinicopathologic study of 40 cases supporting a heterogeneous entity. Am J Surg Pathol 23:1068-1074, 1999.

184. Goldstein NS, Gyorfi T: Focal lymphocytic colitis and collagenous colitis: Patterns of Crohn's colitis? Am J Surg Pathol 23:1075-1081, 1999.

185. Bo-Linn GW, Vendrell DD, Lee E, et al: An evaluation of the significance of microscopic colitis in patients with chronic diarrhea. J Clin Invest 75:1559-1611, 1985.

186. McKenna BJ, Eldeiry D, Odze RD, et al: Apoptotic colopathy: A new variant of microscopic diarrheal disease? Mod Pathol 14:91A, 2001.

187. Peppercorn MA: Drug-responsive chronic segmental colitis associated with diverticula: A clinical syndrome in the elderly. Am J Gastroenterol 87:629-632, 1992.

188. Makapugay LM, Dean PJ: Diverticular disease-associated chronic colitis. Am J Surg Pathol 20:94-102, 1996.

189. Sladen GE, Filipe MI: Is segmental colitis a complication of diverticular disease? Dis Colon Rectum 27:513-514, 1984.

190. Hart J, Baert F, Hanauer S: Sigmoiditis: A clinical syndrome with a spectrum of pathologic features, including a distinctive form of IBD [abstract]. Mod Pathol 8:62A, 1995.

191. Goldstein NS, Leon-Armin C, Mani A: Crohn's colitis-like change in sigmoid diverticulitis specimens is usually an idiosyncratic inflammatory response to the diverticulosis rather than Crohn's colitis. Am J Surg Pathol 24:668-675, 2000.

192. Gledhill A, Dixon MF: Crohn's-like reaction in diverticular disease. Gut 42:349-353, 1998.

193. Burroughs SH, Bowery DJ, Morris-Stiff GJ, et al: Granulomatous inflammation in sigmoid diverticulitis: Two diseases or one? Histopathology 33:349-353, 1998.

194. Glotzer DJ, Glick ME, Goldman H: Proctitis and colitis following diversion of the fecal stream. Gastroenterology 80:438-441, 1981.

195. Komorowski RA: Histologic spectrum of diversion colitis. Am J Surg Pathol 14:548-554, 1990.

196. Harig JM, Soergel KH, Komorowski RA, et al: Treatment of diversion colitis with short-chain fatty acid irrigation. N Engl J Med 320:23-28, 1989.

197. Haque S, Eisen RN, West AB: The morphologic features of diversion colitis: Studies of a pediatric population with no other disease of the intestinal mucosa. Hum Pathol 24:211-219, 1993.

198. Korelitz BI, Cheskin LJ, Sohn N, et al: Proctitis after fecal diversion in Crohn's disease and its elimination with reanastomosis: Implications for surgical management. Gastroenterology 87:710-713, 1984.

199. Fortson WC, Tedesco FJ: Drug-induced colitis: A review. Am J Gastroenterol 79:878-883, 1984.

200. Faucheron JL: Toxicity of non-steroidal anti-inflammatory drugs in the large bowel. Eur J Gastroenterol Hepatol 11:389-392, 1999.

201. Faucheron JL, Parc R: Non-steroidal anti-inflammatory drug-induced colitis. Int J Colorectal Dis 11:99-101, 1996.

202. Lee FD: Importance of apoptosis in the histopathology of drug related lesions in the small intestine. J Clin Pathol 46:118-122, 1993.

203. Puspok A, Kiener H-P, Overhuber B: Clinical, endoscopic, and histologic spectrum of non-steroidal anti-inflammatory drug-induced lesions in the colon. Dis Colon Rectum 43:685-691, 2000.

204. Goldstein NS, Cinenza AN: The histopathology of nonsteroidal anti-inflammatory drug-associated colitis. Am J Clin Pathol 110:622-628, 1998.

205. Bernardino ME, Lawson TL: Discrete colonic ulcers associated with oral contraceptives. Am J Dig Dis 21:503-506, 1976.

206. Gurbuz AK, Gurbuz B, Salas L, et al: Premarin-induced ischemic colitis. J Clin Gastroenterol 19:108-111, 1994.

207. Pawel BR, de Chadarevian JP, Franco ME: The pathology of fibrosing colonopathy of cystic fibrosis: A study of 12 cases and review of the literature. Hum Pathol 28:395-399, 1997.

208. Schwarzenberg SJ, Wielinski CL, Shamieh I, et al: Cystic fibrosis-associated colitis and fibrosing colonopathy. J Pediatr 127:565-570, 1995.

209. Meisel JL, Bergman D, Graney D, et al: Human rectal mucosa: Proctoscopic and morphological changes caused by laxatives. Gastroenterology 72:1274-1279, 1977.

210. Leriche M, Devroede G, Sanchez G, et al: Changes in the rectal mucosa induced by hypertonic enemas. Dis Colon Rectum 21:227-236, 1978.

211. Zwas FR, Cirillo NW, El-Serag HB, et al: Colonic mucosal abnormalities associated with oral sodium phosphate solution. Gastrointest Endosc 43:463-466, 1996.

212. Kiko R, Rutter P, Riddell RH: The solitary ulcer syndrome of the rectum. Clin Gastroenterol 4:505-530, 1975.

213. Shepherd NA: Pathological mimics of chronic inflammatory bowel disease. J Clin Pathol 44:726-733, 1991.

214. Niv Y, Bat L: Solitary rectal ulcer syndrome—clinical, endoscopic, and histologic spectrum. Am J Gastroenterol 81:486-491, 1986.

215. Saul SH: Inflammatory cloacogenic polyp: Relationship to solitary rectal ulcer syndrome/mucosal prolapse and other bowel disorders. Hum Pathol 18:1120-1125, 1987.

216. Kelly JK: Polypoid prolapsing mucosal folds in diverticular disease. Am J Surg Pathol 15:871-878, 1991.

217. Vora IM, Sharma J, Joshi AS: Solitary rectal ulcer syndrome and colitis cystica profunda—a clinico-pathological review. Indian J Pathol Microbiol 35:94-102, 1992.

218. Lee RG: The colitis of Behçet's syndrome. Am J Surg Pathol 10:888-893, 1986.

219. Mir-Madjlessi SH, Farmer RG: Behçet's syndrome, Crohn's disease and toxic megacolon. Cleve Clin Q 39:49-55, 1972.

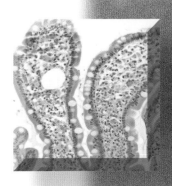

CHAPTER 11

Inflammatory Disorders of the Appendix

ELIZABETH MONTGOMERY • MICHAEL TORBENSON

Normal Histology

Similar to the remainder of the large bowel, the appendix includes mucosa, submucosa, muscularis propria, and serosa. The mucosal architecture also mirrors that seen elsewhere in the large bowel but differs in terms of the abundant, organized lymphoid tissue distributed in a circumferential fashion that more closely resembles the terminal ileum, particularly in young individuals. In contrast to the colon, in which the crypts are more uniformly aligned, appendiceal crypts tend to be irregular and can even be absent adjacent to lymphoid aggregates. The muscularis propria resembles the muscularis propria elsewhere in the gastrointestinal tract, consisting of inner circular and outer longitudinal layers of smooth muscle. The serosa is lined by mesothelium, although the attachment of the mesoappendix lacks a serosa.

Fibrous Obliteration of the Appendiceal Lumen (Neuroma, Neural Hyperplasia)

Obliteration of the appendiceal lumen by spindle cells in a collagenous and myxoid backdrop is found in about a third of excised appendices. Typically the tip of the appendix is affected, but the entire appendix may be involved. Such a process may be confined to the mucosa ("intramucosal variant") or may replace the entire lumen

and underlying crypts. Immunohistochemical staining discloses S100 and neuron-specific enolase-reactive spindle cells (intermingled Schwann cells and axons, respectively), as well as scattered endocrine cells. These phenomena are believed to be proliferative overall, with attendant phases of growth, involution, and finally fibrosis.[1]

Anatomic Abnormalities of the Appendix

The appendix can be characterized by a variety of anatomic abnormalities, including atypical location,[2] duplication,[3,4] and congenital absence.[5] In addition, the appendix can show complete or incomplete septa, which are seen principally in children and young adults and can be associated with acute appendicitis.[6] An abnormally long appendix (normal length is 7 to 10 cm) has been linked to primary acute torsion, although torsion has also been reported in appendices of normal length.[7] Diverticula of the appendix can be congenital (in which case the muscularis propria is part of the diverticular wall) or acquired (in which case the diverticula result from increased intraluminal pressure and mucosal herniation through a defect or weak spot of the muscularis propria, often at the site of a penetrating artery). Acquired diverticula are more common than congenital diverticula and are seen in 1% to 2% of the population.[8] However, the occurrence of acquired diverticula is greatly increased among patients with cystic fibrosis; it can be seen in up to 22% of appendectomy specimens (Fig. 11-1).[8]

General Pathologic Features of Acute and Chronic Appendicitis

Acute appendicitis is a disease of the young, typically presenting in children and adolescents (5 to 15 years of age), although no age group is exempt.[9,10] The pathogenesis of appendicitis is believed (although not by all) to reflect an initial insult to the mucosa resulting from luminal obstruction by a fecalith, a fragment of undigested food, or lymphoid hyperplasia, followed by bacterial infection that progressively spreads from the mucosa into the wall. Imaging methods to detect acute appendicitis have improved over time,[11,12] and laparoscopic appendectomy has emerged as a safe technique.[13] About 70% of patients suspected of appendicitis on clinical and imaging grounds prove to have acute appendicitis on resection.[14,15] Some observers believe that all appendices should be removed during surgery for suspected acute appendicitis, even when grossly normal, because close to 20% of normal-appearing appendices have acute inflammation on microscopic examination.[14,15] A possible exception would be those patients who might require urologic surgery in the future because their appendices may prove useful as urinary conduits.[16] Patients with appendicitis in the setting of human immunodeficiency virus (HIV) infection have similar clinical presentations, although some-times with a less striking elevation in the peripheral white blood cell count. In one surgical series of appendicitis and HIV infection, delays before the time of operation increased the likelihood of perforation.[17]

The appendix may appear grossly normal when inflammation is limited to the mucosa and the submucosa. However, when inflammation extends into the muscularis propria, the appendix frequently becomes swollen and erythematous. When the serosa is affected, the peritoneum is initially dull and gray, then has a purulent exudate. Perforation secondary to mural necrosis (gangrenous appendicitis) can follow, which may lead to abscess formation. At times, an appendix resected in the clinical setting of acute appendicitis is grossly and histologically normal, even after submission of the complete specimen for histologic examination. In these cases, a cause is rarely found, although some possible considerations are listed in Table 11-1.

On microscopic examination, early lesions display mucosal erosions and scattered crypt abscesses. Later, the inflammation extends into the lamina propria, and collections of neutrophils are also seen in the lumen. When the inflammation extensively damages the muscularis propria, mural necrosis can lead to perforation.

As appendices heal, two basic patterns may be seen.[18] In the first, more typical pattern, mixed inflammatory infiltrates range from patchy and mild to diffuse and transmural. In some appendices, there may be intramural or serosal foreign body–type giant cells surrounded by granulation tissue suggestive of previous rupture. Serositis and fibrous adhesions can be present, as can prominent submucosal fibrosis. Mucin extravasation is often seen. A second pattern, which has been called *xanthogranulomatous appendicitis*, features a xanthogranulomatous infiltrate composed of foam cells (Fig. 11-2), scattered multinucleated histiocytes, abundant hemosiderin, and luminal obliteration with spared lymphoid follicles. These latter cases share features with Crohn's disease but differ in that they lack epithelioid granulomas, have fewer lymphoid aggregates, and reveal less profound subserosal fibrosis. However, a patient with features similar to those described earlier was found to have Crohn's disease on follow-up,[19] so careful clinical correlation is always important in such cases.

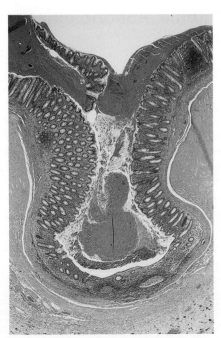

FIGURE 11–1. Acquired appendiceal diverticula in a patient with cystic fibrosis.

TABLE 11–1. Causes to Consider When a Grossly Normal and Histologically Noninflamed Appendix Is Removed From a Patient With Clinical Acute Appendicitis

Other abdominal disease (e.g., endometriosis)
Yersinia ileitis/mesenteric adenitis
Spirochetosis
Cystic fibrosis

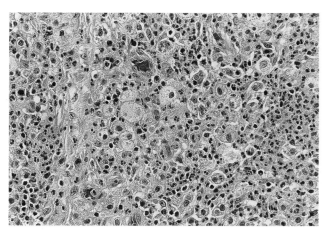

FIGURE 11–2. Healing "chronic" appendicitis with foamy macrophages admixed with neutrophils.

◼ Periappendicitis

Preoperative mechanical manipulation of the appendix alone may result in mild diffuse granulocytic infiltration of the serosa,[20] but when inflammation is accompanied by fibrin deposition and/or adhesions in the absence of luminal active inflammation, this is a potentially clinically significant finding. Periappendicitis alone is found in 1% to 5% of appendices resected for clinically acute appendicitis; a majority of these cases are attributable to salpingitis.[21] In two large series, periappendicitis was attributable to a variety of processes—gonococcal and chlamydial salpingitis, yersiniosis, Meckel's diverticulitis and associated intraperitoneal abscess, urologic disorders, colon neoplasms, infectious colitis, abdominal aortic aneurysm, bacterial peritonitis, and gastrointestinal perforation.[21,22]

◼ Infectious Causes of Acute Appendicitis

Infections of the appendix can be bacterial, viral, fungal, or parasitic in origin. In most cases of acute appendicitis, no organisms are identified by histology, although cultures reveal mixed aerobic and anaerobic isolates in almost all cases. In one study of 41 children with acute appendicitis, an average of 14.1 isolates per specimen were detected.[23] Bacterial isolates are almost always limited to normal flora[23-25] and are generally thought to play a secondary role following mucosal injury. Bacteria belonging to the *Bacteroides fragilis* group are the most frequently isolated anaerobes, and *Escherichia coli* is the most frequently isolated aerobe.[23-25] Bacteria belonging to the *Streptococcus milleri* group are also common aerobes but may be of greater significance because they have been linked to a sevenfold increased risk for abscess formation.[26] Although

specific infectious causes of acute appendicitis are only rarely identified, certain agents can occasionally be implicated and are discussed further in the following sections.

SPECIFIC BACTERIAL INFECTIONS

Actinomyces Species

Actinomyces israelii is a rare cause of appendicitis. *A. israelii* in rare cases can lead to infection of the small intestine, appendix, or colon. Histologically, the long filamentous organisms stain dark blue on routine H&E preparations and are particularly easy to recognize when associated with characteristic sulfur granules. Active inflammation in the mucosal wall is typically present, and fistula formation, rupture of the appendix, and abscess formation may complicate the clinical course.[27] *Actinomyces turicensis* has also been implicated in appendicitis and is frequently accompanied by aerobic bacterial isolates of the *Streptococcus anginosus* group.[28]

Campylobacter Species

Campylobacter jejuni is an uncommon cause of bacterial appendicitis. In one study, *Campylobacter* organisms were detected by immunohistochemical methods in 3 of 116 cases of acute appendicitis.[29] The patients were generally young children who had grossly normal appendices. Histologically, the active inflammatory changes were limited to the mucosa and consisted of cryptitis and surface erosions with focal accumulations of histiocytes that occasionally resulted in a granulomatous appearance.[29]

Clostridium difficile and Shigella Species

C. difficile infections and shigellosis involving the appendix are almost always associated with more general colonic disease, although appendicitis can be a rare clinical presentation. Overall, the histologic findings are identical to those seen in the colon (see Chapter 10).

Malakoplakia

Malakoplakia is most commonly seen in the urinary tract but can occasionally be found in a wide variety of other organs, including the appendix. In one case report, it was associated with ova of the *Taenia* species,[30] but in general, malakoplakia results from an abnormal immune response in which bacteria are incompletely digested and accumulate in histiocytes.[31] The histologic findings typically consist of a diffuse or nodular thickening of the mucosal wall resulting from the accumulation of numerous macrophages, including many that are eosinophilic, with scattered lymphocytes and plasma cells. Most characteristic are the admixed Michaelis-Gutmann bodies, which are round, laminated structures with a targetoid appearance (Fig. 11-3) that can be highlighted with iron or calcium stain.

Spirochetosis

Spirochetosis is caused by *Brachyspira aalborg* and can occasionally be seen in the appendix. In one study, spirochetosis was detected in 1.9% of incidentally removed appendices, 0.7% of appendices in patients with clinical acute appendicitis plus histologic acute appendicitis, and 12.3% of patients with clinical acute appendicitis but no histologic changes.[32] These results suggest that spirochetosis may contribute to clinical symptoms in patients with otherwise normal appendices. Spirochetosis of the small intestine and colon is more commonly found in HIV-infected patients than in non–HIV-infected patients, but little information is available on whether this is also true for the appendix. Overall, adults appear to be more commonly infected than children.[33] Histologically, spirochetosis is characterized by a hazy hematoxylin-positive band of about 3 μm in thickness that lies along the epithelial brush border. Silver stains also highlight the organisms. Typically, no inflammatory response is noted, even though organisms can be seen by electron microscopy within epithelial cells and macrophages.[33]

Tuberculosis

Tuberculosis of the appendix is almost always accompanied by gastrointestinal or pulmonary tuberculosis, although isolated infections have been reported.[34,35] The histologic findings are identical to those seen elsewhere in the body.

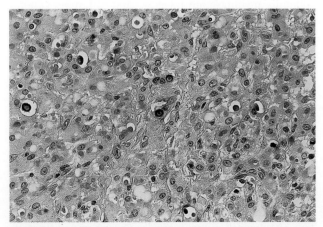

FIGURE 11–3. Malakoplakia showing sheets of histiocytes with admixed Michaelis-Gutmann bodies—round, laminated structures with a targetoid appearance.

Yersinia Species

In one study in which specific cultures for *Yersinia enterocolitica* were obtained, infections were found in approximately 4% of cases of acute appendicitis.[36] In general, *Yersinia* species tend to cause acute enteritis in young children, and terminal ileitis and mesenteric adenitis in older children and young adults. In most cases in the study by Van Noyen and associates, the appendices were grossly normal and either were histologically normal or showed only mild superficial chronic inflammation; only rarely was acute suppurative appendicitis seen.[36] In other cases, *Y. enterocolitica* and *Yersinia pseudotuberculosis* infection can cause granulomatous inflammation with large epithelioid noncaseating granulomas surrounded by prominent lymphoid cuffs.[37] In these cases of granulomatous inflammation, prominent acute inflammation is common and lymphoid hyperplasia is essentially always present.

FUNGAL INFECTIONS

Fungal infections such as aspergillosis and mucormycosis can involve the appendix[38,39] but are almost always part of a systemic infection. Patients are typically immunosuppressed owing to organ transplantation or chemotherapy.

PARASITIC INFECTIONS

Enterobius vermicularis is one of the most common parasites seen in the appendix, especially in temperate climates, with an overall frequency that ranges from 2.4% in Iran[40] to 8.7% in Czechoslovakia.[41] At the Johns Hopkins Hospital, only 4 of 1584 appendices removed over a 17-year period from patients 15 years of age and younger demonstrated *Enterobius* infection. Individuals in late childhood and early adolescence have the highest frequency of infection (ages 5 to 15),[41,42] which can reach as high as 24% in some studies.[41] The worm is most commonly found in the lumen with no mucosal inflammatory response (Fig. 11-4). In one study in which close to 22,000 appendices were evaluated, granulomatous inflammation and increased eosinophils in the lamina propria were quite rare and together were noted in less than 2% of infections.[43] Interestingly, an inverse relationship between active mucosal inflammation and pinworm infection has been noted in several studies.[42,44,45] Mucosal inflammation, when present, has been strongly linked to the presence of parasite ova.[46]

VIRAL INFECTIONS

Viral gastroenteritis does not typically result in appendectomy, although some examples of appendicitis are no doubt caused by viral agents. Viral enteritis classically results in surgical excision of the appendix

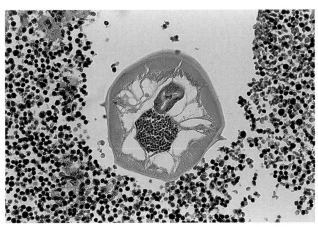

FIGURE 11–4. *Enterobius vermicularis* in the appendiceal lumen. Note the characteristic cuticular crests.

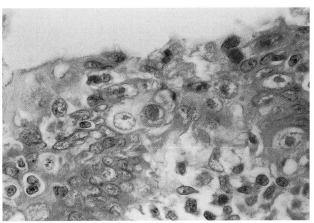

FIGURE 11–5. Adenovirus infection with epithelial cells containing both Cowdry A and Cowdry B inclusions.

when it leads to ileocecal intussusception and ileocolectomy. Intussusception is commonly attributable to lymphoid hyperplasia in the terminal ileum, which can form a "leading edge." It classically occurs in infants and young children. The viral agents most commonly implicated in this setting are rotavirus, echovirus, and adenovirus. The latter is detected most frequently[47,48] and is so named because of its isolation from adenoids. In appendices infected with adenovirus, lymphoid hyperplasia is prominent. Erosions may be identified, but viral inclusions are found in intact mucosal epithelial cells. Zones in which inclusions may be found are selected by scanning at low magnification for areas with frayed-appearing epithelium that show loss of nuclear polarity and an eosinophilic appearance imparted by loss of goblet cell mucin. Such zones are frequently in close association with lymphoid follicles. Intranuclear adenovirus inclusions are typically of the Cowdry B type, consisting of nuclear smudging, although Cowdry A inclusions, featuring sharply demarcated globules surrounded by a clear zone, are found in a minority of cases (Fig. 11-5).

Cytomegalovirus may also be found in the appendices of immunocompromised hosts, in whom it displays the features found in other sites with endothelial cells, rather than epithelial cells, and tends to involve infection. Cytomegalovirus infection may occasionally be responsible for clinical acute appendicitis.[17,49]

■ Chronic Inflammatory Diseases of the Appendix

ULCERATIVE COLITIS

The appendix may play an interesting role in IBD in that an appendectomy has been touted as a protective factor in ulcerative colitis. The prevalence of previous appendectomy is far lower in ulcerative colitis patients than in control groups,[50,51] although this observation

certainly does not necessarily indicate causation. Similar findings have also been observed in a murine model.[52]

Ulcerative appendicitis, the appendiceal counterpart of ulcerative colitis, is typically present in patients with pancolitis[53] but is also common as a "skip lesion" in patients having left-sided or rectal disease,[53-55] occurring in from 20% to more than 80% of such cases. In some cases, the active inflammatory disease in the appendix may be prominent while that in the nearby cecum is mild (discrepancy in disease activity). Ulcerative appendicitis shows the same features as ulcerative colitis. Mucosal-based active inflammation occurs with crypt abscesses, panmucosal plasmacytosis, suppurative luminal exudate, and crypt distortion. Ulcerative appendicitis is distinguished from early acute appendicitis partially on clinical grounds, although early acute appendicitis features less crypt distortion and minimal plasmacytosis. In ulcerative colitis, but not in acute appendicitis, immunostains can show prominent S100 protein–reactive dendritic cells, MAC387-positive dendritic cells, and upregulated HLA class II antigens.[56]

CROHN'S DISEASE

A majority of appendices resected from patients with typical Crohn's disease elsewhere in the gastrointestinal tract are normal, and most patients who present with isolated granulomatous appendiceal disease do not later manifest typical Crohn's disease elsewhere in the gastrointestinal tract. Therefore, many observers believe that there are two diseases: (1) true Crohn's disease of the appendix, and (2) idiopathic granulomatous appendicitis.[57-59] Some studies suggest that appendectomy increases the risk of Crohn's disease, in contrast to ulcerative colitis, which appendectomy has been reported to protect against.[60]

In patients with clinical Crohn's disease, the appendix has the typical histologic features of Crohn's disease seen elsewhere in the GI tract, with fissures, ulcers, active inflammation, and occasional granulomas.[18,57] Dudley and Dean studied the number of granulomas per cross section in appendices resected from patients with typical Crohn's disease and compared this number with cases of isolated "idiopathic granulomatous appendicitis."[57] They found that cases with clinical Crohn's disease had 0.3 granuloma per tissue section, in contrast to about 20 granulomas per tissue section in patients with idiopathic granulomatous appendicitis. Furthermore, none of the patients with idiopathic granulomatous appendicitis had recurrent disease during a mean follow-up period of 4.5 years.

In another series, none of nine patients (identified among 1133 consecutive appendectomy specimens) with idiopathic granulomatous appendicitis developed Crohn's disease in a mean follow-up period of just over 7 years.[61] In contrast, one patient reported in a series by Huang and Appelman with 21 granulomas per cross section later developed Crohn's disease elsewhere in the gut, so the number of granulomas per cross section is not entirely reliable in separation of these entities (Table 11-2).[19] Newer microbiologic techniques may provide some clues to the causes of granulomatous appendicitis. For example, in a 2001 study by Lamps and colleagues, 10 of 40 (25%) cases of granulomatous appendicitis were found to have evidence of pathogenic *Yersinia* species by polymerase chain reaction (PCR).[37]

SARCOIDOSIS

Sarcoidosis of the appendix is rare, although it can manifest as appendicitis. Typical noncaseating epithelioid granulomas can be seen (Fig. 11-6). Of course, this is a clinicopathologic diagnosis rather than one based solely on histology.[62-64]

■ Noninflammatory Abnormalities of the Appendix

CYSTIC FIBROSIS

In cystic fibrosis, the most common histologic finding is enlarged and distended goblet cells that contain normal-appearing mucin, although this can be a subtle finding in many cases. Inspissated eosinophilic mucin in dilated glands can also be seen but is a nonspecific

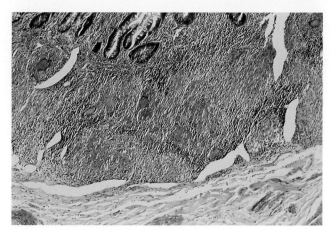

FIGURE 11–6. Sarcoidosis. Clusters of noncaseating epithelioid granulomas are present in the lamina propria.

finding. The most readily identifiable abnormality is usually the thick inspissated eosinophilic mucin in the lumen (Fig. 11-7). This abnormal mucin can cause marked engorgement of the appendix and can lead to a sausagelike appendix. In some cases, the engorged appendix itself can cause clinical symptoms of appendicitis, even though histologic examination reveals no inflammation.[65] Overall, patients with cystic fibrosis have a lower frequency of acute appendicitis (1.5%) than is seen in the general population (approximately 10%).[65] However, the incidence of acquired diverticula is markedly increased (see Fig. 11-1).[8]

INTUSSUSCEPTION OF THE APPENDIX

Intussusception of the appendix is frequently associated with other abnormalities such as endometriosis of the appendix or polypoid lesions at the base of the appendix.[66] Histologically, the mucosa can show changes of prolapse with varying amounts of ingrowth of smooth muscle, mild chronic inflammation, and mild fibrosis.

ENDOMETRIOSIS, DECIDUOSIS, GLIOMATOSIS

Endometriosis is well known to present in a variety of sites and affects the gastrointestinal tract in up to 40% of patients with pelvic endometriosis. The sigmoid

TABLE 11–2. Chronic Inflammatory Disorders of the Appendix

Finding	Idiopathic Granulomatous Appendicitis	Crohn's Disease	Healing Acute Appendicitis
Neutrophilic cryptitis/crypt abscesses	Yes	Yes	Yes
Fissures or fistulas	Occasional fissures	Yes	No
Transmural lymphoid aggregates	Often	Often	Occasionally
Fibrosis	Often	Often	Often
Granulomas	Yes, numerous	Yes, occasional	No, but numerous foam cells may be present

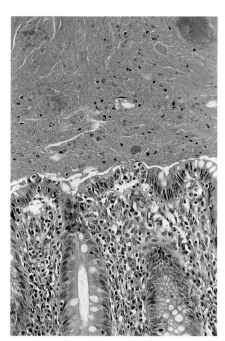

FIGURE 11–7. Cystic fibrosis with intraluminal, thick, inspissated mucin characteristic of cystic fibrosis.

colon is the most common site, but the appendix may be involved in about 15% of cases.[67] Although appendiceal endometriosis can clinically masquerade as acute appendicitis,[67,68] it more typically has a nonspecific presentation,[67-70] although pain may wax and wane with the menstrual cycle. Most examples affect the serosa or muscularis propria and are accompanied by abundant fibrosis and adhesions, although submucosal examples are also reported.[68-70] Endometriosis of the appendix resembles examples found elsewhere, consisting of endometrial-type glands (Fig. 11-8) and stroma associated with hemosiderin deposition and a fibroblastic response. The endometrial-type epithelium changes with the menstrual cycle. A stromal decidual reaction

may be found in endometriotic foci among pregnant patients.[70]

A similar phenomenon, called *deciduosis (ectopic decidua)*, has been found in the appendices of pregnant women. Deciduosis, in contrast to endometriosis, typically presents with signs and symptoms of acute appendicitis.[71] Deciduosis differs from endometriosis in the lack of glands and consists only of large polyhedral cells arranged in sheets in the serosa or outer muscularis propria, although deciduosis has rarely been reported in the mucosa of the gastrointestinal tract.[72] Such cells can sometimes be mistaken for malignant (often epithelial) lesions, but immunohistochemical stains for keratin, CEA, EMA, and S100 protein are negative. The large decidualized cells typically express vimentin and may show desmin or muscle actin positivity.[71]

When present, pelvic gliomatosis can also affect the serosal aspect of the appendix (Fig. 11-9). Gliomatosis peritonei is found in patients with ovarian teratomas and manifests as foci of mature glial tissue deposited ubiquitously over the serosal surfaces.[73] It has also been reported as a rare complication of ventricular shunts,[74] and cases of malignant transformation have been recorded.[75,76]

PIGMENTS, FOREIGN MATERIAL, AND PROCESSING ARTIFACTS

Melanosis involves the appendix in approximately 7% of individuals over the age of 40 and is histologically identical to that seen in the colon[77] with pigmented macrophages containing cytoplasmic material ranging from pale green to dark brown. The pigment is lipofuscin that accumulates as macrophages ingest apoptotic surface epithelial cells.[78] The most common clinical association is laxative abuse in the setting of chronic constipation.

Barium can be present within the lumen of the appendix with no associated mucosal response. How-

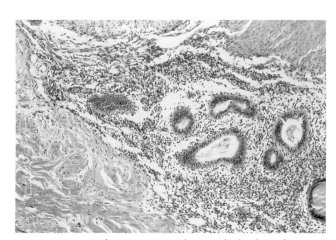

FIGURE 11–8. Endometriosis. Endometrial glands and stroma are present in the muscularis propria.

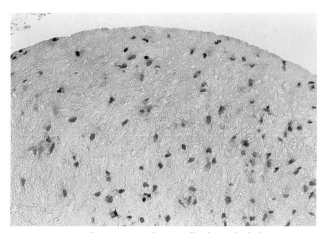

FIGURE 11–9. Gliomatosis. This small plug of glial tissue was adherent to the serosa of the appendix.

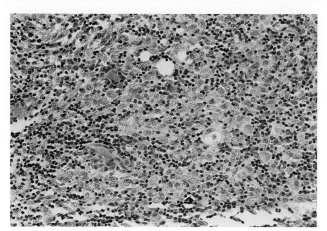

FIGURE 11–10. The granular pigment in the cytoplasm of macrophages is barium.

ever, barium can at times extravasate into the mucosa, where it is phagocytized by macrophages, occasionally resulting in a granulomatous reaction with numerous macrophages and foreign body giant cells. The barium is readily recognized as nonpolarizing crystalline material that is typically light green (Fig. 11-10).

Foreign body appendicitis is rare but always generates considerable interest and has led to large numbers of case reports describing acute appendicitis caused by everything from dog hair to toothpicks to lead shot. A 100-year review of the literature revealed 256 reported cases, with the highest risk associated with stiff or pointed objects.[79] Not all foreign body appendicitis occurs soon after initial ingestion; occasional cases

occur years later.[80] Other foreign material that can be seen in the appendix includes vegetable fragments in the lumen that generally elicit no mucosal response. However, vegetable material may in some cases obstruct the appendix and lead to acute appendicitis. "Foreign" heterotopic bone formation in the appendix is a very rare finding that has been associated with mucin-producing tumors.[81] Finally, foreign bodies in the peritoneum, such as dialysis catheters, can on rare occasions entrap the appendix, leading to appendicitis.[82]

Tissue artifacts can occur at any of the processing steps and are usually readily apparent and cause little confusion. Occasionally, artifacts may be more challenging to recognize. The appendix depicted in Figure 11-11 was inadvertently frozen before it was processed.

References

1. Stanley MW, Cherwitz D, Hagen K, et al: Neuromas of the appendix. A light-microscopic, immunohistochemical and electron-microscopic study of 20 cases. Am J Surg Pathol 10:801-815, 1986.
2. Schumpelick V, Dreuw B, Ophoff K, et al: Appendix and cecum. Embryology, anatomy, and surgical applications. Surg Clin North Am 80:295-318, 2000.
3. Mitchell IC, Nicholls JC: Duplication of the vermiform appendix. Report of a case: Review of the classification and medicolegal aspects. Med Sci Law 30:124-126, 1990.
4. Chew DK, Borromeo JR, Gabriel YA, et al: Duplication of the vermiform appendix. J Pediatr Surg 35:617-618, 2000.
5. Host WH, Rush B, Lazaro EJ: Congenital absence of the vermiform appendix. Am Surg 38:355-356, 1972.
6. de la Fuente AA: Septa in the appendix: A previously undescribed condition. Histopathology 9:1329-1337, 1985.
7. Val-Bernal JF, Gonzalez-Vela C, Garijo MF: Primary acute torsion of the vermiform appendix. Pediatr Pathol Lab Med 16:655-661, 1996.
8. George DH: Diverticulosis of the vermiform appendix in patients with cystic fibrosis. Hum Pathol 18:75-79, 1987.
9. Butler C: Surgical pathology of acute appendicitis. Hum Pathol 12:870-878, 1981.
10. Ferguson E Jr, Pirrung D: Acute appendicitis: Clinical vs. pathologic diagnosis. Am J Proctol 20:269-279, 1969.
11. Rao PM: Presence or absence of gas in the appendix: Additional criteria to rule out or confirm acute appendicitis—evaluation with US. Radiology 217:599-600, 2000.
12. Rettenbacher T, Hollerweger A, Macheiner P, et al: Outer diameter of the vermiform appendix as a sign of acute appendicitis: Evaluation at US. Radiology 218:757-762, 2001.
13. Merhoff AM, Merhoff GC, Franklin ME: Laparoscopic versus open appendectomy. Am J Surg 179:375-378, 2000.
14. Lau WY, Fan ST, Yiu TF, et al: The clinical significance of routine histopathologic study of the resected appendix and safety of appendiceal inversion. Surg Gynecol Obstet 162:256-258, 1986.
15. Grabham JA, Sutton C, Nicholson ML: A case for the removal of the 'normal' appendix at laparoscopy for suspected acute appendicitis. Ann R Coll Surg Engl 81:279-280, 1999.
16. Neulander EZ, Hawke CK, Soloway MS: Incidental appendectomy during radical cystectomy: An interdepartmental survey and review of the literature. Urology 56:241-244, 2000.
17. Binderow SR, Shaked AA: Acute appendicitis in patients with AIDS/HIV infection. Am J Surg 162:9-12, 1991.
18. Carr N, Montgomery E: Patterns of healing in the appendix. The morphologic changes in resolving primary acute appendicitis and a comparison with Crohn disease. Int J Surg Pathol 2:23-30, 1994.
19. Huang JC, Appelman HD: Another look at chronic appendicitis resembling Crohn disease. Mod Pathol 9:975-981, 1996.
20. Sandermann J, Glenthoj A, Nielsen KK: Preoperative mechanical manipulation of the appendix. A cause of periappendicitis? Ann Chir Gynaecol 78:127-129, 1989.

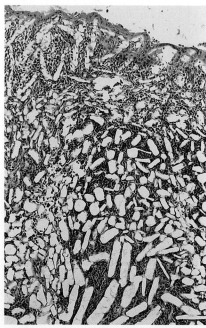

FIGURE 11–11. Empty crystalline spaces found in an appendix that was inadvertently frozen before processing.

21. Bloch AV, Kock KF, Saxtoft Hansen L, et al: Periappendicitis and diagnostic consequences. Ann Chir Gynaecol 77:151-154, 1988.

22. Fink AS, Kosakowski CA, Hiatt JR, et al: Periappendicitis is a significant clinical finding. Am J Surg 159:564-568, 1990.

23. Rautio M, Saxen H, Siitonen A, et al: Bacteriology of histopathologically defined appendicitis in children. Pediatr Infect Dis J 19:1078-1083, 2000.

24. Bennion RS, Baron EJ, Thompson JE, et al: The bacteriology of gangrenous and perforated appendicitis—revisited. Ann Surg 211:165-171, 1990.

25. Jindal N, Kaur GD, Arora S, et al: Bacteriology of acute appendicitis with special reference to anaerobes. Indian J Pathol Microbiol 37:299-305, 1994.

26. Hardwick RH, Taylor A, Thompson MH, et al: Association between *Streptococcus milleri* and abscess formation after appendicitis. Ann R Coll Surg Engl 82:24-26, 2000.

27. Lomax CW, Harbert GM, Thornton WN: Actinomycosis of the female genital tract. Obstet Gynecol 48:341-346, 1976.

28. Sabbe LJ, Van De Merwe D, Schouls L, et al: Clinical spectrum of infections due to the newly described *Actinomyces* species *A. turicensis, A. radingae*, and *A. europaeus*. J Clin Microbiol 37:8-13, 1999.

29. van Spreeuwel JP, Lindeman J, Bax R, et al: *Campylobacter*-associated appendicitis: Prevalence and clinicopathologic features. Pathol Annu 22:55-65, 1987.

30. Jain M, Arora VK, Singh N, et al: Malakoplakia of the appendix. An unusual association with eggs of *Taenia* species. Arch Pathol Lab Med 124:1828-1829, 2000.

31. Lewin KJ, Harell GS, Lee AS, et al: Malacoplakia. An electron-microscopic study: Demonstration of bacilliform organisms in malacoplakic macrophages. Gastroenterology 66:28-45, 1974.

32. Henrik-Nielsen R, Lundbeck FA, Teglbjaerg PS, et al: Intestinal spirochetosis of the vermiform appendix. Gastroenterology 88:971-977, 1985.

33. White J, Roche D, Chan YF, et al: Intestinal spirochetosis in children: Report of two cases. Pediatr Pathol 14:191-199, 1994.

34. al-Hilaly MA, Abu-Zidan FM, Zayed FF, et al: Tuberculous appendicitis with perforation. Br J Clin Pract 44:632-633, 1990.

35. Mittal VK, Khanna SK, Gupta NM, et al: Isolated tuberculosis of appendix. Am Surg 41:172-174, 1975.

36. Van Noyen R, Selderslaghs R, Bekaert J, et al: Causative role of *Yersinia* and other enteric pathogens in the appendicular syndrome. Eur J Clin Microbiol Infect Dis 10:735-741, 1991.

37. Lamps LW, Madhusudhan KT, Greenson JK, et al: The role of *Yersinia enterocolitica* and *Yersinia pseudotuberculosis* in granulomatous appendicitis: A histologic and molecular study. Am J Surg Pathol 25:508-515, 2001.

38. Rogers S, Potter MN, Slade RR: *Aspergillus* appendicitis in acute myeloid leukaemia. Clin Lab Haematol 12:471-476, 1990.

39. ter Borg F, Kuijper EJ, van der Lelie HF, et al: Mucormycosis presenting as an appendiceal mass with metastatic spread to the liver during chemotherapy-induced granulocytopenia. Scand J Infect Dis 22:499-501, 1990.

40. Dalimi A, Khoshzaban F: Comparative study of two methods for the diagnosis of *Enterobius vermicularis* in the appendix. J Helminthol 67:85-86, 1993.

41. Cerva L, Schrottenbaum M, Kliment V: Intestinal parasites: A study of human appendices. Folia Parasitol 38:5-9, 1991.

42. Wiebe BM: Appendicitis and *Enterobius vermicularis*. Scand J Gastroenterol 26:336-338, 1991.

43. Sterba J, Vlcek M: Appendiceal enterobiasis—its incidence and relationships to appendicitis. Folia Parasitol 31:311-318, 1984.

44. Sterba J, Vlcek M, Noll P, et al: Contribution to the question of relationships between *Enterobius vermicularis* (L.) and inflammatory processes in the appendix. Folia Parasitol 32:231-235, 1985.

45. Budd JS, Armstrong C: Role of *Enterobius vermicularis* in the aetiology of appendicitis. Br J Surg 74:748-749, 1987.

46. Williams DJ, Dixon MF: Sex, *Enterobius vermicularis* and the appendix. Br J Surg 75:1225-1226, 1988.

47. Porter HJ, Padfield CJ, Peres LC, et al: Adenovirus and intranuclear inclusions in appendices in intussusception. J Clin Pathol 46:154-158, 1993.

48. Montgomery EA, Popek EJ: Intussusception, adenovirus, and children: A brief reaffirmation. Hum Pathol 25:169-174, 1994.

49. Neumayer LA, Makar R, Ampel NM, et al: Cytomegalovirus appendicitis in a patient with human immunodeficiency virus infection.

50. Anderson RE, Olaison G, Tysk C, Ekbom A: Appendectomy and protection against ulcerative colitis. N Engl J Med 344:808-814, 2001.

51. Scott IS, Sheaff M, Coumbe A, et al: Appendiceal inflammation in ulcerative colitis. Histopathology 33:168-173, 1998.

52. Mizoguchi A, Mizoguchi E, Chiba C, et al: Role of appendix in the development of inflammatory bowel disease in TCR-alpha mutant mice. J Exp Med 184:707-715, 1996.

53. Groisman GM, George J, Harpaz N: Ulcerative appendicitis in universal and nonuniversal ulcerative colitis. Mod Pathol 7:322-325, 1994.

54. Okawa K, Aoki T, Sano K, et al: Ulcerative colitis with skip lesions at the mouth of the appendix: A clinical study. Am J Gastroenterol 93:2405-2410, 1998.

55. Davison AM, Dixon MF: The appendix as a 'skip lesion' in ulcerative colitis. Histopathology 16:93-95, 1990.

56. Waraich T, Sarsfield P, Wright DH: The accessory cell populations in ulcerative colitis: A comparison between the colon and appendix in colitis and acute appendicitis. Hum Pathol 28:297-303, 1997.

57. Dudley TH Jr, Dean PJ: Idiopathic granulomatous appendicitis, or Crohn disease of the appendix revisited. Hum Pathol 24:595-601, 1993.

58. Bak M, Andersen JC: Crohn disease limited to the vermiform appendix. Acta Chir Scand 153:441-446, 1987.

59. Ariel I, Vinograd I, Hershlag A, et al: Crohn disease isolated to the appendix: Truths and fallacies. Hum Pathol 17:1116-1121, 1986.

60. Andersson RE, Olaison G, Tysk C, Ekbom A: Appendectomy is followed by increased risk of Crohn's disease. Gastroenterology 124:40-46, 2003.

61. Richards ML, Aberger FJ, Landercasper J: Granulomatous appendicitis: Crohn disease, atypical Crohn or not Crohn at all? J Am Coll Surg 185:13-17, 1997.

62. Clarke H, Pollett W, Chittal S, et al: Sarcoidosis with involvement of the appendix. Arch Intern Med 143:1603-1604, 1983.

63. Bystrom J: Localized sarcoidosis of the appendix simulating Mb crohn. Report of a case. Acta Chir Scand 134:163-165, 1968.

64. Munt PW: Sarcoidosis of the appendix presenting as appendiceal perforation and abscess. Chest 66:295-297, 1974.

65. Coughlin JP, Gauderer MW, Stern RC, et al: The spectrum of appendiceal disease in cystic fibrosis. J Pediatr Surg 25:835-839, 1990.

66. Jevon GP, Daya D, Qizilbash AH: Intussusception of the appendix. A report of four cases and review of the literature. Arch Pathol Lab Med 116:960-964, 1992.

67. Yantiss RK, Clement PB, Young RH: Endometriosis of the intestinal tract: A study of 44 cases of a disease that may cause diverse challenges in clinical and pathologic evaluation. Am J Surg Pathol 25:445-454, 2001.

68. Langman J, Rowland R, Vernon-Roberts B: Endometriosis of the appendix. Br J Surg 68:121-124, 1981.

69. Uohara JK, Kovara TY: Endometriosis of the appendix. Report of twelve cases and review of the literature. Am J Obstet Gynecol 121:423-426, 1975.

70. Nielsen M, Lykke J, Thomsen JL: Endometriosis of the vermiform appendix. Acta Pathol Microbiol Immunol Scand (A) 91:253-256, 1983.

71. Suster S, Moran CA: Deciduosis of the appendix. Am J Gastroenterol 85:841-845, 1990.

72. Bashir RM, Montgomery EA, Gupta PK, et al: Massive gastrointestinal hemorrhage during pregnancy caused by ectopic decidua of the terminal ileum and colon. Am J Gastroenterol 90:1325-1327, 1995.

73. Harms D, Janig U, Gobel U: Gliomatosis peritonei in childhood and adolescence. Clinicopathological study of 13 cases including immunohistochemical findings. Pathol Res Pract 184:422-430, 1989.

74. Hill DA, Dehner LP, White FV, et al: Gliomatosis peritonei as a complication of a ventriculoperitoneal shunt: Case report and review of the literature. J Pediatr Surg 35:497-499, 2000.

75. Dadmanesh F, Miller DM, Swenerton KD, et al: Gliomatosis peritonei with malignant transformation. Mod Pathol 10:597-601, 1997.

76. Shefren G, Collin J, Soriero O: Gliomatosis peritonei with malignant transformation: A case report and review of the literature. Am J Obstet Gynecol 164:1617-1620; discussion 1620-1621, 1991.

Case report and review of the literature. Arch Surg 128:467-468, 1993.

77. Rutty GN, Shaw PA: Melanosis of the appendix: Prevalence, distribution and review of the pathogenesis of 47 cases. Histopathology 30:319-323, 1997.

78. Walker NI, Smith MM, Smithers BM: Ultrastructure of human melanosis coli with reference to its pathogenesis. Pathology 25:120-123, 1993.

79. Klingler PJ, Seelig MH, DeVault KR, et al: Ingested foreign bodies within the appendix: A 100-year review of the literature. Dig Dis 16:308-314, 1998.

80. Green SM, Schmidt SP, Rothrock SG: Delayed appendicitis from an ingested foreign body. Am J Emerg Med 12:53-56, 1994.

81. Haque S, Eisen RN, West AB: Heterotopic bone formation in the gastrointestinal tract. Arch Pathol Lab Med 120:666-670, 1996.

82. Borghol M, Alrabeeah A: Entrapment of the appendix and the fallopian tube in peritoneal dialysis catheters in two children. J Pediatr Surg 31:427-429, 1996.

POLYPS OF THE GI TRACT

CHAPTER 12

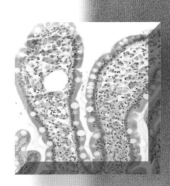

Polyps of the Esophagus

AUDREY LAZENBY

Introduction

In the esophagus, most inflammatory lesions have only slight mucosal irregularity and/or erosions, and most neoplastic processes present at an advanced stage with a gross morphology ranging from strictures to plaquelike masses to fungating ulcers. Polyps—discrete tumorlike protrusions into the lumen—are uncommon in this anatomic site. However, according to Lewin, Riddell, and Weinstein, "most unusual tumors of the esophagus are polypoid; for this reason, when polypoid lesions are encountered, the index of suspicion that an unusual tumor may be present should be high."[1] Thus, although esophageal polyps are rare, they have a high yield of interesting pathology.

Esophageal polyps can be divided into epithelial or mesenchymal, and each grouping further subdivided into benign or malignant. The epithelial character of the polyp is usually apparent at endoscopy or on radiographic study because of mucosal irregularities. Mesenchymal processes, on the other hand, originate in subepithelial tissues and usually simply elevate the overlying mucosa, leaving a smooth mucosal contour.

Benign Epithelial Polyps

(Table 12-1)

INFLAMMATORY POLYPS

Small polyps covered by benign squamous epithelium can be seen throughout the length of the esophagus; the pathogenesis and morphology of these polyps tend to roughly correlate with their site. These squamous polyps

257

TABLE 12-1. Epithelial Polyps of the Esophagus

Benign
- Inflammatory polyp
- Squamous papilloma
- Gastric heterotopia
- Glycogenic acanthosis
- Polypoid dysplasia in Barrett's esophagus

Malignant
- Spindle cell carcinoma
- Conventional squamous cell carcinoma (rarely)*
- Conventional adenocarcinoma (rarely)*
- Melanoma, primary or metastatic

*Most squamous carcinomas or adenocarcinomas of the esophagus present as strictured, ulcerated, or fungating masses. They rarely present as polyps.

can be divided into two main types—inflammatory polyps and papillomas.[1] Inflammatory polyps are the most common of the benign esophageal polyps; they occur primarily in men at the lower esophageal junction and are associated with gastroesophageal reflux.[2-4] These can be conceived of as a response to injury and likely represent healed ulcer sites. Inflammatory polyps may also be seen proximal to the gastroesophageal junction (GEJ), where they are associated with other types of injury such as pill-induced esophagitis, infection, or an anastomotic site.[5] Histologically, these polyps have a smooth, rounded surface contour and consist of irregular tongues of squamous epithelium extending down into an inflamed stroma (Fig. 12-1). They correspond to the endophytic type of polyp described by Odze and associates.[6] Human papillomavirus (HPV) may also be involved in the pathogenesis of some of these types of polyps; Odze and colleagues found HPV to be present in 33% of their endophytic polyps by polymerase chain

reaction (PCR) analysis. They proposed that HPV may be a promoter for epithelial growth in mucosa damaged by irritants.[6]

At the GEJ, polyps composed primarily of hyperplastic foveolae can be found arising in the cardia. Except for a recent pathologic description by Abraham and coworkers,[5] these cardiac-type polyps are most often described in the gastroenterologic or radiologic literature.[7]

SQUAMOUS PAPILLOMAS

The other main type of small squamous polyp is the squamous papilloma.[1,6] Two main histologic patterns correspond to the exophytic and spiked types described by Odze. The exophytic type is more common,[6] and on endoscopy, it looks like a small cauliflower arising in normal squamous mucosa. The cauliflower-like gross appearance can be explained histologically by fingerlike squamous papillae with fibrovascular cores radiating out from a central area (Fig. 12-2). The squamous epithelium of these papillary fingers may have some clear halos around the nuclei but usually lacks the larger, slightly hyperchromatic nuclei; binucleation is typically seen in HPV-infected cervical epithelium. These exophytic, cauliflower-like squamous papillomas occur most frequently at the GEJ, but they also are found in appreciable numbers in the midesophagus and upper esophagus. HPV is strongly associated with this type of polyp (it is identified in 78% of such polyps).[6,8]

The other type of squamous polyp—the spiked polyp—has a verrucoid appearance with a corrugated surface and a prominent granular cell layer. This appears to be the rarest type of squamous polyp and is found most often at the GEJ. Forty percent of these spiked polyps have been found to harbor HPV.[6] It is interesting that Ratoosh and associates described a case of a 60-year-old woman who had a large verrucous

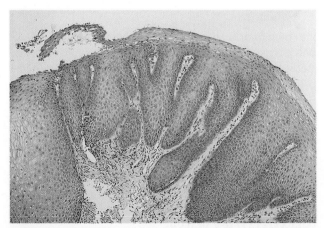

FIGURE 12-1. Inflammatory polyp. These squamous polyps have an endophytic growth pattern characterized by elongated tongues of benign squamous epithelium extending down into underlying stroma. Such polyps are most often located at the gastroesophageal junction and are thought to be a reparative response to injury.

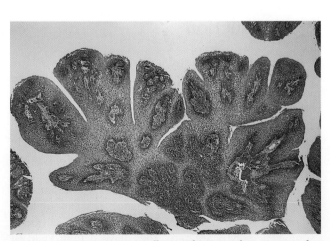

FIGURE 12-2. Squamous papilloma. This type of squamous polyp has an exophytic growth pattern with multiple fibrovascular cores creating a multilobulated appearance. HPV infection is strongly implicated in the pathogenesis of these polyps.

lesion of the distal esophagus and also had multiple warts on her distal fingertips, which she intermittently bit. HPV-45 DNA sequences with 100% identity were found in both the fingertip and esophageal verrucae, suggesting autoinoculation from the nibbled finger warts to the esophagus.[9]

An overwhelming majority of these squamous papillomas are benign. However, one large squamous papilloma has been described as having malignant degeneration with dysplastic and invasive cells extending into the lamina propria. This appears to be the only such case in the literature.[10]

OTHER RARE BENIGN EPITHELIAL POLYPS

Gastric heterotopias, which consist of small congenital islands of gastric mucosa in the upper esophagus, are usually plaquelike. These lesions are rarely the origin for polyps.[11,12] Plaquelike lesions also include common glycogenic acanthosis. Some syndromes, including Cowden syndrome and tuberous sclerosis, are described as having numerous esophageal polyps that appear to be innumerable foci of glycogenic acanthoses.[13,14]

POLYPOID DYSPLASIA IN BARRETT'S ESOPHAGUS

Barrett's esophagus is a columnar metaplasia of the distal esophagus, acquired as an adaptive/healing response to chronic gastroesophageal reflux. Dysplastic changes can arise in the setting of Barrett's esophagus, more commonly in long-segment Barrett's mucosa. These dysplastic lesions may be grossly undetectable or may appear as subtle plaques. Exceptionally, dysplasias have a polypoid configuration (Fig. 12-3). This configuration

was seen in 2% of dysplasias in the series from Boston.[15] The gross and histologic similarities of these polypoid dysplasias to colonic adenomas have led several authors to label these lesions as adenomas.[16] However, it has been clearly established that polypoid dysplasia has clinical, pathologic, and molecular features similar to those of Barrett's-related flat dysplasia.[15]

Polypoid dysplasia is frequently associated with invasive adenocarcinoma. In a study by Odze and colleagues,[15] all of the polypoid dysplasias were found to be associated with carcinoma, including four of five cases with carcinoma in the polyp and a fifth case with carcinoma in flat dysplasia away from the polyp. Because the term *adenoma* connotes a relatively benign lesion, we recommend that such lesions be called polypoid dysplasia.[15] This designation should ensure that these dysplastic lesions are treated appropriately.

■ Malignant Epithelial Polyps

(see Table 12-1)

SPINDLE CELL CARCINOMA

One of the most distinctive polyps in the esophagus is the spindle cell carcinoma, which has numerous synonyms, including carcinosarcoma, pseudosarcoma, polypoid carcinoma, sarcomatoid carcinoma, and spindle cell variant of squamous cell carcinoma.[17] These are bulky intraluminal masses most often seen in the midesophagus of middle-aged to elderly men (80%).[18,19] The most common presenting symptom is dysphagia followed by weight loss and pain.[18] Typical radiologic features include a dilated esophagus expanded by a bulky mass with a smooth or scalloped margin; classic radiologic findings are described as a *cupola sign*.[17,19] These tumors have a biphasic histology with areas of

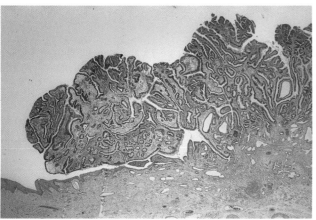
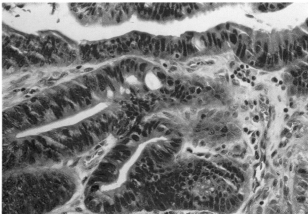

A   **B**

FIGURE 12–3. A, Polypoid dysplasia in Barrett's esophagus. **B,** High-power view reveals the typical histology of high-grade dysplasia with enlarged hyperchromatic nuclei showing focal loss of polarity.

carcinoma and areas of malignant spindle cells. The epithelial character of the spindle cells has been proved by both immunohistochemical and electron micrographic findings.[1,20] The carcinomatous component is usually squamous but can be adenocarcinomatous as well (Fig. 12-4).[21] The carcinomatous component may be seen only at the base of the polyp and is commonly overshadowed by the more abundant spindled component. Lauwers and coworkers have shown that the spindle cell component has a greater proliferative index and increased aneuploidy compared with the carcinomatous component, perhaps giving it a growth advantage and explaining its predominance in most cases.[22] Because these tumors demonstrate greater exophytic growth with less extension into the esophageal wall, they have relatively good survival figures; 50% to 60% of patients are alive at 5 years.[1]

SQUAMOUS CELL CARCINOMA AND ADENOCARCINOMA

In the United States, most squamous cell carcinomas and adenocarcinomas of the esophagus are detected at an advanced stage and have a gross appearance ranging from strictures to irregular masses to ulcers with fungating edges. Only about 15% of esophageal malignancies are described as polypoid, and most of these are the spindle cell carcinomas described previously.[19] Of the advanced tumors, conventional squamous cell carcinoma, small cell (oat cell) carcinoma, and adenocarcinoma are rarely polypoid. Occasional "early" squamous cell carcinomas (defined as having no muscularis propria invasion) have been described as polypoid.[23]

MELANOMA

Primary malignant melanoma of the esophagus is a rare lesion that usually presents as a polypoid mass.[24] These tumors may or may not be pigmented; they show the expected range of histologic patterns, including epithelioid and spindled lesions.[25] Metastatic melanoma may also show a similar polypoid growth, and without a history of melanoma elsewhere, it may be difficult to distinguish between primary and metastatic tumors.[26] Junctional melanocytic activity establishes the primary nature of the melanoma.[27]

■ Benign Mesenchymal Polyps
(Table 12-2)

GRANULAR CELL TUMORS

Granular cell tumors (GCTs) are histologically distinctive benign tumors of Schwann cell origin. They can be seen throughout the body, most commonly on the skin or the tongue. The gastrointestinal tract is an uncommon site for granular cell tumors, but the esophagus is the most common gastrointestinal site. Granular cell tumors, seen primarily in adults (median, 46 to 47 years of age), are more common among women than men, and in the United States, they are more common among blacks than whites. Patients with granular cell tumors are usually asymptomatic; the tumors are most often incidental findings at upper endoscopy.[28-31]

On endoscopy, granular cell tumors can be recognized as yellowish or yellowish-white submucosal lesions that

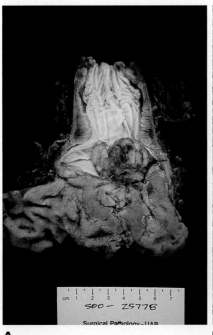
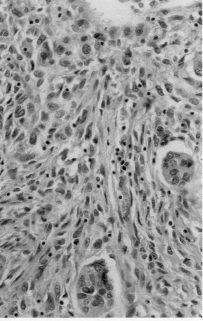

A   **B**

FIGURE 12-4. Spindle cell carcinoma. **A,** This spindle cell carcinoma formed a polypoid intraluminal mass just above the gastroesophageal junction. **B,** Typically, these tumors have a biphasic histology with a predominance of malignant spindle cells and focal areas of carcinoma.

TABLE 12-2. Mesenchymal Polyps of the Esophagus

Benign
- Granular cell tumor
- Leiomyoma
- Giant fibrovascular polyp
- Inflammatory fibroid polyp
- Inflammatory myofibroblastic tumor

Malignant
- Gastrointestinal stromal tumor (GIST)*
- Leiomyosarcoma (rare)

* Most clinically apparent esophageal GISTs are malignant, but a few small incidental GISTs have behaved in a benign fashion.

are firm to the biopsy forceps (Fig. 12-5**A**).[32] These lesions are more common in the distal esophagus and are usually single but can be seen throughout the esophagus; a significant minority can be multiple. In one recent Dutch study by Voskuil and colleagues, 95% of such tumors were single and 75% occurred in the distal esophagus.[30] In this same study, most granular cell tumors were small, with 50% smaller than 5 mm, 25% measuring 5 to 10 mm, and only 18% in the 10- to 30-mm range.[30] Patients with large granular cell tumors can occasionally present with dysphagia. On histology, GCT is seen as subepithelial sheets or nests of cells with abundant granular cytoplasm and small pyknotic nuclei (Fig. 12-5**B**). The cytoplasmic granularity corresponds to vacuoles filled with cellular debris, as shown by elec-

tron microscopy. For unknown reasons, the squamous epithelium over the GCT may become hyperplastic and send irregular tongues down into the granular cells below.[28] This pseudoepitheliomatous hyperplasia may be mistakenly diagnosed by the unwary observer as invasive squamous cell carcinoma. Because GCT is subepithelial, biopsies must include some of these deeper tissues if the pathologist is to be able to make the diagnosis. However, because GCT is so distinctive, even a few of these cells plastered beneath the squamous epithelium are diagnostic. If the diagnosis is in doubt, periodic acid–Schiff (PAS) and S100 stains highlight the neoplastic cells (Fig. 12-5**C**).[29]

Although most granular cell tumors are small, some fill the submucosa, and exceptional cases infiltrate the muscularis propria.[29,33] This infiltrative growth prompts concern of malignancy. One GCT with infiltrative growth, diagnosed as malignant, was incompletely resected, and the patient was reported alive and well 22 years later, suggesting that infiltrative growth does not necessarily imply a malignant neoplasm.[34] Some larger esophageal GCTs have atypical cytologic features, including larger nuclei, prominent nucleoli, and occasional mitotic figures. These cytologic features have been cited as support for a diagnosis of malignant granular cell tumor.[29] Four to eight cases of malignant GCT of the esophagus have been reported, but pathologic details in most of these cases are sketchy.[29,35] Furthermore, few of these reported "malignant" GCTs have resulted in lymph node metas-

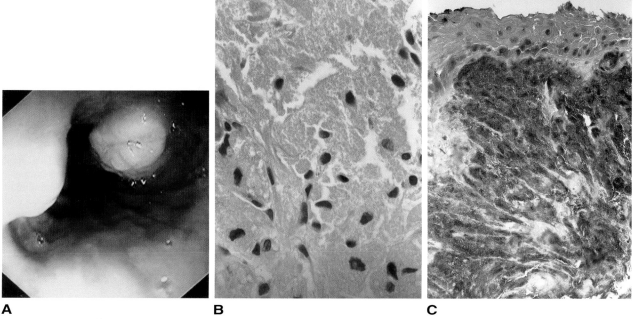

A   **B**   **C**

FIGURE 12–5. Granular cell tumor. **A,** By endoscopy, granular cell tumors are typically seen as small white to yellow subepithelial nodules. (Courtesy of Dr. Christopher Truss.) **B,** By histology, these lesions are composed of large cells with abundant eosinophilic granular cytoplasm and pyknotic nuclei. **C,** If the diagnosis is in question, positive immunoperoxidase stains for S100 can help confirm the diagnosis.

tasis, and no patient has been reported as dying of disease. Thus, the existence of malignant esophageal granular cell tumors remains uncertain.

LEIOMYOMAS

Leiomyomas are the most common of the mesenchymal tumors found in the esophagus. Careful autopsy studies show that 5% to 8% of all esophagi harbor a leiomyoma.[36,37] However, leiomyomas found at autopsy are usually minute. In one Japanese study by Takubo and associates, leiomyomas had a mean size of 2.5 mm and were called *seedling leiomyomas* by the authors.[37] This Japanese study also found that leiomyomas were equally divided between the sexes and were usually single, although 24% of patients had multiple lesions. A vast majority of these seedling leiomyomas were located in the inner circular muscle, but 18% were located in the muscularis mucosae.[37]

Larger leiomyomas do occur and are most often reported in the surgical or radiologic literature. These larger leiomyomas measured from 2 to 10 cm in one series,[38] but massive leiomyomas (larger than 1000 grams) have been reported.[39] Such tumors may be found incidentally on radiographic studies, but patients may present with dysphagia.[38] Most leiomyomas are intramural, but 3% in one series were found to be polypoid.[36] Endoscopic ultrasound may be useful for localizing the layer of the esophagus involved by the intramural mass and for suggesting leiomyoma.[39] Pedunculated leiomyomas, localized to the muscularis mucosae, can be resected endoscopically.[40]

Of 48 esophageal leiomyomas collected in one study from the Armed Forces Institute of Pathology (AFIP) and the Haartman Institute in Helsinki, 79% were found in the distal esophagus, 18% in the midesophagus, and 3% in the proximal esophagus. On gross examination, esophageal leiomyomas are firm in consistency and gray-tan in color; they often have a whorled cut surface similar to their uterine counterparts. On light microscopy, leiomyomas have low cellularity and a pink appearance caused by the abundant fibrillar eosinophilic cytoplasm found in the constituent spindled cells, which have bland nuclei and no or minimal mitotic activity (Fig. 12-6). In equivocal cases, immunohistochemical analysis shows these tumors to be positive for smooth muscle actin, desmin, and high-molecular-weight caldesmon and negative for CD117 (c-*kit*).[41]

GIANT FIBROVASCULAR POLYPS

Fibrovascular polyps are rare but can have a dramatic clinical presentation and a gross appearance; thus, a high percentage of such cases are reported in the literature. In the largest series (16 cases from the AFIP), the mean age of presentation was 56 years, with a range from 32 to 89 years; the sex distribution was relatively equal.[42] These polyps originate high in the esophagus with their pedicles in the region of the cricopharyngeus muscle.[39] From their proximal site of origin, the polyps hang down a considerable distance into the lumen of the distal esophagus, with an average polyp length of 15 cm. Owing to the gigantic size of these polyps, the radiographic findings can be spectacular, with large

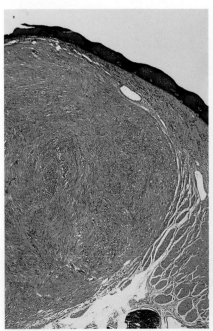 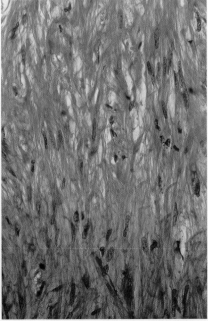

A   **B**

FIGURE 12–6. Leiomyoma. **A,** This esophageal leiomyoma arose from the muscularis mucosae and presented as an intraluminal nodule. **B,** By light microscopy, this leiomyoma is paucicellular, with tumor cells having abundant, fibrillar, brightly eosinophilic cytoplasm.

sausage-shaped structures seen in the esophagus on barium studies.[42] Although most patients present with slowly evolving dysphagia, a significant minority present with acute respiratory distress or even asphyxiation. Respiratory problems are caused by flipping of the polyps into the upper airways when patients vomit, belch, or cough. The clinical stories of some patients are bizarre, with reports of the polyp's "popping out" into the throat, a polyp's sporadically being regurgitated and reswallowed, and patients' having to catch the polyp between the teeth to prevent choking.[43]

On gross examination, these polyps are elongated tubular structures covered by benign squamous epithelium (Fig. 12-7**A**). Although the clinical, radiographic, and gross presentation of these polyps may be dramatic, the histopathology is distinctly dull. The core of the polyp consists only of loose myxoid to collagenized fibrous tissue with varying amounts of adipose tissue (Fig. 12-7**B**).[44] Owing to the considerable adipose tissue present in some cases, these lesions are also reported as lipomas or fibrolipomas.[39] The pathogenesis is thought to be redundant folds in the region of the cricopharyngeus muscle that get pulled down into the distal esophagus by the forces of swallowing. An area known as *Laimer's triangle*, located just below the cricopharyngeal muscle, is described as an area of relative muscular deficiency and is proposed as the site of origin for these polyps.[45] Although no molecular studies have been carried out, it appears that these polyps are not neoplasms but are the result of redundant folds' being stretched to incredible lengths by the actions of swallowing and peristalsis.

RARE MESENCHYMAL POLYPS

Inflammatory fibroid polyps are submucosal lesions characterized by loose stellate cells with a tissue culture appearance with interspersed thin-walled blood vessels and an inflammatory infiltrate containing many eosinophils. These lesions are most often described in the stomach and small bowel, but a handful of cases have been reported in the esophagus.[46] Other rare mesenchymal polyps include inflammatory myofibroblastic tumors[47] and vascular tumors such as hemangiomas[48] and bacillary angiomatosis[49]; the latter has been reported as multiple friable polypoid lesions in the esophagus of an acquired immunodeficiency syndrome (AIDS) patient upon exposure to cats.[49]

Malignant Mesenchymal Tumors (see Table 12-2)

GASTROINTESTINAL STROMAL TUMORS AND LEIOMYOSARCOMAS

Gastrointestinal stromal tumors (GISTs) are mesenchymal tumors currently defined by positivity for CD117 (c-*kit*), which can be determined easily by immunohistochemical staining.[50-52] The protein product of the c-*kit* gene is a transmembrane receptor for a growth factor with an intracytoplasmic tyrosine kinase component.

GISTs are most common in the stomach, followed by the small bowel, with lesser numbers in the rectum. These tumors only rarely arise in the esophagus, with

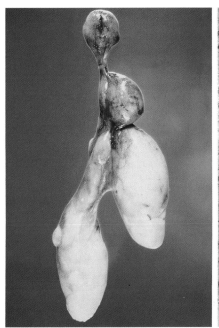
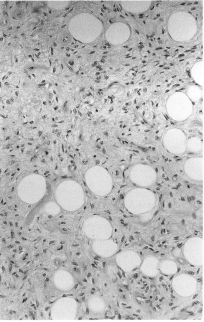

FIGURE 12–7. Giant fibrovascular polyp. **A,** This smooth-surfaced intraluminal polyp hung from a small pedicle and measured approximately 15 cm in length. (Courtesy of Dr. Robert Petras.) **B,** The core of this giant fibrovascular polyp is composed of bland spindle cells, small blood vessels, and fat.

A   **B**

the only series thus far reported by Miettinen and coworkers (see Chapter 22).[41] In their study, esophageal GISTs arose in older patients (median, 63 years), usually in the lower esophagus, with most patients presenting with dysphagia. A majority of esophageal GISTs were intramural, but 17% had intraluminal polypoid growth.

On cut section, these tumors have a soft fish-flesh appearance, often with areas of necrosis. Histologically, most are composed of spindle cells, but almost one quarter comprise epithelioid cells. The low-power pattern of esophageal GIST is varied, ranging from sheets of cells to areas with a neuroid nuclear palisading appearance to areas with marked myxoid change. It is important to note that although most GISTs in sites such as the stomach behave in a benign fashion, more than half of esophageal GISTs are clinically malignant. In the study by Miettinen and associates, most but not all malignant GISTs were greater than 5 cm in size with more than 15 mitotic figures per 50 high-power fields and necrosis.[41]

Esophageal GISTs need to be differentiated from the more common leiomyomas. This distinction can usually be made on gross and microscopic analysis. Leiomyomas are usually small, whorled, and firm on gross examination; on microscopy, they are paucicellular with tumor cells having abundant eosinophilic cytoplasm. GISTs, on the other hand, are usually larger, soft, and "fish-fleshy"; they are more cellular with minimal cytoplasm in individual tumor cells. If in doubt, immunohistochemical studies can aid in this distinction because GISTs are CD117-positive, desmin-negative, and usually smooth muscle actin (SMA)-negative; leiomyomas are the reverse. Also included in the differential are rare esophageal leiomyosarcomas; these are extremely aggressive, with most patients dying within 1 year of presentation. They are composed of malignant spindle cells with eosinophilic cytoplasm and a smooth muscle phenotype (SMA-positive, CD117-negative) and have a high mitotic rate.[41]

References

1. Polyps and tumors. In Lewin KJ, Riddell RH, Weinstein WM (eds): Gastrointestinal Pathology and Its Clinical Implications. New York, Igaku-Shoin, 1992, chapter 12, pp 440-492.
2. Fernandez-Rodriguez CM, Badia-Figuerola N, Ruiz del Arbol L, et al: Squamous papilloma of the esophagus: Report of six cases with long-term follow-up in four patients. Am J Gastroenterol 81:1059-1062, 1986.
3. Quitadamo M, Benson J: Squamous papilloma of the esophagus: Case report and review of the literature. Am J Gastroenterol 50:391-396, 1988.
4. Rabin MS, Bremner CG, Botha JR: The reflux gastroesophageal polyp. Am J Gastroenterol 73:451-452, 1980.
5. Abraham SC, Singh VK, Yardley JH, et al: Hyperplastic polyps of the esophagus and esophagogastric junction: Histologic and clinicopathologic findings. Am J Surg Pathol 25:1180-1187, 2001.
6. Odze R, Antonioli D, Shocket D, et al: Esophageal squamous papillomas. A clinicopathologic study of 38 lesions and analysis for human papillomavirus by the polymerase chain reaction. Am J Surg Pathol 17:803-812, 1993.
7. Croyle P, Nilcaidon H, Gurrarino G: Inflammatory esophagastric junction polyp. Am J Gastroenterol 76:438-440, 1981.
8. Politoske EJ: Squamous papilloma of the esophagus associated with the human papillomavirus. Gastroenterology 102:668-673, 1992.
9. Ratoosh SL, Glombicki AP, Lockhart SG, et al: Mastication of verruca vulgaris associated with esophageal papilloma: HPV-45 sequences detected in oral and cutaneous tissues. J Am Acad Dermatol 36:853-857, 1997.
10. Van Cutsem E, Geboes K, Vantrappen G: Malignant degeneration of esophageal squamous papilloma associated with the human papillomavirus. Gastroenterology 103:1119-1120, 1992.
11. Chatelain D, Flejou JF: Le polype hyperplasique developpe sur heterotopie gastrique. Ann Pathol 18:415-417, 1998.
12. Mion F, Lambert R, Partensky C, et al: High-grade dysplasia in an adenoma of the upper esophagus developing on heterotopic gastric mucosa. Endoscopy 28:633-635, 1996.
13. Hizawa K, Iida M, Matsumoto T, et al: Gastrointestinal manifestations of Cowden's disease. Report of four cases. J Clin Gastroenterol 18:13-18, 1994.
14. Hizawa K, Iida M, Matsumoto T, et al: Gastrointestinal involvement in tuberous sclerosis. Two case reports. J Clin Gastroenterol 19:46-49, 1994.
15. Thurberg BL, Duray PH, Odze RD: Polypoid dysplasia in Barrett's esophagus: A clinicopathologic, immunohistochemical, and molecular study of five cases. Hum Pathol 30:745-752, 1999.
16. Lee RG: Dysplasia in Barrett's esophagus. A clinicopathologic study of six patients. Am J Surg Pathol 9:845-852, 1985.
17. Agha FP, Keren DF: Spindle-cell squamous carcinoma of the esophagus: A tumor with biphasic morphology. Am J Roentgenol 145:541-545, 1985.
18. Iascone C, Barreca M: Carcinosarcoma and pseudosarcoma of the esophagus: Two names, one disease-comprehensive review of the literature. World J Surg 23:153-157, 1999.
19. Olmsted WW, Lichtenstein JE, Hyams VJ: Polypoid epithelial malignancies of the esophagus. Am J Roentgenol 140:921-925, 1983.
20. Kuhajda FP, Sun TT, Mendelsohn G: Polypoid squamous carcinoma of the esophagus. A case report with immunostaining for keratin. Am J Surg Pathol 7:495-499, 1983.
21. Orsatti G, Corvalan AH, Sakurai H, et al: Polypoid adenosquamous carcinoma of the esophagus with prominent spindle cells. Report of a case with immunohistochemical and ultrastructural studies. Arch Pathol Lab Med 117:544-547, 1993.
22. Lauwers GY, Grant LD, Scott GV, et al: Spindle cell squamous carcinoma of the esophagus: Analysis of ploidy and tumor proliferative activity in a series of 13 cases. Hum Pathol 29:863-868, 1998.
23. Tang C-K, Ming S-C: Squamous cell carcinoma and variants of the esophagus. In Ming S-C, Goldman H (eds): Pathology of the Gastrointestinal Tract, 2nd ed. Baltimore, Williams & Wilkins, 1998, chapter 21, pp 475-496.
24. Stranks GJ, Mathai JT, Rowe-Jones DC: Primary malignant melanoma of the oesophagus: Case report and review of surgical pathology. Gut 32:828-830, 1991.
25. Ming S-C: Adenocarcinoma and other epithelial tumors of the esophagus. In Ming S-C, Goldman H (eds): Pathology of the Gastrointestinal Tract, 2nd ed. Baltimore, Williams & Wilkins, 1998, chapter 22, pp 499-521.
26. McDermott VG, Low VHS, Keogan MT, et al: Malignant melanoma metastatic to the gastrointestinal tract. Am J Radiol 166:809-813, 1996.
27. DiCostanzo DP, Urmacher C: Primary malignant melanoma of the esophagus. Am J Surg Pathol 11:46-52, 1987.
28. Johnston J, Helwig EB: Granular cell tumors of the gastrointestinal tract and perianal region: A study of 74 cases. Dig Dis Sci 26:807-816, 1981.
29. Goldblum JR, Rice TW, Zuccaro G, et al: Granular cell tumors of the esophagus: A clinical and pathologic study of 13 cases. Ann Thorac Surg 62:860-865, 1996.
30. Voskuil JH, van Dijk MM, Wagenaar SS, et al: Occurrence of esophageal granular cell tumors in The Netherlands between 1988 and 1994. Dig Dis Sci 46:1610-1614, 2001.
31. Reyes CV, Kathuria S, Molnar Z: Granular cell tumor of the esophagus: A case report. J Clin Gastroenterol 2:365-368, 1980.
32. Brady PG, Nord HJ, Connar RG: Granular cell tumor of the esophagus: Natural history, diagnosis, and therapy. Dig Dis Sci 33:1329-1333, 1988.

33. David O, Jakate S: Multifocal granular cell tumor of the esophagus and proximal stomach with infiltrative pattern: A case report and review of the literature. Arch Pathol Lab Med 123:967-973, 1999.

34. Crawford ES, DeBakey ME: Granular cell myoblastoma: Two unusual cases. Cancer 6:786-789, 1953.

35. Orlowska J, Pachlewski J, Gugulski A, et al: A conservative approach to granular cell tumors of the esophagus: Four case reports and literature review. Am J Gastroenterol 88:311-315, 1993.

36. Postlethwait RW: Benign tumors and cysts of the esophagus. Surg Clin North Am 63:925-931, 1983.

37. Takubo K, Nakagawa H, Tsuchiya S, et al: Seedling leiomyoma of the esophagus and esophagogastric junction zone. Hum Pathol 12:1006-1010, 1981.

38. Bonavina L, Segalin A, Rosati R, et al: Surgical therapy of esophageal leiomyoma. J Am Coll Surg 181:257-262, 1995.

39. Appelman HD: Mesenchymal tumors of the gastrointestinal tract. In Ming S-C, Goldman H (eds): Pathology of the Gastrointestinal Tract, 2nd ed. Baltimore, Williams & Wilkins, 1998, chapter 18, pp 361-398.

40. Kajiyama T, Sakai M, Torii A, et al: Endoscopic aspiration lumpectomy of esophageal leiomyomas derived from the muscularis mucosae. Am J Gastroenterol 90:417-422, 1995.

41. Miettinen M, Sarlomo-Rikala M, Sobin LH, et al: Esophageal stromal tumors: A clinicopathologic, immunohistochemical, and molecular genetic study of 17 cases and comparison with esophageal leiomyomas and leiomyosarcomas. Am J Surg Pathol 24:211-222, 2000.

42. Levine MS, Buck JL, Pantongrag-Brown L, et al: Fibrovascular polyps of the esophagus: Clinical, radiographic, and pathologic findings in 16 patients. Am J Roentgenol 166:781-787, 1996.

43. Owens JJ, Donovan DT, Alford EL: Life-threatening presentations of fibrovascular esophageal and hypopharyngeal polyps. Ann Otol Rhinol Laryngol 103:838-842, 1994.

44. Avezzano EA, Fleischer DE, Merida MA, et al: Giant fibrovascular polyps of the esophagus. Am J Gastroenterol 85:299-302, 1990.

45. Belafsky P, Amedee R, Zimmerman J: Giant fibrovascular polyp of the esophagus. South Med J 92:428-431, 1999.

46. Bosch O, Gonzalez Campos C, Jurado A, et al: Esophageal inflammatory fibroid polyp. Endoscopic and radiologic features. Dig Dis Sci 39:2561-2566, 1994.

47. Pettinato G, Manivel JC, De Rosa N, et al: Inflammatory myofibroblastic tumor (plasma cell granuloma). Clinicopathologic study of 20 cases with immunohistochemical and ultrastructural observations. Am J Clin Pathol 94:538-546, 1990.

48. Araki K, Ohno S, Egashira A, et al: Esophageal hemangioma: A case report and review of the literature. Hepatogastroenterology 46:3148-3154, 1999.

49. Chang AD, Drachenberg CI, James SP: Bacillary angiomatosis associated with extensive esophageal polyposis: A new mucocutaneous manifestation of acquired immunodeficiency disease (AIDS). Am J Gastroenterol 91:2220-2223, 1996.

50. Miettinen M, Sarlomo-Rikala M: Immunohistochemical spectrum of GISTs at different sites and their differential diagnosis with a reference to CD117 (KIT). Mod Pathol 13:1134-1142, 2000.

51. Miettinen M, Sarlomo-Rikala M, Lasota J: Gastrointestinal stromal tumors: Recent advances in understanding of their biology. Hum Pathol 30:1213-1220, 1999.

52. Kindblom LG, Remotti HE, Aldenborg F, et al: Gastrointestinal pacemaker cell tumor (GIPACT): Gastrointestinal stromal tumors show phenotypic characteristics of the interstitial cells of Cajal. Am J Pathol 152:1259-1269, 1998.

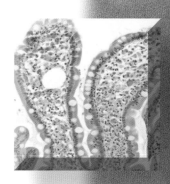

CHAPTER 13

Polyps of the Stomach

JERROLD R. TURNER • ROBERT D. ODZE

Introduction

Gastric polyps are identified in 3% to 5% of patients who have had an upper gastrointestinal endoscopic procedure.[1-3] Polyps may develop as a result of epithelial or stromal cell hyperplasia, inflammation, ectopia, or neoplastic alteration. This chapter classifies gastric polyps according to the predominant cell type (e.g., epithelial, lymphoid, mesenchymal) responsible for polyp growth (Table 13-1).

The importance of clinical-pathologic correlation cannot be overstated in the evaluation of gastric polyps. The anatomic location, endoscopic appearance, number of lesions, and presence or absence of pathology in the surrounding gastric mucosa are critical pieces of information that are usually needed for proper classification of gastric polyps. For example, biopsies obtained from tissue adjacent to an ulcer may show an expanded lamina propria, foveolar hyperplasia, and marked regenerative changes that can mimic a hyperplastic polyp or even an adenoma.

Hyperplastic Polyps

CLINICAL FEATURES

Numerous synonyms, including "inflammatory" polyp, "regenerative" polyp, and "hyperplasiogenous" polyp, have been used to describe hyperplastic polyps. Hyperplastic polyps represent approximately 75% of all gastric polyps. These lesions are believed to develop as a consequence of a mucosal response to tissue injury and inflammation. This sequential process is initiated by gastritis and progresses through phases of foveolar hyperplasia, polypoid foveolar hyperplasia, and ultimately, development of a hyperplastic polyp. Conditions associated with the development of hyperplastic polyps include *Helicobacter pylori* gastritis, chronic non–*H. pylori* gastritis, and gastritis secondary to bile reflux, particularly in patients who have had a Billroth II gastrectomy. In many cases, an underlying cause or associated condition cannot be determined.[4,5] Hyperplastic polyps are detected most often in older patients, with a peak incidence in the sixth and seventh decades of life. They are slightly more common in males.[4-7] Among patients with *H. pylori* infection, regression of hyperplastic polyps has been documented in up to 71% of patients following eradication of the bacterial infection.

PATHOLOGIC FEATURES

Hyperplastic polyps are usually smaller than 1 cm. However, in rare cases, sizes of up to 12 cm may be reached. They occur most commonly in the antrum but can be found anywhere in the stomach. Hyperplastic polyps may develop as a solitary lesion but more frequently occur as multiple polyps, particularly in patients with atrophic gastritis. Grossly, they are typically ovoid and contain a smooth surface contour, although villiform or pedunculated elements may be noted as well. Surface erosion is often present. Rarely, a patient may have more than 50 polyps, in which case a diagnosis of gastric hyperplastic polyposis should be considered, although discrete criteria for this syndrome have not been established.[8]

Microscopically, hyperplastic polyps are characterized by the presence of architecturally distorted,

TABLE 13–1. Classification of Gastric Polyps

Hyperplastic polyps	Hyperplastic polyp
	Polypoid foveolar hyperplasia
	Foveolar polyp
	Gastritis cystica polyposa/profunda
	Ménétrier's disease
Inflammatory polyps	Inflammatory retention polyp
	Polypoid gastritis
Hamartomatous polyps	Fundic gland polyp
	Peutz-Jeghers polyp
	Juvenile polyp
	Cronkhite-Canada syndrome–associated polyp
Heterotopic polyps	Heterotopic pancreatic polyp
	Pancreatic acinar metaplasia
	Brunner's gland hyperplasia
Epithelial polyps	Adenoma
	Polypoid carcinoma
	Carcinoid tumor
	Metastatic carcinoma
Nonepithelial polyps	Inflammatory fibroid polyp
	Gastrointestinal stromal tumor
	Vascular tumor
	Inflammatory myofibroblastic tumor
	Lymphoid hyperplasia
	Lymphoma
Miscellaneous polyps and polyp-like lesions	Xanthoma
	Histiocytosis X
	Granuloma
	Amyloidosis
	Calcium deposits

irregular, cystically dilated, and elongated foveolar epithelium (Fig. 13-1). Crowding of cells and infolding of the epithelium often impart a corkscrew-like appearance to the epithelium. Foveolar cells typically have abundant mucinous cytoplasm but may be mucin depleted focally and contain slightly enlarged and hyperchromatic nuclei with prominent nucleoli, features considered regenerative. Mitotic activity may be brisk in areas of active inflammation and surface ulceration. Pseudogoblet or globoid mucinous cells, which are also frequently present, appear as cells containing apically located nuclei and basally oriented mucous vacuoles. These cells were once considered dysplastic but are now commonly recognized as reactive. Thus, the previously used term *globoid dysplasia* has been discarded in favor of the more descriptive term *dystrophic goblet cell*. Intestinal metaplasia is noted in less than 25% of hyperplastic polyps, but when present it is frequently associated with intestinal metaplasia and chronic gastritis in the surrounding nonpolypoid mucosa. The lamina propria is typically edematous and congested and shows a variable amount of acute and chronic inflammation. The inflammatory infiltrate is usually most prominent in the superficial aspects of the polyp and is often associated with surface erosions. In rare cases, granulation tissue associated with ulcerations may show marked pseudosarcomatous atypical changes in the stromal fibroblasts and endothelial cells that are in fact reactive (see Fig. 13-1**F**). Nodular lymphoid aggregates, with or without germinal centers, may be present as well. Most well-developed hyperplastic polyps also contain thin bundles of smooth muscle that extend upward from the muscularis mucosae toward the polyp surface. *H. pylori* has been documented in up to 76% of hyperplastic polyps.[9,10]

The natural history of hyperplastic polyps is poorly understood, but one report suggests that up to 67% remain stable in size, 27% may enlarge, and 5% shrink.[11] Up to 50% of patients develop recurrent polyps after endoscopic resection.[17,18] Because of the risk of dysplasia in larger polyps, resection is often recommended for all polyps larger than 1.5 cm in greatest diameter.

DYSPLASIA IN HYPERPLASTIC POLYPS

The incidence of dysplasia in hyperplastic polyps ranges from 1% to 20%.[12-15] Although universal agreement has not been reached, it appears that the risk of dysplasia is most related to polyp size; it occurs rarely in polyps smaller than 1.5 cm in diameter. The risk of dysplasia increases progressively with size in polyps that exceed 2 cm. Age is also a risk factor in that both dysplasia- and carcinoma-containing hyperplastic polyps tend to occur in patients older than 50 years of age. Carcinoma is uncommon among hyperplastic polyps but when present is thought to develop from underlying dysplastic epithelium. At least one study has reported that mutations of the *p53* gene may be important in the development of dysplasia and carcinoma in gastric hyperplastic polyps.[16]

The microscopic appearance of dysplasia in hyperplastic polyps is similar to that in other areas of the gastrointestinal tract and is commonly categorized as low- or high-grade dysplasia (Fig. 13-2). In low-grade dysplasia, the epithelium is composed of cells with hyperchromatic elongated nuclei, clumped chromatin, and pseudostratification. These changes always involve the surface epithelium but may also occur in the deep mucosal glands. Multiple nucleoli are not uncommon. Mitotic activity is brisk and may show atypia, particularly at the surface of the polyp. High-grade dysplasia is characterized by a greater degree of nuclear pleomorphism, loss of cell polarity, and more abundant abnormal mitoses than are present in low-grade dyplasia. Architectural alteration may also occur in the form of back-to-back gland formation and full-thickness nuclear stratification. Overall, the architecture is more complex in high-grade dysplasia, with the formation of cribriform profiles and tubular budding. Moreover, features of cellular differentiation, such as cytoplasmic mucin, are progressively lost in high-grade dysplasia.

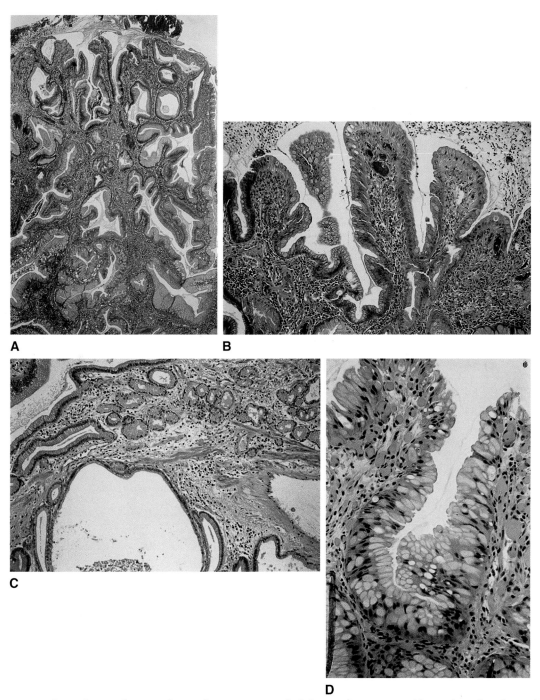

FIGURE 13–1. Gastric hyperplastic polyps. **A,** These polyps are composed of elongated, tortuous, and hyperplastic foveolar epithelium with cystic change. **B,** The lamina propria typically shows an increased amount of acute and chronic inflammation. Villiform surface change is also not uncommon. **C,** A mild amount of muscularis hyperplasia may be seen within the lamina propria, particularly surrounding cystically dilated glands. **D,** The surface and/or foveolar epithelium often shows a proliferation of dystrophic goblet cells, which may give a false appearance of signet ring cell carcinoma in situ.

Continued

The primary differential diagnosis of a hyperplastic polyp with dysplasia is a hyperplastic polyp with marked regeneration but without true dysplasia (Table 13-2). The single most useful discriminating feature is the presence of nuclear atypia at the surface of the lesion. Cytologic atypia limited to the deeper proliferative zones within the polyp and combined with some degree

of surface maturation is more often regenerative than dysplastic (Fig. 13-3). Similarly, in the presence of active inflammation, the degree of atypia may be marked, and a diagnosis of dysplasia should be made with great caution. In contrast, nuclear pleomorphism and loss of cell polarity, particularly in the absence of prominent nucleoli, favor a diagnosis of dysplasia. In addition,

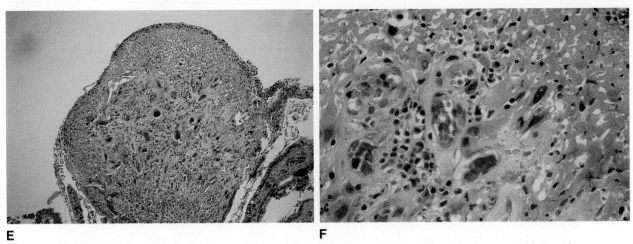

E **F**

FIGURE 13–1, cont'd E, Focal ulceration is not uncommon in hyperplastic polyps. **F,** In this example, a marked "pseudosarcomatous" proliferation of reactive fibroblasts and endothelial cells is seen within granulation tissue.

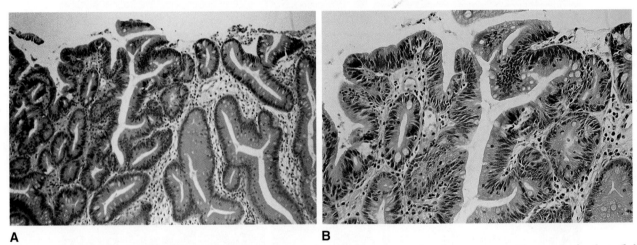

A **B**

FIGURE 13–2. A, Dysplasia arising within a gastric hyperplastic polyp. Medium-power view shows an area of low-grade dysplasia *(left)* adjacent to an area of hyperplastic foveolar epithelium with intestinal metaplasia *(right)*. **B,** Dysplastic epithelium consists of cells with hyperchromatic, elongated, atypical nuclei, increased mitoses, and mucin depletion. Surface maturation is absent. These features are consistent with low-grade dysplasia.

TABLE 13–2. Differentiation Between Dysplasia and Regeneration in Gastric Polyps

	Negative (Regenerative)	Indefinite for Dysplasia	Low-Grade Dysplasia	High-Grade Dysplasia
Surface maturation	Present	Present	Absent	Absent
Increased mitoses	Variable	Variable	Yes	Yes
Atypical mitoses	No	No	Uncommon	Yes
Nuclear shape	Ovoid	Ovoid to elongated	Elongated	Irregular
Chromatin pattern	Hyperchromatic	Hyperchromatic	Irregular, hyperchromatic	Irregular, vesicular
Prominent nucleoli	Present	Variable	Absent	Present, often multiple
Nuclear pseudostratification	Absent	Focal	Mild	Marked
Mucin depletion	Variable	Frequent	Frequent	Frequent
Gland size	Small	Small	Small	Irregular
Budding/branching	Absent	Absent	Focal	Prominent
Cribriform profiles	Absent	Absent	Absent	Frequent
Inflammation	Variable	Present	Absent	Absent

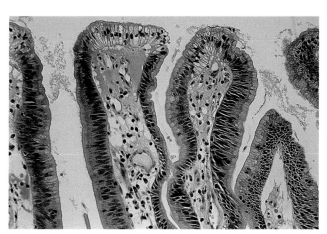

FIGURE 13-3. Marked regeneration in a gastric hyperplastic polyp. In contrast to true dysplasia, regenerating epithelium shows some evidence of surface maturation.

architectural aberration, such as a cribriform growth pattern, strongly suggests dysplasia.

Hyperplastic polyps with dysplasia should also be differentiated from primary gastric adenomas. Adenomas are characterized by the absence of adjacent or underlying hyperplastic foveolar epithelium and cystic change, all of which may be present in hyperplastic polyps.

DIFFERENTIAL DIAGNOSIS

The differential diagnosis of gastric hyperplastic polyps includes polypoid gastritis, polypoid foveolar hyperplasia, gastritis cystica polyposa/profunda, fundic gland polyp, polyps associated with Ménétrier's disease, Cronkhite-Canada syndrome, juvenile polyposis, and Peutz-Jeghers polyposis. Features helpful in this differential are summarized in Table 13-3. Polypoid gastritis and polypoid foveolar hyperplasia are typically smaller than hyperplastic polyps and lack cystically dilated, irregular, and tortuous foveolar epithelium. Additionally, the lamina propria of polypoid foveolar hyperplasia is marked by less inflammation and lacks muscularis hyperplasia.

Gastritis cystica polyposa/profunda is closely related to hyperplastic polyps in both pathogenesis and morphologic appearance (see under Gastritis Cystica Polyposa/Profunda). The surface and intraluminal portions of these two types of lesions may be identical. However, unlike hyperplastic polyps, gastritis cystica polyposa is characterized by the presence of cystically dilated, distorted, and irregularly shaped epithelium and/or glands, located within either the muscularis mucosae or the submucosa. Additionally, polyps related to gastritis cystica polyposa often develop adjacent to stoma sites in patients who have had a partial gastrectomy.

In contrast to hyperplastic polyps, fundic gland polyps contain cystically dilated glands lined predominantly by parietal and chief cells. Occasional cysts may contain mucinous cells as well. Moreover, fundic gland polyps do not normally contain prominent inflammation, ulceration, or marked regenerative changes typical of hyperplastic polyps.

Polyps associated with Ménétrier's disease, Cronkhite-Canada syndrome, and juvenile polyps are histologically similar to hyperplastic polyps. In these instances, appropriate clinical and endoscopic information is essential in order to establish a correct diagnosis.

Peutz-Jeghers polyps of the stomach reveal a characteristic arborizing pattern of smooth muscle that is more extensive than that of hyperplastic polyps. Peutz-Jeghers polyps lack significant stromal inflammation and are usually not associated with an underlying chronic gastritis. However, other features of Peutz-Jeghers polyps are similar to those of hyperplastic polyps.

MORPHOLOGIC VARIANTS

Polypoid Foveolar Hyperplasia

Polypoid foveolar hyperplasia is generally regarded as a precursor to hyperplastic polyps. Similar to hyperplastic polyps, polypoid foveolar hyperplasia is a regenerative lesion associated with chronic gastritis, as well as other types of acute and chronic mucosal injury. For instance, polypoid foveolar hyperplasia often develops at the mucosal edges of surface erosions, ulcers, and carcinomas or adjacent to gastrojejunostomy stomas; it may also be associated with the use of nonsteroidal anti-inflammatory drugs (NSAIDs), with bile reflux, or the use of alcohol.[17-19] Polypoid foveolar hyperplasia may remain stable in size, regress, or grow. The proportion of these lesions that ultimately progress to hyperplastic polyps is unknown.

Pathologically, polypoid foveolar hyperplasia usually appears as a sessile lesion that measures 1 to 2 mm in diameter. Lesions may be single or multiple and are most often found in the antrum. Microscopically, polypoid foveolar hyperplasia is characterized by simple hyperplasia of the gastric foveolar epithelium without cystic change or significant distortion. The foveolar epithelium appears increased in length and shows luminal serration and a corkscrew-like pattern (Fig. 13-4). The foveolae are typically crowded and tightly packed, with little intervening stroma. The epithelium is often mucin depleted and reactive in appearance, with abundant mitotic figures, enlarged nuclei, and prominent nucleoli. Various degrees of intestinal metaplasia may be seen. The lamina propria may have a mild lymphoplasmacytic infiltrate that varies with cause, but smooth muscle proliferation is typically absent, unless bile reflux is present.

TABLE 13–3. Features of Gastric Polyps

Polyp Type	Prevalence	Site	Architecture	Stroma	Adjacent Mucosa	Malignant Potential	Comments
Hyperplastic polyp	75% of gastric polyps	Antrum > body	Elongated, cystic, and distorted foveolar epithelium; often marked regeneration	Inflammation, edema, smooth muscle hyperplasia	Chronic gastritis	<2%	*Helicobacter pylori* often present; dysplasia in 1%–20%; greatest in polyps >2 cm and in patients >50 years
Polypoid gastritis	2nd most common polyp	Antrum > body	Normal architecture ± foveolar hyperplasia	Inflammation	Chronic gastritis	None	*H. pylori* often present, often multiple
Polypoid foveolar hyperplasia	Very common	Antrum > body	Elongated foveolar epithelium; no cysts	Normal lamina propria ± edema	Erosion, chronic gastritis, or normal	None	Increased with NSAIDs, alcohol, bile reflux, post–Billroth II gastrectomy
Fundic gland polyp	Common	Body only	Normal or distorted glands and microcysts lined by parietal and chief cells	Normal ± minimal inflammation	Normal	Rare	May be multiple in FAP; dysplasia in up to 40% of FAP-associated lesions and <1% of sporadic lesions
Adenoma	Common	Antrum > body	Dysplastic intestinal- or gastric-type epithelium; architecture varies with grade	± Inflammation	Chronic gastritis or normal	30% or more	Usually solitary
Gastritis cystica polyposa	Rare	Body > antrum	Entrapped, distorted, cystically dilated glands in muscularis; no atypia	Inflammation, edema, smooth muscle hyperplasia	Chronic atrophic gastritis	None	Most common in post–Billroth II gastrectomy and severe atrophic gastritis
Juvenile polyp	Rare	Body > antrum	Similar to hyperplastic polyp	Inflammation, edema, smooth muscle hyperplasia	Normal	Slight in stomach, greater elsewhere	Clinical history of polyps at other GI sites
Peutz-Jeghers polyp	Very rare	Any site	Normal gastric cell types in arborizing muscle network	Normal lamina propria	Normal	2%–3%	Clinical history of other GI polyps, associated skin changes
Ménétrier's disease	Very rare	Body only	Foveolar hyperplasia, cysts, atrophy of glands	Normal or increased lymphocytes	Antrum normal	Very rare	Diffuse hypertrophy of rugae, hypoproteinemia

FAP, familial adenomatous polyposis; GI, gastrointestinal; NSAIDs, Nonsteroidal anti-inflammatory drugs.

Gastric Foveolar Polyps

Gastric foveolar polyps were originally described by Goldman and Appelman in 1972.[20] It is unclear if these represent a regenerative lesion, a subtype of hyperplastic polyp, or a hamartomatous lesion. The foveolar polyp is not universally accepted as a separate polyp type, perhaps because foveolar hyperplasia occurs so frequently. Foveolar polyps are found primarily in the antrum and are generally smaller than 2 cm in diameter.[20] However, some can reach sizes of up to 8 cm.[6] Gastric foveolar polyps are composed of densely packed foveolar mucinous epithelium that forms an arborizing network. Intestinal metaplasia is noted in approximately

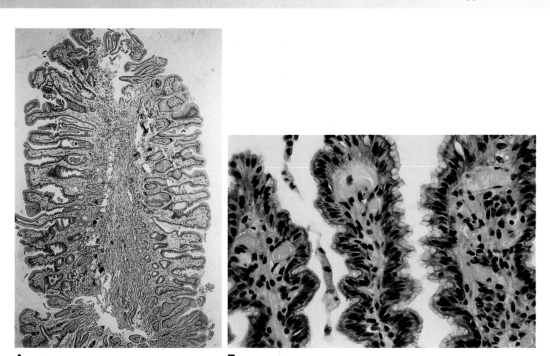

A   **B**

FIGURE 13–4. Polypoid foveolar hyperplasia. **A,** In contrast to hyperplastic polyps, polypoid foveolar hyperplasia shows elongated, hyperplastic, and tortuous foveolar epithelium without significant cystic change or increased inflammation in the lamina propria. **B,** Corkscrew-like appearance to the hyperplastic foveolar epithelium, mucin depletion, and hyperchromaticity of the epithelial nuclei are all features of regeneration. This particular case developed in association with chronic bile reflux gastritis.

33% of cases. Inflammation is conspicuously absent. Notably, of the eight patients originally described,[20] one had coexisting gastric carcinoma, and a second had colonic carcinoma. However, foveolar polyps are not typically associated with an increased risk of malignancy. Foveolar polyps can be differentiated from hyperplastic polyps and polypoid foveolar hyperplasia by the absence of an inflammatory infiltrate and cystic change.

Gastritis Cystica Polyposa/Profunda

Gastritis cystica polyposa/profunda is defined as a hyperplastic polyp that contains foci of misplaced foveolar and/or glandular epithelium in the muscularis mucosae or in deeper portions of the submucosa or the muscularis propria. The lesion is called *polyposa* when an intraluminal polyp is present and *profunda* when the bulk of the lesion is located within the wall of the stomach. These lesions typically occur in patients with chronic bile reflux–induced gastritis as a result of partial gastrectomy.[21-23] Gastritis cystica polyposa is also referred to as *stromal polypoid hypertrophic gastritis* when it occurs in the postoperative gastric remnant. Because of the association with chronic gastritis and partial gastrectomy, it is presumed that gastritis cystica polyposa/profunda is caused by an exuberant reactive proliferation with trauma-induced entrapment of epithelium in deep portions of the gastric wall. However,

the reasons for the development of epithelial cysts within deeper portions of the gastric wall are not clear. Some have suggested that local ischemia or mucosal prolapse is critical to the development of cysts.

Pathologically, polyps of gastritis cystica polyposa/profunda are typically located on the gastric side of gastroenteric anastomoses. Rarely, they develop on a background of chronic gastritis. Grossly, the polyps are indistinguishable from hyperplastic polyps. Lesions may reach up to 3 cm in diameter and are often associated with enlarged rugal folds. The characteristic histologic feature is the presence of entrapped epithelium and/or glands within or beneath the muscularis mucosae of the polyp (Fig. 13-5). The epithelium may be mucinous or glandular, is often cystic, and is usually surrounded by a rim of lamina propria–like stroma. The cysts are usually entrapped within dense disorganized bundles of smooth muscle that extend downward from the muscularis mucosae. Hyperplasia, reactive changes, and mucin depletion within the epithelium are usually marked, imparting an atrophic appearance to the epithelium. Often an associated inflammatory infiltrate composed of neutrophils and mononuclear cells is found within the lamina propria. Superficial erosion and intestinal metaplasia may also occur. Rarely, dysplasia may develop in association with gastritis cystica polyposa/profunda, but it is unclear if the frequency of occurrence is equal to or greater than that with typical hyperplastic polyps.

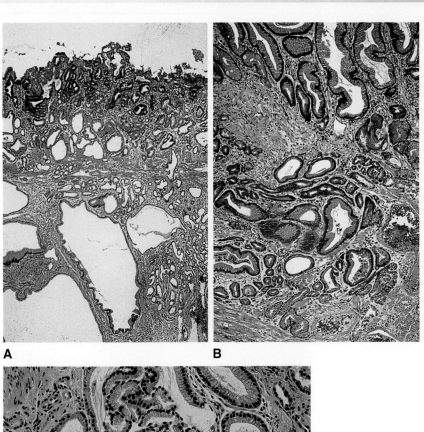

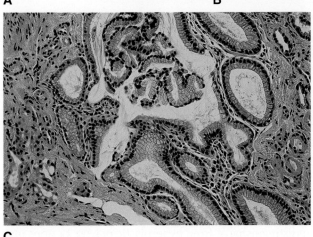

A

B

C

FIGURE 13–5. Gastritis cystica polyposa/ profunda. **A,** This lesion has the mucosal features of a hyperplastic polyp but also shows a proliferation of small to medium-sized glands, with cystic change, within the muscularis mucosae and submucosa. **B,** On deeper sectioning, the misplaced glands in the submucosa connect with the mucosae. **C,** At high power, misplaced glands show a lobular configuration and are composed of cells with basally located regularly sized nuclei. A small rim of lamina propria surrounds the glands.

On occasion, it may be difficult to discriminate between misplaced epithelium in gastritis cystica polyposa/profunda and a well-differentiated invasive adenocarcinoma (Fig. 13-6). Features such as desmoplasia, cellular pleomorphism, irregularity in the size and shape of the glands, atypical mitoses, and the lack of a lamina propria rim surrounding the epithelium in question strongly favor a diagnosis of adenocarcinoma.

▊ Ménétrier's Disease

CLINICAL FEATURES

Ménétrier's disease is a rare disorder characterized by diffuse hyperplasia of the foveolar epithelium of the body and fundus combined with hypoproteinemia due to protein-losing enteropathy. A variety of other symptoms, such as weight loss, diarrhea, and peripheral edema, are also often present. In rare (mostly pediatric) cases, the antrum may be involved. In adults, onset is typically between 30 and 60 years of age, with a male-to-female ratio of 3:1. The syndrome is characterized by pronounced gastrointestinal protein loss and hypoalbuminemia.[24] Although the clinical and pathologic features of Ménétrier's disease in children are essentially similar to those in adults, many children have a history of recent respiratory infection, peripheral blood eosinophilia, and cytomegalovirus infection.[25] It is most important to note that the disease is usually self-limited in children, generally lasting only several weeks.[26,27]

PATHOGENESIS

The cause of Ménétrier's disease is unknown. In children, some cases appear to be associated with

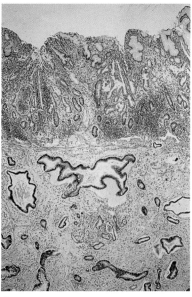

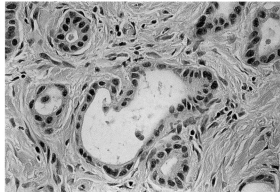

FIGURE 13–6. Well-differentiated adenocarcinoma arising in association with chronic gastritis. In contrast to misplaced glands in gastritis cystica polyposa/profunda, carcinomatous glands are highly irregular in size and shape, show jagged edges, and are arranged in a haphazard nonlobular fashion (**A**). At high power (**B**), malignant glands show a greater degree of cytologic atypia, loss of polarity, and hyperchromaticity and, most importantly, do not contain a rim of lamina propria surrounding the glands. The size and shape of the glands vary significantly.

A　　　　　　　　**B**

cytomegalovirus infection.[25,28] In these cases, spontaneous and treatment-associated remissions may occur.[25,28] In contrast, although *H. pylori* infection and various other conditions have been associated with Ménétrier's disease in adults, antibiotics, acid suppression, octreotide, and anticholinergic agents have had therapeutic benefit in only occasional adult cases.[29,30] One clue to the pathogenesis of this disease relates to the observation that transgenic mice that overexpress transforming growth factor α (TGF-α) in the stomach show many of the clinical and histologic features of Ménétrier's disease, such as marked foveolar hyperplasia, reduced numbers of parietal cells, and decreased acid production.[31,32] In human disease, one study reported cessation of nausea and vomiting, increased serum albumin, and partial restoration of parietal cell mass following experimental treatment of a Ménétrier's disease patient with a monoclonal antibody against the TGF-α cell membrane receptor.[33]

PATHOLOGIC FEATURES

On endoscopic examination, Ménétrier's disease is characterized by diffuse irregular enlargement of the gastric rugae. However, some areas may appear polypoid. Enlarged rugae typically involve the body and fundus but may extend to involve the antrum in rare instances.[34] Histologically, the most characteristic feature of Ménétrier's disease is foveolar mucous cell hyperplasia (Fig. 13-7). The foveolae are elongated and frequently take on a corkscrew-like appearance. Cystic dilatation is also common. Hyperplastic mucous cells are typically fully differentiated without regenerative features or mucin depletion. Inflamma-

tion is usually only modest, and ulcerations are not normally present. Intestinal metaplasia is usually absent. Some cases show marked intraepithelial lymphocytosis. These features are associated with glandular atrophy and hypoplasia of parietal and chief cells.

A diagnosis of Ménétrier's disease may be difficult to make by mucosal biopsy analysis alone because the histologic features can mimic those of a hyperplastic polyp. Thus, clinical information is essential for establishing a correct diagnosis. In addition, Ménétrier's disease must be distinguished from other causes of enlarged gastric rugae, such as chronic gastritis, Zollinger-Ellison syndrome, and infiltration by tumor cells, such as lymphoma. Most of these are easily distinguished by biopsy analysis. For instance, chronic gastritis shows abundant inflammation in the lamina propria without marked foveolar hyperplasia. The absence of foveolar hyperplasia and the presence of parietal cell hyperplasia distinguish the mucosal changes associated with Zollinger-Ellison syndrome from Ménétrier's disease. Lymphoma and other infiltrating tumors may also mimic Ménétrier's disease grossly, but biopsies are diagnostic.

TREATMENT

The treatment of Ménétrier's disease is mainly supportive and is provided in the form of serum albumin and nutritional supplementation. In severe cases, gastrectomy may be necessary.[35] A poorly defined association between Ménétrier's disease and an increased risk of adenocarcinoma has been reported,[36-38] but this remains controversial.

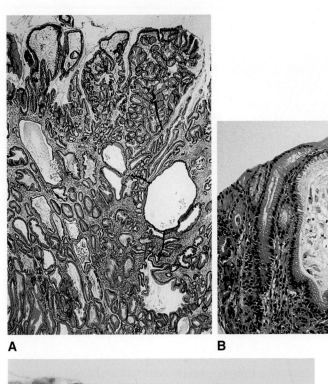

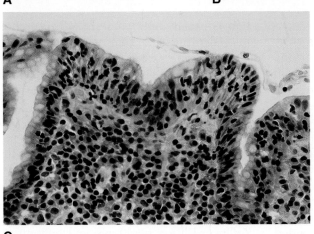

FIGURE 13–7. Ménétrier's disease. **A,** At low microscopic power, a biopsy from Ménétrier's disease may look histologically similar to a hyperplastic polyp, being composed of irregular, tortuous, cystically dilated, and elongated foveolar epithelium. The glandular compartment (*bottom of photo*) shows inflammation and atrophy. **B,** A biopsy from a patient with Ménétrier's disease may look histologically similar to the surface of a hyperplastic polyp. **C,** In some cases of Ménétrier's disease, a marked degree of intraepithelial lymphocytosis simulating lymphocytic gastritis is seen.

◼ Inflammatory Polyps

INFLAMMATORY RETENTION POLYPS

Inflammatory retention polyps are uncommon lesions that typically occur in association with *H. pylori* gastritis. Some cases are associated with hypergastrinemia.[4,5,39] Endoscopically, inflammatory retention polyps are sessile lesions with a smooth surface contour. Microscopically, prominent foveolar cysts filled with retained mucus and variable numbers of neutrophils are the characteristic features. The stroma is often edematous and may contain prominent polymorphonuclear and mononuclear inflammatory infiltrates. Deeper areas of the polyp are typically devoid of epithelium and are characterized by an edematous inflammatory stroma; in some cases a loose proliferation of small blood vessels is seen. Inflammatory retention polyps of the stomach are not particularly well studied and, similar to other inflammatory polyps, may regress following eradication of the underlying gastritis.

POLYPOID GASTRITIS

Polypoid gastritis develops as a result of chronic gastritis; it is characterized by localized lamina propria expansion by inflammatory cells and lymphoid aggregates. Polypoid gastritis typically occurs in patients who are 10 years younger than those with hyperplastic polyps. The major risk factor is *H. pylori* gastritis. Less commonly, polypoid gastritis may develop as a result of atrophic gastritis. Polypoid gastritis is present in approximately 1% of all patients who undergo upper gastrointestinal endoscopy.

Pathologically, these polyps are well-circumscribed nodules that usually measure less than 0.5 cm in diameter. They are most common in the antrum but can be located anywhere in the stomach. Histologically, they are characterized by epithelial regeneration with increased mitotic activity, marked acute and chronic lamina propria inflammation (Fig. 13-8), and nodular lymphoid aggregates. The polymorphic mixed inflammatory infiltrate, which includes neutrophils, plasma cells, and lymphocytes, and the absence of a homogeneous population of atypical lymphocytes and lymphoepithelial lesions are useful features for distinguishing these lesions from lymphoma.

Hamartomatous Polyps

The most common hamartomatous lesions of the stomach are fundic gland polyps. Other less common hamartomatous polyps are usually associated with distinct polyposis syndromes, such as Peutz-Jeghers syndrome, juvenile polyposis, or, rarely, Cronkhite-Canada syndrome. Thus, in most instances, an accurate diagnosis is highly dependent on correlation of the pathologic findings with relevant clinical and endoscopic information.

FUNDIC GLAND POLYPS

Clinical Features

Fundic gland polyps most often occur sporadically but are also common among patients with familial adenomatous polyposis (FAP). Fundic gland polyps are identified in approximately 0.8% of patients who undergo upper gastrointestinal endoscopy. They occur more often in females (female-to-male ratio, 5:1) at an average age of 53 years.[40] Recently, the prevalence of fundic gland polyps has increased dramatically owing to their association with proton pump inhibitor therapy.[41,42] Up to 50% of patients with FAP have fundic gland polyps within oxyntic mucosa.[43-47] These polyps are usually associated with *adenomatous polyposis coli (APC)* gene mutations[46] but not with mutations in beta-catenin, another component of the APC signaling pathway.[48] This contrasts with sporadic lesions, which are associated with activating beta-catenin mutations in more than 90% of cases but with APC gene mutations in less than 10% of cases.[46,48]

Pathologic Features

Fundic gland polyps are smooth, sessile, well-circumscribed lesions that occur exclusively in gastric oxyntic mucosa. They may be single or multiple, particularly in FAP patients. In one study, each FAP patient had an average of four polyps, with a range from 1 to 11.[40] Fundic gland polyps are most often smaller than 1.0 cm, but lesions up to 2 to 3 cm have been reported. Histologically, fundic gland polyps are composed of cystically dilated and architecturally irregular fundic glands (Fig. 13-9). These glands, which may assume a microcystic configuration or may be a disordered arrangement of tortuous glands with prominent budding, are lined by somewhat flattened parietal and chief cells and occasional mucinous foveolar cells. Inflammation is typically absent or minimal. Fundic gland polyps often show surface and foveolar atrophy.

Natural History and Treatment

Although sporadic fundic gland polyps are considered benign lesions with no malignant potential, dysplasia may be present in up to 42% of FAP-associated fundic gland polyps.[49-53] In contrast, dysplasia is found in fewer than 1% of sporadic fundic gland polyps.[51-53] Dysplasia in fundic gland polyps occurs primarily within the foveolar compartment. Similar to dysplasia in adenomas, dysplasia in fundic gland polyps usually reveals elongated hyperchomatic nuclei, increased nucleocytoplasmic ratio, and nuclear pseudostratification that extends to the surface of the polyp (Fig. 13-10). When hyperchromatism and nuclear enlargement are limited to proliferative zones of the polyp, regenerative atypia should be considered as the diagnosis, especially if active inflammation is present.

SYNDROME-ASSOCIATED HAMARTOMATOUS POLYPS

Peutz-Jeghers Polyps

Clinical Features. Peutz-Jeghers syndrome is an autosomal dominant inherited syndrome characterized by the presence of mucocutaneous pigmentation and multiple gastrointestinal hamartomatous polyps. The

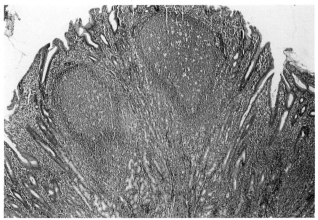

FIGURE 13–8. Polypoid area of gastritis in a patient with chronic active *H. pylori* gastritis. In this case, prominent reactive lymphoid follicles within the mucosa, combined with inflammation in the lamina propria, impart a polypoid appearance to the mucosa.

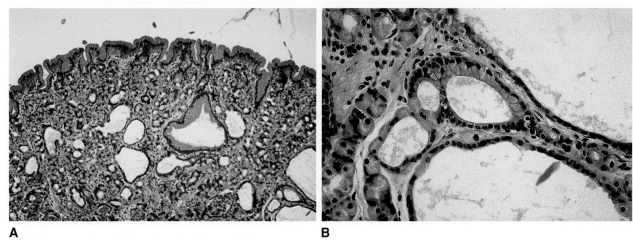

A   **B**

FIGURE 13–9. In contrast to hyperplastic polyps, fundic gland polyps show atrophic foveolar epithelium and a marked increase in the number of oxyntic glands, some with irregular budding, and microcystic change **(A).** At high power **(B),** the microcysts are lined by oxyntic-type cells composed of parietal and chief cells, endocrine cells, and a variable number of mucinous columnar cells *(not seen in this picture).* The degree of inflammation in the lamina propria is typically minimal.

disease occurs equally among males and females and typically presents in the second or third decade of life with abdominal pain, gastrointestinal bleeding, or, less commonly, obstruction. Hamartomatous polyps in Peutz-Jeghers syndrome may occur in any portion of the gastrointestinal tract but are most common in the small intestine. Gastric lesions are present in 25% to 50% of patients. Owing to their small size, gastric Peutz-Jeghers polyps are usually asymptomatic.

Peutz-Jeghers syndrome is caused by a germline mutation in the serine-threonine kinase STK11/LKB1 tumor suppressor gene. The function of this gene product is related to the transforming growth factor-β (TGF-β) signal transduction pathway. Dysplasia and carcinoma are rare in gastric hamartomatous polyps, occurring at an estimated incidence of 2% to 3%.[54]

However, they may develop at a young age. For example, in one series of Peutz-Jeghers syndrome patients with gastric cancer, carcinoma developed at a mean age of 27 years.[55]

Pathologic Features. Gastric Peutz-Jeghers polyps may be sessile lesions but are more commonly pedunculated. They typically measure less than 1 cm in size. However, larger lesions may rarely develop. The gross appearance is similar to Peutz-Jeghers polyps in other portions of the gastrointestinal tract and often includes a velvety papillary or villiform surface. They occur most commonly in the antrum but may occur in any part of the stomach. Microscopically, gastric Peutz-Jeghers polyps show a complex arborizing architecture of smooth muscle. Irregularly organized bundles of smooth muscle extend from the muscularis mucosae into the lamina

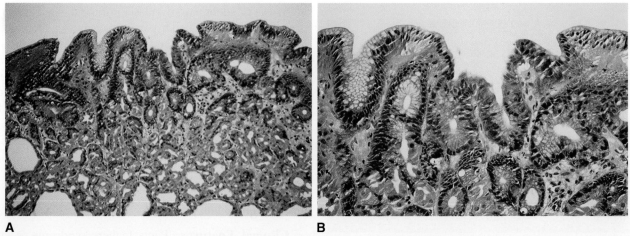

A   **B**

FIGURE 13–10. Dysplasia arising in a fundic gland polyp associated with familial adenomatous polyposis. **A,** The central part of the photograph shows an area of surface and foveolar epithelial atypia consistent with low-grade dysplasia. **B,** The dysplastic epithelium shows a proliferation of cells containing hyperchromatic, pencil-shaped nuclei with clumped chromatin, pseudostratification, and increased mitoses. Dysplastic epithelium may be seen in the glandular or surface compartment of the polyps.

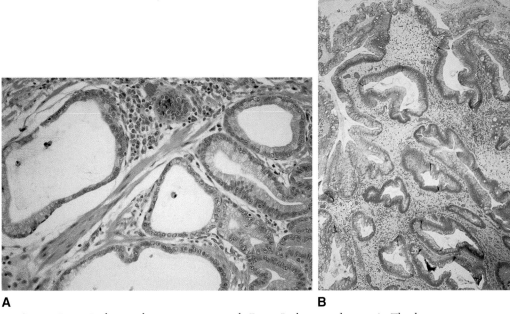

A   **B**

FIGURE 13–11. Gastric Peutz-Jeghers polyp in a patient with Peutz-Jeghers syndrome. **A,** The low-power appearance of a Peutz-Jeghers polyp is similar to that of a hyperplastic polyp. It is composed of an irregular and architecturally distorted proliferation of foveolar epithelium with increased inflammation in the lamina propria. **B,** This Peutz-Jeghers polyp shows a more pronounced muscularis proliferation than is normally seen in hyperplastic polyps.

propria core of papillary projections and extend to the surface of the polyp (Fig. 13-11). Marked surface and foveolar hyperplasia with cystic change is often present. Glandular atrophy commonly is noted, and a mild degree of lamina propria edema, congestion, and inflammation may also be apparent. Morphologic features are essentially similar to those of gastric hyperplastic polyps, with the exception that hamartomatous polyps often have a more fully developed and prominent smooth muscle proliferation. However, this is less well developed than the classic arborizing pattern of small intestinal Peutz-Jeghers polyps. Gastric polyps of Peutz-Jeghers syndrome are usually clinically silent. However, occasional examples of patients who have vomited large polyps, presumably as a result of autoamputation, have been reported.[56] There is presently no consensus on appropriate surveillance or follow-up of gastric Peutz-Jeghers polyps, although general guidelines have been proposed.[57]

Juvenile Polyps

Clinical Features. Sporadic juvenile polyps in the stomach are rare but may occur as part of generalized juvenile polyposis coli or as part of the rare gastric subtype of this polyposis syndrome. Gastric juvenile polyps are present in 15% to 25% of patients with generalized juvenile polyposis coli. Twenty percent to 50% of patients with gastric juvenile polyps have a positive family history

for juvenile polyposis coli. Juvenile polyposis coli is an autosomal dominant condition characterized by a genetic defect and resultant dysregulation of the TGF-β pathway. The mutation most commonly identified thus far involves the gene SMAD4/DPC4, which codes for a cytoplasmic intermediate in TGF-β signaling.[58] However, this mutation is present in only a minority of cases, so other as yet unidentified mutations are likely responsible for this disorder as well.[59] Other implicated genes include *PTEN*, the gene that is mutated in Cowden syndrome.[60]

Pathologic Features. The gross and microscopic features of gastric juvenile polyps resemble those of gastric hyperplastic polyps (Fig. 13-12). In some instances, juvenile polyps may show a less pronounced degree of muscularis hyperplasia and more prominently inflamed lamina propria than hyperplastic polyps. However, because of significant overlap, this is often not helpful in individual cases. The essential features of hyperplastic polyps consist of surface and foveolar hyperplasia, cystic change, edema and inflammation of the lamina propria, smooth muscle hyperplasia, and a variable degree of pyloric or intestinal metaplasia. The polyps may range from a few millimeters to several centimeters in size. Based on histology alone, it is not possible to distinguish an isolated gastric juvenile polyp from a hyperplastic polyp. Therefore, knowledge of the clinical context, including family history, is essential in establishing a correct diagnosis.

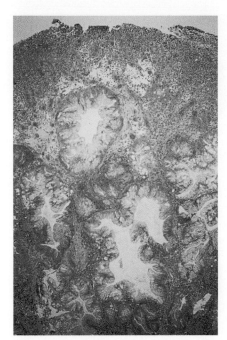

FIGURE 13–12. Gastric juvenile polyp in a patient with generalized juvenile polyposis coli. Similar to hyperplastic polyps and Peutz-Jeghers polyps, juvenile polyps are composed of irregular, dilated, and tortuous foveolar and glandular epithelium with inflammation in the lamina propria. Diffuse ulceration is more common in gastric juvenile polyps than in hyperplastic or Peutz-Jeghers polyps.

Dysplasia and even carcinoma may occur with increased frequency among patients with generalized juvenile polyposis coli. However, dysplasia is rare in gastric polyps. Dysplasia in juvenile polyps appears histologically similar to that which occurs in hyperplastic polyps; it consists of surface and foveolar epithelium that is mucin depleted and contains hyperchromatic elongated nuclei with clumped chromatin, increased nucleocytoplasmic ratio, loss of polarity, and pseudostratification. Lack of surface maturation is a common feature of dysplasia in juvenile polyps. With increasing degrees of dysplasia, the nuclei become larger and show greater overlapping and loss of polarity, and the glands may take on a back-to-back and cribriform growth pattern.

Cronkhite-Canada Syndrome–Associated Polyps

Clinical Features. Cronkhite-Canada syndrome is a nonhereditary generalized polyposis disorder that involves the stomach, small intestine, and colorectum. Unlike most syndromic polyposis disorders, Cronkhite-Canada syndrome typically presents in middle adulthood. It occurs equally among males and females. In addition to the presence of numerous gastrointestinal polyps, patients with this disorder show alopecia, nail atrophy, skin hyperpigmentation, and vitiligo. Common gastrointestinal complaints include diarrhea, weight loss,

abdominal pain, anorexia, weakness, and hematochezia. The etiology of Cronkhite-Canada syndrome is unknown. This disorder is associated with a mortality rate of approximately 50%; most deaths are related to anemia and chronic wasting. Up to 20% of patients may develop gastrointestinal adenocarcinoma, which may occur in any portion of the gastrointestinal tract, including the stomach.[61-63] These cancers occur both in the Cronkhite-Canada polyps and in nonpolypoid areas.

Pathologic Features. Typical advanced cases of Cronkhite-Canada syndrome show diffuse irregular enlargement of the gastric rugae throughout the fundus and antrum (Fig. 13-13). Numerous small to medium-sized polyps that typically measure between 0.5 and 1.5 cm in diameter are superimposed on the enlarged rugae. The endoscopic appearance is similar to that of Ménétrier's disease, except that the entire stomach is involved in Cronkhite-Canada syndrome. Individual polyps may appear as elongated, papillary or villiform lesions or, alternatively, as a sessile cluster of nodules. Helpful in the diagnosis of this disorder is the fact that the interpolypoid mucosa is typically abnormal and shows foveolar hyperplasia, irregularity, and microcystic change.

Microscopically, changes in the stomach involve both the interpolypoid and the polypoid mucosa (Fig. 13-14). Similar features are found in both areas. Similar to Ménétrier's disease, marked surface and foveolar hyperplasia with cystic change and atrophy of the glands are characteristic features. The lamina propria is often edematous and shows a mild to moderate degree of inflammation. Intestinal metaplasia and pyloric metaplasia are uncommon. The surrounding nonpolypoid mucosa shows alternating areas of atrophy and foveolar hyperplasia with cystic change. A single biopsy from a polyp in Cronkhite-Canada syndrome

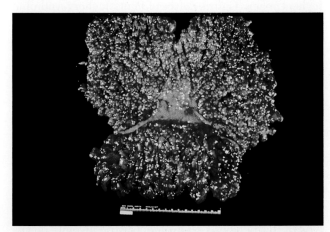

FIGURE 13–13. Resected stomach in a patient with Cronkhite-Canada syndrome. The fundus and the antrum show a carpetlike proliferation of small polyps and enlarged rugae. The disease involves both the fundus and the antrum.

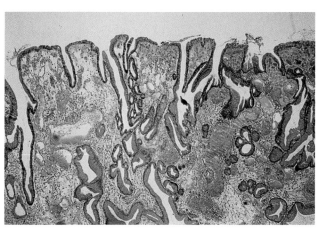

FIGURE 13–14. Both the polypoid and the interpolypoid mucosa show elongated, tortuous, and cystically dilated foveolar epithelium, as well as edema and hemorrhage, in the lamina propria. In contrast to hyperplastic polyps, Cronkhite-Canada syndrome–associated polyps typically do not show prominent inflammation or muscularis hyperplasia.

may look histologically identical to a juvenile polyp or a hyperplastic polyp, or even Ménétrier's disease. However, knowledge of other clinical attributes of this disorder, particularly when combined with diffuse enlargement of the rugae and multiple polyps in all areas of the stomach, is helpful in establishing a correct diagnosis.

▪ Embryonic Rests and Heterotopia

PANCREATIC HETEROTOPIA

Clinical Features

Ectopic rests of pancreatic tissue, called *adenomyomas*, may form during embryonic organogenesis when fragments of pancreas separate during rotation of the foregut. Foci of ectopic pancreatic tissue are most commonly found in the stomach but may occur in the small intestine and colon as well. In one recent series, 4% of all benign gastric polyps were pancreatic heterotopia.[64] Males and females are affected equally, and the average age of diagnosis is 45 years. However, pediatric patients may be affected as well. Heterotopic pancreatic tissue is susceptible to many of the inflammatory disorders that may affect the native pancreas, including pancreatitis and neoplasia, although the latter complication is extremely uncommon.

Pathologic Features

Pancreatic heterotopia most commonly occurs in the prepyloric and antral regions but may also occur rarely in more proximal areas of the stomach. Grossly, the lesions consist of small submucosal protruding nodules that typically measure 1 to 3 cm in diameter. A central dimple or surface erosion, which represents a draining pancreatic duct, is frequently present and is an endoscopic clue to the diagnosis. Ulceration and overt bleeding are frequently associated with pancreatic heterotopia. Clinical symptoms relate to the location and size of the lesion and the presence or absence of ulceration or bleeding.

Microscopically, heterotopic pancreatic tissue may be composed of any of the normal components of pancreatic parenchyma, either in isolation or in combination. Thus, a mixture of exocrine (acinar tissue), endocrine (islet cells), and ductal epithelial elements in combination with pancreatic stroma may be present in various proportions. Histologically, each component is similar to that which occurs in the normal pancreas (Fig. 13-15). Acini typically drain into ducts lined by tall columnar epithelium. However, squamous metaplasia may occasionally be present. Thick disorganized bundles of hyperplastic smooth muscle are often admixed with acini and ducts. Endocrine elements, representing islets of Langerhans, are present in less than 50% of cases. Occasionally, heterotopic pancreatic tissue may show acute and chronic inflammation and necrosis, similar to acute and chronic pancreatitis of the native pancreas. The gastric mucosa overlying the heterotopic pancreas often shows reactive changes, including foveolar hyperplasia, and variable amounts of edema, congestion, and inflammation.

Differential Diagnosis

The differential diagnosis of pancreatic heterotopia includes well-differentiated invasive adenocarcinoma and gastritis cystica polyposa/profunda. This differential diagnosis may be difficult if pancreatic acini and/or endocrine cells are not readily identifiable. However, unlike well-differentiated invasive carcinoma, pancreatic heterotopia does not show significant architectural or cytologic atypia, atypical mitoses, or loss of epithelial polarity. The ducts are often smooth as opposed to irregular in contour, which is typical of invasive carcinoma. Furthermore, foci of pancreatic heterotopia are normally present in an organoid lobulated growth pattern. The smooth muscle proliferation associated with pancreatic heterotopia contrasts with the type of desmoplasia often associated with invasive carcinoma.

Gastritis cystica polyposa/profunda may also have an appearance that is similar to pancreatic heterotopia, but the former is usually associated with more extreme hyperplastic changes, inflammation, and erosions of the overlying mucosa. The submucosal epithelium of gastritis cystica polyposa/profunda is typically mucinous columnar epithelium, with or without gastric glands, in contrast to the pancreatic ductal-type epithelium characteristic of pancreatic heterotopia.

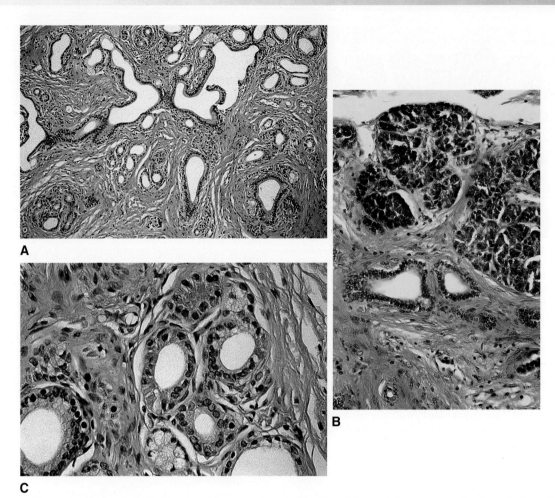

FIGURE 13–15. Pancreatic heterotopia. **A,** Pancreatic heterotopia consists of variably sized ducts, acinar glands, and islet cells within a stroma characterized by muscularis hyperplasia. **B,** Prominent acinar glands, a few ducts, and marked muscularis hyperplasia are evident. **C,** At high power, another area from this case highlights the bland cytologic features of the duct epithelium.

PANCREATIC ACINAR METAPLASIA

Clinical Features

Pancreatic acinar metaplasia may occur in children or adults[65,66] and is detected in approximately 1% of gastric biopsies.[67] In adults, the mean age has been reported to be 52 years, with a range of 18 to 89 years and a male-to-female ratio of 1:1.[68] Pancreatic acinar metaplasia occurs most often in antral and cardiac (gastroesophageal junction) mucosa on a background of either absent or minimal inflammation, often without glandular atrophy or intestinal metaplasia.[66] The cause of pancreatic acinar metaplasia is unknown. Some studies have shown an association with chronic gastritis.[67] However, others have shown no association with esophagitis, intestinal metaplasia, chronic gastritis, or *H. pylori* infection.[68] Thus, this condition has been proposed to represent a congenital rest.[67,68]

Pathologic Features

Pancreatic acinar-like cells are characterized by the presence of fine acidophilic granules in the apical cytoplasm and prominent basophilia of the basal portion of the cells. The cells are usually arranged in small nests or lobules that are often seen in continuity with the surrounding gastric glands (Fig. 13-16).[65] Alternatively, lobules of pancreatic acinar cells may be separated from the surrounding gastric mucosa by connective tissue and smooth muscle.[65] When examined immunocytochemically or by electron microscopy, the cells are indistinguishable from pancreatic acinar cells. They contain exocrine secretory granules that are immunoreactive for exocrine pancreatic markers, such as lipase, trypsinogen, and pancreatic alpha-amylase.[66,67] Occasional cells may also be positive for neuroendocrine markers, such as chromogranin, somatostatin, gastrin, and serotonin, and some cells are positive for both exocrine and neuroendocrine markers.[66]

Differential Diagnosis

The most common differential diagnosis of pancreatic acinar metaplasia is pancreatic heterotopia. The presence of ductal elements, pancreatic stroma, or well-

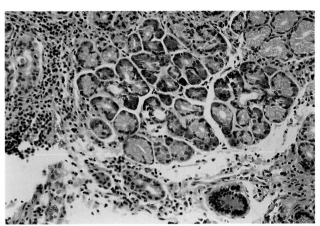

FIGURE 13–16. Pancreatic acinar metaplasia in the gastric cardia of a patient with chronic gastritis. In contrast to pancreatic heterotopia, pancreatic acinar metaplasia is composed of a well-demarcated lobule of pancreatic acinar glands without islets of Langerhans or ducts.

defined islets effectively excludes pancreatic acinar metaplasia. Paneth cell metaplasia may also be considered in the differential diagnosis of pancreatic acinar metaplasia. The well-developed zymogen granules and the prominent small and fine apical granules are distinct from the larger refractile granules of Paneth cells. Immunostains for trypsinogen and lipase can be helpful in difficult cases.

BRUNNER'S GLAND NODULES

Brunner's gland hyperplasia in the proximal duodenum is usually related to chronic duodenitis. In contrast, it is unclear if the presence of Brunner's glands in the prepyloric region represents a hamartomatous process or is the result of proximal extension of hyperplastic duodenal Brunner's glands due to hyperchlorhydria.[64,69,70] Histologically, the lesion is composed of densely packed, cytologically bland Brunner's glands that may form a small submucosal nodule. In rare cases, pyloric obstruction may occur.

▇ Epithelial Polyps

ADENOMAS

Clinical Features

Sporadic adenomas account for 8% to 10% of all gastric polyps. Their incidence increases with patient age.[6,7,12,71] However, there is marked variation in the incidence of adenomas in different populations that generally parallels the incidence of adenocarcinoma. For example, gastric adenomas are more common in the Japanese population in whom the incidence of adenocarcinoma is high.[2,56,72-74] Affected patients are usually in the sixth to seventh decade of life, and the male-to-female ratio is 3:1. Adenomas also occur in association with familial adenomatous polyposis, with an incidence in this patient group of 1% to 15%. Similar to other forms of gastric dysplasia, adenomas often occur on a background of chronic gastritis with atrophy and intestinal metaplasia. This finding has led some authors to speculate that some adenomas may represent polypoid dysplasia that develops as a result of underlying chronic gastritis, similar to polypoid dysplasia in ulcerative colitis.[75] Thus, true sporadic adenomas may be a rare lesion. However, this issue is unresolved and remains to be studied in a rigorous fashion. It is interesting to note that one study has shown that intestinal-type adenomas are more often associated with chronic gastritis compared with lesions that are composed mainly of gastric-type epithelium and therefore may represent polypoid dysplasia.

Adenomas have a high risk of malignancy that is most often related to the size of the lesion, particularly in lesions larger than 2 cm in diameter.[2,12,71] Gastric carcinoma may be present in up to 30% of patients with an adenoma.[11,12,71,76] The molecular features of gastric adenomas are poorly understood. Microsatellite instability is present in a minority of adenomas but occurs more commonly in adenomas that contain carcinoma.[77-79] In contrast, APC mutations occur more commonly in adenomas without carcinoma than in those with carcinoma.[79]

Pathologic Features

Adenomas may occur anywhere in the stomach but are most common in the antrum.[53] More than 80% are solitary,[53] although multiple lesions may occur as well.[80] Grossly, most adenomas are well-circumscribed, sessile, or pedunculated lesions that measure less than 2 cm in diameter. The average size is 1 cm. Rarely, gastric adenomas may be flat or even depressed. Papillary adenomas with a predominantly tubulovillous or villous growth pattern are often larger, with an average diameter of 4 cm, but they may grow to even larger sizes. Papillary adenomas have a velvety surface contour and have a lobulated gross appearance.

Microscopically, most adenomas are composed of columnar intestinal-type epithelium (Fig. 13-17). A brush border is often detectable that confirms intestinal differentiation in the dysplastic epithelium. Goblet cell, Paneth cell, and endocrine differentiation are also commonly present. A small proportion of gastric adenomas are composed predominantly of dysplastic gastric-type mucinous columnar epithelium or a mixture of intestinal and gastric cell types. Adenomas composed of gastric-type epithelium are less likely than those

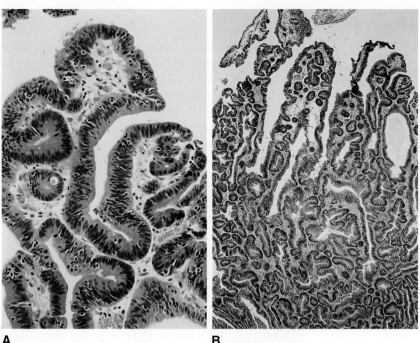

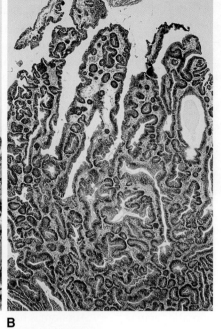

A   **B**

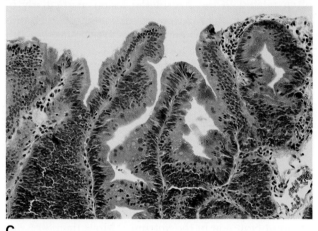

C

FIGURE 13–17. Gastric adenoma. Most gastric adenomas appear histologically similar to their colonic counterparts and are composed of cells with stratification, hyperchromatic pencil-shaped nuclei, and mucin depletion. **A,** This is an intestinal-type adenoma. **B,** This adenoma shows a focus of high-grade dysplasia that is composed of architecturally distorted dysplastic epithelium without obvious invasion into the lamina propria. **C,** This adenoma shows prominent Paneth cell differentiation, which may be marked in some cases.

composed of intestinal-type epithelium to harbor high-grade dysplasia or carcinoma.[53] Chronic gastritis occurs more frequently in association with intestinal-type adenomas than with gastric-type adenomas. Papillary adenomas frequently display a marked degree of pleomorphism and exuberant mitotic activity that is uncommon in flat adenomas.

The classification of adenomas is controversial and differs among pathologists in different parts of the world. Western pathologists typically grade dysplasia in adenomas or in flat mucosa as low or high grade.[81,82] The main advantage of this two-tiered system of classification is that it has a higher degree of interobserver agreement and aligns more precisely with patient management options than do the more complex systems.[82] The main difference in the evaluation of dysplasia between Western and Japanese pathologists is that Western pathologists require lamina propria invasion for the diagnosis of adenocarcinoma,[83] whereas Japanese

pathologists put greater weight on cytologic features in making an assessment of malignancy. Thus, a lesion that would normally be categorized as an adenoma with high-grade dysplasia by Western pathologists might be interpreted as carcinoma by Japanese pathologists.[83] Recognition of this discrepancy between Western and Japanese pathologists in grading gastric dysplasia has led to the establishment of four potential international systems for the classification of dysplasia and early cancer in the stomach (Table 13-4).[81,82,84,85] In these systems, low-grade dysplasia is characterized by hyperchromatic elongated cells with crowding and pseudo-stratification. Mucin depletion is a common feature.[82] The architecture of low-grade dysplasia is often simple; it is composed of multiple small glands with little budding or branching.[81] It is important to note that dysplasia extends to the mucosal surface; this feature can be helpful in the differentiation between regenerative lesions and true dysplasia.

TABLE 13–4. Classification of Gastric Dysplasia

Western Classification	Japanese Classification	Padova Classification	Vienna Classification
Benign reactive	Benign, no atypia Includes intestinal metaplasia, regenerative and hyperplastic epithelium	1. Negative 1.0 Normal 1.1 Reactive 1.2 Intestinal metaplasia 1.2.1 IM, complete type 1.2.2 IM, incomplete type	1. Negative for neoplasia-dysplasia
Indefinite	Benign, with atypia Frequently associated with active inflammation or found within hyperplastic polyp	2. Indefinite for dysplasia 2.1 Foveolar hyperproliferation 2.1 Hyperproliferative intestinal metaplasia	2. Indefinite for neoplasia-dysplasia
Low-grade dysplasia	Borderline, between benign and malignant Dysplastic lesions with architectural and cytologic atypia	3. Noninvasive neoplasia 3.1 Low-grade dysplasia 3.2 High-grade dysplasia 3.2.1 Including suspicious for carcinoma without invasion 3.2.2 Including carcinoma without invasion	3. Noninvasive neoplasia, low grade
High-grade dysplasia	Highly suspicious for carcinoma	4. Suspicious for invasive carcinoma	4. Noninvasive neoplasia, high grade 4.1 High-grade adenoma-dysplasia 4.2 Noninvasive carcinoma (carcinoma in situ) 4.3 Suspicious for invasive carcinoma
Carcinoma	Invasive carcinoma	5. Invasive adenocarcinoma	5. Invasive neoplasia 5.1 Intramucosal carcinoma 5.2 Submucosal carcinoma or deeper

High-grade dysplasia in adenomas is characterized by a more complex architecture and more severe cytologic atypia. This includes irregularly shaped crowded glands with frequent budding and branching. Cribriform profiles may also be noted. Cell nuclei may be elongated and hyperchromatic as in low-grade dysplasia, but they are more frequently ovoid and vesicular with irregular contours, prominent nucleoli, and clumped chromatin. Loss of cellular polarity is also more pronounced in high-grade dysplasia.[81,82]

Differential Diagnosis

The differential diagnosis of a gastric adenoma includes a hyperplastic polyp with dysplasia, fundic gland polyp with dysplasia, and polypoid carcinoma (see under Polypoid Carcinoma). In contrast to adenomas, hyperplastic polyps with dysplasia contain foveolar hyperplasia, cystic change, and inflammation in the underlying polyp. Moreover, dysplasia is often focal in hyperplastic polyps. The presence of cystically dilated fundic glands with specialized parietal and chief cells in the gland compartment beneath the dysplasia is diagnostic of a dysplastic fundic gland polyp.

TREATMENT

Treatment of adenomas is somewhat dependent on the grade of dysplasia. Flat adenomas with low-grade dysplasia are generally treated by complete endoscopic resection and endoscopic surveillance following a careful evaluation of the entire stomach. Adenomas with high-grade dysplasia and lesions that are too large to be removed by endoscopic resection require surgical resection. Although precise guidelines have not been established, future treatment of adenomas may depend on whether the lesion is considered a sporadic adenoma or an area of polypoid dysplasia occurring on a background of chronic gastritis.

POLYPOID CARCINOMA

Polypoid carcinoma, also known as protruded or protuberant-type carcinoma, represents a carcinoma that grows in a polypoid fashion into the gastric lumen. It may be associated with deeply invasive tumor. Polypoid carcinomas represent a minority of gastric cancers, accounting for less than 10% in most series. Similar to other types of gastric cancer, the peak incidence occurs in the sixth decade of life, with a male-to-female ratio of 2 to 3:1. A strong association has been noted with *H. pylori* infection, as well as with other forms of chronic gastritis.

Polypoid carcinomas are most prevalent in the lesser curvature. They are often smaller than 1 cm in diameter. Histologically, polypoid carcinomas often show intestinal-type dysplastic epithelium[53] with high-grade dysplasia and invasion of the lamina propria (Fig. 13-18). Desmoplasia may be noted as well.[53,86]

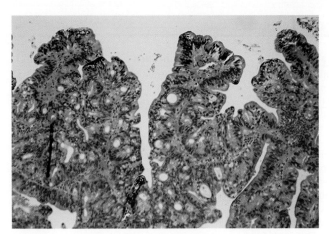

FIGURE 13–18. Polypoid intestinal-type adenocarcinoma. In this case, foci of intramucosal adenocarcinoma are visible above an area of invasive adenocarcinoma (*not seen*).

CARCINOID TUMOR

Up to 30% of gastrointestinal carcinoid tumors occur in the stomach, and the incidence of gastric carcinoid tumors is on the rise. These tumors are discussed more thoroughly in Chapter 21. Carcinoid tumors occur most commonly in the body and fundus and, not uncommonly, may grow as a polypoid lesion. Nodular proliferations of neuroendocrine cells may also be seen. These are called *endocrine hyperplasia* or *endocrine dysplasia* when they measure less than 150 μm in diameter or 150 to 500 μm in diameter, respectively.[87] Nodules that exceed 500 μm in size represent true carcinoid tumors.[87] Any of these lesions may appear polypoid (Fig. 13-19). Treatment for carcinoid tumors is dependent on the cause, size, and multiplicity of lesions and is discussed more thoroughly in Chapter 21.

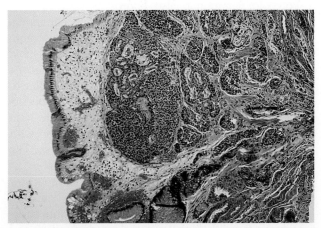

FIGURE 13–19. This photograph shows the intramucosal portion of a well-differentiated carcinoid tumor that presented as a small, sessile, well-circumscribed mucosal nodule.

METASTATIC LESIONS

The stomach may be involved by distant metastasis or by direct extension of tumors from the pancreas, lung, breast, transverse colon, and, in particular, distal esophagus (Fig. 13-20).[88,89] Most metastases to the stomach are located within the submucosa, where the vascular supply is richest. With growth, an ulcerated mucosal mass may form, and, especially in the case of melanoma, ulceration and bleeding may occur.[88,90] In some instances, metastases may appear as irregular polypoid lesions, but this is less common.

◼ Nonepithelial Polyps

INFLAMMATORY FIBROID POLYPS

Clinical Features

Inflammatory fibroid polyps are mesenchymal proliferations composed of a mixture of stromal spindle cells, small blood vessels, and inflammatory cells. They may occur anywhere in the gastrointestinal tract but are most common in the stomach and small intestine. Within the stomach, inflammatory fibroid polyps usually occur during the sixth decade of life, with a slight male predominance. Owing to the small number of cases reported, little additional clinical and epidemiologic information is available. Some have suggested an infectious cause for inflammatory fibroid polyps.[91] However, no causative agent has ever been identified; thus, others believe they are a form of reactive pseudotumor. When small, they may be discovered incidentally at endoscopy. However, large lesions may cause obstructive symptoms such as nausea, vomiting, and abdominal pain. In some cases, inflammatory fibroid polyps may contain a long stalk; these may prolapse through the pyloric sphincter and cause obstruction. Some studies suggest that inflammatory fibroid polyps are more common among patients with atrophic gastritis and pernicious anemia.

Pathologic Features

Inflammatory fibroid polyps are typically small, well-circumscribed, submucosally based, sessile lesions that may show ulceration of the overlying mucosa. Their median size is 1.5 cm, and, although most lesions are smaller than 3 cm in diameter, polyps that measure as large as 5 cm in diameter have been reported. In the stomach, they most commonly arise in the antrum, immediately proximal to or overlying the pyloric sphincter.

Microscopically, inflammatory fibroid polyps typically fill the submucosal space and often show a sharp demarcation at the level of the muscularis propria. Mucosal involvement is common with gastric lesions.

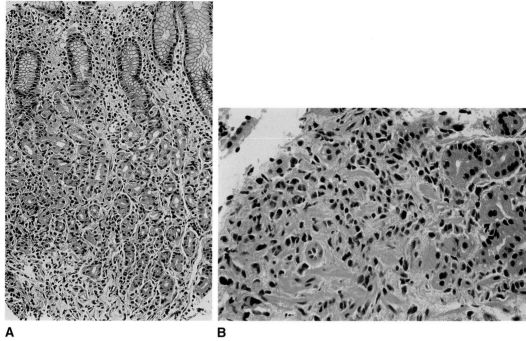

A   B

FIGURE 13–20. Metastatic lobular carcinoma of the breast to the stomach. **A,** At low power, metastatic carcinoma cells may be mistaken for lymphocytes in association with chronic gastritis. **B,** However, at high power, the cells appear highly atypical, are epithelioid in morphology, and show a single-cell file arrangement of cells, unlike lymphocytes.

However, unlike with small intestinal lesions, involvement of the muscularis propria is unusual with gastric polyps. Extension of the tumor into the mucosa causes separation of gastric glands, which results in a disordered and atrophic appearance. Inflammatory fibroid polyps are composed of a loose mixture of spindle-shaped, plump, cytologically bland stromal cells; inflammatory cells; and small, thin-walled blood vessels in an edematous or myxoid background (Fig. 13-21). In the stomach, stromal cells often proliferate in a concentric fashion around small and medium-sized blood vessels.[92,93] Mitotic figures are rare but may occasionally be present within deeper portions of the lesion. Atypical mitoses are never present. Eosinophils are often prominent within the inflammatory component and may also encircle vessels. Larger lesions may show collagen deposition and smooth muscle proliferation, or even giant cell formation.

Immunohistochemically, stromal cells are typically positive for vimentin and CD34.[92] A smaller proportion are also positive for smooth muscle actin, HHF-35, KP-1, and Mac 387.[92] In contrast to stromal tumors of the GI tract, inflammatory fibroid polyps are uniformly negative for CD117 (c-kit).[92]

GASTROINTESTINAL STROMAL TUMORS

Gastrointestinal stromal tumors (GISTs) are discussed in detail in Chapter 22. The stomach is the most

common site of GISTs. Rarely, when these occur in the stomach, they may present as polypoid lesions.

VASCULAR TUMORS

Benign vascular tumors, such as hemangiomas and glomus tumors, that are histologically similar to lesions in other areas of the gastrointestinal tract and skin may occur in the stomach and often present as intraluminal nodules or polyps (Fig. 13-22). These lesions are similar to their counterparts in other areas of the body and are uniformly benign. They can be confused with the more common gastric epithelioid GIST.

INFLAMMATORY MYOFIBROBLASTIC TUMOR

Inflammatory myofibroblastic tumor was originally called *inflammatory pseudotumor* and was described as a tumor of the small intestinal mesentery in preadolescent children.[94] Because of the presence of mature plasma cells and lymphocytes, this lesion has also been referred to as *plasma cell granuloma*. This lesion occurs in young children and adults.[94-96] In the largest reported series of 38 gastrointestinal inflammatory myofibroblastic tumors reported to date, 34% occurred in the stomach.[53,95,96-98] Patients may present with nonspecific symptoms, including fever, growth retardation, and weight loss.[94,95,99] The cause of inflam-

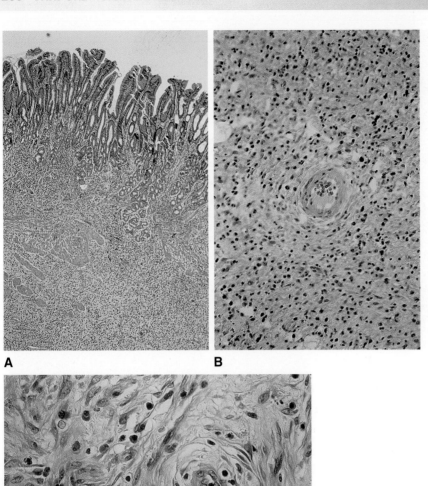

FIGURE 13–21. Gastric inflammatory fibroid polyp. **A,** At low power, a loose mesenchymal proliferation of cells fills the submucosa and muscularis mucosae and penetrates into the basal portion of the mucosa. **B,** The proliferation is composed of bland mesenchymal cells combined with lymphocytes, eosinophils, and small blood vessels. **C,** Mesenchymal cells and eosinophils tend to aggregate in a concentric fashion around blood vessels.

matory myofibroblastic tumor is poorly understood, but this lesion is associated with gastric ulcers, chronic gastritis, NSAID use, and ischemic disease. Abnormalities involving chromosome 2p are present in the majority of cases.[101-105] This gene rearrangement frequently results in a fusion protein that includes anaplastic lymphoma kinase, a putative growth factor receptor.[102-105] Such rearrangements have been reported in up to 60% of inflammatory myofibroblastic tumors[103,106,107] and may be most common in inflammatory myofibroblastic tumors among patients younger than 10 years of age.[103]

Inflammatory myofibroblastic tumors average 8 cm in diameter.[95] They often appear as firm white lesions with infiltrative borders and foci of myxoid change. Histologically, they are composed of spindle cells with features of myofibroblasts, mature plasma cells, and

small lymphocytes (Fig. 13-23).[94] The spindle cells, consistent with their proposed myofibroblastic origin, are often immunohistochemically positive for smooth muscle actin,[95] anaplastic lymphoma kinase,[103,106,107] vimentin, muscle-specific actin, and cytokeratin.[108] Tumors can also be focally positive for CD34 and factor XIIIa.[109] The plasma cell component is polyclonal.[110]

Although they were originally described as benign lesions,[94] it is now clear that inflammatory myofibroblastic tumors can recur locally.[95,97] At present, no specific histologic features associated with recurrence have been described, but several studies suggest that aneuploidy may help identify aggressive lesions.[97,103] An association between clinical outcome and anaplastic lymphoma kinase expression has also been suggested but not confirmed.[103] Owing to the risk of

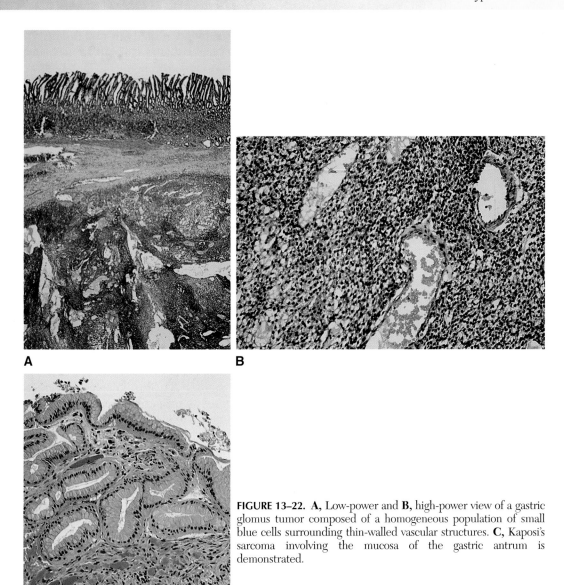

A

B

C

FIGURE 13–22. A, Low-power and **B,** high-power view of a gastric glomus tumor composed of a homogeneous population of small blue cells surrounding thin-walled vascular structures. **C,** Kaposi's sarcoma involving the mucosa of the gastric antrum is demonstrated.

local recurrence, surgical excision and long-term follow-up are indicated in patients with these tumors.[96,97,108]

Lymphoid Polyps

LYMPHOID HYPERPLASIA

Lymphoid hyperplasia with germinal center formation, also known as *follicular hyperplasia* or *chronic* *follicular gastritis*, is typically a manifestation of chronic gastritis, and in particular, of *H. pylori* infection.[111] Consistent with the distribution of disease in *H. pylori* gastritis, reactive lymphoid nodules are most prevalent in the antrum but can also be present in the gastric body. Nodules are often multiple and are generally smaller than 0.3 cm in greatest diameter.[112] They are frequently umbilicated and can be visualized on double-contrast barium studies.[111-113] Eradication of *H. pylori* is associated with a decrease in the prevalence and density of lymphoid follicles.[113]

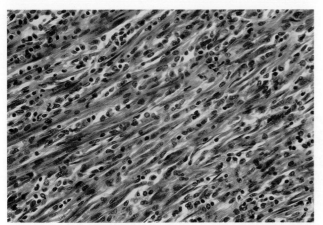

FIGURE 13–23. High-power view of an inflammatory myofibroblastic tumor composed of mildly to moderately atypical mesenchymal cells within a stroma rich in lymphocytes. This tumor should be differentiated from a gastric gastrointestinal stromal tumor.

LYMPHOMA

The gastrointestinal tract is the initial site of presentation in 4% to 20% of all non-Hodgkin's lymphomas.[114] A majority of these cases involve the stomach.[114] Many of these lesions may initially present as polyps, either solitary or multiple. Gastric lymphoma is discussed in detail in Chapter 23.

■ Miscellaneous Polyps and Polyp-like Lesions

XANTHOMAS

Xanthomas are small, sessile, yellow mucosal nodules composed of a loose aggregate of lipid-laden macrophages within the lamina propria (Fig. 13-24). They are most often found in the body and fundus[115,116]; they are typically smaller than 3 mm and are frequently multiple. Xanthomas most commonly develop in association with chronic gastritis, especially following partial gastrectomy. It is believed that they develop as a form of reaction to tissue injury. The differential diagnosis of xanthoma includes benign muciphages, granular cell tumor, and signet ring cell carcinoma. Because xanthomas contain intracellular glycolipids that are lost during tissue processing, the macrophages are negative by the periodic acid–Schiff (PAS) stain, whereas muciphages are typically strongly positive. The cytoplasmic granules of granular cell tumors stain positively by the PAS stain and for the S100 protein by immunohistochemistry. Signet ring cell carcinomas also contain cytoplasmic mucin, which can be demonstrated with PAS or mucicarmine stain; in addition, they can be easily differentiated based on their malignant nuclear cytologic features and cytokeratin immunoreactivity.

HISTIOCYTOSIS X

Histiocytosis X, also known as *Langerhans' cell histiocytosis*, is primarily a disease of young children. Depending on the location of the disease, the terms *eosinophilic granuloma, Hand-Schüller-Christian disease,* or *Letterer-Siwe disease* are also applicable. *Eosinophilic granuloma* is a term that is generally applied to the solitary nodular form of the lesion occasionally found in the stomach.[117,118] When examined histologically, these nodules are composed of tight clusters of cells with finely granular cytoplasm that contain Birbeck granules. Scattered eosinophils may also be present within the nodule, but the mucosa is otherwise intact. The identity of the Langerhans' cells can be confirmed by positive S100 protein and CD1a immunostains and by electron

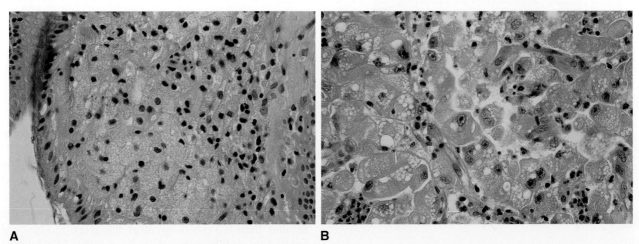

A   **B**

FIGURE 13–24. A, Gastric xanthoma. The mucosa is filled with foamy, lipid-laden macrophages that contain cytologically bland, round, to oval-shaped nuclei without atypia. A mucicarmine stain was negative. **B,** In contrast to **A,** signet ring cell carcinoma shows variably sized mucin-filled cells with a vacuolated appearance and hyperchromatic, atypical, and eccentrically located nuclei with increased mitotic activity. A mucicarmine stain on this tissue was positive.

microscopy showing the characteristic tennis racket–shaped intracytoplasmic Birbeck granules. When present as an isolated gastric nodule, eosinophilic granuloma is typically benign and often regresses without therapy.

GRANULOMAS

Granulomas may occur in the stomach as the result of a number of different causes (see Chapter 5). They occur most frequently in the antrum. Pyloric obstruction may rarely occur as the result of granuloma-associated mucosal thickening.[119] Gastric granulomas may also be associated with systemic granulomatous diseases, including sarcoidosis, Crohn's disease, and, rarely, mycobacterial infection.[120-122] When all apparent causes of granulomatous inflammation have been excluded, a diagnosis of idiopathic granulomatous gastritis may be considered, but this is an uncommon disease. It occurs primarily in older patients and presents clinically as a slowly progressive type of partial gastric outlet obstruction.

AMYLOIDOSIS

Amyloidosis is a heterogeneous group of systemic diseases that is discussed in detail in Chapter 5. When it involves the stomach, amyloidosis may cause ulceration or may form a submucosal nodule or mass. Histologically, amyloid deposits in the stomach are most frequently concentrated in the wall of small to medium-sized blood vessels.[123] Perineural deposits and interstitial deposits may also develop in the submucosa (Fig. 13-25). The condition may be associated with dysmotility, although this complication occurs most frequently in other areas of the gastrointestinal tract. Large interstitial amyloid deposits are often called *amyloidomas*. One group has suggested that AL-type amyloidosis occurs more frequently in the muscularis propria, whereas AA-type

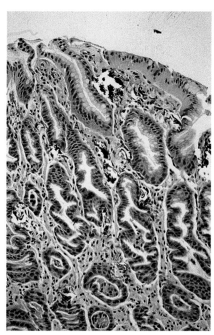

FIGURE 13–26. Gastric antrum shows foveolar hyperplasia, mild chronic inflammation, and heterotopic calcifications in the mucosa as a result of chronic renal failure.

amyloidosis more often involves the lamina propria.[124] Beta$_2$-microglobulin, or dialysis-associated amyloidosis, is most common in patients who have received hemodialysis for 10 or more years.[123] A diagnosis of amyloidosis may be confirmed by the examination of Congo red–stained slides under polarized light.

CALCIUM DEPOSITS

Interstitial calcium deposits within the lamina propria (Fig. 13-26) may rarely give the endoscopic impression of a small white plaque or sessile polyp. These are typically found in patients with end-stage renal disease but may occur in other types of patients as well.[125] The surrounding mucosa may be unremarkable or ulcerated. In the latter case, some have proposed that the ulceration is part of the pathogenesis of the calcium deposits, although direct evidence for this association is lacking.

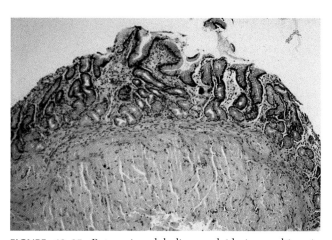

FIGURE 13–25. Beta$_2$-microglobulin amyloidosis resulting in elevation of the mucosa due to a nodular mass of amyloid in the submucosa.

References

1. Ghazi A, Ferstenberg H, Shinya H: Endoscopic gastroduodenal polypectomy. Ann Surg 200:175-180, 1984.
2. Laxen F, Sipponen P, Ihamaki T, et al: Gastric polyps; their morphological and endoscopical characteristics and relation to gastric carcinoma. Acta Pathol Microbiol Immunol Scand [A] 90:221-228, 1982.
3. Rosch W: Epidemiology, pathogenesis, diagnosis and treatment of benign gastric tumours. Front Gastrointest Res 6:167-184, 1980.
4. Varis O, Laxen F, Valle J: *Helicobacter pylori* infection and fasting serum gastrin levels in a series of endoscopically diagnosed gastric polyps. APMIS 102:759-764, 1994.
5. Bonilla Palacios JJ, Miyazaki Y, et al: Serum gastrin, pepsinogens, parietal cell and *Helicobacter pylori* antibodies in patients with gastric polyps. Acta Gastroenterol Latinoam 24:77-82, 1994.

6. Snover DC: Benign epithelial polyps of the stomach. Pathol Annu 20:303-329, 1985.

7. Ming SC: The classification and significance of gastric polyps. Monogr Pathol 18:149-175, 1977.

8. Carneiro F, David L, Seruca R, et al: Hyperplastic polyposis and diffuse carcinoma of the stomach. A study of a family. Cancer 72:323-329, 1993.

9. Abraham SC, Singh VK, Yardley JH, et al: Hyperplastic polyps of the stomach: Associations with histologic patterns of gastritis and gastric atrophy. Am J Surg Pathol 25:500-507, 2001.

10. Ljubicic N, Banic M, Kujundzic M, et al: The effect of eradicating *Helicobacter pylori* infection on the course of adenomatous and hyperplastic gastric polyps. Eur J Gastroenterol Hepatol 11:727-730, 1999.

11. Kamiya T, Morishita T, Asakura H, et al: Long-term follow-up study on gastric adenoma and its relation to gastric protruded carcinoma. Cancer 50:2496-2503, 1982.

12. Orlowska J, Jarosz D, Pachlewski J, et al: Malignant transformation of benign epithelial gastric polyps. Am J Gastroenterol 90:2152-2159, 1995.

13. Zea-Iriarte WL, Sekine I, Itsuno M, et al: Carcinoma in gastric hyperplastic polyps. A phenotypic study. Dig Dis Sci 41:377-386, 1996.

14. Ginsberg GG, Al-Kawas FH, Fleischer DE, et al: Gastric polyps: Relationship of size and histology to cancer risk. Am J Gastroenterol 91:714-717, 1996.

15. Hattori T: Morphological range of hyperplastic polyps and carcinomas arising in hyperplastic polyps of the stomach. J Clin Pathol 38:622-630, 1985.

16. Murakami K, Mitomi H, Yamashita K, et al: p53, but not c-Ki-ras, mutation and down-regulation of p21WAF1/CIP1 and cyclin D1 are associated with malignant transformation in gastric hyperplastic polyps. Am J Clin Pathol 115:224-234, 2001.

17. Koch HK, Lesch R, Cremer M, et al: Polyps and polypoid foveolar hyperplasia in gastric biopsy specimens and their precancerous prevalence. Front Gastrointest Res 4:183-191, 1979.

18. Koga S, Watanabe H, Enjoji M: Stomal polypoid hypertrophic gastritis: A polypoid gastric lesion at gastroenterostomy site. Cancer 43:647-657, 1979.

19. Jablokow VR, Aranha GV, Reyes CV: Gastric stomal polypoid hyperplasia: Report of four cases. J Surg Oncol 19:106-108, 1982.

20. Goldman DS, Appelman HD: Gastric mucosal polyps. Am J Clin Pathol 58:434-444, 1972.

21. Fonde EC, Rodning CB: Gastritis cystica profunda. Am J Gastroenterol 81:459-464, 1986.

22. Franzin G, Novelli P: Gastritis cystica profunda. Histopathology 5:535-547, 1981.

23. Okada M, Iizuka Y, Oh K, et al: Gastritis cystica profunda presenting as giant gastric mucosal folds: The role of endoscopic ultrasonography and mucosectomy in the diagnostic work-up. Gastrointest Endosc 40:640-644, 1994.

24. Jarnum S, Jensen KB: Plasma protein turnover (albumin, transferrin, IgG, IgM) in Menetrier's disease (giant hypertrophic gastritis): Evidence of non-selective protein loss. Gut 13:128-137, 1972.

25. Occena RO, Taylor SF, Robinson CC, et al: Association of cytomegalovirus with Menetrier's disease in childhood: Report of two new cases with a review of literature. J Pediatr Gastroenterol Nutr 17:217-224, 1993.

26. Burns B, Gay BB Jr: Menetrier's disease of the stomach in children. Am J Roentgenol Radium Ther Nucl Med 103:300-306, 1968.

27. Sandberg DH: Hypertrophic gastropathy (Menetrier's disease) in childhood. J Pediatr 78:866-868, 1971.

28. Xiao SY, Hart J: Marked gastric foveolar hyperplasia associated with active cytomegalovirus infection. Am J Gastroenterol 96:223-226, 2001.

29. Bayerdorffer E, Ritter MM, Hatz R, et al: Healing of protein losing hypertrophic gastropathy by eradication of *Helicobacter pylori*—Is *Helicobacter pylori* a pathogenic factor in Menetrier's disease? Gut 35:701-704, 1994.

30. Yeaton P, Frierson HF Jr: Octreotide reduces enteral protein losses in Menetrier's disease. Am J Gastroenterol 88:95-98, 1993.

31. Dempsey PJ, Goldenring JR, Soroka CJ, et al: Possible role of transforming growth factor alpha in the pathogenesis of Menetrier's disease: Supportive evidence from humans and transgenic mice. Gastroenterology 103:1950-1963, 1992.

32. Takagi H, Jhappan C, Sharp R, et al: Hypertrophic gastropathy resembling Menetrier's disease in transgenic mice overexpressing transforming growth factor alpha in the stomach. J Clin Invest 90:1161-1167, 1992.

33. Burdick JS, Chung E, Tanner G, et al: Treatment of Menetrier's disease with a monoclonal antibody against the epidermal growth factor receptor. N Engl J Med 343:1697-1701, 2000.

34. Olmsted WW, Cooper PH, Madewell JE: Involvement of the gastric antrum in Menetrier's disease. Am J Roentgenol 126:524-529, 1976.

35. Scott HW Jr, Shull HJ, Law DH 4th, et al: Surgical management of Menetrier's disease with protein-losing gastropathy. Ann Surg 181:765-767, 1975.

36. Stamm B: Localized hyperplastic gastropathy of the mucous cell- and mixed cell-type (localized Menetrier's disease): A report of 11 patients. Am J Surg Pathol 21:1334-1342, 1997.

37. Stamatakis JD: Menetrier's disease and carcinoma of stomach. Proc R Soc Med 69:264-265, 1976.

38. Wood MG, Bates C, Brown RC, et al: Intramucosal carcinoma of the gastric antrum complicating Menetrier's disease. J Clin Pathol 36:1071-1075, 1983.

39. Covotta A, Paoletti M, Covotta L, et al: Large cystic polyps of the stomach. G Chir 16:107-108, 1995.

40. Marcial MA, Villafana M, Hernandez-Denton J, et al: Fundic gland polyps: Prevalence and clinicopathologic features. Am J Gastroenterol 88:1711-1713, 1993.

41. Choudhry U, Boyce HW Jr, Coppola D: Proton pump inhibitor–associated gastric polyps: A retrospective analysis of their frequency, and endoscopic, histologic, and ultrastructural characteristics. Am J Clin Pathol 110:615-621, 1998.

42. el-Zimaity HM, Jackson FW, Graham DY: Fundic gland polyps developing during omeprazole therapy. Am J Gastroenterol 92:1858-1860, 1997.

43. Watanabe H, Enjoji M, Yao T, et al: Gastric lesions in familial adenomatosis coli: Their incidence and histologic analysis. Hum Pathol 9:269-283, 1978.

44. Burt RW, Berenson MM, Lee RG, et al: Upper gastrointestinal polyps in Gardner's syndrome. Gastroenterology 86:295-301, 1984.

45. Bulow S, Lauritsen KB, Johansen A, et al: Gastroduodenal polyps in familial polyposis coli. Dis Colon Rectum 28:90-93, 1985.

46. Abraham SC, Nobukawa B, Giardiello FM, et al: Fundic gland polyps in familial adenomatous polyposis: Neoplasms with frequent somatic adenomatous polyposis coli gene alterations. Am J Pathol 157:747-754, 2000.

47. Tonelli F, Nardi F, Bechi P, et al: Extracolonic polyps in familial polyposis coli and Gardner's syndrome. Dis Colon Rectum 28:664-668, 1985.

48. Abraham SC, Nobukawa B, Giardiello FM, et al: Sporadic fundic gland polyps: Common gastric polyps arising through activating mutations in the beta-catenin gene. Am J Pathol 158:1005-1010, 2001.

49. Bertoni G, Sassatelli R, Nigrisoli E, et al: Dysplastic changes in gastric fundic gland polyps of patients with familial adenomatous polyposis. Ital J Gastroenterol Hepatol 31:192-197, 1999.

50. Wu TT, Kornacki S, Rashid A, et al: Dysplasia and dysregulation of proliferation in foveolar and surface epithelia of fundic gland polyps from patients with familial adenomatous polyposis. Am J Surg Pathol 22:293-298, 1998.

51. Attard TM, Yardley JH, Cuffari C: Gastric polyps in pediatrics: An 18-year hospital-based analysis. Am J Gastroenterol 97:298-301, 2002.

52. Attard TM, Giardiello FM, Argani P, et al: Fundic gland polyposis with high-grade dysplasia in a child with attenuated familial adenomatous polyposis and familial gastric cancer. J Pediatr Gastroenterol Nutr 32:215-218, 2001.

53. Abraham SC, Montgomery EA, Singh VK, et al: Gastric adenomas: Intestinal-type and gastric-type adenomas differ in the risk of adenocarcinoma and presence of background mucosal pathology. Am J Surg Pathol 26:1276-1285, 2002.

54. Flageole H, Raptis S, Trudel JL, et al: Progression toward malignancy of hamartomas in a patient with Peutz-Jeghers syndrome: Case report and literature review. Can J Surg 37:231-236, 1994.

55. Dodds WJ, Schulte WJ, Hensley GT, et al: Peutz-Jeghers syndrome and gastrointestinal malignancy. Am J Roentgenol Radium Ther Nucl Med 115:374-377, 1972.

56. Lewin KJ, Appelman H: Tumors of the esophagus and stomach. AFIP Atlas of Tumor Pathology Vol 18, 3rd Series, 1996.
57. Wirtzfeld DA, Petrelli NJ, Rodriguez-Bigas MA: Hamartomatous polyposis syndromes: Molecular genetics, neoplastic risk, and surveillance recommendations. Ann Surg Oncol 8:319-327, 2001.
58. Howe JR, Roth S, Ringold JC, et al: Mutations in the SMAD4/DPC4 gene in juvenile polyposis. Science 280:1086-1088, 1998.
59. Houlston R, Bevan S, Williams A, et al: Mutations in DPC4 (SMAD4) cause juvenile polyposis syndrome, but only account for a minority of cases. Hum Mol Genet 7:1907-1912, 1998.
60. Waite KA, Eng C: Protean PTEN: Form and function. Am J Hum Genet 70:829-844, 2002.
61. Sagara K, Fujiyama S, Kamuro Y, et al: Cronkhite-Canada syndrome associated with gastric cancer: Report of a case. Gastroenterol Jpn 18:260-266, 1983.
62. Katayama Y, Kimura M, Konn M: Cronkhite-Canada syndrome associated with a rectal cancer and adenomatous changes in colonic polyps. Am J Surg Pathol 9:65-71, 1985.
63. Rappaport LB, Sperling HV, Stavrides A: Colon cancer in the Cronkhite-Canada syndrome. J Clin Gastroenterol 8:199-202, 1986.
64. Stolte M, Sticht T, Eidt S, et al: Frequency, location, and age and sex distribution of various types of gastric polyp. Endoscopy 26:659-665, 1994.
65. Stachura J, Konturek J, Urbanczyk K, et al: Dispersed and acinar forms of pancreatic metaplasia in human gastric mucosa. Folia Histochem Cytobiol 32:251-255, 1994.
66. Krishnamurthy S, Integlia MJ, Grand RJ, et al: Pancreatic acinar cell clusters in pediatric gastric mucosa. Am J Surg Pathol 22:100-105, 1998.
67. Doglioni C, Laurino L, Dei Tos AP, et al: Pancreatic (acinar) metaplasia of the gastric mucosa. Histology, ultrastructure, immunocytochemistry, and clinicopathologic correlations of 101 cases. Am J Surg Pathol 17:1134-1143, 1993.
68. Wang HH, Zeroogian JM, Spechler SJ, et al: Prevalence and significance of pancreatic acinar metaplasia at the gastroesophageal junction. Am J Surg Pathol 20:1507-1510, 1996.
69. Johnson CD, Bynum TE: Brunner gland heterotopia presenting as gastric antral polyps. Gastrointest Endosc 22:210-211, 1976.
70. Ahnen DJ, Poulsom R, Stamp GW, et al: The ulceration-associated cell lineage (UACL) reiterates the Brunner's gland differentiation programme but acquires the proliferative organization of the gastric gland. J Pathol 173:317-326, 1994.
71. Ming SC, Goldman H: Gastric polyps: A histogenetic classification and its relation to carcinoma. Cancer 18:721-729, 1965.
72. Chua CL: Gastric polyps: The case for polypectomy and endoscopic surveillance. J R Coll Surg Edinb 35:163-165, 1990.
73. Deppisch LM, Rona VT: Gastric epithelial polyps. A 10-year study. J Clin Gastroenterol 11:110-115, 1989.
74. Nakamura T, Nakano G: Histopathological classification and malignant change in gastric polyps. J Clin Pathol 38:754-764, 1985.
75. Torres C, Antonioli D, Odze RD: Polypoid dysplasia and adenomas in inflammatory bowel disease: A clinical, pathologic, and follow-up study of 89 polyps from 59 patients. Am J Surg Pathol 22:275-284, 1998.
76. Itabashi M, Hirota T, Unakami M, et al: The role of the biopsy in diagnosis of early gastric cancer. Jpn J Clin Oncol 14:253-270, 1984.
77. Kim YH, Kim NG, Lim JG, et al: Chromosomal alterations in paired gastric adenomas and carcinomas. Am J Pathol 158:655-662, 2001.
78. Nogueira AM, Carneiro F, Seruca R, et al: Microsatellite instability in hyperplastic and adenomatous polyps of the stomach. Cancer 86:1649-1656, 1999.
79. Lee JH, Abraham SC, Kim HS, et al: Inverse relationship between APC gene mutation in gastric adenomas and development of adenocarcinoma. Am J Pathol 161:611-618, 2002.
80. Watanabe H: Argentaffin cells in adenoma of the stomach. Cancer 30:1267-1274, 1972.
81. Lauwers GY, Riddell RH: Gastric epithelial dysplasia. Gut 45:784-790, 1999.
82. Goldstein NS, Lewin KJ: Gastric epithelial dysplasia and adenoma: Historical review and histological criteria for grading. Hum Pathol 28:127-133, 1997.
83. Lauwers GY, Shimizu M, Correa P, et al: Evaluation of gastric biopsies for neoplasia: Differences between Japanese and Western pathologists. Am J Surg Pathol 23:511-518, 1999.
84. Schlemper RJ, Riddell RH, Kato Y, et al: The Vienna classification of gastrointestinal epithelial neoplasia. Gut 47:251-255, 2000.
85. Rugge M, Correa P, Dixon MF, et al: Gastric dysplasia: The Padova international classification. Am J Surg Pathol 24:167-176, 2000.
86. Park DI, Rhee PL, Kim JE, et al: Risk factors suggesting malignant transformation of gastric adenoma: Univariate and multivariate analysis. Endoscopy 33:501-506, 2001.
87. Solcia E, Fiocca R, Villani L, et al: Hyperplastic, dysplastic, and neoplastic enterochromaffin-like-cell proliferations of the gastric mucosa. Classification and histogenesis. Am J Surg Pathol 19(suppl 1):S1-S7, 1995.
88. Green LK: Hematogenous metastases to the stomach. A review of 67 cases. Cancer 65:1596-1600, 1990.
89. Menuck LS, Amberg JR: Metastatic disease involving the stomach. Am J Dig Dis 20:903-913, 1975.
90. Klausner JM, Skornick Y, Lelcuk S, et al: Acute complications of metastatic melanoma to the gastrointestinal tract. Br J Surg 69:195-196, 1982.
91. Ishikura H, Sato F, Naka A, et al: Inflammatory fibroid polyp of the stomach. Acta Pathol Jpn 36:327-335, 1986.
92. Kolodziejczyk P, Yao T, Tsuneyoshi M: Inflammatory fibroid polyp of the stomach. A special reference to an immunohistochemical profile of 42 cases. Am J Surg Pathol 17:1159-1168, 1993.
93. Kim MK, Higgins J, Cho EY, et al: Expression of CD34, bcl-2, and kit in inflammatory fibroid polyps of the gastrointestinal tract. Appl Immunohistochem Mol Morphol 8:147-153, 2000.
94. Day DL, Sane S, Dehner LP: Inflammatory pseudotumor of the mesentery and small intestine. Pediatr Radiol 16:210-215, 1986.
95. Makhlouf HR, Sobin LH: Inflammatory myofibroblastic tumors (inflammatory pseudotumors) of the gastrointestinal tract: How closely are they related to inflammatory fibroid polyps? Hum Pathol 33:307-315, 2002.
96. Karnak I, Senocak ME, Ciftci AO, et al: Inflammatory myofibroblastic tumor in children: Diagnosis and treatment. J Pediatr Surg 36:908-912, 2001.
97. Biselli R, Ferlini C, Fattorossi A, et al: Inflammatory myofibroblastic tumor (inflammatory pseudotumor): DNA flow cytometric analysis of nine pediatric cases. Cancer 77:778-784, 1996.
98. Riedel BD, Wong RC, Ey EH: Gastric inflammatory myofibroblastic tumor (inflammatory pseudotumor) in infancy: Case report and review of the literature. J Pediatr Gastroenterol Nutr 19:437-443, 1994.
99. Demirkan NC, Akalin T, Yilmaz F, et al: Inflammatory myofibroblastic tumor of small bowel wall in childhood: Report of a case and a review of the literature. Pathol Int 51:47-49, 2001.
100. Griffin CA, Hawkins AL, Dvorak C, et al: Recurrent involvement of 2p23 in inflammatory myofibroblastic tumors. Cancer Res 59:2776-2780, 1999.
101. Amano M, Chihara K, Nakamura N, et al: Myosin II activation promotes neurite retraction during the action of Rho and Rho-kinase. Genes Cells 3:177-188, 1998.
102. Chan JK: Gastrointestinal lymphomas: An overview with emphasis on new findings and diagnostic problems. Semin Diagn Pathol 13:260-296, 1996.
103. Coffin CM, Patel A, Perkins S, et al: ALK1 and p80 expression and chromosomal rearrangements involving 2p23 in inflammatory myofibroblastic tumor. Mod Pathol 14:569-576, 2001.
104. Lawrence B, Perez-Atayde A, Hibbard MK, et al: TPM3-ALK and TPM4-ALK oncogenes in inflammatory myofibroblastic tumors. Am J Pathol 157:377-384, 2000.
105. Stoica GE, Kuo A, Aigner A, et al: Identification of anaplastic lymphoma kinase as a receptor for the growth factor pleiotrophin. J Biol Chem 276:16772-16779, 2001.
106. Cook JR, Dehner LP, Collins MH, et al: Anaplastic lymphoma kinase (ALK) expression in the inflammatory myofibroblastic tumor: A comparative immunohistochemical study. Am J Surg Pathol 25:1364-1371, 2001.
107. Cessna MH, Zhou H, Sanger WG, et al: Expression of ALK1 and p80 in inflammatory myofibroblastic tumor and its mesenchymal mimics: A study of 135 cases. Mod Pathol 15:931-938, 2002.
108. Coffin CM, Watterson J, Priest JR, et al: Extrapulmonary inflammatory myofibroblastic tumor (inflammatory pseudotumor). A clinicopathologic and immunohistochemical study of 84 cases. Am J Surg Pathol 19:859-872, 1995.

109. Hill KA, Gonzalez-Crussi F, Chou PM: Calcifying fibrous pseudo-tumor versus inflammatory myofibroblastic tumor: A histological and immunohistochemical comparison. Mod Pathol 14:784-790, 2001.

110. Pettinato G, Manivel JC, De Rosa N, et al: Inflammatory myofibroblastic tumor (plasma cell granuloma). Clinicopathologic study of 20 cases with immunohistochemical and ultrastructural observations. Am J Clin Pathol 94:538-546, 1990.

111. Ma ZQ, Tanizawa T, Nihei Z, et al: Follicular gastritis associated with *Helicobacter pylori*. J Med Dent Sci 47:39-47, 2000.

112. Torigian DA, Levine MS, Gill NS, et al: Lymphoid hyperplasia of the stomach: Radiographic findings in five adult patients. AJR Am J Roentgenol 177:71-75, 2001.

113. Chen XY, Liu WZ, Shi Y, et al: *Helicobacter pylori* associated gastric diseases and lymphoid tissue hyperplasia in gastric antral mucosa. J Clin Pathol 55:133-137, 2002.

114. Crump M, Gospodarowicz M, Shepherd FA: Lymphoma of the gastrointestinal tract. Semin Oncol 26:324-337, 1999.

115. Isomoto H, Mizuta Y, Inoue K, et al: A close relationship between *Helicobacter pylori* infection and gastric xanthoma. Scand J Gastroenterol 34:346-352, 1999.

116. Javdan P, Pitman ER, Schwartz IS: Gastric xanthelasma: Endoscopic recognition. Gastroenterology 67:1006-1010, 1974.

117. Wada R, Yagihashi S, Konta R, et al: Gastric polyposis caused by multifocal histiocytosis X. Gut 33:994-996, 1992.

118. Hans SS, Hans B, Lee PT, et al: Eosinophilic granulomas of the gastrointestinal tract. Am Surg 43:512-516, 1977.

119. Spinzi G, Meucci G, Radaelli F, et al: Granulomatous gastritis presenting as gastric outlet obstruction: A case report. Ital J Gastroenterol Hepatol 30:410-413, 1998.

120. Wright CL, Riddell RH: Histology of the stomach and duodenum in Crohn's disease. Am J Surg Pathol 22:383-390, 1998.

121. Fireman Z, Sternberg A, Yarchovsky Y, et al: Multiple antral ulcers in gastric sarcoid. J Clin Gastroenterol 24:97-99, 1997.

122. Shapiro JL, Goldblum JR, Petras RE: A clinicopathologic study of 42 patients with granulomatous gastritis. Is there really an "idiopathic" granulomatous gastritis? Am J Surg Pathol 20:462-470, 1996.

123. Jimenez RE, Price DA, Pinkus GS, et al: Development of gastrointestinal beta2-microglobulin amyloidosis correlates with time on dialysis. Am J Surg Pathol 22:729-735, 1998.

124. Yamada M, Hatakeyama S, Tsukagoshi H: Gastrointestinal amyloid deposition in AL (primary or myeloma-associated) and AA (secondary) amyloidosis: Diagnostic value of gastric biopsy. Hum Pathol 16:1206-1211, 1985.

125. Ou Tim L, Hurwitz S, Tuch P: The endoscopic diagnosis of gastric calcification. J Clin Gastroenterol 4:213-215, 1982.

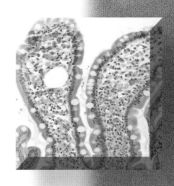

CHAPTER 14

Polyps of the Small Intestine

RHONDA K. YANTISS • DONALD A. ANTONIOLI

Introduction

As a result of the increasing use of minimally invasive endoscopic procedures and advanced techniques in tissue procurement, endoscopic evaluation of the esophagus, stomach, and duodenum has become a mainstay in the management of patients with upper gastrointestinal complaints. In the duodenum, these advances have allowed endoscopists to identify and biopsy a variety of polyps, nodules, excrescences, and subtle abnormalities in the mucosa that had previously been largely unrecognized.[1,2] With the exception of the distal terminal ileum, the remainder of the small intestine is largely unamenable to endoscopic evaluation, so most polypoid lesions of the jejunum and ileum come to clinical attention only when they become symptomatic. The purpose of this chapter is to discuss in terms of their diagnosis and differential diagnosis the important lesions encountered by the surgical pathologist that may cause the clinical impression of a small intestinal polyp (Table 14-1).

Hyperplasia and Heterotopia

BRUNNER'S GLAND HYPERPLASIA

Clinical and Endoscopic Features

Brunner's glands are lobules of tubular and branching glands that are predominantly located in the submucosa of the duodenum, but they may focally extend above the muscularis mucosae into the lamina propria. These glands are composed of neutral mucin-secreting cuboidal to columnar cells with basally located nuclei that are histo-logically indistinguishable from those located in the distal stomach. Occasionally, Brunner's glands extensively involve the lamina propria, creating small polypoid excrescences or imparting a nodular quality to the mucosal surface (Fig. 14-1).[3,4] This phenomenon, called *Brunner's gland hyperplasia*, is most commonly encountered in the duodenal bulb and demonstrates no sex or racial predilection. Although it is usually an incidental finding at endoscopy performed for other indications and has no clinical implications, Brunner's gland hyperplasia may be seen in association with a constellation of other findings (chronic or chronic active duodenitis with incomplete villous shortening, neutrophils, and gastric foveolar cell metaplasia of the villous epithelium) characteristic of peptic duodenitis and has also been associated with end-stage renal disease and uremia.[5-8]

Occasionally, aggregates of hyperplastic Brunner's glands may coalesce to form endoscopically apparent sessile polyps. These lesions are typically small (<1 cm) and clinically insignificant and have been referred to as "Brunner's gland nodules" or "Brunner's gland adenomas."[9-11] Because the biologic nature of these lesions has not been elucidated in the literature and no well-documented cases of either dysplasia or carcinoma arising in this setting have been reported to date, most workers now feel that these lesions represent exuberant Brunner's gland hyperplasia.[9-11] Therefore, we prefer to use the term *Brunner's gland hyperplasia* to describe these lesions because this terminology better reflects the non-neoplastic nature of the entity and diminishes the risk of potential miscommunication between pathologists and clinicians.

TABLE 14-1. Classification of Polypoid Lesions of the Small Intestine

Hyperplasia and heterotopia	Brunner's gland hyperplasia
	Gastric heterotopia
	Pancreatic heterotopia
Inflammatory lesions	Inflammatory polyp NOS ("nodular duodenitis")
	Xanthoma
	Mucosal prolapse polyp
	Crohn's disease–associated inflammatory "pseudopolyp"
	Inflammatory fibroid polyp
Hamartomas	Brunner's gland hamartoma
	Peutz-Jeghers hamartoma
	Juvenile polyp
	Cronkhite-Canada syndrome–associated polyp
	Cowden syndrome–associated polyp
	Other
Benign epithelial neoplasms	Adenoma
Malignant epithelial neoplasms	Adenocarcinoma
Endocrine tumors	Carcinoid tumor
	Somatostatinoma
	Gangliocytic paraganglioma
	Gastrinoma
	Paraganglioma
Mesenchymal tumors	Leiomyoma
	Lipoma
	Hemangioma
	Neurofibroma
	Granular cell tumor
	Ganglioneuroma
	Schwannoma
	Kaposi's sarcoma
	Gastrointestinal stromal tumor
	Leiomyosarcoma
	Other
Lymphoid tumors	Nodular lymphoid hyperplasia
	Diffuse large B-cell lymphoma
	Mantle cell lymphoma (lymphomatoid polyposis)
	Low-grade B-cell lymphoma (follicle center cell, MALT-type, Mediterranean fever)
	T-cell lymphoma (gluten-sensitive enteropathy–associated lymphoma)
Miscellaneous lesions	Endometriosis

Pathologic Features

Brunner's gland hyperplasia is characterized by lobules of glands that are increased in both size and number.[10] These lobules extend from the submucosa into the lamina propria and are separated by thin fibrous septa (Fig. 14-2**A**). Cystically dilated ducts and glands have been reported in Brunner's gland hyperplasia, but this finding is relatively uncommon.[12] The cells constituting the glands are cytologically bland with abundant neutral

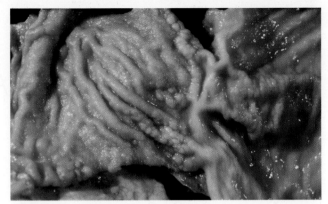

FIGURE 14–1. Brunner's gland hyperplasia. Numerous polypoid excrescences are present within the duodenal bulb, imparting a nodular quality to the mucosal surface.

mucin and small, basally located nuclei with minimal or absent mitotic activity (Fig. 14-2**B**). The diagnosis is straightforward in surgical resection specimens and is a common incidental finding in the duodenum resected for other reasons. However, the diagnostic criteria for Brunner's gland hyperplasia in endoscopically obtained biopsy specimens are somewhat subjective because Brunner's glands may normally be focally present in the lamina propria of the duodenum. At our institutions, we require the presence of lobules of Brunner's glands within the mucosa alone in at least 50% of the length of a biopsy specimen before the diagnosis of hyperplasia is made.

BRUNNER'S GLAND HAMARTOMA

In contrast to Brunner's gland hyperplasia, which usually develops in association with peptic duodenitis, rarely Brunner's glands may grow into a large pedunculated polyp that can produce symptoms of obstruction, intussusception, or melena.[13] These lesions are usually composed of an admixture of fibromuscular and adipose tissue within and surrounding cystically dilated, hyperplastic lobules of Brunner's glands. Based on the combination of mesenchymal and epithelial elements, as well as their large size (>2 cm), many investigators refer to these lesions as *Brunner's gland hamartomas*.[12-14] The distinction between a "hamartoma" and an "adenoma" is also unclear; historically, these terms probably refer to the same entity.

GASTRIC HETEROTOPIA

Congenital rests of gastric mucosa may be seen in many parts of the gastrointestinal tract, including the esophagus, duodenum, small intestine, and Meckel's diverticulum.[15-17] Duodenal gastric heterotopias are most commonly identified in the bulb and are usually incidental, small (<1.5 cm) polypoid nodules that are

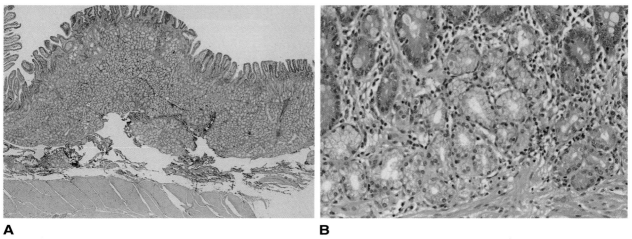

A   **B**

FIGURE 14–2. Brunner's gland hyperplasia. **A,** At low power, lobules of Brunner's glands extend through the muscularis mucosae to fill the lamina propria and are separated by delicate fibrous septa. **B,** High-power examination demonstrates the glands to be composed of cytologically bland, neutral, mucin-containing cells with basal nuclei.

frequently multiple (Fig. 14-3).[18] Gastric heterotopias are benign, non-neoplastic lesions without clinical implications in most instances. However, they may be quite large, causing obstruction or intussusception and rarely may be subject to the same pathologic processes that affect the stomach, such as *Helicobacter pylori* infection.[17,19] Peptic ulceration due to the release of secretions from heterotopic oxyntic glands in the duodenum is rare; it is seen only in cases of extremely large heterotopias because the acidic secretions are quickly diluted by the alkaline duodenal contents derived from the pancreaticobiliary system. However, heterotopic gastric mucosa in Meckel's diverticula may produce peptic ulcerations, which usually occur at the base of the diverticulum. Occasionally, such lesions may present with gastrointestinal bleeding from the ulcer site, particularly if a persistent vitelline artery is present (Fig. 14-4).

Histologically, small intestinal gastric heterotopias contain architecturally normal, tightly packed fundic-type glands composed of chief and parietal cells (Fig. 14-5). Frequently, the intestinal epithelial cells of the overlying surface are replaced by gastric foveolar-type mucinous epithelium, and the adjacent mucosa is usually normal.

Gastric heterotopia should be distinguished from villi containing metaplastic gastric epithelium that may develop in response to long-standing inflammation, such as that seen in chronic duodenitis secondary to peptic injury or Crohn's disease (Table 14-2).[20] In adults, metaplastic foveolar epithelium in the duodenum may be associated with *H. pylori* infection of the stomach.[21,22] The endoscopic appearance is typically that of active injury with mucosal erythema, erosion or ulceration, and loss of the mucosal folds in the proximal duodenum. Duodenal metaplastic gastric epithelium is not associated with oxyntic glands; rather, it consists of columnar cells containing neutral mucin that replace both the absorptive cells and the acid mucin–containing goblet

cells on the villi (Fig. 14-6A). The adjacent duodenal mucosa is abnormal, demonstrating features of chronic or chronic active duodenitis with variable amounts of acute and chronic inflammation in the lamina propria

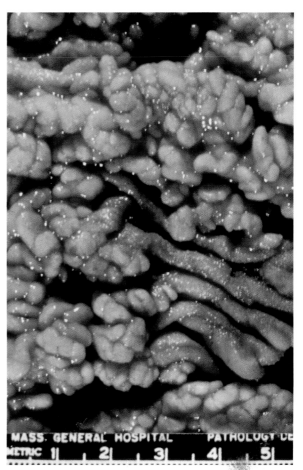

FIGURE 14–3. Gastric heterotopia. Numerous polypoid nodules are present on the mucosal surface and demonstrate a predilection for the duodenal bulb.

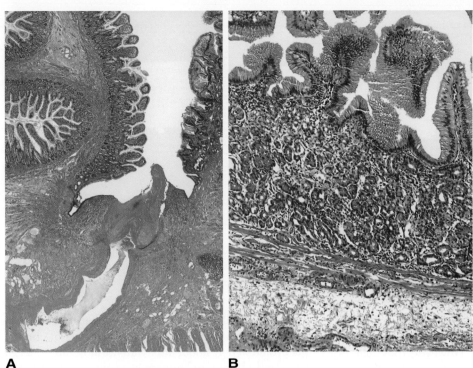

FIGURE 14-4. Meckel's diverticulum with a large ulcer. **A,** A large-caliber artery (vitelline artery) present at the base of an ulcer with an associated intraluminal thrombus. **B,** Acid-producing gastric mucosa is present within the diverticulum adjacent to the ulcer.

A   B

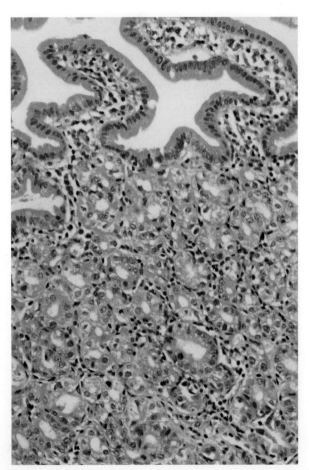

FIGURE 14–5. Gastric heterotopia. Tightly packed aggregates of gastric glands composed of chief and parietal cells fill the lamina propria of the duodenum.

and epithelium, incomplete villous shortening, and regeneration and hyperplasia of the crypts (Fig. 14-6**B**).[5-7] Additionally, Crohn's disease that involves the duodenum or any part of the small intestine may result in pyloric metaplasia of the epithelium; this finding can also be distinguished from heterotopic rests of gastric mucosa by the absence of fundic-type glands.

PANCREATIC HETEROTOPIA

Heterotopic rests of pancreatic tissue are frequently identified in the esophagus, stomach, and duodenum; despite earlier speculation that these lesions resulted from metaplasia in response to chronic injury, they likely represent a congenital abnormality.[23-25] Esophageal rests of pancreatic tissue at the gastroesophageal junction are

TABLE 14-2. Comparison of Gastric Heterotopia and Gastric Metaplasia

	Congenital Rests (Gastric Heterotopia)	Gastric Metaplasia (Foveolar Cell Metaplasia)
Clinical presentation	Usually incidental	Epigastric pain
Endoscopic features	Nodular mucosa	Duodenitis
Microscopic features	Fundic mucosa	Gastric foveolar cells on surface, chronic duodenitis
Clinical implications	None	Chronic duodenitis, *H. pylori* gastritis

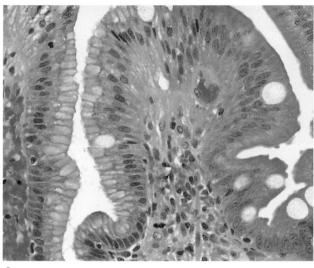

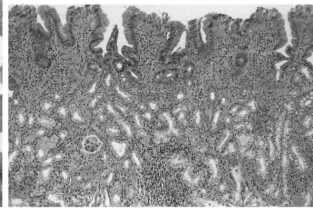

A   **B**

FIGURE 14–6. Chronic duodenitis associated with gastric mucous cell metaplasia. Metaplastic gastric mucous cells are present on the villous surface of the duodenum. **A,** In contrast to the absorptive cells and goblet cells, the metaplastic cells contain small apical vacuoles of faintly eosinophilic neutral mucin, reminiscent of gastric-type foveolar cells. **B,** The adjacent duodenal mucosa demonstrates changes of duodenitis, including Brunner's gland hyperplasia, partial villous shortening, regenerative epithelial changes, and increased inflammation.

endoscopically inapparent, whereas those of the stomach and duodenum characteristically form umbilicated sessile polyps. In the duodenum, heterotopic pancreatic tissue is most commonly located in the periampullary region and may be seen in association other abnormalities, including heterotopic gastric mucosa and Brunner's gland hyperplasia.[26] An association with specific chromosomal abnormalities (trisomies 13 and 18) has also been reported.[27]

Heterotopic pancreatic tissue has a variable gross and microscopic appearance depending on the relative amounts of smooth muscle, fibrous tissue, and acinar or ductal proliferation present. It may present as lobulated tan-yellow nodules indistinguishable from the normal pancreas or as multiloculated cystic lesions (Fig. 14-7).[28] Pancreatic heterotopias are typically composed of admixed lobules of acini, small ductules, and smooth muscle, which are present in variable amounts. Pancreatic islets are seen in one third of cases; however, polyps composed entirely of endocrine cells are uncommon.[29-31] Single lobules of acini are more commonly seen in mucosa-based heterotopias, whereas mural lesions may be histologically indistinguishable from the normal pancreas (Fig. 14-8). In those cases with a minimal or absent acinar component, lesions may entirely comprise large, dilated cysts lined by pancreatic ductal-type cuboidal epithelium associated with a stroma rich in smooth muscle and fibrous tissue (Fig. 14-9**A**).[32-34] The pathogenetic mechanism that underlies the development of this particular form of pancreatic heterotopia is not well understood. Some workers have interpreted these

lesions as simply representing hamartomatous malformations and refer to them as *myoepithelial hamartomas* or *adenomyomas*, but many investigators now feel that they represent an unusual form of chronic pancreatitis involving the heterotopias with progressive ductal dilation secondary to poor drainage of luminal or acinar secretions, resulting in large cysts associated with fibrosis and smooth muscle proliferation (Fig. 14-9**B**).[35]

Unlike gastric heterotopia, which is typically confined to the mucosa, heterotopic pancreatic tissue is frequently found within the duodenal wall, as well as the mucosa. When present in the mucosa, it may form small, inci-

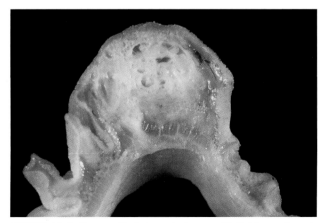

FIGURE 14–7. Pancreatic heteropia (myoepithelial hamartoma). The cut surface is heterogeneous with cystic and solid areas that correspond to cysts lined by biliary-type epithelium enmeshed within a stroma rich in smooth muscle.

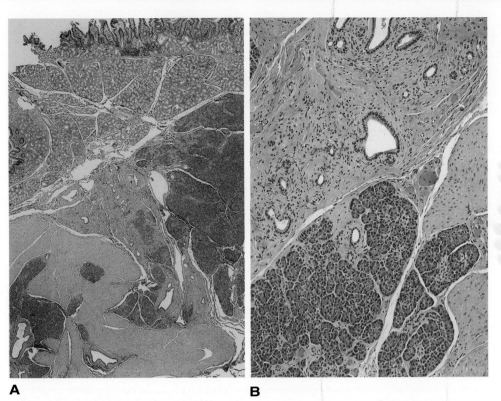

FIGURE 14–8. Pancreatic heterotopia. **A,** Lobules of pancreatic tissue are present within the wall of the duodenum. **B,** The pancreatic acini are indistinguishable from those in the gland proper and are frequently seen in association with dilated ductules.

A   B

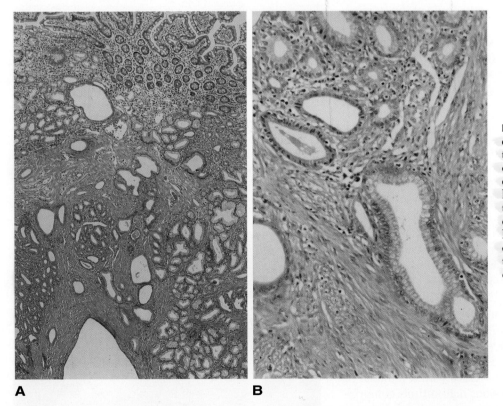

FIGURE 14–9. Pancreatic heterotopia (myoepithelial hamartoma). **A,** Numerous lobules of ductules are present in association with a prominent proliferation of smooth muscle in the submucosa of the duodenum. **B,** The ductules are lined by bland cuboidal and columnar cells containing mucin typical of biliary or pancreatic ductal-type epithelial cells.

A   B

dental polypoid nodules that are of no clinical consequence. However, deeper rests of pancreatic tissue may be associated with marked inflammation and fibrosis secondary to secretions from the pancreatic acini within the heterotopia.[24,36,37] Such lesions are usually symptomatic and may present with gastrointestinal findings, including abdominal pain, gastric outlet obstruction, intussusception, stricture, or bleeding.[38-45] Rare cases of conventional ductal adenocarcinoma arising in pancreatic heterotopias have also been reported.[46-49]

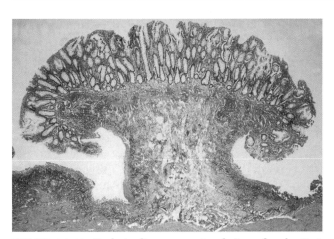

FIGURE 14–10. Crohn's disease–associated "pseudopolyp." A polypoid excrescence of small intestinal mucosa is preserved in an area of the ileum severely affected by active ileitis.

Inflammatory Lesions

A number of non-neoplastic inflammatory lesions may present as polypoid masses in the small intestine, but with the exception of inflammatory "pseudopolyps" associated with Crohn's disease (Fig. 14-10), most are encountered and biopsied during endoscopic evaluation of the duodenum. Lesions such as mucosal prolapse polyps, xanthomas, inflammatory polyps, and inflammatory fibroid polyps have all been reported in this anatomic location (Fig. 14-11).[50-53] These entities do not demonstrate a predilection for the duodenum; most occur more commonly in the remainder of the small intestine, stomach, or colon. Generally, small lesions are discovered incidentally during upper endoscopy performed for other reasons, but large lesions may result in occult blood-positive stool or frank gastrointestinal bleed-

ing. The gross and histologic appearances are indistinguishable from similar lesions found elsewhere in the gastrointestinal tract and are fully discussed in Chapters 12, 13, and 15.

Hamartomas

Most hamartomatous polyps of the small intestine occur in the setting of one of the hamartomatous polyposis syndromes such as Cowden syndrome, Cronkhite-Canada syndrome, Peutz-Jeghers syndrome, or juvenile polyposis; however, they may rarely occur sporadically, in which case they may be extremely large, causing symptoms of intestinal obstruction or intussusception (Fig. 14-12). Hamartomatous polyps of the small intestine represent a heterogeneous group of polypoid lesions characterized by the presence of a variable admixture of epithelial and stromal elements. In some cases, the organization of these elements closely recapitulates that of the normal small intestine (Fig. 14-13), whereas other lesions demonstrate specific histologic and clinical features that aid in their identification. The correct identification and classification of these lesions are critical to the management of the patient in that many polyposis syndromes are associated with the development of gastrointestinal malignancies, as well as extraintestinal manifestations, that may require clinical attention (see Chapters 15 and 19).

PEUTZ-JEGHERS POLYPS

Peutz-Jeghers syndrome is an autosomal dominant hereditary polyposis syndrome resulting from mutations in the *serine threonine kinase (STK) 11* tumor suppressor

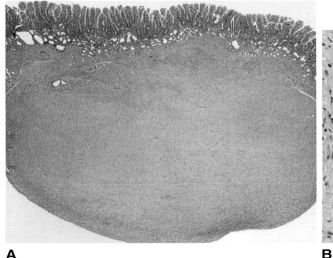

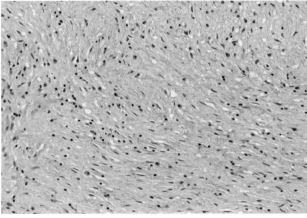

A   **B**

FIGURE 14–11. Inflammatory fibroid polyp of the duodenum. **A,** A well-circumscribed nodule is present in the submucosa of the duodenum. **B,** The tumor is composed of cytologically bland spindle cells enmeshed within a myxoid stroma with prominent eosinophils.

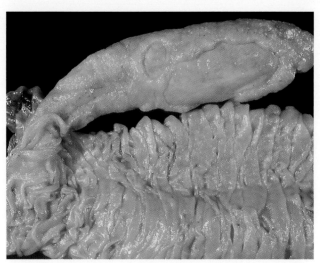

FIGURE 14–12. Hamartoma of the jejunum. A large polypoid lesion lined by ulcerated intestinal mucosa is present within the small intestinal lumen. This patient presented with symptoms of recurrent abdominal pain and occult blood loss.

gene located on chromosome 19p13.3.[54-57] The syndrome is characterized by numerous gastrointestinal hamartomatous polyps, mucocutaneous pigmentation, tumors of the ovary (sex cord–stromal tumor with annular tubules) and testis (large cell–calcifying Sertoli cell tumor), adenoma malignum of the cervix, and an increased risk for the development of breast and pancreatic cancer.[58-64]

Peutz-Jeghers polyps, which are the most common hamartomatous polyps of the small intestine, have a characteristic endoscopic appearance distinct from that

of adenomas. They tend to be irregular, multilobulated lesions that may have a villous appearance but lack the velvety texture typical of adenomas (Fig. 14-14).[4] Histologically, these polyps are composed of an intimate admixture of epithelial elements and smooth muscle fibers that arise from an abnormally prominent muscularis mucosae (Fig. 14-15**A**). The smooth muscle fibers form the cores of arborizing branches lined by intestinal absorptive cells, goblet cells, endocrine cells, and variable numbers of Paneth cells supported by lamina propria tissue (Fig. 14-15**B**).[65] Metaplastic bone formation has also been reported in these polyps.[66] They are frequently associated with mural abnormalities, and up to 10% contain foci of misplaced epithelium within the submucosa, muscularis propria, or subserosa—a phenomenon more frequently encountered in polyps larger than 3 cm in diameter.[67,68] Unlike adenomas with misplaced epithelium, in which epithelial misplacement occurs as a result of mechanical forces, misplaced epithelium in Peutz-Jeghers polyps is likely a developmental phenomenon that reflects the hamartomatous nature of the polyps. As a result, the misplaced epithelium in Peutz-Jeghers polyps is not typically associated with hemosiderin deposits, hemorrhage, or other evidence of trauma. These features, plus the non-neoplastic nature of the epithelium, serve to distinguish this type of polyp from a duodenal adenoma with epithelial misplacement. Furthermore, because the underlying muscularis propria and submucosa are developmentally abnormal in many cases, Peutz-Jeghers polyps are tightly anchored to the underlying bowel wall. Therefore, they rarely undergo auto-

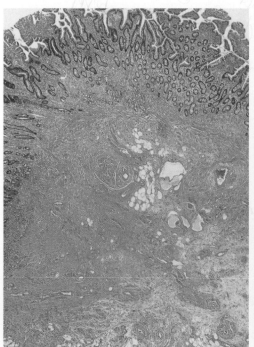

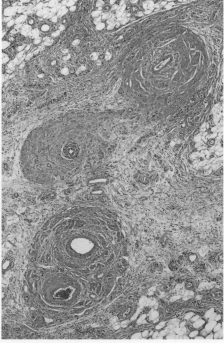

FIGURE 14–13. Hamartoma of the jejunum (case depicted in Fig. 14–12). **A,** The hamartoma is composed of all the normal elements of the mucosa and submucosa, which closely recapitulate those seen in the normal jejunum. However, the villi are haphazardly arranged and the submucosa is fibrotic, containing irregular fascicles of fibromuscular tissue admixed with lobules of mature fat. **B,** Many of the submucosal blood vessels are abnormal and demonstrate irregular and thickened bundles of smooth muscle.

A   **B**

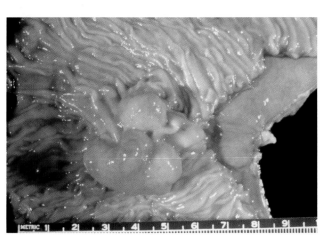

FIGURE 14–14. Peutz-Jeghers polyps of the duodenum. These hamartomatous polyps are endoscopically apparent. They are variable in size and shape and are frequently pedunculated with multinodular, smooth surfaces.

amputation but commonly cause intussusception.[67-71] In fact, recurrent acute abdominal pain secondary to intussusception is the most frequent presenting complaint associated with Peutz-Jeghers polyps.

Although Peutz-Jeghers polyps are classified as hamartomas, patients with the Peutz-Jeghers syndrome are at increased risk for the development of dysplasia and invasive carcinoma in the polyps, as well as in the adjacent mucosa.[61,72-78] Foci of dysplasia and invasive carcinoma are present in 2% to 3% of Peutz-Jeghers polyps and are morphologically similar to those seen in conventional adenomas.[79-81] The diagnosis of invasive adenocarcinoma arising in Peutz-Jeghers polyps may be particularly difficult because these lesions, as noted earlier, are frequently associated with misplaced epithelium deep within the bowel wall. Also, these foci of misplaced epithelium may contain dysplastic epithelium that must be distinguished from invasive adenocarcinoma arising in the polyp. Features that aid in this differential diagnosis include the presence of lamina propria around foci of misplaced epithelium and cytologic and architectural similarities between the misplaced epithelium and the mucosal component of the polyp.[67]

JUVENILE POLYPS

Juvenile polyps of the small intestine are uncommon and usually occur in the setting of extensive involvement of the gastrointestinal tract in patients with a juvenile polyposis syndrome. Their development has been linked to abnormalities in the signaling of transforming growth factor-beta (TGF-β) via genetic alterations in the *SMAD4* gene located on chromosome 18q21.1 or the BMBR1A/ALK3 locus.[82-84] Some workers have suggested a role for a putative tumor suppressor gene located on chromosome 10q22.[85] Like other nonneoplastic polyps at this site, small intestinal juvenile polyps are typically smooth, pedunculated, or sessile mucosal lesions that may be ulcerated and occur

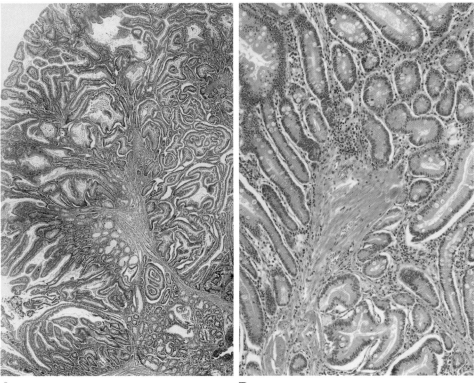

FIGURE 14–15. Peutz-Jeghers polyp of the duodenum. **A,** This polyp is composed of complex, arborizing fronds lined by absorptive cells, goblet cells, and endocrine cells. **B,** On higher power, the stroma is seen to be rich in smooth muscle fibers arising from the muscularis mucosae, which is prominent in these polyps.

A   **B**

primarily in the duodenum. Their histology is diagnostic, featuring cystically dilated glands lined by absorptive, goblet, endocrine, and Paneth cells within a markedly inflamed edematous stroma. They are histologically similar to those seen in the colon (see Chapter 15). Unlike Peutz-Jeghers polyps, juvenile polyps generally lack a prominent smooth muscle component in the stroma.

Because juvenile polyps are usually composed of edematous inflamed loose connective tissue, they tend to be somewhat friable and may ulcerate or undergo autoamputation. As a result, patients typically present with complaints related to bleeding such as occult blood, hematochezia, or anemia. In most instances, polyposis of the small intestine is accompanied by severe disease elsewhere in the gastrointestinal tract, particularly in the colon; therefore, most symptoms reflect disease of the lower gastrointestinal tract. Although the development of dysplasia in juvenile polyps of the colon has been well documented, the rarity of these lesions in the duodenum precludes an adequate assessment of their neoplastic potential in this location.

■ Benign Epithelial Neoplasms

ADENOMAS

Clinical and Endoscopic Features

Adenomas account for approximately 25% of benign neoplasms of the small intestine and have a distinct predilection for the periampullary region.[86] Several investigators have postulated that the periampullary region may be prone to neoplastic transformation because it is chronically irritated by pancreatic juices and bile salts, resulting in long-standing injury to the ampullary mucosa and culminating in epithelial cell dysplasia.[87] Most adenomas occurring in this location are solitary and sporadic; multiple adenomas of the ampulla, periampullary region, and duodenum should prompt suspicion of a hereditary adenomatous polyposis syndrome.[88-90] Patients with small intestinal adenomas usually present between the ages of 30 and 60 years with occult blood-positive stools, luminal obstruction, intussusception, or jaundice secondary to obstruction of the common bile duct.[2] Small adenomas may appear endoscopically as polypoid excrescences or as subtle prominences of the ampulla, whereas larger adenomas, which may be several centimeters in size, appear as velvety flat lesions ("carpet adenomas") that are at significant risk for the development of invasive adenocarcinoma (Fig. 14-16). It is important to note that early adenomas of the ampulla that arise in association with familial adenomatous polyposis may be endoscopically undetectable, similar to the situation one encounters in the colonic mucosa of patients with this syndrome.

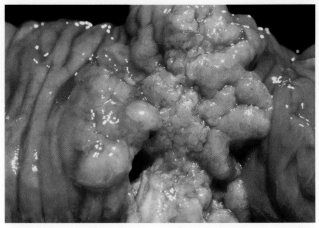

FIGURE 14–16. Villous adenoma of the ampulla. Velvety papillary and polypoid excrescences surround the ampulla.

Pathologic Features

Adenomas of the small intestine are usually sessile and histologically similar to those of the colon. Furthermore, similar to colonic adenomas, small intestinal adenomas that are large (>1 cm) tend to be more villous and contain a higher degree of epithelial cell dysplasia.[91] Approximately 50% of duodenal adenomas have a villous component, consisting of long papillary projections lined by columnar epithelial cells with nuclear stratification. Neoplastic cells are frequently mucin depleted and contain enlarged, hyperchromatic nuclei. Mitotic activity and single necrotic cells are usually present. Notably, numerous Paneth cells and endocrine cells are commonly seen in many small intestinal adenomas.[92]

The criteria for grading dysplasia in small intestinal adenomas are similar to those for colonic adenomas. Low-grade glandular dysplasia is defined as nuclear stratification confined to the lower half of the cells in the absence of complex architectural changes (Fig. 14-17). High-grade glandular dysplasia is characterized by the presence of nuclear stratification involving the entire volume of the cell; severe nuclear changes, including rounded nuclei with irregular contours and open or coarse chromatin and prominent nucleoli; and complex architectural abnormalities such as solid sheets of cells, cribriform spaces, and micropapillary structures (Fig. 14-18). High-grade glandular dysplasia encompasses all of the changes previously called *moderate or severe dysplasia* and *adenocarcinoma in situ*. However, important differences are noted between the colon and the small intestine regarding staging of epithelial neoplasms that infiltrate the lamina propria. In the colon, an adenoma that contains foci of adenocarcinoma that infiltrate but are confined to the lamina propria (intramucosal carcinoma) is staged as an in situ lesion (pTis). In contrast, similar lesions invading the small intestinal mucosa are staged as invasive carcinomas (pT1) because the lamina propria contains extensive lymphatic vessels, whereas

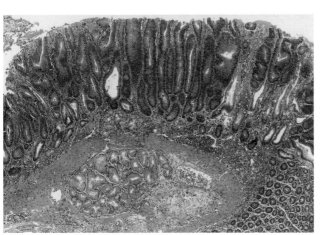

FIGURE 14–17. Ampullary adenoma, low grade. The glands of this adenoma are reminiscent of those seen in colonic adenomas and contain crowded neoplastic cells with enlarged, hyperchromatic nuclei. Adenomatous glands lack severe cytologic or architectural atypia. Periampullary glands are present at the bottom of the field.

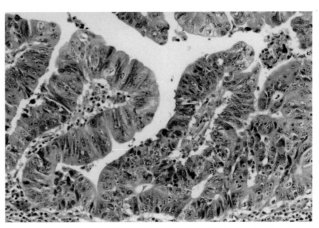

FIGURE 14–18. Ampullary adenoma with high-grade dysplasia/intraepithelial carcinoma. Severe architectural abnormalities, including cribriform glandular spaces, are present. Full-thickness nuclear stratification, single-cell necrosis, and mitotic figures are evident. In contrast to low-grade glandular dysplasia, the cells in this example of high-grade dysplasia contain nuclei with prominent nucleoli, open chromatin, and irregular nuclear membranes.

that of the colon is largely devoid of lymphatic vessels except at the bases of the colonic crypts.[93]

Misplacement of adenomatous epithelium into the submucosa may occur in small intestinal adenoma in a fashion similar to that seen in colonic adenomas; this may cause diagnostic confusion with invasive adenocarcinoma. Helpful distinguishing features of epithelial misplacement include well-circumscribed aggregates of neoplastic epithelium in the submucosa that are cytologically and architecturally similar to the mucosal component of the polyp, the presence of a rim of lamina propria around the misplaced glands, and stromal changes suggestive of mechanical injury such as hemosiderin deposits, fresh hemorrhage, and acellular mucin pools. In addition, the dysplastic epithelium of ampullary adenomas may extend into the underlying ampullary ducts and glands, thereby mimicking invasive adenocarcinoma and resulting in diagnostic confusion (Fig. 14-19**A**). However, in such instances, the lobular architecture of the submucosal glands is maintained, and a desmoplastic stromal response is lacking. Moreover, the adenomatous epithelial cells that involve the ampullary glands are usually morphologically similar to those seen in the surface component of the adenoma (Fig. 14-19**B**).

Risk of Malignancy

Larger adenomas (>4 cm in diameter) and adenomas with high-grade glandular dysplasia are at high risk for invasive adenocarcinoma.[94] In the past, many investigators believed that small intestinal adenomas were more likely than their colonic counterparts to contain foci of invasive carcinoma.[95] However, it appears that much of the literature that suggests a higher malignant potential among small intestinal adenomas likely reflects older data from patients who underwent surgical resection of

symptomatic small intestinal lesions. As a result, many of the tumors evaluated in those studies were large and caused symptoms of biliary or luminal obstruction, gastrointestinal bleeding, and weight loss.

In our institutions, we have noted that endoscopists often encounter and resect numerous smaller, frequently asymptomatic adenomas that are completely benign; thus, in endoscopic series, the malignant potential of small intestinal adenomas may not be as great as was previously reported in surgical series. The available data, however, do suggest that periampullary adenomas present a greater risk for the development of adenocarcinoma than do adenomas elsewhere in the small intestine. For example, Perzin and associates reported that 79% of periampullary adenomas in surgical resection specimens contained foci of invasive adenocarcinoma, compared with 45% of adenomas of comparable size occurring distant from the ampulla.[95] Although the mechanism underlying these apparent differences in biologic behavior is unknown, it is possible that long-term exposure to pancreatic juices, bile salts, or an as yet unrecognized carcinogen, all of which predispose the ampullary mucosa to dysplasia, places the patient at risk for the subsequent development of adenocarcinoma. It is interesting to note that some workers have also identified an association between the occurrence of ampullary adenomas and adenocarcinomas and the presence of pancreatic intraepithelial neoplasia (PanIN) relative to autopsy controls.[96]

As has been noted earlier, adenomas of the duodenum and ampulla are now frequently excised endoscopically, particularly when they are small and confined to the duodenum or ampulla and therefore amenable to local removal or ampullectomy. Given the propensity for these lesions (particularly in the periampullary area) to contain

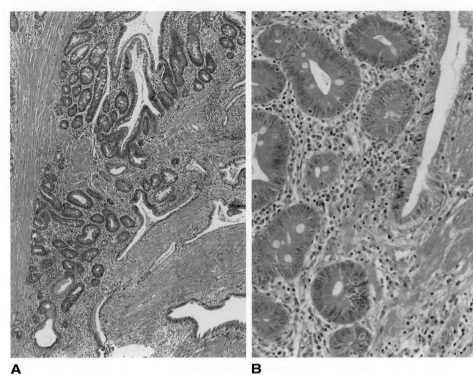

FIGURE 14-19. Ampullary adenoma involving periampullary glands. **A,** Adenomatous epithelium extends into the underlying periampullary glands, which are enmeshed in smooth muscle. **B,** At higher power, an admixture of adenomatous glands and nonneoplastic periampullary glands is seen, associated with a rim of lamina propria.

foci of invasive adenocarcinoma, it is imperative that the surgical pathologist endeavor to ascertain the completeness of the excision whenever possible. Therefore, ampullectomy specimens should be submitted entirely for histologic evaluation, and a definitive statement regarding the adequacy of the surgical margin, as well as the presence or absence of adenocarcinoma, should be made. In those cases that consist entirely of superficial fragments of adenomatous epithelium, the clinician should be made aware that although invasive carcinoma is not present in the specimen, the possibility that the lesion has not been adequately sampled cannot be excluded. Larger adenomas or lesions that are not clearly distinct from the pancreas are not generally amenable to endoscopic resection and thus may require definitive surgical therapy such as a Whipple procedure. In this instance, the lesional tissue should be thoroughly sampled to exclude the possibility of an associated invasive adenocarcinoma.

The evaluation of biopsy or resection specimens of ampullary adenomas may be difficult because many patients present with obstructive jaundice and, as a result, biliary stents have been placed in the common bile duct to relieve the obstruction. These stents cause epithelial injury and erosion of the ductal and periampullary epithelium with concomitant inflammatory, reactive, and regenerative epithelial changes and inflammation of the underlying stroma (Fig. 14-20). This constellation of findings may mimic dysplasia, in situ carcinoma, or even invasive cancer. Therefore, it is imperative that the clinician know the patient's status regarding stenting of the common bile duct so that the specimen can be evaluated properly and the pitfall of overdiagnosing neoplasia can be avoided.

Malignant Epithelial Tumors

ADENOCARCINOMA

Clinical and Endoscopic Features

Small intestinal adenocarcinomas are much less common than adenocarcinomas of the colon. Primary adenocarcinomas of the duodenum account for only 0.3% of gastrointestinal malignancies; however, they account for 50% of adenocarcinomas of the small intestine. A majority of these tumors arise from villous adenomas in the second or third portion of the duodenum near the ampulla; up to 90% of ampullary adenocarcinomas are associated with adenomas. These tumors may arise sporadically or in association with hereditary polyposis syndromes or gluten sensitivity.[88,95,97-104] Owing to their strategic location near the ampulla, these lesions may result in biliary obstruction and jaundice, abdominal pain, or heme-positive stools. They are usually small, polypoid, firm lesions, or they may represent focal areas of induration or ulceration within larger adenomas (Fig. 14-21). In contrast, tumors arising away from the ampulla tend to become symptomatic much later than periampullary lesions and present with intestinal obstruction, pain, anorexia, and gastrointestinal bleeding. These carcinomas are typically large, fungating, or annular masses that obstruct the lumen.[105,106]

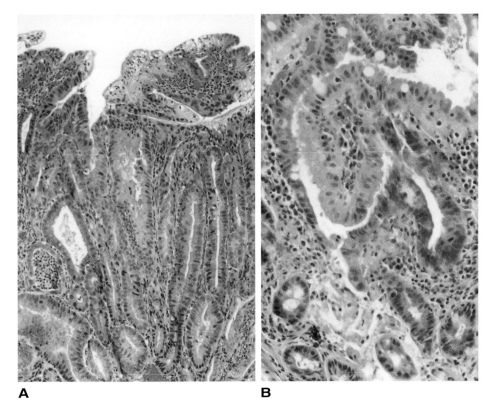

FIGURE 14–20. Regenerative epithelial changes secondary to biliary stenting. **A,** At low power, the duodenal crypts appear crowded and the surface epithelial cells are mucin-depleted. **B,** High-power examination reveals that the duodenal epithelium contains cells harboring enlarged, hyperchromatic nuclei. Numerous mitotic figures are also present.

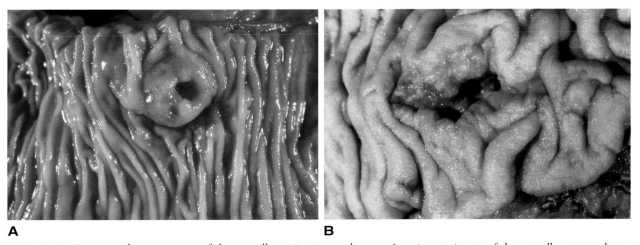

FIGURE 14–21. Invasive adenocarcinoma of the ampulla arising in an adenoma. Invasive carcinoma of the ampulla may produce an indurated polypoid lesion at the ampullary orifice (**A**) or an irregular, ulcerated mass (**B**). Note the presence of thickened duodenal folds indicative of tumor infiltration of the submucosa adjacent to the ulcer (**B**).

Pathologic Features

Adenocarcinomas arising in the small intestinal mucosa may reveal a spectrum of morphologic features. They are typically well to moderately differentiated neoplasms that are morphologically similar to conventional intestinal-type colonic adenocarcinomas in that they are composed of infiltrative glands lined by cytologically malignant cells with enlarged hyperchromatic nuclei, prominent nucleoli, mitotic activity, and frequent single-cell or glandular necrosis (Fig. 14-22). Several morphologic variants of adenocarcinoma may be observed. Well-differentiated carcinoma may assume a villoglandular or papillary architecture, in which case malignant epithelial cells are seen on delicate fibrovascular cores of stroma. Well-differentiated adenocarcinoma may have such bland cytologic and architectural features that, in biopsy specimens, it may easily be confused with adenoma. Appropriate categorization of such well-differentiated tumors requires clinical correlation of

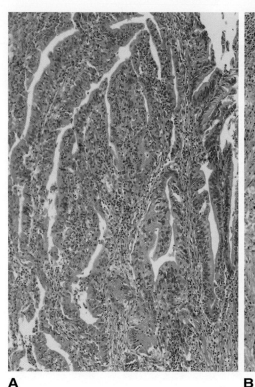

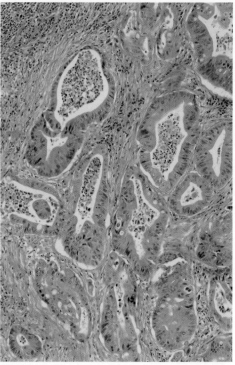

FIGURE 14–22. Invasive adenocarcinoma of the ampulla. **A,** Infiltrating glands are present within the mucosa and submucosa, undermining the noninvasive, adenomatous component of the lesion. The malignant glands contain cells with enlarged, hyperchromatic nuclei and numerous mitotic figures. **B,** Luminal necrosis is also present.

biopsy findings with endoscopic, imaging, and ultrasound studies. Mucinous carcinomas, defined as neoplasms that have mucin lakes containing free-floating malignant cells in clusters that account for more than 50% of the tumor volume, are relatively uncommon. Primary small intestinal undifferentiated carcinomas, choriocarcinomas, small cell carcinomas, mixed adenocarcinomas/endocrine tumors, and signet ring cell carcinomas may also develop but are exceedingly uncommon.[92,107-116]

Ampullary adenocarcinomas arising from the duodenum should be distinguished from adenocarcinomas arising from the biliary epithelium in the region of the ampulla and from ductal carcinomas of the pancreatic head that extend into the duodenum. Such a distinction is clinically important because intestinal-type adenocarcinomas arising in ampullary adenomas tend to have a better prognosis than do pancreaticobiliary adenocarcinomas of this location. Helpful features that suggest a primary duodenal malignancy include epithelial cell dysplasia in the adjacent duodenal mucosa (e.g., remnants of a preexisting adenoma) and the presence of architectural and cytologic features typical of well or moderately differentiated intestinal-type carcinoma. Malignant spindle cells (sarcomatoid carcinoma), squamous differentiation, clear cells, or extremely high-grade cytologic features in the invasive epithelium are uncommon in duodenal adenocarcinomas and are more characteristic of adenocarcinomas of pancreaticobiliary origin. A complete list of the subtypes of invasive adenocarcinoma

encountered in the ampullary region is provided in Table 14-3.

Definitive surgical resection of small intestinal adenocarcinomas is the treatment of choice and the mainstay of therapy.[2] The overall 5-year survival for patients with duodenal adenocarcinoma is less than 20% in most large series; however, patients with periampullary tumors fare better than those with tumors arising elsewhere in the duodenum, with 5-year survival rates ranging up to 52%. This difference in biologic behavior reflects the tendency for periampullary carcinomas to present at a relatively early stage compared with duodenal adenocarcinomas distant from the ampulla. Not surprisingly, the pathologic factors that appear to exert the greatest influence on clinical outcome include local extent of disease, the presence of lymph node metastases, and the grade of differentiation of the tumor.[117,118]

TABLE 14-3. Variants of Adenocarcinoma in the Ampullary Region

Intestinal
Pancreaticobiliary
Poorly differentiated
Signet ring cell
Papillary
Mucinous
Clear cell
Adenocarcinoma with hepatoid features
Adenosquamous carcinoma

Polyposis Syndromes

Virtually all of the hereditary polyposis syndromes may have manifestations in the small intestine (Table 14-4).[54,56-57,65,74-75,83-84,88,89,119-145] Small intestinal and particularly duodenal adenomas in association with familial adenomatous polyposis syndrome, Gardner's syndrome, and Turcot's syndrome are less common than the colonic manifestations of these entities; however, given that many patients now survive for extended periods following prophylactic colectomy, adenomas of the duodenum are encountered in this clinical setting with increasing frequency.[142-144] Adenomas arising in familial adenomatous polyposis demonstrate a predilection for the periampullary region and are usually multifocal. Saurin and colleagues demonstrated that the location of the mutation in the *familial adenomatous*

polyposis (FAP) gene and the age of the patient influence the severity of duodenal polyposis in patients with familial adenomatous polyposis. They found that mutations involving the central portion of the *FAP* gene (codons 279-1309) correlated with increasing numbers of duodenal polyps and with the size of the lesions.[145] Therefore, it appears that different patients with adenomatous polyposis syndromes may be at variable risk for the development of small intestinal neoplasia; this risk is determined in part by the type of mutation noted in the *FAP* gene.

Other workers have also identified progressively enhanced telomerase activity within the non-neoplastic duodenal mucosa, in ampullary adenomas, and in ampullary adenocarcinomas of patients with FAP relative to normal controls.[144] Therefore, increasing levels of telomerase activity may coincide with the stepwise

TABLE 14-4. Clinicopathologic Features of Hereditary Polyposis Syndromes

Syndrome	Inheritance	Genetic Abnormality	Clinical Features	Carcinoma of GI Tract
Familial polyposis coli	Autosomal dominant	FAP gene (tumor suppressor) Chromosome 5q21-22	Adenomas of colon, small intestine, stomach Fundic gland polyps of stomach	Yes
Gardner's syndrome	Autosomal dominant	FAP gene (tumor suppressor) Chromosome 5q21-22	Adenomas of colon, small intestine, stomach, osteoid osteomas of bone, intra-abdominal fibromatosis	Yes
Turcot's syndrome	Autosomal dominant	FAP gene (tumor suppressor) Chromosome 5q21-22 HNPCC mismatch/repair	Adenomas of colon, small intestine, stomach, medulloblastoma (FAP) Glioblastoma multiforme (HNPCC)	Yes
Peutz-Jeghers syndrome	Autosomal dominant	*STK11* (tumor suppressor) Chromosome 19	Hamartomatous polyps of GI tract, sex cord tumor with annular tubules, large cell–calcifying Sertoli cell tumor, adenoma malignum of cervix, breast cancer, mucosal pigmentation	Yes
Juvenile polyposis	Autosomal dominant	*SMAD 4* Chromosome 18q21.1 *BMPR1A* TGF-β signal transduction	Hamartomatous polyps of GI tract, usually colorectal	Yes
Muir-Torre syndrome	Autosomal dominant	Possible mismatch repair genes, *hMLH1, hMLH2*	Adenocarcinoma of the GI tract and gynecologic tract Sebaceous lesions of skin	Yes
Cronkhite-Canada syndrome	No inheritance	Unknown	Inflammatory polyps of GI tract, hair and nail loss, skin hyperpigmentation, protein-losing enteropathy, cachexia	No
Cowden syndrome	Autosomal dominant	Chromosome 10q PTEN gene	Hamartomatous polyps of GI tract, carcinoma of breast and thyroid, gingival hyperplasia	No

FAP, familial adenomatous polyposis; HNPCC, hereditary nonpolyposis colon cancer.

progression of neoplasia in these patients. Of interest, some authors have identified an association between ampullary adenomas and adenocarcinomas and neurofibromatosis type 1.[146] Although hamartomatous polyps may involve the small intestine in hereditary syndromes, the duodenal manifestations of these syndromes (Peutz-Jeghers syndrome, juvenile polyposis syndrome, Cowden syndrome) are much less common than those noted in other parts of the gastrointestinal tract.

Endocrine Tumors

Endocrine tumors throughout the gastrointestinal tract have been called *carcinoid tumors* or *neuroendocrine tumors* to reflect a proposed origin from the neural crest, as well as the morphologic similarities between serotonin-producing neoplasms (true carcinoid tumors) and non–serotonin-producing neoplasms with similar histologic characteristics. However, the postulated origin of these tumors from the neural crest has been refuted, and investigators now believe that these neoplasms are derived from epithelial stem cells rather than from the neural crest.[147] Additionally, the term "carcinoid" is confusing because it has been historically used to describe all neuroendocrine or endocrine neoplasms or hyperplasias, regardless of their anatomic location, morphologic characteristics, or potential for malignant behavior.[148-159]

Recently, other workers have refined its usage to denote a subgroup of epithelial endocrine tumors characterized by serotonin production and to distinguish them from non–serotonin-producing endocrine neoplasms. We regard low-grade epithelial neoplasms with characteristic architectural and cytologic features that suggest endocrine differentiation as "gastrointestinal endocrine tumors" in concordance with the classification scheme currently used to categorize similar tumors in other organ systems such as the pancreas. Such an approach appears to be justified because it has now become clear that distinguishing the different types of endocrine tumors in the gastrointestinal tract has significant clinical implications; many endocrine tumors differ in their biologic behaviors, and they develop only in specific clinical settings (Fig. 14-23).[160-163] Therefore, the pathologist should endeavor to identify any characteristic features that permit accurate classification of these neoplasms.[152]

The gastrointestinal tract is a common location for the development of endocrine tumors. In the small intestine, the greatest proportion of endocrine tumors occur in the ileum, whereas only 2% to 3% occur in the duodenum.[153,164,165] Many small intestinal endocrine tumors form smooth, tan-yellow, submucosal polypoid masses. Incidentally discovered lesions and tumors that become symptomatic secondary to the elaboration of hormones are generally small (<2 cm). Larger lesions may reach several centimeters in diameter and may present with symptoms related to a mass lesion, such as recurrent abdominal pain, painless jaundice, or gastrointestinal bleeding due to ulceration. Serotonin-producing endocrine tumors (true carcinoid tumors) occur for the most part in the distal small intestine and are extremely rare in the duodenum. These lesions, as well as three important types of gastrointestinal endocrine tumors, merit specific mention because they demonstrate a predilection for the duodenum—somatostatinoma, gangliocytic paraganglioma, and gastrinoma.[4] A detailed discussion of other more typical endocrine tumors of the small intestine is provided in Chapter 21.

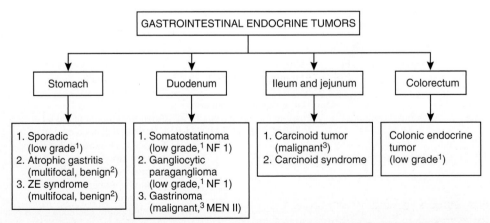

FIGURE 14–23. Diagrammatic representation of classification of gastrointestinal endocrine tumors. [1]Low grade: Usually cured by excision, low risk of metastases, and protracted clinical course despite presence of metastases. [2]Multifocal, benign: Growth hormone–stimulated, usually non-neoplastic proliferation of endocrine cells. [3]Malignant: Significant proportion of tumors associated with regional lymph node or hepatic metastases; despite protracted clinical course, patients may die of disease. ZE, Zollinger-Ellison; NF, neurofibromatosis; MEN, multiple endocrine neoplasia.

CARCINOID TUMOR

Clinical and Endoscopic Features

Ileal endocrine tumors are associated with relatively specific clinical and pathologic features that distinguish them from endocrine tumors that arise elsewhere in the gastrointestinal tract. A large proportion of these tumors elaborate serotonin; therefore, most ileal endocrine tumors are true carcinoid tumors. The presence of metastatic ileal carcinoid tumors in the liver may be heralded by the development of the carcinoid syndrome.[166] Additionally, as a result of the production of serotonin, these tumors are frequently associated with prominent peritumoral or mesenteric fibrosis, which frequently causes symptoms such as recurrent small bowel obstruction and protracted abdominal pain. Approximately one third are associated with synchronous or metachronous malignancies, including gastrointestinal, genitourinary, and gynecologic tract carcinomas.[167-173] Investigators have identified sporadic genetic abnormalities, such as loss of genetic material from chromosomes 18, 11, and 16, and gain of material on chromosomes 4, 17, and 19, in carcinoid tumors; however, no specific unifying genetic alterations have been identified, and the mechanisms underlying their development are largely unknown.[174,175] Unlike some gastric or duodenal endocrine tumors, ileal carcinoid tumors are not associated with hereditary tumor syndromes such as multiple endocrine neoplasia or type 1 neurofibromatosis.[176-178]

Pathologic Features

Ileal carcinoid tumors may have a variable gross appearance, ranging from the presence of polypoid tan-yellow submucosal nodules or annular masses and strictures secondary to the marked degree of fibrosis often characteristic of these lesions (Fig. 14-24). In approximately 20% of cases, the lesions may present as multiple mucosa-based polypoid lesions.[179] The tumors are composed of nests and trabeculae of monotonous epithelial cells arranged in an organoid fashion and enmeshed within a fibrotic stroma (Fig. 14-25). Tumor cells are cytologically bland with abundant amphophilic or faintly eosinophilic cytoplasm, round nuclei with stippled chromatin, and inconspicuous nucleoli. Necrosis, mitotic activity, and severe cytologic atypia are not characteristic of these tumors.

Natural History

Ileal carcinoid tumors generally pursue a more aggressive clinical course than do endocrine tumors that arise elsewhere in the gastrointestinal tract, and they are frequently found to be metastatic to regional lymph nodes or other distant sites at the time of clinical presentation.[149,153,154,157,164,165,179-182] Several pathologic

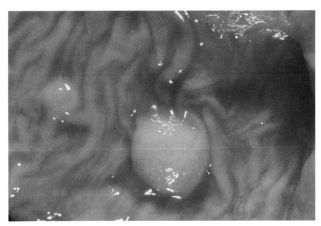

FIGURE 14–24. Carcinoid tumor of the ileum. Carcinoid tumors may form sessile submucosal polypoid masses that are characteristically tan or yellow.

features have been found to be predictive of aggressive clinical behavior. These include depth of tumor invasion, size (>1 cm), regional lymph node metastases, and metastases to the liver.[154,179,183] Other workers have identified several features predictive of aggressive biologic behavior, including female sex, age younger than 50 years, and the presence of the carcinoid syndrome.[179]

SOMATOSTATINOMA

Clinical and Endoscopic Features

Somatostatinomas are gastrointestinal endocrine tumors characterized by the production of somatostatin, a peptide hormone that inhibits secretion of a number of endocrine and exocrine products and diminishes peristaltic contractions in the gallbladder and stom-

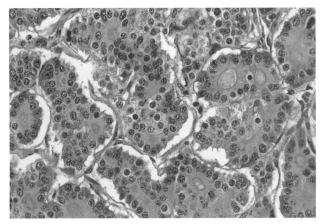

FIGURE 14–25. Carcinoid tumor of the ileum. The tumor is composed of nests, glandular structures, and the trabeculae of cells enmeshed in a loosely fibrotic stroma. The cells are polarized around central lumina and have abundant, faintly eosinophilic cytoplasm and bland, small nuclei with stippled chromatin.

ach.[184] Patients with tumor-related hypersecretion of this hormone suffer from a variety of gastrointestinal complaints such as cholelithiasis (due to suppression of cholecystokinin-pancreozymin release and gallbladder contraction), hyperglycemia (due to inhibition of insulin secretion), and steatorrhea (due to suppressed function of pancreatic enzyme secretion), collectively called the *somatostatinoma syndrome*.[185,186] Somatostatinomas in the pancreas were first described by Larsson and coworkers in 1977; they were later (in 1979) recognized by Kaneka and Murayama as a distinct subtype of duodenal endocrine tumor.[187-189]

Duodenal somatostatinomas are uncommon neoplasms; fewer than 100 cases have been reported in the literature.[190] Several significant clinicopathologic differences between duodenal and pancreatic somatostatinomas have emerged. It is now well established that, in contrast to pancreatic somatostatinomas, a strong association is observed between duodenal somatostatinomas and von Recklinghausen's disease: Approximately 50% of patients with duodenal somatostatinomas have type 1 neurofibromatosis.[161,191-207] Additionally, there is an association between duodenal somatostatinoma and pheochromocytoma in the absence of neurofibromatosis.[161,195,208,209] Other workers have recently suggested a possible association between duodenal somatostatinoma and von Hippel-Lindau disease.[208,210] Moreover, although pancreatic somatostatinomas are associated with elevated serum somatostatin levels (9000 to 13,000 pg/mL; normal, 1 to 12 pg/mL) and with the somatostatinoma syndrome, duodenal tumors do not typically produce marked elevations in circulating hormone levels, and the occurrence of the somatostatinoma syndrome is distinctly uncommon.[185,211]

Pathologic Features

Somatostatinomas have a predilection for the ampulla of Vater, the periampullary region, and the minor papilla; approximately 66% of these tumors occur in these locations (Fig. 14-26).[186,190] As a result, patients with duodenal somatostatinomas typically present with symptoms and signs related to ampullary obstruction, such as bile duct obstruction, abdominal pain, or cholelithiasis.[190,212]

Duodenal somatostatinomas have characteristic morphologic features that aid in their distinction from other endocrine tumors of the duodenum.[189,213] These lesions are composed of nests and trabeculae of cells and acinar structures, lined by polarized cells, with central lumina that frequently contain diastase-resistant proteinaceous secretions (Fig. 14-27). Cytologically, the tumor cells are bland with abundant granular eosinophilic cytoplasm, round smooth nuclei containing stippled chromatin, and small inconspicuous nucleoli (Fig. 14-28). Mitotic activity is minimal and necrosis is generally absent. Slightly more

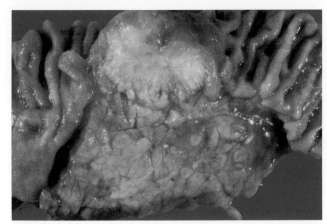

FIGURE 14–26. Periampullary somatostatinoma. The tumor is a relatively well-circumscribed, tan-yellow mass within the submucosa of the periampullary duodenum. The lesion is associated with ulceration of the overlying mucosa.

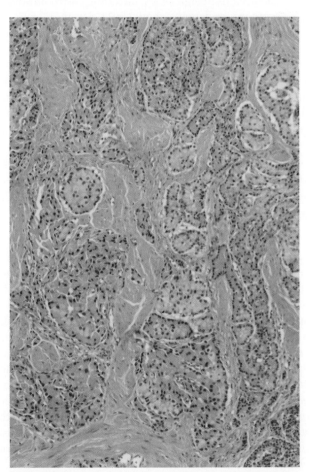

FIGURE 14–27. Periampullary somatostatinoma. The tumor is composed of nests and large aggregates of cells infiltrating the smooth muscle of the sphincter of Oddi. The cells are arranged in glandular structures and are polarized around central lumina.

than two thirds of reported duodenal somatostatinomas contain numerous psammomatous calcifications within the stroma or acini; this feature is helpful to the clinician in correct identification of these lesions (Fig. 14-29).

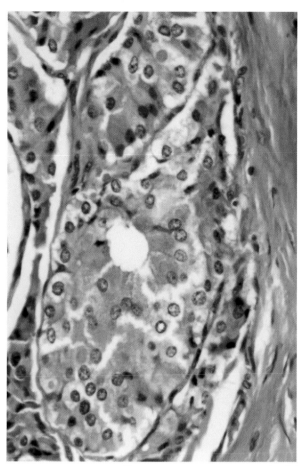

FIGURE 14–28. Periampullary somatostatinoma. A glandular structure is evident in this field. The tumor cells contain abundant eosinophilic cytoplasm and round, bland nuclei with inconspicuous nucleoli.

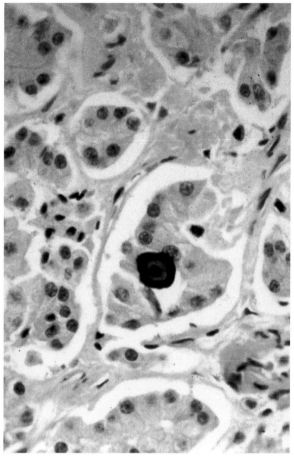

FIGURE 14–29. Periampullary somatostatinoma. Luminal secretions may become inspissated and form dense eosinophilic aggregates or psammomatous calcifications. (Courtesy of Dr. Carolyn C. Compton, Royal Victoria Hospital, Montreal, Canada.)

Psammomatous calcifications are not a feature of pancreatic somatostatinomas.[214,215]

On immunostaining, somatostatinomas demonstrate strong and diffuse cytoplasmic staining for somatostatin and for other endocrine markers such as chromogranin A, neuron-specific enolase, and synaptophysin (Fig. 14-30). Focal positivity for gastrin and calcitonin has been described in nearly 50% of cases,[190] but most tumors do not stain for other peptide hormones such as glucagon, insulin, and serotonin. Despite the presence of glandular structures, these tumors fail to stain for intestinal mucins. Duodenal somatostatinomas are frequently negative for the Grimelius silver stain; modified silver stains (e.g., Hellstrom-Hellman technique, Sevier-Munger method) are required to demonstrate argyrophilic cytoplasmic granules in most instances.[4] However, in the modern era, these stains have been largely replaced by immunohistochemical techniques.

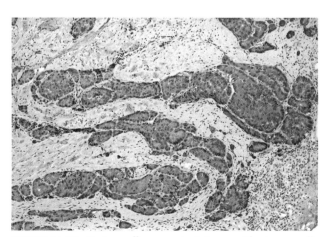

FIGURE 14–30. Periampullary somatostatinoma. The tumor cells demonstrate strong immunohistochemical staining for somatostatin. Notably, these tumors also frequently demonstrate cytoplasmic staining for gastrin.

Natural History

Because duodenal somatostatinomas are uncommon neoplasms, their natural history is not well understood. Many investigators initially believed that these tumors behaved in a benign fashion. However, rare tumors may be clinically aggressive and metastasize. Metastases to regional lymph nodes and the liver are most common, and the risk of metastasis appears to be related to tumor size.[190] Tumors smaller than 2 cm in greatest dimension have a relatively low metastatic potential, whereas those larger than 2 cm in diameter are at risk for associated metastases. These tumors usually pursue a relatively protracted clinical course similar to other gastrointestinal endocrine tumors, despite the presence of metastases.[190,216] Unfortunately, because duodenal somatostatinomas are uncommon neoplasms, data regarding the malignant potential of these lesions are limited. Much of the literature is anecdotal and consists of small series; no large series with long-term clinical follow-up are currently available to address this issue.

GANGLIOCYTIC PARAGANGLIOMA

Clinical and Endoscopic Features

Gangliocytic paragangliomas are rare tumors that demonstrate epithelioid cell, spindle cell, and ganglion cell differentiation. Although endocrine cells may be present, these tumors are typically nonfunctional and present with symptoms secondary to a mass effect. Mucosal erosion with subsequent gastrointestinal bleeding is common; however, these tumors may also cause obstructive jaundice or recurrent abdominal pain.

Gangliocytic paragangliomas demonstrate a predilection for the duodenum and usually involve the second portion, particularly the periampullary region. Endoscopically, these lesions appear as polypoid, largely submucosal nodules ranging from 2 to 4 cm in largest dimension. They usually occur during middle age (mean age, 56 years) but have been reported to occur in younger individuals as well; they have a predilection for males.[217-221] Like somatostatinomas, gangliocytic paragangliomas are associated with type 1 neurofibromatosis.[222]

Pathologic Features

As has been noted earlier, gangliocytic paragangliomas exhibit multidirectional differentiation and are composed of several cell types, including endocrine cells, epithelioid paraganglioma–like cells, spindle cells, and ganglion cells (Fig. 14-31).[223] The endocrine cells are typically arranged in anastomosing cords and trabeculae of small monotonous cells with round nuclei, stippled chromatin, and small nucleoli (Fig. 14-32). These tumor cells stain for neuron-specific enolase, chromogranin A, and somato-

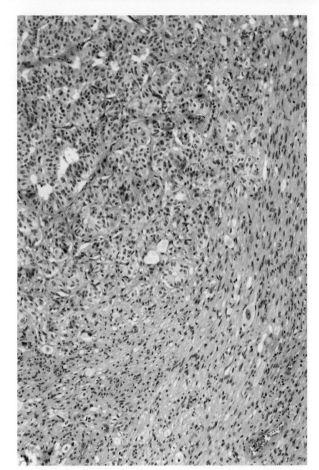

FIGURE 14–31. Gangliocytic paraganglioma. These tumors are composed of an admixture of several different types of cells, including spindle cells *(left)*, epithelioid endocrine cells *(upper right)*, and ganglion cells.

statin and may also demonstrate staining for pancreatic polypeptide, vasoactive intestinal peptide, and other endocrine-associated peptide hormones.[224,225] Other areas of these tumors are reminiscent of a paraganglioma in that they are composed of round nests of nonpolarized polygonal cells enmeshed in a richly vascularized stroma and surrounded by sustentacular cells (Fig. 14-33). These polygonal cells have abundant clear cytoplasm and round nuclei with stippled chromatin and small nucleoli; immunohistochemically, they stain for neurofilament, chromogranin A, and neuron-specific enolase. Spindle cells of gangliocytic paragangliomas are typically long with tapering, faintly eosinophilic cytoplasm, contain elongate nuclei with inconspicuous nucleoli, show minimal or absent mitotic activity, and stain for neurofilament, S100 protein, and neuron-specific enolase (Fig. 14-34; see also Fig. 14-32). Ganglion cells have abundant eosinophilic cytoplasm, large eccentric nuclei, and prominent nucleoli, and they stain for neurofilament, neuron-specific enolase, leu-enkephalin, and occasionally peptide hormones such as pancreatic polypeptide and somatostatin (Fig. 14-35).

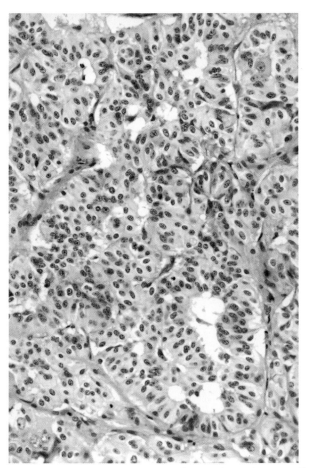

FIGURE 14–32. Gangliocytic paraganglioma. The endocrine cells are arranged in trabeculae, cords, and tubules. The cells have abundant clear cytoplasm and round nuclei with inconspicuous nucleoli.

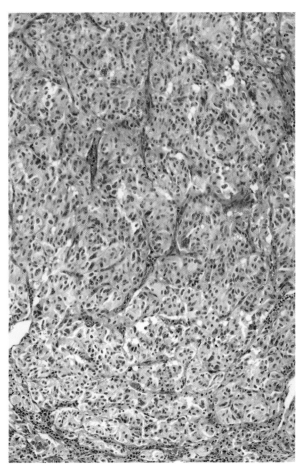

FIGURE 14–33. Gangliocytic paraganglioma. Epithelioid cells arranged in aggregates and nests and associated with a rich capillary network are frequently seen and are reminiscent of the cells seen in conventional paraganglioma. The cells have abundant clear to amphophilic cytoplasm; round, bland nuclei; and frequent degenerative-type nuclear atypia.

The mechanism by which gangliocytic paragangliomas develop is not well understood. Based on their morphologic, immunohistochemical, and ultrastructural characteristics, most investigators believe that these lesions are derived at least in part from progenitor cells of the neural crest.[225,226] The association between von Recklinghausen's disease and gangliocytic paragangliomas is of particular interest because this tumor syndrome is also closely associated with pheochromocytomas, which arise from cells also derived from the neural crest. Further investigations into the role of neurofibromin, the gene product altered in type 1 neurofibromatosis, may offer a unifying hypothesis regarding the development of gangliocytic paragangliomas and pheochromocytomas that arise sporadically and in the setting of von Recklinghausen's disease.

Natural History

A majority of gangliocytic paragangliomas behave in a clinically benign fashion[221]; however, a few reports indicate that rare tumors may metastasize to regional lymph nodes.[227,228] To our knowledge, none of the reported cases of metastatic gangliocytic paraganglioma has resulted in death of the patient. Therefore, a conservative management approach to these tumors is appropriate. Smaller lesions may be adequately treated with snare polypectomy or ampullectomy, but larger lesions of the ampulla may not be amenable to such techniques and thus require surgical intervention.[221]

GASTRINOMA

Clinical and Endoscopic Features

Gastrinomas are gastrin-producing endocrine tumors of the gastrointestinal tract that occur exclusively in the pancreaticoduodenal region. Approximately 50% of gastrin-producing endocrine tumors occur in the pancreas, whereas the remainder develop in the duodenum. Although some gastrinomas reportedly arise in lymph nodes of the pancreaticoduodenal region (gas-

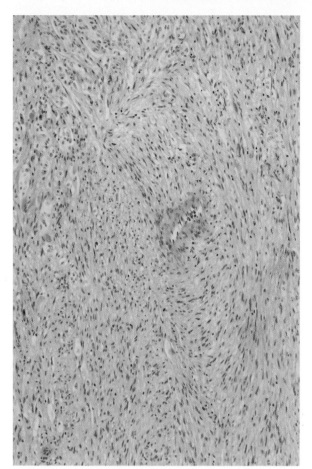

FIGURE 14–34. Gangliocytic paraganglioma. The spindle cells are arranged in intersecting fascicles and contain abundant eosinophilic cytoplasm and elongated nuclei, reminiscent of Schwann cells.

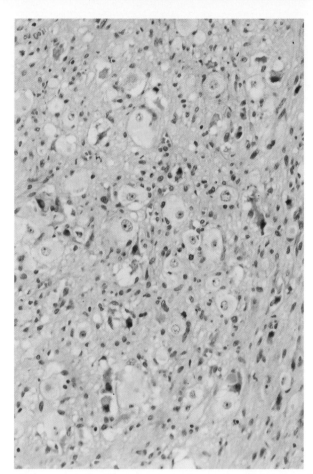

FIGURE 14–35. Gangliocytic paraganglioma. Ganglion cells with abundant eosinophilic cytoplasm, round nuclei, and prominent nucleoli are characteristically interspersed with numerous spindle cells.

trinoma triangle), these lesions most likely represent metastases from undetected lesions within the viscera because investigators have reported lymph node metastases in gastrinomas that range from 2 to 6 mm in diameter.[229-231] In most instances, gastrinomas are functional, resulting in hypergastrinemia and the Zollinger-Ellison syndrome, characterized by multiple duodenal peptic ulcers, prominent gastric rugal folds secondary to an increase in fundic gland mass, and steatorrhea.[232] Most duodenal and pancreatic gastrinomas are sporadic; however, approximately 25% occur in the setting of multiple endocrine neoplasia type 1 (MEN I), in which case they are frequently multifocal.[233]

In contrast to somatostatinomas and gangliocytic paragangliomas, duodenal gastrinomas are typically located in the first or second portion of the duodenum and are uncommonly found in the ampullary region.[234] Most duodenal gastrinomas are small (<2.0 cm) and present with symptoms related to gastrin hypersecretion rather than a mass effect. However, when endoscopically visible, these lesions appear as small umbilicated or ulcerated polyps.[235]

Pathologic Features

Gastrinomas are cellular tumors composed of anastomosing cords, trabeculae, and tubules or glands lined by monotonous cells with eosinophilic cytoplasm and round nuclei containing stippled chromatin and inconspicuous nucleoli (Fig. 14-36). Cells typically harbor perinuclear whorls of filaments that stain strongly for gastrin (Fig. 14-37). Tumor cells also demonstrate staining for endocrine markers such as synaptophysin, chromogranin A, and neuron-specific enolase. Occasionally, gastrinomas may show focal staining for other peptides such as serotonin.

The frequent association between MEN I syndrome and gastrinoma has led many investigators to evaluate the status of the MEN I gene in cases of sporadic gastrinoma. The function of the MEN I gene, located on chromosome 11q13, is currently unknown, but it likely encodes a tumor suppressor gene that serves to regulate the transcription factor JunD.[175,236] Sporadic gastrinomas have also been found to harbor mutations in the MEN I gene in 27% to 37% of cases.[176-178,237-239]

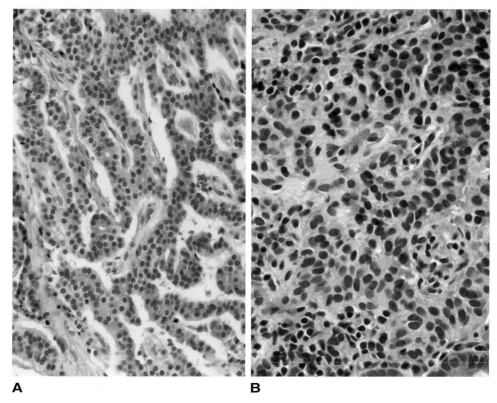

FIGURE 14–36. Duodenal gastrinoma. The tumor is composed of interanastomosing cords and trabeculae of cells with eosinophilic cytoplasm (**A**). The tumor cells are cytologically bland, containing round nuclei with inconspicuous nucleoli (**B**).

A   B

Additional genetic defects such as deletions of the tumor suppressor gene *p16/MTS1*, amplification of either the HER-2/*neu* proto-oncogene (chromosome 17) or chromosome 9q, and deletions of chromosomes 1 and 3p have also been identified in gastrinomas.[240-245]

Natural History

It is important that we distinguish duodenal gastrinomas from other types of gastrointestinal endocrine tumors because this diagnosis has significant clinical implications. In addition to an association between duodenal gastrinomas and the MEN I syndrome, a relatively large proportion of these neoplasms behave in a clinically malignant fashion. Thirty percent to 70% of these tumors metastasize to regional lymph nodes or the liver despite their relatively small size, and most series demonstrate lower than 50% 5-year survival rates.[153,246,247]

■ Mesenchymal Tumors

A variety of benign and malignant mesenchymal tumors in the small intestine, including leiomyomas, lipomas, hemangiomas, neurofibromas, granular cell tumors, ganglioneuromas, schwannomas, Kaposi's sarcoma, and gastrointestinal stromal tumors, have been described, presenting as incidentally discovered polypoid lesions during endoscopy or causing gastrointestinal bleeding due to ulceration or obstructive symptoms due to a strategic anatomic location near the ampulla (Figs. 14-38 and 14-39).[248-254] Most reported cases of duodenal leiomyoma, schwannoma, and neurofibroma in the older literature probably represent gastrointestinal stromal tumors because true smooth muscle and nerve sheath tumors are extremely rare in the duodenum and are more likely to occur elsewhere in the gastrointestinal tract, particularly the

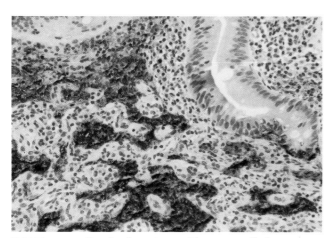

FIGURE 14–37. Duodenal gastrinoma. The tumor cells demonstrate strong cytoplasmic staining for gastrin. They frequently stain for other endocrine markers such as chromogranin, neuron-specific enolase, and synaptophysin as well.

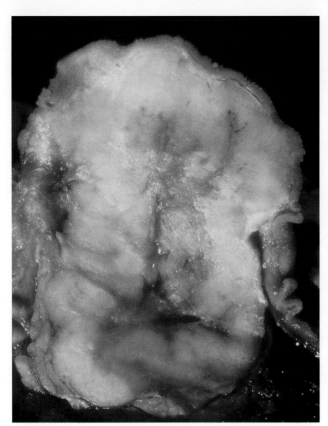

FIGURE 14–38. Gastrointestinal stromal tumor of the ampulla. The tumor is a well-circumscribed, tan, fleshy mass that undermines the duodenal mucosa and infiltrates the duodenal wall. This patient presented with symptoms related to obstruction of the common bile duct.

esophagus, stomach, or colon.[255-257] Histologic features of these tumors are similar to those of lesions occurring in the somatic tissues or elsewhere in the gastrointestinal tract. A complete enumeration of clinical and pathologic features of these tumors is presented in Chapter 22.

Lymphoid Lesions

BENIGN LYMPHOID HYPERPLASIA

The lamina propria of the small intestine normally contains a mild chronic inflammatory infiltrate composed predominantly of mature lymphocytes and scattered plasma cells. In the terminal ileum, nodular aggregates of lymphocytes characteristic of Peyer's patches are a normal finding, and these lymphoid aggregates are composed of mature B and T cells present in the mucosa and submucosa, occasionally in association with germinal centers and lymphoid follicles. The adjacent crypt epithelium and surface enterocytes overlying the Peyer's patches may be infiltrated by mononuclear cells, but this finding should not be interpreted to represent enteritis. Reactive lymphoid hyperplasia in the distal ileum may occur in association with a variety of inflammatory disorders, including several infections (*Salmonella, Yersinia, Mycobacterium*), as well as immune-mediated injury to the small intestine such as that seen in idiopathic inflammatory bowel disease.

Prominent lymphoid nodules may be seen in duodenal biopsies from children, in whom they are usually benign and clinically inconsequential and regress spontaneously over time. However, numerous lymphoid nodules associated with an increased mononuclear cell infiltrate throughout the lamina propria in biopsy specimens taken from adults are usually a pathologic finding.[258]

Increased mononuclear cell inflammation associated with nodular lymphoid hyperplasia may be endoscopically visible as small nodules or polyps on the mucosal surface and can be seen in chronic duodenitis due to peptic disease, celiac disease, or Crohn's disease. In such instances, increased mononuclear cells are frequently present in the overlying epithelium as well and may be asso-

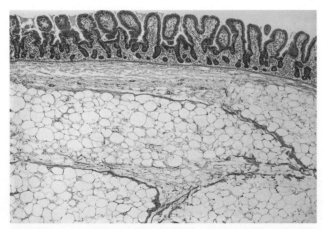

FIGURE 14–39. Lipoma of the duodenum. Mature adipose tissue is present throughout the submucosa, resulting in the formation of a polypoid lesion.

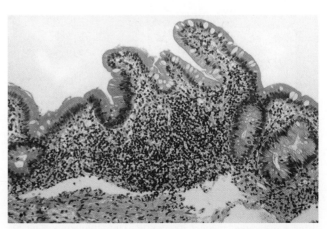

FIGURE 14–40. Reactive lymphoid hyperplasia of the duodenum. Lymphoid aggregates are present within the mucosa of this patient with common variable immunodeficiency (CVID).

ciated with other epithelial changes suggestive of chronic injury such as partial villous shortening, regeneration and hyperplasia of the crypts, and gastric mucus cell metaplasia.

Nodular lymphoid hyperplasia in adults has been associated with deficiencies in humoral immunity, such as selective IgA deficiency and common variable immunodeficiency (CVID), as well as HIV infection (Fig. 14-40).[258-261] Patients with immunoglobulin deficiencies have reduced serum levels of circulating IgA (IgA deficiency) or of IgG, IgM, and IgA (CVID) and are usually young adults (mean age, 30 years). Presenting symptoms range from mild gastrointestinal distress (IgA deficiency) to severe malabsorption and diarrhea, as well as recurrent bacterial infections such as purulent sinusitis, bronchitis, and pneumonia (CVID).[260] The histologic changes are reminiscent of chronic duodenitis and include a prominent mononuclear cell inflammation of the lamina propria, lymphoid nodules, and architectural distortion of the villi. Close examination of biopsy material taken from patients with CVID also reveals the conspicuous absence of plasma cells from the inflammatory infiltrate, a feature that is not seen in other forms of chronic duodenitis. Many patients with IgA deficiency or CVID are also infected with *Giardia lamblia* at the time of diagnosis.[260]

Nodular lymphoid hyperplasia in the absence of an identifiable humoral immunodeficiency has also been directly associated with *Giardia* infection.[261-263] Such patients usually present with complaints of severe diarrhea but have normal serum levels of immunoglobulins. Mucosal biopsies demonstrate lymphoid nodules that are increased in size and number; normal numbers of plasma cells are present. Eradicating *Giardia* from the gastrointestinal tract results in the resolution of gastrointestinal symptoms; however, its effect on the lymphoid hyperplasia is unclear. Some investigators have reported that lymphoid nodules persist despite antibiotic therapy, whereas others suggest that lymphoid hyperplasia regresses following successful treatment of giardiasis.[260,261,263] The association between nodular lymphoid hyperplasia of the duodenum and chronic giardiasis raises the possibility that nodular lymphoid hyperplasia may develop in response to protracted antigenic stimulation resulting from chronic or recurrent giardiasis.[258]

Evidence suggests that nodular lymphoid hyperplasia may represent a premalignant condition, predisposing patients to the development of intestinal lymphomas.[264,265] Although a statistically significant association between nodular lymphoid hyperplasia and lymphoma is lacking, it is interesting that intestinal lymphomas from both immunocompromised and immunocompetent patients frequently demonstrate nodular lymphoid hyperplasia in the adjacent mucosa.[264-267] In such cases, gradual transitions between apparently benign lymphoid tissue and malignant nodules are usually apparent.

Clonality studies have demonstrated monoclonal populations of lymphocytes within morphologically benign lymphoid nodules adjacent to lymphomas and the absence of these cell populations in lymphoid nodules distant from the tumor, indicating that peritumoral lymphoid nodules represent an intermediate stage in the development of lymphoma.[265] Therefore, although the relationship between nodular lymphoid hyperplasia and gastrointestinal lymphoma is not entirely clear, evidence suggests that the presence of persistent nodular lymphoid hyperplasia should raise concerns regarding the development of a lymphoproliferative disorder or malignant lymphoma.

MALIGNANT LYMPHOMA

Lymphomatoid Polyposis

A detailed discussion of hematopoietic malignancies is presented in Chapter 23. However, one unusual form of gastrointestinal lymphoma that merits specific mention is lymphomatoid polyposis. In the small intestine and the colon, lymphomatous polyposis usually occurs as a manifestation of mantle cell lymphoma within the small intestine and colon.[268-270] Patients may present with a variety of complaints, including abdominal pain, obstruction, weight loss, or gastrointestinal bleeding. The endoscopic features of the disease are striking: The mucosal folds are frequently effaced by the presence of innumerable polypoid excrescences, which may appear to carpet the entire mucosal surface, thereby mimicking other disorders such as polyposis syndromes (Fig. 14-41**A**). Histologically, these polyps are composed of nodules of malignant B cells that demonstrate characteristic morphologic and immunophenotypic features (Fig. 14-41**B** and **C**).

Summary

A variety of non-neoplastic and neoplastic lesions may present as clinically apparent polyps of the small intestine, but particularly the duodenum. Although most polypoid lesions of the duodenum are incidental findings encountered at endoscopy, some have important clinical implications. Specific tumors are associated with clinical syndromes that have significant implications for patients and their families, whereas others are premalignant lesions. Therefore, the surgical pathologist should make every effort to correlate the histologic findings observed in the specimen with the clinical impression of a polypoid lesion of the duodenum.

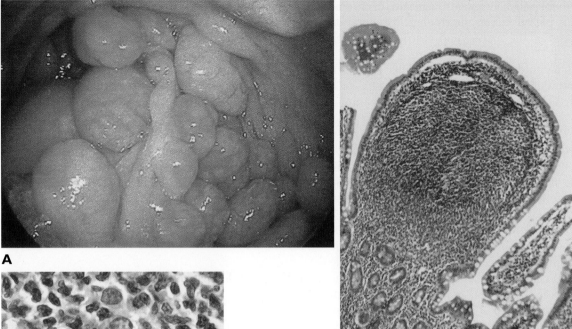

FIGURE 14–41. Lymphomatous polyposis of the duodenum due to mantle cell lymphoma. Innumerable polypoid masses that protrude into the lumen are evident (**A**). Histologically, the polyps are composed of large aggregates of malignant lymphocytes (**B** and **C**). (Courtesy of Dr. Harvey Goldman, Beth Israel Deaconess Medical Center, Boston, Massachusetts.)

References

1. Jepsen JM, Persson M, Jakobsen NO, et al: Prospective study of prevalence and endoscopic and histopathologic characteristics of duodenal polyps in patients submitted to upper endoscopy. Scand J Gastroenterol 29:483-487, 1994.
2. Kim MH, Lee SK, Seo DW, et al: Tumors of the major duodenal papilla. Gastrointest Endosc 54:609-620, 2001.
3. Maratka Z, Kocianova J, Kudrmann J, et al: Hyperplasia of Brunner's glands. Radiology, endoscopy and biopsy findings in 11 cases of diffuse, nodular and adenomatous form. Acta Hepatogastroenterol (Stuttg) 26:64-69, 1979.
4. Attanoos R, Williams GT: Epithelial and neuroendocrine tumors of the duodenum. Semin Diagn Pathol 8:149-162, 1991.
5. Fitzgibbons PL, Dooley CP, Cohen H, et al: Prevalence of gastric metaplasia, inflammation, and Campylobacter pylori in the duodenum of members of a normal population. Am J Clin Pathol 90:711-714, 1988.
6. Shousha S, Parkins RA, Bull TB: Chronic duodenitis with gastric metaplasia: Electron microscopic study including comparison with normal. Histopathology 7:873-885, 1983.
7. Shousha S, Spiller RC, Parkins RA: The endoscopically abnormal duodenum in patients with dyspepsia: Biopsy findings in 60 cases. Histopathology 7:23-34, 1983.
8. Paimela H, Tallgren LG, Stenman S, et al: Multiple duodenal polyps in uraemia: A little known clinical entity. Gut 25:259-263, 1984.
9. deSilva S, Chandrasoma P: Giant duodenal hamartoma consisting mainly of Brunner's glands. Am J Surg 133:240-243, 1977.
10. Franzin G, Musola R, Ghidini O, et al: Nodular hyperplasia of Brunner's glands. Gastrointest Endosc 31:374-378, 1985.
11. Levine JA, Burgart LJ, Batts KP, et al: Brunner's gland hamartomas: Clinical presentation and pathological features of 27 cases. Am J Gastroenterol 90:290-294, 1995.
12. Chatelain D, Maillet E, Boyer L, et al: Brunner gland hamartoma with predominant adipose tissue and ciliated cysts. Arch Pathol Lab Med 126:734-735, 2002.

13. Shemesh E, Ben Horin S, Barshack I, et al: Brunner's gland hamartoma presenting as a large duodenal polyp. Gastrointest Endosc 52:435-436, 2000.

14. Adeonigbagbe O, Lee C, Karowe M, et al: A Brunner's gland adenoma as a cause of anemia. J Clin Gastroenterol 29:193-196, 1999.

15. Shah KK, DeRidder PH: Ectopic gastric mucosa in proximal esophagus. Its clinical significance and hormonal profile. J Clin Gastroenterol 8:509-513, 1986.

16. Jabbari M, Goresky CA, Lough J, et al: The inlet patch: Heterotopic gastric mucosa in the upper esophagus. Gastroenterology 89:352-356, 1985.

17. Tsubone M, Kozuka S, Taki T, et al: Heterotopic gastric mucosa in the small intestine. Acta Pathol Jpn 34:1425-1431, 1984.

18. Tsadilas T: Duodenal polyp composed of ectopic gastric mucosa. Dig Dis Sci 29:475-477, 1984.

19. Vizcarrondo FJ, Wang TY, Brady PG: Heterotopic gastric mucosa: Presentation as a rugose duodenal mass. Gastrointest Endosc 29:107-111, 1983.

20. Elitsur Y, Triest WE: Is duodenal gastric metaplasia a consequence of Helicobacter pylori infection in children? Am J Gastroenterol 92:2216-2219, 1997.

21. Yousfi MM, el-Zimaity HM, Cole RA, et al: Resolution of a metaplastic duodenal polyp after cure of Helicobacter pylori infection. J Clin Gastroenterol 23:53-54, 1996.

22. Khulusi S, Mendall MA, Badve S, et al: Effect of Helicobacter pylori eradication on gastric metaplasia of the duodenum. Gut 36:193-197, 1995.

23. Lai EC, Tompkins RK: Heterotopic pancreas. Review of a 26 year experience. Am J Surg 151:697-700, 1986.

24. Kaneda M, Yano T, Yamamoto T, et al: Ectopic pancreas in the stomach presenting as an inflammatory abdominal mass. Am J Gastroenterol 84:663-666, 1989.

25. Wang HH, Zeroogian JM, Spechler SJ, et al: Prevalence and significance of pancreatic acinar metaplasia at the gastroesophageal junction. Am J Surg Pathol 20:1507-1510, 1996.

26. Tanemura H, Uno S, Suzuki M, et al: Heterotopic gastric mucosa accompanied by aberrant pancreas in the duodenum. Am J Gastroenterol 82:685-688, 1987.

27. Fenoglio-Preiser CM: Gastrointestinal pathology : An atlas and text. Philadelphia, Lippincott-Raven, 1999, pp 603-605.

28. Acea Nebril B, Taboada Filgueira L, Parajo Calvo A, et al: Solitary hamartomatous duodenal polyp; a different entity: Report of a case and review of the literature. Surg Today 23:1074-1077, 1993.

29. Nickels J, Laasonen EM: Pancreatic heterotopia. Scand J Gastroenterol 5:639-640, 1970.

30. Padberg BC, Schroder S: Mucus retention in heterotopic pancreas of the gastric antrum: A lesion mimicking mucinous carcinoma. Am J Surg Pathol 19:1445-1447, 1995.

31. Bussolati G: Heterotopic pancreas. Am J Surg Pathol 20:1427-1428, 1996.

32. Yamagami T, Tokiwa K, Iwai N: Myoepithelial hamartoma of the ileum causing intussusception in an infant. Pediatr Surg Int 12:206-207, 1997.

33. Gal R, Rath-Wolfson L, Ginzburg M, et al: Adenomyomas of the small intestine. Histopathology 18:369-371, 1991.

34. Tanaka N, Seya T, Onda M, et al: Myoepithelial hamartoma of the small bowel: Report of a case. Surg Today 26:1010-1013, 1996.

35. Flejou JF, Potet F, Molas G, et al: Cystic dystrophy of the gastric and duodenal wall developing in heterotopic pancreas: An unrecognised entity. Gut 34:343-347, 1993.

36. Longmire WP, Wallner MA: Pancreatitis occurring in heterotopic pancreatic tissue. Surgery 40:412-418, 1956.

37. Barbosa deCastro JJ, Dockerty MB, Waugh JM: Pancreatic heterotopia: Review of the literature and report of 41 authenticated surgical cases, of which 25 were clinically significant. Surg Gynecol Obstet 82:527-542, 1946.

38. Case records of the Massachusetts General Hospital. Weekly clinicopathological exercises. Case 26-1999. A three-week-old girl with pyloric stenosis and an unexpected operative finding. N Engl J Med 341:679-684, 1999.

39. Thoeni RF, Gedgaudas RK: Ectopic pancreas: Usual and unusual features. Gastrointest Radiol 5:37-42, 1980.

40. Pang LC: Pancreatic heterotopia: A reappraisal and clinicopathologic analysis of 32 cases. South Med J 81:1264-1275, 1988.

41. Daniel T, Natarajan S, Johnston CA: Ectopic pancreas: A rare cause of pyloric stenosis. Int J Pancreatol 27:167-168, 2000.

42. Kawashima H, Iwanaka T, Matsumoto M, et al: Pyloric stenosis caused by noncystic duodenal duplication and ectopic pancreas in a neonate. J Pediatr Gastroenterol Nutr 27:228-229, 1998.

43. Hsia CY, Wu CW, Lui WY: Heterotopic pancreas: A difficult diagnosis. J Clin Gastroenterol 28:144-147, 1999.

44. Hamada Y, Yonekura Y, Tanano A, et al: Isolated heterotopic pancreas causing intussusception. Eur J Pediatr Surg 10:197-200, 2000.

45. Chand EM, Caudell P: Pathologic quiz case. Patient with duodenal strictures and a mass at the head of the pancreas. Arch Pathol Lab Med 125:701-702, 2001.

46. Al Jitawi SA, Hiarat AM, Al-Majali SH: Diffuse myoepithelial hamartoma of the duodenum associated with adenocarcinoma. Clin Oncol 10:289-293, 1984.

47. Zak F: Aberrant pancreatic carcinoma in a jejunal diverticulum. Gastroenterology 30:529-534, 1956.

48. Osanai M, Miyokawa N, Tamaki T, et al: Adenocarcinoma arising in gastric heterotopic pancreas: Clinicopathological and immunohistochemical study with genetic analysis of a case. Pathol Int 51:549-554, 2001.

49. Jeng KS, Yang KC, Kuo SH: Malignant degeneration of heterotopic pancreas. Gastrointest Endosc 37:196-198, 1991.

50. Shekitka KM, Helwig EB: Deceptive bizarre stromal cells in polyps and ulcers of the gastrointestinal tract. Cancer 67:2111-2117, 1991.

51. Kim YI, Kim WH: Inflammatory fibroid polyps of gastrointestinal tract. Evolution of histologic patterns. Am J Clin Pathol 89:721-727, 1988.

52. Ott DJ, Wu WC, Shiflett DW, et al: Inflammatory fibroid polyp of the duodenum. Am J Gastroenterol 73:62-64, 1980.

53. Soon MS, Lin OS: Inflammatory fibroid polyp of the duodenum. Surg Endosc 14:86, 2000.

54. Jenne DE, Reimann H, Nezu J, et al: Peutz-Jeghers syndrome is caused by mutations in a novel serine threonine kinase. Nat Genet 18:38-43, 1998.

55. Amos CI, Bali D, Thiel TJ, et al: Fine mapping of a genetic locus for Peutz-Jeghers syndrome on chromosome 19p. Cancer Res 57:3653-3656, 1997.

56. Hemminki A, Tomlinson I, Markie D, et al: Localization of a susceptibility locus for Peutz-Jeghers syndrome to 19p using comparative genomic hybridization and targeted linkage analysis. Nat Genet 15:87-90, 1997.

57. Trojan J, Brieger A, Raedle J, et al: Peutz-Jeghers syndrome: Molecular analysis of a three-generation kindred with a novel defect in the serine threonine kinase gene STK11. Am J Gastroenterol 94:257-261, 1999.

58. McGarrity TJ, Kulin HE, Zaino RJ: Peutz-Jeghers syndrome. Am J Gastroenterol 95:596-604, 2000.

59. Gilks CB, Young RH, Aguirre P, et al: Adenoma malignum (minimal deviation adenocarcinoma) of the uterine cervix. A clinicopathological and immunohistochemical analysis of 26 cases. Am J Surg Pathol 13:717-729, 1989.

60. Hizawa K, Iida M, Matsumoto T, et al: Cancer in Peutz-Jeghers syndrome. Cancer 72:2777-2781, 1993.

61. Hizawa K, Iida M, Matsumoto T, et al: Neoplastic transformation arising in Peutz-Jeghers polyposis. Dis Colon Rectum 36:953-957, 1993.

62. Scully RE: Sex cord tumor with annular tubules: A distinctive ovarian tumor of the Peutz-Jeghers syndrome. Cancer 25:1107-1121, 1970.

63. Wilson DM, Pitts WC, Hintz RL, et al: Testicular tumors with Peutz-Jeghers syndrome. Cancer 57:2238-2240, 1986.

64. Young RH, Welch WR, Dickersin GR, et al: Ovarian sex cord tumor with annular tubules: Review of 74 cases including 27 with Peutz-Jeghers syndrome and four with adenoma malignum of the cervix. Cancer 50:1384-1402, 1982.

65. Williams GT, Bussey HJ, Morson BC: Hamartomatous polyps in Peutz-Jeghers syndrome. N Engl J Med 299:101-102, 1978.

66. Narita T, Ohnuma H, Yokoyama S: Peutz-Jeghers syndrome with osseous metaplasia of the intestinal polyps. Pathol Int 45:388-392, 1995.

67. Petersen VC, Sheehan AL, Bryan RL, et al: Misplacement of dysplastic epithelium in Peutz-Jeghers polyps: The ultimate diagnostic pitfall? Am J Surg Pathol 24:34-39, 2000.

68. Shepherd NA, Bussey HJ, Jass JR: Epithelial misplacement in Peutz-Jeghers polyps. A diagnostic pitfall. Am J Surg Pathol 11:743-749, 1987.

69. Meshikhes AW, Al-Saif O, Al-Otaibi M: Duodenal and ampullary obstruction by a Peutz-Jeghers polyp. Eur J Gastroenterol Hepatol 12:1239-1241, 2000.

70. Spigelman AD, Arese P, Phillips RK: Polyposis: The Peutz-Jeghers syndrome. Br J Surg 82:1311-1314, 1995.

71. Miyahara M, Saito T, Etoh K, et al: Appendiceal intussusception due to an appendiceal malignant polyp—an association in a patient with Peutz-Jeghers syndrome: Report of a case. Surg Today 25:834-837, 1995.

72. Spigelman AD, Murday V, Phillips RK: Cancer and the Peutz-Jeghers syndrome. Gut 30:1588-1590, 1989.

73. Foley TR, McGarrity TJ, Abt AB: Peutz-Jeghers syndrome: A clinicopathologic survey of the "Harrisburg family" with a 49-year follow-up. Gastroenterology 95:1535-1540, 1988.

74. Giardiello FM, Welsh SB, Hamilton SR, et al: Increased risk of cancer in the Peutz-Jeghers syndrome. N Engl J Med 316:1511-1514, 1987.

75. Giardiello FM, Offerhaus JG: Phenotype and cancer risk of various polyposis syndromes. Eur J Cancer 31A:1085-1087, 1995.

76. Dodds WJ, Schulte WJ, Hensley GT, et al: Peutz-Jeghers syndrome and gastrointestinal malignancy. Am J Roentgenol Radium Ther Nucl Med 115:374-377, 1972.

77. Konishi F, Wyse NE, Muto T, et al: Peutz-Jeghers polyposis associated with carcinoma of the digestive organs. Report of three cases and review of the literature. Dis Colon Rectum 30:790-799, 1987.

78. Narita T, Eto T, Ito T: Peutz-Jeghers syndrome with adenomas and adenocarcinomas in colonic polyps. Am J Surg Pathol 11:76-81, 1987.

79. Flageole H, Raptis S, Trudel JL, et al: Progression toward malignancy of hamartomas in a patient with Peutz-Jeghers syndrome: Case report and literature review. Can J Surg 37:231-236, 1994.

80. Perzin KH, Bridge MF: Adenomatous and carcinomatous changes in hamartomatous polyps of the small intestine (Peutz-Jeghers syndrome): Report of a case and review of the literature. Cancer 49:971-983, 1982.

81. Reid JD: Intestinal carcinoma in the Peutz-Jeghers syndrome. JAMA 229:833-834, 1974.

82. Zhou XP, Woodford-Richens K, Lehtonen R, et al: Germline mutations in BMPR1A/ALK3 cause a subset of cases of juvenile polyposis syndrome and of Cowden and Bannayan-Riley-Ruvalcaba syndromes. Am J Hum Genet 69:704-711, 2001.

83. Howe JR, Ringold JC, Hughes JH, et al: Direct genetic testing for Smad4 mutations in patients at risk for juvenile polyposis. Surgery 126:162-170, 1999.

84. Howe JR, Roth S, Ringold JC, et al: Mutations in the SMAD4/DPC4 gene in juvenile polyposis. Science 280:1086-1088, 1998.

85. Jacoby RF, Schlack S, Cole CE, et al: A juvenile polyposis tumor suppressor locus at 10q22 is deleted from nonepithelial cells in the lamina propria. Gastroenterology 112:1398-1403, 1997.

86. Komorowski RA, Cohen EB: Villous tumors of the duodenum: A clinicopathologic study. Cancer 47:1377-1386, 1981.

87. Yamaguchi K, Enjoji M: Adenoma of the ampulla of Vater: Putative precancerous lesion. Gut 32:1558-1561, 1991.

88. Sarre RG, Frost AG, Jagelman DG, et al: Gastric and duodenal polyps in familial adenomatous polyposis: A prospective study of the nature and prevalence of upper gastrointestinal polyps. Gut 28:306-314, 1987.

89. Spigelman AD, Williams CB, Talbot IC, et al: Upper gastrointestinal cancer in patients with familial adenomatous polyposis. Lancet 2:783-785, 1989.

90. Shemesh E, Bat L: A prospective evaluation of the upper gastrointestinal tract and periampullary region in patients with Gardner syndrome. Am J Gastroenterol 80:825-827, 1985.

91. Schulten MF, Oyasu R, Beal JM: Villous adenoma of the duodenum. A case report and review of the literature. Am J Surg 132:90-96, 1976.

92. Odze RD: Epithelial proliferation and differentiation in flat duodenal mucosa of patients with familial adenomatous polyposis. Mod Pathol 8:648-653, 1995.

93. Fenoglio CM, Kaye GI, Lane N: Distribution of human colonic lymphatics in normal, hyperplastic, and adenomatous tissue. Gastroenterology 64:51-66, 1973.

94. Ryan DP, Schapiro RH, Warshaw AL: Villous tumors of the duodenum. Ann Surg 203:301-306, 1986.

95. Perzin KH, Bridge MF: Adenomas of the small intestine: A clinicopathologic review of 51 cases and a study of their relationship to carcinoma. Cancer 48:799-819, 1981.

96. Agoff SN, Crispin DA, Bronner MP, et al: Neoplasms of the Ampulla of Vater with concurrent pancreatic intraductal neoplasia: A histological and molecular study. Mod Pathol 14:139-146, 2001.

97. Rodriguez-Bigas MA, Vasen HF, Lynch HT, et al: Characteristics of small bowel carcinoma in hereditary nonpolyposis colorectal carcinoma. International Collaborative Group on HNPCC. Cancer 83:240-244, 1998.

98. Kozuka S, Tsubone M, Yamaguchi A, et al: Adenomatous residue in cancerous papilla of Vater. Gut 22:1031-1034, 1981.

99. Fishman MJ, Jeejeebhoy KN, Gopinath N, et al: Small intestinal villous adenoma and celiac disease. Am J Gastroenterol 85:748-751, 1990.

100. Holmes GK, Dunn GI, Cockel R, et al: Adenocarcinoma of the upper small bowel complicating coeliac disease. Gut 21:1010-1016, 1980.

101. Swinson CM, Slavin G, Coles EC, et al: Coeliac disease and malignancy. Lancet 1:111-115, 1983.

102. Yao T, Ida M, Ohsato K, et al: Duodenal lesions in familial polyposis of the colon. Gastroenterology 73:1086-1092, 1977.

103. Levine ML, Dorf BS, Bank S: Adenocarcinoma of the duodenum in a patient with nontropical sprue. Am J Gastroenterol 81:800-802, 1986.

104. Baczako K, Buchler M, Beger HG, et al: Morphogenesis and possible precursor lesions of invasive carcinoma of the papilla of Vater: Epithelial dysplasia and adenoma. Hum Pathol 16:305-310, 1985.

105. Gaddy M, Max MH: Carcinoma of the duodenum. South Med J 78:150-152, 1985.

106. Kutin ND, Ranson JH, Gouge TH, et al: Villous tumors of the duodenum. Ann Surg 181:164-168, 1975.

107. Iwafuchi M, Watanabe H, Ishihara N, et al: Neoplastic endocrine cells in carcinomas of the small intestine: Histochemical and immunohistochemical studies of 24 tumors. Hum Pathol 18:185-194, 1987.

108. Gardner HA, Matthews J, Ciano PS: A signet-ring cell carcinoma of the ampulla of Vater. Arch Pathol Lab Med 114:1071-1072, 1990.

109. Jones MA, Griffith LM, West AB: Adenocarcinoid tumor of the periampullary region: A novel duodenal neoplasm presenting as biliary tract obstruction. Hum Pathol 20:198-200, 1989.

110. London NJ, Leese T, Bingham P, et al: Invasive Paneth cell-rich adenocarcinoma of the duodenum. Br J Hosp Med 40:222-223, 1988.

111. Matthews TH, Heaton GE, Christopherson WM: Primary duodenal choriocarcinoma. Arch Pathol Lab Med 110:550-552, 1986.

112. Shah IA, Schlageter MO, Boehm N: Composite carcinoid-adenocarcinoma of ampulla of Vater. Hum Pathol 21:1188-1190, 1990.

113. Swanson PE, Dykoski D, Wick MR, et al: Primary duodenal small-cell neuroendocrine carcinoma with production of vasoactive intestinal polypeptide. Arch Pathol Lab Med 110:317-320, 1986.

114. Toker C: Oat cell tumor of the small bowel. Am J Gastroenterol 61:481-483, 1974.

115. Zamboni G, Franzin G, Bonetti F, et al: Small-cell neuroendocrine carcinoma of the ampullary region. A clinicopathologic, immunohistochemical, and ultrastructural study of three cases. Am J Surg Pathol 14:703-713, 1990.

116. Lien GS, Mori M, Enjoji M: Primary carcinoma of the small intestine. A clinicopathologic and immunohistochemical study. Cancer 61:316-323, 1988.

117. Talbot IC, Neoptolemos JP, Shaw DE, et al: The histopathology and staging of carcinoma of the ampulla of Vater. Histopathology 12:155-165, 1988.

118. Yamaguchi K, Enjoji M: Carcinoma of the ampulla of vater. A clinicopathologic study and pathologic staging of 109 cases of carcinoma and 5 cases of adenoma. Cancer 59:506-515, 1987.

119. Scott RJ, Meldrum C, Crooks R, et al: Familial adenomatous polyposis: More evidence for disease diversity and genetic heterogeneity. Gut 48:508-514, 2001.

120. Buch B, Noffke C, deKock S: Gardner's syndrome—the importance of early diagnosis: A case report and a review. SADJ 56:242-245, 2001.

121. Burt RW, Berenson MM, Lee RG, et al: Upper gastrointestinal polyps in Gardner's syndrome. Gastroenterology 86:295-301, 1984.

122. Burke AP, Sobin LH: The pathology of Cronkhite-Canada polyps. A comparison to juvenile polyposis. Am J Surg Pathol 13:940-946, 1989.

123. Chi SG, Kim HJ, Park BJ, et al: Mutational abrogation of the PTEN/MMAC1 gene in gastrointestinal polyps in patients with Cowden disease. Gastroenterology 115:1084-1089, 1998.

124. Coburn MC, Pricolo VE, DeLuca FG, et al: Malignant potential in intestinal juvenile polyposis syndromes. Ann Surg Oncol 2:386-391, 1995.

125. Domizio P, Talbot IC, Spigelman AD, et al: Upper gastrointestinal pathology in familial adenomatous polyposis: Results from a prospective study of 102 patients. J Clin Pathol 43:738-743, 1990.

126. Eng C, Peacocke M: PTEN and inherited hamartoma-cancer syndromes. Nat Genet 19:223, 1998.

127. Griffin CA, Lazar S, Hamilton SR, et al: Cytogenetic analysis of intestinal polyps in polyposis syndromes: Comparison with sporadic colorectal adenomas. Cancer Genet Cytogenet 67:14-20, 1993.

128. Haggitt RC, Reid BJ: Hereditary gastrointestinal polyposis syndromes. Am J Surg Pathol 10:871-887, 1986.

129. Hamilton SR, Liu B, Parsons RE, et al: The molecular basis of Turcot's syndrome. N Engl J Med 332:839-847, 1995.

130. Hopkin K: A surprising function for the PTEN tumor suppressor. Science 282:1027-1030, 1998.

131. Jarvinen H, Nyberg M, Peltokallio P: Upper gastrointestinal tract polyps in familial adenomatosis coli. Gut 24:333-339, 1983.

132. Jass JR, Williams CB, Bussey HJ, et al: Juvenile polyposis—a precancerous condition. Histopathology 13:619-630, 1988.

133. Liaw D, Marsh DJ, Li J, et al: Germline mutations of the PTEN gene in Cowden disease, an inherited breast and thyroid cancer syndrome. Nat Genet 16:64-67, 1997.

134. Lynch HT, Smyrk T, McGinn T, et al: Attenuated familial adenomatous polyposis (AFAP). A phenotypically and genotypically distinctive variant of FAP. Cancer 76:2427-2433, 1995.

135. Marsh DJ, Dahia PL, Zheng Z, et al: Germline mutations in PTEN are present in Bannayan-Zonana syndrome. Nat Genet 16:333-334, 1997.

136. Nelen MR, Padberg GW, Peeters EA, et al: Localization of the gene for Cowden disease to chromosome 10q22-23. Nat Genet 13:114-116, 1996.

137. Offerhaus GJ, Giardiello FM, Krush AJ, et al: The risk of upper gastrointestinal cancer in familial adenomatous polyposis. Gastroenterology 102:1980-1982, 1992.

138. Rustgi AK: Hereditary gastrointestinal polyposis and nonpolyposis syndromes. N Engl J Med 331:1694-1702, 1994.

139. Southey MC, Young MA, Whitty J, et al: Molecular pathologic analysis enhances the diagnosis and management of Muir-Torre syndrome and gives insight into its underlying molecular pathogenesis. Am J Surg Pathol 25:936-941, 2001.

140. Spigelman AD, Talbot IC, Penna C, et al: Evidence for adenoma-carcinoma sequence in the duodenum of patients with familial adenomatous polyposis. The Leeds Castle Polyposis Group (Upper Gastrointestinal Committee). J Clin Pathol 47:709-710, 1994.

141. Friedl W, Caspari R, Sengteller M, et al: Can APC mutation analysis contribute to therapeutic decisions in familial adenomatous polyposis? Experience from 680 FAP families. Gut 48:515-521, 2001.

142. Odze R, Gallinger S, So K, et al: Duodenal adenomas in familial adenomatous polyposis: Relation of cell differentiation and mucin histochemical features to growth pattern. Mod Pathol 7:376-384, 1994.

143. Noda Y, Watanabe H, Iida M, et al: Histologic follow-up of ampullary adenomas in patients with familial adenomatosis coli. Cancer 70:1847-1856, 1992.

144. Mizumoto I, Ogawa Y, Niiyama H, et al: Possible role of telomerase activation in the multistep tumor progression of periampullary lesions in patients with familial adenomatous polyposis. Am J Gastroenterol 96:1261-1265, 2001.

145. Saurin JC, Ligneau B, Ponchon T, et al: The influence of mutation site and age on the severity of duodenal polyposis in patients with familial adenomatous polyposis. Gastrointest Endosc 55:342-347, 2002.

146. Costi R, Caruana P, Sarli L, et al: Ampullary adenocarcinoma in neurofibromatosis type 1. Case report and literature review. Mod Pathol 14:1169-1174, 2001.

147. Perry RR, Vinik AI: Endocrine tumors of the gastrointestinal tract. Annu Rev Med 47:57-68, 1996.

148. Kuiper DH, Gracie WA Jr, Pollard HM: Twenty years of gastrointestinal carcinoids. Cancer 25:1424-1430, 1970.

149. Kulke MH, Mayer RJ: Carcinoid tumors. N Engl J Med 340:858-868, 1999.

150. Facer P, Bishop AE, Cole GA, et al: Developmental profile of chromogranin, hormonal peptides, and 5-hydroxytryptamine in gastrointestinal endocrine cells. Gastroenterology 97:48-57, 1989.

151. Lechago J: The endocrine cells of the digestive tract. General concepts and historic perspective. Am J Surg Pathol 11:63-70, 1987.

152. Lechago J: Gastrointestinal neuroendocrine cell proliferations. Hum Pathol 25:1114-1122, 1994.

153. Modlin IM, Sandor A: An analysis of 8305 cases of carcinoid tumors. Cancer 79:813-829, 1997.

154. Moesta KT, Schlag P: Proposal for a new carcinoid tumour staging system based on tumour tissue infiltration and primary metastasis; a prospective multicentre carcinoid tumour evaluation study. West German Surgical Oncologists' Group. Eur J Surg Oncol 16:280-288, 1990.

155. Mulder CJ, Festen HP, Mertens JC, et al: Carcinoid tumor of the ampulla of Vater presenting with biliary obstruction: Report of four cases. Gastrointest Endosc 33:385-387, 1987.

156. Noda Y, Watanabe H, Iwafuchi M, et al: Carcinoids and endocrine cell micronests of the minor and major duodenal papillae. Their incidence and characteristics. Cancer 70:1825-1833, 1992.

157. Saha S, Hoda S, Godfrey R, et al: Carcinoid tumors of the gastrointestinal tract: A 44-year experience. South Med J 82:1501-1505, 1989.

158. Weichert RF 3rd, Roth LM, Krementz ET, et al: Carcinoid-islet cell tumors of the duodenum. Report of twenty-one cases. Am J Surg 121:195-205, 1971.

159. Yoshikane H, Suzuki T, Yoshioka N, et al: Duodenal carcinoid tumor: Endosonographic imaging and endoscopic resection. Am J Gastroenterol 90:642-644, 1995.

160. Rindi G: Clinicopathologic aspects of gastric neuroendocrine tumors. Am J Surg Pathol 19:S20-S29, 1995.

161. Burke AP, Federspiel BH, Sobin LH, et al: Carcinoids of the duodenum. A histologic and immunohistochemical study of 65 tumors. Am J Surg Pathol 13:828-837, 1989.

162. Stamm B, Hedinger CE, Saremaslani P: Duodenal and ampullary carcinoid tumors. A report of 12 cases with pathological characteristics, polypeptide content and relation to the MEN I syndrome and von Recklinghausen's disease (neurofibromatosis). Virchows Arch A Pathol Anat Histopathol 408:475-489, 1986.

163. Madeira I, Terris B, Voss M, et al: Prognostic factors in patients with endocrine tumours of the duodenopancreatic area. Gut 43:422-427, 1998.

164. Godwin JD 2nd: Carcinoid tumors. An analysis of 2,837 cases. Cancer 36:560-569, 1975.

165. Shebani KO, Souba WW, Finkelstein DM, et al: Prognosis and survival in patients with gastrointestinal tract carcinoid tumors. Ann Surg 229:815-821; discussion 822-823, 1999.

166. Beaton H, Homan W, Dineen P: Gastrointestinal carcinoids and the malignant carcinoid syndrome. Surg Gynecol Obstet 152:268-272, 1981.

167. Kothari T, Mangla JC: Malignant tumors associated with carcinoid tumors of the gastrointestinal tract. J Clin Gastroenterol 3(suppl 1): 43-46, 1981.

168. Gerstle JT, Kauffman GL Jr, Koltun WA: The incidence, management, and outcome of patients with gastrointestinal carcinoids and second primary malignancies. J Am Coll Surg 180:427-432, 1995.

169. Rivadeneira DE, Tuckson WB, Naab T: Increased incidence of second primary malignancy in patients with carcinoid tumors: Case report and literature review. J Natl Med Assoc 88:310-312, 1996.

170. Lam KY, Chan AC: Paraganglioma of the urinary bladder: An immunohistochemical study and report of an unusual association with intestinal carcinoid. Aust N Z J Surg 63:740-745, 1993.

171. Tse V, Lochhead A, Adams W, et al: Concurrent colonic adenocarcinoma and two ileal carcinoids in a 72-year-old male. Aust N Z J Surg 67:739-741, 1997.

172. Zucker KA, Longo WE, Modlin IM, et al: Malignant diathesis from jejunal-ileal carcinoids. Am J Gastroenterol 84:182-186, 1989.

173. Mitchell ME, Johnson JA III, Wilton PB: Five primary synchronous neoplasms of the gastrointestinal tract. J Clin Gastroenterol 23:284-288, 1996.

174. Kytola S, Hoog A, Nord B, et al: Comparative genomic hybridization identifies loss of 18q22-qter as an early and specific event in tumorigenesis of midgut carcinoids. Am J Pathol 158:1803-1808, 2001.

175. Tonnies H, Toliat MR, Ramel C, et al: Analysis of sporadic neuroendocrine tumours of the enteropancreatic system by comparative genomic hybridisation. Gut 48:536-541, 2001.

176. Gortz B, Roth J, Krahenmann A, et al: Mutations and allelic deletions of the MEN1 gene are associated with a subset of sporadic endocrine pancreatic and neuroendocrine tumors and not restricted to foregut neoplasms. Am J Pathol 154:429-436, 1999.

177. Debelenko LV, Zhuang Z, Emmert-Buck MR, et al: Allelic deletions on chromosome 11q13 in multiple endocrine neoplasia type 1-associated and sporadic gastrinomas and pancreatic endocrine tumors. Cancer Res 57:2238-2243, 1997.

178. Lips CJ, Landsvater RM, Hoppener JW, et al: Clinical screening as compared with DNA analysis in families with multiple endocrine neoplasia type 2A. N Engl J Med 331:828-835, 1994.

179. Burke AP, Thomas RM, Elsayed AM, et al: Carcinoids of the jejunum and ileum: An immunohistochemical and clinicopathologic study of 167 cases. Cancer 79:1086-1093, 1997.

180. Janson ET, Holmberg L, Stridsberg M, et al: Carcinoid tumors: Analysis of prognostic factors and survival in 301 patients from a referral center. Ann Oncol 8:685-690, 1997.

181. Martensson H, Nobin A, Sundler F: Carcinoid tumors in the gastrointestinal tract—an analysis of 156 cases. Acta Chir Scand 149:607-616, 1983.

182. Soga J: Carcinoids of the small intestine: A statistical evaluation of 1102 cases collected from the literature. J Exp Clin Cancer Res 16:353-363, 1997.

183. Memon MA, Nelson H: Gastrointestinal carcinoid tumors: Current management strategies. Dis Colon Rectum 40:1101-1118, 1997.

184. Lucey MR, Yamada T: Biochemistry and physiology of gastrointestinal somatostatin. Dig Dis Sci 34:5S-13S, 1989.

185. Krejs GJ, Orci L, Conlon JM, et al: Somatostatinoma syndrome. Biochemical, morphologic and clinical features. N Engl J Med 301:285-292, 1979.

186. O'Brien TD, Chejfec G, Prinz RA: Clinical features of duodenal somatostatinomas. Surgery 114:1144-1147, 1993.

187. Larsson LI, Hirsch MA, Holst JJ, et al: Pancreatic somatostatinoma. Clinical features and physiological implications. Lancet 1:666-668, 1977.

188. Kaneko H, Yanaihara N, Ito S, et al: Somatostatinoma of the duodenum. Cancer 44:2273-2279, 1979.

189. Murayama H, Imai T, Kikuchi M, et al: Duodenal carcinoid (apudoma) with psammoma bodies: A light and electron microscopic study. Cancer 43:1411-1417, 1979.

190. Tanaka S, Yamasaki S, Matsushita H, et al: Duodenal somatostatinoma: A case report and review of 31 cases with special reference to the relationship between tumor size and metastasis. Pathol Int 50:146-152, 2000.

191. Griffiths DF, Williams GT, Williams ED: Multiple endocrine neoplasia associated with von Recklinghausen's disease. Br Med J (Clin Res Ed) 287:1341-1343, 1983.

192. Arnesjo B, Idvall I, Ihse I, et al: Concomitant occurrence of neurofibromatosis and carcinoid of the intestine. Scand J Gastroenterol 8:637-643, 1973.

193. Barber PV: Carcinoid tumour of the ampulla of Vater associated with cutaneous neurofibromatosis. Postgrad Med J 52:514-517, 1976.

194. Cantor AM, Rigby CC, Beck PR, et al: Neurofibromatosis, phaeochromocytoma, and somatostatinoma. Br Med J (Clin Res Ed) 285:1618-1619, 1982.

195. Chetty R, Essa A: Heterotopic pancreas, periampullary somatostatinoma and type I neurofibromatosis: A pathogenetic proposal. Pathology 31:95-97, 1999.

196. Dayal Y, Doos WG, O'Brien MJ, et al: Psammomatous somatostatinomas of the duodenum. Am J Surg Pathol 7:653-665, 1983.

197. Dayal Y, Tallberg KA, Nunnemacher G, et al: Duodenal carcinoids in patients with and without neurofibromatosis. A comparative study. Am J Surg Pathol 10:348-357, 1986.

198. Hagen EC, Houben GM, Nikkels RE, et al: Exocrine pancreatic insufficiency and pancreatic fibrosis due to duodenal somatostatinoma in a patient with neurofibromatosis. Pancreas 7:98-104, 1992.

199. Hough DR, Chan A, Davidson H: Von Recklinghausen's disease associated with gastrointestinal carcinoid tumors. Cancer 51:2206-2208, 1983.

200. Johnson L, Weaver M: Von Recklinghausen's disease and gastrointestinal carcinoids. JAMA 245:2496, 1981.

201. Kainuma O, Ito Y, Taniguchi T, et al: Ampullary somatostatinoma in a patient with von Recklinghausen's disease. J Gastroenterol 31:460-464, 1996.

202. Lee HY, Garber PE: Von Recklinghausen's disease associated with pheochromocytoma and carcinoid tumor. Ohio State Med J 66:583-586, 1970.

203. Mao C, Shah A, Hanson DJ, et al: Von Recklinghausen's disease associated with duodenal somatostatinoma: Contrast of duodenal versus pancreatic somatostatinomas. J Surg Oncol 59:67-73, 1995.

204. Frick EJ Jr, Kralstein JR, Scarlato M, et al: Somatostatinoma of the ampulla of vater in celiac sprue. J Gastrointest Surg 4:388-391, 2000.

205. Sawady J, Katzin WE, Mendelsohn G, et al: Somatostatin-producing neuroendocrine tumor of the ampulla (ampullary somatostatinoma). Evidence of prosomatostatin production. Am J Clin Pathol 97:411-415, 1992.

206. Tan CC, Hall RI, Semeraro D, et al: Ampullary somatostatinoma associated with von Recklinghausen's neurofibromatosis presenting as obstructive jaundice. Eur J Surg Oncol 22:298-301, 1996.

207. Warner TF, Baron JJ, Mallin SR, et al: Intestinal development in insulinoma containing Psammoma bodies. Recapitulation of ultrastructural features. Arch Pathol Lab Med 104:432-437, 1980.

208. Griffiths DF, Williams GT, Williams ED: Duodenal carcinoid tumours, phaeochromocytoma and neurofibromatosis: Islet cell tumour, phaeochromocytoma and the von Hippel-Lindau complex: Two distinctive neuroendocrine syndromes. Q J Med 64:769-782, 1987.

209. Griffiths DF, Jasani B, Newman GR, et al: Glandular duodenal carcinoid—a somatostatin rich tumour with neuroendocrine associations. J Clin Pathol 37:163-169, 1984.

210. Karasawa Y, Sakaguchi M, Minami S, et al: Duodenal somatostatinoma and erythrocytosis in a patient with von Hippel-Lindau disease type 2A. Intern Med 40:38-43, 2001.

211. Green BT, Rockey DC: Duodenal somatostatinoma presenting with complete somatostatinoma syndrome. J Clin Gastroenterol 33:415-417, 2001.

212. Case records of the Massachusetts General Hospital. Weekly clinicopathological exercises. Case 15-1989. A 52-year-old man with neurofibromatosis and jaundice. N Engl J Med 320:996-1004, 1989.

213. Marcial MA, Pinkus GS, Skarin A, et al: Ampullary somatostatinoma: Psammomatous variant of gastrointestinal carcinoid tumor—an immunohistochemical and ultrastructural study. Report of a case and review of the literature. Am J Clin Pathol 80:755-761, 1983.

214. Albrecht S, Gardiner GW, Kovacs K, et al: Duodenal somatostatinoma with psammoma bodies. Arch Pathol Lab Med 113:517-520, 1989.

215. Taccagni GL, Carlucci M, Sironi M, et al: Duodenal somatostatinoma with psammoma bodies: An immunohistochemical and ultrastructural study. Am J Gastroenterol 81:33-37, 1986.

216. Schaller P, Schweiger M, Stolte M, et al: [Malignant somatostatinoma—diagnosis after 6 years.] Leber Magen Darm 20:152-156, 1990.

217. Damron TA, Rahman D, Cashman MD: Gangliocytic paraganglioma in association with a duodenal diverticulum. Am J Gastroenterol 84:1109-1114, 1989.

218. Hamid QA, Bishop AE, Rode J, et al: Duodenal gangliocytic paragangliomas: A study of 10 cases with immunocytochemical neuroendocrine markers. Hum Pathol 17:1151-1157, 1986.

219. Kepes JJ, Zacharias DL: Gangliocytic paragangliomas of the duodenum. A report of two cases with light and electron microscopic examination. Cancer 27:61-67, 1971.

220. Sakhuja P, Malhotra V, Gondal R, et al: Periampullary gangliocytic paraganglioma. J Clin Gastroenterol 33:154-156, 2001.

221. Scheithauer BW, Nora FE, LeChago J, et al: Duodenal gangliocytic paraganglioma. Clinicopathologic and immunocytochemical study of 11 cases. Am J Clin Pathol 86:559-565, 1986.

222. Kheir SM, Halpern NB: Paraganglioma of the duodenum in association with congenital neurofibromatosis. Possible relationship. Cancer 53:2491-2496, 1984.

223. Barbareschi M, Frigo B, Aldovini D, et al: Duodenal gangliocytic paraganglioma. Report of a case and review of the literature. Virchows Arch A Pathol Anat Histopathol 416:81-89, 1989.
224. Altavilla G, Chiarelli S, Fassina A: Duodenal periampullary gangliocytic paraganglioma: Report of two cases with immunohistochemical and ultrastructural study. Ultrastruct Pathol 25:137-145, 2001.
225. Perrone T, Sibley RK, Rosai J: Duodenal gangliocytic paraganglioma. An immunohistochemical and ultrastructural study and a hypothesis concerning its origin. Am J Surg Pathol 9:31-41, 1985.
226. Min KW: Gangliocytic paraganglioma of the duodenum: Report of a case with immunocytochemical and ultrastructural investigation. Ultrastruct Pathol 21:587-595, 1997.
227. Inai K, Kobuke T, Yonehara S, et al: Duodenal gangliocytic paraganglioma with lymph node metastasis in a 17-year-old boy. Cancer 63:2540-2545, 1989.
228. Hashimoto S, Kawasaki S, Matsuzawa K, et al: Gangliocytic paraganglioma of the papilla of Vater with regional lymph node metastasis. Am J Gastroenterol 87:1216-1218, 1992.
229. Delcore R Jr, Cheung LY, Friesen SR: Outcome of lymph node involvement in patients with the Zollinger-Ellison syndrome. Ann Surg 208:291-298, 1988.
230. Herrmann ME, Ciesla MC, Chejfec G, et al: Primary nodal gastrinomas. Arch Pathol Lab Med 124:832-835, 2000.
231. Pipeleers-Marichal M, Somers G, Willems G, et al: Gastrinomas in the duodenums of patients with multiple endocrine neoplasia type 1 and the Zollinger-Ellison syndrome. N Engl J Med 322:723-727, 1990.
232. Zimmer T, Stolzel U, Bader M, et al: Brief report: A duodenal gastrinoma in a patient with diarrhea and normal serum gastrin concentrations. N Engl J Med 333:634-636, 1995.
233. Roy PK, Venzon DJ, Feigenbaum KM, et al: Gastric secretion in Zollinger-Ellison syndrome. Correlation with clinical expression, tumor extent and role in diagnosis—a prospective NIH study of 235 patients and a review of 984 cases in the literature. Medicine (Baltimore) 80:189-222, 2001.
234. Capella C, Riva C, Rindi G, et al: Endocrine tumors of the duodenum and upper jejunum. A study of 33 cases with clinico-pathological characteristics and hormone content. Hepatogastroenterology 37:247-252, 1990.
235. Wadas DD, Foutch PG, Manne RK, et al: Endoscopic diagnosis of a duodenal gastrinoma. Gastrointest Endosc 34:430-431, 1988.
236. Agarwal SK, Guru SC, Heppner C, et al: Menin interacts with the AP1 transcription factor JunD and represses JunD-activated transcription. Cell 96:143-152, 1999.
237. Chandrasekharappa SC, Guru SC, Manickam P, et al: Positional cloning of the gene for multiple endocrine neoplasia-type 1. Science 276:404-407, 1997.
238. Bale AE, Norton JA, Wong EL, et al: Allelic loss on chromosome 11 in hereditary and sporadic tumors related to familial multiple endocrine neoplasia type 1. Cancer Res 51:1154-1157, 1991.
239. Zhuang Z, Vortmeyer AO, Pack S, et al: Somatic mutations of the MEN1 tumor suppressor gene in sporadic gastrinomas and insulinomas. Cancer Res 57:4682-4686, 1997.
240. Yu F, Jensen RT, Lubensky IA, et al: Survey of genetic alterations in gastrinomas. Cancer Res 60:5536-5542, 2000.
241. Muscarella P, Melvin WS, Fisher WE, et al: Genetic alterations in gastrinomas and nonfunctioning pancreatic neuroendocrine tumors: An analysis of p16/MTS1 tumor suppressor gene inactivation. Cancer Res 58:237-240, 1998.
242. Evers BM, Rady PL, Sandoval K, et al: Gastrinomas demonstrate amplification of the HER-2/neu proto-oncogene. Ann Surg 219:596-601; discussion 602-604, 1994.
243. Ebrahimi SA, Wang EH, Wu A, et al: Deletion of chromosome 1 predicts prognosis in pancreatic endocrine tumors. Cancer Res 59:311-315, 1999.
244. Chung DC, Smith AP, Louis DN, et al: A novel pancreatic endocrine tumor suppressor gene locus on chromosome 3p with clinical prognostic implications. J Clin Invest 100:404-410, 1997.
245. Speel EJ, Richter J, Moch H, et al: Genetic differences in endocrine pancreatic tumor subtypes detected by comparative genomic hybridization. Am J Pathol 155:1787-1794, 1999.
246. Farley DR, van Heerden JA, Grant CS, et al: Extrapancreatic gastrinomas. Surgical experience. Arch Surg 129:506-511; discussion 511-512, 1994.
247. Modlin IM, Lawton GP: Duodenal gastrinoma: The solution to the pancreatic paradox. J Clin Gastroenterol 19:184-188, 1994.
248. Hirose T, Scheithauer BW, Sano T: Giant plexiform schwannoma: A report of two cases with soft tissue and visceral involvement. Mod Pathol 10:1075-1081, 1997.
249. Bernal A, del Junco GW, Gibson SR: Endoscopic and pathologic features of gastrointestinal Kaposi's sarcoma: A report of four cases in patients with the acquired immune deficiency syndrome. Gastrointest Endosc 31:74-77, 1985.
250. Saltz RK, Kurtz RC, Lightdale CJ, et al: Kaposi's sarcoma. Gastrointestinal involvement correlation with skin findings and immunologic function. Dig Dis Sci 29:817-823, 1984.
251. Imamura K, Fuchigami T, Iida M, et al: Duodenal lipoma—a report of three cases. Gastrointest Endosc 29:223-224, 1983.
252. Onoda N, Kobayashi H, Satake K, et al: Granular cell tumor of the duodenum: A case report. Am J Gastroenterol 93:1993-1994, 1998.
253. Danzig JB, Brandt LJ, Reinus JF, et al: Gastrointestinal malignancy in patients with AIDS. Am J Gastroenterol 86:715-718, 1991.
254. Case records of the Massachusetts General Hospital. Weekly clinicopathological exercises. Case 24-1997. A six-year-old boy with bouts of abdominal pain, vomiting, and a left-sided abdominal mass. N Engl J Med 337:329-336, 1997.
255. Daimaru Y, Kido H, Hashimoto H, et al: Benign schwannoma of the gastrointestinal tract: A clinicopathologic and immunohistochemical study. Hum Pathol 19:257-264, 1988.
256. Miettinen M, Shekitka KM, Sobin LH: Schwannomas in the colon and rectum: A clinicopathologic and immunohistochemical study of 20 cases. Am J Surg Pathol 25:846-855, 2001.
257. Sarlomo-Rikala M, Miettinen M: Gastric schwannoma—a clinicopathological analysis of six cases. Histopathology 27:355-360, 1995.
258. Case records of the Massachusetts General Hospital. Weekly clinicopathological exercises. Case 8-1997. A 65-year-old man with recurrent abdominal pain for five years. N Engl J Med 336:786-793, 1997.
259. Levendoglu H, Rosen Y: Nodular lymphoid hyperplasia of gut in HIV infection. Am J Gastroenterol 87:1200-1202, 1992.
260. deWeerth A, Gocht A, Seewald S, et al: Duodenal nodular lymphoid hyperplasia caused by giardiasis infection in a patient who is immunodeficient. Gastrointest Endosc 55:605-607, 2002.
261. Ward H, Jalan KN, Maitra TK, et al: Small intestinal nodular lymphoid hyperplasia in patients with giardiasis and normal serum immunoglobulins. Gut 24:120-126, 1983.
262. Rambaud JC, De Saint-Louvent P, Marti R, et al: Diffuse follicular lymphoid hyperplasia of the small intestine without primary immunoglobulin deficiency. Am J Med 73:125-132, 1982.
263. Ament ME, Rubin CE: Relation of giardiasis to abnormal intestinal structure and function in gastrointestinal immunodeficiency syndromes. Gastroenterology 62:216-226, 1972.
264. Matuchansky C, Touchard G, Lemaire M, et al: Malignant lymphoma of the small bowel associated with diffuse nodular lymphoid hyperplasia. N Engl J Med 313:166-171, 1985.
265. Matuchansky C, Morichau-Beauchant M, Touchard G, et al: Nodular lymphoid hyperplasia of the small bowel associated with primary jejunal malignant lymphoma. Evidence favoring a cytogenetic relationship. Gastroenterology 78:1587-1592, 1980.
266. Harris M, Blewitt RW, Davies VJ, et al: High-grade non-Hodgkin's lymphoma complicating polypoid nodular lymphoid hyperplasia and multiple lymphomatous polyposis of the intestine. Histopathology 15:339-350, 1989.
267. Castellano G, Moreno D, Galvao O, et al: Malignant lymphoma of jejunum with common variable hypogammaglobulinemia and diffuse nodular hyperplasia of the small intestine. A case study and literature review. J Clin Gastroenterol 15:128-135, 1992.
268. Stessens L, van den Oord JJ, Geboes K, et al: GI lymphomatous polyposis. Gastroenterology 90:2041-2042, 1986.
269. Fernandes BJ, Amato D, Goldfinger M: Diffuse lymphomatous polyposis of the gastrointestinal tract. A case report with immunohistochemical studies. Gastroenterology 88:1267-1270, 1985.
270. Kanehira K, Braylan RC, Lauwers GY: Early phase of intestinal mantle cell lymphoma: A report of two cases associated with advanced colonic adenocarcinoma. Mod Pathol 14:811-817, 2001.

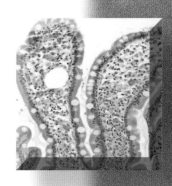

CHAPTER 15

Polyps of the Large Intestine

SUSAN C. ABRAHAM • LAWRENCE J. BURGART
ROBERT D. ODZE

Introduction

Flexible sigmoidoscopy and colonoscopy frequently reveal polypoid lesions that are either biopsied or removed endoscopically. In one study, relatively young (ages 40 to 49 years) and asymptomatic individuals who underwent a screening colonoscopy had a 21% prevalence of epithelial polyps.[1] Broadly speaking, a "polyp" refers to any localized (whether single or multiple) projection above the surrounding colonic mucosa. Epithelial polyps of the colon are customarily categorized into hyperplastic, inflammatory, hamartomatous, and neoplastic (Table 15-1). In addition, polyps may develop from mesenchymal proliferations, benign and malignant hematolymphoid tissue, metastatic tumors, and a wide variety of non-neoplastic substances, such as air. The relative proportions of these various types of polyps depend on the type of population undergoing endoscopy (i.e., age, associated risk factors such as inflammatory bowel disease or polyposis syndrome) and the method (sigmoidoscopy vs. total colonoscopy), but hyperplastic and adenomatous polyps are by far the most common. In one recent large study of 1050 colonic polyps, 95.4% were neoplastic or hyperplastic, 2.8% were inflammatory, and only 1.5% were mesenchymal polyps such as lipomas and leiomyomas.[2]

Epithelial Polyps

HYPERPLASTIC POLYPS

Hyperplastic polyps are small, typically innocuous lesions that may be found throughout the colon of adults but are especially common in the rectum.[3,4] Their prevalence increases with age to up to 30% in asymptomatic individuals older than 50 years of age. Hyperplastic polyps are asymptomatic and thus are usually identified as an incidental finding at the time of endoscopic examination of the colon. Endoscopically, hyperplastic polyps usually cannot be distinguished with certainty from adenomas; therefore, patients typically undergo biopsy and fulguration.[5]

Pathogenesis

The pathogenesis of hyperplastic polyps is essentially unknown.[6] However, one commonly accepted theory suggests that these polyps arise as the result of an increase in crypt epithelial cell turnover combined with delayed migration from the crypt base to the surface of the mucosa. A slower rate of surface cell exfoliation has also been described in hyperplastic polyps, which partially explains the hypermature appearance of the epithelium on histologic evaluation. Some studies also support the concept of early cell maturation along the

TABLE 15–1. Classification of Large Intestinal Polyps

Epithelial polyps
  Hyperplastic
  Inflammatory
    Inflammatory pseudopolyp
    Prolapse-type inflammatory polyp
    Inflammatory myoglandular polyp
  Hamartomas
    Juvenile polyp
    Peutz-Jeghers polyp
    Cowden disease polyp
    Cronkhite-Canada syndrome polyp
  Neoplastic polyps
    Adenomas—tubular, tubulovillous, villous, flat, serrated
    Mixed hyperplastic/adenomatous polyp
    Adenoma and polypoid dysplasia in inflammatory bowel disease
    Adenocarcinoma—polypoid adenocarcinoma and adenocarcinomas arising within an adenoma
    Endocrine (carcinoid) tumor
    Polypoid metastasis
Lymphoid polyp—benign and malignant
Mesenchymal polyps—neurofibroma, ganglioneuroma, leiomyoma, leiomyosarcoma, lipoma, polypoid vascular tumor, granular cell tumor, inflammatory fibroid polyp, polypoid gastrointestinal stromal tumor, etc.
Miscellaneous polypoid lesions—pseudolipomatosis, pneumatosis, endometriosis, xanthoma, inverted appendix, mucosal tags, atheroembolus-associated polyp

crypt axis. Cell kinetic studies have shown that hyperplastic polyps do not in fact reveal epithelial cell hyperplasia.

Recent data suggest that hyperplastic polyps contain various genetic and cell cycle regulatory defects. This has led to the belief that these lesions, particularly those that are larger and/or occur on the right side of the colon, may in fact have a low degree of malignant potential.[6-12] However, this is highly controversial. For instance, hyperplastic polyps have been shown to demonstrate dysregulation of cell proliferation, altered *BCL2* and *BAX* gene expression, loss of a tumor suppression gene on chromosome 1p, TP53 overexpression, a high frequency of K-*ras* mutations, and loss of heterozygosity of the *adenomatous polyposis coli* gene (*APC*), 3p, *TP53*, and *p16* in a small proportion of cases. It has also been revealed that in hyperplastic polyps, *p27* expression is altered. A variety of biochemical and oncofetal blood antigen expression patterns are altered in hyperplastic polyps as well. Furthermore, rarely, adenocarcinoma has been reported to occur in sporadic hyperplastic polyps with adenomatous change.[13] In addition, some studies have shown that hyperplastic polyps may be a high risk indicator for colon carcinoma because some patients share risk factors, such as a diet high in animal fat and alcohol consumption or low folic acid intake, with those who ultimately develop colon cancer. Patients with hyperplastic polyps are also more likely to develop adenomas than are patients without these lesions.

Finally, recent data also suggest that right-sided colonic hyperplastic polyps may give rise to sporadic colorectal carcinomas that show microsatellite instability and a serrated morphologic growth pattern. An increased risk of colon cancer has also been detected in patients with the hyperplastic polyposis syndrome, which at this point has ill-defined clinical pathologic criteria (see under Hyperplastic Polyposis).

Pathologic Features

A vast majority of hyperplastic polyps measure smaller than 5 mm. They are characterized histologically by a "hypermature" appearance and display an irregular sawtooth, or serrated, luminal surface contour (Fig. 15-1). Cross sections of hyperplastic crypts have a stellate appearance reminiscent of a starfish. The superficial portion of a hyperplastic polyp shows hypermucinous cells, which may appear crowded. However, the cells maintain a mature appearance with small nuclei and absence of hyperchromasia or atypia. The deep, regenerative portion of a hyperplastic polyp may be confused with an adenoma because the lower portion of the crypt often appears hyperchromatic compared with surrounding nonlesional colon crypts; however, this is due to the regenerative nature of the cells rather than to any clonal or adenomatous characteristics. The hyperchromatic regenerative zone maintains a rapid, orderly process of maturation to the surface.

On occasion, hyperplastic polyps may become irritated and may contain a variable amount of mononuclear or even neutrophilic inflammation. The subepithelial collagen layer is occasionally thickened and should not be interpreted as representing collagenous colitis.

Hyperplastic polyps may uncommonly show misplacement of epithelium into the submucosa. This phenomenon, which has been referred to as "inverted hyperplastic polyp," may be mistaken for an adenoma with epithelial misplacement or even an invasive adenocarcinoma (see later). Yantiss and associates have provided evidence that this phenomenon is entirely benign and is likely induced by trauma to the overlying polyp,[14] similar to the process of epithelial misplacement in adenomas.

Differential Diagnosis

The basis for differentiating a serrated adenoma from a hyperplastic polyp is primarily the fact that the epithelium in the former is "neoplastic" (dysplastic) and the epithelium in the latter is not (Table 15-2). Serrated adenomas show a lack of surface maturation, which is always present in hyperplastic polyps. Furthermore, adenomas contain mildly enlarged, cigar-shaped nuclei

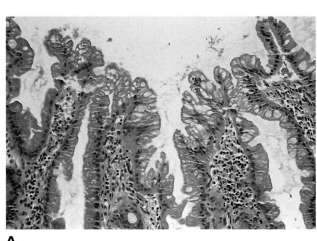 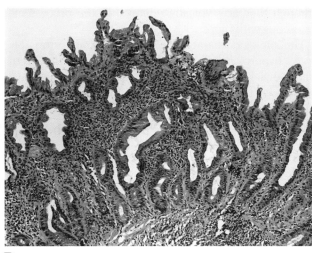

A   **B**

FIGURE 15–1. A, Hyperplastic polyp classically displays mild hyperchromasia in the deep portion of the crypt with hypermucinous maturation at the surface. **B,** Hyperplastic polyps can become inflamed and lose mucin but retain their surface maturation and a serrated architecture.

in contrast to the small, uniform, basally located nuclei typical of hyperplastic polyps. Cautery artifact may artifactually elongate the nuclei of hyperplastic polyps, mimicking pseudostratification. Mucin content and distribution are less helpful in this differential diagnosis because some hyperplastic polyps, particularly those from the right colon, may be somewhat mucin depleted, similar to adenomas.

Serrated adenomas are most often larger than 0.5 cm; they show dilatation of crypts at the base of the mucosa instead of at the surface of the polyp, such as occurs in typical hyperplastic polyps, and they show a higher prevalence of horizontally shaped crypts at the base of the mucosa as well. Scattered endocrine cells are usually not as prominent in serrated adenomas as they are in hyperplastic polyps. However, a key feature of serrated adenomas is their usually marked degree of cytoplasmic eosinophilia, which is present in all layers of the crypt, in contrast to hyperplastic polyps, which more often show mucin preservation. In addition, serrated adenomas may show mitoses at the superficial portion of the polyp instead of only at the base, as is seen in typical hyperplastic polyps.

Hyperplastic polyps should also be distinguished from other entities, such as prolapse-type inflammatory polyps and adenomas with epithelial misplacement, or even adenomas with invasive well-differentiated adenocarcinoma. All of these lesions may contain epithelial elements within the submucosa of the polyp stalk. However, prolapse-type inflammatory polyps are frequently inflamed or even ulcerated, contain markedly regenerative-appearing epithelium, and show characteristic fibromuscular hyperplasia of the lamina propria. In contrast, hyperplastic polyps with misplaced epithelium are largely composed of proliferating crypts without significant inflammation.

In contrast to hyperplastic polyps with misplaced epithelium, adenomas with misplaced epithelium show hyperchromatic, pseudostratified, cigar-shaped atypical nuclei in cells lining the glands in the submucosal space, with frequent mitoses and even single-cell necrosis. However, both types of lesions may show a discrete rim of lamina propria surrounding misplaced glands. In contrast to benign lesions, adenomas with adenocarcinoma typically show irregular infiltrating crypts and desmoplasia, unlike the other lesions discussed earlier.

Natural History and Treatment (see also under Pathogenesis)

Typical hyperplastic polyps do not normally increase in size over time.[14-17] Until recently, small hyperplastic polyps were not thought to require definitive treatment,

Feature	Hyperplastic Polyp	Serrated Adenoma
TABLE 15–2. Hyperplastic Polyp Versus Serrated Adenoma		
Size	<0.5 cm	>0.5 cm
Crypt dilatation	Surface	Base
Surface pseudostratification	–	+→++
Horizontal crypts	+/–	++
Endocrine cells	++	+/–
Nuclear atypia	Mild, base only	Mild→marked, surface and base
Cytoplasmic eosinophilia	+/–	++
Mitoses	+/– Base only	++ Surface and base

+, few; ++, abundant; –, negative.

although they are typically removed in the process of endoscopy with biopsy.

The biologic characteristics and natural history of large hyperplastic-appearing polyps have become controversial in recent years. Hyperplastic polyps that measure greater than 1 cm often form sessile lesions and occur mainly in the right colon. Some of these have been reported to be associated with serrated adenomatous change and even adenocarcinoma.[18-21] Thus, recent data suggest that large hyperplastic polyps should be considered a separate entity, similar to serrated adenomas (discussed later under Serrated Adenoma). Thus, the previously commonly accepted theory that all hyperplastic polyps are benign lesions with no malignant potential has recently come into controversy.[7] As has been mentioned, evidence is rapidly accumulating that supports the theory that some subtypes of hyperplastic polyps may in fact have neoplastic potential.[6]

Hyperplastic Polyposis

Hyperplastic polyposis is a recently described entity (1980) with rapidly evolving diagnostic criteria.[22-24] Although familial clustering has been documented, no consistent pattern of inheritance has been reported.[23] This is probably an underrecognized entity primarily because most patients are asymptomatic unless an associated malignancy develops. It occurs equally among males and females and has been reported in children and young adults as well.[25,26]

The following diagnostic criteria have been suggested[24]: (1) at least five histologically confirmed hyperplastic polyps proximal to the sigmoid colon, of which at least two are greater than 10 mm in diameter, (2) any number of hyperplastic polyps proximal to the sigmoid colon in a subject with a first-degree relative with hyperplastic polyposis, or (3) more than 30 hyperplastic polyps of any size distributed evenly throughout the colon.

Approximately one third of cases have been associated with adenocarcinoma; thus, a definite but poorly defined risk of colorectal carcinoma has been found among patients with this syndrome.[23,24-27] In this syndrome, the largest polyps are often found in the right colon. In one study of 12 patients, seven developed colorectal carcinoma, and five of these cases occurred concurrently at the time of diagnosis of hyperplastic polyposis.[28] Eleven of the 12 subjects also had dysplastic polyps, that is, either serrated or conventional adenomas. Most patients with hyperplastic polyposis who develop colorectal cancer have mixed hyperplastic/adenomatous polyps (see later), or they simply have abundant conventional and numerous hyperplastic polyps. A distinctive genetic pathway for tumors arising in the setting of hyperplastic polyposis

has been recently postulated.[28,29] This is characterized by loss of heterozygosity (LOH) of chromosome 1p, with a lower frequency of K-*ras* mutations and p53 overexpression. Some have shown that microsatellite instability pathways may be important in patients who have carcinomas that arise in this disorder.

INFLAMMATORY POLYPS

Inflammatory polyps are defined as intraluminal projections of mucosa that are formed of a non-neoplastic mixture of stromal and epithelial components and inflammatory cells. These include inflammatory "pseudopolyps" (both related and not related to inflammatory bowel disease [IBD]), prolapse-type inflammatory polyps, and their many variants, as well as inflammatory myoglandular polyps.

Inflammatory Pseudopolyps

Inflammatory pseudopolyps represent areas of inflamed and regenerating mucosa that project above the level of the surrounding mucosa, which is frequently ulcerated. They generally develop as a response to either localized or diffuse inflammatory diseases, such as Crohn's disease or ulcerative colitis, but they also occur in association with other disorders such as ischemic colitis,[30] neonatal necrotizing enterocolitis,[31] and infectious colitis,[32] and they commonly form at the edges of intestinal ulcers and mucosal anastomoses. The pathogenesis is related to full-thickness ulceration of the mucosa, followed by inflammation and regenerative hyperplasia of the intervening nonulcerated epithelium. In rare cases, the patient may have no apparent underlying inflammatory disorder.

PATHOLOGIC FEATURES

Grossly, inflammatory pseudopolyps may be sessile or pedunculated. They are almost always smaller than 2 cm, but so-called giant inflammatory polyps may reach large sizes and cause obstruction.[33] *Filiform polyposis* refers to the presence of numerous dense, filamentous polyps that can project several centimeters above the surrounding mucosa.[34] This form of polyposis is usually associated with IBD or, rarely, juvenile polyposis.

Histologically, some polyps, particularly those adjacent to ulcers or anastomotic sites, are formed entirely or nearly entirely by inflamed granulation tissue (Fig. 15-2). However, most inflammatory pseudopolyps are composed of a mixture of inflamed lamina propria and distorted colonic epithelium; surface erosions may or may not be present (Figs. 15-3 and 15-4). Colonic crypts are often dilated, branched, and hyperplastic, and neutrophilic cryptitis and crypt abscesses may be prominent. In the later stages of development, inflammatory polyps may consist of many finger-like projec-

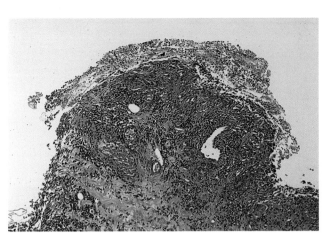

FIGURE 15–2. Granulation tissue polyp. This type of inflammatory pseudopolyp is composed entirely of inflamed granulation tissue and an overlying cap of necroinflammatory exudate. Although they are most common around anastomotic sites, granulation tissue polyps can be present in association with chronic inflammatory bowel disease (as in the illustrated case) or in other conditions that produce mucosal ulceration.

tions of normal or near-normal mucosa surrounding a core of submucosal tissue.

Three potential pitfalls can occur in the histologic evaluation of inflammatory pseudopolyps. First, rarely, dysplasia may develop in these lesions, particularly in those associated with IBD. However, much more commonly, regenerating epithelium, particularly in inflamed or eroded areas, can be extreme, simulating a neoplastic process. Careful attention to surface maturation, which is usually noted in regenerating epithelium and almost never in dysplasia, can help in making this distinction in difficult cases. Second, bizarrely shaped, enlarged, or

multinucleated stromal cells that can mimic sarcoma may develop in inflammatory pseudopolyps.[35] These cells may be spindled or epithelioid in shape and often aggregate at the surface of the polyp in areas of ulceration and granulation tissue reaction (Fig. 15-5).

Finally, in many instances, the histologic appearance of inflammatory pseudopolyps may be indistinguishable from that of juvenile polyps. Distinction between these two types of lesions is based largely on clinical information, such as the age of the patient (almost all such polyps in young children are juvenile polyps), the presence or absence of a clinical history of a hamartomatous polyposis syndrome (juvenile polyposis, Cowden disease, and Bannayan-Riley-Ruvalcaba syndrome can all have juvenile-type polyps), and the presence or absence of an underlying inflammatory injury or chronic disease.

NATURAL HISTORY AND TREATMENT

Inflammatory pseudopolyps tend to persist even after healing of the surrounding mucosa has taken place. They are frequently found in quiescent ulcerative colitis. These polyps are not considered precancerous, and they have no increased tendency for neoplastic transformation. Treatment is usually directed at the underlying inflammatory condition. Rarely, surgical excision is indicated when large or numerous polyps cause symptoms secondary to bleeding or obstruction.[33]

Prolapse-type Inflammatory Polyps

Mucosal prolapse syndrome was proposed by du Boulay and colleagues in 1983 as a unifying term for the clinicopathologic abnormalities underlying solitary rectal ulcer syndrome and related entities.[36] However,

FIGURE 15–3. Inflammatory pseudopolyps in ulcerative colitis. **A,** A colonic resection specimen shows broad, shallow ulcers that are surrounded by raised, erythematous tags of mucosa. (Photograph courtesy of Emma E. Furth, MD, University of Pennsylvania, Philadelphia, PA.) **B,** Inflammatory pseudopolyps in patients with chronic inflammatory bowel disease are frequently composed of a mixture of dense mucosal lymphoplasmacytic infiltrate, mucosal edema, and distorted dilated crypts.

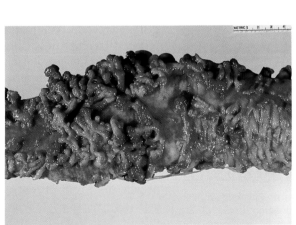

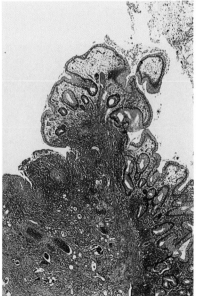

A   **B**

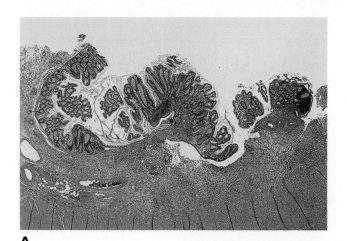

A

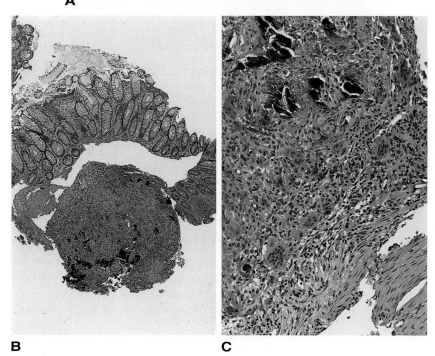

B

C

FIGURE 15–4. Inflammatory pseudopolyps in patients without chronic inflammatory bowel disease. **A,** Raised tags of distorted and edematous mucosa project above adjacent ulcer sites in a patient with colonic ischemia related to use of NSAIDs. Unlike the situation of patients with ulcerative colitis, the mucosa away from the ulcer in this case is normal (left of field). **B,** Inflammatory pseudopolyp at a polypectomy site. A polypoid area was biopsied to rule out residual adenoma. **C,** At higher power, a dense submucosal stromal proliferation contains numerous multinucleated giant cells surrounding areas of stromal calcification.

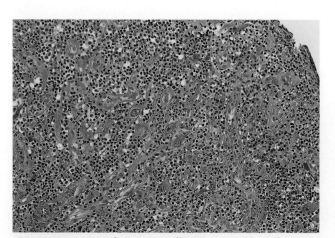

FIGURE 15–5. "Pseudosarcoma cells." Bizarre, enlarged stromal cells may occasionally be seen in granulation tissue of an inflammatory pseudopolyp. Such cells can be confused with sarcoma, carcinoma, or viral infection (e.g., cytomegalovirus).

prolapse-type inflammatory polyps more commonly develop as the result of localized protuberances of mucosa unrelated to the solitary rectal ulcer syndrome. The pathogenesis, in all instances, is related to traction, distortion, and twisting of mucosa caused by peristalsis-induced trauma; this leads to torsion of blood vessels and tissue damage, localized ischemia, and repair in the form of lamina propria fibrosis. Depending on the anatomic location of the injury and the underlying cause, these polyps may be referred to as *inflammatory cloacogenic polyps of the anal transitional zone, inflammatory cap polyps, colitis cystica polyposa,* or *diverticular disease–associated polyps.* All demonstrate some overlapping histologic abnormalities that are usually the result of mucosal prolapse.[37] Inflammatory cap polyps, colitis cystica profunda, and diverticular disease–associated polyps are described in detail in the following sections.

Additionally, solitary or multiple polyps that demonstrate common histopathologic features of mucosal prolapse have been variably called *polypoid prolapsing mucosal folds*[37] or *prolapse-induced inflammatory polyps*.[38] The classic histologic features of prolapse-induced inflammatory polyps include (1) a variable degree of fibromuscular hyperplasia of the lamina propria, (2) thickening, splaying, and vertical extension of the muscularis mucosae into the lamina propria, (3) crypt abnormalities (e.g., elongation, hyperplasia, architectural distortion, and serration), and (4) a variable degree of inflammation and reactive epithelial change (Fig. 15-6).[37,38]

Inflammatory Cap Polyps

Inflammatory cap polyps were first described in abstract form in 1985 by Williams and coworkers.[39] These rare lesions almost always occur in the setting of cap polyposis, in which dozens of these types of polyps develop. There is no sex predilection, and ages range from 17 to 82 years.[40] Clinically, patients with cap polyposis often present with diarrhea, mucoid stools, gastrointestinal bleeding, and/or tenesmus. Occasionally, this is accompanied by severe hypoproteinemia. In fact, a direct loss of protein from cap polyps was confirmed in one 54-year-old woman by scintigraphy with the aid of technetium 99m (Tc99m)-labeled

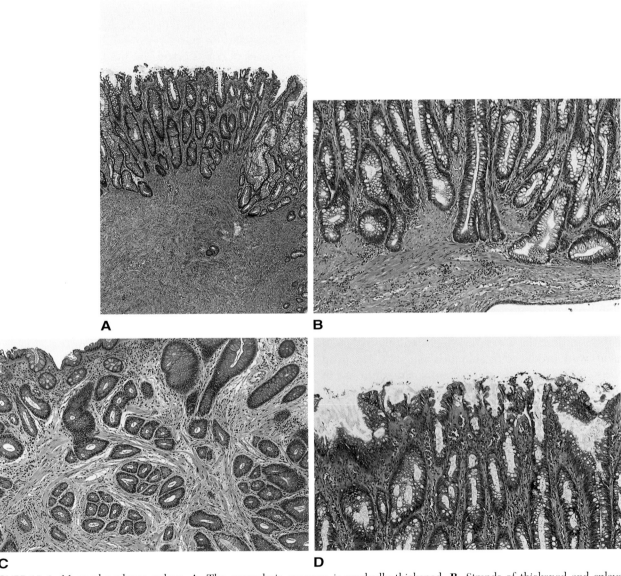

FIGURE 15–6. Mucosal prolapse polyps. **A,** The muscularis mucosae is markedly thickened. **B,** Strands of thickened and splayed muscularis mucosae extend around the crypt bases and into the overlying lamina propria. The crypts themselves assume an angulated and distorted appearance. **C,** When embedded tangentially, prolapse polyps show strands of smooth muscle that appear to encircle colonic crypts, which frequently assume a "diamond" shape. **D,** More superficially, mucosal prolapse polyps often contain regenerative, serrated epithelium that can mimic a hyperplastic polyp or even an adenoma.

diethylenetriaminepentaacetic acid (DTPA) complexed to human serum albumin.[41]

Endoscopically, most cap polyps are small sessile or semipedunculated lesions that range in size from a few millimeters to 2 cm. The most common location is the rectum or rectosigmoid; less commonly, the descending colon is the site.[41-45] Rarely, cap polyps may involve the entire colon and even the stomach.[40,46] Multiple polyps are typically located at the crests of mucosal folds separated by normal or edematous mucosa.

Histologically, cap polyps are non-neoplastic lesions composed of elongated, dilated, or tortuous hyperplastic colonic crypts with abundant inflammation in the lamina propria and a characteristic "cap" of inflamed and ulcerated granulation tissue. Goblet cells of cap polyps have been shown by immunohistochemistry to express nonsulfated mucins.[45] The intervening lamina propria typically contains increased acute and chronic inflammatory cells. The endoscopic "cap" is composed of an inflammatory exudate. Some polyps may contain splayed smooth muscle fibers and/or fibrosis suggestive of mucosal prolapse etiology.[40,43] Many patients with multiple polyps require surgical resection for resolution of their symptoms,[41-45] although some patients improve spontaneously[40] or with *Helicobacter pylori* eradication therapy.[46] Isolated polyps are treated by simple polypectomy.

Colitis Cystica Profunda/Polyposa

CLINICAL FEATURES

Colitis cystica profunda is a rare benign condition characterized by cystic dilatation and misplacement of mature crypts through the muscularis mucosae into the submucosa and/or deeper layers of the bowel wall. The term *colitis cystica polyposa* was first used by Virchow in 1863 to describe a case in which multiple polypoid lesions were produced by submucosal cysts.[47] The term *colitis cystica profunda* subsequently came into use in 1957[48]; most affected patients have both submucosal cysts and associated polypoid lesions. Similar lesions are found in the stomach (gastritis cystica profunda), where they are most frequently associated with post–Billroth II gastrectomies,[49] and in the small bowel (enteritis cystica profunda), where they are often associated with Peutz-Jeghers syndrome.[50]

Rarely, colitis cystica profunda may occur as an isolated lesion (or lesions) in a patient with an otherwise apparently normal colon.[51,52] However, most cases of colitis cystica profunda occur in association with some form of colonic abnormality. The most common association is with the solitary rectal ulcer syndrome,[47,53-55] in which the lesions are rectosigmoid in location. Distal lesions (sometimes called *proctitis cystica profunda*) have also been reported in paraplegics,[56] in patients with self-inflicted rectal trauma,[57] and in patients with postirradiation colonic strictures.[58,59] Less commonly, a diffuse form of colitis cystica profunda occurs in patients with IBD (including ulcerative colitis, Crohn's disease, and unclassified forms[60]) or infectious dysentery.[47]

The pathogenesis of colitis cystica profunda is believed to be related to prolapse and subsequent torsion and trauma of the mucosa and submucosa, leading to vascular compromise and ischemia.[47] In solitary rectal ulcer syndrome, mucosal prolapse results in ischemia and ulceration by virtue of traction exerted on blood vessels.[47] However, in colitis cystica profunda associated with infectious or idiopathic inflammatory bowel disease, the pathologic changes probably occur as a result of misplacement and entrapment of regenerating glands in the submucosa during the process of reepithelialization and tissue healing of ulcers.

Guest and Reznick[47] reviewed the clinical features of 144 cases of colitis cystica profunda. Patients ranged in age from 4 to 76 years (median, 30 years). Males and females were approximately equally affected.[47] The most common presenting symptoms included blood in the stool (68%), mucoid stools (43%), diarrhea (27%), tenesmus (13%), and abdominal discomfort (12%).[47] Rarely, patients presented with obstruction.[51]

PATHOLOGIC FEATURES

Grossly, colitis cystica profunda can be a focal, segmental, or diffuse lesion. Focal or segmental lesions can mimic invasive adenocarcinoma. Transrectal ultrasound and other imaging modalities can aid in this distinction by demonstrating multiple cysts limited to the submucosa and lack of lymph node involvement in the former.[53]

Histologically, the condition is characterized by the presence of multiple cystically dilated, mucin-filled crypts in the submucosa and occasionally in the muscularis propria or serosa. The stroma surrounding misplaced crypts usually consists of lamina propria; this is helpful in distinguishing it from adenocarcinoma, which often has a desmoplastic stroma. Furthermore, misplaced glands in colitis cystica profunda often grow in a lobular configuration without jagged borders or the unusual, irregularly shaped glandular profiles more typical of adenocarcinoma. Misplaced crypts typically show either normal or reactive-appearing colonic epithelium. A mild degree of mucin depletion, pseudostratification, and increased mitotic activity may be noted as well. However, loss of nuclear polarity, increased nucleus-to-cytoplasm ratio, and atypical mitoses should alert one to the possibility of adenocarcinoma. Lamina propria surrounding misplaced glands and lack of dysplastic-appearing epithelium are key features that help distinguish colitis cystica profunda from invasive adenocarcinoma (Table 15-3; Fig. 15-7).

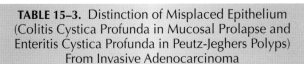

TABLE 15–3. Distinction of Misplaced Epithelium (Colitis Cystica Profunda in Mucosal Prolapse and Enteritis Cystica Profunda in Peutz-Jeghers Polyps) From Invasive Adenocarcinoma

Misplaced epithelium
  Cystically dilated, mucin-filled crypts in submucosa, muscularis propria, serosa
  Normal composition of epithelial cells in misplaced crypts, including brush border
  Lobular arrangement of crypts
  Lack of dysplasia in misplaced crypts
  Lack of desmoplastic response around misplaced crypts
  Presence of lamina propria around misplaced crypts (may show fibrosis or fibromuscular obliteration similar to that of the overlying lamina propria)
  Hemorrhage, congestion, hemosiderin usually present
Invasive adenocarcinoma
  Irregular, nonlobulated crypts with back-to-back configuration
  Variability in size and shape of crypts
  Dysplastic cytologic features
  Atypical mitoses
  Desmoplasia
  Lack of rim of lamina propria surrounding crypts
  Hemorrhage, congestion, hemosiderin variably present

In many patients with rectal prolapse, treatment of the defecation disorder itself (e.g., education to avoid straining at defecation, a high-fiber diet, and bulk laxatives) leads to remission of colitis cystica profunda.[53,55] Some patients require surgical resection because of obstruction,[51] confusion with carcinoma, severe symptoms, or coexistent IBD.[60]

Diverticular Disease–Associated Polyps

Polyps that occur in association with diverticulosis are of two types—inverted diverticula or polypoid prolapsing mucosal folds. Polyps of the former type have been described in patients with inverted Meckel's diverticula of the ileum (wherein they may cause intussusception),[61] isolated inverted colonic diverticula, or inverted sigmoid diverticula in the setting of sigmoid diverticulosis.[62,63] Inverted colonic diverticula usually range from 0.2 to 2 cm in size. They may be sessile or pedunculated but characteristically have the same color as the surrounding mucosa.[60,63] These polyps tend to vanish with gentle pressure either from the biopsy forceps or from air insufflation at endoscopy.[60,63] Bowel perforation may occur as a result of endoscopic polypectomy in cases in which the inverted diverticulum mimics an adenoma.[63,64]

Polypoid prolapsing mucosal folds are the more common form of diverticular disease–associated polyps. Grossly, these appear as bright red, polypoid or slightly elevated patches of mucosa in patients with sigmoid diverticulosis.[65,60] Swollen mucosal folds seen between diverticular ostia may reveal an apical brown discoloration. More advanced lesions characteristically show small, brownish polypoid protrusions of the mucosal folds. Polyps normally range from 0.5 to 3 cm in size.

Histologically, early lesions show vascular congestion, hemorrhage, and hemosiderin deposition. More advanced lesions reveal edema, capillary thrombi, lamina propria fibrosis, and crypt architectural changes such as dilatation and branching. The most advanced, "leaflike" polyps show changes typically seen in mucosal prolapse, such as smooth muscle ingrowth into the lamina propria, crypt hyperplasia, mucin depletion, and serrated hyperplastic changes of the epithelium. Epithelial hyperplasia may be marked and should not be mistaken for an adenoma.[66] Rarely, one may see pseudosarcomatous changes of the stroma, characterized by enlarged and hyperchromatic myofibroblasts that should not be mistaken for malignant sarcoma.[66]

Redundant mucosal folds occur in a large majority (90% to 100%) of patients with advanced sigmoid diverticulosis, although only a minority develop grossly polypoid lesions or frank prolapse-like histologic alterations of the mucosa[67,68] (Fig. 15-8). Thickening of the taenia coli, which leads to shortening of the sigmoid, is believed to be the initiating pathogenetic event in the development of these lesions.

Patients with diverticular disease–associated polyps may develop chronic low-grade blood loss.[69] Treatment is similar to that for diverticulosis in general and in many instances has been shown to result in regression of polyps.[69]

Inflammatory Myoglandular Polyps

Inflammatory myoglandular polyps were described by Nakamura and associates in 1992.[70] They are rare, often underrecognized lesions. Of the 32 cases reported by Nakamura and colleagues, a majority of polyps were solitary and located in the sigmoid colon (18 cases), with the remainder distributed among the transverse colon (8 cases) or descending colon (3 cases) and rectum (3 cases). An inflammatory myoglandular polyp of the terminal ileum has also been reported.[71] The most common symptoms include occult or overt rectal bleeding.[70] Affected patients are predominantly male with a wide age range (15 to 78 years).[70] The pathogenesis of these lesions is controversial. Chronic trauma and mucosal prolapse have been proposed as etiologic possibilities. However, some authors believe that these polyps represent a type of hamartoma.

Grossly, inflammatory myoglandular polyps range in size from 0.4 to 2.5 cm.[70] Most are pedunculated and spherical and contain a smooth surface, either with or without surface erosion. The cut surface typically contains scattered mucin-filled cysts set within a dark brown stroma.[70] Histologically, these polyps are composed of a

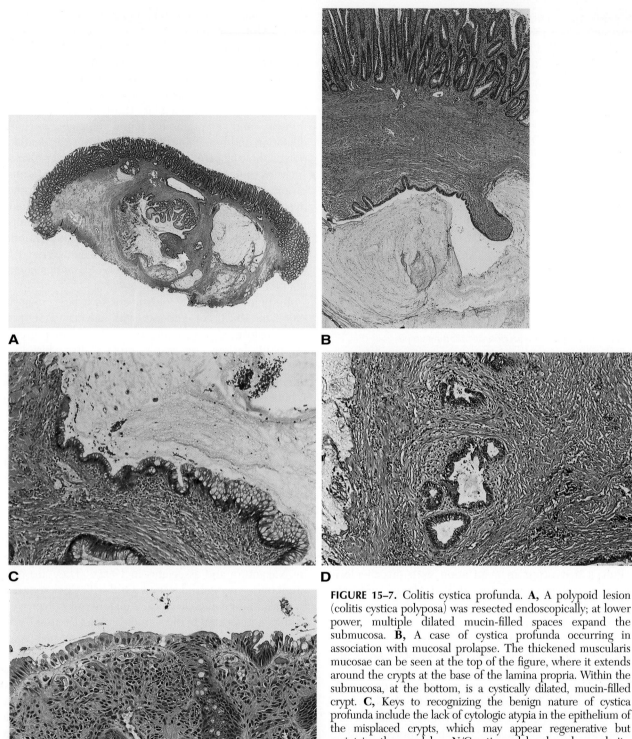

FIGURE 15–7. Colitis cystica profunda. **A,** A polypoid lesion (colitis cystica polyposa) was resected endoscopically; at lower power, multiple dilated mucin-filled spaces expand the submucosa. **B,** A case of cystica profunda occurring in association with mucosal prolapse. The thickened muscularis mucosae can be seen at the top of the figure, where it extends around the crypts at the base of the lamina propria. Within the submucosa, at the bottom, is a cystically dilated, mucin-filled crypt. **C,** Keys to recognizing the benign nature of cystica profunda include the lack of cytologic atypia in the epithelium of the misplaced crypts, which may appear regenerative but maintains the usual low N/C ratio and basal nuclear polarity. **D,** Hemosiderin deposition in the stroma and the presence of lamina propria around misplaced crypts are additional features that separate cystica profunda from infiltrating adenocarcinoma. **E,** One of the most common associations of colitis cystica profunda is with solitary rectal ulcer syndrome (occult rectosigmoid prolapse), in which case the surrounding nonpolypoid mucosa shows characteristic fibromuscular proliferation in the lamina propria.

FIGURE 15–8. Diverticular disease–associated polyps. **A,** Redundant mucosa folds in patients with sigmoid diverticular disease are produced by thickening and shortening of the muscularis propria, as is seen in this section. A more prominent redundant fold at center has the low-power appearance of a pedunculated polyp. **B,** Biopsy specimen of a polyp in a different patient with sigmoid diverticular disease shows features indistinguishable histologically from those of inflammatory pseudopolyps in patients with chronic inflammatory bowel disease, including dense lamina propria chronic inflammation, surface erosion, and distortion of crypts.

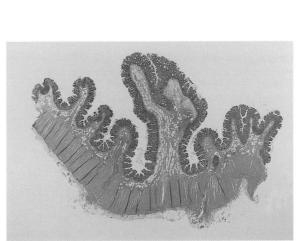

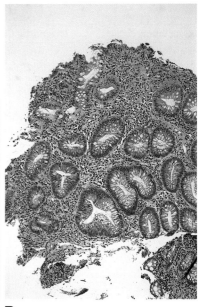

A   **B**

treelike network of radially arranged smooth muscle, similar to Peutz-Jeghers polyps. Hyperplastic and cystically dilated crypts are typical. At the periphery or surface of the polyp, one often finds luminal fibrino-inflammatory exudate and granulation tissue. The surface epithelium may appear regenerative, with a serrated or hyperplastic appearance, and may show mucin depletion. Frequently, hemosiderin deposition is noted within the lamina propria, reflecting areas of mucosal erosion and hemorrhage.[70] The main distinguishing features between inflammatory myoglandular polyps and juvenile polyps include the younger mean age of patients with juvenile polyps and the presence of only a trace amount of smooth muscle within the lamina propria of juvenile polyps. In contrast to inflammatory myoglandular polyps, Peutz-Jeghers polyps do not typically reveal surface erosions or a granulation tissue reaction. However, in some isolated cases, distinction between these entities may not be possible solely on histologic grounds.

HAMARTOMATOUS POLYPS

Hamartomas are defined as overgrowths of cells and tissues native to the anatomic location in which they occur. In the gastrointestinal tract, hamartomas typically incorporate both stromal and epithelial components. Hamartomas are most often solitary but may occur as part of a hamartomatous polyposis syndrome such as Peutz-Jeghers syndrome, juvenile polyposis, Cowden disease, or the Bannayan-Riley-Ruvalcaba syndrome. Because of genotypic and phenotypic overlap between Cowden disease and Bannayan-Riley-Ruvalcaba syndrome, these two conditions may in fact represent

variations of the same entity.[72,73] Cronkhite-Canada syndrome, another form of gastrointestinal polyposis, is believed to have an inflammatory rather than a genetic basis, but it is discussed in this section because of its histologic resemblance to juvenile polyposis.

In aggregate, the hamartomatous polyposis syndromes account for less than 1% of the annual incidence of colorectal carcinoma in the United States and Canada.[72] In addition, isolated sporadic juvenile polyps and (less commonly) Peutz-Jeghers polyps occur, but these have essentially no malignant potential.

Juvenile Polyps and Juvenile Polyposis

CLINICAL FEATURES

Juvenile polyps occur in four distinct settings—sporadic or isolated juvenile polyps of the colon, infantile juvenile polyposis syndrome, juvenile polyposis coli, and generalized juvenile polyposis syndrome (involving the stomach, small bowel, and colon) (Table 15-4). Sporadic or isolated juvenile polyps are the most common type of colon polyp among patients in the first decade of life, but they occur quite commonly in adults as well. One study reported a mean age of occurrence of 5.9 years.[74] Children usually present with either painless rectal bleeding or prolapse of the polyp through the rectum.[74] Adults, if they are symptomatic at all, often present with rectal bleeding.

Juvenile Polyposis Syndrome. Juvenile polyposis syndrome, first described in 1964 by McColl and coworkers,[75] is the most common gastrointestinal hamartomatous polyposis syndrome. Separation of isolated juvenile polyps in childhood from juvenile

TABLE 15–4. Types of Juvenile Polyps

Association	Diagnostic Criteria	Inheritance	Risk of Malignancy
Solitary	<3 Polyps, no family history of juvenile polyposis	None	Essentially none
Juvenile polyposis of infancy	Diarrhea, protein-losing enteropathy, bleeding, rectal prolapse, polyps from stomach through rectum (resembles adult Cronkhite-Canada syndrome)	Autosomal recessive (?)	Usually fatal before age 2 years from non-neoplastic complications
Juvenile polyposis coli	(1) Any number of polyps in a patient with family history, or (2) ≥3 polyps* without family history. Polyps are predominantly colonic; small bowel polyps, if present, are few in number	Autosomal dominant, but family history in only 20% to 50%	68% estimated risk of colorectal carcinoma by age 60
Generalized juvenile polyposis	Polyps throughout stomach, small bowel, and colorectum, usually numbering from 50 to 200	Autosomal dominant, but family history in only 20% to 50%	At least 55% risk of gastrointestinal carcinoma, including stomach, duodenum, jejunum, ileum, and/or colorectum
Familial gastric juvenile polyposis	Multiple polyps limited to the stomach; not well characterized	Unknown whether truly a separate category from generalized juvenile polyposis	Increased risk of gastric carcinoma; ~ 25% risk in one study

*Some investigators use ≥3 polyps, ≥5 polyps, or ≥10 polyps.

polyposis syndrome is important because of their divergent clinical behaviors and neoplastic risks (see under Natural History and Treatment). Criteria for juvenile polyposis syndrome are controversial and are rapidly evolving with the advent of newer molecular diagnostic techniques. However, at this point, the diagnosis should be suggested in any patient with (1) any number of polyps in probands with a family history of juvenile polyposis, (2) polyposis involving the entire gastrointestinal tract, or (3) ≥3 colonic juvenile polyps. (This latter figure has ranged from 3 to 10 polyps according to various diagnostic alorithms.)[76] Hamartomas do not occur outside the gastrointestinal tract, but congenital birth defects are reported in 15% of juvenile polyposis patients; these include malrotation of the gut and cardiac and genitourinary defects.

In 1998, linkage analysis in a large Iowa kindred demonstrated that a gene for familial juvenile polyposis maps to chromosome 18q21.1, a region containing both the *DCC* and the *DPC4/SMAD4* tumor suppressor genes.[77] Germline truncating mutations in *DPC4/SMAD4* were shown shortly thereafter to be responsible for a subset of juvenile polyposis patients.[78] In 2001, germline mutations in the gene encoding bone morphogenic protein receptor 1A, *BMPR1A*, were also reported in juvenile polyposis families lacking *DPC4/SMAD4* mutations.[79] *DPC4/SMAD4* mutations account for 35% to 60% of patients with juvenile polyposis syndrome in North America; *BMPR1A* mutations are found in approximately 40% of patients lacking *DPC4/SMAD4* mutations,[80] suggesting that there is additional (as yet undefined) genetic heterogeneity in juvenile polyposis syndrome. Although it is transmitted in an autosomal dominant fashion, only

20% to 50% of affected patients have a family history of juvenile polyposis.[72]

PATHOLOGIC FEATURES

Isolated juvenile polyps are most common in the rectosigmoid colon (54%). However, 37% of patients have polyps proximal to the splenic flexure.[74] In juvenile polyposis coli (polyps limited to the colon), polyps are most common in the rectosigmoid region and typically number up to 200 (Fig. 15-9). The classic form of juvenile polyp (Fig. 15-10) found most frequently in isolated cases is unilobulated and has a smooth, round surface contour. Histologically, these polyps are characterized by numerous cystic and dilated, often tortuous, crypts, some filled with neutrophils and inspissated mucin (which reflects the older term, *mucous retention polyp*). The intervening lamina propria is edematous and expanded by lymphocytes and plasma cells and occasional neutrophils and eosinophils. Few strands of muscle fibers may be present as well. In ulcerated cases, the epithelium may be markedly regenerative in appearance, simulating dysplasia. In patients with juvenile polyposis syndrome, both classic (typical) and nonclassic (atypical) polyps are usually found. Nonclassic polyps (Fig. 15-11) are often larger, multilobulated, and villiform, often giving the gross appearance of several polyps attached to a single stalk. Histologically, compared with typical cases, they contain less abundant lamina propria and greater epithelial overgrowth, with many elongated, tortuous, and irregularly shaped crypts.[81] The clonal origin of both the epithelium and the fibroblasts in juvenile polyps from *DPC4/SMAD4* mutation carriers was recently shown by means of fluorescence in situ hybridization.[82]

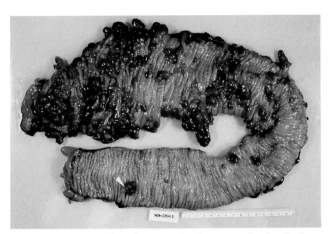

FIGURE 15–9. Juvenile polyposis coli. The resected colon harbors numerous sessile and pedunculated, reddish polyps. These polyps are less numerous than those in familial adenomatous polyposis and are characteristically grouped in the region of the rectosigmoid. (Photograph courtesy of Emma E. Furth, MD, University of Pennsylvania, Philadelphia, PA.)

Syndromic patients may have a combination of other types of polyps as well. Ganglioneuromatous proliferation of mature ganglion cells and nerve bundles may occur in the mucosa and the submucosa of polyps in patients with juvenile polyposis syndrome.[83] Many patients also have separate adenomas or polyps with combined features of a juvenile polyp and an adenoma/dysplasia.[84-86] In fact, true dysplasia (Fig. 15-12) has been detected in up to 30% of polyps of syndromic patients,[81,87] but it is almost never observed in patients with isolated juvenile polyps. Gupta and associates reported dysplasia in only 1 of 331 juvenile polyps from 184 nonpolyposis patients.[74]

NATURAL HISTORY AND TREATMENT

Patients with sporadic juvenile polyps have no increased risk for malignancy.[88,89] Furthermore, they are not predisposed to the development of new juvenile polyps, and they do not require any particular type of follow-up.[89] In contrast, estimates of the risk of gastrointestinal carcinoma in juvenile polyposis syndrome have varied widely. In one large kindred, the risk of upper and/or lower gastrointestinal cancer in affected patients was 55%.[90] In 1995, Desai and colleagues, in a

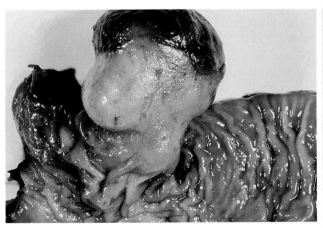

A

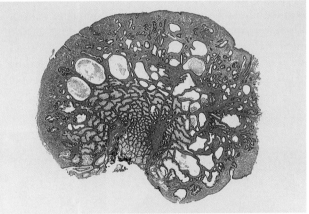

B

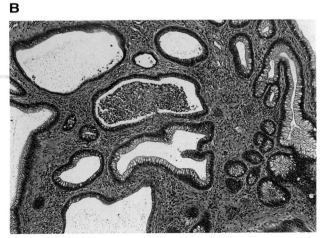

C

FIGURE 15–10. Classic juvenile polyps. **A,** These polyps grossly appear rounded, smooth, and unilobular with an erythematous cap of eroded tissue. (Photograph courtesy of Thomas C. Smyrk, MD, Mayo Clinic, Rochester, MN.) **B,** Their cut surface reveals multiple dilated, mucin-filled crypts, leading to the term "mucus retention polyp." **C,** At higher power, the crypts are dilated and branched. Some, like the one at center, contain crypt abscesses, collections of neutrophils, and/or eosinophils. The surrounding stroma is also expanded and contains numerous mixed inflammatory cells.

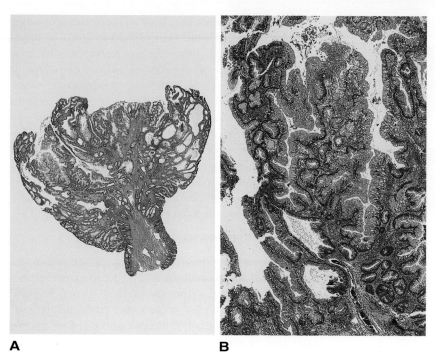

FIGURE 15–11. Atypical juvenile polyp in juvenile polyposis syndrome. **A,** These polyps have a villiform architecture and frequently give the appearance of several polyps attached to the same stalk. **B,** They exhibit more epithelial overgrowth and less abundant stroma in comparison with classic juvenile polyps.

reevaluation of data from the St. Mark's Polyposis Registry, projected an incidence of colorectal carcinoma of 68% through age 60 (see Table 15-3).[91] Surveillance recommendations should take into account the risks of both lower and upper tract cancer, including gastric cancer.[72] Upper and lower endoscopy (including visualization of the entire colon) is usually recommended by age 15 and should be repeated annually. Endoscopic polypectomies and histologic examination of all removed polyps should be performed until the patient is free of polyps, at which point the surveillance interval may be lengthened to 3 years. Consideration should be given to prophylactic gastrectomy or colectomy if diffuse polyposis cannot be controlled by endoscopic polypectomy or if there is a family history of gastrointestinal carcinoma or dysplasia.[92]

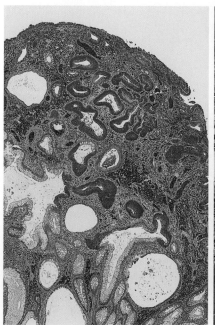
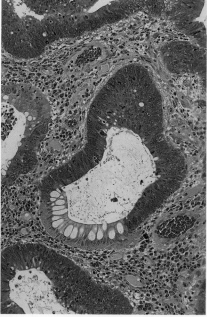

FIGURE 15–12. Dysplasia arising in a juvenile polyp. **A,** A classic juvenile polyp contains an area of hyperchromatic glands at top. **B,** At higher power, the involved crypts, which contain enlarged, hyperchromatic, and crowded nuclei, are cytologically indistinguishable from an adenoma. The crypt at center shows a mixture of dysplastic and nondysplastic epithelium.

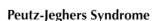

Peutz-Jeghers Syndrome

CLINICAL FEATURES

Peutz-Jeghers syndrome (PJS) is an autosomal dominant syndrome characterized by mucocutaneous pigmentation; distinctive hamartomatous polyps of the small intestine, colon, and stomach; and an increased risk for both intestinal and extraintestinal malignancies (see Chapter 14 for details). Estimates of the incidence of PJS vary widely, from 1 in 8300 births to 1 in 120,000.[93,94] Significant phenotypic variability can occur within PJS kindreds, and patients may not have a family history of PJS. Most patients seek treatment during the second or third decade of life. In one recent study, the average age at presentation was 18 years, with a range from 2 to 62 years.[93] Peutz-Jeghers polyps have also been described in neonates.[95] The main clinical manifestations of PJS include mucocutaneous pigmentation, gastrointestinal polyposis, and an increased risk for gastrointestinal carcinomas, as well as for extraintestinal benign and malignant tumors.

In 1997, the PJS locus was mapped to chromosome 19p13.3; this was achieved through the use of comparative genomic hybridization of PJS polyps in one patient, followed by targeted linkage analysis in 12 affected families.[96] In 1998, two separate reports identified the *LKB1/STK11* gene on 19p13.3 as the main causative gene in PJS.[97,98] Germline mutations in the *LKB1/STK11* tumor suppressor gene, encoding a novel serine threonine kinase, disrupt the function of the protein's kinase domain.[97] Overall, however, *LKB1/STK11* mutations have been found in only approximately 60% of familial and approximately 50% of sporadic cases, suggesting the possibility of genetic heterogeneity in PJS.[99]

PATHOLOGIC FEATURES

Hamartomatous polyps of PJS may occur throughout the gastrointestinal tract but are most common in the small bowel (65% to 95%), followed by the colon (60%) and stomach (20% to 50%).[100] Involved segments of bowel may harbor from 1 to 20 polyps, and these may vary in size from 0.5 to 3 cm. Well-developed polyps located in the small intestine and colon tend to be pedunculated.

Microscopically (Fig. 15-13), the most prominent component is a distinctive, arborizing pattern of smooth muscle derived from the underlying muscularis mucosae. The lamina propria is usually normal in composition and cellularity and does not typically demonstrate increased inflammation. The overlying epithelium is composed of the normal epithelial cells

FIGURE 15–13. Peutz-Jeghers polyps. **A,** Colonic Peutz-Jeghers polyp showing the characteristic overgrowth of epithelium and an arborizing smooth muscle core. **B,** The branching smooth muscle is derived from the muscularis mucosae. **C,** The overlying mucosa is typically non-dysplastic and maintains its normal architecture. Unlike juvenile polyps, the mucosa has a normal ratio of lamina propria to epithelium, and the crypts are not cystically dilated. Cell types normal for that region of the gastrointestinal tract (in this case, goblet cells and absorptive cells) are found within the epithelium.

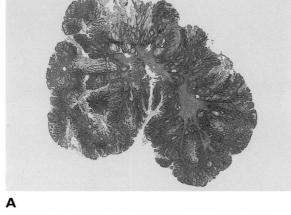

A

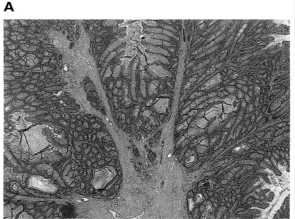

B

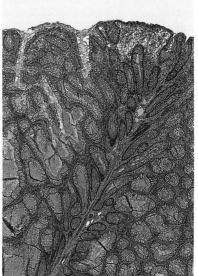

C

typical of the involved segment of the gastrointestinal tract. In most colonic Peutz-Jeghers polyps, the epithelium may show epithelial overgrowth and areas of hyperplasia, but dysplasia is unusual. Nevertheless, nondysplastic epithelium has been shown to be clonal.[96]

Subsequent studies of histologic and molecular alterations have shown that a subset of polyps progress through a hamartoma/adenoma (dysplasia)/carcinoma sequence. Somatic loss of the 19p13.3 allele occurs in a substantial portion of nondysplastic polyps and (in conjunction with germline mutation at this locus) accounts for hamartoma formation,[101,102] whereas dysplasia and carcinoma arise in hamartomas through the acquisition of additional genetic alterations at loci such as *TP53* and *beta-catenin*.[101] Hizawa and coworkers documented adenomatous (dysplastic) foci in 9 of 71 (12.7%) Peutz-Jeghers hamartomas in the gastrointestinal tract.[103] In a study of 52 colonic Peutz-Jeghers polyps, Narita and associates found dysplasia in 3 (5.8%).[104] Intramucosal and invasive carcinomas have been documented in Peutz-Jeghers polyps of the stomach, small bowel, and colon. Carcinomas are more likely to arise in patients with familial PJS. Only a single case report has described the occurrence of carcinoma in a nonsyndromic setting.[105]

Some Peutz-Jeghers polyps show foci of epithelial misplacement, pseudoinvasion, or herniation of benign epithelium into the intestinal wall (all synonymous for the phenomenon of enteritis cystica profunda) (Fig. 15-14). Shepherd and colleagues studied 491 Peutz-Jeghers polyps and reported epithelial misplacement in 10% of small intestinal polyps; however, this phenomenon was never observed in gastric or colonic polyps (see Chapter 13).[106] Polyps with epithelial misplacement are characterized by intramural mucinous cysts that can involve all layers of the bowel wall, including the serosa. Grossly and histologically, these polyps can simulate invasive adenocarcinoma.[107] Helpful histologic discriminators between pseudoinvasion and true carcinoma include the following: (1) lack of cytologic atypia in the deep glands, with a normal composition of epithelial cell types, (2) hemosiderin deposition, and (3) the presence of deep mucinous cysts in pseudoinvasion. Another potential pitfall is the overdiagnosis of misplaced dysplastic epithelium as invasion.[108] Helpful discriminating features in these cases include the presence of both nondysplastic and

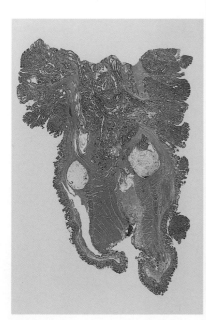

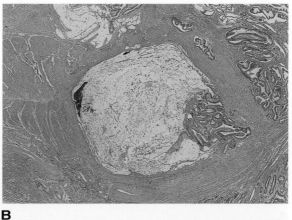

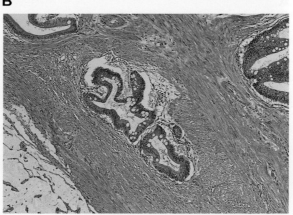

FIGURE 15–14. Epithelial misplacement in Peutz-Jeghers polyps. **A,** At low power, epithelium in the stalk of a Peutz-Jeghers polyp mimics infiltrating carcinoma. At center, dilated glands are found within and deep to the muscularis propria. **B,** A dilated, mucin-filled crypt is seen in the muscularis propria. An epithelial lining with lamina propria is seen at right. **C,** In addition to mucin pools and lamina propria, histologic clues to the benign nature of the misplaced glands include the benign cytology of the involved glands, which contain a normal mix of goblet cells and absorptive cells.

dysplastic epithelium within the dilated misplaced crypts, the presence of lamina propria around the displaced crypts, and the lack of a desmoplastic response in noninvasive cases.

NATURAL HISTORY AND TREATMENT

Non-neoplastic gastrointestinal complications of PJS include gastrointestinal bleeding and abdominal pain related to intussusception or luminal obstruction by large polyps. Intussusception is frequent (occurring in 47% of 222 Japanese PJS patients in a series by Utsunomiya and coworkers) and is most common in the small intestine, owing in part to the pedunculated nature of the small bowel and colonic polyps.[109] Prolapse of pedunculated PJS polyps through the rectum may also occur.[109]

Neoplastic complications of PJS include an increased frequency of both gastrointestinal and extraintestinal neoplasms. Numerous early case reports attested to the increased risk of gastric, small intestinal, and colonic malignancy in PJS, although the absolute risk was debated and was initially thought to be relatively low. Recent studies, however, have confirmed a high risk for cancer development. In a retrospective study from the Mayo Clinic spanning 50 years, 18 of 34 (53%) PJS patients developed noncutaneous cancers, with a mean age of 39.4 years at the time of cancer diagnosis.[110] In particular, the relative risk of gastrointestinal carcinoma (predominantly colon cancers) in this study was 50.5, and in women with PJS, the relative risk of breast and gynecologic cancers was 20.3. In a recent meta-analysis of cancer risk in PJS, Giardiello and associates calculated a cumulative risk for malignancy of 93% in patients 15 to 64 years of age.[111] In that study, the cumulative risk for breast cancer was 54%, colon cancer 39%, pancreatic cancer 36%, gastric cancer 29%, ovarian cancer 21%, and small intestinal cancer 13% (see Table 15-3). Furthermore, significantly increased relative risks were found for cancers of the esophagus (relative risk, 57), stomach (relative risk, 213), small intestine (relative risk, 520), colon (relative risk, 84), pancreas (relative risk, 132), lung (relative risk, 17), breast (relative risk, 15.2), uterus (relative risk, 16), and ovary (relative risk, 27). Although a statistically significantly increased risk for either testicular cancer or cervical cancer could not be demonstrated in Giardiello's study, distinctive tumors in these sites have been reported to occur in PJS.

Surveillance in PJS is indicated for the removal of gastrointestinal polyps and for the early detection of both gastrointestinal and extraintestinal neoplasms.[112] Surveillance recommendations for the gastrointestinal tract include (1) colonoscopy every 1 to 2 years beginning in adolescence and (2) upper endoscopy with either push enteroscopy or double-contrast radiology for imaging of the entire small bowel every 2 years beginning in adolescence. In women, monthly breast self-examinations and annual clinical breast examinations should begin at ages 18 to 20, followed by biannual mammography from ages 25 to 35 and annual mammography after age 40. Minimum gynecologic surveillance recommendations include annual pelvic examinations and Papanicolaou (Pap) smears in women and annular testicular examinations in men. Because of the clearly documented increased risk for pancreatic carcinoma, some authors also advocate yearly pancreatic ultrasound.[113]

Cowden Disease

CLINICAL FEATURES

Cowden disease is an autosomal dominant hamartoma/neoplasia syndrome that bears the family name of the original patient described by Lloyd and Dennis in 1963.[113] In 1996, the susceptibility locus for Cowden disease was mapped to chromosome 10q22-23,[114] and in 1997, germline mutations in the *PTEN* gene on 10q23 were first reported in families with this syndrome.[115,116] Since that time, mutations of the *PTEN* ("phosphatase and tensin homologue, deleted on chromosome ten") tumor suppressor gene have been identified in approximately 80% of patients who meet the strict operational diagnostic criteria set forth by the International Cowden Consortium.[73]

Hamartomas in Cowden disease affect all three germ cell layers but most commonly arise from ectodermal and endodermal elements. Almost all patients (90% to 100%) have mucocutaneous lesions that include trichilemmomas, acral keratoses, and oral papillomas.[73] Breast lesions affect the majority of women and include fibroadenomas, fibrocystic changes, and adenocarcinomas (25% to 50%).[70] Breast carcinoma is occasionally reported in men as well.[117] Thyroid abnormalities, such as goiter and adenoma, are found in one half to two thirds of patients. Thyroid carcinoma occurs in up to 3% to 10% of patients.[73] Macrocephaly, cerebellar gangliocytoma, and genitourinary malformations are also frequent components of Cowden disease. Recently, increased risks for endometrial carcinoma and renal cell carcinoma have been added to the operational criteria for Cowden syndrome.[118]

PATHOLOGIC FEATURES

Gastrointestinal hamartomas are found in only 35% to 40% of patients with Cowden disease. Hamartomatous polyps may affect the stomach, small bowel, and/or colon (Fig. 15-15). The most common esophageal manifestation is glycogenic acanthosis. Most polyps resemble juvenile polyps and consist of cystically dilated, mucin-filled crypts set within an abundant lamina propria.[119,120] Colonic lipomas, fibrolipomas, fibromas,[121] ganglioneuromas, and adenomas[122] have also been

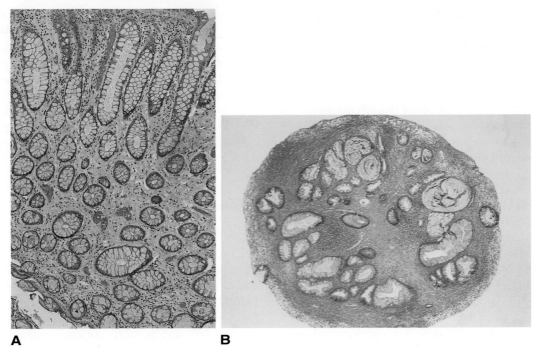

A   **B**

FIGURE 15–15. Cowden disease. **A,** Colonic polyp biopsied from a patient with Cowden disease. There is mild architectural distortion of the crypts, which are arranged in a slightly fibrotic stroma. The epithelium is nondysplastic and contains the usual composition of goblet cells and absorptive cells found in the colon. **B,** In other examples of Cowden disease polyps, the polyps exhibit more prominently dilated glands and are histologically indistinguishable from juvenile polyps.

reported in Cowden disease. Loss of expression of the wild-type *PTEN* allele, coupled with the germline *PTEN* mutation, was demonstrated in both gastrointestinal hamartomas and colonic adenomas of several patients with Cowden disease.[122]

NATURAL HISTORY AND TREATMENT

A definite increased risk of gastrointestinal malignancy has not yet been documented in Cowden disease, but the true risk is unknown because of the rarity of this syndrome. For this reason, endoscopic surveillance of the gastrointestinal tract has been recommended.[72] Perhaps more importantly, screening and surveillance are directed at breast and thyroid malignancies.[72] Recommendations for women include monthly breast self-examinations, annual clinical breast examinations beginning in late adolescence, and mammography beginning at age 25. Annual clinical examination of the thyroid in both sexes should begin in late adolescence with or without parallel use of thyroid ultrasound every 1 to 2 years.[72]

Cronkhite-Canada Syndrome

CLINICAL FEATURES

Cronkhite-Canada syndrome is a nonhereditary polyposis syndrome of unknown etiology (see Chapter 13). Since the first description of this syndrome by Cronkhite and Canada in 1955,[123] hundreds of patients have been reported. Although it is worldwide in its distribution, most cases originate from Japan, Europe, or the United States. Unlike most polyposis syndromes, the mean age of onset is 59 years.[124] Infantile cases of Cronkhite-Canada syndrome are only rarely reported.[125]

Colonic polyps associated with the Cronkhite-Canada syndrome occur in association with distinct ectodermal abnormalities, such as alopecia of both the scalp and body hair, dystrophy of the nails, and skin hyperpigmentation.[123] Skin lesions are usually manifested by the presence of light to dark brown macules on the extremities, face, neck, palms, and soles.[124] Affected patients often present with a variable combination of diarrhea, weight loss, nausea and vomiting, anorexia, and gastrointestinal bleeding. In some cases, diarrhea may result in severe electrolyte abnormalities, with the development of seizures or tetany.[124]

PATHOLOGIC FEATURES

Polyps in Cronkhite-Canada syndrome occur throughout the gastrointestinal tract but spare the esophagus. Histologically, in the colon, they closely resemble juvenile polyps, with cystically dilated, tortuous crypts containing inspissated mucin (Fig. 15-16). The intervening lamina propria is edematous and contains increased numbers of mononuclear cells and eosinophils.

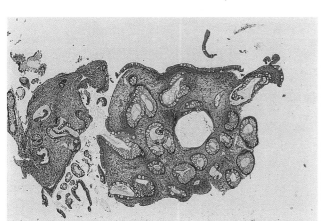

A

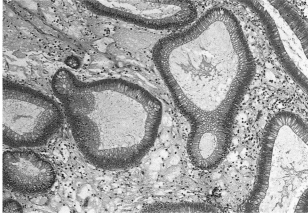

B

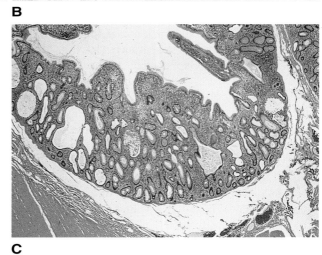

C

FIGURE 15–16. Cronkhite-Canada syndrome. **A,** Biopsy specimen of one of numerous colonic polyps in a patient with Cronkhite-Canada syndrome shows dilated and branched crypts within an expanded lamina propria. **B,** At higher power, cystically dilated glands are filled with mucin; the surrounding lamina propria is edematous and contains increased numbers of mononuclear cells. **C,** Although individual Cronkhite-Canada polyps are histologically indistinguishable from juvenile polyps, biopsy of the intervening nonpolypoid colonic mucosa in a patient with Cronkhite-Canada syndrome shows lamina propria edema and scattered cystically dilated glands.

Burke and Sobin compared the histology of Cronkhite-Canada polyps with that of juvenile polyps.[126] The histologic features of each type are microscopically indistinguishable, although colonic juvenile polyps are more frequently pedunculated.[126] However, in patients with Cronkhite-Canada syndrome, the intervening non-polypoid intestinal mucosa shows pathologic changes such as edema, cystically dilated glands, and increased inflammatory cells (see Fig. 15-16), whereas the intervening mucosa in juvenile polyposis is normal.

NATURAL HISTORY AND TREATMENT

The malignant potential of colonic Cronkhite-Canada polyps is controversial. There have been multiple reports of affected patients who have also had adenoma,[127-130] colorectal carcinoma,[128,129,131] or gastric cancer.[131] Goto and Shimokawa calculated that 18.6% of Japanese Cronkhite-Canada patients suffered from gastrointestinal cancer.[131] Although some authors indicate that dysplastic changes may occur within the polyps,[129,131,132] it is not clear whether these might represent separate incidental adenomas. The mortality rate in Cronkhite-Canada syndrome is high (50% to 60%). Death usually results from malnutrition, gastrointestinal bleeding, or infection. Treatment includes aggressive nutritional

support, antibiotics, corticosteroids, and/or surgical resection of symptomatic segments of the gastrointestinal tract.[124]

NEOPLASTIC POLYPS

Conventional Adenomas

CLINICAL FEATURES

Adenomas are common lesions that are almost always asymptomatic. In fact, most patients present with overt or occult rectal bleeding. Large polyps may lead to iron deficiency anemia. The clinical importance of adenomas is almost entirely related to their well-established premalignant nature. In general, the prevalence of adenomas increases dramatically with age. By the fifth decade of life, approximately 12% of individuals have adenomas, of which about 25% are considered high-risk lesions.[133] After the age of 50, the prevalence of adenomas continues to rise to the point at which they affect approximately 50% of the population in high-risk Western countries, such as the United States.[3,4] An individual's likelihood of developing adenomas is strongly influenced by family history[134,135] and by a variety of nutritional factors.

Adenomatous polyps of the colon may be broadly classified as conventional (tubular, tubulovillous, or villous), serrated, or flat (discussed further in the following section). Some studies suggest that flat adenomas have a higher incidence of high-grade dysplasia and carcinoma and may, therefore, pose a higher risk of malignant degeneration, but this is controversial. Serrated adenomas are discussed later.

PATHOLOGIC FEATURES

Adenomas are morphologically defined as dysplastic clonal proliferations of colonic epithelium (Fig. 15-17). Grossly, adenomas are broadly classified as sessile (without a stalk) or pedunculated (with a stalk). However, intermediate forms between sessile and pedunculated may develop as well. Rarely, adenomas may be multi-lobulated and/or filiform in appearance. However, these features are unusual. Occasionally, surface ulceration may be noted.

Microscopically, adenomas are categorized architecturally as tubular, tubulovillous, or villous (Fig. 15-18). In general, precise histologic criteria for these separate categories vary widely. However, a reasonable rule is that villous lesions should contain at least 75% villi,[136] whereas tubular lesions should contain less than 25% villi. Tubulovillous lesions are, therefore, those that contain between 25% and 75% villous epithelium. The degree of villous differentiation has been shown to increase with increasing size of the adenoma, but this has not proved to be an independent prognostic factor regarding risk of malignancy.[136] Nevertheless, villous lesions are considered advanced for the purposes of

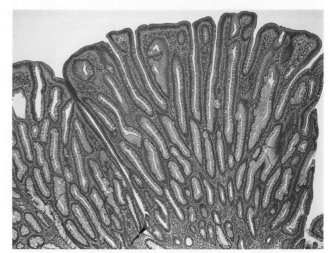

FIGURE 15–17. Tubular adenoma featuring low-grade dysplasia and predominantly tubular architecture. The adenomatous epithelial cells show mild hyperchromasia with enlarged, oval nuclei, which occupies the basal half of the cell cytoplasm. Basal polarization of the nuclei is retained, and no significant pleomorphism occurs. Occasional nondysplastic gland lumina are evident in the deep portion for comparison.

clinical management, as is discussed further in the following sections.

Microscopically, by definition, all adenomas contain at least low-grade (mild) dysplasia. Dysplasia in adenomas is generally classified as of low (mild, moderate) or high grade (severe, including carcinoma in situ) based on a combination of cytologic and architectural features.[136-138] Adenomas that include invasion of the mucosa or the muscularis mucosae (but not beyond) are considered

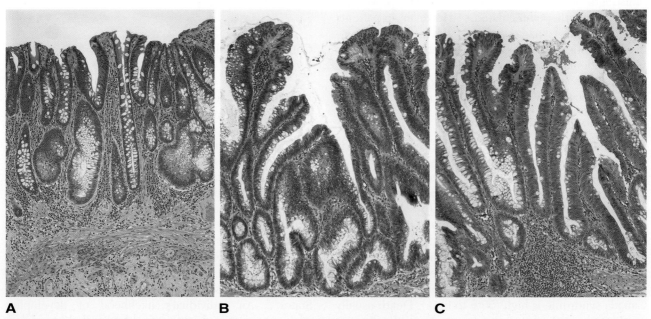

A   **B**   **C**

FIGURE 15–18. Each of these three adenomas displays low-grade dysplasia, but the architecture varies from tubular (**A**) to tubulovillous (**B**) to villous (**C**). The loss of architectural rigidity is a common finding in adenomas.

intramucosal adenocarcinomas. Invasive carcinoma occurs when submucosal stalk invasion is present beyond the muscularis mucosae. This classification system is favored because (1) a decrease in the degree of inter-observer variability has been documented regarding interpretation of dysplasia by pathologists, (2) improved clinical pathologic relevance is seen with regard to surveillance and treatment options, and (3) the term *carcinoma in situ* is often misinterpreted by clinicians as indicative of malignant behavior, and this may lead to an unnecessary colonic resection.

Low-grade dysplasia is defined by the presence of architecturally noncomplex crypts containing nuclei that are pseudostratified, or partially stratified, to the point where the cell nuclei reach only the lower half of the cell cytoplasm. Mitotic activity may be brisk, but atypical mitoses, significant loss of polarity, and pleomorphism are minimal, if present at all. The crypts are arranged in a parallel configuration without significant back-to-back configuration, cribriforming, or complex budding. High-grade dysplasia is defined by marked pseudostratification, or stratification, of neoplastic nuclei that extend toward the luminal half of the cells and usually contain significant pleomorphism, increased mitotic activity, atypical mitoses, and marked loss of polarity. Architectural changes such as back-to-back gland configuration and cribriforming may be noted as well. With progression of neoplasia, glands lose their orderly configuration and become more irregular and complex. In addition, neoplastic nuclei become more "open" in appearance and may contain prominent nucleoli (Fig. 15-19). The nucleus-to-cytoplasm ratio of the cells increases, and loss of polarity becomes marked. In this classification, carcinoma in situ is encompassed and is replaced by the term *high-grade dysplasia*.

Tumors that show single-cell infiltration, small gland proliferation, desmoplasia, or a marked expanding or pushing collection of back-to-back glands with prominent cribriform architecture within the mucosa are considered intramucosal adenocarcinoma (see Fig. 15-19). Differentiation of high-grade dysplasia from intramucosal adenocarcinoma is based on the finding of definite invasion of the lamina propria in the latter compared with the former. Many studies have confirmed that adenomas with high-grade dysplasia or even intramucosal adenocarcinoma have no metastatic potential. Thus, if these lesions are excised with adequate margins, they are adequately treated by polypectomy alone. However, recent data suggest that adenomas with high-grade dysplasia are considered "advanced" lesions, which often leads clinicians to decrease the surveillance interval for affected patients.[139] Advanced lesions, therefore, are adenomas that are large (>1 cm) and contain a villous architecture, or at least high-grade dysplasia.

The lamina propria of adenomas may involve a variable amount of acute and chronic inflammation and eosinophils. Some adenomas, particularly those with high-grade dysplasia or intramucosal adenocarcinoma, may be ulcerated. Paneth cell and/or endocrine cell metaplasia is a common finding and may be marked in certain cases. Rarely, one may see squamous metaplasia in adenomas as well. Some adenomas, particularly those that are pedunculated, may contain dilated and ruptured crypts with mucin extravasation into the lamina propria. Often, these cases are associated with epithelial misplacement into the submucosa. Desmoplasia may occur extremely rarely in cases of adenoma in which carcinoma is limited to the mucosa. However, this feature should make one strongly suspicious of a submucosal invasive tumor.

NATURAL HISTORY

The National Polyp Study,[135,140] a large study initiated in 1990, will provide significant new information in the near future regarding the natural history of adenomas. However, at present, the best predictor for the presence of malignancy within an adenoma at the time of excision is the size of the lesion; in general, villous lesions and/or those with high-grade dysplasia also have an increased risk of adenocarcinoma. In adenomas larger than 2 cm, there is a 10% to 20% risk of carcinoma at the time of removal. Adenomas measuring between 1 and 2 cm have a 5% risk of harboring cancer, and those smaller than 1 cm have a much lower risk of adenocarcinoma (<1%).[141-143]

Degree of dysplasia also represents an independent risk factor for malignancy in adenomas, regardless of size. A vast majority of adenomas display low-grade dysplasia. However, larger lesions have a greater likelihood of harboring high-grade dysplasia.[137,138,144,145] Nevertheless, high-grade dysplasia within a colorectal adenoma does not increase the risk of carcinoma elsewhere in the patient's colon.[144] Because of the time involved for an adenoma to incur sufficient molecular changes to invade through the basement membrane as an adenocarcinoma, most remain benign, slow-growing lesions. The lifetime prevalence of adenoma is approximately 50%, whereas the lifetime prevalence of colorectal adenocarcinoma is approximately 6%. Therefore, it is easy to deduce that only a small minority of polyps ultimately go on to develop adenocarcinoma. Actual longitudinal follow-up data are difficult to obtain because adenomas are typically removed at the time of endoscopic identification.[141] One cohort of 35 patients with an adenoma smaller than 5 mm in diameter was followed for 2 years. In half of these patients, an increase in size of the adenoma occurred; the remainder were unchanged or even slightly regressed.[141,142]

TREATMENT AND SURVEILLANCE ISSUES (Table 15-5)

The appropriate treatment for all colorectal adenomas, regardless of size, architectural type, or degree of dys-

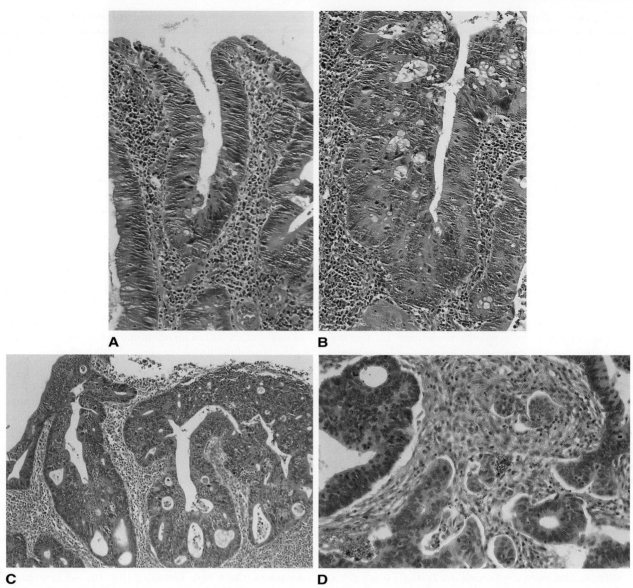

FIGURE 15–19. High-grade dysplasia and intramucosal adenocarcinoma in an adenoma. **A,** Typical focus of high-grade dysplasia (severe dysplasia) shows a marked degree of nuclear hyperchromaticity, pseudostratification, and loss of polarity from the base to the surface of the mucosa. **B,** This lesion is also considered high-grade dysplasia, but in the old nomenclature, it was considered "carcinoma in situ." The cytologic features are similar to those seen in **A;** however, intraluminal cribriforming of the glands is seen without a definite breach of the basement membrane. **C,** This focus of intramucosal adenocarcinoma shows more complex intraluminal cribriforming and large gland formation with the appearance of expanding-type infiltration into the lamina propria without desmoplasia. In intramucosal carcinoma, the nuclei become more rounded, rather than cigar-shaped, and often contain an open chromatin pattern rather than a coarse chromatin pattern. **D,** Another focus of intramucosal adenocarcinoma shows penetration of the lamina propria with small infiltrating glands.

plasia, is complete removal with confirmation of negative mucosal and deep stalk margins.[146,147]

Colorectal adenocarcinoma prevention screening recommendations are based on the distribution of adenomas throughout the colon, the age of the patient, and family history. Although most adenomas occur distal to the splenic flexure, up to 40% occur in the proximal colon. At least one quarter of patients have adenomas that are present only proximal to the splenic flexure.[148-150] Therefore, colonoscopy has virtually replaced all other modalities such as sigmoidoscopy, fecal occult blood testing, and barium enema as the optimal screening tool. The current consensus regarding screening guidelines supports the use of colonoscopy starting at age 50, or at a time 10 years earlier than the age of cancer development in a first-degree family member.[151-158] This should be repeated every 2 to 10 years, depending on the findings of the initial colonoscopy and the patient's family history. See Table 15-5 for details of screening and surveillance.

TABLE 15–5. Guidelines for Adenoma/Carcinoma Surveillance

Average risk (no first-degree relative with colon cancer)
- Colonoscopy at age 50
  If + adenoma or carcinoma, repeat q 3–5 years
  If – adenoma or carcinoma, repeat q 5–10 years
Moderate risk (first-degree relative with colon cancer)
- Colonoscopy 10 years before age of occurrence in relative
  Follow as above
High risk (FAP, HNPCC, chronic ulcerative colitis)
- Colonoscopy q 1–2 years in involved individuals

KEY REPORTING ISSUES

For surgical pathologists, the most important reporting issue, aside from diagnosis, is the status of the polyp margins. Even low-grade adenomas that contain adenomatous tissue at a cauterized margin should be further excised and/or followed closely. Other parameters that should be reported include the architectural type, particularly if the lesion is predominantly villous; the presence or absence of high-grade dysplasia and/or intramucosal adenocarcinoma; and the size of the lesion. Recent data suggest that advanced adenomas (i.e., adenomas >1 cm or those that are predominantly villous or contain high-grade dysplasia) are subtypes that require more aggressive colonoscopic surveillance and that perhaps represent a patient group with an increased risk for further adenomas or adenocarcinoma.[139] For these reasons, the presence of any of these advanced elements should always be included in the surgical pathology report. However, it is also important that the finding of advanced morphologic features not be interpreted as an indication for colectomy; even advanced lesions involve no risk of metastasis in the patient at that time. The presence or absence of intramucosal adenocarcinoma should also be reported, along with the extent of involvement. However, we recommend that documentation of an adenoma with intramucosal adenocarcinoma should always include a statement regarding the absence of invasive cancer in the polyp stalk (i.e., lack of invasive adenocarcinoma), the status of the resection margins, and the overall adequacy of resection and need for further therapy, which in the vast majority of cases is best accomplished with complete polypectomy. In fact, the risk of metastasis in patients with intramucosal adenocarcinoma is virtually zero.

Small diminutive tubular adenomas are usually excised in total with no possibility that the cauterized margins of the specimen will be evaluated. However, this has little clinical relevance for the management of the patient. In contrast, any adenoma larger than 1 cm or that has an easily identifiable stalk should be evaluated regarding the status of the mucosal resection margin and the deep stalk margin.

Adenoma With Epithelial Misplacement (Pseudocarcinoma)

CLINICAL FEATURES

Foci of misplaced epithelium (pseudocarcinoma) and/or mucin extravasation within the submucosa of an adenoma are a rather common finding, particularly in polyps that have a long or pedunculated stalk; this finding often leads to a misdiagnosis of invasive adenocarcinoma.[159-163] This pathologic reaction occurs in 2% to 4% of adenomatous polyps and tends to occur more commonly on the left and, particularly, in the sigmoid colon. It occurs in patients of all ages and is slightly more common among males. Misplaced epithelium in adenomas is believed to occur secondary to twisting and torsion of the polyp stalk, which leads to vascular compromise, breakdown of the muscularis mucosae, and herniation of adenomatous epithelium into the submucosa. Because this reaction occurs more commonly in polyps that have a long stalk, this diagnosis should be made with extreme caution in any sessile polyp.

PATHOLOGIC FEATURES AND DIFFERENTIAL DIAGNOSIS

The intramucosal portion of an adenoma that contains misplaced epithelium may have features that range from low- to high-grade dysplasia, or even intramucosal adenocarcinoma, and may be tubular, tubulovillous, or villous. More often than not, foci of misplaced epithelium include a degree of dysplasia similar to that of the intramucosal portion of the polyp; they usually grow in the submucosa in a lobular configuration or as well-circumscribed aggregates of crypts. Misplaced epithelium is usually surrounded by a distinct rim of lamina propria, is often associated with hemorrhage or hemosiderin deposition, shows no evidence of desmoplasia, and lacks the cytologic and architectural features of invasive carcinoma (Fig. 15-20). Mucin pools, when present in association with misplaced epithelium, are usually either acellular or lined by dysplastic epithelium of a grade similar to that of the surface of the polyp. Furthermore, mucin pools are typically smooth and regular in shape and are usually associated with ruptured crypts with extravasated mucin in the surface of the polyp. In contrast, irregular, jagged mucin pools dissecting through the submucosal stroma and/or associated with cytologically malignant cells floating in the center of the mucin are features that are highly suggestive of adenocarcinoma.

On occasion, misplaced epithelium may be difficult to differentiate from well-differentiated invasive adenocarcinoma[159,160,164] (Table 15-6). Features suggestive of adenocarcinoma include (1) epithelium that contains a greater degree of cytologic and architectural atypia than that of the intramucosal portion of the adenoma, (2) architectural complexity of the glands, such as irregular,

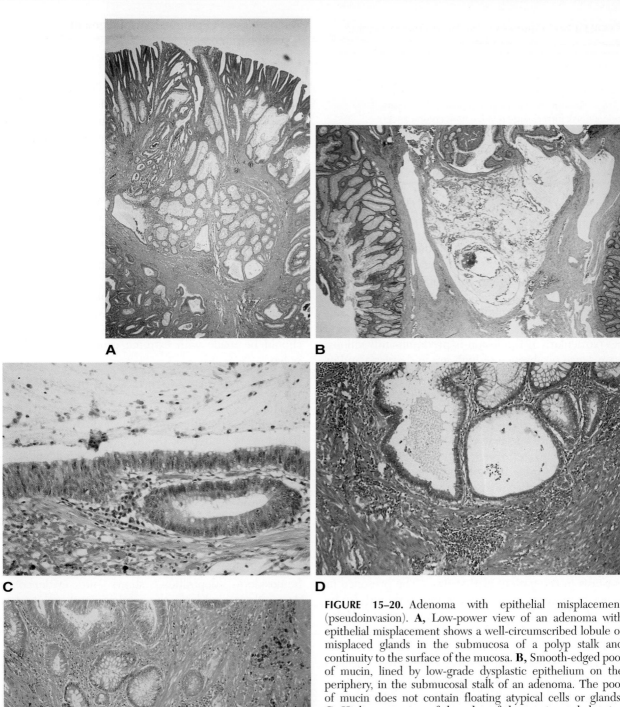

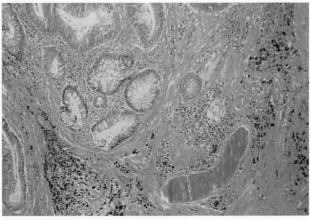

FIGURE 15–20. Adenoma with epithelial misplacement (pseudoinvasion). **A,** Low-power view of an adenoma with epithelial misplacement shows a well-circumscribed lobule of misplaced glands in the submucosa of a polyp stalk and continuity to the surface of the mucosa. **B,** Smooth-edged pool of mucin, lined by low-grade dysplastic epithelium on the periphery, in the submucosal stalk of an adenoma. The pool of mucin does not contain floating atypical cells or glands. **C,** High-power view of the edge of the mucin pool showing low-grade dysplastic epithelium with a small rim of lamina propria–like stroma surrounding an isolated crypt. **D,** Misplaced crypts are present in the submucosa of an adenoma in a smooth, rounded, well-circumscribed lobular configuration. Intervening lamina propria is seen between the crypts, and a small amount of hemosiderin deposition is noted in the left portion of the photograph. **E,** In another area, the misplaced crypts are slightly separated from one another, and marked congestion and hemosiderin deposition are seen around the edges of the misplaced epithelium.

TABLE 15–6. Adenomas With Epithelial Misplacement Versus Adenocarcinoma

Feature	Epithelial Misplacement	Invasive Adenocarcinoma
Pedunculated shape	Usually present	Present or absent
Dysplasia	Similar to polyp surface	Carcinoma-like
Desmoplasia	Absent	Usually present
Hemorrhage/Hemosiderin	Usually present	Usually absent
Lamina propria rim	Usually present	Absent
Architecture	Round, smooth, lobular arrangement of crypts	Irregular, variably sized tortuous crypts, single cells, small clusters of cells
Crypts	Noncomplex	Complex, cribriform, budding
Mucus pools	Round, smooth, lined by dysplastic epithelium at periphery	Irregular, floating cells may be present
Communication to surface	Often present	Present or absent

tortuous, and jagged edges to the crypts, (3) back-to-back gland formation, (4) a nonlobular configuration of crypts, (5) single or small clusters of cells without a surrounding rim of lamina propria, (6) a desmoplastic reaction, and (7) the absence of hemorrhage and/or hemosiderin deposition (Fig. 15-21). Although misplaced benign crypts can often be demonstrated to communicate with the intramucosal portion of the polyp upon deeper sectioning, this feature may be absent in cases of adenocarcinoma.

In diagnostically difficult cases, increased staining of the submucosal epithelium for matrix metalloproteinase-1 (MMP-1) and/or Tp53, combined with decreased staining of the submucosal epithelium for membranous E-cadherin and decreased or irregular collagen deposition surrounding the submucosal glands, may be helpful in establishing a diagnosis of adenocarcinoma.[165,166] For instance, in one study by Yantiss and coworkers, adenomas with invasive adenocarcinoma showed increased MMP-1 staining of the stroma surrounding submucosal epithelium, and increased Tp53 nuclear staining within the submucosal epithelium (91% and 61% of cases, respectively).[165] Cases with carcinoma also showed decreased or discontinuous E-cadherin and collagen IV staining in 65% and 95% of cases, respectively. In contrast, MMP-1 and TP53 were increased in only 48% and 4% of adenomas with misplaced epithelium; they showed complete preservation

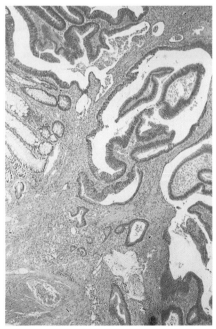
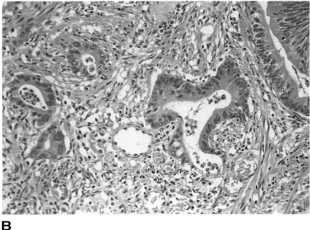

A   **B**

FIGURE 15–21. A, In contrast to adenomas with epithelial misplacement, this adenoma contains invasive well-differentiated adenocarcinoma in the central portion of the polyp stalk. The infiltrating glands are irregular in size and shape, have unusual profiles, and show a lack of lamina propria surrounding the invasive glands; no evidence of hemorrhage or hemosiderin deposition is seen. The infiltrating glands are irregular and jagged in contour and infiltrate in a nonlobular fashion. **B,** High-power view of infiltrating glands shows their irregular profile, surrounding inflammation, and an early desmoplastic reaction.

of membranous E-cadherin staining and basement membrane–associated collagen IV staining in all (100%) cases.

TREATMENT

Adenomas with epithelial misplacement should be excised in total with confirmation that the mucosal and deep cauterized margins are negative, similar to adenomas without epithelial misplacement.[167] For purposes of patient management, pools of mucin at or near the deep, cauterized resection margin, particularly if associated with a rim of dysplastic epithelium, should be considered positive for adenomatous epithelium. Finally, cases in which a definite distinction from adenocarcinoma cannot be made with certainty should probably be considered "atypical" and should be managed with complete polypectomy and/or surgical resection, depending on the presence or absence of favorable prognostic histologic signs (as noted later in the section on malignant polyps) and the clinical circumstances of the patient.

Adenomas (and Polypoid Dysplastic Lesions) in Inflammatory Bowel Disease

GENERAL COMMENTS

Not uncommonly, isolated, well-circumscribed, sessile or pedunculated adenoma-like polypoid dysplastic lesions may occur in patients with ulcerative colitis or Crohn's disease.[168] A common diagnostic dilemma for both clinicians and pathologists is how to differentiate a sporadic adenoma—a lesion that develops coincidentally in a patient with an underlying IBD—from an adenoma-like polypoid dysplastic lesion—a lesion that develops as a pathogenetic consequence of the underlying inflammatory disease.[168,169] The latter lesion is considered a type of dysplasia-associated lesion or mass (DALM), which is discussed more thoroughly in Chapter 10.

Until recently, the distinction between these two types of lesions has been considered clinically important because sporadic adenomas are generally treated by polypectomy and continued surveillance, whereas (adenoma-like) polypoid dysplastic lesions associated with an underlying IBD have generally been regarded as an indication for colectomy in medically fit patients.[168,170,171] However, recent data, based on the results of two important follow-up studies, suggest that IBD patients with an adenoma-like polypoid dysplastic lesion, regardless of whether it represents a sporadic or an IBD-related lesion, may be treated adequately by polypectomy and continued surveillance if there is no evidence of flat dysplasia (either low- or high-grade) in areas of mucosa either close to, or distant from, the dysplastic polyp.[172,173]

In one study, the clinical outcomes of 24 patients with ulcerative colitis who had an adenoma-like polypoid dysplastic lesion were compared with those of 10 ulcerative colitis patients with a coincidental sporadic adenoma (based on the fact that the lesions were located proximal to areas of histologically confirmed colitis) and 49 nonulcerative colitis patients with a sporadic adenoma.[172] After more than 3 years of follow-up, 58% of ulcerative colitis patients with an adenoma-like lesion developed further adenoma-like polyps, which was statistically similar to the 50% of ulcerative colitis patients with a sporadic adenoma and the 39% of nonulcerative colitis patients with sporadic adenoma who developed further adenomas. Only one ulcerative colitis patient with an adenoma-like polyp developed an isolated focus of low-grade dysplasia, and none developed adenocarcinoma. Similar results were found by Rubin and associates in a study of 38 ulcerative colitis patients and 18 Crohn's disease patients with 70 "dysplastic" polyps, all of whom were treated with polypectomy and followed for a mean of 4.1 years.[173] In that study, most patients (52%) did not develop any additional polyps, and none developed either dysplasia or adenocarcinoma.

PATHOLOGIC FEATURES AND DIFFERENTIAL DIAGNOSIS

Grossly, adenomas associated with IBD are endoscopically and histologically identical to those that occur outside the setting of inflammatory disease (see earlier under Conventional Adenomas).[169,174-176] Lesions that occur proximal to histologically confirmed areas of colitis (e.g., right-sided lesions in a patient with left-sided ulcerative colitis) can easily be diagnosed as sporadic adenoma because it is well known that dysplasia related to IBD develops only in areas involved with chronic inflammation.[177,178] However, adenoma-like lesions that occur within areas of colitis may be more difficult to distinguish from true polypoid dysplastic lesions related to the underlying colitis. Several clinical, endoscopic, pathologic, and molecular features may help in distinguishing a sporadic adenoma from an IBD-associated polypoid dysplastic lesion (Table 15-7).[179] Clinically, patients with sporadic adenomas, in contrast to patients with IBD-associated adenoma-like polypoid dysplasia, are typically older (>60 years of age) and have less extensive inflammatory disease, less disease activity, and a shorter duration of disease (generally <10 years). Endoscopically, the lesions may be indistinguishable. However, as has been mentioned, lesions that occur proximal to areas of colitis can reliably be considered sporadic adenomas.

Histologically, IBD-associated adenoma-like polypoid dysplastic lesions often show an increased degree of acute and chronic inflammation in the lamina propria, cryptitis, and crypt abscesses involving dysplastic crypts and a mixture of benign and dysplastic crypts at the

TABLE 15–7. Summary of Differentiating Features Between Sporadic Adenoma and IBD-Associated Polypoid Dysplasia

Feature	Sporadic Adenoma	IBD-Associated Polypoid Dysplasia
Patient age	Older (>60 yr)	Younger (<60 yr)
Extent of disease	Usually subtotal	Usually total
Disease activity	Usually inactive	Usually active
Disease duration	Shorter (<10 yr)	Longer (>10 yr)
Polyp location	Usually nondiseased area (↑ right colon)	Diseased area (↑ left colon)
Associated flat dysplasia	Never	Occasionally
Increased lamina propria and crypt inflammation	Usually absent	Usually present
Villous architecture	Usually absent	Occasionally present
Mixture of benign and dysplastic crypts at surface of polyp	Usually absent	Usually present
Tp53 immunostaining	Usually absent	Usually present
Nuclear beta-catenin immunostaining	Usually prominent	Usually absent
LOH of 3p	Uncommon	Common
LOH of *p16*	Rare	Common

LOH, loss of heterozygosity.

surface of the polyp—features that are not usually seen in sporadic adenomas (Fig. 15-22). In addition, flat dysplasia may be detected in the base of the stalk or in mucosa surrounding the polyp. Stalk dysplasia, if present, should alert the pathologist that dysplasia may be present in the adjacent mucosa and that this is likely to be an IBD-associated lesion rather than a sporadic adenoma. Features such as polyp size, architectural type (tubular, tubulovillous, or villous), and degree of dysplasia, as well as nuclear cytologic features, are not helpful in distinguishing these two groups of lesions.

By immunohistochemistry, IBD-associated adenoma-like polypoid dysplastic lesions have a higher degree of Tp53 and a lower degree of nuclear beta-catenin staining, in contrast to sporadic adenomas.[180,181] Furthermore, their molecular characteristics are different.[178,179,181-184] IBD-associated lesions show a higher prevalence of 3p and p16 mutations, indicating different timing and frequency of molecular defects, in contrast to sporadic adenomas. An interim proposal for the treatment of adenoma-like polypoid dysplastic lesions in IBD is presented in Figure 15-23.

Serrated Adenomas

CLINICAL FEATURES (Table 15-8)

Serrated adenoma is a morphologic subtype of adenomatous polyp that shows dysplastic epithelium in a growth pattern reminiscent of a hyperplastic

polyp.[185,186] Serrated adenomas were first described as a distinct entity in 1990.[187] They show a prominent serrated or sawtooth surface contour and prominent luminal infolding of the epithelium. They account for less than 5% of all adenomas. Serrated adenomas are slightly more common in the left colon.[188] Age of development overlaps with that of conventional adenomas. These polyps are usually sporadic in origin, although in hyperplastic polyposis, a combination of large hyperplastic polyps (see under Sessile Serrated Polyps), serrated adenomas, conventional adenomas, and mixed hyperplastic/adenomatous lesions may be present as well.[189-191]

Recent data suggest that the timing, sequence, and prevalence of certain molecular alterations are different in serrated adenomas compared with conventional adenomas or hyperplastic polyps.[192-197] For instance, *Tp53* mutations are frequent (approximately 50%) in serrated adenomas, particularly among those with high-grade dysplasia, but are virtually never present in hyperplastic polyps. The frequency of K-*ras* mutations in serrated adenomas conflicts with estimates of positivity ranging from 5% to 60%. Similar to hyperplastic polyps, *APC* mutations are extremely uncommon in serrated adenomas compared with conventional adenomas. However, several studies suggest that microsatellite instability is a common genetic pathway of molecular alterations in serrated adenomas; it was present in 53% of polyps in one study.[198] A recent serrated pathway of colonic carcinogenesis has been proposed by Jass and colleagues.[199-201] These authors proposed the development of cancer from microscopic aberrant crypt foci to hyperplastic polyps and eventually serrated adenoma and serrated carcinoma. A large proportion of these tumors show either a low or a high level of microsatellite instability.

A number of histologic and molecular features support this theory. First, transitional histologic forms exist among all lesions, but particularly among hyperplastic polyps, serrated adenomas, and serrated carcinomas (see under Mixed Hyperplastic/Adenomatous Polyps). Aberrant crypt foci are histologically indistinguishable from hyperplastic polyps except for differences in size and configuration.[202] The frequency of K-*ras* mutations is also similar in aberrant crypt foci and hyperplastic polyps. Furthermore, serrated adenomas commonly contain a component of typical benign-appearing hyperplastic epithelium. In fact, a similar pattern of mutations in microsatellite instability markers has been demonstrated in both hyperplastic and adenomatous components of mixed hyperplastic/adenomatous polyps (see under Mixed Hyperplastic/Adenomatous Polyps). One study of sporadic microsatellite unstable cancers revealed a significantly higher incidence of serrated adenomas compared with a control group of microsatellite stable

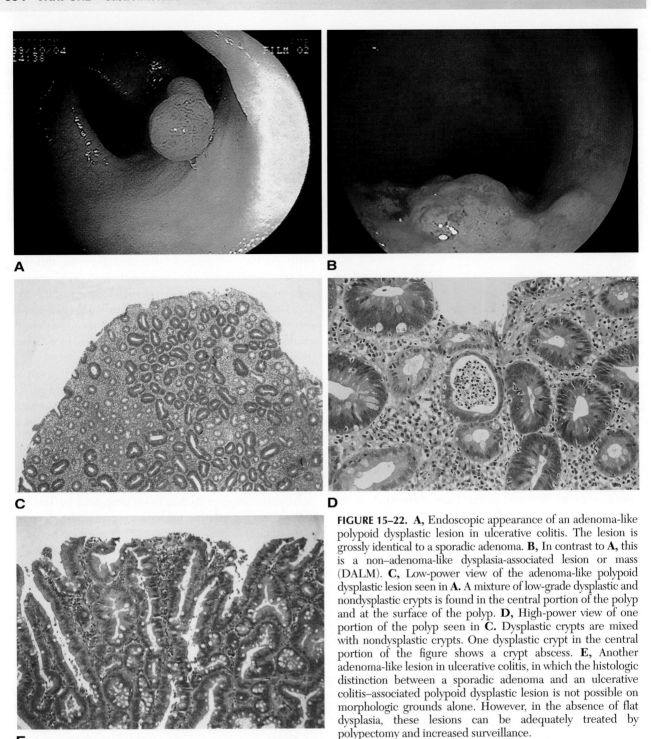

FIGURE 15–22. A, Endoscopic appearance of an adenoma-like polypoid dysplastic lesion in ulcerative colitis. The lesion is grossly identical to a sporadic adenoma. **B,** In contrast to **A,** this is a non–adenoma-like dysplasia-associated lesion or mass (DALM). **C,** Low-power view of the adenoma-like polypoid dysplastic lesion seen in **A.** A mixture of low-grade dysplastic and nondysplastic crypts is found in the central portion of the polyp and at the surface of the polyp. **D,** High-power view of one portion of the polyp seen in **C.** Dysplastic crypts are mixed with nondysplastic crypts. One dysplastic crypt in the central portion of the figure shows a crypt abscess. **E,** Another adenoma-like lesion in ulcerative colitis, in which the histologic distinction between a sporadic adenoma and an ulcerative colitis–associated polypoid dysplastic lesion is not possible on morphologic grounds alone. However, in the absence of flat dysplasia, these lesions can be adequately treated by polypectomy and increased surveillance.

tumors.[203,204] In addition, the adjacent invasive component of these tumors always shows a serrated architecture. It has been suggested that large sessile "serrated" lesions in the proximal colon may be the primary precursor for highly microsatellite unstable tumors. Small serrated lesions, primarily in the left colon and rectum, may be a precursor to tumors with a low-level microsatellite instability.[198,204,205]

PATHOLOGIC FEATURES

Serrated adenomas may be sessile or pedunculated. Occasionally, particularly those in the rectum may take on a predominantly filiform pattern of growth. Serrated adenomas may involve any degree of dysplasia or adenocarcinoma. Dysplasia in serrated adenomas is categorized similarly to conventional adenomas.[185] Overall, at low magnifications, serrated adenomas are

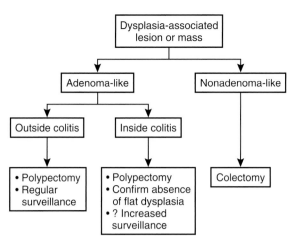

FIGURE 15–23. Treatment of adenoma-like lesions in inflammatory bowel disease.

TABLE 15–8. Differential Features of "Serrated" Lesions

Polyp	Typical Size	Overt Dysplasia	Favored Location	Malignant Potential
Hyperplastic polyp	<5 mm	No	Distal	Minimal
Mixed hyperplastic/ adenoma	>5 mm	Yes	Proximal	Yes
Serrated adenoma	>5 mm	Yes	Distal	Yes
Sessile serrated polyp	>5 mm	No	Proximal	Unknown, probably yes

characterized by a serrated or sawtooth luminal surface contour and prominent infolding of the crypt epithelium (Fig. 15-24). The low-power appearance is that of a hyperplastic polyp. However, upon higher magnification, serrated adenomas are composed of obviously dysplastic epithelium. Nuclei are often pseudostratified and elongated or pencil shaped; they include coarse chromatin and an increased mitotic rate. Lack of surface maturation is a key distinguishing feature from hyperplastic polyps. The cytoplasm of serrated adenomas is often eosinophilic, and often there is tufting of nuclei at the surface of the polyp. Mitoses may be prominent and may be present anywhere along the crypt axis.

As has been mentioned, the natural history of serrated adenomas is unclear. Thus, at present, these lesions should be reported in a manner similar to that of conventional adenomas, with attention to the status of the margin, the degree of dysplasia, the size of the lesion, and the adequacy of excision.

Sessile Serrated Polyps

Lesions with morphologic characteristics that lie between classic hyperplastic polyps and classic serrated adenomas have been referred to as "sessile serrated polyps."[185] However, the biologic characteristics, histologic features, and natural history of this type of polyp have been poorly characterized. These lesions show architectural changes, including crypt dilatation (particularly at the base of the mucosa), branching, and lateral growth along the muscularis mucosae (Fig. 15-25). They tend to contain a higher frequency of Paneth cells and endocrine cells; thus, this has been proposed as a helpful differential feature from classic hyperplastic polyps. Cytologically, the nuclei may appear slightly more

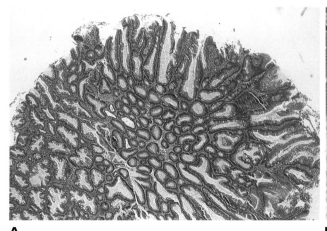

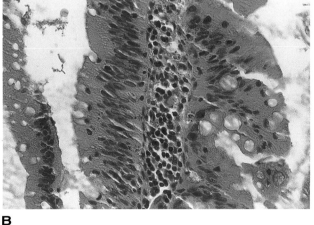

A   **B**

FIGURE 15–24. A, Serrated adenoma features dysplastic epithelium with a "serrated" architecture. Differentiation from a hyperplastic polyp is aided by the presence of nuclear stratification and hypereosinophilic cytoplasm in the adenoma, in contrast to a hyperplastic polyp, which shows neither of these features (**A**). **B,** On high power, the low-grade nature of the dysplasia with retention of goblet cells in this serrated adenoma can complicate the distinction between this lesion and a hyperplastic polyp.

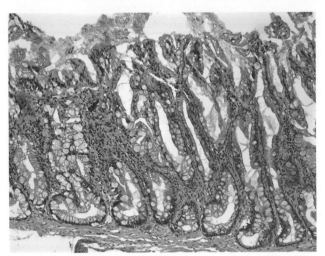

FIGURE 15–25. This is a 1-cm sessile serrated polyp, which demonstrates the architectural changes described in these lesions (see text), including crypt dilatation, branching, and lateral growth along the muscularis mucosae. The degree of cytologic atypia is minimal. It is likely that this lesion represents a very low-grade or "early" serrated adenoma.

atypical than in hyperplastic polyps, with mild pseudo-stratification, loss of polarity, and occasional misplaced mitotic figures. The cytoplasm of these lesions is often mucin depleted and slightly hypereosinophilic. Some authors have shown that these lesions may occur more commonly in the right colon than in the left. Although it is likely that these lesions represent a low-grade, dysplastic form of serrated adenoma, or perhaps a lesion inter-mediate between a hyperplastic polyp and a fully developed serrated adenoma, this has yet to be proved.

Mixed Hyperplastic/Adenomatous Polyps

As has been mentioned in the section on serrated adenomas, mixed hyperplastic/adenomatous polyps are defined as lesions that contain discrete, often adjacent, foci of hyperplastic changes combined with definite dysplastic changes characteristic of an adenoma (Fig. 15-26). The adenomatous component often reveals a serrated contour as well. Thus, most mixed hyperplastic/adenomatous polyps, in fact, represent a combination of a serrated adenoma and an adjacent hyperplastic polyp component.[206-208] The presence of these lesions provides further support for the concept that some hyperplastic polyps may represent a neoplastic precursor to serrated adenomas and serrated carcinomas. It is likely that mixed hyperplastic/adenomatous polyps, sessile serrated polyps, and serrated adenomas represent a spectrum of pathogenetically related lesions.

As has been discussed, recent data suggest that serrated lesions may follow a different molecular pathogenetic pathway of carcinogenesis than is followed by conventional adenomas.[209-216] Frequent CpG island methylation in serrated polyps of the colorectum supports this theory.[205] Target genes for tumorigenesis related to methylation include *hMLH1* (encoding a DNA mismatch repair enzyme) and *O-6-methylguanine-DNA-methyltransferase (MGMT)*. The treatment of choice for mixed hyperplastic/adenomatous polyps is complete removal, as with any other adenoma.[217-219]

Flat Adenomas

Flat adenomas are defined as dysplastic noninvasive lesions without a "polypoid" component.[220-228] They may be slightly raised at the edges, but more typically they have a central depression. Recent studies suggest that flat adenomas are associated with a constellation of molecular abnormalities somewhat different from conventional adenomas.[224-225] The molecular phenotype is thought to be of a more aggressive nature than that of typical adenomas, but this is controversial. Some reports

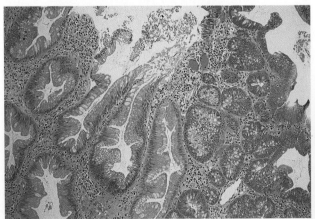

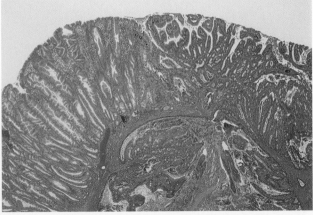

A **B**

FIGURE 15–26. A, Mixed hyperplastic/adenomatous polyps show distinct and separate regions of hyperplastic polyp formation and adenoma with low-grade dysplasia. These mixed polyps may be part of the evolving family of "serrated" lesions that show an increased risk of carcinoma through methylation pathways. **B,** This particular lesion was associated with an underlying invasive adenocarcinoma.

cite an increased prevalence of high-grade dysplasia and a higher rate of progression to adenocarcinoma than are found with conventional adenomas.[221,223,224,227] Of practical clinical importance, these lesions may be difficult to identify endoscopically. An accurate assessment of the prevalence and natural history of these lesions may depend on more extensive studies with the use of chromoscopy and/or high-resolution endoscopy.[222] Lynch and colleagues have described two families with flat adenomatous polyposis.[229-231] The lesions in these patients were predominantly right-sided, but otherwise they did not have features of familial adenomatous polyposis or hereditary nonpolyposis colorectal cancer syndrome (Lynch syndrome). However, familial adenomatous polyposis (FAP) patients do have a higher rate of flat adenoma formation. Flat adenoma may result in the development of flat or depressed invasive adenocarcinoma without evidence of residual overlying or adjacent adenomatous epithelium.

Malignant Epithelial Polyps

CLINICAL FEATURES

A malignant polyp is defined as an adenoma that contains invasive adenocarcinoma (i.e., cancer that extends beyond the muscularis mucosae into the submucosal polyp stalk).[232-234] These are broadly categorized as either polypoid adenocarcinoma, in which the polyp head is totally replaced by cancer with minimal or no evidence of residual adenomatous epithelium, or adenoma with focal adenocarcinoma that invades the submucosal stalk. The pathologic features of these polyps were discussed previously under Adenoma With Epithelial Misplacement (Pseudocarcinoma).[235,236] The adenocarcinoma component of a malignant polyp may be well, moderately, or poorly differentiated, with or without lymphovascular invasion.

TREATMENT

The treatment of a malignant epithelial polyp depends on the type and the growth pattern of the lesion.[234,237] In terms of patient management, polypoid adenocarcinomas (lesions without an adenomatous component) should simply be regarded as a polypoid type of adenocarcinoma. However, the treatment of an adenoma with focal invasive adenocarcinoma is highly dependent on the type of lesion (i.e., whether it is sessile or pedunculated) and on a variety of histologic features (discussed further in the following sections). Adenocarcinoma arising in a sessile adenoma should always be considered a lesion with malignant (metastasizing) potential; thus, a subtotal colectomy is usually recommended for medically fit patients. The risk of metastasis in patients with a sessile adenoma with invasive adenocarcinoma approaches 20%.

In contrast, several studies have evaluated a variety of specific histologic features within pedunculated adenomas with adenocarcinomas that may indicate a poor ("unfavorable") prognosis and hence may not be considered adequately treated by polypectomy alone; more appropriately, a subtotal colectomy and lymph node dissection are usually required. Cooper and coworkers evaluated 140 adenomatous polyps for unfavorable histologic features, which they defined as tumor less than 1 mm from the deep cauterized margin, grade III (poorly differentiated) carcinoma, and/or the presence of lymphovascular invasion. They evaluated patients for recurrence of tumor and/or lymph node metastasis.[234] Nearly 20% of patients with polyps that contained any of these unfavorable histologic parameters had a "poor" outcome compared with none of the patients with polyps without unfavorable histology.

Another study by Volt and associates evaluated unfavorable histologic features in 47 patients with adenoma with invasive adenocarcinoma.[237] In this study, unfavorable histology was regarded as grade III morphology, margins that could not be assessed, or tumor that was found less than 2 mm from the resection margin. Forty-three percent of polyps with unfavorable histology had a poor outcome in contrast to none of the polyps with favorable histology. The results of these studies and of others have been useful in providing criteria that allow pathologists and surgeons to determine if a polypectomy is adequate treatment for malignant polyps. These criteria are summarized in Table 15-9. In brief, polyps with invasive carcinoma that is poorly differentiated, is present less than 1 to 2 mm from the cauterized margins of the specimen, has positive margins, or has definite evidence of lymphovascular invasion are considered unfavorable and should probably be treated with a colectomy in medically fit patients. In contrast, adenomas with intramucosal adenocarcinoma or with moderately well-differentiated adenocarcinoma involving the superficial portion of the polyp stalk in the absence of lymphovascular invasion

TABLE 15–9. Evaluation and Treatment of Adenomas Harboring Adenocarcinoma

	Favorable Histology	Unfavorable Histology
I	Low to moderate grade (moderately well-differentiated)	High grade (grade III of III or IV of IV) (poorly differentiated)
II	No lymphovascular invasion	Lymphovascular invasion
III	Negative margin	Positive polypectomy margin
IV	Invasive tumor >2 mm from margin	Invasive tumor <2 mm from margin
Treatment	Polypectomy	Consider segmental resection

and with negative margins may be considered safely treated by complete polypectomy.

Polypoid Endocrine Tumors

This subject is discussed in detail in Chapters 15 and 21. Polypoid rectal carcinoids tend to be small and are usually adequately treated endoscopically with polypectomy.[238] More proximal carcinoids tend to be aggressive and require more extensive surgery.

Metastasis to the Colon

Metastasis to the colon is discussed in Chapter 19. Metastatic carcinoma, melanoma, or lymphoma can rarely involve the stroma of a tubular adenoma and can be discovered incidentally at the time of an endoscopic polypectomy. Both lobular breast cancer and pulmonary adenocarcinoma have been observed in this setting (personal observation). Peritoneal tumors such as ovarian serous carcinomas can give rise to a submucosal effaced lesion that resembles adenoma or an adenocarcinoma.

Adenomatous Polyposis Syndromes

FAMILIAL ADENOMATOUS POLYPOSIS

FAP is an autosomal dominant condition caused by either inheritance of a mutated *APC* gene (located on chromosome 5q) or a new germline mutation in the same gene (up to one third of cases).[239] Adenomas result from loss of the second *APC* allele within colonic epithelial cells.[240] The *APC* gene serves as a tumor suppressor gene, and its absence allows for additional mutations in other genetic loci such as *K-ras* and *TP53* genes (see Chapter 19). FAP patients develop large numbers of colorectal adenomas during late childhood, adolescence, and early adulthood. FAP has traditionally been defined by the presence of more than 100 adenomatous polyps in the colon, although many patients have several hundreds or thousands of polyps. Adenocarcinoma develops in most patients by the mid-30s, but it can occur as early as age 17. FAP accounts for approximately 1% of colon cancers.

The frequency of FAP is 1 in 8000 to 1 in 14,000 in the general population, with equal sex representation worldwide.[241] FAP patients may express a variety of extraintestinal phenotypes (see later in FAP variants), but all include adenomatous polyps of the gastrointestinal tract. They are predisposed to a high rate of adenocarcinoma (Table 15-10). Upper gastrointestinal adenomas and adenocarcinomas may also develop in FAP patients at a high frequency; they are particularly prominent in the first and second portions of the duodenum and in the periampullary region.[242,243] Unfor-

tunately, periampullary adenomas and adenocarcinomas have recently become the most common causes of morbidity and mortality in FAP patients who have undergone a prophylactic colectomy.[243] The prevalence of noncolonic adenoma in FAP ranges from 9% to 50% in the stomach, and from 50% to 100% in the duodenum. Cyclooxygenase-2 (COX-2) inhibitors have received increased attention lately as a method of decreasing or eliminating rectal adenomas in patients who have had a subtotal colectomy. However, no benefit has been determined for duodenal adenomas or adenomas in ileoanal pouches. Gardner's syndrome, Turcot's syndrome, and attenuated FAP are considered subtypes of FAP; these are discussed further in the following paragraphs.

Screening during adolescence followed by a post-adolescent prophylactic colectomy is the treatment of choice for most patients.

GARDNER'S SYNDROME

This refers to patients with FAP who have extracolonic manifestations.[244,245] The most common extracolonic manifestations include periampullary adenomas and gastric adenomas. Aggressive desmoid tumors (fibromatosis) occur commonly in the abdominal wall and the retroperitoneum. Surgical incisions can also increase the incidence of fibromatosis. Osteomas, dental abnormalities, thyroid carcinoma, and congenital hypertrophy of the retinal pigmented epithelium (CHRPE) can also occur.

TURCOT'S SYNDROME

This term refers to the coexistence of hereditary colon cancer syndrome, such as FAP or hereditary nonpolyposis colorectal cancer (HNPCC), and central nervous system (CNS) tumors.[246-248] Although glioblastomas are the most common primary CNS tumor in FAP patients, other gliomas and medulloblastomas can also occur. This syndrome results from distinct germline defects either in the *APC* gene or in DNA mismatch repair genes.

TABLE 15–10. Magnitude and Age of Cancer Risk in Polyposis Syndromes

Polyposis Syndrome	Risk of Malignancy	Age of Carcinoma Development
Familial adenomatous polyposis	100%	35–45
Hamartomatous polyposis	40%–60%	25—60
Hyperplastic polyposis	Uncertain, >50%	>40
Hereditary nonpolyposis colorectal cancer syndrome	>80%	>35

ATTENUATED FAMILIAL ADENOMATOUS POLYPOSIS

This refers to a hereditary colon cancer syndrome with fewer than 100 colonic polyps (usually fewer than 30).[249,250] When patients present with a suspicious family history and/or mild polyposis, the diagnosis can be further investigated by assaying for mutations in the *APC* gene. In attenuated FAP, as opposed to classic FAP, *APC* mutations tend to occur at the 3-prime aspect of the gene.[250,251] Once the mutations are discovered, these patients require close endoscopic screening for removal of polyps and prevention of adenocarcinoma development. In addition to being fewer in number, adenomas and adenocarcinomas develop at a later stage in life than in classic FAP. These adenomas and adenocarcinomas are otherwise of unremarkable morphology. Upper gastrointestinal lesions and extraintestinal manifestations develop at a rate similar to that in classic FAP.

Hereditary Nonpolyposis Colorectal Cancer Syndrome (Lynch Syndrome)

HNPCC is an autosomal dominant condition caused by inherited defects in at least one of the family of DNA mismatch repair enzymes (hMLH1, hMSH2, hMSH6, hPMS2),[252,253] which lead to microsatellite instability and a rapid accumulation of somatic mutations in genes that control pathways of tumor progression (see also Chapter 19). Most mutations are in the *hMLH1* and *hMSH2* genes and are truncating. As the name implies, these patients do not develop an excess of polyps. However, when adenomas do occur, they carry a significant risk of malignant degeneration. The risk of colon cancer is 80% to 90%. Immunohistochemical staining of an adenoma in an HNPCC patient often demonstrates loss of expression of the inherited faulty mismatch repair protein, indicating that this defect is present at the time of adenoma formation.[254-256] Defective DNA mismatch repair functionality suggests that the adenoma to carcinoma progression could be quite rapid in these patients. It has also been suggested that HNPCC may involve a higher proportion of flat adenomas as well. Patients with HNPCC have a 40% lifetime risk of developing small intestinal carcinoma; the duodenum and the jejunum are the most common sites.

The Amsterdam-2 criteria for HNPCC are as follows[254]: (1) at least three relatives must have an HNPCC-associated cancer, (2) one patient should be a first-degree relative of the other two, (3) at least two successive generations should be affected, (4) at least one tumor should be diagnosed before the age of 50, (5) FAP coli must be excluded, and (6) the tumor should be verified by histopathologic examination.

HNPCC is the most common form of hereditary colon cancer, accounting for approximately 5% of all colon cancers (see Chapter 19). The disorder is characterized by the development of colon cancer at an early age and by a predominance of right-sided cancers. Extracolonic malignancies also occur in a subset of patients (Lynch syndrome II). Recent treatment guidelines have expanded the clinical list of patients for whom genetic counseling and testing for microsatellite instability should be considered. These include individuals with two HNPCC-related cancers, with colorectal or endometrial cancer before age 45, and with colonic adenomas diagnosed before age 40.

The histologic features of colorectal carcinomas in HNPCC are distinctive.[255,257] Sixty percent occur in the proximal colon and are mostly of the mucinous subtype, including signet ring cell carcinoma, or they may appear as medullary carcinomas with a solid growth pattern and prominent tumor-infiltrating lymphocytes. These tumors are often labeled "poorly differentiated." A Crohn's-like lymphoid response is often seen at the leading edges of tumors as well.

Lymphoid Polyps

Lymphomatous polyposis refers to primary clinical presentation of lymphoma in the colon as multiple polyps.[258,259] These are typically smooth, pedunculated polyps found in the right colon and the terminal ileum. Most lymphomatous polyposis cases are due to mantle cell lymphoma, an aggressive variant of low-grade lymphoma. Morphologic and immunophenotypic assessment is needed for accurate subtyping of these cases because a minority are due to low-grade follicular lymphoma or represent another low-grade B-cell subtype.[260,261]

Mesenchymal Polyps

Although a vast majority of colonic polyps are epithelial in origin (or include admixtures of both colonic epithelium and stroma, as in many hamartomatous polyps and inflammatory polyps), some may represent stromal cell proliferations. These include both benign and malignant tumors of adipose tissue (lipomas, liposarcomas, and lipomatous hypertrophy of the ileocecal valve), smooth muscle tissue (true leiomyomas and leiomyosarcomas), vascular tissue (glomus tumors, vascular malformations, lymphangiomas, and angiosarcomas), and neural tissue (ganglioneuromas, neurofibromas, and granular cell tumors), as well as gastrointestinal stromal tumors (GISTs). In addition, mesenchymal polyps of unknown origin such as inflammatory fibroid polyps are found. Some of the more common lesions are described in this section.

GANGLIONEUROMAS

Clinical Features

Ganglioneuromas are mature, benign tumors composed of a proliferation of nerve fibers, Schwann cells, and ganglion cells. They most commonly arise in the posterior mediastinum and the retroperitoneum. Ganglioneuromas of the intestinal tract are considerably less common. Gastrointestinal ganglioneuromas can occur at any level, from the stomach to the anus, and have even been described in the gallbladder. They are most common in the colon and rectum.

Intestinal ganglioneuromas fall into three main groups: (1) solitary polypoid ganglioneuromas, (2) ganglioneuromatous polyposis, and (3) diffuse (transmural) ganglioneuromas. Isolated polypoid ganglioneuromas are most common.[262] These are small sessile or pedunculated polyps, often measuring just a few millimeters, that are endoscopically indistinguishable from adenomas or hyperplastic polyps.[263] No sex predilection has been noted. They do not produce symptoms and are usually detected as an incidental finding at the time of colonoscopy.[263] In ganglioneuromatous polyposis, multiple (dozens to innumerable) polyps are found in the colon. In some patients, polyps are scattered throughout the colorectum, whereas in others, multiple polyps aggregate in a particular segment of the bowel, such as the rectosigmoid or the terminal ileum/right colon region.[262] Unlike solitary ganglioneuromas and ganglioneuromatous polyposis, the epicenter of diffuse ganglioneuromas lies within the muscularis propria, which results in mural thickening and sometimes stricture formation. Affected areas range from 1 to 17 cm in length.[262] Irregular nodular lesions on the mucosal aspect of the bowel can also be seen in cases with transmural involvement.

These categories have different clinical implications. Solitary polypoid ganglioneuromas are not associated with systemic manifestations and do not require long-term follow-up.[263] Ganglioneuromatous polyposis has been associated with multiple cutaneous lipomas and skin tags,[262] Cowden disease,[264] juvenile polyposis,[265] coexistent colonic adenoma or carcinoma,[266] and von Recklinghausen's neurofibromatosis.[266] Diffuse ganglioneuromas occur in patients with multiple endocrine neoplasia (MEN IIb), von Recklinghausen's neurofibromatosis, multiple intestinal neurofibroma, or neurogenic sarcoma.[262,266] Of these, the association between diffuse ganglioneuroma and MEN IIb is particularly strong. Carney and colleagues found that all of their patients with MEN IIb had intestinal ganglioneuromatosis; gastrointestinal symptomatology (including constipation, megacolon, pain, and/or diarrhea) was preceded by endocrine disease in 87%.[267] Smith and coworkers also found diffuse ganglioneuromas in all three pediatric patients with MEN IIb who presented with pseudo-obstruction that mimicked Hirschsprung's disease.[268] Intestinal manifestations preceded the development of medullary thyroid carcinoma in all three cases.

Pathologic Features

Biopsies of ganglioneuromatous polyps reveal a hypercellular and expanded stroma that displaces and distorts colonic crypts. The stroma itself is composed of spindle-shaped cells, which are mainly S100-positive Schwann cells, admixed with variable numbers of ganglion cells (neuron-specific enolase [NSE] -positive) (Fig. 15-27). In the normal colon, ganglion cells are rarely found in the lamina propria. Thus, their presence in mucosal biopsies, particularly when there is more

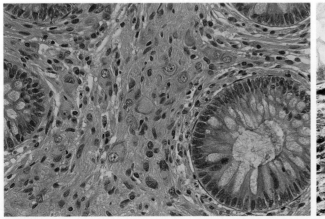
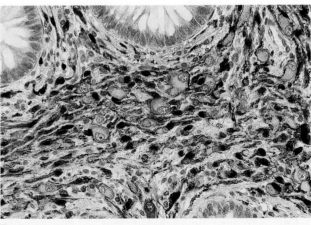

A   **B**

FIGURE 15-27. Mucosal ganglioneuroma (ganglioneuromatous polyp). **A,** At high power, the stromal proliferation is composed of spindle cells and ganglion cells that are either in clusters (as in this case) or in single isolated cells. **B,** S100 immunostain labels the spindled Schwann cells but not the ganglion cells.

than one, should alert one to a possible diagnosis of ganglioneuroma. Occasionally, ectopic ganglion cells may migrate into the lamina propria in response to mucosal injury, such as in Crohn's disease, but these cases lack the characteristic spindle cell proliferation of ganglioneuromas. In some ganglioneuromas the ganglion cell component is readily identifiable, whereas in others it is rare or even absent. A diagnosis of neuroma in these latter cases is more appropriate. Diffuse ganglioneuromas (Fig. 15-28) are centered within the myenteric plexus but also affect all layers of the bowel wall.

NEUROFIBROMAS

Clinical Features

Neurofibromas may occur as isolated lesions or as part of neurofibromatosis type 1 (NF1), or von Recklinghausen's disease. Isolated gastrointestinal neurofibromas outside of the setting of NF1 are exceedingly rare. This is one of the most common genetic diseases, affecting at least 1 in 3000 births. The other form of neurofibromatosis—neurofibromatosis type 2 (NF2)—does not involve the gastrointestinal tract. Patients with NF1 have germline mutations of the *neurofibromatosis 1* tumor suppressor gene on chromosome 17q11.2. Although the syndrome is inherited in an autosomal dominant manner, only approximately half of patients are members of NF1 families (the other half apparently represent sporadic germline mutations).

Diagnostic criteria for NF1 include the presence of at least two of the following features: (1) more than six café-au-lait spots, (2) more than two neurofibromas of any type or more than one plexiform neurofibroma, (3) axillary or groin region freckling, (4) optic glioma, (5) more than two Lisch nodules, (6) a distinctive bony lesion, including dysplasia of the sphenoid bone or dysplasia/thinning of the long bone cortex, and (7) a first-degree relative with NF1.[269] In addition to the dysplastic lesions and benign and malignant tumors that may arise in NF1, these patients also tend to have a stature that is smaller than average, and 40% to 60% suffer from learning disabilities.[269]

Gastrointestinal involvement occurs in up to 25% of patients with NF1. In childhood, severe gastrointestinal complications are rare because neurofibromas generally

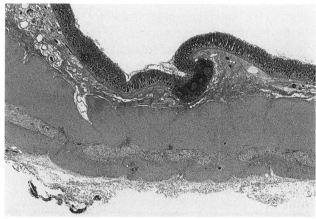

A

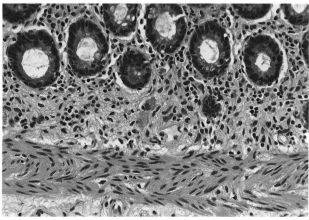

B

C

FIGURE 15–28. Diffuse ganglioneuromatosis. **A,** At low power, the myenteric plexus is diffusely expanded in this patient with MEN IIb. **B,** A cytologically abnormal, double-nucleated ganglion cell within the expanded myenteric plexus attests to the neoplastic nature of the lesion. **C,** The overlying lamina propria in such patients, even if not overly involved by the ganglioneuromatous proliferation, frequently reveals ectopically located ganglion cells.

develop after puberty.[270] Gastrointestinal complaints in both children and adults are most frequently related to the presence of a mass lesion, but severe abdominal pain in the absence of a radiologically identified anatomic lesion has also been described.[270] Mass lesions, or polypoid lesions, in NF1 are of variable types. There is an increased incidence of gastrointestinal stromal tumors,[271-275] diffuse and polypoid ganglioneuromatosis (as described earlier under Ganglioneuromas), gastrointestinal carcinoid tumors (most frequent in the duodenum or periampullary region, often somatostatin-producing lesions),[272,274,276] and gastrointestinal neurofibromas.[277-280] In addition, a possible association between NF1 and duodenal gangliocytic paraganglioma has been described.[281] Finally, there may also be an increased risk for small intestinal adenocarcinoma in NF1.[282]

Symptomatic gastrointestinal neurofibromas in NF1 are unusual and are less commonly reported than GISTs, gastrointestinal ganglioneuromas, or duodenal carcinoids.[277-280] Zöller and associates studied benign and malignant tumors arising over a long-term follow-up in 70 Swedish adults with NF1 and found that only one patient was suspected of having a gastrointestinal neurofibroma; this was based on radiologic evidence of a prepyloric mass and was not confirmed microscopically.[275] Likewise, gastrointestinal neurofibromas were identified by abdominal ultrasound screening in only 4 of 62 asymptomatic adults with NF1 in a study by Wolkenstein and colleagues.[283] Neurofibromas involve (in descending order) the jejunum, stomach, other small intestinal sites such as the ileum and duodenum, colon, and mesentery.[284] In one reported patient with NF1, multiple submucosal neurofibromas involved the common hepatic duct and resulted in a bile duct stricture.[279]

Pathologic Features

These lesions are often plexiform and involve any layer of the bowel wall. Those that arise in the submucosa may extend into the lamina propria and appear polypoid. Their microscopic appearance is similar to that of other extraintestinal neurofibromas (Fig. 15-29). They consist of proliferating bundles of spindle cells with wavy dark nuclei, strands of collagen, varying amounts of myxoid matrix material, and scattered neurites. Both Schwann cells and fibroblasts are present, but S100 usually labels fewer cells than in ganglioneuroma.[280] Submucosal lesions that extend into the muscularis mucosae may splay the overlying crypts and give a low-power appearance of a juvenile polyp.

LEIOMYOMA OF THE MUSCULARIS MUCOSAE

Leiomyomas of the colorectum are benign, true smooth muscle tumors that arise from the muscularis mucosae (see Chapter 22 for details). They constitute the most common type of mesenchymal tumor of the colon[285] and are almost uniformly discovered as incidental polyps in patients undergoing surveillance colonoscopy, or in surgical resection specimens removed for carcinoma. In the largest series of 88 such lesions, Miettinen and coworkers documented a male predominance of 2.4:1 and a median age of 62 years.[286]

Endoscopically, leiomyomas are small, sessile protrusions that appear submucosal in origin. Occasionally, they develop a pedicle and appear pedunculated[286] (Fig. 15-30). Their predominant location is in the rectosigmoid region. Grossly, they are white, firm, well-circumscribed polyps that typically measure several millimeters. However, lesions as large as 2.2 cm have been reported.[286]

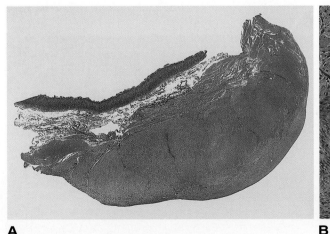

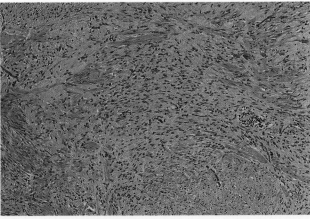

A **B**

FIGURE 15–29. Neurofibroma. **A,** A fusiform enlargement of the muscularis propria is seen in this diffuse neurofibroma. **B,** At higher power, smooth muscle fibers of the muscularis propria are splayed apart by a proliferation of wavy, spindle cells in a fibrotic stroma.

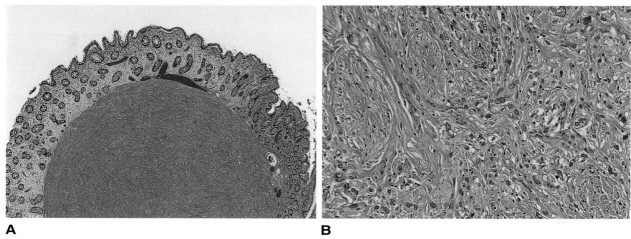

A   **B**

FIGURE 15–30. Leiomyoma. **A,** The polyp is composed of a nodular expansion of the muscularis mucosae, which is sharply demarcated from the overlying, slightly attenuated colonic mucosa. **B,** Occasional leiomyomas contain enlarged and cytologically atypical nuclei, giving the appearance of a "symplastic" leiomyoma. However, more than a rare mitotic figure is never seen in these benign leiomyomas.

Histologically (see Fig. 15-30), they are composed of bundles of mature smooth muscle cells that form a sharply demarcated, nodular expansion of the muscularis mucosae. Smooth muscle cells are more haphazardly arranged than the normal muscularis mucosae, and they merge at the periphery of the leiomyoma with the adjoining muscularis mucosae. In Miettinen's series, only 2 of 88 lesions showed significant cytologic atypia of the smooth muscle cells akin to symplastic leiomyomas of the uterus (see Fig. 15-30), but in only one lesion was there an isolated mitotic figure.[286] The overlying colonic mucosa is usually normal or may be attenuated. In the sigmoid colon (their most common location), leiomyomas outnumber GISTs, but in the rectum, they are either as common as or less common than GISTs.[286] In contrast to GISTs, leiomyomas label strongly and diffusely with smooth muscle actin and desmin and are negative for CD34, CD117, and S100.

Endoscopic polypectomy is sufficient treatment for leiomyomas, which are uniformly clinically benign. Even those tumors with cytologic atypia or mitotic activity need only the assurance of complete endoscopic removal.[286]

LEIOMYOSARCOMAS

True leiomyosarcomas of the colorectum are rare (see Chapter 22 for details); most previously reported cases represent malignant GISTs. Unlike GISTs, true leiomyosarcomas frequently present endoscopically as intraluminal polypoid tumors.[285] In a series of seven cases by Miettinen and associates, the sex distribution and age range were similar to those of leiomyoma, with a male-to-female ratio of 2.5:1 and a median age of 61 years.[287] Colonic leiomyosarcomas are much less common than either leiomyomas or GISTs, and they differ from both of the latter lesions in their more frequent location in the right colon. In contrast to leiomyomas, leiomyosarcomas are of a much larger size (mean of 6.0 cm), often show an ulcerated intraluminal surface, frequently infiltrate into the overlying colonic mucosa, and may show coagulative necrosis.[287] They are predominantly of high-grade histology and are composed of mitotically active spindle cells that resemble smooth muscle cells, with cigar-shaped nuclei and eosinophilic cytoplasm. In Miettinen's series, six of seven cases contained more than 100 mitoses per 50 high-power fields (hpfs).[287] Like leiomyomas, leiomyosarcomas express smooth muscle actin (and often, desmin) and are negative for CD34, CD117, and S100 protein (Fig. 15-31). Therefore, they are not considered variants of GISTs. Most patients die of their disease within 6 months to 3 years, but long-term survival may occur even among patients whose tumors have a high rate of mitotic activity.[287]

Smooth muscle neoplasms graded variably as leiomyosarcomas, leiomyomas, and smooth muscle tumors of uncertain malignant potential also occur in association with human immunodeficiency virus infection or with other immunodeficiency states, including solid organ transplantation and congenital immunodeficiencies. The pathogenesis of these tumors is related in part to Epstein-Barr virus (EBV) infection and subsequent clonal expansion of smooth muscle cells[288,289]; in situ hybridization for EBV sequences is positive in these tumors, as are markers of smooth muscle differentiation such as desmin and smooth muscle actin.[288,289] EBV-associated smooth muscle neoplasms frequently present as gastrointestinal tumors,[289,290] but they also occur in diverse extraintestinal sites such as the lungs,[288,291] liver,[291,292] brain,[293] heart,[294] kidneys,[295] and thyroid,[296] among others. In the gastrointestinal tract, the lesions typically are single or multiple, endoscopically submucosal nodules with central ulceration that measure from less than 1 cm to 4 cm.[297]

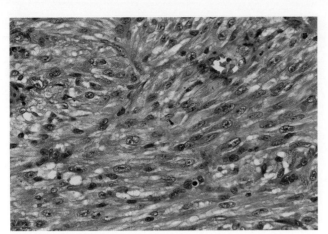

FIGURE 15–31. Leiomyosarcoma. These are more cellular than leiomyomas and contain frequent mitotic figures (*center*).

GASTROINTESTINAL STROMAL TUMORS
(see Chapter 22)

These are uncommon tumors of the colorectum, where they account for only 5% of all GISTs.[286] CD117 expression is found in 76% and CD34 expression in only 59% of colonic tumors,[287] but rectal tumors are characteristically (90%) positive for CD34.[286] Unlike leiomyomas and leiomyosarcomas, colorectal GISTs rarely present as mucosal polyps[286,287] because their epicenters are within the muscularis propria (Fig. 15-32).

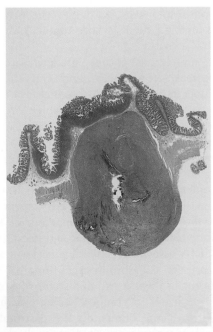

FIGURE 15–32. GIST. Unlike leiomyomas that arise from the muscularis mucosae, the epicenter of GISTs lies within the muscularis propria.

LIPOMAS

Lipomas occur throughout the gastrointestinal tract but are most frequent in the colon,[298] particularly in the ascending colon and cecum (see Chapter 22). In the colon, they represent the most common submucosal mesenchymal tumor[298] and have a predilection for elderly women.[299,300] Their incidence varies from 0.56% in autopsy studies[301] to 0.15% in colonoscopy studies.[302] Although many lipomas are an incidental finding, their tendency to produce symptoms is strongly dependent on their size. Patients with lipomas smaller than 2 cm are rarely symptomatic, whereas larger lesions can result in rectal bleeding, abdominal pain, and a change in bowel habits.[301,303] A significant minority of large lipomas may result in a more dramatic presentation, including intussusception[301,304,305] or luminal obstruction.[304]

Endoscopically, small lipomas are usually soft, sessile polyps that have an intact, smooth overlying mucosa. The mucosa over larger lipomas can be ulcerated and irregular because of mechanical trauma or intussusception.[306] Biopsy forceps that reach through the mucosa can expose endoscopically recognizable, yellow adipose tissue in the submucosa. Most lipomas are solitary. In 25% to 30% of patients, multiple lipomas occur.[301] Rarely, lipomatous polyposis has been reported. In one case, hundreds of lipomas studded the colon of a 51-year-old man, who underwent colectomy because the polyps mimicked FAP.[307] Endoscopic polypectomy or surgical resection is generally indicated for lesions that are symptomatic or larger than 2.5 cm.[308]

Histologically (Fig. 15-33), most lipomas are discrete, although nonencapsulated, lesions that are localized to the submucosa. In rare cases, the lipoma involves the muscularis propria or arises in the subserosal fat.[298] Overlying colonic mucosa can be normal, atrophic, hyperplastic, or ulcerated. It is not unusual to find changes of a hyperplastic polyp overlying submucosal lipomas. Most lipomas are composed of a uniform population of benign-appearing adipocytes. In unusual cases with surface ulceration, there may be atypical hyperchromatic adipocyte nuclei, mitotic activity with occasional atypical mitoses, and cellular fibrosis—changes that are interpreted as reactive.[309]

Lipomatous Ileocecal Valve

True lipomas of the ileocecal valve are well-circumscribed lesions that affect only one of the ileocecal lips.[310] More commonly, there is a diffuse increase in submucosal adipose tissue that causes the ileocecal valve to appear similar to a set of protruding lips. This has been referred to as *lipohyperplasia*, *lipomatosis*, and *lipomatous hypertrophy* of the ileocecal valve. Histologically, deep forceps biopsies show mature adipose tissue within the submucosa, identical to the

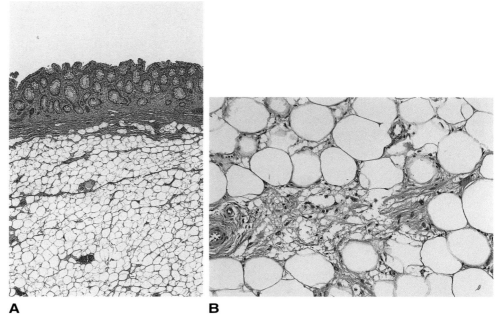

FIGURE 15–33. Lipoma. **A,** A discrete nodule of adipose tissue is localized to the submucosa. The overlying colonic mucosa shows mild crypt distortion due to prolapse and mechanical trauma. **B,** In contrast, this colonic liposarcoma shows a more cellular interstitium and contains lipoblasts.

A   B

histology of a true lipoma. In the past, barium enema examinations sometimes confused these lesions with malignancy.[310] In current practice, lipomatous ileocecal valves are rarely biopsied because their appearance at colonoscopy is characteristic, and they are rarely confused with neoplasms. Most patients do not experience symptoms, but in rare cases, lipomatous hyperplasia may lead to recurrent intussusception[311] or appendicitis.[312] The ileocolonic mucosa overlying the protruding valve can also show nonspecific ulceration related to mechanical trauma.

In one autopsy study, 80.4% of patients had some degree of lipomatous hypertrophy of the ileocecal valve, and it was judged to be marked in 13.7%.[313] The degree of lipohyperplasia correlated with greater body weight and with fatty infiltration into the right ventricle and pancreas.[313]

GRANULAR CELL TUMORS

Granular cell tumors usually arise in the tongue or dermis but can occur in virtually any anatomic site (see Chapters 12 and 22). Within the gastrointestinal tract, granular cell tumors are most common in the esophagus. The colon is the second most common gastrointestinal primary site, followed in descending order by the perianal region, stomach, appendix, and small bowel.[314] Colonic granular cell tumors have a predilection for the right colon and rectum. In most cases, the granular cell tumor is an incidental finding at the time of colonoscopy or surgical resection, although fecal occult blood or rectal bleeding may have precipitated a colonoscopic examination, particularly when the lesion is within the rectum or anus.[315,316] Endoscopically, they typically appear as smooth, sessile sub-

mucosal polyps, ranging in size from a few millimeters to 2 to 3 cm; they are usually covered by an intact colonic mucosa. In 10% of patients, multiple granular cell tumors are present, either in different portions of the gastrointestinal tract or in gastrointestinal plus extraintestinal sites.[314,317]

Histologically (Fig. 15-34), colonic granular cell tumors resemble those in other portions of the gastrointestinal tract. They are poorly circumscribed, unencapsulated tumors composed of plump, rounded or polygonal cells with uniform small nuclei and abundant granular eosinophilic cytoplasm.[318] They are weakly positive with periodic acid–Schiff (PAS) both before and after diastase and uniformly label with both NSE and S100. Their immunohistochemical profile and ultrastructural appearance are now thought to be indicative of neural and, in particular, Schwann cell differentiation. The term *granular cell tumor* thus contrasts with the previous designation of *granular cell myoblastoma*, an appellation that reflected the earlier concept of muscle origin.

Endoscopic polypectomy is the treatment of choice. Only 1% to 2% of granular cell tumors in extraintestinal sites behave in a malignant fashion.[319] Malignant granular cell tumors are extremely difficult to separate histologically from their vastly more common benign counterparts; the distinction is based mostly on clinical evidence of aggressive behavior such as recurrence, rapid growth, or metastasis.[319] Large size (>5 cm), greater cellularity, and mitotic activity (>2 mitoses/10 hpfs) are histopathologic features that raise the suspicion of malignancy.[319] In the largest published series of gastrointestinal granular cell tumors, none of 75 tumors recurred or metastasized.[314]

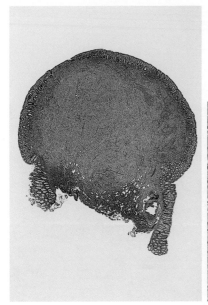

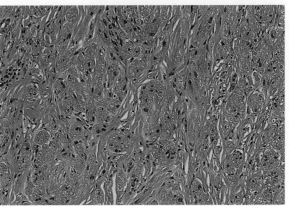

A   **B**

FIGURE 15–34. Granular cell tumor. **A,** This unencapsulated lesion expands the submucosa of the rectum. **B,** The lesional cells are plump, spindle-shaped, and rounded cells with abundant granular cytoplasm.

INFLAMMATORY FIBROID POLYPS

Inflammatory fibroid polyps are histologically and clinically benign lesions that occur throughout the gastrointestinal tract (see Chapters 13 and 14 for details). They are most common in the gastric antrum and the terminal ileum but have been reported in diverse sites, including the esophagus,[319] duodenum,[320] and ileoanal pouch.[321] Inflammatory fibroid polyps occur relatively uncommonly in the colorectum.[322-327] In one study, only 4 (12%) of 33 lesions arose in the colon.[328] Patients of all ages can be affected, and no significant sex predilection has been noted. Although occasional inflammatory fibroid polyps have been reported in patients with Cowden disease,[329] chronic IBD including ulcerative colitis,[321] and Crohn's disease,[330] and in a familial setting spanning three generations,[331] there is in general no specific association between inflammatory fibroid polyps and underlying gastro-intestinal disease. Intestinal lesions most commonly present (in decreasing order) with abdominal pain, bloody stools, weight loss, or diarrhea[322]; those on the ileocecal valve can cause obstruction.[332] A single patient had colocolic intussusception related to inflammatory fibroid polyp of the cecum,[322] but this complication is by far more common with small bowel lesions.

Endoscopically, colonic inflammatory fibroid polyps are usually solitary, sessile polyps that appear sub-mucosally and range in size from 1.5 to 7 cm.[322] In the majority of cases, the overlying colonic mucosa is ulcerated.[323] Histologically (Fig. 15-35), inflammatory fibroid polyps are similar in appearance to those that occur in the small intestine. The epicenter of the tumor is usually in the submucosa, but it can infiltrate into the overlying mucosa and the muscularis propria or serosa.

Some cases are localized entirely within the mucosa. The lesion shows highly vascularized, fibromyxoid stroma that contains abundant inflammatory cells. The vascular network ranges from capillaries to larger, thick- and thin-walled blood vessels, which may be occluded. The inflammatory infiltrate is usually dominated by eosinophils. Lymphocytic aggregates lacking germinal centers may also present, and polyclonal plasma cells, histiocytes, and neutrophils may be seen as well. A characteristic cell type is the stellate or spindle-shaped, bland stromal cell that tends to be arranged in an onionskin pattern around blood vessels and crypts when there is mucosal involvement. Cytologic atypia of the stromal cells is only infrequently present and is at most mild.[333] The stromal cells are reactive for vimentin[334] and CD34 (in 82% to 100% of cases),[333,335] but in contrast to GISTs, they are negative for CD117. Local excision is usually curative.[322-334]

■ Miscellaneous Polypoid Lesions

PNEUMATOSIS COLI

Clinical Features

The hallmark of pneumatosis is the presence of gas within the bowel wall. Radiologically, the gas may appear as either linear streaks or cysts adjacent to the muscularis propria, or a combination thereof. When predominantly cystic, the designation *pneumatosis cystoides intestinalis* is usually applied. The term *pneumatosis coli* refers to either linear or cystic forms that are limited to the wall of the colon. Although frequently cited as a rare diagnosis, pneumatosis is

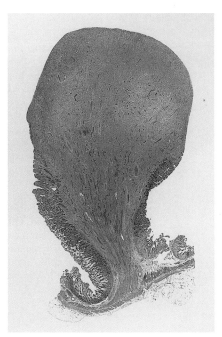

FIGURE 15–35. Inflammatory fibroid polyp. This pedunculated inflammatory fibroid polyp has its epicenter within the submucosa.

often asymptomatic and is likely underreported.[336] Pneumatosis itself is not a single disease entity but rather represents the common end point of multiple pathogenic conditions. It is primary (idiopathic) in only 15% of cases.[337] The other 85% of cases are secondary to diverse predisposing conditions that include trauma from endoscopy or endoscopic polypectomy,[338,339] blunt abdominal trauma,[340] sigmoid volvulus,[341] collagen vascular disease,[342] appendicitis,[343] neonatal necrotizing enterocolitis, adult ischemic bowel disease, infectious colitis such as *Clostridium difficile* colitis,[344] acquired immunodeficiency syndrome (AIDS),[337] idiopathic inflammatory bowel disease, pyloric stenosis, and various pulmonary conditions such as asthma, cystic fibrosis, and emphysema.[345]

Three main (and in some cases, interrelated) mechanisms have been proposed for gas accumulation: (1) In patients with pulmonary disease, air from ruptured pulmonary blebs may pass through the retroperitoneum, along the loose adventitia of mesenteric blood vessels, and into the subserosa of the bowel wall; (2) increased intra-abdominal pressure may force gas through minute defects of the intestinal epithelium, where it accumulates in the loose connective tissue of the submucosa and subserosa; and (3) intestinal necrosis allows gas-forming anaerobic organisms to proliferate within the intestinal wall. Depending on the associated condition, or lack thereof, pneumatosis can be clinically benign or can represent a surgical emergency. The cystic form is often an incidental finding in adults who have clinically benign disease. Linear streaks of gas, in

contrast, usually imply impending bowel perforation resulting from epithelial necrosis. For example, this is the form of pneumatosis typically seen in neonatal necrotizing enterocolitis. One paradoxical exception to the latter rule occurs in patients with AIDS, wherein linear pneumatosis has been reported to follow a benign course, even when associated with infectious colitis.[337]

Of particular relevance to this chapter is the cystic form of pneumatosis coli, which can result in endoscopically (or grossly) polypoid lesions. Whereas in the older literature small intestinal pneumatosis predominated, pneumatosis cystoides coli is now the more common form in adults[345] and usually follows a benign course.[346] Most affected patients are middle-aged, and many are asymptomatic. Symptomatic patients complain of diarrhea, constipation, mucoid stools, bleeding, flatus, abdominal pain, fecal incontinence, or a combination thereof.[346] The necessity for and type of treatment depend on the patient's symptoms and any associated colonic pathology. Rare cases of pneumatosis coli associated with ischemia, perforation, or anaerobic infection are life-threatening and usually require immediate surgery. The cysts of benign pneumatosis cystoides coli resolve spontaneously in up to 50% of cases.[336] Symptomatic patients with pneumatosis cystoides coli can be treated with hyperbaric oxygen[345,347] or symptom-directed therapies such as antidiarrheals or anti-inflammatory drugs.[345] Asymptomatic patients may not require therapy.[348]

Pathologic Features

Grossly, pneumatosis cystoides coli may appear as round polypoid lesions covered by normal mucosa.[347] In one of the largest clinicopathologic series of pneumatosis coli, Gagliardi and associates found that the sigmoid colon was most commonly affected (40%), followed in decreasing order by the rectum, descending colon, transverse and ascending colon, and cecum.[345] Grossly, cystic collections of gas can be found in any layer of the bowel wall, but they predominate in the loose fibrofatty tissues of the submucosa and less prominently in the subserosa. In severe cases, the affected segment may have a spongy appearance caused by the presence of closely packed gas cysts.[343] Microscopically (Fig. 15-36), the cysts appear as empty spaces lined by epithelioid macrophages and multinucleated giant cells that represent a foreign body–type reaction; rarely, foamy macrophages predominate.[345] The macrophage lining cells may be attenuated but can be highlighted by immunohistochemistry for macrophage markers (such as CD68), if necessary. The overlying mucosa may also contain small cystic spaces and epithelioid macrophages or giant cells within the lamina propria. In Gagliardi's series, associated mucosal abnormalities were detected in all cases, including mild atrophy or mild crypt

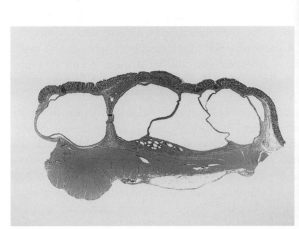

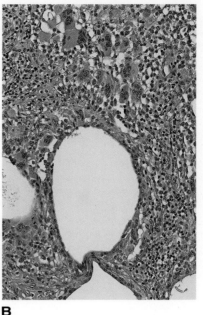

FIGURE 15–36. Pneumatosis coli. **A,** Large cysts characteristically predominate in the submucosa. **B,** Biopsy specimens may contain cystic spaces in both the mucosa and the submucosa; these gas-filled cysts appear "empty" and are lined focally or diffusely by histiocytes and foreign body–type giant cells. Histiocytes lining the gas-filled cysts may be flattened and attenuated. Often, other chronic inflammatory cells, including lymphocytes and plasma cells, are also admixed with the submucosal macrophages.

A   B

distortion in almost all, chronic inflammation in three quarters, and active inflammation in almost one half of patients.[345]

MUCOSAL PSEUDOLIPOMATOSIS

Pseudolipomatosis is a minor procedural complication of endoscopy that results from air insufflation, mild mucosal trauma, and penetration of gas into the lamina propria.[349-351] Most cases involve middle-aged to older adults who undergo colonoscopic screening for rectal bleeding.[350,352,353] Endoscopically, lesions may be solitary or multiple, raised, white to yellow plaques measuring from 1 to 3 cm.[352] Histologically, numerous vacuolated spaces within the lamina propria, measuring from 20 to 240 µm, can be identified.[353] The clear spaces have no epithelial lining but on ultrastructural examination are bounded by collagen and ground substance.[354] Snover and colleagues proposed the term *mucosal pseudolipomatosis* in 1985 based on histochemical and ultrastructural evidence that the vacuoles are composed of trapped gas rather than adipocytes, as was previously believed.[355] Many cases resolve within weeks.[351]

ENDOMETRIOSIS

Clinical Features

Endometriosis is estimated to affect up to 15% of menstruating women.[356] Pelvic involvement is most common, but diverse extrapelvic sites can be affected irrespective of the presence or absence of pelvic disease. The intestinal tract is involved by endometriosis in 15% to 37% of patients with pelvic endometriosis.[357]

Most commonly, the affected site is the rectosigmoid colon, followed by the rectovaginal septum.[358] Any site in the large or small bowel may be affected, but gastric and esophageal involvement does not appear to occur.[357] Although most patients are in their childbearing years, symptomatic sigmoid endometriosis has been documented to occur even in older, postmenopausal women who have not received hormone replacement therapy.[359]

An unknown number of patients with intestinal endometriosis are asymptomatic, but those who come to medical attention suffer from abdominal pain, mass effect, bowel obstruction, rectal bleeding, infertility, diarrhea, or urinary frequency, in decreasing order.[357] Numerous case reports have described patients whose endometriosis clinically and surgically mimicked a primary colonic carcinoma.[360] More commonly, intestinal endometriosis simulates inflammatory bowel diseases such as diverticulitis, appendicitis, or Crohn's disease.[357] Treatment is similar to that for pelvic endometriosis, including pain medication and hormonal therapy; patients with complications such as obstruction, perforation, or a mass lesion that simulates carcinoma may require surgery.

Pathologic Features

The gross features of bowel specimens that come to surgical resection depend on the site of involvement of the bowel wall and the size of the implants. Subserosal endometriotic foci typically elicit a fibrotic response and serosal adhesions. Those in the muscularis propria can elicit smooth muscle hypertrophy akin to that seen in uterine adenomyosis, with irregular mural thickening, strictures, or mass lesions that grossly simulate a stromal tumor. Perhaps more germane to the topic of colonic polyps are the lesions produced by either submucosal or mucosal involvement. In one of the largest systematic studies of intestinal endometriosis, Yantiss and colleagues found that 66% of affected patients had endometriotic foci in either the submucosa or the mucosa, including lamina propria involvement in nearly 30%.[357] These lesions are apt to grossly mimic either primary colon cancer, with production of ischemic mucosal ulceration over a submucosal mass, or an adenomatous polyp.

Histologically (Fig. 15-37), the hallmark of endometriosis is the presence of ectopic endometrial glands and stroma. In the lamina propria, the hyperchromatic columnar nuclei and mucin-depleted cells of endometriotic glands can merge with the adjacent colonic epithelium, creating the appearance of an adenomatous polyp. In fact, dilated and irregularly shaped submucosal endometrial glands can easily cause a misdiagnosis of colonic carcinoma. Recognition of cilia in the endometrial glands and their characteristic surrounding cellular stroma can aid in the distinction between endometriosis and neoplastic colonic epithelium. In difficult cases, a panel of immunohistochemical stains can be useful. Estrogen and progesterone receptors are positive,[356] and CD10 highlights the endometrial stromal cells in 88% of endometriotic foci.[361] Endometrial glands are uniformly CK7+, CK20-, CEA-, whereas colonic epithelium is CK7-, CK20+, and CEA+.[356]

Ectopic endometrial tissue, whether in the lamina propria or in deeper layers of the bowel wall, results in reactive mucosal abnormalities in more than half of affected patients.[357] In Yantiss' study, active chronic inflammatory changes (including crypt architectural distortion, crypt abscesses, and ulceration, similar to the pathologic features of idiopathic chronic IBD) were most common, followed by ischemia and prolapse-type changes.[357]

Up to 1% of women with endometriosis develop endometriosis-associated neoplasms; the ovary is the most common site of malignant transformation, followed by the pelvis and the intestinal tract.[362] Akin to the frequency of benign endometriotic involvement, most such neoplasms develop in the rectosigmoid colon, with fewer in the proximal colon or ileum.[362,363] The entire range of neoplastic and preneoplastic changes of primary uterine pathology have been documented to occur within intestinal sites, including atypical hyperplasia, adenocarcinoma in situ, endometrioid adenocarcinomas, mixed müllerian tumors, and endometrial stromal sarcomas.[362,363] Yantiss and coworkers suggested that "dirty necrosis," higher grade nuclear cytology, and a CK7-/CK20+ cytokeratin profile were most helpful in distinguishing colonic adenocarcinoma from endometrioid adenocarcinoma respectively.[357] Prolonged unopposed estrogen therapy may be a predisposing factor.

BENIGN INFILTRATIVE PROCESSES

Muciphages

Scattered, isolated histiocytes are present in the lamina propria in the majority of colonic biopsy specimens, but they do not tend to form aggregates and therefore usually remain inconspicuous (see Chapter 5). However, biopsy specimens obtained from the rectosigmoid region may show prominent histiocytic aggregates that may impart a nodular or polypoid appearance to the mucosa. In a series of 100 consecutive rectal

FIGURE 15–37. Endometriosis. **A,** A polypoid lesion projects *(at center)* above the surrounding colonic mucosa. In addition, several endometriotic foci can be seen in the muscularis propria, which is characteristically markedly thickened. **B,** Endometriotic glands contain more hyperchromatic nuclei and appear mucin depleted relative to the normal colonic epithelium. They can merge with colonic crypts, giving the appearance of adenoma or dysplasia. Recognition of endometrial stromal cells adjacent to the hyperchromatic glands is key to the correct diagnosis.

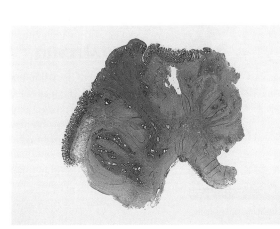

A

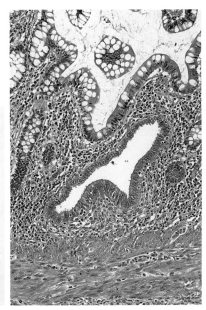

B

biopsy specimens, Bejarano and associates found foamy histiocytes in 40%, and aggregates of large foamy histiocytes were moderate to intense in 23%.[364] In most cases, infiltrates are present in the superficial aspect of the lamina propria, but these can also involve the muscularis mucosae. Immunohistochemical stains reveal these cells to be CD68+ and cytokeratin-negative macrophages. This immunoprofile and the lack of nuclear enlargement or atypia help to distinguish them from signet ring cell carcinomas. In 20% of patients, histiocytic aggregates were the only histologic finding to account for the endoscopic impression of small nodules or polyps.[364]

In most cases, the foamy histiocytes represent muciphages that contain neutral and acidic mucins, mainly sialomucins.[364] Common histologic abnormalities of the associated rectal mucosa include mild to moderate fibrosis of the lamina propria, mild crypt atrophy, and mild chronic inflammation, suggesting that muciphages are the residua of previous mild mucosal injury (Fig. 15-38).[364]

Xanthoma and Xanthogranuloma

In a minority of cases, histiocyte aggregates represent true xanthomas, or localized collections of lipid-containing histiocytes. These cases are not distinguishable from muciphages based on their hematoxylin and eosin–stained appearance. The nature of these histiocytes is revealed by negative mucin histochemical stains, including PAS-diastase, Alcian blue at pH 2.5 and pH 1.0, and mucicarmine. In addition, lipid-containing histiocytes have a characteristic granular, dotlike cytoplasmic labeling for CD68 that contrasts with the usual more clumped cytoplasmic CD68 labeling of muciphages.[364] In contrast to muciphages, true xanthomas are unusual. The most common gastro-

intestinal site of involvement is the stomach. Colorectal xanthomas are almost all located in the sigmoid[365-367] or rectum,[364,365] where they are seen endoscopically as cream-colored to yellow papules or polyps that typically measure from 1 to 4 mm. They are almost all incidental findings at colonoscopy and may be solitary or multiple. Similar to muciphages, histologically, xanthoma cells can involve both the lamina propria and the muscularis mucosae (or even the submucosa if the biopsy is deep enough), but most cases are limited to the lamina propria. Most reported patients with xanthomas are middle-aged, and no clear sex predilection has been noted. Most patients have neither hyperlipidemia nor associated skin lesions.[365]

More extensive xanthomatous or xanthogranulomatous inflammation that involves the deeper layers of the bowel wall, including the muscularis propria, is a rare cause of intestinal obstruction. These cases have been reported in the ileocecal valve[368] and the rectosigmoid colon.[369,370]

Differential Diagnosis of Infiltrative Processes

The finding of histiocytes in the lamina propria may raise a differential diagnosis with lipid storage disease and infection (fungal organisms, acid-fast bacilli, and the Whipple bacillus, among others). In addition, signet ring carcinoma cells can on occasion be confused with histiocytes. Histiocytes are usually readily distinguished from signet ring cell carcinoma by their lack of nuclear enlargement and atypia on routine hematoxylin and eosin staining. In questionable cases, immunohistochemical stains for CD68 and cytokeratin can be performed; histochemical stains for mucin are of no utility in this differential diagnosis because both muciphages and carcinoma cells contain cytoplasmic mucin. Stains for infectious organisms are not usually performed unless the patient is immunosuppressed, the histiocytic aggregates are located proximal to the rectosigmoid, or another clinical indication requires it.

Mucosal infiltrates that are the result of systemic illnesses are explained in detail in Chapter 5.

INVERTED APPENDIX

Appendiceal intussusception is a rare condition, found in only 0.01% of 71,000 appendectomies studied over 40 years in one large series.[371] All ages, from infants to elderly, can be affected, but it is more common in the first decade of life and among males.[372] Anatomically, there are several main types of appendiceal intussusception, which have been reviewed in detail by Langsam and coworkers.[373] Briefly, either the distal or proximal appendix can intussuscept and give rise to a completely or partially inverted appendix that protrudes into the cecum. An inverted appendix must, therefore,

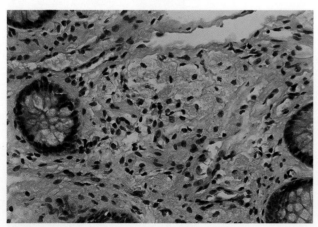

FIGURE 15–38. Muciphages. A cluster of lightly basophilic, foamy macrophages is present in the lamina propria of this rectal biopsy.

be considered in the radiologic and histologic differential diagnosis of polypoid cecal lesions.[374,375]

Most patients with an inverted appendix are symptomatic; their abdominal complaints are nonspecific but can include abdominal pain, nausea and vomiting, and blood in the stool.[372,376-378] Predisposing conditions include abnormal peristalsis (either of the intestine or appendix itself), anatomic abnormalities such as a mobile mesoappendix or a wide appendicular lumen, and mass lesions that form a focal point for intussusception.[372] In the latter category, inverted appendices have been reported in patients with appendiceal mucocele,[376] appendiceal adenoma,[374,375] juvenile polyp,[378] endometriosis,[374] and Peutz-Jeghers syndrome,[379] among others. In some cases, however, the appendix has no apparent abnormality.[377]

Pathologically, the inverted appendix with a mass lesion such as adenoma can appear as a pedunculated polyp in which the inverted appendix forms the "stalk."[379] Histologically, the layers of the appendiceal wall are reversed. The mucosa forms the external layer, and the submucosa and muscularis propria the internal layer. The mucosa may show increased acute and chronic inflammation[372,377] and submucosal fibrosis.[372] In some cases, it is histologically normal.[377] Ischemic changes secondary to inversion can also occur.

MUCOSAL TAG

Small excrescences of histologically normal mucosa are a frequent incidental finding at colonoscopy. Also called *mucosal polyps* by some authors, they represent benign elevations of colonic mucosa. They are most often biopsied to exclude an adenoma or hyperplastic polyp. In one autopsy study of 502 Cretan patients (median age of 65 years), incidental colorectal polyps were identified in 21.1% of cases, and 6.9% of these were "mucosal tags."[380] Even higher frequencies are documented when only diminutive (<5 mm) polyps are considered. Weston and Campbell reported that 17.9% of diminutive polyps represented either mucosal tags or lymphoid follicles,[381] whereas in the study by Hoff and associates, fully 23% of diminutive polyps were mucosal tags.[141] Furthermore, mucosal tags may diminish in size when followed endoscopically.[141]

ATHEROEMBOLUS-ASSOCIATED POLYPS

Some cases of localized colonic ischemia produce the endoscopic appearance of a mass or a polyp. In a study of the histologic features distinguishing ischemia from *C. difficile* colitis, for example, Dignan and Greenson reported that in 7 of 24 patients with ischemic colitis, the endoscopic impression was that of a mass lesion or polyp.[382] Atheroemboli can rarely cause polyp formation through an ischemic mechanism (Fig. 15-39).[383,384]

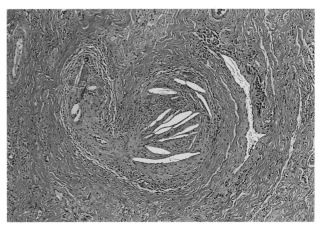

FIGURE 15-39. Atheroemboli-associated polyps. Within the underlying submucosa, an arterial lumen is occluded by atheroembolic material that contains cholesterol clefts.

Submucosal edema that develops in ischemic colitis contributes to this appearance by elevating the overlying ischemic mucosa.[385] Rarely, atheroemboli are seen as an incidental finding in biopsies of adenomatous polyps.[385]

References

1. Imperiale TF, Wagner DR, Lin CY, et al: Results of screening colonoscopy among persons 40 to 49 years of age. N Engl J Med 346:1781-1785, 2002.
2. Khan A, Shrier I, Gordon PH: The changed histologic paradigm of colorectal polyps. Surg Endosc 16:436-440, 2002.
3. Williams AR, Balasooriya BA, Day DW: Polyps and cancer of the large bowel: A necropsy study in Liverpool. Gut 23:835-842, 1982.
4. Vatn MH, Stalsberg H: The prevalence of polyps of the large intestine in Oslo: An autopsy study. Cancer 49:819-825, 1982.
5. Tsai CJ, Lu DK: Small colorectal polyps: Histopathology and clinical significance. Am J Gastroenterol 90:988-994, 1995.
6. Odze RD, Brien T, Brown CA, et al: Molecular alterations in chronic ulcerative colitis-associated and sporadic hyperplastic polyps: A comparative analysis. Am J Gastroenterol 97:1235-1242, 2002.
7. Fenoglio-Preiser CM: When is a hyperplastic polyp not a hyperplastic polyp? Am J Surg Pathol 23:1001-1003, 1999.
8. Otori K, Oda Y, Sugiyama K, et al: High frequency of K-ras mutations in human colorectal hyperplastic polyps. Gut 40:660-663, 1997.
9. Carr NJ, Monihan JM, Nzeako UC, et al: Expression of proliferating cell nuclear antigen in hyperplastic polyps, adenomas and inflammatory cloacogenic polyps of the large intestine. J Clin Pathol 48:46-52, 1995.
10. Kang M, Mitomi H, Sada M: Ki-67, p53, and Bcl-2 expression of serrated adenomas of the colon. Am J Surg Pathol 21:417-423, 1997.
11. Lothe RA, Andersen SN, Hofstad B, et al: Deletion of Ip loci and microsatellite instability in colorectal polyps. Genes Chromosomes Cancer 14:182-188, 1995.
12. Giarnieri E, Nagar C, Valli S, et al: BCL 2 and BAX expression in hyperplastic and dysplastic rectal polyps. Hepatogastroenterology 47:159-162, 2000.
13. Sugimoto K, Kageoka M, Iwasaki H, et al: Adenocarcinoma arising from a hyperplastic polyp with adenomatous foci. Endoscopy 31:S59, 1999.
14. Yantiss RK, Goldman H, Odze RD: Hyperplastic polyp with epithelial misplacement (inverted hyperplastic): A clinicopathologic and immunohistochemical study of 19 cases. Mod Pathol 14:869-875, 2001.

15. Bensen SP, Cole BF, Mott LA, et al: Colorectal hyperplastic polyps and risk of recurrence of adenomas and hyperplastic polyps. Polyps Prevention Study. Lancet 354:1873-1874, 1999.
16. Farraye FA, Wallace M: Clinical significance of small polyps found during screening with flexible sigmoidoscopy. Gastointest Endosc Clin N Am 12:41-51, 2002.
17. Sciallero S, Costantini M, Bertinelli E, et al: Distal hyperplastic polyps do not predict proximal adenomas: Results from a multicentric study of colorectal adenomas. Gastrointest Endosc 46:124-130, 1997.
18. Morimoto LM, Newcomb PA, Ulrich CM, et al: Risk factors for hyperplastic and adenomatous polyps: Evidence for malignant potential? Cancer Epidemiol Biomarkers Prev 11:1012-1018, 2002.
19. Huang EH, Whelan RL, Gleason NR, et al: Increased incidence of colorectal adenomas in follow-up evaluation of patients with newly diagnosed hyperplastic polyps. Surg Endosc 15:646-648, 2001.
20. Burgart LJ, Batts KP, Wang L, et al: Adenocarcinoma involving colonic hyperplastic polyps is associated with loss of DNA repair enzyme MLH-1. Gastroenterology 114:A571, 1998.
21. Tonooka T, Sano Y, Fujii T, et al: Adenocarcinoma in solitary large hyperplastic polyp diagnosed by magnifying colonoscope: Report of a case. Dis Colon Rectum 45:1407-1411, 2002.
22. Williams GT, Arthur JF, Bussey HJ, et al: Metaplastic polyps and polyposis of the colorectum. Histopathology 4:155-170, 1980.
23. Jeevaratnam P, Cottier DS, Browett PJ, et al: Familial giant hyperplastic polyposis predisposing to colorectal cancer: A new hereditary bowel cancer syndrome. J Pathol 179:20-25, 1996.
24. Burt R, Jass JR: Hyperplastic polyposis. In Hamilton SR, Aaltonen LA (eds): WHO International Classification of Tumors: Pathology and Genetics of Tumors of the Digestive System. Berlin, Springer-Verlag, 2000, pp 135-136.
25. Keljo DJ, Weinberg AG, Winick N, et al: Rectal cancer in an 11-year-old with hyperpalastic polyposis. J Pediatr Gastroenterol Nutr 28:327-332, 1999.
26. Bengoechea O, Martinez-Penuela JM, Larrinaga B, et al: Hyperplastic polyposis of the colorectum and adenocarcinoma in a 24-year-old man. Am J Surg Pathol 11:323-327, 1987.
27. Jass JR, Pokos V, Arnold JL, et al: Colorectal neoplasms detected colonoscopically in at risk members of colorectal cancer families stratified by the demonstration of DNA microsatellite instability. J Mol Med 74:547-551, 1996.
28. Leggett BA, Deveraux B, Biden K, et al: Hyperplastic polyposis: Association with colorectal cancer. Am J Surg Pathol 25:117-184, 2001.
29. Rashid A, Houlihan PS, Booker S, et al: Phenotypic and molecular characteristics of hyperplastic polyposis. Gastroenterology 119:323-332, 2000.
30. Levine DS, Surawicz CM, Spencer GD, et al: Inflammatory polyposis two years after ischemic colon injury. Dig Dis Sci 31:1159-1167, 1986.
31. Iofel E, Kahn E, Lee TK, et al: Inflammatory polyps after necrotizing enterocolitis. J Pediatr Surg 35:1246-1247, 2000.
32. De Backer AI, Van Overbeke LN, Mortele KJ, et al: Inflammatory pseudopolyposis in a patient with toxic megacolon due to pseudomembranous colitis. JBR-BTR 84:201, 2001.
33. Nakano H, Miyachi I, Kitagawa Y, et al: Crohn's disease associated with giant inflammatory polyposis. Endoscopy 19:246-248, 1987.
34. Rozenbajgier C, Ruck P, Jenss H, et al: Filiform polyposis: A case report describing clinical, morphological, and immunohistochemical findings. Clin Invest Med 70:520-528, 1992.
35. Jessurun J, Paplanus SH, Nagle RB, et al: Pseudosarcomatous changes in inflammatory pseudopolyps of the colon. Arch Pathol Lab Med 110:833-836, 1986.
36. du Boulay CE, Fairbrother J, Isaacson PG: Mucosal prolapse syndrome—a unifying concept for solitary ulcer syndrome and related disorders. J Clin Pathol 36:1264-1268, 1983.
37. Tendler DA, Aboudola S, Zacks JF, et al: Prolapsing mucosal polyps: An underrecognized form of colonic polyp—a clinico-pathological study of 15 cases. Am J Gastroenterol 97:370-376, 2002.
38. Chetty R, Bhathal PS, Slavin JL: Prolapse-induced inflammatory polyps of the colorectum and anal transitional zone. Histopathology 23:63-67, 1993.
39. Williams GT, Bussey HJR, Morson BC: Inflammatory 'cap' polyps of the large intestine [abstract]. Br J Surg 72(suppl):S133, 1985.
40. Sadamoto Y, Jimi S, Harada N, et al: Asymptomatic cap polyposis from the sigmoid colon to the cecum. Gastrointest Endosc 54:654-656, 2001.
41. Shiomi S, Moriyama Y, Oshitani N, et al: A case of cap polyposis investigated by scintigraphy with human serum albumin labeled with Tc-99m DTPA. Clin Nucl Med 23:521-523, 1998.
42. Oriuchi T, Kinouchi Y, Kimura M, et al: Successful treatment of cap polyposis by avoidance of intraluminal trauma: Clues to pathogenesis. Am J Gastroenterol 95:2095-2098, 2000.
43. Isomoto H, Urata M, Nakagoe T, et al: Proximal extension of cap polyposis confirmed by colonoscopy. Gastrointest Endosc 54:388-391, 2001.
44. Esaki M, Matsumoto M, Kobayashi H, et al: Cap polyposis of the colon and rectum: An analysis of endoscopic findings. Endoscopy 33:262-266, 2001.
45. Buisine MP, Colombel JF, Lecomte-Houcke M, et al: Abnormal mucus in cap polyposis. Gut 42:135-138, 1998.
46. Oiya H, Okawa K, Aoki T, et al: Cap polyposis cured by Helicobacter pylori eradication therapy. J Gastroenterol 37:463-466, 2002.
47. Guest CB, Reznick RK: Colitis cystica profunda; review of the literature. Dis Colon Rectum;32:983-988, 1989.
48. Goodall HB, Sinclair IS: Colitis cystica profunda. J Pathol 73:33-42, 1957.
49. Franzin G, Novelli P: Gastritis cystica profunda. Histopathology 5:535-547, 1981.
50. Dippolito AD, Aburano A, Bezouska CA, et al: Enteritis cystica profunda in Peutz-Jeghers syndrome. Report of a case and review of the literature. Dis Colon Rectum 30:192-198, 1987.
51. Bentley E, Chandrasoma P, Cohen H, et al: Colitis cystica profunda: Presenting with complete intestinal obstruction and recurrence. Gastroenterology 89:1157-1161, 1985.
52. Kim WH, Choe GY, Kim YI, et al: Localized form of colitis cystica profunda—a case of occurrence in the descending colon. J Korean Med Sci 7:76-78, 1992.
53. Valenzuela M, Martin-Ruiz JL, Alvarez-Cienfuegos E, et al: Colitis cystica profunda: Imaging diagnosis and conservative treatment: Report of two cases. Dis Colon Rectum 39:587-590, 1996.
54. Vora IM, Sharma J, Joshi AS: Solitary rectal ulcer syndrome and colitis cystica profunda—a clinico-pathological review. Indian J Pathol Microbiol 35:94-102, 1992.
55. Stuart M: Proctitis cystica profunda. Incidence, etiology, and treatment. Dis Colon Rectum 27:153-156, 1984.
56. Peterkin GA 3rd, Moroz K, Kondi ES: Proctitis cystica profunda in paraplegics. Report of three cases. Dis Colon Rectum 35:1174-1176, 1992.
57. Lifshitz D, Cytron S, Yossiphov J, et al: Colitis cystica profunda: Self-inflicted by rectal trauma? Report of a case. Dig Dis 12:318-320, 1994.
58. Ng WK, Chan KW: Postirradiation colitis cystica profunda. Arch Pathol Lab Med 119:1170-1173, 1995.
59. Gardiner GW, McAuliffe N, Murray D: Colitis cystica profunda occurring in a radiation-induced colonic stricture. Hum Pathol 15:295-298, 1984.
60. Zidi SH, Marteau P, Piard F, et al: Enterocolitis cystica profunda lesions in a patient with unclassified ulcerative enterocolitis. Dig Dis Sci 39:426-432, 1994.
61. Pantongrag-Brown L, Levine MS, Elsayed AM, et al: Inverted Meckel diverticulum: Clinical, radiologic, and pathologic findings. Radiology 199:693-696, 1996.
62. Triadafilopoulos G: Images in clinical medicine. Inverted colonic diverticulum. N Engl J Med 341:1508, 1999.
63. Yusuf SI, Grant C: Inverted colonic diverticulum: A rare finding in a common condition? Gastrointest Endosc 52:111-115, 2000.
64. Hollander E, David G: [Inverted sigmoid diverticulum simulating polyps] [article in Hungarian]. Orv Hetil 134:639-640, 1993.
65. Franzin G, Fratton A, Manfrini C: Polypoid lesions associated with diverticular disease of the sigmoid colon. Gastrointest Endosc 31:196-199, 1985.
66. Kelly JK: Polypoid prolapsing mucosal folds in diverticular disease. Am J Surg Pathol 15:871-878, 1991.
67. Goldstein NS, Ahmad E: Histology of the mucosa in sigmoid colon specimens with diverticular disease: Observations for the interpretation of sigmoid colonoscopic biopsy specimens. Am J Clin Pathol 107:438-444, 1997.
68. Makapugay LM, Dean PJ: Diverticular disease–associated chronic colitis. Am J Surg Pathol 20:94-102, 1996.

69. Mathus-Vliegen EM, Tytgat GN: Polyp-simulating mucosal prolapse syndrome in (pre-) diverticular disease. Endoscopy 18:84-86, 1986.

70. Nakamura S, Kino I, Akagi T: Inflammatory myoglandular polyps of the colon and rectum. A clinicopathological study of 32 pedunculated polyps, distinct from other types of polyps. Am J Surg Pathol 16:772-779, 1992.

71. Griffiths AP, Hopkinson JM, Dixon MF: Inflammatory myoglandular polyp causing ileo-ileal intussusception. Histopathology 23:596-598, 1993.

72. Wirtzfeld DA, Petrelli NJ, Rodriguez-Bigas MA: Hamartomatous polyposis syndromes: Molecular genetics, neoplastic risk, and surveillance recommendations. Ann Surg Oncol 8:319-327, 2001.

73. Waite KA, Eng C: Protean PTEN: Form and function. Am J Hum Genet 70:829-844, 2002.

74. Gupta SK, Fitzgerald JF, Croffie JM, et al: Experience with juvenile polyps in North American children: The need for pancolonoscopy. Am J Gastroenterol 96:1695-1697, 2001.

75. McColl I, Bussey HJR, Veale AMO, et al: Juvenile polyposis coli. Proc R Soc Med 57:896-897, 1964.

76. Giardiello FM, Hamilton SR, Kern SE, et al: Colorectal neoplasia in juvenile polyposis or juvenile polyps. Arch Dis Child 66:971-975, 1991.

77. Howe JR, Ringold JC, Summers RW, et al: A gene for familial juvenile polyposis maps to chromosome 18q21.1. Am J Hum Genet 62:1129-1136, 1998.

78. Howe JR, Roth S, Ringold JC, et al: Mutations in the SMAD4/DPC4 gene in juvenile polyposis. Science 280:1086-1088, 1998.

79. Howe JR, Bair JL, Sayed MG, et al: Germline mutations of the gene encoding bone morphogenetic protein receptor 1A in juvenile polyposis. Nat Genet 28:184-187, 2001.

80. Zhou XP, Woodford-Richens K, Lehtonen R, et al: Germline mutations in BMPR1A/ALK3 cause a subset of cases of juvenile polyposis syndrome and of Cowden and Bannayan-Riley-Ruvalcaba syndromes. Am J Hum Genet 69:704-711, 2001.

81. Woodford-Richens KL, Rowan AJ, Poulsom R, et al: Comprehensive analysis of SMAD4 mutations and protein expression in juvenile polyposis: Evidence for a distinct genetic pathway and polyp morphology in SMAD4 mutation carriers. Am J Pathol 159:1293-1300, 2001.

82. Woodford-Richens K, Williamson J, Bevan S, et al: Allelic loss of SMAD4 in polyps from juvenile polyposis patients and use of fluorescence in situ hybridization to demonstrate clonal origin of the epithelium. Cancer Res 60:2477-2482, 2000.

83. Pham BN, Villanueva RP: Ganglioneuromatous proliferation associated with juvenile polyposis coli. Arch Pathol Lab Med 113:91-94, 1989.

84. Rabin ER, Patel T, Chen FH, et al: Juvenile colonic polyposis with villous adenoma and retroperitoneal fibrosis: Report of a case. Dis Colon Rectum 22:63-67, 1979.

85. Monga G, Mazzucco G, Rossini FP, et al: Colorectal polyposis with mixed juvenile and adenomatous patterns. Virchows Arch A Pathol Anat Histol 382:355-360, 1979.

86. Sharma AK, Sharma SS, Mathur P: Familial juvenile polyposis with adenomatous-carcinomatous change. J Gastroenterol Hepatol 10:131-134, 1995.

87. Wu TT, Rezai B, Rashid A, et al: Genetic alterations and epithelial dysplasia in juvenile polyposis syndrome and sporadic juvenile polyps. Am J Pathol 150:939-947, 1997.

88. Nugent KP, Talbot IC, Hodgson SV, et al: Solitary juvenile polyps: Not a marker for subsequent malignancy. Gastroenterology 105:698-700, 1993.

89. Kapetanakis AM, Vini D, Plitsis G: Solitary juvenile polyps in children and colon cancer. Hepatogastroenterology 43:1530-1531, 1996.

90. Howe JR, Mitros FA, Summers RW: The risk of gastrointestinal carcinoma in familial juvenile polyposis. Ann Surg Oncol 5:751-756, 1998.

91. Desai DC, Neale KF, Talbot IC, et al: Juvenile polyposis. Br J Surg 82:14-17, 1995.

92. Dunlop MG: Guidance on gastrointestinal surveillance for hereditary non-polyposis colorectal cancer, familial adenomatous polyposis, juvenile polyposis, and Peutz-Jeghers syndrome. Gut 51(suppl 5):V21-V27, 2002.

93. Scott RJ, Crooks R, Meldrum CJ, et al: Mutation analysis of the STK11/LKB1 gene and clinical characteristics of an Australian series of Peutz-Jeghers syndrome patients. Clin Genet 62:282-287, 2002.

94. McGarrity TJ, Kulin HE, Zaino RJ: Peutz-Jeghers syndrome. Am J Gastroenterol 95:596-604, 2000.

95. Al Faour A, Vrsansky P, Abouassi F, et al: Peutz-Jeghers colonic tumour in a newborn. Eur J Pediatr Surg 12:138-140, 2002.

96. Hemminki A, Tomlinson I, Markie D, et al: Localization of a susceptibility locus for Peutz-Jeghers syndrome to 19p using comparative genomic hybridization and targeted linkage analysis. Nat Genet 15:5-6, 1997.

97. Jenne DE, Reimann H, Nezu J, et al: Peutz-Jeghers syndrome is caused by mutations in a novel serine threonine kinase. Nat Genet 18:38-43, 1998.

98. Hemminki A, Markie D, Tomlinson I, et al: A serine/threonine kinase gene defective in Peutz-Jeghers syndrome. Nature 391:185-187, 1998.

99. Boardman LA, Couch FJ, Burgart LJ, et al: Genetic heterogeneity in Peutz-Jeghers syndrome. Hum Mutat 16:23-30, 2000.

100. Peter S, Govil S, Ramakrisna BS, et al: Gastrointestinal Peutz-Jeghers syndrome. J Gastroenterol Hepatol 17:1117, 2002.

101. Miyaki M, Iijima T, Hosono K, et al: Somatic mutations of LKB1 and beta-catenin genes in gastrointestinal polyps from patients with Peutz-Jeghers syndrome. Cancer Res 60:6311-6313, 2000.

102. Gruber SB, Entius MM, Petersen GM, et al: Pathogenesis of adenocarcinoma in Peutz-Jeghers syndrome. Cancer Res 58:5267-5270, 1998.

103. Hizawa K, Iida M, Matsumoto T, et al: Neoplastic transformation arising in Peutz-Jeghers polyposis. Dis Colon Rectum 36:953-957, 1993.

104. Narita T, Ohnuma H, Yokoyama S: Peutz-Jeghers syndrome with osseous metaplasia of the intestinal polyps. Pathol Int 45:388-392, 1995.

105. Ichiyoshi Y, Yao T, Nagasaki S, et al: Solitary Peutz-Jeghers type polyp of the duodenum containing a focus of adenocarcinoma. Ital J Gastroenterol 28:95-97, 1996.

106. Shepherd NA, Bussey HJ, Jass JR: Epithelial misplacement in Peutz-Jeghers polyps. A diagnostic pitfall. Am J Surg Pathol 11:743-749, 1987.

107. Westerman AM, Entius MM, de Baar E, et al: Peutz-Jeghers syndrome: 78-year follow-up of the original family. Lancet 353:1211-1215, 1999.

108. Petersen VC, Sheehan AL, Bryan RL, et al: Misplacement of dysplastic epithelium in Peutz-Jeghers polyps: The ultimate diagnostic pitfall? Am J Surg Pathol 24:34-39, 2000.

109. Utsunomiya J, Gocho H, Miyanaga T, et al: Peutz-Jeghers syndrome: Its natural course and management. Johns Hopkins Med J 136:71-82, 1975.

110. Boardman LA, Thibodeau SN, Schaid DJ, et al: Increased risk for cancer in patients with the Peutz-Jeghers syndrome. Ann Intern Med 128:896-899, 1998.

111. Giardiello FM, Brensinger JD, Tersmette AC, et al: Very high risk of cancer in familial Peutz-Jeghers syndrome. Gastroenterology 119:1447-1153, 2000.

112. Hampel H, Peltomaki P: Hereditary colorectal cancer: Risk assessment and management. Clin Genet 58:89-97, 2000.

113. Wirtzfeld DA, Petrelli NJ, Rodriguez-Bigas MA: Hamartomatous polyposis syndromes: Molecular genetics, neoplastic risk, and surveillance recommendations. Ann Surg Oncol 8:319-327, 2001.

114. Nelen MR, Padberg GW, Peeters EA, et al: Localization of the gene for Cowden disease to chromosome 10q22-23. Nat Genet 13:114-116, 1996.

115. Liaw D, Marsh DJ, Li J, et al: Germline mutations of the PTEN gene in Cowden disease, an inherited breast and thyroid cancer syndrome. Nat Genet 16:64-67, 1997.

116. Nelen MR, van Staveren WC, Peeters EA, et al: Germline mutations in the PTEN/MMAC1 gene in patients with Cowden disease. Hum Mol Genet 6:1383-1387, 1997.

117. Fackenthal JD, Marsh DJ, Richardson AL, et al: Male breast cancer in Cowden syndrome patients with germline PTEN mutations. J Med Genet 38:159-164, 2001.

118. Eng C: Will the real Cowden syndrome please stand up: Revised diagnostic criteria. J Med Genet 37:828-830, 2000.

119. Tsuchiya KD, Wiesner G, Cassidy SB, et al: Deletion 10q23.2-q23.33 in a patient with gastrointestinal juvenile polyposis and other features of a Cowden-like syndrome. Genes Chromosomes Cancer 21:113-118, 1998.

120. Cho KC, Sundaram K, Sebastiano LS: Filiform polyposis of the small bowel in a patient with multiple hamartoma syndrome (Cowden disease). Am J Roentgenol 173;501-502, 1999.

121. Solli P, Rossi G, Carbongnani P, et al: Pulmonary abnormalities in Cowden's disease. J Cardiovasc Surg (Torino) 40:753-757, 1999.

122. Chi SG, Kim HJ, Park BJ, et al: Mutational abrogation of the PTEN/MMAC1 gene in gastrointestinal polyps in patients with Cowden disease. Gastroenterology 115:1084-1089, 1998.

123. Cronkhite LW, Canada WJ: Generalized gastrointestinal polyposis: An unusual syndrome of polyposis, pigmentation, alopecia, and onychotrophia. N Engl J Med 252:1011-1015, 1955.

124. Ward EM, Wolfsen HD: Review article: The non-inherited gastrointestinal polyposis syndromes. Aliment Pharmacol Ther 16:333-342, 2002.

125. de Silva DG, Fernando AD, Law FM, et al: Infantile Cronkhite-Canada syndrome. Indian J Pediatr 64:261-266, 1997.

126. Burke AP, Sobin LH: The pathology of Cronkhite-Canada polyps. A comparison to juvenile polyposis. Am J Surg Pathol 13:940-946, 1989.

127. Murata I, Yoshikawa I, Endo M, et al: Cronkhite-Canada syndrome: Report of two cases. J Gastroenterol 35:706-711, 2000.

128. Nakatsubo N, Wakasa R, Kiyosaki K, et al: Cronkhite-Canada syndrome associated with carcinoma of the sigmoid colon: Report of a case. Surg Today 27:345-348, 1997.

129. Malhotra R, Sheffield A. Cronkhite-Canada syndrome associated with colon carcinoma and adenomatous changes in C-C polyps. Am J Gastroenterol 83:772-776, 1988.

130. Kaneko Y, Kato H, Tachimori Y, et al: Triple carcinomas in Cronkhite-Canada syndrome. Jpn J Clin Oncol 21:194-202, 1991.

131. Yamaguchi K, Ogata Y, Akagi Y, et al: Cronkhite-Canada syndrome associated with advanced rectal cancer treated by a subtotal colectomy: Report of a case. Surg Today 31:521-526, 2001.

132. Katayama Y, Kimura M, Konn M: Cronkhite-Canada syndrome associated with a rectal cancer and adenomatous changes in colonic polyps. Am J Surg Pathol 9:65-71, 1985.

133. Imperiale TF, Wagner DR, Lin CY, et al: Results of screening colonoscopy among persons 40 to 49 years of age. N Engl J Med 346:1781-1785, 2002.

134. Fossi S, Bazzoli F, Ricciardiello L, et al: Incidence and recurrence rates of colorectal adenomas in first-degree asymptomatic relatives of patients with colon cancer. Am J Gastroenterol 96:1601-1604, 2001.

135. Winawer SJ, Zauber AG, Gerdes H, et al: Risk of colorectal cancer in the families of patients with adenomatous polyps. National Polyp Study Workgroup. N Engl J Med 334:1339-1340, 1996.

136. Lewin KJ, Riddell RH, Weinstein WM (eds): Gastrointestinal Pathology and Its Clinical Implications. New York, IGAKU-Shoin, 1989, pp 1225-1226.

137. Ikeda Y, Mori M, Shibahara K, et al: The role of adenoma for colorectal cancer development: Differences in the distribution of adenoma with low-grade dysplasia, high-grade dysplasia, and cancer that invades the submucosa. Surgery 131(1 suppl):S105-S108, 2002.

138. Euscher ED, Niemann TH, Lucas JG, et al: Large colorectal adenomas. An approach to pathologic evaluation. Am J Clin Pathol 116:336-340, 2001.

139. Winawer S, Fletcher R, Rex D, et al: Colorectal cancer screening and surveillance: Clinical guidelines and rationale—update based on new evidence. Gastroenterology 124:544-560, 2003.

140. Winawer SJ, Zauber AG, O'Brien MJ, et al: The National Polyp Study. Design, methods, and characteristics of patients with newly diagnosed polyps. The National Polyp Study Workgroup. Cancer 70(5 suppl):1236-1245, 1992.

141. Hoff G, Foerster A, Vatn MH, et al: Epidemiology of polyps in the rectum and colon. Recovery and evaluation of unresected polyps 2 years after detection. Scand J Gastroenterol 21:853-862, 1986.

142. Villavicencio RT, Rex DK: Colonic adenomas: Prevalence and incidence rates, growth rates, and miss rates at colonoscopy. Semin Gastrointest Dis 11:185-193, 2000.

143. Shinya H, Woff WI: Morphology, anatomic distribution and cancer potential of polyps: Analysis of 7000 polyps endoscopically removed. Ann Surg 190:679-683, 1979.

144. Haggitt RC, Glotzbach RE, Soffer EE, et al: Prognostic factors in colorectal carcinomas arising in adenomas: Implications for lesions removed by endoscopic polypectomy. Gastroenterology 89:328-336, 1985.

145. O 'Brien MJ, Winawer SJ, Zauber AG, et al: The National Polyp Study. Patient and polyp characteristics associated with high-grade dysplasia in colorectal adenomas. Gastroenterology 98:371-379, 1990.

146. Bond JH: Polyp guideline: Diagnosis, treatment, and surveillance for patients with colorectal polyps. Am J Gastroenterol 95:3053-3063, 2000.

147. Winawer SJ, Zauber AG: The advanced adenoma as the primary target of screening. Gastrointest Endosc Clin N Am 12:1-9, 2002.

148. Kadakia SC, Wrobleski CS, Kadakia AS, et al: Prevalence of proximal colonic polyps in average-risk asymptomatic patients with negative fecal occult blood tests and flexible sigmoidoscopy. Gastrointest Endosc 44:112-117, 1996.

149. Imperiale TF, Wagner DR, Lin CY, et al: Risk of advanced proximal neoplasms in asymptomatic adults according to the distal colorectal findings. N Engl J Med 343:169-174, 2000.

150. Patel K, Hoffman NE: The anatomical distribution of colorectal polyps at colonoscopy. J Clin Gastroenterol 33:222-225, 2001.

151. Standards of Practice Committee (American Society of Gastrointestinal Endoscopy): Guidelines for colorectal cancer screening and surveillance. Gastrointest Endosc 51:777-782, 2000.

152. Rex DK, Johnson DA, Lieberman DA, et al: Colorectal cancer prevention 2000: Screening recommendations of the American College of Gastroenterology. Am J Gastroenterol 95:868-877, 2000.

153. Frazier AL, Colditz GA, Fuchs CS, et al: Cost-effectiveness of screening for colorectal cancer in the general population. JAMA 284:1954-1961, 2000.

154. Burt RW: Colon cancer screening. Gastroenterology 119:837-853, 2000.

155. Lieberman DA: Cost-effectiveness model for colon cancer screening. Gastroenterology 109:1781-1790, 1995.

156. Lieberman DA, Weiss DG: One-time screening for colorectal cancer with combined fecal occult-blood testing and examination of the distal colon. Veterans Affairs Cooperative Study Group 380. N Engl J Med 345:555-560, 2001.

157. Lieberman DA, Weiss DG, Bond JH, et al: Use of colonoscopy to screen asymptomatic adults for colorectal cancer. Veterans Affairs Cooperative Study Group 380. N Engl J Med 343:162-168, 2000.

158. Loeve F, Brown ML, Boer R, et al: Endoscopic colorectal cancer screening: A cost-saving analysis. J Natl Cancer Inst 92:557-563, 2000.

159. Quizilbash AH, Meghju M, Castelli M: Pseudocarcinomatous invasion in adenomas of the colon and rectum. Dis Colon Rectum 23:529-535, 1980.

160. Muto T, Bussey HJR, Morson BC: Pseudocarcinomatous invasion in adenomatous polyps of the colon and rectum. J Clin Pathol 26:25-31, 1973.

161. Greene FL: Epithelial misplacement in adenomatous polyps of the colon and rectum. Cancer 33:206-217, 1974.

162. Cooper HS, Deppisch LM, Kahn EI, et al: Pathology of the malignant colorectal polyp. Hum Pathol 28:15-26, 1998.

163. Cooper HS: Surgical pathology of endoscopically removed malignant polyps of the colon and rectum. Am J Surg Pathol 7:613-623, 1983.

164. Pascal RR, Hertzler G, Hunter S, et al: Pseudoinvasion with high-grade dysplasia in a colonic adenoma: Distinction from adenocarcinoma. Am J Surg Pathol 14:694-697, 1990.

165. Yantiss RK, Bosenberg MW, Antonioli DA, et al: Utility of MMP-1, p53, E-cadherin, and collagen IV immunohistochemical stains in the differential diagnosis of adenomas with misplaced epithelium versus adenomas with invasive adenocarcinoma. Am J Surg Pathol 26:206-215, 2002.

166. Mueller J, Mueller E, Arras E, et al: Stromelysin-3 expression in early (pT1) carcinomas and pseudoinvasive lesions of the colorectum. Virchows Arch 430:213-219, 1997.

167. Cranley JP, Petras RE, Carey WD, et al: When is endoscopic polypectomy adequate therapy for colonic polyps containing invasive carcinoma? Gastroenterology 91:419-427, 1986.

168. Odze RD: Adenomas and adenoma-like DALMs in chronic ulcerative colitis: A clinical, pathologic, and molecular review. Am J Gastroenterol 94:1746-1750, 1999.

169. Torres C, Antonioli D, Odze RD: Polypoid dysplasia and adenomas in inflammatory bowel disease. Am J Surg Pathol 22:275-284, 1998.

170. Blackstone MO, Riddell RH, Rogers BHG, et al: Dysplasia-associated lesion or mass (DALM) detected by colonoscopy in long-standing ulcerative colitis: An indication for colectomy. Gastroenterology 8:366-374, 1981.

171. Butt JH, Konishi F, Morson BC, et al: Macroscopic lesions in dysplasia and carcinoma complicating ulcerative colitis. Dig Dis Sci 28:18-26, 1983.

172. Engelsgjerd M, Farraye F, Odze RD: Polypectomy may be adequate treatment for adenoma-like dysplastic lesions in chronic ulcerative colitis. Gastroenterology 117:1288-1294, 1999.

173. Rubin PH, Friedman S, Harpaz N, et al: Colonoscopic polypectomy in chronic colitis: Conservative management after endoscopic resection of dysplastic polyps. Gastroenterology 117:1295-1300, 1999.

174. Schneider A, Stolte M: Differential diagnosis of adenomas and dysplastic lesions in patients with ulcerative colitis. Z Gastroenterol 31:653-656, 1993.

175. Medlicott SAC, Jewell LD, Price L, et al: Conservative management of small adenomata in ulcerative colitis. Am J Gastroenterol 92:2094-2098, 1997.

176. Tytgat GNJ, Dhir V, Gopinath N: Endoscopic appearance of dysplasia and cancer in inflammatory bowel disease. Eur J Cancer 31:1174-1177, 1995.

177. Itzkowitz SH, Greenwald B, Meltzer SJ: Colon carcinogenesis in inflammatory bowel disease. Inflamm Bowel Dis 1:142, 1995.

178. Kern SE, Redston M, Seymour AB, et al: Molecular genetic profiles of colitis-associated neoplasms. Gastroenterology 107:420-428, 1994.

179. Odze R, Brown CA, Noffsinger AE, et al: Genetic alterations in chronic ulcerative colitis associated adenoma-like DALMs are similar to non-colitic sporadic adenomas. Am J Surg Pathol 24:1202-1216, 2000.

180. Walsh SV, Loda M, Torres CM, et al: P53 and b catenin expression in chronic ulcerative colitis–associated polypoid dysplasia and sporadic adenomas: An immunohistochemical study. Am J Surg Pathol 2398:963-969, 1999.

181. Yin J, Harpaz N, Tony Y, et al: P53 point mutations in dysplastic and cancerous ulcerative colitis lesions. Gastroenterology 104:1633-1639, 1993.

182. Tarmin L, Yin J, Harpaz N, et al: Adenomatous polyposis coli gene mutations in ulcerative colitis–associated dysplasias and cancers versus sporadic colon neoplasms. J Cancer Res 55:2035-2038, 1995.

183. Fogt F, Vortmeyer AO, Stolte M, et al: Loss of heterozygosity of the von Hippel Lindau gene locus in polypoid dysplasia but not flat dysplasia in ulcerative colitis or sporadic adenomas. Hum Pathol 29:961-964, 1998.

184. Fogt F, Vortmeyer AO, Goldman H, et al: Comparison of genetic alterations in colonic adenoma and ulcerative colitis–associated dysplasia and carcinoma. Hum Pathol 29:131-136, 1988.

185. Torlakovic E, Skovlund E, Torlakovic G, et al: Morphologic reappraisal of serrated colorectal polyps. Am J Surg Pathol 27:65-81, 2003.

186. Jass JR: Serrated adenoma of the colorectum. A lesion with teeth. Am J Pathol 162:705-708, 2003.

187. Longacre TA, Fenoglio-Preiser CM: Mixed hyperplastic adenomatous polyps/serrated adenomas. A distinct form of colorectal neoplasia. Am J Surg Pathol 14:524-537, 1990.

188. Matsumoto T, Mizuno M, Shimizu M, et al: Clinicopathological features of serrated adenoma of the colorectum: Comparison with traditional adenoma. J Clin Pathol 52:513-516, 1999.

189. Hawkins NJ, Gorman P, Tomlinson IP, et al: Colorectal carcinomas arising in the hyperplastic polyposis syndrome progress through the chromosomal instability pathway. Am J Pathol 157:385-392, 2000.

190. Rashid A, Houlihan PS, Booker S, et al: Phenotypic and molecular characteristics of hyperplastic polyposis. Gastroenterology 119:323-332, 2000.

191. Burt RW, Samowits WS: Serrated adenomatous polyposis: A new syndrome? Gastroenterology 110:950-952, 1996-2000.

192. Hiyama T, Yokozaki H, Shimamoto F, et al: Frequent p53 gene mutations in serrated adenomas of the colorectum. J Pathol 186:131-139, 1998.

193. Torlakovic E, Snover DC: Serrated adenomatous polyposis in humans. Gastroenterology 110:748-755, 1996.

194. Iwabuchi M, Sasano H, Hiwatashi N, et al: Serrated adenoma: A clinicopathological, DNA ploidy, and immunohistochemical study. Anticancer Res 20:1141-1147, 2000.

195. Uchida H, Ando H, Maruyama K, et al: Genetic alterations of mixed hyperplastic adenomatous polyps in the colon and rectum. Jpn J Cancer Res 89:2999-2306, 1998.

196. Ajioka Y, Watanabe H, Jass JR, et al: Infrequent K-ras codon 12 mutation in serrated adenomas of human colorectum. Gut 42:680-684, 1998.

197. Dehari R: Infrequent APC mutations in serrated adenomas. Tohoku J Exp Med 193:181-186, 2001.

198. Iino H, Jass JR, Simms LA, et al: DNA microsatellite instability in hyperplastic polyps, serrated adenomas, and mixed polyps: A mild mutator pathway for colorectal cancer? J Clin Pathol 52:5-9, 1999.

199. Jass JR, Young J, Leggett BA, et al: Hyperplastic polyps and DNA microsatellite unstable cancers of the colorectum [review]. Histopathology 37:295-301, 2000.

200. Jass JR: Hyperplastic polyps of the colorectum—innocent or guilty. Dis Colon Rectum 4:163-166, 2001.

201. Jass JR: Serrated route to colorectal cancer: Back street or super highway? [editorial]. J Pathol 193:283-285, 2001.

202. Nucci MR, Robinson CR, Longo P, et al: Phenotypic and genotypic characteristics of aberrant crypt foci in human colorectal tissue. Hum Pathol 28:1396-1407, 1997.

203. Makinen MJ, George SM, Jernvall P, et al: Colorectal carcinoma associated with serrated adenoma—prevalence, histologic featues, and prognosis. J Pathol 193:286-294, 2001.

204. Jass JR, Biden KG, Cummings MC, et al: Characterization of a subtype of colorectal cancer combining features of the suppressor and mild mutator pathways. J Clin Pathol 52:455-460, 1999.

205. Park SJ, Rshid A, Lee JH, et al: Frequent CpG island methylation in serrated adenomas of the colorectum. Am J Pathol 162:815-822, 2003.

206. Torlakovic E, Snover DC: Serrated adenomatous polyposis in humans. Gastroenterology 110:950-952, 1996.

207. Torlakovic E, Skovlund E, Snover DC, et al: Morphologic reappraisal of serrated colorectal polyps. Am J Surg Pathol 27:65-81, 2003.

208. Rex DK, Ulbright TM: Step section histology of proximal colon polyps that appear hyperplastic by endoscopy. Am J Gastroenterol 97:1530-1534, 2002.

209. Jass JR: Serrated adenoma of the colorectum: A lesion with teeth. Am J Pathol 162:705-708, 2003.

210. Jass JR, Whitehall VL, Young J, et al: Emerging concepts in colorectal neoplasia. Gastroenterology 123:862-876, 2002.

211. Burgart LJ: Colorectal polyps and other precursor lesions. Need for an expanded view. Gastroenterol Clin N Am 31:959-970, 2002.

212. Hawkins NJ, Ward RL: Sporadic colorectal cancers with microsatellite instability and their possible origin in hyperplastic polyps and serrated adenomas. J Natl Cancer Inst 93:1282-1283, 2001.

213. Hawkins NJ, Bariol C, Ward RL: The serrated neoplasia pathway. Pathology 34:548-555, 2002.

214. Park S-J, Rashid A, Lee J-H, et al: Frequent CpG island methylation in serrated adenomas of the colorectum. Am J Pathol 162:815-822, 2003.

215. Jass JR, Young J, Leggett BA: Hyperplastic polyps and DNA microsatellite unstable cancers of the colorectum. Histopathology 37:295-301, 2000.

216. Jass JR, Lino H, Ruszkiewicz A, et al: Neoplastic progression occurs through mutator pathways in hyperplastic polyposis of the colorectum. Gut 47:43-49, 2000.

217. Iwabuchi M, Sasano H, Hiwatashi N, et al: Serrated adenoma: A clinicopathological, DNA ploidy, and immunohistochemical study. Anticancer Res 20:1141-1147, 2000.

218. Morita T, Tamura S, Miyazaki J, et al: Evaluation of endoscopic and histopathological features of serrated adenoma of the colon. Endoscopy 33:761-765, 2001.

219. Fogt F, Brien T, Brown CA, et al: Genetic alterations in serrated adenomas: Comparison to conventional adenomas and hyperplastic polyps. Hum Pathol 33:87-91, 2002.

220. Wolber RA, Owen DA: Flat adenomas of the colon. Hum Pathol 22:70-74, 1991.

221. Matsumoto T, Iida M, Kuwano Y, et al: Small nonpolypoid neoplastic lesions of the colon: Endoscopic features with emphasis on their progression. Gastrointest Endosc 41:135-140, 1995.

222. Jaramillo E, Watanabe M, Slezak P, et al: Flat neoplastic lesions of the colon and rectum detected by high-resolution video endoscopy and chromoscopy. Gastrointest Endosc 42:114-122, 1995.

223. Naylor GM, Fujii T, Ishii H, et al: A 0.8-mm depressed adenoma of the colon with high-grade dysplasia. Endoscopy 33:891-893, 2001.

224. Morita T, Tomita N, Ohue M, et al: Molecular analysis of diminutive, flat, depressed colorectal lesions: Are they precursors of polypoid adenoma or early stage carcinoma? Gastrointest Endosc 56:663-671, 2002.

225. Kurahashi T, Kaneko K, Makino R, et al: Colorectal carcinoma with special reference to growth pattern classifications: Clinicopathologic characteristics and genetic changes. J Gastroenterol 37:354-362, 2002.

226. Sato T, Konishi F, Togashi K, et al: Prospective observation of small "flat" tumors in the colon through colonoscopy. Dis Colon Rectum 42:1457-1463, 1999.

227. Kasumi A, Kratzer GL, Takeda M: Observations of aggressive, small, flat, and depressed colon cancer. Report of three cases. Surg Endosc 9:690-694, 1995.

228. Jaramillo E, Watanabe M, Slezak P, et al: Flat neoplastic lesions of the colon and rectum detected by high-resolution video endoscopy and chromoscopy. Gastrointest Endosc 42:114-122, 1995.

229. Lynch HT, Smyrk TC, Lanspa SJ, et al: Phenotypic variation in colorectal adenoma/cancer expression in two families. Hereditary flat adenoma syndrome. Cancer 66:909-915, 1990.

230. Lynch HT, Smyrk T, Lanspa SJ, et al: Flat adenomas in a colon cancer–prone kindred. J Natl Cancer Inst 80:278-282, 1988.

231. Lynch HT, Smyrk TC, Watson P, et al: Hereditary flat adenoma syndrome: A variant of familial adenomatous polyposis? Dis Colon Rectum 35:411-421, 1992.

232. Nascimbeni R, Burgart LJ, Nivatvongs S, et al: Risk of lymph node metastasis in T1 carcinoma of the colon and rectum. Dis Colon Rectum 45:200-206, 2002.

233. Haggitt RC, Glotzbach RE, Soffer EE, et al: Prognostic factors in colorectal carcinomas arising in adenomas: Implications for lesions removed by endoscopic polypectomy. Gastroenterology 89:328-336, 1985.

234. Cooper HS, Deppisch LM, Ghourley WK, et al: Endoscopically removed malignant colorectal polyps: Clinicopathologic correlations. Gastroenterology 108:1657-1665, 1995.

235. Cooper HS: Surgical pathology of endoscopically removed malignant polyps of the colon and rectum. Am J Surg Pathol 7:613-623, 1983.

236. Morson BC, Whiteway JE, Jones EA, et al: Histopathology and prognosis of malignant colorectal polyps treated by endoscopic polypectomy. Gut 25:437-444, 1984.

237. Volk EE, Goldblum JR, Petras RE, et al: Management and outcome of patients with invasive carcinoma arising in colorectal polyps. Gastroenterology 109:1801-1807, 1995.

238. Koura AN, Giacco GG, Curley SA, et al: Carcinoid tumors of the rectum: Effect of size, histopathology, and surgical treatment on metastasis free survival. Cancer 79:1294-1298, 1997.

239. Moisio AL, Jarvinen H, Peltomaki P: Genetic and clinical characterisation of familial adenomatous polyposis: A population based study. Gut 50:845-850, 2002.

240. Robbins DH, Itzkowitz SH: The molecular and genetic basis of colon cancer. Med Clin North Am 86:1467-1495, 2002.

241. Giardiello FM, Brensinger JD, Peterson GM: AGA technical review on hereditary colorectal cancer and genetic testing. Gastroenterology 121:198-213, 2001.

242. Haggitt RC, Reid BJ: Hereditary gastrointestinal polyposis syndromes. Am J Surg Pathol 10:871-887, 1986.

243. Offerhaus GJ, Giardiello FM, Krush AJ, et al: The risk of upper gastrointestinal cancer in familial adenomatous polyposis. Gastroenterology 102:1980-1982, 1992.

244. Wehrli BM, Weiss SW, Yandow S, et al: Gardner-associated fibromas (GAF) in young patients: A distinct fibrous lesion that identifies unsuspected Gardner syndrome and risk for fibromatosis. Am J Surg Pathol 25:645-651, 2001.

245. Lynch HT, Thorson AG, McComb RD, et al: Familial adenomatous polyposis and extracolonic cancer. Dig Dis Sci 46:2325-2332, 2001.

246. Miyaki M, Iijima T, Shiba K, et al: Alterations of repeated sequences in 5' upstream and coding regions in colorectal tumors from patients with hereditary nonpolyposis colorectal cancer and Turcot syndrome. Oncogene 20:5215-5218, 2001.

247. Koot RW, Hulsebos TJ, van Overbeeke JJ: Polyposis coli, cranio-facial exostosis and astrocytoma: The concomitant occurrence of the Gardner's and Turcot syndromes. Surg Neurol 45:213-218, 1996.

248. Cohen SB: Familial polyposis coli and its extracolonic manifestations. J Med Genet 19:193-203, 1982.

249. Hernegger GS, Moore HG, Guillem JG: Attenuated adenomatous polyposis: An evolving and poorly understood entity. Dis Colon Rectum 45:127-134, 2002.

250. Lynch HT, Smyrk T, McGinn T, et al: Attenuated familial adenomatous polyposis (AFAP). A phenotypically and genotypically distinctive variant of FAP. Cancer 76:2427-2433, 1995.

251. Couture J, Mitri A, Lagace R, et al: A germline mutation at the extreme 3' end of the APC gene results in a severe desmoid phenotype and is associated with overexpression of beta-catenin in the desmoid tumor. Clin Genet 57:205-212, 2000.

252. Boardman LA: Heritable colorectal cancer syndromes: Recognition and preventive management. Gastroenterol Clin N Am 31:1107-1131, 2002.

253. Jass JR: Familial colorectal cancer: Pathology and molecular characteristics. Lancet Oncol 1:220-226, 2000.

254. Rodriguez-Bigas MA, Boland CR, Hamilton SR, et al: A National Cancer Institute workshop on hereditary nonpolyposis colorectal cancer syndrome: Meeting highlights and Bethesda guidelines. J NCI 89:1758-1762, 1997.

255. Fran TS: Hereditary cancer syndromes. Arch Pathol Lab Med 125:85-90, 2001.

256. Redston M: Carcinogenesis in the GI tract: From morphology to genetics and back again. Mod Pathol 14:236-245, 2001.

257. Jass JR: Pathology of hereditary nonpolyposis colorectal cancer. Ann N Y Acad Sci 910:62-73, discussion 73-74, 2000.

258. Hashimoto Y, Nakamura N, Kuze T, et al: Multiple lymphomatous polyposis of the gastrointestinal tract is a heterogenous group that includes mantle cell lymphoma and follicular lymphoma: Analysis of somatic mutation of immunoglobulin heavy chain gene variable region. Hum Pathol 30:581-587, 1999.

259. Lavergne A, Brouland JP, Launay E, et al: Multiple lymphomatous polyposis of the gastrointestinal tract. An extensive histopathologic and immunohistochemical study of 12 cases. Cancer 74:3042-3050, 1994.

260. Moynihan MJ, Bast MA, Chan WC, et al: Lymphomatous polyposis. A neoplasm of either follicular mantle or germinal cancer cell origin. Am J Surg Pathol 20:442-452, 1996.

261. Ruskone-Fourmestraux A, Delmer A, Lavergne A, et al: Multiple lymphomatous polyposis of the gastrointestinal tract: Prospective clinicopathologic study of 31 cases. Groupe D'etude des Lymphomes Digestifs. Gastroenterology 112:7-16, 1997.

262. Shekitka KM, Sobin LH: Ganglioneuromas of the gastrointestinal tract. Relation to Von Recklinghausen disease and other multiple tumor syndromes. Am J Surg Pathol 18:250-257, 1994.

263. Srinivasan R, Mayle JE: Polypoid ganglioneuroma of colon. Dig Dis Sci 43:908-909, 1998.

264. Lashner BA, Riddell RH, Winans CS: Ganglioneuromatosis of the colon and extensive glycogenic acanthosis in Cowden's disease. Dig Dis Sci 31:213-216, 1986.

265. Mendelsohn G, Diamond MP: Familial ganglioneuromatous polyposis of the large bowel. Report of a family with associated juvenile polyposis. Am J Surg Pathol 8:515-520, 1984.

266. d'Amore ES, Manivel JC, Pettinato G, et al: Intestinal ganglio-neuromatosis: Mucosal and transmural types. A clinicopathologic and immunohistochemical study of six cases. Hum Pathol 22;276-286, 1991.

267. Carney JA, Go VL, Sizemore GW, et al: Alimentary-tract ganglio-neuromatosis. A major component of the syndrome of multiple endocrine neoplasia, type 2b. N Engl J Med 295:1287-1291, 1976.

268. Smith VV, Eng C, Milla PJ: Intestinal ganglioneuromatosis and multiple endocrine neoplasia type 2B: Implications for treatment. Gut 45:143-146, 1999.

269. Gutmann DH, Aylsworth A, Carey JC, et al: The diagnostic evaluation and multidisciplinary management of neurofibromatosis 1 and neurofibromatosis 2. JAMA 278:1493-1494, 1997.

270. Heuschkel R, Kim S, Korf B, et al: Abdominal migraine in children with neurofibromatosis type 1: A case series and review of gastrointestinal involvement in NF1. J Pediatr Gastroenterol Nutr 33:149-154, 2001.

271. Boldorini R, Tosoni A, Leutner M, et al: Multiple small intestinal stromal tumours in a patient with previously unrecognised neurofibromatosis type 1: Immunohistochemical and ultrastructural evaluation. Pathology 33:390-395, 2001.

272. Karatzas G, Kouraklis G, Karayiannakis A, et al: Ampullary carcinoid and jejunal stromal tumour associated with von Recklinghausen's disease presenting as gastrointestinal bleeding and jaundice. Eur J Surg Oncol 26:428-429, 2000.

273. Artaza T, Garcia JF, González M, et al: Simultaneous involvement of the jejunum and the colon by type-1 neurofibromatosis. Scand J Gastroenterol 34:331-334, 1999.

274. Fernandez MT, Puig L, Capella G, et al: Von Recklinghausen neurofibromatosis with duodenal tumor and submucous leiomyomas of the duodenum. Neurofibromatosis 1:294-298, 1988.

275. Zöller MET, Rembeck B, Odén A, et al: Malignant and benign tumors in patients with neurofibromatosis type 1 in a defined Swedish population. Cancer 79:2125-2131, 1997.

276. Burke AP, Sobin LH, Shekitka KM, et al: Somatostatin-producing duodenal carcinoids in patients with von Recklinghausen's neurofibromatosis. A predilection for black patients. Cancer 1:1591-1595, 1990.

277. Hirata K, Kitahara K, Momosaka Y, et al: Diffuse ganglioneuromatosis with plexiform neurofibromas limited to the gastrointestinal tract involving a large segment of small intestine. J Gastroenterol 31:263-267, 1996.

278. Halkic N, Henchoz L, Gintzburger D, et al: Gastric neurofibroma in a patient with von Recklinghausen's disease: A cause of upper gastrointestinal hemorrhage. Chir Ital 52:79-81, 2000.

279. Taylor MA, Loughrey MB, Toner PG, et al: An unusual cause of biliary stricture in a patient with neurofibromatosis type 1. Eur J Gastroenterol Hepatol 13:199-201, 2001.

280. Kim HR, Kim YJ: Neurofibromatosis of the colon and rectum combined with other manifestations of von Recklinghausen's disease: Report of a case [case report]. Dis Colon Rectum 41:1187-1192, 1998.

281. Castoldi L, De Rai P, Marini A, et al: Neurofibromatosis-1 and ampullary gangliocytic paraganglioma causing biliary and pancreatic obstruction. Int J Pancreatol 29:93-97, 2001.

282. Joo YE, Kim HS, Choi SK, et al: Primary duodenal adenocarcinoma associated with neurofibromatosis type 1. J Gastroenterol 37:215-219, 2002.

283. Wolkenstein P, Freche B, Zeller J, et al: Usefulness of screening investigations in neurofibromatosis type 1. A study of 152 patients. Arch Dermatol 132:1333-1336, 1996.

284. Hochberg FH, Dasilva AB, Galdabini J, et al: Gastrointestinal involvement in von Recklinghausen's neurofibromatosis. Neurology 24:1144-1151, 1974.

285. Miettinen M, Lasota J: Gastrointestinal stromal tumors—definition, clinical, histological, immunohistochemical, and molecular genetic features and differential diagnosis. Virchows Arch 438:1-12, 2001.

286. Miettinen M, Sarlomo-Rikala M, Sobin LH: Mesenchymal tumors of muscularis mucosae of colon and rectum are benign leiomyomas that should be separated from gastrointestinal stromal tumors—a clinicopathologic and immunohistochemical study of eighty-eight cases. Mod Pathol 14:950-956, 2001.

287. Miettinen M, Sarloma-Rikala M, Sobin LH, et al: Gastrointestinal stromal tumors and leiomyosarcomas in the colon. A clinicopathologic, immunohistochemical, and molecular genetic study of 44 cases. Am J Surg Pathol 24:1339-1352, 2000.

288. McClain KL, Leach CT, Jenson HB, et al: Association of Epstein-Barr virus with leiomyosarcomas in children with AIDS. N Engl J Med 332:55-57, 1995.

289. Lee ES, Locker J, Nalesnik M, et al: The association of Epstein-Barr virus with smooth-muscle tumors occurring after organ transplantation. N Engl J Med 332:19-25, 1995.

290. Reyes C, Abuzaitoun O, De Jong A, et al: Epstein-Barr virus—associated smooth muscle tumors in ataxia-telangiectasia: A case report and review. Hum Pathol 33:133-136, 2002.

291. Somers GR, Tesoriero AA, Hartland E, et al: Multiple leiomyosarcomas of both donor and recipient origin arising in a heart-lung transplant patient. Am J Surg Pathol 22:1423-1428, 1998.

292. Kingma DW, Shad A, Tsokos M, et al: Epstein-Barr virus (EBV)—associated smooth-muscle tumor arising in a post-transplant patient treated successfully for two PT-EBV-associated large-cell lymphomas. Case report. Am J Surg Pathol 20:1511-1519, 1996.

293. Mierau GW, Greffe BS, Weeks DA: Primary leiomyosarcoma of brain in an adolescent with common variable immunodeficiency syndrome. Ultrastruct Pathol 21:301-305, 1997.

294. Anguita J, Rico ML, Palomo J, et al: Myocardial Epstein-Barr virus—associated cardiac smooth-muscle neoplasm arising in a cardia transplant recipient. Transplantation 66:400-401, 1998.

295. Creager AJ, Maia DM, Funkhouser WK: Epstein-Barr virus—associated renal smooth muscle neoplasm: Report of a case with review of the literature. Arch Pathol Lab Med 122:277-281, 1998.

296. Tulbah A, Al-Dayel F, Fawaz I, et al: Epstein-Barr virus—associated leiomyosarcoma of the thyroid in a child with congenital immunodeficiency: A case report. Am J Surg Pathol 23:473-476, 1999.

297. Molle ZI, Moallem H, Desai N, et al: Endoscopic features of smooth muscle tumors in children with AIDS. Gastrointest Endosc 52:91-94, 2000.

298. Siegal A, Witz M: Gastrointestinal lipoma and malignancies. J Surg Oncol 47:170-174, 1991.

299. Bruneton JN, Quoy AM, Dageville X, et al: [Lipomas of the digestive tract. Review of the literature apropos of 5 cases]. Ann Gastroenterol Hepatol (Paris) 20:27-32, 1984.

300. Hancock BJ, Vajcner A: Lipomas of the colon: A clinicopathologic review. Can J Surg 31:178-181, 1988.

301. Bromberg SH, Zampieri JC, Cavalcanti LA, et al: [Colorectal lipomas: Anatomoclinical study of 29 cases]. Rev Assoc Med Bras 43:319-325, 1997.

302. Chung YF, Ho YH, Nyam DC, et al: Management of colonic lipomas. Aust N Z J Surg 68:133-135, 1998.

303. Rogy MA, Mirza D, Berlakovich G, et al: Submucous large-bowel lipomas—presentation and management. An 18-year study. Eur J Surg 157:51-55, 1991.

304. Franc-Law JM, Begin LR, Vasilevsky CA, et al: The dramatic presentation of colonic lipomata: Report of two cases and review of the literature. Am Surg 67:491-494, 2001.

305. Alponat A, Kok KY, Goh PM, et al: Intermittent subacute intestinal obstruction due to a giant lipoma of the colon: A case report. Am Surg 64:480, 1998.

306. Notar JR, Masser PA: Annular colon lipoma: A case report and review of the literature. Surgery 110:570-572, 1991.

307. Santos-Briz A, Garcia JP, Gonzalez C, et al: Lipomatous polyposis of the colon. Histopathology 38:81-83, 2001.

308. Ladurner R, Mussack T, Hohenbleicher F, et al: Laparoscopic-assisted resection of giant sigmoid lipoma under colonoscopic guidance. Surg Endosc 17:160, 2003.

309. Snover DC: Atypical lipomas of the colon. Report of two cases with pseudomalignant features. Dis Colon Rectum 27:485-488, 1984.

310. Skaane P, Eide TJ, Westgaard T, et al: Lipomatosis and true lipomas of the ileocecal valve. Rofo Fortschr Geb Rontgenstr Nukelearmedizin 135:663-668, 1981.

311. Walke L, Christie AJ: Lipohyperplasia of ileocecal valve causing recurrent intussusception. Henry Ford Hosp Med J 38:259-261, 1990.

312. Smith SR, Fenton L: Lipohyperplasia of the ileo-caecal valve causing appendicitis. Aust N Z J Surg 70:76-77, 2000.

313. Tawfik OW, McGregor DH: Lipohyperplasia of the ileocecal valve. Am J Gastroenterol 87:82-87, 1992.

314. Johnston J, Helwig EB: Granular cell tumors of the gastrointestinal tract and perianal region: A study of 74 cases. Dig Dis Sci 26:807-816, 1981.

315. Cohen MG, Greenwald ML, Garbus JE, et al: Granular cell tumor—a unique neoplasm of the internal anal sphincter: A report of a case. Dis Colon Rectum 43:1444-1446, 2000.

316. Okano A, Takakuwa H, Nishio A: Granular cell tumor of the rectum. Gastrointest Endosc 54:624, 2001.

317. Melo CR, Melo IS, Schmitt FC, et al: Multicentric granular cell tumor of the colon: Report of a patient with 52 tumors. Am J Gastroenterol 88:1785-1787, 1993.

318. Rossi GB, de Bellis M, Marone P, et al: Granular cell tumors of the colon: Report of a case and review of the literature. J Clin Gastroenterol 30:197-199, 2000.

319. Enzinger FM, Weiss SW: Benign tumors of peripheral nerves. In Enzinger FM, Weiss SW (eds): Soft Tissue Tumors, 3rd ed. St. Louis, Mosby, 1995, pp 821-888.

320. Soon MS, Lin OS: Inflammatory fibroid polyp of the duodenum. Surg Endosc 14:86, 2000.

321. Widgren S, Cox JN: Inflammatory fibroid polyp in a continent ileo-anal pouch after colectomy for ulcerative colitis—case report. Pathol Res Pract 193:643-647; discussion 649-652, 1997.

322. de la Plaza R, Picardo AL, Cuberes R, et al: Inflammatory fibroid polyps of the large intestine. Dig Dis Sci 44:1810-1816, 1999.

323. Nakase H, Mimura J, Kawasaki T, et al: Endoscopic resection of small inflammatory fibroid polyp of the colon. Intern Med 39:25-27, 2000.

324. Aubert A, Cazier A, Baglin AC, et al: [Inflammatory fibroid polyps of the colon][article in French]. Gastroenterol Clin Biol 22:1106-1109, 1998.

325. Shimer GR, Helvig EB: Inflammatory fibroid polyps of the intestine. Am J Clin Pathol 81:708-714, 1984.

326. Pollice L, Bufo P: Inflammatory fibroid polyp of the rectum. Pathol Res Pract 178:508-512, 1984.

327. Ferin P, Skucas J: Inflammatory fibroid polyp of the colon simulating malignancy. Radiology 149;55-56, 1983.

328. Harned RK, Buck JL, Shekitka KM: Inflammatory fibroid polyps of the gastrointestinal tract: Radiologic evaluation. Radiology 182:863-866, 1992.

329. Gooszen AW, Tjon A, Tham RT, et al: Inflammatory fibroid polyp simulating malignant tumor of the colon in a patient with multiple hamartoma syndrome (Cowden's disease). AJR Am J Roentgenol 165:1012-1013, 1995.

330. Williams GR, Jaffe S, Scott CA: Inflammatory fibroid polyp of the terminal ileum presenting in a patient with active Crohn's disease. Histopathology 20:545-547, 1992.

331. Allibone RO, Nanson JK, Anthony PP: Multiple and recurrent inflammatory fibroid polyps in a Devon family ('Devon polyposis syndrome'): An update. Gut 33:1004-1005, 1992.

332. Gutierres AA, Simoneti CA, Braz MA, et al: Intestinal obstruction caused by inflammatory fibroid polyp. Report of a case. Rev Hosp Clin Fac Med São Paulo 52:20-22, 1997.

333. Makhlouf HR, Sobin LH: Inflammatory myofibroblastic tumors (inflammatory pseudotumors) of the gastrointestinal tract: How closely are they related to inflammatory fibroid polyps? Hum Pathol 33:307-315, 2002.

334. Kolodziejczyk P, Yao T, Tsuneyoshi M: Inflammatory fibroid polyp of the stomach. A special reference to an immunohistochemical profile of 42 cases. Am J Surg Pathol 17:1159-1168, 1993.

335. Hasegawa T, Yang P, Kagawa N, et al: CD34 expression by inflammatory fibroid polyps of the stomach. Mod Pathol 10:451-456, 1997.

336. Ryback LD, Shapiro RS, Carano K, et al: Massive pneumatosis intestinalis: CT diagnosis. Comput Med Imaging Graph 23:165-168, 1999.

337. Gelman SF, Brandt LJ: Pneumatosis intestinalis and AIDS: A case report and review of the literature. Am J Gastroenterol 93:646-650, 1998.

338. Jensen R, Gutnik SH: Pneumatosis cystoides intestinalis: A complication of colonoscopic polypectomy. S D J Med 44:177-179, 1991.

339. Gosi G, Huoranszki F: Sigmoidoscopically induced pneumatosis cystoides coli in Crohn's disease manifested by collar subcutaneous emphysema. Endoscopy 33:293, 2001.

340. Jona JZ: Benign pneumatosis intestinalis coli after blunt trauma to the abdomen in a child. J Pediatr Surg 35:1109-1111, 2000.

341. Azimuddin K, Bourne R: Pneumatosis cystoides intestinalis in a case of sigmoid volvulus. Br J Hosp Med 57:468-469, 1997.

342. Lock G, Holstege A, Lang B, et al: Gastrointestinal manifestations of progressive systemic sclerosis. Am J Gastroenterol 92:763-771, 1997.

343. Parra JA, Acinas O, Bueno J, et al: An unusual form of pneumatosis intestinalis associated with appendicitis. Br J Radiol 71:326-328, 1998.

344. Schenk P, Madl C, Kramer L, et al: Pneumatosis intestinalis with *Clostridium difficile* colitis as a cause of acute abdomen after lung transplantation. Dig Dis Sci 43:2455-2458, 1998.

345. Gagliardi G, Thompson IW, Hershman MH, et al: Pneumatosis coli: A proposed pathogenesis based on study of 25 cases and review of the literature. Int J Colorectal Dis 11:111-118, 1996.

346. Snape J, Hulman G, Reddy PR, et al: Pneumatosis coli: An uncommon but treatable cause of faecal incontinence. Int J Clin Pract 52:501-503, 1998.

347. Shimada M, Ina Takahashi H, Horiuchi Y, et al: Pneumatosis cystoides intestinalis treated with hyperbaric oxygen therapy:

Usefulness of an endoscopic ultrasonic catheter probe for diagnosis. Intern Med 40:896-900, 2001.

348. Kianmanesh Rad AR, Vilotte J, Benhamou G: Cystic pneumatosis of the colon. Report of 3 cases and review of the literature. Ann Chir 51:995-1000, 1997.

349. Kavic SM, Basson MD: Complications of endoscopy. Am J Surg 181:313-318, 2001.

350. Kaassis M, Croue A, Carpentier S, et al: A case of colonic pseudolipomatosis: A rare complication of colonoscopy? Endoscopy 29:325-327, 1997.

351. Waring JP, Manne RK, Wadas DD, et al: Mucosal pseudo-lipomatosis: An air pressure–related colonoscopy complication. Gastrointest Endosc 35:93-94, 1989.

352. Witte JT: Colonic mucosal pseudolipomatosis. Gastrointest Endosc 54:750, 2001.

353. Ben Rejeb A, Khedhiri F: Mucosal pseudo-lipomatosis of the colon. Apropos of a case with a review of the literature. Arch Anat Cytol Pathol 37:254-257, 1989.

354. Cook DS, Williams GT: Duodenal 'pseudolipomatosis.' Histopathology 33:394-395, 1998.

355. Snover DC, Sandstad J, Hutton S: Mucosal pseudolipomatosis of the colon. Am J Clin Pathol 84:575-580, 1985.

356. Flieder DB, Moran CA, Travis WD, et al: Pleuro-pulmonary endometriosis and pulmonary ectopic deciduosis: A clinico-pathologic and immunohistochemical study of 10 cases with emphasis on diagnostic pitfalls. Hum Pathol 29:1495-1503, 1998.

357. Yantiss RK, Clement PB, Young RH: Endometriosis of the intestinal tract: A study of 44 cases of a disease that may cause diverse challenges in clinical and pathologic evaluation. Am J Surg Pathol 25:445-454, 2001.

358. Bartkowiak R, Zieniewicz K, Kaminiski P, et al: Diagnosis and treatment of sigmoidal endometriosis—a case report. Med Sci Monit 6:787-790, 2000.

359. Deval B, Rafii A, Felce Dachez M, et al: Sigmoid endometriosis in a postmenopausal woman. Am J Obstet Gynecol 187:1723-1725, 2002.

360. Varras M, Kostopanagiotou E, Katis K, et al: Endometriosis causing extensive intestinal obstruction simulating carcinoma of the sigmoid colon: A case report and review of the literature. Eur Gynaecol Oncol 23:3453-3357, 2002.

361. Sumathi VP, McCluggage WG: CD10 is useful in demonstrating endometrial stroma at ectopic sites and in confirming a diagnosis of endometriosis. J Clin Pathol 55:391-392, 2002.

362. Slavin RE, Krum R, Van Dinh T: Endometriosis-associated intestinal tumors: A clinical and pathological study of 6 cases with a review of the literature. Hum Pathol 31:456-463, 2000.

363. Yantiss RK, Clement PB, Young RH: Neoplastic and pre-neoplastic changes in gastrointestinal endometriosis: A study of 17 cases. Am J Surg Pathol 24:513-524, 2000.

364. Bejarano PA, Aranda-Michel J, Genoglio-Preiser C: Histochemical and immunohistochemical characterization of foamy histiocytes (muciphages and xanthelasma) of the rectum. Am J Surg Pathol 24:1009-1115, 2000.

365. Miliauskas JR: Rectosigmoid (colonic) xanthoma: A report of four cases and review of the literature. Pathology 34:144-147, 2002.

366. Boruchowicz A, Rey C, Fontaine M, et al: Colonic xanthelasma due to glyceride accumulation associated with an adenoma. Am J Gastroenterol 92:159-161, 1997.

367. Weinstock LB, Shatz BA, Saltman RJ, et al: Xanthoma of the colon. Gastrointest Endosc 55:410, 2002.

368. Goodman MD: Segmental xanthomatosis of the ileocecal valve with anatomic and functional obstruction. Arch Pathol Lab Med 121:75-78, 1997.

369. Lo CY, Lorentz TG, Poon CS: Xanthogranulomatous inflammation of the sigmoid colon: A case report. Aust N Z J Surg 66:643-644, 1996.

370. Morimatsu M, Shirozu K, Nakashima T, et al: Xanthogranuloma of the rectum. Acta Pathol Jpn 35:165-171, 1985.

371. Collins DC: 71,000 human appendix specimens: A final report summarizing a 40-year study. Am J Proctol 14:365-381, 1963.

372. Ozuner G, Davidson P, Church J: Intussusception of the vermiform appendix: Preoperative colonoscopic diagnosis of two cases and review of the literature. Int J Colorectal Dis 15:185-187, 2000.

373. Langsam LB, Raj PK, Galang CF: Intussusception of the appendix. Dis Colon Rectum 27:387-392, 1984.

374. Jevon GP, Daya D, Qizilbash AH: Intussusception of the appendix. A report of four cases and review of the literature. Arch Pathol Lab Med 116:960-964, 1992.

375. Kawamura YJ, Toyama N, Kasamatsu T, et al: Intussusception of appendiceal adenoma mimicking invasive carcinoma. Endoscopy 34:749, 2002.

376. Coulier B, Pestieau S, Hamels J, et al: US and CT diagnosis of complete cecocolic intussusception caused by an appendiceal mucocele. Eur Radiol 12:324-328, 2002.

377. Pumberger W, Hormann M, Pomberger G, et al: Sonographic diagnosis of intussusception of the appendix vermiformis. J Clin Ultrasound 28:492-496, 2000.

378. Bailey DJ, Courington KR, Andres JM, et al: Cecal polyp and appendiceal intussusception in a child with recurrent abdominal pain: Diagnosis by colonoscopy. J Pediatr Gastroenterol Nutr 6:818-820, 1987.

379. Miyahara M, Saito T, Etoh K, et al: Appendiceal intussusception due to an appendiceal malignant polyp—an association in a patient with Peutz-Jeghers syndrome: Report of a case. Surg Today 26:834-837, 1995.

380. Weston AP, Campbell DR: Diminutive colonic polyps: Histopathology, spatial distribution, concomitant significant lesions, and treatment complications. Am J Gastroenterol 90:24-28, 1995.

381. Paspatis GA, Papanikolaou N, Zois E, et al: Prevalence of polyps and diverticulosis of the large bowel in the Cretan population. An autopsy study. Int J Colorectal Dis 16:257-261, 2001.

382. Dignan CR, Greenson JK: Can ischemic colitis be differentiated from *C difficile* colitis in biopsy specimens? Am J Surg Pathol 21:706-710, 1997.

383. Cheville JC, Mitros FA, Vanderzalm G, et al: Atheroemboli-associated polyps of the sigmoid colon. Am J Surg Pathol 17:1054-1057, 1993.

384. Gramlich TL, Hunter SB: Focal polypoid ischemia of the colon: Atheroemboli presenting as a colonic polyp. Arch Pathol Lab Med 118:308-309, 1994.

385. O'Brian DS, Jeffers M, Kay EW, et al: Bleeding due to colorectal atheroembolism. Diagnosis by biopsy of adenomatous polyps or of ischemic ulcer. Am J Surg Pathol 15:1078-1082, 1994.

EPITHELIAL NEOPLASMS OF THE GI TRACT

CHAPTER 16

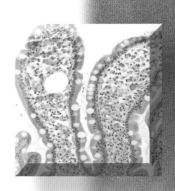

Epithelial Neoplasms of the Esophagus

JONATHAN N. GLICKMAN • ROBERT D. ODZE

Most benign and malignant neoplasms of the esophagus are epithelial in origin (Table 16-1). Overall, esophageal carcinomas account for approximately 5% of all gastrointestinal tract malignant neoplasms and 9% of deaths from gastrointestinal tract cancers in the United States.[1] However, the incidence of esophageal carcinoma has increased dramatically in the United States in the past 30 years, principally because of a marked rise in Barrett's-associated adenocarcinoma,[2] discussed later.

◼ Benign Neoplasms and Tumor-like Lesions

SQUAMOUS PAPILLOMA

Clinical Features

Esophageal squamous papillomas (ESPs) are the most common benign epithelial tumor of the esophagus.[3,4] Studies suggest a prevalence rate of up to 1%. They may affect patients of all ages and both genders. Most ESPs are asymptomatic. However, large lesions may cause epigastric pain, dysphagia, or symptoms related to luminal obstruction.

TABLE 16–1. Classification of Epithelial Tumors of the Esophagus
Tumor-like conditions
Glycogenic acanthosis
Pseudoepitheliomatous hyperplasia
Heterotopia
Cysts/duplications
Pseudodiverticulosis
Fibrovascular polyp
Benign neoplasms
Squamous papilloma
Adenoma (gland/duct)
Barrett's esophagus–associated polypoid dysplasia
Malignant neoplasms
Squamous cell carcinoma, usual type
Squamous cell carcinoma variants
Basaloid carcinoma
Spindle cell carcinoma (carcinosarcoma)
Verrucous carcinoma
Lymphoepithelioma-like carcinoma
Adenocarcinoma, Barrett's esophagus associated
Adenocarcinoma, non-Barrett's associated
Heterotopia associated
Gland/duct type
Adenoid cystic carcinoma
Mixed squamous and glandular tumors
Endocrine tumors
Carcinoid
Small cell carcinoma
Choriocarcinoma
Metastases

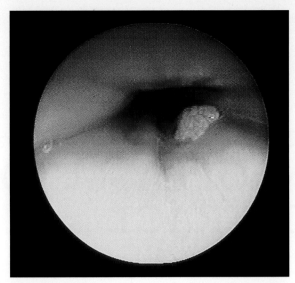

FIGURE 16–1. Endoscopic photograph of an exophytic squamous papilloma of the esophagus showing a well-circumscribed broad-based nodule with a verrucoid irregular surface.

Pathogenesis

The pathogenesis of ESPs is controversial. Whereas several studies have shown a high association with human papillomavirus (HPV) infection, particularly types 6/11, 16, and 18,[3,4] other studies have failed to show a strong association with HPV.[5] Differences in the rate of association with HPV may be due to differences in the techniques used to detect viral antigens or DNA and the possibility that as yet unidentified subtypes of HPV may be involved. In fact, at least one study showed an association between ESPs and rare HPV types such as DL284 and DL436.[4] Others have proposed that these lesions develop as a result of chronic mucosal irritation, perhaps secondary to gastroesophageal reflux disease.

Gross and Microscopic Findings

Grossly, ESPs are usually small, discrete, sessile, soft, tan lesions that range in size from 0.5 to 3 cm; they occur most commonly in the distal esophagus but may develop anywhere in the esophagus (Fig. 16-1). Up to 20% of cases are multiple. Microscopically, three distinct histopathologic types have been recognized: exophytic, endophytic, and spiked (verrucoid) (Fig. 16-2).[3] The exophytic type, which is the most common, is composed of finger-like papillary fronds. The endophytic type shows a smooth round surface contour and an inverted papillomatous proliferation. The least common is the spiked or "verrucoid" type, which has a spiked surface contour, a prominent granular cell layer, and marked hyperkeratosis. All types are characterized by a branched fibrovascular core of lamina propria with a variable degree of acute and chronic inflammation and vascular congestion. The overlying squamous epithelium in all types shows acanthotic, often reactive, epithelium with a prominent basal cell zone and complete surface maturation. Features that are variably present include koilocytosis, parakeratosis, binucleation, dyskeratosis, and prominent granular cell layer.

Differential Diagnosis

Papillomas that are large, are oriented poorly, and show marked reactive changes may, on occasion, be difficult to differentiate from a well-differentiated squamous cell carcinoma or a verrucous carcinoma. However, ESPs lack cytologic atypia, atypical mitoses, and an infiltrative growth pattern characteristic of carcinoma. Furthermore, the gross (endoscopic) appearance of ESPs is distinctive. Papillomas may also be potentially confused with pseudoepitheliomatous hyperplasia occurring adjacent to a healing ulcer or overlying a granular cell tumor. However, the latter type of lesion lacks a fibrovascular core and other features of HPV infection such as koilocytosis. Unlike ESPs, pseudoepitheliomatous hyperplasia often shows abundant inflammation and surface erosion.

Prognosis

Squamous cell papillomas are generally considered benign lesions with little or no malignant potential.[3,6]

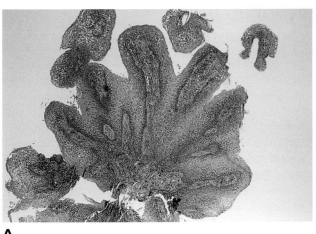

A

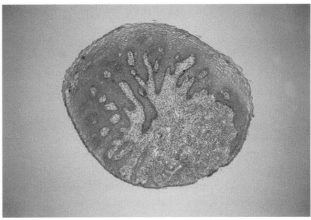

B

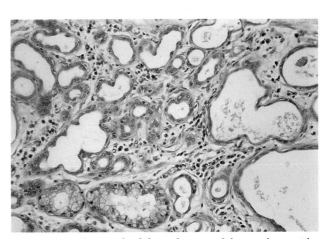

C

FIGURE 16–2. A, Exophytic squamous papilloma of the esophagus. This lesion shows fingerlike projections of acanthotic squamous epithelium covering fibrovascular lamina propria pegs with chronic inflammation. **B,** Endophytic-type squamous papilloma showing an inverted papillomatous surface contour. **C,** Spiked-type squamous papilloma showing prominent spikes of acanthotic epithelium with marked hyperkeratosis and hypergranulosis.

However, rare cases associated with squamous dysplasia, or even squamous cell carcinoma, have been reported.[7]

ADENOMA

Adenomas of the esophagus may develop from the submucosal gland/duct system or, more commonly, from metaplastic columnar epithelium in cases of Barrett's esophagus, in which case the term *polypoid dysplasia* is preferred.

Adenomas that develop from the submucosal glands are rare. They are usually histologically similar to those that arise from the minor salivary glands. This is not surprising because embryologically the esophageal submucosal glands are considered a continuation of the minor salivary glands of the oropharynx. They are usually submucosal and develop as well-circumscribed lesions that resemble pleomorphic adenomas[8] or, more rarely, pancreatic or ovary-like serous cystadenomas.[9]

Microscopically, adenomas that develop from the submucosal gland ducts show a mixture of tubal, cystic, and papillary growth patterns similar to intraductal papillomas of the breast or sialadenoma papilliferum of the salivary glands.[10] The epithelium typically contains two cell

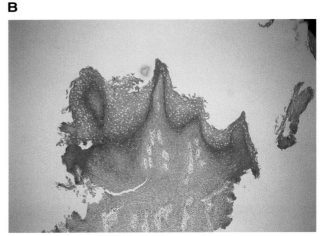

FIGURE 16–3. Benign gland/duct adenoma of the esophagus. The lesion is composed of a proliferation of irregular glands lined by flattened cuboidal to low columnar epithelium focally showing two cell layers. No mitoses or significant atypia is noted.

layers (similar to the normal submucosal gland ducts) with only mild to moderate cytologic atypia and infrequent mitoses (Fig. 16-3). A mixed inflammatory infiltrate may be present. Most of these tumors behave in a benign fashion,[11] although rare carcinomas have been reported.[12]

More commonly, adenoma-like polypoid dysplastic lesions may develop in Barrett's esophagus (see Chapter 7). Endoscopically, these lesions usually appear as well-defined sessile or pedunculated polyps that range in size from 0.5 to 1.5 cm and usually occur in the mid or distal esophagus within areas of Barrett's esophagus (Fig. 16-4). Histologically, these polyps are composed of a tubular or tubulovillous proliferation of low- or high-grade dysplastic epithelium similar in appearance to colonic adenomas. In one study, these lesions showed proliferative and molecular abnormalities (loss of heterozygosity of *APC* and *TP53*) similar to flat dysplasia and thus should probably be treated in a similar fashion.[13] In fact, of the 10 cases reported, 9 were associated with adenocarcinoma, illustrating their high malignant potential.[13]

TUMOR-LIKE LESIONS

Developmental Cysts and Duplications

Congenital cystic lesions and duplications may occur in the esophagus and mimic a malignant tumor because of their mass effect. These lesions are categorized by their site of origin, their embryologic derivation, and the histologic appearance of their lining epithelium. Clinically, they may be asymptomatic or cause symptomatic compression of nearby respiratory or alimentary tract structures.

Bronchogenic cysts result from anomalous budding of bronchial structures derived from the embryonic foregut. They are typically located in the mediastinum or in the wall of the esophagus.[14,15] Grossly, these cysts

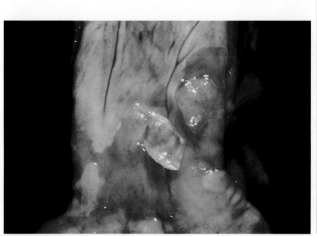

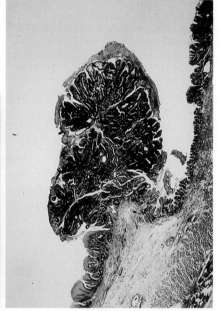

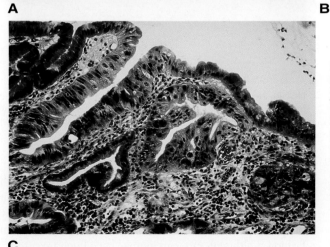

FIGURE 16–4. Polypoid dysplasia in Barrett's esophagus. **A,** Gross image of two well-circumscribed pedunculated polyps situated just above the gastroesophageal junction, and arising on a background of Barrett's mucosa. The squamous mucosa of the normal esophagus is seen just above the polyps. **B,** Low-power photomicrograph of the circumscribed polypoid area of dysplasia seen in part **A.** Note that the polyp is formed of tightly packed convoluted dysplastic glands and is arising from columnar mucosa with intestinal metaplasia. **C,** The polyp is composed of high-grade dysplastic columnar epithelium.

are usually unilocular and do not normally communicate with the esophageal lumen. Microscopically, they are lined by ciliated columnar epithelium and frequently contain cartilage, smooth muscle, and mucous glands in the surrounding cyst-lining tissue.

Intramural cysts most likely develop as a result of abnormal recanalization of the esophageal lumen during embryogenesis. They may produce extrinsic compression and obstruction of the esophageal lumen or trachea. Histologically, unilocular cysts may be lined by respiratory, gastric, oxyntic, squamous, or simple cuboidal epithelium, often with smooth muscle and ganglia in the cyst wall.[14]

Dorsal enteric (neurenteric) cysts occur primarily in the posterior mediastinum of infants and are thought to arise from incomplete closure of the notochordal remnant.[16] These cysts may be associated with additional congenital defects, including spina bifida and vertebral anomalies. Microscopically, they are lined by gastric, intestinal, squamous, or respiratory epithelium and are usually surrounded by all the normal tissue layers of the bowel wall.

Other rare congenital anomalies include esophageal duplications,[17,18] which may be asymptomatic but more often cause dysphagia or respiratory symptoms. Histologically, these cysts may be lined by squamous, gastric, ciliated columnar, or even pancreatic epithelium. The wall consists of admixed fibrous tissue and smooth muscle but does not contain organized layers of muscularis or cartilage.

Developmental cysts and duplications are benign. However, extremely rarely, adenocarcinoma or squamous cell carcinoma may develop from these lesions.[19,20]

Heterotopia

Gastric, thyroid, parathyroid, or even sebaceous tissue may be present in the esophagus (heterotopia) in up to 10% of the general population. Most heterotopias are located in the upper third of the esophagus. Gastric heterotopia is the most common ("inlet patch") and may give rise to symptoms secondary to complications from acid secretion, such as heartburn, dysphagia, ulceration, bleeding, stricture, or perforation.[21] The diagnosis is established by finding gastric glandular and surface epithelium (usually with parietal cells) in the esophagus in patients without intervening Barrett's esophagus. Rarely, adenocarcinoma may develop in gastric heterotopia (Fig. 16-5).[22-24]

Heterotopic sebaceous glands are the second most common form of heterotopia in the esophagus. They usually appear as slightly elevated yellowish lesions, 1 to 2 mm in diameter, and may occur at any level of the esophagus. Microscopically, these lesions show sebaceous cells within the epithelium or in the lamina propria (Fig. 16-6). Sebaceous cells are microvesicular and contain vacuolated cytoplasm filled with lipid substances.

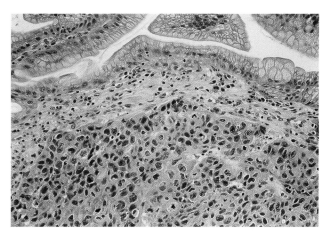

FIGURE 16–5. Poorly differentiated adenocarcinoma *(bottom),* arising in a focus of gastric heterotopia situated in the upper third of the esophagus.

An excretory duct, with or without a connection to the surface epithelium, may be present as well.

It is presumed that all heterotopias are congenital. However, one study suggested that sebaceous glands may represent a metaplastic process because of frequent association with reflux esophagitis and expression of CK14, which has been demonstrated in cell lines thought to represent the progeny of dormant stem cells.[25]

Pseudoepitheliomatous Hyperplasia

Pseudoepitheliomatous hyperplasia is a morphologic pattern of reactive squamous epithelium that occurs

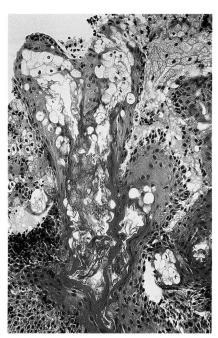

FIGURE 16–6. Sebaceous heterotopia of the esophagus. Protruding from the squamous epithelium is a proliferation of vacuolated sebaceous cells mixed with squamous cells, secretions, and keratin.

most commonly adjacent to healing ulcers. It is characterized by parallel, elongated, and occasionally irregular columns of highly reactive squamous cells, with prominent nucleoli and abundant mitoses that may extend deep into the lamina propria (Fig. 16-7). Its appearance may simulate invasive squamous cell carcinoma. On occasion, this reaction may be endoscopically visible and, as such, may cause diagnostic confusion with a malignant lesion.

Malignant Neoplasms

SQUAMOUS CELL CARCINOMA

Clinical Features

Squamous cell carcinoma is the most common malignant tumor of the esophagus worldwide. In 1997, an estimated 12,300 new cases and 11,500 deaths in the United States were reported.[1] It affects predominantly men (three to four times more often than women) with a peak incidence in the seventh decade of life. There is a marked geographic and ethnic variation in incidence; the highest rates (up to 161 per 100,000 men) occur in China, Iran, South America, and South Africa.[26] In the United States, the disease is approximately five times more common in black men than in white men.[27] Common presenting symptoms include dysphagia and weight loss. A small fraction of patients may also present with hypercalcemia secondary to parathyroid hormone–related protein production by the tumor.[28] In addition, up to 3% of patients with esophageal squamous cell carcinoma also have concurrent head and neck squamous cell carcinoma.[29]

Pathogenesis

The pathogenesis of squamous cell carcinoma is multifactorial and varies significantly among different regions of the world.[30] However, many cases develop without an identifiable cause or predisposing condition. Known risk factors in high-prevalence areas such as China and Iran include consumption of food or water rich in nitrates and nitrosamines, which results in the development of chronic esophagitis. Additional risk factors, common to both Western and developing countries, include tobacco smoke, alcohol, and various vitamin deficiencies. Other predisposing conditions are achalasia,[31-33] Plummer-Vinson syndrome, strictures resulting from acid or lye ingestion, and the rare autosomal dominant condition tylosis palmaris et plantaris.[34] Individuals related to affected family members are also at increased risk for esophageal carcinoma.

HPV infection has been implicated in tumorigenesis. However, its precise role is controversial. HPV DNA has been isolated from esophageal tumors at prevalence rates of 0% to 66%.[35-38] Viral types most commonly identified include HPV types 16 and 18. Varying rates of

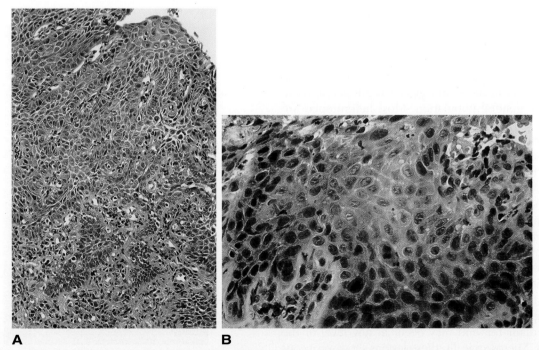

A   **B**

FIGURE 16–7. A, Pseudoepitheliomatous hyperplasia of the esophagus. This marked reactive change is characterized by a proliferation of irregular pegs of squamous epithelium that extend into the underlying lamina propria with a moderate amount of chronic inflammation. On high power **(B),** the epithelium is composed of hyperchromatic cells with a slightly increased N/C ratio. However, no atypical mitoses or significant overlapping of the cells and their nuclei is noted. In addition, no significant loss of polarity is seen.

HPV positivity between different studies may be attributed to differences in the techniques used to detect HPV and to different populations of patients.[37] In one study, tumor samples from various countries were tested for HPV in a single laboratory, and the overall rate of positivity was 14%.[36] Therefore, HPV is most likely a causative factor in only a small fraction of squamous cell carcinomas, particularly those from high-risk areas.

SQUAMOUS DYSPLASIA

Clinical Features

Esophageal squamous cell carcinoma, similar to its counterpart in the skin or cervix, is believed to develop through a progression of premalignant or dysplastic precursor lesions. Dysplasia is defined as the presence of unequivocal neoplastic cells confined to the epithelium. Squamous dysplasia is more common in patients at high risk for squamous cell carcinoma[39] and is adjacent to squamous cell carcinomas in up to 60% to 90% of cases. In addition, dysplasia is frequently multifocal. In one study,[40] severe dysplasia (carcinoma in situ) was found in 14% and mild or moderate dysplasia in 20% of resection specimens with invasive squamous cell carcinoma. Carcinomas associated with dysplasia are also more likely to be multifocal in origin.[41] Dysplasia is generally classified as mild, moderate, or severe (including carcinoma in situ), depending on the degree of involvement of the native squamous epithelium. More recently, a two-tiered system (low-grade and high-grade) is preferred. In this system, low-grade dysplasia includes mild and moderate and high-grade dysplasia includes severe and carcinoma in situ (see later for microscopic description).

Pathologic Features

GROSS PATHOLOGY

Dysplastic epithelium appears erythematous, friable, and irregular in more than 80% of cases.[39] Erosions, plaques, and nodules may also be present. However, dysplasia may appear completely normal endoscopically. Mucosal staining with Lugol's iodine may be helpful to highlight dysplastic mucosa and has been advocated as a means of improving the sensitivity of endoscopic biopsy surveillance in high-risk populations.[42] Dysplastic cells may also be harvested by exfoliative balloon cytology, a technique often used for screening in high-risk areas such as China (see Chapter 2).[43]

MICROSCOPIC PATHOLOGY

Dysplastic squamous epithelium is characterized by a combination of architectural and cytologic abnormalities that vary in extent and severity according to the grade (Fig. 16-8). The epithelium is usually hypertrophic but may be thin or atrophic. Dysplasia may involve the basal layer only or the full thickness of the epithelium.

In 20% of cases, dysplastic epithelium may also spread into esophageal mucosal gland ducts and simulate stromal invasion.[44] Low-grade dysplasia reveals involvement of the basal third to half of the squamous epithelium with neoplastic cells, whereas high-grade lesions show nearly complete or complete involvement of the native squamous epithelium. Dysplastic cells may also occasionally grow as isolated cells in a horizontal "pagetoid" fashion.[45]

Cytologic changes include nuclear hyperchromasia, pleomorphism, increased nucleus-to-cytoplasm ratio, and increased mitotic rate. The chromatin of dysplastic cells is usually coarse and may be associated with thickening of the nuclear membrane. Nucleoli may be present but are not a consistent feature and are not specific because they are also frequently present in reactive squamous epithelium (see later). Architecturally, dysplastic cells display disorganization, loss of polarity, overlapping nuclei, and lack of surface maturation, which are key features in helping to distinguish from non-neoplastic (reactive) processes. Mitotic figures are usually increased in number and may be found at any level of the epithelium. In addition, abnormal (tripolar or disorganized) mitotic figures may be present.

Differential Diagnosis

Squamous dysplasia must be distinguished from reactive epithelial changes associated with esophagitis. Although regenerating squamous cells may show mild nuclear enlargement, hyperchromasia, and expansion of the basal cell layers, they lack significant nuclear pleomorphism, overlapping, or crowding and do not display abnormal mitoses (see Fig. 16-7). Unlike in dysplasia, the chromatin is generally fine and homogeneous, and nucleoli, when present, are small. Architecturally, reactive squamous epithelium often displays some degree of surface maturation. Essential to the diagnosis is the fact that the basal and suprabasal layers maintain their polarity and orderly spacing. Mucosal inflammation frequently accompanies reactive squamous epithelium, and in the presence of inflammation, a diagnosis of dysplasia must be rendered with caution. In biopsy specimens in which the epithelial changes appear sufficiently marked to suggest dysplasia, but in which a reactive process cannot be excluded because of inflammation, a diagnosis of "indefinite for dysplasia" is appropriate. In such cases, follow-up biopsies after treatment of the underlying esophagitis will frequently help resolve the diagnostic uncertainty. Histologic features useful in the differential diagnosis of squamous dysplasia are summarized in Table 16-2. The differential diagnosis of squamous dysplasia and invasive squamous cell carcinoma is discussed later under Invasive Squamous Cell Carcinoma.

In biopsy specimens from patients who have received chemotherapy or radiotherapy, the squamous epithe-

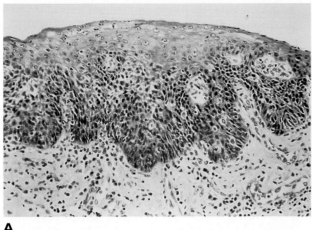

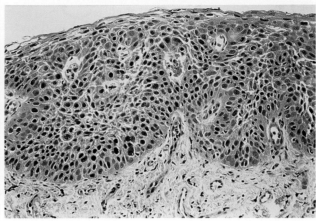

A

B

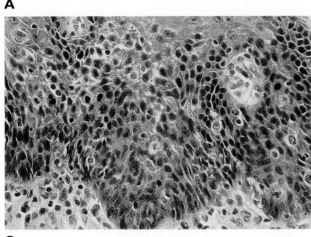

C

FIGURE 16–8. Squamous dysplasia of the esophagus. **A,** Low-grade (mild) squamous dysplasia characterized by a proliferation of neoplastic cells extending about one third up the thickness of the epithelium. **B,** In contrast to **A,** dysplastic cells extend to the surface of the epithelium and are associated with a significant loss of surface maturation (high-grade dysplasia). **C,** In this high-power image, dysplastic cells are noted to have an increased N/C ratio, marked hyperchromatic nuclei, significant loss of polarity, and overlapping of the cells and their nuclei.

lium may contain markedly atypical cells with enlarged hyperchromatic nuclei that raise the possibility of dysplasia. However, unlike in dysplasia, these cells do not have an increased nucleus-to-cytoplasm ratio and often contain a distinctive vacuolization to their cytoplasm. Furthermore, unlike in dysplasia, mesenchymal cells showing similar changes may be present in the lamina propria as well as other stromal changes of chemotherapy or radiotherapy. Thus, awareness of the clinical history is critical.

TABLE 16–2. Features Helpful in Distinguishing Reactive From Dysplastic Squamous Epithelium

Histologic Feature	Reactive	Dysplastic
Nuclear pleomorphism	−	+/++
Increased N/C ratio	+/−	++
Nuclear hyperchromasia	+/−	+
Increased mitotic rate	+/−	+
Abnormal mitoses	−	+
Nuclear crowding, overlapping, disarray	−	+/++
Surface maturation	+	−
Inflammation	++	+/−

N/C, Nucleus-to-cytoplasm.

Biopsy specimens from patients with esophagitis secondary to reflux or other causes may occasionally contain multinucleated epithelial giant cells, which may raise the possibility of dysplasia (Fig. 16-9).[46] In these cases, no other cytologic or architectural features of dysplasia are present, and results of special studies for viral inclusions are negative.

Prognosis and Treatment

Squamous dysplasia frequently occurs adjacent to invasive carcinoma. In addition, patients with squamous dysplasia are at an increased risk for development of squamous cell carcinoma; one study from China showed a 9% incidence of carcinoma during a 15-year period.[47] In another study, 15% of patients with low-grade dysplasia progressed to high-grade dysplasia, whereas 30% of patients with high-grade dysplasia developed invasive carcinoma during an 8-year follow-up period.[48] However, dysplasia may also regress or disappear, although sampling error certainly may account for a normal finding on follow-up biopsy in a patient with dysplasia in a prior biopsy specimen. Therefore, patients with a diagnosis of high-grade squamous dysplasia require thorough endoscopic examination and biopsy to

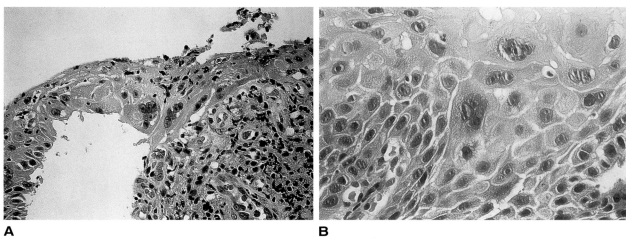

A   **B**

FIGURE 16–9. A, Reactive epithelial giant cell changes noted in the basal portion of the epithelium adjacent to a healing ulcer. **B,** High-power image of another multinucleated epithelial giant cell showing increased nuclear size and prominent nucleoli but a low N/C ratio. These cells are usually located in the basal portion of the epithelium, as is noted in this figure.

exclude invasive squamous cell carcinoma and follow-up to detect an early invasive tumor. In addition, any grade of squamous dysplasia associated with a mass lesion should be considered carcinoma and treated accordingly. Patients with low-grade dysplasia without a mass or associated carcinoma may be managed with repeated biopsies and continued surveillance.

INVASIVE SQUAMOUS CELL CARCINOMA

Squamous cell carcinomas may be separated into early "superficial" and late "advanced" types. Superficial squamous cell carcinomas are defined as those that invade the mucosa and submucosa but do not penetrate the muscularis propria. In most studies, this definition includes tumors with regional lymph node metastasis but not distant metastases.[49-51] These tumors constitute approximately 15% to 20% of all invasive squamous cell carcinomas, with higher prevalence rates in populations that routinely undergo endoscopic surveillance.[26]

Pathologic Features

GROSS PATHOLOGY

Squamous cell carcinomas occur in the middle third of the esophagus in 50% to 60% of cases, the distal third in 30%, and the proximal third in 10% to 20%.[26,52] Superficial tumors most commonly appear as mucosal plaques or slightly elevated flat lesions but may also be ulcerated, polypoid, or even grossly inconspicuous.[50,51] Superficially invasive tumors are more commonly multicentric (up to 20% of cases) compared with advanced tumors. This finding may reflect either synchronous primary tumors occurring in a background of dysplasia[41,53] or the presence of satellite tumor nodules as a result of intramural metastasis.[54]

The gross appearance of advanced tumors may be classified as exophytic or fungating (60% of cases), ulcerating (25% of cases), or infiltrative (15% of cases) (Fig. 16-10)[26]; however, this feature is not a significant prognostic factor. In patients treated with preoperative radiation or chemotherapy, the tumor may be invisible or replaced with a shallow erosion.

MICROSCOPIC PATHOLOGY

Superficially invasive tumors consist of irregular elongated projections of dysplastic epithelium that extend into the lamina propria, muscularis mucosae, or submucosa as isolated cells or clusters of cells with a minimal desmoplastic response (see Fig. 16-9). Invasion of mucosal and submucosal lymphatics is not uncommon and is likely to account for intramural metastasis on occasion. Advanced carcinomas spread through the esophageal wall, either with an infiltrative pattern composed of individual small nests of tumor cells or with an expansile (pushing) growth pattern composed of a solid mass of tumor cells with a smooth advancing edge. A prominent lymphocytic infiltrate occasionally surrounds the tumor.[51,55]

Squamous cell carcinomas show a range of differentiation from well to poor (Fig. 16-11). Well-differentiated tumors show nests of polygonal epithelioid cells with ample eosinophilic cytoplasm, easily recognizable intercellular bridges, and abundant keratinization (squamous pearls), with relatively few compact basaloid cells. Moderately differentiated tumors account for approximately two thirds of squamous cell carcinomas and contain a higher proportion of primitive basaloid cells than well-differentiated tumors do and are typically arranged in irregular nests and trabeculae with only focal keratinization. Poorly differentiated tumors show no evidence of keratinization, grow in solid sheets or as single cells, and may contain large, bizarre pleomorphic

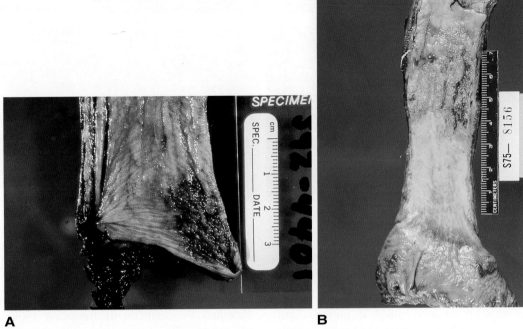

FIGURE 16–10. A, Gross appearance of a superficial squamous cell carcinoma of the esophagus *(right lower corner of the image)*. **B,** Exophytic and ulcerating advanced squamous cell carcinoma of the esophagus is noted in the midportion of the organ.

cells. Squamous cell carcinomas commonly show various degrees of differentiation within a single tumor. Focal glandular or mucinous differentiation (discussed under Carcinoma With Mixed Squamous and Glandular Elements) occurs in up to 20% of cases.[56, 57] If the glandular and squamous components of the tumor are comparable in proportion but intimately mixed, it qualifies as an adenosquamous carcinoma (see under Carcinoma With Mixed Squamous and Glandular Elements). Focal neuroendocrine or small cell differentiation has also been reported.[57,58]

Special studies are rarely required to establish a diagnosis of conventional squamous cell carcinoma but may be useful in small biopsy specimens or when rare tumor cells are present, such as in cases that have received neoadjuvant chemoradiotherapy. By immuno-histochemistry, squamous cell carcinoma cells are positive for broad-spectrum anticytokeratins and for cytokeratins 13, 14, 18, and 19.[59-61] CK7 reactivity is present in up to 29% of cases, but the majority of cases are negative for both cytokeratins 7 and 20.[61,62] Mucin stains may show focal positivity in a high proportion of cases. Focal

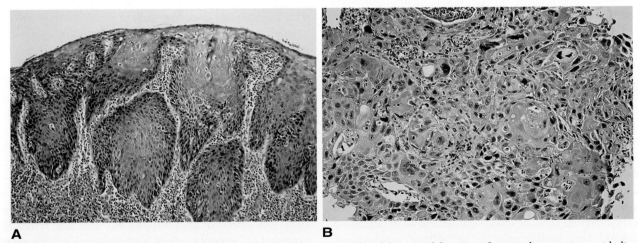

FIGURE 16–11. A, Well-differentiated squamous cell carcinoma characterized by a proliferation of atypical squamous epithelium forming irregular pegs that extend into the underlying lamina propria. This is associated with a mild desmoplastic reaction and chronic inflammation. **B,** Poorly differentiated squamous cell carcinoma characterized by marked nuclear pleomorphism. However, focal areas of cellular keratinization are present.

positivity for neuroendocrine markers such as chromogranin and synaptophysin does not exclude the diagnosis of squamous cell carcinoma if present in a minority of the tumor and if the tumor is otherwise morphologically typical without areas of small cell carcinoma.[63]

Differential Diagnosis

In small poorly oriented biopsy specimens, the distinction between in situ neoplasia (dysplasia) and invasive squamous cell carcinoma may be difficult. Squamous dysplasia, unlike invasive carcinoma, displays smooth-edged papillations with a continuous basement membrane and a connection to the surface epithelium and lacks single-cell infiltration, the presence of irregular discontinuous nests of cells, or a desmoplastic stroma.[64] However, the diagnostic criteria for squamous cell carcinoma differ between Western and Japanese pathologists, such that many lesions considered high-grade dysplasia by Western pathologists are diagnosed as carcinoma by Japanese pathologists solely on the basis of nuclear features.[65]

Invasive squamous cell carcinoma must also be distinguished from non-neoplastic lesions such as pseudo-epitheliomatous hyperplasia and pseudodiverticulosis. Pseudoepitheliomatous hyperplasia, like other reactive squamous proliferations, does not show significant nuclear pleomorphism, loss of polarity, or overlapping of nuclei and always has a connection to the surface epithelium (see Fig. 16-7). Reactive lesions do not show desmoplasia. Pseudodiverticulosis is a rare condition that shows numerous islands of reactive squamous epithelium in the mucosa and submucosa, some of which may be irregular in shape, simulating a carcinoma (Fig. 16-12). This condition is due to extensive squamous metaplasia of the esophageal ducts and glands. Pathologically, these lesions are distinguished from invasive carcinoma by the lack of an infiltrative growth pattern and by the absence of histologic features of dysplastic squamous epithelium.

Biopsy or resection specimens from patients who have been treated with neoadjuvant chemoradiotherapy may contain only scattered atypical cells, in which the distinction between residual carcinoma and reactive mesenchymal cells is occasionally difficult. Carcinoma cells may be identified by positive immunostaining for cytokeratins and an increased nucleus-to-cytoplasm ratio; reactive mesenchymal cells are typically cytokeratin negative and have expanded, often bubbly or "wispy" cytoplasm. Typically, although enlarged, the nucleus-to-cytoplasm ratio of these cells is maintained.

Poorly differentiated tumors may be difficult to recognize as squamous in phenotype, and melanoma or even lymphoma may be suspected on morphologic grounds. Positivity for cytokeratins and negativity for

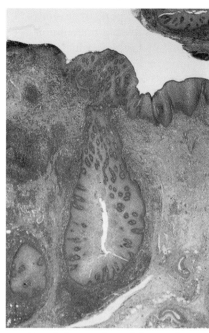

FIGURE 16–12. Pseudodiverticulosis of the esophagus. Low-power image shows a reactive proliferation of squamous epithelium extending into the submucosal gland ducts and associated with a marked chronic inflammatory infiltrate. In contrast to carcinoma, the borders of the squamous proliferation are smooth and do not show atypia or other features of malignancy, such as desmoplasia.

melanocytic and lymphoid markers may help eliminate these alternative diagnoses. In some patients, pulmonary squamous cell carcinoma may involve the esophageal wall by metastasis or direct extension (see later) and may be potentially confused with a primary esophageal tumor. Adjacent squamous dysplasia provides strong evidence for an esophageal origin of the tumor. In addition, approximately 10% to 20% of lung squamous cell carcinomas show nuclear immunostaining for the transcription factor TTF-1, which is not expressed in esophageal epithelium or in tumors derived from it.[66]

Prognosis

Squamous cell carcinomas may invade horizontally but more typically invade vertically through the esophageal wall and, in this manner, may spread to involve contiguous organs such as the trachea, aorta, and pericardium. Intramural metastasis was found in up to 12% of resection specimens in one study.[67] Regional lymph node metastasis is present in approximately 60% of patients at the time of diagnosis, and the positivity rate correlates with depth of invasion (<5% for intramucosal carcinomas and up to 45% for submucosal carcinomas).[52,68] Carcinomas originating in the upper thoracic esophagus are more likely to metastasize to cervical or upper mediastinal nodes, whereas tumors from the middle and lower thirds of the esophagus metastasize to lower mediastinal or perigastric nodes.[52] However, skip nodal metastases are not uncommon in esophageal cancers. Distant metastasis, which most frequently involves the lung or liver, is present in up to 50% of patients at autopsy.[69]

Overall 5-year survival for patients with squamous cell carcinoma approaches 30% to 40% for patients treated with esophagectomy.[52,70] The most significant prognostic factor is tumor stage, which is based on the American Joint Committee on Cancer (AJCC) TNM classification system (Table 16-3).[71,72] Patients with tumors that penetrate into the submucosa have 5-year survival rates in the range of 70%, compared with 40% to 50% and 25% to 30% for patients with tumors that extend into the muscularis propria and adventitia, respectively.[52,73,74] Lymph node metastasis is also an independent predictor of poor survival.[52,73] Some authors have also found that a poor degree of tumor differentiation is an independent prognostic factor,[75] although this is controversial.[73,76] Intramural metastases[67] and lymphovascular invasion[77] have also been found to be predictive of poor survival in some studies but need to

---

TABLE 16–3. AJCC TNM Classification of Esophageal Carcinomas

Primary Tumor (T)
TX	Primary tumor cannot be assessed
T0	No evidence of primary tumor
Tis	Carcinoma in situ
T1	Tumor invades lamina propria or submucosa
T2	Tumor invades muscularis propria
T3	Tumor invades adventitia
T4	Tumor invades adjacent structures

Regional Lymph Nodes (N)
NX	Regional lymph nodes cannot be assessed
N0	No regional lymph node metastasis
N1	Regional lymph node metastasis

Distant Metastasis (M)
MX	Distant metastasis cannot be assessed
M0	No distant metastasis
M1	Distant metastasis
	Tumors of the lower thoracic esophagus:
M1a	Metastasis in celiac lymph nodes
M1b	Other distant metastases
	Tumors of the midthoracic esophagus:
M1a	Not applicable
M1b	Nonregional lymph nodes and/or other distant metastasis
	Tumors of the upper thoracic esophagus:
M1a	Metastasis in cervical nodes
M1b	Other distant metastases

Stage Grouping
Stage 0	Tis	N0	M0
Stage I	T1	N0	M0
Stage IIA	T2	N0	M0
	T3	N0	M0
Stage IIB	T1	N1	M0
	T2	N1	M0
Stage III	T3	N1	M0
	T4	Any N	M0
Stage IV	Any T	Any N	M1
Stage IVA	Any T	Any N	M1a
Stage IVB	Any T	Any N	M1b

Used with the permission of the American Joint Committee on Cancer (AJCC), Chicago, Illinois. The original source for this material is the *AJCC Cancer Staging Manual, Sixth Edition* (2002) published by Springer-Verlag New York, www.springer-ny.com.

---

be tested in a prospective manner. Other parameters, such as tumor size and location, and molecular markers, such as DNA aneuploidy and TP53 status,[70,78] have not been shown to be reliable predictors of survival independent of stage.

VARIANTS OF SQUAMOUS CELL CARCINOMA

Basaloid Squamous Cell Carcinoma

CLINICAL FEATURES

Basaloid (squamous) carcinoma is an unusual variant of squamous cell carcinoma that occurs more commonly in the upper aerodigestive tract, such as the hypopharynx and base of tongue. The true incidence of basaloid squamous carcinoma is unknown, but it has been reported to represent 1% to 11% of squamous cell carcinomas.[79-81] Clinically, these tumors characteristically occur in older men with presenting symptoms of dysphagia and weight loss, similar to conventional squamous cell carcinomas.

PATHOLOGIC FEATURES

Grossly, basaloid squamous carcinomas may be large, bulky, fungating tumors that frequently ulcerate and form strictures. They most commonly arise in the mid and distal esophagus.

Microscopically, these tumors show biphasic or multiphasic differentiation. Thus, it is common to find a mixture of squamous cell carcinoma, adenocarcinoma, small cell carcinoma, or even spindle cell carcinoma along with the basaloid component.[81] For instance, in one study of 18 basaloid carcinomas,[80] 72% of cases showed areas of squamous cell carcinoma, 50% of which also had in situ squamous cell carcinoma. The basaloid component may compose a wide range (5% to 95%) of the tumor. On the basis of these findings, basaloid carcinoma has been proposed to arise from a multipotential stem cell, or basal cell, in the native squamous epithelium. The basaloid component is characterized by a proliferation of oval to round, large, somewhat pleomorphic, basaloid cells with an open pale chromatin pattern, small nucleoli, and scant cytoplasm, arranged in solid or cribriform lobules often showing central necrosis (Fig. 16-13). An in situ or invasive squamous cell carcinoma component is often present, at least focally. Characteristically, the nests of tumor cells show peripheral palisading.

SPECIAL STUDIES

A mucoid matrix that stains positive for PAS and alcian blue may be present in the cribriform spaces of some tumor cell nests. By immunohistochemistry, basaloid carcinomas typically show weak staining for broad-spectrum keratins (in a membrane-type pattern) and absence of staining for neuroendocrine markers,

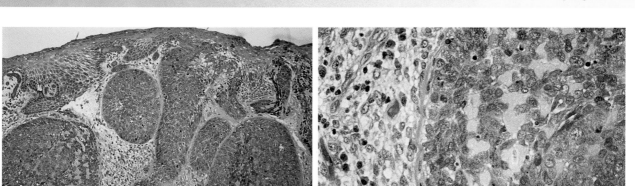

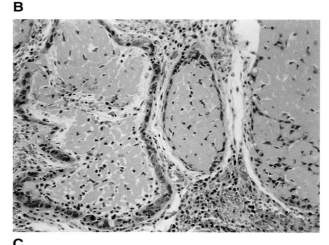

FIGURE 16–13. Basaloid carcinoma of the esophagus. **A,** Low-power image shows a proliferation of well-circumscribed nodules of "basaloid" cells extending beneath mildly dysplastic squamous epithelium. **B,** Basaloid carcinomas are characterized by cells with oval to round nuclei, an open chromatin pattern, small nucleoli, and scant cytoplasm. A mucoid hyaline–like substance is noted in some intercellular spaces. **C,** In some cases, basaloid carcinomas show marked intratumoral necrosis, which gives the false appearance of gland formation and an adenoid-cystic carcinoma–like quality to the tumor nodules.

NSE, and S100. The basal cells stain strongly for CK14 and CK19.[81,82] Some tumors show focal actin and vimentin positivity in the basaloid cells and CEA positivity in the pseudoglandular spaces.

DIFFERENTIAL DIAGNOSIS

The differential diagnosis of basaloid carcinoma includes conventional (pure) squamous cell carcinoma and adenoid cystic carcinoma. Cases with a prominent basaloid mucoid matrix (alcian blue positive, PAS positive) and a pseudoacinar or cribriform pattern closely resemble adenoid cystic carcinomas. Indeed, this is an important distinction because true adenoid cystic carcinomas of the esophagus are less aggressive than basaloid carcinomas (see under Adenoid Cystic Carcinoma). Unlike basaloid carcinomas, adenoid cystic carcinomas form true epithelial lumina, do not coexist with conventional squamous cell carcinoma or squamous dysplasia, and lack significant pleomorphism, mitoses, and necrosis. The basal cells of adenoid cystic carcinoma are smaller and more hyperchromatic and regular than in basaloid carcinoma and stain strongly for S100 and actin, whereas the basal cells of basaloid carcinoma are typically CK14 and CK19 positive.[82] In conventional squamous cell carcinoma, a significant

proportion of tumor cells have eosinophilic cytoplasm, grow in irregular infiltrative clusters rather than in rounded nests, and show focal keratinization. However, as discussed under Adenoid Cystic Carcinoma, the distinction between basaloid and squamous carcinoma may be arbitrary and of little prognostic value. The differential diagnosis of basaloid carcinoma, adenoid cystic carcinoma, and conventional squamous cell carcinoma is summarized in Table 16-4.

PROGNOSIS

Basaloid squamous carcinoma is a highly aggressive tumor that carries a prognosis similar to or possibly even worse than that of pure squamous cell carcinoma.[79] Studies show no differences in overall survival between these two tumor types.[80]

Carcinosarcoma

CLINICAL FEATURES

Carcinosarcoma, also known as polypoid carcinoma, spindle cell carcinoma, and sarcomatoid carcinoma, was first described by Virchow in 1865; it represents approximately 2% of esophageal carcinomas. Similar to squamous cell carcinoma, it predominantly affects

TABLE 16–4. Basaloid Squamous Carcinoma Versus Squamous Cell Carcinoma and Adenoid Cystic Carcinoma

Feature	Basaloid Carcinoma	Squamous Cell Carcinoma	Adenoid Cystic Carcinoma
Age (years)	>60	>60	40-60
Gender	M>F	M>F	F>M
Location middle third	+	+	++
Squamous dysplasia/ carcinoma in situ	+	++	–
Invasive squamous carcinoma	+/–	++	–
Ductal and basaloid cells	–	–	++
True epithelial lumina	–	–	++
Pleomorphism	++	++	–
Increased mitoses	++	++	–
Nuclei			
Open chromatin	+/–	+	–
Dense compact chromatin	–	–	++
Nucleoli	+	+	–
Large nuclei	++	++	–
S100, actin in basal cells	–	–	+
CK19 in basal cells	+	+	–
CEA in ductal cells	–	–	+
Aggressive clinical course	++	++	+/–

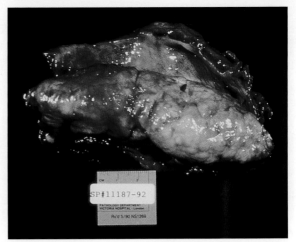

FIGURE 16–14. Gross image of a polypoid carcinosarcoma of the distal esophagus. The lesion protrudes into the lumen of the esophagus and is associated with a gray hemorraghic and necrotic surface.

men (80%) in middle to late adult life (40 to 90 years old).[83] Because of the exophytic intraluminal growth pattern of these tumors, presenting symptoms are commonly related to esophageal obstruction.

PATHOLOGIC FEATURES

Grossly, these tumors may grow to large sizes (1 to 25 cm) and show a predilection for the middle and distal segments of the esophagus. Eighty percent of lesions are polypoid and have an exophytic growth pattern (Fig. 16-14), whereas only 10% of cases show an infiltrative growth pattern.

Microscopically, the tumor is characterized by a combination of epithelial and spindle cell (or mesenchymal) elements (Fig. 16-15). The epithelial element is typically a moderately differentiated to well-differentiated squamous cell carcinoma. In some cases, only in situ carcinoma is present.[84] In fact, some cases show only a small amount of the epithelial component, and this is usually either at the base of the polyp or at the periphery of the invasive tumor. The sarcomatous component is commonly a high-grade spindle cell sarcoma. However, osteosarcomatous, rhabdosarcomatous, or chondrosarcomatous differentiation may be present as well. Immunohistochemically, the epithelial component is typically keratin positive, whereas the sarcomatous component usually stains with vimentin. However, keratin or vimentin may be seen occasionally

in either component of the tumor. By electron microscopy, a mixture of cell types have been identified ranging from pure epithelial cells to cells that show a combination of epithelial and sarcomatous features to cells with pure sarcomatous differentiation.[85] It is these ultrastructural findings, combined with the histologic finding in most cases of areas of transition between epithelial and sarcomatous differentiation, that led to the prevailing theory that these tumors are derived from diverse differentiation (metaplasia) of the carcinomatous element. Interestingly, the two distinct lines of differentiation may show different phenotypic and molecular properties. For instance, in one study of 13 cases, the sarcomatous areas showed higher proliferative indices, higher degree of aneuploidy, and loss of heterozygosity in comparison to the carcinoma component.[86]

DIFFERENTIAL DIAGNOSIS

Esophageal carcinosarcomas must be differentiated from pure sarcomas, either primary to the esophagus or involving the esophagus by direct spread or metastasis. Recognition of the distinctive gross features and pattern of esophageal involvement, as well as the presence of malignant or premalignant epithelial elements, strongly favors carcinosarcoma. Extensive sampling of the tumor and cytokeratin stains may be useful. On occasion, biphasic malignant mesotheliomas may spread from the pleura to involve the esophagus, but these are distinguished by the appropriate clinical history and by the distinctive immunophenotype of mesothelioma (cytokeratin 5/6, WT-1, calretinin positive, CEA and Leu-M1 negative).[87]

PROGNOSIS

Carcinosarcomas are highly aggressive tumors with 5-year survival rates of only 10% to 15%.[83,86] Roughly

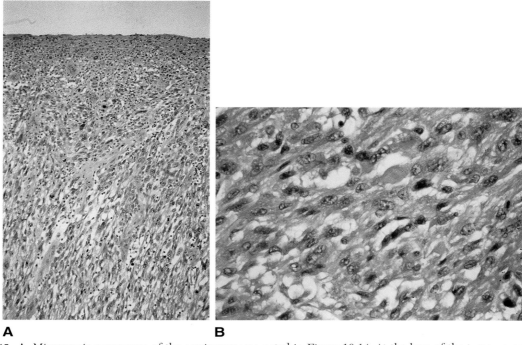

A   **B**

FIGURE 16–15. A, Microscopic appearance of the carcinosarcoma noted in Figure 16-14. At the base of the tumor, a proliferation of epithelioid malignant squamous cells blends imperceptibly with an undifferentiated sarcomatous component noted in the lower portion of the field. **B,** The sarcomatous component of this tumor shows a proliferation of undifferentiated spindle cells with hyperchromatic elongated nuclei.

50% of cases have lymph node metastasis at the time of diagnosis. The sarcomatous component usually exhibits a more aggressive biologic behavior and a higher propensity to metastasize.

Verrucous Squamous Cell Carcinoma

CLINICAL FEATURES

Verrucous carcinoma of the esophagus is an extremely rare (less than 15 cases reported) low-grade malignant neoplasm first described by Ackerman (in the oral cavity) in 1948. Affected patients range from 36 to 76 years of age, and the disease has a male predilection. Unfortunately, these tumors may grow to very large sizes before onset of symptoms and thus cause a long delay in diagnosis. Presenting complaints are usually dysphagia, weight loss, coughing, and hematemesis. The cause has been related to chronic mucosal irritation. A high proportion of cases are associated with chronic caustic injury (lye), achalasia, diverticular disease, or reflux disease.[88]

PATHOLOGIC FEATURES

Pathologically, verrucous carcinomas have an exophytic papillary growth pattern and may occupy the entire circumference of the esophageal lumen. Microscopically, the characteristic features are those of a very well differentiated verrucoid or papillomatous proliferation of squamous cells with minimal cytologic atypia, prominent acanthosis, hyperkeratosis, swollen rete pegs, and inflammation (Fig. 16-16). Invasion is usually difficult to assess and is typically in the form of broad pushing margins.

DIFFERENTIAL DIAGNOSIS

The key differential diagnosis is with benign squamous papilloma (Table 16-5). Clinical and endoscopic findings are usually helpful in differentiating these two tumors, but pathologists should be cautious about making a diagnosis of verrucous carcinoma on biopsy because the superficial aspects of both lesions may be indistinguishable. Grossly, squamous papillomas are small (<3 cm), localized, discrete lesions, whereas verrucous carcinomas more commonly show extensive or circumferential involvement of the esophageal wall. Microscopically, papillomas display koilocytosis and do not show the pushing deep margin, submucosal extension, and mild but definite cytologic atypia of verrucous carcinomas.

PROGNOSIS

Lymph node metastasis may be present rarely, but no cases with distant metastasis have been reported.[89,90] However, these are locally aggressive tumors that often form fistulous tracts with surrounding organs and, as a result, may cause significant morbidity and mortality.[91]

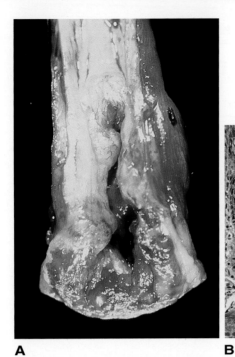

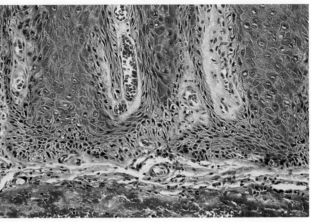

A   B

FIGURE 16–16. Verrucous carcinoma of the esophagus. **A,** In this image, the carcinoma involves the full circumference of the lumen and contains a centrally located fistulous tract. The lesion is hemorrhagic and necrotic in appearance. **B,** At the leading edge of the tumor, a mild degree of atypia is noted in the basal aspect of the carcinoma and is associated with a mild inflammatory response. However, the infiltrating edge is of a pushing, rather than an infiltrating, type.

TABLE 16–5. Esophageal Squamous Papilloma Versus Verrucous Carcinoma

Feature	Papilloma	Verrucous Carcinoma
Clinical behavior	Benign	Aggressive
Size	<3 cm	>3 cm
Polyp	+	–
Circumferential involvement	–	+/–
Ulceration	–	+/–
Stricture	–	+/–
Pushing margin	–	+
Extension into submucosa/muscularis	–	+
Lymph node metastases	–	+
Cytologic atypia	–	+
Koilocytosis	+	–/+

Lymphoepithelioma-like Carcinoma

A small proportion of esophageal carcinomas display an undifferentiated phenotype and are associated with a prominent lymphoid infiltrate, similar to lympho-epitheliomas of the nasopharynx. Most cases have been reported from Japan.[55,92] Their clinical features are similar to squamous cell carcinomas. These tumors are histologically identical to their counterpart in the nasopharynx, showing syncytia of primitive-appearing epithelioid cells surrounded by a dense inflammatory infiltrate including lymphocytes and plasma cells. In one study, only 3% of cases were positive for Epstein-Barr virus by in situ hybridization or immuno-histochemistry.[55] Although these tumors are rare, some authors have suggested that they have a slightly better prognosis than ordinary squamous cell carcinomas do.[92]

ADENOCARCINOMA

More than 95% of esophageal adenocarcinomas develop in association with Barrett's esophagus (BE). Non–BE-associated adenocarcinomas are discussed separately (under Non–Barrett's-Associated Adeno-carcinoma). Adenocarcinomas may also develop from esophageal submucosal glands or ducts or from foci of heterotopic epithelium, but these tumors are extremely rare. Adenocarcinomas that arise at the gastroesophageal junction or gastric cardia are discussed in Chapter 17 but are also discussed briefly here.

Clinical Features

The incidence of adenocarcinoma of the esophagus has increased dramatically in the last two to three decades. This tumor now constitutes approximately 50% of all esophageal carcinomas diagnosed in the United States and is the most common tumor in the distal esophagus.[2,93,94] The incidence of esophageal adeno-carcinoma in American white men was recently esti-mated to be 3.7 per 100,000, with an estimated 13,000 new cases in 2001.[95]

The demographics of patients with adenocarcinoma are similar to those of patients with BE. BE-associated adenocarcinoma affects predominantly older men (mean age, 60 years; M/F ratio, 3:1 to 7:1), and more than 80% of patients are white.[96,97] Depending on the size and location of the tumor, patients may present with dysphagia, odynophagia, or obstruction. Progressive dysphagia and weight loss are ominous signs that are usually associated with advanced disease.

Pathogenesis

The most significant risk factor for adenocarcinoma is BE, defined by the presence of goblet cells anywhere in the tubular esophagus, which develops in approximately 6% to 12% of patients with gastrointestinal reflux disease.[98-100] The overall prevalence of adenocarcinoma in patients with BE has been estimated between 5% and 28%.[101-103] Patients with BE have an estimated 30- to 125-fold increased risk for development of adenocarcinoma compared with the general population.[104,105] Furthermore, some studies suggest that greater lengths of BE are associated with a greater risk of malignancy.[106-109] However, many of the studies that have estimated the risk of adenocarcinoma in patients with BE have been retrospective. More recent prospective studies suggest that the risk of cancer in BE may be overestimated. Indeed, only a small percentage (3% to 5%) of patients with BE develop adenocarcinoma when observed prospectively.[108,110-114] Factors that increase the risk for

development of adenocarcinoma include the presence of dysplasia.[108, 114-116] Alcohol and tobacco use and a positive family history may also contribute to malignant progression.

Pathologic Features

GROSS PATHOLOGY

BE-associated adenocarcinomas are located almost exclusively in the distal third of the esophagus in areas of involvement with BE, with frequent extension into the proximal stomach (Fig. 16-17). They may be classified as polypoid (protruding) (5% to 10%), flat (10% to 15%), fungating (20% to 25%), and infiltrative (40% to 50%).[96] Early carcinomas may be undetectable or appear only as slightly depressed or elevated lesions.[117] Diffusely infiltrative tumors are uncommon. Unfortunately, large tumors may obliterate the underlying or adjacent Barrett's mucosa, particularly those that arise in the distal esophagus at or near the level of the gastroesophageal junction. Patients who have been treated with preoperative chemotherapy or radiation therapy may have little or no gross residual tumor left in their resection specimen. In fact, up to 50% of patients treated with neoadjuvant therapy show either no or only minimal microscopic residual tumor after surgery.[118]

MICROSCOPIC PATHOLOGY

Adenocarcinomas are graded as well, moderately, or poorly differentiated. The AJCC grading system classifies

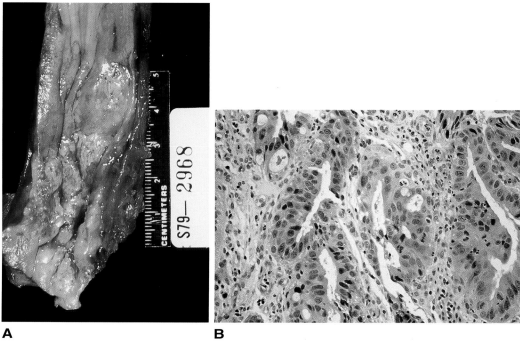

A   **B**

FIGURE 16–17. Barrett's esophagus–associated adenocarcinoma. **A,** An irregular, ulcerating, constricting tumor is present just above the level of the gastroesophageal junction in association with tongues of Barrett's esophagus. **B,** Microscopic appearance of the tumor showing a moderately to well-differentiated adenocarcinoma characterized by gland formation and marked cellular atypia.

tumors by the proportion of the tumor composed of glands.[72] However, the majority of tumors are moderately or well differentiated.[96] Because some tumors show variations in grade within the same tumor, the highest grade is usually recorded for prognostic purposes. Tumors typically spread vertically through the esophageal wall and metastasize to regional lymph nodes, similar to squamous cell carcinomas. Adenocarcinomas are also staged like squamous cell carcinomas by use of the AJCC TNM system (see Table 16-3).

Well-differentiated carcinomas (>95% of tumor composed of glands) are composed almost entirely of irregularly shaped or cystic glandular and tubular profiles that infiltrate the mucosa, submucosa, and muscularis. The tumor cells are cuboidal to columnar and contain irregular nuclei with coarse or vesicular chromatin, prominent nucleoli, and a variable amount of eosinophilic or clear cytoplasm. In moderately differentiated carcinomas (50% to 95% of tumor composed of glands), tumor cells are arranged in solid nests and irregular clusters as well as glands. In these tumors, the tumor cells within the glandular profiles may adopt a cribriform pattern and show considerable stratification. Poorly differentiated carcinomas (5% to 49% of tumor composed of glands) often diffusely infiltrate the esophageal wall with a prominent desmoplastic stroma. The tumor cells are arranged in sheets and poorly formed glandular lumina, and signet ring cells and bizarre pleomorphic tumor cells may be present. Other intestinal cell types, such as Paneth cells and endocrine cells,[119] are present focally in up to 20% of cases.

Approximately 5% to 10% of adenocarcinomas are of the mucinous (colloid) type and are composed of tumor cell clusters floating in pools of mucin. Approximately 5% are composed of signet ring cells.[96] Occasional tumors may show multidirectional differentiation, with coincident areas of glandular, squamous, or neuroendocrine differentiation (see later).

In patients treated with preoperative chemoradiotherapy, residual tumor cells may be present only as individual cells or clusters of cells in association with ulceration, dense fibrosis, or pools of mucin.[120] These cells are frequently pleomorphic, with extreme nuclear irregularity and enlargement, and may be difficult to distinguish from reactive mesenchymal cells. Alternatively, the only sign of treated tumor may be acellular pools of mucin dissecting through the layers of the esophageal wall (Fig. 16-18).

Special Studies

Special studies are usually not necessary to establish a diagnosis of esophageal adenocarcinoma, but they can occasionally be useful in characterizing poorly differentiated lesions, in identifying resections with little or no residual tumor after neoadjuvant therapy, or in distinguishing primary esophageal tumors from metastases. Tumor cells are positive for mucin histochemical stains including mucicarmine, PAS-diastase, and alcian blue, although positive cells may be rare or nonexistent in poorly differentiated tumors. Adenocarcinomas stain positively with broad-spectrum anticytokeratin antibodies and are positive for CK7 and negative for CK20 in 90% of cases.[121] Although detailed studies have not been published, in the authors' experience, these tumors are negative for the lung/thyroid epithelial marker TTF-1. Focal positivity for neuroendocrine markers such as serotonin and somatostatin can be found in up to 80% of cases.[122]

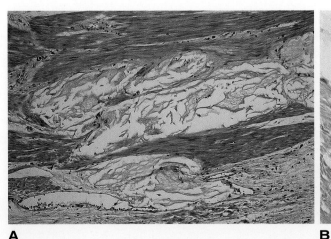
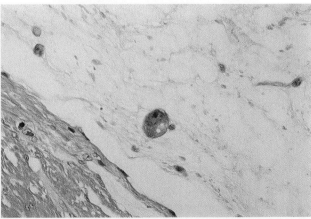

A **B**

FIGURE 16–18. Acellular pools of mucin in the wall of the esophagus in a patient who had neoadjuvant chemoradiotherapy for esophageal adenocarcinoma. **A,** Dissecting pools of mucin are noted within the muscle layers of the wall, but malignant cells are not present. **B,** Occasionally, highly atypical, enlarged, treated tumor cells may be seen floating in pools of mucin.

Differential Diagnosis

Most difficulties regarding the diagnosis of adeno-carcinoma arise in the evaluation of endoscopic biopsy specimens, in which the distinction between high-grade dysplasia and invasive carcinoma may be uncertain. For patients treated with preoperative chemoradiotherapy, cytokeratin immunostaining may be necessary to distinguish rare residual tumor cells from mesenchymal cells showing treatment effect.

In some cases, it may be necessary to distinguish a primary esophageal adenocarcinoma from metastasis or spread from another site, such as stomach, lung, or breast. The presence of BE and dysplastic epithelium adjacent to the carcinoma is convincing evidence that the tumor arises from the esophagus. In addition, primary esophageal adenocarcinomas do not stain for TTF-1 or estrogen receptor,[123] markers of lung and breast tumors, respectively. Distinction of an esophageal adenocarcinoma from a proximal gastric tumor may be difficult, particularly if the tumor has obliterated any underlying Barrett's epithelium. Gastric adenocarcinomas arise in a background of intestinal metaplasia of the gastric mucosa and are positive for CK20 in up to 90% of cases, compared with esophageal adenocarcinomas, which virtually never stain for this antigen.[121,124] However, because these studies did not specifically examine carcinomas arising in the gastric cardia, the cytokeratin immunophenotype of these tumors is uncertain.

Prognosis and Treatment

The majority of esophageal adenocarcinomas show spread into or through the muscularis at the time of clinical presentation. Advanced tumors may spread directly into the mediastinum, aorta, or stomach. Metastasis to regional (periesophageal and perigastric) lymph nodes is present in about 50% to 60% of patients.[96,125] The likelihood of lymph node metastasis is related to tumor depth.[117,126] For instance, in one study of 32 early adenocarcinomas,[117] 0% of tumors limited to the mucosa (T1a) had lymph node metastases, compared with 30% of tumors in the submucosa (T1b). Distant metastases to the liver, lungs, and other portions of the gastrointestinal tract are not uncommon.

Although relatively few large studies have examined prognostic factors in esophageal adenocarcinoma, the most important factor is the AJCC TNM pathologic stage. Patients with tumors limited to the mucosa or submucosa have an 80% to 100% 5-year survival rate, compared with 10% to 20% for patients with tumors that extend into or through the muscularis.[96,97,117,127] Lymph node metastasis is also associated with reduced survival,[96,97] although this effect is not independent of stage. Likewise, other histologic parameters, such as tumor differentiation and lymphovascular or perineural invasion, do not independently predict reduced survival in multivariate analysis.

Adenocarcinomas that have not metastasized to distant sites are treated with esophagectomy. Neoadjuvant chemotherapy or radiotherapy has been advocated as a means of improving resectability and survival, but it has not yet shown a definite survival benefit in some randomized clinical trials.[128]

DYSPLASIA IN BARRETT'S ESOPHAGUS

Clinical Features

There is increasing evidence that esophageal adenocarcinomas arise through progression of premalignant or dysplastic lesions in BE. Dysplasia is defined as unequivocal neoplastic change within the glandular epithelium of BE, without invasion of the lamina propria. The prevalence of dysplasia in patients with BE ranges from 5% to 20% in various reports.[113,115] First, dysplasia is a risk factor for the development of adenocarcinoma (see under Prognosis and Treatment). Furthermore, BE with dysplasia is found adjacent to invasive adeno-carcinomas in more than 90% of cases.[96,117,129]

Pathologic Features

Dysplasia is usually endoscopically indistinguishable from nondysplastic BE and occurs in flat mucosa but may occasionally form a polypoid mass lesion (see under Adenoma). However, extensive areas of dysplasia may impart a soft velvety or raised appearance to the mucosa and may, on occasion, show surface erosion.

Microscopically, dysplastic glandular epithelium shows a range of cytologic and architectural abnormalities and is classified as either low or high grade on the basis of severity of these features (Fig. 16-19; Table 16-6).[130] The architecture of dysplastic epithelium may be normal or show villiform or papillary change with crowded, irregular glands. Cytologic features include decreased mucin production, nuclear hyperchromasia and pleomorphism, increased nucleus-to-cytoplasm ratio, increased mitotic rate with abnormal mitotic figures, and nuclear stratification. All biopsy specimens from BE should be classified as positive or negative for dysplasia on the basis of these criteria. Reactive biopsy specimens may show mucin depletion, mild nuclear enlargement and pseudostratification, and increased mitotic rate but retain surface maturation and do not show significant architectural abnormalities or nuclear pleomorphism. High-grade dysplasia is distinguished from low-grade dysplasia by irregular, crowded glandular profiles with cribriform architecture and by the presence of cells with rounded or irregular pleomorphic nuclei and frequent abnormal mitoses. Some biopsy specimens that show only mild architectural distortion,

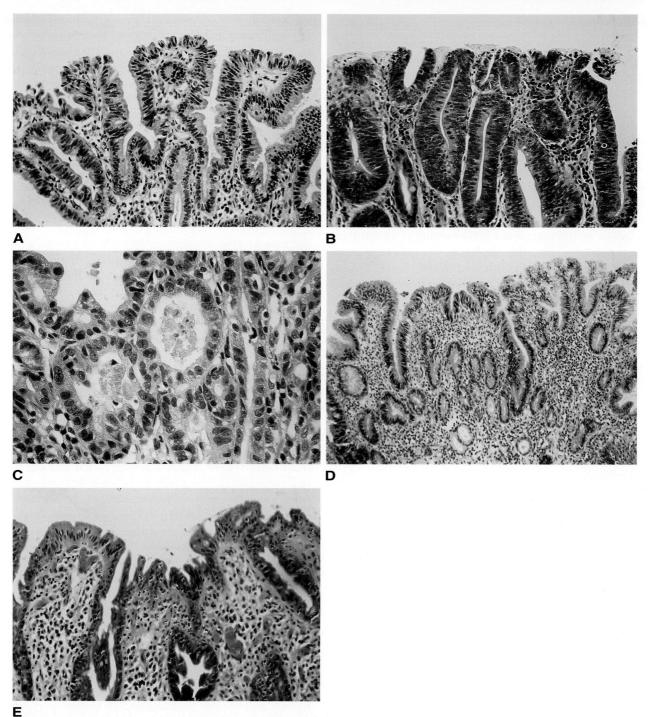

FIGURE 16–19. Dysplasia in Barrett's esophagus. **A,** Typical appearance of low-grade dysplasia characterized by slightly villiform epithelium containing a proliferation of hyperchromatic pencil-shaped nuclei and a distinct lack of surface maturation. In low-grade dysplasia, the dysplastic nuclei occupy predominantly the basal portion of the cell cytoplasm. **B,** High-grade dysplasia shows a more tightly compact arrangement of highly atypical glands with marked hyperchromaticity, pseudostratification, and loss of nuclear polarity. Lack of surface maturation is also apparent in this lesion. **C,** Nonadenomatous variant of high-grade dysplasia shows cuboidal cells in a glandular arrangement with a markedly increased N/C ratio. Most nonadenomatous types of dysplasia are high-grade lesions. **D,** Low-power image of a biopsy from Barrett's esophagus showing columnar atypia considered indefinite for dysplasia. Although the epithelium is slightly villiform and shows cells with pseudostratification and hyperchromaticity, a slight degree of surface maturation is seen focally, and the lesion is associated with a marked degree of acute and chronic inflammation, both within the lamina propria and extending into the epithelium itself. **E,** Marked regeneration (negative for dysplasia) in a biopsy from Barrett's esophagus. The reactive changes are characterized by marked nuclear hyperchromaticity and mucin depletion. However, a slight degree of surface maturation is evident focally, and the cells appear to be tufting at the surface rather than showing loss of polarity. This is the typical appearance of markedly reactive epithelium in association with a fresh ulcer.

TABLE 16–6. Differential Diagnosis of Dysplasia in Barrett's Esophagus

Histologic Feature	Reactive	Indefinite	Low-Grade	High-Grade
Surface maturation	+	+/–	–	–
Villiform architecture	–	+/–	+/–	+/–
Mucin depletion	+/–	+	+	++
Irregular glands	–	+/–	+	++
Glandular crowding	–	+/–	+	++
Cribriform glands	–	–	–	+
Increased N/C ratio	+/–	+	++	+++
Nuclear pseudostratification	+	+	++	+++
Nuclear pleomorphism	–	+/–	+	++
Increased mitotic rate	+	+	+	++
Abnormal mitoses	–	+/–	+	++
Inflammation	++	+	+/–	+/–

N/C, Nucleus-to-cytoplasm.

nuclear stratification, mucin depletion, and increased mitoses but do not meet all the criteria for dysplasia or that occur in the context of significant inflammation are best classified as indefinite for dysplasia (see Fig. 16-19).

Differential Diagnosis

The differential diagnosis of dysplasia in BE includes reactive changes and intramucosal or invasive adeno-carcinoma. Histologic features useful in distinguishing dysplastic and reactive Barrett's epithelium are discussed more thoroughly in Chapter 7. Adenocarcinoma, by definition, is a tumor that shows penetration of the basement membrane. The presence of single cells or clusters of cells without glandular lumina in the lamina propria is strong evidence for adenocarcinoma (Fig. 16-20). In small, superficial biopsy specimens, the distinction

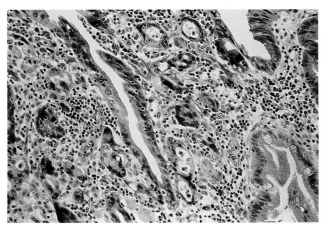

FIGURE 16–20. Well-differentiated intramucosal adenocarcinoma of the esophagus associated with high-grade dysplastic epithelium. The lamina propria shows a proliferation of poorly formed glands, single cells, and clusters of cells infiltrating the lamina propria above the level of the muscularis mucosae.

between high-grade dysplasia and adenocarcinoma may be impossible. However, high-grade dysplasia and adenocarcinoma can be distinguished from low-grade dysplasia and reactive mucosa with a higher degree of reliability.[131-133] Because of the frequent difficulty in classifying dysplastic lesions, confirmation of a diagnosis of dysplasia by pathologists experienced in the evaluation of BE mucosal biopsy specimens is essential. A biopsy specimen with low- or high-grade dysplasia in a patient with a mass lesion should be assumed to represent an adenocarcinoma until proven otherwise.

Ancillary Techniques

Dysplasia shows many of the same molecular alterations found in adenocarcinomas, including increased proliferative indices, aneuploidy, and *TP16* and *TP53* mutations,[134] which may be useful in the differential diagnosis of dysplasia. Indeed, DNA aneuploidy and loss of heterozygosity of the TP53 locus in baseline BE biopsy specimens have been found to be predictive of the development of adenocarcinoma in prospectively observed patients with BE.[115,135,136]

Prognosis and Treatment

In two large prospective studies, 50% to 60% of patients diagnosed with high-grade dysplasia developed adenocarcinoma within 5 years, compared with 8% to 12% of patients with low-grade dysplasia and 4% of patients negative or indefinite for dysplasia.[108,114,115] Patients with high-grade dysplasia have coexisting adenocarcinoma in up to 65% of cases, even when no mass lesion is visible.[137-139] Therefore, either thorough repeated biopsy to detect occult adenocarcinoma or surgical resection is usually recommended for these patients. Alternative therapies for dysplasia include endoscopic mucosal resection[140] and endoscopic mucosal ablation by either photodynamic therapy[141] or laser ablation.[142]

VARIANTS OF ADENOCARCINOMA

Non–Barrett's-Associated Adenocarcinoma

Esophageal adenocarcinomas unrelated to Barrett's esophagus are extremely rare and arise either from foci of gastric heterotopia[22,24] or from the submucosal gland/duct system.[143] Clinically, patients with heterotopia-associated adenocarcinomas are middle-aged, and the presenting symptom is most commonly dysphagia. Morphologically, adenocarcinomas that arise in ectopic gastric mucosa show a range of differentiation and have been reported to show a papillary growth pattern. Adjacent gastric oxyntic mucosa is usually demonstrable, and intestinal metaplasia and dysplasia have been reported adjacent to the adenocarcinoma as well.[23,144] Although these tumors morphologically resemble Barrett's-associated adenocarcinomas (see Fig. 16-12), that diagnosis is ruled out by the proximal location of the tumor and the absence of a segment of Barrett's epithelium between the tumor and the true gastroesophageal junction.

Tumors reported to have arisen within the submucosal gland/duct system are tubular adenocarcinomas with flat or cuboidal tumor cells with eosinophilic cytoplasm, similar to the native esophageal gland ducts (Fig. 16-21).[143] Because of their rarity, little is known about their biologic behavior.

Adenoid Cystic Carcinoma

True adenoid cystic carcinomas of the esophagus are extremely rare.[145] They are histologically and immunophenotypically identical to the salivary gland type of adenoid cystic carcinoma. The great majority of cases previously termed adenoid cystic carcinoma were, most likely, basaloid squamous carcinomas with adenoid cystic carcinoma–like features.[146] True adenoid cystic carcinomas are more common in women, are typically present in middle age, and show no histologic association with squamous cell carcinoma (i.e., are derived from submucosal glands).

Grossly, these tumors form well-circumscribed solid nodules in the submucosa. Adenoid cystic carcinoma is composed of two distinct populations of cells (ductal epithelium and basaloid cells). The basaloid cells are small and hyperchromatic, show no or only minimal pleomorphism, and demonstrate infrequent mitoses and no necrosis (Fig. 16-22). The ductal cells form solid nests or cribriform spaces, often associated with abundant basement membrane material. The overlying squamous epithelium does not exhibit dysplasia.

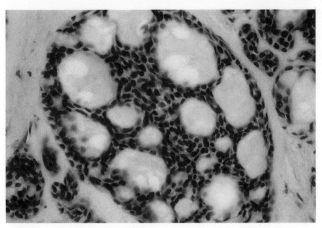

FIGURE 16–22. True adenoid cystic carcinoma of the esophagus. In contrast to basaloid carcinomas, adenoid cystic carcinomas show a proliferation of small hyperchromatic cells with less variation of nuclear size, infrequent mitoses, and no necrosis. The glandular lumina contain a basement membrane–like extracellular material.

Immunohistochemically, adenoid cystic carcinomas show strong keratin and CEA staining in the ductal-type epithelium and weak keratin and strong S100, actin, and vimentin positivity in the basaloid cells.[82]

The principal differential diagnosis of adenoid cystic carcinoma is with basaloid squamous carcinoma (see earlier and Table 16-4).

So few true adenoid cystic carcinomas have been reported that clinical follow-up data are scarce. However, these tumors have a better prognosis than do squamous or basaloid carcinomas, are slow-growing tumors that rarely metastasize, and thus are associated with excellent survival of the patient.[147]

CARCINOMA WITH MIXED SQUAMOUS AND GLANDULAR ELEMENTS

Carcinomas with mixed squamous and glandular elements have been called composite tumor, adenoacanthoma, adenosquamous carcinoma, and mucoepidermoid carcinoma. Esophageal carcinomas (squamous carcinomas and adenocarcinomas) show a high propensity to exhibit divergent differentiation. For instance, composite tumors consisting of two or more cell types, such as squamous cell carcinoma, adenocarcinoma, and small cell carcinoma, are not uncommon.[148] The most widely accepted pathogenetic mechanism is neoplastic transformation of a totipotent primitive stem cell in the basal region of the squamous epithelium that undergoes heterogeneous differentiation within a single tumor. As an extension of this concept, tumors composed of both squamous and glandular (mucinous) differentiation have been variously termed mucoepidermoid carcinoma or adenosquamous carcinoma (Fig.16-23).[149] Unfortunately, there is poor consistency in the literature regarding nomenclature primarily because strict diagnostic

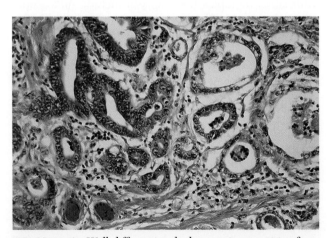

FIGURE 16–21. Well-differentiated adenocarcinoma arising from the submucosal gland/duct system. Some benign and mildly dysplastic glands are noted on the right side in conjunction with invasive glands noted on the left side of the field. In some cases, the glands of the carcinoma may contain two cell layers similar to those of the native gland duct system.

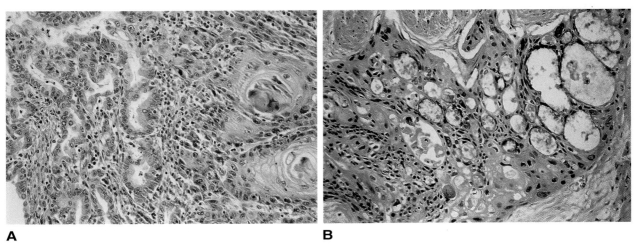

A   **B**

FIGURE 16–23. A, Adenosquamous carcinoma of the esophagus characterized by a proliferation of malignant glands *(left side)* adjacent to malignant squamous epithelium *(right side).* **B,** Mucoepidermoid carcinoma characterized by large aggregates of cells, which have features of malignant squamous cells toward the periphery of the cellular units intimately mixed with centrally located cells that contain mucin.

criteria have not been defined. For instance, although the World Health Organization classification defines mucoepidermoid carcinoma as a tumor composed of an "intimate" mixture of squamous and mucin-secreting elements, and an adenosquamous carcinoma as a tumor that shows the two cellular elements separate from but "intermingled with" each other, clearly some tumors show both of these features in the same case.

In one study,[150] ultrastructural examination of 43 esophageal carcinomas (15 squamous cell carcinoma, 22 adenocarcinoma, 5 small cell carcinoma, 1 adenosquamous carcinoma) showed evidence of multidirectional differentiation in 25% of cases. Tumor cell heterogeneity may also occur in Barrett's-associated adenocarcinomas.[151] In a study by Lam and colleagues,[152] 496 cases of primary esophageal tumors were reviewed. Of these, 11 (2.2%) showed evidence of both squamous cell carcinoma and a mucin-secreting component. The age, sex, and site distribution of these tumors were similar to those of pure squamous cell carcinomas. Histologically, most tumors showed a poorly differentiated squamous cell carcinoma with varying amounts of mucin or glandular differentiation (see Fig. 16-13**B**).

The prognosis of patients with these tumors appears similar to that of patients with pure squamous cell carcinoma.[152] Therefore, it is probably best to consider tumors with mixed squamous and glandular (mucin) differentiation biologically similar to pure squamous cell carcinoma regardless of the terminology used to describe the tumor.

CARCINOID TUMOR

Well-differentiated neuroendocrine tumors (carcinoid tumors) of the esophagus are extremely rare and have

been reported either as isolated polypoid tumors or as incidental findings in esophagectomies for adenocarcinoma.[153,154] Little is known about their biologic behavior. However, they are histologically similar to those that occur in other parts of the gastrointestinal tract.

SMALL CELL CARCINOMA

Poorly differentiated (or undifferentiated) small cell carcinomas of the esophagus account for approximately 1% of esophageal malignant neoplasms.[63,155] In fact, the esophagus is the most common extrapulmonary site for small cell carcinoma. These tumors are most common in middle-aged to elderly individuals (median age, 60 years; range, 40 to 90 years), show a slight (2:1) male predilection, and may present with symptoms of dysphagia or obstruction.

The gross and microscopic features are similar to those that occur in the lung. However, esophageal tumors usually form large exophytic masses. The tumor cells are small to intermediate in size with scant cytoplasm, irregular hyperchromatic nuclei with molding, and frequent single-cell necrosis (Fig. 16-24). In one study of 21 cases,[156] 50% of tumors contained areas of focal squamous or glandular differentiation, and 33% had squamous cell carcinoma in situ. Thus, it is believed that these tumors arise from a multipotential cell in the squamous epithelium. However, others propose that these tumors arise from neuroendocrine (or Merkel) cells in the squamous epithelium, which are present in a high proportion of the general population.[157]

Overall, esophageal small cell carcinomas are highly aggressive neoplasms. Median survival rates for patients are 6 to 12 months or less.[63,155]

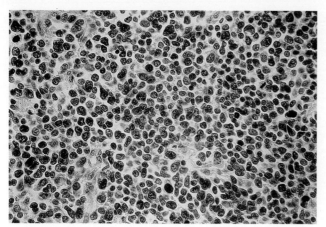

FIGURE 16–24. Typical appearance of a small cell carcinoma of the esophagus, which is histologically identical to small cell carcinomas that occur in the lung. This tumor is characterized by a proliferation of small "blue" cells with marked nuclear hyperchromaticity, lack of nucleoli, nuclear molding, and individual cell necrosis.

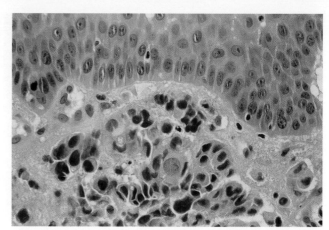

FIGURE 16–26. Metastatic, poorly differentiated carcinoma of the breast to the esophagus. A proliferation of highly atypical cells, some in a single-cell file arrangement, are noted just beneath the epithelium in the upper portion of the lamina propria. The tumor stained positively for ER, PR, and GCDFP.

CHORIOCARCINOMA

Choriocarcinoma of the esophagus is extremely rare and affects adults of both sexes. Of the four cases reported, two developed in association with BE-associated adenocarcinoma.[158,159] Grossly, the tumors are large, exophytic tumors with extensive necrosis, usually located in the distal third of the esophagus. Microscopically, a mixture of cytotrophoblastic and syncytiotrophoblastic giant cells is present, and immunoperoxidase stains for human chorionic gonadotropin are positive in the trophoblastic cells (Fig. 16-25). The primary differential diagnosis is with spread of a mediastinal germ cell tumor and with a squamous cell carcinoma containing pleomorphic giant cells. The prognosis in all reported cases is exceedingly poor, with widespread metastases at presentation and mean survival of a few months.

METASTASES

Metastases to the esophagus are not rare and originate mostly from carcinomas of the lung, breast, and stomach (Fig. 16-26).[160] However, almost any tumor can metastasize to this location. Metastatic lesions typically form nodules within the submucosa but may also produce large symptomatic obstructive lesions. Attention to the clinical history, the distribution of the lesion, and the absence of premalignant squamous or glandular lesions is usually sufficient to distinguish these tumors from a primary esophageal carcinoma. In difficult cases, the use of immunostains for cytokeratins 7 and 20[62] or "organ-specific" markers such as TTF-1 (lung),[66] estrogen receptor (breast), or others may be helpful in suggesting likely primary sites.

References

1. Parker SL, Tong T, Bolden S, et al: Cancer statistics, 1997. CA Cancer J Clin 47:5-27, 1997.
2. Devesa SS, Blot WJ, Fraumeni JF Jr: Changing patterns in the incidence of esophageal and gastric carcinoma in the United States. Cancer 83:2049-2053, 1998.
3. Odze R, Antonioli D, Shocket D, et al: Esophageal squamous papillomas: clinicopathologic study of 38 lesions and analysis of human papillomavirus by the polymerase chain reaction. Am J Surg Pathol 17:803-812, 1993.
4. Lavergne D, DeVilliers EM: Papillomavirus in esophageal papillomas and carcinomas. Int J Cancer 80:680-684, 1999.
5. Carr NJ, Bratthauer GL, Lichy JH, et al: Squamous cell papillomas of the esophagus: A study of 23 lesions for human papillomavirus by in situ hybridization and the polymerase chain reaction. Hum Pathol 25:536-540, 1994.
6. Carr NJ, Moniham JM, Sobin LH, et al: Squamous cell papilloma of the esophagus: A clinicopathologic and follow-up study of 25 cases. Am J Gastroenterol 89:245-248, 1994.
7. Waluga M, Hartleb M, Sliwinski ZK, et al: Esophageal squamous cell papillomatosis complicated by carcinoma. Am J Gastroenterol 95:1592-1593, 2000.
8. Banducci D, Rees R, Bluett MK, et al: Pleomorphic adenoma of the

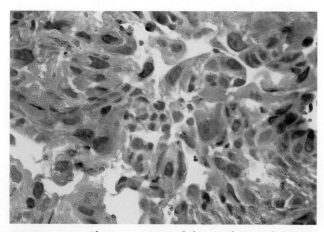

FIGURE 16–25. Choriocarcinoma of the esophagus, showing a proliferation of cytotrophoblastic and syncytiotrophoblastic cells.

cervical esophagus: A rare tumor. Ann Thorac Surg 44:653-655, 1987.

9. Tsutsumi M, Mizunoto K, TsuJ'iuchi T, et al: Serous cystadenoma of the esophagus. Acta Pathol Jpn 40:153-155, 1990.
10. Su JM, Hsu HK, Hsu PI, et al: Esophageal submucosal gland duct adenoma. Am J Gastroenterol 93:461-462, 1998.
11. Rouse RV, Soetikno RM, Baker RJ, et al: Esophageal submucosal gland duct adenoma. Am J Surg Pathol 19:1191-1196, 1995.
12. Takubo K, Esaki Y, Watanabe A, et al: Adenoma accompanied by superficial squamous cell carcinoma of the esophagus. Cancer 71:2435-2438, 1993.
13. Thurberg BL, Duray PH, Odze RD: Polypoid dysplasia in Barrett's esophagus: A clinico-pathologic, immunohistochemical and molecular study of five cases. Hum Pathol 30:745-752, 1999.
14. Harmand D, Grosdidier J, Hoeffel JC: Multiple bronchogenic cysts of the esophagus. Am J Gastroenterol 75:321-323, 1981.
15. Lim LL, Ho KY, Goh PM: Preoperative diagnosis of a para-esophageal bronchogenic cyst using endosonography. Ann Thorac Surg 73:633-635, 2002.
16. Sen S, Bourne AJ, Morris LL, et al: Dorsal enteric cysts—a study of eight cases. Aust N Z J Surg 58:51-55, 1988.
17. McNally J, Charles AK, Spicer RD, Grier D: Mixed foregut cyst associated with esophageal atresia. J Pediatr Surg 36:939-940, 2001.
18. Diaz de Liano A, Ciga MA, Trujillo R, et al: Congenital esophageal cysts—two cases in adult patients. Hepatogastroenterology 46:2405-2408, 1999.
19. Lee MY, Jensen E, Kwak S, et al: Metastatic adenocarcinoma arising in a congenital foregut cyst of the esophagus: A case report with review of the literature. Am J Clin Oncol 21:64-66, 1998.
20. Singh S, Lal P, Sakora SS, Datta NR: Squamous cell carcinoma arising from a congenital duplication cyst of the esophagus in a young adult. Dis Esophagus 14:258-261, 2001.
21. Sanchez-Pemaute A, Hemando F, Diez-Valladares L, et al: Heterotopic gastric mucosa in the upper esophagus ("inlet patch"): A rare cause of esophageal perforation. Am J Gastroenterol 94:3047-3050, 1999.
22. Lauwers GY, Scott GV, Vauthey GN: Adenocarcinoma of the upper esophagus arising in cervical ectopic gastric mucosa: Rare evidence of malignant potential of so-called "inlet patch." Dig Dis Sci 43:901-907, 1998.
23. Berkelhammer C, Bhagavan M, Templeton A, et al: Gastric inlet patch containing submucosally infiltrating adenocarcinoma. J Clin Gastroenterol 25:678-681, 1997.
24. Chistensen WN, Sternberg SS: Adenocarcinoma of the upper esophagus arising in ectopic gastric mucosa. Two case reports and review of the literature. Am J Surg Pathol 11:397-402, 1987.
25. Nakanishi Y, Ochiai A, Shimoda T, et al: Heterotopic sebaceous glands in the esophagus: Histopathological and immunohistochemical study of a resected esophagus. Pathol Int 49:364-368, 1999.
26. Lewin KJ, Appelman HD: Atlas of Tumor Pathology, 3rd Series, Fascicle 18. Tumors of the Esophagus and Stomach. Washington, DC, Armed Forces Institute of Pathology, 1996.
27. Brown LM, Hoover RN, Greenberg RS, et al: Are racial differences in squamous cell esophageal cancer explained by alcohol and tobacco use? J Natl Cancer Inst 86:1340-1345, 1994.
28. Tachimori Y, Watanabe H, Kato H, et al: Hypercalcemia in patients with esophageal carcinoma. The pathophysiologic role of parathyroid hormone–related protein. Cancer 68:2625-2629, 1991.
29. Ina H, Shibuya H, Ohashi I, et al: The frequency of a concomitant early esophageal cancer in male patients with oral and oropharyngeal cancer. Screening results using Lugol dye endoscopy. Cancer 73:2038-2041, 1994.
30. Ribiero U, Posner MC, Safatle-Ribiero AV, et al: Risk factors for squamous cell carcinoma of the oesophagus. Br J Surg 83:1174-1183, 1996.
31. Meijssen MA, Tilanus HW, van Blankenstein M, et al: Achalasia complicated by oesophageal squamous cell carcinoma: A prospective study in 195 patients. Gut 33:155-158, 1992.
32. Streitz JM, Ellis FH, Gibb SP, et al: Achalasia and squamous cell carcinoma of the esophagus: Analysis of 241 patients. Ann Thorac Surg 59:1604-1609, 1995.
33. Sandler RS, Nyren O, Ekblom A, et al: The risk of esophageal cancer in patients with achalasia. A population-based study. JAMA 274:1359-1362, 1995.

34. Marger RS, Marger D: Carcinoma of the esophagus and tylosis. A lethal genetic combination. Cancer 72:17-19, 1993.
35. Turner JR, Shen LH, Crum CP, et al: Low prevalence of human papillomavirus infection in esophageal squamous cell carcinomas from North America: Analysis by a highly sensitive and specific polymerase chain reaction–based approach. Hum Pathol 28:174-178, 1997.
36. Togawa K, Jaskiewicz K, Takahashi H, et al: Human papillomavirus DNA sequences in esophagus squamous cell carcinoma. Gastroenterology 107:128-136, 1994.
37. Poljak M, Cerar A, Seme K: Human papillomavirus infection in esophageal carcinomas: A study of 121 lesions using multiple broad-spectrum polymerase chain reactions and literature review. Hum Pathol 29:266-271, 1998.
38. Chang F, Syrjanen S, Shen Q, et al: Human papillomavirus involvement in esophageal carcinogenesis in the high-incidence area of China. A study of 700 cases by screening and type-specific in situ hybridization. Scand J Gastroenterol 35:123-130, 2000.
39. Dawsey SM, Wang GQ, Weinstein WM, et al: Squamous dysplasia and early esophageal cancer in the Linxian region of China: Distinctive endoscopic lesions. Gastroenterology 105:1333-1340, 1993.
40. Kuwano H, Matsuda H, Matsuoka H, et al: Intra-epithelial carcinoma concomitant with esophageal squamous cell carcinoma. Cancer 59:783-787, 1987.
41. Kuwano H, Ohno S, Matsuda H: Serial histologic evaluation of multiple primary squamous cell carcinomas of the esophagus. Cancer 61:1635-1638, 1988.
42. Dawsey SM, Fleischer DE, Wang GQ, et al: Mucosal iodine staining improves endoscopic visualization of squamous dysplasia and squamous cell carcinoma of the esophagus in Linxian, China. Cancer 83:220-231, 1998.
43. Dawsey SM, Yu Y, Taylor PR, et al: Esophageal cytology and subsequent risk of esophageal cancer. A prospective follow-up study from Linxian, China. Acta Cytol 38:183-192, 1994.
44. Tajima Y, Nakanishi Y, Tachimori Y, et al: Significance of involvement by squamous cell carcinoma of the ducts of esophageal submucosal glands. Analysis of 201 surgically resected superficial squamous cell carcinomas. Cancer 89:248-254, 2000.
45. Chu P, Stagias J, West AB, Traube M: Diffuse pagetoid squamous cell carcinoma in situ of the esophagus: A case report. Cancer 79:1865-1870, 1997.
46. Singh SP, Odze R: Multinucleated epithelial giant cell changes in esophagitis: A clinicopathologic study of 14 cases. Am J Surg Pathol 22:93-99, 1998.
47. Dawsey SM, Lewin KJ, Liu FS, et al: Esophageal morphology from Linxian, China. Squamous histologic findings in 754 patients. Cancer 73:2027-2037, 1994.
48. Qui S, Yang G: Precursor lesions of esophageal cancer in high-risk populations in Henan Province, China. Cancer 62:551-557, 1998.
49. Goseki N, Koike M, Yoshida M: Histopathologic characteristics of early stage esophageal carcinoma. A comparative study with gastric carcinoma. Cancer 69:1088-1093, 1992.
50. Yoshinaka H, Shimazu H, Fukumoto T, Baba M: Superficial esophageal carcinoma: A clinicopathological review of 59 cases. Am J Gastroenterol 86:1413-1418, 1991.
51. Bogomoletz WV, Molas G, Gayet B, Potet F: Superficial squamous cell carcinoma of the esophagus. A report of 76 cases and review of the literature. Am J Surg Pathol 13:535-546, 1989.
52. Ando N, Ozawa S, Kitagawa Y, et al: Improvement in the results of surgical treatment of advanced squamous esophageal carcinoma during 15 consecutive years. Ann Surg 232:225-232, 2000.
53. Morita M, Kuwano H, Yasuda M, et al: The multicentric occurrence of squamous epithelial dysplasia and squamous cell carcinoma in the esophagus. Cancer 74:2889-2895, 1994.
54. Pesko P, Rakic S, Milicevic M, et al: Prevalence and clinicopathologic features of multiple squamous cell carcinoma of the esophagus. Cancer 73:2687-2690, 1994.
55. Mori M, Matsuda H, Kuwano H, et al: Oesophageal squamous cell carcinoma with lymphoid stroma. A case report. Virchows Arch A Pathol Anat Histopathol 415:473-479, 1989.
56. Kuwano H, Nagamatsu M, Ohno S, et al: Coexistence of intra-epithelial carcinoma and glandular differentiation in esophageal squamous cell carcinoma. Cancer 62:1568-1572, 1988.

57. Edwards JM, Hillier VF, Lawson RA, et al: Squamous carcinoma of the oesophagus: Histological criteria and their prognostic significance. Br J Cancer 59:429-433, 1989.

58. Fujiwara Y, Nakagawa K, Tanaka T, et al: Small cell carcinoma of the esophagus combined with superficial esophageal cancer. Hepatogastroenterology 43:1360-1369, 1996.

59. Chu PG, Lyda MH, Weiss LM: Cytokeratin 14 expression in epithelial neoplasms: A survey of 435 cases with emphasis on its value in differentiating squamous cell carcinomas from other epithelial tumours. Histopathology 39:9-16, 2001.

60. Takahashi H, Shikata N, Senzaki H, et al: Immunohistochemical staining patterns of keratins in normal oesophageal epithelium and carcinoma of the oesophagus. Histopathology 26:45-50, 1995.

61. Lam KY, Loke SL, Shen XC, Ma LT: Cytokeratin expression in non-neoplastic oesophageal epithelium and squamous cell carcinoma of the oesophagus. Virchows Arch 426:345-349, 1995.

62. Chu P, Wu E, Weiss LM: Cytokeratin 7 and cytokeratin 20 expression in epithelial neoplasms: A survey of 435 cases. Mod Pathol 13:962-972, 2000.

63. Casas F, Ferrer F, Farrus B, et al: Primary small cell carcinoma of the esophagus: A review of the literature with emphasis on therapy and prognosis. Cancer 80:1366-1372, 1997.

64. Rubio CA, Liu FS, Zhao HZ: Histological classification of intraepithelial neoplasias and microinvasive squamous carcinoma of the esophagus. Am J Surg Pathol 13:685-690, 1989.

65. Schlemper RJ, Dawsey SM, Itabashi M, et al: Differences in diagnostic criteria for esophageal squamous cell carcinoma between Japanese and Western pathologists. Cancer 88:996-1006, 2000.

66. Pelosi G, Fraggetta, Pasini F, et al: Immunoreactivity for thyroid transcription factor-1 in stage I non–small cell carcinomas of the lung. Am J Surg Pathol 25:363-372, 2001.

67. Takubo K, Sasajima K, Yamashita K, et al: Prognostic significance of intramural metastasis in patients with esophageal carcinoma. Cancer 65:1816-1819, 1990.

68. Holscher AH, Bollschweiler E, Schneider PM, Siewert JR: Prognosis of early esophageal cancer. Comparison between adeno- and squamous cell carcinoma. Cancer 76:178-186, 1995.

69. Mandard AM, Chasle J, Marnay J, et al: Autopsy findings in 111 cases of esophageal cancer. Cancer 48:329-335, 1981.

70. Wang LS, Chow KC, Chi KH, et al: Prognosis of esophageal squamous cell carcinoma: Analysis of clinicopathological and biological factors. Am J Gastroenterol 94:1933-1940, 1999.

71. Greene FL, Page DL, Fleming ID, et al, eds: AJCC Cancer Staging Manual, 6th ed. New York, Springer, 2002.

72. Lee RG, Compton CC: Protocol for the examination of specimens removed from patients with esophageal carcinoma. Arch Pathol Lab Med 121:925-929, 1997.

73. Tajima Y, Nakanishi Y, Ochiai A, et al: Histopathologic findings predicting lymph node metastasis and prognosis of patients with superficial esophageal carcinoma: Analysis of 240 surgically resected tumors. Cancer 88:1285-1293, 2000.

74. Sarbia M, Bittinger F, Porschen R, et al: Prognostic value of histopathologic parameters of esophageal squamous cell carcinoma. Cancer 76:922-927, 1995.

75. Torres CM, Wang HH, Turner JR, et al: Pathologic prognostic factors in esophageal squamous cell carcinoma: A follow-up study of 74 patients with or without preoperative chemoradiation therapy. Mod Pathol 12:961-968, 1999.

76. Hambraeus GM, Mercke CE, Willen R, et al: Prognostic factors influencing survival in combined radiotherapy and surgery of squamous cell carcinoma of the esophagus with special reference to a histopathologic grading system. Cancer 62:895-904, 1988.

77. Brucher BL, Stein HJ, Werner M, Siewert JR: Lymphatic vessel invasion is an independent prognostic factor in patients with a primary resected tumor with esophageal squamous cell carcinoma. Cancer 92:2228-2233, 2001.

78. Kanamoto A, Kato H, Tachimori Y, et al: No prognostic significance of p53 expression in esophageal squamous cell carcinoma. J Surg Oncol 72:94-98, 1999.

79. Sarbia M, Verreet P, Bittinger F, et al: Basaloid squamous cell carcinoma of the esophagus: Diagnosis and prognosis. Cancer 79:1871-1878, 1997.

80. Cho KJ, Jang JJ, Lee SS, Zo JI: Basaloid squamous carcinoma of the oesophagus: A distinct neoplasm with multipotential differentiation. Histopathology 36:331-340, 2000.

81. Abe K, Sasano H, Itakura Y, et al: Basaloid-squamous carcinoma of the esophagus. A clinicopathologic, DNA ploidy, and immunohistochemical study of seven cases. Am J Surg Pathol 20:453-461, 1996.

82. Tsubochi H, Suzuki T, Suzuki, S et al: Immunohistochemical study of basaloid squamous cell carcinoma, adenoid cystic and mucoepidermoid carcinoma in the upper aerodigestive tract. Anticancer Res 20:1205-1211, 2000.

83. Iascone C, Barreca M: Carcinosarcoma and pseudosarcoma of the esophagus: Two names, one disease—comprehensive review of the literature. World J Surg 23:153-157, 1999.

84. Uchiyama S, Imai S, Hoshino A, et al: Rapid-growing carcinosarcoma of the esophagus arising from intraepithelial squamous cell carcinoma: Report of a case. Surg Today 30:173-176, 2000.

85. Balercia G, Bhan AK, Dickersin GR: Sarcomatoid carcinoma: An ultrastructural study with light microscopic and immunohistochemical correlation of 10 cases from various anatomic sites. Ultrastruct Pathol 19:249-263, 1995.

86. Lauwers GY, Grant LD, Scott GV, et al: Spindle cell squamous carcinoma of the esophagus: Analysis of ploidy and tumor proliferative activity in a series of 13 cases. Hum Pathol 29:863-868, 1998.

87. Carella R, Deleonardi G, D'Errico A, et al: Immunohistochemical panels for differentiating epithelial malignant mesothelioma from lung adenocarcinoma: A study with logistic regression analysis. Am J Surg Pathol 25:43-50, 2001.

88. Kavin H, Yaremko L, Valaitis J, Chowdhury L: Chronic esophagitis evolving to verrucous squamous cell carcinoma: Possible role of exogenous chemical carcinogens. Gastroenterology 110:904-914, 1996.

89. Tajiri H, Muto M, Boku N, et al: Verrucous carcinoma of the esophagus completely resected by endoscopy. Am J Gastroenterol 95:1076-1077, 2000.

90. Malik AB, Bidani JA, Rich HG, McCully KS: Long-term survival in a patient with verrucous carcinoma of the esophagus. Am J Gastroenterol 91:1031-1033, 1996.

91. Biemond P, ten Kate FJ, van Blankenstein M: Esophageal verrucous carcinoma: Histologically a low-grade malignancy but clinically a fatal disease. J Clin Gastroenterol 13:102-107, 1991.

92. Sashiyama H, Nozawa A, Kimura M, et al: Case report: A case of lymphoepithelioma-like carcinoma of the oesophagus and review of the literature. J Gastroenterol Hepatol 14:534-539, 1999.

93. Blot WJ, Devesa SS, Kneller RW, Fraumeni JF Jr: Rising incidence of adenocarcinoma of the esophagus and gastric cardia. JAMA 265:1287-1289, 1991.

94. Daly JM, Fry WA, Little AG, et al: Esophageal cancer: Results of an American College of Surgeons Patient Care Evaluation Study. J Am Coll Surg 190:562-572, 2000.

95. Bollschweiler E, Wolfgarten E, Gutschow C, Holscher AH: Demographic variations in the rising incidence of esophageal adenocarcinoma in white males. Cancer 92:549-555, 2001.

96. Paraf F, Flejou JF, Pignon JP, et al: Surgical pathology of adenocarcinoma arising in Barrett's esophagus. Analysis of 67 cases. Am J Surg Pathol 19:183-191, 1995.

97. Torres C, Turner JR, Wang HH, et al: Pathologic prognostic factors in Barrett's associated adenocarcinoma: A follow-up study of 96 patients. Cancer 85:520-528, 1999.

98. Spechler SJ: Barrett's esophagus. N Engl J Med 346:836-842, 2002.

99. Falk GW: Barrett's esophagus. Gastroenterology 122:1569-1591, 2002.

100. Hirota WK, Loughney TM, Lazas DJ, et al: Specialized intestinal metaplasia, dysplasia, and cancer of the esophagus and esophagogastric junction: Prevalence and clinical data. Gastroenterology 116:277-285, 1999.

101. Cameron AJ, Lomboy CT, Pera M, Carpenter HA: Adenocarcinoma of the esophagogastric junction and Barrett's esophagus. Gastroenterology 109:1541-1546, 1995.

102. Streitz JMJ, Ellis FHJ, Gibb SP, et al: Adenocarcinoma in Barrett's esophagus. A clinicopathologic study of 65 cases. Ann Surg 213:122-125, 1991.

103. Williamson WA, Ellis FH, Gibb SP, et al: Barrett's esophagus. Prevalence and incidence of adenocarcinoma. Arch Intern Med 151:2212-2216, 1991.

104. Hameeteman W, Tytgat GN, Houthoff HJ, van den Tweel JG: Barrett's esophagus: Development of dysplasia and adenocarcinoma. Gastroenterology 96:1249-1256, 1989.

105. Shaheen NJ, Crosby MA, Bozymski EM, Sandler RS: Is there publication bias in the reporting of cancer risk in Barrett's esophagus? Gastroenterology 119:333-338, 2000.

106. Iftikhar SY, James PD, Steele RJ, et al: Length of Barrett's oesophagus: An important factor in the development of dysplasia and adenocarcinoma. Gut 33:1155-1158, 1992.

107. Rudolph RE, Vaughan TL, Storer BE, et al: Effect of segment length on risk for neoplastic progression in patients with Barrett esophagus. Ann Intern Med 132:612-620, 2000.

108. Weston AP, Badr AS, Hassanein RS: Prospective multivariate analysis of clinical, endoscopic, and histological factors predictive of the development of Barrett's multifocal high-grade dysplasia or adenocarcinoma. Am J Gastroenterol 94:3413-3419, 1999.

109. Avidan B, Sonnenberg A, Schnell TG, et al: Hiatal hernia size, Barrett's length, and severity of acid reflux are all risk factors for esophageal adenocarcinoma. Am J Gastroenterol 97:1930-1936, 2002.

110. van der Burgh A, Dees J, Hop WC, van Blankenstein M: Oesophageal cancer is an uncommon cause of death in patients with Barrett's oesophagus. Gut 39:5-8, 1996.

111. Cameron AJ, Ott BJ, Payne WS: The incidence of adenocarcinoma in columnar-lined (Barrett's) esophagus. N Engl J Med 313:857-859, 1985.

112. O'Connor JB, Falk GW, Richter JE: The incidence of adeno-carcinoma and dysplasia in Barrett's esophagus: Report on the Cleveland Clinic Barrett's Esophagus Registry. Am J Gastroenterol 94:2037-2042, 1999.

113. Conio M, Cameron AJ, Romero Y, et al: Secular trends in the epidemiology and outcome of Barrett's oesophagus in Olmsted County, Minnesota. Gut 48:304-309, 2001.

114. Weston AP, Sharma P, Topalovski M, et al: Long-term follow-up of Barrett's high-grade dysplasia. Am J Gastroenterol 95:1888-1893, 2000.

115. Reid BJ, Levine DS, Longton G, et al: Predictors of progression to cancer in Barrett's esophagus: Baseline histology and flow cytometry identify low- and high-risk patient subsets. Am J Gastroenterol 95:1669-1676, 2000.

116. Miros M, Kerlin P, Walker N: Only patients with dysplasia progress to adenocarcinoma in Barrett's oesophagus. Gut 32:1441-1446, 1991.

117. van Sandick JW, van Lanschot JJ, ten Kate FJ, et al: Pathology of early invasive adenocarcinoma of the esophagus or esophagogastric junction: Implications for therapeutic decision making. Cancer 88:2429-2437, 2000.

118. Dunne B, Reynolds JV, Mulligan E, et al: A pathological study of tumour regression in oesophageal adenocarcinoma treated with preoperative chemoradiotherapy. J Clin Pathol 54:841-845, 2001.

119. Hamilton K, Chiappori A, Olson S, et al: Prevalence and prognostic significance of neuroendocrine cells in esophageal adenocarcinoma. Mod Pathol 13:475-481, 2000.

120. Robey-Cafferty SS, Ajani JA, Ota DM, et al: Histologic observations and P-glycoprotein expression in gastric and esophageal adeno-carcinomas treated with preoperative chemotherapy. Arch Pathol Lab Med 115:807-812, 1991.

121. Ormsby AH, Goldblum JR, Rice TW, et al: The utility of cytokeratin subsets in distinguishing Barrett's-related oesophageal adenocarci-noma from gastric adenocarcinoma. Histopathology 38:307-311, 2001.

122. Griffin M, Sweeney EC: The relationship of endocrine cells, dysplasia and carcinoembryonic antigen in Barrett's mucosa to adenocarcinoma of the oesophagus. Histopathology 11:53-62, 1987.

123. Tot T: The role of cytokeratins 20 and 7 and estrogen receptor analysis in separation of metastatic lobular carcinoma of the breast and metastatic signet ring cell carcinoma of the gastrointestinal tract. APMIS 108:467-472, 2000.

124. Shen B, Ormsby AH, Shen C, et al: Cytokeratin expression patterns in noncardia, intestinal metaplasia-associated gastric adenocarcinoma: Implication for the evaluation of intestinal metaplasia and tumors at the esophagogastric junction. Cancer 94:820-831, 2002.

125. Siewert JR, Stein HJ, Feith M, et al: Histologic tumor type is an independent prognostic parameter in esophageal cancer: Lessons from more than 1,000 consecutive resections at a single center in the Western world. Ann Surg 234:360-367, 2001.

126. Rice TW, Zuccaro GJ, Adelstein DJ, et al: Esophageal carcinoma: Depth of tumor invasion is predictive of regional lymph node status. Ann Thorac Surg 65:787-792, 1998.

127. Rice TW, Blackstone EH, Goldblum JR, et al: Superficial adeno-carcinoma of the esophagus. J Thorac Cardiovasc Surg 122:1077-1090, 2001.

128. Entwistle JW, Goldberg M: Multimodality therapy for resectable cancer of the thoracic esophagus. Ann Thorac Surg 73:1009-1015, 2002.

129. Ruol A, Parenti A, Zaninotto G, et al: Intestinal metaplasia is the probable common precursor of adenocarcinoma in Barrett esophagus and adenocarcinoma of the gastric cardia. Cancer 88:2520-2528, 2000.

130. Haggitt RC: Barrett's esophagus, dysplasia, and adenocarcinoma. Hum Pathol 25:982-993, 1994.

131. Skacel M, Petras RE, Gramlich TL, et al: The diagnosis of low-grade dysplasia in Barrett's esophagus and its implications for disease progression. Am J Gastroenterol 95:3383-3387, 2000.

132. Montgomery E, Bronner M, Goldblum JR, et al: Reproducibility of the diagnosis of dysplasia in Barrett esophagus: A reaffirmation. Hum Pathol 32:368-378, 2001.

133. Reid BJ, Haggitt RC, Rubin CE, et al: Observer variation in the diagnosis of dysplasia in Barrett's esophagus. Hum Pathol 19:166-178, 1988.

134. Jankowski JA, Wright NA, Meltzer SJ, et al: Molecular evolution of the metaplasia-dysplasia-adenocarcinoma sequence in the esophagus. Am J Pathol 154:965-973, 1999.

135. Haggitt RC, Reid BJ, Rabinovitch PS, Rubin CE: Barrett's esoph-agus. Correlation between mucin histochemistry, flow cytometry, and histologic diagnosis for predicting increased cancer risk. Am J Pathol 131:53-61, 1988.

136. Reid BJ, Prevo LJ, Galipeau PC, et al: Predictors of progression in Barrett's esophagus II: Baseline 17p (p53) loss of heterozygosity identifies a patient subset at increased risk for neoplastic progression. Am J Gastroenterol 96:2839-2848, 2001.

137. Reid BJ, Weinstein WM, Lewin KJ, et al: Endoscopic biopsy can detect high-grade dysplasia or early adenocarcinoma in Barrett's esophagus without grossly recognizable neoplastic lesions. Gastro-enterology 94:81-90, 1988.

138. Levine DS, Haggitt RC, Blount PL, et al: An endoscopic biopsy protocol can differentiate high-grade dysplasia from early adeno-carcinoma in Barrett's esophagus. Gastroenterology 105:40-50, 1993.

139. Nigro JJ, Hagen JA, DeMeester TR, et al: Occult esophageal adenocarcinoma: Extent of disease and implications for effective therapy. Ann Surg 230:433-438, 1999.

140. Nijhawan PK, Wang KK: Endoscopic mucosal resection for lesions with endoscopic features suggestive of malignancy and high-grade dysplasia within Barrett's esophagus. Gastrointest Endosc 52:328-332, 2000.

141. Gossner L, Stolte M, Sroka R, et al: Photodynamic ablation of high-grade dysplasia and early cancer in Barrett's esophagus by means of 5-aminolevulinic acid. Gastroenterology 114:448-455, 1998.

142. Sharma P, Bhattacharyya A, Garewal HS, Sampliner RE: Durability of new squamous epithelium after endoscopic reversal of Barrett's esophagus. Gastrointest Endosc 50:159-164, 1999.

143. Endoh Y, Miyawaki M, Tamura G, et al: Esophageal adenocarci-noma that probably originated in the esophageal gland duct: A case report. Pathol Int 49:156-159, 1999.

144. Takagi A, Ema Y, Horii S, et al: Early adenocarcinoma arising from ectopic gastric mucosa in the cervical esophagus. Gastrointest Endosc 41:167-170, 1995.

145. Morisaki Y, Yoshizumi Y, Hiroyasu S, et al: Adenoid cystic carci-noma of the esophagus: Report of a case and review of the Japanese literature. Surg Today 26:1006-1009, 1996.

146. Tsang WY, Chan JK, Lee KC, et al: Basaloid-squamous carcinoma of the upper aerodigestive tract and so-called adenoid cystic carci-noma of the oesophagus: The same tumour type? Histopathology 19:35-46, 1991.

147. Kabuto T, Taniguchi K, Iwanaga T, et al: Primary adenoid cystic carcinoma of the esophagus: Report of a case. Cancer 43:2452-2456, 1979.

148. Kanamoto A, Nakanishi Y, Ochiai A, et al: A case of small polypoid esophageal carcinoma with multidirectional differentiation, including neuroendocrine, squamous, ciliated glandular, and sarcomatous components. Arch Pathol Lab Med 124:1685-1687, 2000.

149. Ter RB, Govil YK, Leite L, et al: Adenosquamous carcinoma in Barrett's esophagus presenting as pseudoachalasia. Am J Gastroenterol 94:268-270, 1999.

150. Newman J, Antonakopoulos GN, Darnton SJ, Matthews HR: The ultrastructure of oesophageal carcinomas: Multidirectional differentiation. A transmission electron microscopic study of 43 cases. J Pathol 167:193-198, 1992.

151. Wilson CI, Summerall J, Willis I, et al: Esophageal collision tumor (large cell neuroendocrine carcinoma and papillary carcinoma) arising in a Barrett esophagus. Arch Pathol Lab Med 124:411-415, 2000.

152. Lam KY, Dickens P, Loke SL, et al: Squamous cell carcinoma of the oesophagus with mucin-secreting component (muco-epidermoid carcinoma and adenosquamous carcinoma): A clinicopathologic study and a review of literature. Eur J Surg Oncol 20:25-31, 1994.

153. Lindberg GM, Molberg KH, Vuitch MF, Albores-Saavedra J: Atypical carcinoid of the esophagus: A case report and review of the literature. Cancer 79:1476-1481, 1997.

154. Hoang MP, Hobbs CM, Sobin LH, Albores-Saavedra J: Carcinoid tumor of the esophagus: A clinicopathologic study of four cases. Am J Surg Pathol 26:517-522, 2002.

155. Lam KY, Law S, Tung PH, Wong J: Esophageal small cell carcinomas: Clinicopathologic parameters, p53 overexpression, proliferation marker, and their impact on pathogenesis. Arch Pathol Lab Med 124:228-233, 2000.

156. Takubo K, Nakamura K, Sawabe M, et al: Primary undifferentiated small cell carcinoma of the esophagus. Hum Pathol 30:216-221, 1999.

157. Harmse JL, Carey FA, Baird AR, et al: Merkel cells in the human oesophagus. J Pathol 189:176-179, 1999.

158. Kikuchi Y, Tsuneta Y, Kawai T, Aizawa M: Choriocarcinoma of the esophagus producing chorionic gonadotropin. Acta Pathol Jpn 38:489-499, 1988.

159. Wasan HS, Schofield JB, Krausz T, et al: Combined choriocarcinoma and yolk sac tumor arising in Barrett's esophagus. Cancer 73:514-517, 1994.

160. Antler AS, Ough Y, Pitchumoni CS, et al: Gastrointestinal metastases from malignant tumors of the lung. Cancer 49:170-172, 1982.

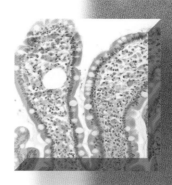

CHAPTER 17

Epithelial Neoplasms of the Stomach

GREGORY Y. LAUWERS

■ Introduction

Although the incidence of gastric cancer has steadily declined during the last few decades, it remains the second most common cancer worldwide, with 800,000 new cases and 650,000 deaths per year.[1] Wide variation among continents and populations is well demonstrated. The highest incidence rates are reported in Asia (Japan), central Europe, and South America.[2] In the United States, gastric cancer is the seventh most frequent cause of cancer-related death. In 2002, approximately 22,000 Americans were diagnosed with gastric carcinoma and about 13,000 died from this disease.[2]

The once well-established characteristics of this disease are being reshaped by two recent trends. First, since the early 1980s, the incidence of proximal tumors has been rising, with carcinomas of the cardia region accounting for close to 30% of gastric cancers.[3,4] During the same period, the increased use of upper endoscopy has led to more frequent detection of early lesions. Early gastric cancers now represent close to 20% of all newly diagnosed cancers in the West and up to 50% in Japan.[5-8] This trend has a dramatic impact on the mortality for what is becoming a curable disease if it is detected at an early stage.

The pathogenesis of gastric carcinoma is a multifactorial process in which both environmental and host-related factors are responsible.[9] This multistep process includes the sequential development of chronic gastritis followed by mucosal atrophy with hypochlorhydria or achlorhydria and intestinal metaplasia, dysplasia, and

ultimately adenocarcinoma.[9,10] Intestinal metaplasia as well as dysplasia and early carcinoma most frequently originates in the neck region of the antral or fundic glands, suggesting that the neck precursor cells of the gastric glands play a unique role in the pathogenesis of gastric cancer.[11]

Geographic variation in incidence, migrant studies, and changes in dietary and sanitary conditions have underscored the role of environmental influences for most gastric carcinomas (i.e., so-called intestinal type).[12-14] Also, the worldwide decrease in rates of this particular type has paralleled the decline in *Helicobacter pylori* infection, suggesting that this bacterium represents the main environmental cause. Over decades, *H. pylori* induces chronic gastritis that gradually develops into atrophic gastritis.[15,16] In turn, there is a significantly increased risk, on the order of fourfold to ninefold, for development of precancerous gastric conditions in infected individuals, especially when *H. pylori* infection occurs in early childhood.[17-19] Chronic acid suppression also increases the risk for development of atrophy in *H. pylori* gastritis, in which it accelerates the progression of gland loss (0.7% in *H. pylori*–negative patients versus 4.7% in *H. pylori*–positive patients).[20]

However, *H. pylori* is not the sole factor responsible for the gastric carcinogenesis. In fact, the majority of *H. pylori*–infected individuals do not develop gastric cancer, whereas up to 20% of patients with gastric cancer are *H. pylori* seronegative. Other environmental and host factors are likely to be important.[21,22] The role of diets rich in salt (dried and salted fish and meats, soy sauce, smoked fish, pickled foods) and low in levels of micronutrients, vitamins, or antioxidants[14] that favor the intraluminal formation of genotoxic agents such as specific N-nitroso compounds (formed by nitrosation of ingested nitrates) has been emphasized.[23-25] In contrast, fresh vegetables, citrus fruits, and ascorbic acid are inversely associated with the development of gastric cancer.[25] Reflux of bile into the stomach is another potential inducer of intestinal metaplasia and has been associated with the development of adenocarcinoma arising in surgical stumps.[26] With regard to host factors, polymorphism of the IL-1 gene is associated with an increased risk for gastric cancer in *H. pylori*–infected individuals. The demonstration of a proinflammatory IL-1 genotype responsible for hypochlorhydria, atrophy, and intestinal-type adenocarcinoma provides a link between an environmental condition and a specific host genetic factor.[27]

In contrast to the intestinal type, diffuse-type gastric cancers, which are diagnosed in younger individuals and observed with an equal incidence in high- and low-risk areas, are regulated to a larger extent by genetic factors.[14,28] The importance of genetic factors is also underscored by the existence of familial clustering of gastric cancer[29] as well as by the high risk of atrophic gastritis in relatives of patients with gastric cancer.[30] (See under Genetic Predisposition and Hereditary Tumor Syndromes.)

Gastric Epithelial Dysplasia

Dysplasia is a noninvasive neoplastic epithelial process considered to be the penultimate stage of gastric carcinogenesis.[31] The presence of high-grade dysplasia, adjacent to 40% to 100% of early gastric cancers and 5% to 80% of advanced carcinomas, supports a direct role in cancer formation.[3,32,33]

Wide variations exist in the prevalence of gastric epithelial dysplasia (GED) worldwide. In nations with high risks for gastric cancer, figures ranging between 9% and 20% are reported. In the West, the prevalence ranges between 0.5% and 3.75%.[33-37] Some conditions are associated with higher rates. In patients with chronic atrophic gastritis or in postgastrectomy patients, it varies from 4% to 30%; GED is found in up to 40% of patients with pernicious anemia.[38-41] GED and adenoma (see definition later) in patients with familial adenomatous polyposis range from 6% to 50% of these patients.[42-44] These lesions occur at a younger age than the sporadic lesions do, and their prevalence increases with age. They are also likely to be smaller and multiple. In patients with Gardner's syndrome, dysplasia and carcinoma are also reported in fundic gland polyps.[44]

The majority of patients are males in their fifth to seventh decades of life, although younger people can be affected.[35-37,45-47] GED is more frequently diagnosed in the antrum and the angulus and typically arises in a background of intestinal metaplasia (usually of the incomplete type).[45,47] It can also develop in apparently histologically normal mucosa.[48] The endoscopic appearance of GED is diverse. Biopsy specimens of ulcers, erosions, atrophic gastritis, polyps, plaques, and scars as well as normal mucosa can show GED.[36,46,47,49,50]

DIAGNOSTIC CRITERIA AND GRADING

When reporting dysplasia, some authors refer to either "adenomatous" dysplasia (or intestinal type, because it resembles colonic adenoma), the most frequent type (Fig. 17-1), or the rarer "foveolar" (or gastric type or type II) dysplasia. This distinction is based on the cellular phenotype; the intestinal type is composed of undifferentiated cells, and the gastric type is composed of cells resembling gastric foveolar cells.[31] In both instances, architectural and cytologic changes are observed. Architectural abnormalities include glandular disarray with dilatation, branching, and intraluminal folding or budding. Intraluminal folding with glandular serration is particularly characteristic of type II dysplasia (Fig. 17-2). Common cytologic features include mucin depletion, cellular crowding, nuclear hyperchromasia, pleomorphism, and stratification. Unlike the cigar-shaped hyperchromatic nuclei of adenomatous dysplasia, the nuclei seen in gastric dysplasia can be vesicular and display less pseudostratification and overlapping. Increased

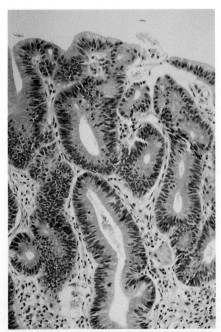

FIGURE 17–1. Low-grade GED, adenomatous type. The lesion is characterized by noticeable glandular disarray and increased cellularity.

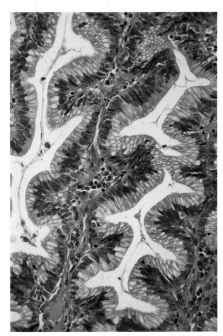

FIGURE 17–2. Gastric-type low-grade GED, showing a distinct serrated appearance and tall foveolar cells.

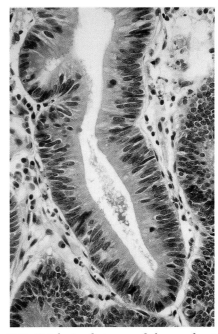

FIGURE 17–3. Cytologic features of low-grade GED with hyperchromatic, cigar-shaped nuclei confined to the basal half of the cells. Mild nuclear pleomorphism can be appreciated.

nucleus-to-cytoplasm ratio and mitotic activity are also variably noted.

A two-tiered grading system of low- and high-grade GED is favored (Table 17-1).[33,46,51-55] In low-grade GED, the glands show only mild architectural disarray (see Fig. 17-1). The cells are closely packed, and the nuclei are confined to the basal half of the cells (Fig. 17-3). High-grade GED is characterized by marked architectural changes such as back-to-back glands and infolding. Larger and irregular nuclei with clumped chromatin and prominent nucleoli are most often seen. The nuclei also frequently extend into the luminal aspect, and their

polarity is partially or totally lost (Fig. 17-4). Frequent mitoses are also characteristic. Of note, high-grade GED also includes the lesion referred to, by some, as carcinoma in situ or intraepithelial carcinoma (pTis), noninvasive lesions showing cytologic changes virtually identical to those found in invasive carcinoma.[31]

TABLE 17–1. Comparison of Features Seen in Low- and High-Grade Gastric Epithelial Dysplasia

Low-Grade Dysplasia	High-Grade Dysplasia
Architectural Features	
Mild to moderate glandular crowding and disarray	Marked glandular disarray with crowding and back-to-back glands
Mild to moderate branching	Moderate to marked branching and frequent budding
Rare glandular budding	Intraluminal folds and cribriforming
Nuclear Features	
Elongated hyperchromatic nuclei	Vesicular round nuclei
Basal location with maintained polarity	Prominent nucleoli
Moderate mitotic activity	Marked increased mitotic activity
	Atypical mitoses

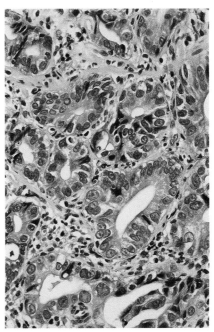

FIGURE 17–4. High-grade GED with markedly disorganized glands lined by large and irregular nuclei. The nuclear polarity is also partially lost, and several mitoses are identified.

GED can be either a flat process or a raised circumscribed lesion protruding above the mucosal surface; in the latter case it is referred to as an adenoma.[55,56] The lesions are slow growing and usually solitary. Adenomas are rare, are preferentially found in the antrum, and represent only about 8% of all gastric polyps.[57,58] They cannot be endoscopically distinguished from other types of polyps unless they display a villous appearance. They are usually sessile and can display a tubular, tubulovillous, or villous architecture.[48,56,59,60] In one series, 93% of adenomas measured less than 2 cm, but importantly, a significant number of cancers are diagnosed in adenomas larger than 2 cm.[57,60,61]

A much rarer type of GED, tubule neck dysplasia (or globoid dysplasia), has been recognized in association with diffuse-type adenocarcinoma.[62] Close observation of the neck region of gastric tubules from which tumor cells seem to bud reveals enlarged clear cells that are similar to their invasive counterpart, with vacuolated nuclei and prominent nucleoli (Fig. 17-5).[62,63] However, tubule neck dysplasia is subtle and not readily recognizable even by morphometric analysis.[64]

DIFFERENTIAL DIAGNOSIS OF GED

It can be difficult to differentiate low-grade dysplasia from reactive or regenerative changes (Table 17-2).[3,55,65,66] In regenerative changes, the cells are frequently cuboidal and appear immature with basophilic cytoplasm because of reduced mucus secretion. The nuclei are frequently large, vesicular, and sometimes pleomorphic. However,

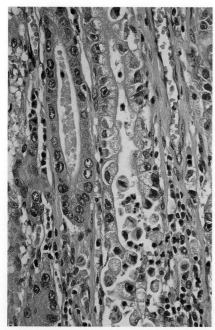

FIGURE 17–5. Tubule neck dysplasia. Note the tubular epithelial lining composed of large globoid cells with clear cytoplasm and atypical vesicular nuclei.

TABLE 17–2. Differentiating Features of Gastric Dysplastic and Regenerative Changes

	Dysplastic Features	Regenerative Changes
Cellular immaturity	Marked	Mild to moderate
Vesicular nuclei	None to moderate	None to moderate
Mucin depletion	Marked	Mild to moderate
Nuclear pleomorphism	Moderate to marked	Mild
Pseudostratification	Mild to marked	None to mild
Surface maturation	Absent	Present
Loss of polarity	Mild to moderate	None to mild
Abnormal mitosis	Mild	None
Architectural disarray	Mild to moderate	None to mild

they are basally or centrally located and arranged in a row, and only mild stratification can be noted. Mitoses are often present, but not on the surface, and abnormal mitoses are absent. Importantly, increased cellular differentiation and maturation are seen toward the luminal surface. Half of the cases diagnosed as hyperplastic or metaplastic lesions by specialists are diagnosed as dysplastic by general pathologists.[49] In cases with interpretative problems, the term *indefinite for dysplasia* is encouraged. Less variation is noted for high-grade lesions. It may be difficult to separate high-grade GED from intramucosal carcinoma. Small glands budding out in the lamina propria are believed to represent early invasion, even in the absence of desmoplasia (Fig. 17-6). In practice, because of the significant clinical implications, it is recommended that a diagnosis of GED be confirmed by a gastrointestinal pathologist.[67,68]

CLINICAL RELEVANCE OF GED

Overall, 57% of the gastric cancers discovered during follow-up of GED are "early" potentially curable cancers, underscoring the importance of endoscopic surveillance.[46,47,49,50,69] Regression of low-grade GED is seen in 40% to 50% of cases, highlighting the fact that many such lesions are truly reactive. However, the possibility remains that a focal lesion either was not sampled by repeated biopsy or had been removed completely by biopsy.[37,46] Persistence of low-grade GED is noted in 20% to 30% of cases, and progression to high-grade GED is observed in up to 15% of cases. After a diagnosis of low-grade GED, a carcinoma can be diagnosed during a mean follow-up period of 10 to 30 months with extremes of 1 month and 39 months.[46,47,49,70] Some report that high-grade GED regresses in about 5% of cases, persists in 15%, and progresses to cancers in 80% to 85%.[37,46] The time frame between a diagnosis of high-grade GED and carcinoma varies between a few

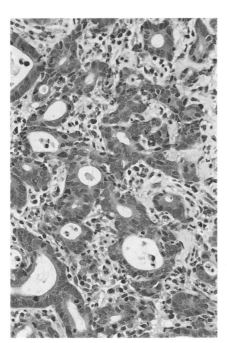

FIGURE 17–6. Intramucosal carcinoma. Despite the cytologic similarities with high-grade GED and the lack of desmoplasia, the glandular budding and anastomosing are sufficient for a diagnosis of carcinoma.

weeks and 39 months, with a mean between 4 and 23 months.[46,47,49,70] After a diagnosis of low-grade GED, endoscopic follow-up is recommended every 3 to 12 months during the first year.[36,37,47,49,50] Because of the close association with adenocarcinoma, surgical resection is suggested when a diagnosis of high-grade GED is rendered and confirmed.[36,46,47,69] However, with the development of endoscopic ultrasonography and endoscopic mucosal resection, a nonsurgical cure for high-grade GED and intramucosal carcinoma can be achieved.[50,71-73]

Gastric Adenocarcinoma

An important epidemiologic shift in the location and frequency of gastric cancer has been noted in the latter half of the 20th century with an increase in incidence of adenocarcinoma of the cardial region. However, much confusion currently exists with regard to this issue. A significant hurdle in the understanding is that there is no clear anatomic landmark or consensus statement to define the gastric cardia either anatomically or histologically. Recent efforts may bring clarity to this subject, and the International Gastric Cancer Association has endorsed a new classification system of these tumors.[74] Type I tumors are defined as those arising in the distal esophagus, type II tumors are those arising in the true gastric cardia, and type III tumors are those arising in the gastric mucosa of the subcardia.

ADENOCARCINOMA OF THE GASTRIC CARDIA

Similar to adenocarcinomas arising in Barrett's esophagus, the incidence of carcinomas of the cardia has been increasing during the past several decades.[4,75] This phenomenon is not reported worldwide, however; publications from Sweden and Japan fail to report similar trends.[76] Some suggest that an increased use of endoscopy with secondary improvement in the diagnosis is responsible for the change in frequency.[77]

Differences between cardial and distal gastric tumors exist. Adenocarcinomas of the cardia are characterized by a higher male-to-female ratio than are distal tumors, and in the United States, they are more frequent in the white population compared with patients of African descent.[78] Whether cardia adenocarcinoma represents the same entity as esophageal adenocarcinoma is still debated.[79-81] Arguments in favor of a single entity include common risk factors and similar age, sex distribution, and phenotype.[80,82] However, obesity, high body mass index, smoking, and alcohol intake have not been universally accepted as risk factors of cardial cancer.[76,82-86]

The carcinogenic sequence of carcinoma of the cardia is not well understood. In some studies, this tumor is significantly associated with older age, *H. pylori* infection, and intestinal metaplasia elsewhere in the stomach.[87-90] However, the relative roles of *H. pylori* and gastroesophageal reflux disease are still debated. It is possible that both factors play a role in the pathogenesis of this disease.[91] Although intestinal metaplasia has been demonstrated adjacent to up to 70% of carcinomas, the risk of malignant transformation appears to be low and has not been well established in prospective series.[92,93] The progression of intestinal metaplasia to dysplasia appears to be slower and less frequent than in Barrett's esophagus, suggesting carcinogenetic differences.[85,88] Currently, intestinal metaplasia of the cardia does not necessitate endoscopic surveillance.

EARLY GASTRIC CANCER

Early gastric carcinomas (EGCs) are defined as invasive adenocarcinomas confined to the mucosa or submucosa with or without lymph node metastasis (Fig. 17-7).[3] Improved techniques and growing number of upper endoscopies worldwide make this lesion encountered more frequently. In Western series, EGCs represent between 15% and 21% of all newly diagnosed cancers; in Japan, they account for 50% of cases.[5-8] The higher prevalence of gastric cancer, a more liberal use of upper endoscopy, and perhaps even a better endoscopic technique may explain the difference. EGC represents an early stage in the development of gastric cancer.[94] During a span of 6 to 88 months, 63% of EGCs progress to advanced carcinomas.[95]

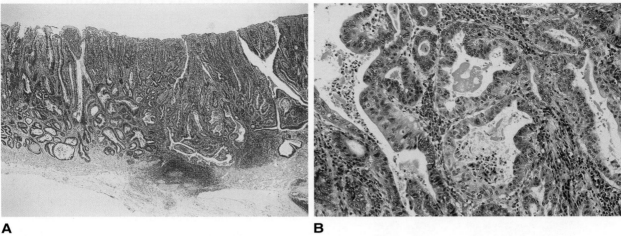

A

B

FIGURE 17–7. Early gastric cancer. **A,** Scanning view shows mucosal thickening. **B,** High magnification demonstrates the malignant glandular proliferation.

Like dysplasia, most EGCs are diagnosed in men older than 50 years. Most patients are asymptomatic, but others may complain of symptoms mimicking peptic ulcer disease.[6,96] The majority of EGCs are small, measuring between 2 and 5 cm and localized on the lesser curvature and around the angulus.[3,97] In 3% to 13% of the patients, multiple tumors are seen and are associated with a worse prognosis.[7,98]

EGCs are divided into three types on the basis of endoscopic macroscopic appearance (Fig. 17-8): protruded (type I), superficial (type II) (Fig. 17-9), and excavated (type III)[99] (see Fig. 17-7). Type II is further subdivided into IIa (elevated type), IIb (flat type), and IIc (depressed type). Superficial EGCs (type II) account for most (80%) of the cases; type IIc is the most common subtype.[100] Type IIb accounts for 58% of tumors measuring less than 5 mm and for none of the larger ones.[101]

Type IIa, in which the lesion is twice as thick as the normal mucosa, and type IIc, which mimics a benign ulcer, are difficult to detect endoscopically and may require multiple biopsies. Subtle diagnostic signs include easy bleeding and irregular interface with the surrounding mucosa.[102,103]

Variants of EGCs have been reported. *Minute* EGCs measure less than 5 mm in diameter, and although the majority of the tumor is limited to the mucosa, submucosal extension is found in up to 15% of cases.[104,105] *Superficial spreading* EGCs are characterized by large serpiginous ulcerations with neoplastic cells spreading over large areas.[3]

The majority of EGCs are well-differentiated glandular carcinomas. Tubular and papillary variants represent 52% and 37% of the cases, respectively, and can be difficult to differentiate from dysplasia (see Fig. 17-7**B**). Signet ring cell carcinoma (Fig. 17-10) and poorly differentiated carcinoma represented 26% and 14% of the cases, respectively, and are usually depressed or ulcerated (types IIc and III).[3,7,100] One should be

FIGURE 17–8. Endoscopic classification of early gastric cancer.

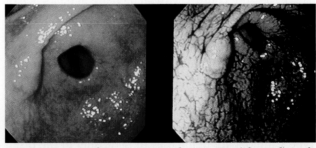

FIGURE 17–9. Endoscopic view of type IIA (elevated) early gastric cancer. The use of dye (chromoendoscopy) greatly improves the detection of the carcinoma. (Courtesy of M. Shimizu, MD, Saitama Medical School, Japan.)

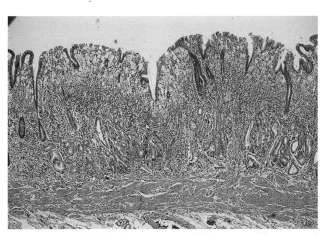

FIGURE 17–10. Early gastric cancer, diffuse type. The tumoral infiltration is limited to the upper half of the mucosa, with preservation of the deep glands.

cautious to differentiate these from gastric xanthomas and poorly differentiated metastatic neoplasms and use immunohistochemistry as necessary.

The prognosis of EGCs is excellent, with a 5-year survival rate greater than 90% in most series.[6-8,96,106] The size and depth of invasion are the two major prognostic indicators; the larger the diameter, the greater the risk of submucosal infiltration.[8,107,108] The risk of invasion should not be overlooked even in very small tumors. In one series, 15.5% of 3- to 5-mm EGCs invaded the submucosa.[105] For intramucosal EGCs, lymph node metastases have been reported in 0% to 7% of cases, and those have a 5-year survival close to 100%.[7,107,108] The rates of lymph node metastases for EGCs extending into the submucosa vary between 8% and 25%, and the 5-year survival is about 80% to 90%.[7,108]

ADVANCED GASTRIC CARCINOMA

Advanced adenocarcinomas invade the gastric wall beyond the submucosa. The majority of the patients are male (M/F ratio of 2:1) in their fifth decade or older. Clinically, the usual complaints range from peptic ulcer symptoms to anemia to weight loss. Hematemesis and symptoms of gastric outlet obstruction are also reported.[3] Another group of patients, typically younger, may present with intra-abdominal dissemination. Among these, female patients may develop the classic metastatic ovarian lesions (Krukenberg tumors), composed of diffuse-type cancer cells.[3]

Most gastric adenocarcinomas are diagnosed in the antrum and antropyloric region, preferentially on the lesser curvature.[109] Approximately half of the gastric adenocarcinomas measure between 2 and 6 cm, and 30% are in the 6- to 10-cm range. Only 15% of gastric carcinomas are larger than 10 cm.[3] Multiple adenocarcinomas are detected in about 5% of patients.[98,110]

Macroscopic Appearance

Advanced gastric carcinomas can display several gross appearances—exophytic, ulcerated, or infiltrative (or combined). Borrmann's classification remains the most widely adopted and divides gastric carcinomas into four types (Fig. 17-11),[111] including polypoid carcinoma (type I), fungating carcinoma (type II), ulcerated carcinoma (type III), and diffusely infiltrative carcinoma (type IV) (Fig. 17-12). Type IV is also known as linitis plastica when it involves the entire stomach (Fig. 17-13). Type II represents 36% of gastric carcinomas and is frequently found in the antrum, along the lesser curvature. Type I and type III represent about 25% of the gastric carcinomas, respectively, and are more common in the corpus, often on the greater curvature.

Histologic Appearance

Gastric adenocarcinomas are characterized by marked heterogeneity at the cellular and architectural level, with frequent overlap between different patterns. Cytologically, a combination of gastric foveolar, intestinal, and endocrine type cells usually composes a tumor.[112,113] Ciliated tumor cells can also be observed.[114] Mucin histochemical and immunohistochemical stains (MUC1, MUC2, MUC5AC, MUC6, CD10) may be useful in highlighting the different components.[48,112,113,115,116] Architecturally, the World Health Organization (WHO) classification recognizes four major types of gastric adenocarcinoma and also acknowledges the Laurén classification. Several rare variants are also included (Table 17-3).[1,48]

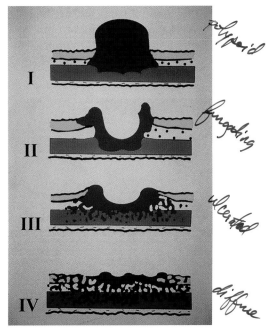

FIGURE 17–11. Borrmann's macroscopic classification of advanced gastric carcinoma.

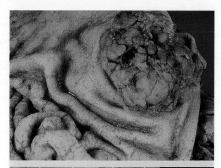

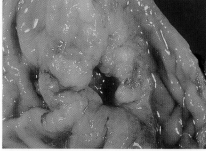

FIGURE 17–12. Growth patterns of gastric carcinoma. *Top*, Polypoid carcinoma, Borrmann's type I. *Bottom*, Ulcerated carcinoma, Borrmann's type III.

TABLE 17–3. WHO Histologic Classification of Malignant Epithelial Gastric Tumors

Adenocarcinoma
  Intestinal type
  Diffuse type
Papillary adenocarcinoma
Tubular adenocarcinoma
Mucinous adenocarcinoma
Signet ring cell carcinoma
Adenosquamous carcinoma
Squamous cell carcinoma
Small cell carcinoma
Undifferentiated carcinoma
Others*

*Rare morphologic variants are classified under this heading.

The three-tiered Laurén classification has been cardinal in helping to understand the role of environmental factors and epidemiologic trends.[117] This scheme recognizes intestinal type, diffuse type, and indeterminate/unclassified type. The relative frequencies are 50% to 67% for the intestinal type, 29% to 35% for the diffuse type, and 3% to 21% for the indeterminate/unclassified type.[117a] The *intestinal-type* adenocarcinomas characteristically form glands of various degrees of differentiation (Fig. 17-14). They are usually diagnosed in older patients, mostly in the antrum, and are linked to chronic *H. pylori* infection with ensuing atrophic gastritis and intestinal metaplasia. The WHO papillary and tubular carcinomas fall into this category. They are both

glandular carcinomas and tend to form polypoid or fungating masses.[48] The *papillary variant* is characterized by epithelial projections scaffolded by central fibrovascular cores (Fig. 17-15). This variant accounts for between 6% and 11% of gastric carcinomas, affects older patients in the proximal stomach, and is frequently associated with liver metastases.[118,119] A higher rate of lymph node metastases (stage for stage) is also reported with papillary adenocarcinoma.[120] The *tubular variant* is composed of distended or anastomosing branching tubules of various sizes (Fig. 17-16). Mucus and cellular and inflammatory debris can be noted intraluminally. In both variants, the cells lining the papillae or the glands can be columnar or cuboidal with various degrees of atypia and mitoses. Combined tubulopapillary variants are also seen.

The Laurén *diffuse-type* adenocarcinomas are composed of single neoplastic cells or small nests diffusely infiltrating through the gastric wall. This type is commonly found in the gastric body and in younger patients. Although it is also associated with *H. pylori* infection, the subsequent carcinogenic sequence is

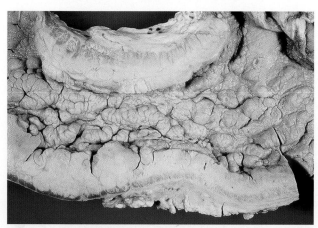

FIGURE 17–13. Infiltrative carcinoma, Borrmann's type IV (linitis plastica). Note the diffusely infiltrated and prominent rugal folds, as well as the markedly thickened gastric wall.

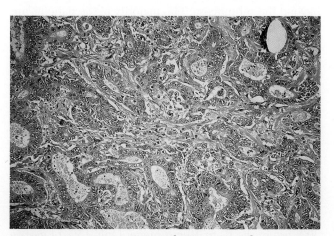

FIGURE 17–14. Laurén's intestinal-type gastric adenocarcinoma formed by infiltrative and anastomosing glands with different degrees of differentiation.

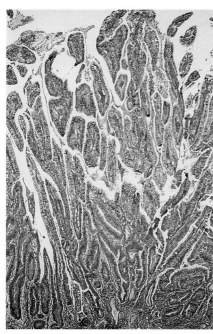

FIGURE 17–15. Papillary-type gastric carcinoma. The projecting and anastomosing fibrovascular cores lined by neoplastic cells are the hallmark of this type.

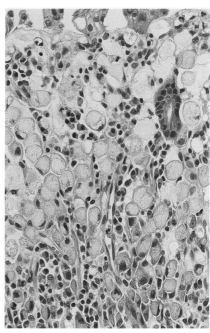

FIGURE 17–17. Signet ring cell carcinoma characterized by prominent intracytoplasmic mucin with eccentric, flattened nuclei.

not well characterized.[31,121] The Laurén *indeterminate/unclassified type* refers to neoplasms that display mixed histologic features. The WHO *signet ring cell carcinomas* are included in the Laurén diffuse type (Fig. 17-17). They are characterized by single infiltrating cells with large distended cytoplasm and peripherally placed crescent-shaped nuclei. Cords, tight clusters, or solid sheets of cells can be seen,[1,48] but well-formed glands are absent. More than 50% of the tumor should be composed of these cells to warrant this classification. Variants including cells resembling histiocytes, deeply eosinophilic cells with neutral mucin, and the anaplastic type with little or no mucin have been observed (Fig.

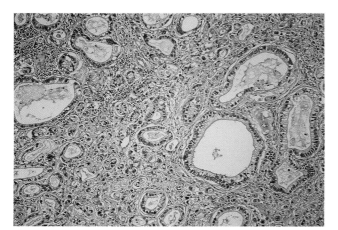

FIGURE 17–16. Tubular adenocarcinoma of the stomach. The neoplasm is composed of well-formed tubules, some cystically dilated.

17-18).[1] Mitoses are characteristically less numerous than in the glandular type.

Mucinous adenocarcinomas, in which pools of extracellular mucin compose at least 50% of the tumor, represent 10% of gastric carcinomas.[48] The cellular component can be formed of glandular structures or irregular cell clusters floating in the abundant mucin.[1]

Undifferentiated carcinomas lack any differentiated features and may resemble lymphomas, squamous cell carcinomas, or sarcomas.[122] They fall into the indeterminate category of the Laurén classification. Immunohistochemistry (positive cytokeratin immunolabeling) may be necessary to confirm their epithelial phenotype.

A three-tiered grading system based on the resemblance with gastric or metaplastic intestinal epithelium is recommended.[1] A well-differentiated adenocarcinoma is composed of well-formed glands or papillae, usually lined by mature cells of either absorptive or goblet cell type. A moderately differentiated carcinoma is characterized by the presence of irregularly branching glands or complex and incomplete papillae. Poorly differentiated carcinomas are formed of ill-formed glands or single infiltrative cells.

On the premise of providing additional prognostic information, several additional classifications have been developed. Ming's two-tiered classification is based on the pattern of growth and invasiveness of the carcinomas.[123] The expanding-type carcinomas represent 67% of gastric cancers and grow by expansion of cohesive tumor masses with a well-defined interface with the stroma (Fig. 17-19**A**). The infiltrative-type carcinomas are char-

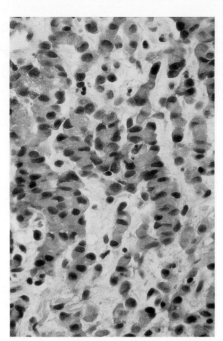

FIGURE 17–18. Mucin-poor, deeply eosinophilic variant of diffuse-type gastric carcinoma forming irregular cords.

acterized by single infiltrative cells, growing independently or aggregated in small nests (Fig. 17-19**B**). Expanding adenocarcinomas are characteristically well-differentiated intestinal-type tumors that have a better prognosis than the infiltrative carcinomas, which are usually composed of diffuse-type adenocarcinomas.[3]

Goseki presented a four-tiered classification based on the degree of tubular differentiation and the amount of mucus production.[124] Retrospective studies have claimed that this scheme provides a more accurate prognosis of advanced gastric adenocarcinomas when added to the TNM system.[125,126]

MORPHOLOGIC SUBTYPES OF GASTRIC ADENOCARCINOMA

Uncommon histologic variants represent about 5% of gastric cancers and include the following subtypes.

Gastric Carcinoma with Lymphoid Stroma

This variety, also reported as medullary carcinoma or lymphoepithelioma-like carcinoma, is characterized by a prominent lymphoid infiltration of the stroma. More than 80% of gastric carcinoma with lymphoid stroma (GCLS) has been associated with Epstein-Barr virus (EBV) infection.[127] When EBV-infected gastric cancer of usual histology is excluded, GCLS represents about 8% of gastric carcinomas.[128,129] GCLS seems to affect males more frequently; in the United States, Hispanics also seem to be preferentially affected.[130,131] The lesions are more common in the proximal stomach and in the gastric remnants.[132,133] GCLS usually has a pushing growth interface and is composed of irregular sheets or syncytia of small polygonal cells, embedded in a prominent lymphocytic infiltrate with occasional lymphoid follicles (Fig. 17-20).[134] Rarely, giant cells are observed.[129] CD8 T lymphocytes form the predominant component of the infiltrate, although B lymphocytes and plasma cells are also present. Intranuclear expression of EBV-encoded nonpolyadenylated RNA-1 can be demonstrated by in situ hybridization. Whether EBV plays a direct role in carcinogenesis or is simply a secondary phenomenon is debated.[134] However, infection appears to occur early in the carcinogenic sequence because EBV can be found in the surrounding dysplastic epithelium.[135] The frequent loss of chromosomes 4p, 11p, and 18q seems to indicate a pathogenetic pathway different from that of usual gastric carcinoma.[128] It was also demonstrated that EBV-positive GCLS represents a CpG island

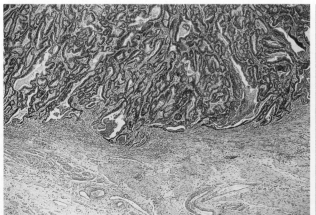 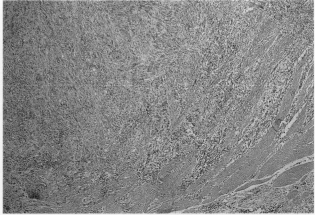

A   **B**

FIGURE 17–19. Ming's classification of gastric carcinoma. **A,** Expanding type, showing a distinct, advancing tumor front. **B,** Infiltrative type with irregular, invasive, single neoplastic cells.

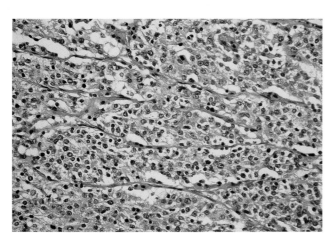

FIGURE 17–20. Gastric adenocarcinoma with lymphoid stroma. This type is composed of irregular sheets of small polygonal cells infiltrated by numerous lymphocytes.

methylator phenotype with frequent aberrant methylation of multiple genes.[136]

The prognosis of GCLS is reportedly better than that of ordinary type with up to 77% survival at 5 years, although this remains controversial.[3,132,137]

Hepatoid and Alpha-Fetoprotein–Producing Carcinomas

The reported incidence of these carcinomas varies from 1.3% to 15% of gastric cancers.[138] The recognition of two histologic types of alpha-fetoprotein–producing tumors may explain the wide variation in incidence. Hepatoid adenocarcinomas are composed of large polygonal cells with prominent eosinophilic cytoplasm resembling hepatocellular carcinoma.[139,140] Hepatoid areas are frequently interspersed within typical adenocarcinomas. Bile and PAS-positive and diastase-resistant intracytoplasmic eosinophilic globules can be seen. The second type is a well-differentiated papillary or tubular adenocarcinoma with clear cytoplasm.[141,142] Combination of both types can be seen. Immunohistochemical and histochemical staining and in situ hybridization have been shown to highlight albumin, alpha-fetoprotein, alpha-1-antichymotrypsin, and bile production.[48] A high level of alpha-fetoprotein can also be detected in the serum of these patients. This subtype is particularly aggressive; a 12% survival rate is reported at 5 years.[48]

Adenosquamous and Squamous Cell Carcinomas

Adenosquamous carcinomas, which account for 0.5% of gastric cancers, are tumors in which the squamous neoplastic component composes at least 25% of the carcinoma.[5] These tumors are usually deeply penetrating, are associated with lymphovascular invasion, and carry a

poor prognosis.[143] Pure squamous cell carcinomas represent between 0.04% and 0.09% of gastric carcinomas and affect men four times as often as women.[48,144,145] The degree of differentiation may vary from moderately differentiated with keratin pearl formation to poorly differentiated (Fig. 17-21). The histogenesis of this tumor is uncertain; the squamous component could arise from squamous metaplasia of adenocarcinomatous cells, from a focus of heterotopic squamous epithelium, or from multipotential stem cells.[144,146] In the cardia, the caudal extension of an esophageal squamous cell carcinoma should be excluded. Gastric squamous cell carcinomas are usually diagnosed at a late stage, and their prognosis is poor.[143,144,146]

Gastric Choriocarcinoma

Pure gastric choriocarcinomas are rare, and most cases demonstrate the combination of syncytiotrophoblastic and cytotrophoblastic elements with an otherwise variably differentiated adenocarcinoma (Fig. 17-22).[147] Yolk sac and hepatoid carcinoma components can also be seen.[148] This neoplasm is characterized by prominent necrosis and hemorrhage at the macroscopic and microscopic level.[149,150] Human chorionic gonadotropin can be detected by immunohistochemistry, and serum levels can be used as a marker of prognosis.[48] These tumors are frequently associated with disseminated hematogenous and lymphatic metastases and have a dismal prognosis.

Gastric Carcinosarcoma

Gastric carcinosarcomas are rare tumors composed of various proportions of adenocarcinomatous and sarcomatous elements. Sarcomatous elements can be composed of uncommitted cells or demonstrate light microscopic or immunohistochemical features of

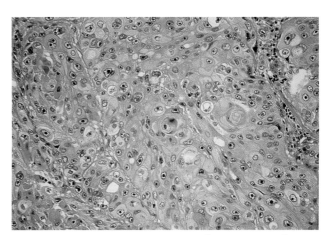

FIGURE 17–21. Gastric squamous cell carcinoma showing moderate differentiation.

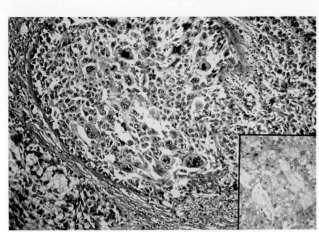

FIGURE 17-22. Gastric choriocarcinoma showing several multinucleated syncytiotrophoblasts. *Inset,* Positive β-HCG immunoreaction. (Courtesy of M. Shimizu, MD, Saitama Medical School, Japan.)

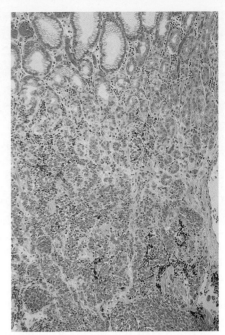

FIGURE 17-23. Gastric small cell carcinoma characterized by sheets and cords of small polygonal cells.

chondrosarcomatous, osteosarcomatous, rhabdomyosarcomatous, or leiomyosarcomatous differentiation.[97,151-153] Tumors with adenosquamous and neuroendocrine components have also been reported.[154,155] Most gastric carcinosarcomas are described as polypoid and associated with a poor outcome. A single case of gastric adenosarcoma, composed of benign tubular and cystic glands embedded in a leiomyosarcomatous stroma, has been reported.[156]

Gastric Small Cell Carcinoma

Approximately 50 cases of small cell carcinoma (oat cell carcinoma or neuroendocrine carcinoma) have been reported.[157] These tumors are frequently diagnosed at an advanced stage; the prognosis is poor, with most patients dying within 1 year of diagnosis.[158,159] Their morphology is reminiscent of their pulmonary counterpart with a sheet-like infiltrative growth pattern and frequent rosette-like arrangement and basal palisading (Fig. 17-23). Immunohistochemically, neuron-specific enolase and chromogranin A are often positive; electron microscopy demonstrates neurosecretory granules.[122,157]

Gastric Parietal Cell Carcinoma and Oncocytic Carcinoma

Fewer than 20 cases of parietal cell carcinoma have been reported. These tumors are composed of solid sheets of polygonal cells with abundant eosinophilic cytoplasm that stains with phosphotungstic acid–hematoxylin. Ultrastructural evaluation reveals abundant mitochondria and intracellular canaliculi.[160-163] It is suggested that they have a better prognosis than the usual gastric adenocarcinomas.[160] Ten cases of oncocytic adenocarcinoma, which are morphologically similar to

parietal cell carcinoma but negative for antiparietal cell antibodies, have been reported.[164]

Gastric Mucoepidermoid and Paneth Cell Carcinoma

Very few cases of these entities have been reported. Mucoepidermoid carcinomas show the typical admixture of mucus-producing and squamous epithelia.[165,166] One case has been shown to arise from submucosal ectopic glands.[165] The prognosis is reportedly poor. Paneth cell carcinomas are characterized by a predominance of Paneth cells characteristically showing eosinophilic cytoplasmic granules, which are positive for lysozyme by immunohistochemistry.[161,162]

Gastric Malignant Rhabdoid Tumor

Approximately 0.1% to 0.2% of gastric carcinomas show areas composed of poorly cohesive cells with round to polygonal nuclei, prominent nucleoli, and eosinophilic or clear cytoplasm.[167,168] These rhabdoid foci can show vimentin, cytokeratin, epithelial membrane antigen, and neuron-specific enolase positivity, but not CEA.[168,169] The prognosis of these tumors is dismal.

Gastric Metastatic Carcinomas

Metastases to the stomach are uncommon and variably reported in less than 2% to 5.4% in autopsy series of cancer patients.[170,171] They present either as large bleeding ulcers mimicking a primary carcinoma (39% of cases) or as submucosal tumors (51% of cases).[171] When diagnosed endoscopically, 65% of gastric metastases are solitary lesions. Malignant melanoma and lung and breast carcinomas are the most commonly recorded primaries.[171-173] However, primary tumors originating from kidney, pancreas, esophagus, and colon have also been reported.[170,171]

The infiltration of the deep layers of the gastric wall and the hyperplastic appearance of the overlying mucosa may mimic a benign hypertrophic gastritis. Submission of multiple deep biopsy specimens, adequate clinical history, and histology resembling the primary neoplasm help secure a correct diagnosis. Metastatic lobular breast carcinoma deserves special attention because its typical single-file growth pattern can mimic linitis plastica (Fig. 17-24). Immunohistochemical staining, such as GCDFP-15, estrogen receptor, and CK7 positivity and CK20 negativity, is useful in establishing the diagnosis.[174,175]

GASTRIC CARCINOMA IN THE SETTING OF SPECIAL CLINICAL CIRCUMSTANCES

Gastric Stump Carcinoma

Gastric surgery is associated with an increased risk for development of gastric cancer, usually after 15 to 25 years.[176,177] Male patients who undergo a Billroth II subtotal gastrectomy have a 3.3-fold higher incidence than in the general population; most carcinomas are diagnosed in the distal residual stomach and pref-

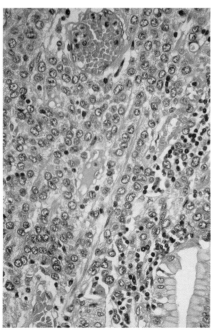

FIGURE 17–24. Metastatic lobular breast carcinoma to the stomach. Note the preservation of the typical single-file infiltrating pattern.

erentially involve the stoma.[178,179] However, dysplasia can be observed elsewhere in the residual pouch in up to 33% of patients.[179] Although similar to the usual gastric carcinomas with regard to morphology, stump carcinomas may follow a different carcinogenic process. Animal models suggest that enterogastric reflux of bile and pancreatic secretions may play an important role in the pathogenesis of these tumors.[180,181] Lesions of the remnant stomach that predate the development of cancer include intestinal metaplasia, atrophy, foveolar hyperplasia, and cystic dilatation of the glands on which dysplasia can develop.[182,183] However, the extent of intestinal metaplasia and *H. pylori* infection in the uninvolved mucosa is significantly reduced compared with usual gastric carcinomas.[179] With regard to operability, because the lymphatic flow has been modified during the initial surgery, the pattern of nodal metastases varies in comparison with primary gastric cancer, and an increased risk of hematogenic and liver metastases is noted.[184]

Gastric Carcinoma in Young Patients

Between 2% and 10% of gastric carcinomas are diagnosed in patients younger than 40 years.[185,186] The presenting symptoms are not different from those in older patients. Interestingly, an equal gender distribution and possibly even a female predominance have been reported.[168,185] Most of the cases are of diffuse type, and these tumors are not associated with intestinal metaplasia. However, *H. pylori* infection (particularly by *cagA*-positive bacteria) is thought to be a risk factor.[186,187] Approximately 10% to 25% of young patients with gastric cancer have a positive family history, suggesting that genetic factors are of etiologic importance.

GENETIC PREDISPOSITION AND HEREDITARY TUMOR SYNDROMES

Familial Diffuse Gastric Carcinoma

Germline mutations in the E-cadherin/*CDH1* gene represent the molecular basis for a familial gastric cancer syndrome.[188-191] In addition to a high susceptibility for development of diffuse gastric carcinoma, an increased risk for lobular breast carcinoma is reported.[190] The penetrance of the gene varies between 70% and 80%, and the average age for the diagnosis of cancer is 37 years.[192] Genetic counseling and testing for E-cadherin germline mutations are recommended for patients with a positive family history, and in such cases, prophylactic gastrectomy, which is associated with prolonged survival, should be considered.[193] Review of these surgical specimens may reveal in situ signet ring cell carcinomas.[193]

Hereditary Nonpolyposis Colorectal Cancer Syndrome

Gastric carcinoma, usually of the intestinal type, is frequent in patients with hereditary nonpolyposis colorectal cancer syndrome, accounting for 5% to 11% of all carcinomas.[194,195] An RER phenotype is noted in 65% of these cases.

Familial Adenomatous Polyposis Coli

Patients with familial adenomatous polyposis coli frequently develop multiple gastric polyps, most commonly fundic gland polyps, which have been shown to be neoplastic in nature with frequent somatic mutations of the *APC* gene.[196] However, the development of carcinoma in these lesions is rare.[44,197-199] Adenomas also arise in these patients but are much less common.

Li-Fraumeni Syndrome

Gastrointestinal tract tumors are relatively infrequent in this syndrome. However, among these patients, gastric carcinomas are more common than colon cancers.[200]

Peutz-Jeghers Syndrome

Patients afflicted with this syndrome develop Peutz-Jeghers polyps but also have an increased risk of gastric cancer. However, the role of germline mutations of the serine/threonine protein kinase STK11, found on chromosome 19p, is not clear.[201]

Hyperplastic Gastric Polyposis

This syndrome is characterized by hyperplastic gastric polyposis, severe psoriasis, and high incidence of gastric cancer of diffuse type.[202,203] It is inherited with an autosomal dominant pattern.

SPREAD, PATHOLOGIC STAGING, AND PROGNOSIS OF GASTRIC ADENOCARCINOMA

Gastric adenocarcinomas can spread by direct extension, metastasis, or peritoneal dissemination. Well-differentiated tumors with an intestinal phenotype preferentially disseminate by liver metastasis; the diffuse carcinomas are more likely to present with peritoneal seeding.[204,205] Carcinomas that display both intestinal and diffuse components have the metastatic abilities of each and have a worse prognosis.[206]

The anatomic spread of gastric cancer (i.e., stage, with special reference to extension to the serosa and lymph nodes) remains the strongest prognostic indicator of this disease. For example, the 5-year survival for carcinoma extending into the muscularis propria is 60% to 80%, but that drops to 50% with serosal involvement.[207] Thus, thorough gross and microscopic examination and ultimately accurate staging are cardinal features of pathologic examination of gastrectomy specimens (Table 17-4). Importantly, the N classification

TABLE 17–4. AJCC TNM Classification of Stomach Carcinomas

Primary Tumor (T)

TX	Primary tumor cannot be assessed
T0	No evidence of primary tumor
Tis	Carcinoma in situ: intraepithelial tumor without invasion of the lamina propria
T1	Tumor invades lamina propria or submucosa
T2	Tumor invades muscularis propria or subserosa*
	T2a Tumor invades muscularis propria
	T2b Tumor invades subserosa
T3	Tumor penetrates serosa (visceral peritoneum) without invasion of adjacent structures**, ***
T4	Tumor invades adjacent structures**, ***

*Note: A tumor may penetrate the muscularis propria with extension into the gastrocolic or gastrohepatic ligaments, or into the greater or lesser omentum, without perforation of the visceral peritoneum covering these structures. In this case, the tumor is classified T2. If there is perforation of the visceral peritoneum covering the gastric ligaments or the omentum, the tumor should be classified T3.
**Note: The adjacent structures of the stomach include the spleen, transverse colon, liver, diaphragm, pancreas, abdominal wall, adrenal gland, kidney, small intestine, and retroperitoneum.
***Note: Intramural extension to the duodenum or esophagus is classified by the depth of the greatest invasion in any of these sites, including the stomach.

Regional Lymph Nodes (N)

NX	Regional lymph node(s) cannot be assessed
N0	No regional lymph node metastasis*
N1	Metastasis in 1 to 6 regional lymph nodes
N2	Metastasis in 7 to 15 regional lymph nodes
N3	Metastasis in more than 15 regional lymph nodes

*Note: A designation of pN0 should be used if all examined lymph nodes are negative, regardless of the total number removed and examined.

Distant Metastasis (M)

MX	Distant metastasis cannot be assessed
M0	No distant metastasis
M1	Distant metastasis

Stage Grouping

Stage 0	Tis	N0	M0
Stage IA	T1	N0	M0
Stage IB	T1	N1	M0
	T2a/b	N0	M0
Stage II	T1	N2	M0
	T2a/b	N1	M0
	T3	N0	M0
Stage IIIA	T2a/b	N2	M0
	T3	N1	M0
	T4	N0	M0
Stage IIIB	T3	N2	M0
Stage IV	T4	N1-3	M0
	T1-3	N3	M0
	Any T	Any N	M1

Used with the permission of the American Joint Committee on Cancer (AJCC), Chicago, Illinois. The original source for this material is the *AJCC Cancer Staging Manual*, Sixth Edition (2002) published by Springer-Verlag New York, www.springer-ny.com.

TABLE 17–5. Genetic Alterations in Gastric Carcinomas and Their Relative Frequency

Genes and Alterations	Well Differentiated	Poorly Differentiated
Telomerase activity	+++	+++
CD44 (abnormal transcript)	+++	+++
TGFA (overexpression)	++	++
DNA repair error	++	++
TP53 (LOH, mutation)	++	++
Beta-catenin (mutation)	+	++
TP16 (reduced expression)	++	+
c-met (amplification)	+	++
VEGF (overexpression)	++	+
EGF (overexpression)	++	+
EGFR (overexpression)	++	+
APC (LOH, mutation)	++	+
DCC (LOH)	++	
BCL2 (LOH)	++	
E-cadherin/CDH1 gene (mutation)		++
K-ras (mutation)	+	+
Cyclin E (amplification)	+	+
c-erbB-2 (amplification)	+	

The number of crosses defines the relative frequency, from + (infrequent) to +++ (very common genetic alteration).

has been revised: a minimum of 15 nodes is required for appropriate staging.[208-210]

The prognosis of advanced adenocarcinomas is poor. The overall survival at 1 year after diagnosis is 63%, and the 5-year survival ranges from 26% to 35% after curative resection.[211] The 10-year relative survival is about 10%. Whether distal adenocarcinomas have a better prognosis compared with carcinomas of the middle third of the stomach is debated.[109,212] After surgery, survival at 5 years for distal carcinomas is 76%, 53%, and 26% for T1, T2, and T3 tumors, respectively. Lymph node status may be the single best indicator of prognosis; for pN1 tumors, the 5-year survival rate is 40%, which drops to 31% for pN2 tumors and 11% for pN3.[212,213] A survival advantage has been associated with female gender and Japanese ethnicity.[109] In addition, variation in tumor location, greater frequency of early-stage carcinomas, and more accurate staging seem to explain the improved survival in Japanese medical centers.[212]

MOLECULAR PATHOLOGY OF GASTRIC EPITHELIAL NEOPLASIA

Genetic alterations responsible for deregulation of cellular proliferation, adhesion, differentiation, signal transduction, and DNA repair play important roles in the development and progression of gastric cancer.[214-218] Although most of the catalogued genetic alterations that have been reported are observed in both intestinal and diffuse types of gastric cancer, it has become apparent that these two histologic subtypes result from different genetic pathways. A thorough review of this extensive subject is beyond the scope of this chapter; however, the major genetic alterations and how they relate to both histologic subtypes are summarized in Table 17-5.

References

1. Fenoglio-Preiser C, Carneiro F, Correa P, et al: Tumours of the stomach. In Hamilton SR, Aaltonen LA (eds): World Health Organization Classification of Tumours: Pathology and Genetics of Tumours of the Digestive System. Lyon, France, IARC Press, 2000, pp 37-52.
3. Lewin KJ, Appleman HD: Carcinoma of the Stomach. Tumors of the Esophagus and Stomach. Atlas of Tumor Pathology, Third Series, Fascicle 18. Washington, DC, Armed Forces Institute of Pathology, 1996, pp 245-330.
4. Blot WJ, Devesa SS, Kneller RW, et al: Rising incidence of adenocarcinoma of the esophagus and gastric cardia. JAMA 265:1287-1289, 1991.
5. Hisamichi S: Screening for gastric cancer. World J Surg 13:31-37, 1989.
6. Sue-Ling HM, Martin I, Griffith J, et al: Early gastric cancer: 46 cases treated in one surgical department. Gut 33:1318-1322, 1992.
7. Everett SM, Axon AT: Early gastric cancer in Europe. Gut 41:142-150, 1997.
8. Folli S, Dente M, Dell'Amore D, et al: Early gastric cancer: Prognostic factors in 223 patients. Br J Surg 82:952-956, 1995.
9. Correa P: Human gastric carcinogenesis: A multistep and multifactorial process—First American Cancer Society Award Lecture on Cancer Epidemiology and Prevention. Cancer Res 52:6735-6740, 1992.
10. Filipe MI, Munoz N, Matko I, et al: Intestinal metaplasia types and the risk of gastric cancer: A cohort study in Slovenia. Int J Cancer 57:324-329, 1994.
11. Hattori T, Sugihara H: The pathological sequence in the development of gastric cancer: I. Scand J Gastroenterol Suppl 214:34-35, 1996.
12. Parkin DM, Laara E, Muir CS: Estimates of the worldwide frequency of sixteen major cancers in 1980. Int J Cancer 41:184-197, 1988.
13. Correa P: A human model of gastric carcinogenesis. Cancer Res 48:3554-3560, 1988.
14. Howson CP, Hiyama T, Wynder EL: The decline in gastric cancer: Epidemiology of an unplanned triumph. Epidemiol Rev 8:1-27, 1986.
15. Siurala M, Sipponen P, Kekki M: Chronic gastritis: Dynamic and clinical aspects. Scand J Gastroenterol Suppl 109:69-76, 1985.
16. Kuipers EJ, Uyterlinde AM, Pena AS, et al: Long-term sequelae of Helicobacter pylori gastritis. Lancet 345:1525-1528, 1995.
17. Forman D, Newell DG, Fullerton F, et al: Association between infection with Helicobacter pylori and risk of gastric cancer: Evidence from a prospective investigation. BMJ 302:1302-1305, 1991.
18. Nomura A, Stemmermann GN, Chyou PH, et al: Helicobacter pylori infection and gastric carcinoma among Japanese Americans in Hawaii. N Engl J Med 325:1132-1136, 1991.
19. Parsonnet J, Friedman GD, Vandersteen DP, et al: Helicobacter pylori infection and the risk of gastric carcinoma. N Engl J Med 325:1127-1131, 1991.
20. Klinkenberg-Knol EC, Nelis F, Dent J, et al: Long-term omeprazole treatment in resistant gastroesophageal reflux disease: Efficacy, safety, and influence on gastric mucosa. Gastroenterology 118:661-669, 2000.
21. Beales IL, Davey NJ, Pusey CD, et al: Long-term sequelae of Helicobacter pylori gastritis. Lancet 346:381-382, 1995.
22. Goodman KJ: Nutritional factors and Helicobacter pylori infection in Colombian children. J Pediatr Gastroenterol Nutr 25:507-515, 1997.
23. Correa P: Diet modification and gastric cancer prevention. J Natl Cancer Inst Monogr 12:75-78, 1992.
24. Kikugawa K, Kato T, Takeda Y: Formation of a highly mutagenic diazo compound from the bamethan-nitrite reaction. Mutat Res 177:35-43, 1987.

25. Mirvish SS, Grandjean AC, Moller H, et al: *N*-Nitrosoproline excretion by rural Nebraskans drinking water of varied nitrate content. Cancer Epidemiol Biomarkers Prev 1:455-461, 1992.

26. Houghton PW, Mortensen NJ, Thomas WE, et al: Intragastric bile acids and histological changes in gastric mucosa. Br J Surg 73:354-356, 1986.

27. El-Omar EM: The importance of interleukin 1beta in *Helicobacter pylori* associated disease. Gut 48:743-747, 2001.

28. Munoz N, Matko I: Histological types of gastric cancer and its relationship with intestinal metaplasia. Recent Results Cancer Res 39:99-105, 1972.

29. Nomizu T, Watanabe I: Clinical investigation of familial clustering of cancer [in Japanese]. Gan No Rinsho 32:485-492, 1986.

30. Cristofaro G, Lynch HT, Caruso ML, et al: New phenotypic aspects in a family with Lynch syndrome II. Cancer 60:51-58, 1987.

31. Lauwers GY, Riddell RH: Gastric epithelial dysplasia. Gut 45:784-790, 1999.

32. Oehlert W, Keller P, Henke M, et al: Gastric mucosal dysplasia: What is its clinical significance? Front Gastrointest Res 4:173-182, 1979.

33. Zhang Y: Typing and grading of gastric dysplasia. In Zhang Y, Kawai K (eds): Precancerous Conditions and Lesions of the Stomach. Berlin, Springer-Verlag, 1993, pp 64-84.

34. Serck-Hanssen A: Precancerous lesions of the stomach. Scand J Gastroenterol 14:104-109, 1979.

35. Camilleri JP, Potet F, Amat C, et al: Gastric mucosal dysplasia: Preliminary results of a prospective study of patients followed for periods of up to six years. In Ming SC (ed): Precursors of Gastric Cancer. New York, Praeger, 1984, pp 83-92.

36. Farinati F, Rugge M, Di Mario F, et al: Early and advanced gastric cancer in the follow-up of moderate and severe gastric dysplasia patients. A prospective study. I.G.G.E.D. Interdisciplinary Group on Gastric Epithelial Dysplasia. Endoscopy 25:261-264, 1993.

37. Bearzi I, Brancorsini D, Santinelli A, et al: Gastric dysplasia: A ten-year follow-up study. Pathol Res Pract 190:61-68, 1994.

38. Stockbrugger RW, Menon GG, Beilby JO, et al: Gastroscopic screening in 80 patients with pernicious anaemia. Gut 24:1141-1147, 1983.

39. Ectors N, Dixon MF: The prognostic value of sulphomucin positive intestinal metaplasia in the development of gastric cancer. Histopathology 10:1271-1277, 1986.

40. Ramesar KC, Sanders DS, Hopwood D: Limited value of type III intestinal metaplasia in predicting risk of gastric carcinoma. J Clin Pathol 40:1287-1290, 1987.

41. Sano R: Pathological analysis of 300 cases of early gastric cancer with special reference to cancer associated to ulcer. Jpn J Cancer Res 11:81-89, 1971.

42. Iida M, Yao T, Itoh H, et al: Natural history of gastric adenomas in patients with familial adenomatosis coli/Gardner's syndrome. Cancer 61:605-611, 1988.

43. Domizio P, Talbot IC, Spigelman AD, et al: Upper gastrointestinal pathology in familial adenomatous polyposis: Results from a prospective study of 102 patients. J Clin Pathol 43:738-743, 1990.

44. Zwick A, Munir M, Ryan CK, et al: Gastric adenocarcinoma and dysplasia in fundic gland polyps of a patient with attenuated adenomatous polyposis coli. Gastroenterology 113:659-663, 1997.

45. You WC, Blot WJ, Li JY, et al: Precancerous gastric lesions in a population at high risk of stomach cancer. Cancer Res 53:1317-1321, 1993.

46. Lansdown M, Quirke P, Dixon MF, et al: High-grade dysplasia of the gastric mucosa: A marker for gastric carcinoma. Gut 31:977-983, 1990.

47. Di Gregorio C, Morandi P, Fante R, et al: Gastric dysplasia. A follow-up study. Am J Gastroenterol 88:1714-1719, 1993.

48. Ming SC: Cellular and molecular pathology of gastric carcinoma and precursor lesions: A critical review. Gastric Cancer 1:31-50, 1998.

49. Fertitta AM, Comin U, Terruzzi V, et al: Clinical significance of gastric dysplasia: A multicenter follow-up study. Gastrointestinal Endoscopic Pathology Study Group. Endoscopy 25:265-268, 1993.

50. Rugge M, Farinati F, Baffa R, et al: Gastric epithelial dysplasia in the natural history of gastric cancer: A multicenter prospective follow-up study. Interdisciplinary Group on Gastric Epithelial Dysplasia. Gastroenterology 107:1288-1296, 1994.

51. Morson BC, Sobin LH, Grundmann E, et al: Precancerous conditions and epithelial dysplasia in the stomach. J Clin Pathol 33:711-721, 1980.

52. Cuello C, Lopez J, Correa P, et al: Histopathology of gastric dysplasias: Correlations with gastric juice chemistry. Am J Surg Pathol 3:491-500, 1979.

53. Jass JR: A classification of gastric dysplasia. Histopathology 7:181-193, 1983.

54. Ming SC, Bajtai A, Correa P, et al: Gastric dysplasia. Significance and pathologic criteria. Cancer 54:1794-1801, 1984.

55. Ming SC: Dysplasia of gastric epithelium. Front Gastrointest Res 4:164-172, 1979.

56. Morson BC, Jass JR: Precancerous lesions of the gastrointestinal tract. In Stomach. London, Baillière Tindall, 1985, pp 5-9.

57. Snover DC: Benign epithelial polyps of the stomach. Pathol Annu 20:303-329, 1985.

58. Orlowska J, Jarosz D, Pachlewski J, et al: Malignant transformation of benign epithelial gastric polyps. Am J Gastroenterol 90:2152-2159, 1995.

59. Nakamura T, Nakano G: Histopathological classification and malignant change in gastric polyps. J Clin Pathol 38:754-764, 1985.

60. Kamiya T, Morishita T, Asakura H, et al: Long-term follow-up study on gastric adenoma and its relation to gastric protruded carcinoma. Cancer 50:2496-2503, 1982.

61. Tomasulo J: Gastric polyps. Histologic types and their relationship to gastric carcinoma. Cancer 27:1346-1355, 1971.

62. Ghandur-Mnaymneh L, Paz J, Roldan E, et al: Dysplasia of nonmetaplastic gastric mucosa. A proposal for its classification and its possible relationship to diffuse-type gastric carcinoma. Am J Surg Pathol 12:96-114, 1988.

63. Grundmann E: Histologic types and possible initial stages in early gastric carcinoma. Beitr Pathol 154:256-280, 1975.

64. Furman J, Lauwers GY, Shimizu M: Gland neck dysplasia in diffuse gastric cancer: A morphometric study [abstract]. Mod Pathol 11:64A, 1998.

65. Antonioli DA: Precursors of gastric carcinoma: A critical review with a brief description of early (curable) gastric cancer. Hum Pathol 25:994-1005, 1994.

66. Lauwers GY, Shimizu M, Correa P, et al: Evaluation of gastric biopsies for neoplasia: Differences between Japanese and Western pathologists. Am J Surg Pathol 23:511-518, 1999.

67. Riddell RH, Goldman H, Ransohoff DF, et al: Dysplasia in inflammatory bowel disease: Standardized classification with provisional clinical applications. Hum Pathol 14:931-968, 1983.

68. Weinstein WM, Goldstein NS: Gastric dysplasia and its management. Gastroenterology 107:1543-1545, 1994.

69. Saraga EP, Gardiol D, Costa J: Gastric dysplasia. A histological follow-up study. Am J Surg Pathol 11:788-796, 1987.

70. Rugge M, Farinati F, Di Mario F, et al: Gastric epithelial dysplasia: A prospective multicenter follow-up study from the Interdisciplinary Group on Gastric Epithelial Dysplasia. Hum Pathol 22:1002-1008, 1991.

71. Ono H, Kondo H, Gotoda T, et al: Endoscopic mucosal resection for treatment of early gastric cancer. Gut 48:225-229, 2001.

72. Hiki Y, Shimao H, Mieno H, et al: Modified treatment of early gastric cancer: Evaluation of endoscopic treatment of early gastric cancers with respect to treatment indication groups. World J Surg 19:517-522, 1995.

73. Takeshita K, Tani M, Inoue H, et al: Endoscopic treatment of early oesophageal or gastric cancer. Gut 40:123-127, 1997.

74. Siewert JR, Stein HJ: Classification of adenocarcinoma of the oesophagogastric junction. Br J Surg 85:1457-1459, 1998.

75. Bosch A, Frias Z, Caldwell WL: Adenocarcinoma of the esophagus. Cancer 43:1557-1561, 1979.

76. Okabayashi T, Gotoda T, Kondo H, et al: Early carcinoma of the gastric cardia in Japan: Is it different from that in the West? Cancer 89:2555-2559, 2000.

77. Allum WH, Powell DJ, McConkey CC, et al: Gastric cancer: A 25-year review. Br J Surg 76:535-540, 1989.

78. Morales TG: Adenocarcinoma of the gastric cardia. Dig Dis 15:346-356, 1997.

79. Cameron AJ, Lomboy CT, Pera M, et al: Adenocarcinoma of the esophagogastric junction and Barrett's esophagus. Gastroenterology 109:1541-1546, 1995.

80. Wijnhoven BP, Siersema PD, Hop WC, et al: Adenocarcinomas of the distal oesophagus and gastric cardia are one clinical entity. Rotterdam Oesophageal Tumour Study Group. Br J Surg 86:529-535, 1999.

81. Clark GW, Smyrk TC, Burdiles P, et al: Is Barrett's metaplasia the source of adenocarcinomas of the cardia? Arch Surg 129:609-614, 1994.

82. Kalish RJ, Clancy PE, Orringer MB, et al: Clinical, epidemiologic, and morphologic comparison between adenocarcinomas arising in Barrett's esophageal mucosa and in the gastric cardia. Gastroenterology 86:461-467, 1984.

83. Brown LM, Swanson CA, Gridley G, et al: Adenocarcinoma of the esophagus: Role of obesity and diet. J Natl Cancer Inst 87:104-109, 1995.

84. Lagergren J, Bergstrom R, Nyren O: Association between body mass and adenocarcinoma of the esophagus and gastric cardia. Ann Intern Med 130:883-890, 1999.

85. Morales TG, Bhattacharyya A, Johnson C, et al: Is Barrett's esophagus associated with intestinal metaplasia of the gastric cardia? Am J Gastroenterol 92:1818-1822, 1997.

86. Chow WH, Blot WJ, Vaughan TL, et al: Body mass index and risk of adenocarcinomas of the esophagus and gastric cardia. J Natl Cancer Inst 90:150-155, 1998.

87. Hackelsberger A, Gunther T, Schultze V, et al: Intestinal metaplasia at the gastro-oesophageal junction: *Helicobacter pylori* gastritis or gastro-oesophageal reflux disease? Gut 43:17-21, 1998.

88. Sharma P, Weston AP, Morales T, et al: Relative risk of dysplasia for patients with intestinal metaplasia in the distal oesophagus and in the gastric cardia. Gut 46:9-13, 2000.

89. Trudgill NJ, Suvarna SK, Kapur KC, et al: Intestinal metaplasia at the squamocolumnar junction in patients attending for diagnostic gastroscopy. Gut 41:585-589, 1997.

90. Morales TG, Bhattacharyya A, Camargo E, et al: Methylene blue staining for intestinal metaplasia of the gastric cardia with follow-up for dysplasia. Gastrointest Endosc 48:26-31, 1998.

91. Goldstein NS, Karim R: Gastric cardia inflammation and intestinal metaplasia: Associations with reflux esophagitis and *Helicobacter pylori*. Mod Pathol 12:1017-1024, 1999.

92. Morales TG, Sampliner RE, Bhattacharyya A: Intestinal metaplasia of the gastric cardia. Am J Gastroenterol 92:414-418, 1997.

93. Ruol A, Parenti A, Zaninotto G, et al: Intestinal metaplasia is the probable common precursor of adenocarcinoma in Barrett esophagus and adenocarcinoma of the gastric cardia. Cancer 88:2520-2528, 2000.

94. Fujita S: Biology of early gastric carcinoma. Pathol Res Pract 163:297-309, 1978.

95. Tsukuma H, Mishima T, Oshima A: Prospective study of "early" gastric cancer. Int J Cancer 31:421-426, 1983.

96. Farley DR, Donohue JH: Early gastric cancer. Surg Clin North Am 72:401-421, 1992.

97. Ming SC, Hirota T: Malignant epithelial tumors of the stomach. In Ming SC, Goldman H (eds): Pathology of the Gastrointestinal Tract, 2nd ed. Baltimore, Williams & Wilkins, 1998.

98. Marrano D, Viti G, Grigioni W, et al: Synchronous and metachronous cancer of the stomach. Eur J Surg Oncol 13:493-498, 1987.

99. Japanese Research Society for Gastric Cancer. Group classification of gastric biopsy specimens. In Nishi M, Omori Y, Miwa K (eds): Japanese Classification of Gastric Carcinoma. Tokyo, Kanehara, 1995, pp 74-76.

100. Xuan ZX, Ueyama T, Yao T, et al: Time trends of early gastric carcinoma. A clinicopathologic analysis of 2846 cases. Cancer 72:2889-2894, 1993.

101. Kurihara M, Shirakabe H, Yarita T, et al: Diagnosis of small early gastric cancer by X-ray, endoscopy, and biopsy. Cancer Detect Prev 4:377-383, 1981.

102. Kobayashi S, Kasugai T, Yamazaki H: Endoscopic differentiation of early gastric cancer from benign peptic ulcer. Gastrointest Endosc 25:55-57, 1979.

103. Blackstone MO: Endoscopic Interpretation: Normal and Pathologic Appearance of the Gastrointestinal Tract. New York, Raven Press, 1984.

104. Kodama Y, Inokuchi K, Soejima K, et al: Growth patterns and prognosis in early gastric carcinoma. Superficially spreading and penetrating growth types. Cancer 51:320-326, 1983.

105. Oohara T, Tohma H, Takezoe K, et al: Minute gastric cancers less than 5 mm in diameter. Cancer 50:801-810, 1982.

106. Itoh H, Oohata Y, Nakamura K, et al: Complete ten-year post-gastrectomy follow-up of early gastric cancer. Am J Surg 158:14-16, 1989.

107. Maehara Y, Orita H, Okuyama T, et al: Predictors of lymph node metastasis in early gastric cancer. Br J Surg 79:245-247, 1992.

108. Yasuda K, Shiraishi N, Suematsu T, et al: Rate of detection of lymph node metastasis is correlated with the depth of submucosal invasion in early stage gastric carcinoma. Cancer 85:2119-2123, 1999.

109. Hundahl SA, Phillips JL, Menck HR: The National Cancer Data Base Report on poor survival of U.S. gastric carcinoma patients treated with gastrectomy: Fifth Edition American Joint Committee on Cancer staging, proximal disease, and the "different disease" hypothesis. Cancer 88:921-932, 2000.

110. Kodera Y, Yamamura Y, Torii A, et al: Incidence, diagnosis and significance of multiple gastric cancer. Br J Surg 82:1540-1543, 1995.

111. Borrmann R: Geshwulste des Magens und Duodenums. In Henke F, Lubarsch O (eds): Handbuch des speziellen Pathologischen Anatomie und Histologie, vol 4. Berlin, Springer-Verlag, 1926, p 865.

112. Fiocca R, Villani L, Tenti P, et al: The foveolar cell component of gastric cancer. Hum Pathol 21:260-270, 1990.

113. Fiocca R, Villani L, Tenti P, et al: Characterization of four main cell types in gastric cancer: Foveolar, mucopeptic, intestinal columnar and goblet cells. An histopathologic, histochemical and ultra-structural study of "early" and "advanced" tumours. Pathol Res Pract 182:308-325, 1987.

114. Chan WY, Hui PK, Leung KM, et al: Gastric adenocarcinoma with ciliated tumor cells. Hum Pathol 24:1107-1113, 1993.

115. Endoh Y, Tamura G, Motoyama T, et al: Well-differentiated adenocarcinoma mimicking complete-type intestinal metaplasia in the stomach. Hum Pathol 30:826-832, 1999.

116. Machado JC, Nogueira AM, Carneiro F, et al: Gastric carcinoma exhibits distinct types of cell differentiation: An immunohisto-chemical study of trefoil peptides (TFF1 and TFF2) and mucins (MUC1, MUC2, MUC5AC, and MUC6). J Pathol 190:437-443, 2000.

117. Laurén P: The two histological main types of gastric carcinoma: Diffuse and so-called intestinal type carcinoma. An attempt at a histo-clinical classification. Acta Pathol Microbiol Scand 64:31-49, 1965.

117a. Cimerman M, Repse S, Jelenc F, et al: Comparison of Laurén's, Ming's and WHO histological classifications of gastric cancer as a prognostic factor for operated patients. Int J Surg 79:27-32, 1994.

118. Uefuji K, Ichikura T, Tamakuma S: Clinical and prognostic characteristics of papillary clear carcinoma of stomach. Surg Today 26:158-163, 1996.

119. Yasuda K, Adachi Y, Shiraishi N, et al: Papillary adenocarcinoma of the stomach. Gastric Cancer 3:33-38, 2000.

120. Hirota T, Itabashi M, Maruyama K: Significance of the histological type of gastric carcinoma as a prognostic factor. Stomach Intestine 26:1149-1158, 1991.

121. Correa P, Tahara E: Pathology of Incipient Neoplasia, 2nd ed. Philadelphia, WB Saunders, 1993.

122. Murayama H, Imai T, Kikuchi M: Solid carcinomas of the stomach. A combined histochemical, light and electron microscopic study. Cancer 51:1673-1681, 1983.

123. Ming SC: Gastric carcinoma. A pathobiological classification. Cancer 39:2475-2485, 1977.

124. Goseki N, Takizawa T, Koike M: Differences in the mode of the extension of gastric cancer classified by histological type: New histological classification of gastric carcinoma. Gut 33:606-612, 1992.

125. Martin IG, Dixon MF, Sue-Ling H, et al: Goseki histological grading of gastric cancer is an important predictor of outcome. Gut 35:758-763, 1994.

126. Songun I, van de Velde CJ, Arends JW, et al: Classification of gastric carcinoma using the Goseki system provides prognostic information additional to TNM staging. Cancer 85:2114-2118, 1999.

127. Matsunou H, Konishi F, Hori H, et al: Characteristics of Epstein-Barr virus–associated gastric carcinoma with lymphoid stroma in Japan. Cancer 77:1998-2004, 1996.

128. zur Hausen A, van Grieken NC, Meijer GA, et al: Distinct chromosomal aberrations in Epstein-Barr virus–carrying gastric carcinomas tested by comparative genomic hybridization. Gastroenterology 121:612-618, 2001.

129. Herrera-Goepfert R, Reyes E, Hernandez-Avila M, et al: Epstein-Barr virus–associated gastric carcinoma in Mexico: Analysis of 135 consecutive gastrectomies in two hospitals. Mod Pathol 12:873-878, 1999.

130. Watanabe H, Enjoji M, Imai T: Gastric carcinoma with lymphoid stroma. Its morphologic characteristics and prognostic correlations. Cancer 38:232-243, 1976.

131. Wang HH, Wu MS, Shun CT, et al: Lymphoepithelioma-like carcinoma of the stomach: A subset of gastric carcinoma with distinct clinicopathological features and high prevalence of Epstein-Barr virus infection. Hepatogastroenterology 46:1214-1219, 1999.

132. Nakamura S, Ueki T, Yao T, et al: Epstein-Barr virus in gastric carcinoma with lymphoid stroma. Special reference to its detection by the polymerase chain reaction and in situ hybridization in 99 tumors, including a morphologic analysis. Cancer 73:2239-2249, 1994.

133. Yamamoto N, Tokunaga M, Uemura Y, et al: Epstein-Barr virus and gastric remnant cancer. Cancer 74:805-809, 1994.

134. Fukayama M, Chong JM, Kaizaki Y: Epstein-Barr virus and gastric carcinoma. Gastric Cancer 1:104-111, 1998.

135. Gulley ML, Pulitzer DR, Eagan PA, et al: Epstein-Barr virus infection is an early event in gastric carcinogenesis and is independent of bcl-2 expression and p53 accumulation. Hum Pathol 27:20-27, 1996.

136. Kang GH, Lee S, Kim WH, et al: Epstein-Barr virus–positive gastric carcinoma demonstrates frequent aberrant methylation of multiple genes and constitutes CpG island methylator phenotype-positive gastric carcinoma. Am J Pathol 160:787-794, 2002.

137. dos Santos NR, Seruca R, Constancia M, et al: Microsatellite instability at multiple loci in gastric carcinoma: Clinicopathologic implications and prognosis. Gastroenterology 110:38-44, 1996.

138. Inagawa S, Shimazaki J, Hori M, et al: Hepatoid adenocarcinoma of the stomach. Gastric Cancer 4:43-52, 2001.

139. Ishikura H, Kirimoto K, Shamoto M, et al: Hepatoid adenocarcinomas of the stomach. An analysis of seven cases. Cancer 58:119-126, 1986.

140. Motoyama T, Aizawa K, Watanabe H, et al: Alpha-fetoprotein producing gastric carcinomas: A comparative study of three different subtypes. Acta Pathol Jpn 43:654-661, 1993.

141. Kodama T, Kameya T, Hirota T, et al: Production of alpha-fetoprotein, normal serum proteins, and human chorionic gonadotropin in stomach cancer: Histologic and immunohistochemical analyses of 35 cases. Cancer 48:1647-1655, 1981.

142. Nagai E, Ueyama T, Yao T, et al: Hepatoid adenocarcinoma of the stomach. A clinicopathologic and immunohistochemical analysis. Cancer 72:1827-1835, 1993.

143. Mori M, Iwashita A, Enjoji M: Adenosquamous carcinoma of the stomach. A clinicopathologic analysis of 28 cases. Cancer 57:333-339, 1986.

144. Marubashi S, Yano H, Monden T, et al: Primary squamous cell carcinoma of the stomach. Gastric Cancer 2:136-141, 1999.

145. Won OH, Farman J, Krishnan MN, et al: Squamous cell carcinoma of the stomach. Am J Gastroenterol 69:594-598, 1978.

146. Yoshida K, Manabe T, Tsunoda T, et al: Early gastric cancer of adenosquamous carcinoma type: Report of a case and review of literature. Jpn J Clin Oncol 26:252-257, 1996.

147. Wurzel J, Brooks JJ: Primary gastric choriocarcinoma: Immunohistochemistry, postmortem documentation, and hormonal effects in a postmenopausal female. Cancer 48:2756-2761, 1981.

148. Garcia RL, Ghali VS: Gastric choriocarcinoma and yolk sac tumor in a man: Observations about its possible origin. Hum Pathol 16:955-958, 1985.

149. Saigo PE, Brigati DJ, Sternberg SS, et al: Primary gastric choriocarcinoma. An immunohistological study. Am J Surg Pathol 5:333-342, 1981.

150. Imai Y, Kawabe T, Takahashi M, et al: A case of primary gastric choriocarcinoma and a review of the Japanese literature. J Gastroenterol 29:642-646, 1994.

151. Cho KJ, Myong NH, Choi DW, et al: Carcinosarcoma of the stomach. A case report with light microscopic, immunohistochemical, and electron microscopic study. APMIS 98:991-995, 1990.

152. Schlemper RJ, Riddell RH, Kato Y, et al: The Vienna classification of gastrointestinal epithelial neoplasia. Gut 47:251-255, 2000.

153. Nakayama Y, Murayama H, Iwasaki H, et al: Gastric carcinosarcoma (sarcomatoid carcinoma) with rhabdomyoblastic and osteoblastic differentiation. Pathol Int 47:557-563, 1997.

154. Sato Y, Shimozono T, Kawano S, et al: Gastric carcinosarcoma, coexistence of adenosquamous carcinoma and rhabdomyosarcoma: A case report. Histopathology 39:543-544, 2001.

155. Tsuneyama K, Sasaki M, Sabit A, et al: A case report of gastric carcinosarcoma with rhabdomyosarcomatous and neuroendocrine differentiation. Pathol Res Pract 195:93-97, 1999.

156. Kallakury BV, Bui HX, delRosario A, et al: Primary gastric adenosarcoma. Arch Pathol Lab Med 117:299-301, 1993.

157. Matsubayashi H, Takagaki S, Otsubo T, et al: Advanced gastric glandular-endocrine cell carcinoma with 1-year survival after gastrectomy. Gastric Cancer 3:226-233, 2000.

158. Hussein AM, Otrakji CL, Hussein BT: Small cell carcinoma of the stomach. Case report and review of the literature. Dig Dis Sci 35:513-518, 1990.

159. Takaku H, Oka K, Naoi Y, et al: Primary advanced gastric small cell carcinoma: A case report and review of the literature. Am J Gastroenterol 94:1402-1404, 1999.

160. Byrne D, Holley MP, Cuschieri A: Parietal cell carcinoma of the stomach: Association with long-term survival after curative resection. Br J Cancer 58:85-87, 1988.

161. Kazzaz BA, Eulderink F: Paneth cell–rich carcinoma of the stomach. Histopathology 15:303-305, 1989.

162. Ooi A, Nakanishi I, Itoh T, et al: Predominant Paneth cell differentiation in an intestinal type gastric cancer. Pathol Res Pract 187:220-225, 1991.

163. Capella C, Frigerio B, Cornaggia M, et al: Gastric parietal cell carcinoma—a newly recognized entity: Light microscopic and ultrastructural features. Histopathology 8:813-824, 1984.

164. Takubo K, Honma N, Sawabe M, et al: Oncocytic adenocarcinoma of the stomach: Parietal cell carcinoma. Am J Surg Pathol 26:458-465, 2002.

165. Hayashi I, Muto Y, Fujii Y, et al: Mucoepidermoid carcinoma of the stomach. J Surg Oncol 34:94-99, 1987.

166. Cremer H, Joneleit V, Seyfarth KA, et al: Mucoepidermoid carcinoma of the stomach. Leber Magen Darm 15:148-151, 1985.

167. Rivera-Hueto F, Rios-Martin JJ, Dominguez-Triano R, et al: Early gastric stump carcinoma with rhabdoid features. Case report. Pathol Res Pract 195:841-846, 1999.

168. Ueyama T, Nagai E, Yao T, et al: Vimentin-positive gastric carcinomas with rhabdoid features. A clinicopathologic and immunohistochemical study. Am J Surg Pathol 17:813-819, 1993.

169. Pinto JA, Gonzalez Alfonso JE, Gonzalez L, et al: Well differentiated gastric adenocarcinoma with rhabdoid areas: A case report with immunohistochemical analysis. Pathol Res Pract 193:801-805, 1997.

170. Niederau C, Sobin LH: Secondary tumors of the stomach. In Hamilton SR, Aaltonen LA (eds): World Health Organization Classification of Tumours. Lyon, France, IARC Press, 2000, pp 66-67.

171. Oda I, Kondo H, Yamao T, et al: Metastatic tumors to the stomach: Analysis of 54 patients diagnosed at endoscopy and 347 autopsy cases. Endoscopy 33:507-510, 2001.

172. Green LK: Hematogenous metastases to the stomach. A review of 67 cases. Cancer 65:1596-1600, 1990.

173. Taal BG, Peterse H, Boot H: Clinical presentation, endoscopic features, and treatment of gastric metastases from breast carcinoma. Cancer 89:2214-2221, 2000.

174. Shimizu M, Matsumoto T, Hirokawa M, et al: Gastric metastasis from breast cancer: A pitfall in gastric biopsy specimens. Pathol Int 48:240-241, 1998.

175. Wang NP, Zee S, Zarbo RJ, et al: Coordinate expression of cytokeratins 7 and 20 defines unique subsets of carcinomas. Appl Immunohistochem 3:99-107, 1995.

176. Toftgaard C: Gastric cancer after peptic ulcer surgery. A historic prospective cohort investigation. Ann Surg 210:159-164, 1989.

177. Safatle-Ribeiro AV, Ribeiro U Jr, Reynolds JC, et al: Morphologic, histologic, and molecular similarities between adenocarcinomas arising in the gastric stump and the intact stomach. Cancer 78:2288-2299, 1996.

178. Safatle-Ribeiro AV, Ribeiro U Jr, Reynolds JC: Gastric stump cancer: What is the risk? Dig Dis 16:159-168, 1998.

179. MacDonald WC, Owen DA: Gastric carcinoma after surgical treatment of peptic ulcer: An analysis of morphologic features and a comparison with cancer in the nonoperated stomach. Cancer 91:1732-1738, 2001.

180. Taylor PR, Mason RC, Filipe MI, et al: Gastric carcinogenesis in the rat induced by duodenogastric reflux without carcinogens: Morphology, mucin histochemistry, polyamine metabolism, and labelling index. Gut 32:1447-1454, 1991.

181. Kaminishi M, Shimizu N, Yamaguchi H, et al: Different carcinogenesis in the gastric remnant after gastrectomy for gastric cancer. Cancer 77:1646-1653, 1996.

182. Offerhaus GJ, van de Stadt J, Huibregtse K, et al: The mucosa of the gastric remnant harboring malignancy. Histologic findings in the biopsy specimens of 504 asymptomatic patients 15 to 46 years after partial gastrectomy with emphasis on nonmalignant lesions. Cancer 64:698-703, 1989.

183. Stael von Holstein C, Hammar E, Eriksson S, et al: Clinical significance of dysplasia in gastric remnant biopsy specimens. Cancer 72:1532-1535, 1993.

184. Ikeguchi M, Kondou A, Shibata S, et al: Clinicopathologic differences between carcinoma in the gastric remnant stump after distal partial gastrectomy for benign gastroduodenal lesions and primary carcinoma in the upper third of the stomach. Cancer 73:15-21, 1994.

185. Koea JB, Karpeh MS, Brennan MF: Gastric cancer in young patients: Demographic, clinicopathological, and prognostic factors in 92 patients. Ann Surg Oncol 7:346-351, 2000.

186. Kokkola A, Sipponen P: Gastric carcinoma in young adults. Hepatogastroenterology 48:1552-1555, 2001.

187. Rugge M, Busatto G, Cassaro M, et al: Patients younger than 40 years with gastric carcinoma: *Helicobacter pylori* genotype and associated gastritis phenotype. Cancer 85:2506-2511, 1999.

188. Guilford P, Hopkins J, Harraway J, et al: E-cadherin germline mutations in familial gastric cancer. Nature 392:402-405, 1998.

189. Gayther SA, Gorringe KL, Ramus SJ, et al: Identification of germline E-cadherin mutations in gastric cancer families of European origin. Cancer Res 58:4086-4089, 1998.

190. Keller G, Vogelsang H, Becker I, et al: Diffuse type gastric and lobular breast carcinoma in a familial gastric cancer patient with an E-cadherin germline mutation. Am J Pathol 155:337-342, 1999.

191. Guilford PJ, Hopkins JB, Grady WM, et al: E-cadherin germline mutations define an inherited cancer syndrome dominated by diffuse gastric cancer. Hum Mutat 14:249-255, 1999.

192. Caldas C, Carneiro F, Lynch HT, et al: Familial gastric cancer: Overview and guidelines for management. J Med Genet 36:873-880, 1999.

193. Huntsman DG, Carneiro F, Lewis FR, et al: Early gastric cancer in young, asymptomatic carriers of germ-line E-cadherin mutations. N Engl J Med 344:1904-1909, 2001.

194. Aarnio M, Salovaara R, Aaltonen LA, et al: Features of gastric cancer in hereditary non-polyposis colorectal cancer syndrome. Int J Cancer 74:551-555, 1997.

195. Mecklin JP, Jarvinen HJ, Peltokallio P: Cancer family syndrome. Genetic analysis of 22 Finnish kindreds. Gastroenterology 90:328-333, 1986.

196. Abraham SC, Nobukawa B, Giardiello FM, et al: Fundic gland polyps in familial adenomatous polyposis: Neoplasms with frequent somatic adenomatous polyposis coli gene alterations. Am J Pathol 157:747-754, 2000.

197. Watanabe H, Enjoji M, Yao T, et al: Gastric lesions in familial adenomatosis coli: Their incidence and histologic analysis. Hum Pathol 9:269-283, 1978.

198. Offerhaus GJ, Entius MM, Giardiello FM: Upper gastrointestinal polyps in familial adenomatous polyposis. Hepatogastroenterology 46:667-669, 1999.

199. Hofgartner WT, Thorp M, Ramus MW, et al: Gastric adenocarcinoma associated with fundic gland polyps in a patient with attenuated familial adenomatous polyposis. Am J Gastroenterol 94:2275-2281, 1999.

200. Kleihues P, Schauble B, zur Hausen A, et al: Tumors associated with p53 germline mutations: A synopsis of 91 families. Am J Pathol 150:1-13, 1997.

201. Entius MM, Westerman AM, van Velthuysen ML, et al: Molecular and phenotypic markers of hamartomatous polyposis syndromes in the gastrointestinal tract. Hepatogastroenterology 46:661-666, 1999.

202. Carneiro F, David L, Seruca R, et al: Hyperplastic polyposis and diffuse carcinoma of the stomach. A study of a family. Cancer 72:323-329, 1993.

203. Seruca R, Carneiro F, Castedo S, et al: Familial gastric polyposis revisited. Autosomal dominant inheritance confirmed. Cancer Genet Cytogenet 53:97-100, 1991.

204. Mori M, Sakaguchi H, Akazawa K, et al: Correlation between metastatic site, histological type, and serum tumor markers of gastric carcinoma. Hum Pathol 26:504-508, 1995.

205. Esaki Y, Hirayama R, Hirokawa K: A comparison of patterns of metastasis in gastric cancer by histologic type and age. Cancer 65:2086-2090, 1990.

206. Carneiro F, Seixas M, Sobrinho-Simoes M: New elements for an updated classification of the carcinomas of the stomach. Pathol Res Pract 191:571-584, 1995.

207. Yoshikawa K, Maruyama K: Characteristics of gastric cancer invading to the proper muscle layer with special reference to mortality and cause of death. Jpn J Clin Oncol 15:499-503, 1985.

208. Hermanek P: The superiority of the new International Union Against Cancer and American Joint Committee on Cancer TNM staging of gastric cancer. Cancer 88:1763-1765, 2000.

209. Hermanek P, Altendorf-Hofmann A, Mansmann U, et al: Improvements in staging of gastric carcinoma from using the new edition of TNM classification. Eur J Surg Oncol 24:536-541, 1998.

210. Greene FL, Page DL, Fleming ID, et al (eds): AJCC Cancer Staging Manual, 6th ed. New York, Springer-Verlag, 2002.

211. Karpeh MS Jr, Brennan MF: Gastric carcinoma. Ann Surg Oncol 5:650-656, 1998.

212. Noguchi Y, Yoshikawa T, Tsuburaya A, et al: Is gastric carcinoma different between Japan and the United States? Cancer 89:2237-2246, 2000.

213. Roder JD, Bottcher K, Busch R, et al: Classification of regional lymph node metastasis from gastric carcinoma. German Gastric Cancer Study Group. Cancer 82:621-631, 1998.

214. Wright PA, Williams GT: Molecular biology and gastric carcinoma. Gut 34:145-147, 1993.

215. Tahara E: Genetic alterations in human gastrointestinal cancers. The application to molecular diagnosis. Cancer 75:1410-1417, 1995.

216. Correa P, Shiao YH: Phenotypic and genotypic events in gastric carcinogenesis. Cancer Res 54:1941s-1943s, 1994.

217. Stemmermann GN: Intestinal metaplasia of the stomach. A status report. Cancer 74:556-564, 1994.

218. Fuchs CS, Mayer RJ: Gastric carcinoma. N Engl J Med 333:32-41, 1995.

CHAPTER 18

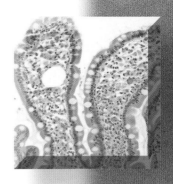

Epithelial Neoplasms of the Small Intestine

AMY NOFFSINGER

Epithelial neoplasms develop far less frequently in the small intestine than in the colon despite the fact that the small intestine has a large epithelial surface area and a high rate of cellular turnover. The reasons for the relative rarity of small bowel adenomas and carcinomas are still unknown, but a number of hypotheses exist to explain this finding.[1,2] First, the transit time of substances through the small intestine is relatively short compared with the colon, which leads to low contact time between the mucosa and the luminal contents. Second, unlike the colon, the small intestine does not contain a large quantity of bacteria. Bacteria are known to convert bile salts into potential carcinogens. Third, the luminal contents in the small intestine are more liquid compared with the colon. As a result, potentially carcinogenic luminal substances are more dilute, and the risk of mechanical trauma is reduced. Fourth, the small intestine is rich in lymphoid tissue, which provides a potentially high level of immunosurveillance against neoplastic cells. Fifth, mucosal enzymes may act to detoxify potentially carcinogenic substances that may be present in the luminal contents.[2]

Epithelial tumors in the small intestine are most commonly located in the duodenum and often in the vicinity of the ampulla of Vater.[3,4] This finding suggests that biliary or pancreatic secretions may play a role in their development, possibly as a result of a carcinogenic effect of bile. Alternatively, the constant influx of alkaline bile or acidic pancreatic juice may cause local cell damage. Epithelial neoplasms also occur in the jejunum and in the ileum less commonly.[5] A number of diseases predispose individual patients to the development of small intestinal adenomas and carcinomas, including familial adenomatous polyposis, Crohn's disease,[6] and gluten-sensitive enteropathy.[7-9] The risk for small intestinal carcinomas may also be increased in individuals with Peutz-Jeghers syndrome,[10,11] juvenile polyposis syndrome,[12,13] and long-standing ileostomies.[14,15]

Small intestinal epithelial tumors are most commonly glandular, although other forms of neoplasia may also arise. Table 18-1 summarizes the World Health Organization (WHO) histologic classification of epithelial tumors of the small intestine.[16]

Adenomatous Polyps

Small intestinal adenomas are rare,[17] accounting for less than 0.05% of all intestinal adenomas. Adenomas peak in incidence in the seventh decade of life but may occur at any age. Most adenomas are asymptomatic and are usually discovered incidentally in individuals who undergo endoscopic examination for other reasons. Adenomas that are symptomatic typically involve the region of the ampulla of Vater and present with biliary colic and obstruction, acute cholangitis, or pancreatitis.[17] Intestinal obstruction, bleeding, nausea, vomiting, anorexia, weight loss, pain, or intussusception may also develop, depending on the size and location of the lesion.

Small intestinal adenomas resemble those that arise in the colon in both their gross and microscopic characteristics (Fig. 18-1). They are usually lobulated and soft; they may be sessile or pedunculated, villous or tubular.

TABLE 18–1. WHO Classification of Epithelial Tumors of the Small Intestine

Adenoma
 Tubular
 Villous
 Tubulovillous
Intraepithelial neoplasia (dysplasia) associated with chronic
  inflammatory diseases
  Low-grade glandular intraepithelial neoplasia (dysplasia)
  High-grade glandular intraepithelial neoplasia (dysplasia)
Carcinoma
 Adenocarcinoma
 Mucinous adenocarcinoma
 Signet ring cell carcinoma
 Small cell carcinoma
 Squamous cell carcinoma
 Adenosquamous carcinoma
 Medullary carcinoma
 Undifferentiated carcinoma
Carcinoid (well-differentiated endocrine neoplasm)
Mixed carcinoid-adenocarcinoma
Gangliocytic paraganglioma
Others

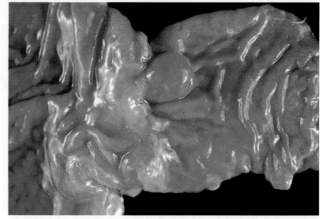

FIGURE 18–1. Duodenal adenoma. Gross photograph showing a pedunculated polypoid lesion projecting into the duodenal lumen. The head of the polyp is smooth and has a somewhat more erythematous appearance than the surrounding non-neoplastic mucosa.

A higher proportion of small intestinal lesions tend to be villous compared with lesions of the colon; this is most likely a reflection of the underlying villous architecture of the small bowel. Tubular adenomas tend to be small, varying in size from 0.5 to 3 cm in maximum diameter. Villous adenomas are often larger, sometimes reaching sizes of 8 cm or more. Small intestinal adenomas are usually single but can be multiple.[18,19] The finding of multiple adenomas in the small intestine is rare in patients without a hereditary polyposis syndrome. As a result, identification of multiple lesions should raise the suspicion of familial adenomatous polyposis (Fig. 18-2).

Histologically, small intestinal adenomas may demonstrate tubular, tubulovillous, or villous growth patterns. They are composed of tall columnar epithelial cells with elongated, crowded, hyperchromatic nuclei arranged in a "picket fence" pattern (Fig. 18-3). Immature goblet cells may be present. In addition, endocrine cells, squamous cells, and, particularly, Paneth cells may be numerous (see Fig. 18-3). Mitoses, normally seen only in the base of the crypts, may occur at all levels of the adenomatous crypts and villi. Normal-appearing lamina propria is usually present between the neoplastic crypts.

Small intestinal adenomas can display varying degrees of dysplasia ranging from low to high grade (carcinoma in situ) and may show intramucosal or invasive carcinoma. As the degree of dysplasia increases, one sees an increased nucleus-to-cytoplasm ratio of the cells, loss of

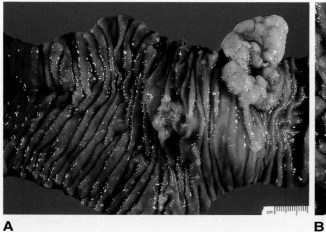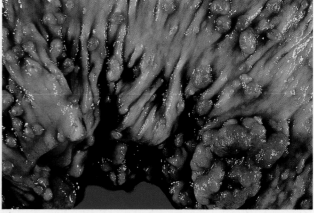

A **B**

FIGURE 18–2. A, Duodenal resection specimen from a patient with familial adenomatous polyposis. Multiple pedunculated and sessile polyps (adenomas) are present. The largest polypoid lesion represents an adenoma with invasive adenocarcinoma. **B,** The colon from the same patient shows multiple adenomatous polyps, as well as an invasive adenocarcinoma *(bottom right)*.

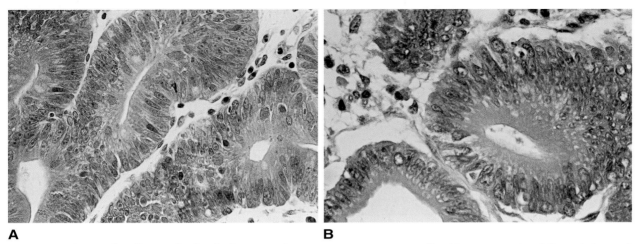

A   **B**

FIGURE 18–3. A, Paneth cells in a duodenal adenoma. Adenomatous crypts contain cells with coarse, eosinophilic, apical vacuoles characteristic of Paneth cells. **B,** This adenoma demonstrates the presence of large numbers of endocrine cells within the glands. These cells have finely granular, eosinophilic cytoplasm. In contrast to Paneth cells, the cytoplasmic granules of endocrine cells are less coarse and are present in a basal location.

cell polarity, and increased mitotic rate. Prominent crypt budding, nuclear stratification, and loss of mucinous differentiation may herald progression to malignancy.

It is important to distinguish regenerative atypia associated with surface erosion from an adenoma. Regenerating cells tend to mature to the surface, whereas adenomas do not. Furthermore, the presence of Paneth or endocrine cells in the superficial portions of the lesion is a finding associated with neoplastic alteration. Prominent acute inflammation with congested capillaries and fibrin deposition, especially when superficial, should alert the examiner to the possibility of regenerative atypia.

Adenomas in Polyposis Syndromes

Familial adenomatous polyposis (FAP) is associated with adenomatous polyps of the intestinal tract as well as with fundic gland polyps of the stomach. In the small intestine, most FAP-associated lesions arise in the duodenum and tend to cluster around the ampulla of Vater.[20-22] They are usually multiple and may be numerous (>20 to 50) in some patients.[23] They are often small, sessile, and tubular, measuring from less than 0.3 to 3 cm in diameter.[22] Ileal adenomas also occur in FAP patients[24] as well as in patients with the hereditary nonpolyposis colon cancer syndrome (HNPCC).[25]

FAP patients with multiple duodenal adenomas have a 100- to 300-fold increased lifetime risk for development of duodenal or periampullary cancer compared with the general population.[26,27] In fact, periampullary adenocarcinoma is the most common extracolonic malignant neoplasm in FAP. As a result, patients with known FAP should undergo endoscopic surveillance for

the purpose of biopsy of grossly normal duodenal and ampullary mucosa to identify early precancerous lesions.[28] Patients who have only a small number of adenomas should be screened every 3 years. In patients with numerous or large lesions, the screening interval should be shortened to 1 year.

Adenocarcinoma

CLINICAL FEATURES AND ASSOCIATIONS

More than half of small intestinal carcinomas arise in the duodenum, even though this organ constitutes only 4% of the entire length of the small intestine.[29] Most carcinomas arise in the region of the ampulla of Vater. A smaller percentage of tumors arise in the jejunum, particularly in the first 30 cm distal to the ligament of Treitz. Ileal carcinomas are the least common, except in patients with Crohn's disease. Small intestinal carcinomas occur more frequently in males than in females and affect blacks more often than whites.[3,30]

Some diseases (e.g., FAP) are associated with an increase in the incidence of small intestinal carcinomas (Table 18-2). Cancers that arise in the upper gastrointestinal tract, and especially in the periampullary region, represent a major cause of death in these patients. Patients with HNPCC also develop small intestinal tumors, often in the jejunum or ileum. Patients with Peutz-Jeghers syndrome demonstrate an approximately 2% risk for development of small intestinal adenocarcinoma, a risk that is less than that of patients with FAP but significantly higher than that seen in the general population.[31,32]

Patients with gluten-sensitive enteropathy have an 80-fold increased incidence of small intestinal adeno-

TABLE 18–2. Conditions Associated With an Increased Risk for Small Intestinal Carcinoma

Sporadic adenomatous polyps
Congenital anomalies
Long-standing ileostomy
Crohn's disease
Gluten-sensitive enteropathy
Alpha chain disease
Familial adenomatous polyposis
Gardner's syndrome
Peutz-Jeghers syndrome
Hereditary nonpolyposis colon cancer syndrome
 (Lynch syndrome)
Juvenile polyposis syndrome

carcinomas.[8] Tumors in these patients often arise in the jejunum.[33]

Ileal adenocarcinomas develop with increased frequency in individuals with long-standing Crohn's disease. However, in these patients, adenocarcinomas typically arise in the setting of dysplasia (flat or polypoid) rather than in preexisting adenomas.

Most small intestinal carcinomas present between 50 and 60 years of age. Tumors that arise in the setting of a hereditary cancer syndrome are generally seen in younger individuals. Patients may present with symptoms of intestinal obstruction, bleeding, intussusception, or perforation. Ampullary carcinomas often present with bile duct obstruction, pancreatitis, and jaundice. Pancreatitis may also develop secondary to pancreatic outflow obstruction.

PATHOLOGIC FEATURES

Small intestinal carcinomas may have a flat, stenotic, ulcerative, infiltrative, or polypoid gross appearance (Fig. 18-4). Tumors typically range from 1.2 to 15 cm in diameter. Larger lesions tend to occur in the more distal portions of the small bowel because lesions in this area often fail to produce symptoms until they are advanced.

Small intestinal adenocarcinomas are similar histologically to those that develop elsewhere in the gastrointestinal tract. However, because small intestinal cancers usually arise from preexisting adenomas, one may see residual adenomatous changes in the adjacent or overlying epithelium, particularly in smaller lesions. More often, the cancer has overgrown the adenomatous component at the time of diagnosis, especially in tumors that arise in sites other than at the ampulla of Vater. Identification of an associated preinvasive lesion allows one to be relatively certain that the tumor is primary to that location. However, some metastatic carcinomas induce significant cytologic atypia in adjacent nonneoplastic small intestinal epithelium that can resemble adenomatous change (Fig. 18-5).

Adenocarcinomas are characterized by cellular and nuclear pleomorphism, loss of epithelial polarity, a gland-in-gland architecture, and invasion into adjacent normal tissues. Most small intestinal adenocarcinomas are moderately differentiated and demonstrate variable degrees of mucin production. About 20% of tumors are poorly differentiated and contain signet ring cells. Other tumors display a prominent extracellular mucinous component. Neoplasms in which more than 50% of the tumor is mucinous should be designated mucinous adenocarcinoma because these tumors tend to have a poorer prognosis than more typical gland-forming lesions have. Neoplastic endocrine cells and Paneth cells are often present. Squamous cells may also be identified but are less common. The presence of endocrine, Paneth, or squamous cells in a carcinoma has no prognostic significance.

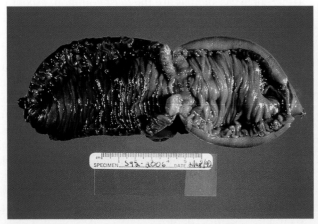

A

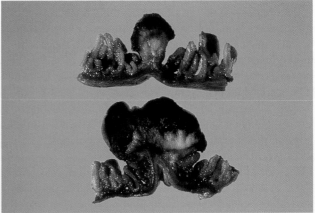

B

FIGURE 18–4. Gross appearance of intestinal adenocarcinoma. **A,** Jejunal resection specimen demonstrating a circumferential adenocarcinoma constricting the small intestinal lumen. **B,** Small intestinal adenocarcinoma demonstrating a polypoid growth pattern. The bulk of the tumor in this case is intraluminal.

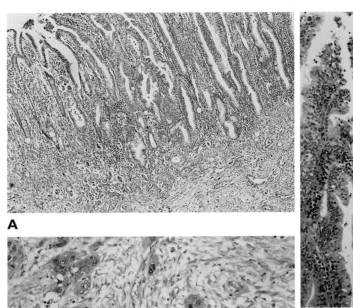

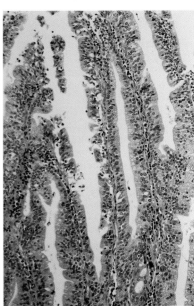

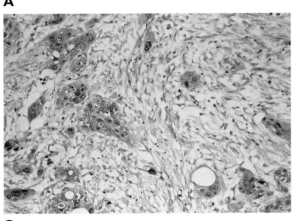

FIGURE 18–5. Metastatic pancreatic carcinoma in the small intestine. **A,** Low-power photomicrograph demonstrating infiltrating nests of cells within the muscularis mucosae and the submucosa. The epithelium within the overlying mucosa appears complex and irregular. **B,** High-power view of the mucosa overlying metastatic pancreatic carcinoma. The epithelium is lined by crowded, mucin-depleted cells with hyperchromatic, somewhat stratified nuclei. The histologic appearance is reminiscent of an adenomatous polyp. **C,** High-power view of metastatic pancreatic adenocarcinoma. Infiltrating clusters of highly atypical cells are present within the wall of the small intestine.

PROGNOSIS

The prognosis of small intestinal carcinomas is poor. This is primarily because patients are often asymptomatic until late in the course of the disease and metastases are often present at the time of diagnosis. Ampulla of Vater tumors generally do better than distal tumors,[34,35] presumably because they become symptomatic early and thus tend to be removed at a less advanced stage of growth. Other prognostic factors include tumor size, surgical resectability of the tumor,[36,37] presence of lymphatic or vascular invasion, depth of invasion into the bowel wall, and presence or absence of invasion into adjacent structures. The TNM staging system for small intestinal carcinoma is outlined in Table 18-3.

◼ Crohn's Disease–Associated Adenocarcinoma

CLINICAL FEATURES

Patients with Crohn's disease are at an increased risk for the development of carcinomas of the colon and small intestine.[38-40] The incidence of small intestinal carcinoma in Crohn's disease is 86-fold greater than that observed in the general population.[6] The cancer risk correlates positively with disease duration and the anatomic extent of the inflammatory process. Risk factors for development of small intestinal carcinoma in individuals with Crohn's disease include surgically excluded loops of small bowel, chronic fistulous disease, and male sex. The mortality in Crohn's disease–associated carcinoma is approximately 80%.

Unlike sporadic small intestinal carcinomas that commonly involve the duodenum, small intestinal carcinomas that develop in Crohn's disease arise in areas involved by inflammatory disease. Thirty percent of tumors arise in the jejunum, and 70% arise in the ileum.

PATHOLOGIC FEATURES OF DYSPLASIA
(see also Chapter 10)

It is now believed that dysplasia precedes cancer development in Crohn's disease, similar to ulcerative colitis.[41-43] However, the diagnosis of dysplasia is sometimes difficult because of recurrent and persistent inflammatory changes associated with the underlying inflammatory bowel disease. Grossly, dysplasia may appear flat or elevated (polypoid). Loss of the normal pattern of mucosal folds may be the only gross manifestation of dysplasia, although a granular or pebbly appearance is not uncommon. On occasion, plaques, nodules, and other irregular polypoid lesions may be identified.

Primary Tumor (T)

TX   Primary tumor cannot be assessed
T0   No evidence of primary tumor
Tis   Carcinoma in situ
T1   Tumor invades lamina propria or submucosa
T2   Tumor invades muscularis propria
T3   Tumor invades through the muscularis propria into the subserosa or nonperitonealized perimuscular tissue (mesentery or retroperitoneum) with extension 2 cm or less*
T4   Tumor perforates the visceral peritoneum or directly invades other organs or structures (includes other loops of small intestine, mesentery, or retroperitoneum more than 2 cm, and abdominal wall by way of serosa; for duodenum only, invasion of pancreas)

*Note: The nonperitonealized perimuscular tissue is, for jejunum and ileum, part of the mesentery and, for duodenum in areas where serosa is lacking, part of the retroperitoneum.

Regional Lymph Nodes (N)

NX   Regional lymph nodes cannot be assessed
N0   No regional lymph node metastasis
N1   Regional lymph node metastasis

Distant Metastasis (M)

MX   Distant metastasis cannot be assessed
M0   No distant metastasis
M1   Distant metastasis

Stage Grouping

Stage 0	Tis	N0	M0
Stage I	T1	N0	M0
	T2	N0	M0
Stage II	T3	N0	M0
	T4	N0	M0
Stage III	Any T	N1	M0
Stage IV	Any T	Any N	M1

Histologically, the diagnosis of dysplasia is based on identification of a combination of architectural and cytologic features.[44] Architectural alterations may result in a configuration that resembles adenomas. Cytologic abnormalities consist primarily of cellular and nuclear pleomorphism, nuclear hyperchromasia, loss of polarity, and nuclear stratification.

Dysplasia is generally classified as low or high grade (including carcinoma in situ). Although invasive carcinoma is more commonly observed in individuals with high-grade dysplasia, it may also be associated with lesser degrees of dysplasia. Low-grade dysplasia is characterized by the presence of tall epithelial cells with elongated hyperchromatic pseudostratified nuclei that fail to differentiate into normal goblet or absorptive cells at the mucosal surface (Fig. 18-6). Dystrophic goblet cells may also be present. In low-grade dysplasia, normal basal polarity of the nuclei is maintained. In contrast, high-grade dysplasia demonstrates true nuclear stratification and a greater degree of cytologic atypia (see Fig. 18-6). In high-grade dysplasia, the nuclei lose their polarity, and instead of being elongated with the long axis of the nucleus perpendicular to the basement membrane, the nuclei become round and develop prominent nucleoli. A type of epithelial alteration that shows elongation and increased tortuosity of hypermucinous epithelium has recently been described in association with Crohn's disease, but its significance is unknown.

PATHOLOGIC FEATURES OF ADENOCARCINOMA

Most carcinomas develop in areas of macroscopically identifiable inflammatory bowel disease. Grossly, they resemble ordinary, sporadic intestinal carcinomas.

Histologically, adenocarcinomas that arise in Crohn's disease resemble sporadic tumors. They may show any degree of differentiation, but in patients with

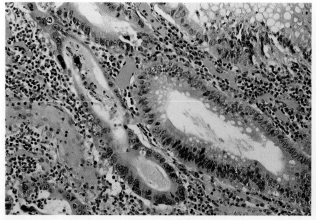
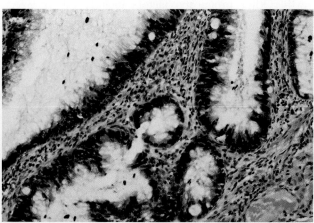

A   **B**

FIGURE 18–6. Dysplasia in Crohn's disease. **A,** Low-grade dysplasia is characterized by nuclear crowding, elongation, and pseudostratification. The epithelium appears similar to that found in adenomatous polyps. **B,** High-grade dysplasia shows more pronounced crowding, hyperchromasia, and loss of polarity and true stratification of the nuclei.

Crohn's disease, there is a higher proportion of poorly differentiated and mucinous tumors compared with the sporadic type.

DIFFERENTIAL DIAGNOSIS

In some cases, Crohn's disease–associated adenocarcinoma may be difficult to distinguish from pseudoinvasion, characterized by misplacement of epithelium in the submucosa or muscularis that develops as a result of recurrent injury, ulceration, and repair.[45] This represents a form of ileitis cystica profunda. Histologically, epithelial misplacement (pseudoinvasion) is characterized by mucus-filled cysts in the submucosa, muscularis propria, or serosa (Fig. 18-7). The cysts are lined by cuboidal to columnar epithelium containing goblet cells, enterocytes, and Paneth cells and are normally associated with a rim of lamina propria. On occasion, the cyst lining may regress from pressure atrophy. Features that help rule out malignancy include the absence of desmoplasia and the presence of a rim of lamina propria surrounding misplaced epithelium. Marked cytologic atypia, desmoplasia, and angular, irregularly shaped glands are characteristics of invasive adenocarcinoma (see Fig. 18-7).

In diagnostically difficult cases, careful sampling and evaluation of the surface epithelium may help resolve the diagnostic dilemma, particularly if dysplastic epithelium is present.

▨ Gluten-Sensitive Enteropathy–Associated Adenocarcinoma

The rate of development of small bowel malignant neoplasms among patients with gluten-sensitive enteropathy is increased 80-fold compared with the general population.[8,46] Adenocarcinoma of the

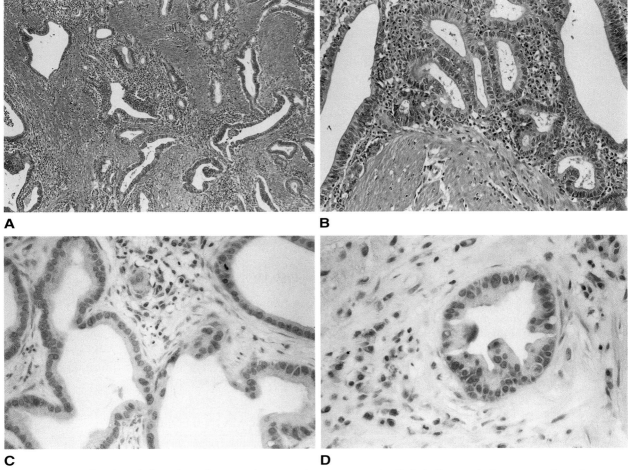

FIGURE 18–7. Misplaced epithelium (pseudoinvasion) versus adenocarcinoma in Crohn's disease. **A,** Low-power view of an area of epithelial misplacement in a patient with Crohn's disease. Irregular-appearing glands are present within the submucosa but are surrounded by a rim of lamina propria. No desmoplasia is noted. **B,** High-power view of misplaced glands surrounded by lamina propria. The glandular epithelium does not appear dysplastic. **C,** A focus of well-differentiated invasive adenocarcinoma from the same patient shown in **A** and **B**. The glands are not surrounded by lamina propria but instead are embedded in a desmoplastic stroma. Mild cytologic atypia is seen. **D,** Higher-power view shows a neoplastic gland surrounded by desmoplastic stroma.

duodenum and proximal jejunum is the most common nonlymphomatous type of malignancy associated with gluten-sensitive enteropathy and accounts for more than 20% of all small bowel malignant neoplasms in patients with this disorder.[46] The risk of cancer is highest after 2 years of disease. The tumors may be multifocal.[46-48] In fact, dysplasia similar to that seen in patients with Crohn's disease[49] may be associated with gluten-sensitive enteropathy adenocarcinomas as well.

Other Types of Carcinoma

HEPATOID CARCINOMA

Rarely, some ampullary cancers may display unusual histologic patterns or produce unusual proteins, such as alpha-fetoprotein (AFP). These tumors are usually moderately to poorly differentiated adenocarcinomas that resemble gastric AFP-producing hepatoid tumors.[50,51] Histologically, they demonstrate solid, papillary, and tubular growth patterns. Clear cell areas may also be present. Alpha-1-antitrypsin immunoreactive hyaline droplets and bile are often found in some cases.[50] In addition to hepatoid areas, one can usually see other areas of the tumor that show evidence of mucin production and other features of adenocarcinoma, such as CEA positivity. Immunohistochemistry for anti– alpha-chymotrypsin, prealbumin, transferrin, and AFP is positive at least focally in most cases.[51] Elevated AFP may also be detectable in the serum of affected patients.

CHORIOCARCINOMA

Primary choriocarcinomas have been reported in the small intestine but are extremely rare.[52,53] Grossly, these tumors often appear hemorrhagic and partially necrotic. Histologically, they are composed of aggregates of relatively uniform, eosinophilic cells with basophilic vesicular nuclei. Multinucleated syncytial cells with irregular cytoplasmic margins and bizarre, anaplastic nuclei are scattered among more uniform smaller cells. Cytotrophoblastic cells are also seen among the syncytial cells. Vascular invasion is often present. Small intestinal choriocarcinomas produce human chorionic gonadotropin and human placental lactogen, both of which can be documented by immunohistochemistry. The majority of reported cases of choriocarcinoma are associated with an adenocarcinoma or anaplastic large cell carcinoma, suggesting that these tumors may arise from multipotential stem cells. Before a diagnosis of primary intestinal choriocarcinoma is established, an ectopic pregnancy, teratoma, or metastatic disease

from an unrecognized primary tumor must be excluded.

SMALL CELL CARCINOMA

Small cell neuroendocrine carcinomas, similar to those in the lung or large intestine, may rarely arise in the small intestine.[54,55] Patients with small cell carcinoma are often elderly men in their fifth to eighth decades of life. These tumors are highly aggressive. Most patients die within 1 year of diagnosis.[55] Histologically, these tumors are composed of small anaplastic cells with hyperchromatic nuclei and scant cytoplasm. The cells form broad sheets, solid nests, and ribbon-like strands. They may resemble lymphoma, a tumor that statistically is much more common in the small intestine than small cell carcinoma. However, immunohistochemistry and special stains can usually help resolve this differential diagnosis. Small cell carcinomas display immunoreactivity for neuron-specific enolase, Leu-7, chromogranin A, neurofilament protein, synaptophysin, and low-molecular-weight cytokeratin CAM 5.2.

ADENOSQUAMOUS CARCINOMA

Primary adenosquamous carcinomas of the small intestine are extremely rare malignant neoplasms composed of a combination of malignant glandular and squamous elements.[56] Both the glandular and squamous components are thought to arise from a single multipotential stem cell presumably located at the base of the crypts.[57,58] Some studies suggest that adenosquamous carcinomas in the colon are more aggressive than pure adenocarcinomas.[57,59] However, whether this also applies to small intestinal adenosquamous carcinomas is unknown.

SQUAMOUS CELL CARCINOMA

Primary squamous cell carcinoma involving the small intestine is extremely rare[60] and usually develops in congenital anomalies such as intestinal duplications and Meckel's diverticula.[61] Squamous cell carcinomas more commonly represent metastasis from other sites, such as the cervix or lung.

CARCINOMA IN ILEOSTOMIES

Adenocarcinomas may arise in ileostomy sites in patients who have undergone bowel resection for FAP or inflammatory bowel disease.[14,62,63] In patients with polyposis, carcinomas develop in adenomatous polyps.[64] Tumors that arise in ileostomies of patients with inflammatory bowel disease occur in those who have had either antecedent backwash ileitis or dysplasia.[14,65] In most cases, the cancers develop many years after creation of the ileostomy.[66]

CARCINOMA IN MECKEL'S DIVERTICULUM

Tumors with varying histology may arise in Meckel's diverticula. Medullary, mucinous, papillary, and anaplastic carcinomas have all been described.[67] Cancer may also develop in heterotopic gastric mucosa and resembles gastric adenocarcinoma.[68,69]

CARCINOMA IN HETEROTOPIC PANCREAS

Pancreatic heterotopia is the most common congenital abnormality to involve the small intestine. Heterotopic pancreas generally remains asymptomatic, although secondary changes can lead to symptom production. A rare complication is the development of adenocarcinoma, which usually arises from the ductular component of the lesion. Histologically, carcinomas that arise in heterotopic pancreas show the full range of histologic changes that occur in ordinary pancreatic carcinomas.[70,71]

METASTATIC CARCINOMA

Metastatic tumors are significantly more common than primary neoplasms in the small intestine.[72,73] Metastatic carcinomas from many sites may affect the small intestine, although melanoma and lung, breast, colon, and renal cell carcinomas are the most common. Tumors from the mesentery, pancreas, stomach, or colon may spread to the small intestine directly. Metastases from carcinomas of the testes, adrenal glands, ovary, stomach, uterus, cervix, and liver have also been reported. Of these, ovarian tumors are most likely to cause widespread serosal implants.

Secondary adenocarcinomas may closely mimic primary small intestinal carcinomas both grossly and microscopically. Grossly, secondary tumors often present as intramural masses; they may form submucosal nodules or plaques or even produce a polypoid structure or sessile mucosal lesion. Patients may present with obstruction, intussusception, or perforation. Napkin ring–like circumferential stenotic lesions may also develop, which can lead to localized serosal retraction and intestinal kinks. Metastatic lesions may also have an infiltrative growth pattern, in which case they may simulate Crohn's disease or an ischemic stricture.

Differentiating metastatic from primary carcinomas of the small intestine is sometimes difficult. When the majority of the neoplastic cells are deep within the wall of the small bowel, and there is little involvement of the mucosa, the lesion is most likely metastatic (Fig. 18-8). Adenomatous or dysplastic change in the epithelium overlying or adjacent to the invasive tumor strongly favors a small intestinal primary. However, secondary

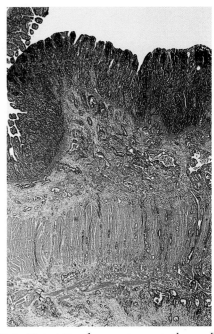

FIGURE 18–8. Metastatic adenocarcinoma in the small intestine. The bulk of the tumor is present within the muscularis propria and the submucosa. The overlying mucosa is inflamed but shows no evidence of precancerous change.

adenocarcinomas, especially pancreatic carcinoma, can rarely induce marked epithelial atypia simulating adenomatous change in epithelium adjacent to carcinoma (see Fig. 18-5). The cells demonstrate cytologic features of malignancy and often appear more disorderly than adenomatous epithelium. However, the pseudostratification of nuclei typical of adenomatous epithelium is usually absent. It is unclear whether this epithelial atypia represents neoplastic transformation of the native intestinal epithelium or pagetoid spread of neoplastic cells.

◼ Gangliocytic Paraganglioma
(see also Chapters 14 and 21)

In 1962, Taylor and Helwig[74] described a cohort of polypoid duodenal tumors that they initially regarded as benign nonchromaffin paragangliomas even though the tumors also contained ganglion cells. Later, Kepes and Zacharias[75] introduced the term *gangliocytic paraganglioma* for this tumor (see also Chapters 14 and 21). Some debate exists as to whether the lesion represents a hamartomatous or neoplastic proliferation of endodermally derived epithelial cells originating from the ventral primordium of the pancreas, combined with neuroectoderm-derived ganglion cells, spindle cells, and Schwann cells. Origin from stray embryonic cells that have migrated into the duodenal wall, recruiting nerves, ganglion cells, and smooth muscle cells, has also been suggested on the basis of the resemblance of these tumors to endodermal-neuroectodermal complexes.

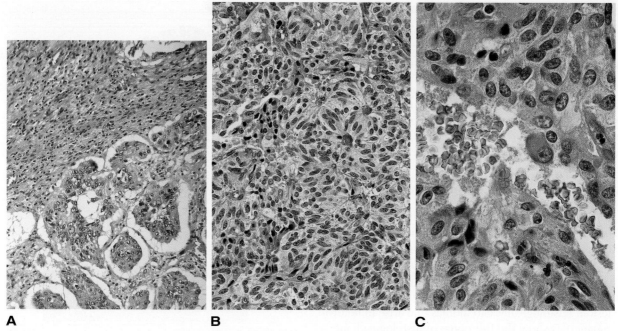

A   **B**   **C**

FIGURE 18–9. Duodenal gangliocytic paraganglioma. **A,** Low-power photomicrograph demonstrating a paragangliomatous pattern of growth. The cells are arranged in clusters and are separated by a rich vascular network. **B,** Higher-power view showing the epithelioid cell component of the tumor. These cells are arranged in trabecular fashion and form rosettelike structures focally. **C,** Scattered ganglion cells are identified within the neoplasm.

Another possibility is that the lesion represents a pancreatic tumor that develops from ganglion–islet cell complexes with secondary involvement of the duodenum.

Most gangliocytic paragangliomas arise in the second portion of the duodenum, especially at the level of the ampulla of Vater. However, some may develop in the jejunum.[74-79] These tumors usually present in the fifth to sixth decades of life, although patients may range in age from 17 to 80 years. The male-to-female ratio is 1.8:1. Most patients present with symptoms similar to those of peptic ulcer disease, including abdominal pain, nausea, vomiting, and upper gastrointestinal tract bleeding. Obstructive jaundice may occur in association with periampullary lesions. The lesions are generally regarded as benign. Lymph node metastasis has been reported,[78] although no deaths have occurred in association with metastasis.

Gangliocytic paragangliomas usually appear grossly as small polypoid submucosal lesions. The overlying mucosal surface is frequently ulcerated. One sees a mixture of histologic patterns that include paraganglioma, neurofibroma with proliferating neural processes and Schwann cells, ganglion cells, and epithelioid cells arranged in clusters, nests, or trabeculae resembling a carcinoid tumor (Fig. 18-9). The neoplasm often extends into the duodenal mucosa.

Most gangliocytic paragangliomas are hormonally inactive. However, immunohistochemical studies have revealed a wide range of polypeptide hormones in the epithelioid cells, such as insulin, glucagon, leu-enkephalin, pancreatic polypeptide, somatostatin, vasoactive intestinal peptide, and serotonin,[76,80] as well as neuron-specific enolase, chromogranin, and synaptophysin. The ganglion cells stain with antibodies against neuron-specific enolase, neurofilament, and synaptophysin. S100 immunoreactivity is often detected in sustentacular cells that typically surround the epithelioid cells of the tumor.[76,77,80]

References

1. Lowenfels AB: Why are small bowel tumors so rare? Lancet 1:24-26, 1973.
2. Wattenberg LW: Studies of polycyclic hydrocarbon hydroxylase of the intestine possibly related to cancer. Cancer 28:99-102, 1971.
3. Thomas RM, Sobin LH: Gastrointestinal cancer. Cancer 75:154-170, 1995.
4. Santoro E, Sacchi M, Scutari F, et al: Primary adenocarcinoma of the duodenum: Treatment and survival in 89 patients. Hepatogastro-enterology 44:1157-1163, 1997.
5. Lien GS, Mori M, Enjoji M: Primary carcinoma of the small intestine: A clinicopathologic and immunohistochemical study. Cancer 61:316-323, 1988.
6. Greenstein AJ, Sachar DB, Smith H, et al: A comparison of cancer risk in Crohn's disease and ulcerative colitis. Cancer 48:2742-2745, 1981.
7. Barry RE, Read AE: Coeliac disease and malignancy. Q J Med 42:665-675, 1973.
8. Nielsen SNJ, Wold LE: Adenocarcinoma of jejunum in association with nontropical sprue. Arch Pathol Lab Med 110:822-824, 1986.
9. Wright DH: The major complications of coeliac disease. Baillieres Clin Gastroenterol 9:351-369, 1995.
10. Hizawa K, Iida M, Matsumoto T, et al: Neoplastic transformation arising in Peutz-Jeghers polyposis. Dis Colon Rectum 36:953-957, 1993.
11. Perzin KH, Bridge MF: Adenomatous and carcinomatous changes in hamartomatous polyps of the small intestine (Peutz-Jeghers syndrome): Report of a case and review of the literature. Cancer 49:971-983, 1982.

12. Howe JR, Mitros FA, Summers RW: The risk of gastrointestinal carcinoma in familial juvenile polyposis. Ann Surg Oncol 5:751-756, 1998.
13. Coburn MC, Pricolo VE, DeLuca FG, et al: Malignant potential in intestinal juvenile polyposis syndromes. Ann Surg Oncol 2:386-391, 1995.
14. Roberts PL, Veidenheimer MC, Cassidy S, et al: Adenocarcinoma arising in an ileostomy. Arch Surg 124:497-499, 1989.
15. Gadacz TR, McFadden DW, Gabrielson EW, et al: Adenocarcinoma of the ileostomy: The latent risk of cancer after colectomy for ulcerative colitis and familial polyposis. Surgery 107:698-703, 1990.
16. Hamilton SR, Aaltonen LA (eds): World Health Organization Classification of Tumours. Pathology and Genetics of Tumours of the Digestive System. Lyon, France, IARC Press, 2000.
17. Perzin KH, Bridge MF: Adenomas of the small intestine: A clinicopathologic review of 51 cases and a study of their relationship to carcinoma. Cancer 48:799-819, 1981.
18. Heiman TM, Cohen LB, Bolnick K, et al: Villous polyposis of the ileum. Am J Gastroenterol 80:983-985, 1985.
19. Nakamura T, Kimura H, Nakao G: Adenomatosis of small intestine: Case report. J Clin Pathol 39:981-986, 1986.
20. Kurtz RC, Sternberg SS, Miller HH, et al: Upper gastrointestinal neoplasia in familial polyposis. Dig Dis Sci 32:459-465, 1987.
21. Iida M, Yao T, Itoh H, et al: Natural history of duodenal lesions in Japanese patients with familial adenomatosis coli (Gardner's syndrome). Gastroenterology 96:1301-1306, 1989.
22. Alexander JR, Andrews JM, Buchi KN, et al: High prevalence of adenomatous polyps of the duodenal papilla in familial adenomatous polyposis. Dig Dis Sci 34:167-170, 1989.
23. Odze R, Gallinger S, So K, et al: Duodenal adenomas in familial adenomatous polyposis: Relation of cell differentiation and mucin histochemical features to growth pattern. Mod Pathol 7:376-384, 1994.
24. Hamilton SR, Bussey HJR, Mendelsohn G, et al: Ileal adenomas after colectomy in nine patients with adenomatous polyposis coli/Gardner's syndrome. Gastroenterology 77:1252-1257, 1979.
25. Jass JR, Stewart SM: Villous adenoma of ileum in Lynch-II syndrome. Histopathology 22:186-187, 1993.
26. Jaegelman DG, DeCosse JJ, Bussey HJR: Upper gastrointestinal cancer in familial adenomatous polyposis. Lancet 1:1149-1151, 1988.
27. Offerhaus GJA, Giardiello FM, Krush AJ, et al: The risk of upper gastrointestinal cancer in familial adenomatous polyposis. Gastroenterology 102:1980-1982, 1992.
28. Kashiwagi H, Spigelman AD, Debinski HS, et al: Surveillance of ampullary adenomas in familial adenomatous polyposis. Lancet 344:1582, 1994.
29. Ross RK, Harnett NM, Bernstein L, et al: Epidemiology of adenocarcinomas of the small intestine: Is bile a small bowel carcinogen? Br J Cancer 63:143-145, 1991.
30. Weiss NS, Yang CP: Incidence of histological types of cancer of the small intestine. J Natl Cancer Inst 78:653-656, 1987.
31. Linos DA, Dozois RR, Dahlin DC, et al: Does Peutz-Jeghers syndrome predispose to gastrointestinal malignancy? A later look. Arch Surg 116:1182-1184, 1981.
32. Lehur P-A, Madarnas P, Devroede G, et al: Peutz-Jeghers syndrome: Association of duodenal and bilateral breast cancers in the same patient. Dig Dis Sci 29:178-182, 1984.
33. Swinson CM, Slavin G, Coles EC, et al: Coeliac disease and malignancy. Lancet 1:111-115, 1983.
34. Sperti C, Pasquali C, Piccoli A, et al: Radical resection for ampullary carcinoma: Long-term results. Br J Surg 81:668-671, 1994.
35. Rotman N, Pezet D, Fagniez PL, et al: Adenocarcinoma of the duodenum—factors influencing survival. Br J Surg 81:83-85, 1994.
36. Griffanti-Bartoli F, Arnone GB, Ceppa P, et al: Malignant tumors in the head of the pancreas and the periampullary region. Diagnostic and prognostic aspects. Anticancer Res 14:657-666, 1994.
37. Matory YL, Gaynor J, Brennan M: Carcinoma of the ampulla of Vater. Surg Gynecol Obstet 177:366-370, 1993.
38. Collier PE, Turowski P, Diamond DL: Small intestinal adenocarcinoma complicating regional enteritis. Cancer 55:516-521, 1985.
39. Ekbom A, Helmick CG, Zack, et al: Survival and causes of death in patients with inflammatory bowel disease: A population-based study. Gastroenterology 103:954-960, 1992.
40. Gillen CD, Andrews HA, Prior P, et al: Crohn's disease and colorectal cancer. Gut 35:651-655, 1994.
41. Craft CF, Mendelsohn G, Cooper HS, et al: Colonic "precancer" in Crohn's disease. Gastroenterology 80:578-584, 1981.
42. Cuvelier C, Bekaert E, Potter C, et al: Crohn's disease with adenocarcinoma and dysplasia. Am J Surg Pathol 13:187-196, 1989.
43. Petras RE, Mir-Madjlessi SH, Farmer RG: Crohn's disease and intestinal carcinoma. A report of 11 cases with emphasis on associated epithelial dysplasia. Gastroenterology 93:1304-1314, 1987.
44. Simpson S, Traube J, Riddell RH: The histologic appearance of dysplasia (precarcinomatous change) in Crohn's disease of the small and large intestine. Gastroenterology 81:492-501, 1981.
45. Aftalion B, Lipper S: Enteritis cystica profunda associated with Crohn's disease. Arch Pathol Lab Med 108:532-533, 1984.
46. Loughran TP, Marshall MD, Kadin MD, et al: T-cell intestinal lymphomas associated with celiac sprue. Ann Intern Med 104:44-47, 1986.
47. Straker RJ, Gunasekaran S, Brady PG: Adenocarcinoma of the jejunum in association with celiac sprue. J Clin Gastroenterol 11:320-323, 1989.
48. Hall MJ, Cooper BT, Rooney N, et al: Coeliac disease and malignancy of the duodenum: Diagnosis by endoscopy, successful treatment of the malignancy, and response to a gluten free diet. Gut 32:90-92, 1991.
49. Bruno C, Batts K, Ahlquist D: Evidence against flat dysplasia as a regional field defect in small bowel adenocarcinoma associated with celiac sprue. Mayo Clin Proc 72:320-322, 1997.
50. Gardiner GW, Lajoie G, Keith R: Hepatoid adenocarcinoma of the papilla of Vater. Histopathology 20:541-544, 1992.
51. Sato Y, Tominaga H, Tangoku A, et al: Alpha-fetoprotein–producing cancer of the ampulla of Vater. Hepatogastroenterology 39:566-569, 1992.
52. Matthews TH, Heaton GE, Christopherson WM: Primary duodenal choriocarcinoma. Arch Pathol Lab Med 110:550-552, 1986.
53. Harada N, Misawa T, Chijiiwa Y, et al: A case of extragenital choriocarcinoma in the jejunum. Am J Gastroenterol 86:1077-1079, 1991.
54. Lee CS, Machet D, Rode J: Small cell carcinoma of the ampulla of Vater. Cancer 70:1502-1504, 1992.
55. Zamboni G, Franzin G, Bonetti F, et al: Small-cell neuroendocrine carcinoma of the ampullary region: A clinicopathologic, immunohistochemical, and ultrastructural study of three cases. Am J Surg Pathol 14:703-713, 1990.
56. Ngo N, Villamil C, Macauley W, et al: Adenosquamous carcinoma of the small intestine: Report of a case and review of the literature. Arch Pathol Lab Med 123:739-742, 1999.
57. Williams GT, Blackshaw AJ, Morson BC: Squamous carcinoma of the colorectum and its genesis. J Pathol 129:209-214, 1987.
58. Crissman JD: Adenosquamous and squamous cell carcinoma of the colon. Am J Surg Pathol 2:47-54, 1978.
59. Petrelli NJ, Valle AA, Weber TK, et al: Adenosquamous carcinoma of the colon and rectum. Dis Colon Rectum 39:1265-1268, 1996.
60. Platt CC, Haboubi NY, Schofield PF: Primary squamous cell carcinoma of the terminal ileum. J Clin Pathol 44:253-254, 1991.
61. Adair HM, Trowell JE: Squamous cell carcinoma arising in a duplication of the small bowel. J Pathol 133:25-31, 1981.
62. Listinsky CM, Halpern NB, Workman RB, et al: Ultrastructural and immunocytochemical features of neuroendocrine carcinoma developing in a prior ileostomy site. Ultrastruct Pathol 18:503, 1994.
63. Suarez V, Alexander-Williams J, O'Connor HJ, et al: Carcinoma developing in ileostomies after 25 or more years. Gastroenterology 95:205-208, 1988.
64. Roth JA, Logu T: Carcinomas arising in an ileostomy. An unusual complication of adenomatous polyposis coli. Cancer 49:2180-2184, 1982.
65. Greenstein AJ, Sachar D, Pucillo A, et al: Cancer in Crohn's disease after diversionary surgery. A report of seven carcinomas occurring in excluded bowel. Am J Surg 135:86-90, 1978.
66. Bedetti CD, DeRisio VJ: Primary adenocarcinoma arising at an ileostomy site: An unusual complication after colectomy for ulcerative colitis. Dis Colon Rectum 29:572-575, 1986.
67. Weinstein EC, Dockerty MB, Waugh L: Neoplasms of Meckel's diverticulum. Int Abstr Surg 116:503-510, 1963.
68. Lin PH, Koffron AJ, Heilizer TJ, et al: Gastric adenocarcinoma of Meckel's diverticulum as a cause of colonic obstruction. Am Surg 66:627-630, 2000.
69. Kusumoto H, Yoshitake H, Mochida K, et al: Adenocarcinoma in Meckel's diverticulum: Report of a case and review of 30 cases in the English and Japanese literature. Am J Gastroenterol 87:910-913, 1992.

70. Brotman SJ, Pan W, Pozner J, et al: Ductal adenocarcinoma arising in duodeno-pyloric heterotopic pancreas. Int J Surg Pathol 2:37-40, 1994.
71. Malchlouf HR, Almeida JL, Sobin LH: Carcinoma in jejunal pancreatic heterotopia. Arch Pathol Lab Med 123:707-711, 1999.
72. De Castro CA, Dockerty MB, Mayo CW: Metastatic tumors of the small intestines. Surg Gynecol Obstet 105:159-165, 1957.
73. Berge T, Lundberg S: Cancer in Malmo 1958-69. Acta Pathol Microbiol Scand S260:140-149, 1977.
74. Taylor HB, Helwig EB: Benign nonchromaffin paragangliomas of the duodenum. Virchows Arch A 335:356-366, 1962.
75. Kepes JJ, Zacharias DDL: Gangliocytic paragangliomas of the duodenum. A report of two cases with light and electron microscopic examination. Cancer 27:61-70, 1971.
76. Hamid QA, Bishop AE, Rode J, et al: Duodenal gangliocytic paraganglioma: A study of ten cases with immunocytochemical markers. Hum Pathol 17:1151-1157, 1986.
77. Perrone T, Sibley RK, Rosai J: Duodenal gangliocytic paraganglioma: An immunohistochemical and ultrastructural study and a hypothesis concerning its origin. Am J Surg Pathol 9:31-41, 1985.
78. Perrone T: Duodenal gangliocytic paraganglioma and carcinoid. Am J Surg Pathol 10:147-149, 1986.
79. Inai K, Kobuke T, Yonehara S, Tokuoka S: Duodenal gangliocytic paraganglioma with lymph node metastasis in a 17-year-old boy. Cancer 63:2540-2545, 1989.
80. Collina G, Maiorana A, Trentini GP: Duodenal gangliocytic paraganglioma. Case report with immunohistochemical study on the expression of keratin polypeptides. Histopathology 19:476-478, 1991.

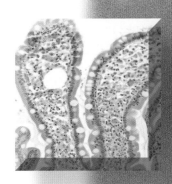

CHAPTER 19

Epithelial Neoplasms of the Large Intestine

MARK REDSTON

The most common neoplasms of the large intestine are adenomas (Table 19-1 discussed in Chapter 15). Malignant epithelial neoplasms of the large intestine can be primary or, less commonly, metastatic. Although there is abundant clinical, morphologic, and genetic evidence to suggest that primary epithelial malignant neoplasms represent a heterogeneous group of tumors, most clinicians consider these neoplasms together under the title "colorectal carcinoma."[1,2] Thus, much of the discussion in this chapter refers to colorectal carcinoma as a generic single disease, recognizing that this is an oversimplification. In practice, about 85% of colorectal carcinomas are typical adenocarcinomas; relatively distinct histologic subtypes form the remainder (see Table 19-1).

▮ Clinical Features

INCIDENCE

Malignant epithelial tumors of the colon and rectum accounted for 8.5% of all cancers worldwide in 2000, with 945,000 new cases diagnosed each year.[3,4] There are marked variations in the age-standardized incidence, with nearly a 20-fold difference between high-risk (developed countries including Europe, the Americas, Australia, and New Zealand) and low-risk regions (Africa and Asia). The likely role of environmental influences, particularly diet, in the genesis of these differences is supported by abundant data.[5] There are also significant global differences in the age at onset of colorectal carcinoma, with a mean age of only 50 years in developing countries.

In the United States, there will be an estimated 105,500 new cases of colon cancer and 42,000 new cases of rectal cancer in 2003.[6] Colorectal carcinoma is the third most common cancer in men and women and the fourth most common cancer overall, representing about 12% of all cancers.[6] It is the second leading cause of cancer death overall, behind only lung cancer.[6] The overall lifetime risk for development of colorectal carcinoma is estimated at nearly 6%.[7] U.S. Surveillance, Epidemiology, and End Results (SEER) Program statistics reveal an incidence of 33.7 per 100,000 for colon carcinoma and 12.8 per 100,000 for rectal carcinoma.[8] Both types of cancer are significantly more common in men (combined incidence of 52.2 per 100,000 in men compared with 37.5 per 100,000 in women).[6] The increased incidence in men is only apparent after the age of 50 years. Paradoxically, because women live longer than men, there are more total cases and cancer deaths in women.[6] Since 1987, the incidence of colon cancer in the United States has been steadily falling.[9] The incidence increases with age, and only about 1% to 2% occur in patients younger than 40 years.

Similar to the global variation in colorectal cancer incidence, there are also significant regional and ethnic differences in incidence within the United States. The incidence varies by about twofold between high-risk regions on the northeast Atlantic coast (Connecticut, Delaware, New Jersey, Pennsylvania, and Rhode Island) and low-risk regions predominantly in the South (Alabama, Georgia, New Mexico, and Utah).[6] There are

441

TABLE 19–1. Classification of Epithelial Neoplasms of the Large Intestine

Category	Neoplasm Subtype
Benign	Hamartoma
	Hyperplastic polyp
	Adenoma
	Mixed hyperplastic–adenomatous polyp
Malignant	Primary colorectal adenocarcinoma
	Other types of primary colorectal carcinoma
	Metastatic carcinoma

TABLE 19–3. Risk Factors for Colorectal Cancer[6]

Factor	Relative Risk
Family history (first-degree)	1.8
Physical activity (<3 hr/wk)	1.7
Inflammatory bowel disease	1.5
Obesity	1.5
Red meat consumption	1.5
Smoking (>1 pk/d)	1.5
Alcohol	1.4
High vegetable consumption (≥5 servings/d)	0.7
Oral contraceptive use (≥5 years)	0.7
Estrogen replacement (≥5 years)	0.8
Multivitamins containing folic acid	0.5

also significant differences related to racial and ethnic backgrounds (Table 19-2). The incidence is highest in blacks and lowest in individuals of Hispanic and Native American origin.[6]

EPIDEMIOLOGIC ASSOCIATIONS

The risk of colorectal cancer is influenced by both endogenous (constitutional) and exogenous (environmental) factors (Table 19-3). For the practicing surgical pathologist, genetic predisposition and long-standing inflammatory bowel disease have the most direct clinical impact, and these are discussed under Genetic Predisposition and under Colitis-Associated Neoplasia.

Among the remaining factors, age (discussed before) is the most powerful risk factor, and colorectal cancer is predominantly a disease of late middle-aged and elderly individuals.[6] Men are at a considerably higher risk than are women (also discussed before), and this sex difference is thought to be related to differences in hormonal milieu.[10]

Diet has been intensively studied, and although there is little doubt that elevated risk is consistently associated with a "Western" type of diet, it has been difficult to tease out which components are most important. Diets with high calorie intake and those rich in meat, particularly animal fat, have been implicated in many studies.[5,11] Possible mechanisms for this effect include the production of heterocyclic amines, stimulation of higher levels of fecal bile acids, production of reactive oxygen species, and elevated insulin levels.[12,13] In addition

TABLE 19–2. Incidence and Mortality Rates of Colorectal Cancer by Race and Ethnicity, 1992–1998, Men and Women Combined*

Race/Ethnic Group	Incidence	Mortality
Black	50.1	22.8
White	42.9	16.8
Asian/Pacific Islander	38.2	10.7
Native American/Alaska Native	28.6	10.3
Hispanic	28.4	10.2

*Rates per 100,000, age-adjusted to the 1970 U.S. standard population.[6]

to high-risk factors, there are inverse associations with vegetable and fiber consumption.[14,15] This effect could be due to anticarcinogens, antioxidants, folate, induction of detoxifying enzymes, binding of luminal carcinogens, fiber fermentation to produce volatile fatty acids, or reduced contact time with epithelium because of faster transit.[14] Several studies have found that high folate intake is associated with a decreased risk of colorectal cancer, providing some of the most direct evidence of dietary risk factor relationships.[16] Finally, alcohol intake has been associated with an increased risk of colorectal cancer as well.[17]

Ingestion of therapeutic agents is linked to colorectal cancer risk. Most notably, there is an inverse association between use of nonsteroidal anti-inflammatory drugs and colorectal cancer risk.[18] Smoking exposure is associated with colorectal cancer, although the relative risk is much less than for many other tobacco-related cancers.[19] In addition, sedentary lifestyle,[20] long-standing inflammatory bowel disease (see under Colitis-Associated Neoplasia),[21] pelvic irradiation,[22] and ureterosigmoidostomy are also associated with an increased risk of colorectal cancer.

Finally, there is evidence to suggest that there are important differences in the epidemiologic risk factors associated with different subtypes of colorectal cancer. There has been a trend in recent years toward the development of more proximal cancers,[8] which may relate to changes in epidemiologic risk factors. Furthermore, there are molecular biologic differences in right- and left-sided colorectal cancers that would support different epidemiologic associations.[23]

GENETIC PREDISPOSITION

Genetic polyposis syndromes account for significantly less than 0.5% of all incident colorectal cancers (Table 19-4) (see Chapters 14 and 15 for details). However, nonpolyposis forms of hereditary colorectal carcinoma have a much higher overall contribution to the causation of colorectal cancer and are discussed later in this chapter.

TABLE 19–4. Classification of Genetic Syndromes Predisposing to Colorectal Cancer

Syndrome	Inherited Gene Defect	Risk in Carriers	Attributable Risk*
Familial adenomatous polyposis	*APC*	>90% by 40 yr	<0.5%
Attenuated familial adenomatous polyposis	*APC*	<90% by 70 yr	<0.5%
Juvenile polyposis syndrome	*SMAD4, BMPRIA*		<<0.5%
Peutz-Jeghers syndrome	*STK/LKB*		<<0.5%
Cowden's syndrome	*PTEN*		<<0.5%
Hereditary non-polyposis colorectal cancer	*MLH1, MSH2, PMS2, MSH6*	50%–90% by 70 yr	2%–3%

*The proportion of colorectal cancer that is attributed to this syndrome.

▮ Essential Pathogenetic Issues

PROGRESSION FROM ADENOMA TO CARCINOMA

It is generally accepted that most colorectal carcinomas arise from adenomas.[24] Residual adenoma is identified in about 10% to 30% of colorectal cancers, presumably being overgrown by the cancer when it is not apparent.[25] Adenomas and carcinomas have a similar distribution in the colorectum, and adenomas usually precede cancer by about 15 years.[26] Endoscopic removal of polyps decreases the incidence of subsequent colorectal cancer in treated subjects.[26]

In the past 10 years, it has also been shown that aberrant crypt foci are likely to be the intermediate step between normal colonic epithelium and grossly apparent adenomatous growth.[27] Aberrant crypt foci are microscopic lesions readily identified by examination of methylene blue–stained, stripped mucosal sheets under a dissecting microscope. They are characterized by a collection of crypts that have increased crypt diameters and increased numbers of lining epithelial cells, giving a serrated or slitlike appearance in methylene blue preparations. Histologic sections of aberrant crypt foci reveal a range of findings from unremarkable or mildly hyperplastic epithelium, to features that are typical of hyperplastic polyps, to the rare occurrence of dysplasia, equivalent to microscopic adenomas incidentally identified in familial adenomatous polyposis. Aberrant crypt foci may also be visualized endoscopically.[28]

With the advent of more careful endoscopic examinations, the finding of very small (<1.0 cm) carcinomas that lack any evidence of residual adenoma has raised the possibility that some cancers may arise de novo.[29] Representing less than 5% of all colorectal carcinomas, these cancers are more likely to be high grade than ex adenoma carcinomas, with lymphatic and blood vessel invasion. Although important for the endoscopist, these lesions probably represent rapid progression from a small adenoma because of the acquisition of high-grade genetic alterations (such as aneuploidy and *TP53* mutations).[29]

GENETIC MODEL OF COLORECTAL CANCER PROGRESSION

Human cancers are characterized by the accumulation of a variety of genetic alterations, including mutations that activate oncogenes and inactivate tumor suppressor genes.[30,31] It is well established that the morphologic progression from adenoma to carcinoma is accompanied by the accumulation of genetic alterations.[32-34] The accumulation of genetic alterations is clearly established in aberrant crypt foci and probably begins in cells without clear morphologic abnormalities.

GENOME INSTABILITY

To accumulate the array of genetic alterations typical of a colorectal cancer, tumor cells must acquire mutations at an increased rate compared with normal crypt epithelial cells.[35] This increased acquisition with tolerance of mutations is a hallmark of colorectal cancers and is referred to as genome instability.[36,37] Genes involved in genome maintenance have been likened to "caretakers" of the genome.[38] There are at least two general forms of genome instability important to colorectal neoplasia. Chromosomal instability is present in up to 85% of colorectal cancers and is characterized by aneuploidy, widespread gains and losses of chromosomal material, and translocations. Microsatellite instability is present in about 10% to 15% of colorectal cancers and is characterized by widespread alterations in the sizes of repetitive DNA sequences. Microsatellite instability is caused by defective DNA mismatch repair (see also under Hereditary Nonpolyposis Colorectal Cancer) (Fig. 19-1).

In a process that may be related to genome instability, colorectal neoplasms also have widespread abnormalities in DNA methylation, particularly hypermethylation of CpG dinucleotides in promoter regions of genes.[39-41] This is a major mechanism of inactivation of tumor suppressor genes such as *TP16* and *CDHI*. In addition, some data suggest that a subset of tumors may be particularly susceptible to DNA methylation (referred to as the CpG island methylator phenotype, or CIMP+).[42] However, possible clinicopathologic associations with this putative pathway are not yet defined.

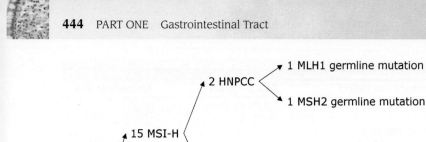

FIGURE 19–1. Breakdown of the molecular pathogenesis of an unselected population of colorectal cancers. The numbers are an approximation based on current knowledge.

WINGLESS SIGNALING ABNORMALITIES

APC was first identified as the gene mutated in individuals with familial adenomatous polyposis.[43] In this syndrome, affected individuals inherit one mutant copy of *APC* that is functionally inactive. In tumorigenesis, the second allelic copy of the gene is also inactivated, fulfilling Knudsen's paradigm for tumor suppressor gene inactivation. *APC* mutations are also present in the majority of sporadic colorectal cancers, and the mutations occur early during neoplastic development, being found in dysplastic aberrant crypt foci.[43] The apparent necessity of *APC* inactivation for the development of early adenomas has resulted in its designation as the "gatekeeper" of colorectal neoplasia.[38] APC is an important component of the Wingless pathway, an evolutionarily conserved signaling cascade critical to embryonic development and intestinal epithelial renewal.[43,44] *APC* mutations abrogate its role in binding beta-catenin, thereby releasing beta-catenin from phosphorylation regulation by GSK3beta and allowing it to accumulate in the nucleus, where it is involved in activating transcription of a number of other downstream targets, including *cyclin D* and c-myc.[43] APC is also involved in cytoskeletal interactions and has been directly implicated in maintaining genome stability.[45]

OTHER GENETIC ALTERATIONS

Activating mutations in K-*ras* are present in about 40% of colorectal carcinomas and were one of the first genetic alterations described in any solid human tumor.[32] These mutations typically occur early, in aberrant crypt foci or small adenomas, and result in constitutive activation of the gene. Mutation and inactivation of the *TP53* gene occurs in about 50% to 70% of carcinomas, often at the transition point of the developing high-grade dysplasia.[46] Among the best known of human tumor suppressor genes, *TP53* is important in the DNA damage response/cell cycle arrest pathway.

SERRATED PATHWAY OF CARCINOGENESIS

Historically, hyperplastic polyps have not been considered a precursor of cancer. However, studies suggest that DNA mismatch repair–deficient colorectal cancers may arise in hyperplastic polyps or serrated adenomas and that hyperplastic polyps contain an array of cell cycle and genetic defects (including loss of *p27* expression, abnormal MIB-1 proliferation indices, K-*ras* mutations, and loss of a variety of chromosomal arms).[39,47-49] For instance, there are well-documented cases with progression from hyperplastic polyp to an MLH1-deficient serrated adenoma and an MLH1-deficient ("serrated") adenocarcinoma in a single lesion.[39,47,48] There is also evidence to suggest that genetic or environmental exposures, such as smoking and estrogen withdrawal, may be associated with the development of serrated pathway carcinomas.[39]

■ Specimen Handling and Gross Features

The principles for handling, evaluating, and processing colorectal specimens for pathologic examination have been well described.[50,51] Tumor location should be specified as to whether it is in the right (cecum, ascending, hepatic flexure, or transverse) or left (splenic flexure, descending, or sigmoid) colon or rectum. Accurately delimiting the proximal extent of the rectum is often difficult. Tumors within the nonperitonealized portion are clearly rectal in origin. All tumors located within 16 cm of the anal verge are also considered rectal in origin. If the tumor is more proximally located and the exact location is unclear, it should be designated rectosigmoid. The point at which the peritoneum no longer surrounds the bowel segment is the true rectosigmoid junction. The taeniae coli also end at the junction of the rectum. When present, the radial margin should be inked fresh. See the section on circumferential resection margin for further discussion of the assessment of rectal specimens.

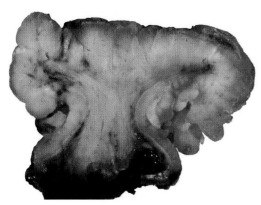

FIGURE 19–2. Invasive adenocarcinoma in a mucosal poly-pectomy specimen. The stalk resection margin is inked blue. Non-neoplastic mucosa is present on both sides of the stalk. A significant component of submucosa forms the central core of the stalk and branches out in the head of the polyp. The left portion of the polyp head is adenomatous and shows a sharply circumscribed interface with the underlying tissue. In the central portion of the polyp, and extending to the right side, the interface with the underlying tissue is obscured owing to the presence of invasive adenocarcinoma that involves the submucosa (AJCC stage T1).

After assessment of the radial margin, fat should be stripped off the colon and placed in Bouin's solution to aid lymph node identification. All grossly negative lymph nodes should be submitted entirely. Grossly positive lymph nodes may be submitted in part. In the case of a large resection specimen that includes multiple sub-segments of the colon or rectum, lymph nodes must be designated regional or nonregional. Definitions are available in the American Joint Committee on Cancer (AJCC) manual. Metastases to nonregional lymph nodes are designated M1.[2]

The macroscopic appearance of colorectal carcinomas is strongly influenced by the timing of the diagnosis in relation to the progression of disease. Some small car-cinomas may be present within larger polypoid adenomas and are often associated with a well-formed stalk (Fig. 19-2). Other small carcinomas are sharply circum-scribed, variably elevated lesions that usually have a flattened center. The consistency varies with the proportion of adenoma, which is softer and more friable than carcinoma.

Large carcinomas take on one of four general gross configurations (Fig. 19-3):

1. Bulky, exophytic, and polypoid tumors. These occur typically in the cecum, rarely result in obstruction, and often become large before clinical presentation.
2. Infiltrative and ulcerating tumors. These cancers are typified by raised, irregular edges and a central, excavated ulceration that may extend to a depth beyond the native muscularis mucosae.
3. Annular and constricting tumors. These tumors produce the characteristic double-contrast "apple-

core" lesion. In association with a functional obstruction, there is often proximal dilatation with attenuation and flattening of the mucosal folds. Associated desmoplasia results in a firm appearance.
4. Diffuse tumors. Analogous to linitis plastica of the stomach, these tumors present with diffuse flattening and thickening of the mucosa initially and of the entire bowel wall with progression.

In all cases, the cut section is usually relatively homo-geneous with admixed areas of necrosis. In addition, there is variable dilatation (secondary to obstruction) and retraction of the serosal surface (usually associated with deep invasion into the muscularis propria or subserosa). These gross appearances are complex, however, and there is much overlap between these patterns. There is no evidence that gross configuration is a prognostic indicator independent of underlying histologic subtype.[52]

Microscopic Features

CRITERIA FOR MALIGNANCY

For reasons that are not entirely clear, although possibly related to the relative paucity of lymphatics, invasion that is confined to the lamina propria and muscularis mucosae is almost never associated with lymph node metastases.[2] Therefore, colorectal carci-nomas are considered to be stage T1 only when they have invaded through the muscularis mucosae into the submucosa.[2] Whereas this may make practical sense for management of patients with colorectal cancer, it has created difficulty with the nomenclature of neoplasms that do not invade into the submucosa. In the AJCC classification, invasion confined to the mucosa is classified as Tis.[2] However, high-grade dysplasia that does not breach the basement membrane is also classified as Tis and is a lesion analogous to carcinoma in situ elsewhere in the body. Furthermore, the term *intramucosal carcinoma* is used by some for both these scenarios (although it seems more fitting for the case of invasion confined to the lamina propria). Until further agreement puts this issue to rest, I prefer to classify lesions confined to the basement membrane as adenomas with high-grade dysplasia and to diagnose invasion con-fined to the mucosa as invasive intramucosal adeno-carcinoma, clearly stating the depth of invasion and that these are classified as Tis.

BIOPSY DIAGNOSIS

Most colorectal carcinomas are diagnosed by endo-scopic biopsy. However, malignancy may be a focal alteration within a larger polypectomy specimen, in

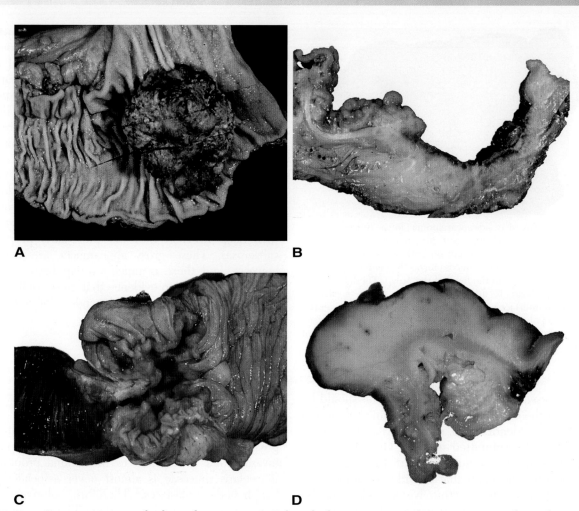

FIGURE 19–3. Gross appearances of colorectal carcinoma. **A,** Polypoid adenocarcinoma with an extensive intraluminal component. **B,** Ulcerating adenocarcinoma. The ulcer base extends beyond the limit of the muscularis propria. Residual adenomatous epithelium is present to the left of the ulcer. **C,** Annular adenocarcinoma. This appearance correlates with an "apple-core" lesion. **D,** Diffuse carcinoma. Prominent infiltration of the mucosa is seen, with expansion of the submucosa, producing a thickened, relatively flat plaque. Microscopic examination revealed a poorly differentiated carcinoma, with undifferentiated and signet ring cell components.

which case the adequacy of endoscopic therapy is determined on the basis of completeness of excision and presence or absence of high-risk factors for lymph node metastases (see Chapter 15).

Biopsy specimens of sessile or flat lesions are usually superficial, often poorly oriented, and often associated with ulceration. The most important aspect of pathologic examination is to determine whether invasion is present. Whereas the presence of single infiltrating cells or small, markedly irregular glands makes the presence of invasion straightforward in many cases (Fig. 19-4), well-differentiated and sometimes even moderately differentiated cancers may not show this pattern. In the absence of these definitive features, diagnosis of invasion relies on identification of desmoplasia. Differentiation between a desmoplastic carcinoma and an ulcerating adenoma can be difficult (Fig. 19-5). The stroma of the ulcerating adenoma is often more cellular, with more abundant microvasculature, inflammatory cells, and plumper-appearing fibroblasts.

If the muscularis mucosae can be identified, it is important to note whether invasion penetrates this layer. In many biopsy fragments, the muscularis mucosae is often difficult to identify clearly. If the biopsy fragments are large and the degree of desmoplasia is well developed, it is usually presumed that the tissue fragment contains submucosa, in which case the carcinoma is at least T1. In smaller fragments, one cannot be as certain, and the possibility must be considered that one is dealing with a polypoid lesion with only superficial invasion (Tis), which may still be amenable to localized excision. In such cases, it is important to note that the biopsy specimens are superficial and that the depth of invasion cannot be accurately determined.

CLASSIFICATION OF HISTOLOGIC SUBTYPES

The vast majority of colorectal cancers are adenocarcinomas (which, by definition, are considered of usual morphology) (Table 19-5). Histologic complexity

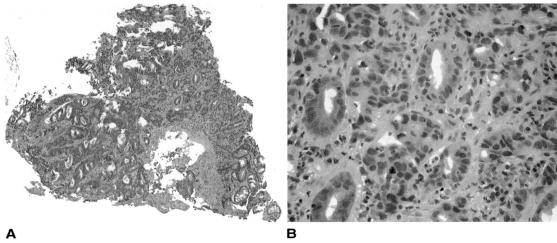

A   **B**

FIGURE 19–4. Biopsy diagnosis of adenocarcinoma. **A,** Low magnification reveals a few non-neoplastic crypts on the right, and a mixture of variably sized glands with moderate atypia and desmoplasia on the left side of the field, indicative of adenocarcinoma. **B,** At high magnification, one can note markedly atypical glands and single cells infiltrating between uninvolved crypts.

is more often related to the presence of small components of different histologic patterns within a typical adenocarcinoma. Whereas there are published criteria for the different subtypes, such as "mucinous" adenocarcinoma (see under Mucinous Adenocarcinoma, Signet Ring Cell Adenocarcinoma, and Undifferentiated Carcinoma), these criteria were developed somewhat arbitrarily and in absentia of our current understanding of the pathogenesis of these tumors. Therefore, in cases in which second elements of differentiation are present but the patterns are insufficient to meet the diagnostic criteria, it is worth commenting on the presence of all components in the final diagnosis (for instance, "moderately differentiated adenocarcinoma, with 10% extracellular mucinous component").

ADENOCARCINOMA, USUAL TYPE

Most adenocarcinomas are moderately well differentiated. Typically, they have medium to large glands, with moderate variability in gland size and configuration, and only moderate amounts of stroma. In well-differentiated tumors, lining cells are usually tall and columnar, becoming increasingly cuboidal or polygonal with decreasing degrees of differentiation. Mitotic figures are usually abundant. Glandular lumina are usually filled with inspissated eosinophilic mucus and nuclear and cellular debris (so-called dirty necrosis) (Fig. 19-6). When "dirty" necrosis is present in a metastasis of

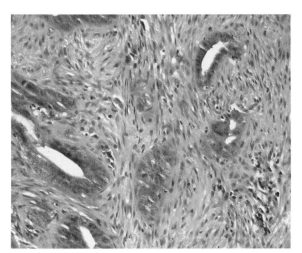

FIGURE 19–5. High magnification of a colonic mass biopsy reveals atypical glands within a desmoplastic stroma, diagnostic of invasion.

TABLE 19–5. Histologic Classification of Colorectal Carcinoma

Histologic Type	Recognized WHO Type[1]	Approximate Frequency (%)
Adenocarcinoma	Yes	85–90
Mucinous (colloid) adenocarcinoma	Yes	8–10
Signet ring cell carcinoma	Yes	2
Medullary carcinoma	Yes	0.5–1.0
Adenosquamous carcinoma	Yes	<1.0
Squamous cell carcinoma	Yes	<1.0
Small cell (neuroendocrine) carcinoma	Yes	<1.0
Undifferentiated carcinoma	Yes	<1.0
Mixed carcinoid-adenocarcinoma	Yes	<1.0
Choriocarcinoma		<0.1
Clear cell carcinoma		<0.1
Microglandular goblet cell carcinoma		<0.1
Carcinomas with melanin production		<0.1
Spindle cell or mesenchymal carcinoma		<0.1

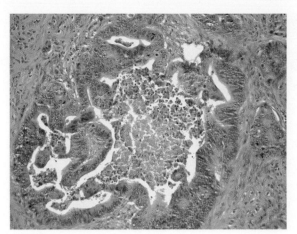

FIGURE 19–6. Typical colorectal adenocarcinoma. A proliferation of complex glandular structures is noted, with infolding and bridging of the epithelium. The cells have cylindrical to ovoid nuclei. The lumen contains abundant eosinophilic and nuclear debris ("dirty" necrosis). This pattern of necrosis is characteristic of colorectal adenocarcinoma.

unknown primary origin, this pattern is often useful to infer a colorectal primary. In general, there tends to be little difference between the superficial and deep portions of the tumor, although the leading edge is often associated with gland rupture and more frequent foci of smaller irregular glands. In addition, some tumors have a prominent papillary component, particularly at the surface. Desmoplasia can be prominent, being reminiscent of cancers of the pancreas and biliary tract. In some instances, the appearance of desmoplasia is due in part to extensive tumor necrosis and hyalinization. In addition to glandular cells, a variable amount of Paneth cells, neuroendocrine cells, squamous cells, melanocytes, and trophoblasts can be found in adenocarcinoma.[66]

GRADING

Grading is one of the most widely used pathologic variables, but it is also one of the most difficult to define accurately. Furthermore, there continues to be controversy as to whether grade is an independent prognostic variable,[53] although most studies show this to be the case.[54,55]

Grading is based primarily on the proportion of the tumor that is composed of glands relative to areas that are solid or composed of nests or cords of cells without lumina. The grading system recommended (Table 19-6) is the one endorsed by the World Health Organization (WHO) and AJCC (Figs. 19-7 and 19-8).[1,2] With use of this system, approximately 10% of adenocarcinomas are well differentiated, 70% are moderately differentiated, and 20% are poorly differentiated.[53]

Overall, poor differentiation is the most reproducibly diagnosed histologic grade and is the most predictive category for survival.[56-58] Unfortunately, many of the studies that show grade to be an independent prognostic variable combine well-differentiated and moderately differentiated tumors in their analyses. As a result, a new two-tiered grading system has been proposed and is currently recommended.[52] In this system, colorectal adenocarcinomas are classified as either low grade (well and moderately differentiated; 50% or more gland formation) or high grade (poorly differentiated; <50% gland formation). Grading of biopsy specimens is often inaccurate and may not reflect the final grade of a resected carcinoma.

Grading of colorectal cancer applies only to adenocarcinoma of the usual type. By definition, signet ring cell carcinomas and small cell carcinomas are considered poorly differentiated. Some also consider all mucinous carcinomas to be poorly differentiated. Grading mucinous cancers on the basis of gland formation and cytologic features is also of questionable practical utility. When there is no or minimal gland formation, cancers are classified as undifferentiated, a distinct histologic subtype that may represent the extreme of poorly differentiated adenocarcinoma (see under Undifferentiated Carcinoma).

FEATURES OF VARIOUS CARCINOMAS

Mucinous Adenocarcinoma

The WHO defines mucinous tumors by the degree of extracellular mucin (tumor composed of ≥50% mucin). The term adenocarcinoma with "mucinous features" or

TABLE 19–6. Grading of Colorectal Adenocarcinomas

Grade	Descriptive Nomenclature	Criteria*	AJCC Recommendation[†]
GX	Grade cannot be assessed		
GI	Well differentiated	>95% gland forming Majority (>75%) of glands are smooth and regular No significant component of high-grade nuclei	Low grade
G2	Moderately differentiated	50%–95% gland forming	Low grade
G3	Poorly differentiated	<50% gland forming	High grade
G4	Undifferentiated	No apparent gland formation[‡]	High grade

*All criteria must be met.
[†]From references 2 and 52.
[‡]Undifferentiated tumors are a distinct subtype.

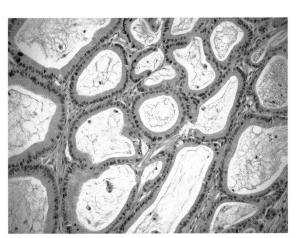

FIGURE 19–7. Well-differentiated adenocarcinoma. The glands are fairly regular in size and shape. The lining cells contain basally oriented nuclei, with only mild atypia.

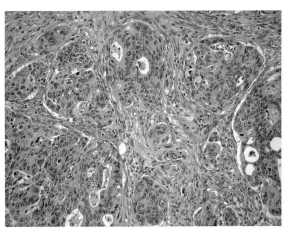

FIGURE 19–8. Poorly differentiated adenocarcinoma. Few glandular lumina are visible; however, most of the tumor is solid. Marked cytologic atypia and abundant mitotic figures are present.

"mucinous differentiation" is often used to describe tumors that have a significant mucinous component (>10%) but less than 50%. Most mucinous adenocarcinomas contain a partial epithelial lining or show free-floating strips of epithelium (Fig. 19-9). One often sees a variable number of cells with a signet ring appearance (Fig. 19-10). When more than 50% of cells have a signet ring cell morphology, the tumor is best classified as "signet ring cell type," even if more than 50% of the tumor is composed of extracellular mucin (Fig. 19-11).

Mucinous adenocarcinomas represent about 10% of all colonic cancers.[59] They are more common in young individuals and in patients with HNPCC, and they are more likely to present at an advanced stage. A number of genetic alterations suggest that the molecular pathogenesis is different from that of usual adenocarcinomas. Defects in DNA mismatch repair and high-frequency microsatellite instability (MSI-H) are more

common in mucinous adenocarcinomas, but this pathologic feature shows a low degree of sensitivity as a marker for this genetic defect.[60] MSI-H mucinous tumors are more often found in younger individuals and are more likely to be exophytic and to have an expanding growth pattern compared with other mucinous cancers.[61] Immunohistochemical staining for *TP53* is less frequently positive (30% vs. >50% in the usual type), suggesting that *TP53* mutations are less frequent or less likely to be stabilizing point mutations.

Mucinous tumors are evenly distributed in the right and left colon and therefore represent a greater proportion of right colon tumors (because there is an overall predominance of left-sided cancers). The tumors tend to be soft, with a gelatinous appearance on cut section, and contain little fibrous tissue, giving the appearance of a "colloid" carcinoma. The appearance is often that of small nodules of mucin.

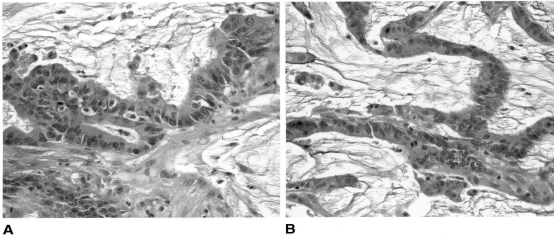

A   **B**

FIGURE 19–9. Mucinous adenocarcinoma. **A,** The characteristic feature is an abundance of pools of mucin. Mucin pools are usually lined by cytologically atypical epithelium with features of adenocarcinoma. **B,** In other areas, the epithelial elements "float" within the mucin.

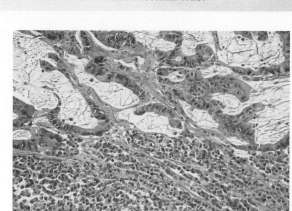

FIGURE 19–10. Mucinous adenocarcinoma with signet ring cell features. This tumor contains a mixture of "mucinous" and signet ring cell adenocarcinoma. However, because the signet ring cells areas constitute less than 50% of the tumor volume, this is best classified as a "mucinous" adenocarcinoma. The presence of signet ring cells in mucinous carcinomas is quite common.

On microscopic examination, mucinous adeno-carcinomas show abundant large glandular structures embedded in pools of mucus that can be highlighted with PAS or alcian blue stains. The margins of the tumor are often infiltrative, which may contribute to the poor prognosis attributed to these tumors. In one series of 132 mucinous carcinomas, adjacent precursor adenomas were identified in 31%, similar to that expected for usual adenocarcinomas.[59] The association between mucinous tumors and survival is somewhat controversial. Whereas many studies have found these tumors to be associated with poor prognosis,[62-64] others have not. Some studies that have examined the behavior of mucinous tumors failed to differentiate those with signet ring cell morphology, which are more aggressive tumors.

Mucinous tumors are more likely to develop peritoneal implants[65] and are more likely to invade adjacent viscera

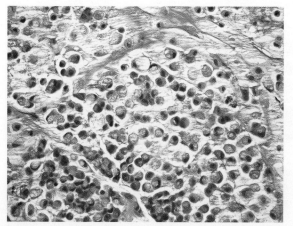

FIGURE 19–11. Signet ring cell adenocarcinoma. The tumor cells display a classic signet ring cell morphology with eccentrically displaced nuclei. Note also the abundant extracellular mucin.

than are usual adenocarcinomas.[66] As a result, they are less likely to undergo curative resection.[65] They are also more likely to have nodal involvement beyond the pericolonic region.[66] Some have advocated more aggressive surgical management for these tumors.[66]

Signet Ring Cell Adenocarcinoma

This is defined as a tumor that is composed of at least 50% signet ring cells. This feature supersedes the presence of extracellular mucin. These tumors make up about 0.5% to 1.0% of all colorectal carcinomas.[67-69] They are slightly more common in men (1.3:1) and occur at a younger age (mean age, 63.5 years).[68] In some studies, more than 50% of tumors are found in individuals younger than 40 years.[70] Signet ring cell carcinoma is also more common in colitis-associated cancers; 30% of tumors occur in patients with ulcerative colitis.[71]

Signet ring cell carcinomas are evenly distributed in the right and left colon and thus constitute a greater fraction of right-sided tumors.[67,68] Synchronous tumors are found in 14% of patients.[67] They are usually ulcerating, and about two thirds have an infiltrative gross appearance.[67,68] A linitis plastica growth pattern occurs in up to 20% of cases.[68]

Histologically, tumor cells show a characteristic mucin vacuole that pushes the nucleus to the periphery of the cell cytoplasm. A subset of signet ring cells are round and contain central nuclei, without an apparent mucin vacuole. Compared with gastric signet ring cell carcinomas, those in the colorectum are more likely to be associated with abundant extracellular mucin and less commonly result in diffuse infiltration of the tissues. Although mucin expression is not helpful in differentiating metastatic gastric from primary colorectal signet ring cell carcinomas, it is useful in differentiating those from the lung, which are MUC1 and TTF-1 positive and MUC2 negative, compared with gastric and colon tumors, which are MUC1 and TTF-1 negative and MUC2 positive.[72]

Similar to mucinous carcinomas, signet ring cell tumors are more likely to present at an advanced stage. Full-thickness penetration of the muscularis propria and peritoneal seeding are more common than in usual adenocarcinomas (36% vs. 12%).[67-70] Some studies report distant metastases in up to 60% of patients at the time of diagnosis.[89,90] As a result, they are less likely to undergo surgical resection (64% vs. 80%).[70] Similar to mucinous carcinomas, signet ring cell carcinomas are associated with a worse outcome. Five-year survival rates of less than 10% have been reported.[68,69] Peritoneal carcinomatosis is seen in virtually all patients who die from their disease, whereas liver metastases are present in less than 50% of cases.[67]

Undifferentiated Carcinoma

The term *undifferentiated carcinoma* is restricted to cancers that contain evidence of epithelial differentiation but without gland formation. Some authors accept less than 5% gland formation as consistent with this diagnosis.[1] Thus, undifferentiated tumors may simply represent an ultra-poorly differentiated adenocarcinoma.

Undifferentiated cancers tend to be bulky and soft owing to their cellularity and relative lack of desmoplasia, and they often show extensive necrosis. Tumors may form sheets of cells, cords, or trabecular structures and often have an infiltrative growth pattern (Fig. 19-12). Anaplasia is variable; some tumors show relatively uniform cytologic features, whereas others show marked nuclear variability.

Although pure undifferentiated cancers are very rare, many tumors contain an undifferentiated component. These tumors are best classified as adenocarcinoma and graded on the basis of overall degree of glandular elements. Nevertheless, the undifferentiated component increases the probability that the tumor contains a DNA mismatch repair deficiency, particularly if it is associated with a prominent tumor-infiltrating lymphocyte reaction (see under Carcinomas With DNA Mismatch Repair Deficiency).

Medullary Carcinoma

Medullary carcinoma is a subtype of colorectal carcinoma that is only recently recognized in the WHO classification. First described by Jessurun and coworkers,[73] this tumor was formerly classified as an undifferentiated carcinoma. It is composed of sheets of polygonal cells with vesicular nuclei, prominent nucleoli, abundant cytoplasm, and marked tumor-infiltrating lymphocytic response (Fig. 19-13).[73] Tumor cells may have an organoid or trabecular architecture, and focal mucin production may be present. This tumor has also been referred to as large cell minimally differentiated carcinoma.[74]

A number of molecular genetic investigations have demonstrated that many (if not most) medullary carcinomas are associated with a characteristic genomic profile. These tumors are less likely to have K-*ras* and *TP53* mutations than are typical colorectal carcinomas, and they are much more likely to harbor defects in DNA mismatch repair (see under Carcinomas with DNA Mismatch Repair Deficiency).[74] In fact, even when present as a small subcomponent of the tumor, this pattern is usually predictive of an underlying mismatch repair deficiency.[60]

Carcinoma With Squamous Metaplasia (Adenoacanthoma)

These types of tumors are extremely rare.[75] In one report, they were defined by the presence of adenocarcinoma elements, with abundant admixed areas of benign-appearing squamous metaplasia. The natural history and treatment are similar to those of pure adenocarcinomas.

Adenosquamous Carcinoma

These are extremely rare neoplasms, although they are three times more common than pure squamous cell carcinomas.[75] They show an even distribution between the right and left colon.[75] The tumors show malignant squamous and glandular elements either as separate components or admixed. These cancers often present at a higher stage; in one study, 50% had metastases at the

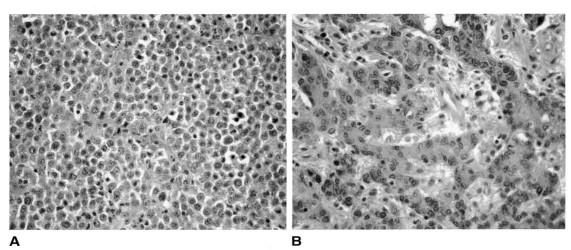

A **B**

FIGURE 19-12. Undifferentiated carcinoma. **A,** This variant is composed of sheets of tumor cells with focal necrosis and no evidence of gland formation. The cells were positive for CK20 and negative for neuroendocrine markers. **B,** This area shows a trabecular pattern of growth and only focal gland formation.

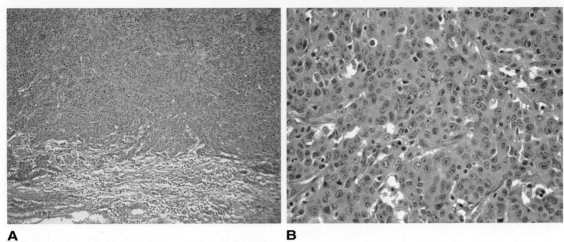

FIGURE 19–13. Medullary carcinoma. **A,** Low magnification reveals a solid and somewhat organoid tumor with a smooth margin of invasion and abundant peritumoral lymphocytes. **B,** The tumor cells contain large vesicular nuclei, prominent nucleoli, and a moderate amount of amphophilic cytoplasm. Numerous tumor-infiltrating lymphocytes are also present. Many, if not most, tumors with this appearance have defective DNA mismatch repair and high-frequency microsatellite instability (MSI-H).

time of diagnosis.[75] Although the overall survival is believed to be low (35% at 5 years), the number of cases studied is too small to determine whether this is independent of tumor stage.[75,76]

Squamous Cell Carcinoma

Primary squamous cell carcinomas of the colorectum are rare tumors; only 69 cases have been reported to 1985.[77] The etiology and histogenesis are poorly understood. Some believe that they arise from areas of squamous differentiation within adenomas. In one series of 11 cases, all tested negative for human papillomavirus (HPV).[75] Interestingly, one case has been described in which squamous metaplasia of the rectum showed concurrent HPV-associated dysplasia and invasive carcinoma, suggesting a pathogenetic role for this virus in this case.[78]

The histopathologic features are similar to those of squamous cell carcinomas that occur elsewhere in the body. Cancers that are in the distal rectum or anorectal region should be differentiated from those that arise in the anus. Supporting the absence of any significant independent prognostic associations, node-negative squamous cell carcinomas are reported to have a 5-year survival of 85%.[75]

Sarcomatoid Carcinoma (Spindle Cell Carcinoma)

Sarcomatoid carcinoma, first reported in 1986,[79] is extremely rare. The tumor is often bulky or fleshy in appearance and shows abundant hemorrhage. Histologic examination reveals a biphasic tumor with combined epithelial and mesenchymal elements that may show areas of transition.[80,81] The spindle cell component may

be undifferentiated or may show osseous or cartilaginous differentiation.[79]

Similar to sarcomatoid carcinomas that occur in other locations, there is usually evidence of keratin and EMA positivity in both the carcinoma and sarcoma components.[79] CEA positivity is usually limited to the adenocarcinoma element, whereas vimentin is usually positive in the sarcoma. Transitional areas may be positive for both cytokeratin and vimentin.[82] Focal S100 and myoglobin positivity has also been described in these tumors.[80] Metastases may show both components or may be composed of only one of the cellular elements.

Choriocarcinoma

Primary choriocarcinomas of the colorectum are limited to scattered case reports.[83] These cancers have occasionally presented with massive gastrointestinal tract bleeding or with massive and sometimes fatal bleeding associated with liver metastases.[84] Microscopic examination reveals a variable admixture of choriocarcinomatous elements and adenocarcinoma. The choriocarcinoma component stains with beta-HCG and alpha-fetoprotein. On occasion, choriocarcinoma elements predominate in metastases in which the primary tumors showed only focal beta-HCG positivity.[85] Increased serum levels of beta-HCG[86] and alpha-fetoprotein[84] have also been reported. These cancers usually show metastasis to liver at diagnosis and thus follow an aggressive clinical course.

Small Cell Carcinoma

These are morphologically identical to small cell carcinomas that occur in the lung. They often arise from an adenoma and not from differentiated neuroendocrine tumors, such as carcinoid tumor. Immunohistochemical staining usually demonstrates positivity for chromogranin and synaptophysin. These tumors are aggressive, usually show liver metastases at the time of presentation, and thus are associated with a poor prognosis.[87]

Mixed (Glandular-Neuroendocrine) Carcinoma

In some cases, the distinct separation between glandular and neuroendocrine tumors becomes blurred by neoplasms that show evidence of dual differentiation. The most subtle forms of these mixed tumors are adenocarcinomas that have interspersed endocrine cells and carcinoid tumors that contain scattered nonendocrine mucin cells. These features are worth noting, but they do not affect tumor behavior or management and therefore do not warrant classification as a distinct entity.

Tumors that show a significant mixture of adenocarcinoma and carcinoid elements are referred to as composite neoplasms.[88] A mixture of adenocarcinoma and well-differentiated carcinoid cells is most common, but a poorly differentiated carcinoid component may occasionally be present. In both forms, the two components are mixed intimately. This contrasts with a tumor collision, in which two separate carcinomas juxtapose each other but do not mix. On occasion, metastases may show only one component. There are insufficient data to comment accurately on clinical behavior.

Tumors that show evidence of neuroendocrine and other forms of differentiation, such as glandular differentiation, in the same cell are called amphicrine neoplasms. By ultrastructural examination, these tumors are characterized by dense-core granules and mucin droplets. There is ongoing controversy about the nature of these neoplasms, and their natural history is unknown.

Other Forms of "Diffuse" Carcinoma

Non–signet ring cell carcinomas may occasionally present with a diffuse pattern of growth similar to linitis plastica. In one study, 15 (0.6%) of 2369 colorectal carcinomas were diffuse; only 7 were signet ring cell type, whereas 8 were the "lymphangiosis" type.[89] The lymphangiosis type of diffuse cancer is typified by gland-forming adenocarcinoma, often of moderate differentiation, with extensive lymphatic and vascular spread.[89,90] As expected, the prognosis of this type of cancer is extremely poor.[89]

Other Rare Subtypes

Melanotic adenocarcinoma of the anorectal junction has been reported rarely, although evidence supports phagocytosis of anal melanocytes rather than true melanocytic differentiation,[91] and clear cell carcinomas have been described. Clear cell carcinomas have clear cytoplasm but lack the presence of cytoplasmic mucin. Strongly positive CEA staining in this tumor is useful to distinguish it from metastatic renal cell carcinomas.[92]

[handwritten: offer DNA analysis on paraffin block but do not order unless requested]

Carcinomas With DNA Mismatch Repair Deficiency

Inactivation of DNA mismatch repair plays an important role in the pathogenesis of 10% to 15% of colorectal cancers. Although some of these tumors are the result of hereditary alterations in one of the mismatch repair genes (see under Hereditary Nonpolyposis Colorectal Cancer), the majority (about 90%) are sporadic, due primarily to promoter methylation and silencing of transcription of *MLH1*. In addition to the characteristic genetic alteration known as high-frequency microsatellite instability (MSI-H), these cancers have a number of specific clinical and pathologic associations that are important to surgical pathologists.[93]

Sporadic mismatch repair–deficient MSI-H colorectal cancers have a marked female predominance (about 4:1), increase in prevalence with age, and are particularly common in women older than 70 years.[94] Most (about 90%) sporadic MSI-H colorectal cancers are located in the right colon, where they constitute about 50% of all right-sided cancers in women older than 70 years.[95] A number of specific pathologic associations have also been described in MSI-H colorectal cancers; these are similar to HNPCC cancers, which are also caused by DNA mismatch repair deficiency (Table 19-7).[60,96-100] MSI-H cancers are more likely to be multiple and to have a polypoid or exophytic growth pattern, often with sharply circumscribed pushing margins and abundant grossly visible necrosis. These tumors are more likely to show mucinous or signet ring cell features, often with microglandular differentiation (Fig. 19-14). Of note, the association between these features and DNA mismatch repair deficiency is present even when less than 50% of the tumor has these histologic features. Therefore, the sensitivity and specificity of these features in the identification of MSI-H cancers vary according to the criteria used.

The host lymphoid response is another feature with striking differences between MSI-H and microsatellite stable cancers. Tumor-infiltrating lymphocytes are highly predictive of MSI-H cancers, particularly in combination with undifferentiated histology (that may or may not be of classic medullary subtype) (Fig. 19-15; see also Fig. 19-13). In one study, the presence of five tumor-infiltrating lymphocytes per 10 high-power fields had a sensitivity of 93% and a specificity of 62% for the detection of MSI-H colorectal cancers.[101] A number

TABLE 19–7. Pathologic Features of MSI-H Colorectal Carcinomas[60,96]

Pathologic Feature	MSI-H (%)	MSI-L/MSS (%)	Positive Predictive Value (%)*
Location in right colon	90	34	32
Exophytic/polypoid	82	54	21
Signet ring cell component	13	5	31
Mucinous type (>50% extracellular mucin)	15	5	35
Mucinous component (>10% extracellular mucin)	22	7	36
Cribriform pattern	13	28	8
Poor differentiation	38	13	34
Medullary type	14	0.4	71
Medullary component (>10%)	25	3	59
Lymphocytosis	21	3	55
Pushing margin	15	8	25 (NS)
Crohn's-like reaction	49	36	19 (NS)
"MSI-H" by pathologist	49	11	44

*Assuming a prevalence of MSI-H of 15%.

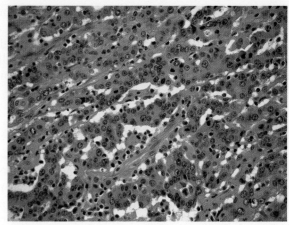

FIGURE 19–15. Cancer with marked tumor-infiltrating lymphocytes. This tumor shows an undifferentiated pattern of growth with focal trabecular architecture. Numerous tumor-infiltrating lymphocytes are seen. This cancer was MSI-H.

of more complex algorithms have been devised in an attempt to determine accurate probabilities that a tumor is MSI-H on the basis of pathologic findings, although the pathologist's overall "opinion" was the most predictive in one study.[61] Finally, compared with MSI-H HNPCC, sporadic MSI-H colorectal cancers are more frequently heterogeneous, poorly differentiated, mucinous, proximally located, and associated with a more prominent tumor-infiltrating lymphocyte reaction.[102]

Clinically, MSI-H colorectal cancers are more likely to present at an advanced T stage but are less likely to have regional lymph node metastases. In fact, most T4 N0 M0 colorectal cancers are DNA mismatch repair deficient.[103] When controlled for stage and other standard prognostic parameters, most studies have found MSI-H colorectal cancers to be associated with improved survival of patients (further discussed under Genetic Markers).[103,104]

COLORECTAL CANCER IN PATIENTS YOUNGER THAN 40 YEARS

Several studies have identified clinical and pathologic differences in colorectal cancers in young patients (younger than 40 years), which make up about 1% to 2% of all colorectal cancers. A family history of

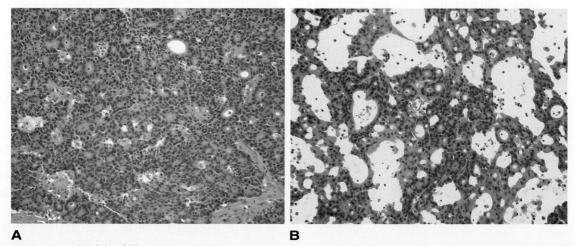

A   **B**

FIGURE 19–14. Microglandular differentiation. **A,** This carcinoma comprises sheets of tumor cells with only focal evidence of glandular lumina. Although some glands are rather well formed, others are rudimentary in appearance. **B,** In a different area, the tumor also shows abundant extracellular mucin production but still maintains a microglandular architecture. These morphologic patterns are more commonly seen in cancers with MSI-H.

colorectal cancer or a clear history of a predisposing condition (such as ulcerative colitis) is found in 21% compared with only 2% of patients older than 40 years.[105] Several studies have also found that they are more likely to present at an advanced stage, with regional or distant metastases.[106,107] Histologically, they are more likely to be mucinous or signet ring cell type.[106,107] In terms of survival, it is generally accepted that young patients with colorectal cancer do poorly, although it is difficult to demonstrate whether this effect is independent of stage, grade, and histologic subtype. In fact, some studies have found no evidence of significant independent survival differences related to young age.[105]

Special Studies

FAT CLEARANCE TECHNIQUES FOR LYMPH NODE DISSECTION

Several procedures have been developed to increase the yield of lymph node dissection. One method involves immersion of the specimen in graded alcohol solutions, followed by xylene, to "clear" the fat. In one study, this increased the average yield of lymph nodes from 6.1 to 12.7 and resulted in upstaging 5 (8.6%) of 58 Dukes' B cancers to Dukes' C.[108] However, this method is time-consuming and expensive and can be performed only after full assessment of the circumferential radial margin. It is therefore not widely recommended or practiced.

SENTINEL LYMPH NODES

The development of distant metastases in 20% to 30% of patients with primary tumors confined to the bowel wall is often cited as evidence of undetectable metastasis at the time of surgical resection and pathologic evaluation. As a result, attempts have been made to better evaluate these patients. One possibility is to identify the sentinel lymph node, that is, the node with the most direct drainage from the tumor, and to subject it to meticulous pathologic evaluation. This approach has received much attention in breast cancer.

To identify the sentinel node in colorectal cancers, the primary tumor is isolated, and blue dye is injected circumferentially around the tumor in the subserosal layer. The first one to four nodes that change color are the sentinel nodes. Evaluation of sentinel nodes includes thin slicing, submission in total, multiple levels, and immunohistochemical analyses. Although there are reports that this adjunctive technique could result in upstaging of tumors,[109] further evaluation is required to assess its clinical usefulness.

IMMUNOPHENOTYPE

Routine examination of colorectal carcinoma specimens does not usually require immunohistochemical studies. These studies are more often required for characterization of distinctive subtypes (such as small cell carcinoma) or for investigation of primary versus metastatic carcinoma. Historically, CEA has been the most commonly used stain for primary colonic cancers. Although it is positive in most colorectal cancers, there is also positivity in a large number of other tumors, relegating it to a supportive but not diagnostic method. More recently, use of cytokeratins 7 and 20 has gained popularity, although again these results yield supportive but not diagnostic findings. A summary of the keratin profile of colorectal adenocarcinoma is presented in Table 19-8.

Differential Diagnosis

METASTASIS VERSUS SYNCHRONOUS PRIMARY CARCINOMA

A small subset of patients with colorectal cancer will have more than one distinct carcinoma. These could represent synchronous primary colorectal carcinomas, or one could be a metastasis from the other. The only definitive diagnostic feature of a primary tumor is the finding of an adjacent in situ adenoma. Thus, synchronous cancers can be definitively diagnosed only if adenomatous epithelium is found in both tumor locations. The absence of mucosal involvement or the presence of extensive mucosal lymphatic involvement is strong evidence in favor of a metastasis. Similarly, the finding of a similar unusual morphologic variant also favors a metastasis, whereas dissimilar morphologic patterns, at least one of which is of an unusual subtype, favor synchronous tumors. For usual adenocarcinomas, a similar morphologic pattern is not helpful because it

TABLE 19–8. CK7/CK20 Profile of Colorectal Cancer[110,217–219]

CK7	CK20	Prevalence in Colorectal Cancer (%)	Differential
Overall results			
+		5–10	
	+	85–100	
Profiles			
+	+	5–10	Pancreas, bile duct, urothelial
+	–	0	Lung, breast, ovary, endometrial
–	+	75–95	Colorectal, gastric
–	–	0–15	Prostate, adrenal, hepatocellular, renal, carcinoid

is, by far, the most predominant pattern in colorectal cancers.

RECURRENT/METASTATIC VERSUS METACHRONOUS CARCINOMA

It is well known that patients with colorectal cancer are at significantly increased risk for the development of new cancers. In these cases, it may be difficult to differentiate a recurrent from a metachronous cancer. If adenoma is identified in the second tumor, a definitive diagnosis of a new primary can be established. If there is an absence of mucosal involvement or there is extensive submucosal-mucosal lymphatic spread in association with multiple tumor nodules, particularly when also present in the original resection, a metastasis should be favored. In the remainder of cases, it is often difficult to be definitive. In the absence of adenoma, recurrence is the favored diagnosis for all cancers that are located at an anastomotic line, even in the absence of other supporting features.

COLORECTAL ADENOCARCINOMA VERSUS ENDOMETRIAL OR OVARIAN ADENOCARCINOMA

The morphologic appearance of some endometrial and endometrioid ovarian carcinomas can have significant overlap with colorectal carcinoma. As a result, it may be difficult to firmly establish the site of origin of tumors that extensively involve the colorectum and other pelvic organs. Similar to the preceding discussion, the presence of adenoma or the absence of mucosal involvement is diagnostic of either a primary colorectal tumor or a noncolorectal primary, respectively.

Immunohistochemical analyses have also proved useful in this setting. Colorectal carcinomas are usually CK7-/CK20+, whereas the majority of endometrial and ovarian cancers are CK7+/CK20-.[110] Nuclear expression of WT1 is often positive in ovarian cancers but negative in colorectal cancers.[111]

Natural History

The overall survival for colorectal carcinoma at 1 and 5 years is 81% and 61%, respectively.[6] As with most solid tumors, survival is stratified according to disease progression, so that the 5-year survival is 89.7% for localized disease, 64.4% for cases with regional metastases, and 8.3% for ones with distant metastases.[6] Pathologic staging in colon cancer (AJCC system) is based on the depth of invasion into the bowel wall and surrounding structures and spread to regional lymph nodes (see Table 19-4). With progression, tumors may penetrate the peritoneal lining, resulting in intra-abdominal spread or invasion into other abdominal and pelvic structures. Spread through lymphatics or blood vessels may occur at any time during the evolution of disease. With further progression, the cancer invades the portal vein tributaries, leading to liver metastases, and the vena cava, leading to lung and bone marrow as well as other distant metastases.

Treatment

Colorectal cancer is traditionally managed by surgical resection plus or minus chemotherapy, depending on the stage of disease progression. In advanced disease (stage IV, Dukes' D, distant metastases), chemotherapy has been used extensively.[112] Until recently, the only agent has been 5-fluorouracil (5-FU). Two new cytotoxic agents—CPT11 (irinotecan), a topoisomerase inhibitor, and oxaliplatin, a third-generation platinum compound—have been shown to be effective in 5-FU–resistant advanced disease.[112] Recent trials also suggest that initial combination therapy with 5-FU leads to improved response rates and more prolonged progression-free survival.[112]

Chemotherapy has also been used in the adjuvant setting for regional metastatic disease (stage III, Dukes' C, lymph node metastases), in which there is proven benefit, with a 5% to 6% absolute survival advantage at 5 years.[113-115] Adjuvant chemotherapy for localized disease (stage II, Dukes' B, nonmetastatic) remains controversial.[116,117] Optimal adjuvant therapy for rectal cancer is even more uncertain, and ongoing trials are comparing combinations of preoperative and postoperative chemotherapy and radiation therapy.[112]

In addition to these agents, a number of other chemotherapeutic and biologic compounds are under investigation and development. This includes inhibition of epidermal growth factor signaling through the epidermal growth factor receptor (antibody C225 and a pharmacologic agent, Iressa), vascular endothelial growth factor inhibitors, cyclooxygenase-2 inhibition, matrix metalloproteinase inhibitors, and immunotherapy.[112]

Prognostic Factors

Guidelines set by the AJCC for the development and evaluation of putative prognostic markers require that they be clinically important and useful in management of patients, independent of other factors, and statistically significant.[118] Prognostic factors are divided into three categories: category I, well supported in literature through outcome studies; category II, well studied biologically or clinically, but clinical utility has not been well established; and category III, studied but not found useful or not adequately studied.

For colorectal carcinoma, the 1999 consensus statement of the College of American Pathologists indicated that pathologic TNM stage, extramural venous invasion, and preoperative CEA level are the most important category I factors.[52] A full list of these and other prognostic factors is presented in Table 19-9.

PATHOLOGIC STAGING

Pathologic stage is the most important predictor of tumor behavior and outcome for the patient. The first staging system was proposed by Dukes,[119] although TNM staging is more widely used now in North America (Table 19-10).

EXTENT OF TUMOR INVASION

Some confusion exists about staging of the extent of tumor invasion in colorectal cancer. The differentiation between high-grade dysplasia and Tis and T1 carcinomas is discussed earlier (see under Criteria for

TABLE 19–9. Prognostic Factors in Colorectal Carcinoma

Factor Classification	Factor
Category I: *clinically proven, prognostically important, generally used*	Local extent of tumor invasion, pT Regional lymph node metastasis, pN Blood or lymphatic vessel invasion Residual tumor, R Preoperative CEA
Category IIA: *extensively studied, prognostically important, further validation required*	Histologic grade Radial margin
Category IIB: *promising in multiple studies, insufficient data for conclusive proof*	Histologic type Histologic features of MSI MSI-H Chromosome 18q/DCC gene loss Tumor border configuration
Category III: *not yet sufficiently studied*	DNA content Other molecular genetic markers Perineural invasion Microvessel density Other protein expression Peritumoral fibrosis Purulent peritumoral inflammatory reaction Foci of neuroendocrine differentiation Nucleolar organizing regions Proliferation indices
Category IV: *well studied, no prognostic significance*	Tumor size Gross configuration

From Compton CC, Fielding LP, Burgart LJ, et al: Prognostic factors in colorectal cancer. College of American Pathologists Consensus Statement 1999. Arch Pathol Lab Med 124:979–994,2000.

TABLE 19–10. AJCC TNM Classification of Colon and Rectal Carcinomas

The same classification is used for both clinical and pathologic staging.

Primary Tumor (T)

TX	Primary tumor cannot be assessed
T0	No evidence of primary tumor
Tis	Carcinoma *in situ:* intraepithelial or invasion of lamina propria*
T1	Tumor invades submucosa
T2	Tumor invades muscularis propria
T3	Tumor invades through the muscularis propria into the subserosa, or into non-peritonealized pericolic or perirectal tissues
T4	Tumor directly invades other organs or structures, and/or perforates visceral peritoneum**, ***

*Note: Tis includes cancer cells confined within the glandular basement membrane (intraepithelial) or lamina propria (intramucosal) with no extension through the muscularis mucosae into the submucosa.

**Note: Direct invasion in T4 includes invasion of other segments of the colorectum by way of the serosa; for example, invasion of the sigmoid colon by a carcinoma of the cecum.

***Tumor that is adherent to other organs or structures, macroscopically, is classified T4. However, if no tumor is present in the adhesion, microscopicaly, the classification should be pT3. The V and L substaging should be used to identify the presence or absence of vascular or lymphatic invasion.

Regional Lymph Nodes (N)

NX	Regional lymph nodes cannot be assessed
N0	No regional lymph node metastases
N1	Metastases in 1 to 3 regional nodes
N2	Metastases in 4 or more regional nodes

Note: A tumor nodule in the pericolorectal adipose tissue of a primary carcinoma without histologic evidence of residual lymph node in the nodule is classified in the pN category as a regional lymph node metastasis if the nodule has the form and smooth contour of a lymph node. If the nodule has an irregular contour, it should be classified in the T category and also coded as V1 (microscopic venous invasion) or as V2 (if it was grossly evident), because there is a strong likelihood that it represents venous invasion.

Distant Metastases (M)

MX	Distant metastasis cannot be assessed
M0	No distant metastasis
M1	Distant metastasis

Used with the permission of the American Joint Committee on Cancer (AJCC), Chicago, Illinois. The original source for this material is the *AJCC Cancer Staging Manual, Sixth Edition* (2002) published by Springer-Verlag New York, www.springer-ny.com.

Malignancy). Invasion into the muscularis propria (T2) is usually readily recognized. Furthermore, the extent of tumor invasion beyond the muscularis propria has been reported to influence prognosis, and an optional substratification of pT3 has been proposed: pT3a to pT3d for invasion less than 1 mm, 1 to 5 mm, more than 5 to 15 mm, or more than 15 mm beyond the border of the muscularis propria, respectively.[120]

As tumors invade deeply beyond the muscularis propria, they either perforate the peritoneum or invade adjacent structures, depending on whether the tumor is within an intra-abdominal (peritonealized) portion of the colorectum or in a retroperitoneal location. The pericolic fibrofatty tissue and peritoneal covering form the serosa. Therefore, stating that "invasion of the serosa" is present may be ambiguous because there are significant differences between invasion into the serosa (T3) and overt perforation of the peritoneum (T4). Thus, it is important to correctly identify tumors that have breached the peritoneal lining (T4). This feature indicates a high risk of intra-abdominal progression. In fact, some studies have shown that localized peritoneal involvement in curative resections has greater prognostic value than does the extent of tumoral invasion or regional lymph node status.[140] Whereas peritoneal involvement was previously subdivided as T4a (direct invasion) and T4b (perforation of free peritoneal surface), all forms of peritoneal invasion are currently simply classified as T4.[2]

Interpretation of the status of invasion of the free peritoneal surface is often difficult. Because of the subjectivity and lack of reproducibility, criteria have been developed.[121] Free tumor cells on the serosal surface, tumor cells at the serosal surface with an associated inflammatory reaction, and even simply mesothelial inflammation or hyperplasia in a region near tumor are all classified as pT4 (peritoneal involvement). This is usually associated with a localized mesothelial proliferative response and often inflammation and fibrin deposition (Fig. 19-16). Tumors that invade the mesocolonic aspect of the bowel will extend deeply into the fibrovascular pedicle, and although they may approach the true resection margin, they do not involve the peritoneum. Care should be taken to explicitly describe the level of invasion and the status of the peritoneal surface; for example, the tumor "invades deeply into pericolic fibrofatty tissues but does not breach the peritoneal surface" (T3).

LYMPH NODE INVOLVEMENT

The total number of lymph nodes sampled is an important determinant of adequacy of pathologic examination. The number of positive nodes identified may depend on the number of nodes examined, although some studies have not found this relationship.[122] More important, the prognosis of node-negative colorectal cancer is directly related to the number of negative lymph nodes identified. This relationship holds true for rectal cancers that have fewer than 14 lymph nodes.[123] Staging criteria are listed in Table 19-10.

Interpretation and classification of tumor deposits in the adventitia without identifiable residual lymph node tissue have also been problematic. In the past, nodules larger than 3 mm were considered to represent lymph node deposits. Foci smaller than 3 mm were classified as "discontinuous tumor extension" (pT3). Currently, tumor deposits in the soft tissue should be classified as lymph node metastases if they are round and smooth (Fig. 19-17). Multiple deposits with smooth contour are scored as multiple separate lymph nodes. If the deposits are irregular, they are best classified as indicative of venous invasion (either V1, microscopic, or V2, macroscopic) (Fig. 19-18).

In some studies, lymph node metastases distant from the primary tumor are associated with a worse outcome. For the TNM classification, the definition of regional lymph nodes varies with the location of the primary tumor, although external iliac and common iliac lymph node metastases are always classified as M1.[2]

Finally, some authors support designating solitary metastases less than 2 mm as micrometastases, although the possible additional prognostic information this might divulge is unknown (Fig. 19-19).[124,125] Nevertheless, these cases should be classified as pN1.[52] Another area of controversy involves the use of ancillary techniques to identify micrometastases in lymph nodes. In one study, micrometastases were identified by polymerase chain

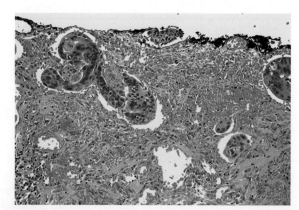

FIGURE 19-16. Peritoneal involvement. The peritoneal surface was inked in the region of the main tumor mass. The tumor is associated with granulation tissue, hemorrhage, and fibrin deposition. A nest of tumor cells is present on the peritoneal surface. In this section, mesothelial proliferation is not apparent.

	Primary	Regional	Distant
TABLE 19-11. Staging of Tumors of the Colon and Rectum[2]			
Stage	**Primary Tumor**	**Regional Lymph Nodes**	**Distant Metastases**
0	Tis	N0	M0
I	T1	N0	M0
	T2	N0	M0
IIA	T3	N0	M0
IIB	T4	N0	M0
IIIA	T1-T2	N1	M0
IIIB	T3-T4	N1	M0
IIIC	Any T	N2	M0
IV	Any T	Any N	M1

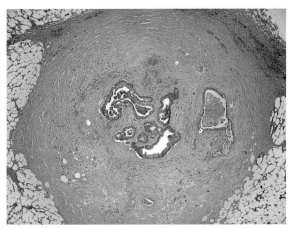

FIGURE 19–17. Pericolic tumor deposit consistent with a lymph node metastasis. Although there is no residual lymph node, the deposit is round and smooth.

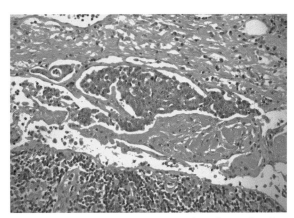

FIGURE 19–19. Micrometastasis. A single subcapsular deposit measures less than 2 mm in size.

reaction analysis of the gene encoding CEA in 14 (54%) of 26 node-negative patients, and the adjusted 5-year survival was 50% versus 91% in patients without micrometastases.[125] However, there are no data yet to support whether these patients will benefit from adjuvant therapy in the same manner as conventional node-positive patients; therefore, further assessment in clinical trials is required before these approaches will come into general use.[58]

HISTOLOGIC GRADE

The importance of histologic grading as a prognostic factor is supported by the consistent finding of independent significance in multivariate analyses.[54,55,58] However, well-differentiated tumors make up a small fraction of most series of cancers that have been studied, and the differences in outcome between well-differentiated and moderately differentiated tumors are not as clearly

demarcated as the differences with poorly differentiated tumors. Therefore, for the purposes of prognostic classification, available evidence supports collapsing the three traditional grades into two tiers (low and high grade).[52]

HISTOLOGIC SUBTYPE

Many historical series have found histologic subtype to be predictive of survival, with poor survival associated with mucinous adenocarcinomas, signet ring cell carcinomas, and undifferentiated carcinomas. However, this is now controversial because of significant advances in our understanding of the molecular basis of colorectal cancer. In particular, it is now recognized that cancers with DNA mismatch repair deficiency have characteristic molecular genetic alterations and are associated with significantly better overall survival.[103] Paradoxically, mucinous, signet ring cell, and undifferentiated cancers are more prevalent in mismatch repair deficiency.[60] At present, the prognosis of these histologic subtypes stratified by mismatch repair status remains unknown.

PROXIMAL AND DISTAL RESECTION MARGINS

The presence of positive margins implies that there is residual tumor in the patient. This has led to the residual tumor classification system (see Table 19-10).[52]

CIRCUMFERENTIAL (RADIAL) RESECTION MARGIN AND TOTAL MESORECTAL EXCISION

Identification of the importance of the circumferential radial margin in colorectal carcinoma has altered the management of this disease. In 1986, Quirke and coworkers[127] first described the importance of lateral spread and the role of involvement of the radial margin in predicting rectal cancer recurrence. By serial

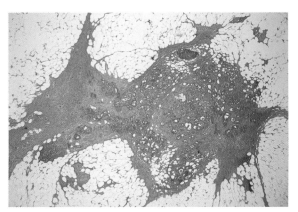

FIGURE 19–18. Pericolic deposit consistent with venous invasion. The deposit is irregular in shape, showing tumor that extends along connective tissue septa. In addition, residual smooth muscle is noted within the deposit, consistent with the wall of a vein.

TABLE 19–12. Relationship Between Outcome and Radial Margin Distance in Rectal Cancer[133]

Distance to Radial Margin (cm)	Local Recurrence (%)	Distant Recurrence (%)	2-Year Survival (%)
<0.10	16.4	37.6	69.7
0.11–0.20	14.9	21.0	84.8
0.21–0.50	10.3	17.2	87.0
0.51–1.0	6.0	8.2	91.2
>1.0	2.4	10.9	92.8

transverse slicing of 52 unopened rectal resection specimens and analysis of whole mount sections, positive lateral resection margins were found in 14 (27%), and 12 of these 14 developed recurrent tumor.[127] These results have been confirmed in larger studies, in which positive radial margins predict not only local recurrence but also survival.[128]

These findings have importance not only for pathologic assessment of rectal cancer but also for surgical management. In fact, Heald and coworkers[129] have long been proponents of total mesorectal excision (TME), which is the sharp dissection of the entire mesorectum along the finely delimited fascial plane. This procedure removes about 2 to 3 cm of perirectal tissue, preserves the pelvic fascia and autonomic plexuses, and is a significant departure from the blunt dissections performed by most general surgeons. The clinical effectiveness of TME has been well established.[130,131] There has also been growing realization that the effectiveness of TME is not simply in prevention of positive margins but in removal of significant unrecognized deposits that are often deep in perirectal adipose tissue.[132]

Results from the Dutch TME trial have found that even when the radial margin is negative, the actual distance from the deepest point of tumor penetration to the margin is predictive of local and distant recurrences (Table 19-12).[133] On this basis, providing an exact

measurement for the distance to tumor is highly recommended in pathology reports (Fig. 19-20). As a result, the Dutch studies have outlined criteria for assessing the completeness of TME specimens.[134] They use a three-grade system based on the gross inspection of the intact specimen. All specimens are photographed before and after sectioning to provide a permanent record. A complete TME shows intact mesorectum with only minor irregularities of a smooth surface, no defects deeper than 5 mm, no coning toward the distal margin, and a smooth circumferential margin on transverse slicing. A nearly complete TME shows moderate bulk to the mesorectum, irregularity to the surface, and moderate coning, but at no site is the muscularis propria visible (except at the insertion of the levator muscles). Finally, an incomplete TME shows little bulk to the mesorectum, defects down into the muscularis propria, and an irregular circumferential margin. In the Dutch series, about 55% of TMEs were complete, 20% were nearly complete, and 25% were incomplete. In cases in which the radial margin was negative, this gross assessment was predictive of recurrence.

INVASION OF ENDOTHELIUM-LINED SPACES

Invasion of lymphatics and veins should be carefully sought and reported as present or absent. Submission of five or more blocks has been found to increase the likelihood of identifying extramural venous invasion.[56] It may not be possible to differentiate lymphatics from small thin-walled postcapillary venules, leading some to favor ambiguous terminology such as "lymphovascular" invasion (Fig. 19-21). Invasion of large veins is usually recognizable and should be clearly indicated when found. The location in the bowel wall in which invasion is found should also be reported because it may have a relationship with outcome. Most studies do not support the use of routine immunohistochemical markers to

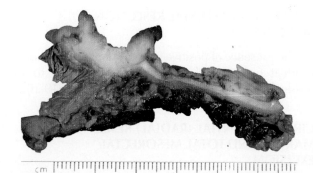

FIGURE 19–20. Radial margin of a rectal cancer. This tumor was located in the upper third of the rectum. The radial resection margin is inked blue. The specimen was opened longitudinally and sectioned transversely. A portion of the specimen has a peritoneal covering (*left side*). Multiple sections should be submitted so that the distance between the tumor and the closest inked margin can be measured.

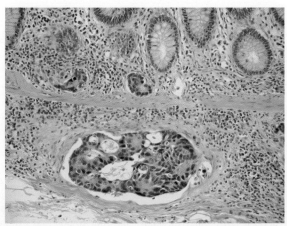

FIGURE 19–21. Lymphovascular invasion. This poorly differentiated adenocarcinoma is present within endothelium-lined spaces.

identify blood vessel invasion, although it may help confirm difficult cases, particularly when there are extensive tissue retraction artifacts. Some pathologists also rely on the so-called isolated artery sign in adventitial tissues, wherein the presence of an artery and a tumor nest without a clearly identifiable vein is interpreted as being highly suggestive of or even diagnostic for venous invasion.

In several but not all studies, lymphatic invasion has been associated with independent prognostic significance, particularly in patients with node-negative disease.[55,135-137] The relationship in individuals with lymph node metastases has not been as clear, and attempts to further stratify the significance by the location of the lymphatics within the bowel wall have also met with variable success.

In contrast, extramural venous invasion has been consistently found to have independent prognostic value, even in the setting of lymph node metastases (Fig. 19-22).[55,135,136,138] In particular, this finding is a marker of increased risk of liver metastases.

HOST LYMPHOCYTIC RESPONSE

There are multiple facets to the inflammatory and immune reaction seen in response to colorectal cancer. These include tumor-infiltrating lymphocytes, peritumoral lymphocytes, peritumoral lymphoid aggregates (which may or may not have germinal centers), reactive regional lymph nodes (particularly paracortical hyperplasia), and neutrophilic infiltrates (usually in association with gland destruction at the leading edge of the tumor).

In general, an intense inflammatory response of any type is associated with improved prognosis.[139] Greatest attention has focused on development of criteria to evaluate and to grade the peritumoral lymphocytic response and the tumor-infiltrating lymphocytes. Graham and Appelman[140] developed the most extensively used criteria for the peritumoral reaction and referred to it as the "Crohn's-like" lymphoid reaction. This classification has three grades: none; mild, defined by occasional aggregates and scattered lymphocytes; and marked, characterized by abundant aggregates, some with germinal centers, and a prominent peritumoral band of lymphocytes (Fig. 19-23). Defined in this way, the Crohn's-like lymphoid reaction has been found to have independent prognostic significance in several studies.[57,141,142]

Tumor-infiltrating lymphocytes have gained attention because of their association with colorectal cancers that contain DNA mismatch repair deficiency.[96] This immune response is characterized by lymphocytes that interdigitate between malignant epithelial cells. Several grading systems are described; the most widely used is a subjective descriptive categorization as none, mild, or marked (similar to the grading for Crohn's-like lymphoid reaction). Other studies have attempted to quantify lymphocytes by counting them in a single high-power field and to develop cutoffs that are highly predictive of DNA mismatch repair deficiency.[60] The role of tumor-infiltrating lymphocytes as an independent prognostic marker is not as well characterized.

INVASIVE MARGIN (LEADING EDGE) OF TUMOR

As in many human cancers, there is variability in the invasive leading edge of colorectal cancers, with smooth, rounded tumors that appear to push into

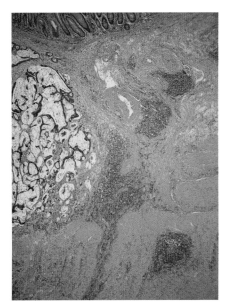

FIGURE 19–23. Crohn's-like lymphoid reaction. Prominent lymphoid aggregates are located at the periphery of the tumor; some of these contain germinal centers. When lymphoid aggregates such as these are numerous, the reaction is classified as "marked."

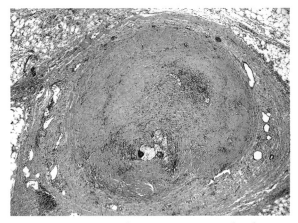

FIGURE 19–22. Extramural venous invasion. This large vein, present in pericolic tissue, is occluded by granulation tissue, inflammatory cells, tumor cells, and mucin. This finding is an adverse prognostic indicator independent of lymph node status.

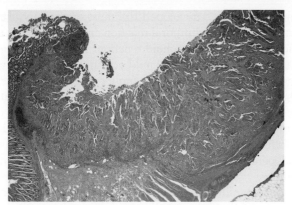

FIGURE 19–24. Pushing or expanding margin of invasion. The invasive tumor edge is smooth and round and well demarcated from the surrounding tissue. Numerous inflammatory cells are located at the edge of the tumor.

adjacent tissue at one end of the spectrum and irregular, infiltrative tumors that aggressively dissect between normal tissue planes at the other end. The importance of this variability was identified in the mid-1980s when it was found to predict prognosis.[57,143] Grading criteria consisting of a two-grade system that includes naked eye and microscopic examination have been defined by Jass.[57] By naked eye examination, infiltrating tumors have ill-defined limits to the invasive border or loss of the host-tumor tissue interface. By microscopic examination, infiltrating tumors show "streaming dissection" of the muscularis propria, dissection of the perimuscular adipose tissue by small glands or irregular clusters of cells, or perineural invasion. Expanding tumors have none of these features (Fig. 19-24). By these criteria, the infiltrating margin was found to be an independent negative prognostic factor.[144] Other classifications have included a mixed category, in which the tumoral edge is not purely pushing or infiltrative. This has utility because tumors that are predominantly pushing or expanding have also been associated with MSI-H cancers.[60,96] Finally, some investigators have described a related feature known as tumor "budding," in which microscopic clusters of undifferentiated cells are identified just ahead of the invasive front of cancer.[145]

OTHER PATHOLOGIC PROGNOSTIC FACTORS

In addition to the features described before, a number of other factors have been examined. Perforation at the site of tumor is also a negative prognostic indicator. Perineural invasion has not been uniformly supported in the literature as an independent prognostic indicator. Angiogenesis has received attention both as a prognostic factor and as a possible therapeutic target. The process of neovascularization is clearly important to tumorigenesis. Microvessel density has been found to be an adverse indicator,[146] but it has not been widely used in clinical practice.

GENETIC MARKERS

In the past two decades, a number of molecular and genetic alterations in colorectal cancer have been touted as possible markers of biologic behavior and outcome. However, many of these studies have not had the power to determine whether the prognostic implications of these alterations are independent of other known clinical and pathologic variables in multivariate analysis. Markers that have been validated or that hold the greatest likelihood of independence are listed in Table 19-13.[58] With the advent of genomic and proteomic profiling technologies, the number of putative markers is likely to significantly increase in coming years.

In brief, the molecular markers that have been most extensively studied and show the most promising results are DNA ploidy (and S phase fraction), *TP53* mutation (or loss of chromosomal region 17p, where it is located), chromosome 18q loss (or *DCC* or *SMAD4* loss, two of the putative target genes in this region), and microsatellite instability. Studies investigating *TP53* have been hampered, in part, by methodologic differences between mutation detection and immunohistochemical analysis of p53 expression.[147] Whereas investigations of p53 expression have been conflicting, studies of *TP53* mutation have mostly shown an association with poor outcome.[147,148] In contrast to the abundance of small molecular studies that have not shown *TP53* significance in multivariate analyses, several studies have found 18q loss, *DCC* loss, and absence of microsatellite instability to be predictive of poor outcome, independent of other standard variables.[103,104,149-152] Finally, poor outcome has also been seen with decreased p27 expression,[153] and although results investigating K-*ras* mutations have been variable, a meta-analysis found that mutations predicted increased recurrence and death.[154] The prognostic significance of microsatellite instability may not be independent in studies that include careful pathologic assessment of lymphoid response, invasion pattern, and vein invasion.[155]

Despite the possible prognostic significance of these molecular alterations, none is used in clinical practice, largely because they do not play a role in treatment decisions. However, there is emerging evidence that some of these markers could be used to predict response to chemotherapeutic agents (discussed next).

TREATMENT AND PREDICTIVE MARKERS

In the adjuvant setting, chemotherapy elicits a 5% to 6% improvement in 5-year survival, which represents a 25% to 35% reduction in the risk for dying of colorectal cancer.[113,116] Whereas this merits generalized use, most patients do not benefit from this therapy. The ability to identify a subset of patients who would most likely benefit from chemotherapy would have significant clinical utility.

To date, there is a paucity of validated or even promising predictive markers. Among these, expression levels of proteins involved in 5-FU metabolism and inhibition of DNA synthesis are most widely studied. One major mechanism of 5-FU activity is thought to be inhibition of thymidylate synthase, an important step in the synthesis of dTTP, one of the building blocks of DNA. Expression levels of thymidylate synthase are thus related to 5-FU effectiveness, and low levels are associated with better responsiveness.[156] Interestingly, a common polymorphism in the promoter region of thymidylate synthase has been associated with constitutive thymidylate synthase levels. Although this may allow a more reliable prediction of treatment response, further validation studies are required. Enzymes involved in catabolism are also important in predicting 5-FU efficacy. For instance, low levels of dihydropyrimidine dehydrogenase, the major enzyme involved in 5-FU breakdown, predict not only good response to 5-FU but also increased toxicity.[157]

Microsatellite instability has also been suggested as a predictor of chemosensitivity; however, it has not been evaluated in controlled trials, and conclusions are not yet possible.[157,158] Early results from ongoing molecular reanalyses of adjuvant chemotherapy trials that included a no-chemotherapy arm suggest that patients with MSI-H tumors may not benefit from chemotherapy.[160] Much attention has also focused on apoptotic abnormalities and how they may affect chemotherapeutic response. For instance, *TP53* mutation has been associated with resistance to chemotherapy.[161,162]

PREOPERATIVE CHEMOTHERAPY AND IRRADIATION OF RECTAL CARCINOMA

The management of rectal cancer has been controversial since the early 1990s, when studies demonstrated that combined modality preoperative therapy (radiation and fluorouracil ± leucovorin) resulted in downstaging and improved local control after resection.[163,164] This preoperative neoadjuvant therapy is the treatment of choice for T3, T4, and node-positive rectal cancers at many centers. Because this protocol is stage specific, accurate radiologic preoperative staging is important in assessment. The role of preoperative therapy in overall survival has not been as clearly delineated, particularly since total mesorectal excision has evolved, and many trials are still ongoing.

The role of the pathologist in examining treated rectal cancers is to carefully evaluate the presence of residual primary tumor and lymph node metastases. Complete pathologic response (no residual tumor on pathologic examination) is seen in 10% to 30%.[165] In one study, only 25% of complete clinical responders had complete pathologic response, whereas an equal number of complete pathologic responders were found in patients with the clinical appearances of residual tumor, usually due to persistent fibrosis or ulceration.[165]

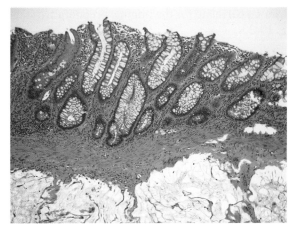

FIGURE 19–25. Rectal adenocarcinoma after preoperative chemoradiation therapy. No residual viable tumor was present. However, on microscopic examination, one sees injured and regenerating epithelium overlying mucin pools.

Pathologic examination reveals variable fibrosis, mucin pools, hemosiderin-laden and foamy macrophages, ulceration or erosion, and reactive epithelial changes (Fig. 19-25). Residual tumor is also variable and may be dispersed anywhere within the rectal wall or perirectal tissues. The pathologic staging is indicated with the prescript *y* to designate that the evaluation was post treatment (ypTNM). Only residual tumor cells are counted in this evaluation.[2,51] I report any tumor cells identified and do not believe it is possible to accurately assess the potential viability of such cells.

Residual mucin pools without epithelium are not classified as viable tumor in staging. Careful attention must be paid to lymph nodes because complete pathologic response of the tumor may be associated with residual lymph node metastases. Note should also be made of the degenerative changes and their location within the wall and regional lymph nodes because this

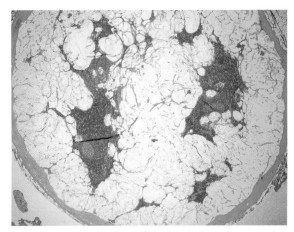

FIGURE 19–26. Perirectal lymph node after preoperative chemoradiation therapy. The lymph node is largely replaced by pools of mucin. Although no residual viable tumor cells are present, the mucin correlates with tumor "necrosis."

provides a correlate for the original preoperative staging (Fig. 19-26).

LIVER METASTASES

About 15% to 25% of patients with colorectal cancer will have liver metastases at the time of presentation, and another 20% will develop metastases after treatment of their primary tumor.[166] Without treatment, the median survival after the detection of liver metastases is approximately 9 months.[167] In selected patients, resection of liver metastases has been shown to improve outcome, with 5-year survival rates between 35% and 40%.[168] Unfortunately, only about 10% to 15% of patients with liver metastases are considered surgical candidates.[169]

In the assessment of a resected liver metastasis, the resection margin status is the most important variable. Improved outcome is reported only for those patients with negative resection margins.[169] Negative margins within 1 cm have also been associated with significantly reduced 5-year survival rates compared with those patients with margins greater than 1 cm.[170]

■ Hereditary Nonpolyposis Colorectal Cancer

Also known as Lynch syndrome I (when confined to colorectum), Lynch II (when associated with extra-colonic cancers), or familial colon cancer, hereditary nonpolyposis colorectal cancer (HNPCC) is characterized by highly penetrant, autosomal dominant–like inheritance of colorectal and other cancers.[171,172] By use of the Amsterdam and Amsterdam II criteria (Table 19-13), which are designed to identify autosomal dominant–like families, this strictly defined syndrome represents about 2% to 3% of all colorectal cancer.[173,174]

It is now known that about two thirds of HNPCC is caused by hereditary defects in one of the DNA mismatch repair genes (Table 19-14).[171] These are ubiquitously expressed genes involved in repair of DNA mismatches that result from misincorporation or slippage events during replication.[175] The mismatch repair genes function in a complex; MSH2 and its binding partners MSH3 and MSH6 mediate recognition of the mismatch. Subsequent recruitment of MLH1, PMS2, and other enzymes leads to excision, repolymerization, and finally ligation of the repaired strand.

In HNPCC caused by DNA mismatch repair defects, colorectal cancers are more likely to occur at a young age, to be multiple, and to be accompanied by cancers of the endometrium, the stomach, and less commonly the ureter, renal pelvis, bladder, pancreas, and biliary tract.[171,172] Some have proposed the term *hereditary mismatch repair deficiency syndrome* to designate the subset of HNPCC caused by these gene defects.[176]

TABLE 19–13. Amsterdam Criteria for Hereditary Nonpolyposis Colorectal Cancer (HNPCC)

Classic ICG-HNPCC Criteria (Amsterdam Criteria I)
There should be at least three relatives with colorectal cancer; all of the following criteria should be present.
One should be a first-degree relative of the other two.
At least two successive generations should be affected.
At least one colorectal cancer should be diagnosed before the age of 50 years.
Familial adenomatous polyposis should be excluded.
Tumors should be verified by pathologic examination.

Revised ICG-HNPCC Criteria (Amsterdam Criteria II)
There should be at least three relatives with an HNPCC-associated cancer (colorectal cancer, cancer of the endometrium, small bowel, ureter, or renal pelvis).
One should be a first-degree relative of the other two.
At least two successive generations should be affected.
At least one should be diagnosed before the age of 50 years.
Familial adenomatous polyposis should be excluded in colorectal cancer case(s), if any.
Tumors should be verified by pathologic examination.

Data from Vasen HF, Mecklin JP, Khan PM, Lynch HT: The International Collaborative Group on Hereditary Non-Polyposis Colorectal Cancer (ICG-HNPCC). Dis Colon Rectum 34:424-425, 1991; and Vasen HF, Watson P, Mecklin JP, Lynch HT: New clinical criteria for hereditary nonpolyposis colorectal cancer (HNPCC, Lynch syndrome) proposed by the International Collaborative Group on HNPCC. Gastroenterology 116:1453-1456, 1999.

Loss of mismatch repair leads to a dramatic increase in mutation rate, which is characterized by frameshift mutations in repetitive DNA sequences known as microsatellites and referred to as microsatellite instability.[93,180] Mutations are also more likely to occur in short repetitive sequences within coding regions of genes, such as *TGFBR2*.[181] Therefore, the molecular pathogenesis of mismatch repair–deficient cancers appears to follow a genetically distinct pathway compared with tumors without mismatch repair deficiency (see under Genome Instability).[180,182]

In addition to identification of patients with HNPCC by family history, mismatch repair–deficient tumors can be identified by genetic and immunohistochemical methods. The frameshift mutations occurring in microsatellites can be identified by extraction of DNA from normal and tumor tissue, amplification of selected micro-

TABLE 19–14. Genetic Basis of Hereditary Nonpolyposis Colorectal Cancer (HNPCC)

High-Frequency Microsatellite Instability (MSI-H)	Gene Mutation
Yes (70%)	*MLH1* (30%)
	MSH2 (30%)
	Other (5%)
	Unknown (5%)
No (30%)	Unknown (30%)

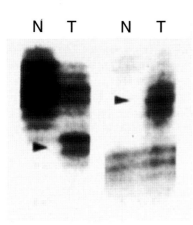

FIGURE 19–27. Molecular analysis for microsatellite instability. Separate DNA samples from normal and tumor tissue have been amplified by polymerase chain reaction at two different loci using radioactively labeled primers, electrophoresed through an acrylamide gel, and exposed to x-ray film. Normal-sized bands are present in the normal (N) and tumor (T) samples, whereas the shifted alleles (indicative of microsatellite instability; *arrowheads*) are present only in the tumor samples.

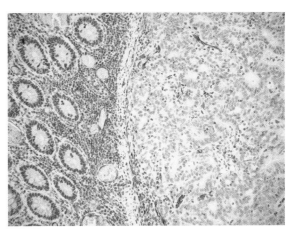

FIGURE 19–28. MLH1 immunohistochemistry. Nuclear expression is strong in crypt epithelial cells and lymphocytes (*left side of field*). In contrast, tumor cells have no apparent nuclear expression (*right side of field*). Within the tumor, focal positivity is noted in tumor-infiltrating lymphocytes.

satellites by polymerase chain reaction (Table 19-15), and analysis of fragment size by gel electrophoresis or automated sequencer (Fig. 19-27).[179] Criteria have been developed to standardize the molecular diagnosis of microsatellite instability (see Table 19-15).[179]

In the setting of HNPCC, most hereditary and second-hit tumor alterations are inactivating chain-terminating mutations. As a result of instability of the truncated mRNA transcript or the protein product, these mutations are associated with complete loss of immunohistochemically detectable mismatch repair protein in tumors (Fig. 19-28).[183-185] The specificity of loss of MLH1 or MSH2 expression for underlying microsatellite instability is virtually 100%.[184] However, mismatch repair protein loss may also occur as a tumor-specific alteration in patients with sporadic colorectal cancer (see under Genome Instability). The sensitivity of immunohistochemistry depends on the underlying mechanism of gene inactivation.[184]

Investigations to characterize and to diagnose hereditary cancers should be undertaken only in the setting of a multidisciplinary cancer genetics program with appropriate counseling of the patient and consent for investigation.

CLINICAL FEATURES

Most patients present with a change in bowel habit, constipation, abdominal distention, hematochezia, or tenesmus (rectosigmoid lesions). Other patients present with only systemic signs and symptoms, including weight loss, malaise, fever, or anemia. Unfortunately, only about 40% of patients present with localized disease.[6] Of the remaining patients, about 40% present with regional metastases and about 20% present with distant metastases. Endoscopy with biopsy is the standard diagnostic approach; computed tomography and magnetic resonance imaging are used to assess depth of invasion, regional spread, and distant metastases.

Several different screening recommendations have been proposed and endorsed by the American Gastro-

TABLE 19–15. Bethesda Criteria for Microsatellite Instability[179]

Loci With Microsatellite Instability*	Classification
≥40%	High-frequency microsatellite instability, MSI-H
10%–30%	Low-frequency microsatellite instability, MSI-L
0%	Microsatellite stable, MSS

*Five microsatellite loci are originally tested. If only one of the five loci has MSI, the result is considered inconclusive, and five additional loci are tested. There are a number of loci specifically recommended in the definition of the criteria.

TABLE 19–16. American Cancer Society Guidelines on Screening and Surveillance for the Detection of Colorectal Adenomas and Cancer[187]

Method	Interval*
Fecal occult blood testing and flexible sigmoidoscopy	Annual occult blood; sigmoidoscopy every 5 years
Flexible sigmoidoscopy	Every 5 years
Fecal occult blood testing	Annual
Colonoscopy	Every 10 years
Double-contrast barium enema	Every 5 years

*Beginning at age 50 years.

enterological Association, American Medical Association, and American Cancer Society (Table 19-16). Screening is clinically effective and cost-effective, yet its use remains relatively low.[186] It has also been established that polypectomy can prevent colorectal cancer, adding a second major benefit to screening.[26] In individuals with a personal or family history of colorectal adenoma or carcinoma, the screening recommendations are modified accordingly.[187]

Finally, it has been estimated that 90% of colorectal cancer deaths are potentially preventable. This includes strategies to diagnose colorectal cancer early and efforts to prevent colorectal cancer by polypectomy. Dietary change and increased exercise alone could have a significant impact on colorectal cancer incidence.[6] In addition, there is abundant evidence suggesting that aspirin-like drugs, postmenopausal hormones, folic acid, calcium, selenium, and vitamin E may help prevent colorectal cancer.[6,18,188,189]

Colitis-Associated Neoplasia

Since the first description of cancer complicating inflammatory bowel disease, numerous studies have demonstrated definite associations between chronic ulcerative colitis and the onset of colonic dysplasia and carcinoma.[190-193] An increased risk of cancer is also seen in patients with Crohn's disease and is similar to ulcerative colitis for a given extent of colonic involvement and severity. The risk of colonic cancer in the setting of chronic colitis is related to early age at onset, increasing duration of disease, severity of disease, and extent of disease within the colon (pancolitis has the greatest risk).[190-193] In addition, the risk rises significantly after 8 to 10 years of disease, increasing at about 0.5% to 1.0% per year and plateauing at about 15% to 20% by 30 years, which is about 20-fold higher than that in the general population.[21,194,195] Several reports have also suggested elevated risk in patients with coexistent sclerosing cholangitis.[196]

In addition to the increased risk of cancer, it is well recognized that cancer is usually preceded by dysplasia, allowing a mechanism for identification and management of patients at a curable stage of their disease (see Chapter 10).

PATHOGENESIS

Several lines of evidence suggest that the molecular pathogenesis of colitis-associated cancer is distinct from sporadic colorectal neoplasia.[192,197] Compared with studies of unselected, apparently sporadic cancers, mutations in APC and K-ras, loss of heterozygosity of

chromosomal arm 18q, BCL2 upregulation, and beta-catenin stabilization are all less frequent in colitis-associated cancer. In contrast, p21 downregulation, p27 downregulation, and p16 hypermethylation are all more frequent. Although there were some early reports that DNA mismatch repair deficiency may play an increased role in colitis-associated neoplasms, this has not been verified. There are also significant differences in the timing of genetic events. Of greatest interest, *TP53* mutations, chromosome 9p loss (site of the gene encoding *p16*), and aneuploidy are much more likely to be present in noninvasive precursor dysplasia than in the sporadic adenomas.[198-201]

In addition to the molecular genetic alterations found in dysplasia, a number of studies have demonstrated clonal genetic alteration in mucosa that is either indefinite or even negative for dysplasia. This includes aneuploidy, *TP53* mutations, K-*ras* mutations, widespread chromosomal instability, and erosion of telomeres.[198,200,202-204]

PATHOLOGIC FEATURES

In the setting of ulcerative colitis, colorectal cancers are usually preceded by dysplasia, an unequivocal neoplastic alteration with cytologic features that resemble adenoma (see Chapter 10).[205] Differentiation of dysplasia from reactive epithelium may be problematic in the presence of significant inflammatory activity, resulting in significant interobserver variation.[206-208] Histologic overlap with sporadic adenoma is also a significant dilemma (see Chapter 10).[209]

A number of features distinguish colitis-associated from sporadic colorectal cancers (Fig. 19-29).[192,210,211] Colitis-associated cancers are often difficult to recognize grossly and are much more likely to present with

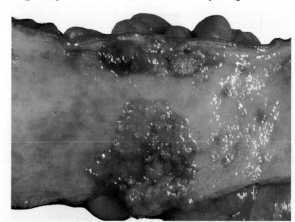

FIGURE 19–29. Adenocarcinoma arising in ulcerative colitis. Severe mucosal flattening and atrophy are evident. The tumor mass is irregular in shape and lies in an area of velvety mucosa (apparent as a slight nodularity to the right of the tumor). Microscopic examination revealed high-grade dysplasia associated with invasive adenocarcinoma. The surrounding flat mucosa also showed extensive low-grade dysplasia.

a linitis plastica pattern of growth.[109] Strictures in ulcerative colitis contain cancer in 24% to 40% of cases.[212] Multiple synchronous cancers are also significantly more frequent in colitis-associated neoplasia. Two primaries occur in about 20% of patients, and three or more primaries in about 10% of patients.[213] Some studies suggest that colitis-associated cancers are more evenly distributed throughout the colon than are sporadic cancers and more likely to present with advanced stage, particularly when they are detected outside of any screening protocol.[192] Signet ring cell carcinomas are significantly more frequent in colitis-associated tumors. One study reported that as many as 30% of signet ring cancers occur in the setting of chronic colitis.[91] Mucinous carcinomas are also reported more frequently in about 20% to 50% (vs. 10% in sporadic).[214,215] However, survival is roughly similar to that of sporadic cancer when controlled for stage and histologic subtype.[215] In fact, the most important prognostic factors are pathologic stage and grade.[216]

Sign-out Checklist

The following list details the features to be considered in colorectal cancer pathologic reports.

Absolutely Necessary Features

1. Specimen type: right hemicolectomy/ segmental resection/ left hemicolectomy/ low anterior resection/ abdominal perineal resection/ subtotal colectomy/ total proctocolectomy
2. Specimen includes: terminal ileum ___ cm/ appendix present/ appendix absent/ colon ___ cm/ rectum ___ cm/ anus
3. Histologic type: adenocarcinoma/ mucinous (>50% mucin)/ signet ring (>50% signet ring)/ undifferentiated (no gland formation)/ "medullary" (solid growth of uniform cells with prominent lymphocytic response)/ small cell (neuroendocrine undifferentiated)/ adenosquamous
4. Grade: GX: cannot be assessed/ G1: well differentiated (>95% gland-forming)/ G2: moderately differentiated (50% to 95% gland-forming)/ G3: poorly differentiated (<50% gland-forming)
5. Tumor site: ileocecal valve/ cecum/ ascending/ hepatic/ transverse/ splenic/ descending/ sigmoid/ rectum
6. Tumor size: greatest diameter ___ cm
7. Depth of invasion: specify deepest tissue layer involved; intraepithelial high-grade dysplasia/ intramucosal invasion/ invades submucosa/ invades muscularis propria/ invades pericolic or perirectal fibrofatty tissue/ invasion into adjacent structures (specify)/ invades through serosal surface (peritoneal covering)

8. Proximal and distal margins: uninvolved/ microscopic residual involvement/ macroscopic residual involvement
9. Radial margins (nonperitonealized rectum): uninvolved, ___ cm from closest margin (specify)/ microscopic residual involvement/ macroscopic residual involvement
10. Angiolymphatic invasion (lymphatic or unknown small endothelium-lined space): absent/ intramural present/ extramural present
11. Venous invasion (definite muscular vein): absent/ intramural present/ extramural present
12. Lymph node ratio: number involved/ number examined (minimum standard 12 to 14 lymph nodes)
13. Distant metastases: present (specify site)
14. AJCC TNM stage: pT__pN__pM__R__
15. Post chemoradiotherapy resection: additional principles
    a. ypTNM: indicates the post-treatment status of tumor
    b. Acellular mucin pools: note specific location in wall/margins
    c. Post chemoradiotherapy inflammatory changes: fibrosis/ telangiectasia/ cellular atypia/ active inflammation/ ulceration
16. Additional pathologic findings: none/ hyperplastic polyp(s)___ (number)/ serrated adenoma(s)___ (number)/ adenoma(s)___ (number)/ diverticular disease/ active colitis/ chronic active colitis

Optional Features (but clinical significance well supported in the literature)

17. Leading edge of tumor: expansile (uniformly smooth)/ mixed/ infiltrative ("streaming dissection")
18. Crohn's-like lymphoid reaction: none/ low grade (occasional peritumoral lymphoid aggregates)/ high grade (two or more lymphoid aggregates with germinal centers per section)
19. Tumor-infiltrating lymphocytes: none/ low grade (3 to 15 per 40× high-power field)/ high grade (>15 per 40× high-power field)

Other Features of Uncertain Clinical Utility

- Depth of invasion: specify the exact distance of invasion; ___ mm into muscularis propria/ ___ mm beyond border of muscularis propria
- Proximal and distal margins: uninvolved, specify exact distance from closest margin, particularly if less than 2 cm
- Perineural invasion: absent/ present
- Tumor perforation: absent/ present (transmural "hole" or inflammatory tract)
- Residual adenoma: none identified/ present
- Regional lymph nodes: specify "micrometastasis" if only one node and focus is less than 2 mm

References

1. Hamilton SR, Aaltonen LA (eds): Pathology and Genetics of Tumours of the Digestive System. World Health Organization Classification of Tumours. Lyon, France, IARC Press, 2000, p 314.
2. Greene FL, Page DL, Balch CM, et al, American Joint Committee on Cancer: AJCC Cancer Staging Manual, 6th ed. New York, Springer-Verlag, 2002, p 435.
3. Potter JD: Colorectal cancer: Molecules and populations. J Natl Cancer Inst 91:916-932, 1999.
4. Parkin DM: Global cancer statistics in the year 2000. Lancet Oncol 2:533-543, 2001.
5. Honda T, Kai I, Ohi G: Fat and dietary fiber intake and colon cancer mortality: A chronological comparison between Japan and the United States. Nutr Cancer 33:95-99, 1999.
6. Cancer Facts and Figures 2002. Atlanta, American Cancer Society, 2003.
7. Burt RW: Colon cancer screening. Gastroenterology 119:837-853, 2000.
8. Thomas RM, Sobin LH: Gastrointestinal cancer. Cancer 75(suppl):154-170, 1995.
9. Garfinkel L, Mushinski M: U.S. cancer incidence, mortality and survival: 1973-1996. Stat Bull Metrop Insur Co 80:23-32, 1999.
10. Allam MF, Lucena RA: Aetiology of sex differences in colorectal cancer. Eur J Cancer Prev 10:299-300, 2001.
11. Truswell AS: Meat consumption and cancer of the large bowel. Eur J Clin Nutr 56(suppl 1):S19-S24, 2002.
12. Bruce WR, Giacca A, Medline A: Possible mechanisms relating diet and risk of colon cancer. Cancer Epidemiol Biomarkers Prev 9:1271-1279, 2000.
13. Sandhu MS, Dunger DB, Giovannucci EL: Insulin, insulin-like growth factor-I (IGF-I), IGF binding proteins, their biologic interactions, and colorectal cancer. J Natl Cancer Inst 94:972-980, 2002.
14. Kim YI: Vegetables, fruits, and colorectal cancer risk: What should we believe? Nutr Rev 59:394-398, 2001.
15. Hill MJ: Vegetables, fruits, fibre and colorectal cancer. Eur J Cancer Prev 11:1-2, 2002.
16. Giovannucci E: Epidemiologic studies of folate and colorectal neoplasia: A review. J Nutr 132(suppl):2350S-2355S, 2002.
17. Seitz HK, Matsuzaki S, Yokoyama A, et al: Alcohol and cancer. Alcohol Clin Exp Res 25(suppl ISBRA):137S-143S, 2001.
18. Chan TA: Nonsteroidal anti-inflammatory drugs, apoptosis, and colon-cancer chemoprevention. Lancet Oncol 3:166-174, 2002.
19. Giovannucci E: An updated review of the epidemiological evidence that cigarette smoking increases risk of colorectal cancer. Cancer Epidemiol Biomarkers Prev 10:725-731, 2001.
20. Boyle P, Langman JS: ABC of colorectal cancer: Epidemiology. BMJ 321:805-808, 2000.
21. Gyde SN, Prior P, Allan RN, et al: Colorectal cancer in ulcerative colitis: A cohort study of primary referrals from three centres. Gut 29:206-217, 1988.
22. Tsunoda A, Shibusawa M, Kawamura M, et al: Colorectal cancer after pelvic irradiation: Case reports. Anticancer Res 17:729-732, 1997.
23. Iacopetta B: Are there two sides to colorectal cancer? Int J Cancer 101:403-408, 2002.
24. Kim EC, Lance P: Colorectal polyps and their relationship to cancer. Gastroenterol Clin North Am 26:1-17, 1997.
25. Fenoglio-Preiser CM, Pascal RR, Perzin KH: Tumors of the Intestines. Atlas of Tumor Pathology, Second Series, Fascicle 27. Washington, DC, Armed Forces Institute of Pathology, 1990.
26. Winawer SJ, Zauber AG, Ho MN, et al: Prevention of colorectal cancer by colonoscopic polypectomy. The National Polyp Study Workgroup. N Engl J Med 329:1977-1981, 1993.
27. Roncucci L, Pedroni M, Vaccina F, et al: Aberrant crypt foci in colorectal carcinogenesis. Cell and crypt dynamics. Cell Prolif 33:1-18, 2000.
28. Takayama T, Katsuki S, Takahashi Y, et al: Aberrant crypt foci of the colon as precursors of adenoma and cancer. N Engl J Med 339:1277-1284, 1998.
29. Mueller JD, Bethke B, Stolte M: Colorectal de novo carcinoma: A review of its diagnosis, histopathology, molecular biology, and clinical relevance. Virchows Arch 440:453-460, 2002.
30. Mendelsohn J, Howley PM, Israel MA, Liotta LA (eds): The Molecular Basis of Cancer, 2nd ed. Philadelphia, WB Saunders, 2001, p 691.
31. Vogelstein B, Kinzler KW (eds): The Genetic Basis of Human Cancer. New York, McGraw-Hill, 1998, p 731.
32. Vogelstein B, Fearon ER, Hamilton SR, et al: Genetic alterations during colorectal-tumor development. N Engl J Med 319:525-532, 1988.
33. Kinzler KW, Vogelstein B: Lessons from hereditary colorectal cancer. Cell 87:159-170, 1996.
34. Fearon ER, Vogelstein B: A genetic model for colorectal tumorigenesis. Cell 61:759-767, 1990.
35. Loeb LA: Mutator phenotype may be required for multistage carcinogenesis. Cancer Res 51:3075-3079, 1991.
36. Lengauer C, Kinzler KW, Vogelstein B: Genetic instability in colorectal cancers. Nature 386:623-627, 1997.
37. Lengauer C, Kinzler KW, Vogelstein B: Genetic instabilities in human cancers. Nature 396:643-649, 1998.
38. Kinzler KW, Vogelstein B: Cancer-susceptibility genes. Gatekeepers and caretakers. Nature 386:761, 763, 1997.
39. Jass JR, Whitehall VL, Young J, Leggett BA: Emerging concepts in colorectal neoplasia. Gastroenterology 123:862-876, 2002.
40. Jubb AM, Bell SM, Quirke P: Methylation and colorectal cancer. J Pathol 195:111-134, 2001.
41. Rountree MR, Bachman KE, Herman JG, Baylin SB: DNA methylation, chromatin inheritance, and cancer. Oncogene 20:3156-3165, 2001.
42. Toyota M, Ahuja N, Ohe-Toyota M, et al: CpG island methylator phenotype in colorectal cancer. Proc Natl Acad Sci U S A 96:8681-8686, 1999.
43. Fodde R: The APC gene in colorectal cancer. Eur J Cancer 38:867-871, 2002.
44. Moon RT, Bowerman B, Boutros M, Perrimon N: The promise and perils of Wnt signaling through beta-catenin. Science 296:1644-1646, 2002.
45. Fodde R, Smits R, Clevers H: APC, signal transduction and genetic instability in colorectal cancer. Nature Rev Cancer 1:55-67, 2001.
46. Leslie A, Carey FA, Pratt NR, Steele RJ: The colorectal adenoma-carcinoma sequence. Br J Surg 89:845-860, 2002.
47. Hawkins NJ, Ward RL: Sporadic colorectal cancers with microsatellite instability and their possible origin in hyperplastic polyps and serrated adenomas. J Natl Cancer Inst 93:1307-1313, 2001.
48. Iino H, Jass JR, Simms LA, et al: DNA microsatellite instability in hyperplastic polyps, serrated adenomas, and mixed polyps: A mild mutator pathway for colorectal cancer? J Clin Pathol 52:5-9, 1999.
49. Odze RD, Brien T, Brown CA, et al: Molecular alterations in chronic ulcerative colitis–associated and sporadic hyperplastic polyps: A comparative analysis. Am J Gastroenterol 97:1235-1242, 2002.
50. Henson DE, Hutter RV, Sobin LH, Bowman HE: Protocol for the examination of specimens removed from patients with colorectal carcinoma. A basis for checklists. Cancer Committee, College of American Pathologists. Task Force for Protocols on the Examination of Specimens from Patients with Colorectal Cancer. Arch Pathol Lab Med 118:122-125, 1994.
51. Compton CC: Updated protocol for the examination of specimens from patients with carcinomas of the colon and rectum, excluding carcinoid tumors, lymphomas, sarcomas, and tumors of the vermiform appendix: A basis for checklists. Cancer Committee. Arch Pathol Lab Med 124:1016-1025, 2000.
52. Compton CC, Fielding LP, Burgart LJ, et al: Prognostic factors in colorectal cancer. College of American Pathologists Consensus Statement 1999. Arch Pathol Lab Med 124:979-994, 2000.
53. Lewin KJ, Ridell RH, Weinstein WM: Gastrointestinal Pathology and Its Clinical Implications. New York, Igaku-Shoin, 1992.
54. Hermanek P, Sobin LH: Colorectal carcinoma. In Hermanek P, Gospodarowicz MK, Henson DE, et al (eds): Prognostic Factors in Cancer. Springer-Verlag, New York, 1995, pp 64-79.
55. Hermanek P, Guggenmoos-Holzmann I, Gall FP: Prognostic factors in rectal carcinoma. A contribution to the further development of tumor classification. Dis Colon Rectum 32:593-599, 1989.
56. Blenkinsopp WK, Stewart-Brown S, Blesovsky L, et al: Histopathology reporting in large bowel cancer. J Clin Pathol 34:509-513, 1981.
57. Jass JR: The grading of rectal cancer: Historical perspectives and a multivariate analysis of 447 cases. Histopathology 10:437-459, 1986.
58. Compton CC: Pathology report in colon cancer: What is prognostically important? Dig Dis 17:67-79, 1999.
59. Symonds DA, Vickery AL: Mucinous carcinoma of the colon and rectum. Cancer 37:1891-1900, 1976.

60. Alexander J, Watanabe T, Wu TT, et al: Histopathological identification of colon cancer with microsatellite instability. Am J Pathol 158:527-535, 2001.
61. Messerini L, Vitelli F, De Vitis LR, et al: Microsatellite instability in sporadic mucinous colorectal carcinomas: Relationship to clinicopathological variables. J Pathol 182:380-384, 1997.
62. Nascimbeni R, Burgart LJ, Nivatvongs S, Larson DR: Risk of lymph node metastasis in T1 carcinoma of the colon and rectum. Dis Colon Rectum 45:200-206, 2002.
63. Connelly JH, Robey-Cafferty SS, Cleary KR: Mucinous carcinomas of the colon and rectum. An analysis of 62 stage B and C lesions. Arch Pathol Lab Med 115:1022-1025, 1991.
64. Consorti F, Lorenzotti A, Midiri G, Di Paola M: Prognostic significance of mucinous carcinoma of colon and rectum: A prospective case-control study. J Surg Oncol 73:70-74, 2000.
65. Umpleby HC, Ranson DL, Williamson RC: Peculiarities of mucinous colorectal carcinoma. Br J Surg 72:715-718, 1985.
66. Yamamoto S, Mochizuki H, Hase K, et al: Assessment of clinicopathologic features of colorectal mucinous adenocarcinoma. Am J Surg 166:257-261, 1993.
67. Anthony T, George R, Rodriguez-Bigas M, Petrelli NJ: Primary signet-ring cell carcinoma of the colon and rectum. Ann Surg Oncol 3:344-348, 1996.
68. Messerini L, Palomba A, Zampi G: Primary signet-ring cell carcinoma of the colon and rectum. Dis Colon Rectum 38:1189-1192, 1995.
69. Psathakis D, Schiedeck TH, Krug F, et al: Ordinary colorectal adenocarcinoma vs. primary colorectal signet-ring cell carcinoma: Study matched for age, gender, grade, and stage. Dis Colon Rectum 42:1618-1625, 1999.
70. Tung SY, Wu CS, Chen PC: Primary signet ring cell carcinoma of colorectum: An age- and sex-matched controlled study. Am J Gastroenterol 91:2195-2199, 1996.
71. Ojeda VJ, Mitchell KM, Walters MN, Gibson MJ: Primary colorectal linitis plastica type of carcinoma: Report of two cases and review of the literature. Pathology 14:181-189, 1982.
72. Hayashi H, Kitamura H, Nakatani Y, et al: Primary signet-ring cell carcinoma of the lung: Histochemical and immunohistochemical characterization. Hum Pathol 30:378-383, 1999.
73. Jessurun J, Romero-Guadarrama M, Manivel JC: Medullary adenocarcinoma of the colon: Clinicopathologic study of 11 cases. Hum Pathol 30:843-848, 1999.
74. Hinoi T, Tani M, Lucas PC, et al: Loss of CDX2 expression and microsatellite instability are prominent features of large cell minimally differentiated carcinomas of the colon. Am J Pathol 159:2239-2248, 2001.
75. Frizelle FA, Hobday KS, Batts KP, Nelson H: Adenosquamous and squamous carcinoma of the colon and upper rectum: A clinical and histopathologic study. Dis Colon Rectum 44:341-346, 2001.
76. Fukui R, Hata F, Yasoshima T, et al: Adenosquamous carcinoma of the colorectum: Report of two cases. J Exp Clin Cancer Res 20:293-296, 2001.
77. Lafreniere R, Ketcham AS: Primary squamous carcinoma of the rectum. Report of a case and review of the literature. Dis Colon Rectum 28:967-972, 1985.
78. Sotlar K, Koveker G, Aepinus C, et al: Human papillomavirus type 16–associated primary squamous cell carcinoma of the rectum. Gastroenterology 120:988-994, 2001.
79. Weidner N, Zekan P: Carcinosarcoma of the colon. Report of a unique case with light and immunohistochemical studies. Cancer 58:1126-1130, 1986.
80. Nakao A, Sakagami K, Uda M, et al: Carcinosarcoma of the colon: Report of a case and review of the literature. J Gastroenterol 33:276-279, 1998.
81. Di Vizio D, Insabato L, Conzo G, et al: Sarcomatoid carcinoma of the colon: A case report with literature review. Tumori 87:431-435, 2001.
82. Isimbaldi G, Sironi M, Assi A: Sarcomatoid carcinoma of the colon. Report of the second case with immunohistochemical study. Pathol Res Pract 192:483-487, 1996.
83. Tokisue M, Yasutake K, Oya M, et al: Coexistence of choriocarcinoma and adenocarcinoma in the rectum: Molecular aspects. J Gastroenterol 31:431-436, 1996.
84. Ostor AG, McNaughton WM, Fortune DW, et al: Rectal adenocarcinoma with germ cell elements treated with chemotherapy. Pathology 25:243-246, 1993.
85. Metz KA, Richter HJ, Leder LD: Adenocarcinoma of the colon with syncytiotrophoblastic differentiation: Differential diagnosis and implications. Pathol Res Pract 179:419-424, 1985.
86. Kiran RP, Visvanathan R, Simpson CG: Choriocarcinomatous metaplasia of a metachronous adenocarcinoma of the colon. Eur J Surg Oncol 27:436-437, 2001.
87. Burke AB, Shekitka KM, Sobin LH: Small cell carcinomas of the large intestine. Am J Clin Pathol 95:315-321, 1991.
88. Klappenbach RS, Kurman RJ, Sinclair CF, James LP: Composite carcinoma-carcinoid tumors of the gastrointestinal tract. A morphologic, histochemical, and immunocytochemical study. Am J Clin Pathol 84:137-143, 1985.
89. Nakahara H, Ishikawa T, Itabashi M, Hirota T: Diffusely infiltrating primary colorectal carcinoma of linitis plastica and lymphangiosis types. Cancer 69:901-906, 1992.
90. Shirouzu K, Isomoto H, Morodomi T, et al: Primary linitis plastica carcinoma of the colon and rectum. Cancer 74:1863-1868, 1994.
91. Chumas JC, Lorelle CA: Melanotic adenocarcinoma of the anorectum. Am J Surg Pathol 5:711-717, 1981.
92. Jewell LD, Barr JR, McCaughey WT, et al: Clear-cell epithelial neoplasms of the large intestine. Arch Pathol Lab Med 112:197-199, 1988.
93. Thibodeau SN, Bren G, Schaid D: Microsatellite instability in cancer of the proximal colon. Science 260:816-819, 1993.
94. Haydon AM, Jass JR: Emerging pathways in colorectal-cancer development. Lancet Oncol 3:83-88, 2002.
95. Jass JR, Smyrk TC, Stewart SM, et al: Pathology of hereditary nonpolyposis colorectal cancer. Anticancer Res 14:1631-1634, 1994.
96. Kim H, Jen J, Vogelstein B, Hamilton SR: Clinical and pathological characteristics of sporadic colorectal carcinomas with DNA replication errors in microsatellite sequences. Am J Pathol 145:148-156, 1994.
97. Ilyas M, Tomlinson IP, Novelli MR, et al: Clinico-pathological features and p53 expression in left-sided sporadic colorectal cancers with and without microsatellite instability. J Pathol 179:370-375, 1996.
98. Jass JR, Do KA, Simms LA, et al: Morphology of sporadic colorectal cancer with DNA replication errors. Gut 42:673-679, 1998.
99. Jass JR: Towards a molecular classification of colorectal cancer. Int J Colorectal Dis 14:194-200, 1999.
100. Chao A, Gilliland F, Willman C, et al: Patient and tumor characteristics of colon cancers with microsatellite instability: A population-based study. Cancer Epidemiol Biomarkers Prev 9:539-544, 2000.
101. Smyrk TC, Watson P, Kaul K, Lynch HT: Tumor-infiltrating lymphocytes are a marker for microsatellite instability in colorectal carcinoma. Cancer 91:2417-2422, 2001.
102. Young J, Simms LA, Biden KG, et al: Features of colorectal cancers with high-level microsatellite instability occurring in familial and sporadic settings: Parallel pathways of tumorigenesis. Am J Pathol 159:2107-2116, 2001.
103. Gryfe R, Kim H, Hsieh ET, et al: Tumor microsatellite instability and clinical outcome in young patients with colorectal cancer. N Engl J Med 342:69-77, 2000.
104. Halling KC, French AJ, McDonnell SK, et al: Microsatellite instability and 8p allelic imbalance in stage B2 and C colorectal cancers. J Natl Cancer Inst 91:1295-1303, 1999.
105. Chung YF, Eu KW, Machin D, et al: Young age is not a poor prognostic marker in colorectal cancer. Br J Surg 85:1255-1259, 1998.
106. Cusack JC, Giacco GG, Cleary K, et al: Survival factors in 186 patients younger than 40 years old with colorectal adenocarcinoma. J Am Coll Surg 183:105-112, 1996.
107. Griffin PM, Liff JM, Greenberg RS, Clark WS: Adenocarcinomas of the colon and rectum in persons under 40 years old. A population-based study. Gastroenterology 100:1033-1040, 1991.
108. Scott KW, Grace RH: Detection of lymph node metastases in colorectal carcinoma before and after fat clearance. Br J Surg 76:1165-1167, 1989.
109. Wood TF, Tsioulias GJ, Morton DL, et al: Focused examination of sentinel lymph nodes upstages early colorectal carcinoma. Am Surg 66:998-1003, 2000.
110. Chu P, Wu E, Weiss LM: Cytokeratin 7 and cytokeratin 20 expression in epithelial neoplasms: A survey of 435 cases. Mod Pathol 13:962-972, 2000.

111. Lee BH, Hecht JL, Pinkus JL, Pinkus GS: WT1, estrogen receptor, and progesterone receptor as markers for breast or ovarian primary sites in metastatic adenocarcinoma to body fluids. Am J Clin Pathol 117:745-750, 2002.

112. Tebbutt NC, Cattell E, Midgley R, et al: Systemic treatment of colorectal cancer. Eur J Cancer 38:1000-1015, 2002.

113. Efficacy of adjuvant fluorouracil and folinic acid in colon cancer. International Multicentre Pooled Analysis of Colon Cancer Trials (IMPACT) investigators. Lancet 345:939-944, 1995.

114. Francini G, Petrioli R, Lorenzini L, et al: Folinic acid and 5-fluorouracil as adjuvant chemotherapy in colon cancer. Gastroenterology 106:899-906, 1994.

115. O'Connell MJ, Laurie JA, Kahn M, et al: Prospectively randomized trial of postoperative adjuvant chemotherapy in patients with high-risk colon cancer. J Clin Oncol 16:295-300, 1998.

116. Efficacy of adjuvant fluorouracil and folinic acid in B2 colon cancer. International Multicentre Pooled Analysis of B2 Colon Cancer Trials (IMPACT B2) Investigators. J Clin Oncol 17:1356-1363, 1999.

117. Wolmark N, Bryant J, Smith R, et al: Adjuvant 5-fluorouracil and leucovorin with or without interferon alfa-2a in colon carcinoma: National Surgical Adjuvant Breast and Bowel Project protocol C-05. J Natl Cancer Inst 90:1810-1816, 1998.

118. Henson DE, Fielding LP, Grignon DJ, et al: College of American Pathologists Conference XXVI on clinical relevance of prognostic markers in solid tumors. Summary. Members of the Cancer Committee. Arch Pathol Lab Med 119:1109-1112, 1995.

119. Dukes C: The classification of cancer of the rectum. J Pathol Bacteriol 35:323-332, 1932.

120. Hermanek P, Henson DE, Hutter RVP, Sobin LH: TNM Supplement. New York, Springer-Verlag, 1993.

121. Shepherd NA, Baxter KJ, Love SB: The prognostic importance of peritoneal involvement in colonic cancer: A prospective evaluation. Gastroenterology 112:1096-1102, 1997.

122. Galvis CO, Raab SS, D'Amico F, Grzybicki DM: Pathologists' assistants practice: A measurement of performance. Am J Clin Pathol 116:816-822, 2001.

123. Tepper JE, O'Connell MJ, Niedzwiecki D, et al: Impact of number of nodes retrieved on outcome in patients with rectal cancer. J Clin Oncol 19:157-163, 2001.

124. Calaluce R, Miedema BW, Yesus YW: Micrometastasis in colorectal carcinoma: A review. J Surg Oncol 67:194-202, 1998.

125. Oberg A, Stenling R, Tavelin B, Lindmark G: Are lymph node micrometastases of any clinical significance in Dukes Stages A and B colorectal cancer? Dis Colon Rectum 41:1244-1249, 1998.

126. Liefers GJ, Cleton-Jansen AM, van de Velde CJ, et al: Micrometastases and survival in stage II colorectal cancer. N Engl J Med 339:223-228, 1998.

127. Quirke P, Durdey P, Dixon MF, Williams NS: Local recurrence of rectal adenocarcinoma due to inadequate surgical resection. Histopathological study of lateral tumour spread and surgical excision. Lancet 2:996-999, 1986.

128. Adam IJ, Mohamdee MO, Martin IG, et al: Role of circumferential margin involvement in the local recurrence of rectal cancer. Lancet 344:707-711, 1994.

129. Heald RJ, Husband EM, Ryall RD: The mesorectum in rectal cancer surgery—the clue to pelvic recurrence? Br J Surg 69:613-616, 1982.

130. MacFarlane JK, Ryall RD, Heald RJ: Mesorectal excision for rectal cancer. Lancet 341:57-60, 1993.

131. Kapiteijn E, Marijnen CA, Nagtegaal ID, et al: Preoperative radiotherapy combined with total mesorectal excision for resectable rectal cancer. N Engl J Med 345:638-646, 2001.

132. Reynolds JV, Joyce WP, Dolan J, et al: Pathological evidence in support of total mesorectal excision in the management of rectal cancer. Br J Surg 83:1112-1115, 1996.

133. Nagtegaal ID, Marijnen CA, Kranenbarg EK, et al: Circumferential margin involvement is still an important predictor of local recurrence in rectal carcinoma: Not one millimeter but two millimeters is the limit. Am J Surg Pathol 26:350-357, 2002.

134. Nagtegaal ID, van de Velde CJ, van der Worp E, et al: Macroscopic evaluation of rectal cancer resection specimen: Clinical significance of the pathologist in quality control. J Clin Oncol 20:1729-1734, 2002.

135. Chapuis PH, Dent OF, Fisher R, et al: A multivariate analysis of clinical and pathological variables in prognosis after resection of large bowel cancer. Br J Surg 72:698-702, 1985.

136. Michelassi F, Block GE, Vannucci L, et al: A 5- to 21-year follow-up and analysis of 250 patients with rectal adenocarcinoma. Ann Surg 208:379-389, 1988.

137. Volk EE, Goldblum JR, Petras RE, et al: Management and outcome of patients with invasive carcinoma arising in colorectal polyps. Gastroenterology 109:1801-1807, 1995.

138. Talbot IC, Ritchie S, Leighton M, et al: Invasion of veins by carcinoma of rectum: Method of detection, histological features and significance. Histopathology 5:141-163, 1981.

139. Nielsen HJ, Hansen U, Christensen IJ, et al: Independent prognostic value of eosinophil and mast cell infiltration in colorectal cancer tissue. J Pathol 189:487-495, 1999.

140. Graham DM, Appelman HD: Crohn's-like lymphoid reaction and colorectal carcinoma: A potential histologic prognosticator. Mod Pathol 3:332-335, 1990.

141. Jass JR: Lymphocytic infiltration and survival in rectal cancer. J Clin Pathol 39:585-589, 1986.

142. Harrison JC, Dean PJ, el-Zeky F, Vander Zwaag R: Impact of the Crohn's-like lymphoid reaction on staging of right-sided colon cancer: Results of multivariate analysis. Hum Pathol 26:31-38, 1995.

143. Carlon CA, Fabris G, Arslan-Pagnini C, et al: Prognostic correlations of operable carcinoma of the rectum. Dis Colon Rectum 28:47-50, 1985.

144. Jass JR, Love SB, Northover JM: A new prognostic classification of rectal cancer. Lancet 1:1303-1306, 1987.

145. Hase K, Shatney C, Johnson D, et al: Prognostic value of tumor "budding" in patients with colorectal cancer. Dis Colon Rectum 36:627-635, 1993.

146. Vermeulen PB, Van den Eynden GG, Huget P, et al: Prospective study of intratumoral microvessel density, p53 expression and survival in colorectal cancer. Br J Cancer 79:16-22, 1999.

147. Houlston RS: What we could do now: Molecular pathology of colorectal cancer. Mol Pathol 54:206-214, 2001.

148. Goh HS, Chan CS, Khine K, Smith DR: p53 and behaviour of colorectal cancer. Lancet 344:233-234, 1994.

149. Jen J, Kim H, Piantadosi S, et al: Allelic loss of chromosome 18q and prognosis in colorectal cancer. N Engl J Med 331:213-221, 1994.

150. Watanabe T, Wu TT, Catalano PJ, et al: Molecular predictors of survival after adjuvant chemotherapy for colon cancer. N Engl J Med 344:1196-1206, 2001.

151. Sankila R, Aaltonen LA, Jarvinen HJ, Mecklin JP: Better survival rates in patients with MLH1-associated hereditary colorectal cancer. Gastroenterology 110:682-687, 1996.

152. Shibata D, Reale MA, Lavin P, et al: The DCC protein and prognosis in colorectal cancer. N Engl J Med 335:1727-1732, 1996.

153. Loda M, Cukor B, Tam SW, et al: Increased proteasome-dependent degradation of the cyclin-dependent kinase inhibitor p27 in aggressive colorectal carcinomas. Nat Med 3:231-234, 1997.

154. Andreyev HJ, Norman AR, Cunningham D, et al: Kirsten ras mutations in patients with colorectal cancer: The multicenter "RASCAL" study. J Natl Cancer Inst 90:675-684, 1998.

155. Gafa R, Maestri I, Matteuzzi M, et al: Sporadic colorectal adenocarcinomas with high-frequency microsatellite instability. Cancer 89:2025-2037, 2000.

156. Aschele C, Lonardi S, Monfardini S: Thymidylate synthase expression as a predictor of clinical response to fluoropyrimidine-based chemotherapy in advanced colorectal cancer. Cancer Treat Rev 28:27-47, 2002.

157. Raida M, Schwabe W, Hausler P, et al: Prevalence of a common point mutation in the dihydropyrimidine dehydrogenase (DPD) gene within the 5'-splice donor site of intron 14 in patients with severe 5-fluorouracil (5-FU)–related toxicity compared with controls. Clin Cancer Res 7:2832-2839, 2001.

158. Elsaleh H, Joseph D, Grieu F, et al: Association of tumour site and sex with survival benefit from adjuvant chemotherapy in colorectal cancer. Lancet 355:1745-1750, 2000.

159. Ricciardiello L, Bazzoli F: The role of genomic instabilities in affecting treatment responses of colorectal cancer. Dig Dis 20:73-80, 2002.

160. Ribic CM, Sargent DJ, Moore MJ, et al: Tumor microsatellite instability (MSI) and the benefit of 5-FU based chemotherapy in stage II and III colon cancer: A pooled molecular reanalysis of randomized chemotherapy trials. American Society of Clinical Oncology, Orlando, Florida, 2002.

161. Ahnen DJ, Feigl P, Quan G, et al: Ki-ras mutation and p53 overexpression predict the clinical behavior of colorectal cancer: A Southwest Oncology Group study. Cancer Res 58:1149-1158, 1998.

162. McGill G, Fisher DE: p53 and cancer therapy: A double-edged sword. J Clin Invest 104:223-225, 1999.

163. Minsky BD, Cohen AM, Kemeny N, et al: Enhancement of radiation-induced downstaging of rectal cancer by fluorouracil and high-dose leucovorin chemotherapy. J Clin Oncol 10:79-84, 1992.

164. Minsky BD, Cohen AM, Kemeny N, et al: Combined modality therapy of rectal cancer: Decreased acute toxicity with the preoperative approach. J Clin Oncol 10:1218-1224, 1992.

165. Hiotis SP, Weber SM, Cohen AM, et al: Assessing the predictive value of clinical complete response to neoadjuvant therapy for rectal cancer: An analysis of 488 patients. J Am Coll Surg 194:131-135; discussion 135-136, 2002.

166. Scheele J, Stangl R, Altendorf-Hofmann A: Hepatic metastases from colorectal carcinoma: Impact of surgical resection on the natural history. Br J Surg 77:1241-1246, 1990.

167. Stangl R, Altendorf-Hofmann A, Charnley RM, Scheele J: Factors influencing the natural history of colorectal liver metastases. Lancet 343:1405-1410, 1994.

168. Fong Y, Cohen AM, Fortner JG, et al: Liver resection for colorectal metastases. J Clin Oncol 15:938-946, 1997.

169. Ruers T, Bleichrodt RP: Treatment of liver metastases, an update on the possibilities and results. Eur J Cancer 38:1023-1033, 2002.

170. Elias D, Cavalcanti A, Sabourin JC, et al: Resection of liver metastases from colorectal cancer: The real impact of the surgical margin. Eur J Surg Oncol 24:174-179, 1998.

171. Lynch HT, Lynch J: Lynch syndrome: Genetics, natural history, genetic counseling, and prevention. J Clin Oncol 18(suppl):19S-31S, 2000.

172. Lawes DA, SenGupta SB, Boulos PB: Pathogenesis and clinical management of hereditary non-polyposis colorectal cancer. Br J Surg 89:1357-1369, 2002.

173. Vasen HF, Mecklin JP, Khan PM, Lynch HT: The International Collaborative Group on Hereditary Non-Polyposis Colorectal Cancer (ICG-HNPCC). Dis Colon Rectum 34:424-425, 1991.

174. Vasen HF, Watson P, Mecklin JP, Lynch HT: New clinical criteria for hereditary nonpolyposis colorectal cancer (HNPCC, Lynch syndrome) proposed by the International Collaborative group on HNPCC. Gastroenterology 116:1453-1456, 1999.

175. Peltomaki P: Deficient DNA mismatch repair: A common etiologic factor for colon cancer. Hum Mol Genet 10:735-740, 2001.

176. Jass JR: Diagnosis of hereditary non-polyposis colorectal cancer. Histopathology 32:491-497, 1998.

177. Ionov Y, Peinado MA, Malkhosyan S, et al: Ubiquitous somatic mutations in simple repeated sequences reveal a new mechanism for colonic carcinogenesis. Nature 363:558-561, 1993.

178. Aaltonen LA, Peltomaki P, Leach FS, et al: Clues to the pathogenesis of familial colorectal cancer. Science 260:812-816, 1993.

179. Boland CR, Thibodeau SN, Hamilton SR, et al: A National Cancer Institute Workshop on Microsatellite Instability for cancer detection and familial predisposition: Development of international criteria for the determination of microsatellite instability in colorectal cancer. Cancer Res 58:5248-5257, 1998.

180. Goel A, Arnold CN, Boland CR: Multistep progression of colorectal cancer in the setting of microsatellite instability: New details and novel insights. Gastroenterology 121:1497-1502, 2001.

181. Markowitz S, Wang J, Myeroff L, et al: Inactivation of the type II TGF-beta receptor in colon cancer cells with microsatellite instability. Science 268:1336-1338, 1995.

182. Redston M: Carcinogenesis in the GI tract: From morphology to genetics and back again. Mod Pathol 14:236-245, 2001.

183. Marcus VA, Madlensky L, Gryfe R, et al: Immunohistochemistry for hMLH1 and hMSH2: A practical test for DNA mismatch repair–deficient tumors. Am J Surg Pathol 23:1248-1255, 1999.

184. Lindor NM, Burgart LJ, Leontovich O, et al: Immunohistochemistry versus microsatellite instability testing in phenotyping colorectal tumors. J Clin Oncol 20:1043-1048, 2002.

185. Thibodeau SN, French AJ, Roche PC, et al: Altered expression of hMSH2 and hMLH1 in tumors with microsatellite instability and genetic alterations in mismatch repair genes. Cancer Res 56:4836-4840, 1996.

186. Frazier AL, Colditz GA, Fuchs CS, Kuntz KM: Cost-effectiveness of screening for colorectal cancer in the general population. JAMA 284:1954-1961, 2000.

187. Smith RA, von Eschenbach AC, Wender R, et al: American Cancer Society guidelines for the early detection of cancer: Update of early detection guidelines for prostate, colorectal, and endometrial cancers. Also: update 2001—testing for early lung cancer detection. CA Cancer J Clin 51:38-75; quiz 77-80, 2001.

188. Stack E, DuBois RN: Role of cyclooxygenase inhibitors for the prevention of colorectal cancer. Gastroenterol Clin North Am 30:1001-1010, 2001.

189. Gwyn K, Sinicrope FA: Chemoprevention of colorectal cancer. Am J Gastroenterol 97:13-21, 2002.

190. Greenson JK: Dysplasia in inflammatory bowel disease. Semin Diagn Pathol 19:31-37, 2002.

191. Eaden JA, Mayberry JF: Colorectal cancer complicating ulcerative colitis: A review. Am J Gastroenterol 95:2710-2719, 2000.

192. Harpaz N, Talbot IC: Colorectal cancer in idiopathic inflammatory bowel disease. Semin Diagn Pathol 13:339-357, 1996.

193. Jain SK, Peppercorn MA: Inflammatory bowel disease and colon cancer: A review. Dig Dis 15:243-252, 1997.

194. Devroede GJ, Taylor WF, Sauer WG, et al: Cancer risk and life expectancy of children with ulcerative colitis. N Engl J Med 285:17-21, 1971.

195. Ekbom A, Helmick C, Zack M, Adami HO: Ulcerative colitis and colorectal cancer. A population-based study. N Engl J Med 323:1228-1233, 1990.

196. Jayaram H, Satsangi J, Chapman RW: Increased colorectal neoplasia in chronic ulcerative colitis complicated by primary sclerosing cholangitis: Fact or fiction? Gut 48:430-434, 2001.

197. Benhattar J, Saraga E: Molecular genetics of dysplasia in ulcerative colitis. Eur J Cancer 31A:1171-1173, 1995.

198. Rubin CE, Haggitt RC, Burmer GC, et al: DNA aneuploidy in colonic biopsies predicts future development of dysplasia in ulcerative colitis. Gastroenterology 103:1611-1620, 1992.

199. Yin J, Harpaz N, Tong Y, et al: p53 point mutations in dysplastic and cancerous ulcerative colitis lesions. Gastroenterology 104:1633-1639, 1993.

200. Brentnall TA, Crispin DA, Rabinovitch PS, et al: Mutations in the p53 gene: An early marker of neoplastic progression in ulcerative colitis. Gastroenterology 107:369-378, 1994.

201. Fogt F, Vortmeyer AO, Goldman H, et al: Comparison of genetic alterations in colonic adenoma and ulcerative colitis–associated dysplasia and carcinoma. Hum Pathol 29:131-136, 1998.

202. Redston MS, Caldas C, Seymour AB, et al: p53 mutations in pancreatic carcinoma and evidence of common involvement of homocopolymer tracts in DNA microdeletions. Cancer Res 54:3025-3033, 1994.

203. Rabinovitch PS, Dziadon S, Brentnall TA, et al: Pancolonic chromosomal instability precedes dysplasia and cancer in ulcerative colitis. Cancer Res 59:5148-5153, 1999.

204. O'Sullivan JN, Bronner MP, Brentnall TA, et al: Chromosomal instability in ulcerative colitis is related to telomere shortening. Nat Genet 32:280-284, 2002.

205. Riddell RH, Goldman H, Ransohoff DF, et al: Dysplasia in inflammatory bowel disease: Standardized classification with provisional clinical applications. Hum Pathol 14:931-968, 1983.

206. Melville DM, Jass JR, Morson BC, et al: Observer study of the grading of dysplasia in ulcerative colitis: Comparison with clinical outcome. Hum Pathol 20:1008-1014, 1989.

207. Eaden J, Abrams K, McKay H, et al: Inter-observer variation between general and specialist gastrointestinal pathologists when grading dysplasia in ulcerative colitis. J Pathol 194:152-157, 2001.

208. Dixon MF, Brown LJ, Gilmour HM, et al: Observer variation in the assessment of dysplasia in ulcerative colitis. Histopathology 13:385-397, 1988.

209. Odze RD: Adenomas and adenoma-like DALMs in chronic ulcerative colitis: A clinical, pathological, and molecular review. Am J Gastroenterol 94:1746-1750, 1999.

210. Shelton AA, Lehman RE, Schrock TR, Welton ML: Retrospective review of colorectal cancer in ulcerative colitis at a tertiary center. Arch Surg 131:806-810; discussion 810-811, 1996.

211. Pohl C, Hombach A, Kruis W: Chronic inflammatory bowel disease and cancer. Hepatogastroenterology 47:57-70, 2000.

212. Lashner BA, Turner BC, Bostwick DG, et al: Dysplasia and cancer complicating strictures in ulcerative colitis. Dig Dis Sci 35:349-352, 1990.

213. Greenstein AJ, Slater G, Heimann TM, et al: A comparison of multiple synchronous colorectal cancer in ulcerative colitis, familial polyposis coli, and de novo cancer. Ann Surg 203:123-128, 1986.

214. Ky A, Sohn N, Weinstein MA, Korelitz BI: Carcinoma arising in anorectal fistulas of Crohn's disease. Dis Colon Rectum 41:992-996, 1998.

215. Sugita A, Greenstein AJ, Ribeiro MB, et al: Survival with colorectal cancer in ulcerative colitis. A study of 102 cases. Ann Surg 218:189-195, 1993.

216. Heimann TM, Oh SC, Martinelli G, et al: Colorectal carcinoma associated with ulcerative colitis: A study of prognostic indicators. Am J Surg 164:13-17, 1992.

217. Kummar S, Fogarasi M, Canova A, et al: Cytokeratin 7 and 20 staining for the diagnosis of lung and colorectal adenocarcinoma. Br J Cancer 86:1884-1887, 2002.

218. Maeda T, Kajiyama K, Adachi E, et al: The expression of cytokeratins 7, 19, and 20 in primary and metastatic carcinomas of the liver. Mod Pathol 9:901-909, 1996.

219. Rullier A, Le Bail B, Fawaz R, et al: Cytokeratin 7 and 20 expression in cholangiocarcinomas varies along the biliary tract but still differs from that in colorectal carcinoma metastasis. Am J Surg Pathol 24:870-876, 2000.

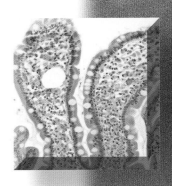

CHAPTER 20

Epithelial Neoplasms of the Appendix

NORMAN J. CARR • THERESA S. EMORY • LESLIE H. SOBIN

Hyperplastic Polyps and Mucosal Hyperplasia

Hyperplastic lesions of the appendiceal mucosa may be divided into two main types—hyperplastic polyps and diffuse hyperplasia.[1] Hyperplastic polyps are localized lesions resembling hyperplastic polyps of the colorectum; they are usually sessile.[2-6] Diffuse hyperplasia is characterized by nonpolypoid growth. Hyperplastic polyps are rare in the appendix, but diffuse hyperplasia is common.[1] Both are often incidental findings, although they can be associated with acute appendicitis.

PATHOLOGIC FEATURES

Histologically, both hyperplastic polyps and diffuse mucosal hyperplasia exhibit elongated tubules with serrated profiles (Figs. 20-1 and 20-2). The muscularis mucosae is intact. Loss of the normal appendiceal lymphoid tissue is often noted.[1]

DIAGNOSIS

The principal differential diagnosis is low-grade adenoma because both serrated adenoma and villous adenoma can mimic hyperplastic lesions. Only lesions with no dysplastic features should be diagnosed as hyperplastic polyps; if nuclear hyperchromasia, pleomorphism, or stratification occurs, the preferred diagnosis is adenoma. Villi or papillary structures suggest adenoma. Hyperplastic lesions, in contrast to adenomas, show a reduction in the proportion of goblet cells. Sometimes, lesions with hyperplastic features in one area and adenomatous features in another occur in the appendix. These can be designated *mixed adenomatous/ hyperplastic polyps* by analogy with similar tumors of the colorectum.[1]

Hyperplasia of the mucosa is significantly associated with adenocarcinoma elsewhere in the large intestine, and the finding of mucosal hyperplasia in an appendectomy is an indication for further tests to exclude colorectal neoplasia.[4]

Adenomas

Appendiceal adenomas occur in adults of all ages.[5] They may be incidental findings or may be discovered in patients with acute appendicitis. Occasionally a palpable mass is found, but such large lesions are more likely to be mucinous tumors of uncertain malignant potential or adenocarcinomas.

PATHOLOGIC FEATURES

The architecture of adenomas of the appendix is usually sessile; pedunculated lesions are rare.[2,5,7] Sometimes, the tumor produces a mucocele by causing cystic dilatation of the appendix.[1,5] Rare sequelae of cystadenomas include porcelain appendix (calcification in the wall) and myxoglobulosis or "caviar appendix" (intraluminal pearl-like spheroids caused by concretions of mucus).[1]

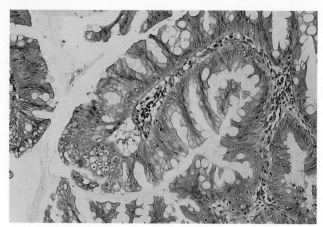

FIGURE 20–1. Hyperplastic polyp. Typical epithelium with serrated profiles.

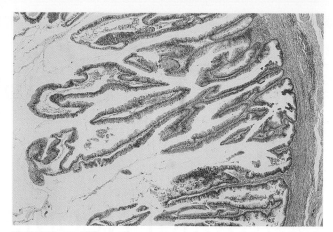

FIGURE 20–3. Villous adenoma.

The terminology recommended for adenomas of the appendix is that of the World Health Organization.[8] Any of the adenomas described in the colon can occur in the appendix. However, compared with adenomas of the colon, adenomas of the appendix are more likely to be villous or serrated (Figs. 20-3 to 20-5).[2,3,5,7,9] Many appendiceal villous and serrated adenomas display minimal cytologic atypia. As they grow, the lining epithelium becomes undulating rather than villous (Figs. 20-6 and 20-7). These undulating adenomas are often grossly cystic, and the term *cystadenoma* may be used. Normal appendiceal lymphoid tissue is frequently lost beneath an adenoma. Fibrosis of the submucosa and the muscularis propria may also be noted.

Adenomas associated with appendiceal dilatation may produce the clinical appearance of a mucocele, that is, an organ distended with mucus. The differential diagnosis in such cases includes simple mucocele (i.e., inflammatory mucocele, appendiceal ectasia). Simple mucoceles are rare lesions defined as dilated appendices caused by inflammation or mucus retention; some occur in patients with cystic fibrosis (mucoviscidosis). Simple mucoceles rarely exceed 2 cm in diameter and

are lined by thin or atrophic mucosa (Fig. 20-8), in contrast to the thickened, raised, or papillary neoplastic epithelium of adenomas and adenocarcinomas.[1] Mucoceles in which there is extensive loss of the epithelium and the cavity is lined by granulation tissue are most likely to be adenocarcinomas. Appendiceal diverticula may simulate cystadenoma. Serrated and villous adenomas with mild dysplasia must be distinguished from hyperplastic lesions of the appendix.

DIAGNOSIS

Appendiceal adenomas are significantly associated with neoplasia elsewhere in the colorectum.[5,10] If a patient has an appendiceal epithelial neoplasm, further investigation to exclude the possibility of a synchronous colorectal carcinoma should be considered.

The limited data available on molecular genetic abnormalities in appendiceal adenomas suggest similarities with colorectal adenomas. K-*ras* mutations have been identified in approximately 70% of appendiceal mucinous adenomas, and loss of heterozygosity has been shown in about half of appendiceal mucinous

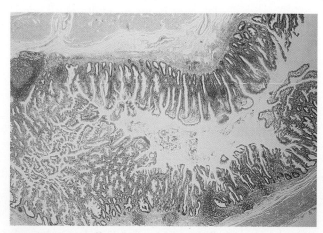

FIGURE 20–2. Diffuse mucosal hyperplasia. This patient had a synchronous adenocarcinoma of the colon.

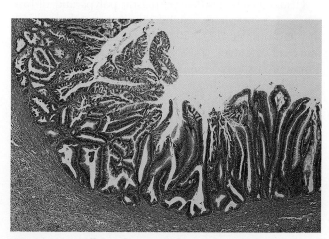

FIGURE 20–4. Villous adenoma with partial serrated pattern.

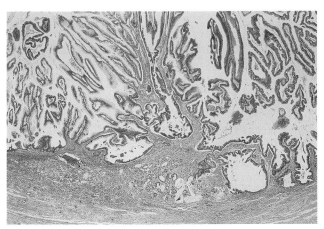

FIGURE 20–5. Invasive adenocarcinoma arising in a villous adenoma.

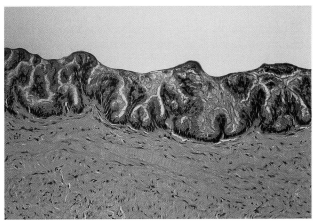

FIGURE 20–7. Undulating area from a cystadenoma.

adenomas at a variety of loci, including the 5q locus linked to the *APC* gene.[11] Adenomas of the appendix show significantly less immunoexpression of Ki67, *TP53*, and BCL2 than do adenomas of the colorectum.[12] It is possible that these differences could be related to the increased proportion of adenomas showing villous or serrated morphology in the appendix; immunohistochemical overexpression of *TP53* is unusual in serrated adenomas and mixed adenomatous/hyperplastic polyps.[6]

Adenocarcinoma

Primary adenocarcinoma of the appendix is unusual, occurring with an age-adjusted incidence of 0.2 per 100,000 per annum in the Surveillance, Epidemiology, and End Results (SEER) study in North America.[13] This rate was constant during the period from 1973 to 1987. A slight male predominance has been noted.[10,13] Adenocarcinomas may be encountered in adults of any age; the median age in the SEER study was about 65 years, although the literature in general suggests a peak age of incidence during the sixth decade.[5,10]

As is true for the rest of the large intestine, an adenoma/carcinoma sequence is assumed to occur in the appendix; the finding of a residual adenoma in some cases of adenocarcinoma supports this hypothesis (see Fig. 20-5).[7] However, some adenocarcinomas appear to arise from goblet cell carcinoid tumors[5,14]; these lesions are not usually associated with an adenoma. Adenocarcinoma of the appendix has been associated with ulcerative colitis and adenomatous polyposis.[15,16]

When compared with adenocarcinomas of the colorectum, adenocarcinomas of the appendix exhibit lower rates of proliferation and apoptosis, consistent with their more indolent behavior.[12] Most appendiceal carcinomas are diploid or near-diploid.[17]

Although the tumor-node-metastasis (TNM) classification of appendiceal adenocarcinomas currently uses the same criteria as for colorectal tumors, appendiceal cases should be separately classified. This is particularly important because of the special nature of pseudomyxoma peritonei, in which malignant cells may be scarce and acellular mucin may seem to have spread farther than the malignant cells.[5]

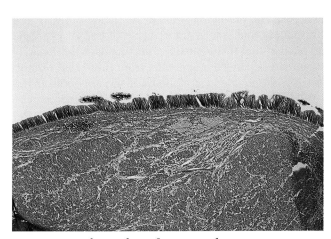

FIGURE 20–6. Flattened area from a cystadenoma.

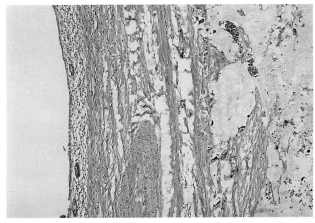

FIGURE 20–8. Simple mucocele. The epithelial lining is flat and atrophic.

CLINICAL FEATURES

Many patients with appendiceal adenocarcinoma present with features of acute appendicitis; these patients are likely to exhibit acute inflammation of the appendix histologically.[5] Others have an abdominal mass.[5,10] Clinically, the tumor may mimic a mass of the uterine adnexa. Spread to the peritoneal cavity may produce large volumes of mucus, causing pseudomyxoma peritonei, and these cases can present with abdominal distention. Sometimes, the pseudomyxoma is first discovered in a hernia sac.[18,19] Rarely, external fistulation occurs.[1,10,20]

PATHOLOGIC FEATURES

In cases of primary adenocarcinoma, the appendix is usually enlarged, deformed, or completely destroyed.[1,5,21] Well-differentiated appendiceal adenocarcinomas are often cystic; such lesions may be called *cystadenocarcinomas*. The appendix may have the appearance of a mucocele, but the term *mucocele* is a gross description only and not a pathologic diagnosis.[1]

Appendiceal adenocarcinomas are graded according to the same criteria as colorectal lesions and are defined as mucinous if more than 50% of the tumor consists of mucin.[8] A majority of appendiceal adenocarcinomas are well differentiated and mucinous (Fig. 20-9)[2,5] and may cause pseudomyxoma peritonei (see below). Rarely, growth of tumor in the retroperitoneum may produce pseudomyxoma retroperitonei.[22] If signet ring cells account for more than 50% of the neoplasm, the term *signet ring cell carcinoma* is appropriate. Nonmucinous adenocarcinomas of the appendix tend to behave similarly to the usual type of carcinoma of the large intestine and do not produce pseudomyxoma peritonei. Other types of carcinoma, for example, small cell carcinoma, may be encountered on rare occasions.[1]

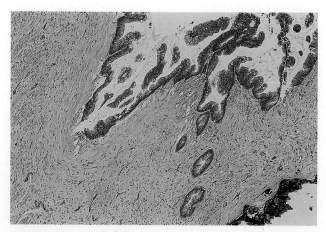

FIGURE 20–9. Well-differentiated mucinous adenocarcinoma (same case as in Fig. 20-12).

DIAGNOSIS

The natural history of appendiceal adenocarcinomas is variable. Well-differentiated lesions producing the clinical picture of pseudomyxoma peritonei tend to remain confined to the abdominal cavity for long periods, often with little or no evidence of lymphatic or hematogenous spread and minimal invasion of underlying viscera.[1] Intestinal obstruction is often the cause of death. Features that have been associated with a poor prognosis in appendiceal adenocarcinoma include advanced stage, high-grade histology, and nonmucinous lesions.[13,23-25] The spread of mucus beyond the right lower quadrant of the abdomen (whether or not cells are identified within it) is an independent prognostic variable, as is the presence of neoplastic cells outside the visceral peritoneum of the appendix.[5] When pseudomyxoma peritonei is present, abdominal distention, weight loss, high histologic grade, and morphologic evidence of invasion of underlying structures have been found to be poor prognostic factors, whereas complete tumor excision is associated with prolonged disease-free survival.[17,21,26] Cytologic examination of aspirated mucus and DNA flow cytometry are unhelpful in predicting prognosis.[17,20]

The main differential diagnosis of well-differentiated appendiceal adenocarcinoma is adenoma. We use the same definition for adenocarcinoma in the appendix as elsewhere in the colorectum; that is, adenocarcinoma is a malignant epithelial neoplasm with invasion beyond the muscularis mucosae.[1,5,8,10] However, in practice, it is not always easy to determine whether invasion has occurred because well-differentiated carcinomas of the appendix can mimic adenomas by invading on a broad front, especially if there is excessive mucus production, rather than showing infiltrative or single-cell invasion. Conversely, in some adenomas, acellular mucin dissects through the wall, mimicking invasion; this feature may be especially prominent if there is inflammation. The dense fibrosis of the appendiceal wall seen in some cystadenomas can be mistaken for a desmoplastic reaction. If acellular mucin is found in the wall, the diagnosis of adenoma should be made only if the muscularis mucosae is intact. The degree of cytologic atypia does not distinguish lesions that have the capacity to spread beyond the appendix from those that do not, because some adenocarcinomas of the appendix are so well differentiated that their dysplastic features may be subtle.[5] The presence of metastatic disease allows the firm designation of malignancy.

TREATMENT

In some cases, it is impossible to determine whether an appendiceal lesion will be cured by local excision (an adenoma) or has the potential to metastasize. We use the term *mucinous tumor of uncertain malignant*

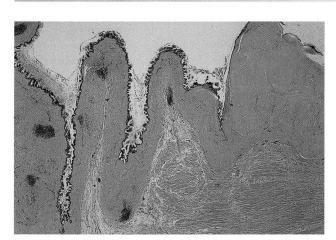

FIGURE 20–10. Mucinous tumor of uncertain malignant potential showing a well-differentiated mucinous epithelium pushing deeply into the appendiceal wall without frank invasion.

potential for such neoplasms.[5] Lesions showing well-differentiated mucinous epithelium pushing deeply into the wall of the appendix but without frank invasion often fall into this category (Fig. 20-10), as do cases in which pools of acellular mucin are present in the wall of the appendix or on its serosal surface. Other authors have suggested the term *low-grade mucinous cystic tumor* for lesions that are not frankly malignant histologically.[18]

It has been recommended that full colonoscopy should be performed in patients with incidentally resected appendiceal adenocarcinoma to exclude the possibility of synchronous lesions.[16]

Pseudomyxoma Peritonei

Pseudomyxoma peritonei is the presence of abundant mucinous material on peritoneal surfaces. It is not a complete histologic diagnosis in itself; the prognosis depends on the nature of the causative lesion. Nevertheless, the term *pseudomyxoma peritonei* is often applied to a distinctive clinical picture produced by well-differentiated mucinous adenocarcinomas in which the growth of malignant cells within the peritoneal cavity causes a slow but relentless accumulation of mucin.

Although most cases of pseudomyxoma peritonei are caused by spread from an appendiceal primary, cases have been reported in association with mucinous carcinomas of other sites, including gallbladder, stomach, colorectum, pancreas, fallopian tube, urachus, lung, and breast.[17,20,26-29] Although the ovary has been thought of as a common primary site, an accumulating body of evidence suggests that this is not the case and that in most cases of pseudomyxoma peritonei with mucinous tumors of both ovary and appendix, lesions are metastatic from an appendiceal primary.[6,21,30-32]

CLINICAL FEATURES

A distinctive feature of pseudomyxoma peritonei is its distribution in the abdomen. The tendency is to spare the peritoneal surfaces of the bowel, whereas large-volume disease is found in the greater omentum ("omental cake"), beneath the right hemidiaphragm, in the right retrohepatic space, at the ligament of Treitz, in the left abdominal gutter, and in the pelvis.[33]

PATHOLOGIC FEATURES

Histologically, malignant cells may be scanty within this mucinous material, and widespread sampling may be required to demonstrate them (Fig. 20-11). When found, they are seen as strips, small groups, acinar structures, or single cells, often with abundant intracellular mucin, sometimes with signet ring morphology (Figs. 20-12 and 20-13). They are frequently well differentiated. Indeed, some authors have suggested that these well-differentiated lesions are derived from adenomas and use the term *adenomucinosis* to distinguish this from peritoneal carcinomatosis.[21,32] However, adenomucinosis can be associated with malignant features such as destruction of the appendix by tumor growth and with metastasis to lymph nodes, mediastinum, pleural cavity, and lung.[21,32,34,35] Therefore, we do not use this term, and we regard cases in which "adenomucinosis" is diagnosed as examples of pseudomyxoma peritonei caused by well-differentiated adenocarcinoma.

Cytologic preparations of pseudomyxomatous material reveal abundant mucin, often with mesothelial cells, histiocytes, and fibroblast-like spindle cells. Epithelial cells with abundant intracellular mucin can be identified in the majority of cases if adequate material is available; they may be present as tight three-dimensional clusters, flat monolayers, strips with basally located nuclei, or single cells.[36] Because of the scarcity

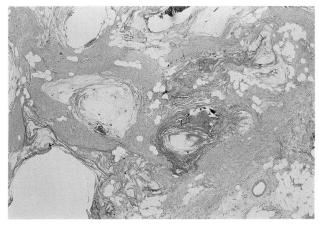

FIGURE 20–11. Pseudomyxoma peritonei showing acellular pools of mucin in fibrotic mesenteric adipose tissue.

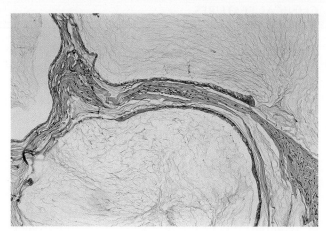

FIGURE 20–12. Pseudomyxoma peritonei showing mucin pools lined by flat glandular epithelium (same case as in Fig. 20-9).

of malignant cells in some cases of pseudomyxoma peritonei, the cytologic demonstration of abundant mucus in patients with abdominal distention, even if no malignant cells are seen, should be taken as presumptive evidence of pseudomyxoma peritonei and should prompt further evaluation.

DIAGNOSIS

In any patient with an intra-abdominal collection of mucus, the source should be identified if possible because the behavior of the lesion will vary according to the nature of the primary. In addition, appropriate staging requires knowledge of the primary site. Therefore, whenever possible, an appendiceal neoplasm should be excluded in all patients with pseudomyxoma peritonei by appendectomy and embedding of the entire appendix for microscopic evaluation.[1]

The differential diagnosis of pseudomyxoma peritonei includes extensive myxoid change within endometriosis[37] or myxoid mesenchymal lesions, such as myxoid leio-

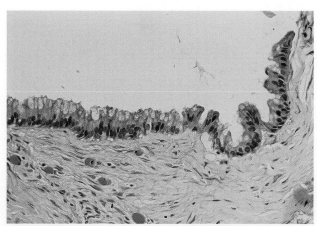

FIGURE 20–13. Pseudomyxoma peritonei associated with well-differentiated mucinous adenocarcinoma of the appendix. Epithelium lining mucinous cyst is minimally atypical.

myosarcoma or aggressive angiomyxoma. If small amounts of mucin adjacent to a ruptured or inflamed viscus are discovered histologically and the mucus does not contain epithelial cells, this may represent simple mucus extravasation rather than neoplasm. If there is any doubt, however, follow-up is indicated.[1]

TREATMENT

The SEER data showed the 5-year survival rates for adenocarcinoma versus mucinous or cystadenocarcinoma to be 95% and 80%, respectively, when no distant metastases occurred. However, when distant metastases were present, the 5-year survival rates were 0% and 51%, respectively.[13] This probably reflects the low aggressive potential of mucinous tumors that spread to the peritoneum.[25] Recent advances in therapy have involved surgery to extirpate all visible peritoneal tumor accompanied by intraperitoneal chemotherapy.[21,32]

■ Goblet Cell Carcinoid

Neuroendocrine neoplasms that arise in the appendix are discussed in Chapter 21, but two distinctive lesions that occur mainly in the appendix—goblet cell carcinoid and tubular carcinoid—are presented in this chapter.

In the World Health Organization histologic classification, goblet cell carcinoids are included as a type of mixed endocrine/exocrine neoplasm because they show features of both endocrine and glandular differentiation.[38] Several synonyms have been applied to them, including *mucinous carcinoid, crypt cell carcinoma,* and *microglandular carcinoma. Adenocarcinoid* has been used for both goblet cell and tubular carcinoids; the term is best avoided to prevent confusion.

CLINICAL FEATURES

Goblet cell carcinoids are encountered almost exclusively in the appendix, although they may be found elsewhere in the gastrointestinal tract on rare occasions. The most frequent clinical presentation is acute appendicitis.[1] Goblet cell carcinoids occur in older patients than do typical appendiceal carcinoids.

PATHOLOGIC FEATURES

It is uncommon for lesions to produce a grossly visible mass. Usually, only a diffuse thickening of the appendiceal wall is observed macroscopically.[14,39,40] Sometimes, the appendix is grossly normal. Sampling of the proximal line of resection is important because extension into the cecum may be evident only microscopically.

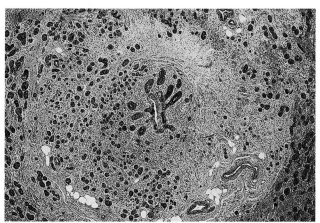

FIGURE 20–14. Goblet cell carcinoid. Typical concentric mural distribution of tumor with compressed but preserved appendiceal lumen. Mucin-positive tumor nests appear green in this Movat stain. (From Capella C, Solcia E, Sobin LH, et al: Endocrine tumours of the appendix. In Hamilton SR, Aaltonen LA [eds]: World Health Organization Classification of Tumours: Pathology and Genetics of Tumours of the Digestive System. Lyon, IARC Press, 2000, p 101, with permission.)

Histologically, the tumor diffusely infiltrates the appendiceal wall (Figs. 20-14 to 20-16).[14,39,40] The typical lesion consists of tight clusters or rosettes of tumor cells; lumen formation is rare. Most cells have a goblet cell or signet ring–like morphology with a small, compressed nucleus and abundant intracytoplasmic mucin. Smaller numbers of endocrine cells with finely granular eosinophilic cytoplasm are normally identifiable. Paneth cells may be found. Sometimes, linear single-file growth is present; such tumors may be likely to metastasize.[41]

DIAGNOSIS

Mucin stains demonstrate the goblet cells and any extracellular mucin (see Fig. 20-14).[42] The endocrine

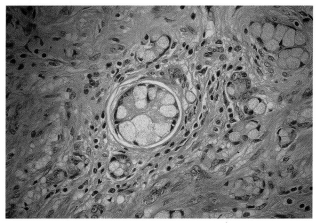

FIGURE 20–16. Goblet cell carcinoid. Goblet cells are arranged as clusters (same case as in Fig. 20-14).

component may be positive for the argyrophil reaction, but this is not invariable.[40] A more reliable way of demonstrating endocrine cells is with the use of immunohistochemistry for chromogranin; these cells may also express other endocrine markers.[14,43] Often, only a minority of the cells are of the endocrine type. Electron microscopy reveals dense core endocrine granules and mucin droplets, occasionally within the same cell.[42,44,45]

The differential diagnosis of goblet cell carcinoid includes metastatic signet ring cell carcinoma and clear cell carcinoid. The latter includes clear cytoplasm that does not contain mucin or glycogen; it is considered to be a variant of classic carcinoid tumor (Fig. 20-17).[41] In addition, goblet cell carcinoids are not to be confused with tubular carcinoids.

TREATMENT

Goblet cell carcinoids are more aggressive than classic carcinoid tumors; they typically act as a low-

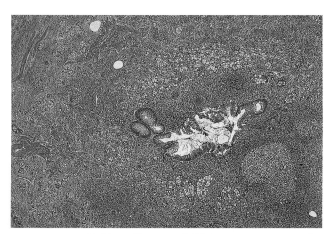

FIGURE 20–15. Goblet cell carcinoid. Without a mucin stain, the intramural nests are less evident (same case as in Fig. 20-14).

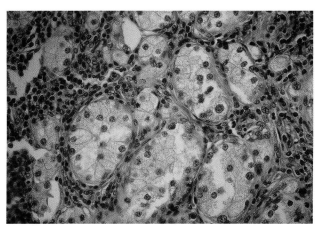

FIGURE 20–17. Clear cell carcinoid. It has superficial resemblance to goblet cell carcinoid, but nuclei are not displaced by cytoplasmic contents. Cells did not stain for mucin.

grade malignancy but tend not to spread as quickly as colonic adenocarcinoma.[40,43,44,46,47] Those involving the appendiceal margin or extending through the appendix into the periappendiceal soft tissue are usually treated with right hemicolectomy.

Some cases of goblet cell carcinoid may be associated with frank adenocarcinoma. In these cases, there is usually no epithelial premalignant lesion, and it can be assumed that such carcinomas arise from the goblet cell carcinoid.[1] The concentric growth pattern typical of goblet cell carcinoid is unusual for adenocarcinoma. The morphology of carcinomas arising from goblet cell carcinoids is sometimes of the signet ring type.

Tubular Carcinoid

Tubular carcinoids are rare. They do not metastasize and most frequently arise at the tip of the appendix in young adults.[14,40]

PATHOLOGIC FEATURES

Grossly, tubular carcinoids produce an ill-defined thickening of the appendiceal wall.[40] Microscopically, they are characterized by discrete tubules, some containing inspissated mucin within their lumina, and short linear structures within an abundant stroma (Figs. 20-18 and 20-19).[14,40,48] Comma-shaped epithelial structures may be seen. The tumor cells have round or oval nuclei with particulate chromatin. The cytoplasm is of variable amount and is eosinophilic. The mucosa is typically intact, although the tumor may appear to arise from crypt bases.

DIAGNOSIS

Although mucin can be demonstrated within the lumina of tubular structures, the cytoplasm is mostly

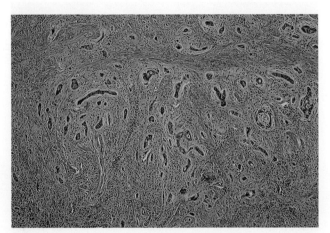

FIGURE 20–18. Tubular carcinoid. Short strips and tubules infiltrate the appendiceal wall.

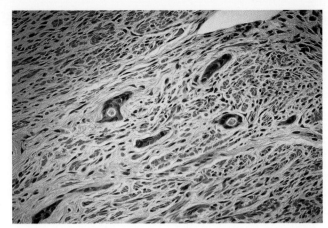

FIGURE 20–19. Tubular carcinoid. Tumor cells are arranged in tubular and atubular nests, bearing some resemblance to metastatic adenocarcinoma.

mucin negative. Immunohistochemically, the tumor cells express a variety of endocrine markers, including chromogranin. They are frequently immunoreactive for glucagon, an unusual feature in other types of carcinoid tumor.[14] Proglucagon *mRNA* can be demonstrated by in situ hybridization.[48]

TREATMENT

It is important that tubular carcinoids be distinguished from goblet cell carcinoids because, in contrast to goblet cell carcinoids, their behavior is benign, and complete excision can be expected to be curative. However, rare lesions have tubular features in some areas but features of goblet cell carcinoid in others[14,40]; such cases should be treated as goblet cell carcinoids. The differential diagnosis of tubular carcinoid also includes metastatic adenocarcinoma; the orderly pattern, lack of cytologic atypia, and absent mitotic activity in tubular carcinoids help in their differentiation.

References

1. Carr NJ, Sobin LH: Unusual tumors of the appendix and pseudomyxoma peritonei. Semin Diagn Pathol 13:314-325, 1996.
2. Higa E, Rosai J, Pizzimbono CA, et al: Mucosal hyperplasia, mucinous cystadenoma, and mucinous cystadenocarcinoma of the appendix: A re-evaluation of the appendiceal 'mucocele.' Cancer 32:1525-1541, 1973.
3. Williams RA, Whitehead R: Non-carcinoid epithelial tumours of the appendix—A proposed classification. Pathology 18:50-53, 1986.
4. Younes M, Katikaneni PR, Lechago J: Association between mucosal hyperplasia of the appendix and adenocarcinoma of the colon. Histopathology 26:33-37, 1995.
5. Carr NJ, McCarthy WF, Sobin LH: Epithelial noncarcinoid tumors and tumor-like lesions of the appendix: A clinicopathologic study of 184 patients with a multivariate analysis of prognostic factors. Cancer 75:757-768, 1995.
6. Rashid A, Houlihan PS, Booker S, et al: Phenotypic and molecular characteristics of hyperplastic polyposis. Gastroenterology 119:323-332, 2000.

7. Qizilbash AH: Mucoceles of the appendix: Their relationship to hyperplastic polyps, mucinous cystadenomas and cystadenocarcinomas. Arch Pathol 99:548-555, 1975.
8. Carr NJ, Arends MJ, Deans GT, et al: Adenocarcinoma of the appendix. In Hamilton SR, Aaltonen LA (eds): World Health Organization Classification of Tumours: Pathology and Genetics of Tumours of the Digestive System. Lyon, IARC Press, 2000, pp 94-98.
9. Williams GR, du Boulay CEH, Roche WR: Benign epithelial neoplasms of the appendix: Classification and clinical associations. Histopathology 21:447-451, 1992.
10. Deans GT, Spence RAJ: Neoplastic lesions of the appendix. Br J Surg 82:299-306, 1995.
11. Szych C, Staebler A, Connolly D, et al: Molecular genetic evidence supporting the clonality and appendiceal origin of pseudomyxoma peritonei in women. Am J Pathol 154:1849-1855, 1999.
12. Carr NJ, Emory TS, Sobin LH: Epithelial neoplasms of the appendix and colorectum: An analysis of cell proliferation, apoptosis, and expression of p53, CD44 and bcl-2. Arch Pathol Lab Med 126:837-841, 2002.
13. Thomas RM, Sobin LH: Gastrointestinal cancer: Incidence and prognosis by histologic type: SEER population-based data, 1973-1987. Cancer 75(suppl):154-170, 1995.
14. Burke AP, Sobin LH, Federspiel BH, et al: Goblet cell carcinoids and related tumors of the vermiform appendix. Am J Clin Pathol 94:27-35, 1990.
15. Odze RD, Medline P, Cohen Z: Adenocarcinoma arising in an appendix involved with chronic ulcerative colitis. Am J Gastroenterol 89:1905-1907, 1994.
16. Parker GM, Stollman NH, Rogers A: Adenomatous polyposis coli presenting as adenocarcinoma of the appendix. Am J Gastroenterol 91:801-802, 1996.
17. Gough DB, Donohue JH, Schutt AJ, et al: Pseudomyxoma peritonei: Long-term patient survival with an aggressive regional approach. Ann Surg 219:112-119, 1994.
18. Young RH, Rosenberg AE, Clement PB: Mucin deposits within inguinal hernia sacs: A presenting finding of low grade mucinous cystic tumours of the appendix. A report of two cases and a review of the literature. Mod Pathol 10:1228-1232, 1997.
19. Esquivel J, Sugarbaker PH: Pseudomyxoma peritonei in a hernia sac: Analysis of 20 patients in whom mucoid fluid was found during a hernia repair. Eur J Surg Oncol 27:54-58, 2001.
20. Hinson FL, Ambrose NS: Pseudomyxoma peritonei. Br J Surg 85:1332-1339, 1998.
21. Ronnett BM, Zahn CM, Kurman RJ, et al: Disseminated peritoneal adenomucinosis and peritoneal mucinous carcinomatosis: A clinicopathologic analysis of 109 cases with emphasis on distinguishing pathologic features, site of origin, prognosis, and relationship to "pseudomyxoma peritonei." Am J Surg Pathol 19:1390-1408, 1995.
22. Matsuoka Y, Masumoto T, Suzuki K, et al: Pseudomyxoma retroperitonei. Eur Radiol 9:457-459, 1999.
23. Cortina R, McCormick J, Kolm P, et al: Management and prognosis of adenocarcinoma of the appendix. Dis Colon Rectum 38:848-852, 1995.
24. Nitecki SS, Wolff BG, Schlinkert R, et al: The natural history of surgically treated primary adenocarcinoma of the appendix. Ann Surg 219:51-57, 1994.
25. Smith JW, Kemeny N, Caldwell C, et al: Pseudomyxoma peritonei of appendiceal origin. Cancer 70:396-401, 1992.
26. Costa MJ: Pseudomyxoma peritonei: Histologic predictors of patient survival. Arch Pathol Lab Med 118:1215-1219, 1994.
27. McCarthy JH, Aga A: A fallopian tube lesion of borderline malignancy associated with pseudomyxoma peritonei. Histopathology 13:223-225, 1988.
28. Kurita M, Komatsu H, Hata Y, et al: Pseudomyxoma peritonei due to adenocarcinoma of the lung: Case report. J Gastroenterol 29:344-348, 1994.
29. Zanelli M, Casadei R, Santini D, et al: Pseudomyxoma peritonei associated with intraductal papillary-mucinous neoplasm of the pancreas. Pancreas 17:100-102, 1998.
30. Prayson RA, Hart WR, Petras RE: Pseudomyxoma peritonei: A clinicopathologic study of 19 cases with emphasis on site of origin and nature of associated ovarian tumors. Am J Surg Pathol 18:591-603, 1994.
31. Young RH, Gilks CB, Scully RE: Mucinous tumors of the appendix associated with mucinous tumors of the ovary and pseudomyxoma peritonei: A clinicopathologic analysis of 22 cases supporting an origin in the appendix. Am J Surg Pathol 15:415-429, 1991.
32. Ronnett BM, Shmookler BM, Diener-West M, et al: Immunohistochemical evidence supporting the appendiceal origin of pseudomyxoma peritonei in women. Int J Gynecol Pathol 16:1-9, 1997.
33. Sugarbaker PH: Pseudomyxoma peritonei: A cancer whose biology is characterized by a redistribution phenomenon. Ann Surg 219:109-111, 1994.
34. Mortman KD, Sugarbaker PA, Shmookler BM, et al: Pulmonary metastases in pseudomyxoma peritonei syndrome. Ann Thorac Surg 64:1434-1436, 1997.
35. Peek DF, Beets GL: Pseudomyxoma peritonei in the peritoneal cavity: Report of a case. Dis Colon Rectum 42:113-116, 1999.
36. Shin HJ, Sneige N: Epithelial cells and other cytologic features of pseudomyxoma peritonei in patients with ovarian and/or appendiceal mucinous neoplasms: A study of 12 patients including 5 men. Cancer 90:17-23, 2000.
37. Clement PB, Granai CO, Young RH, et al: Endometriosis with myxoid change: A case simulating pseudomyxoma peritonei. Am J Surg Pathol 18:849-853, 1994.
38. Capella C, Solcia E, Sobin LH, et al: Endocrine tumours of the appendix. In Hamilton SR, Aaltonen LA (eds): World Health Organization Classification of Tumours: Pathology and Genetics of Tumours of the Digestive System. Lyon, IARC Press, 2000, pp 99-101.
39. Subbuswamy SG, Gibbs NM, Ross CF, et al: Goblet cell carcinoid of the appendix. Cancer 34:338-344, 1974.
40. Warkel RL, Cooper PH, Helwig EB: Adenocarcinoid, a mucin-producing carcinoid tumor of the appendix. Cancer 42:2781-2793, 1978.
41. Burke AP, Sobin LH, Federspiel BH, et al: Appendiceal carcinoids: Correlation of histology and immunohistochemistry. Mod Pathol 2:630-637, 1989.
42. Kanthan R, Saxena A, Kanthan SC: Goblet cell carcinoids of the appendix: Immunophenotype and ultrastructural study. Arch Pathol Lab Med 125:386-390, 2001.
43. Anderson NH, Somerville JE, Johnston CF, et al: Appendiceal goblet cell carcinoids: A clinicopathological and immunohistochemical study. Histopathology 18:61-65, 1991.
44. Edmonds P, Merino MJ, Livolsi VA, et al: Adenocarcinoid (mucinous carcinoid) of the appendix. Gastroenterology 86:302-309, 1984.
45. Isaacson P: Crypt cell carcinoma of the appendix (so-called adenocarcinoid tumor). Am J Surg Pathol 5:213-224, 1981.
46. Park K, Blessing K, Kerr K, et al: Goblet cell carcinoid of the appendix. Gut 31:322-324, 1990.
47. Butler JA, Houshiar A, Lin F, et al: Goblet cell carcinoid of the appendix. Am J Surg 168:685-687, 1994.
48. Shaw PA, Pringle JH: The demonstration of a subset of carcinoid tumours of the appendix by in situ hybridization using synthetic probes to proglucagon mRNA. J Pathol 167:375-380, 1992.

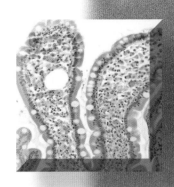

CHAPTER 21

Neuroendocrine Tumors of the GI Tract and Appendix

FIONA GRAEME-COOK

Introduction

The term *gastrointestinal neuroendocrine tumor* (*GI-NET*) refers to a heterogeneous group of tumors. Within this category are all tumors derived from cells of the diffuse gastrointestinal endocrine system or the neuroendocrine system of the gut (GI-NES).

The GI-NES is the largest single endocrine system in the body. It produces more than 30 hormones. The cells produce peptides and amines that regulate motility and digestion and aid in immune surveillance. These cells show remarkable evolutionary preservation; some of the hormones are similar or identical to those found in prevertebrates and protovertebrates.[1] Despite the wide variety of cell types, only a few give rise to tumors. In fact, some cells, such as secretin- and cholecystokinin (CCK)-producing cells, are not associated with tumor formation at all. One possible reason is that the CCK- and secretin-producing cells are not capable of proliferation but appear to differentiate from progenitor cells. Some speculate that these progenitor cells may be responsible for poorly differentiated endocrine carcinomas. Gastrin (G)-producing cells or histamine-producing enterochromaffin-like (ECL) cells, in contrast, show trophic responses to other hormones and neural influences. Unlike classic endocrine organs that act purely through the circulatory system, many GI-NES cells are located near their target cells. In addition to endocrine effects, the GI-NES comprises autocrine, paracrine, and local neuromodulatory effects.

Morphology of Neuroendocrine Cells

Morphologically, only two or three different cell types are recognizable on hematoxylin and eosin–stained tissue sections in normal gastrointestinal mucosa. The distribution of specific cell types determines the neuroendocrine tumor (NET) subtype and behavior (Fig. 21-1).

ENTEROCHROMAFFIN CELLS

Enterochromaffin cells (ECCs) are the most common type of neuroendocrine cell in the gastrointestinal tract. These cells, which are usually located at the base of intestinal crypts, produce serotonin; a subtype also produces substance P.[2] With increased cell turnover, ECCs may be seen at higher levels of the mucosa, but their presence on the surface is highly unusual. ECCs are most numerous in the small intestine and appendix but are also found scattered in the colon, rectum, and stomach, where they are responsible for the development of rare ECC-derived NETs. They are small, polygonal or cone-shaped cells that often communicate with the crypt

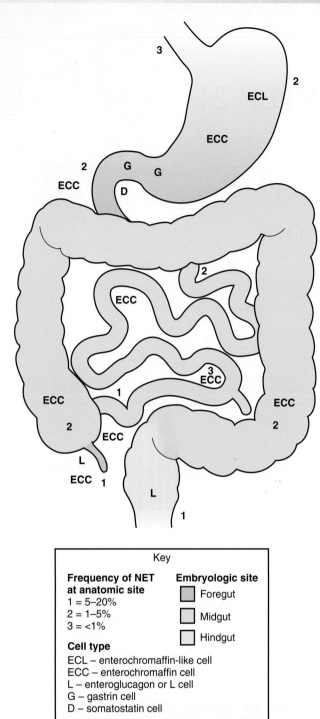

Key

Frequency of NET
at anatomic site
1 = 5–20%
2 = 1–5%
3 = <1%

Embryologic site
☐ Foregut
☐ Midgut
☐ Hindgut

Cell type
ECL – enterochromaffin-like cell
ECC – enterochromaffin cell
L – enteroglucagon or L cell
G – gastrin cell
D – somatostatin cell

FIGURE 21–1. Neuroendocrine tumor (NET) frequency, embryology, and cell of origin, by site.

OPEN NEUROENDOCRINE CELLS

Open neuroendocrine cells, such as gastrin (G) cell, somatostatin (D) cell, L cell, are small and oval and contain cytoplasm that communicates with the lumen of the gland/neck region of the crypts. Their cytoplasm is usually clear; these cells are often mistaken for intraepithelial lymphocytes. However, their nuclear appearance is similar to that of ECCs. It is believed that the function of these cells is related to "tasting" of luminal contents. They respond by releasing hormones either locally or distally during the process of digestion.

CLOSED NEUROENDOCRINE CELLS

ECLs have a morphology similar to G cell morphology, but they do not communicate with the lumina of crypts. They lie close to parietal cells in the body of the stomach. Without communication with the lumina, these cells react to local or circulating hormones or trophic factors.

■ Neuroendocrine Tumor Nomenclature

CLASSIFICATION

Many different classification systems and types of nomenclature have been used for GI-NETs. However, it is now commonly recognized that a classification system based on site, size, depth of invasion, and functionality gives pathologists the best tools for establishing an accurate diagnosis and guiding therapeutic strategies. Present-day knowledge allows us to divide NETs according to cell type and knowledge of cell products. The resultant system is logical both diagnostically and prognostically.[3,4]

The term *NET* is used here to designate any type of carcinoid tumor. The limitations of using the term *carcinoid* as a collective term for all of these tumors are that (1) they are typically derived from many different cell types and (2) the name refers to both benign and malignant tumors. Even tumors that are morphologically identical but arise at different sites can show divergent outcomes (e.g., ileal vs. appendiceal NETs). Use of the term *carcinoid* is increasingly discouraged in favor of the term *NET*.

The term *neuroendocrine* is used rather than the less specific term *endocrine tumor*. This is because GI-NES cells are not purely endocrine but also act in a paracrine and autocrine fashion and communicate closely with neurons of the enteric nervous system (ENS). In contrast to other endocrine cells in the human body, the peptides and amines produced by the GI-NES are frequently found as neurotransmitters and neuromodulators in nerve cells of the central nervous system (CNS) and ENS. These products include substance P (SP) produced by

lumen. Their nucleus is round to oval without an obvious nucleolus and contains finely dispersed chromatin. The cytoplasm is typically filled with fine, eosinophilic-appearing "coppery" granules. ECCs are often oriented with their nuclei toward the crypt lumen and cytoplasm adjacent to the basement membrane. This orientation allows discharge of contents into blood vessels within the basement membrane.

ECC, vasoactive intestinal peptide (VIP), galanin, neuropeptide Y (NPY), peptide YY (PYY) (L cells), and somatostatin (D cells).

The ultrastructural appearance of GI-NES cells is characterized by neurosecretory-like dense core granules and clear vesicles of the synapse type. For these reasons, the term *neuroendocrine* is used in this chapter and is recommended for use by pathologists.

EPIDEMIOLOGY AND CLINICAL FEATURES

NETs are rare tumors, with an annual incidence of 1 to 2:100,000. They represent 2% of all tumors of the GI tract. Gastrointestinal NETs account for 75% of the total proportion of NETs in the body. The ileum, appendix, and rectum are the most common sites, followed by the colon, stomach, and duodenum. Esophageal NETs and NETs within Meckel's diverticulum are extremely rare (Table 21-1).[5] Presenting symptoms are usually nonspecific and consist of abdominal pain, nausea, diarrhea, weight loss, and, rarely, intermittent intestinal obstruction. Almost half of all NETs are discovered incidentally, either at the time of surgery or at autopsy. Because symptoms are generally nonspecific and NETs are rare, they are often misdiagnosed as inflammatory bowel disease or tubo-ovarian disease. Bleeding may occur, particularly with rectal tumors, and rarely, vascular events such as ischemia may develop as well.

The carcinoid syndrome, which is a presenting feature in less than 10% of cases, is caused by high circulating levels of neuroendocrine system (NES) hormones. The features of this syndrome include flushing, diarrhea, asthma, and tricuspid regurgitation. High serotonin (5-HT) levels are usually found as well, but other vasoactive substances, including tachykinins such as SP and histamine (H), also probably contribute to the symptom complex. A large tumor mass is generally needed for the generation of sufficient circulating hormone for the

syndrome to manifest itself. Owing to this fact and to the presence of a high first-pass metabolism rate of hormones in the liver, carcinoid syndrome is most often seen with liver metastasis; rarely, it occurs with bulky retroperitoneal disease.

NATURAL HISTORY

The prognosis for NET is, in general, better than for other types of gastrointestinal tumors, such as adenocarcinoma, gastrointestinal stromal tumor (GIST), and lymphoma. At the time of diagnosis, 50% to 75% are localized, and 25% to 50% have metastasized. Five-year survival rates for NET are about 50%; 5-year survival for localized NET is 80%. This value drops to 50% and 20% with the presence of regional and distant metastases, respectively. The appendix and rectum are the most favorable sites of involvement. Average 5-year survival figures for localized disease, local spread, and distant spread are greater than 95%, 85%, and 34% for appendiceal NETs, and 81%, 47%, and 18% for rectal tumors, respectively (Table 21-2).[5] Incidentally discovered tumors tend to have a better prognosis. This is related mainly to the small tumor size at the time of diagnosis.

NETs most often metastasize initially to regional lymph nodes. Distant metastatic sites include the liver (44%), the lung (14%), the peritoneum (14%), and the pancreas (7%). Rare metastatic sites include the brain and testis. Occasionally, a NET may present as a hepatic metastasis of unknown primary. In these cases, the octreotide scan may help in localization of the primary tumor, which is usually found in the ileum and, rarely, in the jejunum or colon.

Despite the presence of distant metastases, NETs have an indolent biologic behavior; long-term survival is usually possible with metastatic disease, with a reported 53% 5-year survival rate in patients with hepatic metastasis.[6] The presence of lymph node or hepatic metastasis at the time of diagnosis is definite evidence of malignancy, but in the absence of metastasis, it is

TABLE 21–1. Relative Frequency of Gastrointestinal Neuroendocrine Tumors by Site

Site	Percentage*	5-Year Survival (%)
Stomach	4	48
Duodenum	3	–
Jejunum	3	–
Ileum	20	–
Small intestine (all)	29	55
Appendix†	25	85
Colon	10	41
Rectum	17	72

*Total is not 100% because some cases are not always designated by site.
†This number may underrepresent appendiceal NET considered "incidental."
Adapted from Modlin IM, Sandor A: An analysis of 8305 cases of carcinoid tumors. Cancer 79:813-829, 1997.

TABLE 21–2. Staging of Gastrointestinal Neuroendocrine Tumors

Site	Localized Disease	Local Spread	Distant Spread	Total Nonlocalized
Stomach	52%	10%	20%	30%
Small intestine	25%	39%	31%	70%
Appendix*	62%	26%	8%	35%
Colon	22%	33%	37%	71%
Rectum	72%	14%	7%	14%

*The most recent SEER data include staging for tumors designated malignant, so staging for appendiceal NET underrepresents appendiceal NETs that are considered benign or incidental.
Adapted from Modlin IM, Sandor A: An analysis of 8305 cases of carcinoid tumors. Cancer 79:813-829, 1997.

difficult to predict the behavior of individual NETs based purely on morphologic criteria.

As a general principle, NETs smaller than 1 cm, from any anatomic location, usually behave in an indolent fashion with only rare recurrences or distant spread. Tumors that measure larger than 2 cm are usually aggressive. Unfortunately, tumors that measure between 1 and 2 cm are difficult to predict. Brisk mitotic rate, necrosis, and deep tissue invasion are features that indicate malignant behavior.

ETIOLOGY

The pathogenesis of NET is poorly understood. However, an understanding of the physiology of gastric acid synthesis and of the unraveling of the gastrin–histamine–hydrochloric acid–somatostatin pathways has been pivotal to our understanding of gastric NET formation (see below in section on gastric NET). In the stomach, destruction of parietal cells in autoimmune gastritis and the formation of a NET in the setting of hypergastrinemia have provided a good human model of NET tumorigenesis. Mutations in chromosome 11 are now recognized as an important component in the development of Zollinger-Ellison syndrome (ZES) and possibly of sporadic gastric NET. Neurofibromatosis is associated with somatostatin-producing tumors of the duodenum. Rarely, NETs have been reported in familial adenomatous polyposis (FAP) syndromes, but evidence of tumor suppressor pathways linked to FAP has not been found in GI-NET as yet.[7,8] Some preliminary data do not support a role for genomic instability in the pathogenesis of NET.[9]

The role of the GI-NES in inflammatory bowel disease (IBD) has attracted a lot of attention recently, but the topic remains controversial.[10,11] There is also controversy as to whether IBD is associated with hyperplasia of GI-NES cells. Neuroendocrine hyperplasia may occur in IBD, but this finding is not universal.[12,13] Interesting to note are rare case reports of multiple rectal microcarcinoids in association with L-cell hyperplasia,[14] as well as combined adenocarcinoma/neuroendocrine tumors in Crohn's disease. Nevertheless, a strong case for IBD as a risk factor for NET has yet to be proved. GI-NES may contribute to symptoms in patients with IBD. Enteroglucagon, VIP, PYY, and 5-HT have effects on motility and may contribute to the pathophysiology of diarrhea/constipation. The number of VIP-producing nerves is increased in Crohn's disease. The GI-NES may also play a role in inflammation in IBD, as lymphocytes bear receptors for neuropeptides found in ENS and GI-NES cells.[15]

Finally, in approximately 12% of patients with NET, particularly from the rectum, ileum, and appendix, multiple tumors develop. These may be synchronous or metachronous. However, the cause of this phenomenon is poorly understood. It is unclear if these tumors represent separate primaries or if they occur as the result of metastasis of one tumor to another.

CLINICAL MANAGEMENT

Complete surgical resection with negative tissue margins is standard therapy for most NETs. In the case of large appendiceal NETs, a right hemicolectomy may be required. Hepatic metastasis may be managed by partial resection or even liver transplantation. Octreotide chemotherapy, with or without conventional cytotoxic agents, may be used for disseminated disease. Somatostatin has a growth inhibitory effect on many GI-NES cells, including ECCs. ECCs express numerous somatostatin receptors on the cell surface. The use of somatostatin analogues, such as octreotide, has great efficacy in the diagnosis and treatment of NET. Octreotide scanning with radiolabeled octreotide is of great diagnostic value in cases of liver metastasis of unknown primary. Complete regression of hepatic metastasis with octreotide therapy has been reported.[16,17]

MORPHOLOGY

Neuroendocrine tumor cells are typically polygonal with chromatin that is often coarser than that of corresponding benign neuroendocrine cells. Cytologic features of NETs do not vary according to the cell of origin. Distinguishing the cell of origin of an NET is impossible by light microscopy. Tumors that arise from ECCs do not normally contain coppery granules similar to those present in non-neoplastic cells. Mitoses and pleomorphism in NET are unusual features. The hallmarks of NET tumors are their striking degree of monomorphism, uniformity of cell size, and bland cytologic features. However, some particular types of morphologic growth patterns may be characteristic of specific NETs.

Growth Patterns

Type A: Insular or Nested Growth Pattern. Tumor cells grow, without intervening stroma, into large or small islands or nests of cells, sometimes with vague peripheral palisading. Nests often grow with only minimal amounts of fine fibrovascular tissue between the cords of cells. This pattern is seen mostly in ECC tumors (Fig. 21-2).

Type B: Trabecular Growth Pattern. Cells grow in long cords that are usually only 1 cell thick. They may stack together or form long looping ribbons—sometimes called *festoons*. Alternatively, the cords may be short, reminiscent of infiltrating ductal carcinoma of the breast. The cytologic features are bland, and mitoses, atypia, and necrosis are typically absent or minimal. The amount of

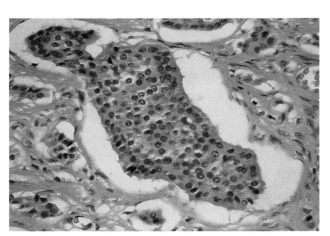

FIGURE 21–2. Type A growth pattern showing a nest of monomorphous, polygonally shaped neuroendocrine cells without mitoses or atypia. Peripheral palisading is present, and the nuclear chromatin is stippled.

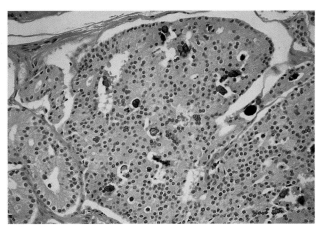

FIGURE 21–4. Type C (glandular or acinar) growth pattern. In this illustration, cribriforming masses of cytologically bland neuroendocrine tumor cells contain psammomatous calcifications within the acinar lumina, characteristic of a D-cell (somatostatin-producing) NET.

stroma is highly variable. In L-cell tumors, in which the type B growth pattern usually predominates, often only a small amount of stroma is seen. However, at the periphery of ECC-NETs, a type B pattern may be associated with dense fibrosis and desmoplasia (Fig. 21-3).

Type C: Acinar Growth Pattern. Small polygonal cells form glandlike lumina and occasionally contain secretions or even psammomatous calcifications. True gland formation does not occur in this growth pattern; the cells do not normally show nuclear orientation at the basement membrane, nor do the gland lumina have the solid configuration of true glands. This growth pattern is characteristic of D-cell tumors and is a common component of many other types of NET (Fig. 21-4).

Type D: Poorly Differentiated Growth Pattern. This pattern shows the nuclear features of an NET but without an organized cellular growth pattern. Generally, these cells show a higher nucleus-to-cytoplasm ratio.

This growth pattern often indicates that the tumor is malignant (neuroendocrine carcinoma). However, it is also seen as a minor component in association with type A and B patterns of growth in colonic NET. Because type D–predominant NETs are usually disseminated at diagnosis, the presence of a type D growth pattern should always be considered an adverse prognostic finding (Fig. 21-5).

COMBINED NEUROENDOCRINE AND GLANDULAR TUMORS

NETs may on occasion be associated with a variable proportion of glandular elements. These "combined" tumors may show a spectrum of combinations from high-grade NET/small cell carcinoma associated with an overlying adenoma at one extreme, to an adenocarcinoma

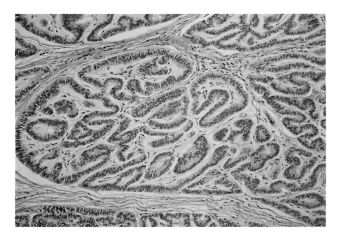

FIGURE 21–3. Type B (ribbon) growth pattern. The tumor cells form long trabeculae of tumor cells that form loops and are separated by fine fibrovascular stroma.

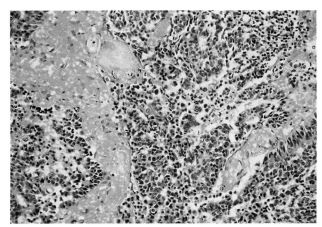

FIGURE 21–5. Type D (poorly differentiated) growth pattern. The tumor cells have a high nucleus-to-cytoplasm ratio and hyperchromatism; they form ill-defined nests and trabeculae.

TABLE 21–3. Spectrum of Neuroendocrine Differentiation and Behavior in Gastrointestinal Tumors

Type	Behavior
Pure neuroendocrine tumors	
Well-differentiated neuroendocrine tumors	
Grade I	Benign
Grade II	Uncertain malignant potential
Well-differentiated neuroendocrine carcinoma	
Grade III	Low malignant potential
Poorly differentiated NET	
Grade IV	High malignant potential
Combined glandular/NET	
Composite	Similar to pure adenocarcinoma (except goblet cell carcinoid)
Amphicrine	Similar to pure adenocarcinoma
Collision	Similar to pure adenocarcinoma
Adenoma/adenocarcinoma with focal neuroendocrine features	Similar to pure adenocarcinoma
Small cell undifferentiated with overlying adenoma or adenocarcinoma	Similar to pure small cell carcinoma

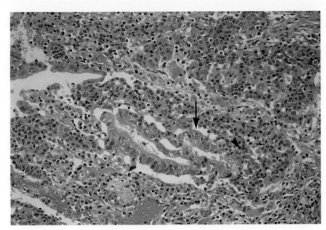

FIGURE 21–6. Composite adenocarcinoma/neuroendocrine tumor. A moderately well-differentiated adenocarcinoma blends with nests of NET. In some areas, individual glands show NET differentiation at one end (*arrow*) and adenocarcinoma at the other (*arrowhead*).

NOMENCLATURE AND SURGICAL SIGNOUT OF NEUROENDOCRINE TUMORS

Tumors that are functional (i.e., they secrete measurable amounts of active hormone) or show end-organ effects of hormone production are generally categorized according to specific cell type (e.g., gastrinoma, somatostatinoma). In contrast, the pathologic term for a non-functional tumor is *NET*. It is important to remember that a tumor with strong immunohistochemical expression of gastrin is not considered a gastrinoma unless it is also clinically functional.

Pathology reports should summarize all of the information necessary for proper clinical management. The pathology report of NET should include the following elements.

Size. Most of the literature pertaining to prognosis in NET is primarily retrospective. Tumor size in most

with only scattered endocrine cells at the other (Table 21-3). The latter is a common finding among gastrointestinal adenocarcinomas. The presence of scattered endocrine cells has no effect on the biologic behavior of typical adenocarcinomas. In the middle of the spectrum are true combined tumors, in which both cellular elements are represented in substantial proportions. Tumors that are composed of endocrine and glandular elements, each of which represent at least one third of the tumor load, may be considered mixed or combined for the purpose of classification. It is interesting to note that metastasis from combined tumors may express either or both types of cellular elements.

Combined tumors may be further subdivided into composite, collision, and amphicrine tumors. All are extremely rare but are most common in the stomach and appendix. Composite tumors are defined as those in which distinct glandular and neuroendocrine elements are intimately admixed (Fig. 21-6). Collision tumors occur when two distinct tumors are found in close proximity to each other but without an intimate admixture of cells. These are exceedingly unusual (Fig. 21-7). Amphicrine tumors are characterized by dual differentiation within individual neoplastic cells. No combined tumors are considered to be grade I from a behavioral point of view. Most of these tumors are grade III or grade IV. However, in the appendix, combined tumors (composite tumors or goblet cell carcinoids) are categorized as grade II.[18-21]

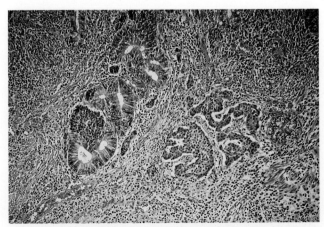

FIGURE 21–7. Collision tumor. Moderately differentiated adenocarcinoma and NET form two distinct growths in close proximity to each other but without an admixture of cell types.

studies is determined in the postformalin fixed state. Significant discrepancies may be noted between fresh and fixed measurements.[22]

Site. Site is an important indicator of malignancy risk (see Table 21-1). The prognosis is worse for colonic NET than for rectal or appendiceal NET, despite their close anatomic proximity.

Depth of Invasion. Nonfunctional NETs that are limited to the mucosa and submucosa are usually low-grade tumors. Tumors that infiltrate the muscularis and serosa often behave in a clinically malignant fashion.

Margins. The state of the surgical resection margins is important.

Multiplicity. Although multiplicity is common in GI-NET (occurs in up to 12% of cases, sometimes with many synchronous NETs), it appears not to have an adverse effect on prognosis. However, this is a controversial and evolving topic.

Disease in Surrounding Mucosa. Disease that occurs in the surrounding mucosa, including atrophic gastritis, inflammatory bowel disease, and any evidence of neuroendocrine hyperplasia, should be included in the pathology report because this will serve to alert the clinician to preexisting conditions such as ZES.

HISTOLOGIC GRADING OF NEUROENDOCRINE TUMORS

Tumor grading provides the clinician with useful prognostic information. The World Health Organization (WHO) classification is summarized in the following sections.[23]

Well-Differentiated Neuroendocrine Tumor

GRADE I (BENIGN BEHAVIOR)

These are nonfunctioning, cytologically bland tumors smaller than 1 cm and confined to the mucosa/submucosa without angioinvasion.

GRADE II (UNCERTAIN MALIGNANT BEHAVIOR)

These are nonfunctioning, cytologically bland tumors that measure 1 to 2 cm and are confined to the mucosa/submucosa. Angioinvasion may be noted (except in the jejunum/ileum).

Well-Differentiated Neuroendocrine Carcinoma

GRADE III (LOW-GRADE MALIGNANCY)

These are nonfunctioning, cytologically bland tumors greater than 2 cm with or without angioinvasion and with extension beyond the submucosa. All functional well-differentiated tumors of any size are included in this category.

Poorly Differentiated Neuroendocrine Carcinoma

GRADE IV (HIGH-GRADE MALIGNANT)

These are cytologically poorly differentiated tumors, functional or nonfunctional, of intermediate- or small-cell type. These tumors have been variously called *neuroendocrine carcinomas*, *atypical carcinoids*, *oat cell carcinomas*, and *small cell carcinomas*. The prognosis is uniformly poor.

Mixed Exocrine/Endocrine Carcinoma

This category includes all combined tumors. The WHO classification and the grading system use similar information in assessing prognosis.[23]

ANCILLARY DIAGNOSTIC AND PROGNOSTIC TOOLS IN NEUROENDOCRINE TUMORS

Electron Microscopy

Electron microscopy (EM) is rarely used as a diagnostic tool, mainly because of the efficacy of immunohistochemistry. However, EM can provide a lot of valuable information in certain clinical situations such as hepatic metastasis from an unknown primary, poorly differentiated small cell tumor, and mucinous ovarian neoplasm of uncertain histogenesis. Neuroendocrine cells contain dense core neurosecretory-type granules that vary in size from 100 to 500 nm. The size of the granule, its density, and the presence of a membrane "halo" can also elucidate the specific cell type (Table 21-4) (Fig. 21-8). The presence of neurosecretory granules in a poorly differentiated small cell tumor is strong evidence of neuroendocrine differentiation. In combined tumors, mucin granules and dense core granules may be found within a single cell.[24-27]

Immunohistochemistry

In most cases, immunohistochemistry is not required for a diagnosis of NET to be established. It is helpful in

TABLE 21–4. Ultrastructural Appearance of Dense Core Granules in Specific Neuroendocrine Cell Types

Cell Type	Granule Size (nm)	Granule Shape	Granule Density
ECC	200–400	Pleomorphic	Dense
D	300–400	Round, uniform	Medium dense
G	180–300	Round, uniform	Flocculent
L	250–300	Round, uniform	Dense
ECL	Variable	Variable	Variable

ECC, enterochromaffin cell; ECL, enterochromaffin-like cell.

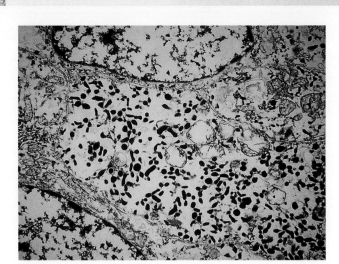

FIGURE 21–8. Electron microscopic appearance of a small intestinal ECC-NET showing multiple pleomorphic dense core granules that measure 200 to 400 nm in diameter.

the investigation of tumors of unknown primary and mixed or poorly differentiated tumors, as well as in confirming the presence of a functional tumor. In addition, limited information regarding prognosis may be obtained by immunohistochemistry. The following is a list of routinely used antibodies for evaluation of possible NET of the gut.

Cytosolic markers include neuron-specific enolase (NSE), PGP9.5, and 7B2. These may be present in cells that contain few, if any, secretory granules; unfortunately, their presence is not limited to endocrine tumors.[28]

Secretory granule markers, that is, chromogranins A and B and secretogranin, are quite specific. They are acidic proteins present in dense core granules. Less differentiated tumors or actively secreting tumors may express little, if any, of these proteins, possibly because of the paucity of granules in these tumors. Chromogranin A is the single best marker. It is expressed only to a small degree, if at all, in hindgut NET (rectal and appendiceal L-cell NET), where chromogranin B and secretogranin are preferentially expressed.[29-31]

Nondense core small vesicle markers include synaptophysin, as well as various antibodies to synaptic vesicle proteins (including antibodies to vesicular membrane transporters [VMATs] -1 and -2), which are integral membrane proteins.[32]

Leu7 (CD57) is a monoclonal antibody raised against a cell membrane glycoprotein from a T-cell leukemia cell line. It also recognizes an epitope on neurosecretory granules.

Although generally a diagnosis of NET can easily be made on hematoxylin and eosin–stained tissue, for circumstances in which it is important to confirm neuroendocrine differentiation, a panel of antibodies, rather than a single antibody, is often most helpful. Antibodies against chromogranin A, NSE, synaptophysin, Leu7 plus or minus serotonin, form a reliable initial neuroendocrine

panel. Strong expression, even in a few cells, is confirmation of at least focal neuroendocrine differentiation. One interesting feature of rectal and ileal NETs is that they may express prostatic acid phosphatase, which is a potential diagnostic pitfall if one is unaware of this fact.[33]

Immunohistochemical staining of keratins may also be helpful in situations related to a metastatic endocrine tumor of unknown primary. Recent studies have shown that cytokeratin 7 is often expressed in NETs that arise from the foregut (stomach, duodenum, pancreas, and lung), whereas cytokeratin 20 is usually positive in tumors from the midgut and the hindgut (small intestine and colorectum).[34]

Cell Proliferation Tests

Mitotic count is notoriously difficult to standardize for a variety of reasons. Variation in the size of the optical field can be obviated by the use of a micrometer. However, other limitations are not as easy to adjust. For instance, the thickness of tissue sections may vary substantially from case to case. In addition, time of tissue fixation is difficult to control, which may result in a 46% reduction in recognizable mitoses after 12 hours. This is due in part to autolytic changes that may obscure distinction between pyknosis and mitosis, but it is also due to completion of mitotic cycles during this time interval. Fortunately, mitotic counts tend not to be independently prognostic in NET.

Proliferating cell nuclear antigen (PCNA) is a 36-kD acidic nuclear protein that is essential for DNA synthesis and accumulates during S phase. MIB-1 antibody reacts with a proliferation-associated antigen that constitutes part of Ki67. Ki67 is expressed in G1 but progressively increases through M phase and is absent in G0 of the cell cycle. These markers may be measured as positive cells per 100 tumor cells. In the pancreas, some correlation has been noted with clinical behavior. PCNA indices greater than 5% have been shown to be more common in cases with extrapancreatic extension. However, data for GI-NET are not as clear. Overall proliferation rates for NETs usually are low, although high proliferation rates may be seen in aggressive tumors. This feature has not been shown to be an independent prognostic factor in most types of GI-NET.[35-37]

Tumor Suppressor Genes

Abnormal *TP53* (formerly *p53*), a cell proliferation regulating nuclear phosphoprotein, has been identified in morphologically atypical α1-NET. Abnormal c-myc, BCL2, and c-erbb2 have been identified in a small percentage of cases of NET.

Membrane glycoproteins such as carcinoembryonic antigen (CEA) and B72.3 also have not been shown to be of prognostic value in GI-NET. Most GI-NETs have the capacity to express CEA, so it is not even a reliable marker for exclusion of glandular differentiation. However, mucin stains are typically negative in GI-NET.

DNA Flow/Image Cytometry

Using the technique of DNA flow or image cytometry, one may analyze NETs for the presence of aneuploidy, which has been shown to be indicative of malignant behavior in some tumor types. The data on its prognostic value are not always encouraging. Most NETs, regardless of their location, size, or degree of malignancy, are euploid. One study of ileal carcinoids showed 80% to be euploid, and this feature was nondiscriminatory with regard to clinical behavior. One study showed aneuploidy to be associated with poor prognosis. At present, ploidy is not routinely recommended for prognosticating NET of the gastrointestinal tract.[38-40]

Esophageal Neuroendocrine Tumors

CLINICAL FEATURES

The esophagus is the rarest site of occurrence of GI-NET, representing only 0.04% in a recent survey of 8305 gastrointestinal cases.[4] Although scattered neuroendocrine cells are present within esophageal mucosal glands in the distal esophagus, no well-developed GI-NES is noted in the esophagus. Esophageal NETs usually occur in older patient groups (generally older than 60 years of age) with a male predominance. The lower third of the esophagus is most often affected, particularly the gastroesophageal junction. Remaining cases occur in the middle to upper third of the esophagus. Esophageal NETs often present with dysphagia and chest pain, or they are discovered incidentally in association with Barrett's esophagus. Survival is related to the particular NET subtype. Primary NETs of the esophagus may be divided into three clinicopathologic groups.

Classic Neuroendocrine Tumors

These are small tumors (<1 cm) that often present as polyps. Only 28 cases have been reported in the English literature. Their morphologic appearance is usually mixed, consisting of nests, cords, and acini. In many cases, they are limited to the mucosa and submucosa and are grade I (well differentiated). These tumors have a good prognosis.[41,42]

High-Grade Neuroendocrine Tumors

This is a more common type of NET of the esophagus. Various synonyms have been used for this tumor, such as *neuroendocrine carcinoma, small* and *large cell types, oat cell carcinoma,* and *atypical carcinoid.* At presentation, these tumors are often larger than 5 cm, and metastasis is found in 75% of cases. Common sites of metastasis include the lymph nodes, liver, bone, and lung.[43] Grossly, they are usually bulky ulcerated tumors. A type D growth pattern is typical. Median survival is extremely poor (mean, 3.1 months).[44]

Combined Adenocarcinoma/Neuroendocrine Tumors

A small number of combined tumors have been reported in association with Barrett's esophagus. It is interesting to note that associated endocrine cell hyperplasia has also been detected in some of these cases. Morphologically, these tumors may be of the collision or composite type; their behavior is usually similar to that of pure adenocarcinomas (Fig. 21-9).[45]

Gastric Neuroendocrine Tumors

Gastric NETs represent 6% of all GI-NETs. However, their incidence appears to be on the rise. Whether this represents a real increase or is a result of more frequent endoscopy is unclear at this time. Furthermore, the influence of widespread use of pharmacologic gastric acid suppression agents in the development of gastric NET is equally uncertain.[46] Localized disease is found in 45% of patients; approximately 20% show regional spread and approximately 20% show distant spread at the time of diagnosis. Although several different α1-NES cell types are located in the stomach, 70% of tumors are derived from a single cell type, the ECLs. Rare tumors may develop from G cells or ECCs.

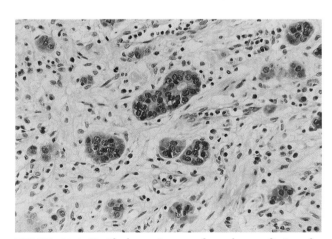

FIGURE 21–9. Residual carcinoma after chemoradiation for Barrett's-associated cancer. Residual malignant cells have "coppery" granules and the nuclear characteristics and immunophenotype of an ECC neuroendocrine tumor.

Gastric NETs (G-NETs) are divided into four general groups. Types 1 and 2 arise in a background of hypergastrinemia; type 1 is associated with chronic atrophic gastritis, and type 2 with ZES/MEN I. NETs of both types 1 and 2 are derived from ECL cells. Types 3 and 4 arise in patients with normal serum gastrin levels. Type 3 comprises sporadic G-NETs. These are generally large, aggressive tumors that are derived mainly from gastric ECCs. Ectopic hormones, such as adrenocorticotropic hormone (ACTH) and growth hormone, may be secreted in these tumors as well. This group also includes the rare antropyloric gastrinomas, which, although aggressive, are usually quite small. Type 4 tumors represent a heterogeneous group of tumors that show evidence of multidirectional differentiation, such as a combination of adenocarcinoma and NET.[47-49]

Another recently described form of gastric NET in Japan is not associated with atrophic gastritis or ZES but instead shows a strong correlation with *Helicobacter pylori* infection. *Helicobacter* infection leads to downregulation of somatostatin-producing D cells. This may lead to elevated gastrin levels, increased acid production, and the potential for ECL NET formation. Experimental evidence has linked *Helicobacter* infection to gastric NETs in gerbils.[50-52]

GENERAL PATHOLOGIC FEATURES

NETs of the stomach may grow as mass lesions or polyps and are multifocal in 10% of cases. The surrounding mucosa often shows atrophic gastritis with patchy intestinal metaplasia. Gastric NETs may arise in the antrum or the body mucosa, depending on the cell of origin. They are rarely associated with the carcinoid syndrome. Morphologically, gastric NETs are usually of the mixed type (ribbons, acini, and solid nests). Types 1 and 2 are usually confined to the mucosa and the submucosa, whereas types 3 and 4 usually show transmural invasion and serosal involvement.

PROGNOSIS

Type 1 tumors are almost invariably of grade I and tend to behave in a relatively indolent fashion. Type 2 NETs, however, have the potential for aggressive behavior and are either grade I or grade II. Type 3 and 4 gastric NETs are usually aggressive tumors. Type 3 tumors develop lymph node metastasis in 60% and liver metastasis in 50% of cases. Type 4 tumors, with mixed adenocarcinoma/NET morphology, are also aggressive tumors. They behave similarly to pure adenocarcinomas. Grade IV tumors (poorly differentiated endocrine carcinomas) are rarely found in the stomach, but when they occur, they are usually of the intermediate-cell type and are exceedingly aggressive (75% mortality within 1 year).

TYPE 1 GASTRIC NEUROENDOCRINE TUMORS
GI-NET associated with type A autoimmune chronic gastritis [CG-A] and pernicious anemia

Atrophic chronic gastritis (autoimmune gastritis) is characterized by circulating autoantibodies directed against microsomes of parietal cells with selective destruction of the acid-producing cells in the body/fundus of the stomach. Parietal cells normally secrete acid in the form of hydrochloric acid, but they also secrete intrinsic factor. Intrinsic factor autoantibodies are present in the serum of 55% to 60% of patients with autoimmune gastritis. Some patients with type A chronic gastritis also develop pernicious anemia due to vitamin B_{12} deficiency. An association between pernicious anemia and GI-NET has been recognized for half a century.

Pathogenesis

Gastrin is the primary neuropeptide involved in gastric acid secretion. It is released from antral and duodenal G cells in response to gastric distention and intraluminal pH increase due to food ingestion. Gastrin has a minor direct effect on parietal cells, causing release of H^+, but it mainly acts by stimulating ECL cells. ECL cells are the main neuroendocrine cells of the stomach, constituting 70% of the total gastric neuroendocrine cells. They are located mainly in the body/fundic glands in close proximity to parietal cells. Recently, an antibody to VMAT-2 has been identified as a marker for ECL cells. ECL cells, which are scattered within the deep portions of the oxyntic mucosa, are of the "closed" type; that is, they do not communicate with the lumina of the glands but are in close contact with the bases of parietal and chief cells. Histamine is the major product of ECL cells. The local release of histamine is responsible for the majority of acid production from adjacent parietal cells by paracrine effect.

An acidic pH within the stomach has an inhibitory effect on gastrin production, which results in feedback inhibition of acid secretion. This occurs via the release of somatostatin, which is produced by D cells. D cells are located throughout the gastrointestinal tract and act as a final common pathway for the inhibition of antral gastrin release, thereby inhibiting acid secretion. Thus, a loss of acid production, such as occurs in chronic atrophic gastritis (autoimmune gastritis), leads to loss of this inhibitory feedback loop, which results in hypergastrinemia and eventually ECL cell hyperplasia and potentially neoplasia.

G cells are normally located in the antrum of the stomach. They are present in the midzone of the mucosa and are more numerous on the greater curve compared with the lesser curve. They are "open-type" neuroendocrine cells; the apical cytoplasm communicates with the lumen of the gland. G-cell hyperplasia may be primary or secondary. The latter is much more common. Counts of 200 to 250 G cells per linear millimeter of mucosa represent a definite increase in cell mass (normal, 50 to 100/mm) and correlate with expansion of the G-cell compartment.[53]

Hypergastrinemia is found in a number of disease states such as atrophic chronic gastritis with corresponding G-cell hyperplasia, ZES, MEN I, and, more recently, pharmacologic acid suppression therapy, particularly with proton pump inhibitors. Laboratory studies have shown that blockage of acid production results in hypergastrinemia, which causes an increased risk of ECL cell hyperplasia, dysplasia, and carcinoid tumor formation in the stomach (see under Pathologic Features).[54-56]

Pathologic Features

Histologically, type 1 tumors are usually associated with a dense lymphoplasmacytic infiltrate in the lamina propria, primarily involving the body/fundus of the stomach, with antral sparing, pyloric or antral metaplasia, and intestinal metaplasia. Ultimately, when the inflammation subsides, complete gastric atrophy with extensive intestinal metaplasia usually remains behind (Figs. 21-10 and 21-11). Despite antral-type glands, G cells are not normally identifiable by immunohistochemistry, which helps confirm that the origin of the mucosa is of the body/fundus type. The antrum typically shows minimal inflammatory changes but usually shows prominent neuroendocrine cells, representing hyperplastic G cells.

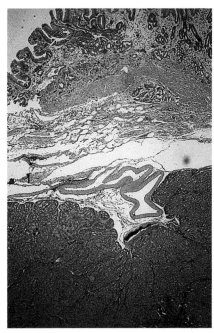

FIGURE 21–11. Type 1 gastric NET underneath atrophic gastric fundic mucosa. The tumor forms a densely cellular lobulated mass with pushing borders that expand the submucosa.

ECL cell hyperplasia is a benign but potentially preneoplastic proliferation. Benign hyperplasia is present in up to 30% of patients with type A chronic atrophic gastritis. It is divided into three morphologic patterns: (1) Diffuse or simple hyperplasia represents an increased number (by more than twofold) of ECL cells in the gastric mucosa (Fig. 21-12). These cells are scattered among the glands diffusely and singly; (2) linear hyper-

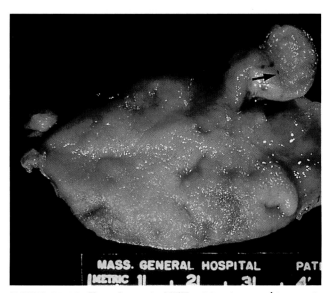

FIGURE 21–10. Type 1 gastric NET arising in atrophic gastric mucosa with dysplastic ECL growth. The tumor forms a pedunculated polyp in the gastric body *(arrow)*. The mucosa is atrophic in appearance with granular and nodular areas corresponding to islands of intestinal metaplasia and ECL dysplasia.

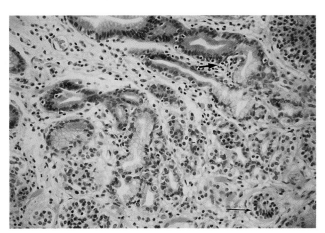

FIGURE 21–12. ECL hyperplasia—simple and linear. Replacing the deep glandular compartment of the gastric body is a proliferation of small cells with clear cytoplasm and round nuclei that appear darker than the surrounding epithelial cell nuclei. These cells are histamine-producing ECL cells. *Thin arrow* indicates an area of increased ECL density. *Thick arrow* indicates a solid line of ECL cells replacing the epithelial cells of one gland (linear hyperplasia).

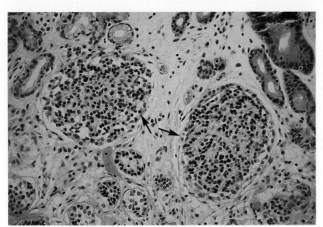

FIGURE 21–13. Micronodular hyperplasia of ECL cells. In this atrophic mucosa, two nodules of ECL cells *(arrows)* have expanded the gland to form nodules that measure less than 150 μm in size.

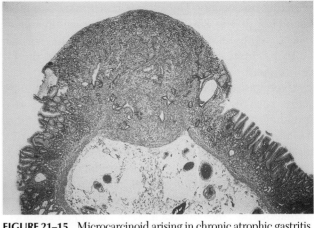

FIGURE 21–15. Microcarcinoid arising in chronic atrophic gastritis. A single mucosal nodule measuring greater than 500 μm (0.5 mm) bulges but does not invade through the muscularis mucosa.

plasia represents a chain-forming proliferation of ECL cells within the glands; and (3) micronodular hyperplasia represents an organized collection of ECL cells that form nodules measuring less than 150 μm (Fig. 21-13). Further NEC proliferation may lead to dysplasia. However, dysplastic nodules are seen in only 6% of cases. In this category, four morphologic groups are recognized. These include (1) enlarging expansive growth pattern (comprising nodules that measure larger than 150 μm), (2) fused micronodules (Fig. 21-14), (3) microinfiltration of the lamina propria, and (4) nodules with surrounding newly formed stroma.

Large micronodules (>150 μm) are often irregular in shape and configuration. Fused micronodules develop when two or more nodules, with a thin strand of connecting ECL cells, fuse together into a single micronodular growth. In the deep lamina propria, multiple small buds may protrude from these nodules, which may impart a false appearance of microinvasion. However, unlike true invasion, fused micronodules are limited to the mucosa in the region of dysplastic foci. Nodules that measure larger than 0.5 mm (>500 μm) but are confined to the mucosa are classified as micro-NET (previously known as microcarcinoidosis) (Fig. 21-15). Dysplastic nodules are most often seen in association with gastric NET that penetrates beyond the muscularis mucosae or shows vascular invasion. Tumors are considered invasive carcinoid tumors, regardless of their size (Table 21-5).[57,58]

NETs that arise in a background of diffuse hyperplasia and dysplasia are usually of low malignant potential. Metastasis occurs in only 14% to 20% of cases, mostly to lymph nodes, but rarely involves the liver as well. Treatment of patients with these tumors is controversial. Spontaneous regression may occur in some cases. Removal of the antrum has been reported to result in rapid regression of hyperplastic ECL cells. However, regression of dysplastic nodules and/or true carcinoid

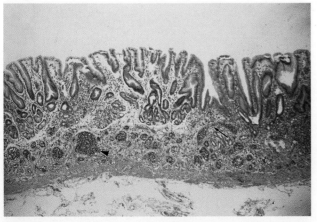

FIGURE 21–14. Dysplastic ECL cell growth pattern in chronic atrophic gastritis. No residual parietal cells are present. The deep lamina propria is cellular owing to the presence of large irregular nodules of ECL cells measuring greater than 150 μm *(arrow)*. There are also areas of fusion of smaller nodules *(arrowhead)*. Multiple small foci of ECL cells represent benign hyperplasia.

TABLE 21–5. Classification of Gastric Neuroendocrine Hyperplasia and Dysplasia

Hyperplasia	Simple
	Linear
	Micronodules (≤150 μm)
Dysplasia	Enlarged micronodules (>150 μm)
	Fused micronodules
	Microinfiltration of lamina propria
	Association with new stroma
Micro-NET	Nodules >500 μm

tumors is less well established with this management technique.[59,60]

TYPE 2 GASTRIC NEUROENDOCRINE TUMORS
ZES/MEN I

Most cases of ZES occur as the result of a functioning pancreatic endocrine tumor. However, some occur secondary to duodenal or gastric gastrinoma. Rarely, primary hyperplasia of antral G cells may cause ZES as well. In these cases, the antral G cells are typically large and clustered and may often form microadenomas, whereas in tumor cases, G cells are either normal or decreased in number. In ZES, the fundic glandular compartment is typically expanded owing to an increase in parietal cell mass. ECCs may also be increased in number but to a smaller degree. In 20% of ZES cases, other endocrine tumors, particularly of the parathyroid and pituitary gland, also develop as a manifestation of MEN I.

Finally, the use of proton pump inhibitors with resultant induction of hypergastrinemia also presents a theoretical risk of carcinoid tumor development. In laboratory rats, high-dose omeprazole has been associated with the development of carcinoid tumors. However, although some humans develop hypergastrinemia and an increase in ECL cells secondary to proton pump inhibitor use, dysplastic nodules and carcinoid tumors have not been reported in the absence of other predisposing conditions such as ZES. As was mentioned previously, ECL-NETs have also been reported in patients with *H. pylori* gastritis.

These NETs often form small mucosal nodules and/or polyps within the body and fundus, although recently, similar tumors have been described in the antrum of ZES patients as well.[54] Histologically, they have a mixed growth pattern, often with closely packed trabeculae and small acini with little stroma. Tumor growth is confined to the mucosa and the submucosa in most cases. VMAT-2 antibody is a good marker for the typing of ECL cells.

TYPE 3 GASTRIC NEUROENDOCRINE TUMORS

The stomach is an extremely uncommon site for NETs derived from ECC. They may arise in any portion of the stomach. At presentation, they are often bulky tumors with local lymph node metastasis. Ectopic hormone production (ACTH, calcitonin) has been reported. Morphologically, these tumors reveal mixed growth patterns. Transmural invasion, serosal involvement, and lymph node metastasis are common at presentation. Smaller tumors may also develop in the antropyloric region and may express gastrin (gastrinoma). Despite

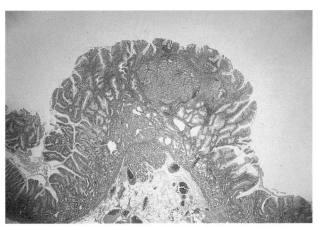

FIGURE 21–16. Small gastrinoma of the pyloric region. A mucosal growth of gastrin-producing neuroendocrine cells expands the mucosa in the pyloroduodenal region. Despite its small size. these proliferations may be functional and biologically malignant.

their small size, these tumors are usually malignant (Fig. 21-16).

TYPE 4 GASTRIC NEUROENDOCRINE TUMORS
Mixed Adenocarcinoma/Neuroendocrine Tumor

This group represents a heterogeneous collection of mixed tumors. Mixed tumors are defined by the presence of a mixture (>30) of glandular and NET components in a single tumor (Figs. 21-17 and 21-18). These tumors can arise from any portion of the stomach. They may be polypoid in appearance and are often large; their behavior tends to be more aggressive than that of pure NETs. Metastases from these tumors may include both cell types or only one. Amphicrine, composite, and collision tumors have also been reported rarely in the stomach (Table 21-6).

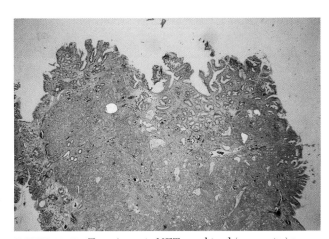

FIGURE 21–17. Type 4 gastric NET: combined (composite) tumor with admixed well-differentiated adenocarcinoma and NET, presenting as a single mucosal polyp in a patient with atrophic gastritis.

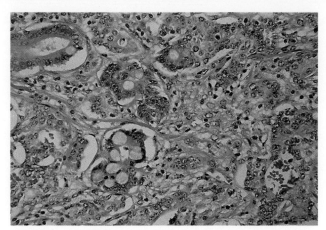

FIGURE 21–18. High-power view of Figure 21-17 showing an intimate admixture of neuroendocrine and glandular components and the very well differentiated nature of the glandular component.

◼ Duodenal Neuroendocrine Tumors

Duodenal NETs represent about 3% of GI-NETs[4] and are the second most common type of malignant tumor in this anatomic area. Duodenal NETs may also be associated with other disorders, such as von Recklinghausen's disease and ZES.[61,62] They often present with bleeding and/or as a polypoid mucosal growth. Ampullary or periampullary tumors usually present with jaundice. Rarely, these tumors are associated with the carcinoid syndrome.

Most duodenal tumors occur in the first or second portion of the duodenum. They may be multicentric, are often small (<1 cm), and are limited to the mucosa/submucosa. However, gangliocytic paragangliomas may occasionally grow to large sizes. Duodenal NETs are generally treated by surgical resection and tend to have an indolent biologic potential. Five distinct subgroups have been described.

GASTRIN-PRODUCING (G-CELL) NEUROENDOCRINE TUMORS

This is the most frequent subtype, representing two thirds of duodenal NETs, and is associated with ZES in one third of cases. Lymph node metastases are found at diagnosis in approximately 30% of cases, even in tumors that are smaller than 1 cm. Tumors not associated with ZES are often indolent and found in older patients. Functional tumors are all regarded as low-grade malignancies and tend to occur in a younger age group. Morphologically, these tumors usually show a mixture of all histologic patterns of growth.

SOMATOSTATIN-PRODUCING (D-CELL) DUODENAL NEUROENDOCRINE TUMORS
(see Chapter 14)

Duodenal somatostatinomas are associated with von Recklinghausen's disease in one third of cases. They are characterized histologically by the presence of pseudo-acini with psammoma bodies. Although somatostatin may be strongly expressed, only rarely is a clinical syndrome associated with somatostatin production (moderate hyperglycemia, cholelithiasis, constipation). Many of these tumors arise in the periampullary region.

SEROTONIN/CALCITONIN-PRODUCING TUMORS

This type of tumor arises from duodenal ECC cells. It is an unusual tumor in that it shows a predominantly type A nested growth pattern combined with immunohistochemical expression of serotonin. Hepatic metastasis may give rise to the carcinoid syndrome (Fig. 21-19).[63]

TABLE 21–6. Classification of Gastric Neuroendocrine Tumors

Benign
Nonfunctioning, cytologically bland tumors up to 1 cm in size limited to mucosa and submucosa, without angioinvasion. Includes most type 1 ECL-NET.

Uncertain Malignant Potential
Nonfunctioning, cytologically bland tumors 1 to 2 cm in size limited to mucosa and submucosa with or without angioinvasion. Includes type 2 gastric NET.

Low-Grade Malignant Potential
Nonfunctioning tumors >2 cm in size with extension beyond submucosa. Includes all sporadic gastric NET and some type 1 or 2 tumors. Includes all functioning tumors of any type and all antropyloric gastrinomas.

High-Grade Malignant Potential
Poorly differentiated functioning or nonfunctioning tumors of intermediate- or small-cell type.

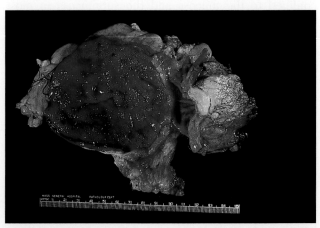

FIGURE 21–19. Duodenal ECC-NET, grade III. A 3-cm tumor mass replaces the duodenal wall and infiltrates underlying pancreatic parenchyma.

POORLY DIFFERENTIATED NEUROENDOCRINE TUMOR

This is a rare type of duodenal NET. It most often occurs in the periampullary region and represents a high-grade NET associated with a dismal prognosis. These tumors usually show transmural invasion and disseminated disease at the time of diagnosis. Survival is usually only 6 to 17 months.[64]

GANGLIOCYTIC PARAGANGLIOMA (see also Chapters 14 and 22)

This tumor arises mainly in the periampullary region. It is formed of ganglion cells intimately mixed with endocrine cells (pancreatic polypeptide [PP] and somatostatin-positive cells) and a stromal element of spindle cells that express neurofilament and S100. It occurs in a younger age group compared with other duodenal NETs. The typical presentation is that of a polypoid mass in the second portion of the duodenum that presents with bleeding. These masses, which may vary in size from 1 to 10 cm, are nonencapsulated, infiltrative tumors. They are histologically variable, showing areas reminiscent of a paraganglioma mixed with endocrine cells and spindle cells and scattered large ganglion cells. Immunohistochemistry confirms the presence of ganglion cells (NSE-positive), S100-positive spindle cells, and keratin-positive endocrine cells. Recurrence and lymph node metastasis are only rarely reported. These tumors are generally considered benign.[65]

■ Jejunal/Ileal Neuroendocrine Tumors (Table 21-7)

CLINICAL FEATURES

Most small intestinal NETs (SI-NETs) are derived from ECC; these account for 30% of all GI-NETs.[4] Almost all SI-NETs produce serotonin and substance P. They are multicentric in 40% of cases, and 17% are associated with multiple separate primary tumors. Their incidence rate increases from the proximal to the distal small intestine. Rarely, they may develop in association with a Meckel's diverticulum.[66]

Symptoms are usually vague. Crampy abdominal pain, nausea, vomiting, and weight loss are the most common presenting complaints. Intermittent small bowel obstruction may occur secondary to tumor fibrosis (Fig. 21-20). Rarely, bleeding, intussusception, or the carcinoid syndrome is the initial presenting finding. Occasionally, they are detected only at autopsy or as an incidental finding, in which case they are usually benign. Rarely, patients with SI-NET present with ischemia as a result of occlusion of vessels by tumor.[67,68] In these cases, one

---

TABLE 21–7. Classification of Small Intestinal Neuroendocrine Tumors

Benign
Nonfunctioning, cytologically bland tumors up to 1 cm in size limited to mucosa and submucosa, without angioinvasion; e.g., small, nonfunctional, gastrin-expressing tumors of the proximal duodenum.

Uncertain Malignant Potential
Nonfunctioning, cytologically bland tumors 1 to 2 cm in size limited to mucosa and submucosa with or without angioinvasion. Includes all gangliocytic paragangliomas of any size without metastasis. Includes intermediate-sized serotonin- or somatostatin-producing tumors.

Low-Grade Malignant Potential
Nonfunctioning tumors >2 cm in size with extension beyond submucosa. Includes all functional tumors such as small gastrinomas and ECC-NET.

High-Grade Malignant Potential
Poorly differentiated functioning or nonfunctioning tumors of intermediate- or small-cell type.

---

may see histologic changes of arterial luminal narrowing, with marked proliferation of elastic tissue, particularly in the adventitia but also in the intima. Veins and capillaries may be affected as well.

Most clinically apparent tumors are larger than 2 cm and show transmural invasion with metastasis at the time of diagnosis.[27] However, metastasis and death from NET can occur as well in cases in which NETs are smaller than 1 cm. For this reason, all NETs of the small intestine are considered to be at least grade II tumors. Five-year survival rates for localized SI-NET approach 65%. However, for NETs with distant spread, this number falls to 20% to 30%.[4,69] Predictors of poor prognosis include distant metastasis, presence of carcinoid syndrome, and female sex.[70]

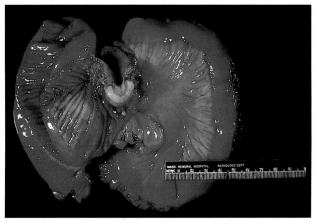

FIGURE 21–20. Ileal ECC-NET, grade III. A 2.5-cm yellow-gray tumor mass infiltrates the small intestinal wall with retraction of the surrounding ileum, causing kinking of the intestinal loop. The tumor appears bisected by hypertrophied muscularis propria.

PATHOLOGIC FEATURES

Grossly, SI-NETs typically appear as firm nodules located immediately below the mucosal surface. Rarely, tumors may be associated with an annular constricting growth pattern caused by the presence of a dense fibrotic stroma often induced by the tumor cells. Trophic factors produced by the tumor may cause hypertrophy of the muscularis propria as well. The tumor is typically pale yellow, and it characteristically shows preservation of the muscularis propria within the tumor mass (Fig. 21-21; see also Fig. 21-20). Lymphatic permeation may be apparent grossly in the form of small miliary-type nodules that extend onto the serosal surface.

Histologically, these tumors are characterized mainly by a type A growth pattern. Thin fibrovascular stroma may be seen between nests of tumor cells. A trabecular or acinar growth pattern (type B or C) is often seen at the periphery of the tumor, either with or without a desmoplastic reaction (Fig. 21-22). Lymphatic permeation may be marked in some cases. Local lymph nodes are almost always involved, and liver metastasis is common.

◼ Colonic Neuroendocrine Tumors (excluding appendix and rectosigmoid)

A colonic NET can be either ECC-derived tumor or a high-grade NET (small cell carcinoma).

ECC-DERIVED TUMOR

Overall, colonic NETs are rare. They account for less than 1% of all colonic tumors and less than 10% of all GI-NETs. Colonic NETs are the most aggressive form

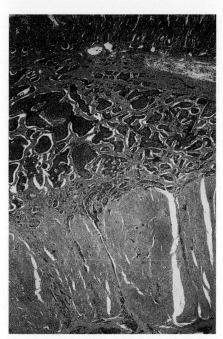

FIGURE 21–22. Ileal ECC-NET. The tumor mass is composed of nests of ECC. Peripherally, a mixture of cords and acini invade through the muscle without fibrosis.

of GI-NET. They rarely present as an incidental finding. Instead, most patients present with nausea, vomiting, weight loss, or an abdominal mass. For unknown reasons, the incidence among women is higher than that among men. These are mainly midgut ECC-derived NETs; they lead to the carcinoid syndrome in only 5% of cases.[4,71,72] Two thirds of colonic NETs arise in the cecum and the right colon. Unfortunately, more than two thirds are metastatic at presentation. The 5-year survival rate for colonic NET with distal spread is only 25% (70% for localized, 40% for regional spread).

Colonic NETs are usually large, bulky, invasive tumors (average size, >5 cm). Histologically, these tumors consist of nests of cells, most with a type A growth pattern similar to that of other ECC tumors, but mixed growth patterns are also common. Some may also show a type D growth pattern. None of the colonic NETs are grade I; all should be considered potentially malignant.

HIGH-GRADE NEUROENDOCRINE TUMOR
Small Cell Carcinoma

This tumor has been variously described as an extra-pulmonary oat cell carcinoma or a small cell neuroendocrine carcinoma. It is considered to be a high-grade neoplasm. These tumors occur in an older age group and do not show the same female predominance as is seen in GI-NET; instead, they show a slight male predominance. Patients usually present with metastatic disease, weight loss, cachexia, and hepatomegaly. The prognosis for patients with these tumors is very poor.

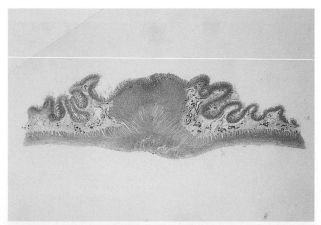

FIGURE 21–21. Ileal ECC-NET. Tumor invades the wall of the bowel and is associated with dense fibrosis in the submucosa, thickening of the muscularis propria, and serosal involvement with fibrosis. Vascular proliferation is prominent in the mucosa and the upper submucosa.

Death usually occurs within 1 year of diagnosis because of distant metastases. In addition to surgery, systemic chemotherapy and radiation, according to a pulmonary small cell protocol, have been used for treatment. However, survival rates are exceedingly poor.[73]

Colorectal small cell neuroendocrine carcinomas are located mainly in the rectosigmoid and the cecum. An overlying adenoma or adenocarcinoma is present in up to 50% of cases (Fig. 21-23).[74] Rarely, squamous elements may be seen as well. Histologic features are similar to those of small cell carcinomas from elsewhere in the body. Mitotic figures and necrosis occur frequently. Vascular involvement is also common.[75]

Rectal Neuroendocrine Tumors

Rectal NETs represent 1% to 2% of all rectal tumors and 17% of all GI-NETs. They occur equally among males and females and are typically diagnosed in the sixth decade of life. They show a low propensity for lymph node involvement (14%) and distal spread; thus, they generally have a good prognosis (72% 5-year survival).[4] Their incidence appears to be on the rise.[76]

Virtually all rectal NETs are derived from hindgut L cells. The classic gross appearance is that of a 1-cm nodule in the midportion of the rectum (4 to 8 cm from the anal verge). They appear as small, yellow, sessile polyps with overlying intact mucosa. Histologically, a ribbon (type B) pattern is typical (Fig. 21-24). These

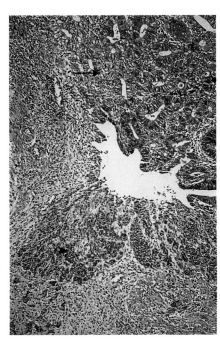

FIGURE 21–23. Colonic NET, grade IV (small cell neuroendocrine carcinoma). The mucosal element of this tumor contains an area of moderately differentiated adenocarcinoma *(arrow)*. The remainder of the tumor showed a type D growth pattern (high-grade NET) *(arrowhead)*.

tumors are usually negative for silver stains and do not normally express chromogranin A; rather, they express chromogranin B and secretogranin. Immunohistochemically, they have also been shown to express enteroglucagon (glicentin), PYY, and pancreatic polypeptide.[77-79]

Small tumors are usually adequately treated by local excision. However, large tumors may have an aggressive course and show both local and distant spread. Features indicative of malignant behavior include size larger than 2 cm, invasion into the muscularis propria, a high mitotic rate, and the presence of necrosis. Invasion of the muscularis propria is often an indication for radical excision.[4]

Appendiceal Neuroendocrine Tumors (Table 21-8)

CLINICAL FEATURES

Appendiceal NETs represent a third of all NETs of the gastrointestinal tract and are the most common type of appendiceal neoplasm (75% of all appendiceal tumors).[80-81] Average age at diagnosis is approximately 20 years younger than that of NETs from other sites. Females predominate, with a male-to-female ratio of 1:3. Appendiceal NETs are also the most common gastrointestinal neoplasm to occur during childhood.[82-84] Many investigators believe that appendiceal NETs are derived from submucosal neuroendocrine cells; they cite the relatively high prevalence of these cells in the tip of the appendix. Others suggest that luminal factors contribute to their formation.[79-81] The prognosis for patients with conventional appendiceal NETs is better than that for all other sites. A majority of appendiceal NETs are localized to the appendix at the time of diagnosis. Eighty percent are smaller than 1 cm and

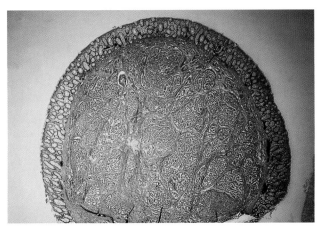

FIGURE 21–24. Rectal NET. A 0.5-cm sessile rectal polyp is composed of a submucosal proliferation of type B–pattern NET. No atypia, mitoses, or muscularis propria invasion was identified.

TABLE 21–8. Classification of Neuroendocrine Tumors of the Appendix
Benign
Nonfunctioning, cytologically bland tumors measuring 1 cm or smaller without extension into mesoappendix—this represents the majority of ECC-NET, all L-cell NET, and most tumors of the appendix.
Uncertain Malignant Potential
Nonfunctioning, cytologically bland tumor measuring 1 to 2 cm with extension into mesoappendix. Includes goblet (crypt) cell carcinoid, as well as ECC tumors with mesoappendix involvement.
Low-Grade Malignant Potential
Nonfunctioning tumors measuring >2 cm deeply invasive into mesoappendix. Functioning tumors of any type.
High-Grade Malignant Potential
Poorly differentiated functioning or nonfunctioning tumors of intermediate- or small-cell type. Combined adenocarcinoma/neuroendocrine tumor.

demonstrate a 5-year survival rate greater than 95%. Lymph node metastasis to regional nodes occurs in approximately 4% of all appendiceal ECC-NETs, usually in tumors larger than 2 cm. Distant metastasis occurs in about 1% of cases, again usually only with larger (>2 cm) tumors. In these rare cases, the carcinoid syndrome has also been reported.

The most common form of clinical presentation is that of an incidental nodule detected at the time of removal of the appendix due to appendicitis. Others may be found incidentally during laparotomy for other reasons. Still others may be found at autopsy. Rarely, they present with an abdominal mass, pain, or the carcinoid syndrome.[85,86] Treatment by appendectomy is curative in most cases, particularly for those smaller than 1 cm. In cases with lymph node involvement, or for those larger than 2 cm or with peritoneal studding, a right hemicolectomy is advised. Certain features, apart from size and invasion, may be associated with more aggressive behavior. In tumors of uncertain malignancy between 1 and 2 cm in size, the presence of deep serosal and mesoappendicular spread and a significant mitotic rate may predict a more aggressive behavior.[69,87]

PATHOLOGIC FEATURES

Appendiceal NETs are divided into three broad histologic types—ECC-derived NETs (conventional carcinoid), NETs with mucin production, and L-cell NETs (tubular NETs).

ECC-Derived Tumor

These represent the most frequent and the best characterized form of appendiceal NET.[1] More than 70% are located in the tip of the appendix and 20% in

the midportion, with the remainder occurring at the proximal end or the base of the appendix.[85,88] Grossly, they are pale yellow and often expand the tip of the appendix as a firm well-circumscribed nodule. Most are smaller than 1 cm. Tumors larger than 2 cm are rare.[87]

Histologically, appendiceal ECC NETs are mainly of the type A growth pattern. At the periphery of the tumor, one often sees a trabecular or type B growth pattern and more pronounced fibrosis with occasional stromal hyalinization. Small tumors are generally confined to the submucosa, but muscularis invasion and lymphatic invasion are quite common, as is extension into the subserosal tissue (Figs. 21-25 and 21-26).[82,89]

Appendiceal Neuroendocrine Tumors With Mucin Production

CLINICAL FEATURES

These tumors represent approximately 40% of all appendiceal NETs reported to the National Cancer Institute surveillance program from 1973 to 1991.[4,81] However, this is probably an overestimate of their true incidence, as all "incidental" appendiceal NETs are excluded from this etiology. They have been reported under a variety of synonyms such as *goblet cell carcinoid, adenocarcinoid, crypt cell carcinoid,* and *mucinous carcinoid.*[90-93] Unfortunately, there has been little uniformity in the reporting and investigation of this group of tumors, so that wide variation has been noted in the literature in their reported histologic features and biologic potential. Furthermore, some

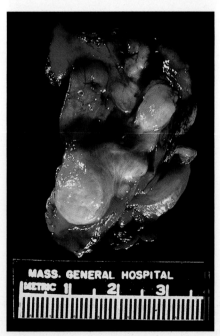

FIGURE 21–25. Appendiceal ECC-NET. A 1-cm nodule with a yellow cut surface is present at the tip of this inflamed appendix.

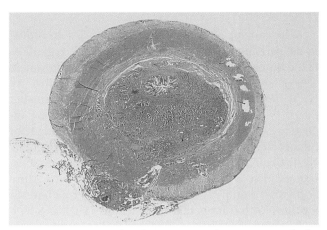

FIGURE 21–26. Appendiceal ECC-NET. The NET expands the submucosa and infiltrates through the wall into the subserosa.

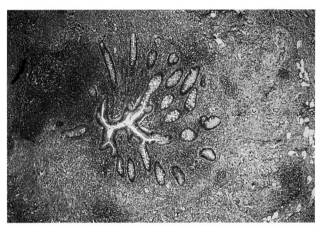

FIGURE 21–28. Low-grade goblet cell (crypt cell) tumor of the appendix in association with Crohn's disease. Ileocecal Crohn's disease involves the tip the appendix. The muscularis propria is infiltrated by a gland-forming neoplasm with goblet cells and endocrine cells.

studies have included mixed adenocarcinoma/carcinoid tumors with the more benign goblet cell carcinoids in their assessment of clinical outcome. In general, the outcome of patients with these tumors has been reported to lie between that of pure adenocarcinoma and conventional ECL-NET. The age at diagnosis is typically slightly older than for conventional ECC-NET (mean, 52 years), and the female-to-male ratio is about equal.

PATHOLOGIC FEATURES

These NETs are characterized by multidirectional cellular differentiation. Two morphologic variants exist, one of which has a poorer prognosis.

The main type (goblet cell or crypt cell carcinoid) is composed of cells with a mixture of all of the normal crypt cell elements, goblet cells, Paneth cells, and even ECCs. These tumors recapitulate the normal crypt architecture (Figs. 21-27 and 21-28). The cytologic

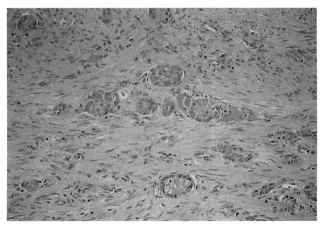

FIGURE 21–27. Goblet cell (crypt cell) tumor of the appendix, grade II. The muscularis propria contains glands showing crypt cell differentiation. Paneth and goblet cells are easily recognized.

features are typically bland, and these tumors do not show malignant cytologic features. Nuclear atypia is typically minimal, and mitoses are normally absent. The nuclei tend to be small without hyperchromasia or large nucleoli. The goblet cells resemble intestinal goblet cells much more than they resemble signet ring cell–type adenocarcinoma. Similar to ECC-NETs, these tumors tend to invade the serosa, lymphatics, and nerves. They are considered a type of low-grade composite tumor. Mucin stains reveal abundant cytoplasmic mucin in goblet cells. By immunohistochemistry, most tumors show only focal neuroendocrine differentiation, which can be confirmed by ultrastructural analysis.[24,94] Rarely, absolutely no evidence of endocrine differentiation is demonstrated in the tumor cells. In these cases, the diagnosis is established based solely on the NET growth pattern, the bland cytologic features, and the absence of a mucosal adenomatous component.[95]

A small subset of mucinous appendiceal NET tumors demonstrate a more aggressive behavior. These tumors show at least focal histologic features of pure conventional glandular differentiation and/or true signet ring cell differentiation with cytologic features of malignancy (mixed adenocarcinoma/NET). Microscopic features that can help distinguish these aggressive tumors from true goblet cell carcinoids include large mucin pools, true gland formation with cribriforming, solid sheets of cells, and signet ring cells with atypical nuclei in the more aggressive type (Fig. 21-29). The presence of cytologic atypia, mitoses, and necrosis indicates aggressive behavior.[96-98] Rarely, tumors of this type may present as ovarian tumors or as bilateral Krukenberg's tumors without an obvious primary. Often the ovarian metastases have more of a signet cell or mucin pool–rich appearance than does the primary tumor.[99,100] The

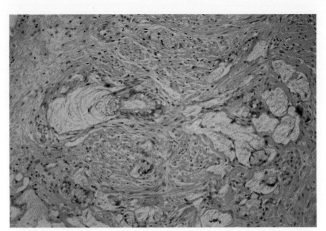

FIGURE 21–29. Combined adenocarcinoma/neuroendocrine tumor of the appendix, grade III. Acellular mucin pools are present. However, others are lined by cytologically malignant glandular epithelium. Scattered clusters of tumor cells without lumina also infiltrate the muscle.

survival rate is similar to that of pure adenocarcinoma of the appendix.

L-Cell Neuroendocrine Tumor

This is an extremely unusual type of appendiceal tumor. These tumors are derived from L cells and are invariably an incidental microscopic finding.[101,102] Many are smaller than 2 mm. Some have questioned whether these growths are in fact truly neoplastic and instead suggest a reactive or a hyperplastic origin. Histologically, they are composed of small acini or tubules, usually dispersed within a loose fibrous stroma that often whorls around teardrop-shaped tubules (Fig. 21-30). Because they are derived from L cells, their immunohistochemical profile reveals enteroglucagon, peptide YY, and pancreatic polypeptide expression but not chromogranin A expression.

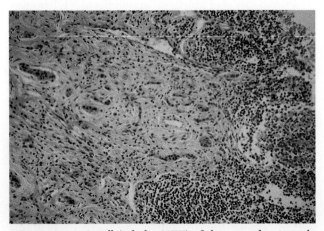

FIGURE 21–30. L cell (tubular NET) of the appendix. A single microscopic focus of small tubules and acini lies within the muscularis mucosae and the submucosa.

MANAGEMENT

Management of appendiceal NET varies according to the particular histologic subtype. However, regardless of the histologic type, the margins of the appendix should always be evaluated and confirmed to be negative. All NETs (except mixed adenocarcinoma/NETs) smaller than 1 cm are considered adequately treated by appendectomy. A right hemicolectomy is recommended for tumors larger than 2 cm and for mixed adenocarcinoma/NETs of any size. The data are unclear for conventional tumors that measure between 1 and 2 cm. More aggressive therapy is advocated for younger patients or for those with tumors that show features such as a high mitotic rate, deep mesoappendiceal invasion, or margin involvement. Any appendiceal tumor with true glandular differentiation (combined adenocarcinoma/NETs) or any type that measures larger than 2 cm should be treated with a right hemicolectomy and lymph node dissection.[91,103]

References

1. Creutzfeldt W: Historical background and natural history of carcinoids. Digestion 55(suppl 3):3-10, 1994.
2. Burke AP, et al: Carcinoids of the jejunum and ileum: An immunohistochemical and clinicopathologic study of 167 cases. Cancer 79:1086-1093, 1997.
3. Kloppel G, et al: Pathology and nomenclature of human gastrointestinal neuroendocrine (carcinoid) tumors and related lesions. World J Surg 20:132-141, 1996.
4. Capella C, et al: Revised classification of neuroendocrine tumors of the lung, pancreas and gut. Digestion 55(suppl 3):11-23, 1994.
5. Modlin IM, Sandor A: An analysis of 8305 cases of carcinoid tumors. Cancer 79:813-829, 1997.
6. Chamberlain RS, et al: Hepatic neuroendocrine metastases: Does intervention alter outcomes? J Am Coll Surg 190:432-445, 2000.
7. Kerfoot BP, et al: Carcinoid tumor in an ileal conduit diversion. J Urol 162:1685-1686, 1999.
8. Frese R, et al: Carcinoid tumor in an ileal neobladder. J Urol 165:522-523, 2001.
9. Ghimenti C, et al: Microsatellite instability and allelic losses in neuroendocrine tumors of the gastro-entero-pancreatic system. Int J Oncol 15:361-366, 1999.
10. Sigel JE, Goldblum JR: Neuroendocrine neoplasms arising in inflammatory bowel disease: A report of 14 cases. Mod Pathol 11:537-542, 1998.
11. Greenstein AJ, et al: Carcinoid tumor and inflammatory bowel disease: A study of eleven cases and review of the literature. Am J Gastroenterol 92:682-685, 1997.
12. Miller RR, Sumner HW: Argyrophilic cell hyperplasia and an atypical carcinoid tumor in chronic ulcerative colitis. Cancer 50:2920-2925, 1982.
13. Gledhill A, et al: Enteroendocrine cell hyperplasia, carcinoid tumours and adenocarcinoma in long-standing ulcerative colitis. Histopathology 10:501-508, 1986.
14. McNeely B, Owen DA, Pezim M: Multiple microcarcinoids arising in chronic ulcerative colitis. Am J Clin Pathol 98:112-116, 1992.
15. Anton PA, Shanahan F: Neuroimmunomodulation in inflammatory bowel disease. How far from "bench" to "bedside"? Ann N Y Acad Sci 840:723-734, 1998.
16. Pelley RJ, Bukowski RM: Recent advances in diagnosis and therapy of neuroendocrine tumors of the gastrointestinal tract. Curr Opin Oncol 9:68-74, 1997.
17. Arnold R, Frank M: Gastrointestinal endocrine tumours: Medical management. Baillieres Clin Gastroenterol 10:737-759, 1996.
18. Hernandez FJ, Reid JD: Mixed carcinoid and mucus-secreting intestinal tumors. Arch Pathol Lab Med 88:489-496, 1969.

19. Mandoky L: Amphicrine tumor. Pathol Oncol Res 5:239-244, 1999.
20. Klappenbach RS, et al: Composite carcinoma-carcinoid tumors of the gastrointestinal tract. A morphologic, histochemical, and immunocytochemical study. Am J Clin Pathol 84:137-143, 1985.
21. Capella C, et al: Mixed endocrine-exocrine tumors of the gastrointestinal tract. Semin Diagn Pathol 17:91-103, 2000.
22. Anderson JR, Wilson BG: Carcinoid tumours of the appendix. Br J Surg 72:545-546, 1985.
23. Creutzfeldt W: Carcinoid tumors: Development of our knowledge. World J Surg 20:126-131, 1996.
24. Cooper PH, Warkel RL: Ultrastructure of the goblet cell type of adenocarcinoid of the appendix. Cancer 42:2687-2695, 1978.
25. Soga J, Yakuwa Y: Bronchopulmonary carcinoids: An analysis of 1,875 reported cases with special reference to a comparison between typical carcinoids and atypical varieties. Ann Thorac Cardiovasc Surg 5:211-219, 1999.
26. Soga J: Gastric carcinoids: A statistical evaluation of 1,094 cases collected from the literature. Surg Today 27:892-901, 1997.
27. Soga J: Carcinoids of the small intestine: A statistical evaluation of 1102 cases collected from the literature. J Exp Clin Cancer Res 16:353-363, 1997.
28. Stachura J, et al: Immunohistology of gastrointestinal carcinoid tumors. Folia Histochem Cytobiol 27:227-231, 1989.
29. Al-Khafaji B, et al: Immunohistologic analysis of gastrointestinal and pulmonary carcinoid tumors. Hum Pathol 29:992-999, 1998.
30. Oberg K: Neuroendocrine gastrointestinal tumours. Ann Oncol 7:453-463, 1996.
31. Fahrenkamp AG, et al: Immunohistochemical distribution of chromogranins A and B and secretogranin II in neuroendocrine tumours of the gastrointestinal tract. Virchows Arch 426:361-367, 1995.
32. Jakobsen AM, et al: Differential expression of vesicular monoamine transporter (VMAT) 1 and 2 in gastrointestinal endocrine tumours. J Pathol 195:463-472, 2001.
33. Sobin LH, et al: Prostatic acid phosphatase activity in carcinoid tumors. Cancer 58:136-138, 1986.
34. Cai YC, et al: Cytokeratin 7 and 20 and thyroid transcription factor 1 can help distinguish pulmonary from gastrointestinal carcinoid and pancreatic endocrine tumors. Hum Pathol 32:1087-1093, 2001.
35. Kawahara M, et al: Immunohistochemical prognostic indicators of gastrointestinal carcinoid tumours. Eur J Surg Oncol 28:140-146, 2002.
36. Sokmensuer C, Gedikoglu G, Uzunalimoglu B: Importance of proliferation markers in gastrointestinal carcinoid tumors: A clinicopathologic study. Hepatogastroenterology 48:720-723, 2001.
37. Li CC, et al: Expression of E-cadherin, b-catenin, and Ki-67 in goblet cell carcinoids of the appendix: An immunohistochemical study with clinical correlation. Endocr Pathol 13:47-58, 2002.
38. Eriksson B, et al: Nuclear DNA distribution in neuroendocrine gastroenteropancreatic tumors before and during treatment. Acta Oncol 28:193-197, 1989.
39. Xu H, Li X, He S: Immunohistochemistry and DNA content of gastro-intestinal carcinoid. Chung Hua Chung Liu Tsa Chih 21:202-204, 1999.
40. Solcia E, et al: Morphological, molecular, and prognostic aspects of gastric endocrine tumors. Microsc Res Tech 48:339-348, 2000.
41. Lindberg GM, et al: Atypical carcinoid of the esophagus: A case report and review of the literature. Cancer 79:1476-1481, 1997.
42. Hoang MP, et al: Carcinoid tumor of the esophagus: A clinicopathologic study of four cases. Am J Surg Pathol 26:517-522, 2002.
43. Doherty MA, McIntyre M, Arnott SJ: Oat cell carcinoma of esophagus: A report of six British patients with a review of the literature. Int J Radiat Oncol Biol Phys 10:147-152, 1984.
44. Soga J: Esophageal endocrinomas, an extremely rare tumor: A statistical comparative evaluation of 28 ordinary carcinoids and 72 atypical variants. J Exp Clin Cancer Res 17:47-57, 1998.
45. Chong FK, Graham JH, Madoff IM: Mucin-producing carcinoid ("composite tumor") of upper third of esophagus: A variant of carcinoid tumor. Cancer 44:1853-1859, 1979.
46. McCloy RF, et al: Pathophysiological effects of long-term acid suppression in man. Dig Dis Sci 40:96S-120S, 1995.
47. Rindi G, et al: Three subtypes of gastric argyrophil carcinoid and the gastric neuroendocrine carcinoma: A clinicopathologic study [comment]. Gastroenterology 104:994-1006, 1993.
48. Thomas RM, et al: Gastric carcinoids. An immunohistochemical and clinicopathologic study of 104 patients [comment]. Cancer 73:2053-2058, 1994.
49. Modlin IM, et al: Gastric carcinoids. The Yale Experience. Arch Surg 130:250-255; discussion 255-256, 1995.
50. Annibale B, et al: Two-thirds of atrophic body gastritis patients have evidence of Helicobacter pylori infection. Helicobacter 6:225-233, 2001.
51. Kagawa J, et al: Enterocromaffin-like cell tumor induced by Helicobacter pylori infection in Mongolian gerbils. Helicobacter 7:390-397, 2002.
52. Sato Y, et al: Gastric carcinoid tumors without autoimmune gastritis in Japan: A relationship with Helicobacter pylori infection. Dig Dis Sci 47:579-585, 2002.
53. Bordi C, et al: Hypergastrinemia and gastric enterochromaffin-like cells. Am J Surg Pathol 19:S8-S19, 1995.
54. Bordi C, et al: The antral mucosa as a new site for endocrine tumors in multiple endocrine neoplasia type 1 and Zollinger-Ellison syndromes. J Clin Endocrinol Metab 86:2236-2242, 2001.
55. Bordi C, et al: Pathogenesis of ECL cell tumors in humans. Yale J Biol Med 71:273-284, 1998.
56. Solcia E, et al: Gastric argyrophil carcinoidosis in patients with Zollinger-Ellison syndrome due to type 1 multiple endocrine neoplasia. A newly recognized association. Am J Surg Pathol 14:503-513, 1990.
57. Solcia E, et al: Hyperplastic, dysplastic, and neoplastic enterochromaffin-like-cell proliferations of the gastric mucosa. Classification and histogenesis. Am J Surg Pathol 19:S1-S7, 1995.
58. Lewin KJ: The endocrine cells of the gastrointestinal tract. The normal endocrine cells and their hyperplasias. Part I. Pathol Annu 21:1-27, 1986.
59. Hirschowitz BI: Pathobiology and management of hypergastrinemia and the Zollinger-Ellison syndrome. Yale J Biol Med 65:659-676; discussion 689-692, 1992.
60. Lewin KJ, et al: The endocrine cells of the gastrointestinal tract. Tumors. Part II. Pathol Annu 21:181-215, 1986.
61. Burke AP, et al: Somatostatin-producing duodenal carcinoids in patients with von Recklinghausen's neurofibromatosis. A predilection for black patients. Cancer 65:1591-1595, 1990.
62. Dayal Y, et al: Duodenal carcinoids in patients with and without neurofibromatosis. A comparative study. Am J Surg Pathol 10:348-357, 1986.
63. Attanoos R, Williams GT: Epithelial and neuroendocrine tumors of the duodenum. Semin Diagn Pathol 8:149-162, 1991.
64. Zamboni G, et al: Small-cell neuroendocrine carcinoma of the ampullary region. A clinicopathologic, immunohistochemical, and ultrastructural study of three cases. Am J Surg Pathol 14:703-713, 1990.
65. Scheithauer BW, et al: Duodenal gangliocytic paraganglioma. Clinicopathologic and immunocytochemical study of 11 cases. Am J Clin Pathol 86:559-565, 1986.
66. McCluggage WG, et al: Small intestinal ulceration secondary to carcinoid tumour arising in a Meckel's diverticulum. J Clin Pathol 52:72-74, 1999.
67. Strobbe L, et al: Ileal carcinoid tumors and intestinal ischemia. Hepatogastroenterology 41:499-502, 1994.
68. Harvey JN, Denyer ME, DaCosta P: Intestinal infarction caused by carcinoid associated elastic vascular sclerosis: Early presentation of a small ileal carcinoid tumour. Gut 30:691-694, 1989.
69. Godwin JD 2nd: Carcinoid tumors. An analysis of 2,837 cases. Cancer 36:560-569, 1975.
70. Talamonti MS, et al: Primary cancers of the small bowel: Analysis of prognostic factors and results of surgical management. Arch Surg 137:564-570; discussion 570-571, 2002.
71. Spread C, et al: Colon carcinoid tumors. A population-based study. Dis Colon Rectum 37:482-491, 1994.
72. Rosenberg JM, Welch JP: Carcinoid tumors of the colon. A study of 72 patients. Am J Surg 149:775-779, 1985.
73. Mills SE, Allen MS Jr, Cohen AR: Small-cell undifferentiated carcinoma of the colon. A clinicopathological study of five cases and their association with colonic adenomas. Am J Surg Pathol 7:643-651, 1983.
74. Hung SS: Small cell carcinoma of the colon. A case report and literature review. J Clin Gastroenterol 11:335-339, 1989.

75. Burke AB, Shekitka KM, Sobin LH: Small cell carcinomas of the large intestine. Am J Clin Pathol 95:315-321, 1991.

76. Tichansky DS, et al: Risk of second cancers in patients with colorectal carcinoids. Dis Colon Rectum 45:91-97, 2002.

77. Burke M, Shepherd N, Mann CV: Carcinoid tumours of the rectum and anus. Br J Surg 74:358-361, 1987.

78. Mani S, et al: Carcinoids of the rectum. J Am Coll Surg 179:231-248, 1994.

79. Soga J: Carcinoids of the rectum: An evaluation of 1271 reported cases. Surg Today 27:112-119, 1997.

80. Connor SJ, Hanna GB, Frizelle FA: Appendiceal tumors: Retrospective clinicopathologic analysis of appendiceal tumors from 7,970 appendectomies. Dis Colon Rectum 41:75-80, 1998.

81. McCusker ME, et al: Primary malignant neoplasms of the appendix: A population-based study from the surveillance, epidemiology and end-results program, 1973-1998. Cancer 94:3307-3312, 2002.

82. Moertel CL, Weiland LH, Telander RL: Carcinoid tumor of the appendix in the first two decades of life. J Pediatr Surg 25:1073-1075, 1990.

83. Skinner MA, et al: Gastrointestinal tumors in children: An analysis of 39 cases. Ann Surg Oncol 1:283-289, 1994.

84. Parkes SE, et al: Carcinoid tumours of the appendix in children 1957-1986: Incidence, treatment and outcome [comment]. Br J Surg 80:502-504, 1993.

85. Moertel CG, et al: Carcinoid tumor of the appendix: Treatment and prognosis. N Engl J Med 317:1699-1701, 1987.

86. Roggo A, Wood WC, Ottinger LW: Carcinoid tumors of the appendix. Ann Surg 217:385-390, 1993.

87. Sandor A, Modlin IM: A retrospective analysis of 1570 appendiceal carcinoids. Am J Gastroenterol 93:422-428, 1998.

88. Dische FE: Argentaffin and non-argentaffin carcinoid tumours of the appendix. J Clin Pathol 21:60-66, 1968.

89. Moertel CG, Dockerty MB, Judd ES: Carcinoid tumors of the vermiform appendix. Cancer 21:270-278, 1968.

90. Haqqani MT, Williams G: Mucin producing carcinoid tumours of the vermiform appendix. J Clin Pathol 30:473-480, 1977.

91. Warkel RL, Cooper PH, Helwig EB: Adenocarcinoid, a mucin-producing carcinoid tumor of the appendix: A study of 39 cases. Cancer 42:2781-2793, 1978.

92. Levendoglu H, Cox CA, Nadimpalli V: Composite (adenocarcinoid) tumors of the gastrointestinal tract. Dig Dis Sci 35:519-525, 1990.

93. Subbuswamy SG, et al: Goblet cell carcinoid of the appendix. Cancer 34:338-344, 1974.

94. Warner TF, Seo IS: Goblet cell carcinoid of appendix: Ultrastructural features and histogenetic aspects. Cancer 44:1700-1706, 1979.

95. Berardi RS, Lee SS, Chen HP: Goblet cell carcinoids of the appendix. Surg Gynecol Obstet 167:81-86, 1988.

96. Burke AP, et al: Goblet cell carcinoids and related tumors of the vermiform appendix. Am J Clin Pathol 94:27-35, 1990.

97. Anderson NH, et al: Appendiceal goblet cell carcinoids: A clinico-pathological and immunohistochemical study. Histopathology 18:61-65, 1991.

98. Carr NJ, Remotti H, Sobin LH: Dual carcinoid/epithelial neoplasia of the appendix. Histopathology 27:557-562, 1995.

99. Edmonds P, et al: Adenocarcinoid (mucinous carcinoid) of the appendix. Gastroenterology 86:302-309, 1984.

100. Hood IC, Jones BA, Watts JC: Mucinous carcinoid tumor of the appendix presenting as bilateral ovarian tumors. Arch Pathol Lab Med 110:336-340, 1986.

101. Iwafuchi M, et al: Immunohistochemical and ultrastructural studies of twelve argentaffin and six argyrophil carcinoids of the appendix vermiformis. Hum Pathol 21:773-780, 1990.

102. Iwafuchi M, et al:. Argyrophil, non-argentaffin carcinoids of the appendix vermiformis. Immunohistochemical and ultrastructural studies. Acta Pathol Japan 37:1237-1247, 1987.

103. Gouzi JL, et al: Indications for right hemicolectomy in carcinoid tumors of the appendix. The French Associations for Surgical Research. Surg Gynecol Obstet 176:543-547, 1993.

NONEPITHELIAL NEOPLASMS OF THE GI TRACT

CHAPTER 22

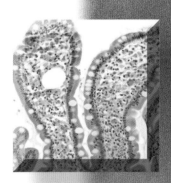

Mesenchymal Tumors of the GI Tract

JOHN R. GOLDBLUM

▍Introduction

Although far less common than epithelial neoplasms, mesenchymal tumors of the gastrointestinal tract are not rare and are divided into two main types. One group of tumors, which accounts for the minority of gastrointestinal mesenchymal tumors, comprises tumors that are histologically identical to their soft tissue counterparts (e.g., lipomas, leiomyomas, hemangiomas), and these are diagnosed according to the same criteria as those that arise in the soft tissue.

The much larger group of gastrointestinal mesenchymal neoplasms is a heterogeneous group of tumors referred to as gastrointestinal stromal tumors (GISTs); these can arise anywhere within the gastrointestinal tract and have distinctive histologic and clinical features that vary according to their primary site of origin.

In the past, cellular spindle cell neoplasms of the gastrointestinal tract have often been referred to as *leiomyomas* or *leiomyosarcomas* because of their purported morphologic resemblance to smooth muscle tumors from nongastrointestinal sites. In 1960, Martin and colleagues identified a group of gastric stromal tumors that were composed mainly of rounded or polygonal cells (epithelioid cells).[1] Two years later, Arthur Purdy Stout coined the term *leiomyoblastoma* to describe tumors composed of epithelioid cells, although this term was not meant to have either a benign or a malignant connotation.[2] With the advent of electron microscopy and immunohistochemistry, an enormous number of publications began to analyze the characteristics of the constituent cells of these tumors. Despite the fact that some GIST cells may show evidence of smooth muscle or neural differentiation, these tumors are not necessarily derived from those cell types. As a result, the noncommittal term *gastrointestinal stromal tumor* has been adopted to describe this heterogeneous group of neoplasms and is currently the preferred term. As is discussed later, regardless of their morphologic features or location within the gastrointestinal tract, the vast majority of GISTs seem to differentiate along the line of interstitial cells of Cajal. These cells are intercalated between autonomic nerves and the muscle layers of the stomach, small bowel, and colon; they play an important role in pacemaker function.

Gastrointestinal Stromal Tumors

CLASSIFICATION AND GENERAL COMMENTS

Since the 1980s, numerous articles have been published in an attempt to correlate histologic features with clinical behavior of GISTs. Although several features consistently correlate with clinical outcome, there are some cases in every study that do not follow the rules. On occasion, even the most histologically benign-appearing tumors have been reported to act in a clinically malignant fashion. Although some authors believe that the vast majority of these tumors can be confidently classified as either benign or malignant based on a constellation of histologic features, others believe that all of these tumors should be considered to be of at least low-grade malignancy.

Given the critical role of accurate and reproducible pathologic diagnosis in ensuring appropriate treatment for patients with GIST in the age of Gleevec (STI-571), the National Institutes of Health (NIH) held a GIST workshop in April of 2001 with the goal of developing a consensus approach to diagnosis and prognostication on the basis of morphologic features.[3] The proposed approach for defining risk of aggressive behavior in GIST by the members of this GIST workshop is summarized in Table 22-1. In brief, these tumors are defined as having very low risk, low risk, intermediate risk, or high risk, based on tumor size (single largest dimension) and mitotic count (number of mitotic figures per 50 high-power fields [hpfs]). Certainly, the latter approach is more reproducible because it relies on two relatively simple objective parameters. However, in my opinion this approach is overly simplistic in that it ignores other well-defined morphologic features that have been repeatedly found to be of prognostic significance in this group of tumors. Moreover, this approach does not account for the differences among GISTs in different anatomic sites.

This chapter focuses on the characteristic morphologic features found in benign and malignant GISTs from various anatomic sites within the gastrointestinal

TABLE 22–1. National Institutes of Health Gastrointestinal Stromal Tumor Workshop 2001: Proposed Approach for Defining Risk of Aggressive Behavior

Risk	Size	Mitotic Count (per 50 hpfs)
Very low risk	<2 cm	<5
Low risk	2–5 cm	<5
Intermediate risk	<5 cm	6–10
	5–10 cm	<5
High risk	>5 cm	>5
	>10 cm	Any mitotic rate
	Any size	>10

Modified from Fletcher CDM, Berman JJ, Corless C, et al. Diagnosis of gastrointestinal stromal tumors: A consensus approach. Hum Pathol 33:459-465, 2002.

tract, with the understanding that a certain subgroup of cases are difficult to classify on the basis of morphologic features alone; their clinical behavior is difficult to predict.

CLINICAL FEATURES

These tumors predominantly arise in middle-aged and elderly individuals. They are rare in young adults and may develop in very young individuals, in which case they may be congenital.[4] The stomach is the most common site; more than two thirds of GISTs arise in this location. Approximately one third of GISTs arise in the small intestine, particularly the duodenum, and less than 10% arise in the esophagus, colon, and anorectum.[5] There does not appear to be a sex predilection, except for those rare gastric epithelioid tumors that arise in the setting of Carney's triad (malignant epithelioid gastric GIST, pulmonary chondroma, and extra-adrenal paraganglioma), nearly all of which occur in females.[6] No risk factors are known for the development of GIST. However, some genetic influence is possible, given the rare reports of familial GIST[7] and syndrome-associated tumors, including those associated with Carney's triad and von Recklinghausen's disease (neurofibromatosis type 1).

The presenting manifestations of GIST are dependent on the site of involvement within the gastrointestinal tract, the size of the tumor, and the precise portion of the gut wall in which the tumor is located. A significant number of benign tumors are asymptomatic and are found incidentally at surgery performed for other reasons, probably because many of these lesions are small. However, even benign tumors can cause symptoms, the most common of which are gastrointestinal bleeding and abdominal pain. Other clinical symptoms or signs include nausea, vomiting, weight loss, and the presence of an abdominal mass. In contrast, malignant tumors are rarely asymptomatic.[8]

Signs and symptoms may lead to endoscopy and biopsy. In some cases, a histologic diagnosis of GIST can be made if a deep biopsy is obtained, or if the neoplasm infiltrates the overlying mucosa. As is discussed later, tumors that infiltrate the mucosa are virtually always malignant, although in general, it is not necessary to distinguish a benign from a malignant GIST on an endoscopic biopsy specimen or for that matter in a frozen section specimen. Radiographic imaging studies, including barium contrast, computed tomography, and endoscopic ultrasound, are commonly used for evaluation and diagnosis of these neoplasms.[9] In addition, some tumors can be diagnosed by fine-needle aspiration cytology, although separation of benign from malignant GISTs is usually not possible with this technique.[10]

GROSS FEATURES

These tumors may develop within any portion of the gut wall, but most are centered within the submucosa or the muscularis propria. Some tumors are predominantly extramural; extremely large tumors may even extend to or infiltrate into adjacent organs.

Most GISTs appear to be well circumscribed, although some may be multinodular. The overlying mucosal surface may be intact or ulcerated, a feature that can be seen in either benign or malignant tumors. On cut section, these tumors lack the characteristic gross appearance of uterine smooth muscle tumors (bulging, whorled cut surface); instead, the cut surface is typically granular and often shows hemorrhage, necrosis, or cystic change (Fig. 22-1). Neither tumor size nor the gross appearance of the neoplasm alone can be used to separate a benign from a malignant GIST.

MICROSCOPIC FEATURES

These tumors show a wide spectrum of histologic features and have distinctive appearances depending on their primary location. Thus, they are discussed separately according to their primary site (stomach, small bowel, anorectum, large bowel, esophagus) and their frequency of occurrence.

Gastric Gastrointestinal Stromal Tumors

Gastric GISTs can be divided into four main tumor types, including benign (cellular spindle cell tumor) and malignant (spindle cell sarcoma) spindle cell tumors and benign and malignant epithelioid tumors. Each of these tumor types has a fairly characteristic morphologic appearance; they usually can be separated from one another by assessment of a combination of histologic features. The classic features of each of these tumor types are summarized in the following sections; this is followed by a discussion of the morphologic parameters useful in predicting clinical behavior.

CELLULAR SPINDLE CELL TUMOR

Also sometimes referred to as *cellular leiomyoma*, this tumor is composed almost exclusively of densely cellular spindle cells that contain abundant pale to eosinophilic fibrillar cytoplasm. The cells vary in size and shape to a minor degree and are typically arranged in either whorls or short fascicles with frequent and prominent nuclear palisading (Fig. 22-2). A characteristic feature is the presence of perinuclear vacuoles that often appear to indent the nucleus. These vacuoles are an artifact of fixation in that they are not present in frozen section specimens. The nuclei are typically uniform with evenly distributed chromatin and inconspicuous nucleoli. Mitotic activity is typically low (<2 mitotic figures/50 hpfs). The cells are often separated by hyalinized, or even calcified, stroma and may show

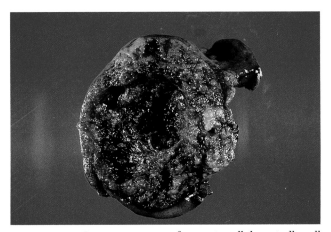

FIGURE 22–1. Gross appearance of a gastric cellular spindle cell tumor. The cut surface is granular and shows foci of hemorrhage. This gross appearance is quite distinct from that seen in typical smooth muscle tumors.

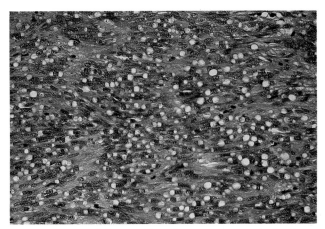

FIGURE 22–2. Cellular spindle cell tumor composed of a dense proliferation of spindle cells with prominent perinuclear vacuolization.

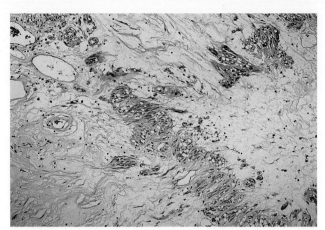

FIGURE 22–3. Cellular spindle cell tumor with extensive stromal liquefactive changes.

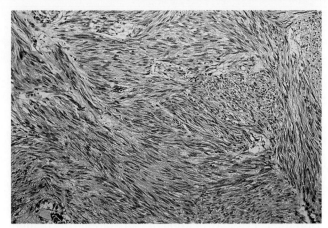

FIGURE 22–5. Gastric spindle cell sarcoma. The tumor is densely cellular and forms tight fascicles of cells. Perinuclear vacuoles are not present.

large areas of liquefactive necrosis. Pools of acellular material may separate perivascular tumor islands (Figs. 22-3 and 22-4).

Tumors that fit this histologic appearance are virtually always benign. In a series of 48 cases with follow-up reported by Appelman and Helwig,[11] only one tumor of this type metastasized. Although the malignant lesion resembled the others, it was 17 cm in greatest dimension and contained an average of 5 mitotic figures/50 hpfs.

SPINDLE CELL SARCOMA

When compared with cellular spindle cell tumors, spindle cell sarcomas are generally larger and more densely cellular. The constituent cells tend to be more crowded because they contain less cytoplasm (Fig. 22-5). The nuclei are more variable with respect to size and shape and are often vesicular (Fig. 22-6). Perinuclear vacuoles are typically absent. Broad areas of tumor cell necrosis are often present. The cells may be

arranged into fascicular and storiform growth patterns. Mitotic figures are usually easily identifiable and typically number greater than 10 mitoses/50 hpfs. With the use of a combination of these features, such tumors can usually be readily distinguished from the cellular spindle cell tumor.[12]

BENIGN EPITHELIOID GASTRIC STROMAL TUMOR

Benign epithelioid stromal tumors are the most common type of GIST in the stomach and are composed predominantly or exclusively of epithelioid cells arranged in sheets (Fig. 22-7). The cells often contain a condensed rim of eosinophilic cytoplasm adjacent to the nucleus with peripheral cytoplasmic clearing that is not usually apparent in frozen section tissue specimens or by ultrastructural examination.[13] In some cases, a majority of the cells contain abundant eosinophilic cytoplasm and show an eccentrically located nucleus (Fig. 22-8). The nuclei are round with small nucleoli,

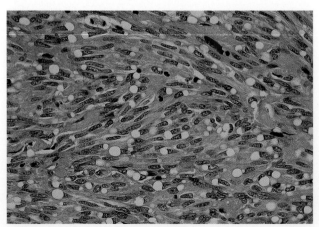

FIGURE 22–4. High-power magnification view of a cellular spindle cell tumor. The cells are cytologically bland. Prominent perinuclear vacuoles are present, which is an artifact of fixation.

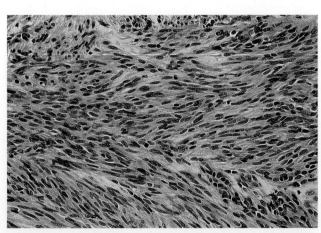

FIGURE 22–6. High-power magnification view of a gastric spindle cell sarcoma. The cells show greater nuclear hyperchromasia and pleomorphism than are seen in benign cellular spindle cell tumors.

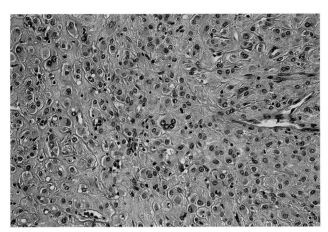

FIGURE 22–7. Benign gastric epithelioid stromal tumor. This low-power view shows the low degree of cellularity of this lesion.

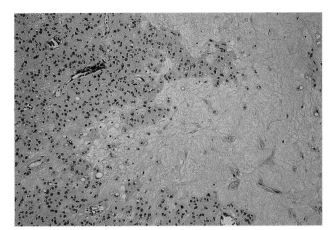

FIGURE 22–9. Benign gastric epithelioid stromal tumor with extensive stromal alterations, leading to a tumor that has the impression of low cellularity.

although scattered multinucleated giant cells or cells with bizarre nuclei may be present. As in cellular spindle cell tumors, mitotic figures are exceedingly rare. Stromal liquefaction, hyalinization, and calcification are often seen as well (Fig. 22-9).

MALIGNANT EPITHELIOID GASTRIC STROMAL TUMOR

The malignant variant of this tumor is composed of cells with significantly less cytoplasm; thus, the cells are more tightly packed, resulting in a highly cellular appearance at low-power magnification (Fig. 22-10). The arrangement of cells often varies between different areas of the tumor. Cells may be arranged in large sheets or in small acinus-like clusters in an acid mucopolysaccharide-rich myxoid stroma (Figs. 22-11 and 22-12). The nuclei are more hyperchromatic than those seen in the benign counterpart and are generally monotonous in appearance. Rarely, malignant epithelioid tumors can be diffusely pleomorphic, but as was

previously mentioned, scattered bizarre cells are more commonly seen in benign epithelioid tumors. The degree of mitotic activity may overlap that seen in the benign counterpart, and unless mitotic figures are numerous, they cannot be used alone to separate benign from malignant epithelioid gastric stromal tumors. It is important to note that areas resembling benign epithelioid tumors are often encountered in these tumors. Therefore, extensive sampling of these lesions is required to help identify the malignant component of the tumor.

A subgroup of gastric epithelioid stromal tumors occurs in patients with Carney's triad; this consists of a combination of malignant gastric epithelioid stromal tumor, a pulmonary chondroma, and a functioning extra-adrenal paraganglioma.[6] These patients tend to be younger (with an average age of approximately 16 years), and the vast majority are female. The gastric tumors are often multifocal and purely epithelioid in histologic appearance with a low risk of metastasis.

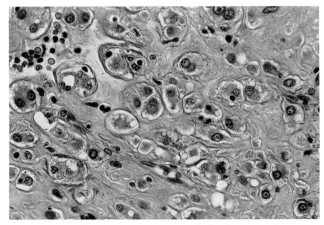

FIGURE 22–8. Benign gastric epithelioid stromal tumor composed of epithelioid cells with abundant eosinophilic cytoplasm. Some of the cells are multinucleated.

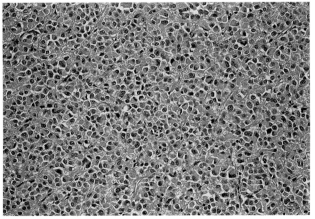

FIGURE 22–10. Malignant gastric epithelioid stromal tumor. The cells have much less cytoplasm than their benign counterpart. A more cellular lesion is recognized at low magnification.

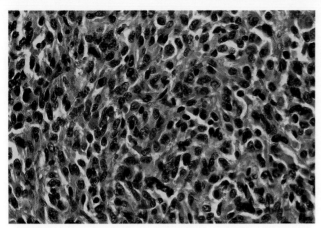

FIGURE 22–11. High-power view of a malignant epithelioid gastric stromal tumor shows the distinctive cytologic features.

However, even among patients who develop metastases, long-term survival is common.

PREDICTORS OF BEHAVIOR IN GASTRIC GIST
(Tables 22-2 and 22-3)

Tumor Size. Although sarcomas tend to be larger than benign stromal tumors, there is significant overlap; thus, size alone cannot be used to distinguish benign from malignant gastric GISTs.[14] However, in gastric stromal tumors that are histologically malignant, tumor size is the single best predictor of metastatic risk. For example, Roy and Sommers studied the relationship between tumor size and metastatic potential in 211 gastric sarcomas.[15] Fifteen percent of sarcomas smaller than 2.5 cm, 29% of those between 2.5 and 5 cm, 65% of those 5 to 10 cm, and virtually all tumors larger than 10 cm metastasized. No other histologic parameter correlated as strongly with metastatic risk or survival. Other studies have also found a relationship between tumor size and patient survival. Appelman and Helwig found that only 1 of 74 (1.5%) benign or malignant gastric epithelioid GISTs smaller than 5.5 cm metas-

TABLE 22–2. Histologic Features of Benign and Malignant Spindle Cell Gastric Stromal Tumors

Feature	Benign	Malignant
Cellularity	High	High
Nuclear atypia	None-minimal	Minimal-marked
Mitotic activity	Typically <2/50 hpfs	Usually >5/50 hpfs
Perinuclear vacuoles	Conspicuous	Usually absent
Mucosal invasion	Absent	May be present
Tumor cell necrosis	Usually absent	Often present

tasized, compared with 9 of 36 (25%) cases that were 6 cm or larger in size.[16] In a study of 44 gastric sarcomas, metastases occurred in 20% of tumors smaller than 6 cm and in 85% of those larger than 6 cm.[12]

Mitotic Count. Virtually all studies have found that higher mitotic counts are associated with decreased patient survival.[17,18] However, it is difficult to compare the results among different studies because different methods of counting mitotic figures were used, including the number of fields counted (10 hpfs vs. 50 hpfs) and the actual size of the hpf. Factors such as type and length of fixation may also account for the variability in mitotic counts between different studies.[19] Similar to the caveat for tumor size, a significant number of clinically malignant tumors have very low mitotic counts (<5/50 hpfs). On the other hand, a vast majority of tumors with high mitotic counts act in a clinically malignant fashion. Thus, this parameter is useful in separating benign from malignant behavior only when mitotic counts are high (minimum of 5/50 hpfs).

Other methods of measuring cellular proliferation in this group of tumors, including nucleolar organizer region content (AgNOR) and antibodies to proliferating cell nuclear antigen (PCNA) and the Ki67 antigen (MIB-1), have been evaluated. Virtually all studies in which these techniques were used have found a correlation between cellular proliferation and prognosis,[20-22] but it is unclear whether these techniques provide any additional prognostic information beyond that obtained through evaluation of mitotic counts. In addition, the lack of uniform technical and quantitative methods applied to the evaluation of these markers limits the degree of certainty regarding their usefulness in clinical practice.[23]

Cellularity. Although it is somewhat subjective, evaluation of cellularity has been found to be an im-

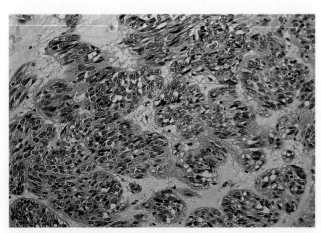

FIGURE 22–12. Malignant epithelioid gastric stromal tumor composed of nests of epithelioid cells in a myxoid stroma.

TABLE 22–3. Histologic Features of Benign and Malignant Epithelioid Gastric Stromal Tumors

Feature	Benign	Malignant
Cellularity	Low	High
Nuclear atypia	None-minimal*	Minimal-marked
Mitotic activity	Typically <2/50 hpfs	Usually >5/50 hpfs
Mucosal invasion	Absent	May be present
Tumor cell necrosis	Absent	Often present

*Scattered multinucleated or bizarre cells are characteristic.

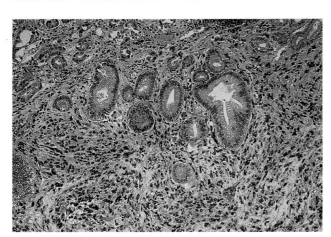

FIGURE 22–13. Malignant gastric spindle cell sarcoma showing an infiltration of neoplastic cells into the overlying mucosa and surrounding gastric glands. This feature correlates strongly with malignancy.

portant parameter in predicting the behavior of gastric stromal tumors. Because mitotic counts are often low in benign and malignant epithelioid gastric stromal tumors, the degree of cellularity is one of the most important features for the recognition of an epithelioid neoplasm as malignant.[16] However, assessing tumor cellularity requires experience in evaluating these tumors. Furthermore, the degree of cellularity may vary significantly within a given tumor. Finally, the criteria for defining a tumor as malignant based on the degree of cellularity are unclear.

Other Parameters. Several additional histologic features should be evaluated in every GIST; these form part of a multiparametric analytic approach to the prediction of the clinical behavior of the tumor. Mucosal invasion, defined as infiltration of tumor cells between mucosal glands, is a highly specific marker of malignant behavior (Fig. 22-13).[12,24] Unfortunately, many malignant tumors do not demonstrate mucosal invasion; thus, this is not a particularly sensitive histologic marker. Furthermore, the presence of mucosal ulceration makes this evaluation of mucosal invasion difficult.

Although tumor cell necrosis is more commonly seen in malignant tumors, large benign tumors may also show tumor cell necrosis. Marked nuclear pleomorphism in a spindle cell lesion suggests a sarcoma. On the other hand, when epithelioid tumors are evaluated, scattered bizarre multinucleated cells are more characteristic of benign lesions. Invasion of adjacent organs, although a rare finding, also correlates with poor outcome. Finally, as has been noted by Cunningham and associates,[25] the presence of metastasis at the time of surgical removal is the single most important prognostic variable. Although it may be intuitively obvious, this information is not always available to the practicing surgical pathologist.

Sarcoma Grading. Aside from the classification scheme proposed by the NIH GIST workshop, no uniform GIST grading scheme is known to be in use. It is unclear whether features commonly used in the grading of soft tissue sarcomas, such as cellularity, nuclear pleomorphism, mitotic count, and tumor cell necrosis, are also useful in the grading of gastric stromal sarcomas. Thus, I do not routinely grade malignant gastric GISTs. Rather, I believe that the size of the tumor is probably the best indicator of metastatic risk in lesions that are histologically malignant.

SUMMARY

The vast majority of gastric stromal tumors can be readily placed into one of the four major subtypes mentioned earlier in this chapter. However, a fraction of cases have features of both benign and malignant tumors; such tumors may be designated as having "borderline" or "indeterminate" malignant potential. Some authors have used the term *borderline malignancy* to describe gastric stromal tumors that are larger than 5 cm but have fewer than five mitoses per 50 hpfs.[26] I believe that this method is overly simplistic; in fact, most tumors that satisfy these criteria are clinically benign. In all likelihood, the NIH GIST classification scheme will become important for the purpose of determining who is likely to benefit from or even receive Gleevec treatment.

Small Bowel Gastrointestinal Stromal Tumors

The small bowel is the second most common site of GISTs; approximately one third arise in this location. Although GISTs may develop anywhere in the small bowel, a disproportionately large number occur in the duodenum. Unlike GISTs of the stomach, those that occur in the small bowel are composed of spindle cells. Epithelioid variants are rare. As a group, a higher percentage of small bowel GISTs are malignant compared with those in the stomach. In fact, small bowel GISTs show a completely different spectrum of histologic features when compared with gastric stromal tumors; thus, they should be evaluated with the use of site-dependent morphologic and prognostic factors (Table 22-4).

TABLE 22–4. Histologic Features of Benign and Malignant Small Bowel Stromal Tumors

Feature	Benign	Malignant
Cellularity	Low	Moderate to high
Organoid pattern	Present	Focal or absent
Epithelioid cells	Absent	May be present
Nuclear atypia	None-mild	Mild-marked
Mitotic figures	<5/50 hpfs	Usually >5/50 hpfs
Mucosal invasion	Absent	May be present
Tumor cell necrosis	Absent	May be present

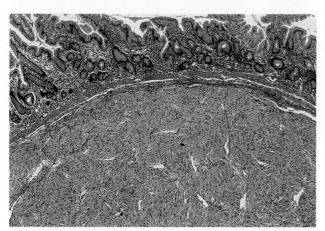

FIGURE 22–14. Low-power magnification of a typical benign small bowel stromal tumor. The tumor pushes the overlying muscularis mucosae but does not appear to penetrate into the mucosa.

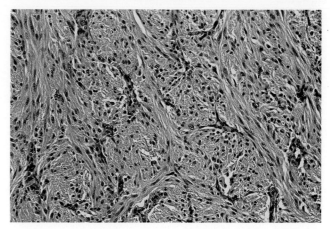

FIGURE 22–16. High-power view of bland spindle cells with eosinophilic fibrillary cytoplasm typical of a benign small bowel stromal tumor.

BENIGN SMALL BOWEL GASTROINTESTINAL STROMAL TUMORS

The classic benign small bowel GIST is small (<5 cm) and is composed of a uniform population of cytologically bland spindle cells with abundant eosinophilic cytoplasm. Overall, these tumors reveal a low degree of cellularity (Figs. 22-14, 22-15, and 22-16). Typically, the tumor cells are divided into groups according to fine fibrovascular septa, which results in an organoid growth pattern (see Fig. 22-15). Eosinophilic collagen globules (so-called skeinoid fibers) are characteristic and often numerous (Fig. 22-17). Mitotic figures are low (<5/50 hpfs), and tumor cell necrosis and mucosal invasion are not noted. Tumors that fulfill these criteria are predictably benign.[27-29]

MALIGNANT SMALL BOWEL GASTROINTESTINAL STROMAL TUMORS

Most malignant small bowel GISTs are composed of a highly cellular proliferation of spindle cells with greater cytologic atypia compared with their benign counterpart (Figs. 22-18 and 22-19). The nuclei are larger and contain coarsely clumped chromatin. Mitotic figures are usually easily found (>5/50 hpfs). The tumor cells are typically arranged into long fascicles, as opposed to the uniform organoid growth pattern commonly seen in benign tumors. Skeinoid fibers are few or completely absent, and many (but not all) malignant small bowel GISTs show at least focal tumor cell necrosis and/or mucosal invasion. In addition, tumors with a conspicuous epithelioid component that accounts for more than 25% of the neoplasm are usually malignant (Fig. 22-20).[27,28] Most small bowel GISTs can be easily categorized as either benign or malignant; as with the stomach, only rare small bowel GISTs fit into the borderline or intermediate malignancy category.

Colonic Gastrointestinal Stromal Tumors

With the exception of the esophagus, the colon is the least common site of GISTs. In fact, few studies that

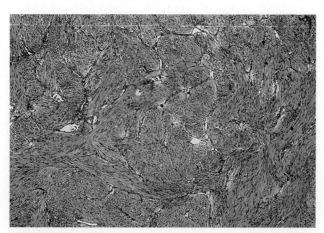

FIGURE 22–15. Organoid growth pattern characteristic of a benign small bowel stromal tumor.

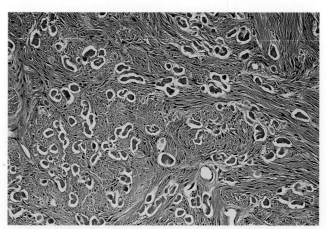

FIGURE 22–17. Benign small bowel stromal tumor containing numerous eosinophilic collagen globules, so-called skeinoid fibers.

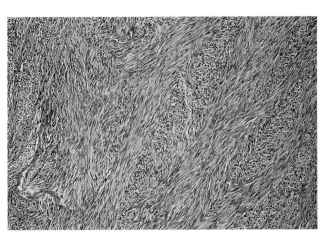

FIGURE 22–18. Malignant small bowel stromal tumor, spindle cell type. The tumor is cellular and composed of fascicles, a feature not seen in its benign counterpart.

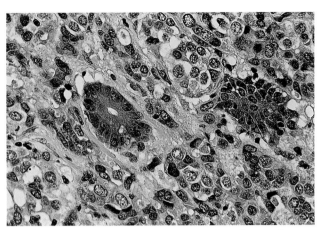

FIGURE 22–20. Malignant epithelioid small bowel stromal tumor showing infiltration of malignant epithelioid cells into the overlying mucosa.

included a significant number of cases have been reported.[30,31] Histologically benign colonic GISTs are exceedingly rare. For example, in the study by Miettinen and colleagues,[31] 4 of 37 colonic GISTs were small, incidental, polypoid serosal protrusions composed predominantly of bland spindle-shaped cells without necrosis with only occasional mitotic figures and skeinoid fibers.

GISTs arising in the colon are more heterogeneous than those found at other sites. These include highly cellular spindle cell tumors, as well as highly pleomorphic sarcomas that resemble malignant fibrous histiocytomas. Despite their morphologic heterogeneity, most colonic GISTs are overtly histologically malignant and behave in a clinically malignant fashion. Most patients present with metastases at the time of clinical presentation and show poor survival.[30,31] In a study by Miettinen and associates,[31] nearly all patients who had a GIST that was 1 cm or larger with more than 5 mitotic

figures per 50 hpfs died of disease, with a median survival of 15 months. Although most patients in their series who had tumors larger than 1 cm, but with 5 or fewer mitotic figures per 50 hpfs, were alive without disease, some of the patients in this category followed a rapidly fatal course. In a study by Tworek and coworkers,[30] an infiltrative growth pattern in the muscularis propria, mucosal invasion, and high mitotic counts (>5 mitotic figures/50 hpfs) correlated significantly with metastasis and death. Coagulative necrosis and dense cellularity were found to be minor criteria in the prediction of an adverse outcome.

Anorectal Gastrointestinal Stromal Tumors

The most common mesenchymal tumor of the anorectum is a benign leiomyoma. This lesion is composed of fully differentiated benign smooth muscle cells derived from the muscularis mucosae and is usually cured by local excision (Fig. 22-21).[32] Aside from leiomyomas, most mesenchymal tumors of the

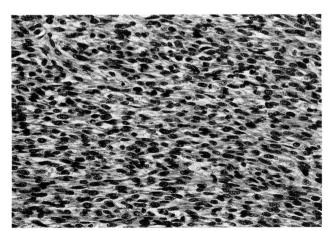

FIGURE 22–19. High-power view of a malignant small bowel stromal tumor, spindle cell type. The cells are strikingly hyperchromatic and show greater pleomorphism than benign small bowel stromal tumors.

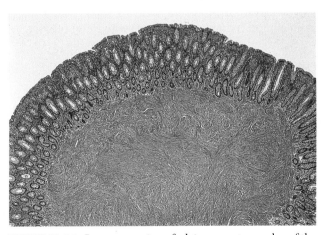

FIGURE 22–21. Low-power view of a leiomyomatous polyp of the rectum.

anorectum are spindle cell tumors that have similar light microscopic, immunohistochemical, and molecular genetic alterations to those of GISTs that arise from other parts of the gastrointestinal tract.[5] Data from most early publications on this group of tumors led to the belief that all anorectal GISTs are malignant regardless of their histologic appearance.[32,33] However, several recent studies have shown that not all anorectal GISTs are necessarily clinically malignant; as with GISTs that develop in other sites, a constellation of features can be used to separate benign from malignant behavior.[34-36]

The most common form of anorectal GIST develops within the muscularis propria and is characterized by fascicles of densely cellular, spindle-shaped cells with elongated, relatively uniform nuclei that often show prominent nuclear palisading. Unlike gastric GISTs, anorectal GISTs only rarely have a predominant epithelioid morphology. Similar-appearing tumors may also arise in the submucosa and, exceptionally, may present as polypoid tumors with mucosal invasion.

Haque and Dean were the first to analyze a large group of these tumors in an attempt to correlate histologic features with clinical outcome.[35] In that study, tumors that were centered in the submucosa revealed little or no infiltration of the muscularis propria, were composed of tightly packed uniform spindle cells with plump nuclei, were arranged in a fascicular or vaguely storiform growth pattern, had very low mitotic counts (<1 mitotic figure/50 hpfs), and behaved in a clinically benign fashion. Malignant tumors tended to be located within the muscularis propria and indicated mild nuclear atypia and higher mitotic counts, typically greater than 5 per 50 hpfs. In a study of 22 anorectal GISTs by Tworek and coworkers,[34] tumor size larger than 5 cm and an infiltrative growth pattern in the muscularis propria correlated with an adverse outcome. However, unlike the study of Haque and Dean, nuclear pleomorphism, necrosis, mitotic count, and intramuscular location did not correlate with clinical behavior. Both studies noted a long latency period before recurrence and/or metastasis, thus emphasizing the need for long-term clinical follow-up in patients with these tumors.

Esophageal Gastrointestinal Stromal Tumors

Benign leiomyomas are the most common type of mesenchymal tumor of the esophagus (Fig. 22-22). Tumors similar to GISTs that arise in other parts of the gastrointestinal tract have not been well characterized in the esophagus, and until a recent report by Miettinen and colleagues,[36] no other studies had reported these tumors as a distinct group.

Esophageal GISTs have a male predilection, and most patients present with dysphagia. These tumors typically arise in the distal esophagus and may involve the esophagogastric junction. Grossly, they have a soft

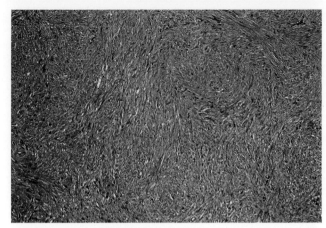

FIGURE 22–22. Esophageal leiomyoma composed of well-differentiated smooth muscle cells.

consistency with a fleshy, variegated cut surface, often with central necrosis and cystic change. Histologically, they are typically highly cellular spindle cell neoplasms composed of mildly atypical nuclei with a wide range of mitotic activity, although most have more than 5 mitotic figures per 50 hpfs. A variety of morphologic patterns may be seen, including sheets of cells, with or without nuclear palisading, myxoid change, and hyaline-like degeneration. Coagulative necrosis and mucosal invasion are noted in a small proportion of cases.

In the study by Miettinen and associates,[37] 9 of 16 patients with follow-up information died of disease, with a median survival of 29 months. All patients who had tumors larger than 10 cm died of disease, whereas none of the patients with tumors smaller than 5 cm died of disease. Additional studies that include a large number of cases with long-term clinical follow-up are required for more precise determination of the parameters of greatest prognostic significance.

IMMUNOHISTOCHEMICAL FEATURES
(Table 22-5)

Published literature on the immunohistochemical findings in GIST has evolved greatly over the past 20 years. Early studies focused on the expression of myogenic and neural antigens; the results from these studies were inconsistent.[38-40] Subsequently, CD34, a hematopoietic stem cell marker, was found to be expressed in a majority (approximately 70%) of GISTs from all sites.[41-44] However, over the past several years, it has become apparent that the cardinal marker is the product of the c-*kit* gene (KIT protein or CD117). Some authors believe that KIT positivity is essential if a diagnosis of GIST in the gastrointestinal tract is to be established.

Virtually all GISTs from all sites, regardless of their particular morphologic features and degree of malignancy, show strong cytoplasmic CD117 staining,

TABLE 22–5. Immunohistochemical Features of Gastrointestinal Stromal Tumors (GISTs) and Comparison of Immunophenotype With Other Gastrointestinal Tract Spindle Cell Tumors

Tumor	KIT (CD117)	CD34	SMA	Desmin	S100
GIST	+	70%	30%-40%	Very rare	Very rare
Schwannoma	–	Antoni B	–	–	+
Fibromatosis	–*	Very rare	+	Very rare	–
Smooth muscle tumor	–	10%-15%	+	+	Very rare

*Most report that fibromatoses are negative for CD117.
Modified from Fletcher CDM, Berman JJ, Corless C, et al. Diagnosis of gastrointestinal stromal tumors: A consensus approach. Hum Pathol 33:459-465, 2002.

sometimes with a prominent membranous reactivity or Golgi zone accentuation (Fig. 22-23).[5,45-48] The *c-kit* gene encodes for a protein that belongs to a family of receptor tyrosine kinases and is a transmembrane growth factor receptor for stem cell factor.[49] CD117 marks interstitial cells of Cajal (ICCs), which are gastrointestinal pacemaker cells that regulate intestinal motility and are normally seen in and around the myenteric plexus, as well as in the outer smooth muscle layer of the gut.[50,51] Because of the similar immunohistochemical and ultrastructural features of ICCs and GISTs, the latter have been proposed to be derived from or to differentiate toward ICCs.[45,46] Given that ICCs have myoid and neural features that can be seen on electron microscopy, this hypothesis helps to explain the many years of conflicting immunohistochemical and ultrastructural data regarding the nature of GIST. An alternative hypothesis is that GISTs originate from primitive stem cells that can differentiate into ICCs and smooth muscle cells.[52] Regardless, the absence of CD117 staining in a tumor suspected of being a GIST should engender serious consideration of an alternative diagnosis. Furthermore, given the therapeutic trials aimed at countering the activation of *c-kit* tyrosine kinase activity with the tyrosine kinase inhibitor Gleevec (STI-571), it has become necessary to document the expression of this antigen in these tumors.[53]

Myoid markers may be identified in a subset of GIST. Up to 20 to 30% of these tumors show positive staining for smooth muscle actin,[5] either focally or diffusely, although expression of this antigen seems to be reciprocally related to CD34 expression. Desmin is found in less than 10% of GIST, and staining is typically limited to scattered tumor cells with a more prominent reaction in tumors with an epithelioid pattern of growth. Caldesmon, an actin-binding cytoskeleton-associated protein, is also detected in a significant subset of GIST.[54]

Neural antigens have also been reported in some of these tumors; S100 protein may be found in up to 10% of GISTs, typically in a focal pattern. These tumors are usually negative for neurofilament protein and glial fibrillary acidic protein. Finally, although scattered tumor cells may stain for cytokeratins, particularly in malignant epithelioid GIST, coexpression with CD117 should prevent confusion with carcinoma.

GENETIC FEATURES

Activating mutations, most commonly in exon 11 of the *c-kit* gene (juxtamembrane domain), result in ligand-independent activation of the kit tyrosine kinase; this appears to be the central event in the pathogenesis of GIST.[55-59] Much less commonly, mutations in exons 9 (extracellular domain) and 13 (kinase domain) may be detected.[60,61] Fortunately, mutations in this gene are not usually found in other tumors that may be potentially confused with GIST, including leiomyosarcomas, fibromatoses, and nerve sheath tumors. Finally, some have found *c-kit* mutations to occur preferentially in malignant GIST[56,60]; Taniguchi and colleagues found these mutations to be of independent prognostic significance.[58] More recently, activating mutations in the *c-kit* gene have become a central target for therapeutic intervention with the use of tyrosine kinase inhibitors (STI-571). Initial results have been promising.[62-66]

Comparative genomic hybridization (CGH) studies have found other genetic alterations in GIST, including losses in chromosomes 14q and 22q.[67-70] El-Rifai and associates found that DNA copy number gains may preferentially occur in malignant GIST.[69] Several other mutations, including losses in 1p[71] and 17p,[72] the site of

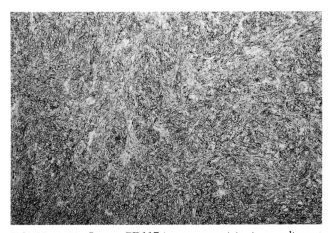

FIGURE 22–23. Strong CD117 immunoreactivity in a malignant small bowel gastrointestinal stromal tumor.

the neurofibromatosis type 1 gene, have also been detected in some cases of GIST.

Gastrointestinal Autonomic Nerve Tumors

Gastrointestinal autonomic nerve tumors (GANTs), or "plexosarcomas," were originally described on the basis of their ultrastructural resemblance to cells of the autonomic nervous system.[73,74] These tumors have a heterogeneous histologic appearance and may arise from any location in the gastrointestinal tract.[75] Characteristic ultrastructural features include complex interdigitating cell processes with bulbous synaptic terminals, neurosecretory granules, rudimentary cell junctions, and intermediate filaments. Although they were originally believed to represent distinct tumors, recent evidence supports the concept that GANTs merely represent a phenotypic variant of GIST. Lee and coworkers found these tumors to be consistently kit-positive, and a substantial percentage were found to harbor GIST-specific gain-of-function mutations in the juxtamembrane domain of the c-*kit* gene.[76] Given that ultrastructural examination of GIST is rarely performed in clinical practice, this type of tumor is believed to be much more common than was previously thought in that it can be recognized and, in fact, is defined only by its characteristic ultrastructural features. Similar to GIST, rare examples of GANT have been associated with Carney's triad[77] and neurofibromatosis type 1.[78] Multiple familial GANT associated with intestinal neuronal dysplasia has also been reported.[79]

Smooth Muscle Tumors

True smooth muscle tumors of the gastrointestinal tract, which are much less common than GISTs, are characterized by positive staining for a variety of muscle markers, including actin and desmin, but are consistently negative for CD117 and almost always for CD34 as well.

Leiomyomas are far more common than leiomyosarcomas. They occur chiefly in the esophagus[37] and colorectum[80] and are exceedingly rare in the stomach and small intestine. Esophageal leiomyomas arise typically in young males (median age, 30 to 35 years), usually in the lower one third of the esophagus. Patients often present with dysphagia.[37] Leiomyomas may on occasion show oval, spherical, or elongated sausage-shaped intramural masses, each measuring less than 3 cm. Rarely, leiomyomas may be found throughout the esophagus, a condition referred to as *esophageal leiomyomatosis*.[81] In the colon and rectum, these lesions develop as small (less than 1 cm) nodules that arise from

the muscularis mucosae. They are typically found incidentally in adults who have undergone endoscopy for other reasons.[80] Leiomyomas are usually excised easily by endoscopic polypectomy. Rarely, leiomyomas may develop as intramural masses in the rectum. In fact, some may be attached to the external rectal wall and resemble uterine leiomyomas; estrogen and progesterone receptors may be positive in this subgroup.[80]

Histologically, gastrointestinal leiomyomas, regardless of their site of origin, are characterized by a proliferation of cytologically bland spindle-shaped cells of low or moderate cellularity; they contain elongated nuclei and eosinophilic fibrillary cytoplasm. Rare cases show nuclear atypia without mitotic activity, reminiscent of symplastic uterine leiomyomas. Calcifications may be noted, particularly in esophageal intramural tumors. All of these tumors, including those with nuclear atypia, behave in a clinically benign fashion.

True leiomyosarcomas of the gastrointestinal tract are exceedingly rare and have been poorly characterized. Immunohistochemically, leiomyosarcomas are actin/desmin-positive and CD117-negative. In fact, most previously published studies of leiomyosarcomas of the gastrointestinal tract include predominantly, or exclusively, GISTs. Like GISTs, these tumors typically occur in older patients and arise as intramural polypoid masses that may involve any portion of the gut wall. There appears to be a female predilection, at least for those that arise in the anorectal region.[34]

Histologically, most leiomyosarcomas are high-grade neoplasms. They show marked nuclear pleomorphism, significant mitotic activity, and necrosis. The cells have elongated cigar-shaped nuclei and contain eosinophilic fibrillary cytoplasm, which allows for their recognition as true smooth muscle tumors; this can be confirmed by immunohistochemistry (actin/desmin-positive; CD117-negative). Given the rarity of these tumors and the fact that many reported series have included GISTs, the clinical behavior of this group of tumors is poorly defined.

Neural Tumors

SCHWANNOMA

Schwannomas are uncommon in the gastrointestinal tract. However, in the tubal gut, they arise most commonly in the stomach[82] and rarely in the esophagus[83] and intestines.[84] They occur mainly during middle to late adulthood with a peak in the sixth decade of life. They are not associated with neurofibromatosis (type 1 or 2).[5,85] Schwannomas typically involve the submucosa and the muscularis propria. The overlying mucosa may be intact or ulcerated. Some have an intraluminal polypoid component as well.

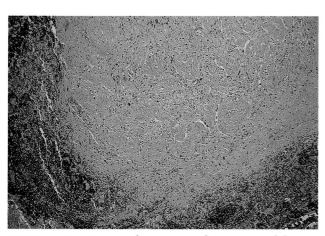

FIGURE 22–24. Gastric schwannoma. The tumor nodules are characteristically surrounded by a cuff of lymphoid cells.

Although grossly well circumscribed, gastrointestinal schwannomas lack a true capsule. Most schwannomas are composed of spindle cells with typical Schwann cell tumor features, including the presence of wavy, or "buckled," nuclei and occasional intranuclear inclusions. Scattered cells with nuclear atypia may be present, but mitotic activity is usually low (<5 mitoses/50 hpfs). Rare cases are composed of epithelioid cells.[84] Cellularity often varies markedly in different portions of the tumor; some areas may be highly cellular and contain aborted fascicles or whorls; other areas may be less cellular and reveal a prominent hyalinized or myxoid stroma. Nuclear palisading and Verocay bodies may be present but are often inconspicuous, as are vascular wall hyalinization and xanthomatous changes (Fig. 22-24). Scattered lymphocytes and plasma cells are often found within the tumor, but many are surrounded by a discontinuous cuff of lymphoid cells with or without germinal center formation (Fig. 22-25). Immunohisto-chemically, schwannomas of the gut show strong S100 protein staining, but muscle markers and CD117 are

negative; some show focal CD34 staining. Tumors such as these behave in a uniformly benign fashion.

NEURAL TUMORS ASSOCIATED WITH NEUROFIBROMATOSIS TYPE 1 AND MULTIPLE ENDOCRINE NEOPLASIA TYPE II (MEN II)

A variety of neural tumors may develop in patients with neurofibromatosis type 1 (von Recklinghausen's disease) and MEN II.[86] Neuromas and ganglio-neuromas arise in either of these syndromes, although sporadic tumors may occur as well. Approximately 10% of patients with von Recklinghausen's disease present with gastrointestinal manifestations,[87] most commonly neurofibromas or plexiform neurofibromas, which on occasion develop into malignant peripheral nerve sheath tumors. These patients can also demonstrate solitary or multiple CD117-positive GISTs, most of which appear histologically and clinically benign.[72,88,89]

GRANULAR CELL TUMORS

Granular cell tumors are composed of nests or sheets of S100-positive plump epithelioid and/or spindle cells with abundant eosinophilic granular cytoplasm that contains numerous phagolysosomes. These tumors, which are usually identified as incidental findings, are most common in the esophagus. In an individual patient, multiple tumor nodules may be seen through-out the gastrointestinal tract.[90,91] Granular cell tumors are usually located in the submucosa but may involve the muscularis propria or the muscularis mucosae and the mucosa. This may result in an elevated lesion that can be detected and possibly removed by endoscopic polypectomy (Figs. 22-26 and 22-27). Virtually all of these lesions behave in a clinically benign fashion. (See Chapters 12 and 16 for more details.)

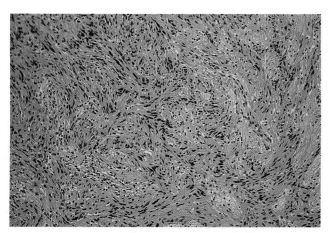

FIGURE 22–25. Gastric schwannoma composed of bland spindle-shaped cells with a vague nuclear palisading.

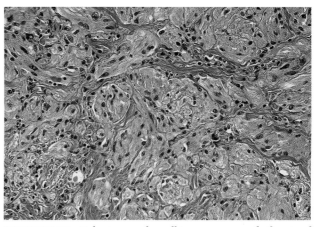

FIGURE 22–26. Colonic granular cell tumor composed of nests of cells with abundant eosinophilic granular cytoplasm.

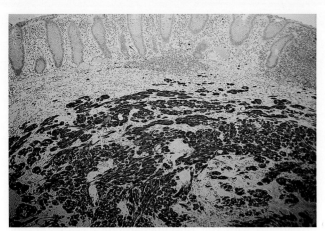

FIGURE 22–27. Diffuse S100 protein immunoreactivity in a colonic granular cell tumor.

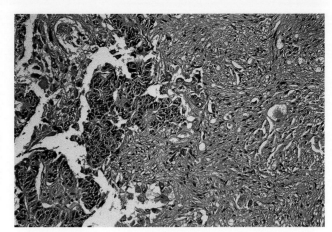

FIGURE 22–29. Gangliocytic paraganglioma composed of an admixture of carcinoid- and ganglioneuroma-like areas.

GANGLIOCYTIC PARAGANGLIOMA

Gangliocytic paraganglioma is a rare tumor that most commonly arises in the duodenum (see also Chapters 18 and 21). It is composed of an admixture of spindle-shaped Schwann cells, ganglion cells, and nests of neuroendocrine cells that resemble a paraganglioma. The tumor affects predominantly adult men. Most patients present with gastrointestinal bleeding.

Histologically, the tumor is composed of epithelioid cells that closely resemble those seen in a paraganglioma; ribbon-like or trabecular growth patterns may be noted (Figs. 22-28 and 22-29). Within the epithelioid areas are ganglion cells that reveal variable degrees of differentiation (Fig. 22-30). In addition, some tumors show a prominent Schwann cell–rich neuromatous stroma.[92] Immunohistochemically, a variety of antigens, including neuron-specific enolase, insulin, glucagon, somatostatin, and serotonin, can be identified in the epithelioid cells. Carcinoid-like areas express chromogranin, and ganglion cells express neuron-specific enolase, synaptophysin, and neurofilament protein. An S100 protein sustentacular network is usually easily demonstrated surrounding epithelioid cell nests (Fig. 22-31). Almost all gangliocytic paragangliomas behave in a clinically benign fashion, although rare cases have metastasized to regional lymph nodes.[93] These tumors are best treated by simple excision.

GANGLIONEUROMA/ GANGLIONEUROMATOSIS

Schwann cell and ganglion cell proliferative lesions may occur within the mucosa throughout the gastrointestinal tract; they may appear as small polypoid lesions. These lesions may be solitary (ganglioneuroma) or multiple (ganglioneuromatosis). The latter condition has been associated with multiple endocrine neoplasia type IIb[94] and type 1 neurofibromatosis (von Recklinghausen's disease).[95] Histologically, the lamina propria is hypercellular and is composed of cytologically

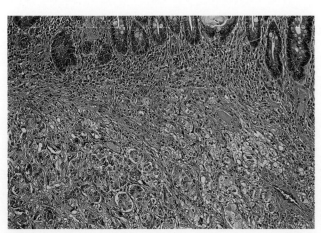

FIGURE 22–28. Low-power view of a duodenal gangliocytic paraganglioma.

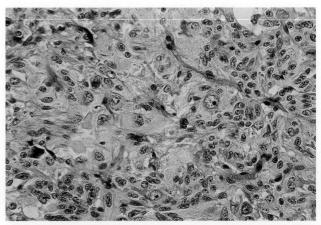

FIGURE 22–30. Gangliocytic paraganglioma with ganglion cells in various stages of differentiation.

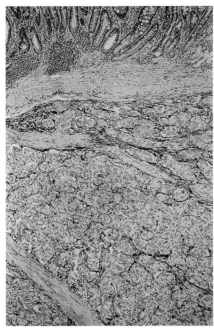

FIGURE 22–31. Gangliocytic paraganglioma showing a strong S100 protein reactivity in the sustentacular network.

bland spindle-shaped cells with "schwannian" features. Ganglion cells may be arranged in clusters but are often isolated and can be difficult to identify in some cases. Crypts are often splayed apart by an expanded lamina propria, which results in a distorted appearance at low magnification.

Lipomatous Tumors

LIPOMATOUS HYPERTROPHY OF THE ILEOCECAL VALVE

Although it is not believed to represent a neoplasm, hypertrophy of mature-appearing fat at the ileocecal valve may result in an elevated mucosal protrusion that often has the endoscopic appearance of a neoplasm (see also Chapter 15). These patients tend to have non-specific symptoms, including constipation and abdominal pain, but it is unclear whether the hypertrophied valve is the cause of clinical symptoms. The etiology of this process is unknown.

LIPOMA AND LIPOSARCOMA

Lipomas are relatively uncommon tumors in the gastrointestinal tract. They are most common in the right colon[96] and usually develop as small mucosa-covered intramural polypoid lesions. Large lesions may be ulcerated and may cause mucosal prolapse–associated changes in the surrounding mucosa. Histologically, these tumors are composed of mature adipocytes that are relatively uniform in size and lack cytologic atypia. They are usually centered in the sub-mucosa and often compress the overlying muscularis mucosae. Clinically, these tumors may cause a variety of symptoms, including abdominal pain, gastrointestinal bleeding, and even symptoms of intestinal obstruction. Rarely, multiple lipomas may develop throughout the gastrointestinal tract in the same patient. Many of these lesions are discovered incidentally.

Liposarcomas are exceptionally rare. Most are retroperitoneal well-differentiated liposarcomas or dedifferentiated liposarcomas that secondarily involve the gastrointestinal tract. Unlike lipomas, well-differentiated liposarcomas are characterized by large atypical hyperchromatic cells. Rarely, these tumors may progress to a high-grade sarcoma that most commonly resembles a pleomorphic/storiform malignant fibrous histiocytoma (dedifferentiated liposarcoma). As a general rule, myxoid/round cell liposarcoma is uncommon in the retroperitoneum; thus, this subtype virtually never involves the gastrointestinal tract. Pleomorphic liposarcoma is also an exceedingly rare tumor; involvement of the gastrointestinal tract has been only infrequently documented.

Vascular Tumors

GLOMUS TUMOR

Glomus tumors are composed of modified smooth muscle cells that represent a counterpart of the peri-vascular glomus body. These tumors most commonly occur in the peripheral soft tissues, especially the distal extremities, but some arise within the gastrointestinal tract, particularly the stomach. In a recent study of gastrointestinal glomus tumors by Miettinen and colleagues,[97] all but 1 of 32 glomus tumors were located in the stomach; the only exception was a cecal tumor. These tumors have a strong predilection for females of a median age of 55 years. Many patients present with gastrointestinal bleeding or ulcer-like symptoms. At the time of excision, most are smaller than 3 cm.

Histologically, glomus tumors resemble their peripheral soft tissue counterparts and are characterized by a proliferation of sharply demarcated, uniform, round glomus cells, often arranged around prominent dilated hemangiopericytoma-like vascular spaces. The tumor cells are round with a centrally located uniform nucleus and pale to clear cytoplasm. Mitotic activity is typically low (fewer than 5 mitoses per 50 hpfs). Focal atypia and vascular invasion may be noted. Immunohistochemically, the neoplastic cells stain for muscle markers such as smooth muscle actin

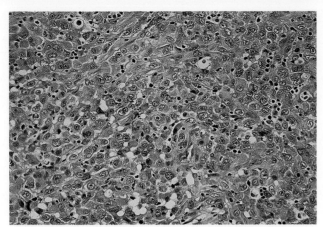

FIGURE 22–32. Epithelioid angiosarcoma of the small bowel composed of sheets of highly malignant epithelioid cells.

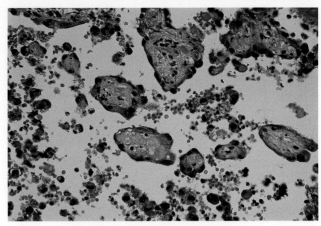

FIGURE 22–33. Colonic epithelioid angiosarcoma. Malignant epithelioid endothelial cells line fibrous cores.

and calponin. Miettinen and associates also noted an elaborate network of pericellular collagen type IV and laminin immunoreactivity in these tumors,[97] which do not express desmin, S100 protein, or CD117.

A vast majority of glomus tumors in the stomach behave in a clinically benign fashion. In the study by Miettinen and coworkers, follow-up revealed only one patient who developed hepatic metastases.[97] In this case, the tumor revealed a low mitotic count as well as spindle cell foci, mild cytologic atypia, and vascular invasion. All other patients in the study remained free of disease during long-term follow-up.

HEMANGIOMAS AND OTHER BENIGN VASCULAR PROLIFERATIONS

Hemangiomas, lymphangiomas, and other benign vascular malformations are relatively common throughout the gastrointestinal tract and resemble their counterparts in the peripheral soft tissues. Some are composed of large cavernous vascular channels, and others contain lobules of small capillary-sized vessels. These vascular proliferations, particularly lymphangiomas and benign vascular malformations (angiodysplasia), may involve large segments of the gastrointestinal tract. The latter can be associated with life-threatening hemorrhage.

ANGIOSARCOMA

Angiosarcoma of the gastrointestinal tract is an exceedingly rare tumor. Most cases have been documented in case reports or small series.[98-100] These tumors are composed of spindle cells that form primitive vascular channels, or epithelioid cells that resemble melanoma, carcinoma, or even mesothelioma (Figs. 22-32 and 22-33). The cells stain positive for vascular endothelial markers, including factor

VIII–related antigen and CD31, but some, especially the epithelioid variants, show significant cytokeratin immunoreactivity. The tendency is toward multifocality, and most patients follow an aggressive clinical course. Outside of the setting of acquired immunodeficiency syndrome, Kaposi's sarcoma of the gastrointestinal tract is exceedingly rare.

References

1. Martin JF, Bazin P, Feroldi J, et al: Tumeurs myoides intramurales de l'estomac. Considerations microscopiques a propos de 6 cas. Ann D'Anat Pathol 5:484-497, 1960.
2. Stout AP: Bizarre smooth muscle tumors of the stomach. Cancer 15:400-409, 1962.
3. Fletcher CDM, Berman JJ, Corless C, et al: Diagnosis of gastrointestinal stromal tumors: A consensus approach. Hum Pathol 33:459-465, 2002.
4. Bates AW, Feakins RM, Scheimberg I: Congenital gastrointestinal stromal tumour is morphologically indistinguishable from the adult form, but does not express CD117 and carries a favourable prognosis. Histopathology 37:316-322, 2000.
5. Miettinen M, Lasota J: Gastrointestinal stromal tumors—definition, clinical, histological, immunohistochemical and molecular genetic features and differential diagnosis. Virchow Arch 438:1-12, 2001.
6. Carney JA: Gastric stromal sarcoma, pulmonary chondroma and extra-adrenal paraganglioma (Carney triad): Natural history, adrenal cortical component and possible familial occurrence. Mayo Clin Proc 74:543-552, 1999.
7. Nashida T, Hirota S, Taniguchi M, et al: Familial gastrointestinal stromal tumours with germline mutation of the KIT gene. Nature Genet 19:323-324, 1998.
8. Appelman HD, Lewin K: Mesenchymal tumors and tumor-like proliferations of the stomach. In Atlas of Tumor Pathology, Third Series, Fascicle 18: Tumors of the Esophagus and Stomach. Washington, DC, Armed Forces Institute of Pathology, 1996.
9. Palazzo L, Landi B, Cellier C, et al: Endosonographic features predictive of benign and malignant gastrointestinal stromal tumours. Gut 46:88-92, 2000.
10. Dodd LG, Nelson RC, Mooney EE, et al: Fine-needle aspiration of gastrointestinal stromal tumors. Am J Clin Pathol 109:439-443, 1998.
11. Appelman HD, Helwig EB: Cellular leiomyomas of the stomach in 49 patients. Arch Pathol Lab Med 101:373-377, 1977.
12. Appelman HD, Helwig EB: Sarcomas of the stomach. Am J Clin Pathol 67:2-10, 1977.
13. Cornog JL: Gastric leiomyoblastoma: A clinical and ultrastructural study. Cancer 34:711-719, 1974.

14. Miettinen M, El-Rifai W, Sobin LH, et al: Evaluation of malignancy and prognosis of gastrointestinal stromal tumors: A review. Hum Pathol 33:478-483, 2002.
15. Roy M, Sommers SC: Metastatic potential of gastric leiomyosarcoma. Pathol Res Pract 185:874-877, 1989.
16. Appelman HD, Helwig EB: Gastric epithelioid leiomyomas and leiomyosarcomas (leiomyoblastomas). Cancer 38:708-728, 1976.
17. Shiu MH, Farr GH, Papachristou DN, et al: Myosarcomas of the stomach: Natural history, prognostic factors and management. Cancer 49:177-187, 1982.
18. Ranchod M, Kempson RL: Smooth muscle tumors of the gastrointestinal tract and retroperitoneum. Cancer 39:255-262, 1977.
19. Baak JPA: Editorial: Mitosis counting in tumors. Hum Pathol 21:683-685, 1990.
20. Yu CCW, Fletcher CDM, Newman PL, et al: A comparison of proliferating cell nuclear antigen (PCNA) immunostaining, nucleolar organizing region (AgNOR) staining, and histologic grading in gastrointestinal stromal tumors. J Pathol 166:147-152, 1992.
21. Amin MB, Ma CK, Linden MD, et al: Prognostic value of proliferating cell nuclear antigen index in gastric stromal tumors: Correlation with mitotic count and clinical outcome. Am J Clin Pathol 100:428-432, 1993.
22. Franquemont DW, Frierson HF: Proliferating cell nuclear antigen immunoreactivity and prognosis of gastrointestinal stromal tumors. Mod Pathol 8:473-477, 1995.
23. Franquemont DW, Geary WA: Gastrointestinal stromal tumors and proliferating cell nuclear antigen: Prognostic challenges [editorial]. Am J Clin Pathol 100:369-370, 1993.
24. Trupiano JT, Stewart RE, Misick C, et al: Gastric stromal tumors: A clinicopathologic study of 77 cases with correlation of features with non-aggressive and aggressive clinical behavior. Am J Surg Pathol 26:705-714, 2002.
25. Cunningham RE, Federspiel BH, McCarthy WF, et al: Predicting prognosis of gastrointestinal stromal tumors: Role of clinical and histologic evaluation, flow cytometry and image cytometry. Am J Surg Pathol 17:588-594, 1993.
26. Ma CK, Amin MB, Kintanar E, et al: Immunohistologic characterization of gastrointestinal stromal tumors: A study of 82 cases compared with 11 cases of leiomyoma. Mod Pathol 6:139-145, 1993.
27. Goldblum JR, Appelman HD: Stromal tumors of the duodenum: A histologic and immunohistochemical study of 20 cases. Am J Surg Pathol 19:71-80, 1995.
28. Brainard JA, Goldblum JR: Stromal tumors of the jejunum and ileum: A clinicopathologic study of 39 cases. Am J Surg Pathol 21:407-416, 1997.
29. Tworek JA, Appelman HD, Singleton TP, et al: Stromal tumors of the jejunum and ileum. Mod Pathol 10:200-209, 1997.
30. Tworek JA, Goldblum JR, Weiss SW, et al: Stromal tumors of the abdominal colon: A clinicopathologic study of 20 cases. Am J Surg Pathol 23:937-945, 1999.
31. Miettinen M, Sarlomo-Rikala M, Sobin LH, et al: Gastrointestinal stromal tumors and leiomyosarcomas in the colon—A clinicopathologic, immunohistochemical and molecular genetic study of forty-four cases. Am J Surg Pathol 24:1339-1352, 2000.
32. Walsh TH, Mann CV: Smooth muscle neoplasms of the rectum and anal canal. Br J Surg 71:597-599, 1987.
33. Golden T, Stout AP: Smooth muscle tumors of the gastrointestinal stromal and retroperitoneal tissues. Surg Gynecol Obstet 73:784-810, 1941.
34. Tworek JA, Goldblum JR, Weiss SW, et al: Stromal tumors of the anorectum: A clinicopathologic study of 22 cases. Am J Surg Pathol 23:946-954, 1999.
35. Haque S, Dean PJ: Stromal neoplasms of the rectum and anal canal. Hum Pathol 23:762-767, 1992.
36. Miettinen M, Furlong M, Sarlomo-Rikala M, et al: Gastrointestinal stromal tumors, intramural leiomyomas and leiomyosarcomas in the rectum and anus: A clinicopathologic, immunohistochemical and molecular genetic study of 144 cases. Am J Surg Pathol 25:1121-1133, 2001.
37. Miettinen M, Sarlomo-Rikala M, Sobin LH, et al: Esophageal stromal tumors: A clinicopathologic, immunohistochemical and molecular genetic study of seventeen cases and comparison with esophageal leiomyomas and leiomyosarcomas. Am J Surg Pathol 24:211-222, 2000.
38. Pike AM, Lloyd RV, Appelman HD: Cell markers in gastrointestinal stromal tumors. Hum Pathol 19:830-834, 1988.
39. Saul SH, Rast ML, Brooks JJ: The immunohistochemistry of gastrointestinal stromal tumors: Evidence supporting an origin from smooth muscle. Am J Surg Pathol 11:464-473, 1987.
40. Franquemont DW, Frierson HF: Muscle differentiation and clinicopathologic features of gastrointestinal stromal tumors. Am J Surg Pathol 16:947-954, 1992.
41. Mikhael AI, Bacchi CE, Zarbo RJ, et al: CD34 expression in stromal tumors of the gastrointestinal tract. Appl Immunohistochem 2:89-93, 1994.
42. Monihan JM, Carr NJ, Sobin LH: CD34 immunoexpression in stromal tumors of the gastrointestinal tract and in mesenteric fibromatoses. Histopathology 25:464-473, 1994.
43. Van de Rijn M, Hendrickson MR, Rouse RV: CD34 expression by gastrointestinal tract stromal tumors. Hum Pathol 25:766-771, 1994.
44. Miettinen M, Virolainen M, Sarlomo-Rikala M: Gastrointestinal stromal tumors: Value of CD34 antigen in their identification and separation from true leiomyomas and schwannomas. Am J Surg Pathol 19:207-216, 1995.
45. Sircar K, Hewlett BR, Huizinga JD, et al: Interstitial cells of Cajal as precursors of gastrointestinal stromal tumors. Am J Surg Pathol 23:377-389, 1999.
46. Kindblom L-G, Remotti HE, Aldenborg F, et al: Gastrointestinal pacemaker cell tumor (GIPACT): Gastrointestinal stromal tumors show phenotypic characteristics of the interstitial cells of Cajal. Am J Pathol 152:1259-1269, 1998.
47. Miettinen M, Sobin LH, Sarlomo-Rikala M: Immunohistochemical spectrum of GISTs of different locations and their differential diagnosis. Mod Pathol 13:536-541, 2000.
48. Sarlomo-Rikala M, Kovatich A, Barusevicius A, et al: CD117: A sensitive marker for gastrointestinal stromal tumors that is more specific than CD34. Mod Pathol 11:728-734, 1998.
49. Kitamura Y, Hirota S, Nashida T: Molecular pathology of c-kit proto-oncogene in development of gastrointestinal stromal tumors. Ann Chir Gynaecol 87:282-286, 1998.
50. Maeda H, Yamagata A, Nishikawa F, et al: Requirement of c-kit for development of intestinal pacemaker system. Development 116:369-375, 1992.
51. Sanders KM: A case for interstitial cells as pacemakers and mediators of neurotransmission in the gastrointestinal tract. Gastroenterology 111:492-515, 1996.
52. Torihashi S, Nishi K, Tokutomi Y, et al: Blockade of KIT signaling induces transdifferentiation of interstitial cells of Cajal to a smooth muscle phenotype. Gastroenterology 117:140-148, 1999.
53. Seymour L: Novel anti-cancer agents in development: Exciting prospects and new challenges. Cancer Treat Rev 25:301-312, 1999.
54. Miettinen M, Sarlomo-Rikala M, Kovatich A, et al: Heavy caldesmon and calponin in smooth muscle tumors and gastrointestinal stromal tumors. Mod Pathol 12:756-762, 1999.
55. Hirota S, Isozaki K, Moriyama Y, et al: Gain-of-function mutations of c-kit in human gastrointestinal stromal tumors. Science 279:577-580, 1998.
56. Ernst SI, Hobbs AE, Przygodzki RM, et al: KIT mutation portends poor prognosis in gastrointestinal stromal/smooth muscle tumors. Lab Invest 78:1633-1636, 1998.
57. Lasota J, Wozniak A, Sarlomo-Rikala M, et al: Mutations in exon 9 and 13 of KIT gene are rare events in gastrointestinal stromal tumors. A study of 200 cases. Am J Pathol 157:1091-1095, 2000.
58. Taniguchi M, Nashida T, Hirota S, et al: Effect of c-kit mutation on prognosis of gastrointestinal stromal tumors. Cancer Res 59:4297-4300, 1999.
59. Heinrich MC, Rubin BP, Longley BJ, et al: Biology and genetic aspects of gastrointestinal stromal tumors: KIT activation and cytogenetic alterations. Hum Pathol 33:484-495, 2002.
60. Lux M, Rubin BP, Biase TL, et al: KIT extracellular and kinase domain mutations in gastrointestinal stromal tumors. Am J Pathol 156:791-795, 2000.
61. Lasota J, Jasinski M, Sarlomo-Rikala M, et al: Mutations in exon 11 of c-kit occur preferentially in malignant versus benign gastrointestinal stromal tumors and do not occur in leiomyomas and leiomyosarcomas. Am J Pathol 154:53-60, 1999.
62. Joensuu H, Roberts PF, Sarlomo-Rikala M, et al: Effect of the tyrosine kinase inhibitor STI571 in a patient with metastatic gastrointestinal stromal tumor. N Engl J Med 344:1052-1056, 2001.

63. Dematteo RP, Heinrich MC, El-Rifai WM, et al: Clinical management of gastrointestinal stromal tumors: Before and after STI-571. Hum Pathol 33:466-477, 2002.

64. Blanke CD, von Mehren M, Joensuu H, et al: Evaluation of the molecularly targeted therapy STI 571 in patients with unresectable or metastatic gastrointestinal stromal tumors expressing KIT [abstract]. Am Soc Clin Oncol Proc 20:2, 2001.

65. Van Oosterom AT, Judson I, Verweij J, et al: STI 571, an active drug in metastatic gastrointestinal stromal tumors (GIST), an EORTC phase I study [abstract]. Am Soc Clin Oncol Proc 20:2, 2001.

66. Van Oosterom AT, Judson I, Verweij J, et al: Safety and efficacy of Imatinib (STI 571) in metastatic gastrointestinal stromal tumors: A phase I study. Lancet 358:1421-1423, 2001.

67. El-Rifai W, Sarlomo-Rikala M, Miettinen M, et al: DNA copy number losses in chromosome 14: An early change in gastrointestinal stromal tumors. Cancer Res 56:3230-3233, 1996.

68. El-Rifai W, Sarlomo-Rikala M, Andersson L, et al: High resolution deletion mapping of chromosome 14 in stromal tumors of the gastrointestinal tract. Genes Chromosomes Cancer 27:387-391, 2000.

69. El-Rifai W, Sarlomo-Rikala M, Andersson L, et al: Prognostic significance of DNA copy number changes in benign and malignant GISTs. Cancer Res 60:3899-3903, 2000.

70. Sarlomo-Rikala M, El-Rifai W, Andersson L, et al: Different patterns of DNA copy number changes in gastrointestinal stromal tumors, leiomyomas and schwannomas. Hum Pathol 29:476-481, 1998.

71. O'Leary T, Ernst S, Przygodzki R, et al: Loss of heterozygosity at 1p36 predicts poor prognosis in gastrointestinal stromal/smooth muscle tumors. Lab Invest 79:1461-1467, 1999.

72. Kindblom LG, Remotti HE, Angervall L, et al: Gastrointestinal pacemaker cell tumor—A manifestation of neurofibromatosis 1. Mod Pathol 12:77A, 1999.

73. Walker P, Dvorak AM: Gastrointestinal autonomic nerve (GAN) tumor: Ultrastructural evidence for a newly recognized entity. Arch Pathol Lab Med 110:309-316, 1986.

74. Herrera GA, Cerezo L, Jones JE, et al: Gastrointestinal autonomic nerve tumors: "Plexosarcomas." Arch Pathol Lab Med 113:846-853, 1989.

75. Lauwers GY, Erlandson RA, Casper ES, et al: Gastrointestinal autonomic nerve tumors: A clinicopathologic, immunohistochemical and ultrastructural study of 12 cases. Am J Surg Pathol 17:887-897, 1993.

76. Lee JR, Joshi V, Griffin JW, et al: Gastrointestinal autonomic nerve tumor: Immunohistochemical and molecular identity with gastrointestinal stromal tumor. Am J Surg Pathol 25:979-987, 2001.

77. Sigal A, Carello S, Caterina P, et al: Gastrointestinal autonomic nerve tumors: A clinicopathologic, immunohistochemical and ultrastructural study of 10 cases. Pathology 26:239-247, 1994.

78. Sakaguchi N, Sano K, Ito M, et al: A case of von Recklinghausen's disease with bilateral pheochromocytoma—Malignant peripheral nerve sheath tumors of the adrenal and gastrointestinal autonomic nerve tumors. Am J Surg Pathol 20:889-897, 1996.

79. O'Brien P, Kapusta L, Dardick I, et al: Multiple familial gastrointestinal autonomic nerve tumors and small intestinal neuronal dysplasia. Am J Surg Pathol 23:198-204, 1999.

80. Miettinen M, Sarlomo-Rikala M, Sobin LH: Mesenchymal tumors of muscularis mucosae of colon and rectum are benign leiomyomas that should be separated from gastrointestinal stromal tumors—a clinicopathologic and immunohistochemical study of eighty-eight cases. Mod Pathol 14:950-956, 2001.

81. Morris CD, Wilkinson J, Fox D, et al: Diffuse esophageal leiomyomatosis with localized dense eosinophilic infiltration. Dis Esoph 15:85-87, 2002.

82. Sarlomo-Rikala M, Miettinen M: Gastric schwannoma—A clinicopathological analysis of six cases. Histopathology 27:355-360, 1995.

83. Prevot S, Bienvenu L, Vaillant JC, et al: Benign schwannoma of the digestive tract: A clinicopathologic and immunohistochemical study of 5 cases, including a case of esophageal tumor. Am J Surg Pathol 23:431-436, 1999.

84. Miettinen M, Shekitka KM, Sobin LH: Schwannomas in the colon and rectum: A clinicopathologic and immunohistochemical study of 20 cases. Am J Surg Pathol 25:846-855, 2001.

85. Daimaru Y, Kido H, Hashimoto H, et al: Benign schwannoma of the gastrointestinal tract: A clinicopathologic and immunohistochemical study. Hum Pathol 19:257-264, 1988.

86. Petersen JM, Ferguson DR: Gastrointestinal neurofibromatosis. J Clin Gastroenterol 6:529-534, 1984.

87. Fuller CE, Williams GT: Gastrointestinal manifestations of type 1 neurofibromatosis (von Recklinghausen's disease). Histopathology 19:1-11, 1991.

88. Schaldenbrand J, Appelman HD: Solitary solid stromal gastrointestinal tumors in von Recklinghausen's disease with minimal smooth muscle differentiation. Hum Pathol 15:229-232, 1984.

89. Walsh NMG, Bodurtha A: Auerbach's myenteric plexus: A possible site of origin for gastrointestinal stromal tumors in von Recklinghausen's neurofibromatosis. Arch Pathol Lab Med 114:522-525, 1990.

90. Johnston J, Helwig EB: Granular cell tumors of the gastrointestinal tract and perianal region: A study of 74 cases. Dig Dis Sci 26:807-816, 1981.

91. Goldblum JR, Rice TW, Zuccaro G, et al: Granular cell tumors of the esophagus: A clinical and pathologic study of 13 cases. Ann Thorac Surg 62:860-865, 1996.

92. Lauwers GY, Goldblum JR, Burgart LJ, et al: Expression of neurotrophin receptors and RET protein in duodenal gangliocytic paraganglioma: A study of 12 cases with histogenetic implications. Am J Surg Pathol (in press).

93. Dookhan DB, Miettinen M, Finkel G, et al: Recurrent duodenal gangliocytic paraganglioma with lymph node metastasis. Histopathology 22:399-405, 1993.

94. Haggitt RC, Reid BJ: Hereditary gastrointestinal polyposis syndromes. Am J Surg Pathol 10:871-887, 1986.

95. Shekitka KM, Sobin LH: Ganglioneuromas of the gastrointestinal tract: Relation to von Recklinghausen disease and other multiple tumor syndromes. Am J Surg Pathol 18:250-257, 1994.

96. Michowitz M, Lazebnik N, Noy S, et al: Lipoma of the colon: A report of 22 cases. Am Surg 51:449-454, 1985.

97. Miettinen M, Paal E, Lasota J, et al: Gastrointestinal glomus tumor: A clinicopathologic, immunohistochemical and molecular genetic study of 32 cases. Am J Surg Pathol 26:301-311, 2002.

98. Taxy JB, Battifora H: Angiosarcoma of the gastrointestinal tract. A report of three cases. Cancer 62:210-216, 1988.

99. Usuda H, Naito M: Multicentric angiosarcoma of the gastrointestinal tract. Pathol Int 47:553-556, 1997.

100. Monihan JM, Meis-Kindblom JM, Kindblom L-G, et al: Angiosarcoma of the gastrointestinal tract: A study of 18 cases [abstract]. Mod Pathol 8:65, 1995.

CHAPTER 23

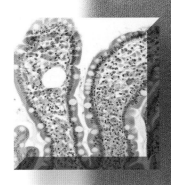

Lymphoid Tumors of the GI Tract

JUDITH A. FERRY

◼ Introduction

The gastrointestinal tract is the most common extranodal site of lymphomas, accounting for 4% to 20% of all non-Hodgkin's lymphomas. The stomach is involved most often, followed by the small intestine and the colon.[1] Lymphoma also occasionally arises in the hepatobiliary tree and rarely in the pancreas. The types of lymphomas encountered in the gastrointestinal tract differ to some extent from those that develop in lymph nodes (Tables 23-1 and 23-2). Whereas lymphomas that arise in lymph nodes and in some extranodal sites are largely idiopathic, in the gastrointestinal tract, the pathogenesis of distinct types of lymphoma is better understood. Predisposing factors include infection, especially *Helicobacter pylori*, celiac disease, inflammatory bowel disease, and a variety of immune deficiency syndromes. The development of some lymphomas appears to be related to chronic antigenic stimulation, inadequate immune regulation, or a combination of these factors.

In 55% to 65% of gastrointestinal lymphomas, the stomach is the primary site. Diffuse large B-cell lymphoma is most frequent, followed closely by marginal zone lymphoma. Lymphoma accounts for 1% to 7% of gastric malignancies.[1] In 20% to 35% of gastrointestinal lymphomas, the small intestine is involved.[1-5] Lymphoma accounts for approximately 25% of small intestinal neoplasms.[1] The most common type is diffuse large B-cell lymphoma, followed by marginal zone B-cell lymphoma (including immunoproliferative small intestinal disease), Burkitt's lymphoma, T-cell lymphoma, mantle cell lymphoma, and follicular lymphoma.[1,2,5-7] The ileum is more commonly affected than the duodenum or the jejunum (see Table 23-2).

The large intestine is the primary site in 7% to 20% of gastrointestinal lymphomas.[3-5] Lymphoma accounts for about 0.5% of malignant neoplasms in the colon.[1,8] The most common lymphoma is the diffuse large B-cell type, followed by marginal zone B-cell lymphoma, mantle cell lymphoma, and rare cases of follicular lymphoma, Burkitt's lymphoma, and peripheral T-cell lymphoma. The cecum is the most common site of involvement, followed by the rectum; other portions of the colon are only rarely affected.[1] Anal lymphomas are rare; they are usually diffuse large B-cell lymphomas (see Table 23-2).[9]

The most common presenting findings associated with gastrointestinal lymphomas are abdominal pain, anorexia or weight loss, obstruction, a palpable mass, diarrhea, nausea or vomiting, fever, perforation, and bleeding. Intussusception may be seen with bulky lymphomas in the ileocecal region. In a few cases, lymphoma may be an incidental finding.[2,4,6,8,10-12] The more common types of lymphoma, based on pathologic subclassification, are discussed individually in the following sections. Lymphoma of the appendix is discussed separately.

TABLE 23–1. Primary Gastrointestinal Tract Lymphoma

B-Cell Lymphoma
Extranodal marginal zone B-cell lymphoma
   Subtype: Immunoproliferative small intestinal disease
Diffuse large B-cell lymphoma
   De novo
   Large cell transformation of marginal zone lymphoma
Mantle cell lymphoma (multiple lymphomatous polyposis)
Burkitt's lymphoma
Follicular lymphoma
Miscellaneous rare types

T/NK-Cell Lymphoma
Enteropathy-type intestinal T-cell lymphoma
Extranodal NK/T-cell lymphoma, nasal type
Peripheral T-cell lymphoma, unspecified type
Miscellaneous rare types

Hodgkin's Disease

Gastric Marginal Zone B-Cell Lymphoma

CLINICAL FEATURES

Gastric marginal zone B-cell lymphoma (low-grade B-cell lymphoma of the mucosa-associated lymphoid tissue [MALT] type) affects men and women equally. Most patients are older adults, with a median age in the seventh decade of life. Infrequently, young adults and adolescents are affected.[13-16] Patients typically present with epigastric pain or dyspepsia, nausea, and vomiting. Bleeding and weight loss may occur but are unusual presenting complaints.[17] In fact, symptoms may resemble those of chronic gastritis or peptic ulcer disease.[18]

Sixty-three percent to 88% of cases are confined to the stomach.[15,19-21] Regional lymph nodes are involved in the remainder of cases. Few patients present with widespread disease.[15,19,21] Widespread disease may involve other extranodal sites such as the intestines, salivary gland, thyroid or orbit, and occasionally, bone marrow.[7,20-23] Gastric lymphomas are indolent and may remain localized for years, even without specific therapy.[7] In 1993, Wotherspoon and colleagues described the remarkable observation of regression of marginal zone B-cell lymphoma upon eradication of *H. pylori* with the use of antibiotics.[24] Since then, many other centers have reported a similar phenomenon, with response rates ranging from 60% to 90%.[17,25,26] However, the interval to histologic regression may be prolonged, with a range of 1 to 25 months and a median of 5 months.[21,25] Features associated with failure of regression include development of a large B-cell lymphoma component, invasion beyond the submucosa, spread beyond the stomach, and chromosomal abnormalities such as t(11;18) and t(1;14).[7,13,21] Surgery, radiation, or chemotherapy may be employed[20,21,25,27,28] for cases that do not respond or relapse, and cure can usually be obtained. The 5-year survival of patients with gastric marginal zone B-cell lymphoma is approximately 90%.[7,14,15,19]

PATHOLOGIC FEATURES

On gross examination, marginal zone lymphoma often consists of erosions, shallow ulcers, mucosal granularity, thickened mucosal folds, or a diffusely infiltrative, ill-defined lesion.[17,18,21,29] It frequently involves the antrum but may be multiple or widespread.[16,18,20,21] Because of the multifocal nature of some cases, residual tumor may be present even when resection margins are negative.[7,16] Some cases grow as localized polypoid tumors, but this is much less common.[7] Most lymphomas are confined to the mucosa or the submucosa. Lymph node involvement is distinctly unusual with superficially invasive lymphomas but is common when lymphoma invades into the muscularis propria.[16]

Microscopic features include a diffuse, or vaguely nodular, infiltrate of marginal zone B cells, which are small or medium-sized cells with slightly irregular nuclei and a distinct rim of clear cytoplasm. In about one third of cases, prominent plasmacytic differentiation occurs

TABLE 23–2. Lymphomas Arising in Gastrointestinal Tract and Hepatobiliary Tree, Including Rare Types

Stomach	Small Intestine	Colon	Anus	Appendix	Liver	Gallbladder	Pancreas
DLBCL	DLBCL	DLBCL	DLBCL	DLBCL	DLBCL	DLBCL	DLBCL
MZL	MZL	MZL		Burkitt's	Burkitt's	MZL	Burkitt's
Burkitt's	Subtype: IPSID	MCL		MZL	MZL		MZL
MCL	Burkitt's	Follicular			HSTCL		
Follicular	ETITL	Burkitt's					
PTCL	MCL	PTCL					
Hodgkin's	Follicular	Hodgkin's					
	PTCL						
	NK cell, nasal type						
	Hodgkin's						

The types of lymphoma are listed according to frequency, with the most common at the top of each column and the least frequent at the bottom.
DLBCL, diffuse large B-cell lymphoma; ETITL: enteropathy-type intestinal T-cell lymphoma; HSTCL, hepatosplenic T-cell lymphoma; IPSID, immunoproliferative small intestinal disease; MCL, mantle cell lymphoma; MZL, extranodal marginal zone B-cell lymphoma; NK cell, natural killer cell; PTCL, peripheral T-cell lymphoma, unspecified type.

in the form of a bandlike infiltrate of plasma cells, often seen in the most superficial portion of the lymphoma. Plasma cells may appear normal or may have cytoplasm with crystalline inclusions or nuclei with Dutcher bodies. Small clusters of neoplastic cells typically infiltrate and disrupt gastric glands to form lymphoepithelial lesions. Reactive lymphoid follicles, often showing infiltration and replacement by neoplastic cells (follicular colonization), are usually present. The cells that colonize the follicles are usually marginal zone–type cells, but plasma cells or large cells may also be found. Even when follicles cannot be seen on routinely stained sections, evidence of preexisting follicles can generally be obtained with the use of antibodies to follicular dendritic cells such as CD21. Small numbers of large cells may be scattered among marginal zone cells (Fig. 23-1).[7,18]

Biopsies also frequently show evidence of gastritis with *H. pylori*. The likelihood that *H. pylori* will be found is greater with lymphomas that are superficial (confined to the mucosa or the submucosa) and of low grade.[30] In addition, the frequency of *H. pylori* positivity varies among studies; although some series report *H. pylori* in 80% to 100% of cases, in others, only a minority of cases have been found to harbor *H. pylori*.[20,28,31]

Complete histologic regression of lymphoma following *H. pylori* eradication therapy is characterized by a lamina propria with a distinctive empty appearance, basal aggregates of small lymphocytes, and scattered plasma cells (Fig. 23-2). Partial regression shows areas of empty lamina propria with foci of atypical lymphoid cells and/or lymphoepithelial lesions.[25]

Early involvement of lymph nodes takes the form of interfollicular or parafollicular aggregates of marginal zone lymphoid cells, progressing to confluent sheets of marginal zone cells with or without monocytoid B cells and follicular colonization.[18] The appearance is indistinguishable from that of nodal marginal zone B-cell lymphoma (Fig. 23-3).

Immunophenotyping shows CD20+, CD5–, CD10–, monotypic surface immunoglobulin (sIg)+ B cells with plasma cells expressing polytypic or monotypic cytoplasmic immunoglobulin (cIg). The Ig is most often

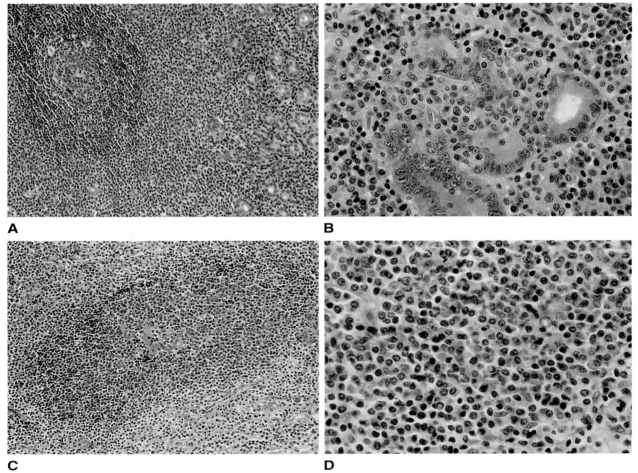

FIGURE 23–1. Gastric marginal zone B-cell lymphoma. **A,** Low power shows a diffuse infiltrate of marginal zone B cells with a reactive follicle (upper left). **B,** Marginal zone cells infiltrate and disrupt gastric glands, forming lymphoepithelial lesions. **C,** A follicle has been replaced by neoplastic cells (follicular colonization). **D,** High power shows that the colonizing cells are plasma cells, some with Dutcher bodies.

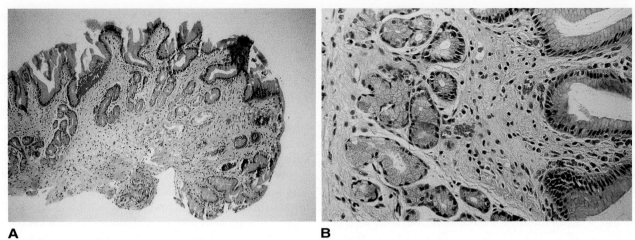

FIGURE 23–2. Gastric mucosa following regression of marginal zone lymphoma. **A,** Low power shows a pale hypocellular lamina propria. **B,** The lamina propria contains loose connective tissue, fibroblasts, and rare lymphocytes.

IgM, but in some cases, it is IgA or IgG. The neoplastic cells are BCL2+, although BCL2 may be lost in colonized follicles. CD43 is coexpressed in up to one third of cases. An immunostain for cytokeratin can be helpful in highlighting lymphoepithelial lesions. The proliferation fraction as measured with the antibody Ki67 is low, although it is characteristically high in residual reactive germinal centers.[16,18,21,32]

Molecular genetic studies show clonally rearranged immunoglobulin heavy and light chain genes. Analysis of heavy chain genes shows somatic hypermutation, consistent with neoplastic cells at a post–germinal center stage of development. *BCL1* and *BCL2* are germline.[7,18] Trisomy 3 is found in about one third of cases.[48] Approximately 30% of marginal zone B-cell lymphomas have a t(11;18)(q21;q21), a translocation involving the *API2* gene on chromosome 11 and the *MLT* gene on chromosome 18, which results in a chimeric transcript that can be detected by reverse transcription–polymerase chain reaction (RT-PCR). This fusion is believed to confer a survival advantage to the neoplastic cells. This translocation may be specific for extranodal marginal zone B-cell lymphoma.[33] Marginal zone lymphomas that fail to regress with therapy to eradicate *H. pylori* usually harbor the t(11;18), although t(11;18) is consistently absent in cases that do regress with such therapy. This translocation also appears to be associated with higher-stage disease.[13]

Another cytogenetic abnormality uncommonly associated with marginal zone lymphoma is t(1;14)(p22;q32). This change results in deregulation of the *BCL10* gene, with resultant loss of its normal proapoptotic activity and acquisition of oncogenic potential.[13] In cases that are histologically negative for lymphoma following *H. pylori* eradication, clonal B cells can be detected by PCR up to several years later.[7,21,25] Microdissection studies suggest that the clonal cells reside in basal lymphoid aggregates.[25]

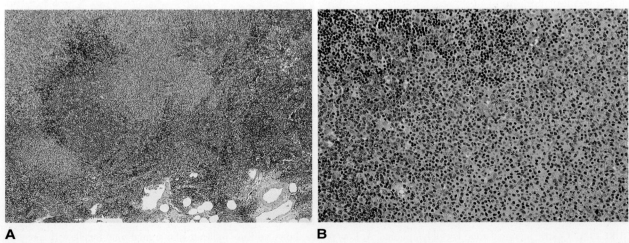

FIGURE 23–3. Perigastric lymph node involved by marginal zone lymphoma. **A,** Large aggregates of neoplastic cells replace much of the lymph node, surrounding and invading a reactive follicle. **B,** Monocytoid B cells with abundant pale cytoplasm encroach on germinal center lymphocytes.

PATHOGENESIS

Marginal zone lymphoma is believed to arise from a background of gastritis with a component of acquired mucosa-associated lymphoid tissue induced by *H. pylori* infection. Persistent infection with chronic antigenic stimulation leads to the appearance of a clonal population of B cells. It is surprising that the B cells do not have specificity for *H. pylori*; instead, they produce antibodies that may be reactive with a variety of autoantigens. It is the T cells within the infiltrate that have strain-specific reactivity for *H. pylori*. In the early phases of disease, the B cells require *H. pylori* and the T cells to proliferate. Accordingly, in this phase, the lymphoma remains localized and may respond to antibiotic therapy directed against *H. pylori*. Over time, the clonal B cells acquire genetic abnormalities such as t(11;18) associated with autonomous growth, leading to a histologically low-grade lymphoma that does not regress with *H. pylori* eradication and that may spread beyond the stomach. Additional genetic abnormalities, such as *TP53* inactivation and allelic loss,[7] *p16* deletion,[34] and c-*myc* translocation,[18,26,34] may occur and lead to large cell transformation.

One important pathogenetic question remains. In some cases, no evidence of *H. pylori* infection can be found.[20,28] In such cases, it is not clear whether infection had been present previously and resolved at a stage after the lymphoma attained autonomous growth, or whether there is another not yet recognized causative agent for gastric marginal zone lymphoma.

DIFFERENTIAL DIAGNOSIS

Marginal Zone Lymphoma Versus Gastritis. On routinely stained sections, the presence of an expansile destructive infiltrate with loss of glands, cytologic atypia of the infiltrating cells (having the appearance of marginal zone B cells rather than normal small lymphocytes), frequent lymphoepithelial lesions, and Dutcher bodies favors lymphoma. Immunohistochemical studies are often of assistance when this question arises in that monotypic Ig light chain expression confirms a diagnosis of lymphoma. A diffuse infiltrate of B cells and coexpression of CD43 by B cells also favor a diagnosis of lymphoma.

Marginal Zone Lymphoma Versus Other Low-Grade Lymphomas. In the stomach, marginal zone lymphoma is much more common than either follicular or mantle cell lymphoma. However, either follicular or mantle cell lymphoma may present in the stomach and mimic marginal zone lymphoma. Marginal zone lymphoma is composed of CD5, CD10– B cells with relatively abundant clear cytoplasm and may show plasmacytic differentiation and an admixture of a few large cells. Mantle cell lymphoma is composed of a monotonous population of small to medium-sized CD5+, cyclin D1+ B cells with scant cytoplasm, without a large cell or plasmacytic component. Follicular lymphoma generally has a more distinct follicular architecture and is composed of CD10+ B cells with nuclei that are usually more irregular and cytoplasm that is usually more scant than those of marginal zone B cells.

Transformation to Large B-cell Lymphoma Versus Marginal Zone Lymphoma with Increased Large Cells. Sheets or confluent clusters of large, transformed cells found outside of follicles in a background of marginal zone lymphoma indicate large cell transformation. Most authorities require clusters of at least 20 large cells for large cell transformation[14,26]; diffusely scattered large cells representing 5% to 10%[14] or even 20%[19] of the total population are not associated with a worse prognosis as long as clusters of large cells are not seen. Others report that patients with 1% to 10% scattered large cells, some of whom also have small clusters of large cells, have a worse chance for survival after long-term follow-up.[26] Before focal large cell transformation is diagnosed, one must exclude the possibility that the large cells are residual reactive germinal center cells or neoplastic large cells colonizing follicles. Immunohistochemical stains to demonstrate a follicular dendritic network can be helpful in the resolution of uncertainties.

Poorly Preserved High-Grade Lymphoma Versus Marginal Zone B-Cell Lymphoma. In a small biopsy with artifactual degenerative change with large B-cell lymphoma or Burkitt's lymphoma, cellular shrinkage and distortion may lead to a false impression of low-grade lymphoma. The presence of apoptotic debris or mitotic figures suggests a higher-grade tumor. Staining with the proliferation marker Ki67 can be quite helpful in distinguishing low- from high-grade lymphoma. Clinical information such as the endoscopic appearance of the tumor can also provide a clue to the diagnosis.[7]

Plasmacytoma Versus Marginal Zone B-Cell Lymphoma. Convincing cases of gastrointestinal plasmacytoma are rare. Most cases reported as such are marginal zone lymphomas with prominent plasmacytic differentiation. The presence of a component of B lymphocytes, lymphoepithelial lesions, and IgM+ neoplastic cells (although marginal zone lymphomas may express other heavy chains) favors lymphoma.

◼ Intestinal Extranodal Marginal Zone B-Cell Lymphoma

CLINICAL FEATURES

This tumor typically arises in older adults with a slight male preponderance[6] and may be located in any portion of the small or large intestine. In the vast majority of cases, disease is localized to the bowel with or without mesenteric nodal involvement, and distant spread is unusual.[10,18,35] A few patients have serum M components.[6]

The prognosis is generally good but is less favorable than that of gastric marginal zone lymphoma.[2,10] In one review, 5-year survival was reported to be between 44% and 75%.[18] More recent studies have reported an even better outcome.

Rare patients with duodenal lymphoma and one patient with a rectal lymphoma of this type have responded to *H. pylori* eradication therapy,[10,36-38] suggesting a pathogenetic link to gastric marginal zone lymphoma.

PATHOLOGIC FEATURES

On gross examination, the lymphomas form polypoid or ulcerated masses,[6,10,11,36] or infrequently they have the appearance of multiple small, slightly raised erosive lesions, akin to early gastric marginal zone lymphoma.[38,39] In most cases, transmural invasion occurs,[6,11,35] but some remain confined to the superficial aspect of the bowel wall.[10] The histologic, immunophenotypic, and genetic features of marginal zone lymphoma in the intestine are similar to those seen in the stomach.[2,6,18,39]

Immunoproliferative Small Intestinal Disease

The frequency of small intestinal lymphoma is higher in the Middle East than in Western countries. The small intestine is the most common primary site for extranodal lymphoma, accounting for 50% of such cases and for 75% of gastrointestinal lymphomas in adults in the Middle East. Approximately half of small intestinal lymphomas are of the distinctive immunoproliferative small intestinal disease (IPSID) type. IPSID is found mainly in the Middle East and in countries around the Mediterranean Sea, but occasional cases in South Africa, the Far East, Europe, and North America have been described. Because of its geographic distribution, IPSID has also been called *Mediterranean lymphoma*.[40,41] IPSID is now considered to be a distinct subtype of extranodal marginal zone B-cell lymphoma.

CLINICAL FEATURES

Most patients are young adults (median age, 25 years); affected patients range from adolescence to middle age with a male-to-female ratio of 1:1. IPSID tends to be associated with lower socioeconomic status. Patients present with abdominal pain, malabsorption, diarrhea, and weight loss of months' to years' duration. Many patients also have digital clubbing.[40,42] Obstruction, bleeding, and perforation are uncommon, in contrast to patients with other types of small intestinal lymphoma.[40] At laparotomy, patients may have one or more recognizable intestinal masses, diffuse mural thickening, and/or luminal dilatation, or they may have normal-appearing bowel. Abnormalities involve the proximal small intestine, the entire small intestine, or rarely, just the ileum, or the small intestine in combination with either stomach or colon.[40] Mesenteric lymph nodes are often enlarged.[18,40-42] Analogous to the situation with gastric marginal zone B-cell lymphoma, in the early phase of the disease the lymphoma may respond to broad-spectrum antibiotics such as tetracycline. Later in the course of disease, when muscle invasion and/or transformation to a high-grade lymphoma occurs, the lymphoma behaves in an aggressive manner.[7] For resectable stage Ie or IIe1 disease, 5-year survival is 40% to 47%. For higher-stage, unresectable disease, 5-year survival has been reported to be as poor as 0% to 25%.[1] However, patients treated with combination chemotherapy have a better outlook, with a complete remission rate of 64%.[42]

In about half of cases, a highly characteristic laboratory abnormality is noted: The serum contains free α heavy chains without associated light chains. Free α heavy chains may also be found in body fluids such as intestinal fluid, urine, and saliva. Secreted α heavy chain is more likely to be found in early stages of IPSID. Cases with this abnormality have been called α heavy chain disease. Closer analysis of this paraprotein reveals that it is an α_1 heavy chain with an internal deletion of V_H (variable region of immunoglobulin heavy chain gene) and $C_H 1$ (first segment, constant region of immunoglobulin heavy chain gene). It has been suggested that IPSID occurs in patients with recurrent or persistent intestinal infection, leading to chronic antigenic stimulation of IgA-secreting lymphoid tissue in this site with a resultant clonal population that acquires mutations leading to the production of α heavy chain with the internal deletion described previously. Subsequently, most cases are characterized by a loss of ability to synthesize light chain.[42]

PATHOLOGIC FEATURES

IPSID is characterized by a dense, continuous, bandlike mucosal lymphoid or lymphoplasmacytic infiltrate that is uninterrupted along the length of the small intestine.[40] The mucosa also shows broad villi and shortened crypts, although intestinal epithelial cells usually remain intact.[41,42] The extent of the infiltrate explains the malabsorption that patients experience. Histologic features are similar to those of marginal zone B-cell lymphoma in other extranodal sites, except that in IPSID, consistently marked plasmacytic differentiation is seen. The following staging system has been proposed to subclassify the infiltrate in IPSID.

Stage A. Lymphoma is confined to the small intestinal mucosa and mesenteric lymph nodes. The infiltrate consists predominantly of plasma cells with smaller numbers of marginal zone B cells. These B cells may be inconspicuous, and an immunostain for CD20 can help with recognition of B cells and of lymphoepithelial lesions.[18] Variable villous atrophy is noted (Fig. 23-4).

Stage B. In addition to the findings characteristic of stage A, the infiltrate has areas of nodularity that correspond to reactive lymphoid follicles colonized by neoplastic cells. Atypical immunoblast-like cells are also found occasionally. The infiltrate invades beyond the muscularis mucosae with total or subtotal villous atrophy.

Stage C. This stage is characterized by high-grade lymphoma with formation of one or more large masses. The lymphoma is composed of large cells, sometimes with the appearance of immunoblasts or plasmacytoid immunoblasts. In other cases, the neoplastic cells are pleomorphic and bizarre.

Immunohistochemical analysis usually shows expression of α heavy chain without light chain, correlating with the serum paraprotein. In a minority of cases, monotypic light chain is expressed. Molecular genetic analysis has shown clonal rearrangement of Ig heavy and light chains, even in early cases responsive to antibiotic therapy. Previously, early phases of IPSID were thought to be inflammatory, but evidence of clonality indicates the neoplastic nature of this process, despite response to antibiotics.[18,43,44]

DIFFERENTIAL DIAGNOSIS

Both IPSID and celiac sprue are characterized by lymphoplasmacytic intestinal mucosal infiltrates and villous atrophy. Patient demographic data should provide a strong clue to the diagnosis in that patients with celiac disease, in contrast to IPSID patients, are predominantly of northwestern European descent and improve on a gluten-free diet. Histologic features in favor of celiac disease include total villous atrophy (in contrast to the villous broadening seen in early-stage IPSID), hyperplastic elongated crypts, intraepithelial lymphocytosis, and surface epithelial damage.[42] High-

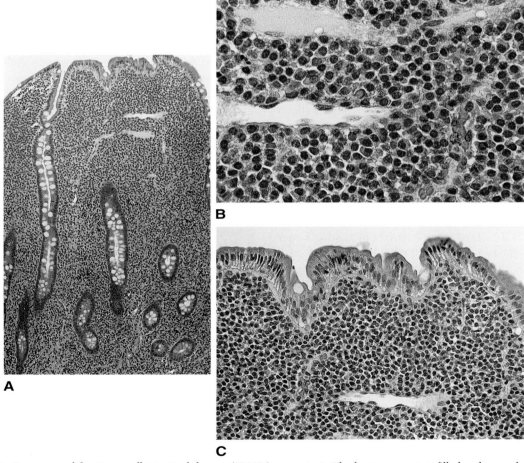

FIGURE 23–4. Immunoproliferative small intestinal disease (IPSID), stage A. **A,** The lamina propria is filled and expanded by a dense cellular infiltrate. **B,** Higher power shows numerous plasma cells, one with a Dutcher body, and scattered small lymphoid cells. **C,** Despite the intensity of the cellular infiltrate, the surface epithelium is well preserved.

grade lymphomas may be found in association with either, but the lymphoma that complicates celiac disease is a T-cell lymphoma prone to cause multifocal perforation.

Distinguishing nonspecific chronic inflammation from early-stage IPSID may be difficult, particularly on a small biopsy. In favor of IPSID is a dense, predominantly plasmacytic infiltrate that distorts the mucosal architecture in a patient with clinical features compatible with IPSID. Immunohistochemical stains that show plasma cells expressing only α heavy chain confirm the diagnosis.

Gastric Diffuse Large B-Cell Lymphoma

CLINICAL FEATURES

Gastric diffuse large B-cell lymphoma is mainly a disease of older adults, with a mean age in the seventh decade; younger adults are affected occasionally. There is a slight male preponderance.[14-16] Patients may have a palpable mass on physical examination.[7] Some arise in association with marginal zone B-cell lymphoma, consistent with large cell transformation of the low-grade lymphoma; others arise de novo. The proportion of cases in the two categories varies among series.[14,15,19,45] In most cases (78% to 95%),[15,19] patients present with stage I or II disease; patients with stage II disease usually outnumber those with stage I, and stage IIe1 is more frequent than IIe2.[14,15,19,45] Patients have been treated with surgery, radiation, chemotherapy, or a combination of these modalities. The 5-year survival is estimated to be 65%.[7] In some series, the subtype of large B-cell lymphoma did not significantly impact prognosis,[19] but in others, it made a substantial difference. In one study, large B-cell lymphoma associated with marginal zone lymphoma had a 5-year survival of 92%, and CD10+ large B-cell lymphoma had a 5-year survival of 89%; however, CD10– large B-cell lymphoma without a low grade component had a 5-year survival of only 30%.[15] In another study, large B-cell lymphoma associated with a component of marginal zone lymphoma or with lymphoepithelial lesions formed by small cells had a 5-year survival of 84% compared with 64% for de novo large B-cell lymphoma. Lymphoepithelial lesions formed by large cells was not associated with a favorable prognosis.[14] Stage is also prognostically important; patients with stage Ie or IIe1 have a better outcome than those with IIe2 or higher.[15,19]

PATHOLOGIC FEATURES

On gross examination, lymphomas are usually solitary, but occasionally, multiple large ulcerated or exophytic lesions are seen that are usually transmurally invasive and may even invade adjacent viscera.[7,45] Microscopic examination reveals a diffuse proliferation of large cells with round, oval, irregular, or lobated nuclei, distinct nucleoli, and a narrow but distinct rim of cytoplasm (Fig. 23-5). Immunophenotyping reveals CD20+ B cells expressing monotypic sIg, and occasionally cIg, and coexpressing CD43 in about half of cases.[19] In contrast to marginal zone lymphomas, the large cell lymphomas that arise from them may be BCL2– and occasionally express BCL6, although they remain CD10–.[15,18] A subset of large B-cell lymphomas are CD10+, BCL6–, suggesting follicle center origin, although most are negative for CD10 and BCL6.[15]

Ig heavy and light chains are clonally rearranged. Complex cytogenetic abnormalities are common.[46] In contrast to nodal large B-cell lymphomas, BCL2 rearrangement is uncommon. Rearrangement of the BCL6 gene is reported to be significantly more common in gastric than in nodal diffuse large B-cell lymphoma. In one study, gastric lymphomas with germline BCL6 had advanced-stage disease more often and showed a trend for decreased chances of complete remission and decreased survival.[47] Frequent (42% of cases) loss of heterozygosity (LOH) on chromosome 6q in sites of putative tumor suppressor genes and a smaller number of cases with LOH of other tumor suppressor genes, including TP53 and APC, have been documented. Amplification of genomic material in the BCL6 locus, the MLL (mixed lineage leukemia) gene, and others was found. A significant association was found between the MLL amplification and LOH of TP53.[46] Despite the high frequency of t(11;18) and trisomy 3 in marginal zone B-cell lymphoma, these appear to be uncommon in diffuse large B-cell lymphoma, suggesting they are not important in the

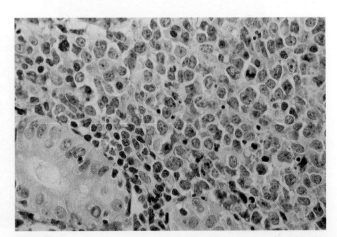

FIGURE 23–5. Gastric diffuse large B-cell lymphoma. The biopsy shows an infiltrate of centroblasts and immunoblasts with oval, vesicular nuclei, prominent nucleoli, and scant cytoplasm, with occasional mitotic figures and interspersed cellular debris.

transformation of marginal zone lymphoma to large B-cell lymphoma.[34,48] One report suggests that trisomies (most often involving chromosomes 12 and 18) are more common among large cell lymphomas that have arisen through transformation of marginal zone lymphoma than among de novo large B-cell lymphomas.[48] A report from Hong Kong documents Epstein-Barr virus (EBV) in a subset of diffuse large B-cell lymphomas.[49]

DIFFERENTIAL DIAGNOSIS

Poorly differentiated carcinoma may be composed of discohesive-appearing cells that form few or no glands; thus, it can be difficult to distinguish from diffuse large B-cell lymphoma. Lymphoid cells may show artifactual vacuolar change and may mimic signet ring cells. Mucin stains and immunohistochemical stains are helpful in establishing a diagnosis.

Intestinal Diffuse Large B-Cell Lymphoma

CLINICAL FEATURES

Most patients with this lymphoma are older adults; a few cases occur in younger adults and children. There is a slight male preponderance among adults, and affected children are almost exclusively boys. Lymphoma in children is virtually only found in the ileocecal area.[6,8,11] In most patients, regional lymph nodes are involved.[6,8] In about half of cases, the lymphoma is confined to the bowel with or without regional lymph node involvement; in the remainder, disease is more widespread.

This type of lymphoma is relatively aggressive. The 5-year survival is estimated to be 25% to 67%.[7,18] In one report, de novo large B-cell lymphoma had a less favorable outcome than large B-cell lymphoma that arose in association with marginal zone B-cell lymphoma.[10]

PATHOLOGIC FEATURES

On gross examination, the tumors tend to be a bit larger than low-grade lymphomas.[10,11] A subset show evidence of perforation.[2] Most are composed of large noncleaved lymphoid cells (centroblasts), often with an admixture of immunoblasts, plasmablasts, and/or multilobated large lymphoid cells; a minority are composed almost exclusively of immunoblasts (Fig. 23-6).[2,6]

In some cases, a component of marginal zone B-cell lymphoma is found, consistent with large cell transformation of low-grade lymphoma. The proportion of cases with an underlying low-grade lymphoma varies greatly in different series, from 10% to more than 50% of large B-cell lymphomas.[2,6,10] The immunophenotypic and genotypic features are similar to those found in gastric diffuse large B-cell lymphoma.

Mantle Cell Lymphoma

CLINICAL FEATURES

Mantle cell lymphoma affects middle-aged to older adults, with almost all patients 50 years of age or older. There is a male preponderance.[11,18,50] The lymphoma often takes the form of innumerable polyps, so-called multiple lymphomatous polyposis. Any portion of the

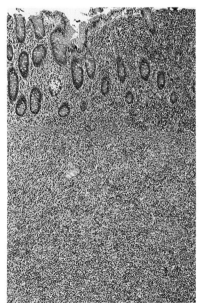

FIGURE 23–6. Diffuse large B-cell lymphoma, arising in the cecum of an HIV-positive patient. **A,** A diffuse infiltrate of lymphoid cells obliterates much of the bowel wall. **B,** The tumor cells are large atypical lymphoid cells with oval or irregular nuclei and prominent nucleoli. Their appearance is consistent with centroblasts.

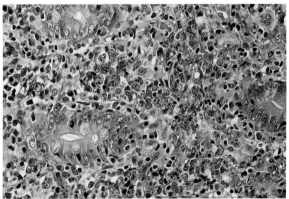

A

B

gastrointestinal tract can be affected, but the ileocecal region tends to contain the largest polyps.[10,18] Mesenteric lymph nodes are usually involved.[18] Staging frequently reveals widespread extraintestinal disease. Although there is usually a response to chemotherapy, relapse is common, and survival is usually less than 5 years. No predisposing factors for the development of mantle cell lymphoma are known.

PATHOLOGIC FEATURES

On gross examination, multiple intestinal polyposis has the appearance of multiple fleshy white nodules, 0.5 to 2 cm in greatest dimension, involving the mucosa, sometimes with superficial submucosal involvement (Fig. 23-7). Less commonly, mantle cell lymphoma takes the form of a discrete mass or an ulcerated lesion.[7]

Microscopic examination shows a bandlike infiltrate or multiple ill-defined nodules of atypical lymphoid cells that are slightly larger and more irregular than normal lymphocytes. They have scant cytoplasm, and nucleoli are not conspicuous. Single epithelioid histiocytes may be scattered among the neoplastic cells. Remnants of reactive follicle centers can be identified within some nodules. The lymphoma tends to displace and obliterate intestinal glands, but formation of true lymphoepithelial lesions is not a feature (Fig. 23-8).[18,50]

Immunophenotyping typically shows CD20+, CD5+, CD43+, CD10–, CD23–, nuclear cyclin D1+ B cells expressing monotypic immunoglobulin, of the IgMD type, with λ being more frequent than κ light chain. With antibodies to follicular dendritic cells such as CD21, a loose, expanded dendritic network is seen. Genetic studies often show t(11;14), a translocation that involves the *BCL1* gene and the Ig heavy chain gene. Expression of a4b7, the mucosal homing receptor, is highly associated with gastrointestinal involvement.[18,51]

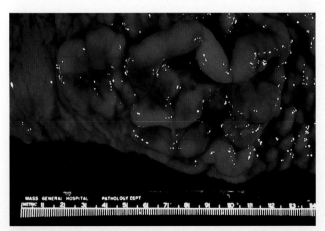

FIGURE 23–7. Multiple lymphomatous polyposis. Gross examination reveals marked expansion of mucosal folds, producing multiple serpiginous and polypoid masses. Microscopic examination revealed mantle cell lymphoma.

DIFFERENTIAL DIAGNOSIS

The main problems in differential diagnosis are that, on occasion, lymphomas other than mantle cell type have been associated with the picture of lymphomatous polyposis, and that not all mantle cell lymphomas take the form of lymphomatous polyposis. Follicular lymphoma[7,10,52] and rarely marginal zone lymphoma[53] can have the appearance of lymphomatous polyposis. Mantle cell lymphoma without the classic polyposis appearance can be mistaken for other low-grade B-cell lymphomas. The problem can be resolved readily in most cases with careful study of routine stained slides augmented by immunohistochemistry. The distinction is important because of the poor outlook of mantle cell lymphoma compared with that of other histologically low-grade lymphomas.

Follicular Lymphoma

It is uncommon for follicular lymphoma to be encountered in the gastrointestinal tract, but several recent studies suggest that follicular lymphoma of the duodenum is a distinct clinicopathologic entity. In 1997, Misdraji and associates reported a case of a 56-year-old woman with follicular lymphoma, grade I of III, arising at the ampulla of Vater, associated with jaundice and clinically mimicking pancreatic carcinoma.[54] The lymphoma formed a 4-cm white-tan mass arising in the wall of the duodenum, surrounding the common bile duct, and invading the head of the pancreas. Peripancreatic lymph nodes showed partial nodal involvement by follicular lymphoma. The patient was treated with radiation and was alive and well 5 months postoperatively. Subsequently, a study from Japan analyzed 222 gastrointestinal lymphomas, among which were 13 duodenal lymphomas and 8 follicular lymphomas. Of the 8 follicular lymphomas, 5 arose in the duodenum, all in its second portion, in the vicinity of the ampulla of Vater. The five patients were all women, aged 37 to 66 years (median, 52), with follicular lymphoma, grade I of III, that produced small polypoid masses and protrusions, or mucosal irregularity. Two patients had partial involvement of regional lymph nodes by follicular lymphoma. All patients were alive and well 2 to 50 months after diagnosis.[5] Recently, Chott and colleagues described 21 intestinal follicular lymphomas, 10 of which arose in the duodenum.[55] All 10 had stage I disease and all were free of extraintestinal disease on follow-up. The patients with nonduodenal follicular lymphomas all had higher-stage disease.[55] In one additional case, a 53-year-old male known to have the hereditary nonpolyposis colorectal cancer syndrome developed duodenal follicular lymphoma, raising intriguing possibilities about the pathogenesis of this disorder.[56]

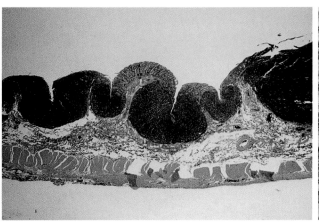

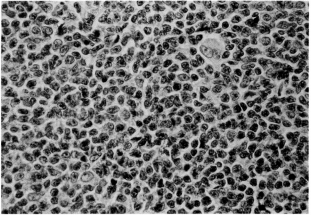

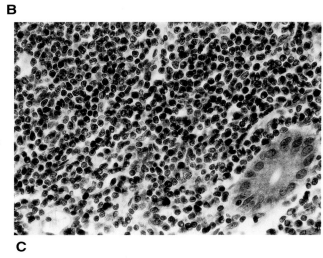

FIGURE 23–8. Multiple lymphomatous polyposis. **A,** Low power. **B,** High power shows small, slightly irregular lymphoid cells with scant cytoplasm and few interspersed single epithelioid histiocytes. **C,** There is staining of the nuclei of many of the atypical cells with an antibody to cyclin D1, confirming a diagnosis of mantle cell lymphoma.

The follicular lymphomas have an immunophenotype similar to that found in nodal follicular lymphomas (CD20+, CD10+, BCL2+, BCL6+) (Fig. 23-9).[5,54,55] Genetic studies using PCR show clonal Ig heavy and light chain genes and *BCL2* rearrangements.[55,56] Thus, a high proportion of duodenal lymphomas are follicular lymphomas, and a high proportion of gastrointestinal follicular lymphomas arise in the duodenum. Duodenal follicular lymphoma appears to have a favorable prognosis.

Follicular lymphoma rarely presents in other sites in the gastrointestinal tract and may form discrete lesions or have the appearance of multiple lymphomatous polyposis.[5,7,10,52] As has been noted earlier, such cases tend to present with more widespread disease than duodenal follicular lymphoma.[7,55]

Burkitt's Lymphoma

CLINICAL FEATURES

Burkitt's lymphoma is a highly aggressive, rapidly growing tumor. In the World Health Organization (WHO) classification of tumors of the hematopoietic and lymphoid tissues,[57] three clinical variants of Burkitt's lymphoma are described: (1) endemic, (2) sporadic, and (3) immune deficiency–associated. Involvement of the ileocecal region is the most common manifestation of sporadic Burkitt's lymphoma. Ileocecal disease is occasionally seen with endemic and immune deficiency–associated Burkitt's lymphoma, although extragastrointestinal presentation is more common. Infrequently, sites in the gastrointestinal tract other than the ileocecal area, including the stomach and more distal portions of the colon, are involved. Burkitt's lymphoma affects children and young adults with a marked male preponderance.[2] Most patients with immune deficiency–associated Burkitt's lymphoma are HIV-positive. In some cases, staging reveals disease beyond the gastrointestinal tract.

PATHOLOGIC FEATURES

On gross inspection, the tumors are usually bulky exophytic lesions, sometimes with ulceration (Figs. 23-10 and 23-11A).[10] Based on histologic features, the WHO classification defines classic Burkitt's lymphoma and two morphologic variants—Burkitt's lymphoma with plasmacytoid differentiation and atypical Burkitt's/Burkitt's-like lymphoma. In classic Burkitt's lymphoma,

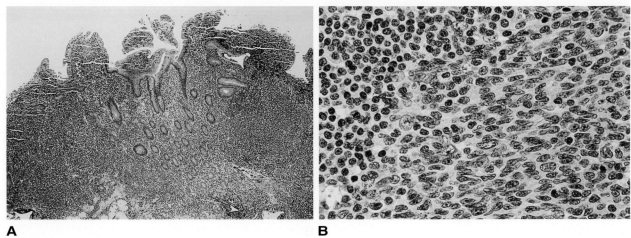

A   **B**

FIGURE 23–9. Follicular lymphoma, grade I of III, duodenum. **A,** The duodenal mucosa contains several large, poorly circumscribed lymphoid follicles. **B,** The lymphoid cells in this follicle are a monomorphous population of centrocytes (small cleaved cells) with only a few large cells. The centrocytes are larger than the small lymphocytes in the adjacent mantle.

microscopic examination reveals a diffuse infiltrate of uniform, medium-sized cells with round nuclei, granular chromatin, three to four small nucleoli, and distinct rims of deeply basophilic cytoplasm. Numerous tingible body macrophages produce a starry-sky pattern. The mitotic rate is high. In the atypical Burkitt's/Burkitt's-like variant, nuclei show greater pleomorphism, and nucleoli are fewer in number but tend to be more prominent (Fig. 23-11**B** through **D**). Burkitt's lymphoma with plasmacytoid differentiation shows some neoplastic cells with eccentric basophilic cytoplasm and often a single central nucleolus. Nuclei may be somewhat pleomorphic. This variant is found most often in immune-deficient patients.

Immunophenotyping reveals monotypic IgM+, CD20+, CD10+, CD5–, BCL2– B cells with a proliferation fraction of nearly 100%. Cytogenetic analysis reveals t(8;14), t(2;8), or t(8;22) corresponding to translocations involving the c-*myc* gene and either the Ig heavy chain gene or the κ or λ light chain gene. EBV

is found in about one third of sporadic Burkitt's lymphomas and in most endemic Burkitt's lymphomas.

■ Enteropathy-type Intestinal T-Cell Lymphoma

An association between malabsorption and intestinal lymphoma has been long recognized. Analysis of these lymphomas suggested that they were a form of malignant histiocytosis; later studies showed the neoplastic cells to be T cells consistent with peripheral T-cell lymphoma,[58,59] now called *enteropathy-type intestinal T-cell lymphoma*[60] (referred to previously as *enteropathy-associated T-cell lymphoma*[61] and *intestinal T-cell lymphoma*).[62] The cell of origin appears to be the intraepithelial T cell.[58]

CLINICAL FEATURES

Enteropathy-type T-cell lymphoma occurs in adults over a wide age range (20 to 80 years; mean or median age in the 50s or 60s) with a slight male preponderance.[63,64] The development of this lymphoma is closely linked to celiac disease, so that, like celiac disease, it is more prevalent among individuals of European descent (in particular, among those from the United Kingdom, especially Ireland and Wales).[63] Patients with enteropathy-type T-cell lymphoma often have a history of celiac disease, which may be of long or short duration.[63] Strict adherence to a gluten-free diet reportedly substantially diminishes the risk for development of lymphoma. Conversely, poor compliance with a gluten-free diet is associated with a significant risk for development of lymphoma.[65]

A subset of patients with enteropathy-type T-cell lymphoma have no previous history of celiac disease; in

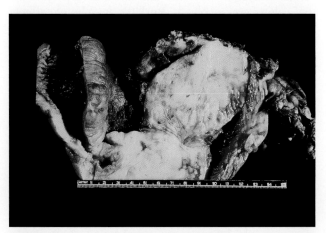

FIGURE 23–10. Burkitt's lymphoma. A large fleshy tumor arises in the ileocecal region.

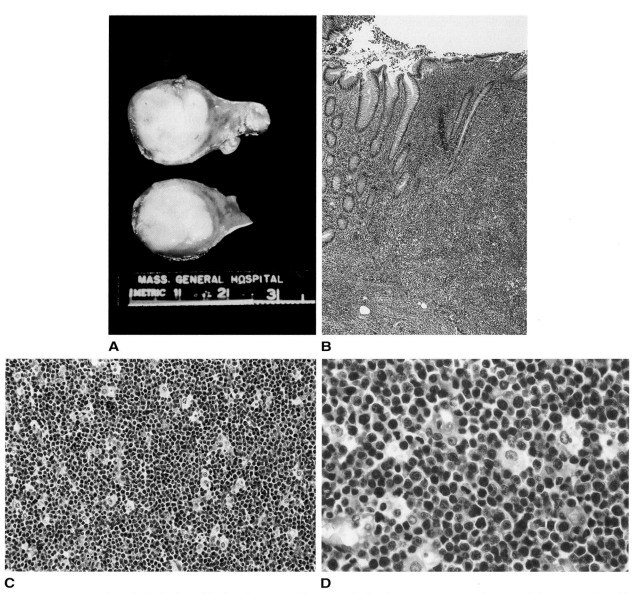

FIGURE 23–11. Atypical Burkitt's/Burkitt's-like lymphoma. **A,** The appendix has been cross-sectioned to reveal that it is replaced by homogeneous white tumor. **B,** A dense, diffuse infiltrate of lymphoid cells involves the appendiceal wall. **C,** A starry-sky pattern is prominent in many areas. **D,** Neoplastic cells are slightly pleomorphic, medium-sized cells with one or more nucleoli and scant to moderate cytoplasm.

some of these cases, histologic evidence of enteropathy is found, suggesting that the patients had subclinical celiac disease. Even when no enteropathy is found, the presence of antibodies to gliadin or endomysium or the HLA phenotype typical of celiac disease (HLA DQA1*0501, DQB1*0201) may be found.[66]

Patients with enteropathy-type T-cell lymphoma present with abdominal pain, weight loss, diarrhea, vomiting, symptoms related to perforation or obstruction, fever, night sweats, or a combination of these findings. Among patients with a history of celiac disease, symptoms often appear to involve worsening of the celiac disease with loss of response to a gluten-free diet.[2,63] Only a small minority have a palpable mass on physical examination, and peripheral lymphadenopathy

is uncommon.[63] Rarely, patients present with evidence of distant spread of disease.[67] The lymphoma affects the jejunum more frequently than the ileum. In some instances, both sites are involved, frequently with involvement of mesenteric lymph nodes. Staging reveals spread in a minority of cases to such sites as the bone marrow or the liver. In the vast majority of cases, lymphoma is confined to the abdomen at the time of presentation. In one series, the Ann Arbor stage was I in 19% of cases, II in 58%, and IV in 23% of cases.[63] Similar results were found in another series: 75% of patients had stage I or II disease.[64]

Among small intestinal lymphomas, enteropathy-type T-cell lymphoma has the worst prognosis.[2] Treatment is complicated by the severe malnutrition that characterizes many of these patients, and fewer than half of patients are able to complete their planned chemotherapeutic regimens.[63,64] Chemotherapy may be complicated by perforation, gastrointestinal bleeding, or sepsis.[63] In one study of 31 patients, 84% died of their lymphoma or of complications of therapy.[63] In another study, median survival was 3 months, and 70% of patients died within 6 months.[64] However, in both of these studies, a few patients treated with chemotherapy were long-term survivors, suggesting that chemotherapy is effective in a subset of cases.[63,64] The perforation associated with intestinal involvement is the most common cause of death, but in some cases, dissemination of disease to lymph nodes and a wide variety of extranodal sites, including liver, spleen, brain, heart, bone marrow, lungs, kidney, thyroid, and other sites, contributes to mortality.[59,63] Unlike B-cell lymphomas, the prognosis for these T-cell lymphomas is independent of the cytology of the neoplastic cells; all behave in an aggressive manner, even when tumor cells are relatively small and uniform.[68]

PATHOLOGIC FEATURES

Within the intestine, lesions may be single or multiple. They take the form of plaques, nodules, or strictures with circumferential ulceration and some-times perforation. Large masses are uncommon (Fig. 23-12).[2,63]

Microscopic examination reveals a dense, diffuse infiltrate of atypical lymphoid cells associated with ulceration and a variable admixture of inflammatory cells, often with many histiocytes. Occasionally, eosinophils are numerous; in such cases, peripheral eosinophilia may be noted.[66] The neoplastic cells may be small, medium-sized, or large and may even have an anaplastic appearance. Careful examination commonly reveals intravascular clusters of tumor cells. Changes of celiac disease, including increased numbers of intraepithelial lymphocytes, villous atrophy, crypt hyperplasia, and a lymphoplasmacytic infiltrate in the lamina propria, are often seen in the mucosa away from the lymphoma (Figs. 23-13 through 15).[42,59,63]

Immunophenotyping shows that neoplastic cells usually express leukocyte common antigen (CD45), cytoplasmic CD3, and CD7 but often lack CD5 and consistently lack CD1 and CD57 (see Fig. 23-13C). CD8 is expressed in some cases, as was noted earlier, but in most cases, both CD4 and CD8 are absent.[61] The T-cell receptor (TCR) α/β receptor is expressed in some cases, indicating origin from α/β T cells. A few cases of γ/δ T-cell origin have been described.[68] CD30 is expressed by some lymphomas with anaplastic morphology, but epithelial membrane antigen (EMA) is

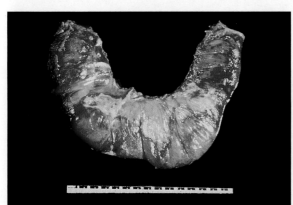

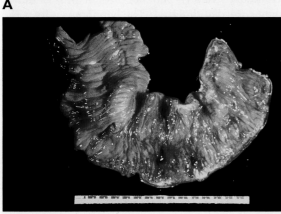

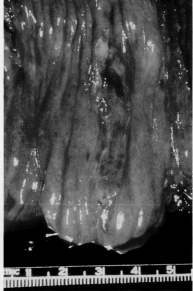

FIGURE 23–12. Enteropathy-type intestinal T-cell lymphoma. **A,** The small intestine is dilated, and its serosal surface is covered by a fibrinopurulent exudate owing to perforation. **B,** The bowel is opened to reveal multiple small ulcerated lesions but no large discrete mass. **C,** Higher power of one of the circumferentially oriented linear ulcers. (**C** Reproduced from Case Records of the Massachusetts General Hospital, Case 53-1987. N Engl J Med 317: 1715–1728, 1987.)

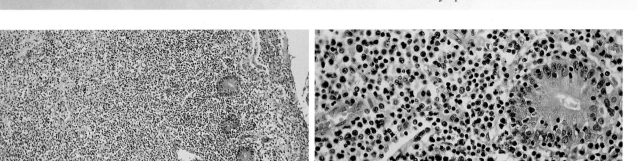

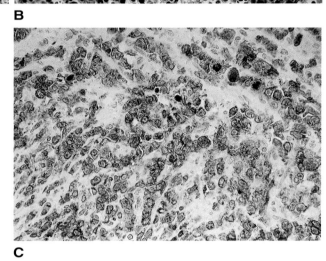

FIGURE 23–13. Enteropathy-associated intestinal T-cell lymphoma. **A,** A diffuse infiltrate of lymphoid cells occupies the bowel wall. **B,** Higher power shows small and medium-sized atypical lymphoid cells. **C,** Neoplastic cells expressed CD3 (immunperoxidase technique on paraffin section).

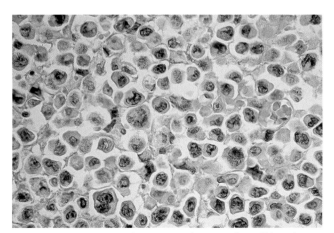

FIGURE 23–14. Enteropathy-associated intestinal T-cell lymphoma. High power shows large bizarre pleomorphic cells; these were positive for CD30 (not shown).

expressed much less often. The neoplastic cells have a cytotoxic phenotype: They express TIA1 and sometimes granzyme B and perforin.[59,61,69] The cytotoxic nature of the neoplastic cells and the intraepithelial cells from which they arise could be responsible for the tissue damage, including villous atrophy, ulceration, and necrosis. In most cases, CD103, the human mucosal lymphocyte antigen (HML-1), is expressed by intestinal intraepithelial lymphocytes and by a subset of lamina propria lymphocytes. Among lymphomas, its expression is nearly unique for enteropathy-type T-cell lymphoma,[70] aside from hairy cell leukemia.

Chott and colleagues have delineated two different types of enteropathy-type T-cell lymphoma based on CD56 expression, and they have identified clinical and pathologic features that correlate with the presence or absence of this antigen.[64] Of the lymphomas, 21% were CD56+; most were composed of a monomorphic population of small to medium-sized cells, but the CD56– lymphomas were usually composed of pleomorphic, medium-sized, or large cells, or anaplastic large cells. The CD56+ cases usually also expressed CD8; the CD56– cases usually lacked both CD4 and CD8. The CD56– cases were more likely to be associated with a history of celiac disease or with histologic features of enteropathy. They also had more conspicuous necrosis and fibrosis and a larger number of admixed inflammatory cells. The CD56– cases have been referred to as *type A*, and the CD56+ cases have been called *type B* (Table 23-3).[64,69]

Molecular genetic studies have shown clonal rearrangement of TCR β and γ chain genes.[64,69,71] No

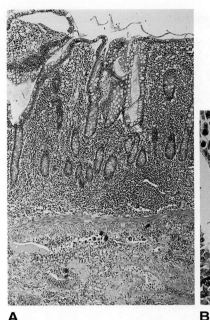

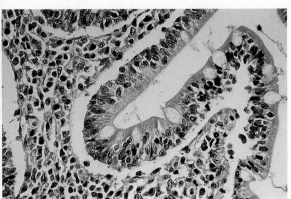

A　　　　　　　　　　**B**

FIGURE 23–15. Enteropathy-type intestinal T-cell lymphoma with changes in surrounding mucosa. **A,** The mucosa shows villous blunting. Tumor cells are seen in the lumen of a small vessel just deep to the muscularis mucosae. **B,** Increased numbers of intraepithelial lymphocytes are seen. The epithelium shows goblet cell loss.

specific cytogenetic abnormality has been recognized. In situ hybridization using probes for Epstein-Barr virus–encoded RNA (EBER) is negative in most European cases, whereas EBV has been detected in all Mexican cases of enteropathy-type T-cell lymphoma in one recent study,[72] as well as among cases arising in immunocompromised patients.

Mesenteric lymph nodes are almost always enlarged, although they are not always involved by lymphoma. In partially involved lymph nodes, the lymphoma may be found in sinuses or in the paracortex.[18] Enlarged nodes free of tumor may show nonspecific reactive changes, edema, or mesenteric lymph node cavitation. In the latter condition, lymph nodes may be markedly enlarged (up to 8 cm) and show cystic change, so that the lymph node consists of thickened capsule and a thin rim of lymphoid tissue surrounding clear or turbid fluid that most likely represents lymph.[73] Mesenteric lymph node cavitation is not specific for enteropathy-type T-cell lymphoma; it may be seen in celiac disease without lymphoma and in refractory sprue. The condition may be related to severe malnutrition. Upon correction of the malnutrition, the lymph node changes may regress; they are reversible with nutritional improvement.[67]

▪ Complicated Celiac Disease: Refractory Sprue and Ulcerative Jejunitis

Refractory sprue and ulcerative jejunitis are serious, potentially fatal complications of celiac disease; they may also be seen in patients with no previous history of celiac disease. Refractory sprue is characterized by

worsening malabsorption and failure to respond to a gluten-free diet. Biopsy shows changes consistent with untreated celiac disease. Ulcerative jejunitis, or ulcerative jejunoileitis, consists of histologically benign mucosal ulcers. Patients with refractory sprue often have ulcerative jejunitis, or vice versa, and either may be associated with enteropathy-type T-cell lymphoma.[58,67]

Normal jejunal intraepithelial lymphocytes are predominantly TCRα/β+, surface CD3 (sCD3)+, CD8+, and CD5dim+. Minor populations also include CD4–, CD8– γ/δ T cells and CD56+ T cells.[64,69] In most patients with refractory sprue, intraepithelial lymphocytes are predominantly sCD3–, cytoplasmic CD3 (cCD3)+, CD4–, and CD8–,[67,69] similar to most enteropathy-type T-cell lymphomas. Molecular genetic analysis has shown that clonal T cells are present in refractory sprue and in ulcerative jejunitis in nearly all cases.[67,69,71,74] In addition, in cases in which lymphoma follows refractory sprue or ulcerative jejunitis, the same clone is found in the lymphoma and in the histologically benign disorders.[71,74]

In one study, some patients with refractory sprue with abnormal intraepithelial lymphocytes had T cells in the peripheral blood with clonal TCR rearrangements identical to those found in the intestine.[67] Patients with normal bowel, other disorders such as Crohn's disease, and celiac disease responsive to a gluten-free diet do not have clonal T cells[67,69,71,74] or increased numbers of CD4–, CD8– T cells.[67,69] Relying solely on increased numbers of CD4–/CD8– T cells to predict the presence of a clonal population of T cells has one pitfall: Enteropathy-type T-cell lymphomas, type B (CD56+, CD8+), do not have an increase in "double-negative" T cells in the surrounding mucosa, but they do have clonal T cells.[69]

TABLE 23–3. Enteropathy-type Intestinal T-Cell Lymphoma and Associated Conditions

Disease	Histology	Immunophenotype	T-Cell Clonality	Prognosis
Celiac disease (untreated)	Increased IELs, villous atrophy, crypt hyperplasia, lymphoplasmacytic infiltrate in lamina propria	IELs: Predominance of CD3+, CD8+, CD103+, TIA-1+ T cells; rare CD4+ cells; rare CD56+ cells; few CD4–/CD8– g/d cells	Polyclonal	Good, with proper diet
Refractory sprue	As for celiac disease	IELs: Predominance of CD3+, CD4–/CD8–, TIA-1+ T cells Lamina propria: Mixture of CD4+ and CD8+ T cells	Almost always monoclonal	Moderately poor; patients may die of malnutrition or may develop lymphoma with same clonal rearrangement as previous refractory sprue
Ulcerative jejunitis	One or more mucosal ulcers with many inflammatory cells	IELs: Predominance of CD3+, CD4-/CD8-, TIA-1+ T cells Ulcer base: Mixture of CD4+ and CD8+ T cells and other inflammatory cells	Monoclonal	Moderately poor; patients may die of malnutrition or perforation, or lymphoma may develop with same clonal rearrangement as previous ulcerative jejunitis
Enteropathy-type intestinal T-cell lymphoma				
Type A	Lymphoma: Medium and large pleomorphic cells or anaplastic large cells	Lymphoma: CD3+, CD4–, CD8–/+, CD103+/–, TIA-1+, CD30+/– cells	Monoclonal	Very poor
	Adjacent mucosa: As for celiac disease	IELs: As for refractory sprue and ulcerative jejunitis	Monoclonal; same clone as the ETITL	
Type B	Lymphoma: Monomorphic medium-sized cells	Lymphoma: CD3+, CD4–, CD8+, CD56+, CD30–, CD103–, TIA-1+	Monoclonal	Very poor
	Adjacent mucosa: As for celiac disease in some; may not show enteropathy	IELs: CD3+, CD4–, CD8+, CD56+ cells	Monoclonal; same clone as the ETITL	

ETITL, enteropathy-type intestinal T-cell lymphoma; IEL, intraepithelial lymphocyte.

This information suggests that refractory sprue and ulcerative jejunitis are neoplastic disorders. Precise classification is difficult, but investigators have suggested that they represent low-grade or cryptic enteropathy-associated T-cell lymphomas.[67] With disease progression, the abnormal T cells may assume the features of an overt, high-grade T-cell lymphoma.[58,67] The optimal treatment for patients with refractory sprue or ulcerative jejunitis is unclear. Most have been treated with a gluten-free diet combined with steroids, other immunosuppressive agents, and/or total parenteral nutrition,[67] but the prognosis remains poor. Treatment with chemotherapy could be considered in certain cases and could possibly prevent progression to overt enteropathy-type T-cell lymphoma (see Table 23-3).

DIFFERENTIAL DIAGNOSIS

Enteropathy-type intestinal T-cell lymphoma usually does not form a large mass, and numerous inflammatory cells may be admixed, obscuring the neoplastic population. These features may lead to diagnosis of an inflammatory ulcer rather than lymphoma. Careful examination of routine sections for atypical cells, augmented by immunohistochemistry, and if necessary molecular genetic studies, should lead to the diagnosis. Any ulcerated lesion occurring in a patient with clinical or histologic evidence of celiac disease should be approached with suspicion.

The differential diagnosis includes diffuse large B-cell lymphoma. In contrast to enteropathy-type T-cell lymphoma, diffuse large B-cell lymphoma tends to be found distally, in the ileum, and is less often multifocal. B-cell lymphomas produce larger, exophytic, or annular masses.[2,61] The villi are normal unless the large B-cell lymphoma has arisen on a background of IPSID. Immunohistochemical studies serve to confirm the diagnosis.

Extranodal natural killer (NK)/T-cell lymphomas occasionally metastasize to the intestine, and lymphomas of this type may even arise in the intestine. The histologic and immunophenotypic features of enteropathy-type T-cell lymphoma overlap with those of extranodal NK/T-cell lymphoma, nasal-type. Features suggesting the latter include CD56 expression, EBV in tumor cells, absence of associated celiac disease, and angiocentric growth. Absence of clonal T cells also provides support for extranodal NK/T-cell lymphoma because most lymphomas in this category are of NK cell origin and do not rearrange their T-cell receptors.

Peripheral T-cell lymphoma of unspecified type may arise in the intestine.[66] The finding of a T-cell lymphoma in the absence of clinical or histologic evidence of enteropathy, antigliadin and antiendomysial antibodies, or human leukocyte antigen (HLA) type associated with celiac disease suggests a diagnosis of peripheral T-cell lymphoma of unspecified type.

Other poorly differentiated malignant tumors such as metastatic melanoma and anaplastic carcinoma may also be considered in the differential diagnosis[61] but are easily distinguished by appropriate immunohisto-chemical panels.

Appendiceal Lymphoma

CLINICAL FEATURES

Appendiceal lymphoma is discussed separately because of its distinctive clinical features. The appendix is a rare primary site for lymphoma. In one series, only 2 of 117 gastrointestinal lymphomas presented with appendiceal involvement.[12] In a series of 27 lymphomas of the colon or appendix, only 1 case of appendiceal lymphoma was found.[75] Lymphoma of the appendix mainly affects children and young adults[75-78]; this is substantially younger than the mean age for lymphoma in other parts of the gastrointestinal tract. There is a slight male preponderance.[78] Almost all patients present with right lower quadrant abdominal pain that mimics acute appendicitis[78]; some have a palpable mass. Most patients have Ann Arbor stage I disease,[75,77-79] although localized disease is important if an appendiceal origin is to be confirmed. Relatively few cases of lymphoma in this site have been studied, but prognosis appears to be good.[78] Patients with low-grade lymphomas have often been treated with resection alone, and patients with higher-grade tumors have usually been

treated with resection combined with radiation or chemotherapy; almost all have remained free of disease at last follow-up.[75-80] It is possible that the favorable outcome is related to the limited nature of the disease in most cases, but lymphoma arising in this site still has a better prognosis than do many other types of gastro-intestinal lymphoma. In most cases, no predisposing factors are known.

PATHOLOGIC FEATURES

The most common type of appendiceal lymphoma is diffuse large cell lymphoma, followed by Burkitt's lymphoma and lymphomas classified as well-differen-tiated lymphocytic type (see Fig. 23-11). In a few cases of large cell lymphoma, B lineage was demonstrated.[6,77] One case of extranodal marginal zone B-cell lymphoma has been reported,[77] and it is possible that cases classified as the well-differentiated lymphocytic type are also marginal zone lymphomas. One case of peripheral T-cell lymphoma has been described[76]; in this case, the diagnosis was confirmed with immunophenotyping and molecular genetic analysis.

Hodgkin's Disease of the Gastrointestinal Tract

The gastrointestinal tract is rarely the primary site for Hodgkin's disease. Less than 0.5% of cases of Hodgkin's disease arise in the gastrointestinal tract.[81] Because of the rarity of Hodgkin's disease in this location, strict criteria for its diagnosis should be used, including (1) absence of peripheral and mediastinal lymph-adenopathy, (2) absence of substantial hepatic or splenic disease, or peripheral blood involvement, (3) predominant gastrointestinal disease, with or without involvement of adjacent lymph nodes, and (4) histologic and immunohistologic features characteristic of Hodgkin's disease.

CLINICAL FEATURES

The disease appears to affect adults over a broad age range, with a male preponderance. In the general population, the sites involved, in descending order, are stomach, small intestine, and colon. A number of patients have had inflammatory bowel disease, almost always Crohn's disease, often for many years, treated with immunosuppressive therapy.[81-83] Hodgkin's disease affects the small intestine, colon, or both in cases as-sociated with inflammatory bowel disease. On occasion, some other form of underlying immunologic abnor-mality or inflammatory condition is found.[81,84] Patients with gastric or duodenal tumors present with upper abdominal pain and have nonhealing ulcers.[85] Those with intestinal tumors have hematochezia, pain, nausea, vomiting, diarrhea, or symptoms related to perforation. In patients with Crohn's disease, the symptoms may resemble exacerbation of the underlying disease.[81,82]

Although by convention the bulk of the tumor is found in the gastrointestinal tract at presentation, staging often reveals regional nodal involvement[82,85] and sometimes foci of distant spread.[81] Patients have a favorable prognosis with good response to therapy in most cases.[81-85]

PATHOLOGIC FEATURES

The tumor tends to involve the full thickness of the bowel wall multifocally, usually resulting in ulceration.[81,83,85] In Crohn's disease patients, preferential involvement of areas with fissures and preexisting severe inflammation is noted.[81,83] Mixed cellularity and nodular sclerosis subtypes have been reported. Immunophenotyping shows that Reed-Sternberg cells and variants are CD15+, CD30+, focally CD20+ or CD20–, CD3–,[81-84,86] CD79a–, and CD45–,[81] typical of Hodgkin's disease elsewhere. Neoplastic cells have been consistently positive for EBV with the use of in situ hybridization[81,83] and immunohistochemistry for latent membrane protein in the small number of cases that have been tested.[81] The neoplastic cells in two cases in patients with Crohn's disease receiving immunosuppressive medication were isolated by means of laser capture microdissection; in both, rearranged immunoglobulin genes were found, consistent with B-cell origin. In one case with stage III disease, a dominant clonal band was found, but in the other, a stage Ie case in which there were small foci of tumor confined to the bowel associated with areas of lymphoid hyperplasia, a polyclonal pattern was detected. The results in these two cases suggest that Hodgkin's disease in immunocompromised patients may show molecular progression, analogous to other immunodeficiency-associated B-cell lymphoproliferative disorders.

In two cases, Hodgkin's disease has been reported to be a component of a composite lymphoma. In one gastric case, the composite lymphoma consisted of Hodgkin's disease and diffuse large B-cell lymphoma. Perigastric lymph nodes contained low-grade follicular lymphoma.[85] In the second, a patient with Crohn's disease developed an ileal composite lymphoma consisting of Hodgkin's disease of the nodular sclerosis type and an anaplastic large cell lymphoma, although detailed immunophenotyping was not performed on the anaplastic large cell lymphoma.[82]

The occurrence of Hodgkin's disease in areas of inflamed bowel suggests that the tumor is pathogenetically related to the chronic inflammatory process. The history of azathioprine or prednisone therapy in most cases and the presence of EBV suggest that immunosuppression plays a role in the genesis of Hodgkin's disease in this setting.[81]

DIFFERENTIAL DIAGNOSIS

The main entity in the differential diagnosis of gastrointestinal Hodgkin's disease is non-Hodgkin's lymphoma. Some cases originally diagnosed as Hodgkin's disease in this site have been classified on review as non-Hodgkin's lymphoma.[85,87] Anaplastic carcinoma may also enter the differential diagnosis. It should be possible to distinguish the two tumors on routine sections, but if immunohistochemistry is employed, it should be noted that, as with Reed-Sternberg cells, gastric carcinoma may be CD15+ and CD45–. An immunohistochemical panel that includes cytokeratin helps in establishing a diagnosis.

■ Gastrointestinal Lymphoma in Abnormal Immune States

HUMAN IMMUNE DEFICIENCY VIRUS INFECTION

Non-Hodgkin's lymphoma is the second most common malignancy in HIV+ patients, following Kaposi's sarcoma. The risk of lymphoma is 50 to 60 times greater than that for individuals without HIV infection.[88,89] Although the frequency of Kaposi's sarcoma and opportunistic infection has decreased dramatically with the advent of highly active antiretroviral therapy (HAART), the incidence of lymphoma shows a less striking decrease. The frequency of lymphoma appears to decrease over time for HIV-positive patients on HAART.[88] The proportion of extranodal lymphomas is higher than in the general population, and the gastrointestinal tract is the extranodal site most often affected, with about one third of all HIV-associated non-Hodgkin's lymphomas arising in this site.[89] Patients are almost all young or middle-aged, homosexual men with a median age of 34[90] and 42[89] in different series. The frequency of lymphoma in different parts of the gastrointestinal tract is the opposite of that in HIV-negative patients: The colon and anorectal area are most often affected, followed by the small intestine, with the stomach least often involved.[89] Grossly, the lymphomas have the appearance of ulcers, masses, or fistulas; the appearance may mimic inflammatory or infectious conditions.

Lymphomas are usually confined to the gastrointestinal tract[89] and are almost all high-grade B-cell lymphomas; diffuse large B-cell lymphoma, often of immunoblastic type, is most common, followed by Burkitt's and Burkitt's-like lymphoma and polymorphous high-grade B-cell lymphoma (see Fig. 23-6). Almost all anorectal cases tested have been EBV+ by in situ hybridization.[90] Rare cases of *H. pylori*+ gastric marginal zone B-cell lymphoma have been reported.[91] Several cases of human herpesvirus 8 (HHV-8)+ large cell lymphoma with features similar to those seen in primary effusion lymphoma have presented with intestinal involvement in HIV+ patients. In two of these patients, lymphomatous effusions later developed.[92,93] The lymphomas can be treated with surgery and chemotherapy, but the prognosis is poor, with many patients dying from lymphoma or other complications of HIV infection.[88,89] It is suggested that the high proportion of anorectal lymphomas may be due to repeated trauma and chronic inflammation with uncontrolled proliferation of EBV+ B cells.[90] In summary, gastrointestinal lymphoma in HIV+ patients affects younger individuals and a higher proportion of male patients, shows preferential involvement of the distal gastrointestinal tract, is more often of high grade, and is more often EBV+ compared with lymphoma in the general population.[89,90]

IATROGENIC IMMUNE SUPPRESSION IN TRANSPLANT RECIPIENTS

Allograft recipients have an increased risk of lymphoproliferative disorders compared with the general population. The post-transplantation lymphoproliferative disorders (PTLDs) have features that differ from those of lymphoma in the nonimmunosuppressed population. PTLDs are characterized by heterogeneous pathologic features, strong association with EBV, variable response to therapy, and an often unpredictable clinical course. The median interval from transplantation to PTLD is typically short, with PTLD often occurring within 6 months in cyclosporine-treated patients. However, PTLD may occur at any time, sometimes many years after transplant. Patients may respond to decreased levels of immunosuppression or may require surgical resection, chemotherapy, and/or radiation. The prognosis is guarded; many patients succumb to PTLD. The risk of PTLD is higher among nonrenal allograft recipients, patients receiving higher levels of immunosuppressive therapy, and patients seronegative for EBV before transplant. Many cases arise in extranodal locations; among patients receiving cyclosporine, the proportion of PTLDs arising in the gastrointestinal tract is particularly high. Up to approximately one third of PTLDs in the setting of cyclosporine-based immunosuppression present with involvement of the gastrointestinal tract. The small intestine is affected more often than the stomach or colon.[94]

In the WHO classification, PTLDs are classified as (1) early lesions, (2) polymorphic PTLDs, (3) monomorphic PTLDs, including plasmacytoma-like lesions,

or (4) Hodgkin's lymphoma/Hodgkin's disease–like lesions.[95] Early lesions resemble lymphoid infiltrates seen in infectious mononucleosis or plasmacytic hyperplasia. They are usually polyclonal, EBV+ B-cell proliferations. Polymorphic PTLDs produce destructive mass lesions and show the full range of B-cell differentiation with lymphocytes, plasma cells, immunoblasts, plasmablasts, and cells resembling follicle center cells (Fig. 23-16). Immunophenotyping reveals B cells expressing either polytypic or monotypic Ig, but genetic studies almost always show clonal B cells infected with EBV. Most cases of monomorphic PTLD have morphologic, immunophenotypic, and genetic features of diffuse large B-cell lymphoma (Fig. 23-17); occasional cases resemble Burkitt's lymphoma or T-cell lymphoma. Monomorphic PTLDs of B lineage are usually EBV+. Plasmacytoma-like and Hodgkin's lymphoma/Hodgkin's disease–like lesions are rare. The polymorphic and monomorphic PTLDs of B lineage are those most likely to be encountered in the gastrointestinal tract.[94-96] A few cases of EBV-negative gastric marginal zone B-cell lymphoma have also been described in allograft recipients (Fig. 23-18).[32,91]

INFLAMMATORY BOWEL DISEASE

Non-Hodgkin's lymphoma is a rare complication of ulcerative colitis. In one series of 117 gastrointestinal lymphomas, one arose in a patient with ulcerative colitis.[12] In series of colorectal lymphoma, from 3% to 15% of cases occurred in ulcerative colitis patients.[8,11,75] Although the risk of lymphoma in ulcerative colitis patients is only slightly increased,[97] lymphoma in this setting does have characteristic features, suggesting it is a distinct entity. Compared with other colonic lymphomas, the lymphomas are more often multiple

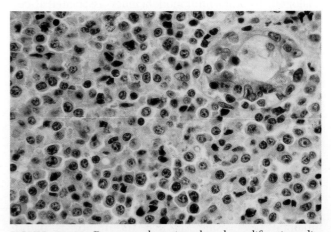

FIGURE 23–16. Post-transplantation lymphoproliferative disorder, polymorphous. This intestinal tumor is composed of a mixture of small and large lymphoid cells, many with plasmacytoid features.

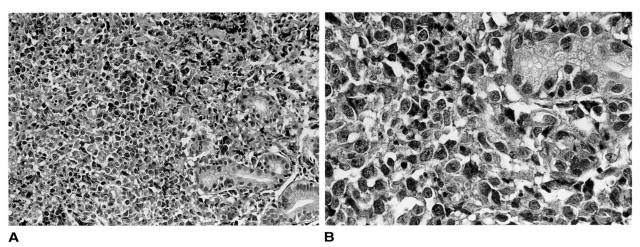

A   **B**

FIGURE 23–17. Post-transplantation lymphoproliferative disorder, monomorphous, involving the stomach. The histologic features are indistinguishable from those of sporadic gastric diffuse large B-cell lymphoma. **A,** Medium power. **B,** High power.

(38% compared with 10% in the general population) and more often distally located in the colon, in contrast to the preferential involvement of the cecum seen without ulcerative colitis.[75,98,99] The lymphomas are almost always found in sites of active inflammation in patients with long-standing ulcerative colitis (mean interval of 12 years to development of lymphoma).[98] In a recent report, the incidence of lymphoma appeared to be increased and the interval to lymphoma appeared decreased (3.1 years) in ulcerative colitis patients treated with immunosuppressive therapy, compared with cases in older reports.[100] This suggests that the immunosuppressive therapy accelerated the development of lymphoma in these susceptible patients. The lymphomas are usually of high grade, and they are often of diffuse large B-cell type.[12,75,100] Rare cases are low- or high-grade polymorphic B-cell lymphomas (possibly of marginal zone type with or without large cell transformation)[87] or marginal zone B-cell lymphomas.[98]

Most are confined to the intestine. Behavior varies according to the grade of the lymphoma. A handful of cases of non-Hodgkin's lymphoma have also been reported in patients with Crohn's disease.[87,100]

X-LINKED LYMPHOPROLIFERATIVE DISORDER

X-linked lymphoproliferative disorder is a rare, X-linked recessive disorder affecting young boys and characterized by a selective immunodeficiency for EBV. Upon exposure to EBV, these children develop severe, often fatal, infectious mononucleosis or malignant lymphoma. Lymphomas affect the gastrointestinal tract in 76% of cases; the ileocecal area is most often affected. They are B-lineage lymphomas that can be classified as Burkitt's lymphoma or diffuse large B-cell lymphoma. Upon testing, EBV has been found in the lymphomas.[101-103]

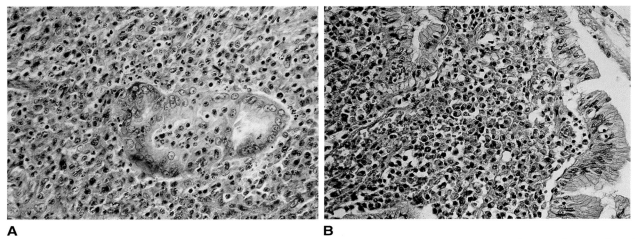

A   **B**

FIGURE 23–18. Gastric marginal zone B-cell lymphoma in a renal allograft recipient. **A,** A diffuse infiltrate of marginal zone cells with lymphoepithelial lesion formation is seen. **B,** The lymphoma shows marked plasmacytic differentiation.

COMMON VARIABLE IMMUNE DEFICIENCY

Common variable immune deficiency (CVID) is typically an adult-onset immunodeficiency syndrome characterized by decreased levels of one or more classes of immunoglobulin and susceptibility to a variety of infections, including *Giardia*. Patients have an increased risk of neoplasia, the most common of which is non-Hodgkin's lymphoma. Rare cases of small intestinal lymphoma, usually of diffuse large B-cell type, have been reported in CVID patients in a background of nodular lymphoid hyperplasia.[104,105]

◼ Miscellaneous Rare Gastrointestinal Lymphomas

Rare cases of other types of lymphoma, including four small intestinal CD30+ T-lineage anaplastic large cell lymphomas, one of which was ALK+,[106] and a rectal anaplastic large cell lymphoma that was CD30+, EMA+, CD45+, and B- and T-cell antigen–negative,[107] have been reported. Cases of primary gastric T-cell lymphoma, including two that were EBV+ and one that was human T-cell lymphotrophic virus (HTLV-I)+, were described in reports from the Far East.[49,108]

◼ Hepatic Lymphoma

PRIMARY HEPATIC LYMPHOMA

Clinical Features

The liver is commonly involved in non-Hodgkin's lymphoma and Hodgkin's disease in cases of widespread disease. Primary hepatic lymphoma—lymphoma arising in and confined to, or nearly entirely confined to, the liver—is an uncommon but well-documented entity that is often associated with an underlying immunologic abnormality. Some authors have suggested that this type of lymphoma has been increasing in frequency,[109,110] although it is also possible that more cases of primary hepatic lymphoma are being recognized. Indeed, in many earlier reports, the diagnosis was made at autopsy.[109] Most cases occur in middle-aged and older adults, but occasional cases in young adults and rare cases in children have been reported. Patients' ages have ranged from 7 to 87, with a median age in the sixth decade. The male-to-female ratio is 2:1 to 3:1. Patients present with right upper quadrant or epigastric pain, nausea, vomiting, anorexia, and/or weakness.

On physical examination, hepatomegaly or a palpable mass is often detected. About half of patients have systemic symptoms (fever, night sweats, or weight loss), but in only a minority is jaundice noted.[111-113] In a few cases of marginal zone B-cell type, the lymphoma was an incidental finding during abdominal surgery per-

formed for other reasons.[114] Lactate dehydrogenase (LDH) is frequently elevated, as are hepatic transaminases; however, alpha-fetoprotein (AFP) and carcinoembryonic antigen (CEA) levels are generally normal or only slightly elevated.[111,115,116]

In up to 40% of cases, patients have some other significant disease, often immune deficiency or chronic stimulation of the immune system.[109,115] These disorders include HIV infection; hepatitis B or hepatitis C virus infection, sometimes associated with chronic active hepatitis, cirrhosis, or hepatocellular carcinoma; iatrogenic immunosuppression in transplant recipients; systemic lupus erythematosus; Felty's syndrome (severe rheumatoid arthritis, neutropenia, and splenomegaly); autoimmune hemolytic anemia; immune thrombocytopenic purpura; primary biliary cirrhosis; previous Hodgkin's disease; active tuberculosis; and others.[109,110,113,115,117-123] Patients who have HIV infection, in contrast to those who are HIV-negative, are younger and are almost exclusively males.[117]

Among the small group of patients with low-grade primary hepatic lymphoma for whom follow-up information is available, some have remained disease-free following resection alone; others have died of unrelated causes.[114,121,124,125] Among patients with intermediate- and high-grade lymphoma, the prognosis is relatively good, with mortality related to complications of surgery or therapy, as well as to progressive disease. In one review of primary hepatic lymphoma, 2-year survival was estimated to be 66%. No patient who survived for 2 years or longer died of lymphoma.[115] Among HIV+ patients, the outcome is worse, with mortality greater than 60%.[110,117]

Pathologic Features

In approximately 70% of cases, the lymphoma forms a large solitary mass. In about 25%, multiple nodules show some tendency to confluence. In about 5% of cases, diffuse hepatic enlargement is seen without a discrete mass.[109,111,115] More than half of the lymphomas are diffuse large B-cell type. The remainder include cases classified as small noncleaved cell lymphoma, extranodal marginal zone B-cell lymphoma, lymphoplasmacytic lymphoma, follicular lymphoma, and peripheral T-cell lymphoma.[109-113,116,118,120,123,124] Almost all lymphomas in HIV+ patients have been of the diffuse large B-cell or small noncleaved cell type.[117] Large B-cell lymphomas are frequently extensively necrotic.[109,111,113] Sclerosis is infrequent. Lymphomas with diffuse hepatic enlargement may show prominent sinusoidal involvement (Fig. 23-19).[111] Marginal zone lymphomas have histologic features similar to those seen in other sites, including the presence of marginal zone cells, monocytoid B cells, reactive follicles, and lymphoepithelial lesions formed with bile duct epi-

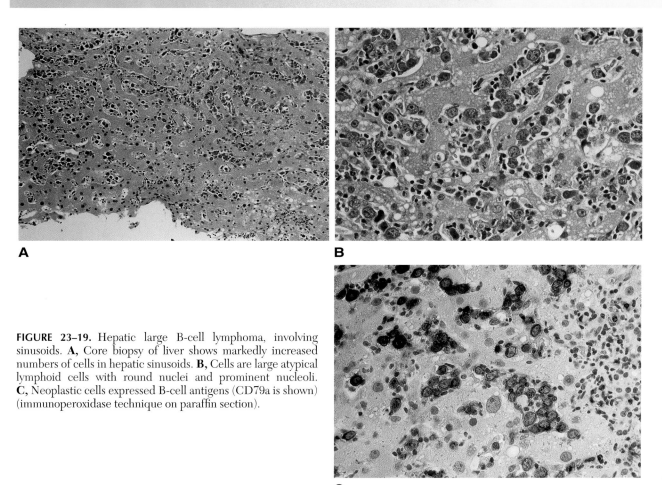

FIGURE 23–19. Hepatic large B-cell lymphoma, involving sinusoids. **A,** Core biopsy of liver shows markedly increased numbers of cells in hepatic sinusoids. **B,** Cells are large atypical lymphoid cells with round nuclei and prominent nucleoli. **C,** Neoplastic cells expressed B-cell antigens (CD79a is shown) (immunoperoxidase technique on paraffin section).

thelium. The marginal zone B cells markedly expand the portal tracts, form intersecting broad serpiginous bands entrapping nodules of hepatocytes, and in some areas, form a diffuse, confluent infiltrate.[114,121,125]

Immunohistochemical features are similar to those seen in other anatomic sites. The large B-cell lymphomas express CD45 and CD20. The marginal zone lymphomas express CD20 and often have a component of plasma cells expressing monotypic cIg. In one case of lymphoplasmacytic lymphoma and in another of marginal zone B-cell lymphoma, patients had monoclonal serum proteins that disappeared postoperatively.[114,124]

Differential Diagnosis

The finding of one or more hepatic lesions raises the question of primary or metastatic carcinoma. The combination of a high LDH and normal CEA and AFP levels, particularly in an immunocompromised patient, may raise the question of lymphoma, but histologic examination is required for a diagnosis to be established.[113,115] In some cases, the differential diagnosis based on histologic features includes poorly differentiated carcinoma,[111] but careful examination of routine

sections and judicious use of immunohistochemical studies are generally sufficient for establishing a diagnosis.

HEPATOSPLENIC γδ T-CELL LYMPHOMA

Clinical Features

Hepatosplenic γδ T-cell lymphoma is a recently described type of lymphoma with distinctive clinical and pathologic features. In contrast to cases included under the category of primary hepatic lymphoma, hepatosplenic γδ T-cell lymphoma typically involves liver, spleen, and bone marrow. Most patients are adolescents or young adult males, with a median age of 25 years.[126] Some are immunosuppressed; this type of lymphoma has been reported in transplant recipients.[127] Patients present with abdominal pain and often have fever, night sweats, or weight loss. The liver and spleen are diffusely enlarged, often strikingly, without conspicuous peripheral lymphadenopathy. The bone marrow is usually involved. Patients may have peripheral blood cytopenias, especially anemia and thrombocytopenia. Circulating tumor cells may be found at presentation, but in some cases, patients develop a leukemic picture late in the course of the disease. Some patients respond to chemotherapy initially, but most have progressive disease with a median survival of 10 months.[126,128-130]

Pathologic Features

The neoplastic cells preferentially involve hepatic sinusoids and splenic red pulp. Neoplastic cells in the marrow are often confined to vascular sinuses and may be inconspicuous on routinely stained sections. Lymphoma may also infiltrate the interstitium of the marrow, and rarely, it forms nodular aggregates or shows diffuse involvement. Immunostains for T cells may be helpful in highlighting abnormal cells in an apparently normal marrow. When lymph nodes are involved, tumor cells tend to be found in sinuses. Neoplastic cells are of medium size (occasionally large) and tend to have oval nuclei with fine chromatin and abundant pale cytoplasm (Fig. 23-20**A** and **B**).[126, 128-130]

Immunohistochemical analysis typically shows CD2+, CD3+, CD5–/+, CD4–, CD8–/+, CD7+/–, γδTCR+, αβTCR– T cells that express the cytotoxic granule–associated protein T-cell intracellular antigen-1 (TIA-1) (Fig. 23-20**C**). Other cytotoxic molecules (granzyme and perforin) are uncommonly detected. Occasionally, NK-associated antigens such as CD16 or CD56 are expressed. Molecular genetic analysis shows clonal T-cell receptor gene rearrangement. The T cells are of the Vδ1 subset.[127] The most common cytogenetic abnormalities include isochromosome 7q and trisomy 8.[127]

HEPATOSPLENIC αβ T-CELL LYMPHOMA

After the recognition of hepatosplenic γδ T-cell lymphoma, cases with similar features, but expressing the αβTCR, were identified. Comparison with the γδ cases shows that the αβ cases have a female preponderance (M/F ratio, 1:4) and affect patients over a wider age range, including children and older adults, with a slightly older median age (36 years). The lymphoma, like the γδ type, is aggressive and carries a poor prognosis. Median survival in one series was less than 6 months. Pathologic features are similar, except that in a minority of cases, hepatic involvement is periportal as well as sinusoidal.[126] A few cases have been positive for EBV.[126] Both αβ and γδ varieties are included in the WHO classification as hepatosplenic T-cell lymphoma.[127a]

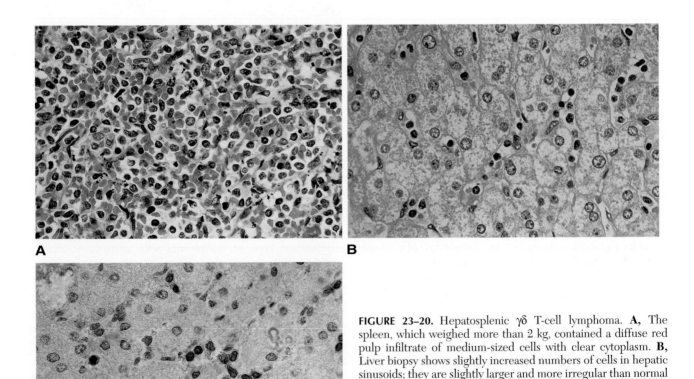

FIGURE 23–20. Hepatosplenic γδ T-cell lymphoma. **A,** The spleen, which weighed more than 2 kg, contained a diffuse red pulp infiltrate of medium-sized cells with clear cytoplasm. **B,** Liver biopsy shows slightly increased numbers of cells in hepatic sinusoids; they are slightly larger and more irregular than normal lymphocytes. **C,** Like the atypical cells in the spleen, they expressed CD3 (immunoperoxidase technique on paraffin section).

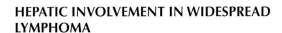

HEPATIC INVOLVEMENT IN WIDESPREAD LYMPHOMA

Some types of lymphoma have characteristic patterns of hepatic involvement, even though they are not confined to the liver at presentation. Diffuse large B-cell lymphoma, for example, most often involves the liver in the form of tumor nodules, with little residual normal parenchyma; it may also predominantly involve the portal tracts with or without sinusoidal infiltration. T cell/histiocyte-rich large B-cell lymphoma (THRBCL), a subtype of diffuse large B-cell lymphoma, often involves the liver and spleen at presentation. In the liver, THRBCL has a characteristic appearance with irregular expansion of the portal tracts by an infiltrate of small lymphocytes, histiocytes, and occasional neoplastic large atypical lymphoid cells, with little or no spread into sinusoids. Other findings include loss of bile ducts in the infiltrate, necrosis or steatosis of hepatocytes adjacent to the lymphoma, bile stasis, and sinusoidal dilatation. Neoplastic cells may be inconspicuous, and the reactive lymphohistiocytic component may damage adjacent parenchyma in a pattern reminiscent of piecemeal necrosis, so that THRBCL may be mistaken for chronic active hepatitis. The combination of large tumor cells in a mixed reactive background may suggest Hodgkin's disease. Immunophenotyping is helpful in establishing a diagnosis by demonstrating CD20+ large B cells in a background of T cells and histiocytes.[131]

Follicular lymphomas show predominantly portal involvement. Hodgkin's disease tends to predominantly involve the portal tracts but may also form solid nodules.[131]

Lymphoma of the Gallbladder

CLINICAL FEATURES

Rare cases of primary lymphoma of the gallbladder have been reported.[132-137] In one series of 54 patients with gastrointestinal lymphoma, only 1 case arose in the gallbladder.[3] Most patients are older adults, with both males and females affected. One patient had a history of HIV infection,[138] and a few have had gallstones.[133,137] Patients present with symptoms that often mimic cholecystitis, cholelithiasis, or choledocholithiasis, such as right upper quadrant pain, nausea, vomiting, or rarely, jaundice.[132]

Follow-up information is available in few cases. Two patients with marginal zone lymphoma were well 6 months and 1 year postoperatively with no additional therapy.[136,137] One patient with diffuse large B-cell lymphoma was alive at 18 months with progressive disease despite combined-modality therapy,[134] and one patient with localized high-grade B-cell lymphoma died of sepsis in the perioperative period.[135]

The cause of lymphoma of the gallbladder is not known, but it has been suggested that lymphomas of the extranodal marginal zone type may arise from chronic follicular cholecystitis, analogous to the pathogenesis of gastric marginal zone B-cell lymphoma.[133,137]

PATHOLOGIC FEATURES

Gross examination of the gallbladder usually shows mural thickening or one or more discrete nodules.[133,134,136] The lymphomas are usually diffuse large B-cell[134] or extranodal marginal zone type.[132,133,136,137]

Lymphoma of the Extrahepatic Biliary Tract

Lymphoma may on occasion involve lymph nodes in the porta hepatis and may compress the extrahepatic biliary tree, resulting in jaundice. Lymphoma arising primarily from the extrahepatic biliary tree is a rare phenomenon; only 13 cases have been reported over the past 20 years. Patients with lymphoma of the biliary tree present with obstructive jaundice, and clinical and radiographic features often suggest carcinoma or sclerosing cholangitis. The lymphomas have been classified according to a variety of different systems, making interpretation of pathology difficult; however, diffuse large B-cell lymphoma appears to be more common than any other type.[139,140]

Pancreatic Lymphoma

CLINICAL FEATURES

Pancreatic lymphoma is a rare disorder, accounting for less than 0.2% of pancreatic malignancies[141] and less than 0.7% of non-Hodgkin's lymphomas.[142] Many of the tumors classified as pancreatic lymphoma involve adjacent structures or show nodal involvement at presentation, and origin from the pancreas is inferred because the bulk of the tumor involves the pancreas. The lymphomas are sometimes confined to the pancreas.[143,143a]

Patients are adults with ages ranging from the third to the ninth decade; the median age is 50 years and the male-to-female ratio is approximately 2:1.[143-150] One patient was HIV-positive,[145] but with this exception, patients have not had conditions that predispose to the development of lymphoma. They present with complaints of abdominal pain, anorexia, nausea, vomiting, weight loss, or malaise, or a combination of these findings.[143,143a,146-151]

On physical examination, patients are often jaundiced, and occasionally, they have a palpable mass.[143,143a,146,147]

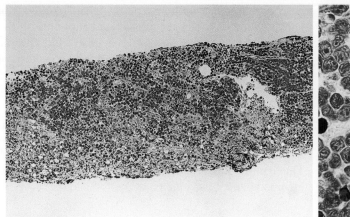

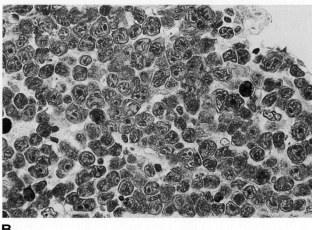

A   **B**

FIGURE 23–21. Pancreatic large B-cell lymphoma. **A,** A needle core biopsy of a pancreatic mass shows a diffuse infiltrate of lymphoid cells. **B,** Higher power shows a monotonous population of large lymphoid cells. Immunohistochemistry demonstrated their B-cell nature, and flow cytometric analysis confirmed the presence of a monotypic population of B cells (data not shown). (**A** and **B**, Giemsa.)

Because signs and symptoms are so similar to those of the much more common pancreatic adenocarcinoma, patients have often undergone laparotomy and resection of tumor; more recently, the trend has been toward making a diagnosis on computed tomography (CT)-guided percutaneous biopsy. The prognosis is difficult to assess because most information is found in individual case reports, and patients have not been treated uniformly. However, more than 50% of patients have succumbed to their lymphoma.[143a]

PATHOLOGIC FEATURES

Tumors take the form of large masses (generally greater than 6 cm) involving the head, body, or tail of the pancreas, or the entire pancreas. Lesions are often cystic or have central necrosis. Invasion into adjacent structures and involvement of abdominal lymph nodes may occur.[143,144,146-150]

Cases reported have been classified according to a variety of classification systems, but most appear to be diffuse large cell lymphomas (Fig. 23-21); a few cases have been classified as small noncleaved cell lymphoma,[145] and one has been classified as marginal zone B-cell lymphoma.[144] Immunophenotyping has been reported in relatively few cases. The lymphomas have almost always been B-lineage tumors,[143a,145,146,150] although T-cell lymphoma has also been reported.[143a,148]

DIFFERENTIAL DIAGNOSIS

Clinically, pancreatic lymphoma may mimic pancreatic adenocarcinoma. On endoscopic retrograde cholangiopancreatography, lymphoma may compress or distort ductal structures, but generally, it does not invade their walls (in contrast to carcinoma).[143] Tissue for pathologic examination establishes the diagnosis.

References

1. Crump M, Gospodarowicz M, Shepherd F: Lymphoma of the gastrointestinal tract. Semin Oncol 26:324-337, 1999.
2. Domizio P, Owen R, Shepherd N, et al: Primary lymphoma of the small intestine. Am J Surg Pathol 17:429-442, 1993.
3. Au E, Ang P, Tan P, et al: Gastrointestinal lymphoma—a review of 54 patients in Singapore. Ann Acad Med Singapore 26:758-761, 1997.
4. Hansen P, Vogt K, Skov R, et al: Primary gastrointestinal non-Hodgkin's lymphoma in adults: A population based clinical and histopathologic study. Intern Med 244:71-78, 1998.
5. Yoshino T, Miyake K, Ichimura K, et al: Increased incidence of follicular lymphoma in the duodenum. Am J Surg Pathol 24:688-693, 2000.
6. Kojima M, Nakamura S, Kurabayashi Y, et al: Primary malignant lymphoma of the intestine: Clinicopathologic and immuno-histochemical studies of 39 cases. Pathol Int 45:123-130, 1995.
7. Chan J: Gastrointestinal lymphomas: An overview with emphasis on new findings and diagnostic problems. Semin Diagn Pathol 13:260-296, 1996.
8. Fan C-W, Changchien C, Wang J-Y, et al: Primary colorectal lymphoma. Dis Colon Rectum 43:1277-1282, 2000.
9. Smith D, Cataldo P: Perianal lymphoma in a heterosexual and nonimmunocompromised patient: Report of a case and review of the literature. Dis Colon Rectum 42:952-954, 1999.
10. Nakamura S, Matsumoto T, Takeshita M, et al: A clinicopathologic study of primary small intestine lymphoma: Prognostic significance of mucosa-associated lymphoid tissue-derived lymphoma. Cancer 88:286-294, 2000.
11. Shepherd N, Hall P, Coates P, et al: Primary malignant lymphoma of the colon and rectum. A histopathological and immunohisto-chemical analysis of 45 cases with clinicopathological correlations. Histopathology 12:235-252, 1988.
12. Lewin K, Ranchod M, Dorfman R: Lymphomas of the gastro-intestinal tract. Cancer 42:693-707, 1978.
13. Liu H, Ruskon-Fourmesstraux A, Lavergne-Slove A, et al: Resistance of t(11;18) + gastric mucosa-associated lymphoid tissue lymphoma to *Helicobacter pylori* eradication therapy. Lancet 357:39-40, 2001.
14. Ferreri A, Freschi M, Dell'Oro S, et al: Prognostic significance of the histopathologic recognition of low- and high-grade components in stage I-II B-cell gastric lymphomas. Am J Surg Pathol 25:95-102, 2001.
15. Takeshita M, Iwashita A, Kurihara K, et al: Histologic and immuno-histologic findings and prognosis of 40 cases of gastric large B-cell lymphoma. Am J Surg Pathol 24:1641-1649, 2000.
16. Yoshino T, Omonishi K, Kobayashi K, et al: Clinicopathological features of gastric mucosa associated lymphoid tissue (MALT)

lymphoma: High grade transformation and comparison with diffuse large B-cell lymphomas without MALT lymphoma features. Clin Pathol 53:187-190, 2000.

17. Yokoi T, Nakamura T, Kasugai K, et al: Primary low-grade gastric mucosa-associated lymphoid tissue (MALT) lymphoma with polypoid appearance. Polypoid gastric MALT lymphoma: A clinicopathologic study of eight cases. Pathol Int 49:702-709, 1999.

18. Isaacson P: Gastrointestinal lymphoma. Hum Pathol 25:1020-1029, 1994.

19. Hsi E, Eisbruch A, Greenson J, et al: Classification of primary gastric lymphomas according to histologic features. Am J Surg Pathol 22:17-27, 1998.

20. Fung C, Grossbard M, Linggood R, et al: Mucosa-associated lymphoid tissue lymphoma of the stomach: Long term outcome after local treatment. Cancer 85:9-17, 1999.

21. Zucca E, Bertoni F, Roggero E, et al: The gastric marginal zone B-cell lymphoma of MALT type. Blood 96:410-419, 2000.

22. Du M, Xu C, Diss T, et al: Intestinal dissemination of gastric mucosa-associated lymphoid tissue lymphoma. Blood 88:4445-4451, 1996.

23. Van Krieken J, Hoeve M: Epidemiological and prognostic aspects of gastric malt-lymphoma. Cancer Res 156:4-8, 2000.

24. Wotherspoon A, Doglioni C, Diss T, et al: Regression of primary low-grade B-cell gastric lymphoma of mucosa-associated lymphoid tissue type after eradication of *Helicobacter pylori*. Lancet 342:575-577, 1993.

25. Thiede C, Wundisch T, Alpen B, et al: Long-term persistence of monoclonal B-cells after cure of *Helicobacter pylori* infection and complete histologic remission in gastric mucosa-associated lymphoid tissue B-cell lymphoma. J Clin Oncol 19:1600-1609, 2001.

26. de Jong D, Boot H, Taal B: Histological grading with clinical relevance in gastric mucosa-associated lymphoid tissue (MALT) lymphoma. Cancer Res 156:27-32, 2000.

27. Gospodarowicz M, Pintilie M, Tsang R, et al: Recent results of cancer research. Cancer Res 156:108-115, 2000.

28. Schechter N, Portlock C, Yahalom J: Treatment of mucosa-associated lymphoid tissue lymphoma of the stomach with radiation alone. J Clin Oncol 16:1916-1921, 1998.

29. Kolve M-E, Fischbach W, Wilhelm M: Primary gastric non-Hodgkin's lymphoma: Requirements for diagnosis and staging. Recent Results Cancer Res 156:63-68, 2000.

30. Nakamura S, Yao T, Aoyagi K, et al: *Helicobacter pylori* and primary gastric lymphoma: A histopathologic and immunohistochemical analysis of 237 patients. Cancer 79:3-11, 1997.

31. Xu W, Ho F, Chan A, et al: Pathogenesis of gastric lymphoma: The enigma in Hong Kong. Ann Oncol 8:41-44, 1997.

32. Hsi E, Singleton T, Swinnen L, et al: Mucosa-associated lymphoid tissue-type lymphomas occurring in post-transplantation patients. Am J Surg Pathol 24:100-106, 2000.

33. Dierlamm J, Baens M, Stefanove-Ouzounova M, et al: Detection of t(11;18)(q21;q21) by interphase fluorescence in situ hybridization using AP12 and MLT specific probes. Blood 96:2215-2218, 2000.

34. Isaacson P: Gastric MALT lymphoma: From concept to cure. Ann Oncol 10:637-645, 1999.

35. Orita M, Yamashita K, Okino M, et al: A case of MALT (mucosa-associated lymphoid tissue) lymphoma occurring in the rectum. Hepatogastroenterology 46:2352-2354, 1999.

36. Kim J, Jung H, Shin K, et al: Eradication of *Helicobacter pylori* infection did not lead to cure of duodenal mucosa-associated lymphoid tissue lymphoma. Scand J Gastroenterol 34:215-218, 1999.

37. Matsumoto T, Iida M, Shimizu M: Regression of mucosa-associated lymphoid-tissue lymphoma of rectum after eradication of *Helicobacter pylori*. Lancet 350:115-116, 1997.

38. Nagashima R, Takeda H, Maeda K, et al: Regression of duodenal mucosa-associated lymphoid tissue lymphoma after eradication of *Helicobacter pylori*. Gastroenterology 111:1674-1678, 1996.

39. Hosaka S, Akamatsu T, Nakamura S, et al: Mucosa-associated lymphoid tissue (MALT) lymphoma of the rectum with chromosomal translocation of the t(11;18)(q21;q21) and an additional aberration of trisomy 3. Am J Gastroenterol 94:1951-1954, 1999.

40. Salem P, El-Hashimi L, Anaissie E, et al: Primary small intestinal lymphoma in adults: A comparative study of IPSID versus non-IPSID in the Middle East. Cancer 59:1670-1676, 1987.

41. Tabbane F, Mourali N, Cammoun M, et al: Results of laparotomy in immunoproliferative small intestinal disease. Cancer 61:1699-1706, 1988.

42. Fine K, Stone M: A-heavy chain disease, Mediterranean lymphoma, and immunoproliferative small intestinal disease. Am J Gastroenterol 94:1139-1152, 1999.

43. Smith W, Price S, Isaacson P: Immunoglobulin gene rearrangement in immunoproliferative small intestinal disease (IPSID). J Clin Pathol 40:1291-1297, 1987.

44. Isaacson P, Dogan A, Price S, et al: Immunoproliferative small intestinal disease: An immunohistochemical study. Am J Surg Pathol 13:1023-1033, 1989.

45. Raderer M, Valencak J, Osterreicher C, et al: Chemotherapy for the treatment of patients with primary high grade gastric B-cell lymphoma of modified Ann Arbor stages IE and IIE. Cancer 88:1979-1985, 1979.

46. Starostik P, Greiner A, Schultz A, et al: Genetic aberrations common in gastric high-grade large B-cell lymphoma. Blood 95:1180-1187, 2000.

47. Liang R, Chan W, Kwong Y, et al: High incidence of BCL-6 gene rearrangement in diffuse large B-cell lymphoma of primary gastric origin. Cancer Genet Cytogenet 97:114-118, 1997.

48. Hoeve M, Gisbertz I, Schouten H, et al: Gastric low-grade MALT lymphoma, high-grade MALT lymphoma and diffuse large B cell lymphoma show different frequencies of trisomy. Leukemia 13:799-807, 1999.

49. Hui P, Tokunaga M, Chan W, et al: Epstein-Barr virus-associated gastric lymphoma in Hong Kong Chinese. Hum Pathol 25:947-952, 1994.

50. O'Briain D, Kennedy J, Daly P, et al: Multiple lymphomatous polyposis of the gastrointestinal tract. Am J Surg Pathol 13:691-699, 1989.

51. Geissmann F, Ruskone-Fourmestraux A, Hermine O, et al: Homing receptor α4β7 integrin expression predicts digestive tract involvement in mantle cell lymphoma. Am J Pathol 153:1701-1705, 1998.

52. Sakata Y, Iwakiri R, Sakata H, et al: Primary gastrointestinal follicular center lymphoma resembling multiple lymphomatous polyposis. Dig Dis Sci 46:567-570, 2001.

53. Auner H, Beham-Schmid C, Lindner G, et al: Successful nonsurgical treatment of primary mucosa-associated lymphoid tissue lymphoma of colon presenting with multiple polypoid lesions. Am J Gastroenterol 95:2387-2389, 2000.

54. Misdraji J, del Castillo C, Ferry J: Follicle center lymphoma of the ampulla of Vater presenting with jaundice. Am J Surg Pathol 21:484-488, 1997.

55. Chott A, Raderer M, Jager U, et al: Follicular lymphoma of the duodenum: A distinct extranodal B-cell lymphoma? Mod Pathol 14:160A, 2001.

56. Rosty C, Briere J, Cellier C, et al: Association of a duodenal follicular lymphoma and hereditary nonpolyposis colorectal cancer. Mod Pathol 13:586-590, 2000.

57. Diebold J: Burkitt lymphoma. In Jaffe E, Harris N, Stein H, et al (eds): Pathology and Genetics of Tumours of Haematopoietic and Lymphoid Tissues. Washington, DC, IARC Press, 2001.

58. Isaacson P: Relation between cryptic intestinal lymphoma and refractory sprue. Lancet 356:178-179, 2000.

59. Isaacson P, Spencer J, Connolly C, et al: Malignant histiocytosis of the intestine: A T-cell lymphoma. Lancet ii:688-691, 1985.

60. Jaffe E, Harris N, Diebold J, et al: World Health Organization classification of neoplastic diseases of the hematopoietic and lymphoid tissues: A progress report. Am J Clin Pathol 111:S8-S12, 1999.

61. Chott A, Vesely M, Simonitsch I, et al: Classification of intestinal T-cell neoplasms and their differential diagnosis. Am J Clin Pathol 111:S68-S74, 1999.

62. Harris NL, Jaffe ES, Stein H, et al: A revised European-American classification of lymphoid neoplasms: A proposal from the International Lymphoma Study Group. Blood 84:1361-1392, 1994.

63. Gale J, Simmonds P, Mead G, et al: Enteropathy-type intestinal T-cell lymphoma: Clinical features and treatment of 31 patients in a single center. J Clin Oncol 18:795-803, 2000.

64. Chott A, Haedicke W, Mosberger I, et al: Most CD56+ intestinal lymphomas are CD8+ CD5- T-cell lymphomas of monomorphic small to medium size histology. Am J Pathol 153:1483-1490, 1998.

65. Holmes GKT, Prior P, Lane MR, et al: Malignancy in coeliac disease—effect of a gluten free diet. Gut 30:333-338, 1989.

66. Kluin P, Feller A, Gaulard P, et al: Peripheral T/NK-cell lymphoma: A report of the IXth workshop of the European Association for Haematopathology. Histopathology 38:250-270, 2001.

67. Cellier C, Delabesse E, Helmer C, et al: Refractory sprue, coeliac disease, and enteropathy-associated T-cell lymphoma. Lancet 356:203-208, 2000.

68. Jaffe E, Krenacs L, Kumar S, et al: Extranodal peripheral T-cell and NK-cell neoplasms. Am J Clin Pathol 111:S46-S55, 1999.

69. Bagdi E, Diss T, Munson P, et al: Mucosal intra-epithelial lymphocytes in enteropathy-associated T-cell lymphoma, ulcerative jejunitis, and refractory celiac disease constitute a neoplastic population. Blood 94:260-264, 1999.

70. Spencer J, Cerf-Bensussan N, Jarry A, et al: Enteropathy-associated T-cell lymphoma (malignant histiocytosis of the intestine) is recognized by a monoclonal antibody (HML-1) that defines a membrane molecule on human mucosal lymphocytes. Am J Pathol 132:1-5, 1988.

71. Ashton-Key M, Diss T, Pan L, et al: Molecular analysis of T-cell clonality in ulcerative jejunitis and enteropathy-associated T-cell lymphoma. Am J Pathol 151:493-498, 1997.

72. Quintanilla-Martinez L, Lome-Maldonado C, Ott G, et al: Primary non-Hodgkin's lymphoma of the intestine: High prevalence of Epstein-Barr virus in Mexican lymphomas as compared with European cases. Blood 89:644-651, 1997.

73. Holmes G: Mesenteric lymph node cavitation in celiac disease. Gut 27:728-733, 1986.

74. Carbonnel F, Grollet-Bioul L, Brouet J, et al: Are complicated forms of celiac disease cryptic T-cell lymphomas? Blood 92:3879-3886, 1998.

75. Glick D, Soule E: Primary malignant lymphoma of colon or appendix. Arch Surg 92:144-151, 1966.

76. Kitamura Y, Ohta T, Terada T: Primary T-cell non-Hodgkin's malignant lymphoma of the appendix. Pathol Int 50:313-317, 2000.

77. Muller G, Dargent J, Duwel V, et al: Leukaemia and lymphoma of the appendix presenting as acute appendicitis or acute abdomen. J Cancer Res Clin Oncol 123:560-564, 1997.

78. Pasquale M, Shabahang M, Bitterman P, et al: Primary lymphoma of the appendix: Case report and review of the literature. Surg Oncol 3:243-248, 1994.

79. Sin I, Ling E, Prentice R: Burkitt's lymphoma of the appendix: Report of two cases. Hum Pathol 11:465-470, 1980.

80. Mori M, Kusunoki T, Kikuchi M, et al: Primary malignant lymphoma of the appendix. Jpn J Surg 15:230-233, 1985.

81. Kumar S, Fend F, Quintanilla-Martinez L, et al: Epstein-Barr virus positive primary gastrointestinal Hodgkin's disease: Association with inflammatory bowel disease and immunosuppression. Am J Surg Pathol 24:66-73, 2000.

82. Kelly, Stuart M, Tschuchnigg M, et al: Primary intestinal Hodgkin's disease complicating ileal Crohn's disease. Aust N Z J Surg 67:485-489, 1997.

83. Li S, Borowitz M: Primary Epstein-Barr virus-associated Hodgkin's disease of the ileum complicating Crohn disease. Arch Pathol Lab Med 125:424-427, 2001.

84. Thomas D, Huston B, Lamm K, et al: Primary Hodgkin's disease of the sigmoid colon. Arch Pathol Lab Med 121:528-532, 1997.

85. Devaney K, Jaffe E: The surgical pathology of gastrointestinal Hodgkin's disease. Am J Clin Pathol 95:794-801, 1991.

86. Vanbockrijck M, Cabooter M, Casselman J, et al: Primary Hodgkin's disease of the ileum complicating Crohn disease. Cancer 72:1784-1789, 1993.

87. Shepherd N, Hall P, Williams G, et al: Primary malignant lymphoma of the large intestine complicating chronic inflammatory bowel disease. Histopathology 15:325-337, 1989.

88. Ole K, Pedersen C, Cozzi-Lepri A, et al: Non-Hodgkin lymphoma in HIV-infected patients in the era of highly active antiretroviral therapy. Blood 98:3406-3412, 2001.

89. Beck P, Gill M, Sutherland L: HIV-associated non-Hodgkin's lymphoma of the gastrointestinal tract. Am J Gastroenterol 91:2377-2381, 1996.

90. Ioachim H, Antonescu C, Giancotti F, et al: EBV-associated anorectal lymphomas in patients with acquired immune deficiency syndrome. Am J Surg Pathol 21:997-1006, 1997.

91. Wotherspoon A, Diss T, Pan L, et al: Low grade gastric B-cell lymphoma of mucosa associated lymphoid tissue in immuno-compromised patients. Histopathology 28:129-134, 1996.

92. Beaty M, Kumar S, Sorbara L, et al: A biphenotypic human herpesvirus 8-associated primary bowel lymphoma. Am J Surg Pathol 23:992-998, 1999.

93. DePond W, Said J, Tasaka T, et al: Kaposi's sarcoma-associated herpesvirus and human herpesvirus 8 (KSHV/HHV8)–associated lymphoma of the bowel: Report of two cases in HIV-positive men with secondary effusion lymphomas. Am J Surg Pathol 21:719-724, 1997.

94. Ferry J, Harris N: Pathology of post-transplant lymphoproliferative disorders. In Solez K, Racusen L, Billingham M (eds): Pathology and Rejection Diagnosis in Solid Organ Transplantation. New York, Marcel Dekker, 1996, pp 277-301.

95. Harris N, Swerdlow H, Frizzera G, Knowles DM: Posttransplant lymphoproliferative disorders. In Jaffe E, Harris N, Stein H, et al (eds): Pathology and Genetics of Tumours of Haematopoietic and Lymphoid Tissues. Washington, DC, IARC Press, 2001.

96. Chadburn A, Cesarman E, Knowles D: Molecular pathology of posttransplantation lymphoproliferative disorders. Semin Diagn Pathol 14:15-26, 1997.

97. Loftus E, Tremaine W, Habermann T, et al: Risk of lymphoma in inflammatory bowel disease. Am J Gastroenterol 95:2308-2312, 2000.

98. Lenzen R, Borchard F, Lubke H, et al: Colitis ulcerosa complicated by malignant lymphoma: Case report and analysis of published works. Gut 36:306-310, 1995.

99. Wagonfeld J, Platz C, Fishman F, et al: Multicentric colonic lymphoma complicating ulcerative colitis. Am J Dig Dis 22:502-508, 1977.

100. Farrell R, Ang Y, Kileen P, et al: Increased incidence of non-Hodgkin's lymphoma in inflammatory bowel disease patients on immunosuppressive therapy but overall risk is low. Gut 47:514-519, 2000.

101. Buckley RH: Breakthrough in the understanding and therapy of primary immunodeficiency. Pediatr Clin North Am 41:665-690, 1994.

102. Harrington DS, Weisenburger DD, Purtilo DT: Malignant lymphoma in the X-linked lymphoproliferative syndrome. Cancer 59:1419-1429, 1987.

103. Tatsumi E, Purtilo DT: Epstein-Barr virus (EBV) and X-linked lymphoproliferative syndrome (XLP). AIDS Research 2:S109-S113, 1986.

104. Sneller MC, Strober W, Eisenstein E, et al: New insights into common variable immunodeficiency. Ann Intern Med 118:720-730, 1993.

105. Castellano G, Moreno D, Galvao O, et al: Malignant lymphoma of jejunum with common variable hypogammaglobulinemia and diffuse nodular hyperplasia of the small intestine. J Clin Gastroenterol 15:128-135, 1992.

106. Carey M, Medeiros L, Roepke J, et al: Primary anaplastic large cell lymphoma of the small intestine. Am J Clin Pathol 112:696-701, 1999.

107. Morphopoulos G, Pitt M, Bisset D: Primary anaplastic large cell lymphoma of the rectum. Histopathology 26:190-192, 1995.

108. Yatabe Y, Mori N, Oka K, et al: Primary gastric T-cell lymphoma. Arch Pathol Lab Med 118:547-550, 1994.

109. Memeo L, Pecorello I, Ciardi A, et al: Primary non-Hodgkin's lymphoma of the liver. Acta Oncol 38:655-658, 1999.

110. Huang C-B, Eng H-L, Chuang J-H, et al: Primary Burkitt's lymphoma of the liver: Report of a case with long-term survival after surgical resection and combination chemotherapy. J Pediatr Hematol Oncol 19:135-138, 1997.

111. Osborne BM, Butler JJ, Guarda LA: Primary lymphoma of the liver. Ten cases and a review of the literature. Cancer 56:2902-2910, 1985.

112. Ryan J, Straus D, Lange C, et al: Primary lymphoma of the liver. Cancer 61:370-375, 1987.

113. Scoazec J, Degott C, Brousse N, et al: Non-Hodgkin's lymphoma presenting as a primary tumor of the liver: Presentation, diagnosis and outcome in eight patients. Hepatology 13:870-875, 1991.

114. Isaacson P, Banks P, Best P, et al: Primary low-grade hepatic B-cell lymphoma of mucosa-associated lymphoid tissue (MALT). Am J Surg Pathol 19:571-575, 1995.

115. Ohsawa M, Aozasa K, Horiuchi K, et al: Malignant lymphoma of the liver. Report of five cases and review of the literature. Dig Dis Sci 37:1105-1109, 1992.

116. Rodriguez J, Rawls D, Speights V: Primary lymphoma of the liver mimicking metastatic liver disease. South Med J 88:677-680, 1995.

117. Scerpella EG, Villareal AA, Casanova PF, et al: Primary lymphoma of the liver in AIDS. Report of one new case and review of the literature. J Clin Gastroenterol 22:51-53, 1996.

118. Kim JH, Kim HY, Kang I, et al: A case of primary hepatic lymphoma with hepatitis C liver cirrhosis. Am J Gastroenterol 95:2377-2380, 2000.

119. Talamo T, Dekker A, Gurecki J, et al: Primary hepatic malignant lymphoma: Its occurrence in a patient with chronic active hepatitis, cirrhosis and hepatocellular carcinoma associated with hepatitis B viral infection. Cancer 46:336-339, 1980.

120. Tsutsumi Y, Deng YL, Uchiyama M, et al: OPD4-positive T-cell lymphoma of the liver in systemic lupus erythematosus. Acta Pathol Japon 41:829-833, 1991.

121. Ye M, Suriawinata A, Black C, et al: Primary hepatic marginal zone B-cell lymphoma of mucosa-associated lymphoid tissue type in a patient with primary biliary cirrhosis. Arch Pathol Lab Med 124:604-608, 2000.

122. Ribas Y, Rafecas A, Figueras J, et al: Post-transplant lymphoma in a liver allograft. Transpl Int 8:488-491, 1995.

123. Bowman SJ, Levison DA, Cotter FE, et al: Primary T cell lymphoma of the liver in a patient with Felty's syndrome. Br J Rheumatol 33:157-160, 1994.

124. Borgonovo G, d'Oiron R, Amato A, et al: Primary lymphoplasma-cytic lymphoma of the liver associated with a serum monoclonal peak of IgG kappa. Am J Gastroenterol 90:137-140, 1995.

125. Maes M, Depardieu J, Hermans M, et al: Primary low-grade B-cell lymphoma of MALT-type occurring in the liver. J Hepatol 27:922-927, 1997.

126. Macon W, Levy N, Kurtin P, et al: Hepatosplenic $\alpha\beta$ T-cell lymphomas. Am J Surg Pathol 25:285-296, 2001.

127. Wu H, Wasik M, Przybylski G, et al: Hepatosplenic gamma-delta T-cell lymphoma as a late onset posttransplant lymphoproliferative disorder in renal transplant recipients. Am J Clin Pathol 113:487-496, 2000.

127a. Jaffe ES, Ralfkiaer E: Hepatosplenic T-cell lymphoma. In Jaffe E, Harris N, Stein H, et al (eds): Pathology and Genetics of Tumours of Haematopoietic and Lymphoid Tissues. Washington, DC, IARC Press, 2001.

128. Wong KF, Chan JKC, Matutes E, et al: Hepatosplenic $\gamma\delta$ T cell lymphoma. A distinctive aggressive lymphoma type. Am J Surg Pathol 19:718-726, 1995.

129. Farcet J, Gaulard P, Marolleau J, et al: Hepatosplenic T-cell lymphoma: Sinusal/sinusoidal localization of malignant cells expressing the T-cell receptor $\gamma\delta$. Blood 75:2213-2219, 1990.

130. Pouderoux P, Gris J, Pignodel C, et al: Primary sinusoidal lymphoma of the liver revealed by autoimmune hemolytic anemia. Gastroenterol Clin Biol 21:514-518, 1997.

131. Dargent J, DeWolf-Peeters C: Liver involvement by lymphoma: Identification of a distinctive pattern of infiltration related to T-cell/histiocyte-rich B-cell lymphoma. Ann Diagn Pathol 2:363-369, 1998.

132. Abe Y, Takatsuki H, Okada Y, et al: Mucosa-associated lymphoid tissue type lymphoma of the gallbladder associated with acute myeloid leukemia. Intern Med 38:442-444, 1999.

133. Bickel A, Eitan A, Tsilman B, et al: Low-grade B cell lymphoma of mucosa-associated lymphoid tissue (MALT) arising in the gallbladder. Hepatogastroenterology 46:1643-1646, 1999.

134. Chatila R, Fiedler P, Vender R: Primary lymphoma of the gall-bladder: Case report and review of the literature. Am J Gastroenterol 91:2242-2244, 1996.

135. Friedman E, Lazda E, Grant D, et al: Primary lymphoma of the gallbladder. Postgrad Med J 69:585-587, 1993.

136. McCluggage W, Mackel E, McCusker G: Primary low grade malignant lymphoma of mucosa-associated lymphoid tissue of gallbladder. Histopathology 29:285-287, 1996.

137. Mosnier J, Brousse N, Sevestre C, et al: Primary low-grade B-cell lymphoma of the mucosa-associated lymphoid tissue arising in the gallbladder. Histopathology 20:273-275, 1992.

138. O'Boyle M: Gallbladder wall mass on sonography representing large-cell non-Hodgkin's lymphoma in an AIDS patient. J Ultrasound Med 13:67-68, 1994.

139. Eliason S, Grosso L: Primary biliary malignant lymphoma clinically mimicking cholangiocarcinoma. Ann Diagn Pathol 5:25-33, 2001.

140. Nguyen G: Primary extranodal non-Hodgkin's lymphoma of the extrahepatic bile ducts. Cancer 50:2218-2222, 1982.

141. Baylor S, Berg J: Cross-classification and survival characteristics of 5,000 cases of cancer of the pancreas. Surg Oncol 5:335-358, 1973.

142. Freeman C, Berg J, Cutler S: Occurrence and prognosis of extranodal lymphomas. Cancer 29:252-260, 1972.

143. Borrowdale R, Strong R: Primary lymphoma of the pancreas. Aust N Z J Surg 64:444-446, 1994.

143a. Nishimura R, Takakuwa T, Hoshida Y, et al: Primary pancreatic lymphoma: Clinicopathological analysis of 19 cases from Japan and review of the literature. Oncology 60:322-329, 2001.

144. Pecorari P, Gorji N, Melato M: Primary non-Hodgkin's lymphoma of the head of the pancreas: A case report and review of literature. Oncol Rep 6:1111-1115, 1999.

145. Jones W, Sheikh M, McClave S: AIDS-related non-Hodgkin's lymphoma of the pancreas. Am J Gastroenterol 92:335-338, 1997.

146. Yusuf S, Harrison J, Manhire A, et al: Primary B-cell immunoblastic lymphoma of pancreas. Eur J Surg Oncol 17:555-557, 1991.

147. Shtamler B, Bickel A, Manor E, et al: Primary lymphoma of the head of the pancreas. J Surg Oncol 38:48-51, 1988.

148. Satake K, Arimoto Y, Fujimoto Y, et al: Malignant T-cell lymphoma of the pancreas. Cancer 6:120-124, 1991.

149. Brown P, Hart M, White T: Pancreatic lymphoma, diagnosis and management. Int J Pancreatol 2:93-100, 1987.

150. Joly I, David A, Payan M, et al: A case of primary non-Hodgkin lymphoma of the pancreas. Pancreas 7:118-120, 1992.

151. Case Records of the Massachusetts General Hospital: Case 11-1985. N Engl J Med 312:706-711, 1985.

ANAL PATHOLOGY

CHAPTER 24

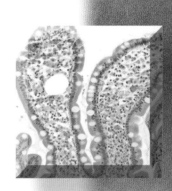

Inflammatory and Neoplastic Disorders of the Anal Canal

CHRISTINE A. IACOBUZIO-DONAHUE

■ Embryology and Anatomy of the Anal Canal

The anal canal forms during the fourth to seventh weeks of gestation following partitioning of the cloaca into the ventral urogenital membrane and a dorsal membrane.[1] The epithelium of the superior two thirds of the primitive anal canal is derived from the endodermal hindgut; the inferior one third develops from the ectodermal proctoderm. The point of fusion of these two epithelial derivatives is indicated by the irregular dentate line, which is located at the inferior limit of the anal valves. The dentate line also indicates the approximate former site of the anal membrane, which ruptures during the eighth week of gestation. The outer layers of the wall of the anal canal are derived from the surrounding splanchnic mesenchyme.

The anal canal is defined surgically by the borders of the internal anal sphincter. The internal sphincter is the most distal portion of the internal circular layer of the muscularis propria, continuous with the muscularis propria of the colorectum. The length of the anal canal ranges from 3 to 4 cm.[2,3] It connects with the rectum superiorly and with the anal skin inferiorly. The surface of the anal canal is lined by vertical mucosal folds called the *anal columns*, or the *columns of Morgagni*; these are separated by the anal sinuses or the sinuses of Morgagni. These columns are connected at the most distal end by a horizontal row of mucosal folds known as the *anal valves.* Anal valves are typically most evident in children but may become more prominent with advancing age.

The location of the anal valves corresponds to the dentate line (also known as the *pectinate line*), located at the midpoint of the surgically defined anal canal. Microscopically, the mucosal lining inferior to the dentate line is of stratified squamous type. This squamous mucous membrane is devoid of hair and other cutaneous appendages. Only where the lower portion of the anal canal ends at the anal verge and the squamous mucosa merges with the true anal skin are hair follicles, sweat glands, and apocrine glands found. The dentate line corresponds generally to the squamocolumnar junction. This is not an abrupt transition but an actual anal transition zone that extends from several millimeters to just over 1 centimeter in length. Microscopically, the anal transition zone varies from lower genitourinary tract–appearing epithelium to stratified squamous, columnar, or cuboidal-type epithelium; islands of colorectal-type mucosa also are frequently present (Fig. 24-1).[1] Immunohistochemical studies for HMB-45 and S100 have also demonstrated the presence of melanocytes within the transitional epithelium, although these are relatively more prominent within the anal squamous zone.[4]

The anal ducts are long tubular structures that closely approach or penetrate into the internal sphincter muscle and may undermine the rectal mucosa. These ducts are lined by transitional or stratified columnar epithelium with mucus-producing cells common at the most terminal portion before opening into the anal crypts. Nodules of lymphoid tissue surrounding these ducts are not uncommon.

The dual origin of the anal canal is indicated by its dual blood supply, venous and lymphatic drainage, and nerve supply.[5,6] The superior two thirds of the anal canal is primarily supplied by the superior rectal artery—a continuation of the inferior mesenteric artery; the venous drainage of the superior anal canal is carried out by the superior rectal veins—tributaries of the inferior mesenteric vein. The lymphatic drainage of the superior two thirds of the anal canal flows eventually to the inferior mesenteric lymph nodes. In contrast, the inferior third of the anal canal is supplied primarily by the inferior rectal arteries, which are branches of the internal pudendal arteries. The venous drainage of this portion of the anal canal goes to the inferior rectal veins, which are tributaries of the internal pudendal veins, and ultimately to the internal iliac veins. Lymphatic drainage moves to the superficial inguinal lymph nodes. The nerve supply of the superior two thirds of the anal canal is provided by the autonomic nervous system; that of the inferior third is supplied by the inferior rectal nerve via the sacral plexus.

These aforementioned differences in embryology, blood supply, drainage, and nervous innervation are clinically relevant, particularly when consideration is given to the spread or staging of tumors that arise in this region.

◼ Tumor-like Lesions of the Anus and Anal Canal

HEMORRHOIDS

The traditional understanding of hemorrhoids is that they represent varicosities of the submucosal plexus of superior hemorrhoidal veins. However, current evidence indicates that hemorrhoids may actually be cushions of fibrovascular and connective tissue normally present within the anal submucosa that serve a protective role during defecation.[7,8] Portal hypertension is not associated with an increased prevalence of hemorrhoids. Rather, hemorrhoidal bleeding in the presence of portal hypertension may be related to severe bleeding that may occur in the presence of coagulopathic disorder rather than simply venous engorgement.

Hemorrhoidal tissue is located above the dentate line on the left lateral, right anterior, and right posterior aspects of the anal canal and is covered by normal rectal or transitional mucosa. Painless bleeding is the most common sign of hemorrhoids; pain may occur if the hemorrhoids become thrombosed or strangulated. With advancing age, the hemorrhoidal tissue may gradually engorge and extend farther into the anal canal, where it

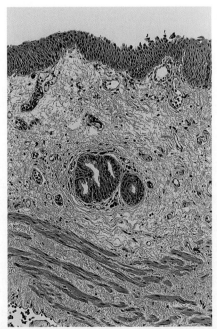

FIGURE 24–1. Normal histologic appearance of the anal transitional zone. The cells are cuboidal with a pseudostratified pattern, similar in appearance to transitional epithelium of the urinary tract. An anal duct is present beneath the surface epithelium and is lined by anal transitional epithelium.

becomes susceptible to the effects of straining at defecation. Clinically prolapsed or thrombosed hemorrhoids may be surgically resected. Microscopically, excised specimens show evidence of dilated thick-walled submucosal vessels and sinusoidal spaces, often with thrombosis and hemorrhage into the surrounding connective tissue (Fig. 24-2). All tissues excised as clinical hemorrhoids should be examined histologically. Although hemorrhoids are common, one must consider infectious processes, Crohn's disease, and a variety of neoplasms in the differential diagnosis.[9]

ANAL TAGS, PAPILLAE, AND FIBROEPITHELIAL POLYPS

Anal tags (fibroepithelial polyps) are projections of anal mucosa with associated submucosal tissue that enlarge in response to congestion, irritation, injury, or infection.[10] The anal mucosa is typically squamous, and the submucosal tissue comprises the loose fibrovascular connective tissue characteristic of this region. Some anal tags may include large, multinucleated, or stellate stromal cells, which are thought to be a reactive process of the stroma.[11,12] Anal tags may have the clinical appearance of a hemorrhoid and are often submitted to the pathologist with this designation.[10] However, unlike hemorrhoids, anal tags do not contain microscopic evidence of dilated or thick-walled vessels, recent or remote hemorrhage, or organizing thrombi. In essence, they are identical to fibroepithelial polyps (acrochordons) of the cutaneous skin (Fig. 24-3).

INFLAMMATORY CLOACOGENIC POLYPS AND MUCOSAL PROLAPSE

Inflammatory cloacogenic polyps (ICPs) are thought to represent part of the continuum of mucosal prolapse disorders of the gastrointestinal tract because the

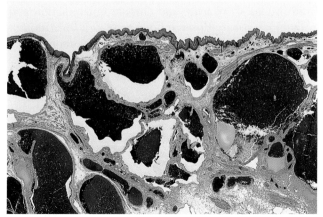

FIGURE 24–2. Low-power view of a hemorrhoid showing vascular dilatation and thrombosis. Chronic inflammation of the intervening stroma is also present.

histologic features of these entities are entirely similar. The unifying concept of all mucosal prolapse disorders is related to chronic mucosal prolapse with associated ischemic and reactive changes of the anal mucosa.[13,14] ICPs occur predominantly in middle-aged patients, although cases of ICP in children have also been described.[15] The most common presentation is rectal bleeding. These polyps are located within the anal canal, may be single or multiple, and are typically sessile. They are variable in size but typically range from 1 to 2 cm grossly. For these reasons, they often clinically mimic hemorrhoids. Simple excision is curative in almost all cases.[14]

The pathogenesis of ICPs is believed to be similar to that of polypoid variants of the solitary rectal ulcer or other mucosal prolapse syndromes.[16] Histologic features include fibrosis of the lamina propria, thickening of the muscularis propria, hyperplasia of the mucosal glands (often with a villus-like configuration), and telangiectasia of the surface vasculature. The muscularis mucosae is thickened and irregular with frequent extension of fibromuscular strands into the lamina propria. The surface epithelium is often a mixture of colorectal and squamous mucosa (Fig. 24-4). Erosion of the surface epithelium is a common finding, and the adjacent epithelium often shows regenerative and/or hyperplastic changes. On low power, ICPs may resemble villous adenomas of the colorectum. However, recognition of the benign epithelial cytology and eroded villiform surface should rule out this possibility.

ANAL FISSURES AND ULCERS

Anal fissures are commonly traumatic lesions, believed to result from tearing of the anal mucosa during the passage of large, firm stools.[17] Anal fissures typically extend from the dentate line to the anal verge in the posterior midline of the anal canal overlying the lower portion of the internal sphincter. Most fissures are superficial and heal quickly. However, they may become chronic, possibly because of the relatively decreased perfusion noted in the posterior anal canal.[18] When fissures become large, deep, and chronic, they are referred to as an *anal ulcer*. Histologically, anal fissures/ulcers are characterized by acute and chronic inflammation and granulation tissue.

Chronic fissures are frequently associated with hypertrophy of the anal papilla at the proximal end of the lesion, called the *sentinel tag*. Histologically, the sentinel tag is similar to other types of fibroepithelial polyp, and it is covered by squamous mucosa. When a fissure is located in an atypical location or fails to heal following treatment, other diagnostic considerations should be entertained. These include inflammatory bowel disease (Crohn's), neoplasm, or infectious processes such as syphilis or tuberculosis.[19,20]

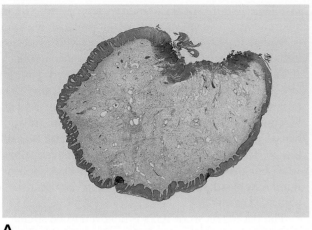

A

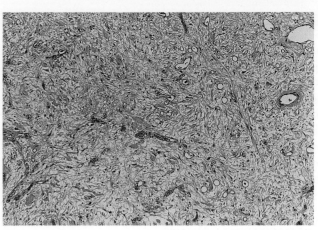

B

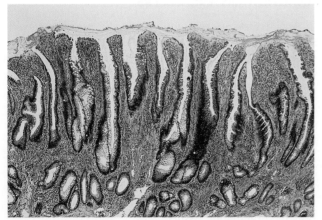

C

FIGURE 24–3. A, Low-power view of an anal tag (fibroepithelial polyp). In this example, the tag is lined by squamous epithelium and is composed of fibrovascular connective tissue. **B,** High-power view of stroma seen in **A. C,** In some anal tags, the stroma may contain numerous stellate-shaped fibroblasts with bizarrely shaped or multiple nuclei. These changes are reactive in nature and are not to be confused with a stromal malignancy.

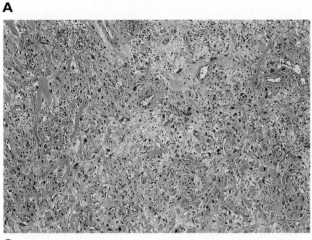

FIGURE 24–4. Epithelial changes characteristic of an inflammatory cloacogenic polyp. Note the villiform appearance, smooth muscle ingrowth into the lamina propria, prominent crypt distortion, and reactive appearance of the epithelium.

ANAL ABSCESSES AND FISTULAS

Anal abscesses and fistulas represent different stages of anorectal suppurative disease. A majority of suppurative processes in this location are believed to result from an infection of an anal duct, which provides a pathway from the anal canal to perineal soft tissues.[21,22] In the acute phase, an abscess may form; the formation of a fistula represents the chronic phase of the infection.

Most anal fistulas or abscesses are idiopathic, although they may occur in patients with Crohn's disease or carcinoma in this region.[23] Histologic specimens taken from fistulas show acute and chronic inflammation and granulation tissue. Foreign body giant cell formation to fecal matter may also be seen in specimens from fistulous tracts of the anus and should not be confused with the sarcoid-like granulomatous reaction typical of Crohn's disease.

Anorectal abscesses may also be found in patients with hydradenitis suppurativa, especially those with diabetes or who are morbidly obese.[24,25] The histologic findings are identical to those in other locations. Wide surgical excision is curative in most cases.

INFLAMMATORY DISORDERS

The histologic features of inflammatory bowel disease are described in detail in Chapters 7 through 11. However, involvement of the anal canal is sufficiently frequent to warrant additional comment here, particularly because neoplastic disorders may present with similar findings in this region.

In ulcerative colitis, involvement of the anus is typically of a nonspecific nature and indistinguishable from such involvement in patients without colitis. Typical findings include superficial inflammation, although anal fissures, abscesses, or fistulas are also found on occasion.

In contrast to ulcerative colitis, the anal canal is involved in approximately 25% of patients with small intestinal Crohn's disease and in 50% to 75% of those with colonic Crohn's disease. Anal findings in Crohn's disease are variable but include anal fissures, fistulas, ulcers, abscesses, and tags.[26] In some cases, anal involvement is the first clinical manifestation of Crohn's disease.

The clinical features of Crohn's disease involving the anus have been well characterized and include the absence of pain and the presence of chronic inflammatory changes, induration of the anal skin, multiplicity of lesions, and skin discoloration.[26] Anal skin lesions include skin tags, fissures, and fistulous openings into or near the anal canal. Anal skin tags are frequent findings and tend to be larger than those from patients without Crohn's disease. Fissures are also common and tend to be large, deep, and located in atypical locations compared with traumatic anal fissures. Fistulas are a component of anal Crohn's disease and may include multiple openings, some at a considerable distance from the anal canal.

Histologically, the diagnosis of anal Crohn's disease may be made based on sarcoid-like granulomatous inflammation close to the anal mucosa, particularly in a young person with no other evident reason for an inflammatory disorder of the anal canal. Patients with tuberculosis of the anal canal may also present with granulomatous inflammation of this region.[19] However, these granulomas are typically caseating, and stains for acid-fast bacilli, if positive, can confirm their infectious etiology.

Benign Tumors of the Anus and Anal Canal

CONDYLOMA ACUMINATUM

Condyloma acuminatum (common genital warts) is a sexually transmitted disease caused by members of the human papillomavirus (HPV) family. It is the most common tumor of the anal and perianal region.[27,28] In this region, the perianal skin is most commonly affected, although condylomas of the anal canal have also been described. Condylomas may be seen in association with penile warts in men or with vulvar warts in

women, but they may also occur as the sole area of infection, particularly among the male homosexual population. Not uncommonly, condylomas occur concomitantly with other sexually transmitted diseases.[29]

Clinically, condylomas are seen as soft, fleshy, tan, gray, or pink papillomatous growths that often occur in groups. Histologically, the papillomatous appearance can also be appreciated. The squamous epithelium shows marked acanthosis but with orderly and progressive maturation of the epithelium. Surface parakeratosis is also present. On higher power, the surface epithelium is seen to contain squamous cells with vacuolated cytoplasm within which an enlarged, irregular, and hyperchromatic nucleus is present. These cells, known as *koilocytes*, are the hallmark of an HPV infection (Fig. 24-5).

Controversy exists as to whether anal condylomas represent a premalignant lesion. Carcinoma in situ and invasive squamous carcinoma have been reported in association with anal condylomas.[30,31] Several types of HPV have been implicated in anogenital lesions, including types 6, 11, 16, and 18. HPV-6 and HPV-11 are most likely to be associated with condyloma acuminatum, whereas HPV-16 and HPV-18 are associated with high-grade dysplasia.[27,29,30] The association between HPV and anal squamous neoplasia is further addressed later in this chapter.

BOWENOID PAPULOSIS

Bowenoid papulosis was initially described as a lesion of the genitalia of young adults. Clinically, it is characterized by multiple small, pigmented papules. In addition to common occurrence on the penis and vulva, anal lesions may also be seen.[32] Despite their benign clinical appearance, the histologic appearance of bowenoid papulosis is similar to that of in situ squamous carcinoma (Bowen's disease). However, in contrast to Bowen's disease, bowenoid papulosis usually presents with more orderly maturation, greater nuclear uniformity, and milder cellular atypia. Clinical follow-up of bowenoid papulosis suggests this is a benign condition. However, because HPV-16 has been demonstrated in these lesions, they are probably best considered a part of the spectrum of intraepithelial neoplasias in this region.[32,33]

ADNEXAL TUMORS

Adnexal tumors of a wide variety have been described in the anal skin.[34] These tumors are most commonly of apocrine gland origin and include such lesions as apocrine gland adenoma or fibroadenoma. Hidradenoma papilliferum, a benign sweat gland tumor usually found in the vulva, may also occur in the anal region (Fig. 24-6).[35]

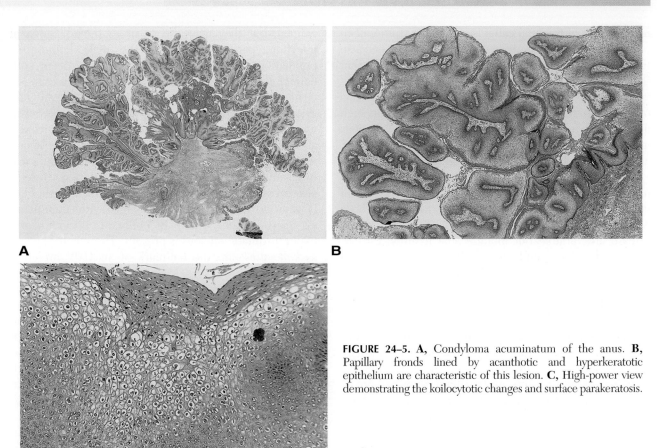

A

B

C

FIGURE 24–5. A, Condyloma acuminatum of the anus. **B,** Papillary fronds lined by acanthotic and hyperkeratotic epithelium are characteristic of this lesion. **C,** High-power view demonstrating the koilocytotic changes and surface parakeratosis.

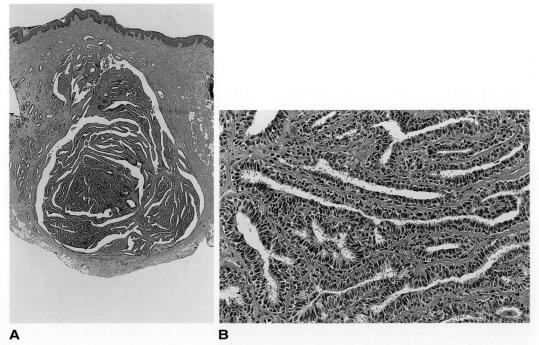

A

B

FIGURE 24–6. A, Hidradenoma papilliferum of the perianal skin. This lesion is identical to its vulvar counterpart. **B,** High-power view demonstrates the glandular appearance and two-cell-layer thickness of the epithelial lining.

GRANULAR CELL TUMORS

Granular cell tumors are common benign tumors that have been described in a variety of locations, including the anal region.[36] Histologically, these lesions are composed of large cells with a characteristic granular cytoplasm that are diastase resistant by periodic acid–Schiff (PAS) stain (Fig. 24-7). These lesions are thought to originate from Schwann cells. Of particular significance is the frequent occurrence of pseudoepitheliomatous hyperplasia of the epithelium overlying the granular cell tumor, which may be mistaken for an infiltrating squamous cell carcinoma.

◼ Malignant Neoplasms of the Anal Canal

Although uncommon, a variety of malignant neoplasms may arise in this location.[37] The World Health Organization recognizes the following anal carcinomas: squamous cell carcinoma (keratinizing, nonkeratinizing, and basaloid/cloacogenic types), adenocarcinoma (rectal type, of anal glands, or within anorectal fistulas), small cell carcinoma, and undifferentiated carcinoma. Each carcinoma is associated with a variety of histologic patterns, which is a reflection of the histologic complexity of the anal canal. However, before a discussion is presented of the histologic varieties of epithelial neoplasms of the anal canal, it should be emphasized that the most important issue is the site of origin of these tumors—that is, the distinction must be made between neoplasms arising above or below the dentate line.

Carcinomas arising above the dentate line are three times more common than neoplasms arising below the dentate line.[38,39] In this region, neoplasms arise from the mucosa of the upper anal canal (the anal transition zone), including those neoplasms designated as *cloacogenic carcinoma*.[40] Often, it is difficult to ascertain the precise origin of the neoplasm both grossly and endoscopically because carcinomas in this location can destroy normal anatomic landmarks. Chemotherapeutic management of anal canal carcinoma may also affect the ability of the pathologist to determine the origin of the neoplasm in that, currently, most patients undergo combination chemoradiation therapy following a diagnostic biopsy, hence avoiding primary surgical removal.[41]

Carcinomas arising above the dentate line are two to three times more common among women than men, with an average age at diagnosis in the sixth decade. Clinical presentations of neoplasms in this location include bleeding, pain, a change in bowel habits, or pruritus ani. The most important prognostic indicators are the depth of invasion and the extent of spread of tumor. Carcinomas arising above the dentate line commonly spread to the lower rectum and involve perirectal and inguinal lymph nodes. The specific histologic type of carcinoma arising in this region is not a significant predictor of survival, although tumor differentiation does correlate with the presence of lymph node metastases.[42] Staging of anal carcinomas should be determined in accordance with the criteria set forth by the American Joint Committee on Cancer (AJCC) (Tables 24-1 and 24-2).[38]

In contrast to the variety of carcinomas arising above the dentate line, virtually all of those that arise below the dentate line are squamous cell carcinomas.[43] Tumors below the dentate line are four times more common among men than women. Coexisting conditions are more common for carcinomas arising in this region and include condyloma, Bowen's disease, chronic fistulas (as in patients with Crohn's disease), chronic pruritus, and a history of radiation treatment.

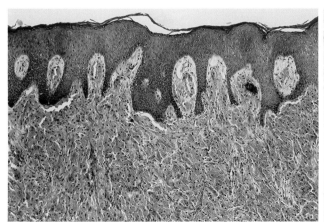
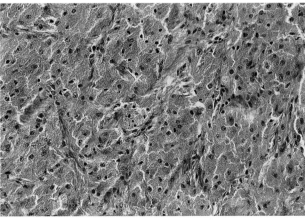

A   **B**

FIGURE 24–7. A, Low-power view of a granular cell tumor arising in the perianal skin. Note the pseudoepitheliomatous changes of the overlying epithelium. **B,** High-power view demonstrating the granular appearance of the cytoplasm and the small hyperchromatic nuclei.

TABLE 24-1. AJCC TNM Classification of Anal Canal Carcinomas

Primary Tumor (T)

TX	Primary tumor cannot be assessed
T0	No evidence of primary tumor
Tis	Carcinoma in situ
T1	Tumor 2 cm or less in greatest dimension
T2	Tumor more than 2 cm but not more than 5 cm in greatest dimension
T3	Tumor more than 5 cm in greatest dimension
T4	Tumor of any size invades adjacent organ(s), e.g., vagina, urethra, bladder*

*Note: Direct invasion of the rectal wall, perirectal skin, subcutaneous tissue, or the sphincter muscle(s) is not classified as T4.

Regional Lymph Nodes (N)

NX	Regional lymph nodes cannot be assessed
N0	No regional lymph node metastasis
N1	Metastasis in perirectal lymph node(s)
N2	Metastasis in unilateral internal iliac and/or inguinal lymph nodes
N3	Metastasis in perirectal and inguinal lymph nodes and/or bilateral internal iliac and/or inguinal lymph nodes

Distant Metastasis (M)

MX	Presence of distant metastasis cannot be assessed
M0	No distant metastasis
M1	Distant metastasis

Used with the permission of the American Joint Committee on Cancer (AJCC), Chicago, Illinois. The original source for this material is the *AJCC Cancer Staging Manual, Sixth Edition* (2002) published by Springer-Verlag New York, www.springer-ny.com.

The clinical presentation of carcinoma in this site ranges from small, firm nodules for early-stage lesions to large, ulcerated tumors for advanced-stage carcinomas. Verrucous forms of squamous carcinoma may also occur at this site. Because carcinomas of the distal anal canal grow more slowly than proximally located tumors and are amenable to earlier diagnosis and treatment, the prognosis is better for carcinomas in this region. Carcinomas arising at the most distal anal margin at the junction of the anal mucosa and hair-bearing skin are staged according to the criteria used for skin cancers.[44] Metastases to inguinal lymph nodes may occur, but visceral metastases are uncommon from squamous cell carcinomas located in this region.

RISK FACTORS AND PREDISPOSING CONDITIONS TO ANAL CARCINOMA

The precursor lesions to anal carcinoma are a subject of ongoing investigation and include condylomas (described previously), squamous cell dysplasias (Bowen's disease), and anal carcinoma in situ (anal canal intraepithelial neoplasia, or ACIN). Risk factors for epithelial carcinomas of the anal canal include receptive anal intercourse, heavy smoking, a history of sexually transmitted diseases, and immunosuppression.[31,45] In women, the presence of lower genital tract squamous neoplasia is also a risk factor, and numerous similarities to the incidence and epidemiology of cervical and vulvar neoplasia have been noted.[45-47]

Similar to its cervical counterpart, ACIN has been identified adjacent to invasive carcinoma of the anal canal and as an incidental finding in resection specimens from this region. ACIN is classified into three groups based on progressively severe cytologic atypia: I (mild dysplasia), II (moderate dysplasia), and III (severe dysplasia or carcinoma in situ). Grade I is considered a low-grade lesion, whereas grades II and III are considered high grade (Fig. 24-8). These preinvasive changes may also occur in associated anal ducts.

In some cases, ACIN may be associated with HPV infection, particularly genotypes 16 and 18 and less commonly genotypes 6 and 11.[31,41,45] Evidence in support of the precursor potential of ACIN involves its close similarity to dysplasias of the uterine cervix, including histologic similarities between the preinvasive and

TABLE 24-2. Stage Groupings Based on AJCC TNM Classification System for Staging Cancer of the Anal Canal

Stage 0	Tis	N0	M0
Stage I	T1	N0	M0
Stage II	T2	N0	M0
	T3	N0	M0
Stage IIIA	T1	N1	M0
	T2	N1	M0
	T3	N1	M0
	T4	N0	M0
Stage IIIB	T4	N1	M0
	Any T	N2	M0
	Any T	N3	M0
Stage IV	Any T	Any N	M1

Used with the permission of the American Joint Committee on Cancer (AJCC), Chicago, Illinois. The original source for this material is the *AJCC Cancer Staging Manual, Sixth Edition* (2002) published by Springer-Verlag New York, www.springer-ny.com.

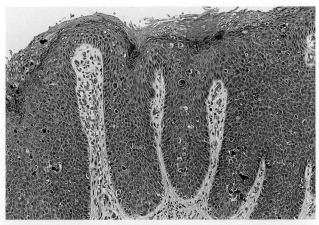

FIGURE 24–8. High-grade anal carcinoma in situ (ACIN III). Note the loss of orderly maturation, abundant mitoses at all levels of the epithelium, and cellular atypia. Pigmented macrophages are also present in this lesion and should not be confused with an anal melanoma.

invasive lesions, a younger average age than its invasive counterpart, and common occurrence adjacent to invasive cancers, particularly those associated with HPV infection and occurring in homosexual men.[45,48] No association has been made between tumor morphology and HPV genotype. The finding of HPV in anal carcinoma is related to the sensitivity of the technique used,[29] but some evidence suggests geographic and/or population differences in the HPV genotypes associated with anal cancers.[49]

Squamous cell dysplasia can be found in tissues removed for a variety of benign conditions.[50,51] Its prevalence within the general population is estimated at 2 to 3 per 1000 individuals, but it may be as prevalent as 4.4% in at-risk populations that include a great proportion of homosexual men.[51] However, in contrast to the documented progression of HPV-associated premalignant conditions of the uterine cervix, the progression of anal intraepithelial to invasive carcinoma appears to be a rare occurrence in that invasive carcinoma in this region is uncommon.

Bowen's disease, a clinicopathologic variant of in situ squamous cell carcinoma, only rarely involves the anal region.[52] When it does occur, it tends to involve the anal margin and adjacent perianal skin as an extension of perineal Bowen's disease. Clinically, Bowen's disease appears as erythematous, scaly plaques that may itch and burn.[52,53] Histologic examination of these plaques reveals a striking disorganization of the squamous epithelium with abundant large, atypical cells and a loss of orderly maturation and polarity. Mitotic figures are frequent and can be seen at all levels of the epithelium. Bowen's disease should be distinguished from the histologically similar but clinically benign bowenoid papulosis.

SQUAMOUS CELL CARCINOMAS

Carcinomas of the anal canal make up 1% to 3% of all distal large bowel cancers,[54] the vast majority of which are squamous cell carcinoma or its histologic variants.[55]

Carcinomas developing above the dentate line are thought to arise from the anal transitional epithelium. A majority of carcinomas arising in this region are typically nonkeratinizing squamous cell carcinomas, although the histologically variable basaloid (cloacogenic or transitional) carcinoma may also arise in this location (Fig. 24-9). A variety of hypotheses regarding the distinct origin of cloacogenic carcinoma have been proposed,

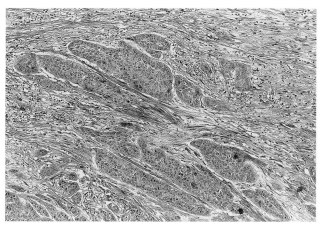
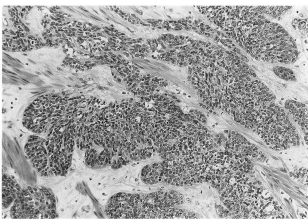

FIGURE 24–9. Morphologic appearances of squamous carcinoma in the anus. **A,** Infiltrating keratinizing squamous carcinoma of the anus. **B,** "Cloacogenic" form of squamous carcinoma comprising small hyperchromatic cells arranged in a trabecular or nested pattern. **C,** In this patient, the cloacogenic carcinoma was arranged in large sheets with a prominent lymphocytic infiltrate.

reflected in part by the specific histologic subtypes that may be observed for this tumor type.[56] These names have included such terms as *basaloid, transitional, nonkeratinizing squamous cell (epidermoid) carcinoma,* and *mucoepidermoid carcinoma* (squamous cell carcinoma with mucinous microcysts). However, the majority opinion for this "cloacogenic" pattern of carcinoma is that it represents a variant of squamous cell carcinoma with the preferred designation of squamous cell carcinoma of basaloid type.[57]

Microscopically, cloacogenic carcinomas frequently show an irregular, angulated, or trabecular pattern. Irrespective of the dominant histologic pattern, foci of squamous differentiation can usually be found. Many different histologic subtypes of this tumor may be seen, particularly at higher powers. Basaloid or transitional patterns consist of nests and trabeculae of small cells without the intercellular bridges typical of conventional squamous cell carcinoma. Some pathologists reserve the term *basaloid* for those carcinomas that show prominent peripheral palisading within tumor nests, similar to cutaneous basal cell carcinomas. In contrast, those without peripheral palisading have been morphologically compared with transitional cell carcinomas of urothelial origin. Some cloacogenic carcinomas are notable for having small cystic foci lined by mucin-producing cells, the reason for the former designation of mucoepidermoid carcinoma. Quite often, a single tumor can show mixtures of a variety of histologic subtypes, including foci of squamous differentiation.

Central necrosis is a common histologic feature. Mitotic figures are also frequently observed, but cellular pleomorphism is not typical. Tumors in this region may extend proximally or distally, often obscuring their precise origin. Often, the adjacent mucosa shows foci of high-grade dysplasia or carcinoma in situ (ACIN) that may extend proximally to the rectal mucosa.

Neoplasms of this type may occasionally arise from the anal duct epithelium, reflecting their common embryologic origin with the anal transitional mucosa. In some instances, in situ carcinoma may occur within both the transitional mucosa and the anal duct epithelium.[58]

Other tumors that rarely arise in the anal canal include verrucous carcinoma and giant condyloma acuminatum.[59] Verrucous carcinoma is a well-differentiated variant of squamous cell carcinoma that most commonly occurs in the oral cavity. These tumors are typically bulky, wartlike growths with a histologically benign appearance. They are locally invasive with a pushing rather than infiltrating tumor margin. Giant condyloma acuminatum, originally described as a tumor of the penis, may occur in the anal canal. These are also large, verrucous growths that are locally invasive. Verrucous carcinoma and giant condyloma acuminatum may in fact be the same lesion. Moreover, it appears that this tumor does not arise from malignant transformation of a condyloma but

may represent a low-grade form of squamous cell carcinoma.

The significance of tumor grading and staging of anal canal carcinomas has been addressed. As has been noted, the degree of differentiation appears to be a more significant factor than the specific histologic subtype of carcinoma. However, it has also been observed that tumors with mucinous microcysts have a poor prognosis. Poorly differentiated basaloid carcinomas of the anal canal must be differentiated from small cell carcinomas that may arise within the rectum and extend into the anal canal. These tumors resemble small cell carcinomas arising in other sites and are similarly aggressive tumors with early dissemination. Distinction often requires immunohistochemical or ultrastructural studies to demonstrate the neuroendocrine differentiation of this tumor type.

Carcinomas arising below the dentate line are virtually all squamous cell carcinomas, although rare tumors with basaloid features may also occur. Carcinomas arising below the dentate line tend to be better differentiated than those that arise above the dentate line and show keratinizing features.[56] In addition, the location of these lesions is exceedingly important because small lesions are more amenable to local excision.

ADENOCARCINOMA

Adenocarcinoma of the anal canal is an uncommon neoplasm; few cases have been described.[60] These tumors may arise from the columnar mucosa of the lower rectum, the mucus-secreting cells of the transition zone, the anal duct glands, or the apocrine glands of the perianal skin.[60] A possible association between anal adenocarcinoma and HPV has been described.[58]

The type of adenocarcinoma that occurs most commonly in the region is a low-lying rectal cancer that extends downward into the anal canal. Differentiation from true anal carcinoma can be made by histologic demonstration of origin in rectal columnar epithelium (Fig. 24-10). Cloacogenic carcinomas, as described above, can sometimes be associated with abundant mucin secretion—a histologic pattern referred to as *mucoepidermoid carcinoma* or *squamous cell carcinoma with mucinous microcysts*. These tumors may arise from the transitional mucosa of the upper anal canal or anal ducts. Recent evidence suggests that mucoepidermoid carcinomas may be histologically distinct from squamous cell carcinomas arising from anal transitional epithelium.[61]

The one true form of primary adenocarcinoma of the anus is believed to arise from anal ducts and is known as *perianal mucinous (colloid) adenocarcinoma*.[62,63] These are extremely rare neoplasms with several clinical and pathologic features in common. First, they are slow-growing tumors frequently associated with long-

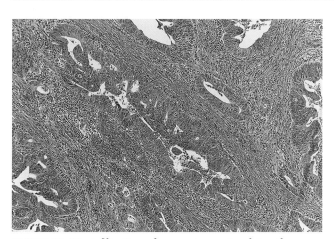

FIGURE 24–10. Infiltrating adenocarcinoma involving the anus. This carcinoma extensively involved the anal canal by direct extension from a rectal primary.

standing fistulas or abscesses, as may be seen in patients with Crohn's disease.[64] Second, they arise in the deep perianal tissues without evidence of surface mucosal involvement. The clinical presentation is often that of a painful mass of the buttock accompanied by a mucin-like discharge. Anorectal bleeding or obstruction is not typical. Histologically, these are well-differentiated adenocarcinomas with abundant mucin production. Multiple deep biopsies are often required for diagnosis because the abundant mucin may make identification of tumor cells difficult.[65,66] Recurrences are common if excision is inadequate, and late metastases to inguinal lymph nodes may occur.

Although the cellular origin of adenocarcinoma is generally agreed upon, the relationship of perianal fistulas and abscesses to the development of carcinoma is uncertain. Some believe that the inflammatory process precedes the neoplasm; others believe that these slow-growing neoplasms undergo fistulization over time. Histochemical studies of mucinous adenocarcinomas associated with chronic anal fistulas have demonstrated that the mucin characteristics are of anal gland origin rather than deriving from rectal mucosa.[67]

PAGET'S DISEASE OF THE ANUS

The most common site of extramammary Paget's disease is the vulva and the contiguous perineal skin that often arises in postmenopausal white women. Involvement of the contiguous perianal skin may also occur, but disease limited to the perianal skin is rare. Anal and perianal Paget's disease may be associated with an underlying carcinoma of the rectum, which may be concurrent with the diagnosis of Paget's disease or may occur later.[68,69]

The clinical appearance of extramammary Paget's disease is well characterized.[69-71] Typical lesions are erythematous patches or plaques that may be scaly,

eroded, or ulcerated. Pruritus is a frequent complaint. Lesions are variable in size, and microscopic evidence of disease may extend beyond the visual limits of involvement. Histologically, Paget's disease is characterized by large, cytologically malignant cells with pale, granular, or vacuolated cytoplasm scattered throughout the epidermis (Fig. 24-11). The cutaneous appendages may also be involved. Paget's cells tend to be more numerous in the basal half of the epidermis. The involved epidermis may show a variety of changes, including hyperkeratosis, parakeratosis, or acanthosis.

The most important differential diagnoses for extramammary Paget's disease are pagetoid malignant melanoma and Bowen's disease.[52] One important feature of Paget's cells is the presence of cytoplasmic acidic mucopolysaccharides that can be demonstrated by a variety of special stains.[72] The presence of melanin pigment within neoplastic cells does not establish a diagnosis of malignant melanoma because melanin can be found in both Paget's cells and the neoplastic keratinocytes of Bowen's disease.[52]

The histopathogenesis of Paget's disease is an area of uncertainty and controversy.[69] The most common conceptions regarding Paget's disease are (1) that it represents migration of Paget's cells into the epidermis from an underlying carcinoma and (2) that Paget's cells develop independently of an underlying carcinoma.[72] Current opinion regards Paget's disease as a form of intraepithelial adenocarcinoma with the ability to progress to invasive disease. However, whereas mammary Paget's disease is virtually always associated with an underlying ductal adenocarcinoma of the breast, a consistent association of extramammary Paget's disease with an underlying carcinoma has not been demonstrated.

The origin of the Paget's cell is also an unresolved issue; some favor an eccrine sweat gland origin, but most support the concept of an apocrine gland origin of

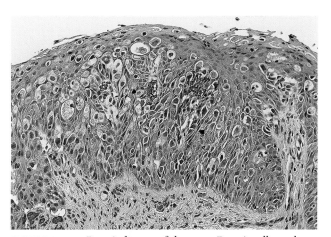

FIGURE 24–11. Paget's disease of the anus. Paget's cells are large and contain a central round nucleus and abundant mucin-filled cytoplasm.

Paget's cells.[73,74] Immunohistochemical demonstration of gross cystic disease fluid protein (GCDFP) expression by Paget's cells, a marker of apocrine epithelium, supports this view. Paget's disease has also been found in association with low-lying rectal carcinoma.[71] Immunohistochemical stains of cytokeratins 7 and 20 in conjunction with GCDFP appear to be useful in distinguishing those cases of perianal Paget's disease that are associated with a regional internal malignancy from those that are not.[75]

MELANOMAS

Melanomas of the anus account for 0.05% of all colorectal malignancies diagnosed each year.[76] Their clinical presentation is not unlike that seen for a variety of benign anal lesions, such as hemorrhoids or anal tags, and is characterized by bleeding, pain, or a mass. These features contribute to the frequently late-stage presentation of anal melanomas.[77,78]

Anal melanomas typically arise as polypoid masses adjacent to or at the dentate line.[76] They are pigmented in 80% of cases, although pigmentation may be obscured by hemorrhage within the lesion. Anal melanomas demonstrate the same immunohistochemical and ultrastructural features as their cutaneous counterparts.[79] However, similar to melanomas arising in other mucous membranes, they are typically of the acrolentiginous type. Invasive melanomas in this region are commonly epithelioid; sarcomatous and desmoplastic melanomas have also been described (Fig. 24-12).

Differentiation of anal melanoma from Paget's disease in this site can be difficult on the basis of histologic criteria alone. As with melanomas occurring elsewhere, histologic features in support of an anal melanoma include melanin production, a nested growth pattern, and asymmetrical junctional changes in association with the appropriate immunohistochemical labeling pattern (positive for S100, HMB-45, and Melan-A; negative for cytokeratins).[79] Junctional changes, although useful when present, may be obscured by ulceration.

The prognosis of anal melanoma is poor, with a 5-year survival rate of approximately 15%.[76,78] The histologic type of anal melanoma is not correlated with survival; however, the thickness of the tumor (as measured from the top of the overlying intact mucosa or ulcerated tumor) does appear to have a relationship to outcome. Anal melanomas that are 2.0 mm or less in thickness have a much better prognosis than those greater than 2.0 mm in thickness.

OTHER RARE NEOPLASMS OF THE ANUS

Basal cell carcinoma of the anus is a rare tumor that arises in the perianal skin. It is similar to cutaneous basal cell carcinoma arising in other sites.[80] The typical gross presentation is that of an ulcerated nodule with raised, pearly margins similar to its cutaneous counterpart. The behavior of basal cell carcinomas of this region is also similar to that of the usual basal cell carcinoma of other sites and is distinctly different from carcinomas of the anal canal. As such, this tumor must be distinguished from the basaloid variant of squamous cell carcinoma. Histologically, anal canal squamous cell carcinoma of the basaloid type has more pronounced cytologic atypia and greater numbers of mitoses.

Other rare tumors of the anal region that have been described include sarcomatoid carcinoma, leiomyosarcoma, gastrointestinal stromal tumor, and embryonal rhabdomyosarcoma. Tumors from other sites, most commonly colorectal carcinoma, may secondarily involve the anus as a result of metastasis or direct extension.[9,81] Rarely, ectopic tissues or acellular material may present as a masslike lesion with associated anorectal bleeding.[82,83] Histologic examination in these cases reveals the benign nature of the lesion.

References

1. Fenger C: Histology of the anal canal. Am J Surg Pathol 12:41-55, 1988.
2. Nivatvongs S, Stern HS, Fryd DS: The length of the anal canal. Dis Colon Rectum 24:600-601, 1981.
3. Rociu E, Stoker J, Eijkemans MJ, et al: Normal anal sphincter anatomy and age- and sex-related variations at high-spatial-resolution endoanal MR imaging. Radiology 217:395-401, 2000.
4. Clemmensen OJ, Fenger C: Melanocytes in the anal canal epithelium. Histopathology 18:237-241, 1991.
5. Godlewski G, Prudhomme M: Embryology and anatomy of the anorectum. Basis of surgery. Surg Clin North Am 80:319-343, 2000.
6. Ayoub SF: Arterial supply to the human rectum. Acta Anat (Basel) 100:317-327, 1978.
7. Hulme-Moir M, Bartolo DC: Hemorrhoids. Gastroenterol Clin North Am 30:183-197, 2001.
8. Morgado PJ, Suarez JA, Gomez LG, et al: Histoclinical basis for a new classification of hemorrhoidal disease. Dis Colon Rectum 31:474-480, 1988.
9. Sawh RN, Borkowski J, Broaddus R: Metastatic renal cell carcinoma presenting as a hemorrhoid. Arch Pathol Lab Med 126:856-858, 2002.

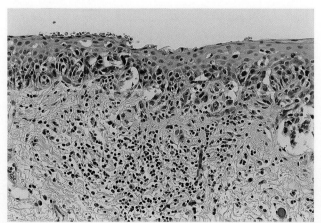

FIGURE 24–12. Melanoma in situ of the anus. Note the epidermotropism, junctional clefting, and lymphocytic infiltrate.

10. Heiken JP, Zuckerman GR, Balfe DM: The hypertrophied anal papilla: Recognition on air-contrast barium enema examinations. Radiology 151:315-318, 1984.
11. Groisman GM, Polak-Charcon S: Fibroepithelial polyps of the anus: A histologic, immunohistochemical, and ultrastructural study, including comparison with the normal anal subepithelial layer. Am J Surg Pathol 22:70-76, 1998.
12. Sakai Y, Matsukuma S: CD34+ stromal cells and hyalinized vascular changes in the anal fibroepithelial polyps. Histopathology 41:230-235, 2002.
13. Saul SH: Inflammatory cloacogenic polyp: Relationship to solitary rectal ulcer syndrome/mucosal prolapse and other bowel disorders. Hum Pathol 18:1120-1125, 1987.
14. Lobert PF, Appelman HD: Inflammatory cloacogenic polyp. A unique inflammatory lesion of the anal transitional zone. Am J Surg Pathol 5:761-766, 1981.
15. Poon KK, Mills S, Booth IW, et al: Inflammatory cloacogenic polyp: An unrecognized cause of hematochezia and tenesmus in childhood. J Pediatr 130:327-329, 1997.
16. Chetty R, Bhathal PS, Slavin JL: Prolapse-induced inflammatory polyps of the colorectum and anal transitional zone. Histopathology 23:63-67, 1993.
17. Fry RD: Anorectal trauma and foreign bodies. Surg Clin North Am 74:1491-1505, 1994.
18. Lund JN, Binch C, McGrath J, et al: Topographical distribution of blood supply to the anal canal. Br J Surg 86:496-498, 1999.
19. Nepomuceno OR, O'Grady JF, Eisenberg SW, et al: Tuberculosis of the anal canal: Report of a case. Dis Colon Rectum 14:313-316, 1971.
20. Chapel TA, Prasad P, Chapel J, et al: Extragenital syphilitic chancres. J Am Acad Dermatol 13:582-584, 1985.
21. Nomikos IN: Anorectal abscesses: Need for accurate anatomical localization of the disease. Clin Anat 10:239-244, 1997.
22. Fucini C, Elbetti C, Messerini L: Anatomic plane of separation between external anal sphincter and puborectalis muscle: Clinical implications. Dis Colon Rectum 42:374-379, 1999.
23. Fry RD, Shemesh EI, Kodner IJ, et al: Techniques and results in the management of anal and perianal Crohn's disease. Surg Gynecol Obstet 168:42-48, 1989.
24. Mitchell KM, Beck DE: Hidradenitis suppurativa. Surg Clin North Am 82:1187-1197, 2002.
25. Wiltz O, Schoetz DJ Jr, Murray JJ, et al: Perianal hidradenitis suppurativa. The Lahey Clinic experience. Dis Colon Rectum 33:731-734, 1990.
26. Solomon MJ: Fistulae and abscesses in symptomatic perianal Crohn's disease. Int J Colorectal Dis 11:222-226, 1996.
27. Luchtefeld MA: Perianal condylomata acuminata. Surg Clin North Am 74:1327-1338, 1994.
28. Wexner SD: Sexually transmitted diseases of the colon, rectum, and anus. The challenge of the nineties. Dis Colon Rectum 33:1048-1062, 1990.
29. Handley JM, Maw RD, Lawther H, et al: Human papillomavirus DNA detection in primary anogenital warts and cervical low-grade intraepithelial neoplasias in adults by in situ hybridization. Sex Transm Dis 19:225-229, 1992.
30. Sobhani I, Vuagnat A, Walker F, et al: Prevalence of high-grade dysplasia and cancer in the anal canal in human papillomavirus-infected individuals. Gastroenterology 120:857-866, 2001.
31. Sonnex C, Scholefield JH, Kocjan G, et al: Anal human papillomavirus infection: A comparative study of cytology, colposcopy and DNA hybridisation as methods of detection. Genitourin Med 67:21-25, 1991.
32. LaVoo JW: Bowenoid papulosis. Dis Colon Rectum 30:62-64, 1987.
33. Gross G, Hagedorn M, Ikenberg H, et al: Bowenoid papulosis. Presence of human papillomavirus (HPV) structural antigens and of HPV 16-related DNA sequences. Arch Dermatol 121:858-863, 1985.
34. Weigand DA, Burgdorf WH: Perianal apocrine gland adenoma. Arch Dermatol 116:1051-1053, 1980.
35. Loane J, Kealy WF, Mulcahy G: Perianal hidradenoma papilliferum occurring in a male: A case report. Ir J Med Sci 167:26-27, 1998.
36. Lack EE, Worsham GF, Callihan MD, et al: Granular cell tumor: A clinicopathologic study of 110 patients. J Surg Oncol 13:301-316, 1980.
37. Beahrs OH, Wilson SM: Carcinoma of the anus. Ann Surg 184:422-428, 1976.

38. Williams GR, Talbot IC: Anal carcinoma—a histological review. Histopathology 25:507-516, 1994.
39. Boman BM, Moertel CG, O'Connell MJ, et al: Carcinoma of the anal canal. A clinical and pathologic study of 188 cases. Cancer 54:114-125, 1984.
40. Klotz RG Jr, Pamukcoglu T, Souilliard DH: Transitional cloacogenic carcinoma of the anal canal. Clinicopathologic study of three hundred seventy-three cases. Cancer 20:1727-1745, 1967.
41. Ryan DP, Compton CC, Mayer RJ: Carcinoma of the anal canal. N Engl J Med 342:792-800, 2000.
42. Shepherd NA, Scholefield JH, Love SB, et al: Prognostic factors in anal squamous carcinoma: A multivariate analysis of clinical, pathological and flow cytometric parameters in 235 cases. Histopathology 16:545-555, 1990.
43. Oliver GC, Labow SB: Neoplasms of the anus. Surg Clin North Am 74:1475-1490, 1994.
44. Chawla AK, Willett CG: Squamous cell carcinoma of the anal canal and anal margin. Hematol Oncol Clin North Am 15:321-344, 2001.
45. Frisch M, Fenger C, van den Brule AJ, et al: Variants of squamous cell carcinoma of the anal canal and perianal skin and their relation to human papillomaviruses. Cancer Res 59:753-757, 1999.
46. Scholefield JH, Sonnex C, Talbot IC, et al: Anal and cervical intra-epithelial neoplasia: Possible parallel. Lancet 2:765-769, 1989.
47. Scholefield JH, Ogunbiyi OA, Smith JH, et al: Anal colposcopy and the diagnosis of anal intraepithelial neoplasia in high-risk gynecologic patients. Int J Gynecol Cancer 4:119-126, 1994.
48. Holly EA, Ralston ML, Darragh TM, et al: Prevalence and risk factors for anal squamous intraepithelial lesions in women. J Natl Cancer Inst 93:843-849, 2001.
49. Scholefield JH, Kerr IB, Shepherd NA, et al: Human papillomavirus type 16 DNA in anal cancers from six different countries. Gut 32:674-676, 1991.
50. Foust RL, Dean PJ, Stoler MH, et al: Intraepithelial neoplasia of the anal canal in hemorrhoidal tissue: A study of 19 cases. Hum Pathol 22:528-534, 1991.
51. Fenger C, Nielsen VT: Dysplastic changes in the anal canal epithelium in minor surgical specimens. Acta Pathol Microbiol Scand [A] 89:463-465, 1981.
52. Papageorgiou PP, Koumarianou AA, Chu AC: Pigmented Bowen's disease. Br J Dermatol 138:515-518, 1998.
53. Stolz E, Vuzevski VD, van der SJ: General perianal skin problems. Neth J Med 37:S43-S46, 1990.
54. Licitra L, Spinazze S, Doci R, et al: Cancer of the anal region. Crit Rev Oncol Hematol 43:77-92, 2002.
55. Quan SH: Anal cancers. Squamous and melanoma. Cancer 70:1384-1389, 1992.
56. Levy R, Czernobilsky B, Geiger B: Cytokeratin polypeptide expression in a cloacogenic carcinoma and in the normal anal canal epithelium. Virchows Arch A Pathol Anat Histopathol 418:447-455, 1991.
57. Vincent-Salomon A, de la Rochefordiere A, Salmon R, et al: Frequent association of human papillomavirus 16 and 18 DNA with anal squamous cell and basaloid carcinoma. Mod Pathol 9:614-620, 1996.
58. Yeong ML, Wood KP, Scott B, et al: Synchronous squamous and glandular neoplasia of the anal canal. J Clin Pathol 45:261-263, 1992.
59. Lu S, Bodemer W, Ostwald C, et al: Anal verrucous carcinoma and penile condylomata acuminata. Dermatology 200:320-323, 2000.
60. Tarazi R, Nelson RL: Anal adenocarcinoma: A comprehensive review. Semin Surg Oncol 10:235-240, 1994.
61. Kondo R, Hanamura N, Kobayashi M, et al: Mucoepidermoid carcinoma of the anal canal: An immunohistochemical study. J Gastroenterol 36:508-514, 2001.
62. Wong NA, Shirazi T, Hamer-Hodges DW, et al: Adenocarcinoma arising within a Crohn's-related anorectal fistula: A form of anal gland carcinoma? Histopathology 40:302-304, 2002.
63. Biggs RL, Lucha PA Jr, Stoll PM: Anal duct carcinoma: Report of case and a survey of the experience of the American Osteopathic College of Proctology. J Am Osteopath Assoc 101:450-453, 2001.
64. Lentini J, Ortiz R, Fornells E: Mucoid adenocarcinoma in anorectal fistula. Am J Proctol 21:103-112, 1970.
65. Navarra G, Ascanelli S, Turini A, et al: Mucinous adenocarcinoma in chronic anorectal fistula. Chir Ital 51:413-416, 1999.
66. Ky A, Sohn N, Weinstein MA, et al: Carcinoma arising in anorectal fistulas of Crohn's disease. Dis Colon Rectum 41:992-996, 1998.

67. Fenger C, Filipe MI: Mucin histochemistry of the anal canal epithelium. Studies of normal anal mucosa and mucosa adjacent to carcinoma. Histochem J 13:921-930, 1981.

68. Lertprasertsuke N, Tsutsumi Y: Latent perianal Paget's disease associated with mucin-producing rectal adenocarcinoma. Report of two cases. Acta Pathol Jpn 41:386-393, 1991.

69. Bouzourene H, Saraga E: Perianal Paget's disease associated with anal canal adenocarcinoma and rectal villous adenoma. Histopathology 31:384-385, 1997.

70. Fazio VW, Tjandra JJ: The management of perianal diseases. Adv Surg 29:59-78, 1996.

71. Kubota K, Akasu T, Nakanishi Y, et al: Perianal Paget's disease associated with rectal carcinoma: A case report. Jpn J Clin Oncol 28:347-350, 1998.

72. Ohnishi T, Watanabe S: The use of cytokeratins 7 and 20 in the diagnosis of primary and secondary extramammary Paget's disease. Br J Dermatol 142:243-247, 2000.

73. Mazoujian G, Pinkus GS, Haagensen DE Jr: Extramammary Paget's disease—evidence for an apocrine origin. An immunoperoxidase study of gross cystic disease fluid protein-15, carcinoembryonic antigen, and keratin proteins. Am J Surg Pathol 8:43-50, 1984.

74. Merot Y, Mazoujian G, Pinkus G, et al: Extramammary Paget's disease of the perianal and perineal regions. Evidence of apocrine derivation. Arch Dermatol 121:750-752, 1985.

75. Goldblum JR, Hart WR: Perianal Paget's disease: A histologic and immunohistochemical study of 11 cases with and without associated rectal adenocarcinomas. Am J Surg Pathol 22:170-179, 1998.

76. Cagir B, Whiteford MH, Topham A, et al: Changing epidemiology of anorectal melanoma. Dis Colon Rectum 42:1203-1208, 1999.

77. Felz MW, Winburn GB, Kallab AM, et al: Anal melanoma: An aggressive malignancy masquerading as hemorrhoids. South Med J 94:880-885, 2001.

78. Rossetti C, Koukouras D, Eboli M, et al: Primary anorectal melanomas: An institutional experience. J Exp Clin Cancer Res 16:81-85, 1997.

79. Ben Izhak O, Levy R, Weill S, et al: Anorectal malignant melanoma. A clinicopathologic study, including immunohistochemistry and DNA flow cytometry. Cancer 79:18-25, 1997.

80. Nielsen OV, Jensen SL: Basal cell carcinoma of the anus—a clinical study of 34 cases. Br J Surg 68:856-857, 1981.

81. Kawahara K, Akamine S, Takahashi T, et al: Anal metastasis from carcinoma of the lung: Report of a case. Surg Today 24:1101-1103, 1994.

82. Matsuo K, Nakamoto M, Yasunaga C, et al: A case of amyloidal anal polyp in long-term hemodialysis. Nephron 79:219-220, 1998.

83. Tekin K, Sungurtekin U, Aytekin FO, et al: Ectopic prostatic tissue of the anal canal presenting with rectal bleeding: Report of a case. Dis Colon Rectum 45:979-980, 2002.

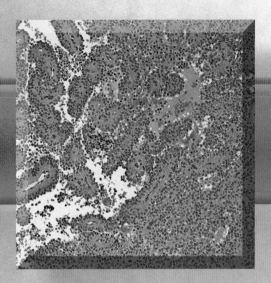

PART TWO

Gallbladder, Extrahepatic Biliary Tract, and Pancreas

CHAPTER 25

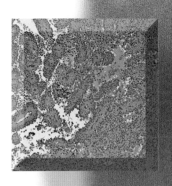

Gallbladder, Extrahepatic Biliary Tract, and Pancreas Tissue Processing Techniques

JAMES M. CRAWFORD

Introduction

Disorders of the biliary tract affect a significant proportion of the world's population. More than 95% of biliary tract diseases are attributable to cholelithiasis (gallstones). In the United States, the annual cost of cholelithiasis and its complications has ranged from $6 billion to $8 billion (in 1998), which represents approximately 1% of the national health care budget. In addition, carcinoma of the pancreas is the fifth most frequent cause of death from cancer in the United States. Its incidence has remained unchanged over the past 50 years. Currently, 28,000 new patients are identified each year, of whom less than 5% survive 5 years.

This chapter presents a practical approach to the processing of surgical specimens of the pancreas, gall-bladder, and extrahepatic biliary tree. Guidelines concerning handling of intraoperative frozen section specimens are also provided.

Pancreas

During pancreatic surgery, two general classes of specimens are obtained. Resection of lesions in the head of the pancreas usually requires a pancreatoduodenectomy (Whipple) resection, which includes a portion of the pancreatic head, the common bile duct, peripancreatic soft tissue and lymph nodes, and a variable portion of the duodenum and gastric antrum. Tumors or lesions in the body or tail of the pancreas are normally resected as a distal pancreatectomy, which usually also includes the spleen and accompanying vessels, as well as peripancreatic soft tissue and lymph nodes. Needle biopsies of the pancreas may be obtained intraoperatively, via endoscopic retrograde cholangiopancreatography (ERCP) (often with brushings), or during radiographic localizing procedures.[1,2] For biopsy specimens of biliary or pancreatic tissue during ERCP, either standard or specially designed small biopsy forceps are used.[3]

Because of rapid evolution in our knowledge of the molecular pathogenesis of pancreatic cancer, preserving fresh frozen tissue for molecular studies is a valuable undertaking. Liquid nitrogen fixation and storage at –80°C is generally sufficient for this purpose. Appropriate tissue specimens should be snap-frozen in liquid nitrogen as soon as possible following surgical excision for preservation of mRNA. Tissue fragments should then be placed in a specimen vial that excludes air; this prevents desiccation during storage.

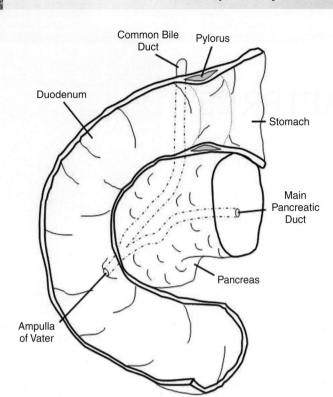

FIGURE 25-1. Typical pancreatoduodenectomy (Whipple) specimen.

PANCREATODUODENECTOMY (WHIPPLE) SPECIMEN

Whipple specimens consist of the proximal duodenum (and the stomach) from the pylorus to the ligament of Treitz, along with the head of the pancreas and the distal extrahepatic biliary tree (Fig. 25-1). The gallbladder is usually also submitted as a separate specimen. In this manner, carcinomas of the common bile duct, ampulla

of Vater, and head of the pancreas are removed with an intent to cure. It is important that proper anatomic orientation be maintained during processing of a Whipple resection specimen.

Upon initial examination, the following anatomic structures should be identified: the common bile duct margin, the pancreatic tissue margin (with the main pancreatic duct), the proximal gut margin (stomach or duodenum), and the distal duodenal margin. The common bile duct, pancreatic, and selected peripancreatic soft tissue margins (anterior, posterior, superior, inferior) should also be inked before processing. Two or more en face sections of the pancreatic resection margin should be obtained, including the pancreatic duct. More sections should be included if there is a suspicion that the margin is positive for tumor. En face sections permit complete assessment of the pancreatic resection margin. Tissue sections that are obtained perpendicular to the margin may permit better visualization of tumor and its relationship to the margin, but this method does not allow sampling of the entire margin. The common bile duct margin, which is usually located posterior to the duodenum, should be cut in cross section and submitted en face for microscopic examination.

When the specimen is fresh, the following protocol for tissue dissection is recommended.[4] The specimen should be opened along the greater curvature of the stomach, the anterior wall of the pylorus, and the greater curvature of the duodenum. The contents of the lumen may be rinsed with saline, and any mucosal lesions, particularly those surrounding the ampulla, should be noted. Photographing lesions is helpful only after the specimen has been fully dissected (Fig. 25-2). A probe may be placed within the common bile duct and advanced toward the ampulla. Similarly, a probe may be placed

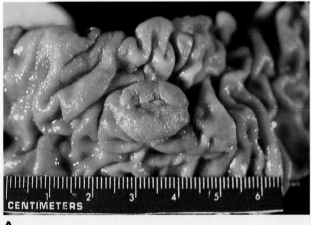

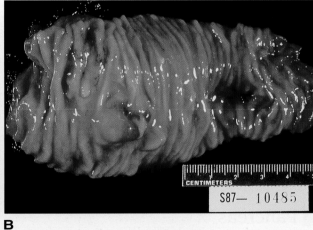

FIGURE 25-2. Pancreatoduodenectomy (Whipple) resection of a periampullary tumor. **A,** Ampulla of Vater, showing a villous adenoma circumferentially involving the ampullary orifice. **B,** Sweep of the duodenum, showing a bulging ampulla of Vater toward the lower left. In this case, a common bile duct cancer subjacent to the ampulla caused its protrusion.

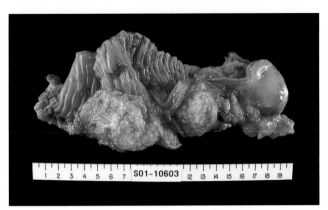

FIGURE 25–3. Pancreatoduodenectomy (Whipple) resection of a pancreatic carcinoma located in the head of the pancreas. An ill-defined mass expands the head of the pancreas in this transected specimen.

within the main pancreatic duct at the pancreatic margin and advanced slowly and carefully toward the ampulla. The ducts may then be opened along the path of the probes with the use of fine blunt scissors. This method of dissection permits evaluation of the relationship of biliary and/or intrapancreatic tumors to the ductal system; it also provides further opportunity for specimen photography (Fig. 25-3) and is helpful for determining the precise anatomic location of the tumor.

The ampulla should always be opened along its posterior aspect owing to the posterior location of the common bile duct. This approach minimizes the amount of duodenal tissue that needs to be transected for exposure of the bile duct. Once the ampulla and common bile duct have been opened entirely, it is usually best to fix the specimen in 10% buffered formalin overnight before further tissue sectioning is performed. Cut sections of the pancreas should be evaluated for color (tan-yellow is normal for pancreas; white is abnormal), consistency (firm is normal, hard is abnormal), texture (fine nodularity is normal, architecture obscured by a dense white infiltrate is abnormal), and the presence of tumors, nodules, cysts, and mass lesions.

Not uncommonly, the extent of pancreatic adenocarcinoma may be difficult to discern on gross examination. Thus, tissue sections should be obtained so that the relationship of the presumed tumor to the pancreatic parenchyma can be defined; these should always include portions of the pancreatic duct, common bile duct, ampulla, duodenum, and pancreatic and common bile duct margins. Perpendicular sections should be obtained through the soft tissue margins—superior, posterior, inferior, and anterior. Additional sections should be obtained from grossly uninvolved pancreas.

For cystic lesions, cystic cavities should be opened and examined closely for areas of thickening, nodularity,

ulceration, tumor, or effacement of adjacent tissue. The walls of the cysts should be sampled generously for histologic analysis, especially for mucinous cystic tumors (see Chapter 31).

All regional lymph nodes should be sampled and separated according to their anatomic location. Lymph nodes sampled may include those superior, posterior, inferior, and anterior to the pancreas, retroperitoneal and lateral aortic areas, hepatic artery area, superior mesenteric area, subpyloric area, and celiac axis area.

DISTAL PANCREATECTOMY

A distal pancreatectomy is generally performed for tumors located in the body/tail of the pancreas. This type of specimen usually includes the tail and a variable portion of the body of the pancreas, the spleen, the splenic vein along the superior aspect of the pancreas, and peripancreatic fat (Fig. 25-4). The following guidelines pertain to dissection and sampling of a distal pancreatectomy specimen.[4]

The specimen should be oriented according to its anterior, posterior, superior, inferior, lateral, and medial aspects, and the organ anatomy (spleen and pancreas), pancreatic resection margin, and main pancreatic duct should be identified. Critical surgical margins should be inked before transection of the specimen is performed (Fig. 25-5). The gross appearance of the specimen should be noted, and the features of the pancreatic corpus should be evaluated as described for Whipple resection specimens. The proximal pancreatic resection margin should be sectioned en face for histologic processing. The pancreas may then be serially sectioned perpendicular to the long axis of the organ. Lesions

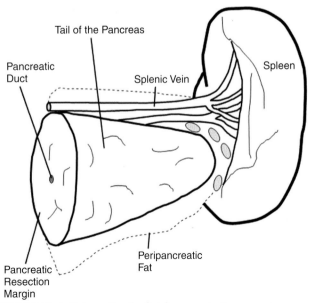

FIGURE 25–4. Schematic of a distal pancreatectomy specimen.

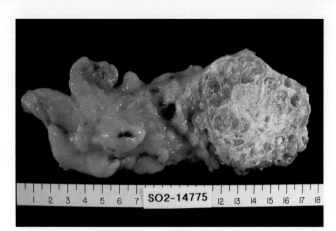

FIGURE 25–5. Distal pancreatectomy, cross section showing a cystic tumor.

should be described in detail, especially regarding their relationship to the tissue margins of the specimen. If not directly involved by tumor, the spleen may be separated from the rest of the specimen and thinly sectioned so that it can be evaluated for the presence of any lesions. The splenic vein, if present, should also be examined for thrombosis or tumor.

Following fixation overnight in 10% buffered formalin, sections of the tumor mass may be taken for histologic analysis; perpendicular sections of the closest approach of the tumor to the soft tissue margins should be obtained as well (superior, posterior, inferior, and anterior). Cystic tumors should be sampled as described earlier for Whipple resection specimens. The peripancreatic soft tissue should then be carefully examined for lymph nodes. Peripancreatic lymph nodes should be submitted separately from splenic lymph nodes. If present in the specimen, perigastric nodes and pericolic

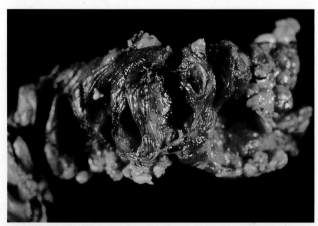

FIGURE 25–6. Acute hemorrhagic pancreatitis. Pancreatoduodenectomy specimen of an acutely hemorrhagic pancreas in a patient who was bleeding heavily from the accessory duct of Santorini. The specimen has been breadloafed to reveal a dusky hemorrhagic pancreatic corpus.

nodes should be submitted separately because if positive for tumor, they represent distant nodal metastasis.

TISSUE PROCESSING FOR PANCREATITIS

Partial resection of the pancreas may be performed as a desperate procedure for patients with acute hemorrhagic pancreatitis. In such instances, the pancreatic corpus is often necrotic and hemorrhagic in appearance (Fig. 25-6). Documentation of the severity and extent of pancreatic injury is the primary goal of tissue processing.

In contrast, partial resection of the pancreas may be performed for cases of chronic pancreatitis as an established procedure for alleviation of intractable pain. The main goals of tissue processing are to establish a diagnosis and the extent of chronic pancreatitis and to exclude carcinoma. Accordingly, attention should be given to the surgical margins of resection, as described earlier, but the primary goal is histologic evaluation of the pancreatic corpus.

Gallbladder

Gallbladders may be removed via open laparotomy or by laparoscopic resection. Those removed for presumed cholecystitis and/or gallstones usually consist only of the gallbladder and a variable portion of the cystic duct. In contrast, a radical resection for gallbladder cancer often includes a substantial portion of the extrahepatic biliary tree and, potentially, the right lobe of the liver.

EVALUATION OF GALLSTONES

There are two main types of gallstones. In the West, about 80% are cholesterol stones. These contain more than 50% crystalline cholesterol monohydrate. The remaining 20% or so are composed predominantly of bilirubin calcium salts and are designated "pigment" stones. There is a greater preponderance of pigmented gallstones in the Orient owing to the prevalence of biliary tract fluke infections in that region of the world.

Cholesterol Stones

Cholesterol is rendered soluble in bile by aggregation with water-soluble bile salts and water-insoluble lecithins, both of which act as detergents. When cholesterol concentrations exceed the solubilizing capacity of bile (supersaturation), cholesterol can no longer remain dispersed, and it nucleates into solid cholesterol monohydrate crystals. Cholesterol gallstone formation involves four simultaneous defects: supersaturation of bile with cholesterol; gallbladder hypomotility, which promotes

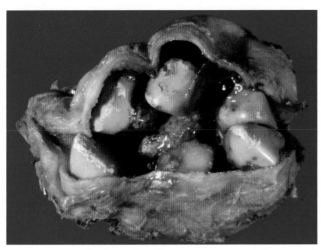

FIGURE 25–7. Cholesterol gallstones in a partially opened gallbladder. The stones are yellow-white, faceted, few in number, and of uniform size.

nucleation; accelerated cholesterol nucleation in bile via alteration in mucoprotein contents; and gallbladder mucus hypersecretion, which traps the crystals and permits their aggregation into stones.[5] Cholesterol stones then grow over the course of many years. As a result, when multiple stones are present, they are generally of similar size and age.[6]

Cholesterol stones arise exclusively in the gallbladder. They are pale yellow and round to ovoid and have a finely granular, hard external surface (Fig. 25-7), which on transection reveals a glistening, radiating, crystalline palisade. With increasing proportions of calcium carbonate, phosphates, and bilirubin, the stones exhibit discoloration and may be lamellar and gray-white to black on transection. Most often, multiple stones that range up to several centimeters in diameter are present. Rarely, a single large stone may fill the fundus or obstruct the gallbladder neck. The surfaces of stones that are multiple may be round or faceted owing to tight apposition.

Cholesterol stones are a "gross only" specimen. Regardless of color, they are hard and difficult to crush (unlike pigmented gallstones). Chemical analysis of stones is not required for clinical care and is of value only for research purposes.

Pigment Stones

Pigment gallstones are formed from a complex mixture of insoluble calcium salts of unconjugated bilirubin along with inorganic calcium salts.[7] Unconjugated bilirubin is normally a minor component of bile, but it increases when infection of the biliary tract leads to release of microbial β-glucuronidases, which hydrolyze bilirubin glucuronides. Thus, infection of the biliary tract, as with *Escherichia coli*, *Ascaris lumbricoides*, or the liver fluke *Opisthorchis sinensis*, increases the likelihood of pigment stone formation. Alternatively, intravascular hemolysis leads to increased hepatic secretion of conjugated bilirubin. Because a low level (about 1%) of bilirubin glucuronides is deconjugated in the biliary tree even under normal circumstances, the aqueous solubility of free bilirubin may easily be exceeded under hemolytic conditions.

Pigment gallstones are trivially classified as "black" and "brown." In general, black pigment stones are found in sterile gallbladder bile, and brown stones are found in infected intrahepatic or extrahepatic ducts. Black pigment stones contain oxidized polymers of calcium salts of unconjugated bilirubin; lesser amounts of calcium carbonate, calcium phosphate, and mucin glycoprotein; and a modicum of cholesterol monohydrate crystals. Brown pigment stones contain pure calcium salts of unconjugated bilirubin, mucin glycoprotein, a substantial cholesterol fraction, and calcium salts of palmitate and stearate. Black stones are rarely larger than 1.5 cm in diameter and are almost invariably present in large numbers (with an inverse relationship between size and number; Fig. 25-8). Their contours are usually spiculated and molded. Brown stones tend to be laminated and soft and may have a soaplike or greasy consistency, resembling fecal material.

Pigment stones are also a "gross only" specimen. Both black and brown stones crumble or crush easily, which provides the primary confirmatory finding for distinguishing true pigment stones from darkly pigmented cholesterol stones (which do not crush).

GALLBLADDER SPECIMEN

Cholecystectomy is performed as treatment for cholelithiasis, cholecystitis, or neoplasia. Cholecystectomy may also be performed as a prophylactic procedure (as in sickle cell disease) or incidentally as part of another

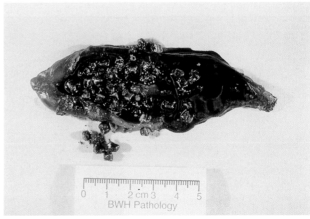

FIGURE 25–8. Pigmented gallstones in an opened gallbladder. The stones are dark black, small and numerous, and do not have uniform shape.

procedure such as a Whipple resection. Gallbladders that are removed by laparotomy are generally intact. However, those removed at laparoscopic cholecystectomy are often torn during the procedure.

The gallbladder should be examined externally and the presence of perforations or tears in the gallbladder specimen noted, because spillage of gallbladder contents (including stones) into the abdominal cavity may have occurred during removal. After the gallbladder has been opened along its length, note should be taken of its contents, that is, volume, color, mucin content, and the presence of sludge or stones. The gallbladder wall thickness and circumference should be measured because these are altered in cholecystitis. The cystic duct is tortuous and often difficult to open, but the presence of stones within the cystic duct and their nature should be noted.

Occasionally, gallstones are returned to the patient. This should be done in a sealed container without formalin because formalin represents a biohazard. If the gallstones have been immersed in formalin, they should be rinsed in water before release. If chemical analysis is requested, the gallstones should be placed in a dry, sterile container and forwarded to the appropriate laboratory for analysis.

The appearance of the gallbladder mucosa should be noted. The normal mucosa has a honeycomb appearance and is tan and velvety in texture. With acute or chronic cholecystitis, the mucosa becomes effaced and loses its velvety appearance; it may be ulcerated and friable in acute cholecystitis or flattened and atrophic in chronic cholecystitis. An incidental finding pertinent to cholesterol biology but not directly related to gallstone formation is cholesterolosis, which results from excessive accumulation of cholesterol esters within the lamina propria of the gallbladder. The mucosal surface may then be studded with minute yellow flecks, producing a "strawberry" appearance (Fig. 25-9).

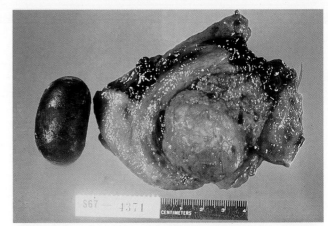

FIGURE 25–10. Opened gallbladder, showing a single cholesterol stone (pigmented darkly due to entrapped bilirubin pigments) and a 5-cm gallbladder adenocarcinoma bulging into the lumen.

Mucosal polyps may be evident as delicate protuberant papillary structures that are easily disrupted. Alternatively, flat areas of mucosal dysplasia or nascent adenocarcinoma may appear as firm, plaquelike elevations of the mucosa or as exophytic tumors (Fig. 25-10), with effacement of the layers of the gallbladder wall in cases of invasive carcinoma. Invasive carcinoma should not be confused with adenomyosis, which is displacement of benign glandular epithelium into the gallbladder wall in association with muscular hypertrophy. Adenomyosis may appear as a dense, focal, tumor-like thickening of the gallbladder wall (Fig. 25-11). Massively dilated Rokitansky-Aschoff sinuses in chronic cholecystitis may impart a tumor-like thickening to the gallbladder wall as well.

Cross sections of the gallbladder fundus and lateral wall should be submitted, along with a section through the neck of the gallbladder and cystic duct. Tumorous lesions should be sampled thoroughly with attention to the surgical margins of the resection specimen. This

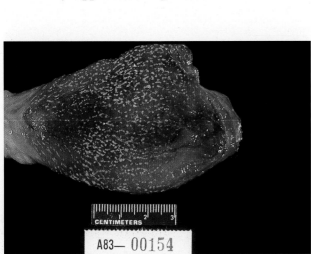

FIGURE 25–9. Gallbladder with cholesterolosis, showing bright yellow flecks scattered throughout the mucosa.

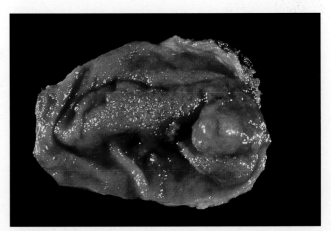

FIGURE 25–11. Gallbladder adenomyoma. The opened gallbladder shows a bulging mural mass in the fundus (*right of image.*)

should include defining the relationship of the tumor to the free serosal surface of the gallbladder and to the hepatic bed (and the hepatic surgical margin, if present), as well as the extent of tumor extension into the extra-hepatic biliary tree. All accompanying lymph nodes should also be submitted for histologic evaluation.

Extrahepatic Biliary Tract

The extrahepatic biliary tract consists of the common bile duct, the cystic duct and gallbladder, and the common hepatic duct. In approximately 60% to 70% of patients, the common hepatic duct bifurcates outside of the liver into the right and left hepatic ducts.[8] The predominant anatomic variation is congenital absence of the right hepatic duct. Instead, in these cases, one finds that the posterior and anterior branches of bile ducts emerging from the right lobe of the liver merge directly with the left hepatic duct.[8] Regardless, the common hepatic duct and its branches lie ventral to the portal vein system. The right bile duct may wrap in an inferior/ventral or superior/dorsal fashion around the right portal vein.

The common bile duct courses through the head of the pancreas before it reaches the ampulla of Vater. In approximately 60% to 70% of individuals, the main pancreatic duct joins the common bile duct and enters the ampulla as a common channel. In the remainder, the two ducts do not join anatomically before reaching the ampulla. Scattered along the intrahepatic and extra-hepatic biliary tract are mucin-secreting submucosal glands. These become particularly prominent near the terminus of the common bile duct, where they appear as microscopic outpouchings that interdigitate with the smooth muscle of the ampullary sphincter.

Two general situations may arise in which part of the extrahepatic biliary tract may be submitted for surgical pathology analysis. The first occurs as a result of resection of a lesion of the biliary tract, as with biliary cancer[9] or a choledochal cyst. More commonly, the biliary tract is submitted as part of a pancreas or liver resection spec-imen. The extrahepatic biliary tract may also be resected following injury. In all instances, reconstruction of the biliary tract is often performed by a Roux-en-Y choledo-chojejunostomy.[10] In an end-to-side or end-to-end fashion, a blind loop of jejunum is anastomosed to a remnant of the bile duct system.

BILIARY TRACT CANCER

Resection specimens for cancer generally consist of a portion of the extrahepatic biliary tract, gallbladder, and accompanying soft tissue and lymph nodes. Anatomic orientation is necessary and should be provided by the surgeon. Consultation with the surgeon is mandatory if there is any uncertainty regarding proper anatomic

orientation. En face sections of the proximal and distal bile duct margins should be obtained. The soft tissue margins should be marked with ink if possible; disruption of anatomic planes during intraoperative dissection may make identification of true soft tissue margins difficult. The biliary system should then be opened in the fresh state to allow inspection of the mucosal aspect of the tumor. The specimen should be fixed in formalin overnight before tissue processing is begun.

Following fixation, cross sections along the length of the biliary tract are optimal for histologic evaluation. These sections should include soft tissue margins (ante-rior, left lateral, posterior, right lateral). Depending on the amount of soft tissue, lymph nodes may be included within cross sections of the biliary tract. If not, they should be dissected out separately and submitted for histologic evaluation. Distinct lymph node groups should be submitted in separate cassettes and separated as follows: periductal, perihilar, peripancreatic, subpyloric, celiac, and preaortic.

A portion of the liver may be resected during resection of an extrahepatic bile duct cancer. The liver should be sampled both for intrinsic damage to the hepatic corpus from biliary obstruction and generously along the liver resection margin for the presence of tumor. Particular attention should be given to intrahepatic invasion of cancer because biliary tract cancer may track extensively along the intrahepatic biliary tree. This may be evident grossly as white, thickened portal tracts. Unfortunately, as a result, hepatic resection margins may include invasive cancer in places where portal tracts have been transected (Fig. 25-12). Thus, generous samples of major portal

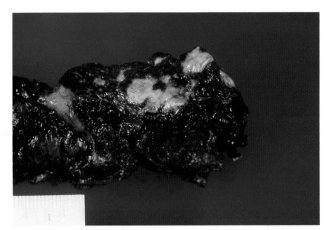

FIGURE 25–12. En face liver surface, representing the resection margin of a left hepatic lobectomy and resection of the upper portion of the extrahepatic biliary tract for Klatskin's tumor. The liver parenchyma is darkly pigmented owing to obstructive cholestasis. Yellow-white portal tracts are massively expanded by invasive bile duct adenocarcinoma (cholangiocarcinoma), tracking up the portal tract system from the main tumor mass located at the confluence of the right and left hepatic bile ducts. Malignant portal tracts were located 5 cm upstream and were not evident on preoperative imaging studies.

tracts at the hepatic resection margin should always be obtained.

CHOLEDOCHAL CYST

Congenital cystic dilatation of the common bile duct (choledochal cyst) may be seen in association with cystic dilatation of the intrahepatic biliary tract (see Chapter 41). Choledochal cysts are classified into four categories: cylindrical dilatation of the common bile duct along some portion of its length, cystic diverticulum off the free portion of the common duct, saccular dilatation of the intrapancreatic portion of the common bile duct (with or without protrusion into the gut lumen at the ampulla of Vater), and various combinations of these.[11,12] Because ascending cholangitis, stone formation, pancreatitis, and biliary tract carcinoma are known complications of choledochal cysts,[13] surgical resection is the preferred method of treatment.

Analysis of the resection specimen requires careful attention to the anatomy of the bile ducts. Unfortunately, the cyst wall is often thin and delicate; thus, the specimen is often disrupted by the surgeon or by the prosecting pathologist. The mucosal surface of the cyst should be examined carefully, and any areas that exhibit plaquelike thickening, a thickened velvety texture, or effacement of the underlying tissue layers should be submitted for histologic examination. Likewise, the proximal and distal bile duct margins (including the region of the ampulla if a Whipple procedure was performed) should be sampled, along with soft tissue margins adjacent to suspicious areas.

EXTRAHEPATIC BILIARY ATRESIA

This condition is discussed further in Chapter 41, particularly with regard to hepatic aspects of the disease. Considerable variability characterizes the anatomy of biliary atresia. When the disease is limited to the common bile duct (type I) or extrahepatic hepatic bile ducts (type II), it is usually surgically correctable. Unfortunately, 90% of patients have type III biliary atresia, in which there is also obstruction of bile ducts at the level of the porta hepatis. This latter group includes "early, severe" biliary atresia, in which the intrahepatic biliary tree does not form properly, resulting in absence of duct patency at the hilum.[14] These cases are noncorrectable surgically except by liver transplantation.

In an infant with type I or type II extrahepatic biliary atresia, biliary tract resection combined with a portoenterostomy is a common surgical procedure (Kasai procedure). Biliary drainage is reestablished by anastomosis of a portion of the jejunum to the hilum of the liver via a Roux-en-Y procedure.[15] The primary responsibility of the pathologist evaluating this type of resection specimen is to obtain cross sections of the resected biliary tree, with particular attention to the most proximal portion. This is because the diameter of residual bile duct lumina at the level of the porta hepatis has been reported to correlate with long-term functionality of the portoenterostomy.[16]

◼ Intraoperative Consultation and Frozen Section Analysis

The extrahepatic biliary tree and pancreas constitute one of the most challenging regions of the body to assess by intraoperative consultation with frozen section analysis. Common situations in which a pathologist may be asked to evaluate a specimen include (1) evaluation of the distal bile duct margin of a partial hepatectomy specimen for biliary tract cancer; (2) evaluation of the proximal bile duct and pancreatic margins of a pancreatoduodenectomy (Whipple) specimen; and (3) evaluation of an intraoperative needle biopsy of the pancreas to distinguish chronic pancreatitis from pancreatic carcinoma. The challenge of diagnosing pancreatic cancer is discussed in detail in Chapter 31. Evaluation of bile duct resection margins is often made difficult by dilatation and inflammation of the proximal common bile duct, which can occur as a result of biliary obstruction. The bile duct epithelium may become inflamed and markedly reactive in appearance, showing loss of epithelial cell maturation, elongation and pseudostratification of epithelial nuclei, and increased mitoses. The peribiliary glands may also become hypertrophied, inflamed, and edematous. Features that favor benign reactive changes include absence of true stratification of the epithelium, gradual transition between atypical areas and epithelial regions that are more clearly reactive in appearance, and the presence of prominent neutrophilic inflammation and/or ulceration.

References

1. Fritscher-Ravens A, Topalidis T, Bobrowski C, et al: Endoscopic ultrasound-guided fine-needle aspiration in focal pancreatic lesions: A prospective intraindividual comparison of two needle assemblies. Endoscopy 33:484-490, 2001.
2. Stasi MD, Lencioni R, Solmi L, et al: Ultrasound-guided fine needle biopsy of pancreatic masses: Results of a multicenter study. Am J Gastroenterol 93:1329-1333, 1998.
3. Jailwala J, Fogel E, Sherman S, et al: Triple-tissue sampling at ERCP in malignant biliary obstruction. Gastrointest Endosc 51:383-390, 2000.
4. Lester SC: Manual of Surgical Pathology. New York, Churchill Livingstone, 2001, pp 198-208.
5. LaMont JT, Carey MC: Cholesterol gallstone formation. 2. Pathobiology and pathomechanics. Prog Liv Dis 10:165-191, 1992.
6. Mok HY, Druffel ER, Rampone WM: Chronology of cholelithiasis: Dating gallstones from atmospheric radiocarbon produced by nuclear bomb explosions. N Engl J Med 314:1075-1077, 1986.
7. Cahalane MJ, Neubrand MW, Carey MC: Physical-chemical pathogenesis of pigment gallstones. Semin Liver Dis 8:317-328, 1988.

8. Nakanuma Y, Hoso M, Sanzen T, et al: Microstructure and development of the normal and pathologic biliary tract in humans, including blood supply. Microsc Res Tech 38:552-570, 1997.

9. Tominaga S, Kuroishi T: Biliary Tract Cancer. Cancer Surveys Volume 19/20: Trends in Cancer Incidence and Mortality. London, UK, Imperial Cancer Research Fund, 1994, pp 125-137.

10. Jones DB, Soper NJ: Complications of laparoscopic cholecystectomy. Ann Rev Med 47:31-44, 1996.

11. Todani T, Watanabe Y, Narasue M, et al: Congenital bile duct cysts: Classification, operative procedures and review of 37 cases including cancer arising from choledochal cyst. Am J Surg 134:263-269, 1977.

12. Todani T, Watanabe Y, Blan WA, et al: Cylindrical dilatation of the choledochus: A special type of congenital bile duct dilatation. Surgery 98:964, 1985.

13. Bloustein PA: Association of carcinoma with congenital cystic conditions of the liver and bile ducts. Am J Gastroenterol 67:40-46, 1977.

14. Desmet VJ: Ludwig symposium on biliary disorders—part I. Pathogenesis of ductal plate abnormalities. Mayo Clin Proc 73:80-89, 1998.

15. Chiba T, Kasai M, Sasano M: Reconstruction of intrahepatic bile ducts in congenital biliary atresia. Tohuku J Exp Med 115:99-104, 1955.

16. Tan CE, Davenport M, Driver M, et al: Does the morphology of the extrahepatic biliary remnants in biliary atresia influence survival? A review of 205 cases. J Pediatr Surg 29:1459-1464, 1994.

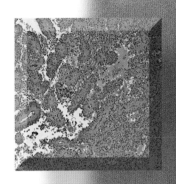

CHAPTER 26

Diagnostic Cytology of the Pancreas and Biliary Tract

BARBARA A. CENTENO

■ Cytology of the Pancreas

Fine-needle aspiration biopsy (FNAB) is the most effective procedure for sampling pancreatic lesions. The most frequent reason for FNAB of the pancreas is evaluation of a pancreatic mass, either benign or malignant. Cystic lesions are frequently aspirated as well.

Contraindications for FNAB of the pancreas are few and include the presence of an uncorrectable bleeding disorder and the lack of a safe needle access route.[1] However, FNAB may be performed in a patient with an uncorrectable bleeding diathesis if the need for a tissue diagnosis is urgent. Also, if the access route cannot be changed by bypassing either a vascular structure or the gastrointestinal tract, use of a small-gauge needle reduces the risk of complications. For endoscopic ultrasound (EUS)-guided FNAB, gastrointestinal obstruction is an absolute contraindication because of the risk of intestinal perforation.[2]

GUIDANCE TECHNIQUES

Guidance techniques include intraoperative palpation and direct visualization, transabdominal ultrasound (TUS), computed tomography (CT), and EUS. In addition, percutaneous techniques have their own advantages and disadvantages.[2] The types of needles and equipment used for aspiration in the pancreas are similar to those used for other deep-seated lesions.

EUS is rapidly becoming the preferred imaging technique because it allows for accurate staging in the process of sampling a pancreatic mass or lymph nodes.[3-6] Briefly, a biopsy needle is passed through the biopsy chamber of an echoendoscope, which consists of a linear array transducer mounted distal to the end of the viewing optical component of the endoscope. Thus, the needle is passed through the gastrointestinal wall into the pancreas under real-time imaging.[7]

Commonly used biopsy needles include the EUSN-1 needle aspiration system (Wilson-Cook Medical Inc., Winston-Salem, NC) and the GIP Medi-Globe (Medi-Globe Corporation, Tempe, AZ). Echoendoscopes are manufactured by both Olympus (Olympus America Inc., Melville, NY) and Pentax (Pentax Precision Instrument Corporation, Orangeburg, NY), the latter of which makes the Pentax FG 32-UA.

DIAGNOSTIC ACCURACY

The sensitivity of percutaneous pancreatic FNAB is approximately 80.5%,[8] and the specificity is over 90%.[9] Numerous papers have recently been published on EUS-guided FNA. Ylagan and associates recently reviewed the literature on EUS-guided FNA of the pancreas and reported on their own series of cases. The sensitivity for EUS-guided FNAB ranges from 64% to 96% in all studies,[10] with most studies reporting a sensitivity of over 80%. Most series report a specificity of 100%.[10]

NORMAL PANCREAS AND CONTAMINANTS

Ductal Cells

The epithelium of the large pancreatic ducts is composed of columnar epithelium arranged in flat, honeycombed sheets of cells. The nuclei are centrally located or may be present in a palisaded, "picket-fence" arrangement in which nuclei are basally located (Figs. 26-1 and 26-2). The main pancreatic ducts may also contain goblet cells. In contrast to the epithelium of the large ducts, intralobular duct epithelium is composed of cuboidal cells with scant basophilic cytoplasm; these cells are usually found in flat sheets (Fig. 26-3) or small clusters or as tubular structures.

Acinar Cells

Aspirates of the normal pancreas consist predominantly of acinar-type epithelium, typically arranged either singly or as small acinar-shaped structures. The cells are pyramidal or triangular and contain abundant granular cytoplasm with numerous intracytoplasmic zymogen granules. The nuclei are round, have a granular chromatin pattern, contain prominent nucleoli, and are either centrally or eccentrically located (Fig. 26-4).

Islet Cells

Islet cells are rarely detected in aspirates of the normal pancreas.[11] When present, they occur as loose aggregates of cells that contain wispy, ill-defined amphophilic cytoplasm and oval nuclei with a stippled chromatin pattern (Fig. 26-5).

Normal Contaminants

Mesothelial cells, hepatocytes, and gastrointestinal epithelium are occasional contaminants in FNAB of the pancreas. Mesothelial cells appear as polygonal cells arranged in flat sheets, showing round to oval nuclei and intercytoplasmic "windows" (Fig. 26-6). Normal hepatocytes are large polygonal cells with dense, sharply defined cytoplasm and round, central or eccentric nuclei with prominent nucleoli.

Gastric or small intestinal epithelium is potentially the most problematic of the contaminants because these cells may be abundant, particularly in aspirates obtained by EUS guidance; therefore, they may be misinterpreted as adenocarcinoma or as a mucinous neoplasm. The surface mucous cells of the gastric epithelium appear as columnar cells arranged in large folded sheets or palisaded rows or as single cells. Intact fragments may reveal the attachment of the surface epithelium to the lamina propria. Typically, a luminal border may be seen along one edge of the cellular aggregates. The sheets are typically monolayered but occasionally may be folded or thick. Gastric pits may appear in some groups of cells as rosettes in the center of a cellular

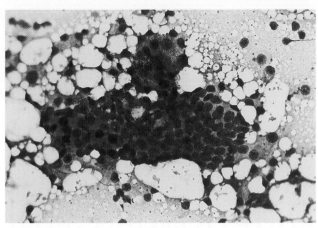

FIGURE 26–2. Large duct epithelium. Flat monolayered sheet of cells with evenly spaced nuclei (Diff-Quik).

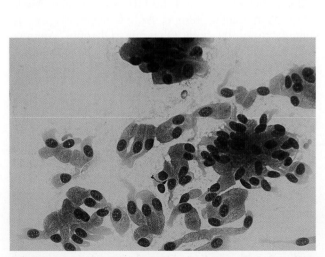

FIGURE 26–1. Large duct epithelium. Columnar epithelium from large pancreatic ducts (Diff-Quik).

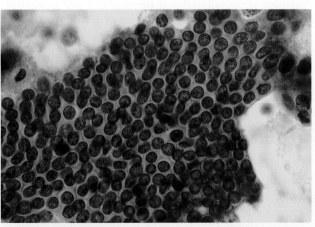

FIGURE 26–3. Small duct epithelium. The cells are arranged in flat monolayered sheets. Nuclei are small, round, and regular in size (Papanicolaou).

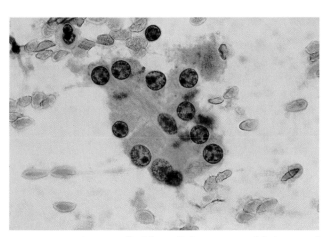

FIGURE 26–4. Acinar cells. The cells have pyramidal shape and contain granular cytoplasm with sharply defined borders. The nuclei are round with smooth borders and prominent nucleoli (Papanicolaou).

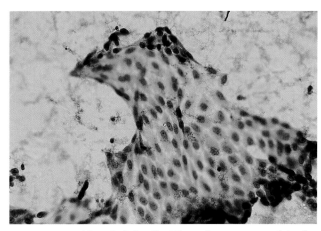

FIGURE 26–6. Mesothelial cells. The cells are arranged in flat sheets and show characteristic intercytoplasmic windows. This feature distinguishes mesothelial cells from normal pancreatic duct cells (Papanicolaou).

sheet. The mucous glands of the cardia or pylorus are indistinguishable from surface mucous cells. Goblet cells are always detected if the needle tract enters non-gastric tissue. Chief and parietal cells may be noted if the needle traverses the fundic region of the stomach. Gastric epithelium is associated with abundant mucus, which may contain degenerated cells if an inflammatory process has occurred (Fig. 26-7).

Small intestinal epithelium has a similar architectural appearance to that of the surface mucus epithelium of the stomach, but the epithelial component is composed of absorptive enterocytes with interspersed goblet cells. The brush border is visible when the cells are seen on edge. Paneth cells are occasionally seen and are identified by the presence of coarse granules in the cytoplasm. Small intestinal epithelium is also associated with mucus.

REACTIVE PROCESSES

The most common reactive processes of the pancreas include acute and chronic pancreatitis. Typical smears of cases with acute pancreatitis are characterized by a dirty, necrotic background; necrotic cells; cellular debris; fat necrosis; and calcifications (Fig. 26-8).[11] Acute inflammation may be prominent. Normal pancreatic elements, when present, show evidence of necrosis and degeneration. Pancreatic ductal epithelium may reveal various degrees of reactive atypia.

In chronic pancreatitis, the cellularity of smears varies greatly depending on the stage of disease. In the earlier stages, which correspond to resolving acute pancreatitis, mononuclear cells with histiocytes, granulation tissue, and early fibrous tissue are present. In the later stages, smears are often scant and contain only ductal epithelium, fibrous tissue, and islet cells (Fig. 26-9).[11]

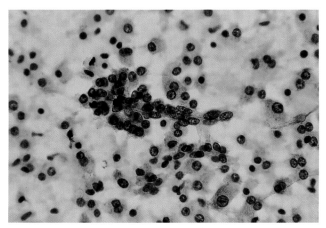

FIGURE 26–5. Loose cluster of islet cells. The cells have a scant amount of amphophilic cytoplasm. The nuclei are oval with finely stippled chromatin pattern (salt-and-pepper)(Papanicolaou).

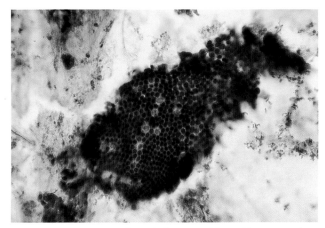

FIGURE 26–7. Intestinal epithelium. Goblet cells are evident within the intestinal epithelium. The sheet of cells is associated with mucin in the background (Papanicolaou).

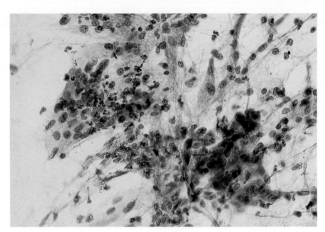

FIGURE 26–8. Acute pancreatitis. The smear is moderately cellular and shows neutrophils infiltrating residual duct cells. A foamy macrophage is also present.

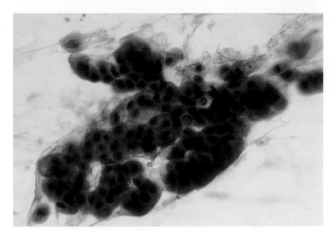

FIGURE 26–10. Reactive changes. This sheet of cells shows a slight increase in the nucleus-to-cytoplasm ratio and slightly enlarged nuclei. However, the sheet is still arranged in a monolayer and is tightly cohesive (Papanicolaou).

In addition to reactive processes, biliary stents and radiation or chemotherapy may cause severe reactive atypia (Fig. 26-10). Nuclear changes may be striking and are characterized by nuclear enlargement, anisocytosis, increased coarseness of the chromatin, including subtle abnormalities of chromatin distribution, and prominent nucleoli. However, in contrast to adenocarcinoma, the cell groups in reactive lesions typically remain cohesive and appear as a monolayer.

DUCTAL ADENOCARCINOMA

Diagnosis of ductal adenocarcinoma of the pancreas based on FNAB samples is usually straightforward. Occasionally, the distinction between benign lesions and adenocarcinoma may be vague. Several studies have evaluated a number of cytomorphologic criteria in pancreatic FNAB specimens in an effort to identify a set of minimal cytologic criteria that could help separate

benign processes from adenocarcinoma.[9,12-14] These features are summarized in Table 26-1.

Overall, many different criteria have been applied, some successfully. However, their usefulness has not been proved in a prospective fashion. Nevertheless, assessment of degree of cellularity, type of architecture, degree of nuclear atypia, presence or absence of single cells, mitoses, and necrosis has been shown to improve diagnostic accuracy and to allow for differentiation of reactive atypia from adenocarcinoma, as well as for the recognition of well-differentiated adenocarcinoma. However, overreliance on a single criterion may lead to decreased sensitivity and specificity; thus, use of a combination of criteria is best when these lesions are evaluated. The cytologic differences between reactive processes and adenocarcinomas are summarized in Table 26-2.

Well-Differentiated Adenocarcinoma

The architectural and nuclear alterations of well-differentiated adenocarcinoma are more subtle compared with those of moderately and poorly differentiated tumors.[13,15,16] Features of well-differentiated adenocarcinomas are summarized below (Figs. 26-11 through 26-16; Box 26-1).

BOX 26–1. Cytologic Features of Well-Differentiated Adenocarcinomas

- Significant nuclear crowding and overlapping
- Cohesive aggregates, lacking feathering at the edges
- Irregular chromatin clearing more common
- Hyperchromasia less common
- Pyramidal and carrot-shaped nuclei containing focal notches, grooves, or convolutions
- Nuclear enlargement (1.5 × RBC on air-dried smears)
- Anisocytosis exceeding 4:1
- Infrequent mitoses

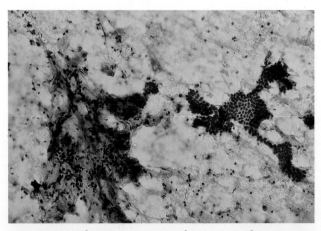

FIGURE 26–9. Chronic pancreatitis. This aspirate is from a patient with late-stage chronic pancreatitis; it shows a fragment of dense fibrous tissue and a cohesive cluster of benign duct cells. The smear lacks intact acinar epithelium (Papanicolaou).

TABLE 26–1. Cytologic Criteria for the Diagnosis of Ductal Adenocarcinoma

Authors	Criteria	Formula
Mitchell and Carney[12]	Disoriented or crowded cell groups Nuclear enlargement Nuclear contour irregularities	Needed all three criteria for diagnosis
Cohen et al[9]	Anisonucleosis (4:1 group) Enlarged nuclei Nuclear molding	Presence of two or more of these criteria was diagnostic
Francillon et al[14]	Irregular nuclear membranes Nuclear enlargement Single malignant cells	Needed all three for diagnosis
Robins et al[13]	**Major:** Nuclear crowding Nuclear contour irregularity Nuclear chromatin irregularity **Minor:** Single cells, necrosis Mitoses Nuclear enlargement (2.5 × RBC)	2 major or 1 major + 2 minor diagnostic

TABLE 26–2. Benign Processes vs. Adenocarcinoma

Feature	Benign Epithelium and Reactive Processes	Adenocarcinoma
Cellularity	Scant (except gastrointestinal contamination)	Moderate to high
Architecture	Flat and cohesive	Irregular
Loss of polarity	Minimal	Prominent
Nuclear crowding	Minimal	Prominent
Nuclear membrane contour	Round, oval	Angulation, elongation, notches, grooves
Chromatin	Fine, granular	Parachromatin clearing
Mitoses	Minimal/normal	Present/atypical
Single atypical cells	Absent	Present
Nuclear enlargement	Minimal	1.5 × RBC or 2–3 × neutrophil
Nuclear size variation	Minimal	4:1

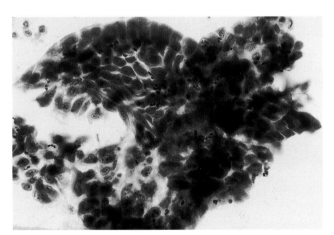

FIGURE 26–11. Radiation-induced changes. The epithelium is gastric in origin. It appears atypical because the cells show an increased nucleus-to-cytoplasm ratio and are hyperchromatic. However, the cells are arranged in a cohesive monolayer, and the nuclei are uniform in size. These features favor a benign process (Papanicolaou).

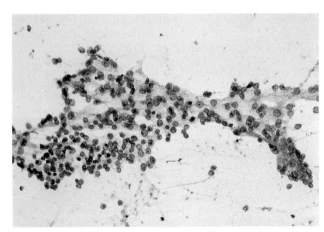

FIGURE 26–12. Adenocarcinoma, well differentiated. In contrast to a benign process in which nuclei tend to be evenly spaced, the nuclei in this case show an uneven distribution (Papanicolaou).

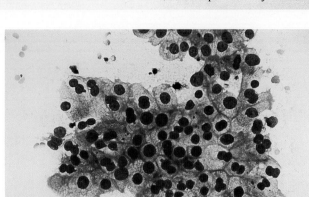

FIGURE 26–13. Adenocarcinoma, well differentiated. The cells are arranged as an exaggerated type of honeycomb sheet. The nuclei show anisocytosis and coarse chromatin but are round in shape (Diff-Quik).

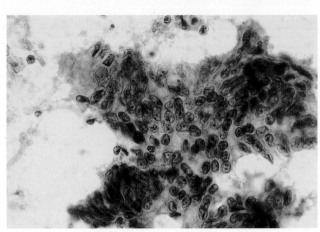

FIGURE 26–15. Adenocarcinoma, well differentiated. This sheet of cells shows crowded and overlapping nuclei, some carrot shaped. The chromatin is pale. These subtle nuclear alterations are characteristic of well-differentiated adenocarcinoma (Papanicolaou).

In general, the degree of cellularity and type of architecture of cell aggregates are helpful in distinguishing benign from malignant epithelium. Patterns typical of malignancy are large folded sheets of cells with nuclear overlapping and crowding, and sheets of cells with an exaggerated honeycomb pattern caused by abundant mucin. In normal ductal or gastrointestinal epithelium, the nuclei are evenly and uniformly spaced, and the cytoplasm is relatively equal in quality and quantity among cells. Dyshesion is not a useful feature because, not uncommonly, sheets of well-differentiated adenocarcinoma are cohesive. However, single epithelial cells with highly atypical cytologic features are diagnostic of malignancy.

Moderately and Poorly Differentiated Adenocarcinomas

Compared with well-differentiated tumors, moderately and poorly differentiated adenocarcinomas are more easily recognized as malignant processes by FNAB (Figs. 26-17 and 26-18; Box 26-2).

Undifferentiated (Anaplastic) Adenocarcinoma

Cytologic features of undifferentiated adenocarcinoma have been poorly described. Smears are typically cellular. Neoplastic cells are often spindly or show multinucleation with bizarre giant cells (Fig. 26-19). Cytophagocytosis, tumor necrosis, and a marked inflammatory infiltrate are additional findings. The cytologic features of undifferentiated carcinoma are summarized in Box 26-3.[17,18]

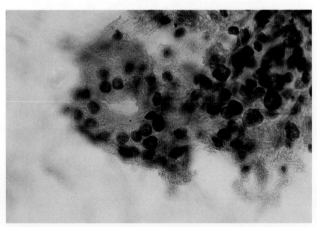

FIGURE 26–14. Adenocarcinoma, well differentiated. This group also shows nuclear crowding and overlapping. An acinar structure is present.

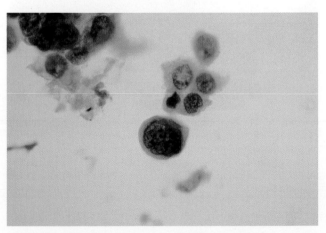

FIGURE 26–16. Adenocarcinoma, well differentiated. The presence of isolated malignant cells is diagnostic (Papanicolaou).

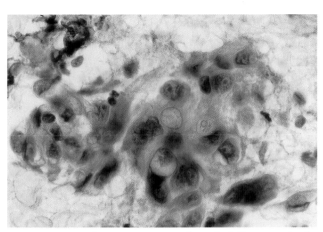

FIGURE 26–17. Adenocarcinoma, moderately differentiated. The cells show enlarged nuclei with anisocytosis. The chromatin is coarse and unevenly distributed. The cells have cytoplasmic mucin vacuoles (Papanicolaou).

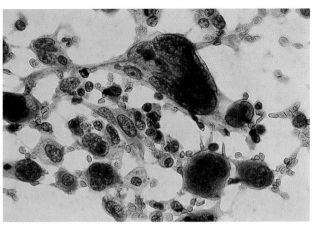

FIGURE 26–19. Adenocarcinoma, undifferentiated. This smear shows a large bizarre multinucleated cell and smaller spindled undifferentiated-appearing malignant cells. A multinucleated osteoclast-type quint cell is present at the bottom of the field (Papanicolaou).

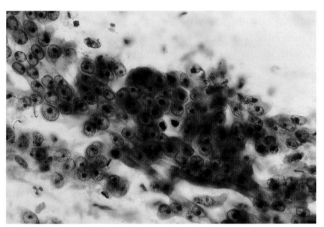

FIGURE 26–18. Adenocarcinoma, poorly differentiated. This group reveals cells with large nuclei and prominent nucleoli. The cells have a scant amount of cytoplasm and are dyshesive, a feature that becomes more prominent with higher-grade tumors (Papanicolaou).

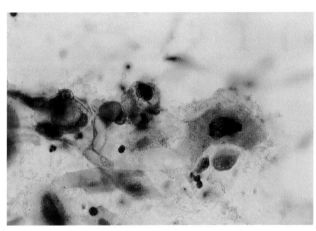

FIGURE 26–20. Adenosquamous carcinoma. This field shows a few keratinized squamous cells mixed with vacuolated glandular cells (Papanicolaou).

BOX 26–2. **Cytologic Features of Moderately and Poorly Differentiated Adenocarcinomas**

- Apparent nuclear irregularities, notched nuclei
- Notched, grooved, or convoluted nuclei
- Greater degree of nuclear enlargement and anisocytosis
- Greater degrees of architectural complexity and cellular dyshesion
- Prominent macronucleoli
- Decreased mucin production
- Increased mitoses and necrosis

BOX 26–3. **Cytologic Features of Undifferentiated Adenocarcinoma**

- Highly cellular
- Bizarre spindle-shaped cells and multinucleated cells
- "Sarcomatoid" cells
- Cytophagocytosis, tumor necrosis, prominent inflammatory infiltrate

Undifferentiated carcinomas are easily recognizable as malignant; however, the morphologic differential diagnosis includes other types of high-grade neoplasm.

Variants of Ductal Adenocarcinoma

Adenosquamous carcinoma is the most common variant of ductal adenocarcinoma, accounting for 3% to 4% of all pancreatic malignancies. Malignant cells that show both glandular and squamous differentiation characterize the smears of aspirates. By convention, to qualify as an adenosquamous carcinoma, the squamous population must account for at least 30% of the lesion (Fig. 26-20).

Signet ring cell carcinomas account for 1% to 3% of malignancies, and mucinous noncystic carcinomas (similar to colloid carcinoma) (Fig. 26-21) account for less than 1% of malignancies.[19] The cytomorphology of these neoplasms is similar to that of malignancies in other sites. Briefly, signet ring cell carcinoma is composed of single malignant cells with a cytoplasmic mucin vacuole that distends and compresses the nucleus. Mucinous noncystic carcinoma shows groups of malignant glands floating in pools of mucin. Identification of these entities is usually straightforward, but the differential diagnosis includes metastasis from other primary sites. A key point regarding mucinous noncystic carcinoma is that it is the most frequent type of invasive carcinoma associated with intraductal papillary mucinous neoplasm.[20]

PANCREATIC CYSTS

When a cytology specimen obtained from a cystic lesion of the pancreas is evaluated, the key differential diagnosis includes mucinous neoplasms versus nonmucinous lesions, pseudocysts versus cystic neoplasms, and benign versus malignant tumors.

Analysis of (1) pancreatic cyst fluid obtained by image-guided FNA for cytology, (2) enzymes, (3) tumor markers, and (4) viscosity has been advocated as a potential means of diagnosing pancreatic cysts preoperatively.[21-23] Cytology can help distinguish mucinous from nonmucinous lesions and can be used to diagnose specific entities and malignant neoplasms when the cell sample is sufficient. However, cytology alone often lacks adequate sensitivity owing to the difficulty inherent in obtaining sufficiently cellular samples.[23-25]

Levels of adequate tumor markers and pancreatic enzymes, as well as cyst fluid viscosity in pancreatic cyst fluid, are assessments by which the diagnostic accuracy of pancreatic cyst fluid analysis[21-23] can be improved over the accuracy of cytology alone. Pancreatic cyst fluid analysis may be evaluated on the basis of the following differential diagnoses.

Mucinous Versus Nonmucinous. Mucinous lesions are characterized by increased viscosity and elevated levels of cyst fluid carcinoembryonic antigen (CEA).[21] These findings alone help exclude serous cystadenoma and pseudocyst from the differential diagnosis. Recently, mucin-like carcinoma antigen[26] and gastric mucin (M1 antigens)[27] have been investigated for their use in diagnosing mucinous lesions; they appear to be specific for the diagnosis of mucinous lesions. Unfortunately, an elevated CEA level is not always indicative of a mucinous neoplasm.

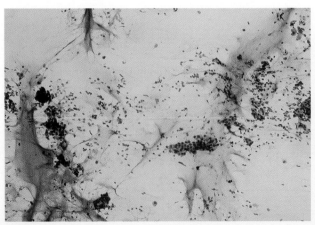 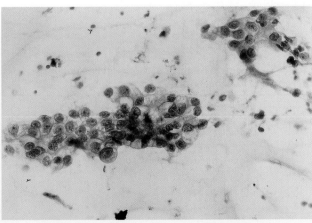

A   **B**

FIGURE 26–21. Mucinous noncystic carcinoma. **A,** At low power, groups of malignant cells appear to be floating with dense mucin (Papanicolaou). **B,** At high power, the cells show minimal nuclear atypia such as nuclear enlargement and coarse chromatin (Papanicolaou).

At the New York Presbyterian-Weill Cornell Center, a patient with a dilated duct caused by obstruction from a pancreatic endocrine tumor had an elevated fluid aspirate CEA level (Barbara A. Centeno, unpublished data). Benign entities such as enteric duplication cysts[28] may also contain elevated CEA levels.

Pseudocysts Versus Cystic Neoplasms. Pseudocysts usually have less relative viscosity than serum and contain low levels of CEA, CA 72-4, and CA 125, as well as a variety of other tumor markers. They typically contain high amylase (usually more than 5000 U/L) and lipase levels.[29]

Benign and Borderline Versus Malignant Mucinous Cystic Neoplasms. Increased levels of CA 72-4 and tissue polypeptide antigen (TPA), which is a proliferation antigen,[21,30] have been shown to correlate with malignancy. CA 15-3 has been shown to correlate with malignancy when its level is greater than 100 ng/mL. However, levels in the lower range overlap with pseudocysts. Benign tumors consistently have levels less than 35 mg/mL. Therefore, when high, CA 15-3 is a specific marker of malignancy, but low levels are nonspecific.[21]

Pancreatic Versus Extrapancreatic Tumors. In the experience of one cytologist, extrapancreatic cysts when compared with pancreatic lesions routinely have amylase and lipase levels below the normal serum level (K. B. Lewandrowski, personal communication). However, this remains to be tested in a systematic fashion.

CA 19-9 has been reported to be useful in the diagnosis of neoplastic cysts,[22] but in our unpublished experience, it has been shown to lack sufficient sensitivity and specificity.[21]

Although cyst fluid analysis can provide valuable additional information, it is recommended that a panel of tests be used[21] and that the results be correlated with all other findings before a treatment plan is instituted.

Non-neoplastic Cysts

Non-neoplastic cysts of the pancreas include inflammatory and infectious "pseudocysts" and congenital cysts. Most of these entities are rare. Pseudocysts are the most common[31] and thus the most clinically relevant. Aspiration of a pseudocyst typically reveals an abundant amount of turbid, brown fluid that contains inflammatory cells (mostly macrophages), fibrin, debris, and bile or hematoidin pigment (Fig. 26-22). This fluid lacks lining epithelial cells but may contain benign cells from adjacent pancreatic parenchyma. The cytologic features of pseudocysts have been described and are listed in Box 26-4.[24]

The differential diagnosis of pseudocysts includes other inflammatory or infectious cysts, as well as true cysts or cystic neoplasms. Secondary bacterial infections may produce cyst fluid that contains abundant neutrophils and proteinaceous background debris.[32] Cultures

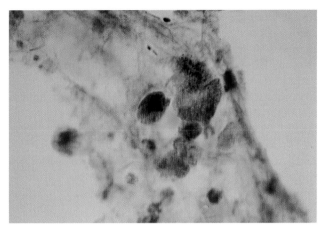

FIGURE 26–22. Pseudocyst. The smear shows abundant fibrillar debris mixed with bile pigment and occasional inflammatory cells (Papanicoloau).

of the fluid are usually positive. The presence of lining epithelium naturally excludes the diagnosis of a pseudocyst.

CYSTIC NEOPLASMS

Cystic neoplasms include serous cystadenomas and mucinous cystic neoplasms. Intraductal papillary-mucinous neoplasms and intraductal papillary-oncocytic neoplasms cause dilatation of the pancreatic ducts that often appears cystic on radiologic studies. Finally, solid neoplasms such as pancreatic endocrine tumors or solid pseudopapillary tumors may undergo cystic degeneration as well.

Serous Cystadenoma/Serous Cystadenocarcinoma

Aspiration of a serous cystadenoma typically provides only a scant amount of fluid. The background is usually watery. The smears are composed of cells that are cuboidal and possess clear cytoplasm arranged in flat, monolayered sheets. The cells contain nuclei that are

BOX 26–4. **Cytologic Features of Pseudocysts**

- Turbid, brown fluid
- Variable numbers of inflammatory cells, including neutrophils and histiocytes
- Granular debris, fibrin, and bile or hematoidin pigment
- Absence of lining epithelial cells
- Normal pancreatic cells, fibroblasts, mesothelial cells, and metaplastic cells

round and uniform in shape; the cytoplasm is fragile and easily stripped from the nuclei, leaving them bare.[24,33] Aspirates may also contain fragments of fibrovascular stroma. The periodic acid–Schiff (PAS) stain with and without diastase may be performed on cytology samples to demonstrate the presence of cytoplasmic glycogen, a characteristic feature of serous cystadenomas (Figs. 26-23 and 26-24; Box 26-5).[24,33]

The diagnosis of cystadenocarcinoma depends primarily on the histologic identification of invasion. No reliable differences have been noted in the cytologic appearance of benign and malignant serous neoplasms.

Mucin-Producing Cystic Neoplasms

Mucinous cystic neoplasms and intraductal papillary-mucinous neoplasms show significant overlap in their

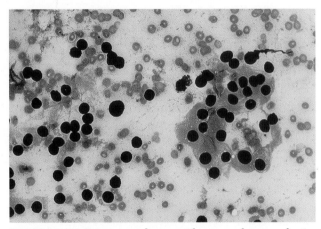

FIGURE 26–23. Serous cystadenoma. The smear shows a cohesive cluster of cells with sharp cytoplasmic borders. The nuclei are round and uniform in shape. Because the cytoplasm is fragile, some nuclei "stripped" of their cytoplasm are present (Diff-Quik).

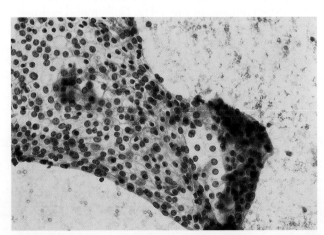

FIGURE 26–24. Serous cystadenoma. Large flat monolayer of epithelial cells of cuboidal shape with clear cytoplasm and round, uniformly spaced nuclei (Papanicolaou).

cytomorphologic features. Occasionally, aspiration of fluid from either of these entities may be difficult because the fluid is often extremely viscous and thus does not readily pass into the needle; this should provide the aspirator with a clue to the diagnosis. Gross examination of the fluid can be extremely helpful. The fluid is highly viscous and may contain floating mucus plugs. A key diagnostic feature on smears is the presence of abundant thick mucin. This mucin usually contains degenerated cellular debris and macrophages (Fig. 26-25). The key diagnostic feature in cytology samples is the presence of mucinous columnar cells. These cells may show a varying degree of architectural and nuclear atypia similar to the high level of heterogeneity of the cyst lining one sees on histopathology (Figs. 26-26 through 26-28). Papillary clusters, nuclear grooves and inclusions, and psammomatous calcifications (Fig. 26-29) are also features of the papillary lesions (Box 26-6).

INVASIVE CARCINOMAS RELATED TO MUCINOUS CYSTIC NEOPLASMS

Aspiration of a solid area of a mucinous cystic neoplasm or intraductal papillary mucinous neoplasm, when visualized under radiologic guidance, may prove diagnostic of adenocarcinoma when the cystic fluid is not.[25,34] Invasion cannot be determined on the basis of evaluation of cystic or ductal fluid only. Nevertheless,

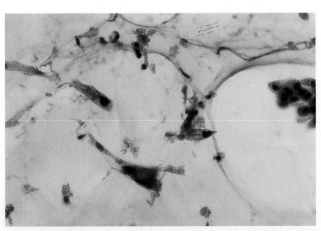

FIGURE 26–25. Mucinous cystic neoplasm. The appearance of the mucin in this case is characteristic. It is pink in color and thick in texture and contains degenerated cells. Also seen are a few degenerated neoplastic mucinous columnar cells (Papanicolaou).

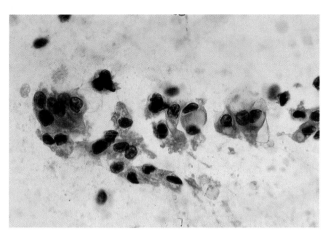

FIGURE 26–26. Mucinous cystadenoma. These cells show a degree of atypia typical of adenomatous lesions. Columnar mucinous cells are relatively dyshesive and contain mucin vacuoles. The nuclei are slightly elongated and irregular in outline and contain nuclear grooves. No mitosis or necrosis is seen in this specimen (Papanicolaou).

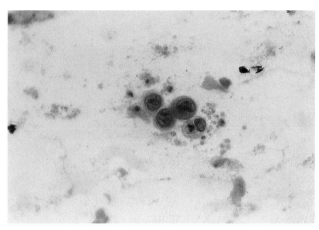

FIGURE 26–28. Intraductal papillary mucinous carcinoma. The presence of isolated single cells with a high N/C ratio and subtle nuclear membrane irregularity is typical of noninvasive carcinoma. The background contains abundant degenerated cellular material (Papanicolaou).

invasive carcinomas are usually identified as malignant. They contain signet ring cells (Fig. 26-30).

Invasive tubular-type carcinomas resemble ductal adenocarcinoma, with abundant necrosis and pleomorphism (see Fig. 26-17). The invasive component most frequently seen in intraductal papillary mucinous neoplasm is a noncystic mucinous carcinoma (see Fig. 26-21).

DIFFERENTIAL DIAGNOSIS OF MUCIN-PRODUCING CYSTIC NEOPLASM

The main differential diagnosis of mucinous cystic neoplasm includes benign gastrointestinal epithelium, retention cysts, and dilated ducts caused by obstruction. Aspirates that are obtained under EUS guidance invariably contain gastric epithelium. Furthermore, the gastric epithelium is often associated with a scant amount of mucin. Further complicating the picture may be the

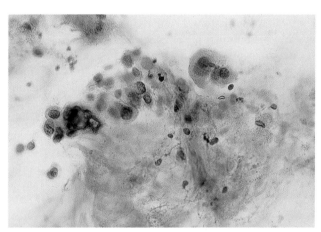

FIGURE 26–29. Intraductal papillary mucinous carcinoma. Psammomatous calcifications may be present occasionally.

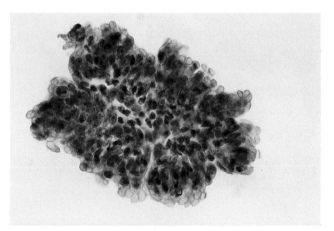

FIGURE 26–27. Intraductal papillary mucinous neoplasm with moderate dysplasia ("borderline" tumor). The sheet of cells shows nuclear crowding and overlapping. The nuclei are enlarged and elongated and have clumped chromatin (Papanicolaou).

BOX 26–6. **Cytologic Features of Mucin-Producing Cystic Neoplasms**

- Highly viscous fluid
- Tenacious mucin in the background
- Mucinous columnar epithelium with a variable degree of architectural and cytologic atypia
- Psammoma bodies (in intraductal papillary mucinous neoplasm)
- Papillary clusters with fibrovascular cores (in intraductal papillary mucinous neoplasm)
- Intranuclear grooves and inclusions (in intraductal papillary mucinous neoplasm)

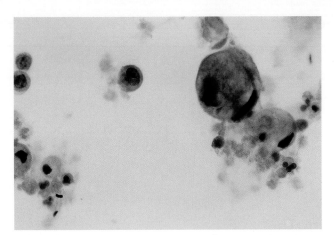

FIGURE 26–30. Invasive mucinous cystadenocarcinoma. Signet ring cells are often associated with invasive mucin-producing cystic neoplasms (Papanicolaou).

presence of cellular debris caused by an inflammatory process that may mimic the contents of mucinous cystic neoplasms. If the aspirated material is highly thick, one can usually feel confident that the aspirate has come from a mucinous and cystic neoplasm because gastrointestinal contents are normally watery and thin. However, fluid from cystic neoplasms may not always be viscous. Therefore, one needs to exercise some caution when evaluating this feature. If the diagnosis is uncertain, the best approach may be to describe the presence of mucinous epithelium and mucin, then provide a differential diagnosis.

Retention cysts are relatively infrequent, small, dilated, cystic segments of pancreatic duct that occur upstream from an area of pancreatic duct obstruction.[31] The diagnosis of a retention cyst is usually made on the basis of clinical data and the finding of a cyst that is connected to a distorted pancreatic ductal system in a patient with a history of chronic pancreatitis. Because they develop from obstructed ducts, the walls of these cysts may be lined by pancreatic ductal epithelium,[31] but inflammation, pressure of cyst contents, and necrosis may ultimately destroy the lining epithelium. Cyst fluid from a retention cyst often includes a variable quantity of inflammatory cells and may contain benign pancreatic ductal epithelium, normal acinar cells, islet cells, or fibroblasts from adjacent parenchyma.[11] The specimen from a retention cyst may also contain abundant inspissated mucus. FNAB findings are similar to those of pseudocysts when the cyst lining epithelium is absent.

The presence of an obstructing mass or a history of pancreatitis may provide evidence that the patient has a dilated duct caused by obstruction. However, patients with intraductal papillary-mucinous neoplasm may also appear to have an obstructing mass and typically also have a history of pancreatitis.[35] Distinction of a dilated duct from an intraductal papillary-mucinous neoplasm may be difficult on cytologic grounds alone because the features have significant overlap.

It is important to remember that accurate diagnosis of mucinous cystic neoplasm often requires correlation among the cytologic, radiologic, and clinical features. For example, if cytologic findings reveal a mucin-producing neoplasm that includes papillary architecture and was obtained from a cyst that connects with a dilated pancreatic duct, a diagnosis of intraductal papillary-mucinous neoplasm should be favored. If the aspirate is obtained from a cystic lesion in the body or tail of the pancreas that does not connect with the main pancreatic duct and is present in a middle-aged female, a diagnosis of mucinous cystic neoplasm should be considered. When the cytologic, radiologic, and clinical features remain uncertain, a diagnosis of mucin-producing cystic neoplasm should be provided, and an appropriate differential diagnosis should be included in the report.

INTRADUCTAL ONCOCYTIC PAPILLARY NEOPLASMS

Intraductal oncocytic papillary neoplasm is a recently described intraductal neoplasm with morphologic and clinical features that overlap with those of intraductal papillary mucinous neoplasms.[20] Cytology smears show a pattern similar to that of intraductal papillary neoplasm. The cells are usually arranged in papillary clusters with background mucin that includes macrophages and cell debris. However, the main distinction is that the cells are oncocytic in appearance (Fig. 26-31).

SOLID-PSEUDOPAPILLARY TUMOR

Solid-pseudopapillary tumor of the pancreas has a characteristic cytologic picture.[36,37] Smears are typically cellular and contain numerous branching papillary-like groups of epithelial cells with a central fibrovascular core. The papillary fronds have three layers—a central

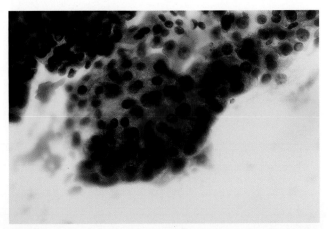

FIGURE 26–31. Intraductal papillary oncocytic neoplasm. The tumor forms papillae similar to those in intraductal papillary-mucinous neoplasms, but the cells are oncocytic in appearance (Papanicolaou).

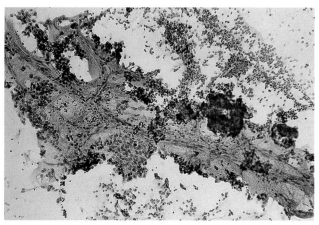

FIGURE 26–32. Solid-pseudopapillary tumor. Clusters of large branching papillae are typical. The papillae have three layers: a central capillary, a mucoid stromal layer surrounding blood vessels, and an outer layer of neoplastic cells.

vessel, a middle mucoid stromal layer, and an outer layer of neoplastic epithelium (Fig. 26-32). The layer of neoplastic epithelium is composed of monomorphic epithelial cells with round to oval nuclei, finely dispersed chromatin, nuclear indentations or grooves, and small nucleoli. The cytoplasm of these cells is basophilic, varies in quantity, and may contain PAS-positive granules. The pathognomonic feature is "balls" of mucoid stroma that may or may not contain a rim of epithelial cells (Fig. 26-33; Box 26-7).[36,37]

CYSTIC PANCREATIC ENDOCRINE TUMORS

Cystic pancreatic endocrine tumors are uncommon, accounting for 3.4% of all cystic neoplasms and 4.3% of all pancreatic endocrine tumors in one series.[38] However, cystic degeneration in large, nonfunctional tumors

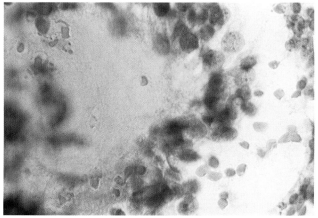

FIGURE 26–33. Solid-pseudopapillary tumor. This smear shows "balls" of mucoid stroma, which are pathognomonic of this tumor. Neoplastic cells tend to surround these structuress (Papanicolaou).

BOX 26–7. **Cytology of Solid-Pseudopapillary Tumor**

- Cellular, branching groups of cells
- Papillary fronds composed of a central fibrovascular core, surrounded by a myxoid layer of stroma and an outer layer of neoplastic cells
- Neoplastic cells with bland nuclei and scant amphophilic cytoplasm that occasionally contain PAS-positive granules
- "Balls" of mucoid stroma +/− rim of neoplastic cells

is a relatively common occurrence.[39] The cytologic features of these tumors are similar to those of their solid counterpart.

RARE PANCREATIC AND EXTRAPANCREATIC CYSTS AND NEOPLASMS

Other lesions such as endothelial tumors (hemangiomas and lymphangiomas, which are rare in this area),[40] rare neoplasms such as acinar cell cystadenocarcinoma,[41,42] and any pancreatic neoplasm that has undergone cystic degeneration should be considered. Peripancreatic and/or retroperitoneal cysts and cystic neoplasms that appear to be pancreatic in origin on radiologic studies account for approximately 21% of lesions that are aspirated percutaneously.[25] These lesions may be misdiagnosed if the possibility of an extrapancreatic cyst is not considered. A few examples of these lesions include hydroureter, adrenal cyst, mesothelial cyst, mesenteric lymphangioma, gastric primary tumor, retroperitoneal leiomyoma, malignant lymphoma in a retroperitoneal lymph node, gastrointestinal stromal tumor, and gastric leiomyosarcoma.[25,43,44]

PANCREATIC METASTASES

The pancreas is the site of metastasis in 3% to 11% of cancer patients with a primary elsewhere.[45-48] FNAB is as useful in the evaluation of secondary pancreatic tumors as it is for primary tumors.[47] Adenocarcinomas, malignant melanoma, and renal cell carcinomas metastatic to the pancreas are discussed in the following sections.

Adenocarcinomas

Cancers of the lung, breast, stomach, and colon are primary tumors that most frequently metastasize to the pancreas. Immunoperoxidase studies may provide helpful information in the differential diagnosis of these tumors. Markers that may be of benefit include CK 7, CK 17, CK 20, TTF-1 and BRST-2, (Table 26-3).[49-54] The differential diagnosis of metastatic lesions is discussed extensively in Chapter 33 and is not discussed further here. Breast, colon, and gastric adenocarci-

TABLE 26–3. Immunoperoxidase Studies for the Differential Diagnosis of Adenocarcinoma

Carcinoma Type	Marker				
	CK 7	CK 17	CK 20	TTF-1	BRST-2
Pancreatic and biliary	+	+/−	+	−	−
Breast primary	+	−	−	−	+
Colon primary	−	−	+	−	−
Lung primary	+	−	−	+	−
Gastric primary	+	−	−	−	−

nomas may be identified because they have morphologic features that make them fairly recognizable. Metastatic pulmonary adenocarcinoma is difficult to distinguish from a pancreatic primary because its morphology is similar. Both sites may demonstrate squamous differentiation; however, this is likely to be more common among lung primaries.

Melanoma

Melanoma is one of the most common types of metastasis to the pancreas.[45-48] Its morphologic features have been well described. Melanin pigment, which is diagnostic, is not always present. In the absence of melanin pigment, helpful diagnostic ancillary studies include immunoperoxidase stains for vimentin, S100, HMB-45, and MART-1.[55]

Renal Cell Carcinoma

Renal cell carcinoma not uncommonly metastasizes to the pancreas.[47,56-66] These metastases are composed of a pleomorphic population of clear cells with central round nuclei and prominent nucleoli. Stripped nuclei, which occur in renal cell carcinoma, are not characteristic of ductal adenocarcinoma of the pancreas.

PANCREATIC ENDOCRINE TUMORS

Collins and Cramer[67] reported their experience with the cytomorphology of pancreatic endocrine tumors. They reported that smears from these tumors, which are cellular and evenly dispersed, are monomorphic and contain round, monotonous-appearing nuclei. The chromatin pattern has a characteristic salt-and-pepper appearance. The cytoplasm is variable in quantity, and because it is fragile, stripped nuclei are common. The cells occur more often singly than in clusters. A plasmacytoid appearance is fairly characteristic. The clear cell variant, which can be recognized on cytologic specimens, contains abundant cytoplasmic lipid[68] (Figs. 26-34 through 26-36; Box 26-8).

The diagnosis of pancreatic endocrine tumors can be confirmed with immunocytochemical studies for chromogranins A, B, and C, neuron-specific enolase,

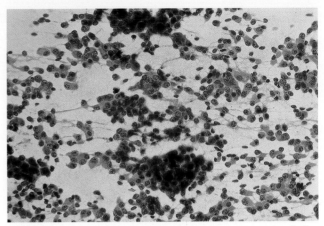

FIGURE 26–34. Pancreatic endocrine tumor. Smears of this tumor are usually cellular and contain evenly dispersed cells. The cells are arranged singly and have abundant well-defined cytoplasm (Papanicolaou).

and synaptophysin, as well as a variety of other regulatory peptides, hormones, and amines. Electron microscopic studies can be used to demonstrate the presence of electron-dense membrane-bound granules,[31] but this is rarely needed.

Benign processes and neoplasms included in the differential diagnosis of pancreatic endocrine tumor include islet cell hyperplasia, solid-pseudopapillary tumor, adenocarcinoma, acinic cell carcinoma, high-grade neuroendocrine carcinoma (small cell carcinoma), non-Hodgkin's lymphoma, and occasionally plasmacytoma and malignant melanoma.

Islet cell hyperplasia, seen in chronic pancreatitis, produces cohesive clusters of islet cells admixed with an exocrine component.[69] Solid-pseudopapillary tumor is characterized by the presence of branching papillary structures with fibrovascular stalks and myxoid stroma—architectural features not usually seen in pancreatic endocrine tumors.

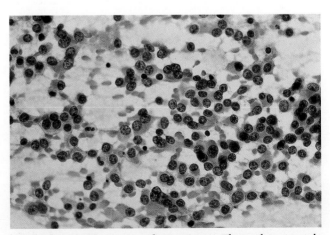

FIGURE 26–35. Pancreatic endocrine tumor. The nuclei are evenly distributed, round, and uniform and contain coarsely clumped chromatin (salt-and-pepper appearance).

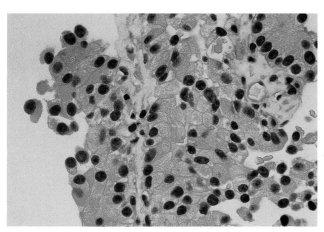

FIGURE 26–36. Pancreatic endocrine tumor, clear cell variant. The cells in this specimen have clear cytoplasm owing to the presence of lipid.

BOX 26–8. **Cytologic Features of Pancreatic Endocrine Tumors**

- Cellular smears; monomorphic, dyshesive cells
- Cells arranged singly or in loose clusters and pseudorosettes
- Naked nuclei
- Cytoplasm basophilic, wispy, and ill-defined, but possibly dense and well defined
- Finely stippled chromatin (a salt-and-pepper appearance)
- Binucleation or multinucleation common
- Plasmacytoid cells with eccentric nucleus and dense cytoplasm
- Cytoplasmic lipid in the clear cell variant

Adenocarcinomas tend to have more cohesive fragments, evidence of glandular differentiation, greater pleomorphism and nuclear atypia, and more extensive mitosis and necrosis compared with pancreatic endocrine tumors. The pseudorosettes of pancreatic endocrine tumors may be mistaken for glands. Occasionally, pancreatic endocrine tumors may have prominent nucleoli, which can cause a mistaken diagnosis of adenocarcinoma. Even when atypia is present, pancreatic endocrine tumors retain the uniformity of their nuclei.

Acinic cell carcinomas are characterized by monomorphic cells with abundant, basophilic cytoplasm that contains zymogen granules.[67]

High-grade neuroendocrine carcinomas have greater nuclear pleomorphism and nuclear molding and more extensive mitosis and necrosis.[70]

Non-Hodgkin's lymphomas are more dyshesive, and the cells have uniformly scant cytoplasm. Lymphoglandular bodies are indicative of a neoplasm with lymphoid differentiation. When these are present, a diagnosis of pancreatic endocrine tumor is excluded.

Plasmacytomas rarely occur in this region.[71] Similar to other lymphomas, plasmacytomas are dyshesive and thus do not produce aggregates or clusters of cells. In difficult cases, ancillary immunohistochemical studies for cytokeratin, chromogranin, and kappa and lambda light chains can be useful. Pancreatic endocrine tumors are positive for cytokeratins and chromogranin, whereas plasmacytomas express light chain.

ACINAR CELL CARCINOMA

The cytologic features of acinar cell carcinoma are not well described.[72-77] At low power, smears resemble pancreatic endocrine tumors because they are richly cellular and show a loosely cohesive population of cells with stripped nuclei. The cells form loose cohesive clusters of large and small acini. Nuclei are euchromatic, round to oval, and centrally or eccentrically located; they contain prominent cherry-red nucleoli (Fig. 26-37). The cytoplasm is scant to moderate in amount, amphophilic and slightly granular in appearance. Romanowsky's stain or a PAS stain (with diastase) can be used to highlight the granularity. Granularity is caused by the presence of cytoplasmic zymogen granules (Box 26-9).

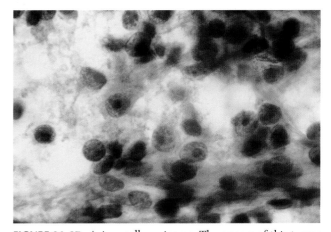

FIGURE 26–37. Acinar cell carcinoma. The smears of this tumor are typically cellular. The cells have overlapping features with endocrine tumors. However, the presence of prominent cherry-red nucleoli, as are seen here, is characteristic (Papanicolaou).

BOX 26–9. **Cytologic Features of Acinar Cell Carcinoma**

- Richly cellular
- Mixture of large and small clusters of cells, single cells, and stripped nuclei
- Uniform cells that resemble normal acinar cells
- Round to oval, central or eccentric euchromatic nuclei with smooth nuclear contours and prominent nucleoli (1 to 2)
- Scant to moderate granular cytoplasm (Romanowsky's stain, PAS with diastase)

On immunohistochemistry, trypsin is consistently expressed by these tumors.[78] Amylase and lipase may be expressed less often.[78-80]

The differential diagnosis of acinar cell carcinoma includes benign pancreatic acini, pancreatic endocrine tumor, solid-pseudopapillary tumor, and pancreatoblastoma.

In contrast to acinar cell carcinoma, benign pancreatic acini typically form more prominent organoid arrangements of acini. Pancreatic endocrine tumors typically lack a prominent cherry-red nucleolus but occasionally form pseudoacinar structures. The architectural features of solid-pseudopapillary tumor, as discussed previously, are fairly unique and easy to differentiate from acinar cell carcinoma. The most difficult lesion to distinguish from acinar cell carcinoma is pancreatoblastoma, which also shows prominent acinar differentiation. Features overlap significantly on smears; however, the diagnosis of pancreatoblastoma may be made when squamous corpuscles, which are most often seen on cell block preparations, are identified.

PANCREATOBLASTOMA

FNA smears of pancreatoblastoma are highly cellular and show a predominantly dissociated smear pattern composed largely of primitive round to oval, and occasionally triangular, epithelial cells with central to eccentric nuclei, evenly distributed coarse chromatin, occasional nucleoli, and delicate, finely granular cytoplasm. Mesenchymal stromal fragments with traversing capillaries, dense acellular stromal fragments, and necrotic debris have also been described (Figs. 26-38 and 26-39; Box 26-10).[81] Identification of squamous corpuscles on smears has not been described; they may be better appreciated on cell block preparations.

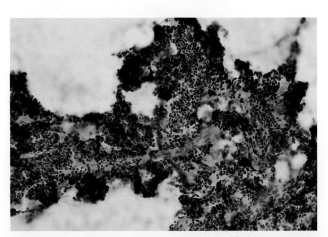

FIGURE 26–38. Pancreatoblastoma. Smears of this tumor are hypercellular and show small undifferentiated cells with scant cytoplasm arranged in large sheets with vascular stroma. Squamous corpuscles are not present in this field (Papanicolaou). (Courtesy of Dr. David Klimstra, Memorial Sloan-Kettering Cancer Center, New York, NY.)

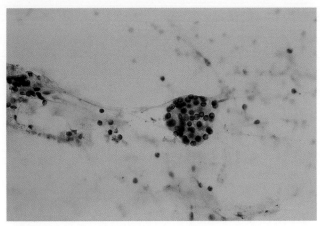

FIGURE 26–39. Pancreatoblastoma. The cells are small and undifferentiated. Stripped nuclei are present in the background (Papanicolaou). (Courtesy of Dr. David Klimstra, Memorial Sloan-Kettering Cancer Center, New York, NY.)

BOX 26–10. **Cytologic Features of Pancreatoblastoma**

- Highly cellular smears
- More frequently single cells than clusters
- Primitive "blastema"-type epithelial cells
- Eccentric nuclei
- Coarse, evenly distributed chromatin
- Delicate cytoplasm
- Stromal fragments
- Squamous cells

The main differential diagnosis is acinar cell carcinoma because of the common finding of acinar cell differentiation in pancreatoblastomas. Squamoid corpuscles are the main diagnostic feature of pancreatoblastoma, but they are not always present. Stromal fragments with traversing capillaries may also raise the possibility of a solid-pseudopapillary tumor.

Cytology of the Biliary Tract

Numerous methods may be used to sample the biliary system. These include aspiration of duodenal contents, direct sampling of biliary secretions, and endobiliary brushing. The most frequent indication is the presence of a stricture or obstruction of the biliary tree. Aspiration of duodenal contents, performed since the 1920s, has low sensitivity.[82] This technique is not popular because it is difficult to perform, cancers are often detected at an advanced stage, detection of neoplastic cells gives no indication of the site of origin of the tumor, and duodenal secretions may degenerate exfoliated tumor cells. The latter of these has caused false-positive diagnoses in a number of patients, including 5% to 10% of controls.

Direct sampling of biliary and pancreatic duct secretions became possible in the 1960s with the introduction of endoscopic retrograde cholangiopancreatography (ERCP) and percutaneous transhepatic cholangiography (PTC). The cumulative sensitivity of this technique for the diagnosis of biliary carcinoma is 66%,[82] and false-positives are rare.

Endobiliary brushing is currently the preferred method of sampling the biliary system in cases of stricture or obstruction because the preparation is usually rich in cells, and cell preservation is excellent if the specimen is fixed immediately.[83] Overall sensitivity is 60%, which is significantly higher than that reported for exfoliative cytology obtained by PTC or ERCP.[82] Prospective studies have also documented a higher level of sensitivity of biliary brushings over exfoliative cytology for the detection of biliary carcinoma.[72,73] Furthermore, the sensitivity of bile duct brushings has been shown to increase after repeated attempts. In fact, the probability of a patient's having a carcinoma is less than 6% after three negative brushings.[74] Furthermore, prospective studies have documented an increase in the sensitivity of biliary sampling when this procedure is used in conjunction with brushings.[75,76]

Most false-negatives occur from sampling error,[77] which may occur when the tumor does not invade biliary mucosa. Examples include lymphomas in periductal nodes, metastatic carcinomas, and pancreatic endocrine tumors or hepatocellular carcinomas without mucosal ulceration. Interpretation errors (17%) and technical errors (17%) are the second most frequent causes of false-negative results. Most interpretation errors result from underinterpretation of adenocarcinoma, which is caused by the difficulty of distinguishing adenocarcinoma from reactive changes.[84] The converse is also true: Reactive changes can mimic adenocarcinoma, leading to false-positives. Degeneration of malignant cells is also a source of false-negatives. Finally, tumors with sclerotic desmoplastic stroma do not exfoliate cells as readily as tumors without desmoplastic stroma; thus, they may not be detected with brushings.

False-positives commonly result from overinterpretation of reactive and degenerative changes[82,85] or adenomatous epithelium from villous tumors of the ampulla[83] or bile duct.[85] Papillary lesions and dysplasia within the biliary ductal system may also cause false-positives.

FNA is of benefit for the diagnosis of cholangiocarcinoma only if the tumor presents as a mass lesion, in which case the cytologic criteria used to diagnose adenocarcinoma of the pancreas may be applied. Unfortunately, cholangiocarcinomas that arise in the common bile duct cannot be distinguished from those of pancreatic origin. Because biliary brushing is the method most frequently used to sample biliary strictures, the remainder of this chapter focuses on exfoliative cytology of the biliary system.

EXFOLIATIVE CYTOLOGY OF THE BILIARY SYSTEM

Normal Biliary Tract

Normal bile duct epithelial cells are tall, columnar, or cuboidal. These cells are typically found in flat, mono-layered sheets in a picket fence arrangement. The cytoplasm of biliary epithelium is cyanophilic; bile fluid in the background usually contains degenerated cells and bile pigment. Brushing samples are usually more cellular than bile fluid.[86] In a situation of inflammation or injury, the epithelial lining may develop mucinous metaplasia or squamous metaplasia (Fig. 26-40).

Reactive Changes

Inflammation of the biliary system results from choledocholithiasis, sclerosing cholangitis, acute cholangitis, infection, calculi, stents, or instrumentation. Unfortunately, the changes induced by inflammation may lead to false-positive diagnosis of carcinoma. Changes induced by inflammation include loss of surface structures, vacuolization of cytoplasm, nuclear enlargement, coarse hyperchromasia, multinucleation, and multinucleolation (Fig. 26-41).[86]

Dysplasia

Dysplasia and carcinoma in situ typically occur on the surface epithelium and either extend downward or project into the lumen.[86] Low-grade dysplasia is characterized by sheets and clusters of cells that show nuclear crowding and overlapping. Nuclear membranes are smooth, and the nucleus-to-cytoplasm ratio is moderate. The chromatin is characteristically clear and granular with mild clumping. Dysplastic cells may have one or two distinct nucleoli. More pronounced nuclear crowding

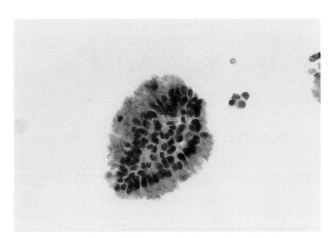

FIGURE 26–40. Normal biliary epithelium. The cells, when seen on edge, are columnar in shape and contain basally located nuclei. They also have abundant cytoplasmic mucin, which is characteristic of mucinous metaplasia (Papanicolaou).

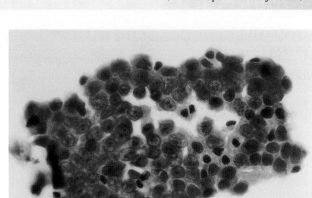

FIGURE 26–41. Reactive changes. This smear is from a patient with a biliary stent. The cells are arranged in a two-dimensional sheet but show nuclear enlargement, increased N/C ratio, and coarse chromatin. Features that favor a benign process are the cohesiveness of the sheet and the lack of anisocytosis (Diff-Quik).

and overlapping occur in high-grade dysplasia. In these cases, nuclear membranes are irregular, the nucleus-to-cytoplasm ratio is significantly increased, chromatin is coarse, and nucleoli are distinct and prominent.[86]

Adenocarcinoma

Adenocarcinoma shows architectural features of high-grade dysplasia but is characterized by a greater number of single cells[86]; thus, smears are highly cellular. The cytologic features of well-differentiated biliary adenocarcinoma overlap with those of well-differentiated pancreatic adenocarcinoma (Fig. 26-42). In higher-grade carcinomas, morphologic features of malignancy are readily apparent (Fig. 26-43). Paradoxically, the cytoplasm

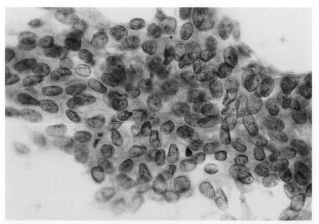

FIGURE 26–42. Adenocarcinoma, well differentiated. The nuclei, which vary slightly in size and shape, are crowded and disoriented and have pale chromatin and grooves. Features shown here are similar to those of well-differentiated adenocarcinoma of the pancreas (Papanicolaou).

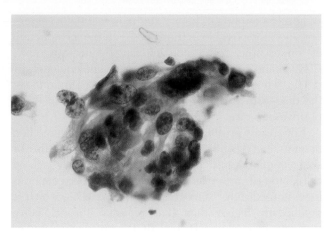

FIGURE 26–43. Adenocarcinoma, moderately differentiated. The nuclei are larger and more hyperchromatic (Papanicolaou).

may be abundant, so that the nucleus-to-cytoplasm ratio does not appear increased. The chromatin is usually coarse, and nucleoli are usually distinct.[86]

Carcinoma with mucinous or papillary differentiation may present a diagnostic pitfall primarily because both of these tumors are often well differentiated.[87] Thus, any mucinous change detected in epithelium needs to be highlighted in the report as possibly representative of a mucinous neoplasm, and further investigation should be recommended. Normal bile epithelium may form pseudopapillary clusters, but cell clusters in papillary lesions are crowded, and nuclei are usually arranged haphazardly. In contrast, the nuclei of papillary lesions are pointy and elongated. Occasionally, the nuclei of benign epithelium may also appear elongated, but again, the architectural arrangement is key. Carcinomas involve a greater degree of architectural abnormality, and hypochromatic transparent nuclei may be present.[87]

Reactive Processes Versus Adenocarcinoma

The differential diagnosis between a reactive process and an adenocarcinoma may be extremely difficult. Many of the features used in biliary samples are similar to those used for pancreatic carcinoma (see Table 26-2). A study from Japan showed that loss of a honeycomb arrangement, an increase in the size of nuclei, loss of polarity, a bloody background, the presence of flat nuclei, and a "cell-in-cell" arrangement are features highly associated with malignancy.[88] Another recent study from Iowa (the Iowa criteria) showed that nuclear molding, chromatin clumping, and an increased nucleus-to-cytoplasm ratio resulted in a sensitivity of 83% and a specificity of 98%.[89] A third method of differentiating reactive processes from adenocarcinoma involves a combination of data from these two studies.

Finally, some investigators are putting greater emphasis on qualitative rather than quantitative criteria. Some series have emphasized that gradation of atypia increases the likelihood of malignancy.[86] One study compared the Japan, Iowa, and Boston criteria (i.e., chromatin clumping, loss of polarity, and nuclear molding) in a series of 165 bile duct brushings. The sensitivities of the Japan and Iowa criteria were lower than those in the original series.[90] This study found that overall assessment of malignancy and evaluation for the presence of chromatin clumping had excellent reproducibility. Indeed, the overall assessment of malignancy was a better predictor of malignancy than was any other criterion, with a sensitivity of 36.2% and a specificity of 95%. Essentially, this study demonstrated that cytologists are capable of determining if the degree of atypia in a sample is representative of malignancy.[90]

References

1. Ryan JM, Hahn PF, Mueller PR: Image-guided pancreatic biopsy: Development, indications and complications. In Centeno BA, Pitman MB (eds): Fine Needle Aspiration Biopsy of the Pancreas. Boston, Butterworth-Heinemann, 1999, pp 1-4.
2. Ryan JM, Hahn PF, Mueller PR: Pancreatic fine needle aspiration biopsy: Imaging, equipment, and technique. In Centeno BA, Pitman MB (eds): Fine Needle Aspiration Biopsy of the Pancreas. Boston, Butterworth-Heinemann, 1999, pp 5-11.
3. Chang KJ: Endoscopic ultrasound-guided fine needle aspiration in the diagnosis and staging of pancreatic tumors. Gastrointest Endosc Clin North Am 5:723-734, 1995.
4. Brugge WR: Pancreatic cancer staging: Endoscopic ultrasonography criteria for vascular invasion. Gastrointest Endosc Clin North Am 5:741-753, 1995.
5. Hawes RH, Zaidi S: Endoscopic ultrasonography of the pancreas. Gastrointest Endosc Clin North Am 5:61-80, 1995.
6. Palazzo L, Roseau G, Gayet B, et al: Endoscopic ultrasonography in the diagnosis and staging of pancreatic adenocarcinoma. Results of a prospective study with comparison to ultrasonography and CT scan. Endoscopy 25:143-150, 1993.
7. Quirk DW, Brugge WR: Endoscopic ultrasonography-directed fine needle aspiration. In Centeno BA, Pitman MB (eds): Fine Needle Aspiration Biopsy of the Pancreas. Boston, Butterworth-Heinemann, 1999, pp 13-16.
8. Bret PM, Nicolet V, Labadie M: Percutaneous fine-needle aspiration biopsy of the pancreas. Diagn Cytopathol 2:221-227, 1986.
9. Cohen MB, Egerter DP, Holly EA, et al: Pancreatic adenocarcinoma: Regression analysis to identify improved cytologic criteria. Diagn Cytopathol 7:341-345, 1991.
10. Ylagan L, Edmundowicz S, Kasal K, et al: Endoscopic ultrasound guided fine-needle aspiration cytology of pancreatic carcinoma. A 3-year experience and review of the literature. Cancer Cytopathol 96:362-369, 2002.
11. Frias-Hidvegi D: Guides to Clinical Aspiration Biopsy: Liver and Pancreas. New York-Tokyo, Igaku-Shoin, 1988.
12. Mitchell ML, Carney CN: Cytologic criteria for the diagnosis of pancreatic carcinoma. Am J Clin Pathol 83:171-176, 1985.
13. Robins DB, Katz RL, Evans DB, et al: Fine needle aspiration of the pancreas. In quest of accuracy. Acta Cytol 39:1-10, 1995.
14. Francillon YJ, Bagby J, Abreo F, et al: Criteria for predicting malignancy in fine needle aspiration biopsies (FNAB) of the pancreas and biliary tree. Acta Cytol 40:1084, 1996.
15. Hejka AG, Bernacki EG: Cytopathology of well-differentiated columnar adenocarcinoma of the pancreas diagnosed by fine needle aspiration. Acta Cytol 34:716, 1990.
16. Lin F, Staerkel G: Cytologic criteria for well-differentiated adenocarcinoma (WDA) of pancreas in fine needle aspiration (FNA) specimens. Cancer Cytopathol 99:44-50, 2003.
17. Silverman JF, Dabbs DJ, Finley JL, et al: Fine-needle aspiration biopsy of pleomorphic (giant cell) carcinoma of the pancreas. Cytologic, immunocytochemical, and ultrastructural findings. Am J Clin Pathol 89:714-720, 1988.
18. Pinto MM, Monteiro NL, Tizol DM: Fine needle aspiration of pleomorphic giant-cell carcinoma of the pancreas. Case report with ultrastructural observations. Acta Cytol 30:430-434, 1986.
19. Klöppel G, Solcia E, Longnecker DS, et al: Histological Typing of Tumours of the Exocrine Pancreas, 2nd ed. Berlin, Springer-Verlag, 1996.
20. Adsay N, Longnecker D, Klimstra D: Pancreatic tumors with cystic dilatation of the ducts: Intraductal papillary mucinous neoplasms and intraductal oncocytic papillary neoplasms. Semin Diagn Pathol 17:16-30, 2000.
21. Lewandrowski K, Lee J, Southern J, et al: Cyst fluid analysis in the differential diagnosis of pancreatic cysts: A new approach to the preoperative assessment of pancreatic cystic lesions. AJR Am J Roentgenol 164:815-819, 1995.
22. Hammel P, Levy P, Voitot H, et al: Preoperative cyst fluid analysis is useful for the differential diagnosis of cystic lesions of the pancreas. Gastroenterology 108:1230-1235, 1995.
23. Pinto M, Meriano F: Diagnosis of cystic pancreatic lesions by cytologic examination and carcinoembryonic antigen and amylase levels of cyst contents. Acta Cytol 35:456-463, 1991.
24. Centeno BA, Lewandrowski KB, Warshaw AL, et al: Cyst fluid cytologic analysis in the differential diagnosis of pancreatic cystic lesions. Am J Clin Pathol 101:483-487, 1994.
25. Centeno BA, Warshaw AL, Mayo-Smith W, et al: Cytological diagnosis of pancreatic cystic lesions: A prospective study of 28 percutaneous aspirates. Acta Cytol 41:972-980, 1997.
26. Sperti C, Pasquali C, Pedrazzoli S, et al: Expression of mucin-like carcinoma-associated antigen in the cyst fluid differentiated mucinous from nonmucinous cysts. Am J Gastroenterol 92:672-675, 1997.
27. Hammel P, Voitot H, Vilgrain V, et al: Diagnostic value of CA 72-4 and carcinoembryonic antigen determination in the fluid of pancreatic cystic lesions. Eur J Gastroenterol Hepatol 10:345-348, 1997.
28. Pins MR, Compton CC, Southern JF, et al: Ciliated enteric duplication cyst presenting as a pancreatic cystic neoplasm: Report of a case with cyst fluid analysis. Clin Chem 38:1501-1503, 1992.
29. Adsay N, Klimstra D, Compton C: Introduction. Cystic lesions of the pancreas. Semin Diagn Pathol 17:1-7, 2000.
30. Yang JM, Southern JF, Warshaw AL, et al: Proliferation tissue polypeptide antigen distinguishes malignant mucinous cystadenocarcinomas from benign cystic tumors and pseudocysts. Am J Surg 171:126-129, 1996.
31. Solcia E, Capella C, Klöppel G: Tumors of the Pancreas, 3rd ed. Washington, DC, Armed Forces Institute of Pathology, 1997.
32. Jorda M, Essenfeld H, Garcia E, et al: The value of fine-needle aspiration cytology in the diagnosis of inflammatory pancreatic masses. Diagn Cytopathol 8:65-67, 1992.
33. Nguyen GK, Suen KC, Villanueva RR: Needle aspiration cytology of pancreatic cystic lesions. Diagn Cytopathol 17:177-182, 1997.
34. Tomaszewska R, Popiela T, Karcz D, et al: Infiltrating carcinoma arising in intraductal papillary-mucinous tumor of the pancreas. Diagn Cytopathol 18:445-448, 1998.
35. Lichtenstein DR, Carr-Locke DL: Mucin-secreting tumors of the pancreas. Gastrointest Endosc Clin North Am 5:237-258, 1995.
36. Cappellari JO, Geisinger KR, Albertson DA, et al: Malignant papillary cystic tumor of the pancreas. Cancer 66:193-198, 1990.
37. Granter SR, DiNisco S, Granados R: Cytologic diagnosis of papillary cystic neoplasm of the pancreas. Diagn Cytopathol 12:313-319, 1995.
38. Iacono C, Serio G, Fugazzola C, et al: Cystic islet cell tumors of the pancreas. A clinico-pathological report of two nonfunctioning cases and review of the literature. Int J Pancreatol 11:199-208, 1992.
39. Buetow PC, Parrino TV, Buck JL, et al: Islet cell tumors of the pancreas: Pathologic-imaging correlation among size, necrosis and cysts, calcification, malignant behavior, and functional status. AJR Am J Roentgenol 165:1175-1179, 1995.
40. Cruickshank AH, Benbow EW: Pathology of the Pancreas, 2nd ed. London, Springer-Verlag, 1995.
41. Cantrell BB, Cubilla AL, Erlandson RA, et al: Acinar cell cystadenocarcinoma of human pancreas. Cancer 47:410-416, 1981.
42. Stamm B, Burger H, Hollinger A: Acinar cell cystadenocarcinoma of the pancreas. Cancer 60:2542-2547, 1987.
43. Sperti C, Cappellazzo F, Pasquali C, et al: Cystic neoplasms of the pancreas: Problems in differential diagnosis. Am Surg 59:740-745, 1993.
44. Malhotra R, Evans R, Bhawan J, et al: A malignant gastric leiomyoblastoma presenting as an infected pseudocyst of the pancreas. Am J Gastroenterol 83:452-456, 1988.

45. Willis RA: The Spread of Tumours in the Human Body, 3rd ed. London, Butterworth, 1973.

46. Cubilla AL, Fitzgerald PJ: The Pancreas. Baltimore, Williams and Wilkins, 1980.

47. Carson HJ, Green LK, Castelli MJ, et al: Utilization of fine-needle aspiration biopsy in the diagnosis of metastatic tumors to the pancreas. Diagn Cytopathol 12:8-13, 1995.

48. Benning TL, Silverman JF, Berns LA, et al: Fine needle aspiration of metastatic and hematologic malignancies clinically mimicking pancreatic carcinoma. Acta Cytol 36:471-476, 1992.

49. Goldstein N, Bassi D: Cytokeratins 7, 17, and 20 reactivity in pancreatic and ampulla of Vater adenocarcinomas: Percentage of positivity and distribution is affected by the cut-point threshold. Am J Clin Pathol 115:695-702, 2001.

50. Wang NP, Zee S, Zarbo RJ, et al: Coordinate expression of cytokeratins 7 and 20 defines unique subsets of carcinomas. Appl Immunohistochem 3:99-107, 1995.

51. Sack M, Roberts S: Cytokeratins 20 and 7 in the differential diagnosis of metastatic carcinoma in cytologic specimens. Diagn Cytopathol 16:132-136, 1997.

52. Blumenfeld W, Turi G, Harrison G, et al: Utility of cytokeratin 7 and 20 subset analysis as an aid in the identification of primary site of origin in cytologic specimens. Diagn Cytopathol 20:63-66, 1999.

53. Chhieng D, Cangierella J, Zakowski M, et al: Use of thyroid transcription factor 1, PE-10, and cytokeratins 7 and 20 in discriminating between primary lung carcinomas and metastatic lesions in fine needle aspiration biopsy specimens. Cancer 25:330-336, 2001.

54. Fiel M, Cernaianu G, Burstein D, et al: Value of GCDFP-15 (BRST-2) as a specific immunocytochemical marker for breast carcinoma in cytologic specimens. Acta Cytol 40:637-641, 1996.

55. Artymyshyn RL: Editorial comments: Extramedullary plasmacytomas versus neuroendocrine tumors—the need for ancillary diagnostic techniques. Diagn Cytopathol 10:374-375, 1994.

56. Biset JM, Laurent F, de Verbizier G, et al: Ultrasound and computed tomographic findings in pancreatic metastases. Eur J Radiol 12:41-44, 1991.

57. Temellini F, Bavosi M, Lamarra M, et al: Pancreatic metastasis 25 years after nephrectomy for renal cancer. Tumori 75:503-504, 1989.

58. Fullarton GM, Burgoyne M: Gallbladder and pancreatic metastases from bilateral renal carcinoma presenting with hematobilia and anemia. Urology 38:184-186, 1991.

59. Rypens F, Van Gansbeke D, Lambilliotte JP, et al: Pancreatic metastasis from renal cell carcinoma. Br J Radiol 65:547-548, 1992.

60. Jenssen E: A metastatic hypernephroma to the pancreas. Acta Chir Scand 104:177-180, 1952.

61. Franciosi RA, Russo JF: Renal cell carcinoma metastasis to the pancreas thirteen years following nephrectomy. Mil Med 134:200-203, 1969.

62. Guttman FM, Ross M, Lachance C: Pancreatic metastasis of renal cell carcinoma treated by total pancreatectomy. Arch Surg 105:782-784, 1972.

63. Saxon A, Gottesman J, Doolas A: Bilateral hypernephroma with solitary pancreatic metastasis. J Surg Oncol 13:317-322, 1980.

64. Yazaki T, Ishikawa S, Ogawa Y, et al: Silent pancreatic metastasis from renal cell carcinoma diagnosed at arteriography. Acta Urol Jpn 27:1517-1522, 1981.

65. Weerdenburg JP, Jurgens PJ: Late metastasis of a hypernephroma to the thyroid and the pancreas. Diagn Imaging Clin Med 53:269-272, 1984.

66. Gohji K, Matsumoto O, Kamidono S: Solitary pancreatic metastasis from renal cell carcinoma. Acta Urol Jpn 36:677-681, 1990.

67. Collins BT, Cramer HM: Fine-needle aspiration cytology of islet cell tumors. Diagn Cytopathol 15:37-45, 1996.

68. Guarda LS, Silva EG, Ordoñez NG, et al: Clear cell islet cell tumor. Am J Clin Pathol 79:512-517, 1983.

69. Nguyen G-K: Cytology of hyperplastic endocrine cells of the pancreas in fine needle aspiration biopsy. Acta Cytol 28:499-502, 1984.

70. Banner BF, Myrent KL, Memoli VA, et al: Neuroendocrine carcinoma of the pancreas diagnosed by aspiration cytology. A case report. Acta Cytol 29:442-448, 1985.

71. Dodd LG, Evans DB, Symmans F, et al: Fine-needle aspiration of pancreatic extramedullary plasmacytoma: Possible confusion with islet cell tumor. Diagn Cytopathol 10:371-374, 1994.

72. Foutch P, Kerr D, Harlan J, et al: A prospective, controlled analysis of endoscopic cytotechniques for diagnosis of malignant biliary strictures. Am J Gastroenterol 86:577-580, 1991.

73. Kurzawinski T, Deery A, Dooley J, et al: A prospective controlled study comparing brush and bile duct exfoliative cytology for diagnosing bile duct strictures. Gut 33:1675-1677, 1992.

74. Rabinovitz M, Zajko AB, Hassanein T, et al: Diagnostic value of brush cytology in the diagnosis of bile duct carcinoma: A study in 65 patients with bile duct strictures. Hepatology 12:747-752, 1990.

75. Ponchon T, Gagnon P, Berger F, et al: Value of endobiliary brush cytology and biopsies for the diagnosis of malignant bile duct stenosis: Results of a prospective study. Gastrointest Endosc 42:565-575, 1995.

76. Pugliese V, Conio M, Nicolo G, et al: Endoscopic retrograde forceps biopsy and brush cytology of biliary strictures: A prospective study. Gastrointest Endosc 42:520-526, 1995.

77. Logrono R, Kurtycz D, Molina C, et al: Analysis of false-negative diagnoses on endoscopic brush cytology of biliary and pancreatic duct strictures: The experience at 2 university hospitals. Arch Pathol Lab Med 124:387-393, 2000.

78. Klimstra DS, Heffess CS, Oertel JE, et al: Acinar cell carcinoma of the pancreas. A clinicopathologic study of 28 cases. Am J Surg Pathol 16:815-837, 1992.

79. Morohoshi T, Held G, Kloppel G: Pancreatic tumors and their histological classification: A study based on 167 autopsy and 97 surgical cases. Histopathology 7:645-661, 1983.

80. Labate AM, Klimstra DL, Zakowski MF: Comparative cytologic features of pancreatic acinar cell carcinoma and islet cell tumor. Diagn Cytopathol 16:112-116, 1997.

81. Silverman JF, Holbrook CT, Pories WJ, et al: Fine needle aspiration cytology of pancreatoblastoma with immunocytochemical and ultrastructural studies. Acta Cytol 34:632-640, 1990.

82. Kurzawinski T, Deery A, Davidson BR: Diagnostic value of cytology for biliary stricture [review]. Br J Surg 80:414-421, 1993.

83. Bardales RH, Stanley MW, Simpson DD, et al: Diagnostic value of brush cytology in the diagnosis of duodenal, biliary, and ampullary neoplasms. Am J Clin Pathol 109:540-548, 1998.

84. Glasbrenner B, Ardan M, Boeck W, et al: Prospective evaluation of brush cytology of biliary strictures during endoscopic retrograde cholangiopancreatography. Endoscopy 31:712-717, 1999.

85. Stewart C, Mills P, Carter R, et al: Brush cytology in the assessment of pancreato-biliary strictures: A review of 406 cases. J Clin Pathol 54:449-455, 2001.

86. Layfield LJ, Wax TD, Lee JG, et al: Accuracy and morphologic aspects of pancreatic and biliary duct brushings. Acta Cytol 39:11-18, 1995.

87. Kocjan G, Smith AN: Bile duct brushing cytology: Potential pitfalls in diagnosis. Diagn Cytopathol 16:358-363, 1997.

88. Nakajima T, Tajima Y, Sugano I, et al: Multivariate statistical analysis of bile cytology. Acta Cytol 38:51-55, 1994.

89. Cohen MB, Wittchow RJ, Johlin FC, et al: Brush cytology of the extrahepatic biliary tract: Comparison of cytologic features of adenocarcinoma and benign biliary strictures. Mod Pathol 8:498-502, 1995.

90. Renshaw AA, Madge R, Jiroutek M, et al: Bile duct brushing cytology. Statistical analysis of proposed diagnostic criteria. Am J Clin Pathol 110:635-640, 1998.

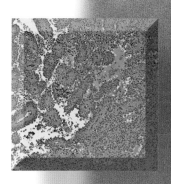

CHAPTER 27

Developmental Disorders of the Pancreas, Extrahepatic Biliary Tract, and Gallbladder

JOSEPH WILLIS

▇ Structural Anomalies of the Pancreas

The pancreas arises from two diverticula, dorsal and ventral, which first appear at approximately the fourth week of gestation. The dorsal bud elongates to form part of the head, body, and tail. The ventral bud develops at the base of the hepatic diverticulum. The left segment of this structure atrophies, and the right rotates posteriorly with the rotation of the duodenum to fuse with the dorsal segment. Portions of pancreas derived from either diverticulum are histologically indistinguishable, although subtle immunohistochemical differences have been noted.[1] Because of the direct association of the development of the common bile duct with the ventral portion of the pancreas, these share a common outflow tract—the ampulla of Vater. When the two pancreatic buds merge at the sixth to seventh weeks, their duct systems also coalesce to form the main pancreatic duct of Wirsung. A remnant of the dorsal bud duct commonly persists as the accessory duct of Santorini with its opening in the minor papilla of the duodenum (Fig. 27-1).[2]

Because pancreatic development is complex, variations in duct anatomy are relatively common, as would be expected. A detailed autopsy study by Berman and associates[3] in which vinyl acetate casts of postmortem pancreas specimens were used revealed the previous pattern of duct arrangement in approximately 90% of specimens. Although a number of ductal anatomic patterns of development were seen, the most common aberrant finding was the insertion of the main pancreatic duct into the common bile duct 5 to 15 mm proximal to the ampulla of Vater. This is known as the "common channel" or the "anomalous pancreaticobiliary junction." In endoscopic retrograde cholangiopancreatography (ERCP) series, this variation in duct anatomy has been noted to occur in 0.9% to 28% of patients (depending on patient selection) and to be associated with an increased prevalence of pancreaticobiliary disease.[4,5]

PANCREAS DIVISUM

The most common congenital anomaly of the pancreas is pancreas divisum; it occurs in 5% to 10% of the population. Although three distinct types are described, the most common, the classic type, arises from lack of fusion of the two embryologic portions of pancreas. As a result, the main portion of the pancreas is drained by a patent duct of Santorini into the minor duodenal papilla. The small size

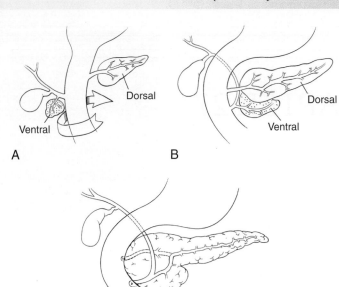

A   B

C

FIGURE 27–1. Embryology of the pancreas. **A,** Separate dorsal and ventral pancreatic anlagen developing from the gut tube at approximately 5 weeks' gestational age. With subsequent midgut rotation, the ventral bud and its closely related biliary ducts migrate posteriorly (*direction indicated by arrow*). **B,** After midgut rotation, the dorsal and ventral anlagen are closely opposed and eventually fuse. Notice the separate dorsal and ventral pancreatic ducts at this time. **C,** Eventually, the pancreatic ducts fuse. The main pancreatic duct is formed from the distal portion of the dorsal duct of the ventral pancreas; it enters the duodenum, along with the common bile duct, at the ampulla of Vater. The proximal portion of the duct of the dorsal pancreas usually becomes obliterated (*dotted line*) but may persist and enter the duodenum separately. (From Dahms BB: Gastrointestinal tract and pancreas. In Gilbert-Barness E [ed]: Potter's Pathology of the Fetus and Infant, vol 1. St. Louis, Mosby, 1997, pp 774-822.)

of this orifice is probably important in the predisposition of pancreatitis in these patients. Pancreas divisum has been identified in 12% to 26% of patients with idiopathic pancreatitis and is sometimes confined to the dorsal portions of the pancreas.[2,6] Most commonly, treatment is conservative. Rarely, surgical resection is necessary.

ANNULAR PANCREAS

Annular pancreas is relatively uncommon; a 20-year review at the Mayo Clinic identified 15 cases.[7] Most commonly, the lesion is composed of a flat band of pancreatic tissue circumferentially surrounding the second part of the duodenum (Fig. 27-2).

Kiernan and colleagues in their extensive review stated that approximately half of all presenting patients are in the pediatric age group; most present during the

neonatal period. Upper gastrointestinal tract obstruction is the most common initial finding. Peptic ulceration, pancreatitis, and other nonspecific symptoms tend to occur in adults.[7]

Pancreatic parenchyma characteristically is found intertwined with the duodenal muscularis mucosae. Only rarely is the anterior wall of the duodenum spared. Most commonly, the ductal system drains around the right side of the duodenum anteriorly to posteriorly to merge with the left duct. However, the right duct may pass anteriorly, or multiple small ducts may penetrate the wall of the duodenum and empty directly into it. A concomitant duodenal atresia/stenosis is often present.[2]

The embryologic sequence that leads to annular pancreas is unclear; several mechanisms have been proposed. One early proposal was that of ventral and dorsal segment hypertrophy encircling the duodenum. Hypertrophy of the dorsal segment would move the main duct anteriorly. Fixation of the tip of the ventral bud before rotation of the duodenum with subsequent persistence of the ventral lobe after rotation is plausible in the majority of cases. Finally, persistence and hypertrophy of the left portion of the ventral bud have been supported in a recent report.[8]

Annular pancreas is often associated with other anomalies, including duodenal bands, intestinal malrotation, Meckel's diverticulum, imperforate anus, cryptorchidism, and heart and spinal cord defects. Down syndrome has been identified in up to 20% of patients. A familial predisposition has also been documented.[9,10]

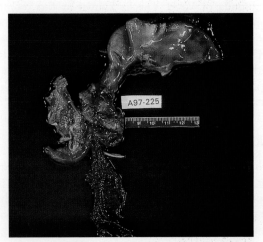

FIGURE 27–2. Annular pancreas at the level of the second part of the duodenum with distended duodenal bulb.

HETEROTOPIC PANCREAS

Pancreatic tissue that lacks anatomic or vascular continuity with the main body of the pancreas has been reported in 1% to 15% of autopsies. A majority are related to the upper portions of the gastrointestinal tract, especially the prepyloric region of the stomach along the greater curvature, although other intra-abdominal sites such as Meckel's diverticulum, liver, gallbladder, small intestine, appendix, colon, and omentum have been identified. Rarely, pancreatic tissue may arise in extra-abdominal sites such as lung and umbilicus.

The age range at initial diagnosis is from a few days old to 84 years. However, most are diagnosed in adulthood and are not suspected preoperatively.[11,12] Grossly, yellow nodules measure 2 mm to 5 cm in diameter. Most are submucosal and thereby enter into the clinical differential diagnosis of a submucosal nodule of the upper gastrointestinal tract. Large submucosal lesions may have a central duct orifice or umbilication. These lesions may also be the cause of biliary obstruction,[13] cholecystitis, or gastric outlet obstruction[11,14] or may present as a mass or polyp at the apex of an intussusception.[15,16]

The exact cause is unclear, but possible mechanisms proposed to explain these diverse anatomic sites of occurrence include failure of part of the ventral bud to undergo atrophy, aberrant migration of ventral bud remnants, metaplasia of multipotent endodermal cells, and, in the duodenum, metaplasia of Brunner's glands.[2]

Histologically, normal pancreatic lobular architecture with acinar and ductal components can be discerned (Fig. 27-3). Up to 84% of pancreatic heterotopias contain islets of Langerhans.[12] Malignant transformation is rare. A recent review of the world literature identified 20 verifiable cases of carcinoma arising in heterotopic pancreas.[17] The histologic spectrum varied among standard-type ductal adenocarcinoma, papillary cystadenocarcinoma, solid and papillary tumor, anaplastic carcinoma, and acinar carcinoma. Rarely, pancreatic endocrine tumors arising in pancreatic heterotopias have been identified.[18]

CONGENITAL CYST OF PANCREAS

Most cysts of the pancreas, even among the pediatric age group, are pancreatic pseudocysts formed secondary to pancreatitis. Congenital cysts are rare and may be solitary or multiple.

Solitary cysts have been identified in all age groups, from fetus to adult, with a predominance among females. These cysts are thought to arise by developmental errors of pancreatic ducts presumably related to localized obstruction of a duct in utero. Pancreatic cysts have been rarely associated with polyhydramnios. Newborns may present with an abdominal mass or upper gastrointestinal or biliary obstruction. An association with other anomalies, including renal tubular ectasia, polydactyly, anorectal malformations, and thoracic dystrophy, has been noted. Multicystic lesions of the pancreas are usually associated with von Hippel–Lindau disease or, rarely, autosomal dominant polycystic kidney disease.

Solitary pancreatic cysts are usually small (1 to 2 cm). Multiple cysts such as those seen in von Hippel–Lindau disease may diffusely efface the pancreas, although the spectrum of changes in these patients is broad. Cysts are lined by non–mucin-producing cuboidal cells with an adjacent fibrous wall.[19,20] These lesions should not be confused with intrapancreatic enteric cysts, which most commonly contain gastric mucosa in the cyst wall, although rarely they may contain small intestinal, ciliated, or respiratory-type epithelium.[21]

COMPLETE AND PARTIAL PANCREATIC AGENESIS

This is a group of rare structural anomalies, many of which go undetected because they may not be associated with pancreatic insufficiency. Complete agenesis of the pancreas is a rare, lethal anomaly sometimes associated with gallbladder agenesis.[22] Partial agenesis, which may be familial, is associated with complete absence of dorsal pancreatic parenchyma and has only rarely been reported.[23] The molecular events governing pancreatic embryogenesis are largely unknown. Recent advances may provide insight into the pathogenesis of some developmental anomalies of the pancreas.[24]

CYSTIC FIBROSIS

Cystic fibrosis (CF) is an autosomal recessive inherited disorder of all ethnicities and is the most common

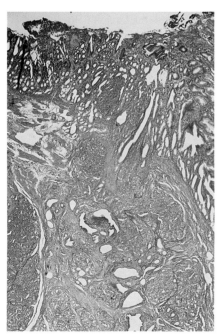

FIGURE 27–3. Antrum of the stomach with heterotopic pancreatic parenchyma.

hereditary disorder among whites, affecting 1 in 2000 members of this population. The genetic abnormality associated with CF is located on chromosome 7q31. This region is responsible for the expression of cystic fibrosis transmembrane conductance regulator protein (CFTR), which functions as a chloride ion channel in epithelial cells. It has been postulated that this defective chloride transport mechanism, which is associated with decreased bicarbonate secretion, causes precipitation of acinar secretions into pancreatic ducts with consequent secondary obstruction.[25] MUC6, a pancreatic mucin, has been implicated in this process.[26]

CF is a multisystem disease with many gastrointestinal tract manifestations[27]; the pancreas was the first organ to be identified as significantly affected in this disease. It is because of the characteristic pathologic findings of pancreatic cysts and fibrosis that this disease was so named.

Clinical and morphologic findings among CF patients are secondary to obstruction of exocrine ducts. This phenomenon has predictable secondary complications in the pancreas, including reduced volume of secretions (causing a relative increase in protein concentration), duct obstruction, and cystic dilatation and acinar atrophy with fibrosis.[28]

Pathologic abnormalities of the pancreas have been recognized at as early as 32 to 38 weeks' gestation and progressively worsen with age. Malabsorption due to pancreatic insufficiency is present in early infancy in 85% of CF patients. Most, though not all, of the remaining patients develop pancreatic insufficiency at some stage during the course of their disease. Newborns with CF have a higher connective tissue–to–acinar gland ratio with more prominent acinar and ductal lumina. Grossly, the parenchyma has a granular appearance secondary to the extensive fibrosis, and cystic spaces are often apparent (Fig. 27-4). The earliest histologic

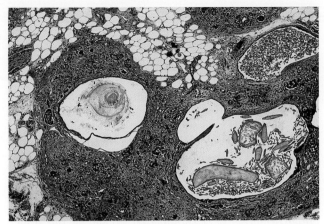

FIGURE 27–5. Marked disruption of the pancreas with cystic dilatation of the ductal system and acini, which contain eosinophilic concentric concretions.

finding is that of abundant eosinophilic concretions in pancreatic ducts (Fig. 27-5). Secondary changes of obstruction include flattening, atrophy, and dilatation of acinar and ductal epithelia. Ductal dilatation with eventual cyst formation and parenchymal fibrosis occurs at an early age in most patients. Continued involution of acinar tissue occurs during childhood, initially with a proliferation of fibroblasts but subsequently by fatty replacement of the entire pancreas (Fig. 27-6). By the end of the first decade, the pancreas is virtually completely replaced by fat even though the normal gross architecture of the organ is maintained.[28]

Islets of Langerhans are usually well preserved initially, but as parenchymal damage progresses, approximately 25% of CF patients, mostly adults, develop insulin-dependent diabetes mellitus, caused by an overall decrease in the number of insulin-producing islet cells.[29]

Sporadic cases of pancreatic adenocarcinoma arising in CF patients have been reported, giving rise to concern of a possible association between these two entities.[30]

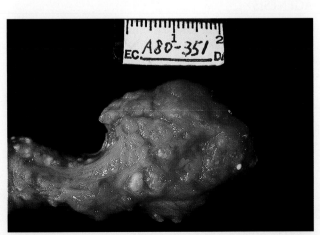

FIGURE 27–4. Pancreas from a 6-year-old patient with cystic fibrosis. Note the accentuation of lobular parenchyma with prominent fibrosis.

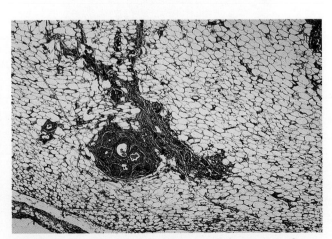

FIGURE 27–6. Diffuse fatty replacement of the pancreas from a 23-year-old patient with cystic fibrosis.

CF patients may also have characteristic liver alterations, including focal or multilobular biliary cirrhosis. The probable cause of most of these lesions is bile duct obstruction resulting from viscid and inspissated biliary secretions. In some cases, common bile duct stenosis occurs as a direct result of pancreatic fibrosis affecting the intrapancreatic biliary tree. This can occur even in CF patients without pancreatic insufficiency.[31] Sclerosing cholangitis, common bile duct strictures, and rarely, extrahepatic cholangiocarcinoma have also been reported.[32]

Increased fecal bile acid loss due to malabsorption renders the bile lithogenic. Thus, at least one third of older CF patients have cholelithiasis. Micro-gallbladders (gallbladder hypoplasia), mucinous metaplasia, and cystic duct stenosis may also occur.[31]

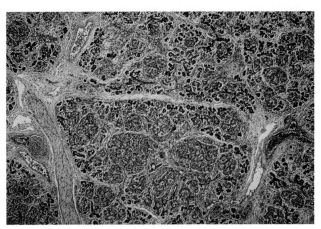

FIGURE 27-7. Beckwith-Wiedemann syndrome characterized by nodular aggregates of pancreatic β cells.

CONGENITAL PANCREATIC EXOCRINE DEFICIENCY (SHWACHMAN-DIAMOND SYNDROME)

Originally described in 1964, this is a rare autosomal recessive inherited multisystem disorder,[33] linked to the centromere region of chromosome 7.[34] Infants usually have low birth weight and commonly fail to thrive; they often have feeding problems, diarrhea, and hypotonia. Virtually all patients are symptomatic by 4 months of age, most with pancreatic insufficiency. After CF, this syndrome accounts for the majority of cases of primary pancreatic insufficiency in childhood.[35] The characteristic finding in the pancreas is diffuse fatty replacement of pancreatic parenchyma early in the disease course. These patients have a high mortality rate resulting from a constellation of problems involving bone marrow abnormalities, including aplasia with a high risk of leukemia, recurrent bacterial infections, myocardial inflammation, and multisystem anomalies.[33,36,37]

Other extremely rare causes of pancreatic exocrine deficiency include Johanson-Blizzard syndrome, exocrine pancreatic dysfunction with refractory sideroblastic anemia, and isolated enzyme deficiencies.[38]

NEONATAL ISLET CELL HYPERTROPHY AND HYPERPLASIA

Marked variation in the size and number of islets of Langerhans in neonates and young adults has been well documented. An assessment of the significance of islet size and number can be made only in conjunction with knowledge of gestational age. Because of this variation, it has been proposed that the definition of islet hypertrophy is a situation in which the percentage of islets larger than 200 μm in diameter exceeds that which would be considered normal when the patient's age is taken into consideration.[39]

The most common cause of islet hypertrophy is maternal diabetes. In addition to hypertrophy and hyperplasia, the islets in infants of diabetic mothers may show increased islet cell volume, pleomorphic nuclei of β cells, fibrosis, and eosinophilic infiltrate with or without Charcot-Leyden crystals.[40-42]

Beckwith-Wiedemann syndrome is a congenital generalized somatic overgrowth syndrome with variable phenotype linked to the imprinted gene cluster on chromosome region 11p15.[43] It is associated with hypoglycemia caused by islet cell hyperplasia and hyperinsulinism in 50% of cases. Islets are enlarged, and smaller clusters of endocrine cells occur in the form of nodular aggregates (Fig. 27-7). Immunohistochemical staining reveals a marked increase in β cells, with a slight increase in α cells. Pancreas polypeptide-producing cells are decreased in number. Rarely, pancreatoblastoma and cystic dysplasia of the pancreas may be noted in these patients.[44,45]

Other causes of islet cell hyperplasia are listed in Table 27-1.

TABLE 27-1. Conditions With Hypertrophy and Hyperplasia of Islets of Langerhans
Infant of diabetic mother
Beckwith-Wiedemann syndrome
Erythroblastosis fetalis
Nesidioblastosis and focal adenomatosis
Zellweger syndrome
Donohue's syndrome
Tyrosinemia
Cyanotic congenital heart disease
Long-term total parenteral nutrition
Multiple endocrine neoplasia type II

From Gilbert-Barness E, Potter EL: Potter's Pathology of the Fetus and Infant. St. Louis, Mosby, 1997.

PERSISTENT HYPERINSULINEMIC HYPOGLYCEMIA OF INFANCY (NESIDIOBLASTOSIS)

Persistent hyperinsulinemic hypoglycemia of infancy (PHHI) is the most common cause of severe, prolonged neonatal hypoglycemia, occurring in 1 of 50,000 births. Although an excellent argument has been made for the designation *PHHI*, the term *nesidioblastosis* is more commonly used.

A number of different etiologic factors can lead to decoupling of β-cell insulin production. The most common are autosomal recessive mutations in SUR 1, the sulfonylurea receptor. Other causes include mutations of the SUR-associated inward rectifier, Kir6.2, and autosomal dominant inherited mutations of glucokinase and glutamate dehydrogenase.[46,47]

The disease is characterized by either diffuse or focal abnormalities of the islets of Langerhans. Histologic features associated with PHHI include enlargement of β-cell nuclei (3 to 4 times normal endocrine nuclei) (Fig. 27-8), ductuloinsular complexes (budding of endocrine cells from duct epithelium) (Fig. 27-9), centroacinar cell proliferation (ductal cells with pale cytoplasm in centroacinar regions), septal islets (islets within fibrous septa), and nesidiodysplasia, a subtle increase in endocrine cell aggregates randomly distributed in pancreatic lobules. The islets are also irregular in size and shape. Adenomatosis, excess islet cell proliferation defined as greater than 40% of a low-power microscopic field, is found less commonly than diffuse islet cell change.[39,40,46,48]

Extensive pancreatic resection is commonly required to control hypoglycemia. Conflicting data have emerged concerning the likelihood of diffuse pancreatic islet cell abnormality in the presence of adenomatosis on a small sample of pancreas taken at intraoperative frozen section before pancreatic resection. One study of 20 infants

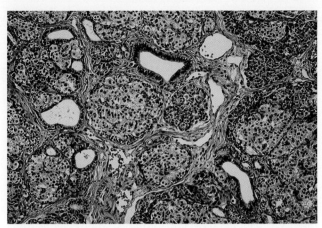

FIGURE 27–9. Ductuloinsular complexes (tubulo–islet cell proliferations) characterized by large aggregates of neuroendocrine cells with intermixed ductal proliferation. Note that some ducts contain intermingled neuroendocrine buds.

found that the taking of multiple frozen sections from different parts of the gland allows for accurate intraoperative diagnosis of focal or diffuse PHHI.[49] These findings are at variance with other published series.[39,46] The possibility that these reported differences are due to different etiologic subsets has been raised.[46]

Extrahepatic Biliary Tract

CHOLEDOCHAL CYST

Cystic dilatation of the biliary tree was described as early as 1723. Not until relatively modern times has there been significant improvement in our understanding of the pathophysiology of the choledochal cyst.

Choledochal cysts are uncommon, occurring in approximately 1 in 100,000 to 150,000 live births. A female-to-male preponderance of 3 to 4:1 has been noted.[50,51] A majority of patients present in infancy and childhood; only 20% to 30% of patients present as adults.[51,52] The cause of choledochal cysts in the majority of patients appears to be an anomalous pancreaticobiliary junction between the common bile duct and the duct of Wirsung. Its sex distribution, a greater incidence among Asian populations, and its rare association with other anomalies suggest a congenital origin.[53-55] Even in adults, choledochal cysts are thought to be mostly congenital in origin. Uncommonly, adults have presented with a dilated common bile duct after extrahepatic biliary tree surgery with normal initial intraoperative cholangiograms. These cases are probably derived, at least in part, from secondary stricture formation, although even in these patients, an anomalous pancreaticobiliary junction is common.[56]

Although five common varieties have been noted, 90% to 95% of choledochal cysts are classified as type 1.[53] This involves a fusiform or saccular dilatation of the

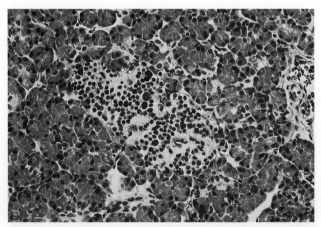

FIGURE 27–8. Persistent hyperinsulinemic hypoglycemia of infancy with enlarged, irregular islets of Langerhans containing β cells with marked nuclear pleomorphism.

common bile duct (Fig. 27-10). Whereas infants usually have complete obstruction of the distal common bile duct, in adults, this is most commonly patent. Rarely, the lesion may be entirely intraduodenal (choledochocele) or may consist of multiple intrahepatic cysts (Caroli's disease). Cystic malformations of the gallbladder probably share a common etiologic basis.

Grossly, a choledochal cyst may contain up to 2 L of bile. The surface is coarsely granular. The wall is fibrotic, and distal narrowing is a common feature. Microscopic findings tend to vary with patient age; intact surface columnar epithelium is characteristic in younger patients, and increasing chronic inflammatory infiltrate and adhesions to adjacent structures are seen in older patients. The cyst wall is composed of dense fibrous tissue with varying amounts of smooth muscle.[53]

Current surgical treatment of choledochal cysts involves complete surgical resection when possible. Previous attempts at various types of surgical drainage procedures, for example, Roux-en-Y cystojejunostomy, are currently not commonly performed owing to high late complication rates.

A significant risk of carcinoma is associated with choledochal cysts; this risk increases with age. The risk in children younger than 10 years old is less than 1%, but risk rises to as high as 14.3% in adults.[57] Reflux of pancreatic enzymes up the common bile duct and abnormal bile composition may predispose to neoplastic changes. For unknown reasons, the neoplasms have a predilection for the posterior wall of the cyst. Most commonly, the tumors are adenocarcinomas (Fig. 27-11), although squamous cell carcinomas and anaplastic carcinomas also occur.[50,58] Other types of neoplasms are extremely rare.[59]

▉ Gallbladder

Surgical pathologists rarely encounter congenital abnormalities of the gallbladder.

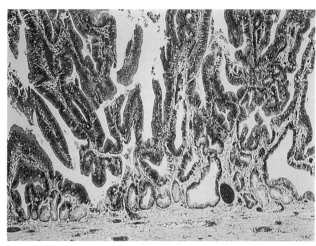

FIGURE 27–11. High-grade dysplasia arising in a choledochal cyst. (From Yazumi S, et al: Intraductal US aids detection of carcinoma in situ in a patient with a choledochal cyst. Gastrointest Endosc 53:233-236, 2001.)

Gallbladder agenesis occurs in approximately 0.1% of the population. In the vast majority of individuals, this is an isolated phenomenon, usually noted incidentally; however, rarely, this condition may be associated with other congenital anomalies. Hypoplastic gallbladder is associated with biliary atresia and cystic fibrosis.

Septation of the gallbladder (Fig. 27-12), most commonly secondary to cholelithiasis, is often diagnosed on preoperative ultrasonography. Rare multiseptate gallbladders present the best evidence for septation as a congenital event.

Septations can occur in the pediatric population and are not associated with gallstones. Each septation may contain a mucosal surface with interdigitating muscle fibers with variable chronic inflammation. Gallbladder septation has been attributed to incomplete cavitation of the developing gallbladder bud.[60]

Acknowledgment: I wish to gratefully acknowledge Dr Beverly Dahms for her editing skills and for allowing me to use some of her case material.

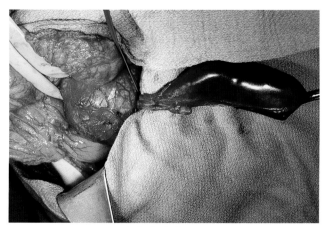

FIGURE 27–10. Type 1 choledochal cyst with fusiform dilatation of the common bile duct and a normal gallbladder.

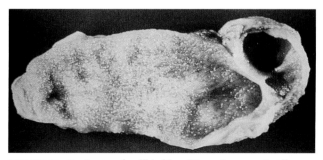

FIGURE 27–12. Septated gallbladder. (From Jessurun J, Albores-Saavedra J: Anderson's Pathology, vol 2. St. Louis, Mosby, 1996.)

References

1. Rahier J, Wallon J, Gepts W, Haot J: Localization of pancreatic polypeptide cells in a limited lobe of the human neonate pancreas: Remnant of the ventral primordium? Cell Tissue Res 200:359-366, 1979.
2. Hill ID, Lebenthal E: Congenital abnormalities of the exocrine pancreas. In Go VLW (ed): The Pancreas: Biology, Pathobiology, and Disease. New York, Raven Press, 1993, p 1029.
3. Berman LC, Prior JT, Abramow SM, et al: A study of the pancreatic duct system in man by the use of vinyl acetate casts of postmortem preparations. Surg Gynecol Obstet 110:391-403, 1960.
4. Egami K, Onda M, Uchida E, et al: Clinicopathological studies on association of gallbladder carcinoma and pancreaticobiliary maljunction. J Nippon Med Sch 65:7-13, 1998.
5. Guelrud M, Morera C, Rodriguez M, et al: Sphincter of Oddi dysfunction in children with recurrent pancreatitis and anomalous pancreaticobiliary union: An etiologic concept. Gastrointest Endosc 50:194-199, 1999.
6. Quest L, Lombard M: Pancreas divisum: Opinio divisa. Gut 47:317-319, 2000.
7. Kiernan PD, ReMine SG, Kiernan PC, et al: Annular pancreas: Mayo Clinic experience from 1957 to 1976 with review of the literature. Arch Surg 115:46-50, 1980.
8. Nobukawa B, Otaka M, Suda K, et al: An annular pancreas derived from paired ventral pancreata, supporting Baldwin's hypothesis. Pancreas 20:408-410, 2000.
9. Hendricks SK, Sybert VP: Association of annular pancreas and duodenal obstruction—evidence for Mendelian inheritance? Clin Genet 39:383-385, 1991.
10. MacFadyen UM, Young ID: Annular pancreas in mother and son. Am J Med Genet 27:987-989, 1987.
11. Case Records of the Massachusetts General Hospital: Weekly clinicopathological exercises. Case 26-1999. A three-week-old girl with pyloric stenosis and an unexpected operative finding. N Engl J Med 341:679-684, 1999.
12. Pang LC: Pancreatic heterotopia: A reappraisal and clinicopathologic analysis of 32 cases. South Med J 81:1264-1275, 1988.
13. O'Reilly DJ, Craig RM, Lorenzo G, et al: Heterotopic pancreas mimicking carcinoma of the head of the pancreas: A rare cause of obstructive jaundice. J Clin Gastroenterol 5:165-168, 1983.
14. Shaib YH, Rabaa E, Feddersen RM, et al: Gastric outlet obstruction secondary to heterotopic pancreas in the antrum: Case report and review of the literature. Gastrointest Endosc (in press).
15. Abel R, Keen CE, Bingham JB, et al: Heterotopic pancreas as lead point in intussusception: New variant of vitellointestinal tract malformation. Pediatr Dev Pathol 2:367-370, 1999.
16. Scholz S, Loff S, Wirth H: Double ileoileal intussusception caused by a giant polypoid mass of heterotopic pancreas in a child. Eur J Pediatr 159:861-862, 2000.
17. Makhlouf HR, Almeida JL, Sobin LH: Carcinoma in jejunal pancreatic heterotopia. Arch Pathol Lab Med 123:707-711, 1999.
18. Ashida K, Egashira Y, Tutumi A, et al: Endocrine neoplasm arising from duodenal heterotopic pancreas: A case report. Gastrointest Endosc 46:172-176, 1997.
19. Kloppel G: Pseudocysts and other non-neoplastic cysts of the pancreas. Semin Diagn Pathol 17:7-15, 2000.
20. Compton CC: Serous cystic tumors of the pancreas. Semin Diagn Pathol 17:43-55, 2000.
21. del Rosario JF, Silverman WB, Ford H, et al: Duplication cyst of the pancreatic duct presenting as pancreatitis. Gastrointest Endosc 47:303-305, 1998.
22. Voldsgaard P, Kryger-Baggesen N, Lisse I: Agenesis of pancreas. Acta Paediatr 83:791-793, 1994.
23. Schnedl WJ, Reisinger EC, Schreiber F, et al: Complete and partial agenesis of the dorsal pancreas within one family. Gastrointest Endosc 42:485-487, 1995.
24. Li H, Arber S, Jessell TM, et al: Selective agenesis of the dorsal pancreas in mice lacking homeobox gene Hlxb9. Nat Genet 23:67-70, 1999.
25. Lebenthal E, Lerner A, Rolston DDK: The pancreas in cystic fibrosis. In Go VLW (ed): The Pancreas: Biology, Pathobiology, and Disease. New York, Raven Press, 1993, pp 1041-1081.
26. Harris A: The duct cell in cystic fibrosis. Ann N Y Acad Sci 880:17-30, 1999.
27. Stern R: Cystic fibrosis and the gastrointestinal tract. In Davis P (ed): Cystic Fibrosis. New York, Marcel Dekker, 1993, pp 401-434.
28. Tomashefski JE, Abramowsky CR, Dahms BB: The pathology of cystic fibrosis. In Davis P (ed): Cystic Fibrosis. New York, Marcel Dekker, 1993, pp 435-489.
29. Abdul-Karim FW, Dahms BB, Velasco ME, et al: Islets of Langerhans in adolescents and adults with cystic fibrosis. A quantitative study. Arch Pathol Lab Med 110:602-606, 1986.
30. Sheldon CD, Hodson ME, Carpenter LM, et al: A cohort study of cystic fibrosis and malignancy. Br J Cancer 68:1025-1028, 1993.
31. Waters DL, Dorney SF, Gruca MA, et al: Hepatobiliary disease in cystic fibrosis patients with pancreatic sufficiency. Hepatology 21:963-969, 1995.
32. Tesluk H, McCauley K, Kurland G, et al: Cholangiocarcinoma in an adult with cystic fibrosis. J Clin Gastroenterol 13:485-487, 1991.
33. Ginzberg H, Shin J, Ellis L, et al: Shwachman syndrome: Phenotypic manifestations of sibling sets and isolated cases in a large patient cohort are similar. J Pediatr 135:81-88, 1999.
34. Goobie S, Popovic M, Morrison J, et al: Shwachman-Diamond syndrome with exocrine pancreatic dysfunction and bone marrow failure maps to the centromeric region of chromosome 7. Am J Hum Genet 68:1048-1054, 2001.
35. Hill RE, Durie PR, Gaskin KJ, et al: Steatorrhea and pancreatic insufficiency in Shwachman syndrome. Gastroenterology 83:22-27, 1982.
36. Klupp N, Simonitsch I, Mannhalter C, et al: Emergence of an unusual bone marrow precursor B-cell population in fatal Shwachman-Diamond syndrome. Arch Pathol Lab Med 124:1379-1381, 2000.
37. Savilahti E, Rapola J: Frequent myocardial lesions in Shwachman's syndrome. Eight fatal cases among 16 Finnish patients. Acta Paediatr Scand 73:642-651, 1984.
38. Durie PR: Inherited and congenital disorders of the exocrine pancreas. Gastroenterologist 4:169-187, 1996.
39. Jaffe R, Hashida Y, Yunis EJ: Pancreatic pathology in hyperinsulinemic hypoglycemia of infancy. Lab Invest 42:356-365, 1980.
40. Dahms BB: Gastrointestinal tract and pancreas. In Gilbert-Barness E (ed): Potter's Pathology of the Fetus and Infant, vol 1. St. Louis, Mosby, 1997, pp 774-822.
41. Barresi G, Inferrera C, De Luca F: Eosinophilic pancreatitis in the newborn infant of a diabetic mother. Virchows Arch A Pathol Anat Histol 380:341-348, 1978.
42. Jaffe R, Hashida Y, Yunis EJ: The endocrine pancreas of the neonate and infant. Perspect Pediatr Pathol 7:137-165, 1982.
43. Itoh N, Becroft DM, Reeve AE, et al: Proportion of cells with paternal 11p15 uniparental disomy correlates with organ enlargement in Beckwith-Wiedemann syndrome. Am J Med Genet 92:111-116, 2000.
44. Drut R, Jones MC: Congenital pancreatoblastoma in Beckwith-Wiedemann syndrome: An emerging association. Pediatr Pathol 8:331-339, 1988.
45. Steigman CK, Uri AK, Chatten J, et al: Beckwith-Wiedemann syndrome with unusual hepatic and pancreatic features: A case expanding the phenotype. Pediatr Pathol 10:593-600, 1990.
46. Jack MM, Walker RM, Thomsett MJ, et al: Histologic findings in persistent hyperinsulinemic hypoglycemia of infancy: Australian experience. Pediatr Dev Pathol 3:532-547, 2000.
47. Glaser B, Kesavan P, Heyman M, et al: Familial hyperinsulinism caused by an activating glucokinase mutation. N Engl J Med 338:226-230, 1998.
48. Goossens A, Gepts W, Saudubray JM, et al: Diffuse and focal nesidioblastosis. A clinicopathological study of 24 patients with persistent neonatal hyperinsulinemic hypoglycemia. Am J Surg Pathol 13:766-775, 1989.
49. Rahier J, Sempoux C, Fournet JC, et al: Partial or near-total pancreatectomy for persistent neonatal hyperinsulinaemic hypoglycaemia: The pathologist's role. Histopathology 32:15-19, 1998.
50. Weyant MJ, Maluccio MA, Bertagnolli MM, et al: Choledochal cysts in adults: A report of two cases and review of the literature. Am J Gastroenterol 93:2580-2583, 1998.
51. Chaudhary A, Dhar P, Sachdev A, et al: Choledochal cysts—differences in children and adults. Br J Surg 83:186-188, 1996.
52. Yamaguchi M: Congenital choledochal cyst. Analysis of 1,433 patients in the Japanese literature. Am J Surg 140:653-657, 1980.
53. O'Neill JA Jr: Choledochal cyst. Curr Probl Surg 29:361-410, 1992.

54. Dudin A, Abdelshafi M, Rambaud-Cousson A: Choledochal cyst associated with rare hand malformation. Am J Med Genet 56:161-163, 1995.

55. Hasegawa T, Kim M, Kitayama Y, et al: Choledochal cyst associated with polycystic kidney disease: Report of a case. HPB Surg 11:185-189, 1999.

56. Hewitt PM, Krige JE, Bornman PC, et al: Choledochal cysts in adults. Br J Surg 82:382-385, 1995.

57. Voyles CR, Smadja C, Shands WC, et al: Carcinoma in choledochal cysts. Age-related incidence. Arch Surg 118:986-988, 1983.

58. Yazumi S, Takahashi R, Tojo M, et al: Intraductal US aids detection of carcinoma in situ in a patient with a choledochal cyst. Gastrointest Endosc 53:233-236, 2001.

59. Patil KK, Omojola MF, Khurana P, et al: Embryonal rhabdomyosarcoma within a choledochal cyst. Can Assoc Radiol J 43:145-148, 1992.

60. Paciorek ML, Lackner D, Daly C, et al: A unique presentation of multiseptate gallbladder. Dig Dis Sci 42:2519-2523, 1997.

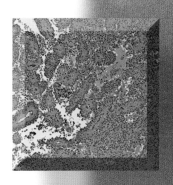

CHAPTER 28

Infectious and Inflammatory Disorders of the Gallbladder and Extrahepatic Biliary Tract

JOSE JESSURUN • STEFAN PAMBUCCIAN

■ Normal Gallbladder and Extrahepatic Bile Ducts

GROSS ANATOMY

The gallbladder is located in a depression on the inferior surface of the right and quadrate hepatic lobes. It is attached to the liver by loose connective tissue containing blood vessels, lymphatics, and occasionally bile ducts; it is attached to the duodenum by a peritoneal fold known as the cholecystoduodenal ligament. From a didactic standpoint, it is useful to divide the organ into three parts. Projecting beyond the liver margin is the blind-ending segment known as the fundus. The central body, or corpus, has a portion that bulges forward toward the upper margin of the first portion of the duodenum, forming the infundibulum or Hartmann's pouch. A short neck continues with the cystic duct.

The gallbladder is irrigated by the cystic artery, which in most cases originates from the right hepatic artery. Its venous blood is carried through small veins that traverse the gallbladder bed and drain into the liver. Lymph drains to one or more lymph nodes at the gallbladder neck; these connect with lymph nodes located near the

hepatic hilum and at the hepatoduodenal ligament. From the anterior and posterior hepatic plexuses, the gallbladder and extrahepatic bile ducts receive sympathetic and parasympathetic nerve fibers.[1]

The cystic duct is a 3-cm tubular structure located in the right free edge of the lesser omentum. At the junction with the gallbladder neck, several mucosal folds project into the lumen, forming the spiral valve of Heister. These valvular infoldings regulate the filling and emptying of the gallbladder in response to pressure changes within the biliary system.

The right and left hepatic ducts arise from the liver and join to form the common hepatic duct, which is joined by the cystic duct to form the common bile duct or the choledochus. This duct, which varies in length from 1.5 to 9.0 cm, empties into the papilla of Vater after proceeding behind the first portion of the duodenum and traversing the head of the pancreas.

The retroduodenal and right hepatic arteries irrigate the supraduodenal segment of the common bile duct and proximal bile ducts. The superior pancreaticoduodenal arteries supply the intraduodenal segments. The venous flow of the common bile duct drains directly into the portal system. Lymphatic drainage occurs into multiple regional lymph nodes of the pancreaticoduodenal and celiac areas and retroperitoneum.

HISTOLOGY

The gallbladder is composed of three layers—mucosa, muscularis, and adventitia.

Mucosa

The mucosa comprises surface epithelium and lamina propria. It projects into the lumen as branching folds that become more prominent when the gallbladder contracts and less prominent when the gallbladder is distended. A single layer of columnar cells with basally oriented nuclei makes up the surface epithelium. The predominant cell has a lightly eosinophilic cytoplasm and a few small, periodic acid–Schiff (PAS)-positive, apical vacuoles. On electron microscopy, these cells are coated with microvilli and display other characteristics of absorptive cells, including basolateral spaces and digitations; they are tightly joined together by apical junctional complexes.[2] Another type of cell occasionally seen in the surface epithelium is a narrow columnar cell with dark eosinophilic cytoplasm, which is referred to as "penciloid" cell. It appears to be more than a compressed common columnar cell in that, ultrastructurally, it contains a greater number of organelles and shows more enzymatic activity than the common columnar cells.[3] The basal cell is a rarely observed type of epithelial cell found in contact with and parallel to the basement membrane. In addition to the epithelial cells, a few T lymphocytes are normally present among the surface columnar cells. Endocrine cells and melanocytes are absent.

Only at the neck of the gallbladder are tubuloalveolar glands composed of mucin-producing cuboidal cells with a clear cytoplasm. These glands are similar to those found in the extrahepatic bile ducts. Their presence in the body or fundus of the gallbladder should be considered abnormal; when present, they represent antral (or gastric) metaplasia resulting from chronic inflammation.

The designation *Rokitansky-Aschoff sinuses* is used to refer to pathologic herniations of the mucosa into and/or through the muscularis. In this sense, they are analogous to intestinal diverticula (pseudodiverticula).

The normal gallbladder epithelium has a low rate of cell renewal; however, the mitotic activity of the epithelium may be stimulated in certain conditions, such as with mechanical distention following ligation of the common bile duct or with neoplastic obstruction. In addition, high DNA synthesis may be stimulated by hormones such as cholecystokinin (CCK), a diet rich in cholesterol or cholic acid, or the presence of gallstones.[4]

The lamina propria is composed of loose connective tissue, nerve fibers, blood vessels, and lymphatics. Small numbers of lymphocytes, IgA-containing plasma cells, mast cells, and macrophages may also be seen.

Muscularis

The muscular layer is a slightly thickened version of the muscularis mucosae of the intestine; it is composed of bundles of loosely arranged smooth muscle separated by fibrovascular connective tissue. Fusiform cells with elongated bipolar or dendritic cytoplasmic projections located close to or in intimate contact with the smooth muscle cells of the muscular layer have recently been recognized in the gallbladder. These cells, which are immunoreactive for CD117 and have been interpreted as interstitial cells of Cajal, may play a role in muscle contraction.[5]

Adventitia

The adventitia is composed of loose connective tissue, blood vessels, lymphatics, nerves, and fatty tissue. Rare paraganglia may be seen adjacent to the vessels. The abdominal side of the adventitia is covered by a serosa. On the hepatic bed, solitary or multiple small bile ducts known as canals of Luschka may be present. The hepatic adventitia may also contain larger accessory biliary ducts. Leakage of bile into the peritoneum may occur if these ducts are left patent after cholecystectomy.

The mucosa of the extrahepatic bile ducts is longitudinally pleated. The predominant epithelial cells are columnar cells similar to those present in the gallbladder. The lamina propria contains scattered collagen and elastic fibers.

The muscularis is not as precisely defined as in the gallbladder and is formed of small bundles of smooth muscle. This layer is commonly absent in the proximal segments and becomes more accentuated in the distal segments. Surrounding the ducts is a layer of loose connective tissue. Small mucous glands, which increase in number distally, open into the lumen as small pits called *the sacculi of Beale.*

EMBRYOLOGY

The gallbladder, bile ducts, liver, and primitive ventral pancreas originate from a diverticulum that appears on the ventral surface of the primitive foregut near the yolk stalk. At 4 weeks' gestation, three separate buds can be recognized: The cranial bud penetrates into the splanchnic mesenchyme of the septum transversum and develops into the liver; the caudal bud becomes the gallbladder; and a smaller basal bud gives rise to the ventral pancreas. Their centrifugal migration causes elongation of those segments originally attached to the foregut, which then become the common hepatic, cystic, and common bile ducts, respectively. Proliferation of epithelial cells transforms these hollow structures into solid cords that reacquire a lumen by cellular vacuolization around 7 weeks' gestation. The extrahepatic segments of the right and left hepatic ducts are recognizable from 12 weeks' gestation. The common hepatic duct and distal parts of both hepatic ducts connect to several ductules in the hilar region. Variations in the remodeling process of these ducts explain the various branching patterns that have been recognized.[6] The lumen of the common bile duct progressively widens during infancy and early childhood, reaching its definitive diameter in adulthood.

PHYSIOLOGY

The liver secretes approximately 1000 mL of bile each day. Bile flow is a consequence of the reciprocal activity of smooth muscle in the gallbladder and the sphincter of Oddi. The ingestion of food induces contraction of the gallbladder and relaxation of the sphincter of Oddi, allowing the release of bile into the duodenum. Fatty meals and to a lesser degree proteins stimulate contraction of the gallbladder smooth muscle, mainly through the action of cholecystokinin, a polypeptide hormone secreted by the proximal small intestine.[1] Cholecystokinin may exert its action through the release of endothelin 1, a small peptide produced by the gallbladder and the bile duct epithelium.[3] Contraction of the gallbladder during the interdigestive period is most likely mediated by motilin, another polypeptide hormone found in the epithelium of the duodenum and jejunum. By contrast, somatostatin, a hormone secreted from the intestine and pancreas after the ingestion of a fatty meal, inhibits gallbladder contraction. Because cholecystokinin and somatostatin are released by the same stimuli, their opposing actions suggest that these hormones balance each other.[7]

During fasting, contraction of the sphincter of Oddi causes the progressive accumulation of bile in the common bile duct. When the pressure in this system exceeds the resting pressure of the gallbladder (approximately 10 mm Hg), bile flows into the latter. Although the capacity of the gallbladder is small (40 to 70 mL), a larger quantity of bile constituents is effectively stored through concentration. Water is absorbed by the epithelial cells through an osmotic gradient generated by a Na^+/K^+ ATPase–mediated sodium-coupled transport of chloride.[8]

In addition to storing bile, the gallbladder secretes mucin via the surface epithelial cells and neck mucous glands. Most of the mucus is neutral and heavily sulfated and contains scarce sialic residues.[9] Recent attention has been focused on these mucosubstances because they may play a role in the formation of gallstones.

▥ Congenital and Developmental Abnormalities

Even though congenital anomalies of the gallbladder are rare, they may represent a challenging group of disorders for the diagnostic radiologist and for the surgeon performing a cholecystectomy.

Congenital malformations include anomalies in shape, number, and position. The most common abnormality in shape is an angulation of the fundus, called a Phrygian cap because of its resemblance to the folded hats worn in the ancient country of Phrygia in Asia Minor. Microscopically, a mucosal fold with some disorientation of the underlying muscle bundles characterizes this abnormality. Although clinically unimportant, it may be mistaken on radiologic examination for a stone or a pathologic septum.[10]

Congenital diverticula of the gallbladder, which are rare, consist of saccular outpouchings of the gallbladder wall. Diverticula are most often single but may occasionally be multiple. They may involve any aspect of the gallbladder and generally come to clinical attention as an incidental finding or when they become infected.

Septation of the gallbladder is characterized by the presence of one or multiple septa dividing the gallbladder lumen into several chambers.[11] This anomaly is most often discovered in adults and probably results from incomplete fusion of the vacuoles, which gives rise to the lumen after the solid stage (see under Embryology). In some cases, the septa may contain muscle fibers that are continuous with those of the outer wall, a finding that has been used as an argument to support a developmental etiology.[12] It is worth noting, however, that inflammatory diseases of the gallbladder can produce internal compartmentalization mimicking congenital septation. Inflammatory septa are usually thicker and made of inflamed fibrous tissue. In some cases, particularly those associated with gallstones, the distinction between inflamed congenital septa and acquired compartmentalization is impossible. Septation of the gallbladder has been associated with intermittent abdominal pain in young adults.[13] Stones are usually absent.

The term *hourglass gallbladder* has been used to describe those cases with a transverse septum that divides the lumen into proximal and distal cavities. Inflammatory changes and stone formation tend to occur more frequently in the distal cavity.

Cystic malformations of the gallbladder may be analogous to the most common choledochal cysts or may arise by occlusion of a diverticulum.[14] In addition, dilatation of the ducts of Luschka may give rise to multilocular cysts around the gallbladder.

Failure of development of the caudal foregut diverticulum results in agenesis of the gallbladder. This developmental abnormality can occur as an isolated phenomenon or can be associated with other anomalies, the most common one being choledocholithiasis. Clinical symptoms of gallbladder agenesis usually present in adults, mimic the symptoms of cholecystitis or cholangitis, and are frequently associated with jaundice.

A hypoplastic gallbladder may occur when the caudal bud undergoes incomplete development, or when the solid stage of the bud is not recanalized. It may be found in association with congenital biliary atresia and in cystic fibrosis. This condition should be differentiated from acquired postinflammatory fibrotic retraction of the gallbladder.[15]

At the opposite end of the spectrum from gallbladder agenesis and hypoplasia is gallbladder duplication, which occurs with excessive budding of the caudal diverticulum. The duplicated cystic ducts most commonly enter the common bile duct separately ("H-type" configuration), or they unite to form a common cystic duct ("Y-type" configuration). Less frequently, they drain independently into the hepatic ducts. Stones, inflammatory conditions, and tumors may preferentially involve one of the gallbladders.[15] A duplicate gallbladder may be an uncommon cause of recurrent acute right upper quadrant abdominal pain after cholecystectomy.[16]

The gallbladder may be located in abnormal sites. It may be found on the left side as the only malpositioned organ or, more commonly, as a part of situs inversus. In other instances, the gallbladder is retroplaced within the falciform ligament or abdominal wall, or it is totally surrounded by liver parenchyma (intrahepatic gallbladder). Another abnormality that may be clinically relevant is the wandering or "floating" gallbladder, so called because it lacks a firm connection to the hepatic parenchyma and is instead completely surrounded by peritoneum. The extreme mobility of this floating gallbladder predisposes to kinking of the cystic duct with subsequent compromise of bile flow or to twisting of the nutrient vessels, resulting in hemorrhagic infarction.[17] A floating gallbladder may also result from agenesis or hypoplasia of the right hepatic lobe.[18]

Biliary cysts and extrahepatic bile duct atresia are the two most common bile duct anomalies that occur during infancy. The latter condition is discussed in detail elsewhere (see Chapter 41).

Common bile duct cysts are rare, with an incidence ranging from 1 in 13,000 to 1 in 2,000,000 live births. Whether these cysts are congenital or acquired is a matter of controversy. In favor of the former hypothesis is the presence of an anomalous pancreaticobiliary junction in 20% of cases and their coexistence with congenital hepatic fibrosis and dilatation of intrahepatic bile ducts. Developmental defects such as failure of canalization of the primordial biliary tree may result in obstruction and secondary dilatation of the common bile ducts. An infectious etiology has also been suggested but not proved.[19]

CHOLEDOCHAL CYSTS

Pathologic Features

The current classification of choledochal cysts is based on the modification by Todani of the scheme proposed by Alonzo-Lej.[20] Type 1 cysts, which are characterized by dilatation of the common bile duct, are the most common type of biliary cysts, accounting for 85% to 90% of these lesions with a 3:1 female predominance (Fig. 28-1). Type 2 cysts have a diverticular outpouching. Type 3 cysts are cystic dilatations of the terminal end of the common bile duct within the duodenal wall. No sex predominance has been noted for types 2 and 3. Type 4 cysts show multiple dilatations of the common bile duct with involvement of the intrahepatic and/or extrahepatic ducts. Type 5 cysts are single or multiple cysts confined to the intrahepatic ducts. When associated with hepatic fibrosis, the disorder is known as Caroli's disease.

Grossly, the wall is thick and fibrotic, and the luminal surface appears irregular. Microscopically, the epithelium may be absent, focally present, and/or attenuated. In uncomplicated cysts, little inflammation occurs. The wall is fibrotic, and the muscle layer, when present, is attenuated or disrupted.

Clinical Features

When symptoms occur during the neonatal period, the clinical picture is similar to that of biliary atresia. Patients present with jaundice, cholestasis, pale stools, and dark urine. Few of them have the classic triad of pain, mass, and jaundice. Two thirds of patients are older than 2 years of age with more insidious symptomatology. Most patients in this group present with a clinical picture of ascending cholangitis with pain, emesis, and jaundice. Less often, they may present with pancreatitis, hepatomegaly, palpable masses, perforation of the cyst, or biliary peritonitis. The diagnosis is confirmed by imaging techniques, which include ultrasound examination and technetium and computed tomographic (CT) scans.

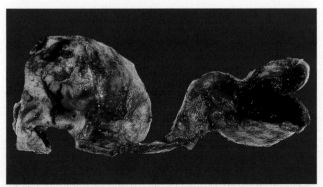

FIGURE 28–1. Choledochal cyst. This type 1 choledochal cyst measured 8 cm. It was excised in conjunction with the gallbladder (*left*).

Even when asymptomatic, choledochal cysts must be surgically treated because untreated cysts may progress to complications that range from cholangitis and pancreatitis to liver abscesses, cirrhosis, and cholangiocarcinoma. The risk of malignant transformation is 14.3% in individuals older than 20 years of age. Adenocarcinomas may develop from the epithelium lining the cyst, pancreas, and gallbladder.[19]

HETEROTOPIAS

Ectopic tissues are rarely found in the wall of the gallbladder. More common in young adults than in children, ectopic gastric mucosa is usually symptomatic and in some cases may lead to perforation and hemorrhage.[21] Microscopically, fundic and antral mucosae are identified in most cases. It is important to recall that antral or pyloric tissue is in most instances metaplastic and is not a "true" heterotopia.

In contrast, ectopic pancreatic tissue is usually an incidental finding in cholecystectomy specimens. Rarely, it has given rise to clinical symptoms of acute pancreatitis.[22] Hepatic and adrenal cortices are incidental microscopic findings.[23]

Gallstones

Gallstones are a common cause of morbidity throughout the world. In the United States, more than 20 million people have gallstones.[24] In 1995, approximately 700,000 cholecystectomies were performed to treat symptomatic gallstone disease or its complications.[25] In the United States, $8 billion to $10 billion—almost 1.5% of health care costs—is spent each year on gallstone disease.[26] Recent technical advances such as shock wave lithotripsy and pharmacologic dissolution of gallstones have become increasingly popular therapeutic alternatives to open or laparoscopic cholecystectomy. Undoubtedly, further improvements in therapy and prevention will derive from a better understanding of the epidemiology and pathophysiology of gallstone formation.

HISTORICAL VIGNETTE

Since antiquity, gallstones have been of interest to physicians. Surprisingly, no mention of gallstone disease in humans is encountered in ancient Greek writings. The first discussion of gallstones as "dried up humors concreted like stones" and their relation to obstruction of the liver is ascribed to the Greek physician Alexander of Tralles (5th century AD). The 14th century physician Gentile da Foligno suggested for the first time the relation of cholecystitis and gallstones based on autopsy findings. Antonio Benivieni succeeded in identifying

gallstones in a patient who was experiencing abdominal pain. His clinical impression was confirmed at autopsy. However, it was Jean Fernel (1581), physician to the King of France, who provided the most accurate clinical description of the symptoms associated with cholelithiasis. Gallstones were removed from a living patient for the first time in 1618 by the German surgeon Wilhelm Fabry. Two and a half centuries later, another German physician, Carl Langenbuch, performed the first cholecystectomy.

The composition of gallstones was unknown until the end of the 17th and 18th centuries. It was through the work of researchers such as Antonio Vallisneri, Pouilletier de la Salle, and Vicq d'Azyr that the chemical composition of gallstones was determined and the fact that there are differences among them was realized.[27]

CLASSIFICATION

Gallstones are composed predominantly of cholesterol, bilirubin, and calcium salts with lesser amounts of other constituents. The most popular classification system, which is based on the relative amount of cholesterol in the stones, includes two primary categories—cholesterol and noncholesterol or pigmented stones (Fig. 28-2). The latter are further classified as either black or brown pigmented stones.[28-30] Cholesterol gallstones account for more than 80% of stones in the industrialized nations and are composed predominantly of cholesterol crystals. Noncholesterol gallstones, in contrast, are much more common in other parts of the world, such as Asia. Black pigmented stones are formed from calcium salts of unconjugated bilirubin in a polymerized matrix. Brown pigmented stones may form within bile ducts (primary bile duct stones) and contain bacterial degradation products of biliary lipids, calcium salts of fatty acids, unconjugated bilirubin, and precipitated cholesterol. Because the pathogenesis and epidemiology of these types of stones are considerably different, they are discussed separately here.

Cholesterol Gallstones

PATHOGENESIS (see also Chapter 25)

The major lipid components of bile are bile salts, phospholipids, and cholesterol. Because cholesterol is virtually insoluble in water, it requires a solubilizing system, which is provided by the detergent phospholipids and bile salts. After being co-secreted by hepatocytes, cholesterol and phospholipids form spherical structures or vesicles that are made of a double layer of phospholipids, of which lecithin (diacylphosphatidylcholines) is the main type. Vesicles are soluble by virtue of the outward orientation of the hydrophilic ("water loving") choline groups, allowing cholesterol to be inserted into

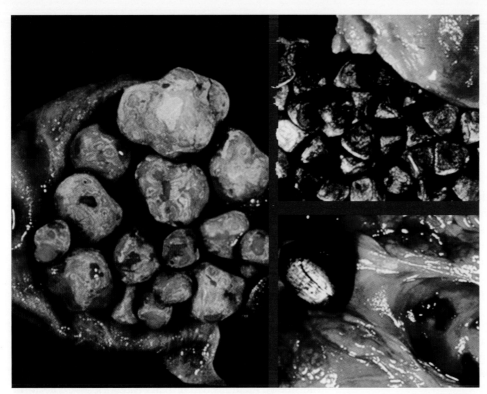

FIGURE 28–2. Gallstones. Cholesterol gallstones *(left panel)*, black stones *(right upper panel)*, and brown stones *(right lower panel)* within bile ducts.

the hydrophobic ("water fearing") milieu provided by the fatty acid chains.[30-32]

Hepatocytes secrete bile acids through a different transport mechanism. Although soluble in water, bile salt monomers self-aggregate into simple micelles once they surpass the so-called critical micellar concentration (0.5 to 5 mM). The amphophilic properties of bile acids render an extremely water-soluble structure resulting from the orientation of the hydrophobic portions away from water and the exposure of hydrophilic surfaces to the aqueous environment. As detergents, bile acids can dissolve portions of vesicles and incorporate them as mixed micelles. The resulting structures are essentially discs composed of cholesterol and phospholipids surrounded by bile acids.[32-34]

As the concentration of cholesterol increases, more of it is carried in vesicles. In addition, increasing cholesterol concentration causes increased cholesterol transfer from vesicles to micelles during the micellation process. The resulting cholesterol-enriched unilamellar vesicles are unstable and fuse into large multilamellar vesicles. When the cholesterol-to-phospholipid ratio exceeds 1, cholesterol crystallizes at their surface. Enhancement of crystallization is influenced by the concentration of solutes in bile in that aggregation occurs more efficiently when cholesterol carriers are close to each other.[31,33,35]

Cholesterol is most soluble in a mixture of lipids containing at least 50% bile acids and smaller amounts of phospholipids. Supersaturation occurs when a solution contains more cholesterol molecules than can be solu-

bilized. Theoretically, bile supersaturation may be due to hypersecretion of cholesterol, hyposecretion of bile acids, hyposecretion of phospholipids, or a combination of these. An increase in biliary cholesterol output—due to either increased synthesis or increased uptake—is the most common cause of supersaturation and subsequent stone formation. Increased uptake by hepatocytes may involve either endogenous cholesterol (transported via low density lipoproteins) or exogenous cholesterol (transported via chylomicrons).

As noted earlier, cholesterol supersaturation may also arise as a consequence of bile acid hyposecretion. However, most patients with gallstones have normal biliary acid secretion. Adequate bile acid secretion depends on the integrity of the enterohepatic circulation. Approximately 90% of bile acids are resorbed from the terminal ileum and returned to the liver via the portal system 3 to 12 times per day. There, the bile acids are reused by the hepatocytes following passive and active reuptake. Theoretically, any interference with this recycling mechanism contributes to bile acid hyposecretion and subsequent cholesterol supersaturation.[32-34]

A study of first-degree relatives of gallstone carriers provided the first clues that bile lipid secretion might be under genetic control.[35] Most recently acquired information in this field is based on animal models. Knockout mice deficient in the multiple drug–resistant gene 2 maintain normal bile acid secretion but are incapable of secreting phospholipids and cholesterol in bile owing to the absence of a protein that "flips" phospholipids from the inner to the outer half of the canalicular membrane.[36] In other mouse models, it has been shown that when these animals are fed a lithogenic diet, gallstones develop in susceptible mice with a frequency that varies according to the presence of the lith-one, lith-two, or lith-three gene, as well as other genes.[26]

Supersaturation of cholesterol is necessary but not sufficient for the formation of cholesterol gallstones. For any given degree of cholesterol saturation, patients with gallstones form cholesterol crystals more rapidly than do individuals without gallstones. This observation led to the idea that stone formation may involve a nucleation process. It has become apparent that the tendency of bile to nucleate its cholesterol depends on the balance between substances that promote and prevent nucleation. Pronucleating substances are mostly heterogeneous mucin gels. Besides mucin, other biliary proteins have been postulated as promoters or inhibitors of cholesterol precipitation in bile.[37-42] However, their participation is most likely nonspecific, and their relevance remains controversial.[43]

Biliary sludge is a viscous gel composed of mucin and microscopic precipitates of multilamellar vesicles, cholesterol monohydrate, and calcium bilirubinate. Because mucin is present at the center of almost all gallstones, it has been suggested that the formation of biliary sludge precedes the formation of macroscopic cholesterol gallstones.[37]

In addition to the possible participation of the epithelium in the secretion of mucin and other pronucleating factors, impaired gallbladder filling and emptying participates in gallstone formation. Stasis of supersaturated bile favors cholesterol crystallization and gallstone formation. Absorption of cholesterol by the gallbladder mucosa is thought to stiffen sarcolemmal membranes and uncouple signal transduction via G proteins, nullifying the intracellular events mediated by the binding of cholecystokinin to its receptor.[44]

EPIDEMIOLOGY

The prevalence of cholesterol gallstones varies greatly according to age, sex, country, and ethnic group. Geographic differences are most likely related to the interaction of genetic and environmental factors. In the United States, it has been estimated that more than 20 million people have gallstones. The incidence of gallstones increases with age. An increased risk for gallstones is associated with multiparity, estrogen replacement therapy, oral contraceptive use, obesity, and rapid weight loss.[45] Whether diabetes predisposes to gallstone formation is still controversial. Substantial evidence suggests that alcohol intake protects against gallstones.[45-46]

In the United States, the highest prevalence of gallstones is observed among Native Americans, with progressively lower risk among whites, blacks, and some Asian groups.[47] Mexican American women also have a higher prevalence of gallstones than do other Hispanic women.[48-49] In other parts of the world, gallstones are extremely common in areas such as Chile and the Scandinavian countries, and they have a much lower incidence in Asia and Africa.[50-51] Epidemiologic data from North America suggest that populations with a high prevalence of gallstones carry dominant Amerindian lithogenic genes transmitted by common ancestral human groups of Asian origin that colonized America more than 20,000 years ago.

In support of this hypothesis, a recent epidemiologic study from Chile found a positive correlation between Native American genes (measured via ABO blood group distribution and determination of mitochondrial DNA polymorphisms) and the prevalence of gallstones in women younger than 35 years of age.[52] In this study, the highest prevalence of gallstone disease was found among native Mapuche Indians (35.2%), followed by residents of urban Santiago (27.5%) and Maoris of Easter Island (20.9%).[52] The high prevalence among Native American and Mexican American women also supports this hypothesis. As has been mentioned, specific genes associated with gallstone susceptibility have been partially characterized in animal models. Undoubtedly, the corresponding human genes and their products will be elucidated over the following decade. Knowledge of the function of the gene products involved in lithogenesis and the potential relevance of genetic polymorphism in their synthesis or functionality will expand our understanding of their complex interactions with environmental (dietary) factors. Based on this information, specific prevention strategies tailored to populations with a high prevalence of cholesterol gallstones will become available.

Pigmented (Noncholesterol) Gallstones

PATHOGENESIS

Pigmented stones are of two types—black and brown. Distinction between these is important because they differ in their etiology, associated clinical conditions, morphology, and chemical composition. Black stones are composed of calcium bilirubinate, phosphate, and carbonate embedded in a glycoprotein matrix; they have a low cholesterol concentration. Brown stones contain calcium salts of bilirubin and fatty acids (palmitate) in a glycoprotein matrix; they have a higher concentration of cholesterol. Calcium carbonate and phosphate are usually not present.[53] Black stones are small, black, and multiple. Brown stones are soft, brownish green, and large.

Because it is a precursor of calcium bilirubinate, unconjugated bilirubin plays a central role in the formation of both brown and black pigmented stones. Unconjugated bilirubin is solubilized by bile salts in mixed micelles; it then combines with calcium to form calcium bilirubinate. Any condition resulting in elevated levels of unconjugated bilirubin can therefore predispose to stone formation. Biliary infections contributing to bile stasis are common causes of brown stones because bacterial overgrowth generates hydrolases that can then form free bile acids from conjugated bile salts. In addition, bacteria elaborate phospholipase A, which cleaves phospholipids to form lysolecithin and free fatty acids. These free fatty acids (mainly palmitic and stearic) combine with the free bile salts generated by the bacterial hydrolases and precipitate as calcium salts. It is not surprising, therefore, that bacteria are found within the matrices of most brown stones.[53]

Black pigmented stone disease is not associated with bacterial infection. An increased concentration of unconjugated bilirubin originates from an increment in the secretion of bilirubin conjugates, as occurs in hemolysis and chronic alcoholism, followed by non-bacterial enzymatic or nonenzymatic hydrolysis. An analogous effect may occur if there is a decrease in the secretion of bile salts, as occurs in patients with cirrhosis, because these compounds are required to solubilize unconjugated bilirubin and buffer ionized calcium.[37] Phospholipids also play an important role in pigment sludge formation. Calcium bilirubinate sludge contains an increased amount of phospholipids, and these compounds are found in the core of pigmented gallstones. Carbohydrate-rich diets stimulate enzymes, such as fatty acid synthetase, that are important in the synthesis of phospholipids. The increased activity of these enzymes may explain the higher hepatic bile phospholipid concentrations found in clinical situations such as total parenteral nutrition.

The gallbladder itself plays a role in lithogenesis. Biliary epithelium functions to acidify bile, thereby increasing the solubility of calcium carbonate. Mucosal inflammation interferes with the ability of the epithelium to perform this acidifying role, resulting in an increased biliary pH and subsequent calcium carbonate precipitation. In addition, reparative metaplastic changes in the mucosa (vide infra) cause an increased concentration of biliary glycoproteins, which in turn promotes gallstone formation.[37]

EPIDEMIOLOGY

Pigmented gallstones occur in patients from all countries. Although they account for only 20% to 25% of stones in the United States, they are the most common type worldwide. Similar to cholesterol gallstones, pigmented stones develop more frequently in women, and their incidence increases with age; however, at variance with the former, race does not appear to be a factor.

Clinical conditions associated with black gallstones include hemolytic anemia, cirrhosis, alcoholism, malaria, pancreatitis, total parenteral nutrition, and advanced age. In addition, black pigmented stones develop more frequently in patients with Crohn's disease, particularly in those with extensive ileitis or who have undergone ileal resection. A predilection for stone formation in this last group of patients stems from the decreased or absent functionality of the terminal ileum, which (as has been discussed) is the site of 90% of bile salt resorption in the normal individual. Any unconjugated bilirubin in normal patients then precipitates in the colon as calcium bilirubinate or another bilirubinate. By contrast, impaired or absent resorptive function in the ileum in patients with Crohn's disease leads to increased levels of bile salts in the colon, where the salts solubilize unconjugated bilirubin.[54] Subsequent increased colonic resorption of this unconjugated bilirubin leads to supersaturation of bile (up to three times normal levels) and stone formation.

PATHOLOGIC FEATURES

Although the "pathology" of gallstones may seem a misnomer, in fact, examination of gallstones by gross inspection is a necessary part of patient care. Cholesterol stones are easily distinguished from pigmented stones; chemical analysis of stone composition is left for research investigations. Cholesterol stones arise in the gallbladder and are composed of cholesterol ranging from 100% pure (which is rare) to around 50% pure. Cholesterol stones are hard and must be fractured before the interior can be examined. Pure cholesterol stones are pale yellow and round to ovoid with a finely granular, hard external surface, which, upon fracture, reveals a glistening, radiating, crystalline palisade. With increasing proportions of calcium carbonate, phosphates, and bilirubin, the stones exhibit discoloration and may be lamellated and gray-white to black on transection. Most often, multiple stones that range up to several centimeters in diameter are present. Rarely, a single, much larger stone may virtually fill the fundus. Surfaces of multiple stones may be rounded or faceted owing to tight apposition.

As has been discussed, pigmented gallstones are classified as black or brown. In general, black pigmented stones are found in sterile gallbladder bile, and brown stones are found in infected intrahepatic or extrahepatic ducts. As mentioned, black pigmented stones contain oxidized polymers of the calcium salts of unconjugated bilirubin; lesser amounts of calcium carbonate, calcium phosphate, and mucin glycoprotein; and a modicum of cholesterol monohydrate crystals. Brown pigmented stones contain pure calcium salts of unconjugated bilirubin, mucin glycoprotein, a substantial cholesterol fraction, and calcium salts of palmitate and stearate. Black stones are rarely larger than 1.5 cm in diameter, are almost invariably present in great number (with an inverse relationship between size and number), and may crumble to the touch. Their contours are usually spiculated and molded. Brown stones tend to be laminated and soft and may have a soaplike or greasy consistency. Mucin glycoproteins constitute the scaffolding and interparticle cement of all stones, whether pigmented or cholesterol.

DIFFERENTIAL DIAGNOSIS

Clinical setting and radiographic findings usually are sufficient to establish whether gallstones are cholesterol stones or pigmented stones; hence, gross examination should serve a confirmatory function. Differential diagnosis of right upper quadrant distress or biliary obstruction is a clinical issue in that other possibilities for biliary obstruction include stricture and tumor.

◼ Cholecystitis

Inflammatory diseases of the gallbladder are a frequent cause of morbidity in Western countries. The term *cholecystitis* encompasses a group of disorders that differ in their pathologic, pathogenetic, and clinical characteristics. As do other organs of the gastrointestinal tract, most inflammatory diseases of the gallbladder show nonspecific histologic features in that they elicit nondistinctive types of cellular infiltrates. However, characterization of inflammatory patterns helps the pathologist to establish a diagnosis and provides insight into the pathogenesis of a disease. In addition, it is through the recognition of differences in inflammatory patterns that clinically useful histologic diagnoses are rendered.

ACUTE CHOLECYSTITIS

Acute cholecystitis is clinically defined as an episode of acute biliary pain accompanied by fever, right upper quadrant tenderness, guarding, persistence of symptoms beyond 24 hours, and leukocytosis.[55] Approximately 90% of cases are associated with gallstones. Ultrasonography demonstrates a thickened gallbladder wall or pericholecystic fluid. The diagnosis is also supported by lack of visualization of the gallbladder during a hepatobiliary scintigram.[56] Because of their unique clinical and/or pathologic characteristics, the following three types of acute cholecystitis are discussed separately here: acute calculous cholecystitis, acute acalculous cholecystitis, and acute emphysematous cholecystitis.

Acute Calculous Cholecystitis

The precipitating event for the development of acute calculous cholecystitis appears to be occlusion of the neck of the gallbladder or cystic duct by a stone. Subsequent increased intraluminal pressure causes dilatation of the gallbladder and edema of its wall. However, outflow obstruction does not always cause acute cholecystitis. Animal models in which the cystic duct has been ligated or obliterated show only shrinkage of the gallbladder, not acute cholecystitis.[57] Other factors contributing to acute cholecystitis may therefore include mucosal ischemia secondary to visceral distention and external compression of the nearby cystic artery by the impacted stone. Formation of inflammatory mediators such as lysolecithin and prostaglandins, and concentrated bile, cholesterol, or gallstones may also contribute to mucosal injury.[58] It has been postulated that trauma to the mucosa caused by stones releases phospholipase from lysosomes residing in mucosal epithelial cells. This enzyme converts lecithin to lysolecithin, which is an active detergent known to be toxic to the mucosa.[59] In addition, phospholipids can damage biliary cells. It has been shown that the bile from patients with gallstones contains lysophosphatidylcholine, which induces mucosal necrosis and inflammation of the gallbladder wall.[60]

When bile cultures are obtained early enough (within 48 hours of onset), bacteria can be identified in 42% to 72% of cases. The predominant organisms are intestinal. These include *Escherichia coli*, other Gram-negative aerobic rods, enterococci, and, in 20% of cases, anaerobes.[61,62] Most authorities agree that the infection is secondary and does not contribute to the onset of acute cholecystitis.

PATHOLOGIC FEATURES

The surgeon identifies acute cholecystitis at the time of laparoscopy or laparotomy through signs of acute inflammation such as omental adhesions to the gallbladder wall, edema, friability, pericholecystic fluid, and frank gangrene. The gallbladder is usually enlarged by a wall that has been thickened by edema, vascular congestion, and hemorrhage, or it may appear necrotic (Fig. 28-3). The serosa is dull and covered with patches of fibrinopurulent exudate. As has been mentioned, a gallstone is frequently found obstructing the outflow pathway. The lumen is filled by pus admixed with thick, cloudy bile. Depending on the severity of the inflammatory response, the mucosal changes range from edema and congestion to widespread ulcers and necrosis. Histologically, an acute inflammatory reaction characterized by edema, vascular congestion, hemorrhage, neutrophilic infiltration, and mucosal necrosis predominates in specimens obtained early in the course of the disease (Fig. 28-4). As the pathologic process evolves, transmural inflammation, secondary acute vasculitis, and mural necrosis follow. Fibrinous pseudomembranes (pseudomembranous cholecystitis) may develop over necrotic-appearing mucosa (Fig. 28-5). As the disease evolves, lymphocytes, plasma cells, macrophages, and numerous eosinophils appear. Granulation tissue and collagen

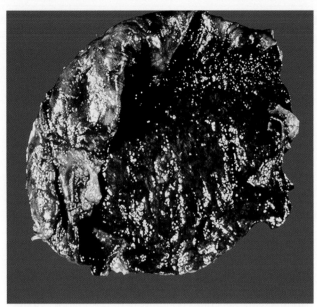

FIGURE 28–3. Acute gangrenous cholecystitis. The gallbladder was distended and contained numerous stones. The mucosa shows a necrotic and hemorrhagic appearance.

deposition replace the previously ulcerated or necrotic tissue. A cholecystectomy for acute cholecystitis should preferably be performed within 2 or 3 days of the onset of symptoms, a time frame that has been referred to as the "golden period."[63,64] After inflammation has been present for longer than 72 hours, the increasing fibrous adhesions and transmural inflammation make cholecystectomy far more laborious and prone to complications.

Complications of acute calculous cholecystitis include empyema, gangrene, and perforation. The latter complication is usually sealed off by the omentum, leading to the formation of pericholecystic adhesions and/or

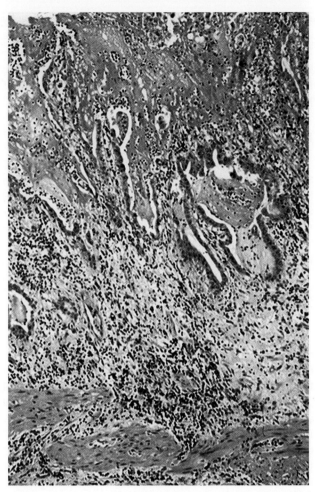

FIGURE 28–5. Acute (pseudomembranous) cholecystitis. Thick fibrinous pseudomembranes are firmly attached to necrotic biliary epithelium and appear to merge with the underlying edematous and inflamed lamina propria.

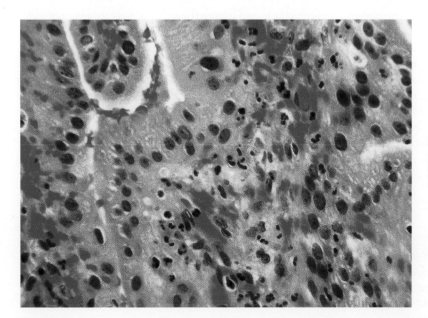

FIGURE 28–4. Acute cholecystitis. In the early phases, neutrophils predominate. As shown in this case, the lamina propria is frequently hemorrhagic.

abscess. In the less fortunate patient, however, life-threatening bacteremia and septic complications may ensue.[55]

CLINICAL CORRELATION

Most patients are women, with a peak incidence at 50 to 70 years of age. Typical symptoms include right upper quadrant pain of recent onset accompanied by abdominal guarding and local tenderness. These symptoms may be deceptively mild or even absent in the elderly. Sometimes, the enlarged gallbladder may be palpated and/or pain may be elicited while the right upper quadrant is palpated when the patient inhales deeply (Murphy's sign). Some patients are febrile and jaundiced, and most show leukocytosis. Because the clinical features are not entirely specific, imaging techniques such as ultrasonography or cholescintigraphy are used to confirm the diagnosis. Preoperative clinical findings of acute cholecystitis are highly reliable for predicting intraoperative gross findings. However, intraoperative findings of acute cholecystitis are commonly found in the absence of preoperative clinical signs. For reasons that are not entirely clear, the correlation between pathologic diagnosis and intraoperative findings is poor.[56]

Acute Acalculous Cholecystitis

This infrequent but clinically serious disease is found in approximately 5% of all patients undergoing cholecystectomy.[65,66] It predominantly affects individuals with other clinicopathologic conditions, including trauma, nonbiliary surgical procedures, sepsis, burns, parenteral nutrition, mechanical ventilation, numerous blood transfusions, and use of narcotics or antibiotics. However, this disorder may occur de novo in patients with no predisposing factors.[67,68]

Its exact pathogenesis is not fully understood, although it appears to be multifactorial.[69] Increased bile viscosity from stasis with subsequent obstruction of the cystic duct has been suggested as a contributing factor and may explain the association of acalculous cholecystitis with a patient history of fasting, narcotic use, dehydration, or anesthesia, all of which result in bile stasis. Undoubtedly, mucosal ischemia plays a major role in patients with underlying cardiovascular disease and in those who develop acute acalculous cholecystitis following trauma, sepsis, or surgical procedures. A high mortality rate of up to 45% characterizes this group of patients. Prostanoid and bile salts also appear to play an important role in the development of acalculous cholecystitis. Prostaglandins are involved in gallbladder contraction, water absorption, and the inflammation and pain associated with gallbladder disease. Different types of prostaglandins have various roles in acute inflammatory conditions of the gallbladder. Prostaglandin E (PGE) levels increase as inflammation increases. In normal gallbladders, the PGE/PGF ratio is 4:1. PGE levels are increased sevenfold in patients with acute acalculous cholecystitis. Tissue anoxia secondary to shock, bacterial contamination and invasion, stasis, and changes in bile salt concentration all participate in injury to the gallbladder mucosa. As a consequence, inflammation, distention, atonicity, and pain develop.[67,69]

In animal models, platelet-activating factor (PAF) has been shown to play a role in the induction of acute acalculous cholecystitis. This substance is released by basophils, eosinophils, neutrophils, macrophages, monocytes, mast cells, vascular endothelial cells, and smooth muscle cells. It increases vascular permeability and induces neutrophil aggregation and degranulation. Indirectly, PAF may cause acalculous cholecystitis by stimulating and releasing interleukin-1, tumor necrosis factor, and interleukin-6. PAF may also be associated with the development of arteriolar thrombosis and ischemia.[69]

PATHOLOGIC FEATURES

Mucosal ischemic changes are frequently observed in acalculous cholecystitis, particularly among postsurgical patients or those hospitalized for trauma or critical illness. However, in general, no specific histologic differences have been noted between acute calculous and acalculous cholecystitis.

Acute Emphysematous Cholecystitis

Acute emphysematous cholecystitis is an uncommon variant of acute cholecystitis caused by bacterial infection with gas-producing organisms. Clinically, this condition is indistinguishable from simple acute cholecystitis, and the distinction is often made with imaging studies. Abdominal radiographs are relatively insensitive in the diagnosis of emphysematous cholecystitis. As a result of the regular use of ultrasonography in suspected hepatobiliary disease, emphysematous cholecystitis is being diagnosed with increased frequency.[70] Delayed diagnosis results in a high incidence of complications such as gangrene and perforation, which explains the much higher overall mortality rate (15% vs. 4.1% for acute calculous cholecystitis). About half of bile cultures are positive for clostridial organisms; others are positive for *E. coli* and *Bacteroides fragilis*.[71] Occlusion of the cystic artery or its branches by atherosclerosis and small vessel disease (both frequent complications of diabetes mellitus) are major contributory factors.[72-73]

PATHOLOGIC FEATURES

During cholecystectomy, the gallbladder may appear distended, tense, and encased by the omentum, fibrous adhesions, and/or a pericholecystic abscess. The necrotic, friable wall frequently causes fragmentation of the gallbladder during its removal. Upon opening, gas and foul-smelling purulent exudate escape from the lumen. Gallstones, frequently of the pigmented type, are found in 70% of cases. The mucosa appears necrotic, congested, and hemorrhagic. Microscopically, the necrotic and acutely inflamed mucosa often contains colonies of Gram-positive bacilli. Gas bubbles are occasionally seen within the wall or in the subserosal connective tissue. Perforation and bile peritonitis may occur in about 10% of cases.

CHRONIC CHOLECYSTITIS

Chronic cholecystitis is almost always associated with gallstones. The pathogenesis of this common disorder is poorly understood. It has been suggested that chronic cholecystitis develops as the result of recurrent attacks of mild acute cholecystitis. However, few patients provide a clinical history supportive of this hypothesis. Inflammatory and reparative changes may be explained in part by repetitive mucosal trauma produced by gallstones, although other factors most likely play a role as well. Because there is a poor correlation between the severity of the inflammatory response and the number and volume of stones, it is possible that the intensity of the inflammatory response of the mucosa caused by gallstones in different populations is genetically determined, as has been demonstrated in other digestive organs.[74]

A potential and currently unproved hypothesis is that a copious inflammatory response in the gallbladder could be a residue of what may have been a "protective effect" for those populations whose ancestors resided in geographic areas with a high incidence of parasitic biliary infections. This energetic inflammatory response of the gallbladder mucosa may have been protective against parasites at one time, but it evolved into a detrimental mechanism in the pathology of gallstone disease. Other scientists have postulated that both cholelithiasis and chronic cholecystitis are caused by an abnormal composition of the bile, leading to stone formation and chemical injury to the mucosa. At variance with the high percentage of positive bile cultures in patients with acute cholecystitis, bacteria, mostly *E. coli* and enterococci, are cultured in less than a third of patients with chronic cholecystitis.[75] A recent study has identified DNA from *Helicobacter* species in biliary tract specimens from a group of Chilean patients with gallbladder disease.[76] However, this association has not been confirmed in other populations with a high incidence of gallstones.[77]

Pathologic Features

The variable appearance of the gallbladder in chronic cholecystitis reflects differences in the degree of inflammation and fibrosis. The gallbladder may be distended or shrunken. Fibrous serosal adhesions suggest previous episodes of acute cholecystitis. On gross examination, the wall is usually thickened, but it may be thin. The mucosa may be intact with preservation or accentuation of its folds, or it may be flattened, as in cases of outflow obstruction. Mucosal erosions or ulcers are frequently found in association with impacted stones (Fig. 28-6). The mere presence of gallstones is neither necessary nor sufficient for the diagnosis of chronic cholecystitis. This diagnosis is based on the following three histologic characteristics: (1) a predominantly mononuclear inflammatory infiltrate in the lamina propria with or without extension to the muscularis and pericholecystic tissues, (2) fibrosis, and/or (3) metaplastic changes.

The degree of the inflammatory reaction is variable. In some cases, the infiltrate is exclusively located in the mucosa; in others, it extends into the muscularis and serosa. The distribution of the infiltrate varies from focal to patchy to diffuse. Commonly, lymphocytes predomi-

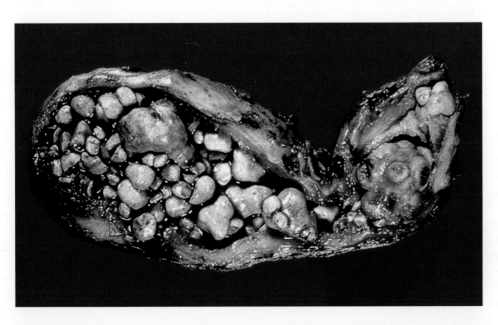

FIGURE 28–6. Chronic calculous cholecystitis. The wall of the gallbladder is thickened, and the lumen contains innumerable cholesterol stones.

nate over plasma cells and histiocytes. It is important to recall that sparse, focally distributed lymphoid cells may be present in normal gallbladders obtained from healthy individuals who died of traumatic causes and whose livers were used for transplantation (Fig. 28-7).[78] Occasional lymphoid follicles arise in a background of chronic inflammation. Most lymphoid follicles are located in the lamina propria, but they may infiltrate the full thickness of the gallbladder wall. When diffuse, the term *follicular cholecystitis* is used to describe this condition (Fig. 28-8).[79] A minor component of eosinophils and neutrophils may also be seen. When neutrophils are predominantly found within the epithelium in a setting of chronic cholecystitis, it is preferable to view them as evidence of "activity" of the inflammatory process rather than as a mixed acute and chronic or subacute condition. We believe that the term *chronic active cholecystitis* better defines these cases (Fig. 28-9).

When bile penetrates into the subepithelial layers through mucosal ulcers or fissures, it frequently elicits an inflammatory reaction characterized by closely packed histiocytes with pale cytoplasm containing abundant brown pigmented granules (Fig. 28-10). In addition to its color, this pigment, referred to as ceroid, is characterized histochemically by its acid fastness and PAS positivity (diastase resistance). A sparse lymphocytic reaction usually accompanies the histiocytes.[80,81] Ceroid granulomas trigger a reparative response, leading to the deposition of dense collagen. Fibrosis eventually replaces those areas previously involved by the inflammatory process and may eventually replace the entire gallbladder. Dystrophic calcifications are often associated with this fibrous tissue, and when diffuse, they give rise to the so-called porcelain gallbladder.[82-83] For unknown reasons, carcinoma of the gallbladder is more frequently associated with this condition than with other forms of chronic

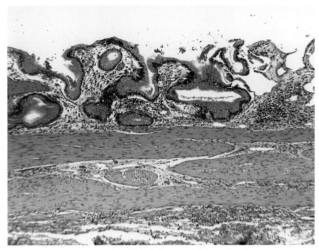

FIGURE 28–7. Normal gallbladder. Focal lymphoid aggregates in the lamina propria such as the one on the right side of this photomicrograph are frequently present in normal gallbladders excised from the livers of donors who died of traumatic injuries.

cholecystitis.[84-85] In addition to ceroid granulomas, foreign body–type granulomas characterized by aggregates of multinucleated giant cells and foamy histiocytes may be seen around clefts containing cholesterol crystals or concretions of bile. Foamy histiocytes are also the predominant cells in xanthogranulomas, usually in association with plasma cells and occasionally with giant cells or ceroid-containing histiocytes (Fig. 28-11). These cells may form tumor-like aggregates that are sometimes confused with neoplasms.[86-89]

A granulomatous reaction of infectious etiology rarely occurs in the gallbladder. As in other organs, special stains aid in identification of the causative organism (Fig. 28-12). As in many other organ systems, chronic injury to the gallbladder mucosa can cause metaplastic

FIGURE 28–8. Chronic follicular cholecystitis. Reactive lymphoid follicles with prominent germinal centers characterize this form of cholecystitis.

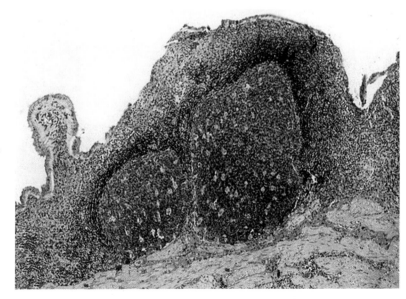

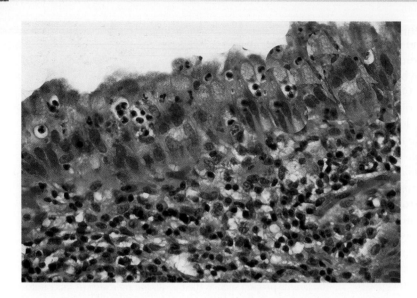

FIGURE 28–9. Chronic active cholecystitis. The dense lymphoplasmacytic infiltrate in the lamina propria defines this process as chronic. Intraepithelial neutrophils are the hallmark of activity.

changes.[90-91] The most common type of metaplasia is of the antral (or pyloric) type, characterized by tubular glands in the lamina propria that are formed by clear cells with abundant mucin vacuoles. These cells are similar to those found in the gastric antrum (Fig. 28-13). The surface epithelium frequently undergoes metaplasia of the superficial gastric type. This change is characterized by focal or diffuse replacement of the columnar epithelium of the gallbladder by taller, mucin-rich, PAS-positive, columnar cells. When the metaplastic pyloric glands proliferate and permeate smooth muscle fibers, their histologic appearance is similar to that of an adenocarcinoma. Rarely, florid pyloric gland metaplasia may show perineural and intraneural invasion. The lobular arrangement of the glands and their bland cytologic features should prevent misinterpretation as adenocarcinoma.[92,93] Less frequently, intestinal metaplasia may occur. It is identified by the appearance of cells with intestinal phenotypes, such as goblet cells, absorptive columnar cells, Paneth cells, and gut endocrine cells. Infrequently, squamous metaplasia may also occur.

Clinical Correlation

Chronic cholecystitis is defined more definitively by its gross and histologic features than by its clinical characteristics. Uncertainty still prevails as to the precise symptom(s) associated with gallstone disease and chronic cholecystitis. Most persons with gallstones never experience pain attacks. The only symptom related to gallstones is episodic upper abdominal pain.[94] Dyspeptic symptoms, belching, bloating, abdominal discomfort, heartburn, and food intolerances are frequently attributed by both patients and physicians to cholelithiasis and chronic cholecystitis. However, most of these symp-

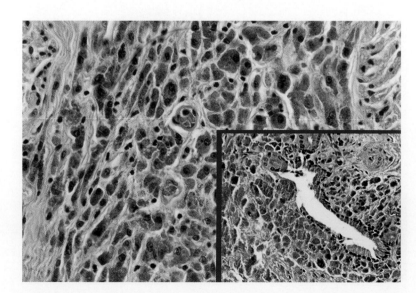

FIGURE 28–10. Ceroid granulomas. Aggregates of histiocytes with a dusky brown pigment are frequently encountered and result from penetration of bile into the lamina propria.

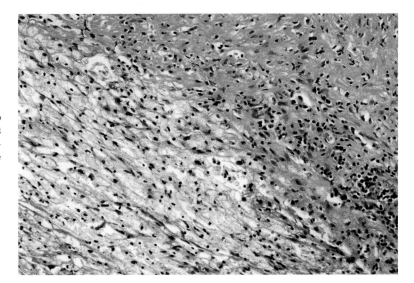

FIGURE 28–11. Xanthogranulomas. In addition to the characteristic aggregates of foamy macrophages that are typical of this lesion, plasma cells, lymphocytes, multinucleated giant cells, and variable fibrosis are commonly present.

toms are probably unrelated to these conditions and frequently persist after cholecystectomy.

In the United States, laparoscopic cholecystectomy has become the preferred treatment for patients with cholelithiasis.[95-96] This minimally invasive surgical procedure offers the advantages of shorter hospitalization, limited postoperative pain, diminished disability, and improved cosmesis. In most instances, the gallbladder is easily removed through the umbilical puncture wound, although difficulties may arise when bile and/or gallstones distend the gallbladder, or when inflammation and fibrosis give rise to a thick, noncollapsible wall. This problem is usually solved by extending the umbilical incision or by removing the bile and stones after the neck of the gallbladder has been pulled through the skin and amputated. Mechanical devices, ultrasound, or laser energy can pulverize large stones.[97] When examining a gallbladder, the pathologist should differentiate the numerous artifacts produced by these procedures from the pathologic changes resulting from disease.

Chronic Acalculous Cholecystitis

About 12% to 13% of patients with chronic cholecystitis do not have gallstones.[98] It has been suggested that postinflammatory stenosis or anatomic abnormalities of the cystic duct might impede normal emptying of the gallbladder. Such patients may pose diagnostic difficulties in that ultrasound scans and oral cholecystograms are often normal. Patients with biliary dyskinesia who may benefit from cholecystectomy are identified by a CCK provocation test. A positive test consists of

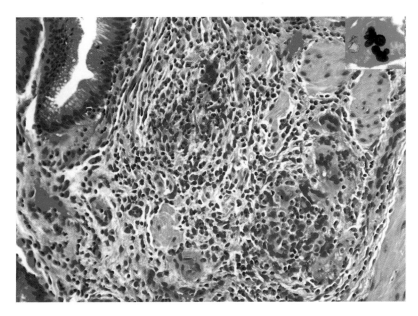

FIGURE 28–12. Granulomatous cholecystitis. These granulomas are composed of epithelioid histiocytes, giant cells, lymphocytes, and numerous eosinophils. Silver stains (*inset*) demonstrated fungal elements. Cultures were positive for the *Trichophyton* species.

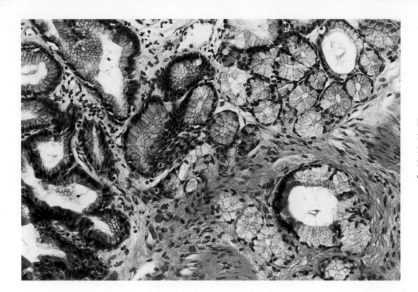

FIGURE 28–13. Antral metaplasia. Composed of mucin-secreting antral-type glands, this is the most common type of metaplasia encountered in cholecystectomy specimens of patients with chronic calculous cholecystitis.

reproduction of pain within 5 to 10 minutes after an IV injection of cholecystokinin.[99] Furthermore, incomplete emptying of the gallbladder can be documented when this test is performed at the same time as oral cholecystography.[100]

PATHOLOGIC FEATURES

At the time of surgery, a normal, distended, or thickened gallbladder may be found. Microscopic examination may reveal an unremarkable appearance, or it may demonstrate changes consistent with outflow obstruction, inflammation, or both. Thickening of the muscularis propria and the presence of Rokitansky-Aschoff sinuses identify outflow obstruction. Gallbladders excised from patients with biliary dyskinesia may show abundant Rokitansky-Aschoff sinuses in the absence of inflammation, a condition that has been referred to as microdiverticulosis or Rokitansky-Aschoff sinusosis.[78] Other patients with this condition may have a normal-appearing gallbladder or nonspecific chronic cholecystitis.

The inflammatory pattern in patients with chronic acalculous cholecystitis is nonspecific. Of interest, inflammatory infiltrates in patients with acalculous cholecystitis contain a higher percentage of eosinophils than do those in patients with gallstones. Referred to as *lymphoeosinophilic cholecystitis,* this type of cholecystitis is diagnosed when eosinophils constitute 50% to 75% of the total number of inflammatory cells. It has been hypothesized that abnormal biliary contents or certain hepatic metabolites may evoke a hypersensitivity reaction in which a large number of eosinophils that cause mucosal damage and gallbladder dysmotility are recruited.[101] True eosinophilic cholecystitis is rare and is characterized histologically by an inflammatory infiltrate composed almost exclusively of eosinophils (Fig. 28-14). Massive eosinophilic infiltrates commonly involve the extrahepatic bile ducts, in addition to the gallbladder.

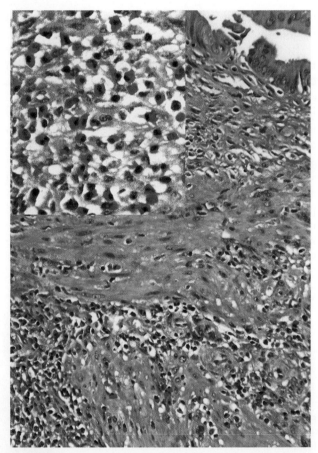

FIGURE 28–14. Eosinophilic cholecystitis. The inflammatory infiltrate is composed almost exclusively of eosinophils. In addition to the gallbladder, the extrahepatic bile ducts are frequently involved. *Inset,* High-power view showing a predominance of eosinophils.

Clinically, these patients may present with obstructive jaundice that mimics a neoplasm.[102]

Another type of chronic cholecystitis that has recently been identified is characterized by diffuse lympho-plasmacytic infiltrates confined to the lamina propria with or without active lesions (intraepithelial neutrophilic infiltrates). In the absence of gallstones, this form of chronic cholecystitis is found in patients with sclerosing cholangitis.[103] However, a recent study has shown that although this inflammatory pattern is highly specific for extrahepatic biliary tract disease, it does not distinguish between primary and secondary cholangiopathies.[104]

Xanthogranulomatous Cholecystitis

This uncommon form of chronic cholecystitis is nearly always associated with stones and is frequently accompanied by fibrosis of variable extent. Its incidence ranges from 0.7% to 1.8% of excised gallbladders, although recent reports demonstrated an incidence of 9.0% in Japan and India.[105,106] The pathogenesis of this condition is uncertain; it has been proposed, however, that xanthogranulomas form as a reaction to the penetration of bile into the gallbladder wall from mucosal ulcers or ruptured Rokitansky-Aschoff sinuses in conjunction with outflow obstruction by calculi and infection.[106,107] Positive bile cultures, mostly for enterobacteria, are found in about 50% of patients.

PATHOLOGIC FEATURES

Areas involved by the xanthogranulomatous process may appear as firm yellow masses that resemble carcinoma clinically and macroscopically.[106] Histologic examination shows rounded to spindle-shaped lipid-laden macrophages, plasma cells, and fibrosis (see Fig. 28-11). Cholesterol clefts, foreign body and Touton-type giant cells, and other inflammatory cells (i.e., lymphocytes,

eosinophils, and neutrophils) are commonly found. Frequently, the xanthogranulomatous reaction occupies a limited area of the gallbladder, and the remainder shows conventional chronic cholecystitis, often with lymphoid follicles.

Xanthogranulomatous inflammation should be differentiated from malakoplakia, which has been reported in the gallbladder.[108] Characteristic microscopic findings of malakoplakia consist of a diffuse proliferation of histiocytes with abundant eosinophilic granular cytoplasm, some of which contains spherules (Michaelis-Gutmann bodies) positive for PAS and von Kossa's (calcium) stain.

CLINICAL CORRELATION

Xanthogranulomatous cholecystitis may be difficult to distinguish from other forms of cholecystitis. However, in contrast to chronic cholecystitis, a history of at least one previous episode of acute cholecystitis is obtained from most patients. Other patients present with a clinical picture suggestive of acute cholecystitis. Imaging studies demonstrate a thickened wall, and gallstones are found in almost all patients. Increased risk for adenocarcinoma of the gallbladder has been reported in patients with xanthogranulomatous cholecystitis[107]; however, recent studies have not confirmed this association.[106]

CHOLECYSTITIS IN PATIENTS WITH AIDS

Acalculous cholecystitis has been cited in several reports as a complication of human immunodeficiency virus (HIV) infection (Fig. 28-15).[109-112] *Cryptosporidium* species are the most commonly identifiable cause of acquired immunodeficiency syndrome (AIDS)-related infection of the extrahepatic bile ducts and gallbladder. These organisms have been found in the bile ducts or stools of 20% to 62% of patients with symptoms of AIDS-related cholangitis. *Crypto-*

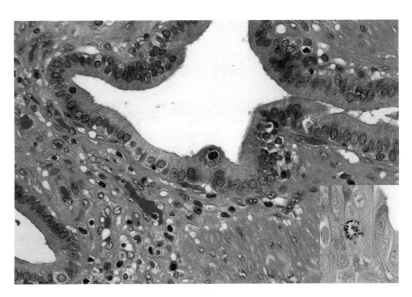

FIGURE 28–15. Cholecystitis in a patient with AIDS. Cytomegalovirus inclusion and microsporidiosis (*insert*, Brown-Brenn stain) were identified in this gallbladder from an HIV-infected patient. This case illustrates the importance of performing special stains to look for multiple causative agents, even when one of them is obvious on initial histologic inspection.

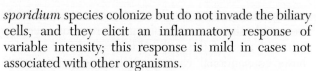

sporidium species colonize but do not invade the biliary cells, and they elicit an inflammatory response of variable intensity; this response is mild in cases not associated with other organisms.

Cytomegalovirus (CMV) is the second most common infection among patients with AIDS-related cholecystitis. It has been estimated that 10% of AIDS patients with CMV develop biliary involvement.[113] This infection is associated with mucosal ulcers and a mixed inflammatory infiltrate. Intranuclear and intracytoplasmic inclusions are found in endothelial and epithelial cells (see Fig. 28-15). Occasionally, CMV and *Cryptosporidium* species infections coexist in the same gallbladder. Rare instances of infection by *Mycobacterium avium* have been reported. The diffuse histiocytic proliferation induced by this organism may mimic xanthogranulomatous cholecystitis and malakoplakia. Other organisms that have been identified in the gallbladder include *Microsporidia*, particularly *Enterocytozoon bieneusi,* and *Isospora* (see Fig. 28-15).[112-114]

DIFFERENTIAL DIAGNOSIS OF CHOLECYSTITIS

The presenting symptomatology of acute cholecystitis overlaps somewhat with the extremely broad differential diagnosis of acute abdominal pain; this provides sufficient challenge to the clinical physician. For the pathologist, critical tasks involve determining (1) whether the gallbladder is inflamed, and (2) whether stones are present; these findings will influence subsequent patient management. It is unusual for a resected gallbladder to be free of stones or inflammation when acute calculous cholecystitis has been diagnosed clinically. This is not true for acute acalculous cholecystitis; for the clinician, it may be extremely difficult to determine that the cause of fever and abdominal pain in a critically ill patient is, in fact, an inflamed gallbladder. For the pathologist, the diagnosis of acute acalculous cholecystitis is readily made.

As a clinical syndrome, chronic cholecystitis is subtle, and so there is greater potential for pathologic analysis to identify an unsuspected process. Most importantly, the presence of a fixed mass in the gallbladder must be excluded because acute or chronic cholecystitis may herald or coexist with a gallbladder malignancy. Fortunate is the patient in whom the neck of the gallbladder is obstructed by a gallstone before a gallbladder malignancy extends beyond the wall of the gallbladder.

Helminth Infestation

Infestation of the gallbladder with *Fasciola hepatica* and *Clonorchis sinensis* induces an inflammatory response rich in lymphocytes and eosinophils and usually accompanied by hyperplasia of metaplastic pyloric-type glands. Granulomatous cholecystitis has been described in association with the ova of *Schistosoma mansoni, Paragonimus westermani,* and *Ascaris lumbricoides.*[115]

Polyarteritis Nodosa and Other Forms of Vasculitis

Histologic changes of classic polyarteritis nodosa are seen in the gallbladder in two clinical settings:[116-118] patients with isolated gallbladder involvement and patients with systemic disease, including scleroderma and systemic lupus erythematosus. The localized form of polyarteritis nodosa may rarely progress to systemic disease, especially in patients with serum autoantibodies (rheumatoid factor, antinuclear antibodies).[118] Other forms of vasculitis include granulomatous vasculitis as described in the gallbladder of patients with Churg-Strauss syndrome or giant cell arteritis. We have seen a case of idiopathic lymphocytic phlebitis confined to the gallbladder. Lesions had the same histologic features as those reported in cases of idiopathic enterocolic lymphocytic phlebitis.[119,120] Lymphocytic vasculitis may also be seen in patients with Behçet's disease (Fig. 28-16).

Cholesterolosis

Cholesterolosis is characterized by aggregates of lipid-containing macrophages in the lamina propria of the gallbladder. Autopsy and surgical studies have demonstrated a prevalence of 12% and 9% to 26%, respectively.[121,122] The cause and pathogenesis of cholesterolosis are poorly understood. Accumulation of cholesterol esters and triglycerides may reflect increased hepatic synthesis of these lipids and/or increased absorption and esterification by the gallbladder. The normal gallbladder can absorb free and nonesterified cholesterol from the bile. Cholesterol is esterified in the endoplasmic reticulum and forms lipid droplets that are released into the intercellular space, where they are phagocytized by macrophages.[123] Patients with cholesterolosis, similar to those with cholesterol stones, have supersaturated bile; as would be expected, these conditions frequently coexist. It is therefore probable that cholesterolosis results from increased cholesterol uptake from supersaturated bile. Another theory postulates that cholesterolosis is caused by defective macrophages, which become incapable of metabolizing and excreting cholesterol absorbed from the bile.[122]

PATHOLOGIC FEATURES

On gross examination, the lipid deposits appear as yellow flecks against a dark green background, thus

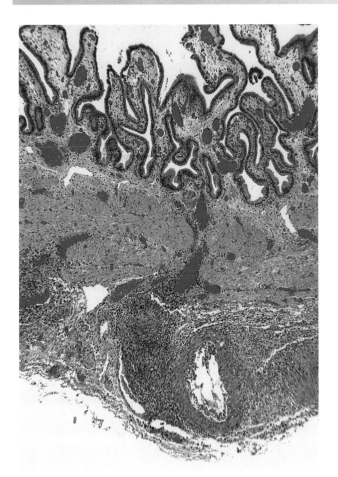

FIGURE 28–16. Lymphocytic phlebitis. Venular lesions identical to the ones present in the gallbladder were also found in sections of the small bowel in this patient with Behçet's disease.

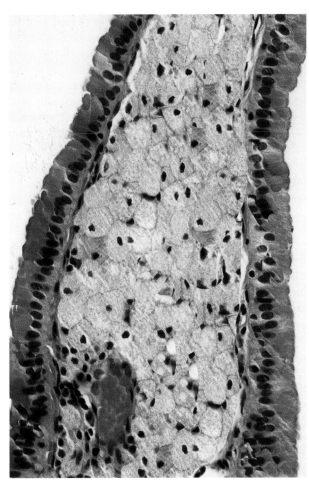

FIGURE 28–17. Cholesterolosis. Numerous foamy macrophages are present within the lamina propria.

earning the sobriquet "strawberry gallbladder." When extensive, these deposits may form polypoid excrescences that project into the lumen. Commonly referred to as *cholesterol polyps* but more properly called *cholesterolosis polyps*, these lesions are generally small but may be large enough to be detected by imaging techniques. Cholesterol gallstones are associated with cholesterolosis in half of surgical cases and in 10% of autopsy series.

Microscopically, the diagnostic feature of cholesterolosis is the accumulation of foamy macrophages within an expanded lamina propria, resulting in thickened folds and/or polyps (Fig. 28-17). The adjacent mucosa may be normal or inflamed; however, inflammation occurs almost exclusively in those patients with coexistent stones.

CLINICAL CORRELATION

Almost a century after the first description of this entity was given, the clinical relevance of cholesterolosis is still debated. Some studies have suggested that cholesterolosis is associated with symptoms in patients having acalculous biliary disease, with colicky abdominal pain and selective food intolerance as the most common complaints. Cholesterolosis is seen in some patients with biliary dyskinesia, in which case the resolution of symptoms following surgery is more likely due to eradication of the dyskinesia than to removal of the cholesterolosis. Recent evidence suggests a possible relationship between cholesterolosis and acute pancreatitis. Temporary impaction of cholesterolosis polyps at the sphincter of Oddi may produce recurrent attacks of acute pancreatitis.[124]

If the prevalence of cholesterolosis as derived from autopsy studies reflects the actual frequency in the general population, it is clear that most individuals with cholesterolosis do not develop severe symptoms. This condition appears to be more prevalent among individuals with morbid obesity.[125]

Hydrops and Mucocele

Gallbladders distended by clear watery fluid (hydrops) or mucus (mucocele) account for 3% of cholecystectomy specimens in adults.[15] In this age group, the most common cause is an impacted stone in the neck of the gallbladder or cystic duct. Less frequent causes include cystic fibrosis, tumors, fibrosis or kinking of the cystic duct, and external compression by inflammatory or neoplastic masses. In children, these conditions are usually acute processes associated with infectious diseases, such as streptococcal infections, mesenteric adenitis, typhoid fever, leptospirosis, and viral hepatitis, or with inflammatory disorders of unknown etiology, such as familial Mediterranean fever and Kawasaki disease. Symptoms may resolve with conservative treatment.[15,126]

PATHOLOGIC FEATURES

The gallbladder is considerably distended and may contain more than 1500 mL of fluid or inspissated mucin. When numerous stones are involved, the wall is usually thickened. By contrast, a thin wall is the rule when a single stone obstructs the cystic duct or in acute childhood cases. Microscopic examination usually reveals a flattened mucosa lined by low columnar or cuboidal cells. As a result of increased intraluminal pressure, Rokitansky-Aschoff sinuses may be plentiful. In some cases, the mucin may reach the peritoneal cavity and simulate mucinous adenocarcinoma. The quantity of inflammatory cells varies from sparse to abundant. Acute cholecystitis with edema of the lamina propria and abundant neutrophils occurs in some patients with Kawasaki disease.[126]

Diverticular Disease

Congenital and traction diverticula are the two types of "true" diverticula that occur in the gallbladder. The congenital lesions have already been discussed. The constituents of their wall differentiate them from the more common acquired pseudodiverticula: True diverticula have all the elements of the normal wall, and pseudodiverticula have little or no smooth muscle. Traction diverticula are caused by the pulling action of post-inflammatory fibrous adhesions anchoring the serosa of the gallbladder to adjacent structures. Erosion by stones, healing fistulas, widespread peritonitis of any cause, or previous intra-abdominal surgery precedes their formation. Traction diverticula are distinguished from congenital outpouchings principally by their relationship with intra-abdominal lesions in the vicinity of the gallbladder and by the predominance of serosal (rather than mucosal) inflammation and fibrosis. In some cases, however, distinction between the two types of true diverticula may be impossible.

Acquired pseudodiverticula are mucosal herniations among the smooth muscle bundles of the wall and should be regarded as prominent Rokitansky-Aschoff sinuses. Almost invariably, these pulsion diverticula are associated with stones and chronic cholecystitis or with outflow obstruction. In analogy to diverticular disease of the colon, the intervening smooth muscle is usually hypertrophied. Mucosal outpouchings and the prominent muscle may form a localized tumor-like lesion that has been referred to as *adenomyoma* (localized adenomyomatous hyperplasia), or they may diffusely thicken the gallbladder wall (diffuse adenomyomatous hyperplasia).[127,128] The epithelium lining the mucosal herniations is usually normal but may rarely show gastric foveolar metaplasia or dysplastic or neoplastic changes. Perineural invasion has rarely been observed in adenomyomatous hyperplasia and should not be confused with adenocarcinoma.[92]

Ischemic Disease

Deprivation of arterial blood flow or obstruction to venous drainage may result in infarction of the gallbladder. Atherosclerosis and its common complication, thrombosis, are the usual causes of obliteration of arterial blood flow. Embolic occlusion may occur as a complication of valvular heart disease or bacterial endocarditis. Another cause of ischemia may be a dissecting aneurysm extending into the celiac artery with occlusion of the origin of the hepatic artery. External compression of the arteries and/or interference with venous drainage may result from impingement on these vessels by stones or tumors or by surgical iatrogenic ligation.[129]

Gallbladders with a great degree of mobility ("floating gallbladders") may twist on their pedicle, a condition known as *torsion* or *volvulus*. As has been mentioned (see under Congenital and Developmental Abnormalities), the floating gallbladder lacks a firm attachment to the liver and is completely surrounded by peritoneum. Torsion in developmentally normal gallbladders may also result from loosening of the suspensory connective tissue, as is seen with aging or shrinkage of the liver (cirrhosis), leading to detachment of the gallbladder from its bed and visceroptosis.[15] As has been mentioned, ischemic lesions may also result from vasculitis.

PATHOLOGIC FEATURES

The gallbladder wall is thickened, and the mucosa is congested or hemorrhagic. Microscopic examination reveals partial or complete loss of the epithelium, edema, and/or hemorrhage in the lamina propria (Fig. 28-18). When occlusion to venous outflow predominates, extensive, often transmural, hemorrhagic infarction occurs. Ischemic lesions associated with primary vasculitis are often focal and confined to the mucosa. In patients with calculous cholecystitis, superimposed ischemic damage caused by secondary vasculitis or small vessel thrombosis is frequently found. Healed ischemic lesions are at least

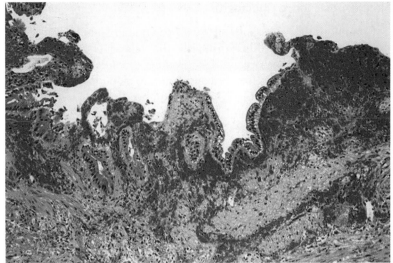

FIGURE 28–18. Ischemic cholangiopathy. Hemorrhage within the lamina propria, epithelial cell necrosis, and paucity of inflammatory cells characterize this condition.

partially responsible for the deposition of fibrous tissue in the so-called sclerosing cholecystitis.

CLINICAL CORRELATION

Most cases occur in patients older than 60 years of age. The preoperative clinical diagnosis is rarely made because symptoms mimic those of acute cholecystitis.

Traumatic Conditions and "Chemical" Cholecystitis

The gallbladder is seldom damaged from abdominal trauma because it is partially protected by the ribs and liver. On occasion, however, blunt abdominal trauma can disrupt a distended gallbladder, causing contusion, laceration, torsion, avulsion, and intraluminal hemorrhage.[130] Penetrating wounds may damage the gallbladder, usually in association with injury to the adjacent organs.

Iatrogenic injury can result from liver biopsy or percutaneous transhepatic cholangiography. Acute cholecystitis with mucosal necrosis followed by fibrosis may occur as a result of repeated infusion of chemotherapeutic agents through a catheter placed in the hepatic artery.[131]

Biliary Fistulas

In most cases, fistulas between the biliary tract and adjacent organs are a consequence of gallstone-associated necrosis and inflammation of the gallbladder and/or bile ducts. Inflammatory adhesions precede their formation; these lesions may form masses that could be confused with a fixed inoperable tumor. A classic cholecystectomy in the presence of fistulas carries a high risk

of injury to the bile ducts. The most common fistulas are cholecystoduodenal, followed by cholecystocolonic and choledochoduodenal.[15] Biliobiliary fistulas may form between the gallbladder and the common bile duct. This complication should be suspected in patients with cholelithiasis and jaundice.[132]

Metachromatic Leukodystrophy

Metachromatic leukodystrophy (MLD) is an inborn error of metabolism associated with deficiency in aryl sulfatase. The disease is characterized by diffuse breakdown of myelin in both the central nervous system and the peripheral nervous system. Microscopic changes in the gallbladder consist of papillary hyperplasia (papillomatosis) and expansion of the lamina propria by macrophages containing the abnormal metachromatic material (sulfatides). This metachromatic material is also found within the epithelial cells and may be responsible for the hyperplastic epithelial changes.[133]

Inflammatory Disorders of the Extrahepatic Bile Ducts

CHOLANGITIS

With the exception of primary sclerosing cholangitis, the pathologic features of most inflammatory conditions of the bile ducts have been poorly studied. Clinically, these conditions mimic obstructive tumors at presentation in that silent cholestasis is common. A useful clinical and pathologic classification of cholangitis groups them into three categories—simple obstructive cholangitis, recurrent pyogenic cholangitis, and primary sclerosing cholangitis.

Simple Obstructive Cholangitis

Conditions that may cause biliary obstruction include those disorders that affect primarily the bile ducts, and diseases of other organs that produce secondary obstruction. Among the former conditions are choledocholithiasis, bile duct cysts, diverticula, tumors, fistulas, and complications from previous surgical procedures (e.g., nonabsorbable sutures, metal clips, plugged T tubes and stents). Extrinsic obstruction of the bile ducts may be a complication of pancreatic tumors, chronic pancreatitis, ampullary lesions, and gallstones within the cystic duct with secondary compression of common bile duct (Mirizzi's syndrome).[134]

In Western countries, migration of cholesterol gallstones from the gallbladder into the bile ducts is the most frequent cause of obstruction.[134,135] As has been mentioned, most cholesterol gallstones do not harbor bacteria and are not associated with infected bile. When bacteria are present, the organisms most commonly found are enteric bacteria such as *E. coli, Streptococcus faecalis,* and *Clostridium, Klebsiella, Enterobacter, Pseudomonas,* and *Proteus* species.[136] The route by which bacteria colonize the biliary system remains unknown. Contamination from an infected gallbladder, duodenal reflux, and lymphatic, hepatic, arterial, or portal venous routes has been proposed. Approximately 15% of patients with cholelithiasis have stones within the bile ducts, of which 15% to 20% are asymptomatic. Because patients with ductal stones may develop severe symptomatic disease, including acute cholangitis, chronic obstruction with hepatic fibrosis, and gallstone pancreatitis, stone removal by endoscopic stone extraction is recommended either at the time of cholecystectomy or after surgery.

Gallstones that form within the bile duct (primary bile duct stones) are usually of the brown pigmented type.[134] At variance with the sterile nature of most cholesterol gallstones, brown stones are frequently associated with infection of and stasis within the biliary tract. Conditions that predispose to primary stone formation include obstructive diseases such as fibrosis secondary to previous biliary surgery, iatrogenic stricture, biliary-enteric anastomosis, sclerosing cholangitis, stenosing papillitis, periampullary duodenal diverticula, parasitic infections, Caroli's disease, indwelling biliary endoprostheses, and use of nonabsorbable suture material or metal clips.[134,137] The bacteria that are most commonly found are β-glucuronidase–producing Gram-negative organisms such as *E. coli* and *B. fragilis.*

PATHOLOGIC FEATURES

In acute cholangitis, the extrahepatic bile ducts show edema and a predominantly neutrophilic infiltrate in the lamina propria that focally infiltrates the epithelium. Also present are ulcers and erosions containing fragments of gallstones. The biliary epithelium shows degenerative and regenerative changes. Extravasation of bile into the lamina propria elicits an intense histiocyte-rich inflammatory reaction that may be followed by fibrosis. As the disorder evolves, lymphocytes and plasma cells become more abundant. However, it must be emphasized that a diffuse, plasma cell–rich infiltrate located predominantly in the mucosa is the histologic hallmark of primary sclerosing cholangitis, a disorder that should be considered in the differential diagnosis, even in the presence of choledocholithiasis.

CLINICAL FEATURES

Classic clinical symptoms associated with acute obstructive cholangitis are known as *Charcot's triad* and consist of intermittent abdominal pain, fever, and jaundice. Its complete form is present in 20% to 70% of cases. Most patients have leukocytosis and abnormal liver function tests, mainly hyperbilirubinemia with elevated alkaline phosphatase and mild to moderate elevation of aminotransferases. Serum amylase is increased in 40% of patients, which does not necessarily indicate concomitant pancreatitis. Blood cultures positive for multiple enteric organisms should be suggestive of biliary sepsis.

A few unfortunate patients develop a severe form of illness with a high mortality known as *acute suppurative* or *toxic cholangitis.* Symptoms typically associated with this condition constitute Reynolds' pentad of abdominal pain, fever, jaundice, shock, and delirium. The risk for progression to toxic cholangitis is apparently increased in patients who do not respond to initial antibiotic management and in those with congenital or malignant obstructions. Acute renal failure and intrahepatic abscess are the two most common complications of acute cholangitis. Renal failure is believed to be attributable to hypoperfusion from sepsis, endotoxemia, and tubular injury from bile pigments.[138-140]

Recurrent Pyogenic Cholangitis

Recurrent attacks of ascending cholangitis due to focal bile duct stricturing and dilatation, intrahepatic and extrahepatic stone formation (in the absence of cholelithiasis), and enteric bacterial infection characterize the syndrome of recurrent pyogenic cholangitis, also known as oriental cholangiohepatitis, intrahepatic pigmented stone disease, and biliary obstruction syndrome of the Chinese. First described among the Chinese population in Hong Kong, it is now recognized as a serious health problem in China, Taiwan, Japan, Korea, Singapore, Vietnam, Malaysia, and the Philippines.[141] This disorder is the main cause of acute abdominal pain in Hong Kong emergency rooms.[142] Sporadic cases have been reported in Europe, South Africa, and Australia. In the United States and Canada, the disease is largely but not exclusively limited to Asian immigrants.[141,143]

The cause of this disease is unknown. The two most popular theories attribute the cause to infection and malnutrition. The former postulates that inflammatory and fibrosing changes are secondary to chronic infestation of the biliary tree with endemic parasites such as *C. sinensis* and *A. lumbricoides*. The interference to bile flow caused by adult flukes or eggs causes stagnation, which leads to secondary bacterial infection, pigmented stone formation, and pyogenic cholangitis.[144] The demonstration of ova or fragments of parasites within stone provides support to this theory. However, patients with recurrent cholangitis have only a slightly higher rate of infestation by *C. sinensis* than the general population in endemic areas where numerous individuals are infected by liver flukes without ever developing cholangitis. In other areas where the parasitic infection is much less common, such as Taiwan, the incidence of recurrent cholangitis and hepatolithiasis is high.

The second theory postulates that recurrent infectious gastroenteritis in malnourished people causes frequent episodes of portal bacteremia. As has been mentioned, bilirubin glucuronide is deconjugated by the β-glucuronidase produced by bacteria. Unconjugated bilirubin precipitates as calcium bilirubinate, which initiates the formation of brown stones.[1] A protein-poor diet is thought to be associated with a deficiency of the natural inhibitors of the enzyme in bile. This theory would explain the much higher incidence of this disease in patients from low socioeconomic classes. However, it does not explain why this disorder is uncommon in other geographic areas where the population also suffers from chronic malnourishment.

PATHOLOGIC FEATURES

Both intrahepatic ducts, defined as those proximal to the confluence of the right and left hepatic ducts, and extrahepatic bile ducts may be affected. The liver may be enlarged and irregularly scarred and may display capsular adhesions. After multiple attacks, it may become shrunken, especially the lateral segment of the left lobe. The intrahepatic bile ducts show alternating areas of stricture and dilatation (Fig. 28-19). An unusual feature is the abrupt tapering toward the periphery of the dilated segments; this contrasts with the diffuse dilatation seen in patients with other causes of obstruction. Within the lumen, pigmented stones and secretions are usually found. In most cases, the extrahepatic ducts are not stenotic except for the most distal segment, where repeated passage of stones through the sphincter of Oddi may cause inflammation and postinflammatory strictures of the papilla, a condition known as stenosing papillitis. The dilated segments are not strictly related to the locations of the stones.[145] Bile duct stones are present in 75% to 80% of cases.

Histologically, portal tracts show the characteristic cluster of changes of bile duct obstruction, that is, proliferation of bile ducts, inflammatory cells (mainly neutrophils), and variable edema. Periductal fibrosis is frequently present. Histologic changes in the extrahepatic ducts include a mixed inflammatory infiltrate with a predominance of neutrophils, variable fibrosis, and epithelial changes ranging from loss of cells to adenomatous hyperplasia. Cholangiocarcinoma develops in 2.4% to 4.9% of patients with recurrent pyogenic cholangitis.[146] It has been suggested that continuous inflammation caused by the concerted action of persistent infection and mechanical irritation by stones lead to adenomatous hyperplasia, dysplasia, and cholangiocarcinoma.[147]

CLINICAL FEATURES

Most cases occur in persons 20 to 40 years of age; no sex predilection has been noted. As has been mentioned,

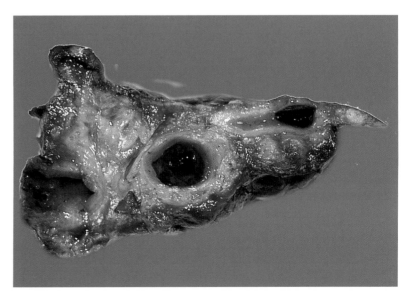

FIGURE 28–19. Recurrent pyogenic cholangitis. A cross section of the left and right hepatic ducts of a patient with recurrent pyogenic cholangitis reveals firm and thickened walls.

a strong association with lower socioeconomic class has been made. Frequently, a history of recurrent attacks is seen, characterized by abdominal pain, nausea, vomiting, fever, shaking chills, and jaundice. Findings on physical examination include epigastric tenderness and rigidity, enlargement of the liver, and a palpable gallbladder. Laboratory findings include leukocytosis and an elevated alkaline phosphatase. Most patients have bile cultures that are positive for enteric bacteria. Imaging studies demonstrate a characteristic pattern consisting of ductal dilatation with tight proximal stenosis, subsequent dilatation, and parenchymal atrophy; this produces the "arrowhead" sign on computed tomographic (CT) scan.[145]

Primary Sclerosing Cholangitis

Primary sclerosing cholangitis (PSC) is a rare disorder with an estimated prevalence of 20 to 60 cases per 1 million people.[148] Persistent chronic inflammation and fibrosis of the intrahepatic and extrahepatic bile ducts characterize this condition. This disorder occurs primarily among young men, with a gradual onset of progressive fatigue and pruritus followed by jaundice and slow progression to cirrhosis. A cholestatic biochemical profile is usually seen. Approximately 70% of patients with PSC have or will develop ulcerative colitis.[148] It is less commonly associated with Crohn's disease. Lending credence to the belief that PSC has an autoimmune pathogenesis is its association with the autoimmune haplotype HLA-A1-B8-DR3 and the presence of auto-antibodies against cross-reactive peptides shared by the colon and biliary epithelial cells.[149] Additional evidence is provided by the presence of antineutrophilic cytoplasmic antibodies (ANCAs) at a high titer in most patients with PSC and its strong association with ulcerative colitis and other autoimmune disorders (e.g.,

insulin-dependent diabetes mellitus, systemic lupus erythematosus, Sjögren's syndrome, celiac disease).[150] It has been suggested that chronic portal bacteremia may play a role in the pathogenesis of this disease. The chronic absorption of toxins and bacterial products in patients with ulcerative colitis may cause the release of inflammatory cytokines in the biliary epithelium. Observations in animal models support this hypothesis. Whether some of these findings have direct pathogenic importance remains to be determined.[151]

PATHOLOGIC FEATURES

The intrahepatic and extrahepatic bile ducts are affected in most patients. The disorder is confined to the intrahepatic biliary tree in about 20% of patients. Intrahepatic and extrahepatic bile ducts show alternating areas of stricture and normal or slightly dilated segments, producing a characteristic "beaded" appearance. These features are better demonstrated by cholangiographic studies than by gross inspection. About one fourth of cases reveal diverticulum-like outpouchings.

Microscopically, cross section of the bile ducts shows expansion of the lamina propria by a plasma cell–rich infiltrate that is diffusely distributed and present even in the segments that are grossly normal (Fig. 28-20). This diffuse mucositis closely mimics the pattern seen in the colonic mucosa in ulcerative colitis. The resemblance is further reinforced by the presence of active lesions characterized by neutrophilic infiltration of the biliary epithelium and glands with formation of microabscesses, erosions, and ulcers. The biliary epithelium shows a variety of changes ranging from atrophy to regenerative hyperplasia and postinflammatory dysplasia.[152,153]

Cholangiocarcinomas develop in 4% to 20% of patients with PSC.[15] Fibrosis is typically present in the strictured segments. Biliary stone disease is commonly present, and if clinical and pathologic features support

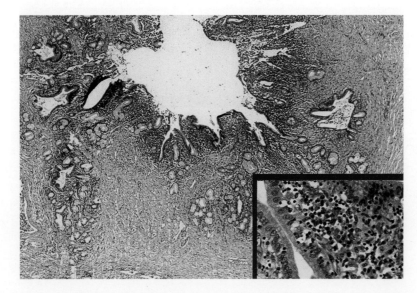

FIGURE 28–20. Primary sclerosing cholangitis. A diffuse mucositis characterizes this disorder. The lamina propria is distended by an inflammatory infiltrate composed of lymphocytes and plasma cells *(inset)*. Intraepithelial neutrophils (active lesions) are commonly present. Partial obliteration of the lumen by fibrous tissue is commonly present in late stages.

the diagnosis of PSC, its presence should not be used as an exclusionary criterion. In contrast, cholelithiasis is usually absent except in patients with cirrhosis. The inflammatory pattern described in the bile ducts is also noted in the gallbladder, a disorder that has been called *diffuse plasmalymphocytic acalculous cholecystitis.* However, as has been mentioned, this inflammatory pattern may be seen in other conditions producing bile duct obstruction.[104] Histopathologic changes that occur in the liver are described elsewhere (see Chapter 35).

CLINICAL FEATURES

As has been mentioned, most patients are men younger than 45 years of age, and half of them have a history of inflammatory bowel disease, usually ulcerative colitis. Other diseases that have been seen in association with PSC include thyroiditis, pancreatitis, insulin-dependent diabetes mellitus, celiac disease, thymoma, the sicca syndrome, retroperitoneal and mediastinal fibrosis, Peyronie's disease, pseudotumor of the orbit, sarcoidosis, histiocytosis X, angioimmunoblastic lymphadenopathy, Weber-Christian disease, rheumatoid arthritis, autoimmune hemolytic anemia, systemic lupus erythematosus, and immune deficiency syndromes.

Approximately 25% of patients are asymptomatic at presentation and are diagnosed by abnormal liver tests and retrograde cholangiopancreatography. Typically, signs and symptoms appear insidiously, the most frequent being fatigue, pruritus, and jaundice. Cholangitis may occur with the development of advanced liver disease and ductal stenosis. Liver function tests reveal a cholestatic profile. Alkaline phosphatase is always elevated three to five times over its normal value. Serum aminotransferase and bilirubin levels are mildly elevated at presentation but increase with disease progression. No consistent serologic markers are useful in the diagnosis of this disorder. Less than half of patients have positive antinuclear and smooth muscle antibodies. Antineutrophilic cytoplasmic antibodies are present in 87% of patients; however, these are not disease specific. Cholangiographic examination demonstrates multifocal strictures involving the intrahepatic and extrahepatic ducts. These strictures are typically short and annular, alternating with normal or dilated segments to produce the characteristic beaded appearance. Outpouchings resembling bile duct diverticula may be noted.

The natural history of PSC has not been clearly defined. Patients with PSC have a variable clinical course: Some remain stable for many years; others progress rapidly to liver failure. In most instances, progressive disease evolves to biliary cirrhosis within 10 to 15 years. The average survival is approximately 10 to 12 years; the most common cause of death is liver failure followed by cholangiocarcinoma. At present, no effective medical treatment is available. Liver transplantation is currently offered to patients with end-

stage disease. PSC recurs in the transplanted liver in up to 20% of patients.[148,149,154]

▇ Parasitic Infestations of the Biliary Tract

CLONORCHIS SINENSIS

It is estimated that 19,000,000 persons worldwide are infected with *C. sinensis;* a majority live in the Far East.[155] Infected persons can harbor the organism inside the biliary system for up to 30 years. Routine stool screening of Chinese immigrants to the United States has demonstrated active infection in 25%.[156] Two intermediate hosts are needed for transmission to humans—various species of snails (not found in the United States) and freshwater fish. Patients acquire this infection by eating raw freshwater fish infected with the metacercariae of this parasite. In humans, these metacercariae excyst in the duodenum, and worms migrate up the bile duct and lodge in the peripheral ducts, where they mature.

Symptoms are related to the fluke burden. Persons with fewer than 100 flukes are usually asymptomatic, whereas those with 100 to 1000 flukes have anorexia, nausea, epigastric pain, and diarrhea. A higher fluke load is accompanied by biliary colic and right upper quadrant tenderness. On cholangiographic studies, the presence of wavy, filamentous filling defects in the bile ducts is pathognomonic for clonorchiasis. Pathologic findings in patients with *C. sinensis* infection vary. Because the parasite does not invade the bile ducts, little inflammatory response is elicited. Initially, the biliary mucosa is edematous with intact or desquamated epithelium. With persistent infection, the epithelium undergoes mucinous metaplasia and becomes hyperplastic. Periductal fibrosis is the hallmark of long-standing infection. At this stage, it is common for organisms to be absent and for mucinous metaplasia to decrease. Uncomplicated lesions contain few or no inflammatory cells. When the condition is complicated by pyogenic cholangitis, a heavy neutrophilic response always occurs and is suggestive of bacterial superinfection, usually by *E. coli.* As a result of disruption of the eggs by inflammatory cells, granulomas rich in eosinophils may form. Secondary biliary cirrhosis is the long-term consequence of chronic cholangitis and fibrosis. Adenomatous hyperplasia may evolve into biliary dysplasia and adenocarcinoma.[24]

ASCARIS LUMBRICOIDES

This nematode is the cause of the most prevalent helminthic infestation in the world. Up to 60% of the population may be infected in endemic areas of South Africa, Asia, India, and South America. In the United States, *A. lumbricoides* account for less than 1% of helminthic infections. Following ingestion of *Ascaris* eggs, the larvae hatch in the jejunum, penetrate into the lymphatic vessels and portal circulation, and migrate through the liver to the lungs. These larvae are then swallowed and mature to adult worms in the gut. The worms may migrate from the intestine into the bile ducts, producing obstruction. Bacterial superinfection may cause recurrent cholangitis. The worms are easily visualized by imaging techniques such as cholangiograms and ultrasound studies.[157,158]

FASCIOLA HEPATICA

F. hepatica is another parasite that can produce biliary obstruction, cholangitis, and rarely, cholecystitis. This infection occurs more frequently in Europe, Asia, Africa, and South America and is acquired by the ingestion of water plants containing encysted metacercariae. In the duodenum, the metacercariae hatch and migrate through the wall of the intestine, penetrate Glisson's capsule, burrow through the parenchyma of the liver, and invade the bile ducts and occasionally the gallbladder. In the acute phase, an inflammatory infiltrate rich in eosinophils may be seen, followed by regenerative hyperplasia of the biliary epithelium and fibrosis.[157,159]

AIDS-Related Lesions

The therapeutic efficacy of current antiretroviral therapy has dramatically improved outcomes for HIV-infected patients. The biliary problems that affect HIV-infected individuals on therapy are identical to those seen in nonimmunosuppressed patients. The most prevalent condition in this population is cholelithiasis. When associated with biliary colic, cholecystectomy may result in pain relief if HIV cholangiopathy is absent. The term *HIV cholangiopathy* has been used to refer to several bile duct lesions unrelated to gallstones, malignant disease, or previous surgery; these lesions, which are most often seen in severely immunosuppressed patients, include papillary stenosis, a sclerosing cholangitis–like disorder, a combination of both, and long extrahepatic bile duct strictures.[160]

PATHOLOGIC FEATURES

Pathologic lesions that characterize these conditions have not been adequately studied. The extrahepatic bile ducts in most cases show nonspecific mixed inflammatory infiltrates and fibrosis. In most instances, no organisms are identified. When present, the organisms that have been reported in the extrahepatic bile ducts include CMV, *Cryptosporidium* and *Isospora* species, *M. avium*, *Pneumocystis carinii*, and *E. bieneusi*. The latter organisms may be seen on hematoxylin and eosin–stained sections within the cytoplasm of biliary cells. However, they are easily missed, even by experienced pathologists. A Giemsa stain may help in their identification; in some cases, electron microscopy is required. In the liver, the portal tracts show increased fibrous tissue and sparse lymphocytic inflammation. Interlobular bile ducts either are absent or show degenerative epithelial changes. Inflammatory cells are characteristically sparse. Lymphoma and Kaposi's sarcoma are rare causes of cholangitis.[160]

CLINICAL FEATURES

Patients with HIV-associated cholangiopathy present with right upper quadrant or epigastric pain and fever. Most have an elevated serum alkaline phosphatase, but only 15% have elevated bilirubin levels. Endoscopic retrograde cholangiopancreatography frequently demonstrates ductal irregularities and a beaded appearance. In patients with papillary stenosis, great relief of pain follows endoscopic sphincterotomy. However, because of ongoing intrahepatic duct disease, serum alkaline phosphatase levels may continue to increase.

The pathogenesis of AIDS-related cholangitis, although unknown, may be similar to that suggested for PSC. The altered immune status of HIV-infected patients may well contribute to the pathogenesis of bile duct damage, as happens in some patients with congenital immune deficiencies. Particularly attractive is the hypothesis that enteric infection in AIDS patients may lead to portal bacteremia, bile duct injury, and destruction. Some cases may be related to either CMV or infection by *Cryptosporidium* species. However, by itself, the *Cryptosporidium* organism is an unlikely candidate because it usually elicits only a mild inflammatory response. Histologic changes associated with CMV infection vary from mild to severe. It is interesting to note that in the neonate, this organism may infect bile duct epithelium and cause obliterative cholangitis and paucity of bile ducts.[161] In addition, its propensity to infect endothelial cells may induce vasculitis and ischemic damage. Infection of the biliary tract with *E. bieneusi* is associated with and may be a cause of AIDS-related cholangitis.[162-164]

Non-neoplastic Biliary Strictures

Non-neoplastic biliary strictures most frequently result from either iatrogenic injury or a blunt or penetrating abdominal trauma. More than 80% of bile duct strictures occur after cholecystectomy. The incidence of this complication is roughly 2 per 1000 operations. Inadvertent damage of the bile ducts may occur as a result of failure to recognize unexpected anatomic varia-

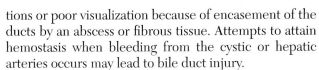

tions or poor visualization because of encasement of the ducts by an abscess or fibrous tissue. Attempts to attain hemostasis when bleeding from the cystic or hepatic arteries occurs may lead to bile duct injury.

Even in expert hands, extreme friability of acutely inflamed tissues makes dissection of Calot's triangle a formidable task. A classic cholecystectomy in the presence of a biliobiliary fistula carries a high risk of injury to the right or common hepatic duct. Ischemia contributes to the formation of postoperative fistulas. Damage to the vessels that nourish the bile ducts may result in necrosis and fibrous occlusion of the ducts. Other conditions that affect the biliopancreatoduodenal area that may give rise to postinflammatory bile duct strictures include subhepatic abscess, chronic duodenal ulcer, chronic pancreatitis, and granulomatous lymphadenitis. Knowledge of the location of the stricture is essential in planning the type of surgical repair required and predicting the outcome.[165-167]

References

1. Frierson HF Jr: The gross anatomy and histology of the gallbladder, extrahepatic bile ducts, Vaterian system, and minor papilla. Am J Surg Pathol 13:146-162, 1989.
2. Gilloteaux J: Introduction to the biliary tract, the gallbladder, and gallstones. Microsc Res Tech 38:547-551, 1997.
3. Albores-Saavedra J, Henson DE, Klimstra D: Tumors of the gallbladder, extrahepatic bile ducts and ampulla of Vater. Third Edition, Fascicle A23. Washington, DC, Armed Forces Institute of Pathology, 2000.
4. Lamonte J, Willems G: DNA synthesis, cell proliferation index in normal and abnormal gallbladder epithelium. Microsc Res Tech 38:609-615, 1997.
5. Ortiz-Hidalgo C, deLeon B, Albores-Saavedra J: Stromal tumor of the gallbladder with phenotype of interstitial cells of Cajal. A previously unrecognized neoplasm. Hum Pathol (in press).
6. MacSween RNM, Scothorne RJ: Developmental anatomy and normal structure. In MacSween RNM, Anthony PP, Scheuer PJ, et al (eds): Pathology of the Liver, 3rd ed. Edinburgh, Churchill Livingstone, 1994, pp 1-49.
7. Fisher RS, Rock E, Levin G, et al: Effects of somatostatin on gallbladder emptying. Gastroenterology 92:885-890, 1987.
8. Frizzell RA, Heintze K: Transport functions of the gallbladder. In Javitt NB (ed): Liver and Biliary Tract Physiology. International Review of Physiology, vol 21. Baltimore, University Park Press, 1980.
9. Madrid JF, Hernandez F, Ballesta J: Characterization of glycoproteins in the epithelial cells of human and other mammalian gallbladders. Microsc Res Tech 38:616-630, 1997.
10. Williams I, Slavin G, Cox A, et al: Diverticular disease (adenomyomatosis) of the gallbladder: A radiological-pathological survey. Br J Radiol 59:29-34, 1986.
11. Esper E, Kaufman DB, Crary GS, et al: Septate gallbladder with cholelithiasis: A cause of chronic abdominal pain in a 6-year-old child. J Pediatr Surg 27:1560-1562, 1992.
12. Haslam RH, Gayler BW, Ebert PA: Multiseptate gallbladder. A cause of recurrent abdominal pain in childhood. Am J Dis Child 112:600-603, 1966.
13. Bhagavan BS, Amin PB, Land AS, et al: Multiseptate gallbladder. Embryogenetic hypotheses. Arch Pathol 89:382-385, 1970.
14. Lobe TE, Hayden CK, Merkel M: Giant congenital cystic malformation of the gallbladder. Pediatr Surg 21:447-448, 1986.
15. Weedon D: Pathology of the Gallbladder. New York, Masson, 1984.
16. Shapiro T, Rennie W: Duplicate gallbladder cholecystitis after open cholecystectomy. Ann Emerg Med 33:584-587, 1999.
17. Chiavarini RL, Chang SF, Westerfield JD: The wandering gallbladder. Radiology 115:47-48, 1975.
18. Maeda N, Horie Y, Shiota G, et al: Hypoplasia of the left hepatic lobe associated with floating gallbladder. A case report. Hepatogastroenterology 45:1100-1103, 1998.
19. RHA S-Y, Stovroff MC, Glick PL, et al: Choledochal cysts: A ten year experience. Am Surg 62:30-34, 1996.
20. Todani T, Watanabe Y, Narusue M, et al: Congenital bile duct cyst classification, operative procedures, and review of 37 cases including cancer arising from a choledochal cyst. Am J Surg 134:263-269, 1977.
21. Boyle L, Gallivan MVE, Chun B, et al: Heterotopia of gastric mucosa and liver involving the gallbladder. Report of two cases with literature review. Arch Pathol Lab Med 116:138-142, 1992.
22. Qizilbash AH: Acute pancreatitis occurring in heterotopic pancreatic tissue in the gallbladder. Can J Surg 19:413-414, 1976.
23. Busuttil A: Ectopic adrenal within the gallbladder wall. J Pathol 113:231-233, 1974.
24. Everhart JE: Gallstones. In Everhart JE (ed): Digestive Diseases in the United States: Epidemiology and Impact. Washington, DC, US Government Printing Office, 1994, pp 647-690.
25. Diehl AK: Gallstone disease in Mestizo Hispanics. Gastroenterology 115:1012-1015, 1998.
26. Lammert F, Carey MC, Paigen B: Chromosomal organization of candidate genes involved in cholesterol gallstone formation: A murine gallstone map. Gastroenterology 120:221-238, 2001.
27. Hendry A, O'Leary JP: The history of cholelithiasis. Am Surg 64:801-802, 1998.
28. Cooper AD: Epidemiology, pathogenesis, natural history and medical therapy of gallstones. In Sleisenger MH, Fordtran JS (eds): Sleisenger and Fordtran Gastrointestinal Disease. Philadelphia, Saunders, 1990, pp 1788-1804.
29. Ostrow JD: The etiology of pigment gallstones. Hepatology 4:215S-222S, 1984.
30. Dowling RH: Review: Pathogenesis of gallstones. Aliment Pharmacol Ther 14:39-47, 2000.
31. Moser AJ, Abedin MZ, Roslyn JJ: The pathogenesis of gallstone formation. Adv Surg 26:357-386, 1993.
32. Bowen JC, Brenner HI, Ferrante WA, et al: Gallstone disease. Pathophysiology, epidemiology, natural history, and treatment options. Med Clin North Am 76:1143-1157, 1992.
33. Everson GT: Gallbladder function in gallstone disease. Gastroenterol Clin North Am 20:85-110, 1991.
34. Paumgartner G, Sauerbruch T: Gallstones: Pathogenesis. Lancet 338:1117-1121, 1991.
35. Gilat T, Feldman C, Halpern Z, et al: An increased familial frequency of gallstones. Gastroenterology 84:242-246, 1982.
36. Smit JJ, Schrinkel AH, Oude Elferink RP, et al: Homozygous disruption of the murine mdr2 P-glycoprotein gene leads to a complete absence of phospholipid from bile and to liver disease. Cell 75:451-462, 1993.
37. Donovan JM, Carey MC: Physical-chemical basis of gallstone formation. Gastroenterol Clin North Am 20:47-66, 1991.
38. Bennion LJ, Grundy SM: Effects of obesity and caloric intake on biliary lipid metabolism in man. J Clin Invest 56:996-1011, 1975.
39. Holan KR, Holzbach RT, Hermann RE, et al: Nucleation time: A key factor in the pathogenesis of cholesterol gallstone disease. Gastroenterology 77:611-617, 1979.
40. Harvey PR, Strasberg SM: Will the real cholesterol-nucleating and -antinucleating proteins please stand up? Gastroenterology 104:646-650, 1993.
41. Ohya T, Schwarzendrube J, Busch N, et al: Isolation of a human biliary glycoprotein inhibitor of cholesterol crystallization. Gastroenterology 104:527-538, 1993.
42. Abei M, Kawczak P, Nuutinen H, et al: Isolation and characterization of a cholesterol crystallization promoter from human bile. Gastroenterology 104:539-548, 1993.
43. Wang DQ, Cohen DE, Lammert F, et al: No pathophysiologic relationship of soluble biliary proteins to cholesterol crystallization in human bile. J Lipid Res 40:415-425, 1999.
44. Yu P, Chen Q, Harnett K, et al: Direct G-protein activation reverses impaired CCK-signaling in human gallbladders with cholesterol stones. Am J Physiol 269:G659-G665, 1995.
45. Maclure KM, Hayes KC, Colditz GA, et al: Dietary predictors of symptom-associated gallstones in middle-aged women. Am J Clin Nutr 52:916-922, 1990.

46. Everhart JE, Khare M, Hill M, et al: Prevalence and ethnic differences in gallbladder disease in the United States. Gastroenterology 117:632-639, 1999.
47. Weiss KM, Ferrell RE, Hanis CL, et al: Genetics and epidemiology of gallbladder disease in New World native peoples. Am J Hum Genet 36:1259-1278, 1984.
48. Maurer KR, Everhart JE, Ezzati TM, et al: Prevalence of gallstone disease in Hispanic populations in the United States. Gastroenterology 96:487-492, 1989.
49. Maurer KR, Everhart JE, Knowler WC, et al: Risk factors for gallstone disease in the Hispanic populations of the United States. Am J Epidemiol 131:836-844, 1990.
50. Mendez-Sanchez N, Jessurun J, Ponciano-Rodriguez G, et al: Prevalence of gallstone disease in Mexico. A necropsy study. Dig Dis Sci 38:680-683, 1993.
51. Simonovis NJ, Wells CK, Feinstein AR: In-vivo and post-mortem gallstones: Support for validity of the "epidemiologic necropsy" screening technique. Am J Epidemiol 133:922-931, 1991.
52. Miquel JF, Covarrubias C, Villaroel L, et al: Genetic epidemiology of cholesterol cholelithiasis among Chilean Hispanics, Amerindians, and Maoris. Gastroenterology 115:937-946, 1998.
53. Trotman BW: Pigment gallstone disease. Gastroenterol Clin North Am 20:111-126, 1991.
54. Fevery J: Pigment gallstones in Crohn's disease. Gastroenterology 116:1492-1494, 1999.
55. Sen M, Williamson RCN: Acute cholecystitis: Surgical management. Baillieres Clin Gastroenterol 5:817-840, 1991.
56. Fitzgibbons RJ Jr, Tseng A, Wang H, et al: Acute cholecystitis. Does the clinical diagnosis correlate with the pathological diagnosis? Surg Endosc 10:1180-1184, 1996.
57. Salomonowitz E, Frick MP, Simmons RL, et al: Obliteration of the gallbladder without formal cholecystectomy. A feasibility study. Arch Surg 119:725-729, 1984.
58. Sjodahl R, Wetterfors J: Lysolecithin and lecithin in the gallbladder wall and bile; their possible roles in the pathogenesis of acute cholecystitis. Scand J Gastroenterol 9:519-555, 1974.
59. Pellegrini CA, Way LW: Acute cholecystitis. In Way LW, Pellegrini CA (eds): Surgery of the Gallbladder and Bile Ducts. Philadelphia, Saunders, 1987.
60. Neiderhiser DH: Acute acalculous cholecystitis induced by lysophosphatidylcholine. Am J Pathol 124:559-563, 1986.
61. Claesson BE, Holmlund DE, Matzsch TW: Microflora of the gallbladder related to duration of acute cholecystitis. Surg Gynecol Obstet 162:531-535, 1986.
62. Adam A, Roddie ME: Acute cholecystitis: Radiological management. Baillieres Clin Gastroenterol 5:787-816, 1991.
63. Hawasli A: Timing of laparoscopic cholecystectomy in acute cholecystitis. J Laparoendosc Surg 4:9-16, 1994.
64. Rattner DW, Ferguson C, Warshaw AL: Factors associated with successful laparoscopic cholecystectomy for acute cholecystitis. Ann Surg 217:233-236, 1993.
65. Babb RR: Acute acalculous cholecystitis: A review. J Clin Gastroenterol 15:238-241, 1992.
66. Frazee RC, Nagorney DM, Mucha P Jr: Acute acalculous cholecystitis. Mayo Clin Proc 64:163-167, 1989.
67. Sjodahl R, Tagesson C, Wetterfors J: On the pathogenesis of acute cholecystitis. Surg Gynecol Obstet 146:199-202, 1978.
68. Parithivel VS, Gerst PH, Banerjee S, et al: Acute acalculous cholecystitis in young patients without predisposing factors. Am Surg 65:366-368, 1999.
69. Kaminski DL, Andrus CH, German D, et al: The role of prostanoids in the production of acute acalculous cholecystitis by platelet-activating factor. Ann Surg 212:455-461, 1990.
70. Gill KS, Chapman AH, Weston MJ: The changing face of emphysematous cholecystitis. Br J Radiol 70:986-991, 1997.
71. Garcia-Sancho RL, Rodriguez-Montes JA, Fernandez-de-Lis S, et al: Acute emphysematous cholecystitis. Report of twenty cases. Hepatogastroenterology 46:2144-2148, 1999.
72. Mentzer RM Jr, Golden GT, Chandler JG, et al: A comparative appraisal of emphysematous cholecystitis. Am J Surg 129:10-15, 1975.
73. Lee BY, Morilla CV: Acute emphysematous cholecystitis: A case report and review of the literature. N Y State J Med 92:406-407, 1992.
74. El-Omar EM, Carrington M, Chow WH, et al: Interleukin-1 polymorphisms associated with increased risk of gastric cancer. Nature 404:398-402, 2000.
75. Bergan T, Dobloug I, Liavag I: Bacterial isolates in cholecystitis and cholelithiasis. Scand J Gastroenterol 14:625-631, 1979.
76. Fox JG, Dewhirst FE, Shen Z, et al: Hepatic Helicobacter species identified in bile and gallbladder tissue from Chileans with chronic cholecystitis. Gastroenterology 114:755-763, 1998.
77. Mendez-Sanchez N, Pichardo R, Gonzalez J, et al: Lack of association between Helicobacter sp colonization and gallstone disease. J Clin Gastroenterol 32:138-141, 2001.
78. Coad JE, Carlon J, Jessurun J: Microdiverticulosis (Rokitansky-Aschoff "sinusosis") in patients with biliary dyskinesia (BD). Modern Pathol 12:73A, 1999.
79. Albores-Saavedra J, Gould E, Manivel-Rodriguez C, et al: Chronic cholecystitis with lymphoid hyperplasia. Rev Invest Clin (Mex) 41:159-164, 1989.
80. Hanada M, Tujimura T, Kimura M: Cholecystic granulomas in gallstone disease. A clinicopathologic study of 17 cases. Acta Pathol Jpn 31:221-231, 1981.
81. Amazon K, Rywlin AM: Ceroid granulomas of the gallbladder. Am J Clin Pathol 73:123-127, 1980.
82. Ashur H, Siegal B, Oland Y, et al: Calcified gallbladder (porcelain gallbladder). Arch Surg 113:594-596, 1978.
83. Weiner PL, Lawson TL: The radiology corner. Porcelain gallbladder. Am J Gastroenterol 64:224-227, 1975.
84. Berk RN, Armbuster TG, Saltzstein SL: Carcinoma in the porcelain gallbladder. Radiology 106:29-31, 1973.
85. Polk HC Jr: Carcinoma and the calcified gall bladder. Gastroenterology 50:582-585, 1966.
86. Roberts KM, Parson MA: Xanthogranulomatous cholecystitis: Clinicopathological study of 13 cases. J Clin Pathol 40:412-417, 1987.
87. Howard TJ, Bennion RS, Thompson JE Jr: Xanthogranulomatous cholecystitis: A chronic inflammatory pseudotumor of the gallbladder. Am Surg 57:821-824, 1991.
88. Goodman ZD, Ishak KG: Xanthogranulomatous cholecystitis. Am J Surg Pathol 5:653-659, 1981.
89. Dao AH, Wong SW, Adkins RB Jr: Xanthogranulomatous cholecystitis. A clinical and pathologic study of twelve cases. Am Surg 55:32-35, 1989.
90. Kozuka S, Hachisuka K: Incidence by age and sex of intestinal metaplasia in the gallbladder. Hum Pathol 15:779-784, 1984.
91. Albores-Saavedra J, Nadji M, Henson DE, et al: Intestinal metaplasia of the gallbladder: A morphologic and immunocytochemical study. Hum Pathol 17:614-620, 1986.
92. Albores-Saavedra J, Henson DE: Adenomyomatous hyperplasia of the gallbladder with perineural invasion. Arch Pathol Lab Med 199:117-176, 1995.
93. Albores-Saavedra J, Henson DE: Pyloric gland metaplasia with perineural invasion of the gallbladder. A lesion that can be confused with adenocarcinoma. Cancer 86:2625-2631, 1999.
94. Diehl AK: Symptoms of gallstone disease. Baillieres Clin Gastroenterol 6:635-657, 1992.
95. Soper NJ, Flye MW, Brunt LM, et al: Diagnosis and management of biliary complications of laparoscopic cholecystectomy. Am J Surg 165:663-669, 1993.
96. Deziel DJ, Millikan KW, Economou SG, et al: Complications of laparoscopic cholecystectomy: A national survey of 4,292 hospitals and an analysis of 77,604 cases. Am J Surg 165:9-14, 1993.
97. Fitzgibbons RJ Jr, Annibali R, Litke BS: Gallbladder and gallstone removal, open versus closed laparoscopy, and pneumoperitoneum. Am J Surg 165:497-504, 1993.
98. Raptopoulos V, Compton CC, Doherty P, et al: Chronic acalculous gallbladder disease: Multiimaging evaluation with clinical-pathologic correlation. AJR Am J Roentgenol 147:721-724, 1986.
99. Sykes D: The use of cholecystokinin in diagnosing biliary pain. Ann R Coll Surg Engl 64:114-116, 1982.
100. Griffen WO Jr, Bivins BA, Rogers EL, et al: Cholecystokinin cholecystography in the diagnosis of gallbladder disease. Ann Surg 191:636-640, 1980.
101. Dabbs DJ: Eosinophilic and lymphoeosinophilic cholecystitis. Am J Surg Pathol 17:497-501, 1993.
102. Rosengart TK, Rotterdam H, Ranson JH: Eosinophilic cholangitis: A self-limited cause of extrahepatic biliary obstruction. Am J Gastroenterol 85:582-585, 1990.
103. Jessurun J, Bolio-Solis A, Manivel JC: Diffuse lymphoplasmacytic acalculous cholecystitis: A distinctive form of chronic cholecystitis

associated with primary sclerosing cholangitis. Hum Pathol 28:512-517, 1998.

104. Abraham SC, Cruz-Correa M, Argani P, et al: Diffuse lympho-plasmacytic chronic cholecystitis is highly specific for extrahepatic biliary tract disease but does not distinguish between primary and secondary cholangiopathies. Mod Pathol 16:270A, 2003.

105. Hanada K, Nakata H, Nakayama T, et al: Radiologic findings in xanthogranulomatous cholecystitis. Am J Radiol 148:727-730, 1987.

106. Dixit VK, Prakash AN, Gupta A, et al: Xanthogranulomatous cholecystitis. Dig Dis Sci 43:940-942, 1998.

107. Gockel HP: Xanthogranulomatous cholecystitis. Fortschr Roentgenstr 140:223-224, 1994.

108. Charpentier P, Prade M, Bognel C, et al: Malacoplakia of the gallbladder. Hum Pathol 14:827-828, 1983.

109. Kavin H, Jonas RB, Chowdhury L, et al: Acalculous cholecystitis and cytomegalovirus infection in the acquired immunodeficiency syndrome. Ann Intern Med 104:53-54, 1986.

110. Blumberg RS, Kelsey P, Perrone T, et al: Cytomegalovirus- and *Cryptosporidium*-associated acalculous gangrenous cholecystitis. Am J Med 76:1118-1123, 1984.

111. Lebovics E, Dworkin BM, Heier SK, et al: The hepatobiliary manifestations of human immunodeficiency virus infection. Am J Gastroenterol 83:1-7, 1988.

112. Nash JA, Cohen SA: Gallbladder and biliary tract disease in AIDS. Gastroenterol Clin North Am 26:323-335, 1997.

113. Forbes A, Blanshard C, Gazzard B: Natural history of AIDS-related sclerosing cholangitis: A study of 20 cases. Gut 34:116-121, 1993.

114. Garcia GR, Meza H, Sadowinski-Pine S: Colecistitis acalculosa por *Microsporidium* en un paciente con SIDA. Patologia 31:37-39, 1993.

115. Yellin AE, Donovan AJ: Biliary lithiasis and helminthiasis. Am J Surg 142:128-134, 1981.

116. Nohr M, Lausstsen J, Falk E: Isolated necrotizing panarteritis of the gallbladder. Case report. Acta Chir Scand 155:485-587, 1989.

117. Ito M, Sano K, Inaba H, et al: Localized necrotizing arteritis. A report of two cases involving the gallbladder and pancreas. Arch Pathol Lab Med 115:780-783, 1991.

118. Burke AP, Sobin LH, Virmani R: Localized vasculitis of the gastro-intestinal tract. Am J Surg Pathol 19:338-349, 1995.

119. Sarage EP, Costa J: Idiopathic entero-colic lymphoyctic phlebitis. A cause of ischemic intestinal necrosis. Am J Surg Pathol 13:303-308, 1989.

120. Tuppy H, Haidenthaler A, Schandalik R, et al: Idiopathic enterocolic lymphocytic phlebitis: A rare cause of ischemic colitis. Mod Pathol 13:897-899, 2000.

121. Salmenkivi K: Cholesterosis of the gallbladder. Surgical consider-ations. Int Surg 45:304-309, 1966.

122. Jacyna MR, Bouchier IAD: Cholesterolosis: A physical cause of "functional" disorder. Br Med J (Clin Res Ed) 295:619-620, 1987.

123. Satoh H, Koga A: Fine structure of cholesterolosis in the human gallbladder and the mechanism of lipid accumulation. Microsc Res Tech 39:14-21, 1997.

124. Parrilla-Paricio P, Garcia-Olmo D, Pellicer-Franco E, et al: Gall-bladder cholesterolosis: An etiological factor in acute pancreatitis of uncertain origin. Br J Surg 77:735-736, 1990.

125. Aidonopoulos AP, Papavramidis ST, Zaraboukas TG, et al: Gall-bladder findings after cholecystectomy in morbidly obese patients. Obes Surg 4:8-12, 1994.

126. Suddleson EA, Reid B, Woolley MM, et al: Hydrops of the gall-bladder associated with Kawasaki syndrome. J Pediatr Surg 22:956-959, 1987.

127. Williams I, Slavin G, Cox A, et al: Diverticular disease (adeno-myomatosis) of the gallbladder: A radiological-pathological survey. Br J Radiol 59:29-34, 1986.

128. Berk RN, van der Vegt JH, Lichtenstein JE: The hyperplastic cholecystoses: Cholesterolosis and adenomyomatosis. Radiology 146:593-601, 1983.

129. Matz LR, Lawrence-Brown MM: Ischaemic cholecystitis and infarction of the gallbladder. Aust N Z J Surg 52:466-471, 1982.

130. Salman AB, Yildirgan MI, Celebi F: Posttraumatic gallbladder torsion in a child. J Pediatr Surg 31:1586, 1996.

131. Carrasco CH, Freeny PC, Chuang VP, et al: Chemical cholecystitis associated with hepatic artery infusion chemotherapy. AJR 141:703-706, 1983.

132. Rao PS, Tandon RK, Kapur BM: Biliobiliary fistula: Review of nine cases. Am J Gastroenterol 83:652-657, 1988.

133. Oak S, Rao S, Karmarkar S, et al: Papillomatosis of the gallbladder in metachromatic leukodystrophy. Pediatr Surg Int 12:424-425, 1997.

134. Liu TH, Moody FG: Pathogenesis and presentation of common bile duct stones. Semin Laparosc Surg 7:224-231, 2000.

135. Thompson JE Jr, Tompkins RK, Longmire WP Jr: Factors in management of acute cholangitis. Ann Surg 195:137-145, 1982.

136. Lee DW, Chung SC: Biliary infection. Baillieres Clin Gastroenterol 11:707-724, 1997.

137. Cuschieri A: Ductal stones: Pathology, clinical manifestations, laparoscopic extraction techniques, and complications. Semin Laparosc Surg 7:246-261, 2000.

138. O'Connor MJ, Schwartz ML, McQuarrie DG, et al: Acute bacterial cholangitis: An analysis of clinical manifestation. Arch Surg 117:437-441, 1982.

139. Boey JH, Way LW: Acute cholangitis. Ann Surg 191:264-270, 1980.

140. Lipsett PA, Pitt HA: Acute cholangitis. Surg Clin North Am 70:1297-1312, 1990.

141. Harris HW, Kumwenda ZL, Sheen-Chen SM, et al: Recurrent pyogenic cholangitis. Am J Surg 176:34-37, 1998.

142. Carmona RH, Crass RA, Lim RC Jr, et al: Oriental cholangitis. Am J Surg 148:117-124, 1984.

143. Wilson MK, Stephen MS, Mathur M, et al. Recurrent pyogenic cholangitis or "oriental cholangiohepatitis" in occidentals: Case reports of four patients. Aust N Z J Surg 66:649-652, 1996.

144. Seel DJ, Park YK: Oriental infestational cholangitis. Am J Surg 146:366-370, 1983.

145. Lim JH: Oriental cholangiohepatitis: Pathologic, clinical, and radio-logic features. AJR Am J Roentgenol 157:1-8, 1991.

146. Koga A, Ichimiya H, Yamaguchi K, et al: Hepatolithiasis associated with cholangiocarcinoma. Possible etiologic significance. Cancer 55:2826-2829, 1985.

147. Nakanuma Y, Terada T, Tanaka Y, et al: Are hepatolithiasis and cholangiocarcinoma aetiologically related? A morphological study of 12 cases of hepatolithiasis associated with cholangiocarcinoma. Virchows Arch A Pathol Anat Histopathol 406:45-58, 1985.

148. Zein CO, Lindor KD: Primary sclerosing cholangitis. Semin Gastrointest Dis 12:103-112, 2001.

149. Mitchell SA, Chapman RW: Primary sclerosing cholangitis. Clin Rev Allergy Immunol 18:185-214, 2000.

150. Seibold F, Slametschka D, Gregor M, et al: Neutrophil auto-antibodies: A genetic marker in primary sclerosing cholangitis and ulcerative colitis. Gastroenterology 107:532-536, 1994.

151. Lichtman SN, Okoruwa EE, Keku J, et al: Degradation of endogenous bacterial cell wall polymers by the muralytic enzyme mutanolysin prevents hepatobiliary injury in genetically susceptible rats with experimental intestinal bacterial overgrowth. J Clin Invest 90:1313-1322, 1992.

152. Ludwig J: Surgical pathology of the syndrome of primary sclerosing cholangitis. Am J Surg Pathol 13:43-49, 1989.

153. Harrison RF, Hubscher SG: The spectrum of bile duct lesions in end-stage primary sclerosing cholangitis. Histopathology 19:321-327, 1991.

154. Stiehl A, Benz C, Sauer P: Primary sclerosing cholangitis. Can J Gastroenterol 14:311-315, 2000.

155. Lin AC, Chapman SW, Turner HR, et al: Clonorchiasis: An update. South Med J 80:919-922, 1987.

156. Schwartz DA: Cholangiocarcinoma associated with liver fluke infection: A preventable source of morbidity in Asian immigrants. Am J Gastroenterol 81:76-79, 1986.

157. Leung JW, Yu AS: Hepatolithiasis and biliary parasites. Baillieres Clin Gastroenterol 11:681-706, 1997.

158. Choi TK, Wong J: Endoscopic retrograde cholangiopancreatography and endoscopic papillotomy in recurrent pyogenic cholangitis. Clin Gastroenterol 15:393-415, 1986.

159. Carpenter HA: Bacterial and parasitic cholangitis. Mayo Clin Proc 73:473-478, 1998.

160. Nash JA, Cohen SA: Gallbladder and biliary tract disease in AIDS. Gastroenterol Clin North Am;26:323-335, 1997.

161. Finegold MJ, Carpenter RJ: Obliterative cholangitis due to cyto-megalovirus: A possible precursor of paucity of intrahepatic bile ducts. Hum Pathol 13:662-665, 1982.

162. Cavicchi M, Pialoux G, Carnot F, et al: Value of liver biopsy for the rapid diagnosis of infection in human immunodeficiency virus-infected patients who have unexplained fever and elevated serum

levels of alkaline phosphatase or gamma-glutamyl transferase. Clin Infect Dis 20:606-610, 1995.

163. Pol S, Romana CA, Richard S, et al: Microsporidia infection in patients with the human immunodeficiency virus and unexplained cholangitis. N Engl J Med 328:95-99, 1993.

164. Pol S, Romana C, Richard S, et al: Enterocytozoon bieneusi infection in acquired immunodeficiency syndrome-related sclerosing cholangitis. Gastroenterology 102:1778-1781, 1992.

165. Standfield NJ, Salisbury JR, Howard ER: Benign non-traumatic inflammatory strictures of the extrahepatic biliary system. Br J Surg 76:849-852, 1989.

166. Lillemoe KD: Benign post-operative bile duct strictures. Baillieres Clin Gastroenterol 11:749-779, 1997.

167. Lillemoe KD, Pitt HA, Cameron JL: Postoperative bile duct strictures. Surg Clin North Am 70:1355-1380, 1990.

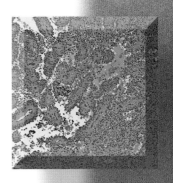

CHAPTER 29

Benign and Malignant Tumors of the Gallbladder and Extrahepatic Biliary Tract

LINDA A. MURAKATA • JORGE ALBORES-SAAVEDRA

◼ Normal Gallbladder and Extrahepatic Bile Ducts

Located beneath the right lobe of the liver, the gallbladder is a pear-shaped organ attached to the inferior surface of the liver bed by connective tissue that merges with the interlobular connective tissue of the liver. The free surface of the gallbladder is covered by serosa that continues over the liver surface. On rare occasions, the gallbladder may be completely buried within the liver parenchyma, or it may be suspended freely by a mesentery from the cystic duct and subject to torsion. Hartmann's pouch, a diverticulum located near the cystic duct, is currently believed to be the result of chronic inflammation.[1,2]

The gallbladder is divided into three zones—the neck, the fundus, and the body. The wall of the gallbladder is composed of four layers.

1. The *mucosa* consists of a single layer of columnar epithelium sitting directly on a basement membrane, and the lamina propria (there is no formal muscularis mucosae).

2. A *smooth muscle layer*, which is irregular and sometimes discontinuous and contains a small quantity of collagen, reticulin, and elastic fibers. Fusiform cells with elongated bipolar or dendritic cytoplasmic projections located very close to, or in intimate contact with, smooth muscle cells of the muscle layer have recently been recognized in the gallbladder as well. These cells, which are immunoreactive for CD117, have been interpreted as interstitial cells of Cajal and may play a role in muscle contraction or may act as mediators of neurotransmission.[2-4]

3. The *perimuscular connective tissue*, or subserosa, which contains large blood vessels, lymphatics, and nerves.

4. The *serosa*.

Luschka's ducts are often seen in specimens adjacent to the liver bed and are considered accessory or residual bile ducts and ductules. Fragments of hepatic parenchyma are sometimes seen near the ducts, and a dense collagen collar may surround the ducts. Small paraganglia may be found in the subserosal tissues close to nerves and ganglion cells. Ganglion cells, which are found scattered in all layers, are increased in the neck region. Lobules of intramural mucous glands are normally found in the neck of the gallbladder but are not considered normal in other locations.

The mucosa forms undulating branching folds that change in height and width as the lumen fills and empties with bile. An overextended lumen causes stretching of the mucosa and the muscle layer, leading to flattening of the folds and the development of gaps between muscle bundles. With continued filling of the lumen, pressure tends to push the mucosa down between the gaps in the muscle, where with contraction, the mucosa becomes trapped, forming Rokitansky-Aschoff sinuses. These sinuses may extend into the subserosa.[1,2]

The epithelium contains the following four types of cells: (1) ordinary tall columnar cells with basal nuclei and occasional small apical vacuoles; (2) occasional dark, thin "pencil" cells, which are thought to represent contracted columnar cells; (3) small "cask"-shaped cells (stem cells), which contain a dark oval nucleus and lie adjacent to the basement membrane; and (4) small, round cells with clear scant cytoplasm, which represent intraepithelial T lymphocytes.[1,2,5] Argentaffin cells are present in the mucous glands of the neck, but endocrine cells are not normally found in the fundus or body of the gallbladder.[2,6]

The lamina propria is composed of loose connective tissue containing small blood vessels, lymphatics, elastic fibers, and a few scattered lymphocytes, plasma cells, mast cells, and macrophages. Neutrophils are an abnormal finding unless they are contained within the blood vessels.[1,2]

The cystic duct and the extrahepatic bile ducts are lined by the same type of columnar epithelium that lines the gallbladder, but it usually contains less mucin. The lining may be flat or pleated, and it lies directly in contact with the stroma of the wall. At the junction of the cystic duct and the neck are thin groups of smooth muscle that form the spiral valve of Heister.

The wall of the gallbladder is composed of dense connective tissue with collagen, thin groups of smooth muscle, and some elastic fibers. Farther away from the cystic duct, the smooth muscle becomes thinner and may be absent altogether. Small groups of mucous glands are embedded in the wall of the extrahepatic bile ducts and drain into the sacculi of Beale, which are invaginations of the surface epithelium.

The subserosal tissue contains adipose tissue, nerves, occasional ganglion cells, large blood vessels, and lymphatics, but lymphocytes and plasma cells are usually sparse or absent.[1,2]

Benign Epithelial Tumors of the Gallbladder

ADENOMA

Clinical Features

Adenomas, which are usually found incidentally in cholecystectomy specimens, are generally asymptomatic, unless they are multiple, fill the gallbladder, or become detached, which can lead to obstruction of bile flow. Distention of the gallbladder with adenomas or bile produces symptoms of chronic cholecystitis. Pedunculated adenomas may undergo torsion and infarction or act as a "ball-in-valve," causing intermittent obstruction. In the extrahepatic bile ducts, patients present early with symptoms of obstruction. Although adenomas are rare among children, age in a series of 37 patients ranged from 17 to 79 years; the mean age was 58 years, and 70% of patients were female.[2,7]

Pathologic Features

This benign neoplasm arises from the surface mucosa and grows outward into the lumen to form a polyp or nodule. Adenomas may be pedunculated or sessile,[8] single or multiple; they are usually smaller than 2 cm. Malignant potential increases with the size of the lesion (>2 cm). Large adenomas resemble colonic adenomas and have a cauliflower-like appearance. They occur more commonly in the body or fundus of the gallbladder and less commonly in the bile ducts. Gallstones occur in 50% to 65% of cases.[9-12] Patients with Peutz-Jeghers or Gardner's syndrome may also manifest gallbladder adenomas.[13,14]

Histologically, adenomas, by definition, exhibit at least mild dysplasia and are divided into three types—tubular, papillary, and tubulopapillary. These are further divided according to the type of glandular epithelium into various subtypes—intestinal, pyloric, or biliary. Various types of metaplastic change may also be seen in adenomas, such as gastric foveolar metaplasia; intestinal metaplasia with goblet cells, Paneth cells, and endocrine cells; and pyloric metaplasia.[2,9,10,11] Metaplastic spindle-squamoid morulae, which are rare and frequently multifocal, are typically located between mucin-depleted pyloric-type glands. The spindle-squamoid cells are cytologically bland with eosinophilic cytoplasm. No intercellular bridges or keratinization is found.[15] Rarely, adenomas may extend into, or arise from, Rokitansky-Aschoff sinuses, a finding that should not be mistaken for carcinoma.

TUBULAR ADENOMA, PYLORIC GLAND TYPE

This is the most common type of gallbladder adenoma. It is typically pedunculated with a short stalk and is composed of tightly packed pyloric or antral-type

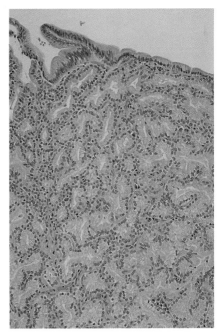

(mucous) glands that are histologically similar to mucous glands of the stomach or Brunner's glands of the duodenum (Fig. 29-1). These glands are typically composed of short round tubules, and they are lined by a single layer of cells with small, dark, or vesicular nuclei that are basal in location (Fig. 29-2). Often, one sees a continuous layer of cuboidal epithelium covering the surface of the adenoma in continuity with the normal gallbladder mucosa. The amount of stroma is variable and is usually inconspicuous. In some cases, the stroma may be loose and edematous and may contain acute and chronic inflammatory cells. Scattered aggregates of foamy macrophages may also be present near the surface of the adenoma. Cystic dilatation in which the lumina of the glands may include serous or purulent material is not uncommon. Granulation tissue and surface erosion may be associated with reactive epithelial atypia and loss of cytoplasmic mucin. Dysplasia may arise from either the surface epithelium or the pyloric-type glands. Metaplastic cells are often admixed with mucous cells, Paneth and endocrine cells, and rarely, squamoid spindle cell morulae.[2,9-11,15,16] A small proportion of pyloric gland adenomas may progress to carcinoma.

TUBULAR ADENOMA, INTESTINAL TYPE

This type closely resembles colonic adenomas (Figs. 29-3 and 29-4). It is composed of tubular-shaped glands lined by columnar cells that are pseudostratified with elongated hyperchromatic nuclei (see Fig. 29-3). Nucleoli are usually inconspicuous. Mucin production is minimal. Dysplasia is often diffusely distributed throughout the adenoma and is usually of a higher grade than in the pyloric gland type. Occasionally, the base of the adenoma may contain metaplastic pyloric-type glands. Metaplastic tissue is seen frequently and may be composed of a mixture of goblet, Paneth, and endocrine cells. A continuous layer of columnar epithelium, which usually covers the

FIGURE 29–2. Tubular adenoma, pyloric gland type. Higher magnification of closely packed tubular glands lined by columnar cells with mucin-containing cytoplasm and homogeneous round basal nuclei. The surface is covered by biliary-type mucosa with focal pseudostratified nuclei.

surface of the adenoma, is generally continuous with the normal non-neoplastic mucosa. Malignant transformation is uncommon.[2,9-11]

PAPILLARY ADENOMA, INTESTINAL TYPE

This variant consists of papillary or villous structures lined by columnar epithelium that contains cells with elongated, hyperchromatic, and pseudostratified nuclei (Fig. 29-5). The central core of the adenoma is composed of fibrovascular tissue with scattered chronic inflammatory cells, fibroblasts, and smooth muscle cells. Foamy histiocytes are rarely encountered. Dysplasia is usually of a

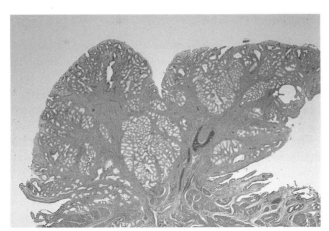

FIGURE 29–1. Tubular adenoma, pyloric gland type. The tumor shows well-defined lobules of pyloric glands.

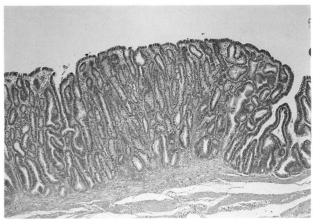

FIGURE 29–3. Tubular adenoma, intestinal type. Sessile adenoma with long tubular glands lined by intestinal-type epithelium.

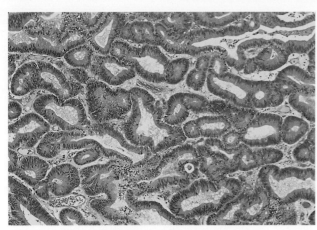

FIGURE 29–4. Tubular adenoma, intestinal type. Higher magnification of tubular glands lined by tall columnar cells with elongated hyperchromatic nuclei similar to colonic adenomas.

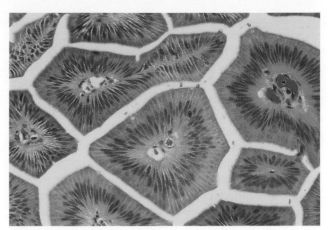

FIGURE 29–6. Papillary adenoma, biliary type. Columnar biliary-type cells showing elongated pseudostratified nuclei consistent with mild dysplasia.

higher grade than that seen in biliary-type papillary adenomas. Cellular mucin is usually minimal in quantity. Mitoses are frequent. Metaplastic tissues such as goblet, Paneth, and endocrine cells are also common among these lesions. A small proportion of gallbladder adenocarcinomas may arise from papillary adenomas of the intestinal type.[2,9-11]

PAPILLARY ADENOMA, BILIARY TYPE

This type of adenoma is very rare; it morphologically resembles papillary hyperplasia but with mild dysplasia (Fig. 29-6). The tumor is characterized by a single layer of tall columnar epithelium that lines papillary structures. Cells include elongated nuclei that are pseudostratified and contain vacuolated cytoplasm. Metaplastic epithelium is rarely found in these lesions. Malignant transformation has not been described.[2,9-11]

TUBULOPAPILLARY ADENOMA

These lesions contain a mixture of at least 20% tubular and papillary structures. This subtype may also exhibit a combination of any of the previously mentioned metaplastic or dysplastic changes.[2,9]

Special Studies

The glandular epithelium of adenomas is predominantly cytokeratin 7 (CK 7) positive. Foci of cytokeratin 20 (CK 20) immunoreactivity occur frequently in areas of intestinal metaplasia with goblet cells and in pyloric gland metaplasia. Epithelial markers, including epithelial membrane antigen, Ber-EP4, and carcinoembryonic antigen (CEA), are also usually positive. Endocrine cells are typically immunoreactive with neuroendocrine markers such as chromogranin, synaptophysin, and serotonin and occasionally with peptide hormones, including somatostatin, pancreatic polypeptide, and gastrin.

Differential Diagnosis

Pyloric gland adenomas may be mistaken for heterotopic gastric mucosa, but the latter usually contains fundic-type glands with chief and parietal cells. Foci of pyloric gland metaplasia may also form a polypoid lesion, but the lack of dysplasia provides evidence against a diagnosis of adenoma.

Intestinal-type adenomas should be differentiated from intestinal-type adenocarcinomas, which show an invasive growth pattern and a greater degree of cytologic atypia.[2,10]

PAPILLOMATOSIS (ADENOMATOSIS)

Papillomatosis is more common in the extrahepatic bile ducts than in the gallbladder and is composed of

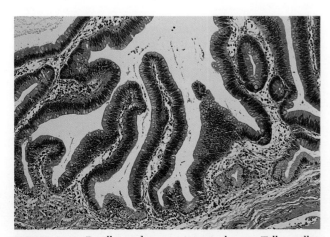

FIGURE 29–5. Papillary adenoma, intestinal type. Tall papillae are lined by columnar cells with pseudostratified hyperchromatic cells, scattered goblet cells, and Paneth cells.

multiple papillary adenomas, or it manifests as a diffuse growth that may extend into the Rokitansky-Aschoff sinuses and the intrahepatic bile ducts. Papillary structures may branch or form complex glands that are lined by tall columnar cells admixed with metaplastic tissue (Fig. 29-7). High-grade dysplasia is often present. Thus, distinguishing this lesion from papillary carcinoma may be impossible. Most patients are between 50 and 60 years of age. Both sexes are affected equally. The potential for malignant transformation is much greater with this lesion than with solitary adenomas.[2,9,17-19]

CYSTADENOMA

Clinical Features

Cystadenomas are multiloculated epithelial neoplasms that occur more frequently in extrahepatic bile ducts than in the gallbladder. Affected patients may be asymptomatic or may present with signs and symptoms of obstructive jaundice. Malignant transformation is not uncommon; thus, incomplete removal may result in local recurrence.[2,9]

Pathologic Features

Cystadenomas may reach up to 20 cm in greatest dimension. The cut surface often shows multilocular cysts containing serous or mucinous fluid. The walls of these cysts may vary in thickness from 0.3 to 3 cm in diameter and often reveal a finely granular or trabeculated surface. Occasionally, small polypoid excrescences may protrude into the lumen.[2,9]

Microscopically, the cystic loculi are usually lined by a single layer of cuboidal or columnar cells, resembling either biliary or foveolar gastric epithelium. A highly cellular mesenchymal tissue that closely resembles ovarian

stroma is always present underneath the epithelial layer (Fig. 29-8). Dense fibrous tissue forms the outer wall of the tumor. The amount of mesenchymal stroma may vary from area to area, and in some places, the epithelium may lie directly on fibrous tissue. Foci of intestinal metaplasia with Paneth and endocrine cells may be present in the epithelium as well.[2,9,20-25]

Special Studies

The epithelium is immunoreactive for pancytokeratin (AE1/AE3) CK 7, with focal CK 20 positivity in areas of intestinal metaplasia, epithelial membrane antigen (EMA), and CEA. Endocrine cells are immunohistochemically reactive for neuroendocrine markers such as chromogranin, synaptophysin, and serotonin and occasionally for peptide hormones. The mesenchymal stroma is immunoreactive for vimentin and may reveal focal reactivity for muscle-specific actin. Estrogen and progesterone receptors have been detected in the mesenchymal stroma but not in the surface epithelium. The tumor-associated antigen CA 19-9 has recently been reported to be elevated in patients with this type of lesion.[26]

◼ Premalignant Epithelial Lesions of the Gallbladder

DYSPLASIA

Dysplasia is often unrecognizable in gross specimens, unlike the adenomas just described. Foci suspicious for dysplasia may appear granular, slightly raised, thickened, or depressed. Microscopically, dysplasia in the gallbladder is characterized by uniformity of atypical cells rather than by the heterogeneity seen in

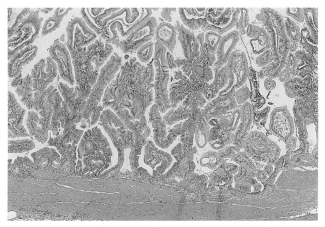

FIGURE 29–7. Papillomatosis. Tall branching papillae diffusely line the wall of the gallbladder and are lined by dysplastic columnar epithelium.

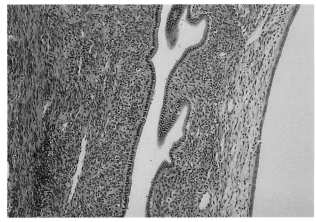

FIGURE 29–8. Cystadenoma. The cyst wall is lined by biliary-type epithelium and contains a subepithelial layer of dense mesenchymal stroma.

reactive epithelial lesions. Cells show uniform hyperchromasia, nuclear stratification, and atypia, with an increased nucleus-to-cytoplasm ratio. Dysplasia may be patchy or multifocal. In fact, multiple grades of dysplasia are often noted in the same specimen. Thus, extensive sampling is necessary when a focus of dysplasia is discovered.

One does not usually see a sharp area of transition between normal and dysplastic cells. Occasionally, the abruptness of the transition can be striking when one progresses from normal to dysplastic epithelium. Nuclear atypia and loss of polarity may be minimal in low-grade lesions and almost impossible to differentiate from severe reactive atypia. Metaplastic goblet cells, Paneth cells, and endocrine cells may also be present.[2,27-30]

Criteria for grading dysplasia are the same as those applied to the colon (Table 29-1). Mild dysplasia reveals basal elongated nuclei that involve the basal portion of the cell cytoplasm; moderate dysplasia (Fig. 29-9) includes elongated nuclei that extend into the luminal portion of the cell cytoplasm; in severe dysplasia, the nuclei reach the surfaces of cells; and in carcinoma in situ, marked alteration in nuclear size and shape is seen, with overlapping, crowding, and loss of polarity (Fig. 29-10).[2,9,27-31] The growth pattern demonstrates increasing complexity, with gland-in-gland (cribriform) formations and papillary or villous structures. Dysplasia may also be classified as low grade (which includes mild and moderate dysplasia) or high grade (which involves severe dysplasia and carcinoma in situ).

Dysplastic epithelium may extend along the mucosal surface and into Rokitansky-Aschoff sinuses and metaplastic glands, where it is sometimes mistaken for invasion.[27-31] In fact, desmoplasia may not be present in areas of invasive carcinoma. Occasionally, the stromal reaction surrounding ruptured and inflamed glands may simulate desmoplasia.

Reactive atypia may be difficult to distinguish from mild dysplasia in severely inflamed gallbladders or extrahepatic bile ducts. It is helpful to consider the background mucosa and the presence of ulceration, erosion, acute inflammation, necrosis, infarction, and suppuration; when all of these changes are seen, one should consider a reactive process.

Carcinoma in Situ

Cells show marked nuclear atypia with frequent mitoses, increased nucleus-to-cytoplasm ratio, hyper-

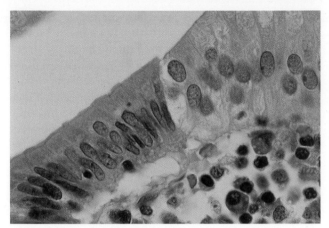

FIGURE 29–9. Moderate dysplasia. Dysplastic epithelium *(left)* shows elongated hyperchromatic nuclei and is located adjacent to normal biliary epithelium *(right)*.

chromasia, loss of polarity, overlapping, and crowding. Carcinoma in situ may arise in flat mucosa or in an adenomatous polyp. The cells may form a single layer or complex (back-to-back) and villous structures (see Fig. 29-10). Cells with giant or bizarre nuclei and prominent nucleoli may also be noted.[31-34] A rare variant of in situ carcinoma is composed of signet ring cells that are cytokeratin and CEA positive.[2]

A lesion is no longer classified as in situ when the lamina propria is invaded; instead it is intramucosal carcinoma. Budding and/or microgland formation may be seen within the lamina propria. Desmoplasia is not a reliable indication of invasion because it is usually not present when invasion occurs. A variable mixture of chronic inflammatory cells, including lymphocytes, plasma cells, and macrophages, may be seen in the lamina propria. Occasionally, lymphoid follicles with germinal centers and xanthogranulomatous and acute inflammation may occur with early invasive tumors.

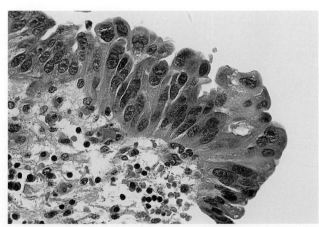

FIGURE 29–10. Carcinoma in situ. A single layer of highly dysplastic cells with overlapping, crowded, hyperchromatic nuclei and prominent nucleoli.

TABLE 29–1. Grading Dysplasia in the Gallbladder	
Low Grade	**High Grade**
Mild dysplasia	Severe dysplasia
Moderate dysplasia	Carcinoma in situ

■ Malignant Epithelial Tumors of the Gallbladder

ADENOCARCINOMA

Clinical Features

Patients with gallbladder carcinoma usually present with right upper quadrant abdominal pain or other non-specific symptoms resembling those of cholecystitis, such as weight loss, malaise, pruritus, anorexia, nausea, and vomiting. Gallstones are associated with carcinoma in more than 80% of cases; the incidence is higher among women than men (3:1).[2,10] Cancer of the gallbladder and extrahepatic bile ducts occurs in an older age group (average age, 72.2 years). The youngest person ever reported was an 11-year-old Native American girl.[1,35] The incidence of gallbladder carcinoma varies among ethnic groups and parts of the world, as it does within the same country. In the United States, Native and Hispanic Americans have a higher rate of gallbladder cancer than blacks or whites. One study reported incidence rates of 21 per 100,000 female Native Americans and 1.4 per 100,000 white females.[1,2,10] In the general population of the United States, gallbladder carcinoma accounts for 0.49% of cancers among females and 0.17% of cancers among males. The 5-year survival rate for patients with adenocarcinoma is 13%.[36] Extrahepatic bile duct carcinoma shows no variation in incidence; it represents 0.16% of all cancers in males and 0.15% of all cancers in females in the general population of the United States.[2]

An association between carcinoma of the gallbladder and an anomalous connection between the choledochus and the pancreatic duct has been reported.[2,10,37-39] Adenocarcinoma in association with "porcelain" gallbladder occurs in approximately 20% of cases.[1,2]

Pathologic Features

Most gallbladder and extrahepatic bile duct malignancies are well to moderately differentiated adenocarcinomas (Table 29-2). Sixty percent arise in the fundus, 30% in the body, and 10% in the neck of the gallbladder.[2,10,40] Grossly, carcinomas may appear as raised mucosal plaques, focal indentations, or areas of thickening, polyps, or large fungating intraluminal masses.

Microscopically, gallbladder adenocarcinomas resemble those that arise in other parts of the body. Table 29-2 shows the distribution of histologic types among 386 patients with carcinoma of the gallbladder. Most are composed of tubular glands lined by pseudostratified cuboidal to columnar cells. Nuclei are often pleomorphic and hyperchromatic with prominent nucleoli. Many mitotic figures and, occasionally, bizarre cells are typically seen. Mucin is often noted within cells and in the

TABLE 29–2. Distribution of Histologic Types in 386 Patients With Malignant Tumors of the Gallbladder

Histologic Type	Number of Patients (%)	Males	Females
Adenocarcinoma, well to moderately differentiated	186 (48.2)	31	155
Undifferentiated spindle and giant cell carcinoma	51 (13.2)	14	37
Adenosquamous carcinoma	37 (9.58)	2	35
Poorly differentiated adenocarcinoma, small cell type	25 (6.48)	3	22
Small cell carcinoma	18 (4.66)	2	16
Papillary adenocarcinoma	17 (4.40)	1	16
Mucinous carcinoma	16 (4.14)	5	11
Carcinoma in situ	14 (3.63)	1	13
Signet ring cell carcinoma	10 (2.59)	3	7
Squamous cell carcinoma	4 (1.04)	1	3
Intestinal-type adenocarcinoma	4 (1.04)	1	3
Adenocarcinoma with choriocarcinoma-like areas	1 (0.26)	0	1
Carcinosarcoma	1 (0.26)	0	1
Carcinoid tumor	1 (0.26)	1	0
Malignant fibrous histiocytoma	1 (0.26)	0	1
Total	**386**	**65**	**321**

Data from Albores-Saavedra J, Henson DE, Klimstra DS: Tumors of the Gallbladder, Extrahepatic Bile Ducts, and Ampulla of Vater. AFIP Atlas of Tumor Pathology, 3rd series, Washington, DC, AFIP, 2000, p 65.

lumina of the glands. Paneth cells, goblet cells, and, occasionally, endocrine cells are revealed in up to one third of tumors.[2,36,40]

Adenocarcinomas may be divided into well, moderately, and poorly differentiated types. Well-differentiated adenocarcinoma, which resembles biliary epithelium, comprises at least 95% well-formed glands. Moderately differentiated adenocarcinoma shows between 40% and 95% gland formation. Less than 40% glands defines poorly differentiated adenocarcinoma.[2] Poorly differentiated tumors form sheets, nests, and cords of tumor cells with varying amounts of desmoplastic stroma. Desmoplasia is frequently absent or scanty in intramucosal tumors, but it may become more prominent in tumors that infiltrate the muscle layer and the subserosal connective tissue. In mucinous variants, extracellular mucin, mucin pools within the subserosal connective tissue, and mucinous material with dilated glands are noted.[2,36,40] Tumors are best classified on the basis of the poorest degree of differentiation. Unusual and rare histologic types of adenocarcinoma may display cribriform patterns of growth, angiosarcoma-like areas, choriocarcinoma-like areas, signet ring cells, pseudosarcomatous growth patterns, abundant clear cells or small cells, and undifferentiated areas.[2,41]

Mucin positivity is demonstrated by d-PAS (PAS with diastase), mucicarmine, and Alcian blue stains. Tumor cells are typically immunoreactive for pancytokeratin and CK 7, and they often show dual immunoreactivity for CK 7 and (focally) CK 20. Other positive immunohistochemical stains include CA 19-9, CEA, and EMA. Endocrine cells are immunoreactive for chromogranin, synaptophysin, serotonin, and peptide hormones.[2,36] Metaplastic pyloric-type glands are usually immunoreactive with CK 20.

Histologic Subtypes

PAPILLARY ADENOCARCINOMA

This is a type of well-differentiated adenocarcinoma that is composed of villous or papillary structures that sometimes branch or form fronds lined by highly atypical epithelium with little or no fibrovascular core (Fig. 29-11). The tumor may be a single polypoid or sessile lesion; it may be multifocal or diffuse. The cells are cuboidal or columnar and contain variable atypia, hyperchromatic nuclei with prominent nucleoli, mitotic figures, and a high nucleus-to-cytoplasm ratio. Variable quantities of mucin production, intestinal metaplasia with goblet cells, endocrine cells, and Paneth cells may also be seen. The tumor tends to grow intraluminally and may become very large before invading deeper layers of the wall.[2,10]

ADENOCARCINOMA, INTESTINAL TYPE

This variant of well-differentiated adenocarcinoma comprises many tubular glands lined by tall columnar cells with abundant goblet cells and occasional Paneth cells, along with endocrine cells (Fig. 29-12). Endocrine cells are seen in approximately one third of tumors. Goblet cell numbers are variable, but they may fill entire glands. Columnar cells containing hyperchromatic, basally located nuclei are often pseudostratified. The cytoplasm of cells may be distended with mucin. Mitotic activity is typically low, and necrotic material may be seen as well.[2,10,42,43] Another variant that closely resembles colonic mucosa contains benign-appearing columnar epithelium and a well-defined brush border.

ADENOCARCINOMA, GASTRIC FOVEOLAR TYPE

A rare malignant neoplasm composed of glands lined by gastric foveolar-type epithelium (tall columnar cells, basal nuclei, and cytoplasm almost entirely filled with mucus) has been reported (Fig. 29-13). This tumor can occur in the gallbladder or in the extrahepatic bile ducts.

ADENOCARCINOMA, CLEAR CELL TYPE

This is a very rare variant composed of water-clear cells that contain abundant cytoplasmic glycogen and well-defined cell membranes (Fig. 29-14). This tumor grows in sheets, nodules, papillary structures, and cords. Clear cells with a glandular pattern may also predominate in some conventional adenocarcinomas or squamous cell carcinomas.[41,44,45] Transition zones from dysplastic surface epithelium to carcinoma are helpful in distinguishing a primary clear cell carcinoma of the gallbladder from metastatic renal cell carcinoma.

Rarely, hepatoid differentiation has been reported in this variant; these areas show positive immunoreactivity with HepPar-1 (hepatocyte immunostain).[46] In addition, canaliculi and bile production have been detected in hepatoid cells on electron microscopy. Canaliculi can also be seen with the polyclonal CEA immunostain; these may be focally positive for alpha-fetoprotein.[41,47,48]

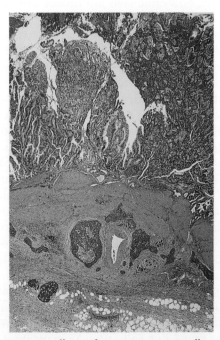

FIGURE 29–11. Papillary adenocarcinoma. Papillary adenoma *(left)* and adenocarcinoma *(right),* showing invasion through the muscle layer and into the subserosal connective tissue.

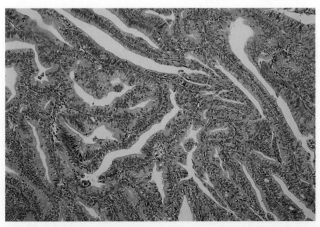

FIGURE 29–12. Adenocarcinoma, intestinal type. High magnification of intestinal-type epithelium showing a complex growth pattern and back-to-back glands.

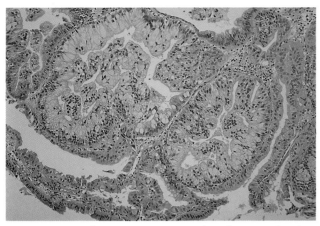

FIGURE 29–13. Adenocarcinoma, gastric foveolar type. Abundant cytoplasmic mucinous epithelium with scattered goblet cells and a crowded complex growth pattern.

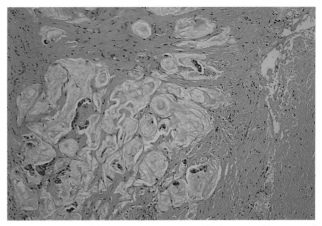

FIGURE 29–15. Mucinous carcinoma. High magnification of stromal mucin pools containing single cells and groups of malignant cells.

ADENOCARCINOMA, MUCINOUS TYPE

A pure mucinous carcinoma is defined as a tumor that contains more than 50% extracellular mucin.[2] It commonly appears as a gelatinous mass in the wall of the gallbladder. This tumor may display one of two histologic patterns—pools of mucin with free-floating tumor cells in the center or pools of mucin partially lined by malignant epithelium (Fig. 29-15). Malignant cells are mucin-producing columnar cells or cells that contain a single large, cytoplasmic vacuole that compresses the nucleus to the side of the cell (signet ring cell). Fibrous stroma often surrounds pools of mucin.[2] Occasionally, classic well- or moderately differentiated adenocarcinoma is also present. Other variant cell types, such as squamous cell carcinoma, clear cell carcinoma, and undifferentiated carcinoma, may also be noted.

Occasionally, differentiating clear cell carcinoma from metastatic renal clear cell carcinoma or hepatocellular clear cell carcinoma may be difficult histo-

logically. A battery of immunohistochemical stains, together with clinical exclusion of other possible primary sites, is often helpful.[49]

Mucinous carcinomas are usually immunoreactive for both CK 7 and CK 20. In addition, they show positivity for pancytokeratin, polyclonal CEA, and EMA. Mucin may be highlighted with d-PAS, mucicarmine, or Alcian blue stain.

Natural History and Prognosis

The prognosis for gallbladder carcinoma is best predicted on the basis of pathologic stage at the time of surgical resection, rather than according to histologic subtype. Table 29-3 shows the tumor-node-metastasis (TNM) classification used to stage carcinoma of the gallbladder. In general, adenocarcinomas that are discovered incidentally in cholecystectomy specimens have a better prognosis than those that present symptomatically, mainly because the latter are usually already advanced, in which case most patients die within a year of diagnosis. Papillary carcinomas and carcinomas that do not penetrate the muscle layer have a better prognosis and an increased chance of cure by resection alone. Patients with unsuspected carcinoma have a 5-year survival of 14.9% (in a 215-patient subgroup of 6222 cases), as opposed to 4.1% (6222 total cases reviewed in 1978) when the tumor is symptomatic.[2,10,36] Tumor usually spreads via lymphatics and blood vessels.

PURE SIGNET RING CELL CARCINOMA

In this variant, signet ring cells, which are the predominant (>90%) cell type, reveal a growth pattern (linitis plastica appearance) similar to that seen in its gastric counterpart. This variant accounts for 3% of all malignant gallbladder tumors.[2] Cells contain a large mucin vacuole that displaces the nucleus to one side of

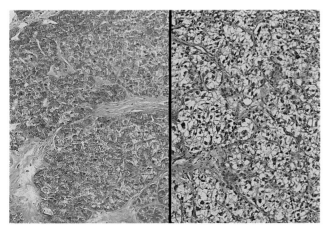

FIGURE 29–14. Clear cell carcinoma. Sheets of clear cells containing abundant glycogen are demonstrated with a periodic acid–Schiff stain *(left)* and after digestion with diastase *(right)*.

TABLE 29–3. TNM Classification of Tumors of the Gallbladder			
Clinical			
TX	Primary tumor cannot be assessed		
T0	No evidence of primary tumor		
TIS	Carcinoma in situ		
T1	Tumor invades lamina propria or muscle layer		
	T1a	Tumor invades lamina propria	
	T1b	Tumor invades muscle layer	
T2	Tumor invades perimuscular connective tissue; no extension beyond serosa or into liver		
T3	Tumor perforates serosa or directly invades into one adjacent organ or both (extension ≤2 cm into liver)		
T4	Tumor extends >2 cm into liver and/or into two or more adjacent organs		
NX	Regional lymph nodes cannot be assessed		
N0	No regional lymph node metastasis		
N1	Regional lymph node metastasis		
	N1a	Metastasis in cystic duct, pericholedochal cyst, and/or hilar lymph nodes	
	N1b	Metastasis in peripancreatic (head only), periduodenal, periportal, celiac, and/or superior mesenteric lymph nodes	

pTNM Pathological Classification of Gallbladder Cancer (Pathologic: pT, pN, and pM categories correspond to T, N, and M categories.)

Stage Grouping

Stage 0	Tis	N0	M0
Stage I	T1	N0	M0
Stage II	T2	N0	M0
Stage III	T1	N1	M0
	T2	N1	M0
	T3	Any N	M0
Stage IV	T4	Any N	M0
	Any T	Any N	M1

Summary

T1	Gallbladder wall	
	T1a	Mucosa
	T1b	Muscle
T2	Perimuscular connective tissue	
T3	Serosa and/or one organ, liver <2 cm	
T4	Two or more organs, or liver >2 cm	
N1a	Hepatoduodenal ligament	
N1b	Other regional	

Adapted from Albores-Saavedra J, Henson DE, Sobin LH, et al: WHO International Histological Classification of Tumours, Histological Typing of Tumours of the Gallbladder and Extrahepatic Bile Ducts, 2nd ed. Berlin, Springer-Verlag, 1991, pp 23-28.

the cell cytoplasm. The tumor grows in nests, cords, sheets, or incomplete glandular structures. Occasionally, chromogranin-positive endocrine cells, as well as scattered Paneth cells, are noted in the tumor (Fig. 29-16). Occasionally, conventional adenocarcinoma is seen admixed with signet ring cells; if the former makes up the majority of the tumor volume when only a small focus of signet ring cells is seen, it is best classified as a conventional adenocarcinoma.[2,41] If neoplastic signet ring cells do not invade below the surface mucosa or its intramural invaginations, it should be considered an in situ lesion. Signet ring cells are typically also immunoreactive for CK 7, CK 20, pancytokeratin, and polyclonal CEA.

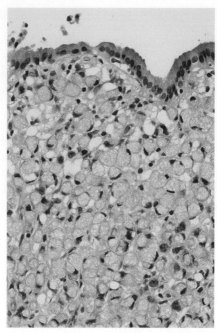

FIGURE 29–16. Signet ring cell carcinoma. Each sheet of signet ring cells contains a large cytoplasmic mucinous vacuole that displaces the nucleus to the side of the cell cytoplasm.

ADENOSQUAMOUS CARCINOMA

When two separate malignant glandular and squamous components occur in varying amounts, the term _adenosquamous carcinoma_ is used (Fig. 29-17). Both components tend to reveal a moderate degree of differentiation. In addition, squamous pearls and mucin are often present. The squamous cell component grows in nests and cords, often surrounded by a dense desmoplastic stroma. This variant represents about 7% to 9% of all carcinomas of the gallbladder. Rarely, spindle cells and osteoclast-like giant cells have been observed in the

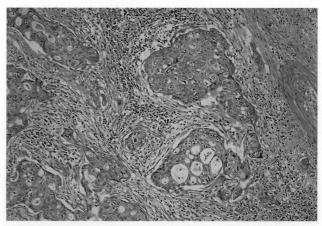

FIGURE 29–17. Adenosquamous carcinoma. Infiltrating nests of squamous epithelium _(upper right)_ and mixed squamous and glandular _(lower left)_ malignant epithelium.

stroma of these tumors.[2,50-52] Cytokeratin 903 (high-molecular-weight cytokeratin) is a marker for mature squamous epithelium. CK 7, CK 20, EMA, Ber-EP4, and CEA are usually positive in the adenocarcinoma component.

PURE SQUAMOUS CELL CARCINOMA

This is a rare tumor that accounts for only about 1% of all gallbladder carcinomas; it is usually associated with gallstones. The tumor is composed of malignant squamous cells with varying degrees of differentiation. Ultrastructurally, well-developed desmosomes and tonofilaments join individual tumor cells. Keratinization may be seen focally, along with areas of clear cells rich in glycogen. Tumor cells typically grow in nests, islands, and cords separated by dense fibrous stroma. Focal spindle cell transformation may occur as well. If a spindle cell pattern predominates, differentiation from a primary sarcoma or a malignant fibrous histiocytoma may be difficult. However, immunohistochemical stains for cytokeratin and other epithelial markers are helpful in the differential diagnosis.[2,53]

Because pure squamous cell carcinomas are rare, adequate sampling of the tumor is necessary before this diagnosis is established. However, the presence of a minor glandular component (less than 5% to 10% of the tumor volume) is permissible.[2] In addition, the surface mucosa may reveal varying degrees of dysplasia or squamous metaplasia adjacent to the tumor. Cytokeratin 903 (high-molecular-weight cytokeratin) and CEA may exhibit focal immunoreactivity.

SMALL CELL CARCINOMA (OAT CELL CARCINOMA)

Small cell carcinomas of the gallbladder are extremely rare, occurring mainly in elderly women with cholelithiasis.[2,54,55] In 29 cases reported by Albores-Saavedra and associates,[41] most patients were women in the sixth or seventh decade of life. All patients presented with symptoms of cholecystitis with gallstones. Seventy-five percent of patients initially had direct extension into the liver and regional lymph node metastases. Of 23 patients who were followed, 22 died as a direct result of their tumors. Paraneoplastic syndromes may be associated with small cell carcinoma of the gallbladder, and Cushing's syndrome has been reported as well in three patients with this type of tumor.[2,54,56]

Histologic features of small cell carcinoma of the gallbladder are similar to those of small cell carcinoma of the lung, pancreas, or intestine. They occur more commonly in the gallbladder than in the extrahepatic bile ducts. Cells are small and round or fusiform; they contain finely stippled chromatin, inconspicuous nucleoli, and sparse eosinophilic cytoplasm. A high mitotic rate, single-cell

necrosis, and nuclear "molding" are also common features. Tumor cells are usually arranged in compact sheets or in trabeculae, nests, and festoons. Occasionally, tumor cells form rosettes or tubules. Necrosis is common and can be extensive. This tumor is often associated with dysplastic epithelium or even an adenoma. Combined small cell carcinomas and adenocarcinomas, as well as small cell carcinomas with focal squamous differentiation, have also been documented.[2,41,57] Extremely rarely, neuroendocrine tumors are of the large cell type and similar to the large cell neuroendocrine carcinoma of the lung.[58]

In special studies, neurosecretory granules are demonstrated by electron microscopy. Immunoreactivity for neuroendocrine markers is usually only focal, unlike in carcinoid tumors, which show diffuse positivity. Positive immunohistochemical markers include neuron-specific enolase, chromogranin A, synaptophysin, Leu7, serotonin, somatostatin, and adrenocorticotropic hormone (ACTH). Epithelial markers such as EMA, AE1/AE3, CAM 5.2, and CEA may be positive as well.

CYSTADENOCARCINOMA

Cystadenocarcinomas are usually the result of malignant transformation of a benign cystadenoma.[2,20] This tumor is more common in the extrahepatic bile ducts than in the gallbladder.[23] Cystadenocarcinomas are composed of multiloculated cysts, lined by dysplastic columnar to cuboidal epithelium; they contain mucinous or serous fluid (Fig. 29-18). The subepithelial stroma is composed of highly cellular mesenchyme that resembles ovarian stroma, which is immunoreactive for estrogen and progesterone receptor markers. Epithelial cells are usually pseudostratified and hyperchromatic and are noted to have prominent nucleoli and occasional mitoses.

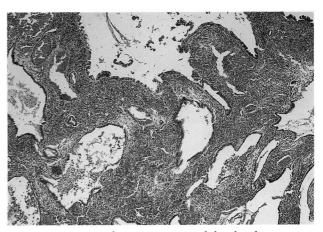

FIGURE 29–18. Cystadenocarcinoma. Multiloculated tumor containing small glandular structures in the wall. Locules are lined by dysplastic biliary epithelium with a subepithelial mesenchymal stroma.

Complex growth patterns involving cribriform and solid papules are typically an indication of malignant transformation. Multiple papillary structures may also grow into the lumen without wall invasion. Invasion should be suspected when small microglands are noted within the walls of cysts, either with or without a desmoplastic reaction (Fig. 29-19).[21,24]

UNDIFFERENTIATED CARCINOMA

This type of tumor is more common in the gallbladder than in the extrahepatic bile ducts. It accounts for only 10.4% of all gallbladder carcinomas.

Undifferentiated carcinomas are composed of malignant spindle, polygonal, and giant epithelial cells without obvious gland formation.[59,60] However, occasional foci of squamous differentiation or adenocarcinoma may be found in rare cases. Although it is occasionally mistaken for a primary sarcoma, keratin expression in spindle cells of this tumor is helpful in revealing this diagnosis. Rarely, osteoclast-like giant cells may be a prominent feature in this type of tumor.[2,41,61]

Four histologic variants of undifferentiated carcinoma of the gallbladder are seen.

Spindle and Giant Cell Type. This is the most common variant and is composed of a mixture of spindle cells, giant cells, and polygonal epithelioid cells (Fig. 29-20). It is sometimes referred to as *sarcomatoid carcinoma*. Large polygonal cells are often pleomorphic and reveal large pleomorphic nuclei, nucleoli, and bizarre shapes. Bizarre mitotic figures are frequently present. Cytoplasmic mucin droplets may be seen in the large cells. Multinucleated giant cells resembling osteoclasts may be scattered within the tumor. Furthermore, foci of conventional adenocarcinoma or squamous carcinoma may be noted. Cytokeratin and EMA are more likely to be seen in this variant than in other types of undifferentiated carcinoma.[61,62]

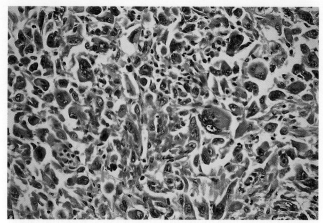

FIGURE 29–20. Undifferentiated carcinoma, spindle and giant cell type. High magnification of large, bizarre cells shows multinucleation, macronucleoli, and a proliferation of smaller spindle-shaped and round cells.

Small Cell Type. This variant of undifferentiated carcinoma may be distinguished from pure small (oat) cell carcinoma by the following features: The cells (1) are slightly larger and may contain mucin; (2) comprise vesicular nuclei with prominent nucleoli; (3) do not form ribbons, festoons, and pseudorosettes; and (4) lack spindle cells and secretory granules.[2,41,59]

Lobular Type. This variant, which grows in nests or lobules, resembles lobular carcinoma of the breast. The cells are homogeneous, small, and round, with inconspicuous nucleoli.

Osteoclast-like Giant Cell Type. This variant exhibits a mixture of spindle cells, sheets of large oval to round cells, and numerous osteoclast-like multinucleated giant cells (Fig. 29-21). The tumor resembles giant cell tumor of bone. Osteoclast-like giant cells are typically immunoreactive for CD68 (a histiocytic marker), and the

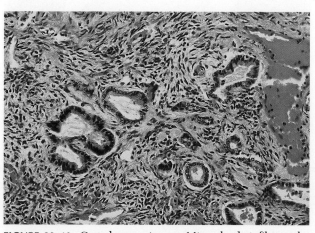

FIGURE 29–19. Cystadenocarcinoma. Microglands infiltrate the wall of the cyst.

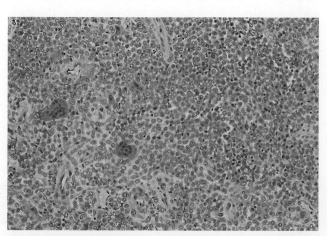

FIGURE 29–21. Undifferentiated carcinoma with osteoclast-like giant cells. Several multinucleated osteoclast-like cells are admixed with small round to oval cells.

round cells are reactive for epithelial markers (EMA, cytokeratin). These tumors in rare cases are found in the extrahepatic bile ducts and ampulla of Vater, where they sometimes form bone.[61]

PORCELAIN GALLBLADDER WITH ADENOCARCINOMA

Porcelain gallbladder usually develops as an end result of severe xanthogranulomatous inflammation. It is found in less than 0.1% of cholecystectomy specimens and may involve the entire gallbladder or only portions of the wall. Carcinoma is present in approximately 20% of porcelain gallbladders, and gallstones occur in up to 95% of cases.[2] Grossly, the gallbladder wall is rigid and does not collapse upon opening of the specimen (Fig. 29-22). The lumen may contain thick, tan-yellow, paste-like material or "milky-limey" fluid.[1] Sectioning of the wall may be difficult and requires decalcification before processing is begun. The histology of the gallbladder wall varies, but typically, the surface epithelial layer and muscle layer are almost entirely absent and have been replaced by dense fibrous tissue. Aggregates of chronic inflammatory cells, typically plasma cells, are sometimes "sandwiched" between layers of fibrous tissue; occasionally, residual foci of xanthogranulomatous inflammation are seen. Calcified areas may form broad bands or may be focally deposited within layers of fibrous tissue.

When carcinoma is present, atypical glandular structures are randomly distributed in the fibrous wall (Fig. 29-23). The extent of carcinoma varies from only a few malignant glands encased in dense fibrous tissue to large foci admixed with chronic inflammatory cells and loose connective tissue. Thus, the entire gallbladder should be carefully examined.

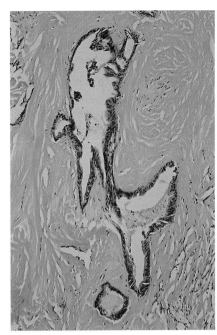

FIGURE 29–23. Porcelain gallbladder with adenocarcinoma. High magnification of a highly angulated gland lined by neoplastic columnar epithelium and encased in dense fibrous stroma.

■ Endocrine Tumors of the Gallbladder and Extrahepatic Biliary Tract

CARCINOID TUMOR AND VARIANTS

Clinical Features

Carcinoid tumor is sometimes discovered incidentally in routine cholecystectomy specimens, but more often, patients present with cholecystitis-like symptoms. When it occurs in the extrahepatic bile ducts, the sudden onset of biliary colic or painless jaundice may be the initial presentation.

Carcinoid tumors of the gallbladder and extrahepatic bile ducts have been rarely associated with von Hippel–Lindau disease, Zollinger-Ellison syndrome, multiple endocrine neoplasia (MEN I), and carcinoid syndromes.[2,63] Several patients with liver metastases developed the carcinoid syndrome. Gastrin-secreting carcinoids may cause the Zollinger-Ellison syndrome.[64,65] Classic carcinoids of the gallbladder rarely invade or metastasize; they have an extremely favorable prognosis compared with atypical carcinoids, the latter of which show a higher degree of cytologic atypia and necrosis and a greater risk of metastasis.[58,66]

Carcinoids account for less than 1% of all carcinoid tumors of the body. In a study of 8305 carcinoid tumors from various sites, only 19 (0.2%) were removed from the gallbladder and only 1 (0.01%) was taken from the biliary tree.[67] In another study by Godwin,[68] 2837

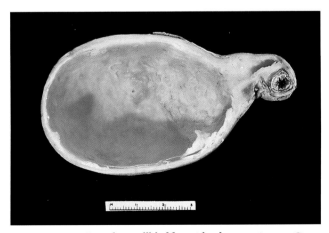

FIGURE 29–22. Porcelain gallbladder with adenocarcinoma. Gross example of a bisected porcelain gallbladder.

carcinoid tumors from the files of the National Cancer Institute of the United States were analyzed; only one involved the gallbladder, and one the bile duct. The average age at presentation is 60 years, which is lower than the average age for all carcinomas of the gallbladder. The female-to-male ratio in most series is 1.2:1.[67] The gallbladder and extrahepatic bile ducts are derived from the endodermal lining of the foregut; thus, these tumors are categorized as foregut carcinoids. Scattered chromogranin-positive cells are normally found in the neck of the gallbladder and in nonneoplastic epithelium that exhibits hyperplastic or metaplastic changes.

Pathologic Features

Carcinoid tumors are usually nodular or polypoid lesions that protrude into the lumen. They may be located anywhere in the gallbladder or extrahepatic bile ducts. Their cut surface is typically white-tan or yellow. These tumors are often fairly well demarcated from the normal gallbladder wall.[2]

Although gallbladder carcinoids are more diverse morphologically than carcinoid tumors of the pancreas, their growth pattern still consists primarily of trabeculae, nests, or solid areas with or without tubular formation (Fig. 29-24).[2] The cells are usually homogeneous in appearance and show mild nuclear pleomorphism, inconspicuous nucleoli, rare mitoses, and eosinophilic cytoplasm. Fibrous tissue may surround nests of tumor cells. Carcinoid tumors that occur in association with

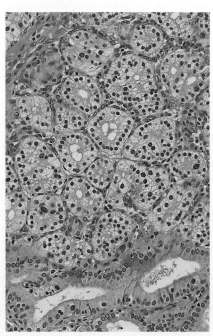

FIGURE 29–24. Tubular carcinoid tumor. Tubules are lined by cuboidal cells with clear cytoplasm and small round nuclei.

von Hippel–Lindau disease consist predominantly of tubular structures lined by clear cells that are inhibin positive.[69]

A tubular variant composed primarily of small, round tubules of bland, homogeneous, cuboidal cells with finely granular chromatin and inconspicuous nucleoli may be mistaken for adenocarcinoma.[2] The cytoplasm may be eosinophilic or clear, and the lumina of the tubules may contain extracellular mucin (see Fig. 29-24).

Some cases show a mixture of adenocarcinoma and carcinoid tumor (mixed carcinoid/adenocarcinoma) components. The adenocarcinoma may arise from the surface epithelium with carcinoid tumor below it, or intermingling of both components may be seen in the same lesion. Mixed carcinoid/adenocarcinomas should be differentiated from adenocarcinoma with neuroendocrine features, the latter of which shows scattered chromogranin-positive cells within malignant glands. Mixed tumors behave similarly to pure adenocarcinomas in that they are more aggressive than pure carcinoid tumors.[70,71]

Grimelius and immunohistochemical stains for chromogranin A, neuron-specific enolase, and occasionally cytokeratin and synaptophysin are positive in carcinoid tumors. In addition, immunoreactivity may be seen with serotonin, somatostatin, and other peptide hormones (e.g., gastrin, human pancreatic polypeptide). Neurosecretory intracytoplasmic granules can be demonstrated on electron microscopy.[2]

PARAGANGLIOMA

These rare benign lesions are usually discovered incidentally in cholecystectomy specimens. Although most are asymptomatic, they may occasionally cause acute cholecystitis secondary to hemorrhage[72] or common bile duct obstruction.[73]

Paragangliomas typically measure less than 1 cm in greatest dimension, are well to poorly demarcated, and are located predominantly in perimuscular connective tissue (Fig. 29-25). Rarely, paragangliomas may be found in the lamina propria or in the extrahepatic bile ducts.

Microscopically, the tumor is believed to arise from normal paraganglia; thus, it is composed of chief and sustentacular cells.[2,74,75] Chief cells are polygonal and form nests ("zellballen") separated by thin fibrous septa containing capillaries. Cells contain eosinophilic or clear cytoplasm and round hyperchromatic nuclei. Sustentacular cells are round or stellate, and they surround chief cells. Mitoses are typically absent.

The S100 protein immunostain is positive in sustentacular cells (Fig. 29-26). In contrast, chief cells are argyrophilic and stain for neuron-specific enolase and chromogranin A. Peptide hormones have not been identified in these lesions.[2]

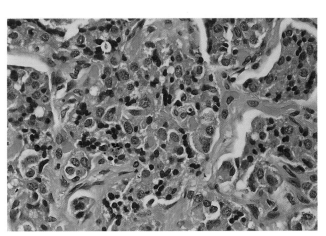

FIGURE 29–25. Paraganglioma. Polygon-shaped chief cells admixed with stellate sustentacular cells and capillaries.

■ Benign Nonepithelial Tumors of the Gallbladder

LEIOMYOMA

This is a rare, benign smooth muscle tumor that arises from the normal muscle layers of the gallbladder.[2,11,76,77] Although it is usually solitary, one case of multiple leiomyoma of the gallbladder was recently reported in a young child infected with human immunodeficiency virus (HIV).[78] Another child with severe combined immunodeficiency after bone marrow transplant developed innumerable Epstein-Barr virus–associated leiomyomas of the gallbladder.[78a] This tumor is grossly and histologically similar to smooth muscle tumors that arise in other organs. It is composed of interlacing fascicles of uniform spindle-shaped cells with plump oval nuclei and blunt ends. Mitoses are absent or rare. Epithelioid leiomyomas consist of nests of round or polygonal cells admixed with spindle cells. These tumors are immunoreactive for smooth muscle actin, muscle-specific actin, vimentin, and rarely, desmin.

Extremely rarely, a benign stromal tumor with an interstitial cell of Cajal phenotype may develop in the gallbladder wall.[79] The cells of this tumor are immunoreactive for vimentin, CD34, and CD117 (c-*kit*).[79]

LIPOMA

Lipomas are exceedingly rare in the gallbladder, and only occasional cases have been reported. They may be associated with MEN.[11,80-83] These benign tumors, which are composed of mature adipose tissue, may be found in the wall or attached to the adventitia of the gallbladder. Lipomas of the common duct have also rarely been reported.[84]

HEMANGIOMA

Only four cases of cavernous hemangioma of the gallbladder have been reported in the English literature.[85,86] Hemangiomas may arise in the wall or from the external surface of the gallbladder (Fig. 29-27).[11,87] The lesion is composed of communicating vascular spaces of variable sizes that are lined by a single layer of benign endothelial cells immunoreactive for CD31, CD34, and factor VIII–related antigen. The vascular spaces are typically filled with blood but may contain recent or organized thrombi.

LYMPHANGIOMA

This rare lesion resembles hemangiomas histologically, but the vascular spaces contain lymph fluid instead of red blood cells (Fig. 29-28). The spaces are of variable size, or they may be cystically dilated. The single layer of endothelium, which rests on a basement membrane, shows an immunoreactivity pattern similar to that of hemangioma.[88-90]

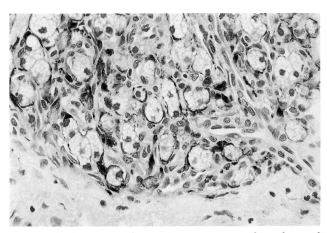

FIGURE 29–26. Paraganglioma. An S100 immunohistochemical stain highlights sustentacular cells that surround chief cells.

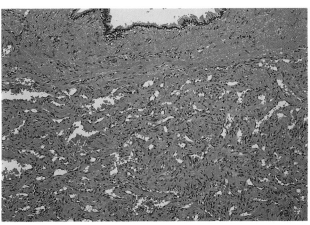

FIGURE 29–27. Hemangioma. Low-magnification view of a benign vascular proliferation in the subserosa.

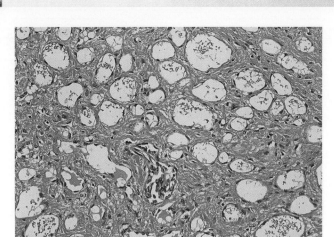

FIGURE 29–28. Lymphangioma. Lymphatic spaces are lined by flattened endothelium; the lumen contains lymph fluid with occasional red blood cells.

OSTEOMA

Single or multiple osteoma of the gallbladder is an extremely rare neoplasm.[91] Osseous metaplasia may occur within a cholesterol polyp[92] (Fig. 29-29).

GRANULAR CELL TUMOR

This benign tumor is more common in the extrahepatic bile ducts than in the gallbladder, and it frequently causes obstruction with mucocele or hydrops when located in the neck or cystic duct. Granular cell tumors may be single or multicentric and coexist with granular cell tumors in other locations of the body.[2,93-97] They are typically located underneath the mucosa (Fig. 29-30). They are poorly demarcated and yellow and usually measure less than 2 cm in greatest dimension. Microscopically and immunohistochemically, they are similar to tumors that occur in other parts of the gastrointestinal tract[93] (Fig. 29-31).

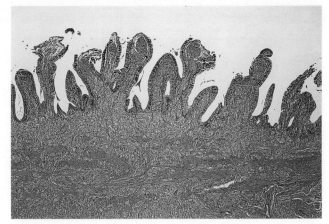

FIGURE 29–30. Granular cell tumor. The gallbladder wall and villi contain an eosinophilic cellular infiltrate.

NEUROGENIC TUMORS

Neurogenic tumors such as neurofibromas, schwannomas (either with or without neurofibromatosis), and ganglioneuromas, the latter often associated with MEN syndrome type IIb, may rarely occur in the gallbladder or the extrahepatic biliary tree. These are histologically and immunohistochemically similar to those that occur in other soft tissues of the body (Figs. 29-32, 29-33, and 29-34).[98-106]

■ Malignant Mesenchymal Tumors of the Biliary Tract

RHABDOMYOSARCOMA (SARCOMA BOTRYOIDES)

Embryonal rhabdomyosarcoma is an extremely rare tumor. However, it is the most common biliary tract malignancy among children. A majority of cases involve the extrahepatic bile ducts. However, rarely, they occur

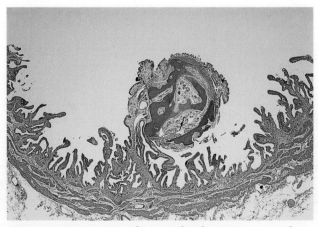

FIGURE 29–29. Osteoma. This is a polyp that contains metaplastic bone.

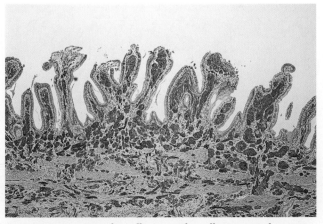

FIGURE 29–31. Granular cell tumor. The cells are strongly reactive for S100 protein (S100 protein immunostain).

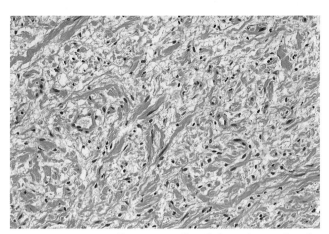

FIGURE 29–32. Neurofibroma. Spindle cells have elongated nuclei and are set in a mucopolysaccharide-rich, collagenous stroma.

in the gallbladder as well.[2,107] Children usually present with obstructive jaundice, hepatomegaly, and abdominal pain and range in age from 16 months to 11 years.[2,108,109]

These tumors may be sessile or pedunculated. They often reveal a gelatinous appearance, forming soft, polypoid, grapelike structures that protrude into the lumen.[20] The gallbladder may become distended with "milky white" bile because of obstruction by the tumor, and the wall of the bile ducts may be distended and thickened as well. Microscopically, malignant cells are typically located beneath a single layer of biliary epithelium and are composed of small, round blue cells (primitive mesenchymal cells) that contain a variable amount of eosinophilic cytoplasm. Rhabdomyoblasts and fusiform cells that form the cambium layer may be seen as well (Fig. 29-35). A myxoid stroma composed of loose connective tissue, collagen fibers, undifferentiated stellate cells, and delicate blood vessels is also typically noted.[20,110]

Tumor cells with abundant eosinophilic cytoplasm (rhabdomyoblasts) are typically immunoreactive for anti-

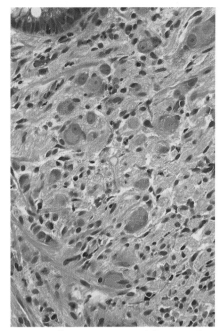

FIGURE 29–34. Ganglioneuroma. A proliferation of ganglion cells are scattered in the lamina propria.

myoglobin, myosin, desmin, and muscle-specific actin, whereas keratin is normally negative. Electron microscopy shows cross-striations in less than half of cells.[20]

MALIGNANT FIBROUS HISTIOCYTOMA

Currently, six cases of primary malignant fibrous histiocytoma (MFH) of the gallbladder have been documented in the English literature.[2,111-113] These tumors are composed of spindle-shaped fibroblasts, myofibroblasts, undifferentiated cells, and histiocyte-like cells. The spindle cells may be arranged randomly or may appear in a storiform growth pattern. Histiocyte-like cells are

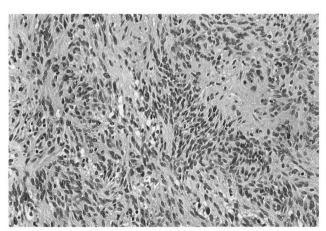

FIGURE 29–33. Schwannoma. Fascicles of spindle cells contain plump oval nuclei and a variable amount of collagen in the stroma.

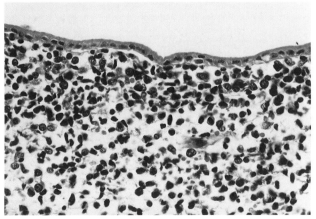

FIGURE 29–35. Rhabdomyosarcoma. Small, round blue cells with scant eosinophilic cytoplasm are concentrated beneath normal biliary epithelium.

typically round and small and contain a variable amount of cytoplasm. Large, bizarre, multinucleated forms may be present as well. Metaplastic bone and cartilage may be noted in pleomorphic MFH. Immunostains are used to exclude other neoplasms, such as melanoma, lymphoma, and carcinoma. KP-1 and CD68 are expressed in some cells but are also expressed by nonhistiocytic tumors, including lymphoma, malignant melanoma, and some carcinomas. The prognosis for MFH is dismal. Recurrence rates are extremely high.

ANGIOSARCOMA

Between 1989 and 1994, six case reports of angiosarcoma of the gallbladder were documented.[2,114-118] Two were reported to display an epithelioid growth pattern, and one contained a synchronous squamous cell carcinoma. These tumors occur in older individuals, usually older than 60 years of age, and may metastasize to the liver, omentum, and other organs. They are histologically identical to those that arise in other organs (Fig. 29-36) and show immunohistochemical reactivity for various endothelial markers, such as CD34, CD31, and factor VIII–related antigen.

LEIOMYOSARCOMA

This rare tumor of smooth muscle origin is more common among women than men.[2,108,119-123] Patients may present with symptoms that resemble cholecystitis or cholelithiasis. Leiomyosarcoma has a poor prognosis. It may be apparent on ultrasound or computed tomographic (CT) scan as an irregularly thickened area or as an intraluminal polyp. Histology and immunohistochemical features are similar to those of smooth muscle tumors in other locations, and both epithelioid and spindle cell patterns of growth may be exhibited (Fig. 29-37).

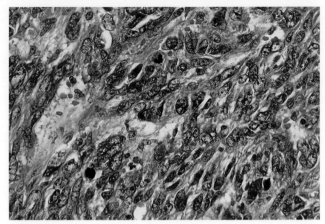

FIGURE 29–37. Leiomyosarcoma. High magnification shows many mitotic figures, pleomorphic hyperchromatic nuclei, and high cellularity.

Rarely, a malignant spindle cell tumor, similar to a gastrointestinal stromal tumor, with an interstitial cell of Cajal phenotype has been reported in the gallbladder as well.[124]

KAPOSI'S SARCOMA

Most cases of Kaposi's sarcoma that involve the gallbladder or extrahepatic bile ducts are discovered as incidental findings at autopsy in acquired immunodeficiency syndrome (AIDS) patients.[2,20,125] One patient with AIDS developed Kaposi's sarcoma in the absence of a cutaneous lesion.[126] The lesions were hemorrhagic in appearance and involved the subserosa and muscle layers of the gallbladder wall. The pathologic features of Kaposi's sarcoma are the same as those of tumors in other locations in the gastrointestinal tract.[2,20] The tumor is composed of spindle-shaped cells with numerous vascular slits, extravasated red blood cells, and hyaline globules. The spindle cells are immunohistochemically reactive for CD34 and CD31, and the hyaline globules may be highlighted with d-PAS and Masson's trichrome stain.

▮ Miscellaneous Tumors

CARCINOSARCOMA (MALIGNANT MIXED TUMOR)

By definition, this neoplasm contains at least two malignant components—carcinoma and sarcoma. It occurs in both the gallbladder and the bile ducts,[2,20] but most cases reported in the recent literature have involved the gallbladder.[127-129]

Pathologically, they are usually polypoid or pedunculated neoplasms that protrude into the lumen of the gallbladder and measure from 3 to 25 cm in greatest dimension. Cystic changes and foci of calcification have

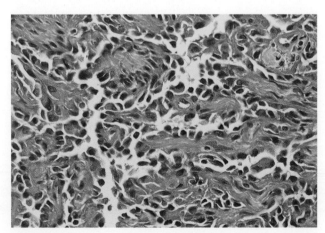

FIGURE 29–36. Angiosarcoma. Large, plump, highly atypical endothelial cells surround a fibrovascular core.

also been described. Microscopically, the carcinomatous component can be glandular or squamous or both. However, moderately to poorly differentiated adenocarcinoma usually dominates the epithelial component. The glands may form cords, trabeculae, sheets, or nests of cells with a pseudoadenoid cystic or lacy growth pattern. The glands are typically surrounded by a malignant stroma containing undifferentiated spindle cells, blood vessels, and collagen. Keratinization and squamous pearls are occasionally seen. The sarcomatous component may contain areas of chondrosarcoma, osteosarcoma, or rhabdomyosarcoma (Fig. 29-38).[2,130] These latter features help distinguish a true carcinosarcoma from an undifferentiated spindle and giant cell carcinoma.

One study reported a small component of small cell carcinoma in one of nine cases of carcinosarcoma of the gallbladder.[131] Epithelial markers for cytokeratin, EMA, and CEA help separate the carcinomatous component from sarcomatous areas. The presence of mesenchymal elements helps in differentiating carcinosarcoma from undifferentiated carcinoma, spindle cell carcinoma, and giant cell carcinoma. Carcinosarcomas are aggressive neoplasms whose natural history is similar to that of pure carcinomas.[130]

MALIGNANT MELANOMA

Primary malignant melanoma of the gallbladder is extremely rare and is difficult to distinguish from metastatic melanoma unless there is a history of a previously excised primary melanoma from the skin, eye, or other site.[132] Melanocytes are present in normal gallbladder epithelium, as demonstrated by electron microscopy, and these are believed to represent the origin of primary malignant melanoma.[133] "Junctional" activity is reported to occur in both primary and metastatic tumors; therefore, this is not a reliable feature for establishing a diagnosis of a primary tumor (Fig. 29-39).[134,135] Patients may

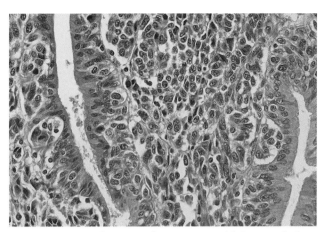

FIGURE 29–39. Malignant melanoma. Normal biliary epithelium is infiltrated by melanoma cells, which resembles "junctional" activity. The lamina propria is filled with melanoma cells.

be asymptomatic or may present with symptoms that mimic acute cholecystitis. These tumors often grow as well-circumscribed polypoid or pedunculated lesions. Histologically, their appearance is similar to that of cutaneous melanomas. Melanin pigment may be found in some tumor cells. Large tumors are frequently eroded. Occasional foci of junctional activity may be identified adjacent to normal surface epithelial cells.

Immunohistochemically, melanomas are reactive for S100 protein, HMB-45 antigen, and Melan-A.[2,135] They are negative for cytokeratin, which may aid in distinguishing melanoma from poorly differentiated adenocarcinoma and from spindle and giant cell undifferentiated carcinoma.

LYMPHOMA

Primary and secondary lymphomas are more common in the gallbladder than in the extrahepatic bile ducts. Most primary gallbladder lymphomas are low-grade, B-cell, mucosa-associated lymphoid tissue lymphomas (*MALTomas*) (Fig. 29-40).[136-139] Other less common types of lymphoma include large B-cell, small lymphocytic, follicular, and T-cell lymphoblastic lymphoma.[140] One case was recently reported of primary Hodgkin's lymphoma limited to the gallbladder,[141] and angiotropic intravascular lymphoma has been reported in one patient as well.[142] *Helicobacter* species, although associated with the development of MALToma in the stomach, have not been linked with gallbladder malignancies.[143-145]

◼ Secondary Tumors of the Gallbladder and Extrahepatic Biliary Tract

Metastases to the gallbladder are rare and are usually discovered incidentally. Most metastases occur via peritoneal spread from the gastrointestinal tract, pancreas,

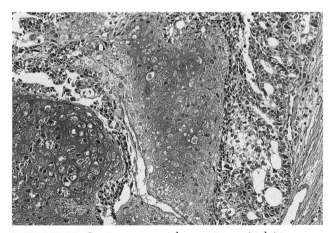

FIGURE 29–38. Carcinosarcoma. Adenocarcinoma (*right*) is accompanied by malignant cartilage (*left*).

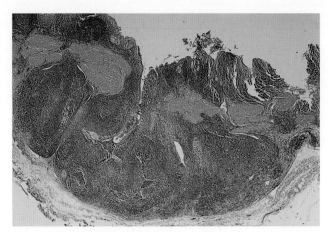

FIGURE 29–40. Malignant lymphoma, MALToma. A small monotonous B-cell lymphocytic infiltrate involves the full thickness of the gallbladder wall and contains scattered residual follicles.

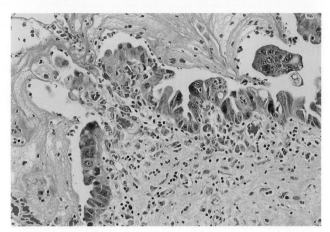

FIGURE 29–41. Regenerative atypia. Regenerating epithelium is composed of a heterogeneous population of cells with ample cytoplasm and occasional nucleoli. The background shows acute and chronic inflammation and a pseudomembrane attached to the surface.

ovary, bile duct, or breast carcinoma. Hematogenous metastases are less common. These usually involve malignant melanoma and carcinomas of the kidney, lung, breast, esophagus, and nasopharynx.[2,146-151] Overall, malignant melanoma is the most common metastatic tumor; it accounts for more than 50% of all gallbladder metastases.[146-148]

Tumor-like Lesions of the Gallbladder

REGENERATIVE ATYPIA

Injury and subsequent repair to the epithelium in chronic cholecystitis can be notable, especially when associated with gallstones. Regeneration of injured tissue may result in regrowth of architecturally abnormal epithelium that may resemble malignancy. In some cases, regenerative epithelium is histologically similar to low-grade dysplasia; as a result, it may not be possible for these two lesions to be differentiated. A helpful clue is provided by assessment of the pattern of cellular growth. An organized homogeneous proliferation of atypical cells with enlarged hyperchromatic nuclei, loss of polarity, and pleomorphism is distinctive for dysplasia, whereas reactive epithelium more often appears as a heterogeneous population of columnar and cuboidal cells with ballooned cytoplasm and prominent nucleoli (Figs. 29-41 and 29-42).[1,2,20] Mitotic activity is seen in both entities and is not a reliable indicator of malignancy. However, atypical mitoses are characteristic of dysplasia. One should always exercise caution when evaluating atypical cells adjacent to areas of ulceration and/or acute inflammation because regeneration may be marked. Furthermore, regenerating epithelium, and even dysplasia, may extend deep into the epithelium of Rokitansky-Aschoff sinuses, simulating an invasive tumor.

CHOLECYSTITIS WITH LYMPHOID HYPERPLASIA

It is not unusual for prominent lymphoid follicles to be seen in chronic cholecystitis. In severe cases, reactive lymphoid follicles with germinal centers may occupy a large portion of the mucosa or may extend into the subserosa, resembling malignant lymphoma (Fig. 29-43).[2,138,152] The mucosa may appear granular, or it

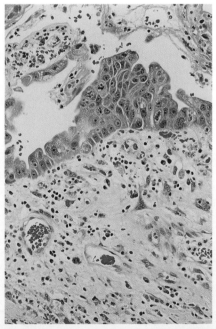

FIGURE 29–42. Regenerative atypia. The lamina propria is edematous and congested. Acute and chronic inflammation is seen. The surface epithelium shows enlarged cells with prominent nucleoli and crowding. An inflammatory exudate and degenerating strips of epithelium are extruded into the lumen.

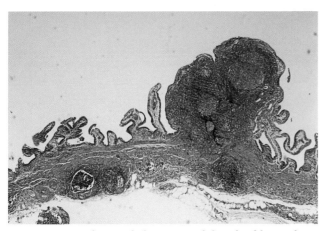

FIGURE 29–43. Chronic cholecystitis with lymphoid hyperplasia. Variably sized lymphoid follicles with germinal centers extend from the mucosa to the subserosa.

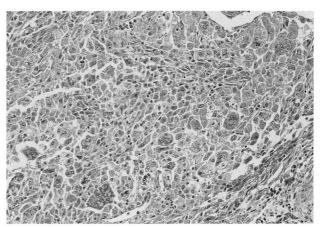

FIGURE 29–44. Xanthogranulomatous cholecystitis. Pigment-laden macrophages with engulfed and free-floating bile pigment.

may contain small polyps and nodules that are tan, measure from 2 to 9 mm, and are covered by intact mucosa.[153] Histologically, one sees a polyclonal lymphoid infiltrate in the lamina propria, along with reactive lymphoid follicles that vary in size and occasionally extend into the subserosa.[2,152]

A key to a benign diagnosis is the fact that many of the follicles contain germinal centers with B lymphocytes, tingible body macrophages, and dendritic reticulum cells. Unfortunately, reactive follicles are also a characteristic feature of MALT lymphomas. The latter can be distinguished by the presence of lymphoepithelial lesions, centrocyte-like cells (CCLs), plasma cells, and lymphoid follicles that are colonized by CCLs[136] (see Chapter 23). In fact, some suggest that long-standing chronic cholecystitis with lymphoid hyperplasia may be the initial stage of development of MALT lymphoma.

XANTHOGRANULOMATOUS CHOLECYSTITIS

Xanthogranulomatous cholecystitis is an uncommon inflammatory response to foreign material. It is present in about 2% of cholecystectomy specimens, mainly from middle-aged women with symptoms of cholecystitis.[2,11] In some cases, the lesions may be poorly demarcated, or they may form discrete nodules that range in size from a few millimeters to larger than 2.5 cm in diameter.[154-159] Microscopically, the nodules contain variable proportions of foamy histiocytes, ceroid-laden macrophages, acute and chronic inflammatory cells, and fibroblastic scarring (Fig. 29-44) (see Chapter 28 for details).[154-156] Ulceration of the overlying mucosa is common, and scattered foreign body giant cells, cholesterol clefts, microabscesses, and remnants of epithelium are also occasionally seen.[2,154-156] The content of the histiocytic cells may be highlighted with Oil Red O stain or the

d-PAS stain.[2,154] Histiocyte immunostains include KP-1 (CD68), lysozyme, and Mac 386. In rare instances, sinus tracts may form between adjacent organs such as small bowel and mesentery.[2] In these cases, spindle cells may predominate, especially if the inflammatory reaction is old, and a storiform pattern of growth may be noted. However, the lack of nuclear atypia and the absence of mitotic activity help in excluding a diagnosis of sarcoma.[2]

Xanthogranulomatous cholecystitis may coexist with a malignant tumor.[160] In one study, adenocarcinoma was detected in 8 of 40 cases of xanthogranulomatous cholecystitis; 26 had cholelithiasis and 6 had choledocholithiasis.[154]

Finally, in rare instances, malakoplakia of the gallbladder, another type of inflammatory reaction (see Chapter 28), may progress into a mass lesion, grossly simulating a malignant tumor.[161-163] Malakoplakia histologically resembles xanthogranulomatous cholecystitis with the exception that the histiocytes contain variably sized, laminated, calcified microspherules referred to as *Michaelis-Gutmann bodies* (Fig. 29-45). This condition is due to an acquired defect in monocyte bactericidal activity related to lysosomal degradation.

MUCOCELE (HYDROPS)

Mucocele of the gallbladder develops as a result of obstruction of the gallbladder neck by gallstones, polyps, or neoplasms. Mucin accumulates in the lumen, leading to marked distention (Fig. 29-46). Rarely, mucus may dissect through the wall into the subserosal connective tissue, thereby resembling a mucinous carcinoma. Muciphages are occasionally seen within pools of mucin and may be mistaken for signet ring tumor cells, but the lack of nuclear atypia and positivity for macrophage markers (CD68, KP-1, and lysozyme) facilitate the diagnosis.[2]

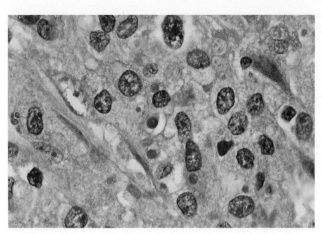

FIGURE 29–45. Malakoplakia. Intramural lesion composed of histiocytes containing small, round, blue calcified concretions (Michaelis-Gutmann bodies).

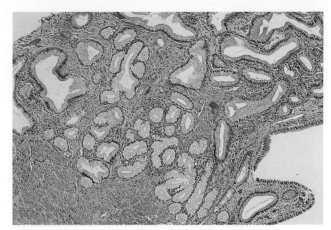

FIGURE 29–47. Pyloric gland metaplasia. Proliferation of benign branching mucous glands that fill the lamina propria.

PYLORIC GLAND METAPLASIA, INTESTINAL METAPLASIA, AND SQUAMOUS METAPLASIA

Metaplastic changes that arise on a background of chronic cholecystitis and cholelithiasis are part of the spectrum of "hyperplastic cholecystoses." Similar lesions occur in the extrahepatic bile ducts in association with chronic inflammation or tumor.[2,164]

Pyloric gland metaplasia, or mucous gland metaplasia, is the most common metaplastic lesion associated with gallstones (Fig. 29-47).[2,165] The glands are lined by columnar cells with vacuolated cytoplasm and contain nonsulfated acid mucin. The nuclei of pyloric glands are basally located and flattened. Scattered endocrine and

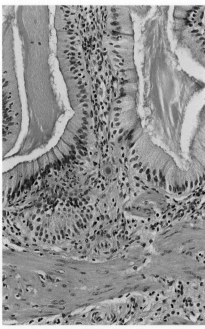

FIGURE 29–46. Mucocele. Villi are lined by mucinous epithelium.

Paneth cells may be present as well within the epithelium. Pyloric glands may form small lobular structures when they proliferate, or they may appear as small clusters throughout the lamina propria. In fact, florid proliferations of pyloric glands may appear "masslike," causing diffuse thickening of the mucosa. Rarely, glands may extend into the subserosal tissues and may appear to involve nerve bundles. A recent report of four patients with florid pyloric gland metaplasia showed perineural and intraneural involvement by benign metaplastic glands in all cases.[166] Pyloric gland metaplasia may coexist with other types of metaplastic reactions and even dysplasia or carcinoma.

Intestinal metaplasia also arises on a background of chronic cholecystitis. The frequency of intestinal metaplasia increases with age and duration of gallstones. Histologically, glands are lined by tall columnar cells with a brush border and exhibit an intestinal phenotype (Fig. 29-48).[2] One may see variable proportions of goblet cells, Paneth cells, and endocrine cells admixed with columnar cells. Goblet cells usually outnumber the other cellular components.[6] Intestinal metaplasia has a high propensity for the development of dysplasia.[2] In fact, intestinal metaplasia is often seen adjacent to invasive adenocarcinoma.

Squamous metaplasia is a rare form of metaplastic reaction. It is also typically associated with cholelithiasis and cholecystitis. Normal columnar epithelium is replaced by mature, stratified squamous epithelium either with or without keratinization and a granular layer.[2] The significance of squamous metaplasia is unknown.

PAPILLARY HYPERPLASIA

When associated with chronic cholecystitis, cholelithiasis, inflammatory bowel disease, or primary sclerosing cholangitis, papillary hyperplasia is considered a secondary lesion.[1,2,9,167,168] It is usually associated with gallstones.[2] Patients present with symptoms of biliary

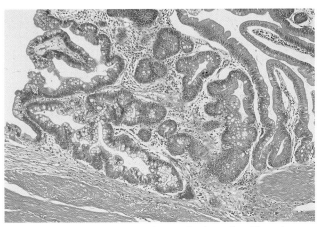

FIGURE 29–48. Intestinal metaplasia. Glands are lined by columnar epithelium with goblet cells.

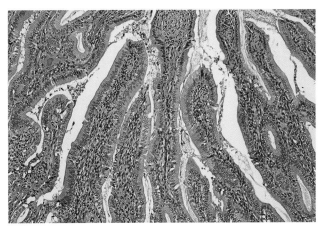

FIGURE 29–50. Papillary hyperplasia. The villi are lined by benign-appearing nondysplastic columnar epithelium.

colic and a thickened gallbladder wall on radiographic studies. Papillary lesions may be diffuse, segmental, or focal and may extend into the bile ducts.[2,20] In one reported case of primary papillary hyperplasia, a young girl without gallstones had papillary hyperplasia of the entire gallbladder and cystic and common bile ducts.[169]

Microscopically, the epithelial cells that line the papillae are similar to those in the normal gallbladder and bile duct epithelium (Figs. 29-49 and 29-50). Occasional Paneth cells or goblet cells may be interspersed among biliary-type epithelial cells.[1,2,9] Certain diseases such as ulcerative colitis and primary sclerosing cholangitis exhibit mucus-type cells as well.[2,20] In this setting, columnar cells may show mild nuclear atypia, but dysplasia is extremely uncommon.

ADENOMYOMATOUS HYPERPLASIA

This is a distinctive lesion that frequently involves the wall and subserosa of the gallbladder[2,11,20,169-171] and is composed of invaginated surface epithelium (diverticula) intermingled with hyperplastic smooth muscle. It is more common among women than men and is frequently associated with gallstones. Patients may be asymptomatic or may present with symptoms of chronic cholecystitis.[2] Grossly, this condition may be localized, segmental, or diffuse. The localized form is commonly seen in the fundus, where it is referred to as *adenomyoma*.[1,2,20,170] Fundic adenomyomas may appear as intramural nodules with umbilication of the overlying mucosa. Transection of the nodules reveals multiple cystic spaces that communicate with the main lumen through a central channel. The glands become cystic when the channel is obstructed with inflammation, calculi, or inspissated material. Segmental and diffuse adenomyomatous hyperplasia reveals many cystically dilated ductal structures found predominantly in perimuscular connective tissue (Fig. 29-51). Microscopically, the cells that line the glands are biliary-type columnar cells identical to those in the surface epithelium. Gastric mucinous epithelium may be present as well. A variable amount of chronic inflammation may be present, as well as pyloric, intestinal, and endocrine metaplasia.[2]

When cysts become infected, a purulent exudate may fill the lumen; upon rupture, this develops into an intramural abscess. Branching and horizontal extensions of the glands along tissue planes are not uncommon. In addition, secondary gland formation may occur with mucous metaplasia. In the subserosa, benign glands from invaginated epithelium may involve nerve bundles and may thereby be mistaken for invasive carcinoma.[170,172] Carcinoma arising in adenomyomatous hyperplasia is extremely rare.[173-175] Adenomyomatous hyperplasia may also occur in the extrahepatic bile ducts.[176]

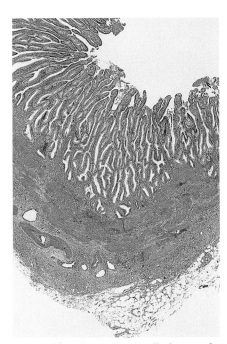

FIGURE 29–49. Papillary hyperplasia. Tall, thin nondysplastic villi protrude into the lumen of the gallbladder.

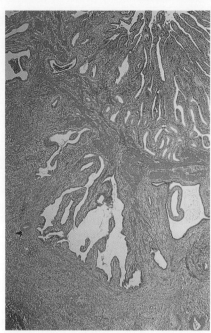

FIGURE 29–51. Adenomyomatous hyperplasia. The surface shows papillary hyperplasia with glands that extend deep into the subserosal connective tissue accompanied by smooth muscle.

CHOLESTEROL POLYP

Cholesterol polyp is a type of lesion that may cause symptoms of right upper quadrant pain and indigestion. Grossly, these polyps range in size from 0.1 to 0.5 cm. They may be single or multiple, and occasionally they become detached from the mucosa and float freely in the lumen.[11] Cholesterol polyps develop as aggregates of foamy histiocytes within the lamina propria of the villi. With further accumulation of histiocytes, the lamina propria becomes expanded, forming a polyp (Fig. 29-52). In some cholesterol polyps, foamy histiocytes are replaced by a fibrous stroma with only scant remnants of foamy cells. Large cholesterol polyps may be detected by cholecystogram or sonogram; they appear as mulberry-like punctate structures with a high echo.[2,177,178] Polyps may be highlighted by d-PAS or by the Oil Red O stain.

HETEROTOPIA (ECTOPIA, CHORISTOMA)

Heterotopia is the appearance of normal tissue in an abnormal anatomic location.[20] It may appear as an intramural nodule or polyp that bulges into the lumen of the gallbladder, and it can range from 1.0 to 2.5 cm in diameter.[11] Symptoms include right upper quadrant pain, nausea, and vomiting. Many heterotopic lesions are located in the neck or cystic duct and can cause obstruction, whereas lesions in the fundus or body of the gallbladder may be asymptomatic. Serosal lesions also occur. Rarely, the various heterotopias that may

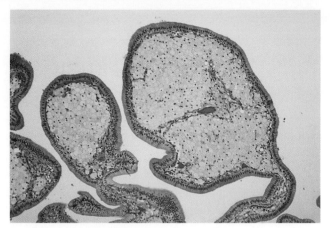

FIGURE 29–52. Cholesterol polyp. The villi are expanded with foamy macrophages.

involve the gallbladder or biliary tract include gastric, pancreatic, hepatic, thyroid, and adrenal cortical tissue[2,11,179-190] (Figs. 29-53 and 29-54).

CILIATED FOREGUT CYST

Ciliated foregut cysts rarely occur in the gallbladder/biliary tree region, but when present they may be located in the serosa or in tissue adjacent to the gallbladder.[191] These cysts are usually solitary and unilocular. They arise from the embryologic foregut. The cyst wall comprises four characteristic layers: (1) an inner layer of ciliated pseudostratified columnar cells and mucous cells, (2) subepithelial loose connective tissue, (3) one to three

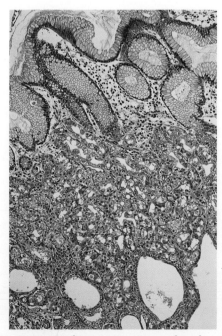

FIGURE 29–53. Gastric heterotopia. Gastric foveolar-type glands and glands composed of chief and parietal cells are present.

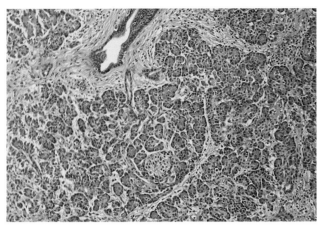

FIGURE 29–54. Pancreatic heterotopia. Normal pancreatic tissue is composed of both exocrine and endocrine cells and is present in the wall of the gallbladder.

layers of smooth muscle, and (4) an outer fibrous wall (Figs. 29-55 and 29-56). These benign cysts do not have malignant potential.

Benign Tumors of the Extrahepatic Bile Ducts

BILE DUCT ADENOMA

Adenomas are more common in the gallbladder than in the bile ducts. They may be single or multiple, and they may involve long segments of the extrahepatic bile ducts (Figs. 29-57 and 29-58). They also have been reported in Gardner's syndrome[192] and familial adenomatosis coli.[193,194] Clinically, adenomas may cause obstructive jaundice. Distention of the duct by the tumor may also result in biliary colic and pain.[2]

Pathologically, bile duct adenomas resemble colonic adenomas. They are classified as tubular, papillary, and

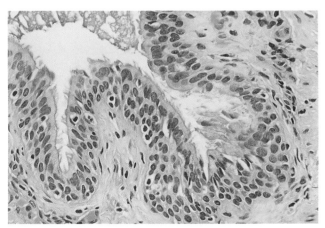

FIGURE 29–55. Ciliated foregut cyst. The cyst lining is composed of pseudostratified cells, many of which have surface cilia. Below is loose connective tissue.

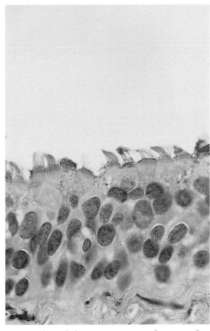

FIGURE 29–56. Ciliated foregut cyst. High magnification shows long, thin cilia attached to a terminal bar.

mixed tubulopapillary types and are further subclassified histologically into intestinal and biliary types.[2,9,20] Papillary adenomas are more common than tubular or mixed types. Adenomas that contain pyloric-type glands are rarely encountered.[2,195-198] By definition, the epithelium of adenomas contains at least low-grade dysplasia. Low-grade dysplasia includes mild and moderate dysplasia, whereas high-grade dysplasia includes severe dysplasia and carcinoma in situ. Most adenomas contain intestinal-type epithelium, with Paneth, endocrine, and goblet cell differentiation.[2,9,199] Because adenomas are uncommon in the bile ducts, most cases of bile duct carcinoma are not believed to arise from adenomas, nor is there evidence of preexisting adenomas in most cases of resected extrahepatic bile duct carcinoma.[2] Dysplasia and carcinoma in situ arising in flat mucosa probably account for most cases of invasive carcinoma. Some cases occur in association with primary sclerosing cholangitis and ulcerative colitis.[200]

BILIARY PAPILLOMATOSIS

This rare lesion involves both the intrahepatic bile ducts and the extrahepatic bile ducts.[2,9,17-19] It is characterized by multiple papillary (villous) excrescences that cause dilatation of the bile ducts (Fig. 29-60). In addition, the ducts may contain mucinous material, cellular debris, and blood. These lesions have a high rate of recurrence[19] and progression to malignancy.[17] Microscopically, the papillary lesions contain a fibrovascular stalk and are covered by tall columnar epithelium with complex, branching patterns of growth.[2,9] The nuclei

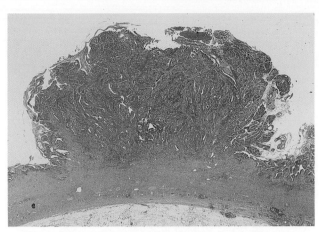

FIGURE 29–57. Common bile duct adenoma. A sessile adenoma is lined by dysplastic intestinal-type epithelium.

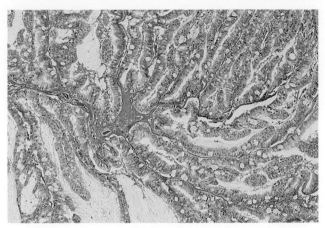

FIGURE 29–59. Biliary papillomatosis. Long, thin papillary structures diffusely line the wall of the bile duct.

are typically basally located, nucleoli are usually small or inconspicuous, and cytoplasmic mucin is noted in variable amounts. Nuclear atypia and mitotic figures are uncommon. Some authors suggest that papillomatosis is an entity with a broad morphologic spectrum; thus, some cases should be classified as intraductal papillary carcinoma, similar to those that occur in the pancreas.[2]

BILIARY CYSTADENOMA

Although most cystadenomas arise in the liver, they occasionally develop in the gallbladder, extrahepatic bile ducts, pancreas, and retroperitoneum.[2,9,20-22,24] Cyst-

adenomas are more common among middle-aged women, who present with symptoms of abdominal pain, jaundice, and a palpable mass.[2] In addition, serum CA 19-9 levels may be elevated.[26]

Grossly, cystadenomas are well-demarcated lesions that measure from 1.5 to 20 cm, are typically multiloculated but may also be unilocular, and often contain serous or mucinous fluid that is rich in CEA. The walls of the cyst vary in thickness and may be fibrotic. The inner surface may be smooth, granular, or trabeculated. Polypoid structures may protrude into the lumina of the loculi.

Microscopically, these lesions are composed of a single layer of cuboidal to columnar, biliary-type epithelium; rarely, foci of gastric foveolar-type epithelium may be noted as well. A subepithelial layer of mesenchymal stroma (ovarian-like) is present in 85% to 90% of cases, and the outer wall consists of hyalinized fibrous tissue (Figs. 29-60 and 29-61).[2,9,20-22,24] Occasionally, the cyst wall reveals chronic inflammation, foamy histiocytes, pigment-laden macrophages, hemosiderin deposits, and multinucleated foreign body giant cells. Metaplastic

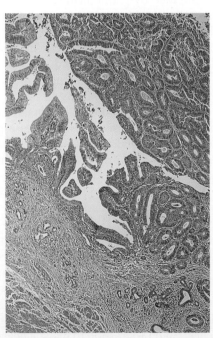

FIGURE 29–58. Common bile duct adenoma. The adenoma is lined by intestinal-type epithelium. In this photograph there are microglands invading the lamina propria (intramucosal adenocarcinoma).

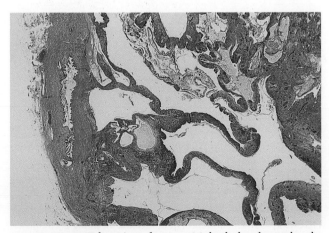

FIGURE 29–60. Biliary cystadenoma. Multiple locules with subepithelial mesenchymal stroma line the wall of the bile duct.

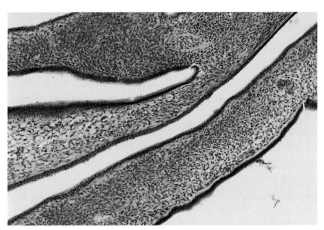

FIGURE 29–61. Biliary cystadenoma. High magnification of the cyst wall shows ovarian-type mesenchymal stroma situated directly beneath the surface biliary epithelium.

foci containing Paneth, endocrine, and goblet cells are noted in 20% of tumors.[2] Dysplasia has been reported in up to 13% of cystadenomas. However, malignant transformation has not been reported in lesions that occur in the extrahepatic bile ducts.[24] Immunohistochemical stains are typically positive for cytokeratin, EMA, CEA, and CA 19-9 in the biliary epithelium. However, the ovarian-like stroma often reveals positivity for vimentin, muscle-specific actin, and desmin. Estrogen and progesterone receptors have also been reported in mesenchymal stromal cells of cystadenomas.[2,26,201]

BILIARY GRANULAR CELL TUMOR

Generally, granular cell tumors occur most commonly in the common bile duct, followed by the cystic duct and the hepatic ducts.[2,93] Ninety percent arise in females and 65 percent in blacks, with a mean age of 34 years.[2,94] Presenting symptoms include abdominal pain and jaundice. Grossly, these tumors are usually poorly demarcated, yellow-tan, firm lesions. Microscopically, they appear similar to those that occur elsewhere in the gastrointestinal tract. They are composed of large polygonal and occasionally, spindle-shaped cells with abundant granular eosinophilic cytoplasm and small round to oval nuclei. The cells may infiltrate the wall or form nests and clusters of cells that may obliterate the lumen. The overlying epithelium is usually normal in appearance but may exhibit mild hyperplasia.[2,93,94,97] Hyperplasia and reactive atypia of the intramural glands also occur. By immunohistochemistry, granular cell tumors are positive for inhibin alpha and S100.[2,93] Malignant granular cell tumors have been reported but not in the extrahepatic bile ducts.[2]

MISCELLANEOUS BENIGN TUMORS

Paragangliomas, leiomyomas, lipomas, and adenomyomas occurring in the extrahepatic bile ducts have all been described, mostly as single case reports. For further discussion of this topic, see under Endocrine Tumors of the Gallbladder and Extrahepatic Biliary Tree and under Nonepithelial Tumors.

▇ Malignant Tumors of the Extrahepatic Bile Ducts

CARCINOMA

Clinical Features

Adenocarcinoma of the extrahepatic bile ducts generally occurs in older people with an average age of 68.4 years. It occurs almost equally among both sexes and also equally among blacks and whites.[202] In Japan, males outnumber females by a ratio of 1.9 to 1. Most patients manifest obstructive jaundice, weight loss, elevated serum bilirubin, and right upper quadrant pain. In the United States, the ratio of gallbladder cancer to bile duct cancer is 2:1, but the incidence increases with age.

Carcinoma may develop anywhere in the bile ducts. However, 49% of cases occur in the upper third or hilar area, 25% in the middle third, and 19% in the lower third. Diffuse involvement occurs in 7% of cases.[2,202] Risk factors include primary sclerosing cholangitis, choledochal cysts, an anomalous pancreaticobiliary junction with reflux,[203] cholelithiasis, gallbladder carcinoma, cigarette smoking, infection with liver flukes (*Clonorchis sinensis* or *Opisthorchis viverrini*),[204,205] and use of oral contraceptives.[10] Adenocarcinoma represents the largest group of bile duct carcinomas. However, many different histologic types may occur (Table 29-4).[2]

TABLE 29–4. Histologic Types in 143 Cases of Extrahepatic Bile Duct Carcinomas*

Histologic Type	Number of Patients	Percent
Adenocarcinoma, well to moderately differentiated	108	76
Adenosquamous carcinoma	8	5.5
Papillary adenocarcinoma	6	4.1
Undifferentiated carcinoma	6	4.1
Adenocarcinoma, intestinal type	4	2.7
Adenocarcinoma, clear cell type	4	2.7
Small cell carcinoma	3	2
Mucinous carcinoma	2	1.3
Signet ring cell carcinoma	1	0.7
Adenocarcinoma, foveolar type	1	0.7
Total	143	100

*Cases obtained from the General Hospital of Mexico City, Mexico City, Mexico; Jackson Memorial Hospital, Miami, FL; University of Texas Southwestern Medical Center, Dallas, Texas; and personal consultation files (JA-S).
From Albores-Saavedra J, Delgado R, Henson DE: Well differentiated adenocarcinoma, gastric foveolar type, of the extrahepatic bile ducts: A previously unrecognized and distinctive morphologic variant of bile duct carcinoma. Ann Diagn Pathol 3:75-80, 1999.

Pathologic Features

Carcinomas often appear grossly as firm, ill-defined, tan-white areas with thickening, induration, ulceration, or stricturing of the wall. The mucosa may be granular, friable, or necrotic.[2,206]

Histologically, bile duct carcinomas are similar to those that develop in the gallbladder.[2,202,207-210] Adenocarcinomas are often desmoplastic, frequently involve the full thickness of the wall, and reveal perineural and intraneural invasion. Well-differentiated adenocarcinomas lined by cells with minimal atypia, basal nuclei, inconspicuous nucleoli, and a low nucleus-to-cytoplasm ratio may have a deceptively bland appearance. Dysplasia is often noted in adjacent noncancerous epithelium. However, an infiltrative pattern of growth, best seen with the use of cytokeratin stains, and evidence of perineural involvement are helpful features in establishing a correct diagnosis (Fig. 29-62). Adenocarcinomas are usually mucin positive and exhibit both intracellular and extracellular mucin production. Pancytokeratin, EMA, CA 19-9, CK 7, and dual CK 7/CK 20 immunoreactivity is present in normal and malignant glands. In addition, glands are usually CEA positive. In about a third of well- to moderately differentiated adenocarcinomas, endocrine cells are also present and can be demonstrated immunohistochemically with stains for chromogranin, synaptophysin, and serotonin or peptide hormones such as somatostatin, gastrin, and pancreatic polypeptide.[2]

Prognosis

The histologic grade of extrahepatic bile duct carcinomas has been shown to correlate with prognosis. These tumors are graded as well-differentiated, moderately differentiated, poorly differentiated, or undifferentiated. Papillary carcinomas, which may be invasive or noninvasive, have the most favorable prognosis. According to a National Cancer Institute study, the 5-year survival for these is 22%, compared with 8% for conventional adenocarcinomas.[2,202] Minimally invasive and noninvasive papillary carcinomas tend to behave similar to in situ carcinomas,[209] whereas widely invasive papillary carcinomas are associated with poor prognosis.[211] Perineural, vascular, and lymphatic invasion also correlates with decreased survival rates. The extent of disease should be reported with the use of the TNM staging system (Table 29-5).[2,20]

TABLE 29-5. TNM Classification of Tumors of the Extrahepatic Bile Ducts

Primary Tumor (T)			
TX	Primary tumor cannot be assesse		
T0	No evidence of primary tumor		
Tis	Carcinoma in situ		
T1	Tumor invades subepithelial connective tissue or fibromuscular layer		
	T1a	Tumor invades subepithelial connective tissue	
	T1b	Tumor invades fibromuscular layer	
T2	Tumor invades perifibromuscular connective tissue		
T3	Tumor invades adjacent structures: liver, pancreas, duodenum, gallbladder, colon, and stomach		
Regional Lymph Nodes (N)			
NX	Regional lymph nodes cannot be assessed		
N0	No regional lymph node metastasis		
N1	Metastasis in cystic duct, pericholedochal cyst, and/or hilar lymph nodes (i.e., in the hepatoduodenal ligament)		
N2	Metastasis in peripancreatic (head only), periduodenal, periportal, celiac, superior mesenteric, posterior mesenteric, and posterior pancreaticoduodenal lymph nodes		
Distant Metastasis (M)			
MX	Distant metastasis cannot be assessed		
M0	No distant metastasis		
M1	Distant metastasis		
Stage Grouping			
Stage 0	Tis	N0	M0
Stage I	T	N0	M0
Stage II	T2	N0	M0
Stage III	T1	N1, N2	M0
	T2	N1, N2	M0
Stage IVA	T3	Any N	M0
Stage IVB	Any T	Any N	M1

Adapted from Albores-Saavedra J, Henson DE, Sobin LH, et al: WHO International Histological Classification of Tumours, Histological Typing of Tumours of the Gallbladder and Extrahepatic Bile Ducts, 2nd ed. Berlin, Springer-Verlag, 1991, pp 25-26.

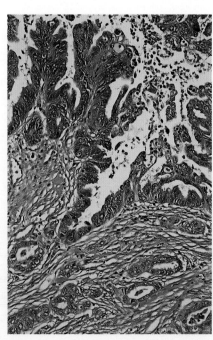

FIGURE 29-62. Adenocarcinoma, common bile duct. Papillary adenocarcinoma with invasion into the wall.

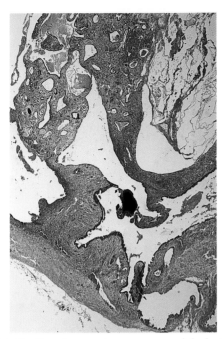

FIGURE 29–63. Cystadenocarcinoma, common bile duct. Multiple loculi are lined by dysplastic epithelium and highly cellular thickened walls. Invasive tumor was present elsewhere in this case.

CYSTADENOCARCINOMA

Cystadenocarcinomas occur more often in the extrahepatic bile ducts than in the gallbladder and are composed of multiloculated cysts lined by malignant columnar epithelium with a characteristic subepithelial mesenchymal stroma (Fig. 29-63).[2,21,23,24] It has been suggested that this malignant tumor originates from previously benign cystadenomas. Both benign and malignant epithelium may exist in the same locule. For further discussion, see under Malignant Epithelial Tumors of the Gallbladder.

CARCINOID TUMOR

Carcinoid tumor of the extrahepatic bile ducts represents only 0.1% to 0.2% of all gastrointestinal carcinoids.[2,210] No particular sex predilection has been noted, and the average age is 40 years. Abdominal pain and jaundice are typical presenting symptoms caused by early obstruction of the lumen. These tumors often appear as small, circumscribed, yellow nodules composed of small, uniform cells with homogeneous nuclei and inconspicuous nucleoli. The cells form nests, cords, or trabeculae that are surrounded by fibrous stroma and can involve the full thickness of the wall. Rarely, the tumor may be polypoid or pedunculated. Perineural and intraneural invasion is common.[210,212,213] Similar to other foregut carcinoids, the cells are immunoreactive with chromogranin and synaptophysin and sometimes with serotonin. However, they rarely express positivity for peptide hormones such as somatostatin, gastrin, cholecystokinin, and pancreatic polypeptide.[214-217] Although carcinoid tumors are regarded as low-grade malignancies, they can metastasize to lymph nodes and liver.

EMBRYONAL RHABDOMYOSARCOMA

The common bile duct is the most common location for this tumor, which is the most common neoplasm of bile ducts in children.[218-221] Patients may present with intermittent jaundice, abdominal distention, fever, and anorexia. Pathologic features are discussed under Malignant Mesenchymal Tumors of the Biliary Tract.

■ Tumor-like Lesions of the Extrahepatic Bile Ducts

HYPERPLASIA OF INTRAMURAL GLANDS OF EXTRAHEPATIC BILE DUCTS

In contrast to pyloric, intestinal, and squamous metaplasia, which are incidental microscopic findings, hyperplasia of intramural glands of the extrahepatic bile duct can lead to biliary obstruction and be symptomatic. Hyperplasia of intramural glands of the extrahepatic bile ducts is a reactive process that lacks specificity. It can be seen in primary sclerosing cholangitis, other nonspecific inflammatory lesions, and malignant epithelial neoplasms. Florid intramural gland hyperplasia can be confused with adenocarcinoma, especially when the reactive glands show perineural and intraneural invasion.[222]

CONGENITAL CYST

Congenital cysts and fusiform dilatations of the extrahepatic bile ducts are located predominantly in the common bile duct (choledochal cyst), where they are classified according to their shape and location.[223] Diagnosis is based primarily on the appearance of the bile ducts as assessed by imaging studies or by gross inspection because, histologically, they have no distinctive features (Fig. 29-64). Choledochal cysts have a female predominance. The most common clinical presentations involve abdominal pain and jaundice.[10,224,225] An anomalous pancreaticobiliary junction is reported in 64% to 97% of patients with choledochal cysts.[226] It is postulated that reflux of pancreatic enzymes into the bile duct weakens the wall by damaging intercellular junctions of the surface epithelium.[1] In addition, reflux of pancreatic enzymes can cause chronic inflammation with fibrosis and surface erosion. Many cysts contain calculi and mucobiliary material and are characterized by bacterial overgrowth. Over time, metaplastic transformation, dysplasia, and carcinoma may develop.

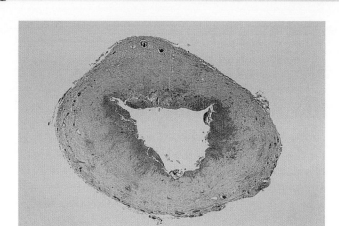

FIGURE 29–64. Choledochal cyst. Cross section shows fibrosis and thickening of the cyst wall. The surface is eroded and hemorrhagic.

Up to 15% of patients with choledochal cysts may develop carcinoma.[203,227-230] However, the incidence of carcinoma in choledochal cysts varies with age. It is estimated to be less than 0.1% in children under 10 years of age, 6.8% between 10 and 20 years of age, and 15% in patients older than 20 years of age.[2] Adenocarcinoma is the most common malignant tumor in choledochal cysts, but carcinoid tumors and rhabdomyosarcomas have also been reported.[203,227-230]

AMPUTATION (TRAUMATIC) NEUROMA

This is a lesion that develops as a result of cholecystectomy. It is typically located in the stump of the cystic duct. Histologically, amputation neuromas are similar to neuromas that occur at other locations. They are nodular and are composed of distorted nerve fibers separated by variable amounts of fibrous tissue.[231-238]

References

1. Weedon D: Pathology of the Gallbladder, 1st ed. Masson Monographs in Diagnostic Pathology. New York, Masson Publishers USA, 1984.
2. Albores-Saavedra J, Henson DE, Klimstra DS: Tumors of the Gallbladder, Extrahepatic Bile Ducts, and Ampulla of Vater. 3rd series. Fascicle 27. Washington, DC, Armed Forces Institute of Pathology, 2000.
3. Huizinga JD: Pathophysiology of gastrointestinal motility related to interstitial cells of Cajal. Am J Physiol 275:6381-6386, 1998.
4. Kindblom LG, Remoti HE, Aldenborg F, et al: Gastrointestinal pacemaker cell tumor (GIPACT). Gastrointestinal stromal tumors show phenotypic characteristics of the interstitial cells of Cajal. Am J Pathol 152:1259-1269, 1998.
5. Togari C, Okada T: The minute structure of the epithelium of the human gallbladder. Okajimas Folia Anat Jpn 25:1-12, 1953.
6. Albores-Saavedra J, Nadji M, Henson DE, et al: Intestinal metaplasia of the gallbladder: A morphologic and immunocytochemical study. Hum Pathol 17:614-620, 1986.
7. Mogilner JG, Dharan M, Siplovich L: Adenoma of the gallbladder in childhood. J Pediatr Surg 26:223-224, 1991.
8. Sato H, Mizushima M, Ito J, Doi K: Sessile adenoma of the gallbladder. Reappraisal of its importance as a precancerous lesion. Arch Pathol Lab Med 109:65-69, 1985.
9. Albores-Saavedra J, Vardaman C, Vuitch F: Non-neoplastic polypoid lesions and adenomas of the gallbladder. Pathol Ann 28:145-177, 1993.
10. Owen DA, Kelly JK: Neoplasms of the gallbladder. In Pathology of the Gallbladder, Biliary Tract and Pancreas, 1st ed. Philadelphia, WB Saunders, 2001, pp 286-310.
11. Christensen AH, Ishak KG: Benign tumors and pseudotumors of the gallbladder: Report of 180 cases. Arch Pathol 90:423-432, 1970.
12. Lin G, Hagerstrand I: Multiple adenomas of the gallbladder. Acta Pathol Microbiol Immunol Scand [A] 91:475-476, 1983.
13. Wada K, Tanaka M, Yamaguchi K, et al: Carcinoma and polyps of the gallbladder associated with Peutz-Jeghers syndrome. Dig Dis Sci 32:943-946, 1987.
14. Tantachamrun T, Borvonsombat S, Theetranont C: Gardner's syndrome associated with adenomatous polyp of the gallbladder. J Med Assoc Thai 62:441-447, 1979.
15. Nishihara K, Yamaguchi K, Hashimoto H, et al: Tubular adenoma of the gallbladder with squamoid spindle cell metaplasia. Report of 3 cases with immunohistochemical study. Acta Pathol Jpn 41:41-45, 1991.
16. Kushima R, Remmele W, Stolte M, et al: Pyloric gland type adenoma of the gallbladder with squamoid spindle cell metaplasia. Pathol Res Pract 192:963-969, 1996.
17. Bottger TK, Sorger E, Junzinger T: Progressive papillomatosis of the intrahepatic and extrahepatic bile ducts. Acta Chir Scand 155:125-129, 1989.
18. Eiss S, Dimaio D, Caedo JP: Multiple papillomas of the entire biliary tract: Case report. Ann Surg 152:320-324, 1960.
19. Hubens G, Delvaux G, Willems G, et al: Papillomatosis of the intra- and extrahepatic bile ducts with involvement of the pancreatic duct. Hepatogastroenterology 38:413-418, 1991.
20. Albores-Saavedra J, Henson DE, Sobin LH: Histological Typing of Tumours of the Gallbladder and Extrahepatic Bile Ducts, 2nd ed. Berlin, Springer-Verlag, 1991.
21. Ishak KG, Willis GW, Cummins SD, et al: Biliary cystadenoma and cystadenocarcinoma: Report of 14 cases and review of the literature. Cancer 38:322-338, 1977.
22. Akwari OE, Tucker A, Seigler HF, et al: Hepatobiliary cystadenoma with mesenchymal stroma. Ann Surg 211:18-27, 1990.
23. O'Shea JS, Shah D, Cooperman AM: Biliary cystadenocarcinoma of extrahepatic duct origin arising in previously benign cystadenoma. Am J Gastroenterol 82:1306-1310, 1987.
24. Devaney K, Goodman ZK, Ishak KG: Hepatobiliary cystadenoma and cystadenocarcinoma: A light microscopic and immunohistochemical study of 70 patients. Am J Surg Pathol 18:1078-1091, 1994.
25. Simmons T, Miller C, Pesigan A, et al: Cystadenoma of the gallbladder. Am J Gastroenterol 84:1427-1430, 1989.
26. Thomas JA, Scriven MW, Puntis MC, et al: Elevated CA19-9 levels in hepatobiliary cystadenoma with mesenchymal stroma. Two case reports with immunohistochemical confirmation. Cancer 70:1841-1846, 1992.
27. Albores-Saavedra J, Alcantra-Vazquez A, Cruz-Ortiz H, et al: The precursor lesions of invasive gallbladder carcinoma. Hyperplasia, atypical hyperplasia and carcinoma-in-situ. Cancer 45:919-927, 1980.
28. Yamagiwa H: Mucosal dysplasia of gallbladder. Isolated and adjacent lesions to carcinomas. Jpn J Cancer Res 80:238-243, 1989.
29. Yamagiwa H: Dysplasia of gallbladder. Its pathological significance. Acta Pathol Jpn 37:747-754, 1987.
30. Ojeda VJ, Shilkin KB, Walters MN-I: Premalignant epithelial lesions of the gallbladder: A prospective study of 120 cholecystectomy specimens. Pathology 17:451-454, 1985.
31. Yamamoto M, Nakajo S, Tahara E: Dysplasia of the gallbladder. Its histogenesis and correlation to gallbladder adenocarcinoma. Pathol Res Pract 185:454-460, 1989.
32. Albores-Saavedra J, Angeles-Angeles A, Manrique J, et al: Carcinoma in situ of the gallbladder: A clinicopathologic study of 18 cases. Am J Surg Pathol 8:323-333, 1984.
33. Yamaguchi K, Enjoji M: Carcinoma-in-situ of the gallbladder with superficial extension into the Rokitansky-Aschoff sinuses and mucous glands. Gastroenterol Jpn 27:765-772, 1992.
34. Nakajo S, Yamamoto M, Tahara E: Morphometric analysis of gallbladder adenoma and adenocarcinoma: With reference to histogenesis and adenoma-carcinoma sequence. Virchows Arch [A] 417:49-56, 1990.

35. Rudolph R, Cohen JJ: Cancer of the gallbladder in an 11 year old Navajo girl. J Pediatr Surg 7:66-67, 1972.
36. Hensen DE, Albores-Saavedra J, Corle D: Carcinoma of the gallbladder. Histologic types, stage of disease and survival rates. Cancer 70:1493-1497, 1992.
37. Miyazaki K, Date K, Imanmura S, et al: Familial occurrence of anomalous pancreaticobiliary duct union associated with gallbladder neoplasms. Am J Gastroenterol 84:176-181, 1989.
38. Kinoshita H, Nagata E, Hirohashi K, et al: Carcinoma of the gallbladder with an anomalous connection between the choledochus and the pancreatic duct. Cancer 54:762-769, 1984.
39. Tanaka K, Nishimura A, Yamada K, et al: Cancer of the gallbladder associated with anomalous junction of the pancreaticobiliary duct system without bile duct dilatation. Br J Surg 80:622-624, 1993.
40. Sumiyoshi K, Nagai E, Chigiiwa K, et al: Pathology of carcinoma of the gallbladder. World J Surg 15:315-321,1991.
41. Albores-Saavedra J, Molberg K, Henson DE: Unusual malignant epithelial tumors of the gallbladder. Semin Diagn Pathol 13:326-338, 1996.
42. Albores-Saavedra J, Henson DE, Angeles-Angeles A: Enteroendocrine cell differentiation in carcinoma of the gallbladder and mucinous cystadenocarcinoma of the pancreas. Pathol Res Pract 183:169-175, 1989.
43. Albores-Saavedra J, Nadji M, Henson DE: Intestinal type adenocarcinoma of the gallbladder. A clinicopathologic and immunohistochemical study of seven cases. Am J Surg Pathol 10:19-25, 1986.
44. Vardaman C, Albores-Saavedra J: Clear cell carcinoma of the gallbladder and extrahepatic bile ducts. Am J Surg Pathol 19:91-99, 1995.
45. Bittinger A, Altekruger I, Barth P: Clear cell carcinoma of the gallbladder. A histological and immunohistochemical study. Pathol Res Pract 191:1259-1265, 1995.
46. Maitra A, Murakata LA, Albores-Saavedra J: Immunoreactivity for hepatocyte paraffin 1 antibody in hepatoid adenocarcinomas of the gastrointestinal tract. Am J Clin Pathol 115:689-694, 2001.
47. Watanabe M, Hari Y, Najimi T, et al: Alpha-fetoprotein producing carcinoma of the gallbladder. Dig Dis Sci 38:561-564, 1993.
48. Sugaya Y, Sugaya H, Kuronuma Y, et al: A case of gallbladder carcinoma producing both alpha-fetoprotein (AFP) and carcinoembryonic antigen (CEA). Gastroenterol Jpn 24:325-331, 1989.
49. Murakata LA, Ishak KG, Nzeako UC: Clear cell carcinoma of the liver: A comparative immunohistochemical study with renal clear cell carcinoma. Mod Pathol 13:874-881, 2000.
50. Suster S, Huszar M, Herczeg E, et al: Adenosquamous carcinoma of the gallbladder with spindle cell features. A light microscopic and immunocytochemical study of a case. Histopathology 11:209-214, 1987.
51. Nishihara K, Nagai E, Iumi Y, et al: Adenosquamous carcinoma of the gallbladder. A clinicopathological immunohistochemical and flow cytometric study of twenty cases. Jpn J Cancer Res 85:389-399, 1994.
52. Nishihara K, Takashima M, Haraguchi M, et al: Adenosquamous carcinoma of the gallbladder with gastric foveolar-type epithelium. Pathol Int 45:250-256, 1995.
53. Hanada M, Shimizu H, Takami M: Squamous cell carcinoma of the gallbladder associated with squamous metaplasia and adenocarcinoma in situ of the mucosal columnar epithelium. Acta Pathol Jpn 36:1879-1886, 1986.
54. Albores-Saavedra J, Soriano J, Larraza-Hernandez O, et al: Oat cell carcinoma of the gallbladder. Hum Pathol 15:639-646, 1984.
55. Maitra A, Tascilar M, Hruban RH, et al: Small cell carcinoma of the gallbladder. A clinicopathologic, immunohistochemical, and molecular pathology study of 12 cases. Am J Surg Pathol 25:595-601, 2001.
56. Nishihara K, Tsuneyoshi M: Small cell carcinoma of the gallbladder: A clinicopathological, immunohistochemical and flow cytometrical study of 15 cases. Int J Oncol 3:901-908, 1993.
57. Nishihara K, Naga E, Tsuneyoshi M, et al: Small-cell carcinoma combined with adenocarcinoma of the gallbladder. A case report with immunohistochemical and flow cytometric studies. Arch Pathol Lab Med 118:177-181, 1994.
58. Papotti M, Cassoni P, Sapino A: Large cell neuroendocrine carcinoma of the gallbladder. Report of two cases. Am J Surg Pathol 24:1424-1428, 2000.
59. Albores-Saavedra J, Cruz-Ortiz H, Alcantara-Vazques A, et al: Unusual types of gallbladder carcinoma. A report of 16 cases. Arch Pathol Lab Med 105:287-293, 1981.
60. Guo KJ, Yamaguchi K, Enjoji M: Undifferentiated carcinoma of the gallbladder. A clinicopathologic, histochemical, and immunohistochemical study of 21 patients with a poor prognosis. Cancer 61:1872-1879, 1988.
61. Diebold-Berger S, Vaiton JC, Pache JC, et al: Undifferentiated carcinoma of the gallbladder. Report of a case with immunohistochemical findings. Arch Pathol Lab Med 119:279-282, 1995.
62. Nishihara K, Tsuneyoshi M: Undifferentiated spindle cell carcinoma of the gallbladder: A clinicopathologic, immunohistochemical and flow cytometric study of 11 cases. Hum Pathol 24:1298-1305, 1993.
63. Barone GW, Schaefer RF, Counce JS, et al: Gallbladder and gastric argyrophil carcinoid associated with a case of Zollinger-Ellison syndrome. Am J Gastroenterol 87:392-394, 1992.
64. Slany J, Wonger R, Kuhlmayer R: Multiple primary carcinoid of the gallbladder, pancreas and ileum with cardiac metastases. Z Gastroenterol 7:213-219, 1969.
65. Salimi Z, Sharafuddin M: Ultrasound appearance of primary carcinoid tumor of the gallbladder associated with carcinoid syndrome. J Clin Ultrasound 23:435-437, 1995.
66. Papotti M, Galliano D, Monga G: Signet-ring cell carcinoid of the gallbladder. Histopathology 71:255-259, 1990.
67. Modin IM, Sandor A: An analysis of 8305 cases of carcinoid tumors. Cancer 79:813-829, 1997.
68. Godwin JD II: Carcinoid tumors: An analysis of 2837 cases. Cancer 36:560-569, 1975.
69. Sinkre PA, Murakata L, Rabin L: Clear cell carcinoid tumor of the gallbladder: Another distinctive manifestation of von Hippel-Lindau disease. Am J Surg Pathol 25:1334-1339, 2001.
70. Wada A, Ishiguro S, Tateishi M, et al: Carcinoid tumor of the gallbladder associated with adenocarcinoma. Cancer 51:1911-1917, 1983.
71. Fish DE, Al-Izzi M, George PP, et al: Combined endocrine cell carcinoma and adenocarcinoma of the gallbladder. Histopathology 17:471-472, 1990.
72. Cho YU, Kim JY, Choi SK, et al: A case of hemorrhagic gallbladder paraganglioma causing acute cholecystitis. Yonsei Med J 42:352-356, 2001.
73. Caceres M, Mosquera LF, Shih JA, et al: Paraganglioma of the bile duct. South Med J 94:515-518, 2001.
74. Fine G, Raju UB: Paraganglia in the human gallbladder. Arch Pathol Lab Med 104:265-268, 1980.
75. Miller TA, Weber TR, Appelman HD: Paraganglioma of the gallbladder. Arch Surg 105:637-639, 1972.
76. Arbab AA, Brasfield R: Benign tumors of the gallbladder. Surgery 61:535-540, 1967.
77. Huff DS, Lischner HW, Go HC, et al: Unusual tumors in two boys with Wiskott-Aldrich-like syndrome. Lab Invest 40:305, 1979.
78. Toma P, Loy A, Pastorino C, et al: Leiomyomas of the gallbladder and splenic calcifications in an HIV-infected child. Pediatr Radiol 27:92-94, 1997.
78a. Monteforte-Muñoz H, Kapoor N, Albores-Saavedra J: Epstein-Barr virus-associated leiomyomatosis and post-transplant lymphoproliferative disorder in a child with severe combined immunodeficiency. Case report and review of the literature. Ped Development Pathol. In press.
79. Ortiz-Hidalgo C, DeLeon Bojorge B, Albores-Saavedra J: Stromal tumor of the gallbladder with phenotype of interstitial cells of Cajal. Am J Surg Pathol 24:1420-1423, 2000.
80. Barber KW, ReMine WH, Harrison EG, et al: Benign neoplasms of extrahepatic bile ducts, including papilla of Vater. Arch Surg 81:479-484, 1960.
81. Hofmann M, Schilling T, Heilmann P, et al: Multiple endocrine neoplasia associated with multiple lipomas. Med Klin 93:546-549, 1998.
82. Takagi I, Watanabe T, Shibamoto Y, et al: Lipoma of the gallbladder. Ryoikibetsu Shokogun Shirizu 9:514-515, 1996.
83. Furukawa H: Leiomyoma, lipoma, myxoma, and fibroma of the gallbladder. Ryoikibetsu Shokogun Shirizu 9:333-334, 1996.
84. Barber KW, ReMine WH, Harrison EG, et al: Benign neoplasms of extrahepatic bile ducts, including papilla of Vater. Arch Surg 81:479-484, 1960.
85. Mayorga M, Hernando M, Val-Bernal JF: Diffuse expansive cavernous hemangioma of the gallbladder. Gen Diagn Pathol 142:211-215, 1997.

86. Jones WP, Keller FS, Odrezin GT, et al: Venous hemangioma of the gallbladder. Gastrointest Radiol 12:319-321, 1987.

87. Furukawa H, Kanai Y, Mukai K, et al: Arteriovenous hemangioma of the gallbladder: CT and pathologic findings. AJR Am J Roentgenol 168:1383, 1997.

88. Amadori G, Micciolo R, Poletti A: A case of intra-abdominal multiple lymphangiomas in an adult in whom the immunological evaluation supported the diagnosis. Eur J Gastroenterol Hepatol 11:347-351, 1999.

89. Ohba K, Sugauchi F, Orito E, et al: Cystic lymphangioma of the gallbladder: A case report. J Gastroenterol Hepatol 10:693-696, 1995.

90. Choi JY, Kim MJ, Chung JJ, et al: Gallbladder lymphangioma: MR findings. Abdom Imaging 27:54-57, 2002.

91. Chen KTK: Osteomas of the gallbladder. Arch Pathol Lab Med 118:755-756, 1994.

92. Ortiz-Hidalgo C, Baquera-Heredia J: Osseous metaplasia in polypoid cholesterolosis. Am J Surg Pathol 24:895, 2000.

93. Murakata LA, Ishak KG: Expression of inhibin-alpha by granular cell tumors of the gallbladder and extrahepatic bile ducts. Am J Surg Pathol 25:1200-1203, 2001.

94. Aisner SC, Khaneja S, Ramirez O: Multiple granular cell tumors of the gallbladder and biliary tree. Arch Pathol Lab Med 106:470-471, 1982.

95. Lindberg G, Saboorian H, Housini I, et al: The clinicopathologic spectrum of granular cell tumors (abstract). Lab Invest 74:9A, 1996.

96. Yamaguchi K, Kuroki S, Daimaru Y, et al: Granular cell tumor of the gallbladder. Report of a case. Acta Pathol Jpn 35:687-691, 1985.

97. Yamashina M, Stemmerman GN: Granular cell tumor: Unusual cause for mucocele of gallbladder. Am J Gastroenterol 79:701-703, 1984.

98. Acebo E, Fernandez FA, Val-Bernal JF: Solitary neurofibroma of the gallbladder. A case report and review of the literature. Gen Diagn Pathol 143:337-340, 1998.

99. Morizumu H, Sano T, Hirose T, et al: Neurofibroma of the gallbladder seen as a papillary polyp. Acta Pathol Jpn 38:259-268, 1988.

100. Eggleston JF, Goldman RL: Neurofibroma and elastosis of the gallbladder. Report of an unusual case. Am J Gastroenterol 77:335-337, 1982.

101. Perentes E, Nakagawa Y, Ross GW, et al: Expression of epithelial membrane antigen in perineurial cells and their derivatives. An immunohistochemical study with multiple markers. Acta Neuropathol 75:160-165, 1987.

102. Oden B: Neurinoma of the common bile duct. Acta Chir Scand 108:393-397, 1955.

103. Rutgeerts P, Hendricks H, Geboes K, et al: Involvement of the upper digestive tract by systemic neurofibromatosis. Gastrointest Endosc 1:22-25, 1981.

104. Lukash WM, Morgan RI, Sennett CO, et al: Gastrointestinal neoplasms in von Recklinghausen's disease. Arch Surg 92:905-908, 1966.

105. Chetty R, Clark SP: Cholecystitis, cholelithiasis, and ganglioneuromatosis of the gallbladder: An unusual presentation of MEN type 2b. J Clin Pathol 46:1061-1063, 1993.

106. Carney JA, Sizemore GW, Hayles AM: Multiple endocrine neoplasia, type 2b. Pathobiol Annu 8:105-153, 1978.

107. al-Jaberi TM, al-Masri N, Tbukhi A: Adult rhabdomyosarcoma of the gallbladder: Case report and review of published works. Gut 35:854-856, 1994.

108. Willen R, Willen H: Primary sarcoma of the gallbladder. A light and electron-microscopical study. Virchows Arch A Pathol Anat Histol 396:91-102, 1982.

109. Mihara S, Matsumoto H, Tokunaga F, et al: Botryoid rhabdomyosarcoma of the gallbladder in a child. Cancer 49:812-818, 1982.

110. Aldabagh SM, Shibata CS, Taxy JB: Rhabdomyosarcoma of the common bile duct in an adult. Arch Pathol Lab Med 110:547-550, 1986.

111. Gruttadauria S, Doria C, Minervini MI, et al: Malignant fibrous histiocytoma of the gallbladder: Case report and review of the literature. Am Surg 67:714-717, 2001.

112. Tomono H, Fujioka S, Kato K, et al: Malignant fibrous histiocytoma of the gallbladder. Hepatogastroenterology 45:1468-1472, 1998.

113. Kristofferson AO, Domellof L, Emdin SO, et al: Malignant fibrous histiocytoma of the gallbladder: A case report. J Surg Oncol 23:56-59, 1983.

114. Kumar A, Singh MK, Kapur BM: Synchronous double malignant tumors of the gallbladder. A case report of squamous cell carcinoma with an angiosarcoma. Eur J Surg Oncol 20:63-67, 1994.

115. White J, Chan YF: Epithelioid angiosarcoma of the gallbladder. Histopathology 24:269-271, 1994.

116. Byers RJ, McMahon RF: Epithelioid angiosarcoma of the gallbladder. Histopathology 25:502-503, 1994.

117. Hittmair A, Sandbichler P, Totsch M, et al: Primary angiosarcoma of the gallbladder. Case report with review of the literature. Pathologe 23:279-281, 1991.

118. Kawai T, Hirose Y, Ainota T, et al: A case of hemangiosarcoma of the gallbladder. Nippon Shokakibyo Gakkai Zasshi 86:2611-2616, 1989.

119. Danikas D, Theodorou SJ, Singh R, et al: Leiomyosarcoma of the gallbladder: A case report. Am Surg 67:873-874, 2001.

120. Zeig DA, Memon MA, Kennedy DR, et al: Leiomyosarcoma of the gallbladder—a case report and review of the literature. Acta Oncol 37:212-214, 1998.

121. Kumar S, Gupta A, Shrivastava UK, et al: Leiomyosarcoma of the gallbladder: A case report. Indian J Pathol Microbiol 36:78-80, 1993.

122. Fotiadis C, Gugulakis A, Nakopoulou L, et al: Primary leiomyosarcoma of the gallbladder. Case report and review of the literature. HPB Surg 2:211-214, 1990.

123. Yasuma T, Yanaka M: Primary sarcoma of the gallbladder—report of three cases. Acta Pathol Jpn 21:285-304, 1971.

124. Mendoza-Marin M, Hoang MP, Albores-Saavedra J: Malignant stromal tumor of the gallbladder with interstitial cells of Cajal phenotype. Arch Pathol Lab Med 126:481-483, 2002.

125. Lesman AJ, Golub R, Giron JA, et al: Primary Kaposi's sarcoma of the gallbladder in AIDS. J Clin Gastroenterol 17:352-353, 1993.

126. Enad JG, Lapa JC, Jaklic B, et al: Kaposi's sarcoma of the gallbladder. Mil Med 157:559-561, 1992.

127. Eriguchi N, Aoyagi S, Hara M, et al: A so-called carcinosarcoma of the gallbladder in a patient with multiple anomalies—a case report. Kurume Med J 46:175-179, 1999.

128. Rys J, Kruczak A, Iliszko M, et al: Sarcomatoid carcinoma (carcinosarcoma) of the gallbladder. Gen Diagn Pathol 143:321-325, 1998.

129. Fagot H, Fabre JM, Ramos J, et al: Carcinosarcoma of the gallbladder. A case report and review of the literature. J Clin Gastroenterol 18:314-316, 1994.

130. Ishihara T, Kawano H, Takahashi M, et al: Carcinosarcoma of the gallbladder. A case report with immunohistochemical and ultrastructural studies. Cancer 66:992-997, 1990.

131. Henson DE, Albores-Saavedra J, Corle D: Carcinoma of the gallbladder. Histologic types, stage of disease and survival rates. Cancer 70:1493-1497, 1992.

132. DeSimone P, Mainente P, Bedin N: Gallbladder melanoma mimicking acute acalculous cholecystitis. Surg Endosc 14:593, 2000.

133. Laitio M: Melanogenic metaplasia of the gallbladder epithelium. Acta Chir Scand 141:57-60, 1975.

134. Higgins CM, Strutton CM: Malignant melanoma of the gallbladder—does primary melanoma exist? Pathology 27:312-314, 1995.

135. Ricci R, Maggiano N, Martini M, et al: Primary malignant melanoma of the gallbladder in dysplastic naevus syndrome. Virchows Arch 438:159-165, 2001.

136. McCluggage WG, Mackel E, McCusker G: Primary low grade malignant lymphoma of mucosa-associated lymphoid tissue of gallbladder. Histopathology 29:285-287, 1996.

137. Bickel A, Eitan A, Tsilman B, et al: Low-grade B cell lymphoma of mucosa-associated lymphoid tissue (MALT) arising in the gallbladder. Hepatogastroenterology 46:1643-1646, 1999.

138. Tomori H, Nagahama M, Miyazato H, et al: Mucosa-associated lymphoid tissue (MALT) of the gallbladder: A clinicopathological correlation. Int Surg 84:144-150, 1999.

139. Abe Y, Takatsuki H, Okada Y, et al: Mucosa-associated lymphoid tissue type lymphoma of the gallbladder associated with acute myeloid leukemia. Intern Med 38:442-444, 1999.

140. Papalampros E, Kalovidouris A, Pangalis GA: Primary non-Hodgkin's lymphoma of the gallbladder. Leuk Lymphoma 40:123-131, 2000.

141. Orton DF, Saigh JA: CT of Hodgkin's lymphoma limited to the gallbladder. Abdom Imaging 21:238-239, 1996.

142. Laurino L, Melato M: Malignant angioendotheliomatosis (angiotropic lymphoma) of the gallbladder. Virchows Arch [A] 417:243-246, 1990.

143. Myung SJ, Kim MH, Shim KN, et al: Detection of *Helicobacter pylori* DNA in human biliary tree and its association with hepatolithiasis. Dig Dis Sci 45:1405-1412, 2000.

144. Mendez-Sanchez N, Pichardo R, Gonzalez J, et al: Lack of association between *Helicobacter* spp. colonization and gallstone disease. J Clin Gastroenterol 32:138-141, 2001.

145. Arnaout AH, Abbas SH, Shousha S: *Helicobacter pylori* is not identified in areas of gastric metaplasia of gallbladder. J Pathol 160:333-334, 1990.

146. Dong XD, DeMatos P, Prieto VG, et al: Melanoma of the gallbladder. A review of cases seen at Duke University Medical Center. Cancer 85:32-39, 1999.

147. Lang RG, Bailey EM, Sober AJ: Acute cholecystitis from metastatic melanoma to the gallbladder in a patient with a low risk melanoma. Br J Dermatol 136:279-282, 1997.

148. McFadden PM, Krementz ET, McKinnon WM, et al: Metastatic melanoma of the gallbladder. Cancer 44:1802-1808, 1979.

149. Coskun F, Cetinkaya M, Cengiz O, et al: Metastatic carcinoma of the gallbladder due to renal cell carcinoma in the ectopic kidney (letter). Acta Chir Belg 95:56-58, 1995.

150. Pagano S, Ruggeri P, Franzoso F, et al: Unusual renal cell carcinoma metastasis to the gallbladder. Urology 45:867-869, 1995.

151. Nagler J, McSherry CK, Miskovitz P: Asymptomatic metachronous metastatic renal cell adenocarcinoma to the gallbladder. Report of a case and guidelines for evaluation of intraluminal polypoid gallbladder masses. Dig Dis Sci 39:2476-2479, 1994.

152. Albores-Saavedra J, Gould E, Manivel-Rodriguez C, et al: Chronic cholecystitis with lymphoid hyperplasia. La Rev Invest Clin (Mex) 41:159-164, 1989.

153. Yamaguchi K, Enjoji M: Gallbladder polyps: Inflammatory, hyperplastic and neoplastic types. Surg Pathol 1:203-213, 1988.

154. Goodman ZG, Ishak KG: Xanthogranulomatous cholecystitis. Am J Surg Pathol 5:653-659, 1991.

155. Guo KJ, Yamaguchi K, Izomi Y, et al: Xanthogranulomatous cholecystitis: A clinicopathologic study of 68 cases. Surg Pathol 1:241-248, 1988.

156. Roberts KM, Parsons MA: Xanthogranulomatous cholecystitis: Clinicopathological study of 13 cases. J Clin Pathol 40:412-417, 1987.

157. Kim PN, Lee SH, Gong GY, et al: Xanthogranulomatous cholecystitis: Radiologic finding with histologic correlation that focuses on intramural nodules. Am J Roentgenol 172:949-953, 1999.

158. Ros PR, Goodman ZD: Xanthogranulomatous cholecystitis versus gallbladder carcinoma. Radiology 203:10-12, 1997.

159. Yoshida J, Chijiiwa K, Shimura H, et al: Xanthogranulomatous cholecystitis versus gallbladder cancer: Clinical differentiating factors. Am Surg 63:367-371, 1997.

160. Lozez JI, Elizalde JM, Calvo MA: Xanthogranulomatous cholecystitis associated with gallbladder adenocarcinoma. A clinicopathologic study of 5 cases. Tumori 77:358-360, 1991.

161. Hide G, Desai S, Bloxham CA: Malakoplakia of the gallbladder: Imaging and histological features. Clin Radiol 56:326-328, 2001.

162. Charpentier P, Prade M, Bognel C, et al: Malacoplakia of the gallbladder. Hum Pathol 14:827-828, 1983.

163. Hanada M, Tujimura T, Kimura M: Cholecystic granulomas in gallstone disease. A clinicopathologic study of 17 cases. Acta Pathol Jpn 31:221-231, 1981.

164. Hoang MP, Murakata LA, Padilla-Rodriguez AL, et al: Metaplastic lesions of the extrahepatic bile ducts: A morphologic and immunohistochemical study. Mod Pathol 14:1119-1125, 2001.

165. Laitio M: Goblet cells, enterochromaffin cells, superficial gastric-type epithelium and antral-type glands in the gallbladder. Beitr Pathol Bd 156:343-358, 1975.

166. Albores-Saavedra J, Henson DE: Pyloric gland metaplasia with perineural invasion of the gallbladder. A lesion that can be confused with adenocarcinoma. Cancer 86:2627-2631, 1999.

167. Albores-Saavedra J, Nadji M, Henson DE, et al: Intestinal metaplasia of the gallbladder. A morphologic and immunocytochemical study. Hum Pathol 17:614-620, 1986.

168. Yamamoto M, Nakajo S, Ito M, et al: Primary mucosal hyperplasia of the gallbladder. Acta Pathol Jpn 38:393-398, 1988.

169. Albores-Saavedra J, Defortuna SM, Smothermon WE: Primary papillary hyperplasia of the gallbladder and cystic and common bile ducts. Hum Pathol 21:228-231, 1990.

170. Woodard BH: Adenomyomatous hyperplasia of the human gallbladder. South Med J 75:533-535, 1982.

171. Albores-Saavedra J, Henson DL: Adenomyomatous hyperplasia of the gallbladder with perineural invasion. Arch Pathol Lab Med 119:1173-1176, 1995.

172. Kasahara Y, Sonobe N, Tomiyoshi H, et al: Adenomyomatosis of the gallbladder. A clinical survey of 30 surgically treated patients. Arch Jpn Chir 61:190-198, 1992.

173. Lauwers GY, Wahl SJ, Scott GV, et al: Papillary mucinous adenoma arising in adenomyomatous hyperplasia of the gallbladder. J Clin Pathol 48:965-967, 1995.

174. Aldridge MC, Gruffaz F, Castaing D: Adenomyomatosis of the gallbladder. A premalignant lesion? Surgery 109:107-110, 1991.

175. Ootani T, Shirai Y, Tzukada K, et al: Relationship between gallbladder carcinoma and segmental type of adenomyomatosis of the gallbladder. Cancer 69:2647-2652, 1992.

176. Katoh T, Nakai T, Hayashi S, et al: Noninvasive carcinoma of the gallbladder arising in localized type adenomyomatosis. Am J Gastroenterol 83:670-674, 1988.

177. Ulich TR, Kollin M, Simmons GE, et al: Adenomyoma of the papilla of Vater. Arch Pathol Lab Med 111:388-390, 1987.

178. Price RJ, Stewart TE, Foley D, et al: Sonography of polypoid cholesterolosis. Am J Radiol 139:1197-1198, 1982.

179. Ukai K, Akita Y, Mizuno S, et al: Cholesterol polyp of the gallbladder showing rapid growth and atypical changes. A case report. Hepatogastroenterology 39:371-373, 1992.

180. Boyle L, Gallivan MVE, Chun B, et al: Heterotopia of gastric mucosa and liver involving the gallbladder. Arch Pathol Lab Med 116:138-142, 1992.

181. Vallera DU, Dawson PJ, Path FR: Gastric heterotopia in the gallbladder. Case report and review of literature. Pathol Res Pract 188:49-52, 1992.

182. Uchiyama S, Imai S, Suzuki T, et al: Heterotopic gastric mucosa of the gallbladder. J Gastroenterol 30:543-546, 1995.

183. Leyman P, Saint-Marc O, Hannoun L, et al: Heterotopic gastric mucosa presenting as gallbladder polyps. Acta Chir Belg 96:128-129, 1996.

184. Inoue Y, Shibata T, Miinobu T, et al: Heterotopic gastric mucosa in the gallbladder: Sonographic and CT findings. Abdom Imaging 25:198-200, 2000.

185. Hamazaki K, Fujiwara T: Heterotopic gastric mucosa in the gallbladder. J Gastroenterol 35:376-381, 2000.

186. Xeropotamos N, Skopelitou AS, Batsis C, et al: Heterotopic gastric mucosa together with intestinal metaplasia and moderate dysplasia in the gallbladder: Report of two clinically unusual cases with literature review. Gut 48:719-723, 2001.

187. Martinez-Urratia MJ, Vasques EJ, Larrauri J, et al: Gastric heterotopy of the biliary tract. J Pediatr Surg 25:356-357, 1990.

188. Kondi-Paphiti A, Antoniou AG, Kotsis T, et al: Aberrant pancreas in the gallbladder wall. Eur Radiol 7:1064-1066, 1997.

189. Murakami M, Tsutsumi Y: Aberrant pancreatic tissue accompanied by heterotopic gastric mucosa in the gallbladder. Pathol Int 49:580-582, 1999.

190. Bhana BD, Chetty R: Heterotopic pancreas—an unusual cause of cholecystitis. S Afr J Surg 37:105-107, 1999.

191. Inceoglu R, Dosluoglu HH, Kullu S, et al: An unusual cause of hydropic gallbladder and biliary colic-heterotopic pancreatic tissue in the cystic duct: Report of a case and review of the literature. Surg Today 23:532-534, 1993.

192. Matsuoka J, Tanaka N, Kojima K, et al: A case of traumatic neuroma of the gallbladder in the absence of previous surgery and cholelithiasis. Acta Med Okayama 50:273-277, 1996.

193. Erwald R: Gardner's syndrome with adenoma of the common bile duct: A case report. Acta Chir Scand 520:63-68, 1984.

194. Jarvinen H, Nyberg M, Peltokallio P: Biliary involvement in familial adenomatosis coli. Dis Colon Rectum 26:525-528, 1983.

195. Parker MC, Knight M: Peutz-Jeghers syndrome causing obstructive jaundice due to polyp in common bile duct. J Roy Soc Med 76:701-703, 1983.

196. Helling TS, Strobach RS: The surgical challenge of papillary neoplasia of the biliary tract. Liver Transpl Surg 2:290-298, 1996.

197. Buckley JG, Salimi Z: Villous adenoma of the common bile duct. Abdom Imaging 18:245-246, 1993.

198. Jennings PE, Rode J, Coral A, et al: Villous adenoma of the common hepatic duct: The role of ultrasound in management. Gut 31:558-560, 1990.

199. Loh A, Kamar S, Dickson GH: Solitary benign papilloma (papillary adenoma) of the cystic duct: A rare cause of biliary colic. Br J Clin Pract 48:167-168, 1994.

200. Ferrell LD, Beckstead JH: Paneth-like cells in an adenoma and adenocarcinoma in the ampulla of Vater. Arch Pathol Lab Med 115:956-958, 1991.

201. Wheeler DA, Edmondson HA: Cystadenoma with mesenchymal stroma (CMS) of the liver and bile ducts: A clinicopathologic study of 17 cases, 4 with malignant change. Cancer 56:1434-1445, 1985.

202. Vuitch F, Battifora H, Albores-Saavedra J: Demonstration of steroid hormone receptors in pancreato-biliary mucinous cystic neoplasms (abstract). Lab Invest 68:114A, 1993.

203. Oguchi Y, Okada A, Nakamura T, et al: Histopathologic studies of congenital dilatation of the bile duct as related to an anomalous junction of the pancreaticobiliary ductal system: Clinical and experimental studies. Surgery 103:168-173, 1988.

204. Carriaga MT, Henson DE: Liver, gallbladder, extrahepatic bile ducts, and pancreas. Cancer 75:171-190, 1995.

205. Sher L, Iwatsuki S, Lebeau G, et al: Hilar cholangiocarcinoma associated with clonorchiasis. Dig Dis Sci 34:1121-1123, 1989.

206. Haswell-Elkins MR, Staarug S, Elkins DB: *Opisthorchis viverrini* infection in Northeast Thailand and its relationship to cholangiocarcinoma. J Gastroenterol Hepatol 7:538-548, 1992.

207. Todoroki T, Okamura T, Fukao K, et al: Gross appearance of carcinoma of the main hepatic duct and its prognosis. Surg Gynecol Obstet 150:33-40, 1980.

208. Henson DE, Albores-Saavedra J, Corle D: Carcinoma of the extrahepatic bile ducts: Histologic types, stage of disease, grade, and survival rates. Cancer 70:1498-1501, 1992.

209. Albores-Saavedra J, Murakata L, Krueger JE, et al: Non-invasive and minimally invasive papillary carcinomas of the extrahepatic bile ducts. Cancer 89:508-515, 2000.

210. Yamaguchi K, Enjoji M, Nakayama F: Cancer of the extrahepatic bile duct: A clinicopathologic study of immunohistochemistry for CEA, CA 19-9, and p21. World J Surg 12:11-17, 1988.

211. Hoang MP, Murakata L, Katabi N, et al: Invasive papillary carcinomas of the extrahepatic bile ducts: A clinicopathologic and immunohistochemical study of 13 cases. Mod Pathol 15:1251-1258, 2002.

212. Bergdahl L: Carcinoid tumor of the biliary tract. Aust N Z J Surg 46:136-138, 1976.

213. Chamberlain RS, Blumgart LH: Carcinoid tumors of the extrahepatic bile duct. A rare cause of malignant biliary obstruction. Cancer 86:1959-1965, 1999.

214. Rugge M, Sonego F, Militello C, et al: Primary carcinoid tumor of the cystic and common bile ducts. Am J Surg Pathol 16:802-807, 1992.

215. Maitora A, Krueger JE, Tascilar M, et al: Carcinoid tumors of the extrahepatic bile ducts: A study of seven cases. Am J Surg Pathol 24:1501-1510, 2000.

216. Goodman ZD, Albores-Saavedra J, Lundblad DM: Somatostatinoma of the cystic duct. Cancer 53:498-502, 1984.

217. Yoshida T, Matsumoto T, Morii Y, et al: Carcinoid somatostatinoma of the papilla of Vater: A case report. Hepatogastroenterology 45:451-453, 1998.

218. Davis GL, Kissane JM, Ishak KG: Embryonal rhabdomyosarcoma (sarcoma botryoides) of the biliary tree: Report of five cases and a review of the literature. Cancer 24:333-342, 1969.

219. Akers DR, Needham ME: Sarcoma botryoides (rhabdomyosarcoma) of the bile ducts with survival. J Pediatr Surg 6:474-479, 1971.

220. Ruymann FB, Raney B, Crist WM, et al: Rhabdomyosarcoma of the biliary tree in childhood: A report from the intergroup Rhabdomyosarcoma Study. Cancer 56:575-581, 1985.

221. Aldabagh SM, Shibata CS, Taxy JB: Rhabdomyosarcoma of the common bile duct in an adult. Arch Pathol Lab Med 110:547-550, 1986.

222. Katabi N, Albores-Saavedra J: The extrahepatic bile duct lesions in end-stage primary sclerosing cholangitis. Am J Surg Pathol 27:349-355, 2003.

223. Vick DJ, Goodman ZD, Deavers MT, et al: Ciliated hepatic foregut cyst. A study of six cases and review of the literature. Am J Surg Pathol 123:1115-1117, 1999.

224. Todani T, Watanabe Y, Narusue M, et al: Congenital bile duct cysts: Classification, operative procedures and review of thirty-seven cases, including cancer arising from choledochal cyst. Am J Surg 134:263-269, 1977.

225. Katyal D, Lees GM. Choledochal cysts: A retrospective review of 28 patients and a review of the literature. Can J Surg 35:584-588, 1992.

226. O'Neill JA Jr: Choledochal cyst. Curr Probl Surg 29:361-410, 1992.

227. Voyles CR, Smadja C, Shands C, et al: Carcinoma in choledochal cysts. Age-related incidence. Arch Surg 118:986-988, 1983.

228. Holzinger F, Baer HU, Schilling M, et al: Congenital bile duct cyst: A premalignant lesion of the biliary tract associated with adenocarcinoma. A case report. Z Gastroenterol 34:382-385, 1996.

229. Komi N, Tamura T, Miyoshi Y, et al: Nationwide survey of cases of choledochal cyst. Analysis of coexistent anomalies, complications and surgical treatment in 645 cases. Surg Gastroenterol 3:69-72, 1984.

230. Komi N, Tamura T, Miyoshi Y, et al: Histochemical and immunohistochemical studies in development of biliary carcinoma in forty-seven patients with choledochal cyst—special reference to intestinal metaplasia in the biliary duct. Jpn J Surg 15:273-278, 1985.

231. Patil KK, Omojola MF, Khurana P, et al: Embryonal rhabdomyosarcoma within a choledochal cyst. Can Assoc Radiol J 43:145-148, 1992.

232. Larson DM, Storsteen KA: Traumatic neuroma of the bile ducts with intrahepatic extension causing obstructive jaundice. Hum Pathol 15:287-290, 1984.

233. Sano T, Hirose T, Kagawa N, et al: Polypoid traumatic neuroma of the gallbladder. Arch Pathol Lab Med 109:574-576, 1985.

234. Elhag AM, al Awadi NZ: Amputation neuroma of the gallbladder. Histopathology 21:586-587, 1992.

235. Sieratzki JS: Traumatic neuroma. Hum Pathol 17:866, 1986.

236. Takahara N, Saito S, Yoshida M, et al: A case of amputation neuroma of the biliary tract with obstructive jaundice. Gastroenterol Jpn 16:521-526, 1981.

237. Arai A: A case of obstructive jaundice by neuromas in the common bile duct. Acta Hepatol Jpn 25:813-817, 1984.

238. Peison B, Benisch B: Traumatic neuroma of the cystic duct in the absence of previous surgery. Hum Pathol 16:1168-1169, 1985.

CHAPTER 30

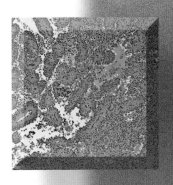

Inflammatory, Infectious, and Other Non-neoplastic Disorders of the Pancreas

BRUCE M. WENIG • CLARA S. HEFFESS

Introduction

The classification of non-neoplastic disorders of the pancreas is listed in Table 30-1. These include inflammatory and infectious processes, congenital abnormalities, anatomic variations in the normal distribution of the pancreatic duct system, hereditary diseases, and acquired diseases. Inflammatory conditions of the pancreas are the most common of these disorders. This chapter focuses primarily on inflammatory conditions that surgical pathologists are most likely to encounter in practice; also included is a discussion of less common inflammatory, infectious, and acquired diseases of the pancreas.

Inflammatory Disorders of the Pancreas

ACUTE PANCREATITIS

Acute pancreatitis is an acute inflammatory disorder associated with abdominal pain and elevated pancreatic enzymes in blood or urine.[1] Acute pancreatitis is divided into acute interstitial pancreatitis and acute hemorrhagic pancreatitis. *Acute interstitial pancreatitis* is defined as the presence of acute intrapancreatic inflammation with or without peripancreatic inflammation but without disruption of the pancreatic microvasculature (pancreas remains well perfused). Acute interstitial pancreatitis is generally considered to represent a clinically "mild" form of pancreatitis. It is not associated with local or systemic complications and is usually successfully managed medically. This disorder has an excellent prognosis with extremely low mortality rates. *Acute hemorrhagic pancreatitis* is defined by disruption of the pancreatic microcirculation that results in necrotizing pancreatitis. Acute hemorrhagic pancreatitis is considered to represent clinically a "severe" form of pancreatitis. It is more often associated with local or systemic complications and often requires surgical intervention. This condition is associated with higher rates of morbidity and mortality.

Clinical Features

Acute pancreatitis is an uncommon condition. Its incidence is difficult to determine precisely because the

TABLE 30-1. Classification of Non-neoplastic Lesions of the Pancreas

Congenital Abnormalities of the Exocrine Pancreas
Aplasia and hypoplasia (congenital short pancreas)
Duct abnormalities
Pancreas divisum
Annular pancreas
Congenital cysts
  Solitary
  Multiple
Choledochal cyst

Hereditary Diseases
Cystic fibrosis
Diabetes mellitus*
Shwachman-Diamond syndrome
Johanson-Blizzard syndrome
Sideroblastic anemia and exocrine pancreatic insufficiency
Enzymatic deficiencies
Hereditary pancreatitis

Infectious Diseases
Bacteria, fungi, viruses, protozoa, others

Pancreatitis
Acute interstitial pancreatitis
Acute hemorrhagic pancreatitis
Chronic pancreatitis

Acquired Lesions/Diseases
Age-related alterations
Heterotopic pancreas
Pseudocysts
True (non-neoplastic) cysts
  Lymphoepithelial cyst
  Enterogenous cyst
  Endometrial cyst
  Parasitic cyst
Hamartoma
Inflammatory pseudotumor

*Not strictly a hereditary disease.

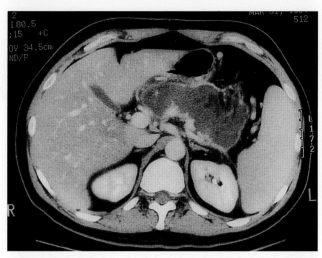

FIGURE 30–1. CT scan of acute pancreatitis showing generalized enlargement of the pancreas.

distinction between acute and chronic pancreatitis is not always possible on clinical grounds. Furthermore, patients with mild to moderate levels of disease are not always recognized clinically. Features of acute pancreatitis vary according to the underlying cause. Choledocholithiasis represents the single most common cause of acute pancreatitis; women are affected more often than men, and the age of peak incidence is between 50 and 60 years.[2] In contrast, acute pancreatitis secondary to alcohol consumption is more common among men than among women. Most often, acute pancreatitis has a rapid onset and is accompanied by upper abdominal pain, epigastric tenderness,[3] and other commonly associated signs and symptoms such as nausea, vomiting, and low-grade fever.

In severe hemorrhagic pancreatitis, blood may dissect into the retroperitoneal space in the flank or periumbilical area, resulting in a bluish discoloration referred to as Grey Turner's or Cullen's sign, respectively; this finding usually occurs a few days after the onset of disease.[3] Acute attacks of pancreatitis tend to be recurrent.[3] Radiologic features include generalized enlargement of the pancreas (Fig. 30-1). Abnormal laboratory studies include elevated serum amylase (hyperamylasemia) and lipase, transient hyperglycemia, and hypertriglyceridemia in the presence of normal or near-normal serum cholesterol levels.[3,4] Hypocalcemia occurs in approximately 25% of cases.[5] Patients with acute pancreatitis are usually treated by medical management, including supportive care with fluid replacement, relief of pain with parenteral injections of meperidine, and reduction of pancreatic secretions by avoidance of oral alimentation until the inflammation has subsided. Superimposed infection, seen much more frequently in acute hemorrhagic pancreatitis than in acute interstitial pancreatitis, requires appropriate antibiotic therapy.[6] The mortality rate for acute pancreatitis averages from 9% to 10%.[7,8] In general, patients with pancreatic necrosis have a higher mortality rate than do those with interstitial pancreatitis.[9] Systemic complications of acute pancreatitis, seen more often with acute hemorrhagic pancreatitis, include cardiovascular collapse, respiratory failure, renal failure, and sepsis.[9] Prognostic predictors of severity in acute pancreatitis include Acute Physiology and Chronic Health Evaluation (APACHE-II) and Ranson's signs.[9-11]

Pathogenesis

The causes of acute pancreatitis are listed in Table 30-2. Biliary tract disease and alcohol account for 80% to 90% of cases of acute pancreatitis.[2] Another 10% are the result of other causes, such as hyperlipidemia, various drugs (particularly those associated with acquired immunodeficiency syndrome [AIDS] treatment), infections, autoimmune disease, hypercalcemia, duct obstruction, and impaired pancreatic perfusion.[2,12] Infectious agents include various viruses, parasites, and bacteria (see under Infectious Diseases of the Pancreas).[3,13] Further, several autoimmune diseases, such as systemic

TABLE 30-2. Etiology of Acute Pancreatitis
Obstruction
Biliary tract stones
Anatomic anomalies (e.g., pancreas divisum, choledochal cysts, others)
Neoplasms (e.g., pancreatic carcinoma, ampullary or periampullary neoplasms)
Ethanol abuse
Drug-associated
Metabolic
Hyperlipidemia
Hypercalcemia
Others
Infection
Viral (e.g., HIV)
Parasitic (e.g., ascariasis)
Bacteria (e.g., *Mycoplasma* species)
Trauma
Autoimmune
Familial
Pregnancy
Miscellaneous
Idiopathic

lupus erythematosus (SLE), have been associated with acute pancreatitis.[2] A small proportion of cases are idiopathic.[2]

Recent studies have shown a possible molecular basis for acute pancreatitis. Abnormalities in intracellular transport of calcium and secretion of enzymes may play a role in the development of acute pancreatitis as well.[14,15] Trypsinogen activation is considered to be a key step in acute pancreatitis.[16] The activation of pancreatic enzymes before their secretion from acinar cells is felt to represent one of the most commonly reported theories for the pathogenesis of acute pancreatitis.[17]

Pathologic Features

GROSS PATHOLOGY

The pancreas typically appears swollen, pale, and indurated. On cut section, lobules appear separated by edematous interstitial tissue; purulent material may be present. Fat necrosis may be evident as white opaque areas within peripancreatic tissue. Hemorrhage is a feature associated with acute hemorrhagic pancreatitis. In hemorrhagic pancreatitis, sharply defined areas of relatively normal-appearing pancreas may persist between areas of red to reddish black necrotic tissue.

MICROSCOPIC PATHOLOGY

In general, acute pancreatitis is a clinical diagnosis. Thus, biopsy material is seldom obtained from patients with this disorder. Nevertheless, necrosis is a constant feature. It may involve a small part of the gland, most of the gland, or, rarely, the entire gland.

Acute interstitial pancreatitis is characterized by a diffuse acute inflammatory cell infiltrate, consisting primarily of polymorphonuclear leukocytes in the interstitial tissue, edema, and a fibrinous exudate. Focal or diffuse ductular dilatation may also occur. Secondary metaplastic changes, such as mucous cell metaplasia, hyperplasia, and squamous metaplasia, may be noted as well. Vascular thrombosis and acute necrotizing arteritis are not features of interstitial pancreatitis.

The essential feature of hemorrhagic pancreatitis is necrosis. It may involve all components of the pancreas, including the acini and ducts, interstitial tissue, vascular structures, nerves, islets of Langerhans, and adipose tissue (Fig. 30-2). Necrosis tends to be patchy, seldom involves the entire gland, and may be present in a periductal or perilobular distribution. The degree of inflammation varies with the duration of illness. In early

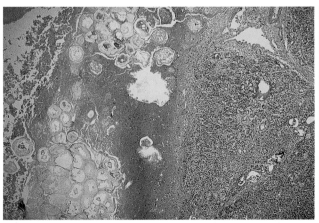
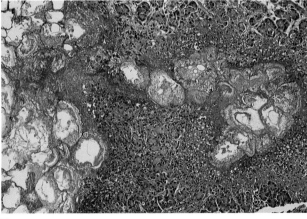

A **B**

FIGURE 30–2. Acute pancreatitis. **A,** The necrosis tends to be patchy and seldom involves the entire gland. To the left is marked necrosis of the pancreas; toward the right, focal necrosis is seen within intact pancreatic parenchyma. **B,** Higher magnification shows patchy intra-acinar necrosis with a minimal amount of inflammation.

stages of disease or when survival is short, a relatively minimal number of (acute) inflammatory cells are seen; over time, the amount of polymorphonuclear leukocyte infiltration becomes marked, especially in the interlobular septa. Vascular thrombosis and acute necrotizing arteritis may be noted as well.

Acute pancreatitis may be associated with fat necrosis, pseudocysts, and pancreatic abscess formation, all of which are related to the release of digestive enzymes from acinar cells. The release of lipase results in fat necrosis in peripancreatic tissues and subcutaneous fat. Pseudocysts represent extrapancreatic collections of pancreatic juice that result from duct rupture (described later in the section on chronic pancreatitis). Abscesses may develop and consist of necrotic connective tissue containing activated digestive enzymes and a mixed bacterial flora; this complication is associated with significant morbidity and mortality. Complete restitution of the pancreatic parenchyma may occur when the episode of pancreatitis has subsided or resolved.

CHRONIC PANCREATITIS

Chronic pancreatitis is defined as a progressive inflammatory disease of the pancreas characterized by the clinical triad of diabetes, steatorrhea, and radiographic evidence of calcification, along with permanent impairment of function and irreversible morphologic changes.[18-20]

The most common cause of chronic pancreatitis is alcohol ingestion, which accounts for approximately 70% of cases.[21-23] The next most frequent type is idiopathic chronic pancreatitis.[21,23] It is interesting to note that only a small percentage of patients (approximately 4%) with chronic pancreatitis have disease due to choledocholithiasis.[21]

Several classification schemes for chronic pancreatitis have been proposed, including the Marseille classification of 1963, the revised Marseille classification of 1984, the Marseille-Rome classification of 1988, the Cambridge classification of 1984, the more recently proposed Zurich classification (1997), and the Japan Pancreas Society classification (1997).[19,20] However, despite many attempts at classification of chronic pancreatitis, at present no single widely accepted system adequately addresses the clinical status, cause, pathogenesis, structure, or function.[19-21] The Marseille and Marseille-Rome classifications are considered inadequate and outdated[19,20]; the Cambridge classification uses imaging features for grading and disease severity but does not distinguish the different forms of chronic pancreatitis according to cause and clinical outcome.[19,20] The Zurich classification specifically addresses the alcoholic form of chronic pancreatitis (Table 30-3) but in a complex way that considers diagnosis, cause, clinical staging, and pain profile individually. Thus, this classification scheme is also

not widely accepted.[20] The Japan Pancreas Society classification (Table 30-4) attempts to standardize diagnostic criteria but lacks causative and pathogenetic features; it is only partially useful in a clinical setting.[20]

Alcohol- and Obstruction-Related Chronic Pancreatitis

CLINICAL FEATURES

The incidence of chronic pancreatitis has been stated to vary geographically, but this is in dispute in that some early studies found no geographic discrepancy in the incidence of this disease.[21,24] Chronic pancreatitis is more common among men than among women and is most frequent in the fourth to sixth decades of life. However, its incidence among women is increasing, likely owing to increasing alcohol consumption in this population.[25]

TABLE 30-3. Zurich Classification of Chronic Pancreatitis

Definite Alcoholic Chronic Pancreatitis
In addition to the typical history or a history of excessive alcohol intake (>80 g/day), one or more of the following criteria establish the diagnosis:
    Calcification in pancreas
    Moderate to marked ductal lesions ("Cambridge" criteria)
    Marked exocrine insufficiency (steatorrhea >7 g fat/24 hr), normalized or markedly reduced by enzyme supplementation
    Typical histology of an adequate surgical specimen

Probable Alcoholic Chronic Pancreatitis
In addition to the typical history or a history of excessive alcohol intake (>80 g/day), the diagnosis of probable chronic pancreatitis is likely if one or more of the following criteria are present (*Note:* These diagnostic criteria may also be used for nonalcoholic chronic pancreatitis):
    Mild ductal alterations ("Cambridge" criteria)
    Recurrent or persistent pseudocysts
    Pathologic secretin test
    Endocrine insufficiency

Etiologic Factors
Alcohol
Nonalcohol
    Tropical (nutritional)
    Hereditary
    Metabolic
    Idiopathic
    Autoimmune
    Miscellaneous (e.g., radiation injury, phenacetin abuse)
    "Anatomic" chronic pancreatitis (i.e., associated with anatomic abnormalities: obstructive pancreatitis, pancreas divisum, post-traumatic pancreatic duct scars, periampullary duodenal wall cysts)

Clinical Staging
Early stage: recurrent attacks of clinical alcoholic acute pancreatitis without evidence of abnormalities of chronic pancreatitis
Late stage: any evidence of probable or definite chronic pancreatitis

TABLE 30-4. Japan Pancreas Society Classification of Chronic Pancreatitis

Definite Chronic Pancreatitis

Imaging
  Ultrasonography: pancreatic stones evidenced by intrapancreatic hyperreflective echoes with acoustic shadows behind
  CT: pancreatic stones evidenced by intrapancreatic calcifications
ERCP
  Irregular ductal dilatation of pancreatic branches of variable intensity with scattered distribution throughout the pancreas; or
  Irregular dilatation of the main pancreatic duct and branches proximal to complete or incomplete obstruction of the main pancreatic duct (with pancreatic stones or protein plugs)
Secretin test: abnormally low bicarbonate concentration combined with either decreased enzyme output or decreased secretory volume
Histologic evaluation of biopsy, surgical excision or autopsy: destruction or loss of exocrine parenchyma with irregular fibrosis and patchy fibrosis of interlobular spaces; intralobular fibrosis alone is not specific for chronic pancreatitis
Other: protein plugs, pancreatic stones, dilatation of the pancreatic ducts, hyperplasia and metaplasia of the ductal epithelium, and cyst formation

Probable Chronic Pancreatitis

Imaging
  Ultrasonography: intrapancreatic coarse hyperreflectivities, irregular dilation of pancreatic ducts, or pancreatic deformity with irregular contours
  CT: pancreatic deformity with irregular contours
ERCP: irregular ductal dilatation of the main pancreatic duct alone; intraductal filling defects suggestive of noncalcified pancreatic stones or protein plugs
Secretin test
  Abnormally low bicarbonate concentration alone; or
  Decreased enzyme output plus decreased secretory volume
Histologic evaluation: intralobular fibrosis with one of the following findings: loss of exocrine parenchyma, isolated islets of Langerhans, or pseudocysts

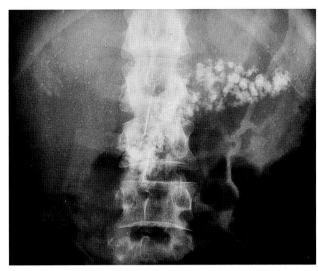

FIGURE 30–3. Pancreatic calcifications, as demonstrated in this abdominal x-ray, are diagnostic of chronic pancreatitis.

elevated amylase concentration in the ascitic fluid, gastrointestinal bleeding, peptic ulceration, metastatic fat necrosis (leakage of lipase into the circulation), and cirrhosis (in alcohol-related pancreatitis).[21]

Elevated serum levels of CA 19-9 may occur in patients with chronic pancreatitis in the absence of a pancreatic adenocarcinoma.[26-28] Calcifications may be detected in 30% to 70% of patients at clinical presentation by radiographic evaluation (Fig. 30-3).[21]

RISK OF PANCREATIC CANCER

The incidence of pancreatic cancer in patients with chronic pancreatitis varies from 0% to 30%.[29] Lowenfels and associates[30] showed that chronic pancreatitis, regardless of its cause, is a risk factor for the development of pancreatic cancer. This cancer occurs more frequently in chronic hereditary pancreatitis syndromes than in those related to chronic alcohol ingestion.[31,32] The development of pancreatic cancer in the setting of chronic pancreatitis is likely the result of multiple interrelated factors associated with chronic pancreatitis, including alcohol and smoking. Evidence in the literature conflicts regarding the presence of K-*ras* mutations in chronic pancreatitis.[33-35] Although K-*ras* mutations in chronic pancreatitis may play a role in the development of carcinoma, it is likely that other interrelated molecular biologic alterations contribute to the development of carcinoma in the setting of chronic pancreatitis; these include *p16 (INK4)*, *DPC4*, and *BRCA2* gene mutations or microsatellite instability.[36,37]

PATHOGENESIS

The causes of chronic pancreatitis are listed in Table 30-5. In urban areas of the United States, Europe, and South Africa, chronic pancreatitis is most often caused by alcohol abuse. In conjunction with alcohol abuse, tobacco

The most common form of chronic pancreatitis is related to long-term alcohol ingestion. More than 80% of patients present with abdominal pain (intermittent or chronic) and weight loss. Chronic pancreatitis may result in symptoms of pancreatic exocrine insufficiency, particularly when the disorder is caused by chronic alcohol abuse. Malabsorption, including steatorrhea and azotorrhea, may occur; however, with rare exceptions, steatorrhea and azotorrhea do not occur until pancreatic enzyme secretion (lipase and trypsin, respectively) has been reduced by 90%.[21] Chronic pancreatitis may also cause pancreatic endocrine insufficiency. Diabetes is commonly seen with pancreatitis but usually is not noted until the disease is advanced.

Other clinical manifestations of chronic pancreatitis may include a pancreatic mass, pseudocyst or abscess formation, pancreatic ascites or pleural effusion with

TABLE 30-5. Etiology of Chronic Pancreatitis
Alcohol
Idiopathic disease
Nutritional deficiencies
Hereditary factors
Cystic fibrosis
Trauma
Hypercalcemia
Chronic renal failure
Vascular disease
Hyperlipidemia
Gallstones
Others

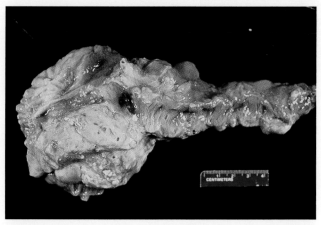

FIGURE 30–4. Chronic pancreatitis with segmental involvement of the head, causing dilatation of the ducts.

smoking may be an additive factor in chronic pancreatitis; smoking increases the risk of chronic pancreatitis almost tenfold.

PATHOLOGIC FEATURES

Multiple attempts have been made to subclassify chronic pancreatitis according to the degree and extent of anatomic change in the pancreas (e.g., segmental vs. diffuse) (Table 30-6).[38] However, most subclassification schemes are not reproducible. Hence, most authorities do not find any usefulness in subclassifying chronic pancreatitis on the basis of anatomic changes.[23,39] In fact, the cause of chronic pancreatitis (e.g., alcohol, idiopathic, obstruction) cannot be classified reliably and reproducibly on the basis of morphologic findings alone because histologic patterns of disease overlap considerably.

GROSS PATHOLOGY

Chronic pancreatitis may involve the pancreas in a focal, segmental, or diffuse manner. Involved areas of pancreas are typically enlarged (either in part or in toto)

TABLE 30-6. Marseille (1984) Morphologic Classification of Chronic Pancreatitis*
Histologic features seen in all etiologies include
Irregular sclerosis with loss and destruction of exocrine parenchyma—focal, segmental, or diffuse
Dilatation of ductal system associated with strictures and stones
Possible presence of inflammatory cells
Relative sparing of islets of Langerhans
Subclassification based on histologic findings include
Chronic pancreatitis with focal necrosis
Chronic pancreatitis with segmental or diffuse fibrosis
Chronic pancreatitis with and without calculi
Obstructive chronic pancreatitis (listed as a distinct form) characterized by
Ductal dilatation proximal to occlusion of major duct
Diffuse atrophy of acinar parenchyma
Uniform fibrosis with calculi uncommon

*Not reproducible, therefore not in use. Chronic pancreatitis (e.g., alcoholic, idiopathic, obstructive) cannot be classified on the basis of morphology.

and indurated ("rock hard") and reveal abundant fibrosis (Fig. 30-4). Involved ducts may be distorted and show irregular cystic dilatation; they may also contain calcified protein plugs (calculi). With progression of disease, the entire gland undergoes atrophy. The pancreas in advanced chronic pancreatitis is typically hard and shrunken. Extrapancreatic pseudocysts of variable size may be present, some measuring up to 10 cm in greatest dimension. They often appear grossly as thick-walled fibrous cysts filled with necrotic hemorrhagic debris.

MICROSCOPIC PATHOLOGY

The histologic features of chronic pancreatitis are similar regardless of the specific cause, with the exception of cases secondary to duct obstruction (e.g., stones, fibrosis, or tumor), in which the affected tissue is usually more evenly involved than in alcohol-related cases and the process is typically less severe, with the ductal epithelium less likely to undergo morphologic alterations (e.g., hyperplasia, metaplasia, atrophy).[40] In contrast to acute pancreatitis, which is usually characterized by complete restitution of pancreatic parenchyma following resolution of inflammation, in chronic pancreatitis, the morphologic alterations are permanent.

Essential histologic features of chronic pancreatitis include preservation of the normal lobular architecture of the acini, irregular loss of acinar and ductal tissue combined with various types of duct alterations, a variable degree of chronic inflammation, and fibrosis (Fig. 30-5). Preservation of the lobular architecture of the pancreas is perhaps the most important feature and represents a helpful diagnostic feature in differentiating chronic pancreatitis from duct-type adenocarcinoma. However, preserved lobules may be normal or may reveal various degrees of atrophy, depending on the degree of progression of disease.

Even in advanced disease, the lobular pattern tends to be well preserved. Duct and acinar cell atrophy,

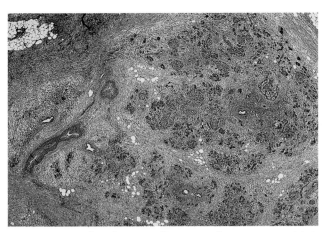

FIGURE 30–5. A key diagnostic feature in chronic pancreatitis is retention of the normal lobular architecture of the gland. Additional features include loss of acinar and ductal tissue, ductal dilatation, chronic inflammation, and fibrosis. Fibrosis, a common feature in chronic pancreatitis, is often irregular in distribution and can be seen in periductal, intralobular, and interlobular areas.

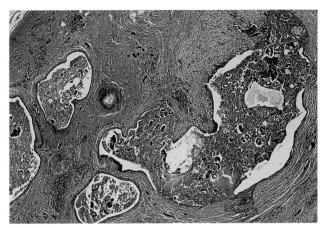

FIGURE 30–7. Ductal dilatation (ectasia) with inspissated secretions in this case of pancreatitis.

which may be irregular in distribution, is always present (Fig. 30-6). Various duct alterations include dilatation and ectasia, cyst formation, and the presence of inspissated secretions or calculi (Fig. 30-7). Saccular dilatation of large ducts is not uncommon (Fig. 30-8). Duct epithelial alterations include atrophy, hyperplasia (pseudopapillary or papillary), and metaplasia (e.g., mucous cell, pyloric gland, or squamous). In mucous cell metaplasia, the ducts are lined by tall columnar cells that contain mucin (mucus-rich cells) in the apical region of the cytoplasm; the nuclei are typically small and uniform and well aligned along the basal aspect of the epithelium (see Fig. 30-8). In addition, reactive duct epithelial changes and intraductal neoplasia (dysplasia) may occur. Reactive changes consist of cells with nuclear enlargement and greater irregularity in

size, shape, and chromatin distribution compared with normal duct cell nuclei (Fig. 30-9). Various degrees of pancreatic intraepithelial neoplasia (dysplasia) may be noted and are described in greater detail in Chapter 31. Mitotic activity may be increased. However, the cytologic features that characterize adenocarcinoma, such as nuclear pleomorphism, nuclear crowding, nuclear stratification, increased nucleus-to-cytoplasm ratio, prominent nucleoli, and mitotic figures, are typically not present.

A variable degree of chronic inflammation is normally present as well in chronic pancreatitis. The inflammatory infiltrate is usually a minor component of the process but occasionally may be prominent. A marked eosinophilic infiltrate may raise the possibility of eosinophilic pancreatitis (see under Eosinophilic Pancreatitis). Perineural and intraneural inflammation and perineural fibrosis are characteristic features of chronic pancreatitis. Hyperplasia and hypertrophy of the nerves and fibrosis are also common findings. Fibrosis is often irregular in distribution and may be seen in periductal, intralobular, and interlobular areas.

The islets of Langerhans are relatively resistant to the effects of chronic pancreatitis. In the early stages of chronic pancreatitis, the islets of Langerhans are usually normal in appearance or show only minimal morphologic alteration. In more advanced stages of disease, islet alterations include reduction in number and progressive atrophy. Insulin-producing cells tend to be lost preferentially. Occasionally, islet cell hyperplasia may be seen. Glucagon and pancreatic polypeptide–producing cells are also usually increased, but somatostatin cells typically remain constant in number.[41] With increasing degrees of acinar atrophy, the islets may appear to be numerous and hyperplastic, possibly suggesting an endocrine neoplasm (Fig. 30-10). In contrast to hyperplastic islets, neoplastic islets have associated intratumoral fibrosis or sclerosis, or they may have an amyloid-rich

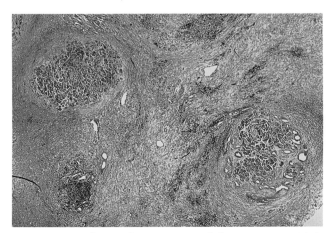

FIGURE 30–6. Along with progression of chronic pancreatitis is marked lobular atrophy of the exocrine pancreas.

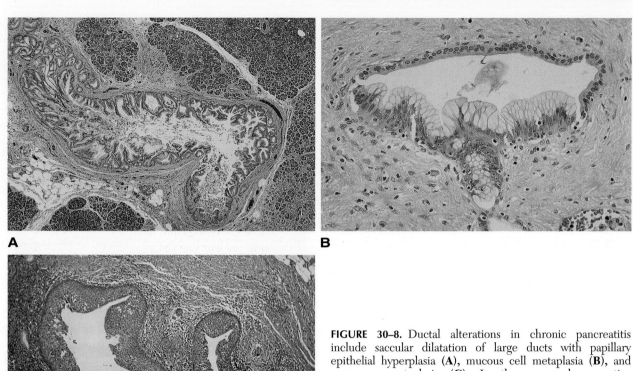

FIGURE 30–8. Ductal alterations in chronic pancreatitis include saccular dilatation of large ducts with papillary epithelial hyperplasia (**A**), mucous cell metaplasia (**B**), and squamous metaplasia (**C**). In these examples, reactive epithelial changes are present, but there is no cytologic atypia.

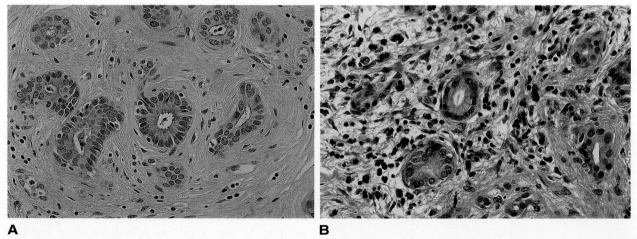

FIGURE 30–9. The cytologic changes in chronic pancreatitis include nuclear enlargement with a greater degree of irregularity in size, shape, and chromatin distribution compared with normal duct cell nuclei; these cytologic changes occur regardless of the extent of inflammation, which may be minimal (**A**) or moderate (**B**). However, cytologic features of adenocarcinoma are not present. The latter include marked nuclear pleomorphism with nuclear crowding, nuclear stratification, increased nucleus-to-cytoplasm ratio, prominent nucleoli, and mitotic figures.

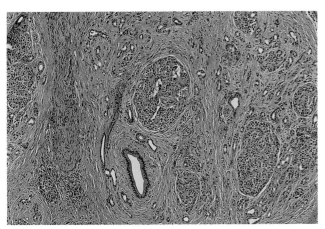

FIGURE 30–10. As a result of atrophy of the exocrine component of the pancreas, the islets of Langerhans appear hyperplastic in chronic pancreatitis, possibly leading to diagnostic consideration of an endocrine neoplasm. In this field, a hypertrophic nerve is present *(left)*, adding difficulty to the diagnosis of this case.

stroma. With severely progressive disease, eventual loss of islet tissue may be noted as well.

Some patients with chronic pancreatitis develop pseudocysts. Pseudocysts are lined by fibrous tissue, inflammation, and granulation tissue, but they do not contain an epithelial lining.

Patients with acute exacerbation of chronic pancreatitis often have a prominent polymorphonuclear leukocytic infiltrate and necrosis (intraparenchymal and in peripancreatic adipose tissue).

INTRAOPERATIVE CONSULTATION (FROZEN SECTION) FOR CHRONIC PANCREATITIS

Pathologists are often consulted in the operating room to help differentiate chronic pancreatitis from ductal adenocarcinoma by intraoperative (frozen section) analysis. Hyland and colleagues[42] compared the frozen section features of chronic pancreatitis with those of pancreatic adenocarcinoma and identified many histologic and cytologic criteria that can help distinguish these two disorders.

Histologic features suggestive of chronic pancreatitis include interlobular ducts that are round or tubular without branching or outpouchings; these are usually lined by one or two layers of columnar epithelium. Intralobular ducts are typically small and round to ovoid and are lined by a single layer of cuboidal to low columnar cells. Duct distribution is usually regular; necrotic glandular debris is always absent, and perineural invasion is never identified (Fig. 30-11). Cytologic features of benign disease (chronic pancreatitis) include a maximum nuclear size variation of 3:1, absence of mitoses, and the absence of enlarged, irregular nucleoli.

In contrast, histologic features of adenocarcinoma include an overall increase in the number of glandular

structures in both the intralobular and interlobular areas. Malignant ducts are normally larger than benign ducts, are more irregularly distributed, and often show irregular branching. Characteristic features of malignancy include malignant glands with partial or incomplete lumen formation, solid nests of cells without lumina, cribriform glandular patterns, single cell filing, isolated individual malignant cells in the stroma, and ducts that show an incomplete epithelial lining.

According to Hyland and coworkers,[42] necrotic material may be seen within glandular lumina in up to 70% of cases of adenocarcinoma. Neurotropism (perineural and intraneural invasion) may occur in up to 28% of cases. Cytologically, adenocarcinomas show great variation in nuclear size ($\geq$4:1) and increased numbers of both normal and abnormal mitotic figures. Atypical mitoses and large irregular nuclei are seen in up to 48% of malignant cases.

DIFFERENTIAL DIAGNOSIS

Chronic pancreatitis may clinically and histopathologically simulate a malignant neoplasm. Furthermore, the morphologic changes of chronic pancreatitis may be noted in malignant cases. Table 30-7 illustrates the key diagnostic features (e.g., clinical, radiologic, gross, microscopic) that can help distinguish chronic pancreatitis from ductal adenocarcinoma in resection specimens. Clinically, some studies have suggested that a marked elevation of serum CA 19-9 levels to greater than 300 UI/mL is helpful in differentiating benign from malignant disease,[43,44] but other reports have not found similar results.[27,45] For instance, in chronic pancreatitis, a false-positive elevation of serum CA 19-9 may be due to structural changes that occur in the pancreas, such as calcification, pancreatic duct stenosis, or obstruction.[46] Serum tissue polypeptide-specific antigen (TPS) has also been used as a complement to CA 19-9. Slesak and associates[47] reported that the median levels of TPS and CA 19-9 for pancreatic carcinoma were significantly higher than those for chronic pancreatitis ($P < .0001$). In fact, Slesak and colleagues[47] suggest that TPS may be more useful than CA 19-9 in differentiating carcinoma from chronic pancreatitis. These authors found elevated levels of CA 19-9 preoperatively in 70% of patients with pancreatic carcinoma but in only 19% of chronic pancreatitis patients. Elevated TPS levels were detected in 100% of patients with pancreatic carcinoma, but they were found in only 22% of patients with chronic pancreatitis. Similarly, CA 242 levels have been shown to be useful in this differential diagnosis. Structural alterations that cause false-positive elevations of CA 19-9 in patients with chronic pancreatitis appear to have no influence on CA 242 levels.[46] Mixed results have been reported regarding the use of *TP53* tumor suppressor gene mutations[48] and K-*ras* mutations[49-51] in differentiating benign from malignant disease.

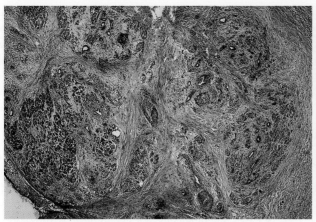

A

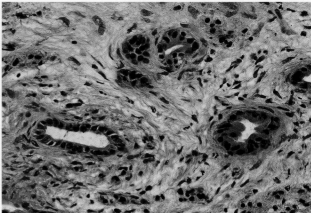

B

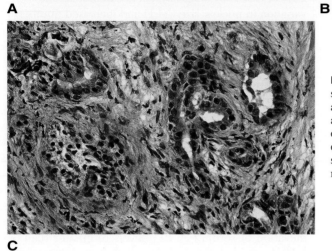

C

FIGURE 30–11. Intraoperative consultation (frozen section) specimen of a patient with chronic pancreatitis. **A,** The lobular architecture of the pancreas is preserved. **B** and **C,** The ducts are round or tubular; they are nonbranching or contain small outpouchings and are circumferentially lined by an intact layer of cuboidal to low columnar cells in which the maximal nuclear size variation is 3:1 without enlargement, irregular-appearing nucleoli, or mitotic figures.

TABLE 30-7. Chronic Pancreatitis Versus Ductal Adenocarcinoma

Features	Chronic Pancreatitis	Ductal Adenocarcinoma
Clinical symptoms	Abdominal pain (>80%) and weight loss	Jaundice, epigastric pain, weight loss
Radiology	Calcifications on abdominal films	Mass-deforming contours of gland; severe ductal abnormalities (strictures longer than 10 mm and duct irregularities) with pancreatitis; cancers in head may obstruct pancreatic and common bile ducts, resulting in "double duct sign" by ERCP; abrupt cutoff to the main pancreatic duct by ERCP
Location	Occurs anywhere in the pancreas as focal, segmental, or diffuse involvement	Head more often than body and tail
Gross features	Involved pancreas is enlarged (either in part or in toto) and indurated with associated sclerosis; fibrous strands in end stage	Mass lesion, solitary and poorly demarcated
Histology	Preservation of lobular architecture; irregular loss of acinar and ductal tissue with ductal dilatation, cyst formation; inspissated secretions, or calculi; ductal epithelial alterations (atrophy, hyperplasia, or metaplasia) with minimal atypia; variable inflammation; fibrosis; islets unaltered in early stages but abnormal in later stages of disease (reduction in number and progressive atrophy)	Loss of lobular architecture; invasive growth by neoplastic ducts and/or individual tumor cells with desmoplastic reaction; ducts or glands composed of atypical columnar or cuboidal cells with enlarged, irregular nuclei, prominent nucleoli, and mitoses; neurotropism; variable mucin production; minor alterations of islets

Other Types of Chronic Pancreatitis

HEREDITARY PANCREATITIS

Hereditary pancreatitis is defined as a recurrent inflammatory condition of the pancreas that occurs in at least two generations of blood-related family members in whom no other risk factors for chronic pancreatitis have been identified.[52,53] It is an autosomal dominant condition with 80% penetrance and variable expression, and it occurs with equal frequency among men and women. Characteristically, symptoms occur within the first decade of life. The clinical presentation is similar to that of other types of chronic pancreatitis and includes epigastric pain, nausea, and vomiting. With increasing age, attacks usually become less severe. Laboratory findings include elevated serum pancreatic amylase and lipase with an increased amylase-to-creatinine clearance ratio. Associated abnormalities may include hyperlipemia, hypercalcemia, increased serum immunoglobulin concentrations, and increased frequency of HLA types B12, B13, and BW40.

Complications are similar to those seen in non-hereditary forms of chronic pancreatitis and include pancreatic calcification, diabetes mellitus, exocrine pancreatic insufficiency, pseudocysts, abscess formation, and pancreatic carcinoma; less frequently, portal or splenic vein thrombosis, jaundice, and pancreatic ascites may occur. Mutations in the cationic trypsinogen gene on the short arm of chromosome 7 (7q35) have been implicated as a potential cause of hereditary pancreatitis.[54-57] Three point mutations (R117H, N21I, A16V) within the cationic trypsinogen gene have been identified in patients with hereditary pancreatitis.[58-61] The pathologic features (gross and microscopic) of hereditary pancreatitis are indistinguishable from those of other more common causes of chronic pancreatitis (see under Chronic Pancreatitis).

AUTOIMMUNE PANCREATITIS

Autoimmune pancreatitis includes autoimmune-related pancreatitis, nonalcoholic duct destructive chronic pancreatitis, and lymphoplasmacytic sclerosing pancreatitis. This is a category of chronic pancreatitis that has poorly defined clinical and pathologic criteria and whose classification has not been refined.[62] The concept of autoimmune pancreatitis was first introduced in a patient with pancreatitis and hypergammaglobulinemia.[63] Since this initial report, it has been well established that pancreatitis may occur in association with systemic autoimmune diseases, such as Sjögren's syndrome, primary sclerosing cholangitis, primary biliary cirrhosis, chronic idiopathic inflammatory bowel disease (ulcerative colitis and Crohn's disease), systemic lupus erythematosus, diabetes mellitus, and others.[19,23,62,64-69] Given the association of chronic pancreatitis with these other autoimmune diseases, an autoimmune mechanism for chronic

pancreatitis was originally proposed.[62] However, the clinical and pathologic findings associated with autoimmune pancreatitis may also be noted in patients without systemic autoimmune disease, thus leading to the concept of a primary autoimmune-related pancreatitis.[69]

The clinical and pathologic features of autoimmune-related pancreatitis overlap with those of entities referred to as nonalcoholic duct destructive chronic pancreatitis and lymphoplasmacytic sclerosing pancreatitis. Some authors advocate separating cases of chronic pancreatitis without evidence of autoimmunity from autoimmune-related cases (even if steroid therapy is effective)[61]; other authorities are less clear about this separation and indicate that no significant differences in pancreatic pathology have been found between patients with or without known autoimmune disease.[23] At present, the relationship of autoimmune pancreatitis to nonalcoholic duct destructive chronic pancreatitis and lymphoplasmacytic sclerosing pancreatitis remains unresolved. Because of their many shared features and the lack of clear evidence that these are distinct entities, they are included under a single heading. Nevertheless, sclerosing changes of the extrapancreatic bile ducts and pancreas, similar to those seen in primary biliary cirrhosis, have also been reported as lymphoplasmacytic sclerosing pancreatitis,[70] sclerosing pancreatocholangitis,[71] and inflammatory pseudotumor associated with sclerosing cholangitis.[63]

CLINICAL FEATURES

Autoimmune pancreatitis, autoimmune-related chronic pancreatitis, and nonalcoholic duct destructive chronic pancreatitis are uncommon disorders without a known prevalence. The sex predilection is essentially unknown, but some studies show a slight male predominance.[23,68,69,72] These diseases typically occur during the second to eighth decades of life.[23,68,69,72] Clinical findings include mild epigastric discomfort, abdominal pain, and obstructive (painless) jaundice.[23,62,66,68,69,72] Some patients may present with weight loss, polydipsia, and polyuria.[66,72] In some patients, pancreatic disease may be incidentally detected at the time of evaluation of another disease process.[23,62]

Typical laboratory findings include increased levels of serum pancreatic enzymes, hypergammaglobulinemia, and the presence of autoantibodies (including antinuclear antibody [ANA]), antilactoferrin (ALF), anticarbonic anhydrase II (ACA-II), and rheumatoid factor.[66,68,69] Antibodies against α-fodrin, which may be involved in Sjögren's syndrome, may be present as well.[66,73] Antimitochondrial (M2) antibodies of the type that is elevated in primary biliary cirrhosis are rarely found in autoimmune pancreatitis.[66,69] Patients with stenosis of the common bile duct may have abnormalities of serum bilirubin and hepatobiliary enzymes. Antineutrophil cytoplasmic autoantibodies (ANCAs) are usually absent.[23,72]

Pancreatic and biliary imaging studies may show a diffusely enlarged pancreas with a "sausage-like" appearance and a capsule-like rim.[69,74] Segmental or diffuse narrowing of the main pancreatic duct may be detected by endoscopic retrograde cholangiopancreatography (ERCP).[75,76] Furthermore, sclerosing changes of the extrapancreatic bile ducts similar to those seen in primary sclerosing cholangitis may be noted.[66-71] Obstructive jaundice due to stenosis of the intrapancreatic common bile duct occurs in autoimmune pancreatitis but is rarely seen in other types of pancreatitis.[62]

Some patients improve spontaneously with no treatment.[23,66,69,72,78] In patients with common bile duct stenosis unresponsive to steroid therapy, surgery is often necessary for symptomatic relief.[23,77-80] Overall, the long-term prognosis is unknown. For patients with a known autoimmune disease, the prognosis may depend on the severity of complications.

PATHOGENESIS

The pathogenesis of autoimmune pancreatitis is unclear. In some cases, an association is found with other autoimmune diseases (secondary autoimmune pancreatitis),[62] including Sjögren's syndrome,[64] primary sclerosing cholangitis,[65,70] primary biliary cirrhosis,[65] idiopathic inflammatory bowel disease (ulcerative colitis and Crohn's disease),[62] systemic lupus erythematosus, diabetes mellitus,[62] and retroperitoneal fibrosis.[71,81] These findings support the hypothesis that an autoimmune mechanism may be involved in the pathogenesis in some patients with pancreatitis.[62] In these instances, antigens may be found in the pancreas that are common to other exocrine organs, such as the salivary glands, biliary tract, and renal tubules.[62] Increased levels of activated CD4+ and CD8+ T cells bearing HLA-DR in peripheral blood lymphocytes and in the pancreas have been reported in patients with autoimmune pancreatitis,[68] lending support to an autoimmune mechanism.

However, the pathogenesis in cases not associated with a systemic autoimmune disease ("primary autoimmune pancreatitis")[62] is unclear. Furthermore, some patients initially diagnosed with primary autoimmune pancreatitis have been shown to develop systemic autoimmune disease.[19,69]

PATHOLOGIC FEATURES

Gross Pathology. Macroscopic features vary from case to case. Some show diffuse firm enlargement of the pancreas without a distinct mass.[72] Others show alternating firm and edematous areas without a mass lesion.[72] Finally, some patients present with a white, masslike lesion that may be localized (e.g., head).[23] On ERCP, segmental duct stenosis of the main pancreatic duct may be seen.[23,66,72] Sclerosing alterations of extrapancreatic ducts may also occur.

Microscopic Pathology. The histologic features of this group of lesions are similar regardless of the presence of an associated autoimmune disease.[23] The most important striking changes include a dense lymphocytic or lymphoplasmacytic inflammatory infiltrate with or without lymphoid follicle formation surrounding medium-sized to large interlobular ducts (Fig. 30-12). Immunohistochemical evaluation of the lymphocytic cell infiltrate shows a predominance of T cells (positive for CD3 and UCHL-1) with fewer B cells (positive for L26).[23,66,72] The T-cell infiltrate includes cells positive for both CD4 and CD8.[23,66] Inflammation may also involve the main pancreatic duct. The extent of the inflammatory infiltrate is usually moderate to severe; it may be unevenly distributed, showing areas of dense inflammation alternating with less inflamed and uninvolved regions. In addition, the inflammatory infiltrate may include variable numbers of eosinophils, neutrophils, macrophages, and dendritic cells.[23] Furthermore, periductal inflammation often extends into the duct epithelium, causing degenerative changes

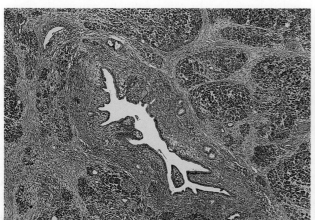 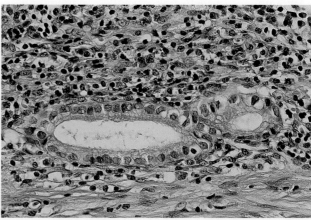

A **B**

FIGURE 30–12. A, Dense periductal inflammatory cell infiltrate in a case of "autoimmune" pancreatitis. **B,** The inflammatory cell component includes mature lymphocytes and plasma cells. In addition, reactive ductal epithelial changes are seen.

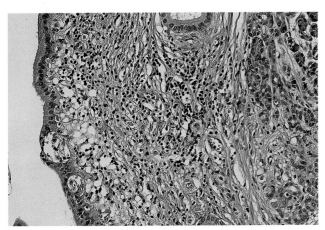

FIGURE 30–13. Periductal inflammation focally infiltrates the duct epithelium in this case of autoimmune pancreatitis.

(Fig. 30-13). In advanced cases, the ducts may show prominent periductal fibrosis, which may lead to duct obstruction and chronic pancreatitis of the distal pancreas. Perilobular fibrosis is often more extensive than intralobular fibrosis,[23] and it may involve the contiguous (peripancreatic) soft tissues.

Another characteristic feature is phlebitis of small to medium-sized veins (Fig. 30-14).[23,62] Obliterative phlebitis may also involve the portal vein.[62,71,75] Calcification, pseudocyst formation, protein plugging of the ducts, and fat necrosis, which are all common features in alcohol-related chronic pancreatitis, are not normally present in autoimmune or nonalcoholic duct destructive chronic pancreatitis.[23,66,72]

DIFFERENTIAL DIAGNOSIS

The differential diagnosis of autoimmune pancreatitis includes lymphoproliferative disorders (e.g., malignant lymphoma, plasmacytoma) and chronic pancreatitis of other causes.[66,69,74,76] In contrast to patients with alcohol-related pancreatitis, patients with nonalcoholic

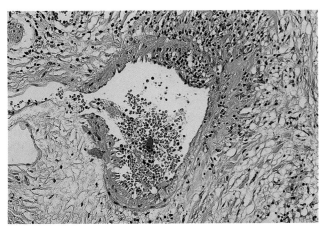

FIGURE 30–14. Phlebitis of medium-sized vein is often seen in autoimmune pancreatitis. In addition to the lymphoplasmacytic cell infiltrate, scattered eosinophils are present.

duct destructive pancreatitis do not usually show calcifications or pseudocyst formation. The contrasting histologic features between alcoholic and nonalcoholic chronic pancreatitis are further detailed in Table 30-8. Malignant lymphomas of the pancreas are uncommon and usually occur secondary to primary retroperitoneal tumors, although primary pancreatic lymphomas occur rarely as well. In contrast to lymphomas, which are composed of a monomorphic population of cells that is documented by immunohistochemical and molecular analyses, the cells in autoimmune pancreatitis are heterogeneous (admixture of different cell types) and polyclonal in origin.

DIABETES MELLITUS

Diabetes mellitus is defined as a state of chronic hyperglycemia due to insulin deficiency (absolute or relative); it occurs as a consequence of severe loss of islet B cells and/or peripheral resistance to the effects of insulin.

Clinical Features

The classification of diabetes mellitus includes type 1 (early-onset insulin-dependent diabetes, or juvenile diabetes) and type 2 (insulin-independent diabetes, or mature-onset diabetes). Type 1 diabetes classically occurs in children and juveniles who are prone to ketoacidosis and are dependent on insulin therapy. Type 2 diabetes classically occurs in adults and is treated by diet and/or hypoglycemic medication. The lack of insulin, either absolute or relative, results in inadequate glucose utilization, which leads to a diabetic syndrome characterized by glucosuria accompanied by loss of water and dehydration; weight loss due to loss of glucose and utilization of fat and protein energy reserves; and increased breakdown of neutral fat, leading to increased circulating free fatty acids (hyperlipidemia and hyper-cholesterolemia) that are oxidized by the liver into ketone bodies, potentially resulting in ketoacidosis. The combination of these may ultimately cause diabetic coma. Sustained hyperglycemia affects virtually every organ (multisystemic effects), which can result in macroangiopathy, atherosclerosis with increased risk of myocardial infarction, cerebral vascular accident (CVA, or stroke), gangrene of distal (lower) extremities, micro-angiopathy, diabetic glomerulosclerosis (Kimmelstiel-Wilson glomerulosclerosis), diabetic retinopathy, diabetic polyneuropathy, and susceptibility to infection (pyogenic and fungal) caused by alterations in leukocyte function.

Pathogenesis

Type 1 diabetes is associated with autoimmunity and genetic predisposition in which there is severe loss of

TABLE 30-8. Histologic Findings in Nonalcoholic Versus Alcoholic Chronic Pancreatitis

Histology	Nonalcoholic	Alcoholic
Involved ducts	Medium-sized interlobular ducts	Large interlobular ducts
Periductal inflammation	Dense, infiltrating epithelium	Mild, scattered without infiltration
Lymphocytes	Abundant (T cells > B cells)	Sparse (T cells)
Eosinophils	Present	Absent
Plasma cells	Present	Present
Neutrophils	Present	Present in association with calculi
Macrophages	Present	Rare
Dendritic cells	Present	Rare

Adapted from Ectors N, Maillet B, Aerts R, et al: Nonalcoholic duct destructive chronic pancreatitis. Gut 41:263-268, 1997.

islet B cells. Other possible pathogenetic considerations in the development of type 1 diabetes include viral and toxic effects of drugs or chemicals. Type 2 diabetes is associated with obesity, heredity (family history of diabetes), peripheral insulin resistance, and impaired B-cell function.

Pathologic Features

GROSS PATHOLOGY

In type 1 diabetes, if the disease is of recent onset, the pancreas shows little alteration. Long-standing disease may result in atrophy of the pancreas with fibrosis. In type 2 diabetes, few, if any, gross alterations of the pancreas are seen.

MICROSCOPIC PATHOLOGY

Microscopically, in type 1 diabetes, the islets show distinctive changes, even in cases of recent onset. The islets are composed of narrow cords of small cells within a fibrous stroma (islet fibrosis).[82] These islets are irregular in shape and may show continuity between the endocrine and acinar cells. An inflammatory cell infiltrate, composed predominantly of mature lymphocytes, is often present in some but not all islets. This finding is called *insulitis*. The inflammatory cell infiltrate can be focal and mild, or it can be florid, obscuring the normal microanatomy of the involved islet(s). Insulitis is restricted to islets that contain B cells and is more frequent among patients younger than 10 years of age. Islet amyloidosis is a rare feature in type 1 diabetes. Alterations in the exocrine pancreas include acinar cell atrophy and interacinar and interlobular fibrosis. Vascular changes include atherosclerosis of large arteries and diabetic microangiopathy of smaller arterioles.

In type 2 diabetes, the islets are usually normal in appearance. In some type 2 diabetics, little, if any, morphologic difference is noted compared with islets in nondiabetic patients. However, in some patients, up to a 50% reduction in islet cell mass can occur owing to a decrease in the total number of insulin-producing B

cells. Islet amyloidosis (islet hyalinization) is a common feature in type 2 diabetes. Amyloidosis in type 2 diabetes remains localized to the pancreas (localized amyloidosis) and is restricted to islets that are composed exclusively of B cells. Islet amyloidosis is considered diagnostic of type 2 diabetes, but it is not pathognomonic for diabetes. For instance, islet amyloidosis develops commonly among patients older than 50 years of age. It affects approximately 50% of diabetic patients over 70 years of age. Amyloid deposits stain with thioflavine T but only weakly with Congo red. Additional alterations in type 2 diabetes include islet fibrosis and fatty infiltration of the pancreas. Insulitis is a rare feature of type 2 diabetes.

EOSINOPHILIC PANCREATITIS

Eosinophilic pancreatitis is a rare condition characterized by a prominent eosinophilic infiltrate in the pancreas that may result in the development of a mass lesion or a common bile duct obstruction.[83-86] Pancreatic eosinophilia may be seen in a wide variety of diseases, including parasitic infection, pancreatic allograft rejection,[87] hypersensitivity reactions to medication,[88] milk allergy,[89] inflammatory myofibroblastic tumor,[90,91] pseudocyst formation in chronic pancreatitis[92,93] as part of the inflammatory component in lymphoplasmacytic sclerosing pancreatitis,[94] and cancer. Primary eosinophilic pancreatitis is extraordinarily rare.

Clinical Features

The clinical presentation varies depending on the circumstances in which pancreatic eosinophilia occurs. Patients may present with abdominal pain and obstructive jaundice. Patients with eosinophilic pancreatitis often have systemic manifestations, including peripheral eosinophilia, elevated serum immunoglobulin E (IgE) levels, and eosinophilic infiltrates in other organs. Some patients have hypereosinophilic syndrome,[95] including an elevated eosinophil count (more than 1500 cells/mm^3) of at least 6 months' duration, allergies (e.g., asthma, rhinitis), and multiorgan system involvement, including the skin, heart, and gastrointestinal tract, with no other identifiable causes of eosinophilia.

Pathologic Features

Pathologically, the pancreas may be enlarged and fibrotic. Extent and intensity of the eosinophilic infiltrate vary according to the setting in which the disease occurs. Eosinophils may diffusely infiltrate the pancreas and surround the ducts and acini, often within septa, and may involve blood vessels (e.g., phlebitis, arteritis) as well.

Infectious Diseases of the Pancreas

CLINICAL FEATURES

Infection as a cause of pancreatic disease in immune competent hosts is uncommon. The incidence of acute pancreatitis caused by infectious agents is difficult to estimate in that many cases are mild or subclinical.[13] A wide variety of infections have been associated with acute pancreatitis (see under Etiology). Clues to the infectious nature of pancreatitis are based on the characteristic signs and symptoms associated with the particular infectious agent.[13] Immune suppressed patients (e.g., AIDS, organ transplant) have a higher incidence of acute pancreatitis compared with the general population.[2,13,95-98]

ETIOLOGY

Infectious pancreatitis may be caused by a variety of pathogens, including viruses, parasites, bacteria, and fungi. Viral infections include mumps, rubella, Coxsackie B virus, Epstein-Barr virus (EBV), cytomegalovirus (CMV), herpes simplex virus, hepatitis A and B, and human immunodeficiency virus (HIV).[2] Parasitic infections associated with acute pancreatitis include *Ascaris lumbricoides*,[99] *Clonorchis sinensis*,[2] *Strongyloides stercoralis*,[13] and *Echinococcus granulosus*.[13] Among the bacteria that may cause pancreatitis are *Mycoplasma pneumoniae*, *Salmonella typhi*, *Campylobacter jejuni*, *Yersinia enterocolitica*, *Actinomyces* and *Nocardia* species, *Mycobacterium tuberculosis*, and *Mycobacterium avium-intracellulare* complex, as well as *Legionella*, *Leptospira*, and other species.[2,13] Potential fungal infections include *Aspergillus* species, *Cryptococcus neoformans*, *Coccidioides immitis*, *Paracoccidioides brasiliensis*, *Histoplasma capsulatum*, and *Pneumocystis carinii*.[2] In AIDS patients, a majority of cases of acute pancreatitis are due to dissemination of opportunistic infections, such as CMV.[2,96] Other causes include *Cryptococcus* species, *Toxoplasma gondii*, *Cryptosporidium* species, *M. tuberculosis*, and *M. avium* complex.[2]

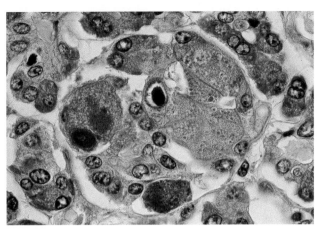

FIGURE 30–15. Cytomegalovirus infection of pancreatic acinar tissue shows characteristic intranuclear inclusions.

PATHOLOGIC FEATURES

The pathologic features of infectious pancreatitis vary according to the type of pathogen involved. For instance, CMV inclusions are typically found in mesenchymal cells and may be seen in epithelial cells (Fig. 30-15). Granulomas may occur in mycobacterial or fungal infection.[100] Depending on the cause, the granulomatous process may be necrotizing (caseating) or non-necrotizing and may present anywhere within the pancreatic parenchyma. The absence of an identifiable microorganism by light microscopy and/or histochemical stain does not exclude an infectious cause.

Microbiologic cultures of suspected cases of infectious pancreatitis are usually necessary to establish a diagnosis. The most common parasitic pancreatitis is caused by the nematode *A. lumbricoides*.[13] This large worm may enter the pancreas via the pancreatic duct, causing necrosis, abscess formation, granulomatous inflammation, and fibrosis. *A. lumbricoides* eggs and larvae may be identified. In the absence of an identified infectious cause for a particular granulomatous infiltrate, other uncommon possible causes include pancreatic involvement by sarcoidosis,[100,101] which appears as noncaseating granuloma, or an autoimmune disease such as Crohn's disease[102] or rheumatoid arthritis, the latter of which is characterized by a rheumatoid nodule (Fig. 30-16).

Non-neoplastic Cystic Lesions of the Pancreas

PSEUDOCYSTS

Pancreatic pseudocyst, the most common type of cystic lesion in the pancreas, represents a localized collection of secretions that develop as a result of inflammation. By definition, these cysts do not contain an epithelial lining.[103]

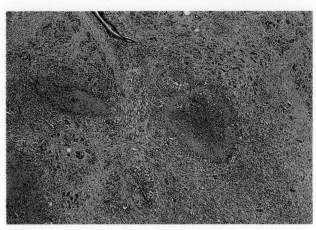

FIGURE 30–16. Rare example of granulomatous pancreatitis in a patient with rheumatoid arthritis characterized by the presence of rheumatoid nodules.

Clinical Features

Pseudocysts occur most commonly as a result of pancreatitis (acute or chronic) or trauma, but they may rarely be seen in association with a neoplasm as a result of duct obstruction. Pseudocysts related to alcoholic pancreatitis are more common among men than among women. In non–alcohol-related disorders, a more equal sex distribution is seen. Pseudocysts occur predominantly in adults but may occur in children and young adults as well, particularly as a result of trauma or in association with hereditary pancreatitis.[104] Most patients present with abdominal pain.[104] Pancreatic pseudocysts may grow to large sizes and present as a palpable abdominal mass.[104] They may occur in any portion of the pancreas and may be multiple (Fig. 30-17).

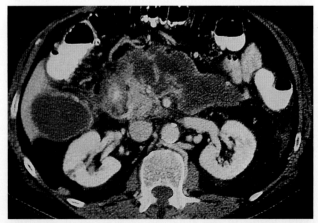

FIGURE 30–17. Pancreatic pseudocysts in acute pancreatitis. This computed tomographic scan was taken several weeks after the initial attack and shows multiple well-delineated cystic lesions in the head, body, and tail.

Pathogenesis, Natural History, and Treatment

Pseudocysts usually develop as a consequence of severe acute alcoholic pancreatitis. Thus, a majority of pseudocysts are associated with alcoholism. Other causes include biliary disease (gallstones), nonoperative and operative trauma, drugs, hyperlipidemia, and hereditary pancreatitis; they may also be idiopathic.[104] In acute pancreatitis, pseudocysts develop as sequelae of extensive necrosis (liquefaction) involving peripancreatic tissues (e.g., fat), alone or in combination with intrapancreatic parenchymal necrosis that results from activated pancreatic enzymes.[103] In chronic pancreatitis and in duct obstruction related to cancer, pseudocysts are formed when strictures, inspissated secretory protein, or intrapancreatic calcifications cause obstruction, leading to dilatation, loss of the epithelial lining, and enlargement.[104]

Pseudocysts may resolve spontaneously, remain stable in size, or grow progressively.[104] The treatment for pseudocysts includes medical management, surgery or surgical drainage, and percutaneous external drainage or endoscopic internal drainage. External drainage is preferred when the cyst wall is not thick enough to allow for the creation of an anastomosis. Internal drainage with a roux-en-Y anastomosis to the jejunum (cystojejunostomy) or to the posterior wall of the stomach (cystogastrostomy) or to the duodenum (cystoduodenostomy) is common.[104] Complications of pancreatic pseudocysts include infection, hemorrhage, rupture, and obstruction. Infection of the peritoneal cavity may lead to purulent peritonitis or sepsis, which are the most common causes of death from acute pancreatitis.[103] Hemorrhage results from erosion of the pseudocyst into vascular structures and is associated with increased morbidity and mortality. Acute rupture (perforation) is uncommon, but if it occurs in the abdomen, it may result in signs and symptoms of acute peritonitis. Rupture is associated with higher mortality rates.[104]

Pathologic Features

GROSS PATHOLOGY

Pseudocysts are usually unilocular lesions with a ragged inner surface and a thick fibrotic wall (Fig. 30-18). Their contents include thick or thin, turbid or milky, clear or blood-tinged fluid. A high intracystic amylase level is typical. Most pseudocysts develop in the body and tail; approximately one third are localized to the head of the pancreas.[104] Pancreatic pseudocysts vary in size; the largest are associated with alcoholic pancreatitis and with others located outside of the pancreas.[103]

MICROSCOPIC PATHOLOGY

Microscopically, pseudocysts are by definition devoid of an epithelial lining. The lining of the pseudocyst is

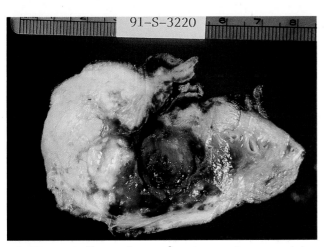

FIGURE 30–18. Pancreatic pseudocyst appearing as an intrapancreatic unilocular hemorrhagic cystic lesion.

typically composed of granulation tissue, inflammatory cells, and fibrous tissue (Fig. 30-19). With progression, the wall of the pseudocyst becomes usually densely fibrotic and shows a lower degree of vascularity. In addition, pancreatic parenchyma may be present in or adjacent to the fibrous wall of the pseudocyst; this may be atrophic in appearance or may show evidence of resolving pancreatitis. Most notably, liquefactive necrosis is absent, a feature that helps to separate pseudocysts from pancreatic abscesses.

Pseudocysts may or may not show evidence of communication with the main pancreatic duct system. Generous sampling of the wall of a presumed pseudocyst is necessary for preventing a missed diagnosis of mucinous or serous neoplasm; such neoplasms may on occasion contain only minimal focal areas of nondenuded epithelium.

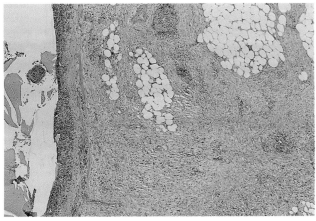

FIGURE 30–19. Pancreatic pseudocyst. The cyst lining is composed of granulation tissue and inflammatory cells without a discrete epithelial lining. A thickened fibrotic wall with prominent vascularity is present.

Differential Diagnosis

Pseudocysts must be differentiated from true, epithelially lined cystic lesions, including cystic neoplasms of the pancreas (Table 30-9). Histologic differentiation between pseudocysts and true cysts resides in the identification of an epithelial lining. In contrast to pseudocysts, true cysts of the pancreas have an identifiable epithelial lining. Microcystic adenomas are lined by cuboidal to flattened epithelial cells with round nuclei, inconspicuous nucleoli, and clear to occasionally eosinophilic cytoplasm. Histochemical stains show the presence of diastase-sensitive, periodic acid–Schiff–positive intracytoplasmic material indicative of glycogen. Pancreatic mucinous cystic neoplasms are lined by columnar, mucus-producing cells, and "ovarian-type" stroma can be seen. Histochemical stains show the presence of mucicarmine and diastase-resistant, periodic acid–Schiff–reactive intracytoplasmic material indicative of mucin (see Chapter 31 for details).

LYMPHOEPITHELIAL CYSTS

Lymphoepithelial cysts are benign squamous epithelium–lined cystic lesions that have some features of cutaneous epidermal inclusion cysts.[105,106]

Clinical Features

Lymphoepithelial cysts of the pancreas are rare lesions, representing approximately 0.5% of all pancreatic cysts.[106] They predominantly affect adult men and may be asymptomatic, or they may be discovered incidentally or at autopsy.[105] Common symptoms include vague intermittent abdominal pain, persistent diarrhea, weight loss, intermittent nausea and vomiting, and an abdominal mass. Lymphoepithelial cysts may be located anywhere in the pancreas (head, body, or tail), or they may be extrapancreatic, that is, connected to the pancreas by a short stalk of normal pancreatic tissue.[105] Treatment for pancreatic lymphoepithelial cyst is surgical resection, which is curative.

Pathogenesis

Proposed origins for lymphoepithelial cysts include development from epithelial remnants within peripancreatic lymph nodes, from squamous metaplasia of the pancreatic ducts with subsequent cystic transformation, or from a branchial cleft cyst that was misplaced and fused with the pancreas during embryogenesis.[106] Some authors have suggested that lymphoepithelial cysts may represent a teratoma, or they may develop as a result of elaboration of growth factors by lymphoid cells.[105]

TABLE 30-9. Cystic Lesions of the Pancreas

Features	Pseudocyst	Microcystic Adenoma	Mucinous Cystic Neoplasm
Sex/Age	M>F; wide age range	F>M; 5th–7th decades	F>M; middle-aged
Clinical signs and symptoms	Generally found in the setting of chronic pancreatitis, often associated with biliary tract disease and alcoholism	Found incidentally at autopsy or presents as an abdominal mass with or without associated pain; tumors in pancreatic head may cause biliary tract or gastrointestinal obstruction, resulting in jaundice	Intermittent or continuous abdominal pain or discomfort; enlarging abdominal mass
Radiology	Well-defined fibrous capsules; low-density fluid centers	Multicystic, honeycomb-appearing mass; most cysts < 2 cm in diameter; small calcifications and central stellate scar common	Large, multicystic masses, may be unilocular, without honeycomb appearance; cysts measure >2 cm in diameter; prominent internal septations; absent central scar; enhancement of solid components after contrast
Location in pancreas	Anywhere in pancreas	Anywhere (even distribution)	More common in tail and body
Gross features	Thick-walled; adherent to surrounding structures; hemorrhagic fluid contents rich in pancreatic enzymes	Well-circumscribed; spongy and honeycomb appearance; central, often calcified, scar; clear, watery fluid contents, occasionally hemorrhagic	Encapsulated mass with smooth surface; unilocular or multilocular with smooth cyst lining, but papillary excrescences are common; occasional calcifications at periphery; thick, mucoid, or gelatinous fluid content; necrosis and hemorrhage may occur
Histology	Absence of an epithelial lining; fibrous wall with chronic inflammation and necrotic debris	Cysts lined by cuboidal to flattened cells with round nuclei, inconspicuous nucleoli, and clear to occasionally eosinophilic cytoplasm; tiny papillae may be present; hypocellular stroma	Cysts lined by columnar, mucus-producing cells aligned in a single row; may form papillae; cellular atypia, including nuclear pleomorphism, and nuclear stratification may be seen; hypercellular "ovarian-type" stroma
Histochemistry	Absence of mucus production	Glycogen is present in epithelial cells (PAS+; d-PAS–)	Epithelial cells are mucin+ (mucicarmine+; PAS+; d-PAS+)
Adjacent pancreas	Healing pancreatitis common	Normal appearance; uncommon atrophic changes secondary to tumor compression or to obstruction	Normal appearance; occasional atrophic changes secondary to obstruction
Treatment and prognosis	Pain medications; pancreatic enzyme replacement; surgery as last resort; morbidity high but mortality low	Surgery generally curative	Surgical resection; generally has an indolent course, with cure following resection; because of metastatic capability of all histologic types, considered as a malignant neoplasm

PAS, periodic acid–Schiff without diastase digestion; d-PAS, periodic acid–Schiff with diastase digestion.

Pathologic Features

GROSS PATHOLOGY

Lymphoepithelial cysts are well-demarcated, often encapsulated, spherical to egg-shaped lesions that can measure from 2 to 17 cm in greatest diameter. These lesions have a tendency to be multilocular (60% of cases).[105] The cyst wall lining is typically thin and smooth to granular in texture. The cyst contents are often caseous in appearance, semisolid in texture, and gray-white to tan in color.

MICROSCOPIC PATHOLOGY

Microscopically, lymphoepithelial cysts are lined by a stratified squamous epithelial cell layer either with or without prominent keratinization; undulated or invaginated architecture may be detected (Fig. 30-20). A transitional type of epithelium, as well as a flattened, cuboidal epithelium, may be focally present in some cases. Occasionally, sebaceous or mucinous cell differentiation may be noted. However, epidermal appendages are not a feature of this lesion. Most notably, abundant mature lymphocytes are found in the cyst wall and often form lymphoid aggregates with germinal centers. The lymphoid component may be exuberant.[105] Epimyoepithelial cell islands, similar to those seen in benign lymphoepithelial lesions of the salivary glands, may be present in some cases as well. Typically, a thin rim of pancreatic tissue, including ducts, acini, and islets, is often present immediately outside the lymphocytic layer. In fact, the pancreatic

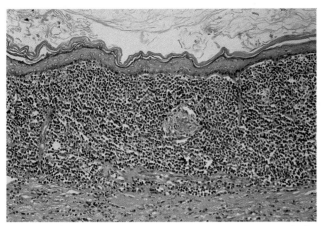

FIGURE 30–20. Pancreatic lymphoepithelial cyst lined by keratinizing squamous epithelium, including a granular cell layer; the cyst wall consists of a mature lymphocytic cell infiltrate with an associated lymphoid aggregate.

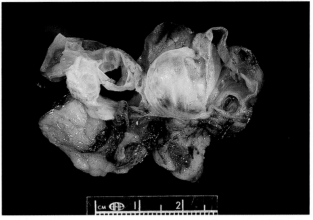

FIGURE 30–21. Pancreatic retention cyst characterized by the presence of a cystically dilated segment of pancreatic duct. This type of cyst develops as a consequence of duct obstruction.

parenchyma may show atrophic changes. Granulomas, collections of foamy histiocytes, and fat necrosis may be identified focally. Lymphoepithelial cysts do not normally show an acute inflammatory cell infiltrate or a granulation tissue reaction.

Differential Diagnosis

The differential diagnosis of pancreatic lympho-epithelial cyst includes cystic neoplasms, pseudocysts, other squamous epithelial cell–lined pancreatic cystic lesions such as dermoid cysts (monodermal teratoma), and epidermoid cysts within accessory splenic tissue.[105] Dermoid cysts occur more often in young patients and with an equal sex predilection. Histologically, dermoid cysts show adnexal tissue, sebaceous glands, and acute inflammation in the cyst wall—features that are not normally seen in lymphoepithelial cysts. Epidermoid cysts in intrapancreatic accessory splenic tissue also occur in a younger population with an equal sex predilection. Histologically, these lesions show splenic tissue within the cyst wall.[106]

OTHER CYSTS

Other unusual types of pancreatic cysts include enterogenous or enteric duplication cysts and endometrial cysts, retention cysts, congenital (dysgenetic) cysts, acinar cell transformations, periampullary duodenal wall cysts, and parasitic cysts.[103] Enterogenous cyst is a type of congenital malformation that essentially represents a gastrointestinal or enteric duplication cyst. It occurs early in life. Patients may be asymptomatic or may present with symptoms of gastric acid secretion or pancreatitis. These cysts originate from either the midgut or the foregut and characteristically include a well-developed bilayered muscular wall. The lining

epithelium may include gastric-type, intestinal-type, serous, mucous, or ciliated epithelium.[103] Those that occur in the duodenal wall next to the pancreas may communicate with the pancreatic duct system.

Endometrial cysts are rare lesions that reveal the same characteristic histologic features of endometriotic cysts in other organs. Endometrial glands and stroma with associated hemorrhage are the pathognomonic features.

Retention cyst is a lesion that shows a cystically dilated segment of pancreatic duct that develops as a consequence of obstruction (Fig. 30-21). The lining of retention cysts comprises normal ductal columnar epithelium. Part of the epithelium may be replaced by inflammation and necrosis.

Congenital (dysgenetic) cysts are intrapancreatic cystic lesions that do not communicate with the duct system and are lined by a single layer of flat epithelium. These cysts are lined by a single layer of cuboidal/columnar or flattened epithelium with a fibrous wall; stratified squamous epithelium may be seen. The epithelial cystic lining may be obliterated by inflammation or infection.

Congenital cysts may be multiple when associated with von Hippel-Lindau disease.[107] Acinar cell transformation is a type of multiloculated cystic change of the pancreas in which the cystic spaces are lined by non-neoplastic acinar cells. Echinococcal (hydatid) cysts may rarely occur in the pancreas as well.[103]

▇ Congenital and Hereditary Abnormalities of the Exocrine Pancreas

Congenital abnormalities of the pancreas include pancreas divisum, annular pancreas, aplasia, hypoplasia and dysplasia of the pancreas, variations in pancreatic ductal anatomy, choledochal cysts, and congenital cysts that may rarely occur in the pancreas and cause diagnostic confusion. These lesions are discussed more thoroughly in the following paragraphs.

PANCREAS DIVISUM

Pancreas divisum is the embryologic defect that results from incomplete fusion of the dorsal and ventral pancreatic ductal systems, leading to a pancreas with two separate drainage systems. Pancreas divisum represents the most common congenital anomaly of the pancreas (3% to 10% incidence).[28] The incidence of this lesion increases to 50% among patients who undergo ERCP for evaluation of "idiopathic" pancreatitis. Symptoms generally begin in the third to fifth decades of life,[108] but the defect may also be an incidental finding. Some patients present with recurrent attacks of epigastric pain and bouts of acute pancreatitis. Pancreatitis, when present, most often affects the dorsal derivative, but the ventral portion may be affected as well. Pseudocysts may be noted in some cases at the time of clinical presentation. However, the mechanism of pancreatitis in pancreas divisum remains unknown. For patients with severe attacks, various procedures such as endoscopic balloon dilatation, papillotomy, and stenting have been used. In refractory cases, direct duct drainage or distal pancreatic resection, with or without distal drainage into a Roux-en-Y loop, is usually performed.

The pathologist usually plays little or no role in the diagnosis of this condition because it is characteristically a radiographic diagnosis. ERCP with injection of contrast material, which is the best diagnostic procedure, reveals separate ventral and dorsal pancreatic ducts.[109]

ANNULAR PANCREAS

Annular pancreas is an embryologic abnormality in which the ventral primordium of the pancreas fails to rotate properly, which results in complete or incomplete bands of pancreatic tissue surrounding the second portion of the duodenum. Annular pancreas may present itself anytime after birth. In the neonatal period, annular pancreas usually occurs in association with polyhydramnios. Patients present with failure to tolerate feedings, persistent bile-stained vomiting, and distention of the upper abdomen.[110] In adults, symptoms include epigastric or upper abdominal pain, gastric outlet obstruction, pancreatitis, pancreatic mass, gastric/duodenal ulcer, nausea and vomiting, weight loss, and upper gastrointestinal bleeding.[110-114] In one recent study, three of seven patients (40%) were first diagnosed intraoperatively.[111]

In neonates, plain abdominal films show a characteristic "double bubble" sign indicative of duodenal obstruction. In older children and adults, upper gastrointestinal contrast studies demonstrate an annular filling defect across the second portion of the pancreas, symmetrical dilatation of the proximal duodenum, and reverse peristalsis of the duodenal segment proximal to the annulus.[112]

Annular pancreas may be associated with several other congenital anomalies, suggesting that the defect occurs early in embryogenesis. Associated malformations include intestinal malrotation, cardiac defects, Meckel's diverticulum, imperforate anus, duodenal bands, spinal defects, and cryptorchidism.[112] A high incidence of annular pancreas is found in patients with Down syndrome as well.[110] Proposed mechanisms for the development of annular pancreas include (1) hypertrophy of both ventral and dorsal anlagen, resulting in complete constriction around the duodenum; (2) persistence and enlargement of the left bud of the paired ventral primordium; and (3) fixation of the ventral bud tip before rotation, resulting in persistence of the ventral bud around the duodenum.[112] Grossly and histologically, annular pancreas comprises normal pancreatic tissue, which may show focal areas of inflammation (pancreatitis), and is presumably related to duct obstruction.

PANCREATIC DISEASE RELATED TO CYSTIC FIBROSIS

Cystic fibrosis is an inherited multisystemic disease characterized by pancreatic insufficiency, chronic pulmonary disease, and failure to thrive. Synonyms include *fibrocystic disease of the pancreas, mucoviscidosis,* and *pancreatic fibrosis.*

Clinical Features

It is the most common inherited disease among the white population of North America and Europe. Cystic fibrosis occurs in 1 of 2000 whites but in only 1 of 17,000 blacks.[82] The hallmarks of cystic fibrosis include pancreatic insufficiency (steatorrhea), elevated sweat electrolytes (sodium and chloride), pulmonary involvement, increased viscosity of pancreatic and bronchial tree secretions, meconium ileus, and failure to thrive.

Pathologic Features

Pathologically, the pancreas in cystic fibrosis is usually small, hard, and nodular and may show an increased quantity of fat and multiple cysts. The histologic changes of cystic fibrosis vary according to the stage of disease. Early alterations include dilated (ectatic) ducts with intraluminal eosinophilic secretions or concretions (Fig. 30-22). These secretions, which represent mucoprotein, react with stains for acid mucopolysaccharides. Desquamated epithelial cells and inflammatory cells are usually admixed with intraluminal secretions. The concretions are deeply eosinophilic and

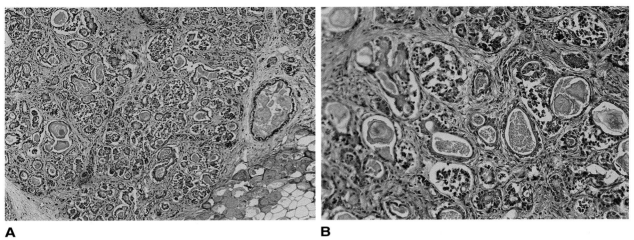

A   **B**

FIGURE 30–22. Pancreatic changes associated with cystic fibrosis. **A,** Dilated (ectatic) ducts with intraluminal eosinophilic secretions or concretions; the secretions represent mucoprotein. Fat necrosis *(lower right)* is noted. **B,** In the course of the disease ductal, acinar, and islet cell atrophy can be seen. The intraluminal concretions are eosinophilic and appear focally laminated.

may be laminated or calcified. Additional changes in the course of the disease include intralobular fibrosis, interlobular fibrosis with associated ductular ectasia, microcysts, and ductal and acinar cell atrophy (see Fig. 30-22). The acinar cells may become flattened to form a thin epithelial cell wall. An inflammatory cell infiltrate that includes polymorphonuclear leukocytes may be seen in the intralobular fibrous tissue in and around the ducts and acini. Marked interstitial lymphocytic infiltration is noted. Intraductal papillary hyperplasia and goblet cell metaplasia may be observed on occasion. With progression of disease, liposclerosis, ductal obliteration, and endocrine (islet cell) atrophy develop.

HETEROTOPIC PANCREAS AND OTHER ANOMALIES

Other congenital anomalies of the pancreas are uncommon and include agenesis, aplasia, hypoplasia and dysplasia, various malformations of the pancreatic duct system, choledochal cysts, congenital cysts, and heterotopia.[82] Of these, pathologists most often encounter pancreatic heterotopia.

Pancreatic heterotopia is defined as pancreatic tissue that lacks anatomic and vascular continuity with the main pancreas. Synonyms include *ectopic, aberrant,* or *accessory pancreas.* The incidence of pancreatic heterotopia is 0.55% to 15% among autopsy specimens.[82] In approximately 70% of patients with pancreatic heterotopia, the pancreas is located in the upper gastrointestinal tract, specifically (in descending order of frequency) in the duodenum, stomach (usually within 5 cm of the pylorus), and jejunum. Other intra-abdominal sites of involvement include the liver, gall-bladder and bile ducts, distal small intestine, appendix, colon, omentum, abdominal wall, Meckel's diverticulum, and spleen. Extra-abdominal pancreatic hetero-

topia are rare and include foci in bronchogenic cysts, pulmonary sequestration, and the umbilicus.

Most patients with heterotopic pancreas are asymptomatic. However, occasionally, symptoms related to pancreatic heterotopia occur; these include abdominal distention, epigastric pain, dyspepsia, nausea, and vomiting. The radiographic and endoscopic appearances are characteristic and include a well-defined dome-shaped filling defect that is smaller than 1 cm and reveals central umbilication. In the stomach, the most common location is along the greater curvature of the antrum or in the prepyloric region.

Pancreatic heterotopias are usually discrete, irregular, firm, yellow nodules that measure 0.2 to 4 cm in diameter. In most cases, the heterotopic nodule is found in the submucosa, but it may be seen in the subserosal tissue or in the muscularis propria. Microscopically, ductal and acinar cell components are present in most cases. The ducts may be the dominant component because acinar tissue may be sparse and difficult to detect. Islets of Langerhans are identified in only one third of cases. Rarely, heterotopic pancreas may reveal features of pancreatitis (acute or chronic); it may rarely develop into exocrine or endocrine neoplasms.

▪ Age-Related Alterations of the Pancreas

A variety of morphologic alterations occur in the pancreas with advancing age. These findings are unrelated to any specific clinical features. Histologic alterations with increasing age include fatty replacement, which is also referred to as *lipomatosis of the pancreas.* In this condition, the pancreas shows near-total atrophy of the exocrine component, as well as panlobular replacement of acinar cells by fat (Fig. 30-23). Pancreatic

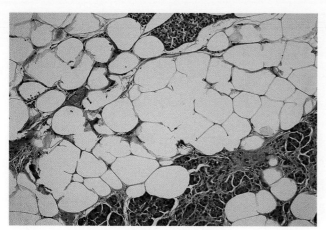

FIGURE 30–23. Pancreatic lipomatosis (fatty replacement) in a patient with diabetes mellitus.

islets are usually spared the effects of aging; thus, they stand out on a background of exocrine pancreatic atrophy. Some cases develop secondary ductal mucinous metaplasia without atypia. Despite atrophy of the exocrine pancreas, clinical pancreatic insufficiency usually does not occur.[115] Normally, the adult pancreas decreases in weight, but with advancing age and lipomatosis, the weight of the gland increases. Lipomatosis of the pancreas also occurs in obesity, in adult-onset diabetes mellitus, and in severe generalized lipomatosis. Lipomatous atrophy (Shwachman-Diamond syndrome) shows similar histopathologic features as lipomatosis but is part of a systemic syndrome characterized by pancreatic insufficiency (steatorrhea, diarrhea, and failure to thrive in infancy), neutropenia, recurrent infection, and a variety of skeletal and dermatologic abnormalities.[116] It is the second most common cause of pancreatic insufficiency, second only to cystic fibrosis.[117]

Ductal changes related to aging include dilatation of major and small peripheral ducts with an increase in the quantity of inspissated secretions, periductal fibrosis, and enlargement of duct epithelial cells, including mucous cell hyperplasia (also known as *mucoid transformation, mucinous hyperplasia, goblet cell metaplasia,* and *nonpapillary hyperplasia*).[40,118] Other metaplastic changes include squamous metaplasia, papillary hyperplasia, and pyloric gland metaplasia. In this instance, the mucus is periodic acid–Schiff–positive and Alcian blue–negative at pH 2.5, which is indicative of sialomucins rather than sulfomucins. These ductal changes, which may also be seen in chronic pancreatitis, with steroid use, or in association with pancreatic ductal carcinoma, ductal obstruction of any cause, and diabetes mellitus,[119] are most often found in the pancreatic head.

Acinar cell changes include decreased or absent basophilia, a decrease in the quantity of zymogen granules, reduction in cell size, alterations in nuclear size and shape (enlargement, pyknosis, variations in shape), cytoplasmic vacuolization, and acinar dilatation (acinar ectasia)[118]; the last is characterized by inspissated secretions in the acini accompanied by acinar dilatation with reduction in the height of the acini, loss of zymogen granules, and normal basal basophilia.[118] Similar acinar cell changes may also be seen in association with acute duct obstruction, heavy cigarette smoking, excessive alcohol use, chronic renal failure (uremia), dehydration, and other metabolic disturbances; in children treated with chemotherapy for cancer; and as a result of severe bacterial infection.[40]

Centroacinar cell and intercalated duct changes related to aging include dilatation of centroacinar cells (Fig. 30–24) and increased numbers of centroacinar cells and intercalated ducts. These centroacinar cells and intercalated duct changes can also be seen in metabolic disturbances such as uremia and dehydration, in hypergastrinemia, in insulin-producing pancreatic endocrine neoplasms, and following obstruction of the major pancreatic ducts.[40]

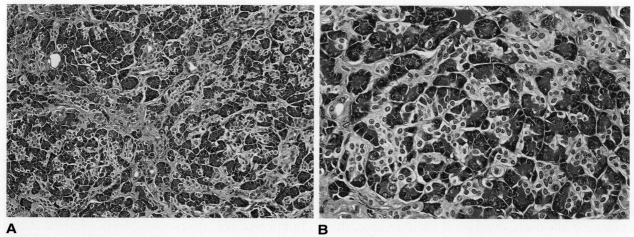

A   **B**

FIGURE 30–24. Age-related alterations. **A,** An increase in the number of centroacinar cells is seen. **B,** Interspersed acinar cells show a decrease in cytoplasmic basophilia and a decrease in the number of zymogen granules.

References

1. Bradley EL III: A clinically based classification system for acute pancreatitis. Arch Surg 128:586-590, 1993.
2. Sakorafas GH, Tsiotou AG: Etiology and pathogenesis of acute pancreatitis. Current concepts. J Clin Gastroenterol 30:343-356, 2000.
3. Levitt MD, Eckfeldt JH: Diagnosis of acute pancreatitis. In Go VLW, DiMagno EP, Gardner JD, et al (eds): The Pancreas: Biology, Pathobiology and Disease, 2nd ed. New York, Raven Press, 1993, pp 613-635.
4. Kessler JI, Miller M, Barza D, et al: Hyperlipidemia in acute pancreatitis. Am J Med 42:968-976, 1967.
5. Weir GC, Lesser PB, Drop LJ, et al: The hypocalcemia of acute pancreatitis. Ann Intern Med 83:185-189, 1975.
6. Golub R, Siddiqi F, Pohl D: Role of antibiotic in acute pancreatitis: A meta-analysis. J Gastrointest Surg 2:496-503, 1998.
7. Steinberg W, Tenner S: Acute pancreatitis. N Engl J Med 330:1198-1210, 1994.
8. Lowham A, Lavelle J, Leese T: Mortality from acute pancreatitis. Int J Pancreatol 25:103-106, 1999.
9. Banks P: Medical management of acute pancreatitis and complications. In Go VLW, DiMagno EP, Gardner JD (eds): The Pancreas: Biology, Pathobiology and Disease, 2nd ed. New York, Raven Press, 1993, pp 593-611.
10. Wrobleski DM, Barth MM, Oyen LJ: Necrotizing pancreatitis: Pathophysiology, diagnosis, and acute care management. AACN Clin Issues 10:464-477, 1999.
11. Ranson JHC, Rifkind KM, Roses DF, et al: Prognostic signs and the role of operative management in acute pancreatitis. Surg Gynecol Obstet 139:69-81, 1974.
12. Runzi M, Layer P: Drug-associated pancreatitis: Facts and fiction. Pancreas 13:100-109, 1996.
13. Parenti DM, Steinberg W, Kang P: Infectious causes of acute pancreatitis. Pancreas 13:356-371, 1996.
14. Niederau C, Luthen R: Events inside the pancreatic acinar cell in acute pancreatitis: Role of secretory blockade, calcium release, and dehydration in the initiation of trypsinogen activation and autodigestion. In Lankisch PG, DiMagno EP (eds): Pancreatic Disease: State of the Art and Future Aspects of Research. Berlin, Springer, 1999, pp 14-23.
15. Luthen R, Grendell JH, Niederau C, et al: Trypsinogen activation and glutathione content are linked to pancreatic injury in models of biliary acute pancreatitis. Int J Pancreatol 24:193-202, 1998.
16. Luthen R, Grendell JH, Haussinger D, et al: Trypsinogen activation occurs inside the acinar cell early in the course of acute cerulein-induced pancreatitis. Pancreas 17:38-43, 1998.
17. Niederau C, Schulz HU: Current conservative treatment of acute pancreatitis: Evidence of animal and human studies. Hepatogastroenterology 6:538-549, 1993.
18. Sarner M: Pancreatitis definitions and classification. In Go VLW, DiMagno EP, Gardner JD, et al (eds): The Pancreas: Biology, Pathobiology and Disease, 2nd ed. New York, Raven Press, 1993, pp 575-580.
19. Etemad B, Whitcomb DC: Chronic pancreatitis: Diagnosis, classification and new genetic developments. Gastroenterology 120:682-707, 2001.
20. Uomo G: How far are we from the most accurate classification system for chronic pancreatitis? J Pancreas 3:62-65, 2002.
21. DiMagno EP, Layer P, Clain JE: Chronic pancreatitis. In Go VLW, DiMagno EP, Gardner JD, et al (eds): The Pancreas: Biology, Pathobiology and Disease, 2nd ed. New York, Raven Press, 1993, pp 665-706.
22. Worning H: Incidence and prevalence of chronic pancreatitis. In Berger HG, Büchler M, Ditschuneit H, et al (eds): Chronic Pancreatitis. Berlin, Springer-Verlag, 1990, pp 35-40.
23. Ectors N, Maillet B, Aerts R, et al: Non-alcoholic duct destructive chronic pancreatitis. Gut 41:263-268, 1997.
24. O'Sullivan JN, Nobrega FT, Morlock CG, et al: Acute and chronic pancreatitis in Rochester, Minnesota, 1940 to 1969. Gastroenterology 62:373-379, 1972.
25. Riela A, Zinmeister AR, Melton LJ, et al: Trends in the incidence and clinical characteristics of chronic pancreatitis. Pancreas 5:727, 1990.
26. Minghini A, Weirter LJ Jr, Perry RR: Specificity of elevated CA 19-9 levels in chronic pancreatitis. Surgery 124:103-105, 1997.
27. Tolliver BA, O'Brien BL: Elevated tumor-associated antigen CA 19-9 in a patient with an enlarged pancreas: Does it always imply malignancy? South Med J 90:89-90, 1997.
28. Frey CF: The surgical treatment of chronic pancreatitis. In Go VLW, DiMagno EP, Gardner JD, et al (eds): The Pancreas: Biology, Pathobiology and Disease, 2nd ed. New York, Raven Press, 1993, pp 707-740.
29. Ammann RW, Knoblauch M, Mohr P, et al: High incidence of extrapancreatic carcinoma in chronic pancreatitis. Scand J Gastroenterol 15:395-399, 1980.
30. Lowenfels AB, Maisonneuve P, Cavallini G, et al: Pancreatitis and the risk of pancreatic cancer. N Engl J Med 328:1433-1437, 1993.
31. Paolini O, Hastier P, Buckley M, et al: The natural history of hereditary chronic pancreatitis: A study of 12 cases compared to chronic alcoholic pancreatitis. Pancreas 17:266-271, 1998.
32. Madrazo-de la Garza JA, Hill ID, Lebenthal E: Hereditary pancreatitis. In Go VLW, DiMagno EP, Gardner JD, et al (eds): The Pancreas: Biology, Pathobiology and Disease, 2nd ed. New York, Raven Press, 1993, pp 1095-1101.
33. Rivera JA, Rall CJN, Graeme-Cook F, et al: Analysis of K-ras oncogene mutations in chronic pancreatitis with ductal hyperplasia. Surgery 121:42-49, 1997.
34. Hsiang D, Friess H, Buchler MW, et al: Absence of K-ras mutations in the pancreatic parenchyma of patients with chronic pancreatitis. Am J Surg 174:242-246, 1997.
35. Luttges J, Diederichs A, Menke MAOH, et al: Ductal lesions in patients with chronic pancreatitis show K-ras mutations in a frequency similar to that in normal pancreas and lack nuclear immunoreactivity for p53. Cancer 88:2495-2504, 2000.
36. Cottliar AS, Fundia AF, Moran C, et al: Evidence of chromosome instability in chronic pancreatitis. J Exp Clin Cancer Res 19:513-517, 2000.
37. Gerdes B, Ramaswamy A, Kresting M, et al: p16 alterations in chronic pancreatitis—indicator for high-risk lesions for pancreatic cancer. Surgery 129:490-497, 2001.
38. Singer MV, Gyr K, Sarles H: Revised classification of pancreatitis: Report of the second international symposium on the classification of pancreatitis in Marseilles, France, March 28-30, 1984. Gastroenterology 89:865-870, 1984.
39. Lack EE, Legg MA: Pancreatitis and its sequelae. In Silverberg SG, DeLellis RA, Frable WJ (eds): Principles and Practice of Surgical Pathology and Cytopathology. New York, Churchill Livingstone, 1997, pp 2025-2028.
40. Oertel JE, Oertel YC, Heffess CS: Pancreas. In Sternberg SS (ed): Diagnostic Surgical Pathology, 3rd ed. New York, Raven Press, 1999, pp 1469-1507.
41. Bommer G, Friedl U, Heitz PU, et al: Pancreatic PP cell distribution and hyperplasia. Immunocytochemical morphology in the normal human pancreas, in chronic pancreatitis and pancreatic carcinoma. Virchows Arch (A) 387:319-331, 1980.
42. Hyland C, Kheir SM, Kashlan MB: Frozen section diagnosis of pancreatic carcinoma. A prospective study of 64 biopsies. Am J Surg Pathol 5:179-191, 1981.
43. Nouts A, Levy P, Violet H, et al: Diagnostic value of serum CA 19-9 antigen in chronic pancreatitis and pancreatic adenocarcinoma. Gastroenterol Clin Biol 22:152-159, 1998.
44. Tanaka N, Okada S, Ueno H, et al: The usefulness of serial changes in serum CA 19-9 levels in the diagnosis of pancreatic cancer. Pancreas 20:378-381, 2000.
45. Riker A, Bartlett D: Pancreaticoduodenectomy for chronic pancreatitis: A case report and literature review. Hepatogastroenterology 46:2005-2010, 1999.
46. Furuya N, Kawa S, Hasebe O, et al: Comparative study of CA242 and CA19-9 in chronic pancreatitis. Br J Cancer 73:372-376, 1996.
47. Slesak B, Harlozinska-Szmyrka A, Knast W, et al: Tissue polypeptide specific antigen (TPS), a marker for differentiation between pancreatic carcinoma and chronic pancreatitis. A comparative study with CA 19-9. Cancer 89:83-88, 2000.
48. Raedle J, Oremek G, Welker M, et al: p53 autoantibodies in patients with pancreatitis and pancreatic carcinoma. Pancreas 13:241-246, 1996.
49. Berndt C, Haubold K, Wenger F, et al: K-ras mutations in stools and tissue samples from patients with malignant and nonmalignant pancreatic tissues. Clin Chem 44:2103-2107, 1998.

50. Theodor L, Melzer E, Sologov M, et al: Detection of pancreatic carcinoma: Diagnostic value of K-ras mutations in circulating DNA from serum. Dig Dis Sci 44:2014-2019, 1999.

51. Queneau PE, Adessi GL, Thibault P, et al: Early detection of pancreatic cancer in patients with chronic pancreatitis: Diagnostic utility of a K-ras point mutation in the pancreatic juice. Am J Gastroenterol 96:700-704, 2001.

52. Gross JB: Hereditary pancreatitis. In Go VLW (ed): The Exocrine Pancreas: Biology, Pathobiology and Diseases. New York, Raven Press, 1986, pp 829-839.

53. Whitcomb DC: Hereditary pancreatitis: New insights into acute and chronic pancreatitis. Gut 45:317-322, 1999.

54. Le Bodic L, Bignon JD, Raguenes O, et al: The hereditary pancreatitis gene maps to long arm of chromosome 7. Hum Mol Genet 5:549-554, 1996.

55. Whitcomb DC, Preston RA, Ashton CE, et al: A gene for hereditary pancreatitis maps to chromosome 7q35. Gastroenterology 110:1975-1980, 1996.

56. Pandya A, Blanton SH, Landa B, et al: Linkage studies in a large kindred with hereditary pancreatitis confirms mapping of the gene to a 16 cm region on 7q. Genomics 38:227-230, 1996.

57. Whitcomb DC, Gorry MC, Preston RA, et al: Hereditary pancreatitis is caused by a mutation in the cationic trypsinogen gene. Nat Genet 14:141-145, 1996.

58. Truninger K, Kock J, Wirth HP, et al: Trypsinogen gene mutations in patients with chronic or recurrent acute pancreatitis. Pancreas 22:18-23, 2001.

59. Gorry MC, Gabbaizedeh D, Furey W, et al: Mutations in the cationic trypsinogen gene are associated with recurrent acute and chronic pancreatitis. Gastroenterology 113:1063-1068, 1997.

60. Perrault J: Hereditary pancreatitis. Gastroenterol Clin North Am 23:743-752, 1994.

61. Comfort M, Steinberg A: Pedigree of a family with hereditary chronic relapsing pancreatitis. Gastroenterology 21:54-63, 1952.

62. Okazaki K, Chiba T: Autoimmune related pancreatitis. Gut 51:1-4, 2002.

63. Sarles H, Sarles JC, Camatte R, et al: Observation on 205 confirmed cases of acute pancreatitis, recurring pancreatitis, and chronic pancreatitis. Gut 6:545-559, 1965.

64. Montefusco PP, Geiss AC, Bronzo RL, et al: Sclerosing cholangitis, chronic pancreatitis, and Sjögren's syndrome: A syndrome complex. Am J Surg 147:822-826, 1984.

65. Epstein O, Chapman RWG, Lake-Bakaar G, et al: The pancreas in primary biliary cirrhosis and primary sclerosing cholangitis. Gastroenterology 83:1117-1182, 1982.

66. Uchida K, Okazaki K, Konishi Y, et al: Clinical analysis of autoimmune-related pancreatitis. Am J Gastroenterol 95:2788-2794, 2000.

67. Kino-Ohsaki J, Nishimori I, Okazaki K, et al: Serum antibodies to carbonic anhydrase I and II in patients with idiopathic pancreatitis and Sjögren's syndrome. Gastroenterology 110:1579-1586, 1996.

68. Okazaki K, Uchida K, Ohana M, et al: Autoimmune-related pancreatitis is associated with autoantibodies and Th1/Th2-type cellular immune response. Gastroenterology 118:573-581, 2000.

69. Okazaki K, Uchida K, Chiba T: Recent concept of autoimmune-related pancreatitis. J Gastroenterol 36:293-302, 2001.

70. Kawaguchi K, Koike M, Tsuruta K, et al: Lymphoplasmacytic sclerosing pancreatitis with cholangitis: A variant of primary sclerosing cholangitis extensively involving pancreas. Hum Pathol 22:387-395, 1991.

71. Horiuchi A, Kawa S, Hamano H, et al: Sclerosing pancreato-cholangitis responsive to corticosteroid therapy: Report of 2 case reports and review. Gastrointest Endosc 53:518-522, 2001.

72. Scully KA, Li SC, Hebert JC, et al: The characteristic appearance of non-alcoholic duct destructive chronic pancreatitis. A report of 2 cases. Arch Pathol Lab Med 124:1535-1538, 2000.

73. Haneji N, Hamano H, Yanagi K, et al: Identification of α-fodrin as a candidate autoantigen in primary Sjögren's syndrome. Science 276:604-607, 1998.

74. Irie H, Honda H, Baba S, et al: Autoimmune pancreatitis: CT and MR characteristics. Am J Roentgenol 170:1323-1327, 1998.

75. Yoshida K, Toki F, Takeuchi T, et al: Chronic pancreatitis caused by an autoimmune abnormality. Proposal of the concept of autoimmune pancreatitis. Dig Dis Sci 40:1561-1568, 1995.

76. Toki F, Kozu T, Oi I: An unusual type of chronic pancreatitis showing diffuse irregular narrowing of the entire main pancreatic duct on ERC. A report of 4 cases. Endoscopy 24:640, 1992.

77. Ito T, Nakano I, Kayanagi S, et al: Autoimmune pancreatitis as a new clinical entity. Three cases of autoimmune pancreatitis with effective steroid therapy. Dig Dis Sci 42:1458-1468, 1997.

78. Okazaki K: Autoimmune-related pancreatitis. Curr Treat Option Gastroenterol 4:369-375, 2001.

79. Tanaka S, Kobayashi T, Nakanishi K, et al: Corticosteroid-responsive diabetes mellitus associated with autoimmune pancreatitis. Lancet 356:910-911, 2000.

80. Taniguchi T, Seko S, Okamoto M, et al: Association of autoimmune pancreatitis and type 1 diabetes: Autoimmune exocrinopathy and endocrinopathy of the pancreas. Diabetes Care 23:1592-1594, 2000.

81. Chutaputti A, Burrell MI, Boyer JL: Pseudotumor of the pancreas associated with retroperitoneal fibrosis: A dramatic response to corticosteroid therapy. Am J Gastroenterol 90:1155-1158, 1995.

82. Wenig BM, Heffess CS, Adair CF: Non-neoplastic lesions of the pancreas. In Wenig BM, Heffess CS, Adair CF (eds): Atlas of Endocrine Pathology. Philadelphia, WB Saunders, 1997, pp 181-206.

83. Flejou JF, Potet F, Bernades P: Eosinophilic pancreatitis: A rare manifestation of digestive allergy? Gastroenterol Clin Biol 13:731-733, 1989.

84. Bastid C, Sahel J, Choux R, et al: Eosinophilic pancreatitis: Report of a case. Pancreas 5:104-107, 1990.

85. Barthet M, Hastier P, Buckley MJ, et al: Eosinophilic pancreatitis mimicking pancreatic neoplasia: EUS and ERCP findings—is nonsurgical diagnosis possible? Pancreas 17:419-422, 1998.

86. Eusher E, Vaswani K, Frankel W: Eosinophilic pancreatitis: A rare entity that can mimic a pancreatic neoplasm. Ann Diagn Pathol 4:379-385, 2000.

87. Drachenberg CB, Abruzzo LV, Klassen DK, et al: Epstein-Barr virus–related posttransplantation lymphoproliferative disorder involving pancreas allografts: Histological differential diagnosis from acute allograft rejection. Hum Pathol 29:569-577, 1998.

88. Robbie MJ, Scurry JP, Stevenson P: Carbamazepine-induced severe systemic hypersensitivity reaction with eosinophilia. Drug Intell Clin Pharm 22:783-784, 1988.

89. de Diego Lorenzo A, Robles Fornieles J, Herrero Lopez T, et al: Acute pancreatitis associated with milk allergy. Int J Pancreatol 12:319-321, 1992.

90. Ryan KG: Eosinophilic infiltration of duodenum and pancreatic head: Report of a case studied arteriographically. Surgery 77:321-324, 1977.

91. Walsh SV, Evangelista F, Khettry U: Inflammatory myofibroblastic tumor of the pancreaticobiliary region: Morphologic and immuno-cytochemical study of three cases. Am J Surg Pathol 22:412-418, 1998.

92. Hashimoto F: Transient eosinophilia associated with pancreatitis and pseudocyst formation. Arch Intern Med 140:1099-1100, 1980.

93. Tokoo M, Oguchi H, Kawa S, et al: Eosinophilia associated with chronic pancreatitis: An analysis of 122 patients with definitive chronic pancreatitis. Am J Gastroenerol 87:455-460, 1992.

94. Ito T, Nakano I, Koyanagi S, et al: Autoimmune pancreatitis as a new clinical entity. Three cases of autoimmune pancreatitis with effective steroid therapy. Dig Dis Sci 42:1458-1468, 1997.

95. Fauci AS, Harley JB, Roberts WC, et al: The idiopathic hyper-eosinophilic syndrome. Clinical, pathophysiologic, and therapeutic considerations. Ann Intern Med 97:78-92, 1982.

96. Dassopoulos T, Ehrenpreis ED: Acute pancreatitis in human immunodeficiency virus–infected patients: A review. Am J Med 107:78-84, 1999.

97. Parthivel VS, Yousuf AM, Albu E, et al: Predictors of severity of acute pancreatitis in patients with HIV infection or AIDS. Pancreas 19:133-136, 1999.

98. Manocha AP, Sossenheimer M, Martin SP, et al: Prevalence and predictors of severe acute pancreatitis in patients with acquired immune deficiency syndrome (AIDS). Am J Gastroenterol 94:784-789, 1999.

99. Mackrell PJ, Lee K, Garcia N, et al: Pancreatitis secondary to *Ascaris lumbricoides* infection. Surgery 129:511-512, 2001.

100. Stürmer J, Becker V: Granulomatous pancreatitis—granulomas in chronic pancreatitis. Virchows Arch Pathol Anat (A) 410:327-338, 1987.

101. Gaur S: Sarcoidosis manifested as hypercalcemic pancreatitis. South Med J 94:939-940, 2001.

102. Gschwantler M, Kogelbauer G, Klose W, et al: The pancreas as a site of granulomatous inflammation in Crohn's disease. Gastroenterology 108:1246-1249, 1995.

103. Kloppel G: Pseudocysts and other non-neoplastic cysts of the pancreas. Semin Diagn Pathol 17:7-15, 2000.

104. Maule WF, Reber HA: Diagnosis and management of pancreatic pseudocysts, pancreatic ascites, and pancreatic fistulas. In Go VLW, DiMagno EP, Gardner JD, Lebenthal E, Reber HA, Scheele GA (eds): The Pancreas: Biology, Pathobiology and Disease, 2nd ed. New York, Raven Press, 1993, pp 741-750.

105. Adsay NV, Hasteh F, Cheng JD, et al: Squamous-lined cysts of the pancreas: Lymphoepithelial cysts, dermoid cysts (teratomas), and accessory-splenic epidermoid cysts. Semin Diagn Pathol 17:56-65, 2000.

106. Adsay NV, Hasteh F, Cheng JD, et al: Lymphoepithelial cysts of the pancreas: A report of 12 cases and a review of the literature. Mod Pathol 15:492-501, 2002.

107. Neumann HP, Dinkel E, Brambs H, et al: Pancreatic lesions in the von Hippel-Lindau syndrome. Gastroenterology 101:465-471, 1991.

108. Varshney S, Johnson CD: Pancreas divisum. Int J Pancreatol 2:135-141, 1999.

109. Morgan DE, Logan K, Baron TH, et al: Pancreas divisum: Implications for diagnostic and therapeutic pancreatography. AJR Am J Roentgenol 173:193-198, 1999.

110. Kiernan PD, ReMine SG, Kiernan PC, et al: Annular pancreas: Mayo clinic experience from 1957-1976 with review of the literature. Arch Surg 115:46-50, 1980.

111. Urayama S, Kozarek R, Ball T, et al: Presentation and treatment of annular pancreas in an adult population. Am J Gastroenterol 90:995-999, 1995.

112. Hill ID, Lebenthel E: Congenital abnormalities of the exocrine pancreas. In Go VLW, DiMagno EP, Gardner JD, et al (eds): The Pancreas: Biology, Pathobiology and Disease, 2nd ed. New York, Raven Press, 1993, pp 1029-1040.

113. Schlinkert RT, Burns B, Argueta R, et al: Insulinoma in a patient with annular pancreas. Mayo Clin Proc 65:518-520, 1990.

114. Kamisawa T, Tabata I, Isawa T, et al: Annular pancreas associated with carcinoma in the dorsal part of pancreas divisum. Int J Pancreatol 17:207-211, 1995.

115. Robson HN, Scott GBD: Lipomatous pseudohypertrophy of the pancreas. Gastroenterology 23:74-81, 1953.

116. Goeteyn M, Oranje AP, Vuzevski VD, et al: Ichthyosis, exocrine pancreatic insufficiency, impaired neutrophil chemotaxis, growth retardation, and metaphyseal dysplasia (Shwachman syndrome). Arch Dermatol 127:225-230, 1991.

117. Tada H, Ri T, Yoshida H, et al: A case report of Shwachman syndrome with increased spontaneous chromosome breakage. Hum Genet 77:289-291, 1987.

118. Oertel JE: The pancreas. Nonneoplastic alterations. Am J Surg Pathol 13(suppl 1):50-65, 1989.

119. Allen-Mersh TG: What is the significance of pancreatic ductal mucinous hyperplasia? Gut 26:825-833, 1985

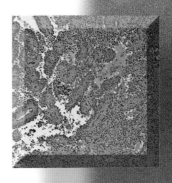

CHAPTER 31

Benign and Malignant Tumors of the Pancreas

DAVID S. KLIMSTRA • N. VOLKAN ADSAY

Introduction

Tumors of the pancreas present a variety of challenges to the surgical pathologist. The most common pancreatic tumor, ductal adenocarcinoma, is notoriously difficult to diagnose. The relative inaccessibility of the pancreas means that the diagnosis of this deadly tumor type must often be made on the basis of minimal pathologic material. Also challenging is the accurate classification of other less common tumors that may occur in the pancreas, many of which are less aggressive than ductal adenocarcinoma. Variants of ductal adenocarcinoma, cystic and intraductal tumors, acinar tumors, and endocrine tumors are all described, but their relative rarity means that pathologists may be unaware of their diagnostic features.

The increased use of sensitive imaging techniques, such as spiral computed tomographic (CT) scans, endoscopic ultrasound, and magnetic resonance cholangiopancreatography (MRCP), has contributed to an increase in detection of some less common pancreatic tumors. In addition, advances in surgical techniques and better postoperative care have allowed pancreatectomy to become a more commonplace operation with decreased morbidity and mortality. Furthermore, because of an enhanced detection of pancreatic tumors (and often at earlier stages in their evolution), the past three decades have witnessed the characterization of several previously unrecognized categories of neoplasia in the pancreas. The classification of pancreatic tumors and our understanding of the mechanisms of pancreatic neoplasia have improved significantly. In the following sections, the pathology of tumors and tumor-like lesions that occur in the pancreas is presented. Emphasis is given to the more common and clinically important tumors.

The classification of pancreatic tumors is listed in Table 31-1.[1] This current classification is based on three general features: the line of cellular differentiation,[2] gross configuration (solid vs. cystic), and for an important subgroup of potentially noninvasive tumors, degree of atypia (benign vs. borderline vs. carcinoma).

The line of differentiation refers to the cellular phenotype of the tumor. Most pancreatic tumors recapitulate one or more of the normal epithelial cell lines of the pancreas—ductal, acinar, or endocrine. Defining pathologic features of each of these normal cell types are reflected, to varying degrees, in their corresponding tumors (Table 31-2).

Ductal differentiation in pancreatic neoplasia is defined as the recapitulation of characteristics of normal ducts, that is, gland or tubule formation and mucin production. Mucin, which can be demonstrated histochemically with stains such as periodic acid–Schiff (PAS), mucicarmine, or high-iron diamine and Alcian blue, is regarded as a hallmark of ductal differentiation in the pancreas. Immunohistochemical markers of ductal differentiation such as CA 19-9, carcinoembryonic antigen (CEA), B72.3, DUPAN-2, and MUC1,[3-5] many of which detect mucin-related antigens or oncoproteins, are often helpful.[2,6] In addition, mutation at codon 12 of the K-*ras* oncogene is common (>90%) in ductal adenocarcinoma (and usually is not seen in

TABLE 31-1. Classification of Pancreatic Neoplasms

Ductal Adenocarcinoma
Tubular (conventional) ductal adenocarcinoma
Colloid (mucinous noncystic) carcinoma
Medullary carcinoma
Squamous cell carcinoma
Adenosquamous carcinoma
Undifferentiated carcinoma
   Anaplastic giant cell carcinoma
   Sarcomatoid carcinoma
   Carcinosarcoma
   Osteoclastic giant cell carcinoma
Mixed ductal/endocrine carcinoma

Serous Tumors
Microcystic serous cystadenoma
Macrocystic serous cystadenoma
Solid serous adenoma
Serous cystadenocarcinoma

Mucinous Cystic Tumors
Mucinous cystadenoma
Mucinous cystic neoplasm, borderline
Mucinous cystadenocarcinoma
   In situ
   Invasive

Intraductal Tumors
Intraductal papillary-mucinous neoplasm
   Intraductal papillary-mucinous adenoma
   Intraductal papillary-mucinous neoplasm, borderline
   Intraductal papillary-mucinous carcinoma
      In situ
      Invasive
Intraductal oncocytic papillary neoplasm

Acinar Cell Tumors
Acinar cell carcinoma
Acinar cell cystadenoma
Acinar cell cystadenocarcinoma
Mixed acinar/endocrine carcinoma
Mixed acinar/ductal carcinoma
Mixed acinar/endocrine/ductal carcinoma

Pancreatoblastoma

Pancreatic Endocrine Tumors
Microadenoma
Low-grade pancreatic endocrine neoplasm
   Functioning
      Insulinoma
      Glucagonoma
      Somatostatinoma
      VIPoma
   Nonfunctioning
      PPoma
      Not otherwise specified
High-grade neuroendocrine carcinoma
   Small cell carcinoma
   Large cell neuroendocrine carcinoma

Solid-Pseudopapillary Tumor

Mesenchymal Tumors

Lymphoma

Secondary Tumors

nonductal tumors) and may be considered as evidence of ductal differentiation in certain situations.

Endocrine differentiation is defined as the production of peptide hormones or bioamines by tumor cells.[2] In addition, endocrine tumors often have an organoid growth pattern and a characteristic appearance of the chromatin. Endocrine differentiation is most commonly documented by immunohistochemistry, and general endocrine markers (e.g., chromogranin and synaptophysin) are considered the most specific. Other markers include neuron-specific enolase, Leu7 (CD57), and neural cell adhesion molecule (CD56), but the specificity of these markers is questionable. The production of specific peptides or bioamines may also be demonstrable in pancreatic endocrine tumors but is not necessary diagnostically. Electron microscopy may be used to identify dense core secretory granules, but this technique has been largely supplanted by immunohistochemistry.

Pancreatic tumors with acinar differentiation are less common than tumors that exhibit other lines of differentiation,[2] despite the preponderance of acinar cells among the epithelial elements of the gland. In addition to having characteristic light microscopic features, acinar cell neoplasms produce pancreatic enzymes that can be detected immunohistochemically. Antibodies against trypsin, chymotrypsin, and lipase are a few of these.[7,8] Enzyme-containing zymogen granules can also be demonstrated with the PAS stain (resistant to diastase), which reveals small, positive cytoplasmic granules. Zymogen granules can be visualized ultrastructurally as well, and a second granule type, the irregular fibrillary granule, is also highly specific for acinar tumors.

Many primary tumors of the pancreas have a characteristic radiographic and macroscopic appearance. Thus, most can be divided into primarily solid or primarily cystic categories (Table 31-3). Several tumors are inherently cystic, with each locule lined by neoplastic epithelial cells. Other tumors develop cystic change through a process of degeneration or necrosis; this feature is characteristic of some entities but may affect solid tumors as well. Finally, intraductal tumors often appear cystic owing to massive dilatation of the native pancreatic ducts.

The concept of "borderline malignant potential" has recently been applied to certain pancreatic tumors.[1] Although most pancreatic tumors can be divided into frankly benign and malignant categories, some exhibit a range of atypia and fall between these two extremes. Mucinous cystic neoplasms and intraductal papillary mucinous neoplasms, in particular, may be "borderline" in the WHO classification of pancreatic tumors (see Table 31-1).[9,10] This concept has also been proposed for a subset of pancreatic endocrine neoplasms, as well as for solid-pseudopapillary tumors.

TABLE 31-2. Characteristics of Pancreatic Epithelial Cell Lines

Cell Line	Light Microscopy	Histochemistry	Immunohistochemistry	Ultrastructure	Genetic Changes
Ductal	Glands, papillae, lumina, mucin	Mucin stains positive	Glycoprotein markers (B72.3, CEA, DUPAN2, MUC1, CA 19-9)	Mucigen granules	K-ras, TP53, DPC4, p16
Acinar	Solid sheets, nests, acini; granular eosinophilic cytoplasm; prominent nucleoli	DPAS-positive granules	Enzyme markers (trypsin, lipase, chymotrypsin)	Zymogen granules, irregular fibrillary granules	APC/beta-catenin
Endocrine	Nested, trabecular, gyriform patterns; cytologic uniformity; "salt-and-pepper" chromatin	Argyrophil (Grimelius)-positive granules	Neuroendocrine markers (chromogranin, synaptophysin, Leu7, neuron-specific enolase, and CD56)	Neurosecretory granules	*menin* gene, p16

■ Ductal Adenocarcinoma and Its Variants

The ductal system of the pancreas, which is responsible for carrying acinar secretions to the duodenum, is perhaps the smallest epithelial component of the pancreas. However, most pancreatic tumors (>90%) are of ductal origin, and a majority of these (80% to 90%) are ductal adenocarcinomas.[11] It is this type of neoplasm that imbues "pancreatic cancer" with such a dismal outlook, and the diagnosis of ductal adenocarcinoma remains problematic for pathologists.

Pancreatic carcinomas of ductal type can be separated into several categories:

1. Conventional ductal adenocarcinoma (tumors that form small tubular glands with luminal and intracellular mucin and are associated with marked stromal desmoplasia).
2. Unusual histologic patterns of conventional ductal adenocarcinoma (e.g., foamy gland pattern, large duct pattern, vacuolated pattern, lobular carcinoma-like pattern).
3. Other carcinomas of ductal origin (e.g., colloid carcinoma, adenosquamous carcinoma, squamous cell carcinoma, medullary carcinoma, and un-

differentiated carcinomas). Most tumors in this last category usually have an associated component of conventional ductal adenocarcinoma, which provides evidence of their ductal origin.

DUCTAL ADENOCARCINOMA

Conventional Ductal Adenocarcinoma, Tubular Adenocarcinoma

Clinical Features

This is the most common pancreatic tumor and is one of the deadliest of all human cancers. Affected patients are usually between 60 and 80 years old; occurrence in those younger than 40 is exceptional.[12] Patients usually present with jaundice (resulting from invasion and obstruction of the common bile duct) or nonspecific symptoms such as back pain and weight loss. The cause of ductal adenocarcinoma is complex and is probably multifactorial. Smoking and high intake of dietary fat are considered risk factors. Whether acquired chronic pancreatitis and diabetes mellitus constitute risk factors is a subject of ongoing debate, although patients with hereditary chronic pancreatitis are at increased risk. Whereas most ductal adenocarcinomas are sporadic, families with pancreatic cancer have also been recorded. In a small subset of cases, a genetic association with disorders such as Peutz-Jeghers syndrome, breast and ovarian carcinomas (related to the *BRCA2* gene), or familial atypical multiple melanoma syndrome (FAMMM, possibly caused by *p16* mutation) has been documented.[13]

Most ductal adenocarcinomas (>75%) are solid tumors and develop in the head of the pancreas.[14] Possibly because of the lack of a capsule around the organ, ductal adenocarcinomas typically invade surrounding structures, especially the common bile duct and the duodenum. Ductal adenocarcinomas that occur in the tail of the pancreas often spread to surrounding organs (e.g.,

TABLE 31-3. Solid and Cystic Pancreatic Tumors

Typically Solid Tumors	Typically Cystic Tumors
Ductal adenocarcinoma (and variants)	Serous cystic tumor
Pancreatic endocrine neoplasm	Mucinous cystic tumor
Acinar cell carcinoma	Intraductal papillary-mucinous tumor
Pancreatoblastoma	Solid-pseudopapillary tumor Lymphoepithelial cyst

spleen, kidney, stomach, and colon).[14] A large portion of cases (close to 80%) are unresectable at the time of diagnosis,[15] mostly owing to encasement of major mesenteric vessels[16] or because of metastasis to the liver, peritoneum, or other distant sites. Ductal adenocarcinoma often disseminates early in the course of the disease. In fact, if a solid pancreatic tumor measures larger than 5 cm and is still resectable, it is unlikely to be a ductal adenocarcinoma.

Pathologic Features

GROSS PATHOLOGY

Grossly, most ductal adenocarcinomas are solid, firm, infiltrative tumors. The cut surface is often gritty or slightly gelatinous. Less commonly, areas of necrosis may be present. It is often difficult to distinguish carcinoma from adjacent areas of fibrosing chronic pancreatitis. For tumors in the head of the gland, direct invasion of the common bile duct and duodenum is common. Recognition that the center of the tumor is within the head of the pancreas is helpful in distinguishing pancreatic ductal adenocarcinomas from primary carcinomas of the common bile duct, duodenum, or ampulla of Vater.[17] Some ductal adenocarcinomas exhibit cystic change, resulting from degeneration, necrosis, or cystic dilatation of either obstructed ducts or the neoplastic glands ("large duct pattern"; see under Morphologic Patterns). Rarely, one may find a preexisting benign cystic or intraductal tumor associated with a ductal adenocarcinoma.

MICROSCOPIC PATHOLOGY

Microscopically, in its conventional form, ductal adenocarcinoma is characterized microscopically by small tubular structures lined by cuboidal cells within abundant desmoplastic stroma.[18,19] In well-differentiated ductal adenocarcinoma, the growth pattern and cytologic appearance of the cells may be deceptively benign, closely mimicking ductules in chronic pancreatitis (Fig. 31-1). The cells lining the malignant tubules typically form a single regular layer, but stratification and irregular papillae may be prominent in some cases. The cytoplasm may be abundant and generally contains mucin; clear cell change is also common. The nuclei may retain basal orientation within the cells, but loss of polarity in at least some of the glands is typical. The nuclei vary in size, shape, and intracellular location between cells within each gland (Fig. 31-2). In fact, a greater than threefold difference in size between adjacent nuclei is highly suggestive of carcinoma. Perineural invasion and vascular invasion are common. In some cases, tumor cells infiltrate adjacent normal islets. In more poorly differentiated ductal adenocarcinomas, neoplastic glands are admixed with small cell clusters with ill-formed lumina, pleomorphic nuclei, and more mitotic figures.

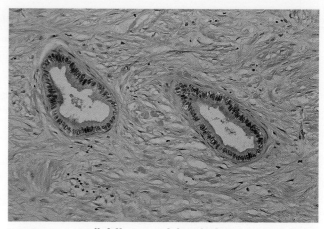

FIGURE 31–1. Well-differentiated ductal adenocarcinoma. Some infiltrating carcinomas consist of remarkably well-formed glands and exhibit relatively minimal cytologic atypia, mimicking benign ductules.

The periphery of ductal adenocarcinomas is often indistinct, such that neoplastic glands may be present well beyond the apparent gross extent of the tumor. The current grading scheme for pancreatic ductal adenocarcinoma (Kloppel's grading scheme, also endorsed by the World Health Organization [WHO]) entails evaluation of glandular differentiation, mucin production, mitosis, and nuclear atypia.[20] This scheme correlates well with prognosis but is rather cumbersome and hence is not widely used. The American Joint Committee on Cancer (AJCC) staging system for pancreatic adenocarcinoma is shown in Table 31-4.

Chronic pancreatitis (i.e., interstitial fibrosis, atrophy, and inflammation) is often present in the pancreas adjacent to ductal adenocarcinoma. The distinction of chronic pancreatitis from carcinoma is discussed later (see under Differential Diagnosis). In addition, the lining of native pancreatic ducts may show proliferative changes that are now referred to as *pancreatic*

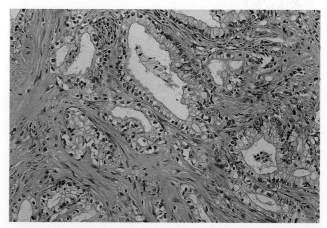

FIGURE 31–2. Cytologic features of ductal adenocarcinoma. The nuclei show variability in size, shape, and location within the glands.

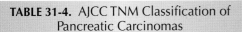

intraepithelial neoplasia (see under Pancreatic Intraepithelial Neoplasia). Squamous, transitional,[21] and rarely, oncocytic metaplasia[22-24] may be noted in nonneoplastic ducts.

Mucin histochemistry and immunohistochemical markers of ductal differentiation (glycoproteins) invariably show at least focal positivity in ductal adenocarcinomas. In addition, stains for cytokeratins 7, 8, 18, and 19 and epithelial membrane antigen (EMA) are usually positive, and cytokeratin 20 is detected in about half of cases. Stains for chromogranin or synaptophysin demonstrate a minor endocrine cell component associated with the neoplastic glands. Some of these endocrine cells are non-neoplastic islet cells entrapped within the tumor, but neoplastic endocrine cells also occur within ductal adenocarcinomas. Mutation in codon 12 of the K-*ras* oncogene is detected in more than 90% of ductal adenocarcinomas, and *TP53* mutation in 50%.[25,26] Most ductal adenocarcinomas also have abnormalities in *p16*, which occur through either mutation or hypermethylation of the promotor region of DNA.[13] Loss of Smad4 (DPC4) is also common and is found in 55% of invasive ductal adenocarcinomas. Many other molecular abnormalities may occur in ductal adenocarcinoma,[13] but this constellation of genetic changes is characteristic, and these four abnormalities are largely restricted to ductal-type tumors in the pancreas.

Differential Diagnosis

The main issue in the differential diagnosis of conventional ductal adenocarcinoma is the distinction of a well-differentiated carcinoma from benign ductules associated with chronic pancreatitis. Ductal adenocarcinoma may be deceptively benign-appearing, and ductules in chronic pancreatitis may appear infiltrative. Most importantly, on low-power examination, the ductules in chronic pancreatitis retain the original lobular configuration that characterizes the normal pancreas. Each lobular cluster of ductules comprises a central larger, slightly dilated duct surrounded by small, round ductules (Fig. 31-3A). The stroma within the

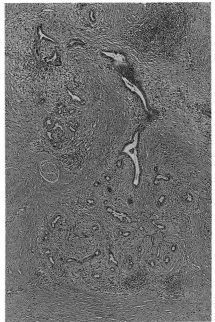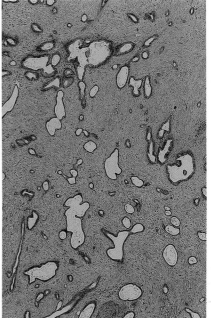

A   **B**

FIGURE 31-3. Comparison between atrophic chronic pancreatitis and well-differentiated ductal adenocarcinoma. In these low-power images, the example of chronic pancreatitis (**A**) shows retention of the lobular architecture of the gland with larger dilated central ducts surrounded by smaller round ductules. The stroma separating each lobule is somewhat more dense than the intralobular stroma. In contrast, adenocarcinoma (**B**) shows a haphazard arrangement of neoplastic glands, lacking a lobular configuration.

lobule is less dense than that between lobules. In contrast, invasive glands of ductal adenocarcinoma lack a lobular pattern and are distributed haphazardly (Fig. 31-3**B**). The contours of individual units are irregular and often sharply angulated. Cytologically, nuclear enlargement, nuclear contour irregularities, and loss of polarity are important clues to the diagnosis of carcinoma. Dense cytoplasmic acidophilia is more commonly seen in carcinoma than in benign conditions. Unlike other sites in which reactive stromal cells may display tremendous atypia, it is uncommon to see pleomorphism and bizarre nuclei in the stroma in inflammatory conditions of the pancreas; individual atypical cells in the stroma of the pancreas are more likely to be cancer cells, especially if they have dense acidophilic cytoplasm. The location of atypical glands is also helpful in that perineural invasion and immediate juxtaposition of glands to adipocytes both are usually diagnostic of carcinoma.

Invasive ductal adenocarcinoma also needs to be differentiated from noninvasive pancreatic intraepithelial neoplasia (see under Pancreatic Intraepithelial Neoplasia) that may display cytologic abnormalities of invasive carcinoma. The number, distribution, and location of the units (in relation to the lobular architecture) are helpful in this distinction. Also, the presence of desmoplastic stroma and irregularity of ductal contours are characteristic of invasive carcinoma. Because pancreatic ducts do not have a basal cell or myoepithelial layer, no immunohistochemical stains can help in determination of whether a particular atypical gland is invasive.

Another pitfall in the differential diagnosis of ductal adenocarcinoma is the aggregation of islets that occurs in atrophic chronic pancreatitis (Fig. 31-4). Clustered islets form small, irregular nests or chains of cells that may have an infiltrative appearance. Sometimes these cells are arranged around small nerves, simulating

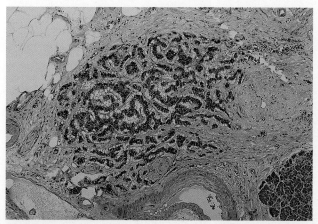

FIGURE 31–4. Pancreatic atrophy with aggregation of islets. The endocrine cells in this focus exhibit a trabecular configuration, suggesting that they originated from the diffuse islets in the posterior head of the pancreas. The pseudoinfiltrative nature of these endocrine cells may simulate an invasive carcinoma.

perineural invasion. Uniformity of the cells, the presence of round nuclei, lack of glandular lumina, and the presence of neuroendocrine-type chromatin help point toward a benign diagnosis.

Prognosis and Treatment

As has been mentioned, the prognosis for pancreatic ductal adenocarcinoma is dismal.[27] It is the fourth leading cause of death from cancer in the Western world. Overall 5-year survival is less than 5%, and median survival is about 9 months. Surgical resection is the best hope for a relatively long survival, but only about 20% of ductal adenocarcinomas are resectable at the time of diagnosis; the remainder are either locally advanced (mostly invading neighboring large mesenteric vessels) or metastatic (usually to the liver or peritoneum). In addition to high-resolution CT scanning, laparoscopy is increasingly used before laparotomy to identify radiographically occult metastatic disease. The median survival of resected cases is 12 to 18 months, with a reported 5-year survival rate as high as 20%; however, survival beyond 7 to 8 years is exceedingly rare.[28] Some authors advocate adjuvant therapy (chemotherapy and radiation) after surgery. Those cases that are unresectable are generally treated with chemotherapy. Current chemotherapy protocols mostly include gemcitabine and cisplatin.[29]

Morphologic Patterns

Ductal adenocarcinoma of the pancreas includes, in addition to its conventional pattern, several morphologic variations, which are described here. The clinical and biologic characteristics of these patterns do not differ significantly from those of conventional ductal adenocarcinoma. They are often found focally within otherwise typical ductal adenocarcinoma.

FOAMY GLAND PATTERN

This is a subtle, well-differentiated carcinoma that mimics benign glands.[30] In this variant, infiltrating well-formed glands are lined by columnar cells that have abundant pale cytoplasm. The nuclei are typically well polarized but wrinkled in appearance, with indentations caused by the cytoplasmic contents (Fig. 31-5). The most characteristic features that help distinguish this variant from benign mucinous ducts include foamy, microvesicular, pale cytoplasm with vesicles that are small, fine, and evenly sized; and a chromophilic condensation in the apical edge of the cytoplasm that forms a thin, well-delineated band reminiscent of a brush border. Although this apical condensation is strongly positive with mucin markers, the microvesicular component of the cytoplasm is negative (in contrast to benign mucinous ducts, which are often PAS-positive). This

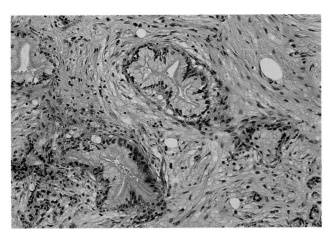

FIGURE 31–5. Ductal adenocarcinoma with foamy gland pattern. The tumor exhibits well-formed ductal structures, simulating a low-grade intraductal proliferation. Abundant, foamy cytoplasm with a thick apical cytoplasmic condensation is seen. Only subtle nuclear abnormalities are present.

staining pattern parallels that of small nonmucinous intralobular ducts, which have apical mucin granules that do not form a distinct band but rather show a gradual acquisition. *TP53* is also often abnormally expressed in the nuclei of malignant glands.

LARGE DUCT PATTERN

Occasionally, invasive tubular adenocarcinomas show a microcystic appearance caused by ectasia of infiltrating neoplastic glands (Fig. 31-6).[31] For unclear reasons, this phenomenon may be particularly pronounced in regions of tumor that infiltrate the muscularis propria of the duodenum. Although microcystic glands may be detected grossly, cystic change is generally not pronounced enough to be detected radiographically.

The cytologic appearance of the epithelium may be deceptively bland. Tumors with a large duct pattern have only a slightly longer survival rate compared with conventional ductal adenocarcinoma. Thus, it is important that cystic dilatation of an invasive gland not be mistaken for a noninvasive unit characteristic of a mucinous cystadenocarcinoma or intraductal neoplasm; the latter have a better prognosis. Features that favor large duct–type adenocarcinoma include clustering of glands, irregularity in the contour of the ducts, and a desmoplastic stroma. Intraluminal necrotic debris with neutrophils is often noted.

VACUOLATED PATTERN

In this pattern, a gland-in-gland architecture is noted, in which tumor cells form cribriform nests punctuated by multiple large vacuoles (or microcysts) that contain cellular debris and mucin. Apparently, these vacuoles are formed by merging multiple intracytoplasmic lumina. Focally vacuolated cells have the morphologic features of adipocytes or signet ring cells.[32,33] This pattern may be helpful in the differential diagnosis of metastatic tumors of unknown origin because it is seen only rarely in other adenocarcinoma types.

LOBULAR CARCINOMA–LIKE PATTERN

Occasionally, ductal adenocarcinoma can display a pattern that is similar to that of mammary lobular carcinoma.[34] Instead of forming tubules, the tumor cells form cords and may achieve an Indian file appearance (Fig. 31-7). Targetoid patterns as well as individual cell infiltration may also be noted, often with signet ring cell formation.[32] This growth pattern may mimic the diffuse type of gastric adenocarcinoma. Often, it is associated with the more conventional tubular pattern found elsewhere in the tumor.

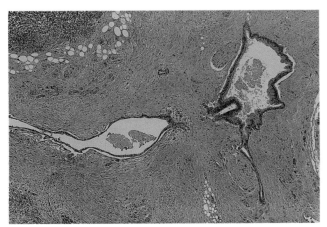

FIGURE 31–6. Ductal adenocarcinoma with a large duct pattern. The invasive neoplastic glands are ectatic, resembling dilated native ducts, but the configuration is irregular and smaller. More typical infiltrating glands are also present.

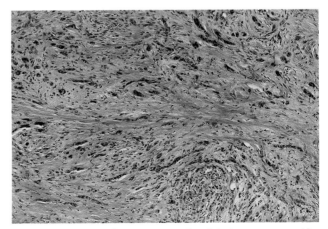

FIGURE 31–7. Ductal carcinoma with a lobular carcinoma–like pattern. Small neoplastic cells are arranged in thin cords without lumen formation, resembling the pattern of mammary lobular carcinoma.

SOLID NESTED PATTERN

Pancreatic ductal adenocarcinomas may infiltrate in a nested pattern without prominent gland formation, thereby mimicking a neuroendocrine neoplasm or squamous cell carcinoma. Most cases, however, contain foci of more typical ductal (tubular) adenocarcinoma. In some cases, cells in this pattern display abundant acidophilic cytoplasm and a single prominent nucleolus. This creates a picture reminiscent of hepatocellular carcinoma (hepatoid pattern) or oncocytic tumors.[35-37] However, the immunohistochemical staining pattern is different from that of hepatocellular carcinoma. In some cases, cells in the nested pattern show clear cytoplasm, resembling renal cell carcinoma, which has prompted some authors to refer to this variant as clear cell carcinoma.[38-40]

OTHER PANCREATIC CARCINOMAS OF DUCTAL ORIGIN

Colloid Carcinoma

Colloid carcinoma is a type of tumor that is clinically and biologically distinct from the other tumors previously discussed.[41,42] Whereas the tumor types discussed earlier are clinically aggressive, colloid carcinoma has a protracted clinical course. Colloid carcinoma, also referred to as mucinous noncystic carcinoma, is characterized by stromal pools of mucin containing scant malignant epithelial cells arranged as strips, stellate or cribriform clusters, small round tubules, or individual signet ring cells (Fig. 31-8). Colloid carcinoma is often associated with intraductal papillary-mucinous neoplasms or mucinous cystic neoplasms. Colloid carcinomas appear to have a more favorable clinical course than other invasive carcinomas of ductal type. In a recent report, the 5-year survival in resected cases of colloid carcinoma was 55%, as opposed to 12% to 15% for ductal adenocarcinoma. Some patients died of thromboembolic complications. In the same study, all patients who died had a history of an incisional biopsy, raising the possibility that disruption of the integrity of the tumor may cause dissemination of tumor cells and mucin.

Medullary Carcinoma

Medullary carcinoma in the pancreas has been described only recently.[43,44] As in the breast and the large intestine, medullary carcinoma is defined as a tumor with pushing borders that displays syncytial growth of poorly differentiated epithelial cells, mostly devoid of a desmoplastic reaction but often accompanied by an inflammatory infiltrate (Fig. 31-9). Experience with these tumors is too limited to allow accurate determination of the prognosis, but it does not appear to be significantly different from that of conventional ductal adenocarcinoma. In contrast to conventional ductal adenocarcinoma, some medullary carcinomas are associated with genetic alterations commonly seen in medullary carcinomas of the colon (microsatellite instability).[43] In fact, some cases are characterized by a personal or family history of colon cancer, raising the possibility of an inherited cancer syndrome.

Squamous Cell Carcinoma and Adenosquamous Carcinoma

These tumors may also occur in the pancreas[45-47] and constitute approximately 2% of all pancreatic cancers.[48] They appear to be somewhat more prevalent in the tail of the organ.[14] Some cases have the appearance of adenoacanthomas, whereas others may be well differentiated with keratinization, poorly differentiated without keratinization, or basaloid in appearance. Pure squamous

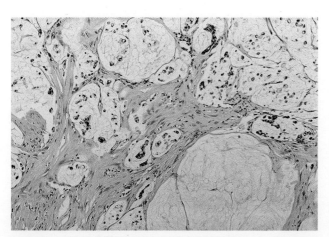

FIGURE 31-8. Colloid carcinoma (mucinous noncystic carcinoma). The tumor is composed of large stromal mucin lakes in which are suspended relatively scant strips and clusters of cells. Individual cells have a signet ring cell configuration.

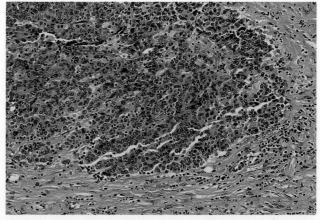

FIGURE 31-9. Medullary carcinoma. The tumor is poorly differentiated, lacks gland formation, and displays a pushing growth pattern at the periphery. The tumor cells are large and appear syncytial. A lymphocytic infiltrate is seen between the cells.

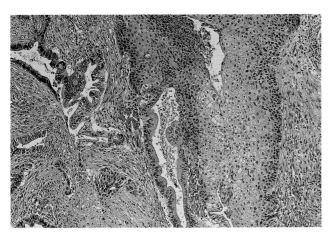

FIGURE 31–10. Adenosquamous carcinoma. The tumor contains neoplastic glands resembling conventional ductal adenocarcinoma, as well as large nests with squamous differentiation.

cell carcinoma (without a glandular component) is exceedingly rare. Most cases reveal a glandular component (i.e., adenosquamous carcinoma) on careful examination (Fig. 31-10). The clinical outcome of these tumors is similar to that of conventional ductal adenocarcinomas and is possibly worse.

Undifferentiated Carcinoma

As can occur in other organs, the pancreas can give rise to a family of tumors that show little morphologic evidence of epithelial differentiation. In theory, an undifferentiated carcinoma could arise from any of the epithelial cell lines in the pancreas, but most un-

differentiated carcinomas are believed to be ductal-type neoplasms. In most instances, evidence for ductal origin comes from the frequent association of undifferentiated carcinoma with a better-differentiated component of ductal adenocarcinoma.[49] In some cases, mutations in oncogenes (such as K-*ras*) typical of ductal-type carcinomas have been identified.[50,51] Several histologic types of undifferentiated carcinomas exist, including spindle cell (sarcomatoid) carcinoma, carcinosarcoma, anaplastic giant cell carcinoma,[52,53] and osteoclastic giant cell carcinoma (see Osteoclastic Giant Cell Carcinoma). The histologic features of the first three overlap, with sarcomatoid components consisting of either anaplastic giant cells or spindle cells (Fig. 31-11), sometimes with heterologous stromal differentiation (e.g., bone, cartilage, skeletal muscle).[54] The designation *carcinosarcoma* is used when a separate glandular component is present, resulting in a biphasic appearance. In some cases, the undifferentiated elements retain immunohistochemical positivity for epithelial markers such as keratin or EMA. In others, all epithelial features are absent, even at immunohistochemical and ultrastructural levels. If these tumors lack an associated glandular component, they are essentially indistinguishable from undifferentiated sarcomas; cases revealing differentiation along a definable mesenchymal line may be classified as primary sarcomas of the pancreas, even though they may have originated from epithelial precursors. With the exception of osteoclastic giant cell carcinoma, the prognosis for undifferentiated carcinomas is extremely poor, possibly even worse than that for conventional ductal adenocarcinoma.

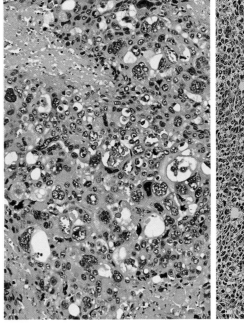
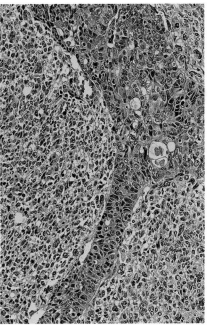

FIGURE 31–11. Undifferentiated carcinoma. Patterns of undifferentiated carcinoma include anaplastic giant cell carcinoma (**A**) with enormous tumor cells growing in solid sheets and having markedly atypical nuclei, as well as carcinosarcoma (**B**) in which the tumor exhibits a biphasic pattern of glandular epithelium and sarcomatoid elements.

A   B

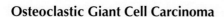
Osteoclastic Giant Cell Carcinoma

Undifferentiated Carcinoma With Osteoclastic Giant Cells

This type of undifferentiated carcinoma of the pancreas shares histologic features with a family of poorly differentiated tumors, including carcinomas of most epithelial organs, sarcomas, and even melanoma. In all of these situations, undifferentiated tumors that contain neoplastic plump spindle cells and non-neoplastic osteoclastic giant cells occur.[55-58] In the pancreas, many cases of osteoclastic giant cell carcinoma contain separate glandular components, and associated preinvasive neoplasia such as a mucinous cystic neoplasm[49,59] or pancreatic intraepithelial neoplasia may also be found. The neoplastic elements are moderately to markedly atypical, dyscohesive, somewhat epithelioid spindle cells. Sprinkled among the neoplastic cells are variable numbers of osteoclasts. These cells contain multiple nuclei and little atypia (Fig. 31-12**A**). Some cases include anaplastic giant tumor cells in addition to osteoclasts. The osteoclasts have phagocytic capability and may contain engulfed neoplastic cells. The giant cells are indeed of histiocytic origin as demonstrated by immunohistochemical staining for CD68 (Fig. 31-12**B**) and other histiocytic markers.[60,61] The neoplastic cells are generally totally undifferentiated at the immunohistochemical level, keratin expression being restricted to any associated glandular components. It is interesting to note that mutations in the K-*ras* oncogene have been detected in the neoplastic elements of osteoclastic giant cell carcinomas.[61] Some cases of this tumor follow a less aggressive clinical course than the undifferentiated nature of the tumor would suggest, but osteoclastic giant cell carcinomas are certainly not indolent neoplasms; most examples lead to death of the patient within 2 years.

PANCREATIC INTRAEPITHELIAL NEOPLASIA

Precursors of pancreatic ductal adenocarcinoma have been recognized as proliferative changes in the epithelium of the ducts. Many of these lesions have long been recognized and designated by descriptive terminology.[62-65] Some lesions with minimal cytologic atypia were not regarded to be neoplastic and were designated hyperplasia or metaplasia, but molecular findings have established most ductal proliferative lesions as neoplastic.[66] Thus, the entire spectrum of ductal proliferative lesions is now referred to as pancreatic intraepithelial neoplasia (PanIN),[67] including PanIN1A, PanIN1B, PanIN2, and PanIN3.

The earliest form of this process is the change previously designated *mucinous metaplasia* (or *mucous cell hypertrophy*) (Fig. 31-13**A**). Because some of these lesions have been shown to harbor mutations in the K-*ras* oncogene,[68,69] they are regarded as the earliest part of the neoplastic transformation and are graded as PanIN1. When the cells are tall, columnar, and mucinous, with well-polarized nuclei with no atypia or loss of polarity and no papillary or micropapillary formations, the lesion is considered PanIN1A. In PanIN1B, the nuclei begin to stratify at the basal aspect of the epithelium, and papillary or micropapillary projections are often found. When stratification becomes more prominent with some loss of polarity, and cells begin to show cytologic atypia, the process is graded as PanIN2 (atypical hyperplasia) (Fig.

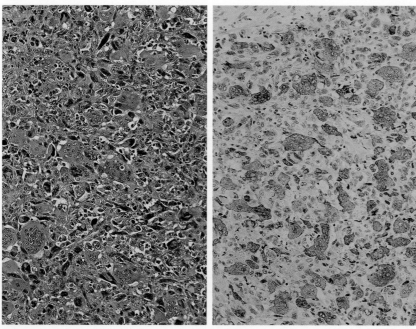

A **B**

FIGURE 31–12. Osteoclastic giant cell carcinoma (undifferentiated carcinoma with osteoclastic giant cells). This tumor contains neoplastic undifferentiated cells that vary from epithelioid to spindle in shape, mixed with varying numbers of non-neoplastic multinucleated osteoclasts (**A**). Immunohistochemical staining for CD68 (**B**) demonstrates the histiocytic nature of the osteoclastic giant cells.

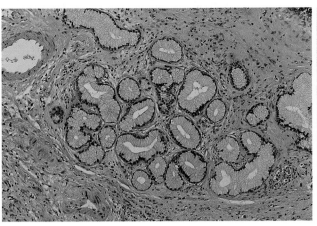

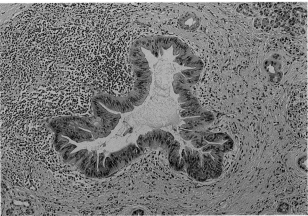

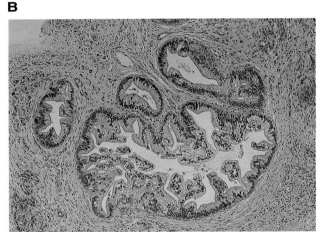

FIGURE 31–13. Pancreatic intraepithelial neoplasia (PanIN). In PanIN1A (**A**), small ductules are lined by tall columnar mucinous epithelial cells without loss of polarization or nuclear atypia. PanIN2 (**B**) also shows tall columnar cells along with full-thickness nuclear pseudostratification and mild to moderate nuclear atypia. PanIN3 (**C**) exhibits more substantial cyto-architectural abnormalities, including complete loss of polarity with budding of unsupported epithelial tufts into the gland lumen. Marked nuclear atypia is also present.

31-13**B**). PanIN3 (carcinoma in situ or severe dysplasia) shows significant loss of polarity, tufting of cells into the lumen, irregularity of nuclei, presence of mitotic figures, and necrosis (Fig. 31-13**C**). Most molecular abnormalities identified in established invasive ductal adenocarcinomas have been found in PanIN as well, with some changes occurring early in the sequence (K-*ras* mutations) and others occurring later (*DPC4* and *TP53* mutations).[68,70]

PanINs are relatively frequent incidental findings, with nearly half of older adults having foci of PanIN1.[71] PanINs are significantly more common among pancreata with invasive ductal carcinomas, and foci of PanIN found in association with other tumor types or in pancreata without tumors are most often of low grade.[71] Because of the difficulty of detecting PanINs without resection of the pancreas, the natural history is essentially unknown; only rare cases have been documented in which a PanIN lesion was identified before the development of invasive carcinoma.[72] Although it is difficult to determine their biologic significance, foci of PanIN2 and PanIN3 identified in resected pancreata should be recorded, especially in cases lacking invasive carcinoma. Ideally, detection of pancreatic cancer at the PanIN3 stage would provide an opportunity for cure that is usually lost once patients develop clinical symptoms.

■ Cysts and Cystic Tumors

Cystic tumors of the pancreas are less common than ductal adenocarcinomas, representing 5% to 10% of all pancreatic neoplasms (see Table 31-3), but they constitute an important subset in that many cystic tumors are benign or, at worst, low-grade indolent malignancies.[73,74] Cystic lesions are detected more commonly owing to the increased use of sensitive imaging techniques. Most true cystic tumors of the pancreas are either serous cystadenomas or mucinous cystic neoplasms, but a number of other less common cystic tumors also occur. A radiographically cystic appearance may occur in typically solid tumors and in intraductal neoplasms.

SEROUS CYSTIC TUMORS

Clinical Features

Serous cystic tumor represents the most common true cystic tumor of the pancreas.[75-78] Serous cystadenomas are usually microcystic; thus, this term has been used synonymously with microcystic adenoma, although a macrocystic (oligocystic) type of serous cystadenoma exists as well.[79,80] Microcystic serous cystadenomas are composed of numerous small cysts, each ranging from less than 1 mm to about 1 cm, ultimately forming a well-delineated tumor mass. Microcystic serous cystadenomas usually present as a relatively large mass (measuring up to 25 cm), mostly in the body or tail of the pancreas, and develop predominantly in females (female-to-male ratio, 3:1). The mean age of patients is 66 years. Patients with von Hippel-Lindau syndrome may have histologically similar cysts (often multiple),[81-83] although most patients with microcystic serous cystadenoma have no other associated diseases. Other types of concurrent pancreatic tumors, including ductal adenocarcinoma[84] and pancreatic endocrine neoplasm, have been described in patients with microcystic serous cystadenoma.[85]

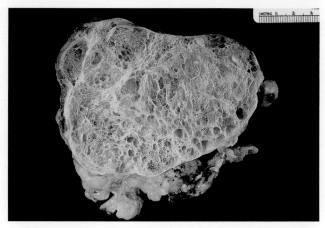

FIGURE 31–14. Gross appearance of microcystic serous cystadenoma. The lesion is well circumscribed and is composed of small cysts (each measuring less than 1 cm) separated by thin, translucent septa.

Pathologic Features

GROSS PATHOLOGY

Grossly, microcystic serous cystadenomas are usually well circumscribed and often contain a central fibrous scar. The innumerable cysts produce the appearance of a sponge (Fig. 31-14). In some regions, the cysts may be so small that the tumor grossly appears to have a solid configuration.

MICROSCOPIC PATHOLOGY

Microscopically, the cysts of microcystic serous cystadenomas are lined by a single layer of cuboidal cells with clear cytoplasm, well-defined cytoplasmic borders, and small, round nuclei that contain dense,

homogeneous chromatin (Fig. 31-15). The cytoplasmic clearing is due to glycogen; mucin is not generally present. In rare cases, the cells are more columnar and have abundant, acidophilic, granular cytoplasm. In some areas, blunt papillary projections may be found, but well-formed or complex papillae are unusual. The stroma between the cysts is hyalinized and may contain entrapped islets. Degenerative changes, including hemorrhage and macrocystic degeneration, may be prominent.

The cytologic features of serous tumors of the pancreas are present not only in microcystic serous cystadenomas but also in the less common serous tumors—macrocystic

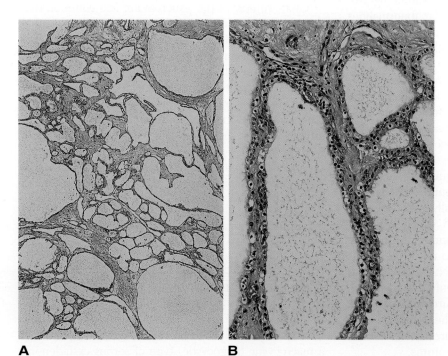

A   **B**

FIGURE 31–15. Microcystic serous cystadenoma. At low power (**A**), each small cyst is lined by a flattened layer of epithelium. Cytologically (**B**), lining cells show clear cytoplasm and small, uniform, hyperchromatic nuclei.

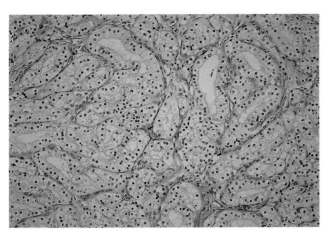

FIGURE 31–16. Solid serous adenoma. There is no cyst formation; back-to-back glands exhibit the same cytologic features as the cystic members of the serous tumor family.

serous cystadenoma and solid serous adenoma.[86] Macrocystic serous cystadenomas occur more commonly among males. The boundaries of the tumor are often poorly defined, and the cysts range in size from 1 to several centimeters. Microscopically, the lining of the cysts is identical to that found in the microcystic type, with glycogen-rich clear cells arranged in a single flat layer without atypia or mucin production. The solid serous adenoma, in contrast, shows the complete absence of cystic change. It is characterized by a back-to-back arrangement of small glands with the cytologic features of a typical serous tumor (Fig. 31-16).

Both histologically and immunophenotypically, serous adenomas appear to recapitulate centroacinar cells.[77] They express low-molecular-weight keratins (in addition to broad-spectrum keratins), EMA, and melanoma antigen recognized by T cells (MART-1).[87] HMB-45 is negative. Ductal mucin markers (B72.3, MUC1, CA 19-9, and CEA) are either negative or only focally positive. Molecular alterations include those associated with the *VHL* gene (chromosome 3p25) and 10q.[88]

Differential Diagnosis

The differential diagnosis includes other cystic tumors of the pancreas (see under Differential Diagnosis of Cystic and Intraductal Lesions). In addition, the clear cell nature of the cytoplasm raises the possibility of metastatic renal cell carcinoma, a tumor that may involve the pancreas as the sole site of metastasis and may show cystic changes. The presence of more solid and acinar regions and of greater nuclear atypia, along with a sinusoidal vascular pattern, favors a diagnosis of renal cell carcinoma.

Most serous tumors of the pancreas are benign. Serous cystadenocarcinoma of the pancreas is extremely rare.[89-94] Most malignant serous tumors exhibit the typical microscopic pattern of microcystic serous cystadenoma,

with no morphologic findings that suggest malignancy. In these cases, the diagnosis of cystadenocarcinoma is based on the presence of metastases that also appear benign histologically. In fact, some have questioned the malignant potential of these rare cases, suggesting instead that they develop as a form of parasitic growth of a benign tumor or as a multicentric tumor. Suffice it to say that in the absence of demonstrable metastases, a typical example of a serous tumor can be considered benign. In fact, if a definitive diagnosis can be achieved preoperatively and the tumor is asymptomatic, observation is a viable option in the management of patients with serous tumors.[95]

MUCINOUS CYSTIC NEOPLASMS

Clinical Features

Mucinous cystic neoplasms represent the other significant cystic tumor of the pancreas.[96-101] In contrast to most serous cystadenomas, mucinous cystic neoplasms are consistently macrocystic; when defined strictly, they have distinctive clinicopathologic characteristics. They are seen almost exclusively in women during the fifth to sixth decades of life (mean age, 50), and the tumor is nearly always located in the tail of the pancreas. Presenting symptoms are nonspecific and usually result from the effects of an enlarging mass.

Pathologic Features

GROSS PATHOLOGY

Macroscopically, mucinous cystic neoplasms exhibit large, multilocular cysts surrounded by a thick fibrotic capsule (Fig. 31-17). The mean size of these tumors is greater than 10 cm. Unless fistulas have formed, these

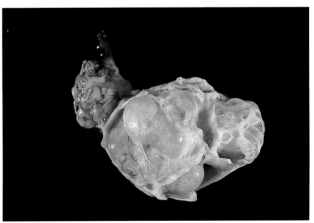

FIGURE 31–17. Gross appearance of a mucinous cystic neoplasm. The circumscribed tumor involves the tail of the pancreas and contains numerous large (1- to 5-cm) cysts. Septa are fibrotic and show no gross evidence of solid tumor nodules in this particular example.

tumors do not communicate with the pancreatic ductal system. The septa between individual cysts are usually thin and may show velvety papillations; some appear trabeculated and thickened. The cyst contents are often mucoid, but a more watery consistency may be noted. Solid areas within the cyst should be sampled extensively because they may harbor an invasive component.

MICROSCOPIC PATHOLOGY

Histologically, pancreatic mucinous cystic neoplasms are similar to ovarian mucinous tumors. The lining epithelium generally consists of tall, columnar cells with abundant apical mucin, although cuboidal cells lacking obvious mucin may also be present (Fig. 31-18). Intestinal-type epithelium with goblet cells may be noted as well, and endocrine cells and Paneth cells can sometimes be detected. The epithelium displays a wide range of cytologic atypia similar to that seen in analogous ovarian tumors. Some mucinous cystic tumors are largely bland in appearance, containing mostly uniform, basally oriented nuclei and displaying minimal architectural complexity, whereas other tumors exhibit abundant papillary formations, pseudostratified hyperchromatic nuclei, and a cribriformed architecture. Findings of severe epithelial atypia may be focal, and numerous sections are required for proper evaluation of these tumors (Fig. 31-19).

The resemblance to ovarian tumors includes the presence of a distinctive subepithelial stroma (referred to as ovarian-like). This stroma is a consistent feature of these tumors, and some authors require its presence for the establishment of a diagnosis. In addition to densely cellular spindle cell elements, the stroma contains nests of epithelioid cells—changes suggestive of luteinization (Fig. 31-20). Occasionally, large circumscribed regions of stromal hyalinization resembling corpora albicantia

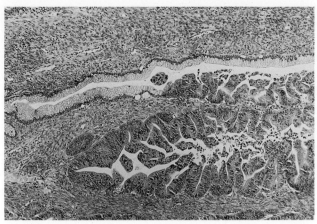

FIGURE 31–19. Mucinous cystic neoplasm. Cytoarchitectural atypia may be focal, with an abrupt transition from benign-appearing mucinous epithelium. In this case, marked nuclear atypia and complete loss of polarity are noted with no evidence of invasive carcinoma (in situ mucinous cystadenocarcinoma).

may be seen. Occasionally, this stroma shows sarcomatous transformation.[102-104] The stromal cells frequently express estrogen and progesterone receptors as well as inhibin,[105] the last being intensely expressed in the epithelioid, lutea-like cells. A satisfactory explanation for the presence of ovarian-like stroma in mucinous cystic neoplasms has yet to be put forward.

Invasive carcinoma may develop within mucinous cystic neoplasms. In cases with cellular atypia, this is of particular concern. In such instances, the solid areas of the tumor and the interface with adjacent tissues should be sectioned carefully. Invasive carcinoma is often focal and may be detected only after careful examination and extensive sampling. Invasive carcinoma arising in mucinous cystic neoplasms usually resembles conventional tubular-type ductal adenocarcinoma, but other types

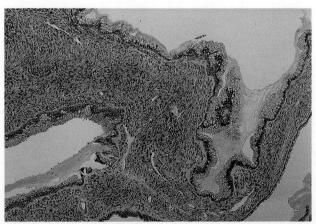

FIGURE 31–18. Mucinous cystic neoplasm. The epithelial lining is composed of tall, columnar, mucin-containing cells. In this region, no significant nuclear atypia, loss of polarity, or architectural complexity (mucinous cystadenoma) is seen. The subepithelial stroma is hypercellular, resembling the stroma of the ovary.

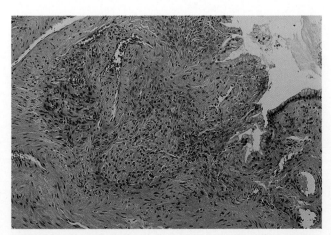

FIGURE 31–20. Stroma of mucinous cystic neoplasm. In addition to the hypercellular spindle cell component, clusters of epithelioid cells resembling the luteinized stroma of the ovary are seen.

may also occur, such as sarcomatoid carcinoma or colloid carcinoma (Fig. 31-21).

According to the WHO,[9,10] mucinous cystic neoplasms are classified as mucinous cystadenomas if minimal cytoarchitectural atypia is seen in the lining epithelium. Those with moderate atypia are considered mucinous cystic tumors of borderline malignant potential. Mucinous cystic neoplasms with severe atypia (but no invasive carcinoma) are considered in situ mucinous cystadenocarcinomas. Finally, cases with invasive carcinoma are classified as invasive mucinous cystadenocarcinomas. The extent of invasion (intratumoral or extratumoral) should also be determined.

The clinical relevance of this classification system is subject to debate. Some authors have reported recurrence or metastasis from tumors that lack invasive carcinoma (or even significant atypia)[96,97]; these authors suggest that even mucinous cystadenomas have latent malignant potential. Other investigators have suggested that these rare occurrences can be explained on the basis of inadequate sampling of the primary tumor, with failure to identify a component of invasive carcinoma. When mucinous cystic neoplasms are thoroughly sectioned, most studies have found no recurrences in cases that lack invasive carcinoma.[99-101] Thus, exhaustive (if not complete) histologic examination of apparently benign mucinous cystic neoplasms would be required for establishment of a benign diagnosis. DNA ploidy analysis may also correlate with prognosis.[106] Overall, the rate of malignant behavior in mucinous cystic neoplasms is approximately 10%, and it has been suggested that invasive carcinomas that arise in them are less aggressive than conventional ductal adenocarcinomas. Nevertheless, surgical resection is recommended for all patients with mucinous cystic neoplasms.

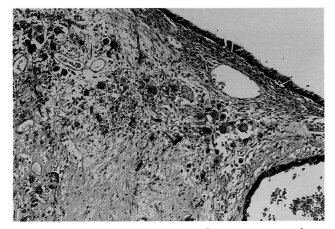

FIGURE 31–21. Invasive mucinous cystadenocarcinoma. Within a septum of this tumor is a component of undifferentiated anaplastic giant cell carcinoma, one of several types of invasive carcinoma that may arise in mucinous cystic neoplasms.

Differential Diagnosis

The differential diagnosis for mucinous cystic neoplasms is discussed later (see under Differential Diagnosis of Cystic and Intraductal Lesions). Sometimes mucinous cystic neoplasms may develop extensive denudation of the lining epithelium, with the underlying stroma showing hemorrhage, fibrosis, and inflammation. Biopsy specimens from these regions reveal an appearance similar to that of a pseudocyst. Recognition of the clinical setting (e.g., young woman, usually without a history of pancreatitis or other cause for a pseudocyst and having an otherwise normal-appearing pancreas) can direct the surgeon and pathologist to examine other regions of the cyst to find the characteristic mucinous lining. Also, elements of ovarian-like stroma may persist in denuded areas. Immunohistochemical demonstration of hormone receptors in these stroma cells is confirmatory. One other important consideration is to avoid the use of the term *mucinous cystadenocarcinoma* for ductal adenocarcinomas showing ectatic glands (large duct pattern) unless evidence indicates that the tumor arose in a preexisting mucinous cystic neoplasm.

CYSTIC CHANGE IN SOLID TUMORS

Cystic Change in Ductal Adenocarcinoma

This uncommon phenomenon appears to occur via three mechanisms.[107] A large, radiographically detectable cyst may form because of central necrosis of the tumor.[108] This can be clinically challenging, but the presence of residual carcinoma at the periphery of the cystic cavity is usually easily recognizable histologically. In other cases, ductal adenocarcinoma can lead to cystic dilatation of obstructed ducts. This is often associated with reactive atypia of the ductal epithelium, which may resemble intraductal papillary mucinous neoplasms. A large duct (microcystic) pattern of ductal adenocarcinoma occurs in which the infiltrating tubular units are larger than those of most ductal adenocarcinomas, sometimes achieving the size of grossly visible cysts.[31] The cystic glands may appear not to be invasive, mimicking foci of PanIN or even intraductal papillary mucinous neoplasm, especially when the change occurs within the pancreatic parenchyma.

Cystic Pancreatic Endocrine Neoplasm

This is a rare neoplasm that usually consists of a single unilocular cyst that occupies the majority of the tumor.[107] The cysts in pancreatic endocrine neoplasms are lined by a cuff of well-preserved endocrine tumor with overlying fibrin; the cyst cavity is filled with clear fluid instead of necrotic debris. Presumably, the cystic change is degenerative. Some of these neoplasms may reach a significant size (up to 25 cm). The pathologic diagnosis of cystic endocrine neoplasm is relatively simple if attention is paid to the cytologic features of the tumor cells.

Cystic Acinar Tumors

Acinar cell cystadenoma and acinar cell cystadenocarcinoma are discussed in later sections.

LYMPHOEPITHELIAL CYST

This tumor is seen predominantly, but not exclusively, in men in the fifth and sixth decades of life.[109] It does not appear to be associated with autoimmune conditions, human immunodeficiency virus infection, lymphoma, or carcinoma, all of which have been documented to occur in lymphoepithelial cysts of the salivary glands. The cyst contents may vary from serous to caseous depending on the degree of keratin formation. The cyst wall and trabecula are usually thin. The inner lining of the cyst is smooth with occasional nodularity. The lymphoid tissue is not prominent grossly because it often is limited to a thin band surrounding the epithelium.

Microscopically, these cysts are lined by stratified squamous epithelium that may or may not reveal prominent keratinization (Fig. 31-22). In some areas, the lining epithelium may be transitional in appearance, and in others, it may be cuboidal or focally denuded. Sebaceous elements and mucinous cells are exceedingly uncommon, and their presence should suggest a diagnosis of teratoma. The cyst wall and trabecula are made up of dense lymphoid tissue composed of mature T lymphocytes. Germinal centers formed by B cells are abundant in some cases. The number of lymphocytes found within the epithelium is usually not significant.

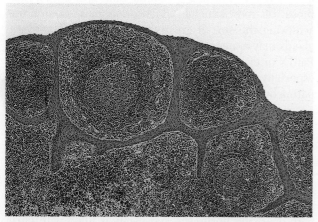

FIGURE 31–22. Lymphoepithelial cyst. The wall of the cyst is lined by squamous epithelium without keratinization in this region. Underlying the epithelium is a dense band of lymphocytes containing germinal centers.

Solid lymphoepithelial islands (i.e., microscopic clusters of epithelial cells admixed with lymphocytes, akin to the so-called epimyoepithelial islands in salivary glands) may be present. The uninvolved pancreas is unremarkable in most cases.

MISCELLANEOUS EPITHELIAL CYSTS

Dermoid Cysts

These are exceedingly rare in the region of the pancreas.[110] They are reported in young patients (second and third decades of life) and are morphologically similar to teratomas that develop in other sites.

Epidermoid Cysts in Intrapancreatic Accessory Spleen

These are also rare lesions[110] that are seen in younger patients (second and third decades of life). They occur almost exclusively in the tail of the pancreas, a location at which accessory splenic tissue is not uncommon. These cysts are lined with attenuated squamous cells surrounded by normal-appearing splenic tissue.

Paraduodenal Wall Cyst

These cysts occur as a consequence of chronic fibrosing inflammation in the periampullary region.[111] Accessory pancreatic ducts may form a cyst in the duodenal wall that can mimic duodenal duplication. The cyst wall is lined partially by ductal epithelium and partly by inflammation and granulation tissue.

Others

Other rare cysts that can occur in the pancreas include parasitic cysts, endometriotic cysts, and congenital foregut (intestinal-type) cysts.

▓ Intraductal Tumors

Intraductal tumors have rapidly become one of the most widely studied groups of pancreatic neoplasms.[112-114] These tumors have distinctive clinical and radiographic findings. In addition, they are usually readily treatable by surgery. Many cases appear radiographically cystic, and the distinction of an intraductal tumor from a true cystic neoplasm can be difficult.[30] Most importantly, intraductal tumors reflect a spectrum of neoplastic progression that ranges from the earliest neoplastic changes to invasive carcinoma; however, unlike PanIN lesions associated with conventional ductal adenocarcinomas, intraductal tumors are clinically detectable, providing an excellent model of preinvasive neoplasia in the pancreas.[115]

INTRADUCTAL PAPILLARY-MUCINOUS NEOPLASMS

Clinical Features

Intraductal papillary-mucinous neoplasms are characterized by an intraductal proliferation of mucinous cells, usually arranged in a papillary pattern.[114,116-123] The papillae formed range from microscopic to large nodular masses. This proliferation is usually associated with intraluminal mucin deposition that leads to cystic dilatation of the ducts and, at times, to mucin extrusion through the ampulla of Vater—an endoscopic finding that is virtually diagnostic of these tumors.[124,125] Depending on the location of the primary process and subsequent mechanical changes in the ducts, intraductal papillary-mucinous neoplasms may present as multilocular cystic masses or as abundant papillary nodules. This spectrum is reflected in the variety of designations that have been used for these tumors before they came to be categorized under one heading. Previous names included *mucinous duct ectasia (ductectatic mucinous cystadenoma)*,[98,126-129] *mucin-producing tumor*,[130,131] *villous adenoma of the pancreatic duct*,[132,133] and *intraductal papillary tumor*.[134]

Intraductal papillary-mucinous neoplasms account for approximately 5% of pancreatic neoplasms; however, they are now reported in increasing numbers and may be more common than was previously recognized. Patients with intraductal papillary-mucinous neoplasms are usually in their seventh or eighth decades of life and have nonspecific symptoms. A history of pancreatitis is noted in some cases. Endoscopic findings (mucin extrusion through the ampulla of Vater) and radiographic findings (ectasia of the ducts) are diagnostic features of these tumors, which occur mostly (80%) in the head of the pancreas.

Pathologic Features

GROSS PATHOLOGY

Careful macroscopic examination is imperative for documentation of the intraductal nature of the tumor. The extent of ductal dilatation and the amount of gross papilla formation may vary from case to case and even regionally within a given case (Fig. 31-23). In some cases, the tumor involves predominantly the major pancreatic ducts (main duct type), and in others, it is limited to the secondary ducts (branch duct type), particularly in the uncinate process. Some studies claim this distinction is of clinical importance because main duct–type tumors have a greater likelihood of harboring intraductal or invasive carcinoma. Intraductal papillary-mucinous neoplasms may be localized or multicentric; rarely, the entire ductal system of the organ may be involved. Thorough sampling of the specimen for an invasive carcinoma, which is present in about 35% of cases, is vital.

MICROSCOPIC PATHOLOGY

Microscopically, the cystic ducts of these tumors contain mucinous cells with various degrees of atypia (Fig. 31-24). Two distinct papillary patterns have been described: (1) the intestinal type (85% of cases), which is morphologically similar to villous adenomas of the gastrointestinal tract or to gastric foveolar cells, and (2) the pancreaticobiliary type (15% of cases), in which the papillae are more complex and contain cuboidal cells with prominent nucleoli (Fig. 31-25).[115,116] The immunophenotypes of these two patterns were found to reveal significant differences. Expression of MUC1 (mammary-type mucin) is more common in the pancreaticobiliary pattern; in contrast, MUC2 is more commonly expressed in the intestinal type.

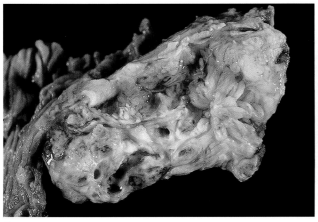 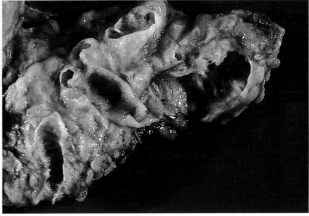

A   **B**

FIGURE 31–23. Gross appearance of an intraductal papillary-mucinous neoplasm. The pancreatic ducts are significantly dilated. In some examples, obvious gross papilla formation is noted **(A)** with extensive involvement of the main pancreatic ducts and cystic dilatation of branch ducts. In other examples **(B)**, intraductal papillae are inconspicuous, and the lesion appears largely as cystic dilatation of branch ducts.

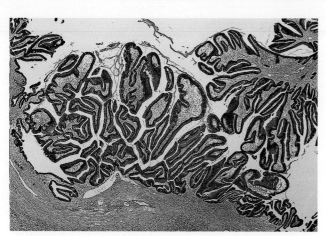

FIGURE 31–24. Intraductal papillary-mucinous neoplasm. At low power, the ducts are filled with variably complex papillary projections lined by tall, columnar, mucinous epithelial cells.

Similar to mucinous cystic neoplasms, intraductal papillary mucinous neoplasms are classified as adenoma, borderline, or carcinoma. The morphologic progression within this spectrum exactly parallels that seen in pancreatic intraepithelial neoplasia. Invasive carcinoma, present in a third of cases, is of either the colloid[41] or the tubular (ordinary ductal) type (Fig. 31-26).[116,135] When present, invasive carcinoma may be focal (or multifocal), or it may represent the majority of the gross tumor mass.

Intraductal papillary-mucinous neoplasms form a distinct pathway of carcinogenesis in the pancreas, displaying molecular alterations different from those of conventional ductal adenocarcinomas. DPC4 is retained, and K-*ras* mutation, TP53 overexpression, and MUC1 expression are less common.[13,115,135-137] Intraductal papillary-mucinous neoplasms are also distinct from other types of preinvasive neoplasia.[115]

Prognosis and Treatment

The overall 5-year survival for intraductal papillary-mucinous neoplasms is good, with more than 75% of patients being free of disease. Even patients with an associated invasive carcinoma do well, especially if the carcinoma is of the colloid type. Cases with a significant component of invasive tubular carcinoma may follow an aggressive course, similar to that of conventional ductal carcinoma arising without a preexisting intraductal tumor. Intraductal papillary-mucinous neoplasms appear to be both a precursor and a marker of invasive carcinoma,[116] which may occur within or away from the intraductal component.[138] The multicentric nature of intraductal papillary mucinous neoplasms raises the question of total pancreatectomy as an option in the management of these tumors. However, most cases managed by conservative resection of the gross disease (usually a pancreatoduodenectomy) will not experience local recurrence, even if the intraductal component extends to the pancreatic ductal margin. Additional long-term follow-up is needed to determine the optimal management of cases with a positive ductal margin; different approaches that are being applied in different institutions are largely individualized to the patient. It is

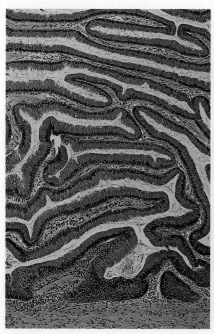
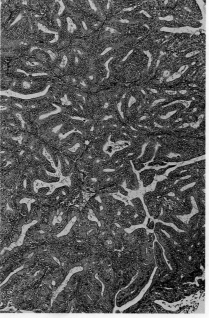

A **B**

FIGURE 31–25. Intraductal papillary-mucinous neoplasm. Different types of papillae may be found. Most cases exhibit intestinal-type papillae **(A),** which may resemble either the papillae of villous adenomas of the large bowel or, as in this example, gastric foveolar cells. Some intraductal papillary-mucinous neoplasms exhibit pancreatobiliary papillae **(B)** in which the lining epithelium shows marked architectural complexity with cribriforming and micropapilla formation; nuclei are round and lack the pseudostratification of intestinal-type tumors.

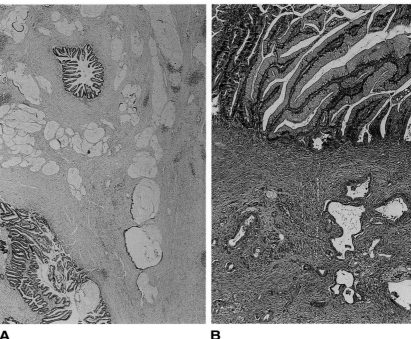

FIGURE 31–26. Intraductal papillary-mucinous carcinoma, invasive. Two distinct types of invasive carcinoma may arise from intraductal papillary-mucinous neoplasms. Colloid carcinomas **(A)** consist of paucicellular stromal mucin pools with strips and clusters of floating epithelial cells. In other cases, the invasive component is of the tubular type **(B),** resembling conventional ductal adenocarcinomas.

A   **B**

agreed, however, that patients with invasive carcinoma should be treated similarly to those with ordinary ductal adenocarcinoma.

Differential Diagnosis

The differential diagnosis of intraductal papillary-mucinous neoplasms and mucinous cystic neoplasms is discussed later (see under Differential Diagnosis of Cystic and Intraductal Lesions). These tumors also should be distinguished from microscopic proliferative lesions involving the native pancreatic ducts. PanIN, small incidental ectatic ducts,[139] and retention cysts (secondary cystic dilatation of obstructed ducts) are also intraductal processes that may involve mucinous cells and formation of papillae. Small, intraductal papillary-mucinous neoplasms are essentially indistinguishable from large foci of PanIN; criteria to separate these two related preinvasive neoplasms have yet to be defined, perhaps awaiting further information about the biologic and genetic differences between these two processes. However, PanINs are usually incidental microscopic lesions that are unlike intraductal papillary-mucinous neoplasms, which form radiographically or macroscopically detectable masses or cysts. Some authors apply an arbitrary size criterion of 1 cm in this distinction.

One challenge in the diagnosis of intraductal papillary-mucinous neoplasms is the recognition of focal invasive colloid carcinoma and its distinction from mucin leakage into the stroma, presumably from ruptured ducts. Mucin leakage into the stroma is an unexpectedly rare event in these tumors. When it happens, it is usually

limited. The mucin is located adjacent to an involved duct and is devoid of any free-floating epithelial cells. If present, epithelium is usually seen in continuity with the epithelium of the intraductal component. Finally, mucin leakage is more likely to produce an inflammatory reaction than occurs with the mucin of invasive colloid carcinoma.

INTRADUCTAL ONCOCYTIC PAPILLARY NEOPLASMS

Intraductal oncocytic papillary neoplasm is a recently described tumor[140] with many clinicopathologic similarities to the intraductal papillary-mucinous neoplasm.[112] Grossly, these tumors exhibit cystic dilatation of the ducts, many of which contain large, tan, and friable nodular proliferations. The tumors are usually relatively large (mean, 5.2 cm) at the time of diagnosis. Histologically, they are characterized by an intraductal papillary growth pattern frequently associated with mucin production, as well as multilocular cystic transformation of the ductal system similar to intraductal papillary-mucinous neoplasms. However, in intraductal oncocytic papillary neoplasms, the cells are oncocytic in appearance and are characterized by a distinctive papillary pattern, consisting of exuberant, arborizing papillae lined by one to five cell layers of cuboidal cells (Fig. 31-27). The nuclei contain single prominent and eccentric nucleoli. One distinctive feature that appears to be relatively specific for these tumors is the presence of mucin-containing intraepithelial lumina that appear as round, punched-out spaces within the epithelium, leading to a cribriform architecture. Invasive carcinomas may occur

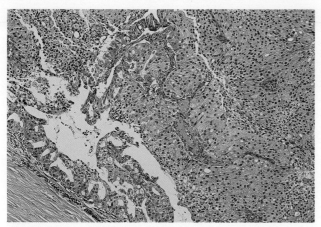

FIGURE 31–27. Intraductal oncocytic papillary neoplasm. These intraductal tumors exhibit markedly comple papillae, with cribriformed areas and fusion of papillae to form solid sheets. The tumor cells also exhibit intracellular lumina and contain abundant eosinophilic cytoplasm.

in association with intraductal oncocytic papillary neoplasms; some examples, similar to colloid carcinomas arising in intraductal papillary-mucinous neoplasms, produce abundant extracellular mucin. However, most invasive carcinomas retain oncocytic features, a highly unusual pattern for invasive carcinoma in the pancreas. Because of limited experience, behavioral differences between intraductal papillary-mucinous neoplasms and intraductal oncocytic papillary neoplasms have not been elucidated. Preliminary evidence suggests differences in molecular alterations; for instance, intraductal oncocytic papillary neoplasms lack mutations in the K-*ras* oncogene.

Most intraductal oncocytic papillary neoplasms are in situ carcinomas; complete resection is warranted whenever possible. Neoplasms with invasive carcinoma should be treated similarly to ordinary ductal adenocarcinoma, although they seem to be less aggressive, possibly because the invasive component is often limited.

Although intraductal oncocytic papillary neoplasms are distinct from intraductal papillary-mucinous neoplasms with intestinal-type papillae, those with pancreaticobiliary-type papillae form a transitional group between these two entities. Intraductal oncocytic papillary neoplasms can be distinguished from all intraductal papillary-mucinous neoplasms by their marked architectural complexity, distinctive intraepithelial lumina, and predominance of oncocytic cells.

Differential Diagnosis of Cystic and Intraductal Lesions

Because of radiographic similarities among many of the cystic and intraductal tumors of the pancreas, it is appropriate for the clinician to consider their differential diagnosis together. In the differential diagnosis of this group of tumors, clinical, radiologic, and macroscopic findings are crucial. Analysis of cyst fluid for tumor markers has been used as a diagnostic aid, successfully in some cases, in the preoperative evaluation of cystic pancreatic lesions.[73,80,141]

Almost all microcystic tumors of the pancreas are serous cystadenomas and are therefore benign. Thus, the size of the cyst is critical. Radiographically, a central stellate scar is also typical of serous cystadenoma. These tumors lack mucinous epithelium, so the finding of columnar, mucin-containing cells in a cystic lesion rules out a serous tumor. Macrocystic serous cystadenomas may grossly simulate either mucinous cystic neoplasms or intraductal papillary-mucinous neoplasms (especially the branch duct type), but the clear cell epithelial lining that lacks mucin allows their distinction.

A greater problem involves the distinction of mucinous cystic neoplasms from intraductal papillary-mucinous neoplasms; both lesions may appear macrocystic and both contain mucinous epithelium. Helpful criteria are summarized in Table 31-5. Mucinous cystic neoplasms are seen predominantly in middle-aged women in the tail of the pancreas, whereas intraductal papillary-mucinous neoplasms affect both sexes, arise in older patients, and are located predominantly in the head of the organ. Involvement of the pancreatic ducts is the hallmark of intraductal papillary-mucinous neoplasms, whereas mucinous cystic neoplasms do not communicate with the ductal system unless fistulas have formed. Microscopically, tributary ducts and the absence of ovarian-like stroma help to differentiate the cystically dilated duct of an intraductal papillary-mucinous neoplasm from de novo true cysts of a mucinous cystic neoplasm. The cytoarchitectural features of these two entities extensively overlap, but extensive formation of papillae is less common in mucinous cystic neoplasms. Finally, the cellular ovarian-like stroma is highly specific for mucinous cystic neoplasms.

TABLE 31-5. Features of Mucinous Cystic Neoplasms and Intraductal Papillary-Mucinous Neoplasms

Feature	Intraductal Papillary-Mucinous Neoplasm	Mucinous Cystic Neoplasm
Age	50–75 years	40–50 years
Sex	Male > Female	Female preponderance
Location	Head > tail	Tail >>>> head
Intraductal	Yes	No
Cyst configuration	Multiple	Single, multilocular
Papilla formation	Usually extensive	Usually minimal
Ovarian-like stroma	Absent	Present

Acinar Cell Carcinoma, Pancreatoblastoma, and Related Entities

Defined by the presence of enzyme production by neoplastic cells, acinar differentiation is the predominant feature of a number of uncommon pancreatic tumors, including acinar cell carcinoma, pancreatoblastoma, and many of the carcinomas with mixed differentiation. These tumors all differ substantially from the more common ductal adenocarcinoma at histologic, immuno-histochemical, and molecular levels.

ACINAR CELL CARCINOMA

Clinical Features

Acinar cell carcinomas of the pancreas[7,142,143] are uncommon, accounting for no more than 1% to 2% of all pancreatic carcinomas. Most patients are adults in their seventh decade of life, and there is a male predominance. Pediatric cases have also been described but are rare.[144,145] The presenting symptoms are generally nonspecific, and in contrast to ductal adenocarcinoma, jaundice is rare. A minority of patients may develop a syndrome consisting of lipase hypersecretion,[146,147] characterized by subcutaneous (and intraosseous) fat necrosis, polyarthralgia, and occasionally eosinophilia associated with markedly elevated serum lipase levels.[146-148] Thrombotic endocarditis may be seen.[149] Most patients with acinar cell carcinoma have metastases early in the course of disease. Regional spread to the lymph nodes and liver is most common, but some patients also develop distant metastases. The long-term survival for acinar cell carcinoma is poor, with few patients living longer than 5 years. However, several studies have confirmed that the clinical course is less rapidly fatal than that of ductal adenocarcinoma, and survival for 2 to 3 years in the presence of hepatic metastases may occur.[150]

Pathologic Features

GROSS PATHOLOGY

Grossly, acinar cell carcinomas are usually large, solid, well-circumscribed tumors that sometimes show extensive necrosis or cystic degeneration. The absence of a prominent stromal reaction imparts a soft consistency to most cases.

MICROSCOPIC PATHOLOGY

Microscopically, acinar cell carcinomas are generally highly cellular lesions that form large nodules of tumor cells and lack the desmoplastic fibrous stroma so

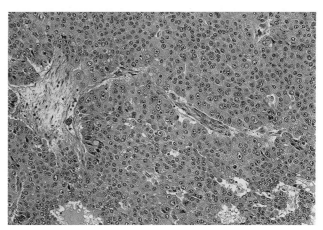

FIGURE 31–28. Acinar cell carcinoma. These tumors commonly exhibit a solid growth pattern with sheets and nests of cells having moderate amounts of amphophilic cytoplasm and minimal lumen formation.

characteristic of ductal adenocarcinoma. In fact, many cases have almost no stroma within the tumor nodules, other than thin fibrous bands accompanying the capillaries. The cells are monotonous in appearance and are arranged in solid sheets and nests punctuated by acinar and small glandular spaces (Fig. 31-28). Occasionally, a trabecular pattern may occur, mimicking the architecture of endocrine tumors. The cells exhibit evidence of basal polarization, even in solid areas (Fig. 31-29). The cytoplasm is moderate to focally abundant and characteristically shows eosinophilic granularity in the apical regions, reflecting aggregates of zymogen granules. However, in many examples of acinar cell carcinoma, the granules are difficult to appreciate. The nuclei are usually only moderately atypical, although occasional anaplasia may be encountered. Prominent single nucleoli are a helpful clue to diagnosis (Fig. 31-30).[151]

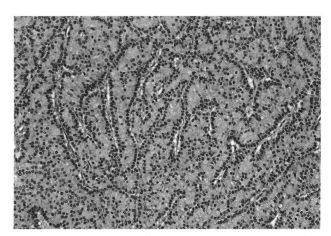

FIGURE 31–29. Acinar cell carcinoma. In some examples, pronounced basal polarization of the nuclei occurs where the tumor cell nests interface with the minimal vascular stroma.

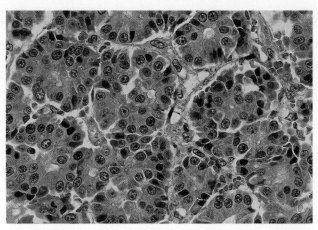

FIGURE 31–30. Acinar cell carcinoma. At high power, the acinar structures of this tumor are evident, with pinpoint lumina and basally located nuclei. Prominent nucleoli are also a characteristic feature.

Documentation of enzyme production is often helpful in confirming a diagnosis of acinar cell carcinoma. Zymogen granules stain with PAS and are resistant to diastase. In a well-granulated case, this stain may be adequate to support the diagnosis (provided the possibility of mucin granules is excluded). However, a much more sensitive and specific way to detect acinar differentiation is by immunohistochemical staining for specific enzymes (e.g., trypsin, lipase, and chymotrypsin); 95% of acinar cell carcinomas express one or more enzymes by this technique. Finally, ultrastructural demonstration of zymogen granules can also be used to establish a diagnosis.[7,152] The morphology of these granules varies somewhat from that of zymogen granules in non-neoplastic acini, but they are usually sufficiently large to be distinguished from neurosecretory granules in endocrine tumors. A second granule type, the irregular fibrillary granule, is found in pancreatic acinar tumors and appears to be even more specific than classic zymogen granules for an acinar cell lineage.[7]

Limited information is available about genetic changes in acinar cell carcinomas.[153] In contrast to ductal adenocarcinomas, acinar cell carcinomas lack abnormalities in K-ras, TP53, p16, or Smad4.[143] The abnormalities that have been detected involve the adenomatous polyposis coli (APC)/beta-catenin pathway and are present in 23.5% of cases. Also, allelic losses on chromosome 11p are present in 50% of cases.

The differential diagnosis of acinar cell carcinoma is largely pancreatic endocrine neoplasm, and in some cases, these two tumors may be nearly indistinguishable. Pancreatoblastoma and solid-pseudopapillary tumor must also be considered. The distinguishing features of these solid, cellular pancreatic tumors are discussed in the following section.

CYSTIC ACINAR NEOPLASMS

Pancreatic acinar neoplasms are generally solid tumors, but cystic changes may occur occasionally owing to degeneration or necrosis. A small number of fundamentally cystic acinar neoplasms exist, including acinar cell cystadenoma[154,155] and acinar cell cystadenocarcinoma.[156,157] In both entities, the cysts are relatively small and are lined by cytologically characteristic acinar cells. The benign variant is often microscopic and incidental, although more extensive involvement of the gland may occur rarely. Cases of acinar cell cystadenocarcinoma show a high degree of cytologic atypia, commonly invade into adjacent structures, and have a prognosis similar to that of solid acinar cell carcinoma. Enzymes can be detected by immunohistochemistry in the cells that line both types of acinar cystic tumors.

PANCREATOBLASTOMA

Pancreatoblastoma is uncommon but represents the most frequent pancreatic tumor of early childhood.[158,159] Most cases occur in the first decade of life, with a mean age of 4 years. Some cases are congenital, and an association with the Beckwith-Wiedemann syndrome has been described.[160] Rarely, pancreatoblastomas occur in adults.[159,161]

Pancreatoblastoma is defined as an epithelial tumor that exhibits acinar differentiation, often with a lesser degree of endocrine and ductal differentiation, and is associated with squamoid corpuscles. As an acinar neoplasm, pancreatoblastoma shares the solid, highly cellular appearance of acinar cell carcinomas. The tumor is generally lobulated, with lobules separated by hypercellular stromal bands. In some cases, the stroma itself appears neoplastic, and heterologous bone and cartilage formation may occur. The epithelial cells are arranged in solid sheets and as small acini and contain a modest amount of cytoplasm and prominent nucleoli.

The squamoid corpuscle is the histologic hallmark of pancreatoblastoma. These structures may be loose aggregates of larger spindled cells, or they may be more frankly squamous, even with keratinization (Fig. 31-31). The exact nature of squamoid corpuscles is unclear. They do not appear to exhibit a reproducible line of differentiation.

Acinar differentiation is found in nearly all cases of pancreatoblastoma, as demonstrated by histochemical[162] and immunohistochemical positivity for pancreatic enzymes (e.g., trypsin and chymotrypsin) or the presence of zymogen granules and irregular fibrillary granules by electron microscopy. In addition, it is common for variable amounts of endocrine and ductal differentiation to be detected by immunohistochemistry, but this is usually a minor component of the tumor.[159] Alpha-fetoprotein production has been reported (also in cases of acinar cell carcinoma in childhood) and is

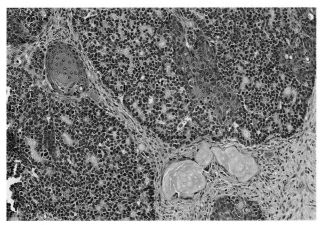

FIGURE 31–31. Pancreatoblastoma. Solid nests with acinar lumina are formed from small cells with hyperchromatic nuclei. Several squamoid corpuscles composed of larger cells with less dense nuclei are seen; focal keratinization is evident in this example.

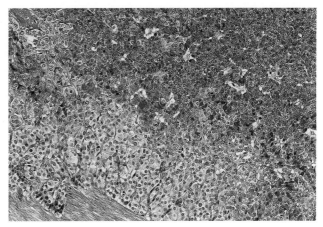

FIGURE 31–32. Mixed acinar-endocrine carcinoma. Periodic acid–Schiff stain after diastase pretreatment. In this example, two morphologically separate cell populations are identifiable; the dPAS-positive elements represent the acinar component, and the pale-staining peripheral elements represent the endocrine component.

detectable both in the serum and by immunohisto-chemistry.[163,164] The data on genetic alterations in pancreatoblastoma are rather limited, but findings are similar to those in acinar cell carcinoma.[165] Typical genetic changes of ductal adenocarcinoma are absent, but alteration in the APC/beta-catenin pathway is even more common in pancreatoblastoma than in acinar cell carcinoma.

The behavior of pancreatoblastoma differs in infants versus adults. In childhood, most cases that are detected before the development of metastases are curable by surgery. In addition, marked responses to preoperative chemotherapy have been achieved.[145,166] For cases with metastases, the prognosis is poor, although newer chemotherapy combinations hold some promise for long-term survival in these patients. In adults, almost all cases of pancreatoblastoma are fatal.

The differential diagnosis includes other solid, cellular tumors of the pancreas (see Differential Diagnosis of Solid Cellular Tumors). In particular, pancreatoblastoma shares many features of acinar cell carcinoma,[142] to the point that some observers consider pancreatoblastoma a pediatric form of acinar cell carcinoma. Because both tumors show similar lines of differentiation, it is the characteristic histologic features of pancreatoblastoma (especially the squamoid corpuscles) that help to distinguish them.

"MIXED" ACINAR NEOPLASMS

Scattered endocrine cells are present in up to 40% of acinar cell carcinomas.[167] In fact, minor elements of ductal differentiation can also be detected by staining for mucin or for glycoproteins such as CEA. In addition, some tumors contain more substantial amounts of two (or even all three) different cell types.[167-169] Mixed

carcinomas have been arbitrarily defined as those having at least 25% of each line of differentiation.[167,169] Different combinations occur, including mixed acinar-endocrine, mixed acinar-ductal, mixed ductal-endocrine, and mixed acinar-endocrine-ductal carcinomas.[170] The mixed ductal-endocrine tumors are discussed in the following section; most of the other mixed tumors exhibit predominantly acinar differentiation. In rare cases, histologically separate elements of each line of differentiation are found (Fig. 31-32). Usually, however, transitional features are apparent throughout the tumor, with only the morphology raising the suggestion of mixed differentiation. In these instances, immunohisto-chemistry is needed to recognize the type and extent of each line of differentiation (Fig. 31-33).

Because mixed tumors contain elements associated with different genetic abnormalities, the molecular phenotype of these tumors may be interesting but has yet to be evaluated. Most examples containing substantial acinar elements appear to behave clinically like acinar cell carcinomas (for instance, most mixed acinar-endocrine carcinomas are more aggressive than comparable pancreatic endocrine neoplasms). Thus, for treatment purposes, these tumors are best classified as variants of acinar cell carcinoma unless data emerge that define a distinctive biology for them.

■ Endocrine Tumors

Pancreatic endocrine neoplasms constitute a major class of pancreatic tumors with distinctive histologic features and clinical characteristics, including a variety of peptide-mediated paraneoplastic syndromes. Approximately 5% to 8% of clinically relevant pancreatic tumors

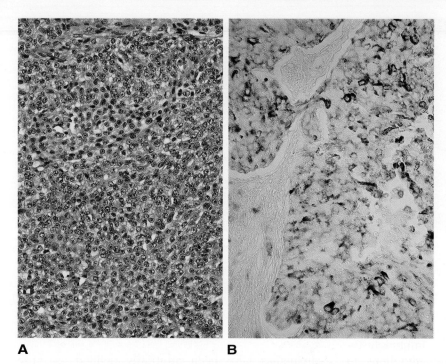

A   **B**

FIGURE 31–33. Mixed acinar-endocrine carcinoma. In most examples of mixed tumors, the dual cell population is difficult to recognize on routine microscopy (**A**). Immunohistochemical staining (**B**) demonstrates that each component represents more than 25% of the tumor cell population (double immunohistochemical staining for trypsin [blue reaction product] and chromogranin [brown reaction product]).

are pancreatic endocrine neoplasms. However, microscopic, clinically undetectable pancreatic endocrine neoplasms (microadenomas) are commonly found at autopsy. A majority of pancreatic endocrine neoplasms are low- to intermediate-grade tumors that exhibit well-developed endocrine differentiation. This category is sometimes referred to as *differentiated endocrine neoplasms*. Rarely, the pancreas gives rise to high-grade ("undifferentiated") neuroendocrine carcinomas with a high proliferative rate and distinctive cytologic features that distinguish them from other types of pancreatic carcinoma.

PANCREATIC ENDOCRINE NEOPLASMS

Clinical Features

Pancreatic endocrine neoplasms may occur at any age but are more common among middle-aged adults (mean age, 55 to 60 years).[171] Traditionally, they are divided into functional and nonfunctional categories, depending on the presence of an associated paraneoplastic syndrome. Based on the type of syndrome present, functional tumors have been designated as insulinoma, glucagonoma, gastrinoma, somatostatinoma, VIPoma, or carcinoid tumor. A majority (65% to 75%) of pancreatic endocrine neoplasms are clinically functional, but a sizable proportion of pancreatic endocrine neoplasms are not associated with a clinically evident paraneoplastic syndrome. These tumors are designated "nonfunctional" pancreatic endocrine neoplasms, although evidence of peptide or bioamine production may be

found if serologic assays or immunohistochemical studies are performed. Thus, it would be more accurate to designate clinically nonfunctional pancreatic endocrine neoplasms as "nonsyndromic," but the traditional terminology remains. Patients with nonfunctional pancreatic endocrine neoplasms usually present with nonspecific symptoms related to the presence of the mass, although biliary obstruction and jaundice may occur with tumors in the head of the pancreas. In some cases, the symptoms of metastatic disease cause the patient to seek medical attention.

One of the most challenging issues regarding pancreatic endocrine neoplasms is the prediction of biologic behavior. A number of different classification schemes have been proposed in an effort to separate benign from malignant tumors.[169,172-175] Although many features are more common in clinically aggressive tumors, some apparently malignant pancreatic endocrine neoplasms are cured by resection, whereas apparently benign cases may recur or metastasize. Certainly, it is well accepted that tumors smaller than 0.5 cm (defined as microadenomas) are clinically benign, although such tumors are rarely detectable unless they are functional.

Some authorities do not classify clinically relevant pancreatic endocrine neoplasms as benign or malignant but prefer to characterize prognostic factors that may help predict the postsurgical outcome.[173] One of the reasons for specifying the functional nature of pancreatic endocrine neoplasms is that a specific prognosis has been ascribed to each different variety. Most importantly, insulinomas pursue an indolent clinical course in 90% of cases and have often been regarded as benign. In contrast, most other functional pancreatic endocrine neoplasms recur or metastasize in 50% to 70% of cases. It is likely that the favorable outcome of patients with insulinomas is due in part to the relatively small size at which these tumors are typically detected, relative to other functional neoplasms.

Tumor size is indeed an important prognostic factor in all types of pancreatic endocrine neoplasms. Tumors smaller than 2 cm, in general, have a low risk for malignant behavior. Other pathologic prognostic factors include mitotic rate, presence of necrosis, vascular invasion, and extrapancreatic invasion. As has been proposed for carcinoid tumors and atypical carcinoid tumors of the lung, a recently proposed classification divides pancreatic endocrine neoplasms into low- and intermediate-grade groups based on the mitotic rate and the presence of necrosis. In this system, pancreatic endocrine neoplasms with two or more mitoses per 50 high-power fields or with necrosis are considered of intermediate grade. Although the low-grade group is still not considered totally benign, the difference in recurrence-free survival between these two groups is highly significant. Other ancillary methods such as DNA ploidy analysis have some value in predicting behavior.[176,177] The Ki67 labeling index seems to be promising.[178]

Pancreatic endocrine neoplasms are generally considered indolent tumors. For insulinomas and other small examples of pancreatic endocrine neoplasm, this is true. However, many other functional and most nonfunctional pancreatic endocrine neoplasms have the potential for aggressive behavior. Metastases, most commonly to the regional lymph nodes and liver, are frequent. Although pancreatic endocrine neoplasms progress slowly, they are rarely curable once they metastasize. Survival for years (or even decades) may be possible in the presence of metastatic disease, but most chemotherapeutic options are ultimately unsuccessful. For functional tumors, surgical resection or embolization of metastases or treatment with somatostatin analogues may help reduce hormone-related symptoms.

Although many pancreatic endocrine neoplasms are sporadic, these tumors, along with parathyroid and anterior pituitary endocrine lesions, represent one of the major components of the multiple endocrine neoplasia I (MEN I) syndrome. MEN I patients often have multiple pancreatic endocrine neoplasms,[179] including both functional (insulinoma and gastrinoma especially) and nonfunctional types. A dominantly inherited defect in the *menin* gene has been described in these patients; spontaneous *menin* gene abnormalities also occur in sporadic pancreatic endocrine neoplasms.[180] Patients with von Hippel-Lindau syndrome also develop pancreatic endocrine neoplasms,[82,83] some of which have clear cell features (see Fig. 31-38).

Pathologic Features

Pancreatic Endocrine Microadenomas. These lesions, which measure smaller than 0.5 cm, are commonly found at autopsy. They may also be incidental findings in patients with other types of pancreatic tumors. Histologically, they resemble large pancreatic endocrine neoplasms with nests and trabeculae of uniform endocrine cells, usually without stromal fibrosis (Fig. 31-34). Mitoses are generally not detectable. Microadenomas can be distinguished from enlarged but non-neoplastic islets based on alterations in the proportion and distribution of peptide cell types that occur in pancreatic endocrine neoplasms. Many microadenomas show a predominance of α cells.

Differentiated Pancreatic Endocrine Neoplasms. Grossly, most pancreatic endocrine neoplasms are relatively well-circumscribed, homogeneous tumors (Fig. 31-35). A soft consistency is common, but some cases have dense sclerosis. Occasional pancreatic endocrine neoplasms grossly invade adjacent structures.

Histologically, pancreatic endocrine neoplasms are usually characterized by a proliferation of round, uniform cells with a moderate amount of cytoplasm and a "salt-and-pepper" chromatin pattern. These cells are usually clustered in distinct nests separated by small vessels, and they may form trabecular, gyriform, or rosette-like patterns (Fig. 31-36). Some cases have glandular lumina. The stroma varies from minimal to abundant but is rarely desmoplastic. Hyalinized, amyloid-like stroma is typical (Fig. 31-37), and true congophilic amyloid may be present. Psammoma bodies may be found in some pancreatic endocrine neoplasms. Most cases show minimal nuclear pleomorphism and indistinct nucleoli. Mitotic figures are usually difficult to find. The presence of scattered mitoses suggests that a formal mitotic count should be performed, and no differentiated pancreatic endocrine neoplasm should have more than 10 mitoses

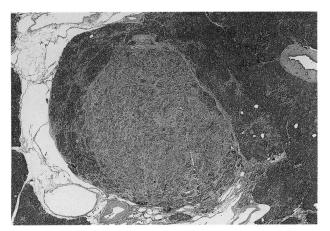

FIGURE 31–34. Endocrine microadenoma. This 0.3-cm endocrine neoplasm is cytoarchitecturally similar to larger pancreatic endocrine neoplasms but is defined as a microadenoma based primarily on its size (smaller than 0.5 cm).

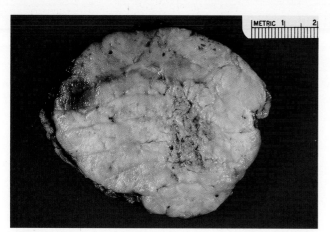

FIGURE 31–35. Gross appearance of pancreatic endocrine neoplasm. Many examples are relatively well circumscribed and exhibit lobules of soft, tan, homogeneous tissue.

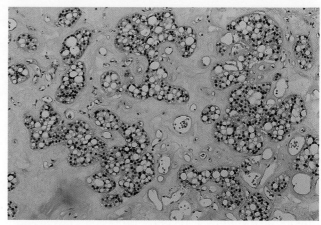

FIGURE 31–37. Pancreatic endocrine neoplasm with stromal hyalinization. Some cases exhibit pronounced collagenization of the stroma that focally resembles amyloid. This example also shows unusual vacuolization of the tumor cells.

per 10 high-power fields (the definition of a high-grade neuroendocrine carcinoma). Necrosis is also uncommon; when present, it is usually infarct-like.

Relative to differentiated endocrine tumors of other organs, differentiated pancreatic endocrine neoplasms have an exceptional range of histologic variation. Massive

cystic degeneration may result in an appearance simulating a lymphoepithelial cyst or pseudocyst. The cytoplasm may exhibit[181] clear cell change (Fig. 31-38), especially in patients with von Hippel–Lindau syndrome. A lipid-rich variant with vesicular cytoplasm has also been reported,[182] as have oncocytic varieties.[183-188] Some

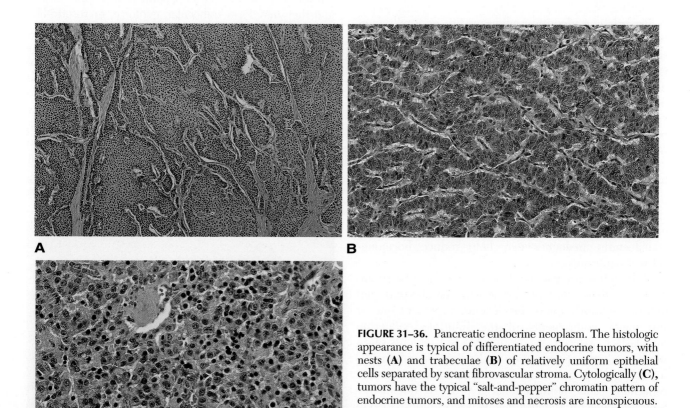

A

B

C

FIGURE 31–36. Pancreatic endocrine neoplasm. The histologic appearance is typical of differentiated endocrine tumors, with nests **(A)** and trabeculae **(B)** of relatively uniform epithelial cells separated by scant fibrovascular stroma. Cytologically **(C)**, tumors have the typical "salt-and-pepper" chromatin pattern of endocrine tumors, and mitoses and necrosis are inconspicuous.

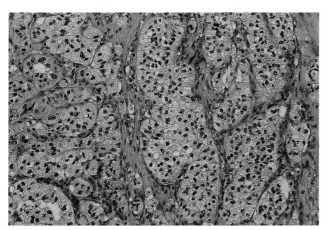

FIGURE 31–38. Pancreatic endocrine neoplasm with clear cell features. Tumor cells exhibit numerous small, clear, cytoplasmic vacuoles, resulting in a foamy appearance.

cases display widespread glandular differentiation with abundant lumina lined by endocrine cells. Although most examples are cytologically bland, some pancreatic endocrine neoplasms have macronucleoli, and others exhibit striking nuclear pleomorphism (Fig. 31-39). Pleomorphic pancreatic endocrine neoplasms are commonly mistaken for adenocarcinomas or other high-grade tumors,[189] but in these former cases the enlarged nuclei are accompanied by abundant cytoplasm (cytomegaly). Furthermore, mitotic activity is not usually increased, and the prognosis is similar to that of conventional examples.

Immunohistochemistry is invaluable in establishing a diagnosis of pancreatic endocrine neoplasm. General endocrine markers such as chromogranin and synaptophysin are usually positive. In some pancreatic endocrine neoplasms, staining for chromogranin may be less intense and widespread than that for synaptophysin. Other general markers (e.g., neuron-specific

enolase, Leu7, CD56) are also generally expressed but are less specific. Staining for peptide hormones may be of interest, and in some (but not all) functional tumors, it is possible to document the production of the specific hormone responsible for the syndrome. It is important to remember, however, that functional tumors are defined clinically and not by immunohistochemistry. A clinically nonsyndromic pancreatic endocrine neoplasm that stains for insulin could be considered a β-cell tumor; it should not be designated as an insulinoma with the associated favorable prognosis. In fact, the immunohistochemically defined peptide profile of pancreatic endocrine neoplasms does not have prognostic significance, and many pancreatic endocrine neoplasms stain for several different peptides in varying amounts.[190] Thus, staining for peptides is largely performed for academic interest only.

Electron microscopy is also useful for confirming the endocrine nature of pancreatic endocrine neoplasms. Secretory granules are usually easy to find and are distributed evenly throughout the cytoplasm. In some cases, the morphology of the granules resembles that of the corresponding peptide granule types in non-neoplastic islet cells; however, often the appearance is nonspecific.

Molecular alterations identified in pancreatic endocrine neoplasms are significantly different from those in ductal adenocarcinoma, with the exception of occasional *p16* abnormalities.[191,192]

Differential Diagnosis

The differential diagnosis largely includes the other solid, cellular pancreatic tumors (see under Differential Diagnosis of Solid Cellular Tumors). Cases with gland formation or nuclear pleomorphism may resemble ductal adenocarcinoma. It is important that the typical endocrine cytology and growth patterns be recognized in these cases, as well as the absence of mitoses. Once the possibility of an endocrine neoplasm is considered, immunohistochemical staining for chromogranin and synaptophysin is usually diagnostic.

HIGH-GRADE NEUROENDOCRINE CARCINOMAS

Primary high-grade neuroendocrine carcinomas are rare in the pancreas, constituting less than 5% of pancreatic endocrine neoplasms and affecting primarily older adult patients.[193-195] These rare tumors may exhibit large, pleomorphic nuclei (large cell neuroendocrine carcinoma), but they more commonly resemble small cell carcinomas such as those that arise in the lung.[196-198] More important than the degree of nuclear atypia in pancreatic neuroendocrine carcinomas is the presence of a diffusely infiltrative growth pattern, numerous

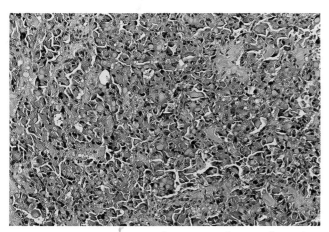

FIGURE 31–39. Pancreatic endocrine neoplasm with nuclear pleomorphism. This case exhibits enlarged, bizarre nuclei in cells also showing abundant cytoplasm. There is no increase in mitotic rate to suggest a higher-grade tumor.

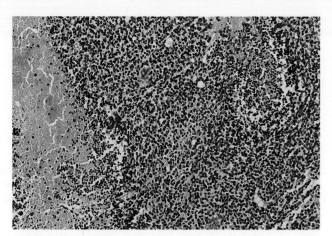

FIGURE 31–40. High-grade neuroendocrine carcinoma. This tumor shows a monotonous proliferation of small cells cytologically resembling small cell carcinoma. Abundant necrosis and innumerable mitotic figures are seen.

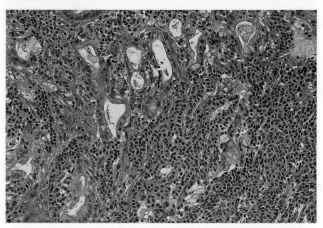

FIGURE 31–41. Mixed endocrine-ductal carcinoma. Two morphologically separate elements are present—one consisting of solid sheets of endocrine cells, the other consisting of cytologically more atypical ductal structures containing obvious intracellular mucin.

mitotic figures (more than 10 per 10 high-power fields), and abundant tumor necrosis (Fig. 31-40). In cases with the typical cytologic features of small cell carcinoma, it is not necessary that endocrine differentiation be documented, but for large cell neuroendocrine carcinomas, positive immunohistochemical staining for chromogranin or synaptophysin should be obtained to confirm the diagnosis. These tumors are highly aggressive. They exhibit early dissemination and a rapidly fatal course. Owing to the rarity of small cell carcinoma of the pancreas, a metastasis from the lung (or other sites) must be excluded before a specific case is accepted as primary to the pancreas. Another entity to consider is primitive neuroectodermal tumor (PNET), a tumor that shares some of the cytologic features of small cell carcinoma; it occurs in younger patients, however, and stains immunohistochemically for CD99.[199]

MIXED ENDOCRINE NEOPLASMS

Pancreatic endocrine neoplasms often exhibit focal glandular formation, focal luminal mucin positivity, or immunohistochemical staining for glycoproteins such as CEA or CA 19-9. These features, which signify a component of ductal differentiation, may be widespread,[200,201] but none has been shown to have clinical significance. Because the designation of a tumor as a mixed ductal/endocrine carcinoma suggests a more aggressive prognosis (caused by the ductal adeno-carcinoma component),[202,203] the definition of mixed ductal/endocrine carcinoma requires more than simple ductal differentiation in a typical pancreatic endocrine neoplasm. True mixed ductal/endocrine carcinomas contain morphologically separate elements of ductal adenocarcinoma and pancreatic endocrine neoplasm (Fig. 31-41); each component has the histologic and immunohistochemical features of the corresponding

"pure" tumor entity. These tumors are extremely uncommon, and many cases reported in the literature do not meet these criteria. The clinical behavior is unknown, although a tumor with a significant component of ductal adenocarcinoma would likely behave aggressively.

Mixed acinar/endocrine neoplasms are discussed earlier in the acinar tumor section.

Solid-Pseudopapillary Tumor

CLINICAL FEATURES

Solid-pseudopapillary tumor[204] is a tumor of uncertain differentiation.[205] This is reflected in the various descriptive names previously used for this tumor, such as *solid and cystic tumor*, *solid and papillary epithelial neoplasm*, and *papillary-cystic tumor*.[206-209] Clinically, solid-pseudopapillary tumors are significantly more common in women than in men (male-to-female ratio, 1:9). They have been reported in all age groups,[145] but the mean age is 30 years.[210] Occurrence in the first decade, however, is rare. Symptoms are nonspecific, and some cases are detected incidentally following trauma or during gynecologic or obstetric examinations. Often, solid-pseudopapillary tumors reach very large sizes before coming to clinical detection; the average solid-pseudopapillary tumor measures larger than 10 cm.

PATHOLOGIC FEATURES

Essentially, solid-pseudopapillary tumors are solid tumors that undergo cystic degeneration as they increase in size. Grossly, the color varies from yellow-brown to hemorrhagic. Most are soft and friable, but some are densely fibrotic. When present, the cysts are irregular

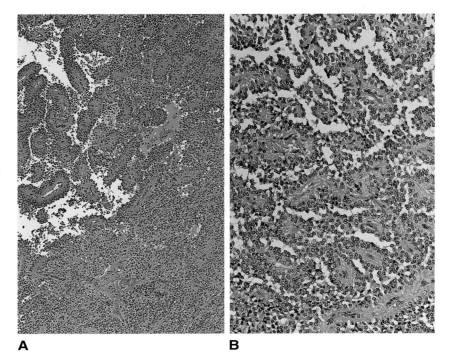

FIGURE 31–42. Solid-pseudopapillary tumor. The solid, cellular regions of this tumor are punctuated by numerous small vessels. In some areas, the tumor cells between the vessels are dyscohesive and have degenerated, resulting in pseudopapillae (**A**). At higher magnification (**B**), the central vessel of each pseudopapilla can be seen with a rim of cytoplasm separating it from surrounding nuclei. Nuclei are oval and bland with longitudinal grooves.

A   **B**

and are lined by shaggy debris. Extreme cystic change may simulate the appearance of a pseudocyst.

The diagnosis of solid-pseudopapillary tumor is essentially based on routine histology or cytopathology.[211] Its basic architecture comprises solid cellular nests with abundant small vessels. As cells situated away from the vessels degenerate, a cuff of remaining cells surrounding each vessel gives rise to pseudopapillary structures (Fig. 31-42). True luminal spaces are not found, although cytoplasmic vacuolization may be prominent. Variable degrees of stromal hyalinization may be present, and some cases exhibit balls of stroma within tumor cell nests, resulting in a cylindromatous pattern. The cytoplasm is usually moderate in amount and eosinophilic and may appear oncocytic in some cases.[212,213] Eosinophilic "hyaline globules" are typically found in the cytoplasm, usually within clusters of adjacent cells (Fig. 31-43). The nuclei are relatively uniform and typically contain longitudinal grooves. Despite the grossly circumscribed appearance of solid-pseudopapillary tumors, microscopic infiltrative growth is common, especially into the adjacent non-neoplastic pancreas.

Despite intensive study, the line of differentiation of solid-pseudopapillary tumor is still unknown. Some cases appear to exhibit endocrine differentiation based on consistent staining for CD56 (neural cell adhesion molecule) and occasional staining for synaptophysin, but chromogranin is always negative. Both acinar and ductal markers are also consistently negative. In fact, the absence of keratin expression in more than half of cases is unusual for any of the epithelial tumors or normal epithelial cells encountered in the pancreas. The only other consistently

positive immunohistochemical stains are vimentin, alpha-1-antitrypsin (Fig. 31-44) (and alpha-1-antichymotrypsin), nuclear beta-catenin, and CD10, none of which is specific for any particular line of differentiation. By electron microscopy, the most striking finding is the presence of large electron-dense granules, generally containing complex internal membranous and granular inclusions.[204,214] Initially interpreted to represent zymogen granules or neurosecretory granules,[188] these structures resemble complex secondary lysosomes, and they contain alpha-1-antitrypsin immunohistochemically. In keeping with their female predilection, solid-pseudopapillary

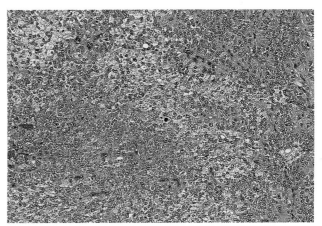

FIGURE 31–43. Solid-pseudopapillary tumor. Some cells show foamy cytoplasm, and others contain numerous large hyaline globules.

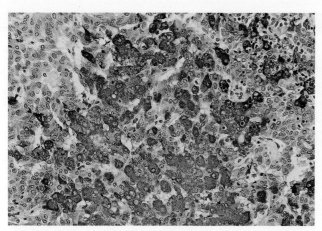

FIGURE 31–44. Solid-pseudopapillary tumor: Immunohistochemical staining for alpha-1-antitrypsin. Intense positivity is seen in clusters of cells, corresponding to the cells containing hyaline globules.

tumors often express progesterone receptors, but estrogen receptor expression is not typical.[204,215] Of note, solid-pseudopapillary tumors often harbor beta-catenin mutations, so most tumors show nuclear beta-catenin staining by immunohistochemistry.[216]

PROGNOSIS AND TREATMENT

Although the line of differentiation exhibited by solid-pseudopapillary tumors is uncertain, the entity can be readily diagnosed microscopically and has a characteristic biology. These tumors are regarded as malignant, but metastases occur in only 10% to 15% of cases.[204,217,218] In almost every instance, metastases occur to either the liver or the peritoneum; nodal metastases are rare. Most patients who do not have metastases on first presentation will not develop them after complete surgical resection.[219] It is interesting to note that even patients with metastatic disease often survive for many years (even decades) with few symptoms. In fact, only rare deaths have been attributed to the direct effect of solid-pseudopapillary tumor.

DIFFERENTIAL DIAGNOSIS

The differential diagnosis of solid-pseudopapillary tumors is discussed in the following section. In addition to primary pancreatic tumors, solid-pseudopapillary tumors must be distinguished from adrenal cortical tumors, which also may exhibit a pseudopapillary pattern due to degeneration. Both of these share vimentin positivity, frequent keratin negativity, and occasional staining for synaptophysin. Staining of adrenal cortical tumors for inhibin and identification of the alpha-1-antitrypsin–positive globules in solid-pseudopapillary tumors are helpful.

■ Differential Diagnosis of Solid Cellular Tumors

The group comprising acinar cell carcinoma, mixed acinar tumors, pancreatoblastoma, pancreatic endocrine neoplasms, and solid-pseudopapillary tumor shares a relatively solid, cellular appearance, distinct from conventional ductal adenocarcinoma and cystic neoplasms. Thus, these entities commonly cause diagnostic difficulties. Certain clinical features (e.g., age, sex) are helpful (Table 31-6) in diagnosis. In childhood, pancreatoblastoma is most common in those younger than 10 years of age, but solid-pseudopapillary tumors are more prevalent among teenagers. The latter tumor is much more frequent in females, whereas all other solid, cellular tumors affect both sexes. Some histologic findings are also highly suggestive of a diagnosis, such as squamoid corpuscles in pancreatoblastoma (see Table 31-6). However, immunohistochemistry, which is the most helpful diagnostic technique, is essential in many instances.[7,8,159,167,204] With the combination of intermediate filament markers, endocrine and enzyme markers, and selected other stains, most cases can be accurately characterized (Table 31-7). In fact, some of these stains are required for the diagnosis of mixed tumors.

TABLE 31-6. Clinical and Pathologic Features of Solid, Cellular Pancreatic Tumors

Feature	Acinar Cell Carcinoma	Mixed Acinar-Endocrine Carcinoma	Pancreatoblastoma	Pancreatic Endocrine Neoplasm	Solid Pseudopapillary Tumor
Age (yr)	50–80	18–75	0–9	30–80	15–45
Sex	Male > Female	Male > Female	Male > Female	Male = Female	Female >>> Male
Symptoms	Pain, lipase hypersecretion	Pain	Pain	Pain, endocrine paraneoplastic syndrome	Pain
Histology	Solid nests, acini, scant stroma	Solid nests, acini, variable stroma	Solid nests, acini, squamoid corpuscles, cellular stroma	Solid nests, trabeculae, hyalinized stroma	Pseudopapillae, no lumina, variable stroma

TABLE 31-7. Immunohistochemical Findings of Solid Cellular Pancreatic Tumors

Parameter	Acinar Cell Carcinoma	Mixed Acinar-Endocrine Carcinoma	Pancreatoblastoma	Pancreatic Endocrine Neoplasm	Solid Pseudopapillary Tumor
Keratin	++	++	++	++	−/+
Vimentin	−	−	−	−	++
Trypsin*	++	++	++	−	−
Chromogranin	−	++	+	++	−
Synaptophysin	−	++	+	++	+
CD56	−	++	+	++	++
Alpha-1-antitrypsin	+	+	+	−/+	++
CEA	−	−	+	+	−
CD10	no data	no data	no data	no data	++
Beta-catenin (nuclear)	no data	no data	no data	no data	++

*Also chymotrypsin.
−, usually negative; −/+ , usually negative, may be positive; +, often positive; ++, consistently positive.

Mesenchymal and Lymphoid Tumors

Primary mesenchymal tumors are rare in the pancreas. A review of the literature reveals occasional examples of most of the common soft tissue tumor types, especially those that typically involve adjacent structures, such as the retroperitoneum or the duodenum. In fact, some pancreatic mesenchymal tumors probably arise from adjacent tissues and thus only secondarily involve the pancreas.

Examples of benign pancreatic soft tissue tumors include schwannoma and lymphangioma.[220] This latter entity may simulate a serous cystadenoma, but it has aggregates of lymphocytes in the walls of the cysts. Lymphangiomas must also be distinguished from lymphoepithelial cysts; immunohistochemical staining for epithelial and vascular markers is helpful in problematic cases. Solitary fibrous tumors may arise in the pancreas. These are histologically typical, with alternating areas of hypocellular and hypercellular spindle cell elements, variable collagenation, and hemangiopericytoma-like vascular spaces. Entrapped non-neoplastic pancreatic parenchyma may be extensive (Fig. 31-45). Another recently described pancreatic tumor is the benign sugar tumor, a smooth muscle neoplasm of perivascular epithelioid cell origin related to renal angiomyolipoma and pulmonary sugar tumor (Fig. 31-46).[221] As in these other entities, pancreatic sugar tumors express HMB-45 immunohistochemically.

Most types of soft tissue sarcomas also have been reported in the pancreas, including liposarcoma, leiomyosarcoma, synovial sarcoma, and malignant fibrous histocytoma; of these, leiomyosarcoma is probably the most frequent. Gastrointestinal stromal tumors may also

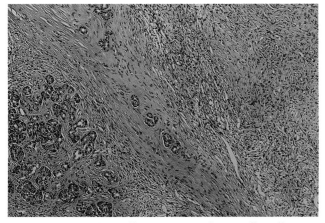

FIGURE 31–45. Solitary fibrous tumor. This spindle cell tumor exhibits variable cellularity and ectatic, hemangiopericytoma-like vasculature. The tumor surrounds clusters of non-neoplastic acini.

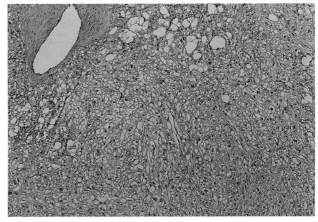

FIGURE 31–46. Sugar tumor. This tumor is composed of epithelioid spindle cells with cytoplasmic vacuolization and focally prominent vessels, resembling cellular angiomyolipoma of the kidney.

involve the pancreas and presumably originate from the duodenum. Critical to the diagnosis of a primary pancreatic sarcoma is exclusion of a sarcomatoid carcinoma[54] or carcinosarcoma. Because some of these fundamentally epithelial tumors may exhibit heterologous mesenchymal differentiation, it is important to look for epithelial differentiation by immunohistochemistry in the more generic spindle cell elements.

Primitive neuroectodermal tumors also rarely affect the pancreas.[199] Most patients are relatively young. The histologic appearance resembles that of pancreatic endocrine neoplasms, although primitive neuroectodermal tumors generally are more infiltrative and have smaller cells than do differentiated pancreatic endocrine neoplasms (Fig. 31-47). A confounding feature in the differential diagnosis is that pancreatic primitive neuroectodermal tumors commonly express keratin in a strong, diffuse manner. Furthermore, differentiated pancreatic endocrine neoplasms may express CD99 (similar to islet cells). Thus, confirmation of the diagnosis of pancreatic primitive neuroectodermal tumor with the demonstration of characteristic (11;22) chromosomal translocation is helpful.

Involvement of the pancreas by lymphoma is not uncommon in patients with widespread disease and may occur as either primary involvement of the organ or by direct extension from adjacent lymph nodes. However, a primary origin of lymphoid neoplasms in the pancreas is rare. A number of previously reported cases are plasmacytomas, but other types of non-Hodgkin's lymphoma may also arise in the pancreas.

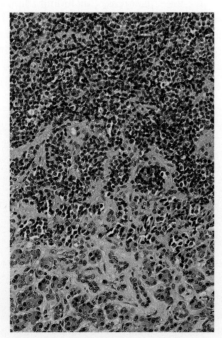

FIGURE 31–47. Primitive neuroectodermal tumor. Dense cellularity and uniform small round cells characterize pancreatic primitive neuroectodermal tumors.

Tumor-like Lesions

Various types of inflammatory processes may result in the development of a pancreatic mass.[222] In some studies, 5% of pancreatectomies performed with a preoperative diagnosis of carcinoma later proved to be non-neoplastic on pathologic examination.[222] These cases of "pseudotumoral pancreatitis" may have a number of different causes. In some cases, ordinary chronic pancreatitis[223] (alcohol or gallstone related) may have an exaggerated focus of fibrosis mimicking carcinoma. In others, pancreatitis and pseudotumor formation may represent autoimmune disease or a manifestation of multifocal fibrosclerosis. Some cases exhibit morphologic findings of inflammatory myofibroblastic tumor ("inflammatory pseudotumor"). In a small proportion of cases, periampullary and duodenal pathology (possibly congenital or heterotopia related) can lead to scarring of the ampulla or common bile duct. These cases may also reveal cystic dystrophy (an exaggerated form of which is referred to as *paraduodenal wall cyst*) and adenomyomatous hyperplasia in the ampullary and accessory ampullary regions of the pancreas.

One subset of cases deserves special mention. *Lymphoplasmacytic sclerosing pancreatitis*[224,225] is the term that has been recently applied to a form of chronic pancreatitis sometimes associated with autoimmune disease or multifocal fibrosclerosis (e.g., retroperitoneal fibrosis, mediastinal fibrosis, Riedel's thyroiditis, inflammatory pseudotumor of the orbit). In these cases, a dense lymphoplasmacytic inflammatory infiltrate centered on medium to large ducts is seen, along with duct epithelial destruction, inflammatory aggregates within and around small veins ("periphlebitis"), fibrosis, and atrophy (Fig. 31-48). Many patients with this histologic type of pancreatitis do not have an associated documented autoimmune disease,[224] and it remains to be determined whether there are different causes for this disorder. Documented cases are important because the radiographic findings, including bile duct involvement with biliary obstruction, closely mimic those of pancreatic carcinoma.[226] If a diagnosis of lymphoplasmacytic sclerosing pancreatitis is suspected, serum levels of IgG4 may be elevated. Favorable response to steroid therapy has been described.

Secondary Tumors

Secondary tumors of the pancreas are rare.[227-230] In one study,[228] an analysis of 4955 autopsies showed that of 190 primary tumors that involved the pancreas, 82 were secondary. At autopsy, lung cancer was the most common source of metastasis to the pancreas, followed by lymphoma and then carcinomas of the gastroin-

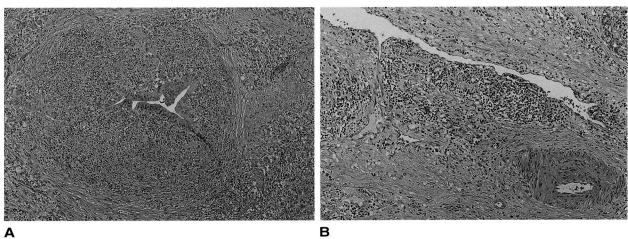

FIGURE 31–48. Lymphoplasmacytic sclerosing pancreatitis. Dense inflammation is centered around pancreatic ducts **(A)** and is composed predominantly of lymphocytes, plasma cells, and scattered eosinophils. Involvement of the walls of small veins ("periphlebitis") is a typical feature of this type of pancreatitis **(B).**

testinal tract, kidney, and breast. These cases are rarely biopsied because they usually occur in patients with widespread disease.

On the other hand, among surgical specimens, lymphomas are the most common secondary tumor of the pancreas, followed by gastric adenocarcinoma and renal cell carcinoma. A majority of gastric carcinomas involve the pancreas by direct extension. Lymphomas and renal cell carcinomas are more prone to preoperative misdiagnosis as primary pancreatic carcinoma. Pancreatic metastases from renal cell carcinoma may be solitary and may form polypoid lesions in the ampulla or in the pancreatic ducts. They may present years (even decades[231]) after the original diagnosis; furthermore, the pancreas may be the only site of recurrence. Resection of these secondary tumors, especially renal cell carcinomas, is associated with relatively good survival rates.[232,233] Secondary tumors in the pancreas may mimic primary neoplasia not only clinically but also microscopically; some may even grow within the ducts.

▨ Gross Evaluation and the Surgical Pathology Report

Standard information that should be included in surgical pathology reports regarding pancreatic ductal adenocarcinoma includes the following[234]: (1) general characteristics of the tumor (location, type, and grade), (2) pathologic degree of invasiveness (vascular and perineural invasion), (3) pathologic parameters of staging (size; extrapancreatic extension; presence or absence and degree of involvement of the common bile duct, duodenum, and other organs; and lymph node status), and (4) significant other findings such as associated lesions, incidental lesions, findings in uninvolved pancreas, and precursor lesions. The margins to be evaluated in a pancreatoduodenectomy specimen are the common bile duct and the pancreatic (ductal), retroperitoneal (posterior, uncinate), and mucosal (gastric/duodenal and distal) margins.[235] The posterior margin is of special importance because it is an important determinant of outcome.[236]

For tumors such as intraductal papillary-mucinous neoplasms or mucinous cystic tumors, the characteristics (e.g., size, extent) of the in situ and, if present, invasive components should be reported separately.

References

1. Solcia E, Capella C, Kloppel G: Tumors of the pancreas. In Armed Forces Institute of Pathology. Atlas of Tumor Pathology, vol 20. Washington, DC, American Registry of Pathology, 1997.
2. Klimstra DS: Cell lineage in pancreatic neoplasms. In Sarkar F, Dugan MC (eds): Pancreatic Cancer: Advances in Molecular Pathology, Diagnosis and Clinical Management. Natick, Mass, BioTechniques Books, 1998.
3. Lyubsky S, Madariaga J, Lozowski M, et al: A tumor-associated antigen in carcinoma of the pancreas defined by monoclonal antibody B72.3. Am J Clin Pathol 89:160-167, 1988.
4. Suriawanata A, Klimstra D: Distinguishing bile duct adenoma, hamartoma and ductular proliferation from metastatic pancreatic adenocarcinoma of the liver by immunohistochemistry [abstract]. Mod Pathol 15:294A, 2002.
5. Tempero M, Takasaki H, Uchida E, et al: Co-expression of CA 19-9, DU-PAN-2, CA 125, and TAG-72 in pancreatic adenocarcinoma. Am J Surg Pathol 13:89-95, 1989.
6. Kim JH, Ho SB, Montgomery CK, et al: Cell lineage markers in human pancreatic cancer. Cancer 66:2134-2143, 1990.
7. Klimstra DS, Heffess CS, Oertel JE, et al: Acinar cell carcinoma of the pancreas. A clinicopathologic study of 28 cases. Am J Surg Pathol 16:815-837, 1992.
8. Morohoshi T, Kanda M, Horie A, et al: Immunocytochemical markers of uncommon pancreatic tumors. Acinar cell carcinoma, pancreatoblastoma, and solid cystic (papillary-cystic) tumor. Cancer 59:739-747, 1987.
9. Kloppel G, Luttges J: WHO classification 2000: Exocrine pancreatic tumors. Verh Dtsch Ges Pathol 85:219-228, 2001.
10. Kloppel G, Solcia E, Longnecker DS, et al: World Health Organization International Histologic Classification of Tumors. Histologic Typing of Tumors of the Exocrine Pancreas, vol 2. Geneva, Springer, 1996.

11. Klimstra DS, Adsay NV: Pancreas cancer—pathology. In Kelsen DP, Daly JM, Kern SE (eds): Gastrointestinal Oncology: Principles and Practices. Philadelphia, Lippincott Williams & Wilkins, 2002.

12. Pernick NL, Eldean ZS, Kabbani W, et al: Pancreatic ductal adenocarcinoma in young patients [abstract]. Mod Pathol 14:201A, 2001.

13. Hruban RH, Iacobuzio-Donahue C, Wilentz RE, et al: Molecular pathology of pancreatic cancer. Cancer J 7:251-258, 2001.

14. Brennan MF, Moccia RD, Klimstra D: Management of adenocarcinoma of the body and tail of the pancreas. Ann Surg 223:506-511, 1996; discussion 511-512.

15. Conlon KC, Dougherty E, Klimstra DS, et al: The value of minimal access surgery in the staging of patients with potentially resectable peripancreatic malignancy. Ann Surg 223:134-140, 1996.

16. Harrison LE, Klimstra DS, Brennan MF: Isolated portal vein involvement in pancreatic adenocarcinoma: A contraindication for resection. Ann Surg 224:342-349, 1996.

17. Albores-Saavedra J, Henson DE, Klimstra DS: Tumors of the gallbladder, extrahepatic bile ducts, and ampulla of Vater. In Armed Forces Institute of Pathology, Atlas of Tumor Pathology, vol 3. Washington, DC, American Registry of Pathology, 2000.

18. Chen J, Baithun SI: Morphological study of 391 cases of exocrine pancreatic tumours with special reference to the classification of exocrine pancreatic carcinoma. J Pathol 146:17-29, 1985.

19. Cubilla AL, Fitzgerald PJ: Morphological patterns of primary non-endocrine human pancreas carcinoma. Cancer Res 35:2234-2248, 1975.

20. Luttges J, Schemm S, Vogel I, et al: The grade of pancreatic ductal carcinoma is an independent prognostic factor and is superior to the immunohistochemical assessment of proliferation. J Pathol 191:154-161, 2000.

21. Klimstra DS: Pancreas. In Sternberg SS (ed): Histology for Pathologists. New York, Lippincott-Raven, 1997.

22. Chiu T: Focal eosinophilic hypertrophic cells of the rat pancreas. Toxicol Pathol 15:1-6, 1987.

23. Frexinos J, Ribet A: Oncocytes in human chronic pancreatitis. Digestion 7:294-301, 1972.

24. Tasso F, Sarles H: [Canalicular cells and oncocytes in the human pancreas. Comparative study on the normal condition and in chronic pancreatitis]. Ann Anat Pathol 18:277-300, 1973.

25. Barton CM, Staddon SL, Hughes CM, et al: Abnormalities of the p53 tumour suppressor gene in human pancreatic cancer. Br J Cancer 64:1076-1082, 1991.

26. Hameed M, Marrero AM, Conlon KC, et al: Expression of p53 nucleophosphoprotein in in situ pancreatic ductal adenocarcinoma: An immunohistochemical study of 100 cases. Lab Invest 70:132A, 1994.

27. Evans DB, Abruzzese JL, Rich TA: Cancer of the pancreas. In Devita VT, Hellman S, Rosenberg SA (eds): Cancer: Principles and Practice of Oncology. Philadelphia, Lippincott Williams & Wilkins, 2001.

28. Conlon KC, Klimstra DS, Brennan MF: Long-term survival after curative resection for pancreatic ductal adenocarcinoma. Clinico-pathologic analysis of 5-year survivors. Ann Surg 223:273-279, 1996.

29. Philip PA, Zalupski MM, Vaitkevicius VK, et al: Phase II study of gemcitabine and cisplatin in the treatment of patients with advanced pancreatic carcinoma. Cancer 92:569-577, 2001.

30. Adsay V, Logani S, Sarkar F, et al: Foamy gland pattern of invasive ductal adenocarcinoma of the pancreas: A deceptively benign appearing variant. Am J Surg Pathol 24:493-504, 2000.

31. Andea A, Lonardo F, Adsay V: Microscopically cystic and papillary "large-duct-type" invasive adenocarcinoma of the pancreas: A potential mimic of intraductal papillary mucinous and mucinous cystic neoplasms [abstract]. Mod Pathol (in press).

32. Chow LT, Chow WH: Signet-ring mucinous adenocarcinoma of the pancreas. Chin Med Sci J 9:176-178, 1994.

33. McArthur CP, Fiorella R, Saran BM: Rare primary signet ring carcinoma of the pancreas. Mol Med 92:298-302, 1995.

34. Adsay V, Kabbani W, Sarkar F, et al: Infiltrating "lobular-type" carcinoma of the pancreas: A morphologically distinctive variant of ductal adenocarcinoma of the pancreas mimicking lobular carcinoma of the breast [abstract]. Mod Pathol 12:159A, 1999.

35. England DW, Kurrein F, Jones EL, et al: Pancreatic pleural effusion associated with oncocytic carcinoma of the pancreas. Postgrad Med J 64:465-466, 1988.

36. Huntrakoon M: Oncocytic carcinoma of the pancreas. Cancer 51:332-336, 1983.

37. Zerbi A, De Nardi P, Braga M, et al: An oncocytic carcinoma of the pancreas with pulmonary and subcutaneous metastases. Pancreas 8:116-119, 1993.

38. Kanai N, Nagaki S, Tanaka T: Clear cell carcinoma of the pancreas. Acta Pathol Japon 37:1521-1526, 1987.

39. Luttges J, Vogel I, Menke M, et al: Clear cell carcinoma of the pancreas: An adenocarcinoma with ductal phenotype. Histopathology 32:444-448, 1998.

40. Taziaux P, Dallemagne B, Delforge M, et al: [An unusual case of clear-cell carcinoma of the pancreas]. J Chir 131:86-89, 1994.

41. Adsay NV, Pierson C, Sarkar F, et al: Colloid (mucinous noncystic) carcinoma of the pancreas. Am J Surg Pathol 25:26-42, 2001.

42. Cubilla LA, Fitzgerald PJ: Tumors of the exocrine pancreas. In Armed Forces Institute of Pathology. Atlas of Tumor Pathology, vol 19. Washington, DC, Armed Forces Institute of Pathology, 1984.

43. Goggins M, Offerhaus GJ, Hilgers W, et al: Pancreatic adeno-carcinomas with DNA replication errors (RER+) are associated with wild-type K-ras and characteristic histopathology. Poor differentiation, a syncytial growth pattern, and pushing borders suggest RER+. Am J Pathol 152:1501-1507, 1998.

44. Wilentz RE, Goggins M, Redston M, et al: Genetic, immuno-histochemical, and clinical features of medullary carcinoma of the pancreas: A newly described and characterized entity. Am J Pathol 156:1641-1651, 2001.

45. Kardon DE, Thompson LD, Przygodzki RM, et al: Adenosquamous carcinoma of the pancreas: A clinicopathologic series of 25 cases. Mod Pathol 14:443-451, 2001.

46. Motojima K, Tomioka T, Kohara N, et al: Immunohistochemical characteristics of adenosquamous carcinoma of the pancreas. J Surg Oncol 49:58-62, 1992.

47. Yamaguchi K, Enjoji M: Adenosquamous carcinoma of the pancreas: A clinicopathologic study. J Surg Oncol 47:109-116, 1991.

48. Adsay V, Sarkar F, Vaitkevicius V, et al: Squamous cell and adenosquamous carcinomas of the pancreas: A clinicopathologic analysis of 11 cases [abstract]. Mod Pathol 13:179A, 2000.

49. Lane RB Jr, Sanguenza OP: Anaplastic carcinoma occurring in association with a mucinous cystic neoplasm of the pancreas. Arch Pathol Lab Med 121:533-535, 1997.

50. Gocke CD, Dabbs DJ, Benko FA, et al: KRAS oncogene mutations suggest a common histogenetic origin for pleomorphic giant cell tumor of the pancreas, osteoclastoma of the pancreas, and pancreatic duct adenocarcinoma. Hum Pathol 28:80-83, 1997.

51. Hoorens A, Prenzel K, Lemoine NR, et al: Undifferentiated carcinoma of the pancreas: Analysis of intermediate filament profile and Ki-ras mutations provides evidence of a ductal origin. J Pathol 185:53-60, 1998.

52. Paal E, Thompson LD, Frommelt RA, et al: A clinicopathologic and immunohistochemical study of 35 anaplastic carcinomas of the pancreas with a review of the literature. Ann Diagn Pathol 5:129-140, 2001.

53. Tschang TP, Garza-Garza R, Kissane JM: Pleomorphic carcinoma of the pancreas: An analysis of 15 cases. Cancer 39:2114-2126, 1977.

54. Alguacil-Garcia A, Weiland LH: The histologic spectrum, prognosis, and histogenesis of the sarcomatoid carcinoma of the pancreas. Cancer 39:1181-1189, 1977.

55. Klimstra DS, Rosai J: Osteoclastic giant cell tumor of the pancreas. Pathol Res Pract 189:232-233, 1993.

56. Lewandrowski KB, Weston L, Dickersin GR, et al: Giant cell tumor of the pancreas of mixed osteoclastic and pleomorphic cell type: Evidence for a histogenetic relationship and mesenchymal differentiation. Hum Pathol 21:1184-1187, 1990.

57. Molberg KH, Heffess C, Delgado R, et al: Undifferentiated carcinoma with osteoclast-like giant cells of the pancreas and periampullary region. Cancer 82:1279-1287, 1998.

58. Watanabe M, Miura H, Inoue H, et al: Mixed osteoclastic/pleomorphic-type giant cell tumor of the pancreas with ductal adenocarcinoma: Histochemical and immunohistochemical study with review of the literature. Pancreas 15:201-208, 1997.

59. Posen JA: Giant cell tumor of the pancreas of the osteoclastic type associated with a mucous secreting cystadenocarcinoma. Hum Pathol 12:944-947, 1981.

60. Dworak O, Wittekind C, Koerfgen HP, et al: Osteoclastic giant cell tumor of the pancreas. An immunohistological study and review of the literature. Pathol Res Pract 189:228-231, 1993; discussion 232-234.

61. Westra WH, Sturm P, Drillenburg P, et al: K-ras oncogene mutations in osteoclast-like giant cell tumors of the pancreas and liver: Genetic evidence to support origin from the duct epithelium. Am J Surg Pathol 22:1247-1254, 1998.

62. Brockie E, Anand A, Albores-Saavedra J: Progression of atypical ductal hyperplasia/carcinoma in situ of the pancreas to invasive adenocarcinoma. Ann Diagn Pathol 2:286-292, 1998.

63. Klimstra DS, Hameed M, Marrero AM, et al: Ductal proliferative lesions associated with infiltrating ductal adenocarcinoma of the pancreas. Int J Pancreatol 16:224-225, 1994.

64. Kozuka S, Sassa R, Taki T, et al: Relation of pancreatic duct hyperplasia to carcinoma. Cancer 43:1418-1428, 1979.

65. Sommers SC, Murphy SA, Warren S: Pancreatic duct hyperplasia and cancer. Gastroenterology 27:629-640, 1954.

66. Klimstra DS, Longnecker DS: K-ras mutations in pancreatic ductal proliferative lesions. Am J Pathol 145:1547-1550, 1994.

67. Hruban RH, Adsay NV, Albores-Saavedra J, et al: Pancreatic intraepithelial neoplasia: A new nomenclature and classification system for pancreatic duct lesions. Am J Surg Pathol 25:579-586, 2001.

68. Lemoine NR, Jain S, Hughes CM, et al: Ki-ras oncogene activation in preinvasive pancreatic cancer. Gastroenterology 102:230-236, 1992.

69. Yanagisawa A, Ohtake K, Ohashi K, et al: Frequent c-Ki-ras oncogene activation in mucous cell hyperplasias of pancreas suffering from chronic inflammation. Cancer Res 53:953-956, 1993.

70. Moskaluk C, Hruban RH, Kern SE: p16 and K-ras gene mutations in the intraductal precursors of human pancreatic adenocarcinoma. Cancer Res 57:2140-2143, 1997.

71. Andea A, Munn T, Sarkar F, et al: A study of pancreatic intraepithelial neoplasia (PanIN) in malignant and benign pancreata [abstract]. Mod Pathol (in press).

72. Brat DJ, Lillemoe KD, Yeo CJ, et al: Progression of pancreatic intraductal neoplasias to infiltrating adenocarcinoma of the pancreas. Am J Surg Pathol 22:163-169, 1998.

73. Adsay NV, Klimstra DS, Compton CC: Cystic lesions of the pancreas. Semin Diagn Pathol 17:1-6, 2000.

74. Albores-Saavedra J, Choux R, Gould EW, et al: Cystic tumors of the pancreas. Pathol Annu 2:19-51, 1994.

75. Alpert LC, Truong LD, Bossart MI, et al: Microcystic adenoma (serous cystadenoma) of the pancreas. A study of 14 cases with immunohistochemical and electron-microscopic correlation. Am J Surg Pathol 12:251-263, 1988.

76. Compagno J, Oertel JE: Microcystic adenomas of the pancreas (glycogen-rich cystadenomas): A clinicopathologic study of 34 cases. Am J Clin Pathol 69:289-298, 1978.

77. Compton CC: Serous cystic tumors of the pancreas. Semin Diagn Pathol 17:43-56, 2000.

78. Pyke CM, van Heerden JA, Colby TV, et al: The spectrum of serous cystadenoma of the pancreas. Clinical, pathologic, and surgical aspects. Ann Surg 215:132-139, 1992.

79. Egawa N, Maillet B, Schroder S, et al: Serous oligocystic and ill-demarcated adenoma of the pancreas: A variant of serous cystic adenoma. Virchows Arch 424:13-17, 1994.

80. Lewandrowski K, Warshaw A, Compton C: Macrocystic serous cystadenoma of the pancreas: A morphologic variant differing from microcystic adenoma. Hum Pathol 23:871-875, 1992.

81. Girelli R, Bassi C, Falconi M, et al: Pancreatic cystic manifestations in von Hippel-Lindau disease. Int J Pancreatol 22:101-109, 1997.

82. Hough DM, Stephens DH, Johnson CD, et al: Pancreatic lesions in von Hippel-Lindau disease: Prevalence, clinical significance, and CT findings. AJR Am J Roentgenol 162:1091-1094, 1994.

83. Neumann HP, Dinkel E, Brambs H, et al: Pancreatic lesions in the von Hippel-Lindau syndrome. Gastroenterology 101:465-471, 1991.

84. Nodell CG, Freeny PC, Dale DH, et al: Serous cystadenoma of the pancreas with a metachronous adenocarcinoma. AJR Am J Roentgenol 162:1352-1354, 1994.

85. Keel SB, Zukerberg L, Graeme-Cook F, et al: A pancreatic endocrine tumor arising within a serous cystadenoma of the pancreas. Am J Surg Pathol 20:471-475, 1996.

86. Perez-Ordonez B, Naseem A, Lieberman PH, et al: Solid serous adenoma of the pancreas. The solid variant of serous cystadenoma? Am J Surg Pathol 20:1401-1405, 1996.

87. Yantiss K, Compton C: The utility of MART-1 staining in the distinction between serous cystadenomas and other solid and/or cystic tumours of the pancreas [abstract]. Histopathology 41:126, 2002.

88. Moore PS, Zamboni G, Brighenti A, et al: Molecular characterization of pancreatic serous microcystic adenomas: Evidence for a tumor suppressor gene on chromosome 10q. Am J Pathol 158:317-321, 2001.

89. George DH, Murphy F, Michalski R, et al: Serous cystadenocarcinoma of the pancreas: A new entity? Am J Surg Pathol 13:61-66, 1989.

90. Haarmann W, Mittelkotter U, Smektala R: Monstrous recurrence of serous cystadenocarcinoma of the pancreas. Zentralbl Chir 122:122-125, 1997.

91. Kamei K, Funabiki T, Ochiai M, et al: Multifocal pancreatic serous cystadenoma with atypical cells and focal perineural invasion. Int J Pancreatol 10:161-172, 1991.

92. Ohta T, Nagakawa T, Itoh H, et al: A case of serous cystadenoma of the pancreas with focal malignant changes. Int J Pancreatol 14:283-289, 1993.

93. Widmaier U, Mattfeldt T, Siech M, et al: Serous cystadenocarcinoma of the pancreas. Int J Pancreatol 20:135-139, 1996.

94. Yoshimi N, Sugie S, Tanaka T, et al: A rare case of serous cystadenocarcinoma of the pancreas. Cancer 69:2449-2453, 1992.

95. Balcom IJ, Fernandez-Del Castillo C, Warshaw AL: Cystic lesions in the pancreas: When to watch, when to resect. Curr Gastroenterol Rep 2:152-158, 2000.

96. Compagno J, Oertel JE: Mucinous cystic neoplasms of the pancreas with overt and latent malignancy (cystadenocarcinoma and cystadenoma). A clinicopathologic study of 41 cases. Am J Clin Pathol 69:573-580, 1978.

97. Thompson LDR, Becker RC, Pryzgodski RM, et al: Mucinous cystic neoplasm (mucinous cystadenocarcinoma of low malignant potential) of the pancreas: A clinicopathologic study of 130 cases. Am J Surg Pathol 23:1-16, 1999.

98. Warshaw AL: Mucinous cystic tumors and mucinous ductal ectasia of the pancreas. Gastrointest Endosc 37:199-201, 1991.

99. Wilentz RE, Albores-Saavedra J, Hruban RH: Mucinous cystic neoplasms of the pancreas. Semin Diagn Pathol 17:31-43, 2000.

100. Wilentz RE, Talamani MA, Albores-Saavedra J, et al: Morphology accurately predicts behavior of mucinous cystic neoplasms of the pancreas. Am J Surg Pathol 23:1320-1327, 1999.

101. Zamboni G, Scarpa A, Bogina G, et al: Mucinous cystic tumors of the pancreas: Clinicopathological features, prognosis, and relationship to other mucinous cystic tumors. Am J Surg Pathol 23:410-422, 1999.

102. Garcia Rego JA, Valbuena Ruvira L, Alvarez Garcia A, et al: Pancreatic mucinous cystadenocarcinoma with pseudosarcomatous mural nodules. A report of a case with immunohistochemical study. Cancer 67:494-498, 1991.

103. van den Berg W, Tascilar M, Offerhaus GJ, et al: Pancreatic mucinous cystic neoplasms with sarcomatous stroma: Molecular evidence for monoclonal origin with subsequent divergence of the epithelial and sarcomatous components. Mod Pathol 13:86-91, 2000.

104. Wenig BM, Albores-Saavedra J, Buetow PC, et al: Pancreatic mucinous cystic neoplasm with sarcomatous stroma: A report of three cases. Am J Surg Pathol 21:70-80, 1997.

105. Ridder GJ, Maschek H, Flemming P, et al: Ovarian-like stroma in an invasive mucinous cystadenocarcinoma of the pancreas positive for inhibin. A hint concerning its possible histogenesis. Virchows Arch 432:451-454, 1998.

106. Southern JF, Warshaw AL, Lewandrowski KB: DNA ploidy analysis of mucinous cystic tumors of the pancreas. Correlation of aneuploidy with malignancy and poor prognosis. Cancer 77:58-62, 1996.

107. Adsay NV, Klimstra DS: Cystic forms of typically solid pancreatic tumors. Semin Diagn Pathol 17:66-81, 2000.

108. Adsay NV, Andea A, Weaver D, et al: Centrally necrotic invasive ductal adenocarcinomas of the pancreas presenting clinically as macrocystic lesions [abstract]. Mod Pathol 13:1125A, 2001.

109. Adsay NV, Hasteh F, Cheng JD, et al: Lymphoepithelial cysts of the pancreas: A report of 12 cases and a review of the literature. Mod Pathol 15:492-501, 2002.

110. Adsay NV, Hasteh F, Cheng JD, et al: Squamous-lined cysts of the pancreas: Lymphoepithelial cysts, dermoid cysts (teratomas) and accessory-splenic epidermoid cysts. Semin Diagn Pathol 17:56-66, 2000.

111. Kloppel G: Pseudocysts and other non-neoplastic cysts of the pancreas. Semin Diagn Pathol 17:1-7, 2000.

112. Adsay NV, Longnecker DS, Klimstra DS: Pancreatic tumors with cystic dilatation of the ducts: Intraductal papillary mucinous neoplasms and intraductal oncocytic papillary neoplasms. Semin Diagn Pathol 17:16-30, 2000.

113. Klimstra DS: Pancreatic intraductal neoplasms. Adv Anat Pathol 4:233-238, 1997.

114. Kloppel G: Clinicopathologic view of intraductal papillary-mucinous tumor of the pancreas. Hepatogastroenterology 45:1981-1985, 1998.

115. Adsay NV, Merati K, Andea A, et al: The dichotomy in the preinvasive neoplasia to invasive carcinoma sequence in the pancreas: Differential MUC1 and MUC2 expression supports the existence of two separate pathways of carcinogenesis. Mod Pathol 15:1087-1095, 2002.

116. Adsay V, Conlon K, Zee SY, et al: Intraductal papillary mucinous neoplasms of the pancreas: An analysis of in-situ and invasive carcinomas associated with 28 cases. Cancer 94:62-77, 2002.

117. Azar C, Van de Stadt J, Rickaert F, et al: Intraductal papillary mucinous tumours of the pancreas. Clinical and therapeutic issues in 32 patients. Gut 39:457-464, 1996.

118. Fukishima N, Mukai K, Kanai Y, et al: Intraductal papillary tumors and mucinous cystic tumors of the pancreas: Clinicopathologic study of 38 cases. Hum Pathol 28:1010-1017, 1997.

119. Loftus EV Jr, Olivares-Pakzad BA, Batts KP, et al: Intraductal papillary-mucinous tumors of the pancreas: Clinicopathologic features, outcome, and nomenclature. Members of the Pancreas Clinic and Pancreatic Surgeons of Mayo Clinic. Gastroenterology 110:1909-1918, 1996.

120. Longnecker DS: Observations on the etiology and pathogenesis of intraductal papillary-mucinous neoplasms of the pancreas. Hepatogastroenterology 45:1973-1980, 1998.

121. Paal E, Thompson LD, Przygodzki RM, et al: A clinicopathologic and immunohistochemical study of 22 intraductal papillary mucinous neoplasms of the pancreas, with a review of the literature. Mod Pathol 12:518-528, 1999.

122. Sessa F, Solcia E, Capella C, et al: Intraductal papillary-mucinous tumours represent a distinct group of pancreatic neoplasms: An investigation of tumour cell differentiation and K-ras, p53 and c-erbB-2 abnormalities in 26 patients. Virchows Arch 425:357-367, 1994.

123. Shimizu M, Manabe T: Mucin-producing pancreatic tumors: Historical review of its nosological concept. Zentralbl Pathol 140:211-223, 1994.

124. Cellier C, Cuillerier E, Palazzo L, et al: Intraductal papillary and mucinous tumors of the pancreas: Accuracy of preoperative computed tomography, endoscopic retrograde pancreatography and endoscopic ultrasonography, and long-term outcome in a large surgical series. Gastrointest Endosc 47:42-49, 1998.

125. Yamaguchi K, Tanaka M: Mucin-hypersecreting tumor of the pancreas with mucin extrusion through an enlarged papilla. Am J Gastroenterol 86:835-839, 1991.

126. Agostini S, Choux R, Payan MJ, et al: Mucinous pancreatic duct ectasia in the body of the pancreas. Radiology 170:815-816, 1989.

127. Itai Y, Ohhashi K, Nagai H, et al: "Ductectatic" mucinous cystadenoma and cystadenocarcinoma of the pancreas. Radiology 161:697-700, 1986.

128. Nagai E, Ueki T, Chijiiwa K, et al: Intraductal papillary mucinous neoplasms of the pancreas associated with so-called "mucinous ductal ectasia." Histochemical and immunohistochemical analysis of 29 cases. Am J Surg Pathol 19:576-589, 1995.

129. Yanagisawa A, Ohashi K, Hori M, et al: Ductectatic-type mucinous cystadenoma and cystadenocarcinoma of the human pancreas: A novel clinicopathological entity. Jpn J Cancer Res 84:474-479, 1993.

130. Ohhashi K, Murakami Y, Takekoshi T, et al: Four cases of mucin producing cancer of the pancreas on specific findings of the papilla of Vater. Prog Dig Endosc 20:348-351, 1982.

131. Yamada M, Kozuka S, Yamao K, et al: Mucin-producing tumor of the pancreas. Cancer 68:159-168, 1991.

132. Payan MJ, Xerri L, Moncada K, et al: Villous adenoma of the main pancreatic duct: A potentially malignant tumor? Am J Gastroenterol 85:459-463, 1990.

133. Rogers PN, Seywright MM, Murray WR: Diffuse villous adenoma of the pancreatic duct. Pancreas 2:727-730, 1987.

134. Morohoshi T, Kanda M, Asanuma K, et al: Intraductal papillary neoplasms of the pancreas. A clinicopathologic study of six patients. Cancer 64:1329-1335, 1989.

135. Luttges J, Zamboni G, Longnecker D, et al: The immuno-histochemical mucin expression pattern distinguishes different types of intraductal papillary mucinous neoplasms of the pancreas and determines their relationship to mucinous noncystic carcinoma and ductal adenocarcinoma. Am J Surg Pathol 25:942-948, 2001.

136. Iacobuzio-Donahue CA, Klimstra DS, Adsay NV, et al: Dpc-4 protein is expressed in virtually all human intraductal papillary mucinous neoplasms of the pancreas: Comparison with conventional ductal adenocarcinomas. Am J Pathol 157:755-761, 2000.

137. Terada T, Ohta T, Nakanuma Y: Expression of oncogene products, anti-oncogene products and oncofetal antigens in intraductal papillary-mucinous neoplasm of the pancreas. Histopathology 29:355-361, 1996.

138. Miyakawa S, Horiguchi A, Hayakawa M, et al: Intraductal papillary adenocarcinoma with mucin hypersecretion and coexistent invasive ductal carcinoma of the pancreas with apparent topographic separation. J Gastroenterol 31:889-893, 1996.

139. Kimura W, Nagai H, Kuroda A, et al: Analysis of small cystic lesions of the pancreas. Int J Pancreatol 18:197-206, 1995.

140. Adsay NV, Adair CF, Heffess CS, et al: Intraductal oncocytic papillary neoplasms of the pancreas. Am J Surg Pathol 20:980-994, 1996.

141. Alles AJ, Warshaw AL, Southern JF, et al: Expression of CA 72-4 (TAG-72) in the fluid contents of pancreatic cysts. A new marker to distinguish malignant pancreatic cystic tumors from benign neoplasms and pseudocysts. Ann Surg 219:131-134, 1994.

142. Hoorens A, Gebhard F, Kraft K, et al: Pancreatoblastoma in an adult: Its separation from acinar cell carcinoma. Virchows Arch 424:485-490, 1994.

143. Hoorens A, Lemoine NR, McLellan E, et al: Pancreatic acinar cell carcinoma. An analysis of cell lineage markers, p53 expression, and Ki-ras mutation. Am J Pathol 143:685-698, 1993.

144. Osborne BM, Culbert SJ, Cangir A, et al: Acinar cell carcinoma of the pancreas in a 9-year-old child: Case report with electron microscopic observations. South Med J 70:370-372, 1977.

145. Shorter NA, Glick RD, Klimstra DS, et al: Malignant pancreatic tumors in childhood and adolescence: The Memorial Sloan-Kettering experience, 1967 to present. J Pediatr Surg 37:887-892, 2002.

146. Burns WA, Matthews MJ, Hamosh M, et al: Lipase-secreting acinar cell carcinoma of the pancreas with polyarthropathy. A light and electron microscopic, histochemical, and biochemical study. Cancer 33:1002-1009, 1974.

147. Klimstra DS, Adsay NV: Acinar cell carcinoma of the pancreas: A case associated with lipase hypersecretion syndrome. Pathol Case Rev 6:121-126, 2001.

148. Radin DR, Colletti PM, Forrester DM, et al: Pancreatic acinar cell carcinoma with subcutaneous and intraosseous fat necrosis. Radiology 158:67-68, 1986.

149. Webb JN: Acinar cell neoplasms of the exocrine pancreas. J Clin Pathol 30:103-112, 1977.

150. Holen K, Klimstra D, Hummer A, et al: Clinical characteristics and outcomes from an institutional series of acinar cell carcinoma of the pancreas. J Clin Oncol 20:4673-4678, 2002.

151. Labate AM, Klimstra DL, Zakowski MF: Comparative cytologic features of pancreatic acinar cell carcinoma and islet cell tumor. Diagn Cytopathol 16:112-116, 1997.

152. Buchino JJ, Castello FM, Nagaraj HS: Pancreatoblastoma. A histochemical and ultrastructural analysis. Cancer 53:963-969, 1984.

153. Abraham SC, Wu TT, Hruban RH, et al: Genetic and immuno-histochemical analysis of pancreatic acinar cell carcinoma: Frequent allelic loss on chromosome 11p and alterations in the APC/beta-catenin pathway. Am J Pathol 160:953-962, 2002.

154. Albores-Saavedra J: Acinar cystadenoma of the pancreas: A previously undescribed tumor. Ann Diagn Pathol 6:113-115, 2002.

155. Zamboni G, Terris B, Scarpa A, et al: Acinar cell cystadenoma of the pancreas: A new entity? Am J Surg Pathol 26:698-704, 2002.
156. Cantrell BB, Cubilla AL, Erlandson RA, et al: Acinar cell cystadenocarcinoma of human pancreas. Cancer 47:410-416, 1981.
157. Stamm B, Burger H, Hollinger A: Acinar cell cystadenocarcinoma of the pancreas. Cancer 60:2542-2547, 1987.
158. Horie A, Haratake J, Jimi A, et al: Pancreatoblastoma in Japan, with differential diagnosis from papillary cystic tumor (ductuloacinar adenoma) of the pancreas. Acta Pathol Japon 37:47-63, 1987.
159. Klimstra DS, Wenig BM, Adair CF, et al: Pancreatoblastoma. A clinicopathologic study and review of the literature. Am J Surg Pathol 19:1371-1389, 1995.
160. Drut R, Jones MC: Congenital pancreatoblastoma in Beckwith-Wiedemann syndrome: An emerging association. Pediatr Pathol 8:331-339, 1988.
161. Palosaari D, Clayton F, Seaman J: Pancreatoblastoma in an adult. Arch Pathol Lab Med 110:650-652, 1986.
162. Cooper JE, Lake BD: Use of enzyme histochemistry in the diagnosis of pancreatoblastoma. Histopathology 15:407-414, 1989.
163. Cingolani N, Shaco-Levy R, Farruggio A, et al: Alpha-fetoprotein production by pancreatic tumors exhibiting acinar cell differentiation: Study of five cases, one arising in a mediastinal teratoma. Hum Pathol 31:938-944, 2000.
164. Morohoshi T, Sagawa F, Mitsuya T: Pancreatoblastoma with marked elevation of serum alpha-fetoprotein. An autopsy case report with immunocytochemical study. Virchows Arch A Pathol Anat Histopathol 416:265-270, 1990.
165. Abraham SC, Wu TT, Klimstra DS, et al: Distinctive molecular genetic alterations in sporadic and familial adenomatous polyposis-associated pancreatoblastomas: Frequent alterations in the APC/beta-catenin pathway and chromosome 11p. Am J Pathol 159:1619-1627, 2001.
166. Vannier JP, Flamant F, Hemet J, et al: Pancreatoblastoma: Response to chemotherapy. Med Pediatr Oncol 19:187-191, 1991.
167. Klimstra DS, Rosai J, Heffess CS: Mixed acinar-endocrine carcinomas of the pancreas. Am J Surg Pathol 18:765-778, 1994.
168. Nonomura A, Kono N, Mizukami Y, et al: Duct-acinar-islet cell tumor of the pancreas. Ultrastruct Pathol 16:317-329, 1992.
169. Yantiss RK, Chang HK, Farraye FA, et al: Prevalence and prognostic significance of acinar cell differentiation in pancreatic endocrine tumors. Am J Surg Pathol 26:893-901, 2002.
170. Ulich T, Cheng L, Lewin KJ: Acinar-endocrine cell tumor of the pancreas. Report of a pancreatic tumor containing both zymogen and neuroendocrine granules. Cancer 50:2099-2105, 1982.
171. Heitz PU, Kasper M, Polak JM, et al: Pancreatic endocrine tumors. Hum Pathol 13:263-271, 1982.
172. Capella C, Heitz PU, Hofler H, et al: Revised classification of neuroendocrine tumors of the lung, pancreas and gut. Digestion 55:11-23, 1994.
173. Hochwald SN, Zee S, Conlon KC, et al: Prognostic factors in pancreatic endocrine neoplasms: An analysis of 136 cases with a proposal for low-grade and intermediate-grade groups. J Clin Oncol 20:2633-2642, 2002.
174. La Rosa S, Sessa F, Capella C, et al: Prognostic criteria in nonfunctioning pancreatic endocrine tumours. Virchows Arch 429:323-333, 1996.
175. Lam KY, Lo CY: Pancreatic endocrine tumour: A 22-year clinico-pathological experience with morphological, immunohistochemical observation and a review of the literature. Eur J Surg Oncol 23:36-42, 1997.
176. Bottger T, Seidl C, Seifert JK, et al: Value of quantitative DNA analysis in endocrine tumors of the pancreas. Oncology 54:318-323, 1997.
177. Tomita T: DNA ploidy and proliferating cell nuclear antigen in islet cell tumors. Pancreas 12:36-47, 1996.
178. Pelosi G, Bresaola E, Bogina G, et al: Endocrine tumors of the pancreas: Ki-67 immunoreactivity on paraffin sections is an independent predictor for malignancy: A comparative study with proliferating-cell nuclear antigen and progesterone receptor protein immunostaining, mitotic index, and other clinicopathologic variables. Hum Pathol 27:1124-1134, 1996.
179. Donow C, Pipeleers-Marichal M, Schroder S, et al: Surgical pathology of gastrinoma. Site, size, multicentricity, association with multiple endocrine neoplasia type 1, and malignancy. Cancer 68:1329-1334, 1991.
180. Debelenko LV, Zhuang Z, Emmert-Buck MR, et al: Allelic deletions on chromosome 11q13 in multiple endocrine neoplasia type 1-associated and sporadic gastrinomas and pancreatic endocrine tumors. Cancer Res 57:2238-2243, 1997.
181. Guarda LA, Silva EG, Ordonez NG, et al: Clear cell islet cell tumor. Am J Clin Pathol 79:512-517, 1983.
182. Ordonez NG, Silva EG: Islet cell tumour with vacuolated lipid-rich cytoplasm: A new histological variant of islet cell tumour. Histopathology 31:157-160, 1997.
183. Carstens PH, Cressman FK Jr: Malignant oncocytic carcinoid of the pancreas. Ultrastruct Pathol 13:69-75, 1989.
184. Gotchall J, Traweek ST, Stenzel P: Benign oncocytic endocrine tumor of the pancreas in a patient with polyarteritis nodosa. Hum Pathol 18:967-969, 1987.
185. Nguyen-Ho P, Nguyen GK, Jewell LD: Oncocytic neuroendocrine carcinoma of the pancreas. Report of a case with needle aspiration cytology, immunocytochemistry and electron microscopy. Acta Cytol 38:611-613, 1994.
186. Pacchioni D, Papotti M, Macri L, et al: Pancreatic oncocytic endocrine tumors. Cytologic features of two cases. Acta Cytol 40:742-746, 1996.
187. Radi MJ, Fenoglio-Preiser CM, Chiffelle T: Functioning oncocytic islet-cell carcinoma. Report of a case with electron-microscopic and immunohistochemical confirmation. Am J Surg Pathol 9:517-524, 1985.
188. Sadoul JL, Saint-Paul MC, Hoffman P, et al: Malignant pancreatic oncocytoma. An unusual cause of organic hypoglycemia. J Endocrinol Invest 15:211-217, 1992.
189. Zee S, Hochwald SN, Conlon K, et al: Pleomorphic pancreatic endocrine neoplasms (PENs): A variant commonly confused with adenocarcinoma [abstract]. Mod Pathol 2001:1212A, 2001.
190. Liu TH, Zhu Y, Cui QC, et al: Nonfunctioning pancreatic endocrine tumors. An immunohistochemical and electron microscopic analysis of 26 cases. Pathol Res Pract 188:191-198, 1992.
191. Lee CS: Lack of p53 immunoreactivity in pancreatic endocrine tumors. Pathology 28:139-141, 1996.
192. Pellegata NS, Sessa F, Renault B, et al: K-ras and p53 gene mutations in pancreatic cancer: Ductal and nonductal tumors progress through different genetic lesions. Cancer Res 54:1556-1560, 1994.
193. Corrin B, Gilby ED, Jones NF, et al: Oat cell carcinoma of the pancreas with ectopic ACTH secretion. Cancer 31:1523-1527, 1973.
194. Hobbs RD, Stewart AF, Ravin ND, et al: Hypercalcemia in small cell carcinoma of the pancreas. Cancer 53:1552-1554, 1984.
195. Tranchida P, Hasteh F, Sarkar F, et al: Poorly differentiated neuroendocrine (small cell) carcinomas of the pancreas: An analysis of 8 examples of a debated entity [abstract]. Mod Pathol 13:190A, 2000.
196. O'Connor TP, Wade TP, Sunwoo YC, et al: Small cell undifferentiated carcinoma of the pancreas. Report of a patient with tumor marker studies. Cancer 70:1514-1519, 1992.
197. Ordonez NG, Cleary KR, Mackay B: Small cell undifferentiated carcinoma of the pancreas. Ultrastruct Pathol 21:467-474, 1997.
198. Reyes CV, Wang T: Undifferentiated small cell carcinoma of the pancreas: A report of five cases. Cancer 47:2500-2502, 1981.
199. Movahedi-Lankarani S, Hruban RH, Westra WH, et al: Primitive neuroectodermal tumors of the pancreas: A report of seven cases of a rare neoplasm. Am J Surg Pathol 26:1040-1047, 2002.
200. Kamisawa T, Fukayama M, Tabata I, et al: Neuroendocrine differentiation in pancreatic duct carcinoma: Special emphasis on duct-endocrine cell carcinoma of the pancreas. Pathol Res Pract 192:901-908, 1996.
201. Kloppel G: Mixed exocrine-endocrine tumors of the pancreas. Semin Diagn Pathol 17:104-108, 2000.
202. Kashiwabara K, Nakajima T, Shinkai H, et al: A case of malignant duct-islet cell tumor of the pancreas: Immunohistochemical and cytofluorometric study. Acta Pathol Jpn 41:636-641, 1991.
203. Schron DS, Mendelsohn G: Pancreatic carcinoma with duct, endocrine, and acinar differentiation. A histologic, immuno-cytochemical, and ultrastructural study. Cancer 54:1766-1770, 1984.
204. Klimstra DS, Wenig BM, Heffess CS: Solid-pseudopapillary tumor of the pancreas: A typically cystic tumor of low malignant potential. Semin Diagn Pathol 17:66-81, 2000.
205. Kissane JM: Pancreatoblastoma and solid and cystic papillary tumor: Two tumors related to pancreatic ontogeny. Semin Diagn Pathol 11:152-164, 1994.

206. Kloppel G, Morohoshi T, John HD, et al: Solid and cystic acinar cell tumour of the pancreas. A tumour in young women with favourable prognosis. Virchows Arch [Pathol Anat] 392:171-183, 1981.

207. Lieber MR, Lack EE, Roberts JR Jr, et al: Solid and papillary epithelial neoplasm of the pancreas. An ultrastructural and immunocytochemical study of six cases. Am J Surg Pathol 11:85-93, 1987.

208. Pettinato G, Manivel JC, Ravetto C, et al: Papillary cystic tumor of the pancreas. A clinicopathologic study of 20 cases with cytologic, immunohistochemical, ultrastructural, and flow cytometric observations, and a review of the literature [published erratum appears in Am J Clin Pathol 99:764, 1993] [see comments]. Am J Clin Pathol 98:478-488, 1992.

209. Stommer P, Kraus J, Stolte M, et al: Solid and cystic pancreatic tumors. Clinical, histochemical, and electron microscopic features in ten cases. Cancer 67:1635-1641, 1991.

210. Adair CF, Wenig BM, Heffess CS: Solid and papillary cystic carcinoma of the pancreas: A tumor of low malignant potential [abstract]. Int J Surg Pathol 2:326, 1995.

211. Pelosi G, Iannucci A, Zamboni G, et al: Solid and cystic papillary neoplasm of the pancreas: A clinico-cytopathologic and immuno-cytochemical study of five new cases diagnosed by fine-needle aspiration cytology and a review of the literature. Diagn Cytopathol 13:233-246, 1995.

212. Goldstein J, Benharroch D, Sion-Vardy N, et al: Solid cystic and papillary tumor of the pancreas with oncocytic differentiation. J Surg Oncol 56:63-67, 1994.

213. Lee WY, Tzeng CC, Jin YT, et al: Papillary cystic tumor of the pancreas: A case indistinguishable from oncocytic carcinoma. Pancreas 8:127-132, 1993.

214. Balercia G, Zamboni G, Bogina G, et al: Solid-cystic tumor of the pancreas. An extensive ultrastructural study of fourteen cases. J Submicrosc Cytol Pathol 27:331-340, 1995.

215. Ladanyi M, Mulay S, Arseneau J, et al: Estrogen and progesterone receptor determination in the papillary cystic neoplasm of the pancreas. With immunohistochemical and ultrastructural observations. Cancer 60:1604-1611, 1987.

216. Abraham SC, Klimstra DS, Wilentz RE, et al: Solid-pseudopapillary tumors of the pancreas are genetically distinct from pancreatic ductal adenocarcinomas and almost always harbor beta-catenin mutations. Am J Pathol 160:1361-1369, 2002.

217. Nishihara K, Nagoshi M, Tsuneyoshi M, et al: Papillary cystic tumors of the pancreas. Assessment of their malignant potential. Cancer 71:82-92, 1993.

218. Sclafani LM, Reuter VE, Coit DG, et al: The malignant nature of papillary and cystic neoplasm of the pancreas. Cancer 68:153-158, 1991.

219. Martin RC, Klimstra DS, Brennan MF, et al: Solid-pseudopapillary tumor of the pancreas: A surgical enigma? Ann Surg Oncol 9:35-40, 2002.

220. Paal E, Thompson LD, Heffess CS: A clinicopathologic and immuno-histochemical study of ten pancreatic lymphangiomas and a review of the literature [published erratum appears in Cancer 83:824, 1998]. Cancer 82:2150-2158, 1998.

221. Zamboni G, Pea M, Martignoni G, et al: Clear cell "sugar" tumor of the pancreas. A novel member of the family of lesions characterized by the presence of perivascular epithelioid cells. Am J Surg Pathol 20:722-730, 1996.

222. Adsay NV, Tranchida P, Hasteh F, et al: Pseudotumoral pancreatitis. A clinicopathologic analysis of 33 patients with mass-forming pancreatitis with emphasis on the probable mechanisms [abstract]. Mod Pathol 13:179A, 2000.

223. Kloppel G, Maillet B: Chronic pancreatitis: Evolution of the disease. Hepatogastroenterology 38:408-412, 1991.

224. Ectors N, Maillet B, Aerts R, et al: Non-alcoholic duct destructive chronic pancreatitis. Gut 41:263-268, 1997.

225. Suriawanata A, Cubukcu-Dimopula O, Weber S, et al: Histopathology of lymphoplasmacytic sclerosing pancreatitis [abstract]. Mod Pathol 15:294A, 2002.

226. Klimstra DS, Conlon KC, Adsay NV: Lymphoplasmacytic sclerosing pancreatitis with pseudotumor formation. Pathol Case Rev 6:94-99, 2001.

227. Ferrozzi F, Bova D, Campodonico F, et al: Pancreatic metastases: CT assessment. Eur Radiol 7:241-245, 1997.

228. Nassar H, Sarkar F, Das S, et al: Secondary tumors of the pancreas [abstract]. Mod Pathol 12:165A, 1999.

229. Opocher E, Galeotti F, Spina GP, et al: [Diagnosis of secondary tumors of the pancreas. Analysis of 13 cases]. Minerva Med 73:577-581, 1982.

230. Roland CF, van Heerden JA: Nonpancreatic primary tumors with metastasis to the pancreas. Surg Gynecol Obstet 168:345-347, 1989.

231. Temellini F, Bavosi M, Lamarra M, et al: Pancreatic metastasis 25 years after nephrectomy for renal cancer. Tumori 75:503-504, 1989.

232. Hiotis SP, Klimstra DS, Conlon KC, et al: Results after pancreatic resection for metastatic lesions. Ann Surg Oncol 9:675-679, 2002.

233. Nassar H, Sakr W, Grignon D, et al: Metastatic renal cell carcinoma in the pancreas and periampullary region [abstract]. Mod Pathol 13:118A, 2000.

234. Albores-Saavedra J, Heffess C, Hruban RH, et al: Recommendations for the reporting of pancreatic specimens containing malignant tumors. The Association of Directors of Anatomic and Surgical Pathology. Am J Clin Pathol 111:304-307, 1999.

235. Luttges J, Zamboni G, Kloppel G: Recommendation for the examination of pancreaticoduodenectomy specimens removed from patients with carcinoma of the exocrine pancreas. A proposal for a standardized pathological staging of pancreaticoduodenectomy specimens including a checklist. Dig Surg 16:291-296, 1999.

236. Luttges J, Vogel I, Menke M, et al: The retroperitoneal resection margin and vessel involvement are important factors determining survival after pancreaticoduodenectomy for ductal adenocarcinoma of the head of the pancreas. Virchows Arch 433:237-242, 1998.

PART THREE

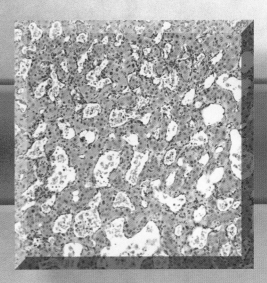

Liver

PART THREE

Liver

CHAPTER 32

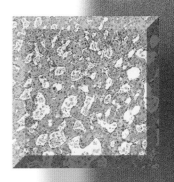

Liver Tissue Processing Techniques

LILIAN B. ANTONIO • ARIEF SURIAWINATA • SWAN N. THUNG

◾ Liver Biopsy Specimens

Often, crucial diagnoses of liver diseases rely on the examination of needle liver biopsy specimens. One limitation, however, is that the specimen represents a small portion of the entire organ. Hence, there is a premium on the performance of a skilled, trained physician to obtain an adequate core biopsy specimen and well-trained personnel to process the specimen. In this chapter, details specific to the processing and staining of liver biopsy specimens are given as a guideline for achieving optimal material for diagnostic interpretation. Actual interpretation is discussed in following chapters; specifics for processing pediatric liver biopsy specimens are given in Chapter 41.

SPECIMEN HANDLING

At the time of the biopsy procedure, the needle liver biopsy specimen is immediately examined for adequacy. It should be at least 1.5 cm in total length; otherwise, another pass is recommended. Adequate size of the specimen minimizes sampling error.[1,2] The specimen is then discharged into a Petri dish lined with lens paper, which has been wetted with normal saline solution to prevent the fresh tissue from sticking onto the lens paper. Gross characteristics of the tissue, such as color, consistency, and tendency to fragment or to float in the fixative solution, are documented by the performing physician. Tumors or granulomas, for example, can be recognized as white areas in an otherwise reddish brown tissue. Gray-black discoloration is seen in Dubin-Johnson syndrome, rusty brown in hemochromatosis, green in cholestasis, yellow in steatosis, and variegated or dark brown in melanoma. Fragmented specimens, especially when a Menghini needle is used, often indicate cirrhosis. Artifacts from squeezing or drying of the specimen should be avoided.

The routine fixative for liver biopsies is 10% neutral buffered formalin (NBF). Based on the clinical diagnosis or possible differential diagnoses, the clinician determines which additional procedures are required: fixation in 3% buffered glutaraldehyde for electron microscopy; fresh, unfixed tissue for viral and mycobacterial cultures; rapid freezing in liquid nitrogen or a mixture of dry ice and isopentane for fat stains, certain immunohistochemical and enzyme activity studies,[3] quantitative studies of hormone receptors, and isolation of genomic and viral DNA and RNA for molecular analyses[4] (see Chapter 41); and fixation in 1% periodic acid in 10% neutral buffered formalin at 4°C for 48 hours for evaluation of glycogen storage diseases.[5] It is imperative that needle liver biopsy specimens be placed immediately in the desired fixatives, because the foundation of a good histologic preparation is rapid and complete fixation.

The following information may be used as a guideline for achieving good preservation of tissue. First, the volume of the fixative should be at least 15 to 20 times the volume of the tissue.[6] Second, sufficient time must be allowed for fixation before processing is begun. Formalin penetrates most tissues at about 0.5 mm per hour at room temperature, and 4 hours are needed for penetration of 2 mm of tissue. Fixation may be shortened by application of heat, pressure, vacuum, agitation, or microwave techniques. Fragmentation of the central portion of liver biopsy sections along the long axis is a sign of insufficient time for fixation. Conversely, formalin exposure does not result in "overfixation," that is, hardening of tissue. However, prolonged formalin exposure (i.e., longer than 24 hours) may reduce the availability of antigen sites for immunohistochemical studies. Tissues may afterward be stored in 10% NBF or in 70% alcohol.[7]

PROCESSING TECHNIQUES

Rush liver biopsy specimens are manually processed to shorten the time schedule and meet the needs of critically ill patients; regular specimens are processed in an automated tissue processor.

Manual Method

The liver cores are removed from the specimen container, and their macroscopic appearance is noted. They are then arranged parallel to each other on a lens paper that has been wetted with formalin before wrapping, or they are inserted directly into a cassette cushioned with a foam biopsy pad. The foam biopsy pad is presoaked in 10% NBF to prevent the cassette from floating. The use of lens paper is preferred to a foam biopsy pad, which can carry more than 2 to 3 mL of fluid into the next container. Curved forceps are commonly used to handle these delicate and fragile specimens. Crushing artifacts, however, may occur with forceps use. In our laboratory, such artifacts are prevented by the use of a plastic pipette, the tip of which is cut to a desirable size to permit free passage of tissue fragments. The bulb of the plastic pipette is compressed before it is introduced into the specimen container. By aiming the tip at one end of the liver core, gentle release of the compressed bulb sucks the core up the shaft of the pipette, permitting gentle release of the specimen onto the lens paper. Rinsing the pipette between specimen handlings helps to prevent cross contamination.

Successfully obtaining good sections from well-processed tissue results from proper orientation in the paraffin mold. Paraffin-infiltrated tissues, especially when composed of multiple core fragments, have to be arranged at the same plane, parallel to the longer side of the mold.

Automated Method

Although processing differs in terms of the schedules and the chemicals used from one laboratory to another, it always follows the same principles: fixation, dehydration, clearing, and infiltration. With the availability of modern state-of-the-art tissue processors, processing can be carried out with one, two, or three combinations of the following features—agitation, heat, pressure, and vacuum—to shorten processing time. Paraffin temperature is kept between 58°C and 60°C (Table 32-1).

The application of microwave in histologic techniques has significantly reduced processing time to as little as 15 minutes for a tiny biopsy specimen or a 60- to 90-minute cycle for a larger biopsy specimen. This technique has been a valuable adjunct in histotechnology.[8]

Slide Preparation

The number of sections routinely cut from a block varies from one laboratory to another. In our laboratory

TABLE 32-1. Schedule for Liver Tissue Processing

Solution	Core Biopsy Specimens (2 × 0.1 × 0.1 cm in greatest dimension)		Resection Specimens (2 × 2 × 0.3 cm in greatest dimension [ideal size])
	A: Manual	B: Automatic	C: Automatic
10% NBF	—	30 min	60 min
10% NBF (37°C)	30–60 min	30 min (P/V)	90 min (P/V)
70% alcohol	10 min	10 min	60 min
80% alcohol	10 min	10 min	—
95% alcohol	10 min	—	60 min
95% alcohol	—	10 min	60 min
100% alcohol × 2	10 min (one change)	10 min	60 min
Xylene × 3	5 min (2 changes)*	10 min (P/V)	45 min (35°C)
Paraffin, 58°C × 2	15 min	10 min (P/V)	30 min (P/V)
Paraffin, 58°C × 2	—	10 min (P/V)	30 min (P/V)

Notes: Specimens received have been partially fixed in 10% NBF before processing.
P/V, pressure/vacuum; NBF, neutral buffered formalin.
*Check for tissue translucency before transferring to paraffin.
For schedule A, 10% NBF, 70% alcohol, and one solution of xylene are changed every other day; 80% alcohol is discarded on a daily basis, and the remaining alcohol solutions are rotated. Absolute alcohol should be changed on a daily basis. Test paraffin by dipping a gloved finger into the paraffin bath. If the solidified paraffin is white and firm, it is satisfactory. If it is glossy and soft, it has been saturated with xylene.
For schedules B and C, one solution of 10% NBF, xylene, and paraffin are changed every other day. The first change of each group solution is discarded, and the remaining group solutions are rotated accordingly. The last changes for each group solution are all fresh solutions. For the alcohol series, 70% alcohol is discarded every other day and fresh solution is prepared; discard 80% alcohol (for schedule B) and the first 95% alcohol (for schedule C). The remaining alcohol solutions are rotated. The last change of absolute alcohol should be fresh. These schedules work well in our laboratory.

at Mount Sinai Medical Center in New York, seven slides are serially sectioned from each block; each slide is 3 to 5 μm thick. Each slide contains one or two sections. Slides 1, 3, and 5 are stained with hematoxylin and eosin (H&E). Slides 2, 4, and 6 are polylysine slides and are left unstained for additional histochemical or immunohistochemical stains that are requested when needed. Slide 7 is stained with Masson's trichrome. Stains routinely applied to liver biopsy specimens also vary according to the laboratory. The minimum should be H&E and a reliable method for connective tissue, which in our laboratory is the Masson trichrome.

EXPECTED OUTCOME

A quantitative study of liver biopsy specimens was performed by Crawford and associates,[9] based on liver biopsy specimens from 16 patients undergoing liver biopsy for screening procedures (age 49 ± 14 years, ± mean SD) that were found to be normal by histologic examination. A Menghini cutting needle (14 gauge; internal diameter, 1.6 mm) was used for this 1998 study, which was a diameter somewhat larger than needles used currently. The average aggregate length of the liver tissue was 1.8 ± 0.8 cm (area, 16.4 ± 10.7 mm²). Although the liver tissue originally extruded from the biopsy needle may not have been fragmented, by the time histologic sections were placed on a glass slide, 7 ± 3 tissue fragments were found per biopsy. In addition, partial tears in the region of terminal hepatic veins at the edges of the specimen were routinely observed. Portal triads containing at least one profile each of a portal vein, a hepatic artery, and an interlobular bile duct numbered 11 ± 6 per biopsy (range, 3 to 23). This translates into 0.8 ± 0.5 portal triads per linear centimeter of tissue. Portal dyads, which did not contain one of these profiles (usually the portal vein), numbered 8 ± 5 (range, 1 to 18); 6 ± 6% of portal tracts did not contain bile ducts. Because of the multiplicity of profiles within portal tracts, however, the average number of profiles per portal tract collectively was 6 ± 5 (range, 1 to 35). Notably, 2.3 ± 2.2 interlobular bile ducts were seen per portal tract, compared with 2.6 ± 2.3 hepatic arteries and 0.7 ± 0.7 portal veins. Conversely, on a per-specimen basis, 38% of portal tracts did not contain a portal vein, 7% did not contain a bile duct, and 9% did not contain a hepatic artery. The average minimum external diameter of interlobular bile ducts was 13 ± 4 μm, of hepatic arteries 12 ± 5 μm, and of portal veins 35 ± 25 μm. Bile ducts larger than 30 μm in diameter were rare; only one each in two biopsies were observed. The most important finding was that portal tracts almost always contained a bile duct–hepatic artery pair of approximately equal diameter.

Although the liver biopsy technique, especially the choice of needle and hence needle diameter, does influence the sampling of liver tissue, these parameters provide an idea of expected outcome for percutaneous liver biopsy specimens. It is obvious but important to note that the number of portal tracts is proportional to the total length of the specimen obtained.

Liver Resection Specimens

Partial liver resections are usually performed to remove focal lesions. The characteristics of the lesions and of the surrounding liver parenchyma are described (see Chapter 42). The gross presence or absence of involvement of the resection margins by the lesion and the presence or absence of significant fibrosis of the liver parenchyma or cirrhosis are noted. Representative sections are taken. As has been mentioned, for additional tests that must be considered, fresh tissue or tissue in fixatives other than formalin must be submitted.

Explanted livers during liver transplantation or retransplantation are examined carefully (see Chapter 39). This examination includes a thorough examination of the hilar region for patency of the hepatic artery, portal vein, and bile duct. Following the gross examination, several sections from the hilum are taken in a plane perpendicular to the long axis of the major hilar structures at 4- to 6-mm intervals.[10] Horizontal cross sections of the liver across each of the hepatic lobes reveal the openings of the hepatic veins, which are examined for their patency. The entire liver is then sectioned in a parallel plane at 0.5-cm intervals. This thin sectioning is necessary so that small hepatocellular carcinomas and/or dysplastic nodules, which may contain focal hepatocellular carcinoma, are not missed. All distinct nodules and lesions are sampled. In addition, routine sectioning consisting of five sections each from the right and the left lobes and one section from the caudate lobe is also performed.[11]

Considering that formalin will only penetrate superficially into a liver specimen, dissection and serial sectioning of the organ must be performed while the organ is fresh. Preferably, this is done soon after receipt of the liver specimen in the dissection suite. Key samples for histology and special studies should be obtained immediately. The tissue slabs can then be fixed overnight in formalin before the complement of "routine" sections is obtained.

Histochemistry

The following details the principles for processing paraffin sections for histochemistry, with abbreviations and acronyms as given.

DPHW: deparaffinize, hydrate, water
DPHA: deparaffinize, hydrate, alcohol

1. Deparaffinize tissue sections in four changes of xylene.
2. Hydrate through descending grades of alcohol.
3. Wash well in water (W), or keep slides in 70% alcohol (A).

DHCM: dehydrate, clear, and mount

1. Dehydrate through ascending grades of alcohol.
2. Clear in four changes of xylene.
3. Mount in an appropriate medium. If not indicated, use synthetic medium.

DIW: deionized water
D/W: distilled water

ROUTINE HEMATOXYLIN AND EOSIN STAINING

H&E stain allows an accurate histologic diagnosis in almost all liver biopsy specimens. Other advantages offered by this stain are that it is quick and inexpensive, and it can be easily used with good results.

APPLICATION

Well-fixed, paraffin-embedded sections, unfixed frozen sections, and smears

SOLUTIONS

Harris hematoxylin is available through Diagnostic Solutions Inc. (Yonkers, NY).

Acidified Harris hematoxylin is prepared by adding 15 mL of glacial acetic acid to 500 mL of filtered Harris hematoxylin. The addition of acid reduces the bluish coloration of goblet cell mucin while it increases the sharpness of nuclear staining.[12]

Ammonia water is prepared by adding 18 drops of concentrated ammonium hydroxide to 500 mL of DIW.

1% Alcoholic eosin stock solution is available through Richard-Allan Scientific Inc. (Kalamazoo, MI).

Acidified alcoholic eosin working solution is prepared by mixing 50 mL of 1% alcoholic eosin with 150 mL of 80% alcohol and 1 mL of glacial acetic acid.

PROCEDURE

1. DPHW.
2. Stain in acidified Harris hematoxylin for 8 minutes. Wash in running tap water.
3. Differentiate in 0.5% hydrochloric acid in 70% alcohol for 3 to 4 dips. Immediately wash in running tap water. Check under the microscope for proper differentiation.
4. Use ammonia water for 10 dips. Wash well in lukewarm tap water.
5. Rinse in 95% alcohol.
6. Counterstain in acidified alcoholic eosin for 20 seconds.
7. Differentiate in 95% alcohol for 10 dips.
8. DHCM.

RESULTS

Nuclei = clear blue
Cytoplasm = pink

SPECIAL STAINS

In addition to the routinely performed H&E stain, other histochemical or so-called special stains are frequently requested to confirm structures or findings seen or suspected on the H&E slide. Several special stains that have been found to be most helpful in liver pathology are discussed in this chapter (Table 32-2).

TABLE 32-2. List of Selected Special Stains Frequently Used in Liver Specimens

Special Stains	Fixatives	Uses
Connective and Muscle Tissues		
Masson's trichrome	Bouin's is preferred, 10% NBF	Muscle, keratin, cytoplasm, megamitochondria = red Collagen = blue Mallory's hyaline = red or blue
Sirius red	10% NBF	Collagen = red Mallory's hyaline = reddish-orange
Gordon and Sweets reticulin	10% NBF	Reticulin = black Collagen = rose color
PTAH	10% NBF	Fibrin, nuclei, cytoplasm, mitotic figures, mitochondria = blue Collagen = red
Microorganisms		
Ziehl-Neelsen stain	10% NBF or Helly's fluid	*Mycobacterium*, lipofuscin, ceroid = red Background = light blue
Shikata's orcein	10% NBF	Elastic fibers, hepatitis B surface antigen, copper-binding protein = dark brown
Victoria blue	10% NBF	Elastic fibers, hepatitis B surface antigen, copper-binding protein, lipofuscin, mast cell = blue Cytoplasm, nuclei = red
Ammoniacal silver stain	10% NBF	Fungi, bacteria, mucin, glycogen, melanin = black Background = green
Pigments and Minerals		
Perls' iron	10% NBF	Iron (ferric state) = blue
Hall's stain	10% NBF, Bouin's, or Carnoy's Helly's and Zenker's are unsuitable	Bilirubin = green Muscle and cytoplasm = yellow Collagen = red
Rhodanine	10% NBF	Copper = reddish-orange
Glycogen		
PAS	10% NBF, absolute alcohol 10% formol–alcohol	Glycogen, atypical *Mycobacterium*, fungi = magenta
d-PAS	10% NBF, absolute alcohol 10% formalin–alcohol	Glycoprotein, basement membrane, alpha-1-antitrypsin = magenta Glycogen = digested, no magenta color
Amyloid		
Congo red	10% NBF, absolute alcohol, or Bouin's solution	Amyloid = pink to red Nuclei = blue Elastic fiber = pink
Lipids		
Oil Red O	Frozen section fixed in 10% NBF	Fat = red Nuclei = blue

NBF, Neutral buffered formalin; d-PAS, periodic acid–Schiff reagent with diastase digestion; PAS, periodic acid–Schiff reagent; PTAH, phosphotungstic acid hematoxylin.

Masson's Trichrome Stain (Fig. 32-1)[13-15]

APPLICATION

Formalin- or Bouin-fixed, paraffin-embedded sections

SOLUTIONS

Modified Weigert's iron hematoxylin stock solution

Solution A is prepared by dissolving 2 g of hematoxylin powder (Color Index 75290) in 100 mL of 90% alcohol.

Solution B is prepared by adding 4 mL of 62% aqueous solution of ferric chloride to 95 mL of D/W. One mL of concentrated hydrochloric acid is added drop by drop.

Working solution is prepared by mixing 25 mL of solution A and 25 mL of solution B.

Biebrich scarlet–acid fuchsin solution is prepared by mixing 45 mL of 1% aqueous solution of Biebrich scarlet, 5 mL of 1% aqueous solution of acid fuchsin, and 0.5 mL of glacial acetic acid.

Phosphomolybdic-phosphotungstic acid solution is prepared by dissolving 2.5 g of phosphotungstic acid and 2.5 g of phosphomolybdic acid in 100 mL of D/W.

Aniline blue solution is prepared by dissolving 10 g of aniline blue powder in 400 mL of D/W. Eight mL of glacial acetic acid is also added.

PROCEDURE

1. DPHW.

2. Sections are treated with Bouin fixative solution for 1 hour at 56°C (or overnight at room temperature). Allow to cool, and wash in running tap water until yellow color disappears.

3. Stain in modified Weigert's iron hematoxylin solution for 5 minutes. Wash well in water. Differentiate in 0.5% hydrochloric acid in 70% alcohol for 3 to 4 dips.

4. Wash well in running tap water for 10 minutes.

5. Stain in Biebrich scarlet–fuchsin solution for 2 minutes. Rinse in D/W.

6. Differentiate in phosphomolybdic-phosphotungstic acid for 15 minutes.

7. Without rinsing, stain in aniline blue for 20 minutes. Rinse briefly in D/W.

8. Differentiate in 1% aqueous acetic acid for 3 minutes.

9. DHCM.

RESULTS

Nuclei = black

Collagen and mucus = blue

Mallory's hyaline = red or blue

Cytoplasm, keratin, muscle fiber, megamitochondria = red

NOTES

The use of double-strength Weigert's iron hematoxylin improves the shelf life of working solution from a few days to a week. Differentiation after staining with this solution is recommended to clear the cytoplasm of the excess hematoxylin stain.

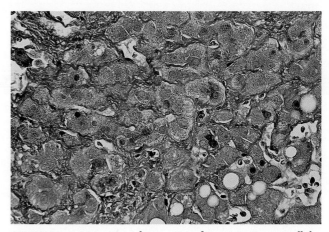

FIGURE 32–1. Masson's trichrome stain demonstrating pericellular "chicken wire" fibrosis in a patient with alcoholic liver disease.

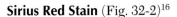

Sirius Red Stain (Fig. 32-2)[16]

APPLICATION

Formalin-fixed, paraffin-embedded sections

SOLUTIONS

0.1% Sirius red F3B solution is prepared by dissolving 0.1 g of Sirius powder (Pfaltz & Bauer, Waterbury, CT) in 100 mL of saturated aqueous solution of picric acid.

0.2% light green SF stock solution is prepared by dissolving 0.2 g of light green SF powder in 100 mL D/W, acidified with 0.2 mL of glacial acetic acid.[17]

Light green working solution is prepared by diluting 10 mL of the light green stock solution in 40 mL of D/W.

PROCEDURE

1. DPHW.
2. Stain in 0.1% Sirius red solution for 30 minutes.
3. Rinse slides briefly in tap water for 3 to 6 dips to remove excess stain.
4. Counterstain in light green working solution for 3 to 4 dips.
5. DHCM.

RESULTS

Collagen = red

Mallory's hyaline = reddish orange

Background = green

NOTE

Counterstaining with light green gives better contrast.

Perls' Iron Stain (Fig. 32-3)[18,19]

APPLICATION

Well-fixed, paraffin-embedded sections and smears

SOLUTION

Nuclear fast red solution is prepared by dissolving 0.1 g of nuclear fast red in 100 mL of 5% aqueous aluminum sulfate. The solution is brought to boil, then is cooled and filtered; a grain of thymol is added as a preservative.

PROCEDURE

1. DPHW.
2. Place slides in an equal volume of aqueous solutions of 2% aqueous potassium ferrocyanide and 2% hydrochloric acid for 10 minutes at room temperature. Rinse in D/W.
3. Counterstain in 0.1% nuclear fast red solution for 5 minutes. Wash thoroughly in running tap water for 2 minutes.
4. DHCM.

RESULTS

Hemosiderin and some oxides and salts of iron = blue

Nuclei and cytoplasm = pink to red

NOTES

1. Avoid glassware, chemicals, or water contaminated with iron.[20]
2. Counterstain should be light. This enables evaluation of other pigments such as bile and lipofuscin.
3. Avoid any metallic forceps.

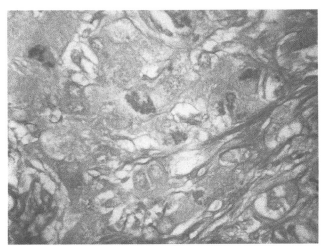

FIGURE 32–2. Sirius red stain, collagen red, and Mallory's hyaline in the cytoplasm of hepatocytes (reddish-orange).

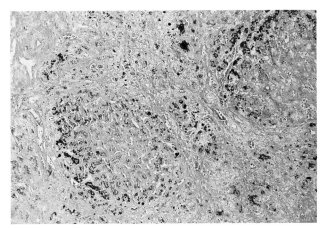

FIGURE 32–3. Perls' iron stain showing coarse and fine iron granules in hepatocytes of the cirrhotic liver of a patient with hereditary hemochromatosis.

Periodic Acid–Schiff–Hematoxylin Without (PAS) and With (d-PAS) Diastase Digestion

(Figs. 32-4 and 32-5)[21,22]

APPLICATION

Formalin, absolute alcohol, or formalin/alcohol-fixed, paraffin-embedded sections, and smears

SOLUTIONS

Diastase is available through EM Science (Gibbstown, NJ).

Schiff reagent is available through Fisher Scientific (Fair Lawn, NJ).

PROCEDURE

1. DPHW two sets of test and control slides. Label slides as follows:

   PAS: one set of test and control slides (hold in D/W).

   d-PAS: one set of test and control slides.

2. Incubate slides labeled d-PAS in 1% aqueous diastase for 1 hour at 37°C. Wash in lukewarm running tap water for 5 minutes.

3. Oxidize both sets of slides in 0.5% aqueous periodic acid for 10 minutes. Wash well in D/W.

4. Place in Schiff reagent for 15 minutes. Rinse in three changes of water.

5. Place in 0.3% aqueous borate solution for 15 seconds.

6. Rinse in four changes of water.

7. Stain in acidified Lillie-Mayer hematoxylin for 45 seconds.

8. Rinse in three changes of water.

9. Place in 0.3% aqueous borate solution for 10 seconds.

10. Rinse in four changes of water.

11. DHCM.

RESULTS

PAS slides:

   Glycogen in cytoplasm of hepatocytes = magenta

   Nuclei = blue

d-PAS slides:

   Magenta granular deposits of glycogen seen on PAS slides are absent.

   Glycoproteins (e.g., basement membrane), alpha-1-antitrypsin globules, ceroid pigments in macrophages, and Kupffer cells = magenta.

   Nuclei = blue

NOTES

1. The use of sulfurous rinse, which is often recommended, is not necessary.

2. In place of 1% aqueous diastase for 1 hour, 0.5 g of diastase in 50 mL of phosphate buffer for 2 hours at 37°C can be used, which gives consistent results in our laboratory.

3. Thorough washing for 5 to 10 minutes in water instead of the use of borate solution may follow Schiff reagent.

4. In our laboratory, we counterstain with acidified Harris hematoxylin for 1 minute and dip in ammonia water for 10 dips followed by thorough washing in water. This replaces the use of acidified Lillie-Mayer hematoxylin and borate solutions.

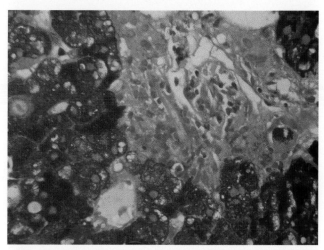

FIGURE 32–4. Glycogen in the cytoplasm of periportal hepatocytes stained magenta following periodic acid–Schiff (PAS) reaction.

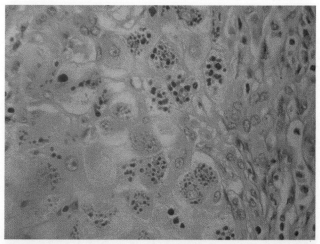

FIGURE 32–5. Diastase digestion abolishes the glycogen, and the PAS reaction reveals the undigestible alpha-1-antitrypsin globules.

Ziehl-Neelsen Method for Acid-Fast Bacilli[23]

APPLICATION

Well-fixed, paraffin-embedded sections and smears

SOLUTIONS

Ziehl-Neelsen carbol fuchsin is available through Poly Scientific (Bay Shore, NY). Filter the solution before use.

Methylene blue stock solution is prepared by dissolving 0.25 g of methylene blue in 100 mL of D/W acidified with 1 mL of glacial acetic acid.

PROCEDURE

1. DPHW.
2. Stain in carbol fuchsin for 30 minutes. Wash well in running tap water.
3. Decolorize in 1% hydrochloric acid in 70% alcohol until the sections are pale pink. Wash well in running tap water.
4. Counterstain with methylene blue. Rinse in D/W. Sections should be pale blue in color.
5. DHCM.

RESULTS

Acid-fast bacilli, lipofuscin, and ovum of *Schistosoma mansoni* = bright red

Background = pale blue

NOTES

1. To visualize the presence of lipofuscin, use 5 to 10 dips in saturated picric acid as counterstain.
2. The use of 0.5% hydrochloric acid in 70% alcohol for decolorizing works equally well.

Brown-Hopps Gram's Stain[24]

APPLICATION

Formalin-fixed, paraffin-embedded sections and smears

SOLUTIONS

Gram's iodine is prepared by dissolving 3 g of potassium iodide and 1.5 g of iodine crystals in 100 mL of D/W. Then add the remaining 350 mL of D/W.

0.25 % stock basic fuchsin solution is prepared by dissolving 0.25 g of basic fuchsin in 100 mL of D/W.

Working basic fuchsin solution is prepared by diluting 4 mL of the stock solution with 50 mL of D/W.

Gallego's differentiating solution is prepared by mixing 50 mL of D/W, 1 mL of 37% to 40% formaldehyde, and 0.5 mL of glacial acetic acid.

Picric acid–acetone is a mixture of 20 mL of saturated aqueous solution of picric acid and 500 mL of acetone.

PROCEDURE

1. DPHW.
2. Stain with 1% aqueous crystal violet solution for 2 minutes. Rinse slides in D/W.
3. Mordant with Gram's iodine for 5 minutes. Rinse in D/W.
4. Individually blot and decolorize slide quickly in acetone.
   NOTE: Immediate rinsing of slides in water is important to stop the decolorizing effect of acetone.
5. Counterstain with basic fuchsin for 5 minutes. Rinse in D/W.
6. Differentiate with Gallego's solution for 5 minutes. Rinse slides in D/W.
7. Individually blot slide, dip once in acetone quickly.
8. Dip in picric acid–acetone three times.
9. Dip once in acetone quickly.
10. Clear in xylene.
11. Mount.

RESULTS

Gram-positive = blue to blue-black

Gram-negative and nuclei = red

Background = yellow

NOTES

1. Steps 7, 8, 9, and 10 are continuous processes. Do not stop between steps until the last change of xylene. Immediate clearing is important to stop the decolorizing effect of acetone.
2. The original procedure uses picric acid powder in the preparation of picric acid–acetone. We use a substitute of saturated aqueous picric acid solution for easier handling of this highly explosive chemical.
3. To obtain a deeper red color counterstain, the volume of the diluted basic fuchsin is increased from 2 to 4 mL.

Victoria Blue Stain (Fig. 32-6)[25]

APPLICATION

Formalin-fixed, paraffin-embedded sections

SOLUTION

Victoria blue solution is prepared by boiling a mixture of 4 g of dextrine, 16 g of Victoria blue powder (Sigma, St. Louis, MO), and 32 g of resorcin in 1600 mL of DIW. Boil 200 mL of 29% aqueous ferric chloride in a separate container. Combine the two mixtures, and boil further for 3 minutes. Cool, and then filter the precipitate. The precipitate is dried in a 50°C oven. Dissolve the precipitate completely in 3200 mL of 70% alcohol. Add 32 mL of concentrated hydrochloric acid drop by drop. Then, finally add 48 mL of phenol. Mix well. The solution is stable for 2 years.

PROCEDURE

1. DPHA.
2. Tissue sections are oxidized in an equal volume of aqueous solutions of 0.3% potassium permanganate and 0.3% sulfuric acid for 5 minutes. Rinse briefly in D/W.
3. Reduce in 4% aqueous sodium metabisulfite for 1 minute. Rinse in D/W for 5 minutes.
4. Leave tissue sections in Victoria blue solution overnight. Incubation may range from 5 hours to 2 to 3 days.
5. Differentiate in 70% alcohol for 3 to 5 minutes until the background becomes clear. Slides can remain in 70% alcohol up to 1 day. Rinse in D/W.
6. Stain in 0.1% aqueous nuclear fast red for 5 minutes.
7. Wash thoroughly in running water. Rinse in D/W.
8. DHCM.

RESULTS

Hepatitis B surface antigen, elastic fibers, lipofuscin, mast cells, copper binding protein, mucin in the goblet cells = blue

Cytoplasm, nuclei = red

NOTES

Treating sections with acidified potassium permanganate intensifies Victoria blue staining. This is more reliable than orcein stain.

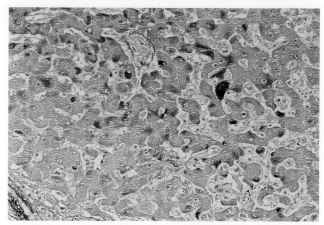

FIGURE 32–6. Hepatitis B surface antigen (HBsAg) stained blue with Victoria blue.

Hall's Stain for Bilirubin[26]

APPLICATION

Formalin-fixed, paraffin-embedded sections

SOLUTIONS

Fouchet's reagent is prepared with 25.0 g of trichloroacetic acid and 100.0 mL of distilled water, to which is added 10.0 mL of 10% ferric chloride.

10% Ferric chloride solution is prepared by dissolving 10.0 g of ferric chloride in 100.0 mL of distilled water.

Van Gieson's solution is prepared by mixing 2.5 mL of 1% aqueous acid fuschin with 97.5 mL of saturated aqueous picric acid.

PROCEDURE

1. DPHW.
2. Expose to Fouchet's reagent for 5 minutes. Wash in running water, then in distilled water.
3. Expose to Van Gieson's solution for 5 minutes.
4. DHCM.

RESULTS

Hall's stain oxidizes bilirubin to biliverdin, which appears olive drab green to emerald green depending on the concentration of bilirubin

Collagen = red

Smooth muscle fibers = yellow

Gordon and Sweet's Stain for Reticular Fibers[27,28]

APPLICATION

Formalin-fixed, paraffin-embedded sections

SOLUTION

Ammoniacal silver solution is prepared by adding concentrated ammonium hydroxide drop by drop to 5 mL of 10% silver nitrate, until the precipitate that forms is completely dissolved. Do not add excess ammonium hydroxide. Add 5 mL of 3% aqueous sodium hydroxide. Redissolve the formed precipitate with concentrated ammonium hydroxide until the solution retains an opalescence. If opalescence is absent, add a few drops of 10% silver nitrate to produce a light precipitate. Make up the volume to 50 mL with D/W. Use chemically cleaned glassware only. Refrigerate. Filter the solution before use.

PROCEDURE

1. DPHW.
2. Oxidize in 1% aqueous potassium permanganate for 5 minutes. Wash well in water.
3. Bleach in 1% aqueous oxalic acid for 1 minute or until the sections turn white. Wash well in running water for 3 minutes.
4. Treat with 2.5% aqueous iron alum for at least 15 minutes. Wash well in D/W.
5. Incubate in ammoniacal silver nitrate solution for 2 minutes. Wash well in D/W.
6. Reduce in 10% aqueous formalin solution for 2 minutes. Wash well in D/W.
7. Tone in 0.2% aqueous gold chloride solution for 10 minutes. Wash well in D/W.
8. Treat with 5% aqueous sodium thiosulfate solution for 1 minute. Wash well in D/W.
9. DHCM.

RESULTS

Reticular fibers = black

Collagen = rose color

NOTES

1. Stain with iron alum for less than 5 minutes if paler nuclear staining is desired.
2. It has been suggested that diastase digestion of heavy glycogen deposits before reticulum staining reduces background staining.
3. This provides a sensitive low-power indication of structural changes.

Modified Shikata's Orcein Stain (Fig. 32-7)[29]

APPLICATION

Formalin-fixed, paraffin-embedded sections

SOLUTIONS

Shikata's orcein stain solution is prepared by dissolving 1 g of orcein powder (Sigma, St. Louis, MO) in 100 mL of 70% alcohol. Add 1 mL of concentrated nitric acid. Leave this solution at room temperature for 24 hours before use. The solution is then kept in the refrigerator and is good for 3 months.

Acidified potassium permanganate is prepared by dissolving 0.15 g of potassium permanganate in 50 mL D/W. Add 0.1 mL of concentrated sulfuric acid. Prepare fresh before use. Discard after use.

PROCEDURE

1. DPHW.
2. Oxidize in freshly prepared acidified potassium permanganate for 5 minutes. Wash in water.
3. Bleach in 2% aqueous solution of oxalic acid for 1 minute or until the sections turn white. Wash well in water.
4. Rinse briefly in 70% alcohol.
5. Place in modified Shikata's solution for 10 minutes.
6. Remove excess stain in 70% alcohol.
7. DHCM.

RESULTS

Shikata's stain demonstrates the same structures stained with Victoria blue stain

Hepatitis B surface antigen, elastic fibers, copper binding protein = dark brown

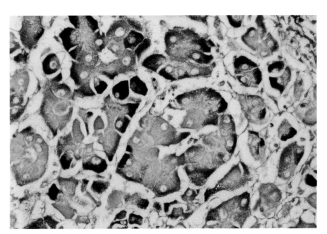

FIGURE 32–7. HBsAg containing ground-glass hepatocytes stained brown with Shikata's orcein stain.

Modified Puchtler's Congo Red Stain for Amyloid[30]

Formalin- or absolute alcohol–fixed, paraffin-embedded, 6- to 12-µm sections

Sodium chloride–alcohol solution is prepared by dissolving 2.5 g of sodium chloride in 50 mL of D/W, then adding 50 mL of absolute alcohol.

Sodium hydroxide 1% is prepared by dissolving 1 g of sodium hydroxide in 100 mL of D/W.

Congo red solution is prepared by dissolving 0.1 g of Congo red (Color Index 22120) in 50 mL of sodium chloride–alcohol solution; 0.5 mL of 1% aqueous sodium hydroxide is then added. Filter the solution before use.

1. DPHW.
2. Stain in modified Weigert's iron hematoxylin for 10 seconds.
3. Wash in tap water. Rinse in D/W.
4. Place in 0.5% hydrochloric acid in 70% alcohol for 5 seconds.
5. Wash in running tap water for 1 minute. Rinse in D/W.
6. Place in 95% alcohol for 5 seconds.
7. Stain in Congo red for 20 minutes.
8. DHCM.

Amyloid = red

Nuclei = black

Erythrocytes = pale orange

Eosinophil granules = reddish orange

1. Eliminate background staining by using modified Weigert's iron hematoxylin.
2. Staining of elastic, collagen, and muscle is suppressed by incorporating sodium chloride in the preparation of Congo red stain.

Ammoniacal Silver Nitrate for Demonstrating Fungi and *Pneumocystis carinii*[31]

Formalin-fixed, paraffin-embedded sections on charged slides

Ammoniacal silver solution is prepared by mixing 10 mL of 10% silver nitrate and 5 mL of 4% lithium hydroxide monohydrate. Concentrated ammonium hydroxide is added drop by drop with constant shaking until the precipitate just dissolves. Adjust the volume with distilled water to 1000 mL. The solution is good for at least a month when refrigerated.

Fast green stock solution is prepared by dissolving 0.2 g of fast green FCF (for coloring food) in 100 mL of D/W. Acidify with 0.2 mL of glacial acetic acid.

Fast green working solution is prepared by diluting 10 mL of the fast green stock solution with 35 mL of D/W.

1. DPHW.
2. Place 45 mL of 5% aqueous chromic acid in a Coplin jar, and microwave at power level 1 (60 W) for 3 minutes. Mix with a plastic pipette. Place the slides into this solution for 3 minutes. Wash thoroughly in D/W.
3. Treat with 1% sodium bisulfite for 30 seconds. Wash thoroughly in D/W.
4. Microwave 40 mL of cold ammoniacal silver in a loosely capped plastic Coplin jar at power level 7 (420 W) for 1 minute. Mix. Immediately place the slides into this hot solution. Reheat at power level 2 (120 W) for 30 seconds. Mix with a plastic pipette. Leave the slides in this solution for 1 to 2 minutes or until the sections appear medium brown. Wash well in D/W.
5. Tone in 0.2% aqueous gold chloride solution for 30 seconds. Wash well in D/W.
6. Place in 2% aqueous sodium thiosulfate solution for 30 seconds. Wash well in D/W.
7. Counterstain with working fast green solution for 30 seconds. Wash in D/W.
8. DHCM.

Fungi, mucin, glycogen, melanin = black

Background = green

Pneumocystis carinii = sharply delineated in black

NOTES

1. The use of chemically cleaned glassware is important to reduce background staining. Overnight soaking in household bleach in the amount of ¾ cup of bleach solution to a gallon of water may be used instead of potassium dichromate–sulfuric acid glassware cleaning solution.

2. In our laboratory, the stock ammoniacal silver nitrate is prepared as follows: Mix 10 mL of 10% silver nitrate and 1 mL of 10% potassium hydroxide. Dissolve the precipitate by adding concentrated ammonium hydroxide drop by drop, leaving just a few grains of precipitate. To use this ammoniacal silver nitrate solution, the working solution is prepared by heating 50 mL of DIW at full power for 35 seconds and by adding 18 drops of the stock solution. Mix. Place slides (six slides, including control); reheat at full power for 25 seconds. Mix. Let stand for 30 seconds to 1 minute or until the sections turn medium brown. This works well in our laboratory.

3. Teflon-coated or plastic forceps are preferred.

4. Variant silver stains such as Gomori silver stain (GMS) also works well.

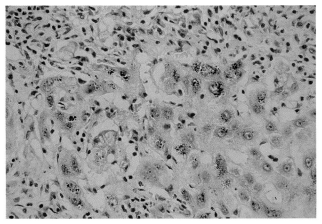

FIGURE 32–8. Orange copper granules in periportal hepatocytes demonstrated by rhodanine stain.

Rhodanine Copper Stain (Fig. 32-8)[32]

APPLICATION

Formalin-fixed, paraffin-embedded, 6- to 10-µm sections on charged slides

SOLUTIONS

Rhodanine stock solution is prepared by dissolving 0.2 g of *p*-dimethylaminobenzalrhodanine (DMABR) (Mallinckrodt Inc., Paris, KY) in 100 mL of absolute alcohol.

Rhodanine working solution is prepared by diluting 6 mL of DMABR stock solution with 94 mL of DIW. Shake stock solution well before using.

Mayer's hematoxylin is available through Poly Scientific.

Diluted Mayer's hematoxylin is prepared by mixing 25 mL of D/W and 25 mL of the stock solution of Mayer's hematoxylin.

PROCEDURE

1. DPHW.
2. Incubate in rhodanine working solution at 37°C for 18 hours.
3. Wash well in D/W.
4. Stain in diluted Mayer's hematoxylin for 10 minutes. Rinse in D/W.
5. Quickly rinse in 0.5% aqueous sodium borate. Rinse in D/W.
6. DHCM.

RESULTS

Copper = bright red to red yellow

Nuclei = blue

NOTES

To shorten the staining time, our laboratory applies the following steps:

1. Microwave 40 mL of rhodanine working solution containing slides in a loosely capped plastic Coplin jar at power level 8 (950 W) for 30 seconds. Mix. Place the Coplin jar in a 56°C water bath for 1 hour.

2. Counterstaining using Harris hematoxylin for 1 minute is also satisfactory.

3. The use of ammonia water for 2 to 3 dips instead of 0.5% sodium borate works equally well. (See H&E stain for preparation of ammonia water.)

Selected Special Procedures

IMMUNOHISTOCHEMISTRY[33,34]

This immunologic reaction is performed in liver specimens for (1) localization of viral antigens, (2) identification and classification of tumors, (3) prognostic factors in malignant tumors, (4) lymphoma/leukemia immunophenotyping, (5) identification of bile duct epithelium, and (6) demonstration of excess protein in hepatocytes. The availability of better and more specific antibodies and continuous improvements in techniques through the years have resulted in immunohisto-chemistry becoming a routine procedure in a histo-pathology laboratory; interpretation is much easier for the pathologist as well. Another advantage of this method is that it can be applied to routinely processed material.

Prolonged fixation in formalin may reduce the availability of antigen-binding sites. When fixed speci-mens are not to be embedded in paraffin right away, they may be stored in 70% alcohol. Several modifications in staining procedures are available, but the most commonly used are the peroxidase-antiperoxidase (PAP)[35] and the avidin-biotin peroxidase complex (ABC) methods.[36] Optimal dilutions of the antibodies and inclusion of positive and negative controls are important.

Troubleshooting

A. Control and test slides exhibit overstaining in the following conditions:
   1. Concentration of the primary and/or the labeled secondary antibody is too high.
   2. Incubation time of antibodies and/or substrate is longer than recommended.
   3. Reaction temperature exceeds the optimum limit.
B. Control and test slides produce weak staining in the following situations:
   1. Concentration of primary and/or labeled secondary antibody is too low.
   2. Preservative such as sodium azide or thimerosal is present.
   3. Excessive dilution of reagents occurs because of incomplete removal of rinse buffers from slides.
   4. Dissolution of end products occurs owing to in-correct use of counterstain and mounting media.
   5. Substrate is too old.
C. Control and test slides are negative under the following conditions:
   1. Target tissue antigen is not present.
   2. Tissues are allowed to dry during staining.
   3. Sequential procedural steps are not strictly followed.

D. Control slides are positive while test slides are negative in the following situations:
   1. Target antigen is absent from the tissue.
   2. Tissues are autolyzed owing to delayed fixation.
   3. Drying of tissue sections occurs in temperatures above 60°C.
   4. Overfixation with formalin has occurred.
   5. Denaturation effect of fixative or embedding method is seen on antigens.
E. Nonspecific background staining and artifacts include the following:
   1. Endogenous peroxidase or endogenous biotin is present in tissue sections. Hepatocytes are rich in endogenous biotin.
   2. Inadequate rinse occurs between steps.
   3. Concentrations of primary antibody, link, and/or label are too high.
   4. Reaction time for substrate is too long.
   5. Tissues have soluble antigens.
   6. Overoxidized hematoxylin is used.

Frequently Performed Immunohistochemistry Procedures in Liver Pathology

DETECTION OF VIRAL ANTIGENS

- Hepatitis B virus (HBV) surface antigen (HBsAg) and core antigen (HBcAg) (Figs. 32-9 and 32-10): to confirm HBV infection and to evaluate the status of HBV replication, especially in combined hepatitis viral infections[37,38]
- Hepatitis delta virus (HDV): to confirm HDV coinfection or superinfection in HBV-infected patients[39]
- Nonhepatotropic viruses (e.g., cytomegalovirus [CMV], herpes simplex, Epstein-Barr virus [EBV], adenovirus) in infants and immunosuppressed patients[40]

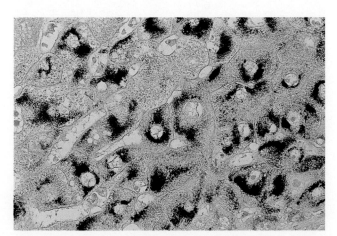

FIGURE 32–9. Immunoperoxidase stain showing HBsAg-positive hepatocytes (methylene blue counterstain).

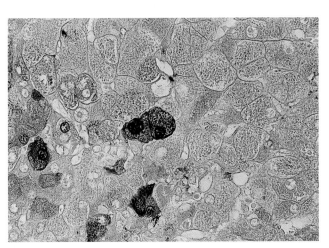

FIGURE 32–10. Immunoperoxidase stain showing nuclear and cytoplasmic HBcAg (methylene blue counterstain).

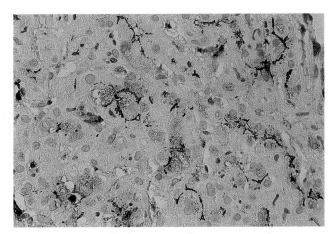

FIGURE 32–11. Canalicular pattern of CEA staining, characteristic for hepatocellular carcinoma (immunostain using polyclonal anti-CEA; counterstain with hematoxylin).

IDENTIFICATION AND CLASSIFICATION OF TUMORS

- To confirm the diagnosis of hepatocellular carcinoma (HCC)[41]: alpha-fetoprotein (AFP)-positive in about 40%, positive canalicular carcinoembryonic antigen (CEA) staining using polyclonal antibody (Fig. 32-11), and negative for cytokeratins 7 and 20 (CK7 and CK20)
- Hepatoblastoma positive for AFP in all cases
- To differentiate cholangiocarcinoma from metastatic adenocarcinoma (Fig. 32-12): CK7, CK20, TTF1, BRST-2, prostate-specific antigen, estrogen and progesterone receptors for metastatic breast carcinoma, and so forth[42]

IDENTIFICATION OF BILE DUCT EPITHELIUM

- In bile duct paucity syndromes with antibodies to biliary cytokeratins 7, 8, 18, and 19 of the catalogue of Moll[43]
- To confirm the degree of bile ductular proliferation in bile duct diseases[44]

PROGNOSTIC FACTORS

- To differentiate HCC from high-grade dysplastic nodule or hepatocellular adenoma: AFP, Ki67, or proliferating cell nuclear antigen (PCNA) (Fig. 32-13) and smooth muscle actin (Fig. 32-14) to identify neovascularization in HCC[45-47]
- To determine the aggressiveness of the tumor: PCNA, Ki67

LYMPHOMA/LEUKEMIA PHENOTYPING

- To differentiate and/or confirm post-transplant lymphoproliferative disease (PTLD) from EBV hepatitis or acute rejection[48]
- To confirm and classify lymphoma

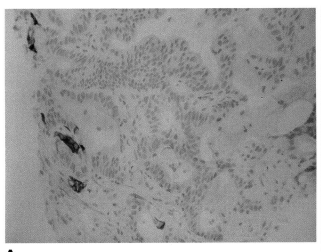
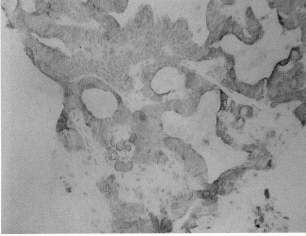

A   **B**

FIGURE 32–12. A, CK7-negative and **B,** CK20-positive tumor cells, consistent with metastatic colon carcinoma to the liver. Bile ductules in **A** are positive for CK7 (immunostain; counterstain with hematoxylin).

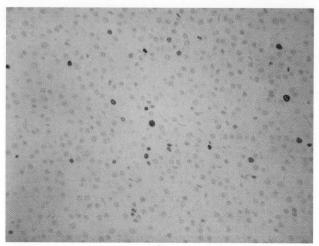

FIGURE 32–13. Ki67 staining in nuclei of a well-differentiated hepatocellular carcinoma is used to assess the degree of tumor proliferation (immunostain; counterstain with hematoxylin).

STORAGE DISEASES

- To demonstrate alpha-1-antitrypsin (A1AT) in A1AT deficiency (Fig. 32-15) and fibrinogen in fibrinogen storage disease

ELECTRON MICROSCOPY

Electron microscopy (EM) is not routinely performed on all liver specimens. It has a limited but well-defined place in liver pathology. Submitting tissue in glutaraldehyde for EM has to be considered in diseases of inborn errors of metabolism,[49] in viral infection not otherwise identified by light microscopy or serology, in tumors of unknown histogenesis, in certain drug-induced liver injury such as occurs with amiodarone, and in diseases of unclear etiology.[50,51] For this purpose,

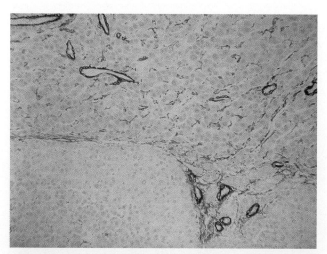

FIGURE 32–14. Immunostain of a high-grade dysplastic nodule showing smooth muscle actin–positive neoarterioles in the well-differentiated hepatocellular carcinoma but not in the area of small cell change (*bottom left*) (counterstain with hematoxylin).

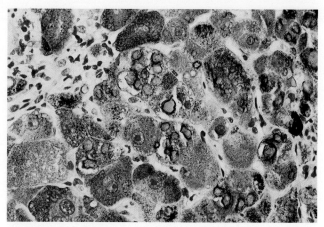

FIGURE 32–15. Hepatocytes filled with alpha-1-antitrypsin (A1AT) granules and globules in the liver of a patient with A1AT deficiency (immunostain; counterstain with hematoxylin).

small pieces of up to 5 mm from the liver core should be immersed immediately in ice cold 3% glutaraldehyde. Reprocessing of formalin-fixed, paraffin-embedded tissue for ultrastructural examination, although not optimal, is often satisfactory, particularly for viral identification.

SOLUTIONS

3% glutaraldehyde fixative is prepared by mixing the following solutions: 12 mL of 25% aqueous purified glutaraldehyde (EM grade); 5 mL of 2 M sodium cacodylate, stock solution; 5 mL of 2 M sucrose, stock solution; 70 mL of D/W. Adjust the pH to 7.2 with 2 M HCl. Adjust the volume to 100 mL with D/W. This solution is good for 1 to 2 weeks if refrigerated.

Buffer solution for washing is prepared by mixing the following solutions: 5 mL of 2 M sodium cacodylate, stock solution; 5 mL of 2 M sucrose, stock solution. Adjust the volume to 70 mL with D/W. Adjust the pH to 7.2 with 2 M HCl. The final volume is 100 mL with D/W.

1% osmium tetroxide fixative is prepared by dissolving 2 g of osmium tetroxide in water with 100 mL of s-Collidine buffer.

s-Collidine buffer is prepared by mixing the following solutions: 2.7 mL of 2,4,6-collidine; 50 mL of D/W; 8 mL of 1M HCl. Adjust pH to 7.4. The final volume is 100 mL with D/W.

PROCEDURE

1. Immerse pieces in ice cold 3% glutaraldehyde on a sheet of dental wax.
2. Divide the tissue into small cubes less than 1 mm across.

3. Fix in larger volume of fixative for 2 to 24 hours, 0°C to 4°C. This has to be done with great care to avoid compression artifacts.

4. Wash in at least two changes of buffered washing solution for 1 hour at 0°C to 4°C. Tissue can be kept in this solution for many days.

5. Postfix in osmium tetroxide solution for 1 hour at 0°C to 4°C.

6. Dehydrate and embed.

IN SITU HYBRIDIZATION

This method has been applied to liver tissue for the identification of hepatitis A, B, C, and D viruses, as well as CMV and EBV. These viruses, however, can be easily identified by immunohistochemistry, which has become a routine procedure in most laboratories and provides more or less the same sensitivity as in situ hybridization.[48] In situ hybridization is performed in our laboratory for the detection of EBV RNA in paraffin sections of liver with possible EBV hepatitis, or with PTLD with the use of fluorescein-conjugated peptide nucleic acid (PNA) probe (EBER) followed by PNA ISH Detection Kit (DAKO, Carpinteria, CA).

POLYMERASE CHAIN REACTION

The polymerase chain reaction (PCR) can be applied to fresh, unfixed liver tissue or to formalin-fixed paraffin block.[19,48,52] It provides a sensitive diagnostic and research tool in viral infections and genetic diseases. This procedure requires a special laboratory with experienced individuals to run it; it cannot be performed in a histopathology laboratory.

References

1. Snover DC: Biopsy Diagnosis of Liver Disease: Technical Aspects of the Evaluation of Liver Biopsies. Baltimore, Williams and Wilkins, 1992, pp 2-22.
2. Barwick K, Rosai J: Liver. In Rosai J (ed): Ackerman's Surgical Pathology, 7th ed, vol 1. St. Louis, CV Mosby, 1989, pp 675-735.
3. Thung SN, Gerber MA: Enzyme pattern and marker antigens in nodular regenerative hyperplasia of the liver. Cancer 47:1796-1799, 1981.
4. Shieh YSC, Shim KS, Lampertico P, et al: Detection of hepatitis C virus sequences in liver by the polymerase chain reaction. Lab Invest 65:408-411, 1991.
5. Kinsley D, Everds N, Arp L, et al: Optimization of techniques for the preservation of glycogen in paraffin embedded mouse liver. J Histotech 23:51-55, 2000.
6. Sheehan DC, Hrapchak BB: Fixation. In Sheehan L, Hrapchak BB (eds): Theory and Practice of Histotechnology, 2nd ed. Columbus, Battelle Press, 1980, pp 40-58.
7. Hoyer PE, Lyon H, Moller MP, et al: Tissue processing III: Fixation general aspects. In Lyon H (ed): Theory and Strategy in Histochemistry. Berlin, Springer-Verlag, 1991, pp 171-186.
8. Rohr RL, Layfiled LJ, Wallin D, et al: A comparison of routine and rapid microwave tissue processing in a surgical pathology laboratory. Am J Clin Pathol 115:703-708, 2001.
9. Crawford AR, Lin XZ, Crawford JM. The normal adult human liver biopsy: A quantitative reference standard. Hepatology 28:323-331, 1998.
10. Demetris AJ, Jaffe R, Starzl TE: A review of adult and pediatric post-transplant liver pathology. Pathol Annu 2:346-386, 1987.
11. Theise ND, Schwartz M, Miller C, et al: Macrogenerative nodules and hepatocellular carcinoma in forty-four sequential adult liver explants with cirrhosis. Hepatology 16:949-955, 1992.
12. Thompson SW: Microscopic Demonstration of Morphologic Components of Animal Tissues: Selected Histochemical and Histopathological Methods. Springfield, IL Charles C Thomas, 1966, pp 749-873.
13. Churukian CJ: Masson trichrome stain. Manual of the Special Stains Laboratory. Rochester, NY, University of Rochester Medical Center, Biological Stain Commission, 2000, pp 81-83.
14. Prophet EB, Mills B, Arrington S, et al: Masson trichrome stain. In Armed Forces Institute of Pathology Staff: AFIP Laboratory Methods in Histotechnology. Washington, DC, American Registry of Pathology, 1992, pp 132-133.
15. Luna LG: Connective tissues, muscle, and muscle entities. In Luna LG: Histopathologic Methods and Color Atlas of Special Stains and Tissue Artifacts. Gaithersburg, MD, American Histolabs, 1992, pp 399-459.
16. Junqueiria LCU, Bignolas G, Brentani RR: Picrosirius staining plus polarization microscopy; a specific method for collagen detection in tissue section. Histochem J 11:447-455, 1979.
17. Vacca LL: Grocott's methenamine silver. In Vacca LL: Laboratory Manual of Histochemistry. New York, Raven Press, 1985, pp 358-361.
18. Alan S: Pigments and minerals. In Bancroft J, Alan S (eds): Theory and Practice of Histological Techniques, 3rd ed. Edinburgh, Churchill Livingstone, 1990, pp 245-267.
19. Fiel MI, Schiano TD, Bodenheimer HC, et al: Genotypic, biochemical, and histological analyses for hereditary hemochromatosis in liver transplant patients. Liver Transpl Surg 5:50-56, 1999.
20. Horobin RW, Bancroft JD: Perl's Prussian blue for ferric iron. In Horobin RW, Bancroft JD: Troubleshooting Histology Stains. New York, Churchill Livingstone, 1998, pp 160-163.
21. Cook HC: Carbohydrates. In Bancroft JD, Alan S (eds): Theory and Practice of Histological Technique, 3rd ed. Edinburgh, Churchill Livingstone, 1990, pp 177-213.
22. Churukian CJ: Microwave periodic acid with diastase for selective elimination of glycogen. Manual of the Special Stains Laboratory. Rochester, NY, University of Rochester Medical Center, Biological Stain Commission, 2000, pp 54-55.
23. Luna LG: Bacteria, fungi, and spirochetes. In Luna LG: Histopathologic Methods and Color Atlas of Special Stains and Tissue Artifacts. Gaithersburg, MD, American Histolabs, 1992, pp 180-229.
24. Carson FL: Microorganisms. In Carson FL: Histotechnology: A Self-instructional Text. Chicago, ASCP Press, 1990, pp 187-208.
25. Tanaka K, Mori W, Suwa K: Victoria blue nuclear fast red stain for HBs antigen detection in paraffin section. Acta Pathol Jpn 31:93-96, 1981.
26. Hall MJ: Method for bilirubin staining. Am J Clin Pathol 34:313-316, 1960.
27. Bradbury P, Gordon K: Connective tissues and stains. In Bancroft JD, Alan S (eds): Theory and Practice of Histological Technique, 3rd ed. Edinburgh, Churchill Livingstone, 1990, pp 119-142.
28. Carson FL: Connective and muscle tissues. In Carson FL: Histotechnology: A Self-instructional Text. Chicago, ASCP Press, 1990, pp 39-165.
29. Shikata T, Izawa T, Yoshiwara N, et al: Staining methods of Australia antigen in paraffin section. Jpn J Exp Med 44:25-36, 1974.
30. Churukian CJ: Modified Puchtler Congo red amyloid method. Manual of the Special Stains Laboratory. Rochester, NY, University of Rochester Medical Center, Biological Stain Commission, 2000, pp 70-71.
31. Churukian CJ: Microwave Ammoniacal Silver Method for Demonstrating Fungi and Pneumocystis carinii: Manual of the Special Stains Laboratory. Rochester, NY, University of Rochester Medical Center, Biological Stain Commission, 2000, pp 24-26.
32. Sheehan DC, Hrapchak BB: Pigments and minerals. In Sheehan DC, Hrapchek BB: Theory and Practice of Histotechnology, 2nd ed. Columbus, OH Battelle Press, 1980, pp 214-232.
33. Bratthauer GL: Immunocytochemical methods and protocols. In Javois LC (ed): Methods in Molecular Biology, 2nd ed., NJ, Humana, 1999, pp 181-222.

34. Taylor CR, Cote RJ: Immunomicroscopy: A Diagnostic Tool for the Surgical Pathologist (Major Problems in Pathology, vol 19), 2nd ed. Philadelphia, WB Saunders, 1994.

35. Sternberger LA: Immunocytochemistry. Englewood Cliffs, NJ, Prentice Hall, 1974, pp 129-134.

36. Hsu SM, Raine L, Franger H: Use of avidin-biotin peroxidase complex (ABC) in immunoperoxidase techniques. A comparison between ABC and unlabeled antibody (PAP) procedures. J Histochem Cytochem 29:557-580, 1981.

37. Gerber MA, Thung SN: The localization of hepatitis virus in tissues. Int Rev Exp Pathol 29:49-76, 1979.

38. Guido M, Rugge M, Fattovich G, et al: Intrahepatic expression of hepatitis B virus antigens. Effect of concommitant hepatitis C virus infection. Med Pathol 12:599-603, 1999.

39. Thung SN, Gerber MA: Immunohistochemical study of delta antigen in an American metropolitan population. Liver 3:392-397, 1983.

40. Theise N, Conn M, Thung SN: Localisation of CMV antigens in liver allografts. Hum Pathol 24:103-108, 1992.

41. Thung SN, Gerber MA, Sarno E, et al: Distribution of five antigens in hepatocellular carcinoma. Lab Invest 41:101-105, 1979.

42. Fucich LF, Cheles MK, Thung SN, et al: Primary versus metastatic hepatic carcinoma. An immunohistochemical study of 34 cases. Arch Pathol Lab Med 118:927-930, 1994.

43. Moll R, Franke WW, Schiller D, et al: The catalog of human cytokeratins: Pattern of expression in normal epithelia, tumors and cultured cells. Cell 31:11-24, 1982.

44. Thung SN: The development of ductular structures in diseased liver. An immunohistochemical study. Arch Pathol Lab Med 114:407-411, 1990.

45. Theise ND, Fiel IM, Hytiroglou P, et al: The presence of macroregenerative nodules in cirrhosis is not associated with elevated serum or stainable tissue alpha-fetoprotein. Liver 15:30-34, 1995.

46. Park Y-N, Yang C-P, Fernandez GJ, et al: Neoangiogenesis and sinusoidal "capillarization" in dysplastic nodules of liver. Am J Surg Pathol 22:656-662, 1998.

47. Theise ND, Marcelin K, Goldfisher M, et al: Low proliferative activity in macroregenerative nodules: Evidence for an alternate hypothesis concerning human hepatocarcinogenesis. Liver 16:134-139, 1996.

48. Lones MA, Shintaku IP, Weiss LM, et al: Post-transplant lymphoproliferative disorders (PTLDs) in liver allograft biopsies; a comparison of three methods for the demonstration of Epstein-Barr virus. Hum Pathol 28:533-539, 1997.

49. Ishak KG, Sharp HL: Metabolic errors and liver disease. In MacSween RNM, Anthony PP, Scheuer PJ, et al (eds): Pathology of the Liver, 3rd ed. Edinburgh, Churchill Livingstone, 1994, pp 123-218.

50. Scheuer PJ, Lefkowitch JH: Electron microscopy and other techniques. In Scheuer PJ, Lefkowitch JH (eds): Liver Biopsy Interpretation. London, WB Saunders, 2000, pp 344-356.

51. Phillips MJ, Poncell S, Patterson J, et al: The Liver. An Atlas and Text of Ultrastructural Pathology. New York, Raven Press, 1987.

52. Saito K, Sullivan D, Haruna Y, et al: Detection of hepatitis C virus RNA sequences in hepatocellular carcinoma and its precursors by microdissection PCR. Arch Pathol Lab Med 121:400-403, 1997.

CHAPTER 33

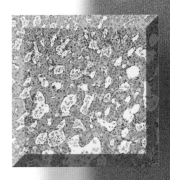

Diagnostic Cytology of the Liver

MARTHA BISHOP PITMAN

Introduction

Fine-needle aspiration biopsy (FNAB) is the diagnostic procedure of choice in the diagnosis of liver lesions both large and small; in most cases, it is performed to confirm a suspected malignancy. In the experienced hands of both the radiologist and the cytopathologist, the procedure is considered safe, efficacious, accurate, and cost-effective.[1-8] When FNAB provides an early diagnosis, the total number of tests, especially invasive tests, is reduced, and the length of the hospital stay may be decreased.[9] Indeed, the procedure is often performed on an outpatient basis. Historically, percutaneous computed tomography (CT) and ultrasound (US)-guided biopsies have been the techniques of choice. Endoscopic ultrasound (EUS)–guided FNAB is a new technique that is gaining favor for use with lesions accessible by this technique.[10-13]

The primary contraindications for percutaneous FNAB include an uncorrectable bleeding diathesis, the lack of a safe access route (e.g., biopsy through a large vascular structure), and an uncooperative patient in whom awkward positioning or maintenance of strict breath control is necessary to ensure proper needle placement in the lesion.[1,3-7,14] FNAB may proceed in the presence of an uncorrectable bleeding diathesis, however, if the need for a tissue diagnosis is urgent. For EUS-guided FNAB, gastrointestinal obstruction is an absolute contraindication because of the risk of intestinal perforation.[10]

Complications of FNAB are uncommon.[15] Bleeding may occur, particularly in the case of a vascular lesion; the risk of bleeding is often dependent on the size of the needle used, with risk of bleeding increasing with needle size. Seeding of the biopsy tract with tumor cells is extremely rare if a small (<22 gauge), noncutting needle is used.[15] With larger needles, especially the Vim-Silverman needle, seeding is more common.[16-18]

Prebiopsy assessment of patients undergoing FNAB includes, as for all deep FNAB procedures, evaluation of the coagulation system to identify patients at risk for excessive bleeding. In addition, a preprocedure analysis is performed to determine the optimal imaging modality, the size and location of the lesion(s), and the degree of tumor vascularity. Body habitus and other specific patient requirements must be considered. Finally, and importantly, the procedure itself is discussed with the patient; a clear explanation is provided of the degree of pain to be expected and the likely outcome of the procedure. Obtaining full patient cooperation by reducing patient anxiety increases the likelihood of success.

Liver FNAB is mostly percutaneous and employs interventional imaging techniques for localization, most commonly US and CT. EUS-guided FNAB is used primarily for lesions in the left lobe of the liver with the needle easily traversing the stomach or small intestinal wall.[11,19-21] Among the factors influencing the choice of guidance system are the size and location of the lesion and the experience and preferences of the operator.[14] US enables rapid localization, flexible patient positioning, and variable imaging of the lesion; in addition, of course, it can be performed without radiation. US is generally used to provide initial guidance, particularly with multiple lesions and/or large, relatively superficial lesions. CT has a number of advantages for aspiration biopsy. It facilitates optimal resolution of smaller lesions or lesions not visible on US, allows accurate localization of the needle tip immediately before sampling, and provides improved definition of tissue components and vascularity. No potential impediments such as drains, bone, and gas are transmitted. CT also precisely demonstrates the anatomic relationships of a given lesion. Multiple biopsies can generally be performed with minimal morbidity.

Transabdominal or percutaneous FNAB techniques include individual puncture, coaxial biopsy, and tandem needle biopsy techniques.[14] Individual puncture is used with real-time US only and requires considerable experience and skill. Coaxial biopsy allows for precise needle placement with the use of a stiff cannula for guidance; this can be performed with either US or CT. Both US and CT can also be used for the tandem needle biopsy technique; a reference needle serves as a guide for the biopsy needle, allowing multiple aspirations to be performed without repeat imaging (Fig. 33-1).[22]

Optimal aspiration results include both smears and cell block preparations in all FNABs of the liver. Smears are made from the aspiration part of the biopsy with the use of a small needle (<22 gauge), which provides a rapid means of evaluating the specimen, not only for cellular adequacy but frequently for diagnosis. Multiple aspiration biopsies can be performed with minimal morbidity. Cell blocks are obtained from needle rinsings,

any tissue fragments that are gathered, and dedicated core needle biopsies with the use of a spring-loaded 18- to 20-gauge core needle biopsy gun, such as the ASAP Biopsy System (MediTech/Boston Scientific Corp, Watertown, MA) or the Coaxial Temno Biopsy System (Allegiance Healthcare Corp, McGaw Park, IL). This material provides a formalin-fixed, paraffin-embedded tissue sample from which special stains and immuno-histochemical studies can be readily obtained. It also provides, in many cases, the architecture necessary for a specific diagnosis, particularly with benign liver lesions.

As with any other form of biopsy, sampling error can occur. Sampling error results most often from inexact needle localization, which sometimes reflects the fact that the sought-after lesion is smaller than 1 cm; it may also occur in bigger lesions, possibly indicating that large areas of necrosis or fibrosis or a prominent inflammatory rim is present. For these reasons, the supplemental use of FNAB with concomitant core biopsy improves accuracy, specificity, and sensitivity.[23,24]

Core biopsy specimens can be used for rapid interpretation when the core is touched to a glass slide in a touch prep fashion (Fig. 32-2).[25] Despite the presence of thick, three-dimensional tissue fragments and the probability of some air-drying artifact caused by the inherent time delay in preparation of the slide, architectural clues may still be readily apparent to aid in rapid diagnosis (Fig. 33-3).

The cytopathologist is an important part of the overall team approach to FNAB of the liver. The presence of a cytopathologist at the time of the biopsy procedure increases the overall accuracy of the procedure.[26-28] The time of the actual biopsy, when additional tissue is still

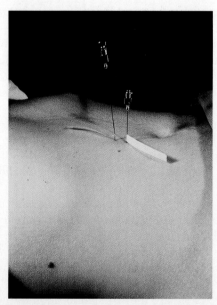

FIGURE 33–1. Tandem needle biopsy technique in fine-needle aspiration biopsy of the liver. A reference needle is used to guide the biopsy needle, allowing for multiple aspirations without repeat imaging. (Courtesy of Dr. Peter Mueller, Department of Radiology, Massachusetts General Hospital, Boston.)

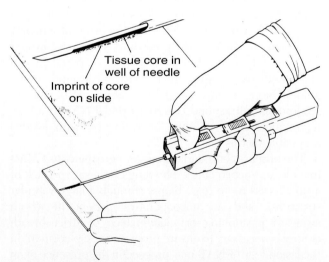

FIGURE 33–2. Touch prep technique of a core biopsy for rapid diagnosis at the time of fine-needle aspiration biopsy. A core of tissue is touched to the slide while it is still in the biopsy gun. (From Hahn PF, Eisbenberg PJ, Pitman MB, et al: Cytopathologic touch preparations [imprints] from core needle biopsies: Accuracy compared with that of fine-needle aspirates. AJR 165:1277-1279, 1995.)

Tissue core in well of needle

Imprint of core on slide

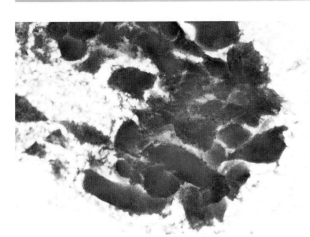

FIGURE 33–3. A touch imprint of a core biopsy taken during fine-needle aspiration biopsy. Despite thickness and three-dimensionality of the tissue groups, a trabecular architecture with peripheral endothelial wrapping is obvious, leading to a rapid interpretation of hepatocellular carcinoma (objective magnification 5×).

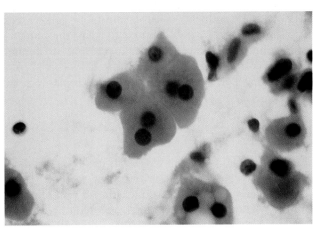

FIGURE 33–4. Normal hepatocytes demonstrating a polygonal shape, abundant granular cytoplasm, focal steatosis, and one or two round to oval centrally placed nuclei, with an even chromatin pattern and small nucleoli (Papanicolaou, objective magnification, 40×).

readily available, is the best time for evaluating the specimen for adequacy and for triaging the tissue for special studies such as flow cytometry or electron microscopy studies. If a cytopathologist or a technologist is not available to assist in the preparation of the specimen, it is imperative that the radiologist learn how to make proper smears. The most highly cellular specimen is useless if it has been inadequately prepared for optimal interpretation. The advent of liquid-based cytology (Thin Prep, Cytyc Corp, Roxborough, MA; Autocyte, Tripath Imaging Corp, Burlington, NC) has provided an alternative means of specimen preparation, but it is recommended only as an adjunct to smears or for use by practitioners with a low success rate in obtaining primary smears.

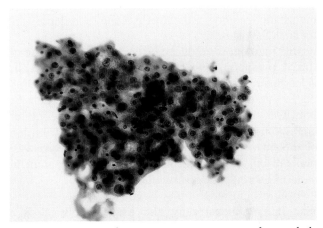

FIGURE 33–5. Benign hepatocytes present in a jagged, irregularly shaped cluster without peripherally wrapping endothelium (Papanicolaou, objective magnification 5×).

■ Benign Conditions

NORMAL MORPHOLOGY

When a normal liver is aspirated, the smears are dominated by benign hepatocytes. Scattered bile duct epithelial cells are also present. The normal hepatocyte is a large polygonal cell with abundant granular cytoplasm, one or two round to oval, centrally placed nuclei with an even chromatin pattern, and occasionally prominent nucleoli. These may be present singly, in small clusters (Fig. 33-4), or in larger flat sheets, which have an irregular jagged edge (Fig. 33-5). Normal bile duct epithelial cells are smaller than hepatocytes and may have a varied appearance. They are most often present as flat, monolayered, typically glandular-appearing sheets of epithelial cells (Fig. 33-6). They may also be present in an on-edge picket-fence arrangement, or in small acinar

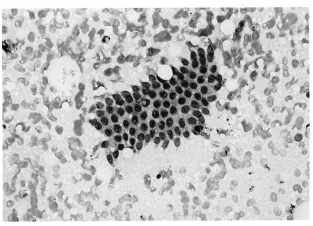

FIGURE 33–6. Benign bile duct epithelial cells present in a flat, monolayered, honeycombed sheet, with evenly spaced, round, regular nuclei (Diff-Quik, objective magnification 25×).

structures. Endothelial cells of sinusoidal spaces and Kupffer cells are rarely appreciated in the normal aspirate and are only sporadically present in benign non-neoplastic and neoplastic entities. Endothelial cells are discussed in greater detail under Hepatocellular Carcinoma.

PIGMENTS

Pigments and inclusions may be as readily recognized in cytology preparations as in histologic sections. Lipofuscin pigment, which constitutes the debris of intracellular lysosome breakdown, increases with age. It is a fine, golden, granular, relatively nonrefractile pigment that is typically concentrated around the nucleus (Fig. 33-7). This pigment is generally common in the aspirate of the adult liver, and its absence should increase suspicion of a tumor, especially in the setting of a mass lesion. One pitfall to keep in mind is that lipofuscin pigment stains darkly with a Fontana-Masson stain, creating a potential diagnostic pitfall and a diagnosis of metastatic melanoma; the liver is a common depository for such metastases.[29]

Bile pigment is produced by hepatocytes; because of this, its presence within the cytoplasm of malignant cells is pathognomonic for hepatocellular carcinoma (Fig. 33-8). Bile is variable in color, texture, size, and density, but it is recognized by its coarse, irregular, rather amorphous, nonrefractile appearance. The distribution of the pigment depends on the degree of cholestasis; pools of bile within canalicular spaces are apparent in cases of extrahepatic obstruction (Fig. 33-9).

Iron or hemosiderin may be present in hepatocytes, bile duct epithelial cells, and Kupffer cells. It is a coarse, brown-black, refractile pigment on standard Papanicolaou stain (Fig. 33-10). Malignant hepatocytes

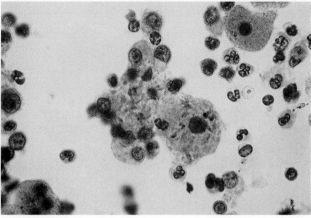

FIGURE 33–8. Cytoplasmic bile pigment, although variable in color, texture, size, and density, is recognized by its coarse, irregular, rather amorphous, nonrefractile appearance (Papanicolaou, objective magnification 20×).

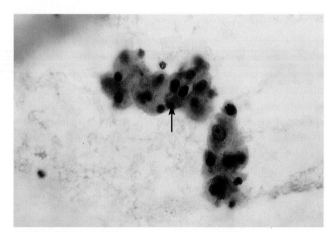

FIGURE 33–9. Canalicular bile plugs (*arrow*) can be appreciated in cases of extrahepatic obstruction (Papanicolaou, objective magnification 40×).

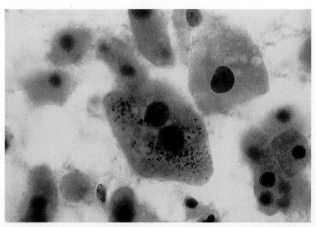

FIGURE 33–7. Lipofuscin pigment is present as a fine, golden, granular, relatively nonrefractile pigment typically concentrated around the nucleus (Papanicolaou, objective magnification 63×).

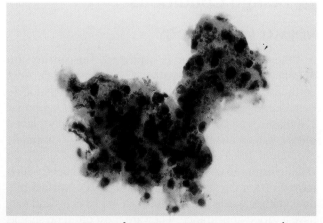

FIGURE 33–10. Hemosiderin pigment appears as coarse, brown-black, refractile pigment on the standard Papanicolaou stain, seen here in benign hepatocytes (Papanicolaou, obejctive magnification 63×).

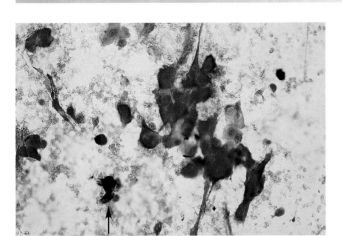

FIGURE 33–11. Hepatocellular carcinoma arising in the setting of hemochromatosis. Malignant hepatocytes fail to stain blue with a special stain for iron, contrasting nicely with the small, blue-stained, benign hepatocytes *(arrow)* (Prussian blue, objective magnification 10×).

lose their ability to retain iron, and in the setting of cirrhosis from hemachromatosis, wherein reactive hepatocyte atypia may be marked, use of a special stain for iron (e.g., Prussian blue) to highlight cells or clusters of cells without staining is helpful (Fig. 33-11). This is a useful ancillary tool for the identification of well-differentiated hepatocellular carcinoma.[30]

STEATOSIS

Fatty change in hepatocytes, although common in many liver conditions (especially toxic/metabolic injury as seen in alcohol abuse), may be the reason for the appearance of a mass lesion on radiologic studies.[31] Cytologically, as in histology, fat is present as single large vacuoles (macrovesicular steatosis) or multiple small vacuoles (microvesicular steatosis) (Fig. 33-12).

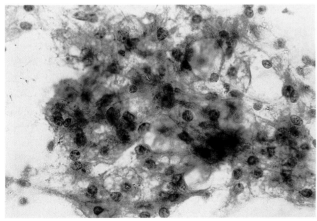

FIGURE 33–12. Fatty change in hepatocytes is readily appreciated on cytology as either single large vacuoles (macrovesicular) or small multiple vacuoles (microvesicular) (Papanicolaou, objective magnification 20×).

INFECTION

Abscess formation in the liver is often suspected radiologically from the characteristic double-target sign on CT.[32] Pyogenic abscess is the most common, and percutaneous biopsy is performed for tissue confirmation, culture, and drainage. Smears are dominated by acute inflammatory cells and cellular debris. Cultures are helpful for the identification of bacterial organisms, but special stains of smears, such as Brown-Brenn or Brown-Hopps, are not helpful in my experience. Uniquely characteristic organisms, such as the "sulfur granules" of actinomyces (Fig. 33-13**A**) and ecchinococcal hooklets in hydatid disease (Fig. 33-13**B**), may be readily identified on smears.

Granulomatous inflammation may be related to infection such as that associated with fungal or acid-fast organisms, but the presence of granulomas on a liver aspirate is in no way diagnostic of an infectious etiology. Granulomas may be related to many conditions, including primary hepatobiliary disorders such as primary biliary cirrhosis, sarcoidosis, and tumors such as lymphoma and metastatic carcinoma. Cytologically, granulomas are composed of clusters of epithelioid histiocytes that have oval to elongated, sometimes twisted, nuclei and visible but indistinct cytoplasm (Fig. 33-14). Special stains such as Gomori's methenamine silver (GMS) and Ziehl-Neelsen for acid-fast bacillus (AFB) stain can be performed on smears; however, these are easier to perform on cell block preparations and tend to be more helpful than special stains for bacteria.

BILE DUCT ADENOMA AND HAMARTOMA

Both bile duct adenoma and hamartoma may present as a mass lesion mimicking a neoplasm, most commonly a metastasis; as a result, both may be encountered on FNAB.[33,34] Aspiration of these lesions is identical, producing a predominant population of benign-appearing bile duct epithelial cells (Fig. 33-15**A**). Cell block preparations are helpful in rendering a specific diagnosis (Fig. 33-15**B**) (Box 33-1).

HEMANGIOMA

Although they are generally asymptomatic, these mass lesions are picked up incidentally during workup for other conditions, including staging of malignancy; they can be difficult to distinguish radiologically from a metastasis.[35,36] Cytologically, aspirate smears are often disappointing and are frequently considered unsatisfactory or nondiagnostic owing to the predominance of blood or the presence of nonspecific connective tissue. It is this loose, rather than dense, fibrous-type connective tissue associated with blood and few to no background hepatocytes that should alert the pathologist to the diagnosis of hemangioma in the proper clinical setting

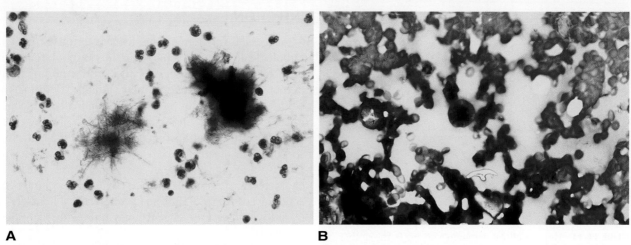

A **B**

FIGURE 33–13. A, Fibrillar, star-shaped "sulfur granules" are characteristic of *Actinomyces* species on cytology preparations (Papanicolaou, 10×). **B,** Refractile hooklets from echinoccal protoscoleces may be identified in aspirated fluids from hydatid cysts (Diff-Quik, objective magnification 40×). (Courtesy of Drs. Uma Handa and Harsh Mohan, Department of Pathology, Government Medical Center, Chandigarh, India.)

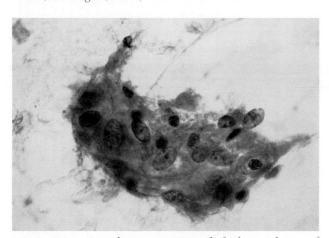

FIGURE 33–14. Granulomas are composed of cohesive clusters of epithelioid histiocytes with oval to elongated, often twisted nuclei and indistinct but visible cytoplasm (Papanicolaou, objective magnification 63×).

(Fig. 33-16**A**). Again, cell block preparation of a core needle biopsy is crucial if a specific diagnosis is to be made accurately (Fig. 33-16**B**) (Box 33-2).

ANGIOMYOLIPOMA

The histologic and cytologic features of this tumor are similar in the liver and the kidney. Varying combinations of fat, smooth muscle, and vessels are present, and the diagnosis is relatively straightforward when the fatty component is readily recognized (Fig. 33-17).[37-39] Diagnostic difficulty arises when the fatty component is scant or focal and is not sampled, leading the pathologist down the differential diagnostic path of spindle cell lesions of the liver. Rarely, solid epithelioid areas mimicking carcinoma can create a diagnostic

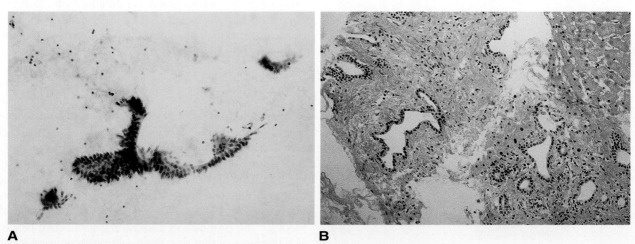

A **B**

FIGURE 33–15. A, Bile duct hamartoma. Aspirate smears are dominated by benign-appearing bile duct epithelial cells with uncharacteristically scant numbers of associated hepatocytes (Papanicolaou, objective magnification 2.5×). **B,** Bile duct hamartoma. Cell block preparations of core needle biopsies show the characteristic angulated proliferation of variably dilated bile ductules in a fibrotic background, allowing for a specific diagnosis (objective magnification 10×).

Box 33–1. **Bile Duct Hamartoma**

- Greater than normal number of groups or sheets of benign-appearing bile duct epithelium
- Uncharacteristically few hepatocytes in the background

Box 33–2. **Hemangioma**

- Bloody, scantily cellular smears
- Loose connective tissue; generally few to no hepatocytes
- Smears commonly nondiagnostic; specific diagnosis dependent on cell block

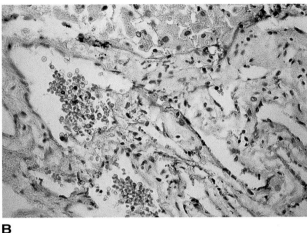

FIGURE 33–16. A, Hemangioma. The presence of loose rather than dense fibrous connective tissue associated with blood and few to no background hepatocytes, although considered nondiagnostic and often unsatisfactory for diagnosis, is a typical finding in the aspiration of hepatic hemangioma (Papanicolaou, objective magnification 2.5×). **B,** Hemangioma. Cell block preparation of a core needle biopsy allowed for a specific diagnosis of hepatic hemangioma (objective magnification 20×).

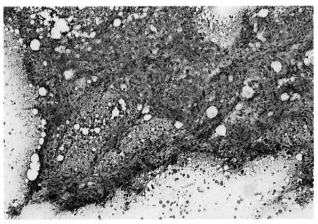

FIGURE 33–17. Angiomyolipoma. A combination of vessels, smooth muscle, and adipocytes allows for a specific diagnosis on fine-needle aspiration biopsy (Diff-Quik, objective magnification 2.5×).

Box 33–3. **Angiomyolipoma**

- Interlacing complex of smooth muscle, fat, and blood vessels
- Smooth muscle may dominate smears and can demonstrate atypia (pitfall)
- Solid epithelioid areas can also be present (pitfall)
- Immunocytochemistry stain to be used for confirmation: HMB-45

pitfall.[40] Positive staining with HMB-45 confirms the diagnosis (Box 33-3).[41]

BENIGN HEPATOCYTIC NODULES AND MASSES

Benign hepatocytic nodules and mass lesions, both non-neoplastic and neoplastic (e.g., macroregenerative nodule, dysplastic nodule, focal nodular hyperplasia,

and hepatocellular adenoma), are discussed together here because they share many cytologic features and distinction between them on smear cytology alone is not possible. In addition, all of these lesions share the same differential diagnosis, namely well-differentiated hepatocellular carcinoma.

The initial approach to evaluating smears of a liver aspirate, and one of the most important, should include a low-power overall scan of the smear for smear pattern, especially in the differential diagnosis of benign versus malignant hepatocytic lesions. Benign reactive and neoplastic processes share the presence of variably cellular (but not densely cellular) smears composed of benign-appearing hepatocytes present in irregularly shaped, jagged-edged clusters without associated peripherally wrapping endothelial cells (Fig. 33-18).

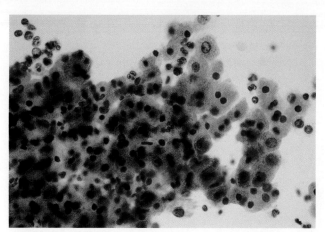

FIGURE 33–18. Benign reactive and regenerative hepatocytic processes are composed of irregularly shaped, jagged-edged clusters without associated peripherally wrapping endothelial cell (Papanicolaou, objective magnification 25×).

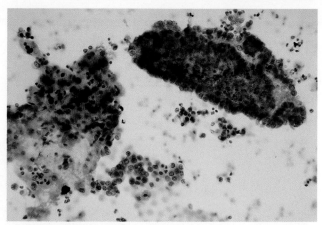

FIGURE 33–20. Proliferative and reactive bile duct epithelial cells *(upper right corner)* in the presence of irregular jagged clusters of hepatocytes are a feature of a reactive process and suggestive of cirrhosis (Papanicolaou, objective magnification 10×).

Proliferating or arborizing vessels (transgressing endothelial cells) may occasionally be present, but this feature is much more common in hepatocellular carcinoma (see Fig. 33-28).[2,4,42] Nodules of cirrhosis may produce smooth-edged–appearing clusters but do not demonstrate endothelial cell wrapping (Fig. 33-19). Reactive and proliferative bile duct epithelial cells may also be seen; their presence should greatly raise one's threshold of suspicion for a malignant diagnosis (Fig. 33-20).

Large regenerative nodules, most commonly arising in a background of cirrhosis and to a greater degree than in focal nodular hyperplasia and hepatocellular adenoma, have a tendency to include reactive hepatocytes, which can demonstrate significant nuclear atypia (large cell change, also called large cell dysplasia) (Fig. 33-21). The key to recognition of these cells as benign is their sporadic placement in a background of

otherwise typically reactive-appearing hepatocytes. Additional features of reactivity include an apparent hepatocytic pleomorphism rather than monomorphism (Fig. 33-22), an increased number of binucleated cells (which tend to be decreased in hepatocellular carcinoma), a relatively low nucleus-to-cytoplasm ratio, smooth nuclear membranes, prominent nucleoli (not macronucleoli) (Fig. 33-23), and the presence of reactive bile duct cells. Bile duct cells should not be seen in a pure aspirate of hepatocellular carcinoma; this is an important clue that can lead to the correct diagnosis.

In most instances, the clinical differential diagnosis is narrow—for example, a prominent nodule in a background of cirrhosis (is it hepatocellular carcinoma?) or a mass lesion in a noncirrhotic liver (is it malignant, primary, or metastatic?). To the pathologist, an aspirate

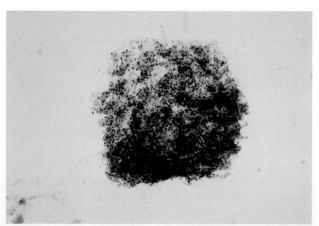

FIGURE 33–19. Nodules of cirrhosis may produce smooth-edged clusters, but peripheral wrapping edothelial cells are not present (Papanicolaou, objective magnification 10×).

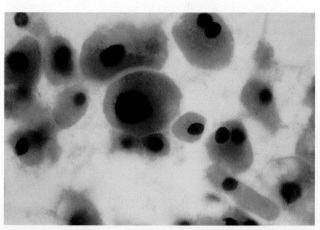

FIGURE 33–21. Hepatocytes that demonstrate significant atypia or large cell change (large cell dysplasia) are recognized as benign by their sporadic placement among otherwise benign and reactive-appearing hepatocytes (Papanicolaou, objective magnification 63×).

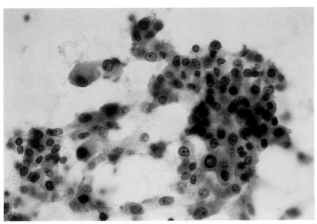

FIGURE 33–22. Reactive hepatocytes demonstrate cellular and nuclear pleomorphism (in contrast to the monomorphism demonstrated by hepatocellular carcinoma) (Papanicolaou, objective magnification 25×).

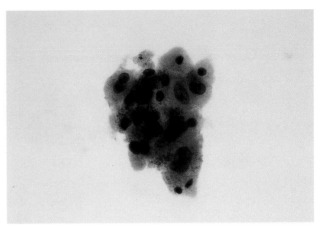

FIGURE 33–23. Binucleated hepatocytes are common in reactive hepatocellular proliferations, whereas they are decreased in hepatocellular carcinoma (Papanicolaou, objective magnification 40×).

smear composed of obvious hepatocytes narrows the differential diagnosis to a benign or malignant hepatocytic process, which, in essence, is all that is necessary for proper clinical management. Because of the overlap in components of these various benign entities on smear cytology, cell blocks as well as radiologic and clinical correlation are crucial in making a specific diagnosis. The smallest fragment of tissue may be all that is necessary to render a specific diagnosis (Figs. 33-24 and 33-25). This readily available tissue may be used for the few ancillary tests that can aid in the benign versus malignant differential diagnosis (Box 33-4).

■ Malignant Neoplasms

PRIMARY NEOPLASMS

Hepatocellular Carcinoma

The cytologic diagnosis of hepatocellular carcinoma can be separated into two main categories, that is, low-grade (well differentiated) and high-grade tumors (moderately and poorly differentiated).

WELL-DIFFERENTIATED HEPATOCELLULAR CARCINOMA

As has been mentioned in the discussion of benign hepatocytic proliferations, well-differentiated hepatocellular carcinoma is a tumor that looks hepatocytic but does not look obviously malignant. Given that the tumor cells of well-differentiated hepatocellular carcinoma are so similar to normal liver, the smear pattern proves to be a critical feature in assessment of these tumors.[2,4,42-46]

The three basic smear patterns include a cohesive, nested, and trabecular pattern with peripherally wrapping endothelial cells; loosely cohesive sheets with transgressing endothelial cells and vessels; and a dispersed small cluster/single-cell pattern.

Box 33–4. Benign and Reactive Hepatocytic Nodules

- Hepatocytes in jagged, irregular clusters or arranged singly
- No peripherally wrapping endothelial cells
- Clusters may have transgressing endothelial cells
- Mild pleomorphism of cell and nuclear size; sporadically placed large, atypical cells (dysplastic hepatocytes/large cell change)
- Many binucleated hepatocytes
- Variably prominent nucleoli but no macroeosinophilic nucleoli
- Cytoplasm is generally abundant and granular but may show fatty change, lipofuscin pigment, or iron deposition
- Reticulin stain shows retained framework of one to two cell layers on cell block

The most specific is the peripherally wrapping endothelial pattern.[2,4,46,47] In this pattern, the endothelial cells of the sinusoids wrap around smooth-edged, rounded nests and thickened hepatic trabeculae (Figs. 33-26 and 33-27). Endothelial cell nuclei may not be apparent in every plane of focus, but the presence of even one or two nuclei at the edge is sufficient. Although this pattern is found in less than half of tumors,[2,4] when present, it has been found to be specific for the diagnosis of hepatocellular carcinoma. This pattern has proved to be one of the most important diagnostic clues in separating reactive non-neoplastic and benign neoplastic proliferations from well-differentiated hepatocellular carcinoma.[4,42]

The other pattern of endothelial proliferation has been called *transgressing*,[4] *arborizing*,[48] or *central*.[2] A complex network of small vessels is present in a loosely cohesive sheet of hepatocytes (Fig. 33-28). The appearance is similar to that of proliferating capillaries in other processes, such as granulation tissue, suggesting that these endothelial cells are associated with basement

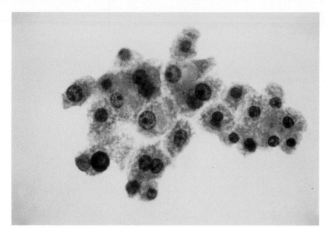

FIGURE 33–24. Reactive hepatocytes demonstrate a low nucleus-to-cytoplasm ratio and nuclei with smooth nuclear membranes and prominent nucleoli (but not macronucleoli) (Papanicolaou, objective magnification 63×).

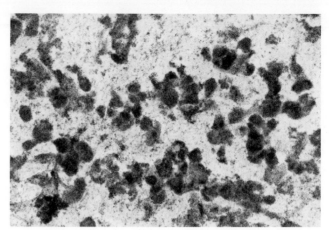

FIGURE 33–26. The peripherally wrapping endothelial cell pattern demonstrates endothelial cells of sinusoids wrapping around smooth-edged, rounded nests and thickened hepatic trabeculae of hepatocytes (rapid hemotoxylin and eosin, objective magnification 2.5×).

membranes, a feature of abnormal sinusoids seen in hepatocellular carcinoma.[49,50] This pattern is not as specific for hepatocellular carcinoma as is the peripherally wrapping endothelial pattern, but it is highly associated with this diagnosis. It is rarely seen in cases of cirrhosis and hepatitis.[4]

The dispersed small cluster/single-cell pattern, which is completely nonspecific, may be seen in all types of hepatocellular proliferations (Fig. 33-29). One variant of hepatocellular carcinoma that is particularly prone to a dispersed smear pattern is the fibrolamellar type. The dense lamellar fibrosis that separates loosely cohesive sheets of malignant hepatocytes is not easily aspirated with a fine needle, yielding not only a dispersed cell pattern but frequently a paucicellular smear. The peripherally wrapping endothelial pattern has not been described, but the transgressing pattern may be seen. Fibrolamellar hepatocellular carcinoma is composed of

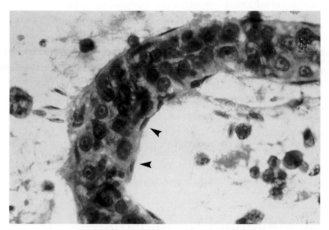

FIGURE 33–27. Peripherally wrapping endothelium may be identified as one or two endothelial cell nuclei (*arrowheads*) splayed across a rounded nest or thickened trabeculum of hepatocytes (Papanicolaou, objective magnification 63×).

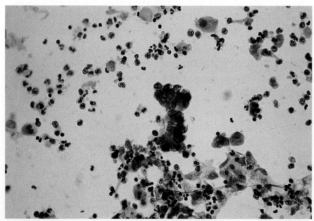

FIGURE 33–25. Abundant inflammation and reactive bile duct epithelial cells support a benign diagnosis (Papanicolaou, objective magnification 20×.) (Courtesy of Dr. Wanda Szyfelbein, MGH, Boston.)

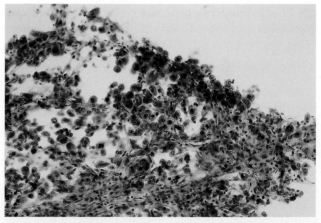

FIGURE 33–28. The transgressing endothelial pattern demonstrates an arborizing, proliferating, or transgressing meshwork of capillaries in a loosely cohesive sheet or aggregate of neoplastic hepatocytes (objective magnification 10×).

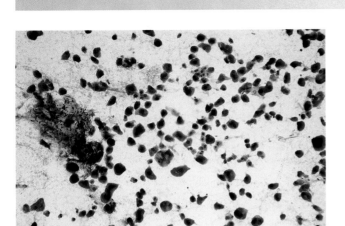

FIGURE 33–29. The dispersed, small cluster, single-cell pattern of hepatocellular carcinoma shows malignant hepatocytes as predominantly large polygonal single cell with frequent naked nuclei (Papanicolaou, objective magnification 5×).

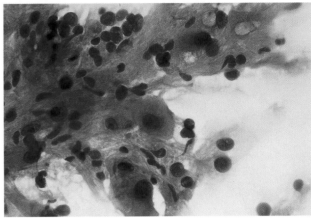

FIGURE 33–30. Fibrolamellar hepatocellular carcinoma is uniquely characterized by large polygonal hepatocytes with a deceptively low nucleus-to-cytoplasm ratio, dense oxyphilic cytoplasm, frequent intranuclear inclusions, and intracytoplasmic pale bodies. (Papanicolaou, objective magnification 40×.) (Courtesy of Dr. Edmond Cibas, Brigham & Women's Hospital, Boston.)

large malignant hepatocytes with a deceptively low nucleus-to-cytoplasm ratio, abundant dense oxyphilic-type cytoplasm, and numerous intranuclear inclusions and intracytoplasmic pale bodies (Fig. 33-30).[51-54]

Because the smear pattern is not helpful in all cases, other features need to be assessed. Many studies have evaluated the cytomorphologic features of hepatocellular carcinoma.[3,5,43-46,48,55-65] Such features as increased nucleus-to-cytoplasm ratio, trabecular formation, the presence of bile, atypical naked nuclei, and a loss of polarity within cell groups have all been described as important features of hepatocellular carcinoma.[5,43,44,61] Most of these studies included all grades of hepatocellular carcinoma, somewhat skewing the criteria. For example, the presence of bile is not a helpful finding in the benign versus malignant differential diagnosis, and in my experience, the presence of atypical naked nuclei[62] is a more reliable feature for the primary versus metastatic differential diagnosis than for the benign versus malignant differential. In addition, some of the described features can be difficult to appreciate, especially when the population is a pure hepatocellular carcinoma population and normal hepatocytes are not present for comparison (e.g., with a smaller than normal cell size in well-differentiated hepatocellular carcinoma).

Individual cellular features that support a malignant diagnosis include the presence of cellular monotony with a uniformly elevated nucleus-to-cytoplasm ratio (e.g., all cells appear to have the same degree of atypia) (Fig. 33-31) and macroeosinophilic nucleoli on Papanicolaou stain (Fig. 33-32).[4,5,42,64,66] A concomitant absence of lipofuscin pigment within cells is also supportive of a malignant diagnosis. Hyaline globules such as alpha-1-antitrypsin and alpha-fetoprotein are common but are not specific for hepatocellular carcinoma or malignancy.

Ancillary studies are relatively limited in the diagnosis of well-differentiated hepatocellular carcinoma. One of the most helpful tests involves the use of the reticulin stain.[1,42,58,67] This stain can be used on either smears or cell block preparations. An abnormal reticulin staining pattern, usually the absence of reticulin staining (Fig. 33-33), is highly associated with hepatocellular carcinoma.[1,42,58,67] A pitfall in interpretation of the reticulin stain is the presence of marked steatosis, which can cause a false-negative result. Although the endothelial cell marker CD34 is negative in normal hepatic sinusoids and stains vessels diffusely in hepatocellular carcinoma, the use of this marker provides no added value over the easily performed (and less expensive) reticulin stain in the benign versus malignant differential diagnosis.[68] An iron stain such as the

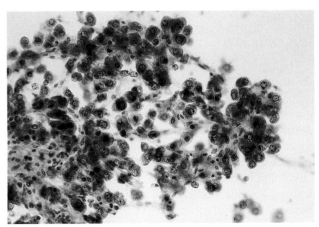

FIGURE 33–31. Well-differentiated hepatocellular carcinoma demonstrates the cellular monotony of a uniform population of cells with an elevated nucleus-to-cytoplasm ratio (Papanicolaou, objective magnification 25×).

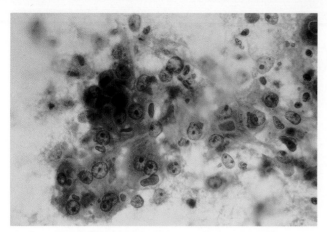

FIGURE 33–32. Macroeosinophilic nucleoli are a feature of hepatocellular carcinoma but are not present in all cases (rapid hematoxylin and eosin, objective magnification 63×).

Prussian blue stain can highlight the normal, hemosiderin-laden hepatocytes as bright blue, leaving unstained the malignant hepatocytes that have lost their ability to retain iron (see Fig. 33-11).

Immunocytochemistry is of much more limited use. Alpha-fetoprotein staining is helpful if positive, but a negative stain in no way rules out the presence of a tumor. Approximately 40% of tumors are associated with a positive stain.[69] One must also keep in mind that alpha-fetoprotein may occasionally be positive in reactive processes,[70] so a positive stain does not in itself diagnose malignancy. Serum levels of alpha-fetoprotein greater than 500 ng/mL are highly associated with hepatocellular carcinoma, but not all tumors are associated with elevated levels (particularly the fibrolamellar variant).[51] Highlighting the abnormal sinusoids with CD34[68,71] or laminin[50] does not improve on the diagnostic information of the reticulin stain. Other stains for keratin, carcinoembryonic antigen, and alpha-1-antitrypsin are nondiscriminatory, as is electron microscopy (Boxes 33-5 and 33-6).[44,72]

HIGH-GRADE HEPATOCELLULAR CARCINOMA

High-grade hepatocellular carcinoma displays features of obvious malignancy—for example, smears of high cellularity with cellular crowding and nuclear overlapping, nuclear membrane abnormalities, hyperchromasia, and macronucleoli—which are many of the same features used to assess malignancy in a histologic preparation. Moderately differentiated hepatocellular carcinoma has relatively good hepatocellular preservation yet obvious malignant features, a morphology that makes it one of the easier grades to diagnose (Fig. 33-34). Poorly differentiated hepatocellular carcinoma is a tumor that is obviously malignant but has poor hepatocellular preservation and is difficult to distinguish from any other poorly differentiated tumor (Fig. 33-35).

Box 33–5. Well-differentiated Hepatocellular Carcinoma

- Low-power smear pattern with smooth-edged clusters and thickened trabeculae with peripherally wrapping endothelial cells (virtually pathognomonic)
- Low-power smear pattern with more than focal, loosely cohesive sheets of hepatocytes with transgressing vessels (highly suspicious finding)
- Monotonous uniform hepatocytic cell population with subtle malignant features
- Acinar cell formation in clusters
- Increased nucleus-to-cytoplasm ratio compared with normal hepatocytes
- Macroeosinophilic nucleoli
- Reduced number of binucleated cells
- Background free of bile duct epithelial cells
- Reticulin stain demonstrates reticulin loss and loss of the normal hepatic plate architecture (e.g., ≥3 cells thick)
- Iron stain fails to stain tumor in cases of hemochromatosis
- AFP is helpful if strongly positive, but often it is not

Box 33–6. Fibrolamellar Hepatocellular Carcinoma

- Population of large hepatocytes arranged singly and in loose clusters
- Smears may be paucicellular owing to fibrosis
- Transgressing vessels may be seen
- Deceptively low nucleus-to-cytoplasm ratio
- Large, variably atypical nuclei with prominent nucleoli and frequent intranuclear inclusions
- Cytoplasm is characteristically abundant and oncocytic-appearing

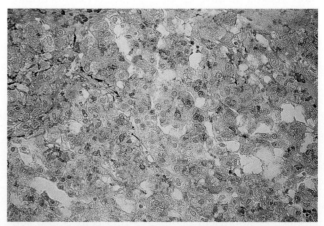

FIGURE 33–33. Reticulin staining on cell block preparations of hepatocellular carcinoma shows an abnormal reticulin staining pattern, mostly an absence of staining, in contrast to the maintained 1- or 2-cell-layer-thick black-staining hepatic framework of benign processes (not shown) (objective magnification 20×).

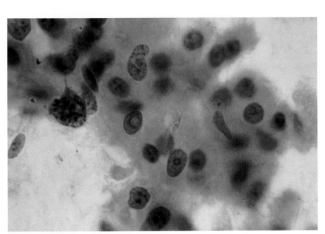

FIGURE 33–34. Moderately differentiated hepatocellular carcinoma maintains some hepatic preservation while displaying obvious malignant features (Papanicolaou, objective magnification 63×).

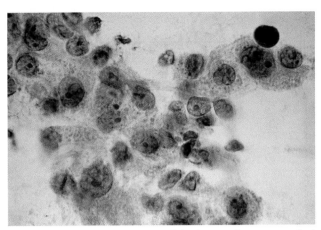

FIGURE 33–36. Intracytoplasmic bile (orange-brown in color) is identified in this cluster of malignant epithelial cells, pathognomonic of hepatocellular carcinoma (Papanicolaou, objective magnification 40×).

Smear patterns, especially the peripherally wrapping endothelial pattern, are equally important in the diagnosis of high-grade tumors. The presence of peripherally wrapping endothelial cells around the smooth-edged nests and trabeculae of cells eliminates the need for any confirmatory ancillary studies in most cases (see Fig. 33-27). This pattern is not a feature of other malignancies, in my experience. Tumors with a similar pattern are rare, and the pattern is usually only really appreciated on cell block preparations (see under Metastatic Neoplasms). The peripheral pattern is not a feature of metastatic renal cell carcinoma—a morphologic mimicker of hepatocellular carcinoma[73]—but the transgressing pattern is the most common pattern of renal cell carcinoma both in the kidney and in metastatic deposits (see Box 33-20).[73]

Although it is found in less than half of cases, the presence of bile production by malignant tumor cells is a pathognomonic finding for the diagnosis of hepatocellular carcinoma; when this is detected, no further studies should be necessary (Fig. 33-36).[2,56,64] Hall's stain (see Chapter 32) can be used to confirm the nature of the pigment as bile. The presence of intracytoplasmic mucin generally excludes hepatocellular carcinoma (except in the rare case of a combined hepatocellular cholangiocarcinoma), and its detection should focus the differential diagnosis on adenocarcinoma.

In addition to the fibrolamellar variant, morphologic variants to be noted include clear cell and acinar variants. The acinar cell variant is more of a diagnostic challenge on cell block preparations when the frequently back-to-back acini give the appearance of an adenocarcinoma (Fig. 33-37). There should be no mucin in the lumen of the acini or within the cytoplasm of the cells, and the

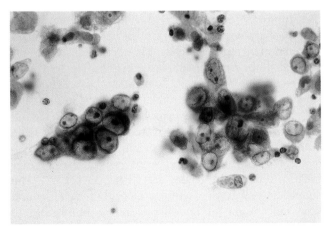

FIGURE 33–35. Poorly differentiated hepatocellular carcinoma displays an obviously malignant high-grade tumor without hepatic preservation and is difficult to distinguish from any other poorly differentiated tumor (Papanicolaou, objective magnification 40×).

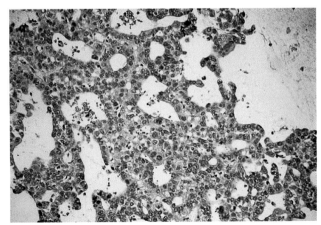

FIGURE 33–37. The acinar variant of hepatocellular carcinoma is apparent on cell block preparations, where numerous variably sized glandular spaces mimic the appearance of adenocarcinoma. Endothelial nuclei on the exterior of the cell clusters help confirm this as a form of hepatocellular carcinoma (objective magnification 10×).

Box 33–7. **Moderately Poorly Differentiated Hepatocellular Carcinoma**

- Peripherally wrapping endothelial smear pattern is virtually pathognomonic
- Transgressing vessels are suggestive but cannot distinguish hepatocellular from renal cell carcinoma
- Presence of intracytoplasmic bile is pathognomonic
- Polygonal cells with central nuclei and prominent nucleoli with visible, granular to clear cytoplasm in moderately differentiated tumors; scant to no cytoplasm in poorly differentiated tumors
- Immunophenotype: low-MW cytokeratin (Cam 5.2), polyclonal CEA, and CD10 (canalicular), HepPar-1-positive; AFP variable; high-MW cytokeratin (AE1)-usually negative

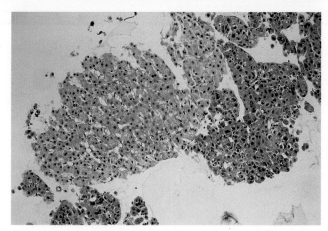

FIGURE 33–39. Cell block preparations of poorly differentiated hepatocellular carcinoma often demonstrate a more apparent hepatocytic morphology of tumor cells than may be apparent on smears (objective magnification 10×).

acini should be separated by similarly malignant cells with no true cribriforming. Immunohistochemical stains (Box 33-7) are helpful in establishing the correct diagnosis.

The clear cell variant introduces clear cell tumors metastatic from other sites (especially from the kidney) into the differential diagnosis. As has been mentioned, the peripherally wrapping endothelial pattern is a distinguishing finding excluding renal cell carcinoma, but the transgressing pattern is not. Morphologically, the clear malignant hepatocytes are large polygonal cells with central nuclei, large nucleoli, and abundant clear, vacuolated cytoplasm filled with glycogen (Fig. 33-38)[74,75]; these are impossible to distinguish from clear cells of renal cell carcinoma. Immunostains are usually required for diagnosis (see Box 33-20).

Cell block preparations may provide additional architectural and morphologic clues; it is not uncommon

for hepatocytic features to be more apparent in the cell block than on smear cytology (Fig. 33-39), potentially precluding the need for confirmatory studies.

The basic immunocytochemical panel in the differential diagnosis of hepatocellular carcinoma and metastatic carcinoma includes alpha-fetoprotein, low-molecular-weight (Cam 5.2) and high-molecular-weight (AE1) cytokeratin (CK), polyclonal carcinoembryonic antigen (CEA), and, more recently, antihepatocyte antibody (hepatocyte paraffin 1 [HepPar-1])[76-78] MOC-31,[79,80] and canalicular neprilysin (CD10) staining.[81] For a more detailed discussion and illustrations of hepatocellular carcinoma immunostaining, see Chapter 42.

Hepatoblastoma

Recapitulating the histomorphology of hepatoblastoma (see Chapter 42), the FNAB smears of this tumor can have a varied appearance according to the cell type of the tumor.[82,83] Smears of the epithelial or mixed epithelial and mesenchymal type of hepatoblastoma are dominated by epithelial cells. These epithelial cells may be fetal, embryonal, or anaplastic in type. The fetal-type cell resembles the normal hepatocyte but is generally smaller (Fig. 33-40). The nuclei are central, round, and bland-appearing, and the cytoplasm may contain fat and glycogen, unlike the embryonal cell type.[84,85] The embryonal cell is primitive and undifferentiated with hyperchromatic nuclei and scant cytoplasm that may form rosettes and trabeculae (Fig. 33-41).[85,86] The anaplastic cell type resembles any other small, round blue cell tumor of childhood and is impossible to distinguish from neuroblastoma or Wilms' tumor on the basis of morphology alone.[87] The mesenchymal component, if present, occurs as cellular, spindle cell–type mesenchyme, but heterologous elements, including

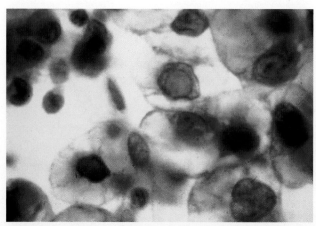

FIGURE 33–38. Clear cell hepatocellular carcinoma demonstrates polygonal cells with abundant vacuolated cytoplasm mimicking other clear cell tumors, especially renal cell carcinoma (Papanicolaou, objective magnification 63×). (From Pitman MB, Szyfelbein WM: Fine Needle Aspiration Biopsy of the Liver. London, Hodder Arnold, 1994, p 66.)

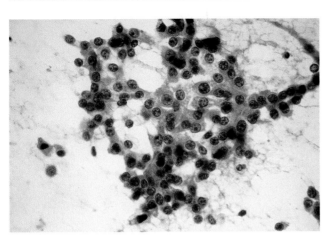

FIGURE 33–40. Hepatoblastoma, fetal type. The fetal-type cells resemble the normal hepatocyte but are generally smaller with central, round, and bland nucleoli (Papanicolaou, objective magnification, 25×).

osteoid, cartilage, skeletal muscle, and particularly extramedullary hematopoiesis, may also be noted.[84-86] A myxoid matrix has been described.[88]

The primary differential diagnosis rests most frequently between the fetal-type hepatoblastoma and hepatocellular carcinoma, and between embryonal or anaplastic hepatoblastoma and other pediatric small, round blue cell tumors.[88,89] No cytomorphologic feature alone can aid in the narrowing of either differential diagnosis; ancillary studies and clinicopathologic correlation are required to do this. Of course, HepPar-1 positivity supports a hepatic primary over other small, round blue cell tumors of nonhepatic origin,[76-78,89] but this stain cannot separate hepatoblastoma from hepatocellular carcinoma. Cytokeratin staining can be helpful in that tumor cells of most hepatoblastomas stain with high-

Box 33–8. **Hepatoblastoma**

- Epithelial dominant smears; some mesenchymal (spindle cell) component and/or heterologous elements may be seen, especially extramedullary hematopoiesis
- Epithelial cells may be small hepatocytic cells (fetal type), smaller pleomorphic cells (embryonal type), or smaller still undifferentiated blue cells (anaplastic type)
- Epithelial cells may be present in cohesive, crowded clusters, cords, ribbons, or rosettes
- Immunophenotype: positive for low-MW and high-MW cytokeratin (Cam 5.2 and AE1), polyclonal CEA (carcinoembryonic antigen) with variable canalicular/cytoplasmic staining, HepPar-1

molecular-weight CK,[90] whereas tumor cells of most hepatocellular carcinomas do not.[91] Both tumors stain with low-molecular-weight CK (Cam 5.2).[90] Polyclonal CEA stains hepatoblastomas with a variable and inconsistent canalicular and/or cytoplasmic pattern, depending on the type of hepatoblastoma.[89] This stain does not distinguish hepatoblastoma from hepatocellular carcinoma but can help in the distinction between a primary and a metastatic tumor (Box 33-8).

Cholangiocarcinoma

The most common histologic appearance of cholangiocarcinoma is a well- to moderately differentiated adenocarcinoma that forms tubules infiltrating a sclerotic stroma.[93] Although this morphology is characteristic of cholangiocarcinoma and can distinguish cholangiocarcinoma from hepatocellular carcinoma, it is not specific for cholangiocarcinoma and cannot separate this tumor from metastatic adenocarcinoma.

Aspirate smears generally produce a readily recognizable adenocarcinoma with nonspecific features. A low-power smear pattern demonstrating irregular, variably sized sheets of atypical to malignant-appearing glandular cells that resemble bile duct epithelium is suggestive of a primary adenocarcinoma (Fig. 33-42). Clusters of tumor cells may resemble hepatocellular carcinoma; however, no intracytoplasmic bile is seen, intracytoplasmic mucin may be noted, and no peripherally wrapping endothelial cells are seen around cell clusters (Fig. 33-43).[4]

Cell block preparations are particularly helpful in this diagnosis because the characteristic common histologic pattern described previously may be recognized (Fig. 33-44) and may reveal a peritumoral portal tract with the usual finding of in situ carcinoma or dysplasia (Fig. 33-45). Cell blocks also provide easily accessible tissue for immunohistochemical stains that may help in the differential diagnosis (see Chapter 42) (Box 33-9).

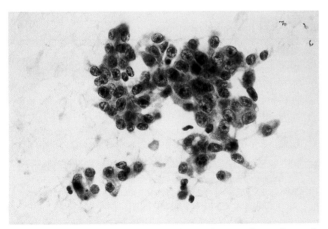

FIGURE 33–41. Hepatoblastoma, embryonal type. The embryonal-type cell is more primitive than the fetal cell type and undifferentiated with hyperchromatic nucleoli and scant cytoplasm (Papanicolaou, objective magnification, 25×).

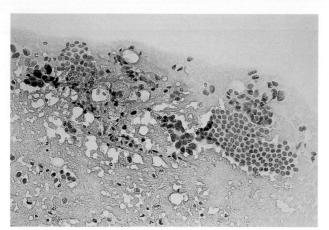

FIGURE 33–42. Cholangiocarcinoma. This low-power smear pattern demonstrates irregular, variably sized sheets of atypical to malignant-appearing glandular cells that resemble bile duct epithelium, admixed with sheets of benign bile duct epithelium (rapid hematoxylin and eosin, objective magnification 2.5×).

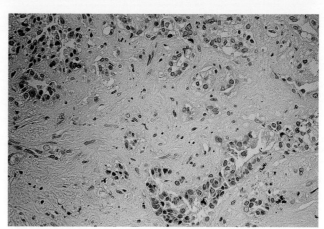

FIGURE 33–44. Cholangiocarcinoma. Cell block preparations of tissue fragments may demonstrate the characteristic sclerosis of this tumor (objective magnification 10×).

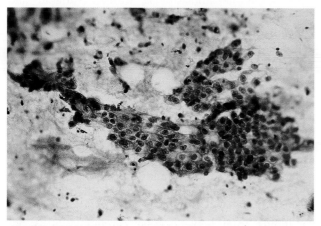

FIGURE 33–43. Cholangiocarcinoma. Clusters of tumor cells may resemble hepatocellular carcinoma. The absence of peripherally wrapping endothelium, the absence of intracytoplasmic bile, and the presence of intracytoplasmic mucin support a diagnosis of adenocarcinoma (Papanicolaou, objective magnification 10×).

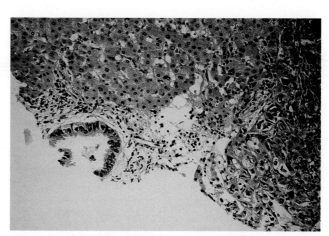

FIGURE 33–45. Cholangiocarcinoma. A cell block of a core needle biopsy shows a peritumoral portal tract containing in situ cholangiocarcinoma (objective magnification 20×).

Angiosarcoma

Aspirate smears are bloody and may be paucicellular.[93] Malignant endothelial cells can be seen interdigitating among reactive hepatocytes. These malignant endothelial cells have elongated, spindle-shaped hyperchromatic nuclei that are easier to appreciate in small clusters (Fig. 33-46) than in large clusters, where they tend to blend into the hepatocytes (Fig. 33-47). Tumor cells should stain positively for factor VIII, CD31, CD34, or *Ulex europaeus* lectin[94,95] (Box 33-10).

Box 33–9. Cholangiocarcinoma

- Glandular cells in flat, angulated sheets
- Can see exaggerated honeycombed pattern caused by mucinous cytoplasm
- Nuclei are variably atypical, depending on grade, but most are of relatively low grade
- A range of atypia may be seen, from borderline malignant-appearing to obviously malignant-looking
- Impossible to definitely distinguish from other adenocarcinomas on the basis of morphology alone
- Cell blocks can help by demonstrating sclerotic stroma and possibly a portal tract with in situ cholangiocarcinoma

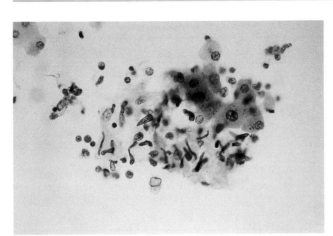

FIGURE 33–46. Angiosarcoma. Malignant endothelial cells with elongated spindle-shaped hyperchromatic nuclei are easiest to appreciate in small clusters (Papanicolaou, objective magnification 10×).

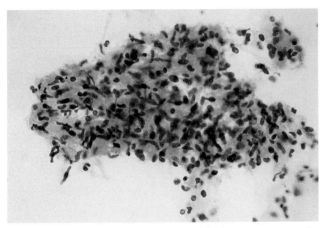

FIGURE 33–47. Angiosarcoma. Larger cell clusters appear to be hypercellular, and individual malignant endothelial cells are more difficult to separate from the reactive hepatocytes than in smaller clusters (Papanicolaou, objective magnification 25×).

Box 33–10. **Angiosarcoma**

- Atypical to overtly malignant endothelial cells interspersed with hepatocytic clusters
- Spindle cell sarcoma, possibly with blood lakes
- Immunocytochemistry stains: factor VIII, CD31, CD34, *Ulex europaeus* lectin

Embryonal Sarcoma (Box 33-11)

Embryonal sarcoma produces aspirate smears that recapitulate the varied histologic pattern of this tumor.[96-98] Smears are generally hypercellular and are composed of large, anaplastic cells (Fig. 33-48), multinucleated tumor giant cells, and atypical spindled cells. Intracytoplasmic globules that are periodic acid–Schiff (PAS)-positive but –diastase resistant may be seen (Fig. 33-49).

Box 33–11. **Embryonal Sarcoma**

- Hypercellular smears
- Large, pleomorphic anaplastic cells with multinucleated giant cells and atypical spindled cells
- Intracytoplasmic globules that are PAS-positive, diastase-resistant

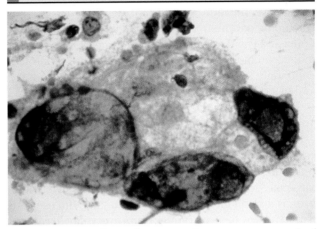

FIGURE 33–48. Embryonal sarcoma. Smears are composed of large, anaplastic, often multinucleated tumor giant cells (rapid hematoxylin and eosin, objective magnification 100× oil).

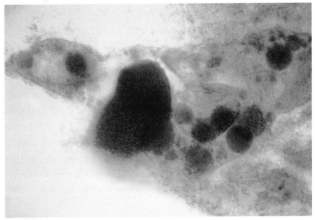

FIGURE 33–49. Embryonal sarcoma. Tumor cells may also contain PAS-positive diastase-resistant intracytoplasmic globules (PAS with diastase, objective magnification 100× oil).

METASTATIC NEOPLASMS

The distinction between primary and metastatic malignancy in the liver is of both therapeutic and prognostic significance. A vast majority of malignancies in the liver are metastases,[99] and as such, the most common purpose for FNAB is the evaluation of suspected metastatic disease. In most cases, the patient has a known history of a primary tumor. This history is vital in evaluating the morphology and in determining whether it is compatible with that primary site. Metastatic tumors tend to recapitulate their appearance in the primary organ, and specific tumor types such as small cell carcinoma and lymphoma generally maintain a consistent cytologic appearance. Adenocarcinoma, although frequently recognizable as an entity, presents the greatest difficulty for those attempting to make a specific diagnosis as to site of origin. Fortunately, it is the recognition of adenocarcinoma alone that affects patient management and prognosis.[100]

Metastatic tumors commonly encountered in FNAB of the liver include those from the pancreas (adenocarcinoma and neuroendocrine), stomach (adenocarcinoma and gastrointestinal stromal tumors), breast, lung (adenocarcinoma, small cell carcinoma, and much less commonly, squamous cell carcinoma), skin (melanoma), and bladder. Lymphoma is also commonly seen.

Less common but diagnostically more challenging are metastases from the kidney and adrenal gland, often exhibiting morphologic overlap with hepatocellular carcinoma. Sarcomas are the least encountered tumor type; the most common type of sarcoma is leiomyosarcoma, generally from the uterus.[99] The liver, however, is a frequent depository of metastatic disease, and almost every type of tumor from every site has been described there. More information on the epidemiology and general characteristics of metastatic tumors can be found in Chapter 42.

The cytologic features helpful in the diagnosis of a variety of metastatic tumors are presented here with accompanying supportive ancillary tests and illustrations (Boxes 33-12 through 33-23; Figs. 33-50 through 33-61) but without further discussion.

Adenocarcinoma from the colon is the most common metastasis to the liver.[99] The presence of an adenocarcinoma with a "dirty necrosis" background is sufficient for a diagnosis of adenocarcinoma consistent with colon primary in a patient with a history of colon cancer; the presence of these features should direct the clinician to evaluate the colon first in a patient with an unknown primary.

If lymphoma is suspected on rapid interpretation, a dedicated aspirate should be requested for flow cytometry analysis (i.e., the aspirate is not expressed onto a slide, but rather the aspirated tissue is rinsed into buffered normal saline, cytolyte solution, or RPMI). The combination of cytologic evaluation and flow cytometry immunophenotyping is often sufficient for a subclassified diagnosis of non-Hodgkin's lymphoma.[101-105]

Hepatoid yolk sac tumor is another tumor that can demonstrate a peripherally wrapping endothelial pattern similar to hepatocellular carcinoma and adrenal carcinoma, although I have not seen a case in which this was present on the smears; it was seen only on the cell block preparations. Patients with this germ cell tumor invariably have a history of such a tumor, and confirmation of metastasis can be achieved with positivity of tumor cells for placental alkaline phosphatase, a marker that is negative in primary hepatic tumors.[106]

Spindle cell tumors in the liver are relatively

Box 33–12. Adenocarcinoma (General)

- Polygonal to columnar glandular cells arranged in flat, monolayered sheets, in three-dimensional clusters, or singly
- Lumina within clusters may be seen in some cases
- Nuclei are variably atypical, ranging from bland in low-grade tumors to extremely atypical and obviously malignant in high-grade tumors
- Cytoplasm is delicate and frequently vacuolated, sometimes wispy
- Intracytoplasmic mucin may be seen; mucicarmine or other mucin stains can help identify focal mucin production

Box 33–13. Colonic Adenocarcinoma (Fig. 33-50)

- Cigar-shaped, often palisaded nuclei
- Variably prominent nucleoli with no macroeosinophilic nucleoli
- Dirty necrosis in the background (important)
- Immunocytochemistry: CK20+, CK7–, CEA+

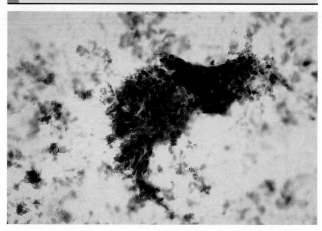

FIGURE 33–50. Metastatic colon adenocarcinoma. Cigar-shaped, often palisaded nuclei are present. Glandular cell clusters appear in a background of distinctive dirty necrosis (Papanicolaou, objective magnification 10×).

Box 33–14. Breast Carcinoma, Ductal Type (Fig. 33-51)

- Often low-grade with a monomorphous cell population
- Flat, angulated groups
- Single flame- or cone-shaped cells
- Target cells (cells with intracytoplasmic lumen)
- Cell-in-cell arrangement
- Immunocytochemistry
  - Estrogen/progesterone: ± but nonspecific
  - Gross cystic disease protein-15 is supportive if positive

uncommon.[35] In the metastatic category, gastrointestinal stromal tumors and leiomyosarcomas are the most important to distinguish for therapeutic purposes.[107,108]

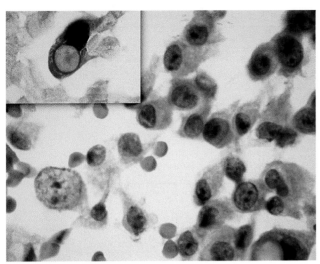

FIGURE 33–51. Metastatic breast carcinoma, ductal type. Distinctive flame- or cone-shaped cells in a dyshesive single-cell pattern with scattered "target cells" *(lower right and inset)* demonstrating intracytoplasmic lumina are characteristic of breast carcinoma (Papanicolaou, objective magnification 40×).

Box 33–15. **Squamous Cell Carcinoma** (Fig. 33-52)

- Relatively uncommon metastasis to the liver
- Large polygonal cells singly and in clusters
- Usually high-grade with large, hyperchromatic nuclei and irregular nuclear membranes
- Cytoplasm is dense and nonvacuolated as opposed to that of adenocarcinoma
- Keratinizing squamous cells stain orangeophilic on Papanicolaou stain, but this feature may not be noted

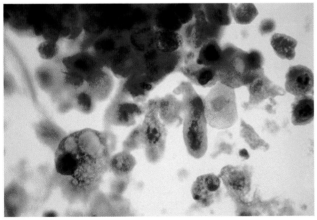

FIGURE 33–52. Metastatic squamous cell carcinoma. This uncommon metastasis to the liver is characterized by large polygonal cells with dense nonvacuolated cytoplasm and occasionally keratinized cells that stain orangeophilic on Papanicolaou stain (objective magnification 40×). (A hepatocyte with fat droplets is also present.)

Box 33–16. **Small Cell Undifferentiated Carcinoma** (Fig. 33-53)

- Small pleomorphic blue cells with little to no cytoplasm in clusters and arranged singly
- Nuclei are hyperchromatic with coarse, stippled chromatin
- Nuclear molding is common and characteristic
- Necrosis and apoptosis are common
- Smear or crush artifact is invariably present because of the fragile nature of the cells

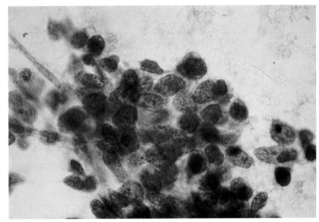

FIGURE 33–53. Metastatic small cell undifferentiated carcinoma. Small blue pleomorphic cells with little to no cytoplasm are present in clusters, demonstrating hyperchromatic, often molded nuclei with stippled chromatin (Papanicolaou, objective magnification 63×).

Box 33–17. **Neuroendocrine Tumors*** (Figs. 33-54 and 33-55)

- Small uniform blue cells with visible cytoplasm that tends to be scant and more evenly perinuclear in carcinoid tumors and more abundant and eccentric in PET
- Nuclei with coarse, stippled chromatin; more obvious in carcinoids than in PET
- Nucleoli generally not present in carcinoid tumors but visible in PET
- No nuclear molding, much less crush artifact, and no significant necrosis/apoptosis compared with small cell undifferentiated carcinoma

*For instance, metastatic pancreatic endocrine tumor (PET) and carcinoid tumor.

Box 33–18. **Non-Hodgkin's Lymphoma** (Fig. 33-56)

- Mostly large B-cell lymphoma
- Dyshesive, single-cell population; may have pseudogroups (e.g., artifactual clustering)
- Lymphoglandular bodies (globules of stripped cytoplasm) in the background
- Coarse, frequently peripherally clumped chromatin
- Nucleoli may be present
- Cytoplasm is scant to invisible but may be abundant in anaplastic large cell lymphoma

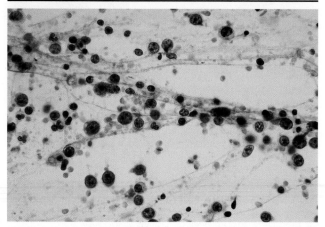

FIGURE 33–56. Non-Hodgkin's lymphoma. Most commonly a large B-cell lymphoma, the smears are characterized by a dyshesive single-cell pattern of large cells with peripherally clumped chromatin, scant to no cytoplasm, occasionally prominent nucleoli, and scattered lymphoglandular bodies (stripped cytoplasmic fragments) in the background (Papanicolaou, objective magnification 40×).

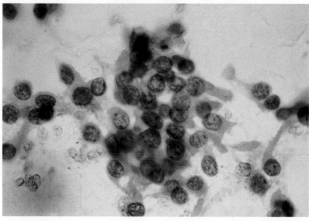

FIGURE 33–54. Metastatic carcinoid tumor. Small uniform blue cells with scant cytoplasm, coarse stippled chromatin, no necrosis, no nuclear molding, and generally no nucleoli are characteristic (Papanicolaou, objective magnification 63×).

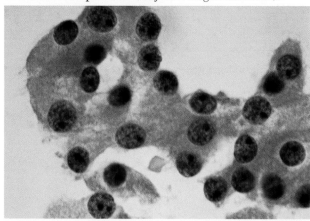

FIGURE 33–55. Metastatic pancreatic endocrine tumor (PET). Uniform tumor cells often demonstrate plasmacytoid features with eccentric nuclei, a more open stippled chromatin pattern, and frequently prominent nucleoli (Papanicolaou, objective magnification 40×). (Courtesy of Dr. Vikram Deshpande, MGH, Boston.)

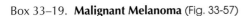

Box 33–19. **Malignant Melanoma** (Fig. 33-57)

- Large polygonal cells arranged singly and in clusters; may also be spindled or small blue cells with scant cytoplasm
- Central to eccentric nuclei with large nucleoli
- Intranuclear inclusions common
- Cytoplasm is commonly abundant, nongranular, and frequently nonpigmented
- Fontana-Masson stain stains cytoplasmic melanin pigment black but also stains lipofuscin (pitfall)
- Immunocytochemistry: S100, HMB-45, MART-1, and Melan-A–positive; keratin-negative

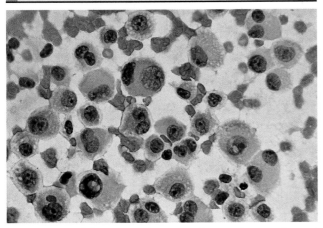

FIGURE 33–57. Metastatic malignant melanoma. Large polygonal cells both singly and in clusters may be polygonal or spindled with large macroeosinophilic nucleoli and frequent intranuclear inclusions (Papanicolaou, objective magnification 40×).

Box 33–20. **Renal Cell Carcinoma** (Fig. 33-58)

- Large polygonal cells arranged singly and in clusters
- Transgressing endothelial pattern is the most common vascular pattern, but peripherally wrapping endothelial pattern is not a feature
- Round central nuclei with prominent macronucleoli ("owl's eye") in typical clear/granular cell type; papillary renal cell carcinoma (RCC) type does not demonstrate prominent nucleoli
- Intranuclear inclusions can be seen and are frequent in chromophobe type
- Cytoplasm is commonly abundant and clear or granular; excessive and "balloon-like" in chromophobe RCC and scant, often with hemosiderin in papillary RCC
- Immunocytochemistry: keratin, vimentin, CD10, and EMA (epithelial membrane antigen)–positive; CEA-negative

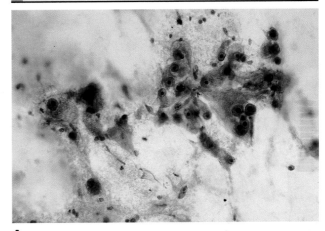

A

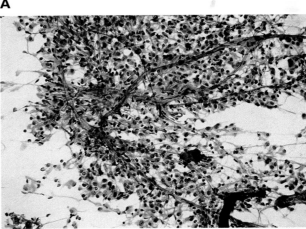

B

FIGURE 33–58. A, Metastatic renal cell carcinoma. The classic appearance of renal cell carcinoma is that of large polygonal cells with clear to granular cytoplasm, central nuclei, and large macroeosinophilic nucleoli (Papanicolaou, objective magnification 40×). **B,** The transgressing endothelial pattern is the most common vascular pattern of renal cell carcinoma and cannot be used as a feature to distinguish hepatocellular carcinoma from metatastatic renal cell carcinoma (Papanicolaou, objective magnification 5×).

Box 33–21. **Adrenal Carcinoma** (Fig. 33-59)

- Medium-sized polygonal cells arranged singly and in clusters
- No transgressing endothelial pattern but peripherally wrapping endothelial pattern may be seen on cell block
- Nuclei are variably atypical with hyperchromasia and pleomorphism; nucleoli do not tend to be macro-eosinophilic as in hepatocellular carcinoma
- Immunocytochemistry: keratin, EMA, CEA–negative; vimentin, synaptophysin, inhibin, Melan-A–positive

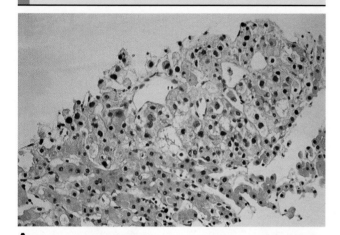

A

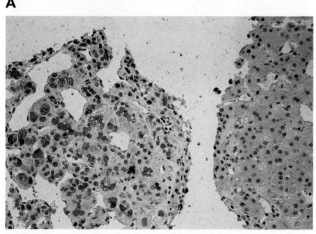

B

FIGURE 33–59. A, Metastatic adrenal carcinoma. This cell block preparation demonstrates the remarkable morphologic similarity between hepatocellular carcinoma and metastatic adrenal cell carcinoma, with large polygonal cells forming pseudoacini (objective magnification 10×). **B,** Immunohistochemical stain for Melan-A helps to distinguish metastatic adrenal cell carcinoma (positive) from hepatocellular carcinoma (negative) (avidin-biotin antiperoxidase, objective magnification 10×).

Box 33–22. **Gastrointestinal Stromal Tumor** (Fig. 33-60)

- Monomorphic spindle cells in loose groups and arranged singly; occasional epithelioid features
- Prominent vascular pattern
- Relatively bland nuclei without overt hyperchromasia or pleomorphism
- Delicate cytoplasmic processes
- Little to no crush artifact
- Immunophenotype: c-*kit* (CD117)–positive; smooth muscle actin–variably positive; desmin–negative

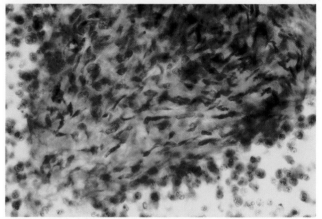

FIGURE 33–60. Metastatic gastrointestinal stromal tumor. Monomorphic spindle cells with delicate cytoplasmic processes demonstrating little to no crush artifact help to separate this tumor from metastatic leiomyosarcoma (Papanicolaou, objective magnification 40×).

Box 33–23. **Leiomyosarcoma** (Fig. 33-61)

- Pleomorphic spindle cells in tightly cohesive three-dimensional groups and syncytia; occasional epithelioid features
- No prominent vascular pattern
- Hyperchromatic, pleomorphic nuclei with crush artifact common
- Wiry, refractile cytoplasmic processes and/or stroma
- Immunophenotype: Desmin and smooth muscle actin positive; c-*kit* negative

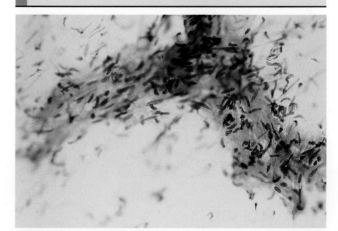

FIGURE 33–61. Metastatic leiomyosarcoma. Pleomorphic spindle cells and tightly cohesive groups without a prominent vascular pattern demonstrate wiry refractile cytoplasmic processes as opposed to those of a gastrointestinal stromal tumor (as seen in Fig. 33-60) (Papanicolaou, objective magnification 40×).

References

1. Bergman S, Graeme-Cook F, Pitman MB: The usefulness of the reticulin stain in the differential diagnosis of liver nodules on fine-needle aspiration biopsy cell block preparations. Mod Pathol 10:1-7, 1997.

2. Kung ITM, Chan SK, Fung KH: Fine-needle aspiration in hepatocellular carcinoma: Combined cytologic and histologic approach. Cancer 67:673-680, 1991.

3. Pisharodi LR, Lavoie R, Bedrossian CWM: Differential diagnostic dilemmas in malignant fine-needle aspirates of liver: A practical approach to final diagnosis. Diagn Cytopathol 12:364-371, 1995.

4. Pitman MB, Szyfelbein WM: The significance of endothelium in the FNA diagnosis of hepatocellular carcinoma. Diagn Cytopathol 12:208-214, 1995.

5. Suen KC: Diagnosis of primary hepatic neoplasm by fine needle aspiration biopsy cytology. Diagn Cytopathol 2:99-109, 1986.

6. Welch TJ, Sheedy PF, Johnson CD, et al: CT-guided biopsy: Prospective analysis of 1,000 procedures. Radiology 171:493-496, 1989.

7. Whitlatch S, Nunez C, Pitlik DA: Fine needle aspiration biopsy of the liver. A study of 102 consecutive cases. Acta Cytol 28:719-725, 1984.

8. Centeno BA, Pitman MB: Fine Needle Aspiration Biopsy of the Pancreas. Boston, Butterworth-Heinemann, 1999.

9. Bret PM, Fond A, Casola G, et al: Abdominal lesions: A prospective study of clinical efficacy of percutaneous fine-needle biopsy. Radiology 159:345-346, 1986.

10. Quirk DW, Brugge WR: Endoscopic ultrasonography-directed fine needle aspiration. In Centeno BA, Pitman MB (eds): Fine Needle Aspiration Biopsy of the Pancreas. Boston, Butterworth-Heinemann, 1999, pp 13-16.

11. Nguyen P, Feng JC, Chang KJ: Endoscopic ultrasound (EUS) and EUS-guided fine-needle aspiration (FNA) of liver lesions. Gastrointest Endosc 50:357-361, 1999.

12. Caletti G, Fusaroli P: Endoscopic ultrasonography. Endoscopy 33:158-166, 2001.

13. Fritscher-Ravens A, Broering DC, Sriram PV, et al: EUS-guided fine-needle aspiration cytodiagnosis of hilar cholangiosarcoma: A case series. Gastrointest Endosc 52:534-540, 2000.

14. Pitman MB, Szyfelbein WM: Fine Needle Aspiration Biopsy of the Liver. Boston, Butterworth-Heinemann, 1994, p 88.

15. Smith EH: Complications of percutaneous abdominal fine-needle biopsy. Radiology 178:253-258, 1991.

16. Vergara V, Garripoli A, Marucci MM, et al: Colon cancer seeding after percutaneous fine needle aspiration of liver metastasis. J Hepatol 18:276-278, 1993.

17. Yamada N, Shinzawa H, Ukai K, et al: Subcutaneous seeding of small hepatocellular carcinoma after fine needle aspiration biopsy. J Gastroenterol Hepatol 8:195-198, 1993.

18. Hamazaki K, Matsubara N, Mori M, et al: Needle track implantation of hepatocellular carcinoma after ultrasonically guided needle liver biopsy: A case report. Hepatogastroenterology 42:601-606, 1995.

19. Giovanni M, Seitz J, Monges G: Fine needle aspiration cytology guided by endoscopic ultrasonography: Results in 141 patients. Endoscopy 27:171-177, 1995.

20. Bentz JS, Kochman ML, Faigel DO, et al: Endoscopic ultrasound-guided real-time fine-needle aspiration: Clinicopathologic features of 60 patients. Diagn Cytopathol 18:98-109, 1998.

21. Wiersema MJ, Kochman ML, Cramer HM, et al: Endosonography-guided real-time fine-needle aspiration biopsy. Gastrointest Endosc 40:700-707, 1994.

22. Wittenberg J, Mueller PR, Ferrucci JT, et al: Percutaneous core biopsy of abdominal tumors using 22 gauge needles: Further observations. AJR Am J Roentgenol 139:75-80, 1982.

23. Isler RJ, Ferucci JT, Wittenberg J, et al: Tissue core biopsy of abdominal tumors with a 22 gauge cutting needle. AJR Am J Roentgenol 136:725-728, 1981.

24. Bell DA, Carr CP, Szyfelbein WM: Fine needle aspiration cytology of focal liver lesions. Results obtained with examination of both cytologic and histologic preparations. Acta Cytol 30:397-402, 1986.

25. Hahn PF, Eisenberg PJ, Pitman MB, et al: Cytopathologic touch preparations (imprints) from core needle biopsies: Accuracy compared with that of fine-needle aspirates. AJR Am J Roentgenol 165:1277-1279, 1995.

26. Austin JHM, Cohen MB: Value of having a cytopathologist present during percutaneous fine-needle aspiration biopsy of lung: Report of 55 cancer patients and metaanalysis of the literature. AJR Am J Roentgenol 160:175-177, 1993.

27. Miller DA, Carrasco CH, Katz RL, et al: Fine needle aspiration biopsy: The role of immediate cytologic assessment. AJR Am J Roentgenol 147:155-158, 1986.

28. Pak HY, Yokota S, Teplitz RL, et al: Rapid staining techniques employed in fine needle aspirations of the lung. Acta Cytol 25:178-184, 1981.

29. Brennick JB, O'Connell JX, Dickersin GR, et al: Lipofuscin pigmentation (so-called) "melanosis" of the prostate. Am J Surg Pathol 18:446-454, 1994.

30. Terada T, Nakanuma Y: Iron-negative foci in sideriotic macroregenerative nodules in human cirrhotic liver. A marker of incipient neoplastic lesions. Arch Pathol Lab Med 113:916-920, 1989.

31. Layfield LJ: Focal fatty change of the liver: Cytologic findings in a radiographic mimic of metastases. Diagn Cytopathol 11:385-387, 1994.

32. Leiman G, Leibowitz CB, Dunbar F: Fine-needle aspiration of the liver: Out of the ivory tower and into the community. Diagn Cytopathol 5:35-39, 1989.

33. Cho C, Rullis I, Rogers LS: Bile duct adenomas as liver nodules. Arch Surg 113:272-274, 1978.

34. Iha H, Nakashima Y, Fukukura Y, et al: Biliary hamartomas simulating multiple hepatic metastasis on imaging findings. Kurume Med J 43:231-235, 1996.

35. Guy CD, Yuan S, Ballo MS: Spindle-cell lesions of the liver: Diagnosis by fine-needle aspiration biopsy. Diagn Cytopathol 25:94-100, 2001.

36. Layfield LJ, Mooney EE, Dodd LG: Not by blood alone: Diagnosis of hemangiomas by fine-needle aspiration. Diagn Cytopathol 19:250-254, 1998.

37. Sawai H, Manabe T, Yamanaka Y, et al: Angiomyolipoma of the liver: Case report and collective review of cases diagnosed from fine needle aspiration biopsy specimens. J Hepatobiliary Pancreat Surg 5:333-338, 1998.

38. Cha I, Cartwright D, Guis M, et al: Angiomyolipoma of the liver in fine-needle aspiration biopsies: Its distinction from hepatocellular carcinoma. Cancer 87:25-30, 1999.

39. Blasco A, Vargas J, deAgustin P, et al: Solitary angiomyolipoma of the liver. Report of a case with diagnosis by fine needle aspiration biopsy. Acta Cytol 39:813-816, 1995.

40. Mai KT, Yazdi HM, Perkins DG, et al: Fine needle aspiration biopsy of epithelioid angiomyolipoma. A case report. Acta Cytol 45:233-236, 2001.

41. Sturtz CL, Dabbs DJ: Angiomyolipomas: The nature and expression of the HMB45 antigen. Mod Pathol 7:842-845, 1994.

42. deBoer WB: Cytodiagnosis of well differentiated hepatocellular carcinoma: Can indeterminate diagnoses be reduced? Cancer Cytopathol 87:270-277, 1999.

43. Cohen MB, Egerter DP, Holly EA, et al: Pancreatic adenocarcinoma: Regression analysis to identify improved cytologic criteria. Diagn Cytopathol 7:341-345, 1991.

44. Silverman JF, Geisinger KR: Ancillary studies in FNA of liver and pancreas. Diagn Cytopathol 13:396-410, 1995.

45. Sóle M, Calvet X, Cuberes T, et al: Value and limitations of cytologic criteria for the diagnosis of hepatocellular carcinoma by fine needle aspiration biopsy. Acta Cytol 37:309-316, 1993.

46. Tao LC, Ho CS, McLoughlin MJ, et al: Cytologic diagnosis of hepatocellular carcinoma by fine needle aspiration biopsy. Cancer 53:547-552, 1984.

47. Cohen MB, Haber MM, Holly EA, et al: Cytologic criteria to distinguish hepatocellular carcinoma from nonneoplastic liver. Am J Clin Pathol 95:125-130, 1991.

48. Noguchi S, Yamamoto R, Tatsuta M, et al: Cell features and patterns in fine-needle aspirates of hepatocellular carcinoma. Cancer 58:321-328, 1986.

49. Haratake J, Hisaoka M, Yamamoto O, et al: An ultrastructural comparison of sinusoids in hepatocellular carcinoma, adenomatous hyperplasia, and fetal liver. Arch Pathol Lab Med 116:67-70, 1992.

50. Williams SS, Pitman MB, Szyfelbein WM, et al: Laminin immunostaining differentiates well-differentiated hepatocellular carcinoma from benign tissue in FNAB of liver. Mod Pathol 13:58A, 2000.

51. Craig JR, Peters RL, Edmondson HA, et al: Fibrolamellar carcinoma of the liver: A tumor of adolescents and young adults with distinctive clinico-pathologic features. Cancer 46:372-379, 1980.

52. Farhi DC, Shikes RH, Murari PJ, et al: Hepatocellular carcinoma in young people. Cancer 52:1516-1525, 1983.

53. Hodgson HJF: Fibrolamellar cancer of the liver. J Hepatol 5:241-247, 1987.

54. Perez-Guillermo M, Masgrau NA, Garcia-Solano J, et al: Cytologic aspect of fibrolamellar hepatocellular carcinoma in fine-needle aspirates. Diagn Cytopathol 21:180-187, 1999.

55. Ali MA, Akhtar M, Mattingly RC: Morphologic spectrum of hepatocellular carcinoma in fine needle aspiration biopsies. Acta Cytol 30:294-302, 1986.

56. Bottles K, Cohen MB, Holly EA, et al: A step-wise logistic regression analysis of hepatocellular carcinoma. Cancer 62:558-563, 1988.

57. Domagala W, Lasota J, Weber K, et al: Endothelial cells help in the diagnosis of primary versus metastatic carcinoma of the liver in fine needle aspirates. An immunofluorescence study with vimentin and endothelial cell-specific antibodies. Anal Quant Cytol Histol 11:8-14, 1989.

58. Gagliano EF: Reticulin stain in the fine needle aspiration differential diagnosis of liver nodules. Acta Cytol 39:596-598, 1995.

59. Greene CA, Suen KC: Some cytologic features of hepatocellular carcinoma as seen in fine needle aspirates. Acta Cytol 28:713-718, 1984.

60. Nguyen GK: Fine-needle aspiration biopsy cytology of hepatic tumors in adults. Pathol Annu 21:321-349, 1986.

61. Pedio G, Landolt V, Zöbeli L, et al: Fine needle aspiration of the liver: Significance of hepatocytic naked nuclei in the diagnosis of hepatocellular carcinoma. Acta Cytol 32:437-442, 1988.

62. Pilotti S, Rilke F, Claren R, et al: Conclusive diagnosis of hepatic and pancreatic malignancies by fine needle aspiration. Acta Cytol 32:27-38, 1988.

63. Salomao DR, Lloyd RV, Goellner JR: Hepatocellular carcinoma: Needle biopsy findings in 74 cases. Diagn Cytopathol 16:8-13, 1997.

64. Wee A, Nilsson B, Chan-Wilde C, et al: Fine needle aspiration biopsy of hepatocellular carcinoma. Some unusual features. Acta Cytol 35:661-670, 1991.

65. Longchampt E, Patriarche C, Fabre M: Accuracy of cytology vs. microbiopsy for the diagnosis of well-differentiated hepatocellular carcinoma and macroregenerative nodule. Definition of standardized criteria from a study of 100 cases. Acta Cytol 44:515-523, 2000.

66. Cappellari JO, Geisinger KR, Albertson DA, et al: Malignant papillary cystic tumor of the pancreas. Cancer 66:193-198, 1990.

67. Ljung BM, Ferrell LD: Fine-needle aspiration biopsy of the liver: Diagnostic problems. In Williams R (ed): Pathology: State of the Art Reviews. Philadelphia, Hanley & Belfus, 1996, pp 365-388.

68. de Boer WB, Segal A, Frost FA, Sterrett GF: Can CD34 discriminate between benign and malignant hepatocytic lesions in fine-needle aspirates and thin core biopsies? Cancer 90:273-278, 2000.

69. Imoto M, Nishimura D, Fukuda Y, et al: Immunohistochemical detection of alpha-fetoprotein, carcinoembryonic antigen and ferritin in formalin-paraffin sections from hepatocellular carcinoma. Am J Gastroenterol 80:902-906, 1985.

70. Roncalli M, Borzio M, DeBiagi G, et al: Liver cell dysplasia and hepatocellular carcinoma: A histological and immunohistochemical study. Histopathology 9:209-221, 1985.

71. Kong CS, Appenzeller M, Ferrell LD: Utility of CD34 reactivity in evaluating focal nodular hepatocellular lesions sampled by fine needle aspiration biopsy. Acta Cytol 44:218-222, 2000.

72. Johnson DE, Powers CN, Rupp G, et al: Immunocytochemical staining of fine-needle aspiration biopsies of the liver as a diagnostic tool for hepatocellular carcinoma. Mod Pathol 5:117-123, 1992.

73. Weir M, Pitman MB: The vascular architecture of renal cell carcinoma in fine-needle aspiration biopsies. An aid in its distinction from hepatocellular carcinoma. Cancer Cytopathol 81:45-50, 1997.

74. Donat EE, Anderson V, Tao L-C: Cytodiagnosis of clear cell hepatocellular carcinoma. A case report. Acta Cytol 35:671-675, 1991.

75. Gupta RK, Al Ansari AG, Gauck R: Aspiration cytodiagnosis of clear cell hepatocellular carcinoma in an elderly woman. A case report. Acta Cytol 38:467-469, 1994.

76. Minervini MI, Demetris AJ, Lee RG, et al: Utilization of hepatocyte-specific antibody in the immunocytochemical evaluation of liver tumors. Mod Pathol 10:686-692, 1997.

77. Leong AS-Y: Hep Par 1 and selected antibodies. Histopathology 33:318-324, 1998.

78. Zimmerman RL, Burke MA, Young NA, et al: Diagnostic value of hepatocyte paraffin 1 antibody to discriminate hepatocellular carcinoma from metastatic carcinoma in fine-needle aspiration biopsies of the liver. Cancer 93:288-291, 2001.

79. Niemann TH, Hughes JH, DeYoung BR: MOC-31 aids in the differentiation of metastatic adenocarcinoma from hepatocellular carcinoma. Cancer 87:295-298, 1999.

80. Porcell AI, DeYoung BR, Proca DM, et al: Immunohistochemical analysis of hepatocellular and adenocarcinoma in the liver: MOC31 compares favorably with other putative markers. Mod Pathol 13:773-778, 2000.

81. Borscheri N, Roessner A, Rocken C: Canalicular immunostaining of neprilysin (CD10) as a diagnostic marker for hepatocellular carcinomas. Am J Surg Pathol 25:1297-1303, 2001.

82. Haas JE, Muczynski KA, Krailo M, et al: Histopathology and prognosis in childhood hepatoblastoma and hepatocarcinoma. Cancer 64:1082-1095, 1989.

83. Ersoz C, Zorludemir U, Tanyeli A, et al: Fine needle aspiration cytology of hepatoblastoma. A report of two cases. Acta Cytol 42:799-802, 1998.

84. Wakely PE, Silverman JF, Geisinger KR, et al: Fine needle aspiration biopsy cytology of hepatoblastoma. Mod Pathol 3:688-693, 1990.

85. Us-Krasovec M, Pohar-Marinsek Z, Golouh R, et al: Hepatoblastoma in fine needle aspirates. Acta Cytol 40:450-456, 1996.

86. Dekmezian R, Sneige N, Popok S, et al: Fine-needle aspiration cytology of pediatric patients with primary hepatic tumors: A comparative study of two hepatoblastomas and a liver-cell carcinoma. Diagn Cytopathol 4:162-168, 1988.

87. Kaw YT, Hansen K: Fine needle aspiration cytology of undifferentiated small cell ("anaplastic") hepatoblastoma. A case report. Acta Cytol 37:216-220, 1993.

88. Cangiarella J, Greco MA, Waisman J: Hepatoblastoma. Report of a case with cytologic, histologic and ultrastructural findings. Acta Cytol 38:455-458, 1994.

89. Fasano M, Theise ND, Nalesnik M, et al: Immunohistochemical evaluation of hepatoblastomas with use of the hepatocyte-specific marker, hepatocyte paraffin 1, and the polyclonal anti-carcino-embryonic antigen. Mod Pathol 11:934-938, 1998.

90. Van Eyken P, Sciot R, Callea F, et al: A cytokeratin-immunohisto-chemical study of hepatoblastoma. Hum Pathol 21:302-308, 1990.

91. Johnson DE, Herndier BG, Medeiros LJ, et al: The diagnostic utility of the keratin profiles of hepatocellular carcinoma and cholangiocarcinoma. Am J Surg Pathol 12:187-197, 1988.

92. Anthony PP: Tumours and tumour-like lesions of the liver and biliary tract. In Macsween RNM, Burt AD, Portman BC, et al (eds): Pathology of the Liver, 3rd ed. Edinburgh, Churchill Livingstone, 1994, p 670.

93. Liu K, Layfield LJ: Cytomorphologic features of angiosarcoma on fine needle aspiration biopsy. Acta Cytol 43:407-415, 1999.

94. Saleh HA, Tao LC: Hepatic angiosarcoma: Aspiration biopsy cytology and immunocytochemical contribution. Diagn Cytopathol 18:208-211, 1998.

95. Boucher LD, Swanson PE, Stanley MW, et al: Cytology of angiosarcoma. Findings in fourteen fine-needle aspiration biopsy specimens and one pleural fluid specimen. Am J Clin Pathol 114:210-219, 2000.

96. Sharifah NA, Muhaizan WM, Rahman J, et al: Fine needle aspiration cytology of undifferentiated embryonal sarcoma of the liver: A case report. Malays J Pathol 21:105-109, 1999.

97. Pollono DG, Drut R: Undifferentiated (embryonal) sarcoma of the liver: Fine-needle aspiration cytology and preoperative chemotherapy as an approach to diagnosis and initial treatment. A case report. Diagn Cytopathol 19:102-106, 1998.

98. Garcia-Bonafe M, Allende H, Fantova MJ, et al: Fine needle aspiration cytology of undifferentiated (embryonal) sarcoma of the liver. A case report. Acta Cytol 41:1273-1278, 1997.

99. Edmondson HA, Craig JR: Neoplasms of the liver. In Schiff L, Schiff ER (eds): Diseases of the Liver. Philadelphia, JB Lippincott, 1987, pp 1109-1116.

100. Samaratunga H, Wright G: Value of fine needle aspiration biopsy cytology in the diagnosis of discrete hepatic lesions suspicious for malignancy. Aust N Z J Surg 62:540-544, 1992.

101. Dong HY, Harris NL, Preffer FI, et al: Fine-needle aspiration biopsy in the diagnosis and classification of primary and recurrent lymphoma: A retrospective analysis of the utility of cytomorphology and flow cytometry. Mod Pathol 14:472-481, 2001.

102. Young NA, Al-Saleem TI, Ehya H, et al: Utilization of fine-needle aspiration cytology and flow cytometry in the diagnosis and subclassification of primary and recurrent lymphoma. Cancer 84:252-261, 1998.

103. Moriarty AT, Wiersema L, Synder W, et al: Immunophenotyping of cytologic specimens by flow cytometry. Diagn Cytopathol 9:252-258, 1993.

104. Lui K, Mann KP, Vitellas KM, et al: Fine-needle aspiration with flow cytometry immunophenotyping for primary diagnosis of intra-abdominal lymphomas. Diagn Cytopathol 21:98-104, 1999.

105. Robins DB, Katz RL, Swan F, et al: Immunotyping of lymphoma by fine-needle aspiration. A comparative study of cytospin preparations and flow cytometry (see comments). Am J Clin Pathol 101:569-576, 1994.

106. Morinaga S, Nishiya H, Inafuku T: Yolk sac tumor of the liver combined with hepatocellular carcinoma. Arch Pathol Lab Med 120:687-690, 1996.

107. Rader AE, Avery A, Wait CL, et al: Fine-needle aspiration biopsy diagnosis of gastrointestinal stromal tumors using morphology, immunocytochemistry, and mutational analysis of c-kit. Cancer 93:269-275, 2001.

108. Wieczorek TJ, Faquin WC, Rubin BP, et al: Cytologic diagnosis of gastrointestinal stromal tumor with emphasis on the differential diagnosis with leiomyosarcoma. Cancer 93:276-287, 2001.

CHAPTER 34

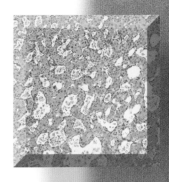

Acute and Chronic Hepatitis

LAURA W. LAMPS • KAY WASHINGTON

Introduction

A wide variety of infectious agents may involve the liver. The most common are probably the known hepatotropic viruses—hepatitis A, B, C, D, and E. Many other viruses such as cytomegalovirus (CMV) and Epstein-Barr virus (EBV) may cause hepatic injury as part of a systemic infection. Although some infectious agents produce characteristic morphologic patterns of injury, in many cases, the findings are relatively nonspecific, and proper interpretation of the liver biopsy depends on adequate clinical information. Knowledge of the patient's travel history and immunologic status and serologic studies are often necessary.

Viral Hepatitis

Viral hepatitis may be defined as hepatocyte necrosis and hepatic inflammation resulting from systemic viral infection and leading to a characteristic constellation of clinical and morphologic features. Most cases are caused by one of four well-known hepatotropic viruses (hepatitis A, B, C, or E); hepatitis B infection may be further complicated by coinfection or superinfection with hepatitis D. Other viruses such as CMV and EBV may cause hepatic injury and inflammation as part of a systemic illness, but the hepatitis is usually overshadowed by clinical manifestations of involvement of other organ systems. Other agents of viral hepatitis are postulated, based in part on the continued, albeit rare, occurrence of post-transfusion hepatitis despite screening of blood donors for known infectious agents.

Viral hepatitis is divided into acute and chronic forms, based on evidence of chronicity. By convention, the term *chronic hepatitis* is used when hepatic necrosis and inflammation are present for at least 6 months, as documented by histology or by sustained elevations in serum transaminase levels.

CLINICAL FEATURES

Acute Viral Hepatitis. Acute viral hepatitis is often asymptomatic and remains undiagnosed; it is often recognized only in retrospect when serologic testing reveals past infection. In many patients, symptoms are mild and nonspecific and include malaise, fatigue, low-grade fever, and flulike complaints. Asymptomatic or mild, inapparent cases of acute viral hepatitis are more common among children; adults are more likely to be symptomatic.

Symptomatic acute viral hepatitis is generally preceded by a prodrome phase that lasts from a few days to several weeks and is characterized by nonspecific symptoms such as nausea and vomiting, myalgias, anorexia, and malaise. Once jaundice appears, constitutional symptoms typically begin to wane. Physical examination is notable only for jaundice and hepatomegaly; the liver may be tender to palpation in some patients. Serum transaminases, the key indicators of hepatocellular injury, are elevated, usually in the range of 5- to 10-fold above normal. Alkaline phosphatase is only mildly elevated; conjugated hyperbilirubinemia is present in some but not all patients. Full recovery usually occurs within weeks, but in some cases, convalescence may be prolonged. Treatment is generally supportive.

In a small minority of cases of acute viral hepatitis (<1%), fulminant hepatic failure may occur, as evidenced by the rapid development of liver failure. Although acute liver failure may also result from other causes such as ischemic injury and exposure to toxins, in most countries, the most common cause is acute viral hepatitis.[1] The clinical course is characterized by coagulopathy and encephalopathy; mortality may exceed 80% without liver transplantation.

Chronic Viral Hepatitis. The distinction between acute and chronic viral hepatitis is based on a minimum duration of 6 months for chronic hepatitis. As with acute hepatitis, chronic hepatitis has a wide spectrum of clinical manifestations, ranging from asymptomatic infection to decompensated cirrhosis. Many patients are asymptomatic or have only mild, nonspecific complaints such as fatigue. Findings on physical examination are few but include hepatomegaly and stigmata of chronic liver disease such as palmar erythema. Patients with advanced cirrhosis may also exhibit ascites and varices. Serum transaminase levels fluctuate but are chronically elevated, usually in the 2- to 10-fold range, although a substantial number of patients with mild chronic hepatitis C have persistently normal transaminase levels. Alkaline phosphatase and bilirubin levels are usually normal to mildly elevated unless hepatic decompensation occurs.

HEPATITIS VIRUSES

Hepatitis A

Hepatitis A, a small, 27-nm, nonenveloped, single-stranded RNA virus in the Picornaviridae family (Table 34-1), is the most common cause of acute viral hepatitis in the United States, accounting for roughly 50% of cases.[2] Large epidemics occur approximately every 10 years. Infection rates are higher in settings associated with poor sanitation or overcrowding, such as in developing countries and institutions for persons with developmental disabilities. Outbreaks in day care centers where children wear diapers have been recognized since the 1970s.[3]

The major route of transmission for hepatitis A is oral ingestion of fecally excreted virus through person-to-person contact or ingestion of contaminated food or water. Rarely, hepatitis A may be transmitted by transfusion.[3] Approximately 50% of patients have no identified source of infection.

Hepatitis A virus is transported across intestinal epithelium and travels to the liver via the portal system, where it is taken up by hepatocytes. Virus replicates in hepatocytes, is excreted into bile, and is shed in the stool. Hepatitis A virus is not directly cytopathic; a cell-mediated immune mechanism is probably responsible for hepatocyte injury. The virus is resistant to bile lysis because it has no envelope, thus resulting in efficient fecal-oral transmission. Four genotypes have been recognized but only one serotype. The mean incubation period for hepatitis A is 28 days (range, 15 to 40 days). Diagnosis is confirmed by detection of immunoglobulin M (IgM) antibodies to hepatitis A; these are detectable in serum 1 to 2 weeks after exposure and persist for 3 to 6 months.[4] Hepatitis A virus immunoglobulin G (IgG) is detectable 5 to 6 weeks after exposure and persists for years, probably conferring lifelong protection.

Clinical symptoms of hepatitis A are generally mild, and many cases are asymptomatic. The most important factor in assessment of disease severity is age; only 30% of children are symptomatic, compared with 70% of adults. The overall case fatality rate associated with fulminant hepatitis A is low (0.3%), but hepatitis A may produce substantial morbidity in elderly patients or those with preexisting chronic liver disease.[3] The onset of classic hepatitis A is generally abrupt with fever, headache, malaise, and nonspecific gastrointestinal symptoms, generally followed a week later by jaundice. Symptoms usually resolve within 8 weeks. A relapsing variant is recognized, and, in up to 10% of patients, the disease has a prolonged cholestatic course; however, chronic disease never occurs.

TABLE 34–1. Viral Hepatitis

	Hepatitis A	Hepatitis B	Hepatitis C	Hepatitis D	Hepatitis E
Type of virus	RNA, picornavirus	DNA, hepadnavirus	RNA, flavivirus	RNA, defective virus	RNA, calicivirus
Route of infection	Fecal-oral	Parenteral, perinatal, sexual	Parenteral; rarely sexual; sporadic	Parenteral	Fecal-oral
Chronic infection	No	Up to 10%	85%	5% with hepatitis B virus coinfection; up to 70% with superinfection of patient with hepatitis B virus	No

Hepatitis B

Hepatitis B has a partially double-stranded circular DNA genome and is classified in the Hepadnaviridae family. The complete viral particle, the Dane particle, consists of an outer envelope surrounding a core containing DNA, the hepatitis B core antigen (HBcAg), and DNA-dependent polymerase. The envelope contains the hepatitis B surface antigen (HBsAg). Complete and incomplete viral particles circulate in the blood of infected patients; HBsAg can circulate in large quantities as incomplete tubular or spherical structures lacking DNA. The genome of hepatitis B virus also codes for a variant of HBcAg with "pre-core" region. The longer polypeptide is secreted into blood as hepatitis Be antigen (HBeAg). Viral DNA may become incorporated into the host DNA in infected hepatocytes, particularly in patients infected at a young age, and such patients are at high risk for subsequent development of hepatocellular carcinoma.

Hepatitis B is transmitted by exposure to infected body fluids, through intravenous drug use, sexual contact, or occupational activity. Perinatal transmission is common (90%) if the mother is HBeAg-positive, indicating highly infectious disease with active viral replication, and less frequent (10%) if the mother is HBsAg-positive. In high-prevalence areas, the infection is often acquired by maternal-neonatal transmission, resulting in a high rate of chronic disease. In areas of lower prevalence, hepatitis B is a disease of young adults who acquire the disease through parenteral or sexual exposure. Post-transfusion hepatitis B is virtually nonexistent in the United States owing to routine screening of blood donors.

Hepatitis B is responsible for up to 40% of cases of acute hepatitis in the United States. Clinical symptoms of acute hepatitis occur in approximately 30% of infected adults but in only 10% of children younger than 4 years old; these generally appear 45 to 180 days after exposure.[5] Fulminant hepatic failure occurs in about 1% of cases of acute hepatitis B. Acute liver failure may also occur in patients with chronic hepatitis B virus with mutations in the viral precore or core promoter regions.[5] Chronic hepatitis develops in 10% of patients. The rate of progression to cirrhosis depends on the activity of the hepatitis; 50% of patients with chronic hepatitis with marked activity progress to cirrhosis within 4 years. The annual rate of probability of development of cirrhosis is estimated as 12% for patients with chronic hepatitis B. Hepatocellular carcinoma develops in 2.4% of patients with chronic hepatitis B annually and in 0.5% of patients with chronic hepatitis without cirrhosis.[5]

Hepatitis C

Hepatitis C is a spherical, enveloped, single-stranded RNA virus, measuring approximately 50 μm in diameter. It is classified as a separate genus in the Flaviviridae family. The genome for hepatitis C is characterized by sequence heterogeneity, caused by pressure from the host immune system; this feature allows the virus to escape immune surveillance and establish chronic infection. Six major genotypes are recognized; the most common are 1a, 1b, 2a, and 2b.

Hepatitis C is transmitted primarily through parenteral exposure; intravenous drug users and patients with hemophilia have a particularly high prevalence of infection. Intranasal cocaine use and sexual promiscuity appear to be independent risk factors for acquisition of the infection,[6] although the risk associated with sexual transmission is low compared with that associated with human immunodeficiency virus (HIV) or hepatitis B.[7] Although it was initially identified as the etiologic agent of transfusion-acquired non-A, non-B hepatitis, the incidence of post-transfusion hepatitis C has decreased dramatically with implementation of donor screening; the risk of infection with hepatitis C virus is now estimated at 0.01% to 0.001% for each unit of blood transfused.[7] Rates of perinatal transmission are estimated at 5% to 6%.

Hepatitis C accounts for approximately 15% of cases of acute hepatitis in the United States,[2] but the acute infection is usually asymptomatic and is rarely recognized; only one third of patients exhibit jaundice or symptoms. The incubation period is 7 weeks, with a range of 2 to 30 weeks, based on study of transfusion-acquired cases.[8] Fulminant hepatitis is rare. Chronic infection is a much more common problem, occurring in at least 85% of infected patients. Most patients with chronic hepatitis C have few if any symptoms, and serum transaminase levels are often only mildly elevated, fluctuating from 1.5 to 10 times the upper limit of normal; up to 30% have normal levels at any one time.[9] Host and viral factors associated with progressive disease include age older than 40 years at exposure, immunodeficiency, high degrees of viral heterogeneity, genotype 1, male sex, and extended duration of infection.[9] Alcohol is known to potentiate viral replication and is associated with greater activity and fibrosis.[10] Diagnostic tests currently in use include polymerase chain reaction (PCR) for detection of circulating viral RNA and a third-generation enzyme immunoassay for detection of anti–hepatitis C virus antibodies.

The natural history of hepatitis C infection has proved difficult to study owing in part to the inability of clinicians to accurately determine the onset of infection. In most patients, the disease is thought to have an indolent course for one to two decades; cirrhosis develops in 20% to 30% of patients in studies with 10 to 20 years of follow-up.[11] Currently, chronic hepatitis C accounts for 30% of liver transplants performed in the United States. The annual risk for hepatocellular carcinoma in hepatitis C virus–related cirrhosis is estimated at 1% to 4%[9]; genotype 1b has been implicated in the pathogenesis of hepatocellular carcinoma in this disease.

Hepatitis C infection is associated with a variety of systemic manifestations and is now thought to be responsible for most cases of essential mixed cryoglobulinemia.[12] Hepatitis C is also strongly associated with porphyria cutanea tarda (PCT) in the United States, although marked geographic variation has been noted in the prevalence of hepatitis C virus in patients with PCT.[13] Homozygosity for the Cys282Tyr mutation in the hemochromatosis gene and hepatitis C viral infection are significant risk factors for the expression of PCT; heavy alcohol use is often a contributing factor.[14] The characteristic birefringent yellow-brown needle-shaped crystals described in PCT are rarely found in routinely processed liver biopsy specimens, however, because of their high solubility in water; alcohol fixation is required.

Hepatitis D

Hepatitis D (delta agent) is a small, defective RNA virus that requires HBsAg for packaging and transmission before it can cause infection and disease. It is spread through the same routes as hepatitis B virus and may present as coinfection or superinfection with hepatitis B virus. Hepatitis D viral infection can cause acute or chronic hepatitis; superinfection may cause fulminant hepatic failure. Hepatitis D superinfection should be suspected in patients with hepatitis B virus who have severe exacerbation of disease activity; the finding of anti–hepatitis D IgM in a patient who is seropositive for HBsAg is diagnostic. Three genotypes are recognized.[15] Histologic features of hepatitis D viral infection are not distinctive, but hepatitis D virus is associated with more pronounced necroinflammatory activity and more rapid progression than are generally seen with hepatitis B virus alone. Microvesicular fat may be present in severe cases.[16] Delta antigen, which may be demonstrated by immunohistochemical means, is primarily located in hepatocyte nuclei.[15]

Hepatitis E

Hepatitis E is a small, nonenveloped, single-stranded RNA virus structurally similar to the caliciviruses but more closely resembling rubella in its genomic structure.[17] Two main geographically distinct strains—Asian and Mexican—are recognized.[18] Hepatitis E is endemic in the Indian subcontinent, where it causes up to 70% of sporadic acute viral hepatitis; it is also endemic in southeast and central Asia and Mexico. Fecal-oral transmission occurs, usually through ingestion of contaminated water. Hepatitis E causes a mild acute hepatitis lasting 1 to 4 weeks in most patients but is particularly severe in pregnant women, in whom it carries a high mortality rate of up to 25%. The incubation period is 4 to 5 weeks.

Two histopathologic patterns are described. Approximately half of patients have typical changes resembling those of other causes of acute hepatitis. In the remaining patients, a cholestatic form of the disease occurs, characterized by canalicular bile plugs and cholestatic regenerative rosette formation.[19] Massive or submassive necrosis occurs in severe cases. Chronic infection does not occur. Serologic assays for anti–hepatitis E IgG and IgM and reverse transcriptase PCR assays are useful for confirming diagnosis.[18]

The GBV-C virus, also known as hepatitis G, is a recently discovered flavivirus from the same family as hepatitis C. This virus has been found in 1.4% of volunteer blood donors in the United States and can be transmitted by blood transfusion.[20] It does not worsen the course of concurrent hepatitis C and does not cause hepatitis by itself. Indeed, because it is not hepatotropic, this nonpathogenic virus appears to be misnamed. Similarly, a newly discovered DNA virus, the TT virus, was originally suspected to cause transfusion-associated hepatitis but was later found in more than 90% of Japanese blood donors, casting doubt on its causative role in disease.[21] A related single-stranded circular DNA virus, the SEN virus, has also been found in patients with transfusion-associated hepatitis, although causality has not been established.[22]

ACUTE HEPATITIS

Pathologic Features

MICROSCOPIC PATHOLOGY

Acute hepatitis is seldom seen in liver biopsy specimens because the diagnosis is usually readily established by noninvasive means. When liver tissue is available for examination, the necroinflammatory process involves all areas of the lobule and is not confined to portal regions. The combination of hepatocyte loss and regeneration and a mononuclear inflammatory infiltrate leads to lobular disarray, reflecting disruption of the normal orderly architecture of the liver cell plates (Fig. 34-1).

Hepatocellular changes include ballooning degeneration—in which the affected cells are swollen and pale staining, with clumping of cytoplasm around the nucleus—and various forms of hepatocyte necrosis. Ballooned hepatocytes often undergo lytic necrosis, which generally does not result in an identifiable necrotic cell. Rather, these areas are marked by small foci of parenchymal collapse with associated clusters of mononuclear inflammatory cells. Alternatively, hepatocytes may undergo acidophilic changes, in which the cell becomes shrunken, angular, and hypereosinophilic with a densely staining pyknotic nucleus. Such cells may change into acidophilic bodies (apoptotic bodies)—small, mummified, rounded cell remnants—and may extrude nuclear fragments. Apoptotic bodies often are

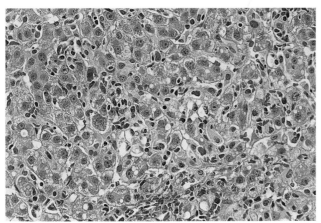

FIGURE 34–1. Acute viral hepatitis. Lobular disarray is due to hepatocyte necrosis, hepatocellular regeneration, Kupffer cell hyperplasia and hypertrophy, and a diffuse, predominantly mononuclear inflammatory infiltrate.

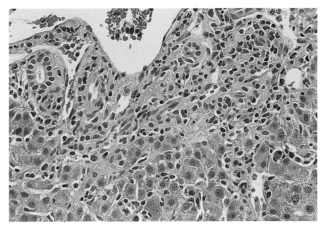

FIGURE 34–3. Acute viral hepatitis. The portal inflammatory infiltrate is primarily mononuclear cells, with scattered neutrophils and eosinophils. Inflammation spills over into the adjacent parenchyma.

not associated with inflammatory cells and are usually phagocytosed by Kupffer cells within a matter of hours. Hence, identification of apoptotic bodies indicates recent cell death. Individual or small clusters of necrotic hepatocytes are collectively referred to as *spotty hepatocyte necrosis*. Regeneration of remaining hepatocytes contributes to the "busy" appearance of the lobule as the liver cell plates are irregularly thickened. Nonspecific hepatic steatosis may also be seen.

Canalicular cholestasis is usually not prominent in acute hepatitis, but in some cases, it may be so pronounced that the histologic changes suggest biliary obstruction. In this variant, known as *acute cholestatic hepatitis*, prominent bile ductular proliferation with associated neutrophils in portal areas further leads to confusion with biliary obstruction. Ballooning degeneration and regenerating "cholestatic" rosettes or hepato-

cyte "pseudoglands" may be seen in the lobule (Fig. 34-2). Acute cholestatic hepatitis typically has a prolonged clinical course.

The inflammatory infiltrate in acute hepatitis is primarily mononuclear and is composed of lymphocytes, macrophages, scattered eosinophils, and occasional plasma cells and neutrophils, as is shown in Figure 34-3 for a portal tract. In contrast to chronic hepatitis, in which portal inflammation usually predominates, in acute hepatitis, the inflammatory infiltrate is generally not concentrated in portal tracts but is spread throughout the lobule. Sinusoidal mononuclear cells are often prominent. Kupffer cells are more numerous than usual, are hypertrophic, and may contain phagocytized cellular debris and prominent lipofuscin. Although the necroinflammatory process is panlobular, inflammation and necrosis may be more pronounced in centrilobular areas in acute hepatitis. Bridging necrosis may be seen in more severe cases, with a zone of necrosis extending from portal tract to terminal hepatic vein (Fig. 34-4), and may be associated with a more protracted clinical course.

Special studies such as immunohistochemistry for viral antigens are generally not useful in the evaluation of acute hepatitis because virus is rapidly eliminated from liver cells and is not detectable with the use of immunostains. Serologic studies are generally readily available and are more reliable.

MASSIVE AND SUBMASSIVE NECROSIS

In severe cases of acute hepatitis, portions of lobules (submassive necrosis) or entire contiguous lobules (massive necrosis) may undergo necrosis. Submassive necrosis usually involves zone 3 but may extend to zone 2 as well. Extensive destruction of hepatic parenchyma results in the clinical syndrome of fulminant hepatic failure. On gross examination, the liver with massive

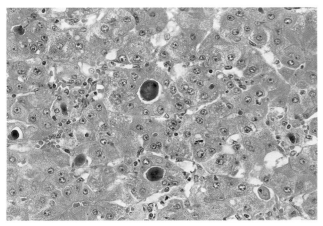

FIGURE 34–2. Acute viral hepatitis. Hepatocyte regeneration is in the form of cholestatic rosettes, with hepatocytes surrounding a central bile plug.

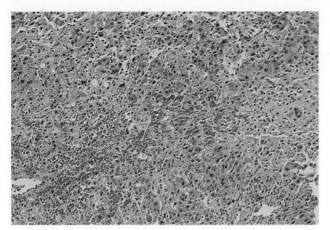

FIGURE 34–4. Acute viral hepatitis with portal-central bridging necrosis. A zone of confluent necrosis extends from a portal tract (*right*) to a central vein (*lower left*).

necrosis appears shrunken and flaccid with wrinkling of the capsular surface and a mottled parenchyma. Regenerating nodules of hepatocytes, often bile stained, are irregularly distributed and may form nodular masses. Necroinflammatory activity is variable, even among patients with a similar clinical course.[23] Proliferating bile ductules with associated neutrophils are prominent in periportal areas (Fig. 34-5). The histologic features of submassive and massive hepatic necrosis are not specific for acute viral hepatitis but may be the result of a variety of insults, such as toxic injury, severe drug reaction, and Wilson's disease. Trichrome stain for connective tissue is useful in distinguishing massive hepatic necrosis from cirrhosis by demonstrating the lack of dense collagen deposition in massive necrosis. Reticulin stain is also helpful in demonstrating the collapsed reticulin framework of the liver.

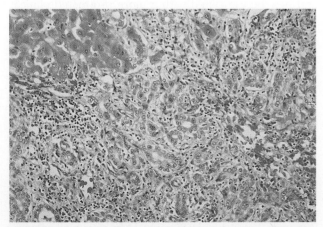

FIGURE 34–5. Acute viral hepatitis. Massive necrosis, defined as destruction of contiguous lobules, often exhibits marked bile ductular proliferation.

Prognostic Factors

Histopathologic features of acute hepatitis predictive of progression to chronicity have been difficult to elucidate, based in part on the rarity of liver biopsy in acute hepatitis. Interface hepatitis is probably not a reliable predictive feature in that it may be seen in cases of acute hepatitis A that do not progress to chronic hepatitis. Similarly, bridging necrosis is predictive of progression to chronic hepatitis in some studies[24] but not in others.[25] Although approximately one third of patients with acute viral hepatitis in one series exhibited bridging necrosis on biopsy, these patients could not be clearly distinguished from patients with less severe necroinflammatory histologic activity, and on follow-up, they had completely recovered.[26] In patients with massive hepatic necrosis, a liver biopsy specimen may not be representative of the overall status of the liver, given the heterogeneity of regeneration and necrosis from region to region.

Differential Diagnosis

The two major entities that may be confused with acute viral hepatitis are chronic hepatitis and drug-induced hepatitis. If the lobular inflammatory component of chronic hepatitis is prominent, it may be confused with acute hepatitis. In particular, autoimmune hepatitis may have a prominent lobular component and may prove difficult to distinguish from acute viral hepatitis. Again, serologic tests are helpful, but autoimmune markers such as antinuclear antibody are not always positive early in the course of autoimmune hepatitis. Concentration of the inflammatory infiltrate in portal areas, with formation of dense lymphoid aggregates, favors chronic hepatitis. Fibrosis is also an indicator of chronicity.

Drug reaction may be indistinguishable from acute viral hepatitis; prominent eosinophils and granulomas, sinusoidal dilatation, and fatty changes suggest drug reaction, but they are not pathognomonic. Kupffer cell nodules are commonly seen in resolving acute hepatitis and should not be mistaken for non-necrotizing granulomas.

CHRONIC HEPATITIS

Pathologic Features

Chronic hepatitis is generally defined as liver disease with persistent necroinflammatory activity lasting longer than 6 months. Regardless of cause, chronic hepatitis is characterized by a combination of portal inflammation, interface hepatitis, parenchymal inflammation, necrosis, and, in many cases, fibrosis. This histologic pattern of injury is not specific for viral hepatitis but may be seen in autoimmune hepatitis, metabolic disorders such as

Wilson's disease, alpha-1-antitrypsin deficiency, and drug reactions and as an idiopathic finding.

PORTAL INFLAMMATION

In most cases of chronic hepatitis, a prominent inflammatory infiltrate involves the portal tracts. This infiltrate consists primarily of lymphocytes, with a variable number of plasma cells. Scattered macrophages, neutrophils, and eosinophils may be found in some cases but are typically a minor component of the infiltrate. Lymphoid follicles may be present, particularly in hepatitis C, and germinal centers may be seen (Fig. 34-6). Bile ductular proliferation may be noted at the periphery of the portal tracts but is typically not prominent. As in any lesion with bile ductular proliferation, neutrophils may be associated with proliferating ductular epithelium as a result of cytokine release by biliary epithelium[27] and should not be interpreted as evidence of acute cholangitis.

Interface hepatitis, also known as *piecemeal necrosis* or *periportal necrosis*, is an important feature of chronic hepatitis, although it is focal or not present in cases with minimal necroinflammatory activity. Often, all portal tracts in a biopsy specimen are not equally involved by the process, and variation within the liver may result in sampling error. Interface hepatitis has two morphologic components—a mononuclear inflammatory infiltrate involving hepatocytes at the limiting plate, and degenerative changes in hepatocytes. The lymphocytes and plasma cells of the inflammatory periportal infiltrate are closely associated with degenerating hepatocytes at the limiting plate (Fig. 34-7), to the point that indentation of the cytoplasm of the hepatocyte occurs, or even engulfment of the inflammatory cell by the hepatocyte. Hepatocytes in areas of interface hepatitis necrosis often undergo ballooning degeneration and appear pale and swollen with clumping of cytoplasm. Apoptotic

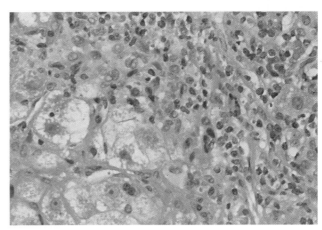

FIGURE 34–7. Chronic viral hepatitis. Interface hepatitis produces a ragged limiting plate, with hepatocellular ballooning degeneration in this example.

bodies may also be seen in areas of active interface hepatitis. The periportal parenchyma is gradually destroyed and replaced by fibrosis; this irregular expansion of the portal tracts and periportal regions by fibrous tissue leads to entrapment of single hepatocytes and small clusters of hepatocytes.

LOBULAR NECROINFLAMMATORY ACTIVITY

Hepatocyte necrosis in chronic hepatitis is variable in severity but usually spotty, and the lobular disarray often seen in acute hepatitis is not a prominent feature. Apoptotic hepatocytes (acidophil bodies) are often more numerous in periportal areas but are also scattered within the lobule (Fig. 34-8). Mononuclear inflammatory cells cluster around injured hepatocytes and may obscure focal hepatocyte necrosis (Fig. 34-9). Kupffer cells in these areas of spotty hepatocyte necrosis may contain phagocytosed cellular debris. Ballooning degeneration of hepatocytes, which may be seen in

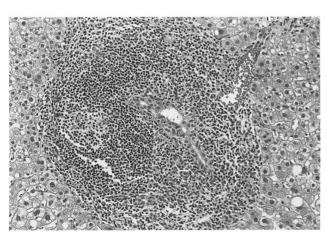

FIGURE 34–6. Chronic viral hepatitis. Mononuclear portal inflammation is variable; lymphoid aggregates, sometimes with terminal centers, are common in hepatitis C.

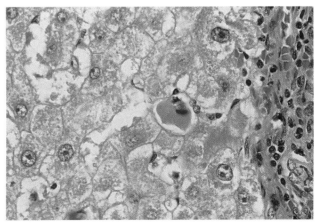

FIGURE 34–8. Chronic viral hepatitis. An acidophilic body with partially extruded nucleus is present in the sinusoid.

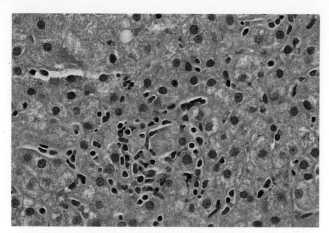

FIGURE 34–9. Chronic viral hepatitis. A cluster of mononuclear inflammatory cells is indicative of lytic hepatocyte necrosis.

exacerbations of chronic viral hepatitis, may be associated with zone 3 cholestasis. Regeneration of hepatocytes is recognizable by the formation of liver cell plates that are two cells thick and by the formation of regenerating rosettes of hepatocytes.

FIBROSIS

Progressive fibrosis at the limiting plate as a result of continued necroinflammatory activity leads to stellate enlargement of the portal tract. Deposition of collagen and other extracellular matrix materials in the space of Disse, at the leading edge of the periportal fibrosis results in capillarization of the sinusoids. Portal-portal fibrous septa are the result of linkage of adjacent fibrotic portal tracts (Fig. 34-10). Portal-central fibrous bridges can also develop, generally from superimposed episodes of severe lobular necroinflammatory activity involving zone 3. Central-central bridges are formed via the same mechanisms but are less common in chronic hepatitis. The end result of bridging fibrosis, if peri-

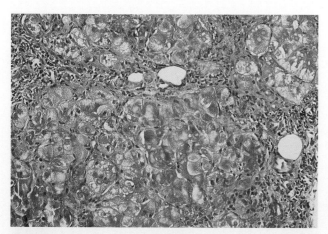

FIGURE 34–10. Chronic viral hepatitis. Shown is portal-portal bridging fibrosis in long-standing chronic hepatitis C. Focally, interface hepatitis continues along the fibrous septa.

septal activity continues, is cirrhosis (usually macronodular or mixed micronodular/macronodular).

Nomenclature and Scoring

In the past, the term *chronic active hepatitis* was used to describe biopsy specimens with interface hepatitis, and *chronic persistent hepatitis* was applied to biopsies with portal inflammation without significant periportal/piecemeal necrosis. This distinction was thought to be important because chronic persistent hepatitis was considered a relatively benign process that occurred without progression to significant liver disease. The identification of hepatitis C, with recognition of the waxing and waning nature of the disease and the prolonged time to progression to cirrhosis in many cases, has led to the abandonment of this nomenclature. In current practice, the recommended terminology is simply *chronic hepatitis*,[28] with inclusion of a statement in the pathology report regarding severity of necroinflammatory activity (grade), extent of fibrosis (stage), and etiology (if known or inferred).[29]

Many different systems for scoring necroinflammatory activity and fibrosis have been developed. The Knodell system, published in 1981, has served as a prototype for semiquantitative scoring of liver biopsy specimens.[30] With modifications, this system is still widely used, especially in therapeutic trials comparing changes in necroinflammatory activity in pretreatment and post-treatment liver biopsy specimens.[31,32] In the Knodell system, periportal necrosis with or without bridging necrosis, intralobular necrosis and inflammation, portal inflammation, and fibrosis are all assigned numeric values, which are added together to obtain the hepatitis activity index (HAI), ranging from 0 to 22. An obvious criticism of this practice is the inclusion of fibrosis (stage) as a determinant of activity (grade). In practice, the HAI is often modified so that bridging necrosis is dissociated from interface hepatitis, and only the elements relating to grade are summed to produce the modified HAI (mHAI), with scores ranging from 0 to 18; stage is reported separately.[33] An alternative grading system used by the French METAVIR Cooperative Study Group evaluates only two features (periportal necrosis and lobular necroinflammatory activity) instead of three; portal inflammation is excluded because of its strong correlation with piecemeal necrosis and because it is considered a prerequisite for the diagnosis of chronic hepatitis, even without activity.[34]

These semiquantitative grading schemes, although useful for evaluating the effects of a particular treatment in a clinical trial setting, are probably not necessary for routine reporting of liver biopsy specimens. For diagnostic purposes, simpler schemes are sufficient for everyday practice, and several such schemes have been

TABLE 34–2. Scoring System for Grading Necroinflammatory Activity in Chronic Hepatitis[36]

Description	Score	Lymphocytic Piecemeal Necrosis/Interface Hepatitis	Lobular Inflammation and Necrosis
No activity; may have portal inflammation only	0	None	None
Minimal	1	Minimal; patchy	Minimal, with occasional spotty necrosis
Mild	2	Mild; involves some or all portal tracts	Mild, with little hepatocellular injury
Moderate	3	Moderate; involves all portal tracts	Moderate, with hepatocellular degeneration
Severe	4	Severe activity ± bridging fibrosis	Severe, with prominent, diffuse hepatocellular damage

TABLE 34–3. Scoring System for Staging of Chronic Hepatitis[36]*

Degree of Fibrosis	Score	Features
No fibrosis	0	Normal
Portal fibrosis	1	Fibrous portal expansion, confined to enlarged portal zones
Periportal fibrosis	2	Periportal expansion; rare portal-portal septa may be seen
Septal fibrosis	3	Architectural distortion (bridging or septal fibrosis) without obvious cirrhosis
Cirrhosis	4	Cirrhosis

*See also Table 35-6.

proposed.[35-38] Most use four or five categories (0 through 3 or 0 through 4) for necroinflammatory activity and five (0 through 4)[36] to seven (0 through 6)[33] for stage of fibrosis. A system employing scales of 0 to 4 is shown in Tables 34-2 and 34-3 and in Figures 34-11 and 34-12.[36] A verbal descriptor (inactive to severe) and a corresponding number are assigned for each feature evaluated. When discrepancies occur between lobular and portal/periportal activity, overall grade is determined by the more severe lesion. Stage is best evaluated on trichrome stain in that delicate septa of early

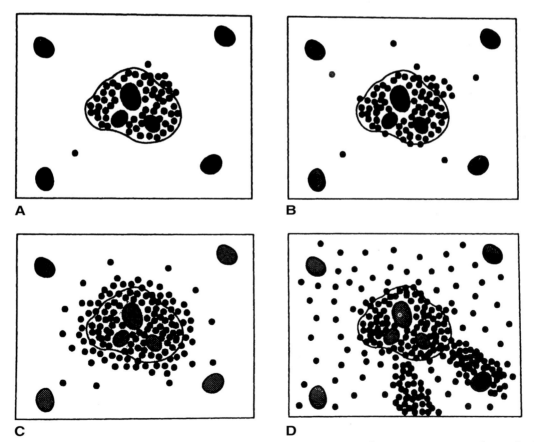

FIGURE 34–11. A grading scheme for increasing severity of portal and lobular necroinflammatory activity in chronic hepatitis[35] (see Table 34-2). **A,** Minimal activity. **B,** Mild activity. **C,** Moderate activity. **D,** Severe activity. (From Batts KP, Ludwig J: Chronic hepatitis. An update on terminology and reporting. Am J Surg Pathol 19:1409-1417, 1995.)

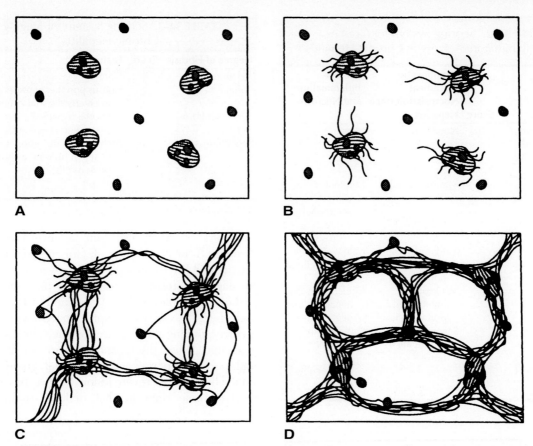

A

B

C

D

FIGURE 34–12. Staging scheme for assessment of progression of fibrosis in chronic hepatitis[35] (see Table 34-3). **A,** Portal fibrosis. **B,** Periportal fibrosis. **C,** Septal fibrosis. **D,** Cirrhosis. (From Batts KP, Ludwig J: Chronic hepatitis. An update on terminology and reporting. Am J Surg Pathol 19:1409-1417, 1995.)

bridging fibrosis may be inapparent on hematoxylin and eosin stain.

Histopathology of Specific Types of Chronic Hepatitis

CHRONIC HEPATITIS B

Ground-glass cells containing abundant hepatitis B surface antigen in smooth endoplasmic reticulum may be recognized on hematoxylin and eosin–stained section (Fig. 34-13). These are not present in all cases, however, and are more likely to be numerous in biopsy specimens with little necroinflammatory activity. HBcAg accumulation in hepatocyte nuclei produces a "sanded" appearance, but such changes are difficult to recognize on routine stains. Identification of cytoplasmic HBsAg may be facilitated by use of one of the Shikata stains such as Victoria blue, orcein, or aldehyde fuchsin, or by immunohistochemical stain (Fig. 34-14). HBcAg accumulation may be identified with the use of immunohistochemical stains (Fig. 34-15), and cytoplasmic or membranous expression of this antigen correlates with high levels of necroinflammatory activity.[39]

DELTA VIRUS

Sanded hepatocyte nuclei may be seen in hepatitis B with delta virus infection. Delta antigen may be demonstrated within nuclei of hepatocytes by immunohistochemical stains. Overall, the histopathology resembles hepatitis B without delta infection, but the necroinflammatory activity is often more severe.

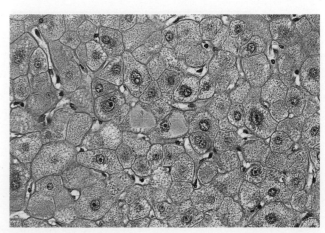

FIGURE 34–13. Ground-glass hepatocytes in chronic hepatitis B contain hepatitis B surface antigen.

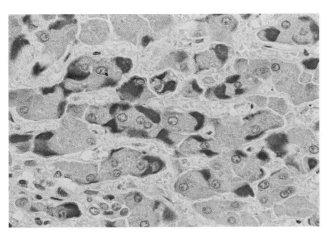

FIGURE 34–14. Positive cytoplasmic staining for hepatitis B surface antigen, with perinuclear cytoplasmic crescent-shaped staining (immunoperoxidase stain).

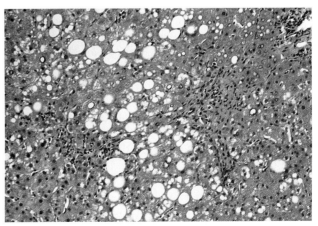

FIGURE 34–16. Chronic hepatitis C. The bile duct is infiltrated and almost obscured by mononuclear inflammatory cells.

HEPATITIS C

Histologically, chronic hepatitis caused by hepatitis C tends to be mild. Characteristic features include portal lymphoid aggregates and follicles, bile duct infiltration by lymphocytes, and steatosis.[40,41] Dense aggregates of lymphocytes in portal tracts are a distinctive but not pathognomonic feature of hepatitis C and are readily apparent on low-power examination (see Fig. 34-6). The bile duct injury in hepatitis C is rarely severe, and duct loss is not a feature. The biliary epithelium of affected ducts may be focally disrupted and, in addition to infiltration by lymphocytes, reveals reactive changes such as vacuolation of epithelium and nuclear crowding and enlargement (Fig. 34-16). Steatosis in hepatitis C is usually macrovesicular and focal rather than panlobular and may be associated with severe necroinflammatory activity (Fig. 34-17). Non-necrotizing granulomas occur in a small percentage of cases, but other concurrent causes of granulomas must be excluded.[42] Mallory's hyaline–like cytoplasmic inclusions are also reported,[43] but these may very well represent cytoplasmic clumping in ballooned hepatocytes simulating Mallory's hyaline. Immunoperoxidase staining for hepatitis C virus has been reported in paraffin-embedded tissue, but available stains are difficult to interpret and are not in widespread use.[44]

Double infection with hepatitis B and hepatitis C is not rare, occurring in more than 10% of hepatitis B patients.[45] In some patients, superinfection is associated with viral interference, with the more recently acquired virus suppressing replication of the preexisting virus. If co-replication of both hepatitis C and hepatitis B does occur, as is evidenced by the presence of nucleic acids of both hepatitis B and hepatitis C, the liver disease is likely to be more active and to show faster progression. The histologic features of hepatitis C are often predominant in liver biopsies.

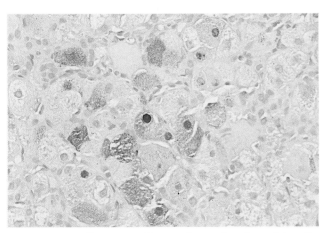

FIGURE 34–15. Positive nuclear and cytoplasmic staining for hepatitis B core antigen signifies active viral replication (immunoperoxidase stain).

FIGURE 34–17. Chronic hepatitis C. Macrovesicular hepatic steatosis is a common feature in hepatitis C infection and often correlates with increased necroinflammatory activity.

Prognostic Factors

Factors associated with progression of chronic hepatitis to cirrhosis may be divided into those related to the specific virus, host-related factors, and extraneous factors such as alcohol use. For hepatitis C, development of chronic hepatitis does not appear to be related to the amount of virus in the initial exposure. Viral genotype may be important in progression of hepatitis C infection, with genotype 1 associated with more severe disease than genotype 2[9,46]; however, other studies have not confirmed this association.[47] Host-related factors for disease severity are incompletely defined, but age at infection and sex appear to be relevant in that males and older persons are more likely to exhibit progression of fibrosis.[47] Alcohol consumption increases replication of hepatitis C and is associated with more severe disease.[10] In general, grade of hepatic necroinflammatory activity in the liver biopsy correlates with serum hepatitis C virus RNA levels,[48] and rate of progression to cirrhosis correlates with high-grade activity and advanced stage in initial biopsy specimens.[49] Hepatic steatosis is also associated with increased disease severity and is more commonly seen in infections with genotype 3b.[50]

Accumulation of iron in hepatocytes and Kupffer cells in hepatitis C may influence disease course and response to therapy in an adverse manner.[51] It should be noted, however, that many patients with chronic hepatitis, including hepatitis C, have abnormal serum iron studies but normal or scant iron accumulation in liver biopsy.

DIFFERENTIAL DIAGNOSIS OF CHRONIC AND ACUTE HEPATITIS

The morphologic pattern of chronic hepatitis may be seen in a variety of conditions and is not specific for viral hepatitis. Distinction from acute hepatitis rests on the focality of lobular inflammation and a predominance of portal changes in chronic hepatitis; portal fibrosis in particular is a helpful feature that indicates chronicity. In some cases, distinction of acute and chronic hepatitis may not be possible on morphologic grounds, but a duration of longer than 6 months is an indication of chronic disease.

Early in the course of the disease, portal lymphocytic inflammation of primary biliary cirrhosis (PBC) may resemble chronic viral hepatitis, particularly hepatitis C. Interface hepatitis may also be seen in primary biliary cirrhosis and cannot be used to distinguish PBC from chronic hepatitis. Loss of interlobular bile ducts is the most helpful distinguishing feature in that bile duct loss occurs in PBC but not in chronic hepatitis. Bile ducts are infiltrated by lymphocytes in chronic hepatitis C but are not destroyed. Chronic cholestasis is not a feature of precirrhotic chronic hepatitis; demonstration of increased copper or copper-binding protein by use of copper or

Shikata's stain may be helpful in some cases. Portal granulomas are also not common in chronic hepatitis and should suggest primary biliary cirrhosis in the appropriate clinical setting. Knowledge of viral serologic studies and the anti–mitochondrial antibody status may be necessary if the distinction is to be made.

Primary sclerosing cholangitis (PSC) in its early stages may also overlap morphologically with chronic hepatitis in that both may reveal a portal lymphocytic infiltrate with interface activity; this distinction may be particularly difficult in childhood PSC. Again, bile duct loss should suggest the possibility of a chronic biliary process; alkaline phosphatase levels are generally higher in PSC, but cholangiography is usually necessary for the diagnosis of PSC to be established. In patients with ulcerative colitis and a liver biopsy specimen with a pattern of inflammation suggesting chronic hepatitis, the possibility of PSC should be strongly considered.

Chronic viral hepatitis may be indistinguishable from autoimmune hepatitis on morphologic grounds. The presence of numerous plasma cells both in the portal inflammation infiltrate and in the lobule is suggestive of autoimmune hepatitis, but clinical correlation is necessary to distinguish these entities. Bile duct infiltration by lymphocytes is also seen in autoimmune hepatitis and cannot be used as a distinguishing feature from hepatitis C.

Wilson's disease also has a chronic hepatitis pattern of injury on liver biopsy specimen and should be considered in biopsy specimens from young patients with negative viral serologies. Serum ceruloplasmin and quantitative copper studies on liver tissue are necessary for definitive diagnosis. Alpha-1-antitrypsin deficiency may also reveal a chronic hepatitis pattern of injury; accumulation of periodic acid–Schiff (PAS)-positive, diastase-resistant cytoplasmic globules in hepatocytes is generally evident in liver biopsy specimens from adults.

Mild lobular hepatitis with spotty hepatocyte necrosis and a scant mononuclear inflammatory infiltrate may be seen as a nonspecific finding in a variety of systemic and immune-mediated disorders, as well as in patients with intra-abdominal inflammatory processes. These changes may mimic mild acute or chronic hepatitis but are considered a reactive process. In some cases with morphologic changes of chronic hepatitis on liver biopsy specimens, no cause is apparent after extensive serologic and clinical testing has been done; these cases may be labeled *cryptogenic* or *idiopathic*.

Other Viral Infections of the Liver

A wide variety of viruses other than hepatitis A, B, and C may affect the liver, with results ranging from mild, transient transaminase elevations to dramatic and fatal hepatic necrosis. These viruses are often seen in neonates or in immunocompromised persons as a part of disseminated infection.

EPSTEIN-BARR VIRUS

The liver is affected in more than 90% of cases of EBV-related mononucleosis. Hepatic involvement is indicated by elevated aminotransferases,[52] often accompanied by other symptoms of mononucleosis. Jaundice occurs in only a minority of patients. Fulminant liver failure secondary to EBV infection has been described, particularly in immunocompromised children[53] but also in healthy ones. Fulminant hepatic failure due to EBV may not be accompanied by the typical features of mononucleosis.

The most characteristic histologic feature in essentially healthy patients infected with EBV is a diffuse lymphocytic sinusoidal infiltrate in a single-file "string-of-beads" pattern, occasionally containing atypical lymphocytes (Fig. 34-18). Focal apoptotic hepatocytes and steatosis may be seen; cholestasis is not typical.[52,54] Small Kupffer cell clusters and, rarely, discrete noncaseating granulomas or fibrin-ring granulomas can be seen. Progression to chronic hepatitis or cirrhosis is rare. EBV hepatitis may also develop after solid organ transplantation, particularly liver. The histologic picture may be more severe in this context, with a marked portal and periportal inflammatory infiltrate containing numerous atypical lymphocytes, immunoblasts, and plasma cells and revealing mild bile duct damage and prominent necrosis.[55]

Confirmatory tests include serologic, immunohistochemical, and in situ hybridization studies. The differential diagnosis predominantly includes other viruses, most importantly CMV infection. Hepatic involvement by leukemia or lymphoma must also be excluded when atypical lymphocytes are numerous. Human

herpesvirus-6 has been implicated in a similar mononucleosis-like illness with hepatic involvement[56] as well.

CYTOMEGALOVIRUS

Patients with CMV hepatitis may show an increase in transaminases and/or a cholestatic pattern of enzyme elevation. The clinical and histologic features of CMV hepatitis vary according to the immune status of the host.

CMV Infection in Otherwise Healthy Patients

Primary CMV infections in healthy people are usually self-limited, although a mononucleosis-like syndrome may occur in a minority. CMV hepatitis in immunocompetent persons is often part of a multiorgan infectious process.[57] Rare cases of fulminant liver failure have been described, but chronic liver disease does not develop in this population. Neither viral inclusions nor immunohistochemically demonstrable CMV antigen is generally seen in these patients.[58]

CMV Infection in Immunocompromised Patients

CMV infection of the liver is more commonly seen in immunocompromised persons and is a particular problem for transplant patients. CMV infection is the single most important pathogen in solid organ transplant patients of all types.[59] It may be acquired through primary infection, reactivation, or superinfection by a new strain in a previously seropositive patient.[59] Infection occurs approximately 2 to 16 weeks following solid organ transplantation, and symptoms range from mild to life threatening. Although any organ may be involved in these patients, hepatic involvement may predominate; in liver transplant patients particularly, the allograft is the most common site of involvement.[59]

In immunocompromised patients, CMV hepatitis is characterized by the cytopathic effects of the virus.[60,61] Infected cells are markedly enlarged and contain the characteristic "owl's eye" inclusions visible on routine hematoxylin and eosin sections (Fig. 34-19). Inclusions may be seen in any cell type within the liver, either intracytoplasmic or intranuclear. Infected cells are often surrounded by neutrophilic microabscesses, with or without admixed mononuclear cells, but they may display only minimal accompanying inflammation. Numbers of inclusions vary widely, and typical neutrophilic microabscesses centered on injured and dying hepatocytes should trigger suspicion of CMV infection. Other associated features include hepatocyte apoptosis and focal necrosis; a portal and lobular

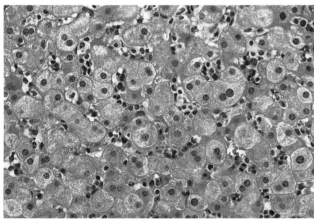

FIGURE 34–18. A diffuse lymphocytic sinusoidal infiltrate in a single-file "string-of-beads" pattern characterizes EBV infection.

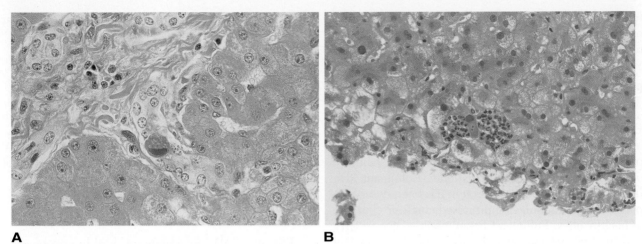

A   **B**

FIGURE 34–19. A, A biliary epithelial cell contains a large "owl's eye" inclusion with minimal inflammatory infiltrate. **B,** A neutrophilic microabscess surrounds a CMV-infected hepatocyte in a liver transplant patient.

mononuclear cell infiltrate; and, rarely, granulomas, including fibrin-ring granulomas.[62,63] Chronic liver disease does not ensue.

CMV Infection in the Neonate

Liver involvement is a common feature of neonatal/perinatal CMV infection. Affected infants usually have marked hepatosplenomegaly and jaundice. Histologically, the liver biopsy specimen reveals opportunistic CMV infection, with variable numbers of typical inclusions. A wide range of other alterations may be seen, including portal inflammation, marked cholestasis, giant cell transformation, focal necrosis, and prominent extramedullary hematopoiesis.[64] Bile duct damage and obliteration are rarely seen, although CMV (as well as several other viruses) has been associated with biliary atresia and paucity of intrahepatic bile ducts. In rare cases, portal or sinusoidal fibrosis may develop.

Useful diagnostic aids include viral culture, PCR assays, in situ hybridization, and CMV serologic studies/antigen tests.[59] Isolation of CMV in culture, however, does not imply active infection because the virus may be excreted for months to years after a primary infection has resolved.[65]

The differential diagnosis in healthy persons is primarily that of similar viral infections, particularly EBV. The differential diagnosis in immunocompromised patients primarily includes other viral infections as well, such as herpesvirus and adenovirus; other causes of microabscess such as ischemia should be considered, particularly in transplant patients.[66] In the neonate, the differential diagnosis includes other causes of neonatal hepatitis, as well as congenital disorders of bile ducts as mentioned earlier.

HERPESVIRUS

Herpes simplex virus hepatitis is usually seen in immunocompromised patients as part of disseminated infection, although it can occur in otherwise healthy persons.[68] Hepatic manifestations may dominate the clinical picture, however. Neonates, children who are malnourished or recovering from other infections (particularly measles), pregnant women, and immunocompromised persons are at significant risk for serious infection.[67] Clinically, patients are febrile, and some have concomitant oral or mucosal herpetic lesions, pharyngitis, headache, abdominal pain, or myalgias. Transaminases are elevated (often markedly), and hepatomegaly is frequently present. A rapidly progressive course with high mortality is common, and early liver biopsy may be invaluable for diagnosis.

Grossly, livers are enlarged and mottled and reveal multiple foci of necrosis, often surrounded by a zone of hemorrhage.[67,68] Histologically, randomly distributed zones of necrosis range from focal to visible with the naked eye. Portal tracts may be spared. The necrotic zones are often circumscribed by congestion and extravasated red blood cells.[67,68] Typical viral inclusions, both Cowdry type A and ground-glass cells, are found within hepatocyte nuclei at the periphery of necrotic areas (Fig. 34-20). Inclusions may be single or multiple. Inflammation is generally minimal.[67,68] Viral culture is the most valuable aid to diagnosis; immunohistochemistry and in situ hybridization may also be used.

The differential diagnosis predominantly includes other viral infections such as CMV and adenovirus, but these viruses do not cause the typical necrotic pattern of herpes simplex virus. Although viral hemorrhagic fevers may cause focal necrosis, widespread zonal necrosis and nuclear inclusions are absent. The varicella-zoster herpesvirus produces histologic lesions identical to those seen

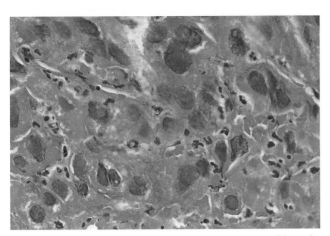

FIGURE 34–20. Herpes simplex. Viral inclusions are visible within dead hepatocytes at the periphery of necrotic areas; multinucleated infected hepatocytes may be seen.

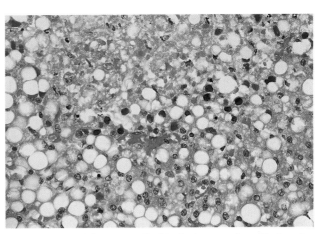

FIGURE 34–21. Adenovirus. Viral inclusions are found in hepatocytes at the edge of randomly distributed areas of necrosis. Infected cells are slightly enlarged, with dark homogeneous "smudged" nuclei.

in herpes simplex virus, but varicella patients generally exhibit a rash.[67,68] Ischemia or toxic injury may cause widespread necrosis, although it is often more zonally distributed in these conditions, and viral inclusions would not be seen.[68]

ENTERIC VIRUSES

This group of viruses rarely affect the liver, but fatal hepatic necrosis often results. Adenovirus is most commonly implicated, generally in immunocompromised patients (particularly children). Clinically, patients are febrile with hepatomegaly and markedly elevated transaminases. Concomitant pneumonia and diarrhea reflect disseminated infection.[69] Grossly, livers are enlarged and mottled with foci of necrosis. Histologic features may be similar to those of herpes infection with widespread random zones of necrosis. Although intranuclear viral inclusions may be seen, they are dark and homogeneous, unlike herpes inclusions (Fig. 34-21). Some cases exhibit randomly distributed, circumscribed inflammatory lesions consisting of mononuclear cells and granulocytes with rare inclusions at the edges of the inflammatory lesions; necrosis may be much less prominent in these cases. Granulomas have been rarely described.[70]

Useful diagnostic aids include immunohistochemistry, stool or tissue examination by electron microscopy, and viral culture. The differential diagnosis is primarily that of other viral infections, particularly herpes. Coxsackieviruses and echoviruses may exhibit a similar histologic picture, but inclusions are seldom seen.

VIRAL HEMORRHAGIC FEVERS

The geographic distributions, modes of transmission, and clinical courses of this diverse group of viruses are extremely variable (Table 34-4).[71,72] Death from liver failure is rare with the exception of yellow fever. Liver pathology is similar regardless of the type of virus; useful adjunctive tests include serologic studies and immunohistochemistry, although these are not widely available. Patients present with a viral prodrome consisting of fever, headache, and myalgia, followed by hemorrhagic manifestations. Elevated transaminases and hepatomegaly are common. Histologically, viral hemorrhagic fevers feature foci of coagulative necrosis with minimal inflammation. Necrosis is usually multifocal and is randomly distributed rather than massive. Some foci of necrosis may be surrounded by macrophages.[72,73] Steatosis is variable, and cholestasis is

TABLE 34–4. Viral Hemorrhagic Fevers

Disease	Geographic Distribution	Transmission/Reservoir	Selected Signs and Symptoms	Mortality
Dengue fever	Africa, Asia, tropical Americas, Caribbean	Mosquito/human	Viral prodrome and rash	<20%
Yellow fever	Africa, South America	Mosquito/human	Viral prodrome with vomiting, jaundice; elevated bilirubin	10%–50%
Lassa fever	West Africa	Person-to-person and body fluid/rat	Viral prodrome; vomiting, cough, abdominal pain	<25%
Marburg fever	Central/southern Africa	Unknown	Viral prodrome, nausea, vomiting, diarrhea	?25%
Ebola fever	Central Africa	Unknown	Similar to Marburg virus	>80%

not usually prominent. Adjacent intact hepatocytes may reveal regenerative changes and ballooning. Inclusions are not typically seen.

Other viruses that cause hepatitis include measles (rubeola), rubella, and parvovirus, which may affect the liver in the context of hydrops fetalis. Primary HIV infection has been noted to cause liver involvement similar to that seen in EBV-related mononucleosis, as well as neonatal hepatitis.[74]

The virus-associated (reactive) hemophagocytic syndrome (VAHS) is strongly associated with viral infection, particularly EBV, although other viruses have also been implicated.[75-77] Patients present with fever, hepatomegaly, splenomegaly, peripheral blood cytopenias, and lymphadenopathy; many patients report a viral-like prodrome. Among adults, patients are often immunocompromised; children with VAHS do not usually have underlying immune deficiencies. Most patients recover spontaneously. Histologic features include cytologically benign hemophagocytic histiocytes within both portal tracts and sinusoids. Kupffer cells may be hypertrophic and may reveal hemophagocytosis as well as siderosis. Focal hepatocyte necrosis may be noted.

Bacterial Infections of the Liver

PREDOMINANTLY SUPPURATIVE BACTERIAL INFECTIONS

Suppurative hepatic inflammation is usually accompanied by hepatocyte necrosis; lesions may range from microscopically visible microabscesses to pyogenic abscesses seen with the naked eye. A general discussion of suppurative hepatic abscess is presented here, followed by a more detailed discussion of some specific suppurative infections.

Pyogenic Bacterial Abscess

Pyogenic abscesses are caused by a wide range of bacteria. Most patients are older adults who present with nonspecific symptoms, including abdominal pain, hepatomegaly, malaise, and fever. Jaundice is rare. Transaminases are usually elevated but with a disproportionately high level of alkaline phosphatase.

In general, pyogenic abscesses are secondary infections seeded from other sites, particularly the biliary tree and gastrointestinal tract. They are often polymicrobial; commonly implicated bacteria include *Escherichia coli*, *Staphylococcus aureus*, and *Streptococcus*, *Klebsiella*, *Proteus*, *Pseudomonas*, *Bacteroides*, and *Fusobacterium* species. Less common yet noteworthy pathogens include *Aeromonas*, *Actinomyces*, *Nocardia*, *Salmonella*, and *Yersinia* species, as well as

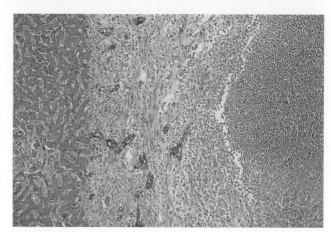

FIGURE 34–22. Hepatic abscess. A suppurative center is surrounded by granulation tissue and fibrosis in this *Staphylococcus* species–related pyogenic abscess.

Haemophilus influenzae.[78-80] Predisposing conditions include diabetes, intra-abdominal malignancies, cholangitis, idiopathic inflammatory bowel disease, appendicitis, and diverticulosis.[81,82] Tumors, cysts, and infarctions may also become secondarily infected, leading to abscess formation.

Abscesses may be multiple or solitary and are more common in the right lobe.[81] Sizes range from microscopic to larger than 3 cm.[82] As with abscesses elsewhere in the body, these consist of central suppurative inflammation and necrosis, surrounded by organizing inflammation and fibrosis (Fig. 34-22). The fibrous rind may be prominent and may contain bizarre reactive fibroblasts and atypical reactive lymphocytes. Granulomatous reactions are occasionally seen. Nonspecific reactive changes, including cholestasis, portal inflammation, ductular proliferation, and venulitis, are noted in the surrounding liver. If the primary site of infection is the biliary tree, changes of acute cholangitis may occur. Organisms are occasionally detectable with special stains.

If a surgical drainage procedure or aspiration is undertaken, culture of the resultant purulent material is of paramount importance. Otherwise, blood cultures may be valuable in isolating the causative organism. The differential diagnosis primarily includes other causes of hepatic abscess, such as amebae, hydatid disease, and necrotic tumors.

Tularemia

Francisella tularensis is a Gram-negative coccobacillus that is endemic in many areas of North America. It is transmitted to humans from rodents.[83] Hepatic involvement may be subclinical and often involves disseminated infection. Patients have elevated transaminases, hepatomegaly, and, rarely, jaundice. Histologically, typically suppurative microabscesses appear with occasional surrounding macrophages; as the lesions evolve, they may become more granulomatous.[83] Organisms are rarely seen on special stains; thus, cultures and serologic tests are useful diagnostic modalities.

Listeria monocytogenes

Hepatic listeriosis may be seen in both neonates and adults; in the latter group, it is frequently a feature of disseminated infection in immunocompromised patients and diabetic patients. Histologically, scattered microabscesses are seen, often with small granulomas. Sometimes, an exclusively microgranulomatous pattern and, rarely, true epithelioid granulomas may be present.[84] Occasionally, short, pleomorphic, Gram-positive rods may be identified, but blood culture is the most important diagnostic adjunct. DNA probes and immunohistochemistry may be useful but are not widely available.

THE LIVER IN SEPSIS

Sepsis and bacteremia cause a wide spectrum of hepatic injury. Both cholestatic and hepatitic patterns of enzyme elevations may be seen. Histologically, some cases reveal predominantly neutrophilic inflammation (both portal and lobular) with microabscesses. Other cases exhibit cholestatic features, with centrilobular canalicular cholestasis, ductular cholestasis with ductular proliferation, inspissated bile, and a periductular neutrophilic infiltrate (Fig. 34-23). The biliary ductal epithelium may be flattened and atrophic with vacuolation and necrosis. Focal necrosis of hepatocytes, mild portal inflammation, Kupffer cell hyperplasia, and fatty changes may also be seen.[85-87] Venous congestion and ischemic necrosis can be prominent in cases of septic shock.

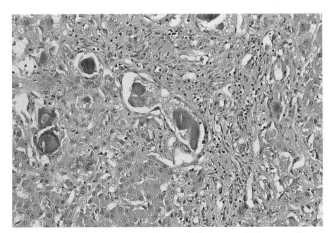

FIGURE 34–23. Sepsis. Ductular proliferation, cholestasis-dense inspissated bile, and flattened, atrophic biliary epithelium are features often seen in sepsis.

PREDOMINANTLY GRANULOMATOUS BACTERIAL INFECTIONS

Hepatic granulomas are reportedly present in 2% to 10% of all liver specimens examined in general practice. However, the causes of many of these granulomas remain elusive. The following section focuses on infectious causes of granulomas, but the clinician must also be aware of noninfectious entities in the differential diagnosis, such as sarcoidosis, PBC, adverse drug reaction, berylliosis, Hodgkin's disease, and foreign body reaction.[88] The morphology of granulomas may provide a clue to diagnosis (Table 34-5).

The distinctive hepatic fibrin-ring granuloma (Fig. 34-24) bears special mention. Although they have been classically described in association with Q fever, these lesions are nonspecific and have been observed in the context of numerous diseases, including leishmaniasis, boutonneuse fever, Hodgkin's disease, allopurinol reaction, toxoplasmosis, CMV infection, mononucleosis, and typhoid fever.[89]

Mycobacterium tuberculosis

Liver involvement is seen in almost all cases of miliary tuberculosis and is common both in localized extrapulmonary tuberculosis and in association with pulmonary tuberculosis. Signs and symptoms of liver disease may be the dominant or presenting features of tubercular infection. Although liver involvement is often asymptomatic, hepatomegaly, right upper quadrant pain, and fever may be seen. Ascites and jaundice are less frequent. Patients may have elevated bilirubin and transaminases, along with a disproportionately high alkaline phosphatase.[90] Confluent granulomas can lead to hepatic masses (tuberculomas) and periportal lymphadenopathy.[90,91]

The histologic hallmark of hepatic tuberculosis is the epithelioid granuloma, which is often accompanied by caseation and giant cells (Fig. 34-25). Granulomas are usually small but may coalesce to form nodules or masses with central liquefactive necrosis.[91] Older lesions may reveal fibrosis, calcification, and occasionally associated amyloid.[92] These are often accompanied by reactive hepatitis. It is often difficult to detect mycobacteria on special stains; thus, culture and PCR assays may be of value.

Mycobacterium avium-intracellulare

MAI infection is most commonly associated with, but not limited to, patients with acquired immunodeficiency syndrome (AIDS). The liver is involved in more than 50% of disseminated cases. Histologically, most liver biopsies exhibit some degree of granulomatous inflammation (Fig. 34-26). Some patients, particularly the immunocompetent, have discrete epithelioid

TABLE 34–5. Classification of Granulomatous Lesions in the Liver by Histologic Pattern

Fibrin-Ring Granuloma	Microgranulomas	Stellate Microabscess With Granulomatous Inflammation	Foamy Macrophage Aggregates	Predominantly Suppurative, Without or With Granulomatous Inflammation	Epithelioid Granuloma, Infectious Causes	Epithelioid Granuloma, Other Causes
Q fever	*Listeria* species (rare)	Actinomycosis	*Rhodococcus equi*	Tularemia	*M. tuberculosis* (usually caseating)	Drug reaction
Toxoplasmosis	Usually nonspecific reaction to liver injury	*Nocardia* species	Whipple's disease	Listeriosis	Brucellosis	Foreign body reaction
Salmonella species		*Bartonella* species	*MAI* (immune compromised patients)	Melioidosis	*MAI* (immune competent patients)	Sarcoidosis
CMV		Tularemia	Lepromatous leprosy		*Listeria* species (rare)	Autoimmune diseases
EBV		*Candida* species	Histoplasmosis		Tuberculoid leprosy	Primary biliary cirrhosis
Leishmaniasis		Other fungi	Leishmaniasis		Tertiary syphilis	Hodgkin's disease
Drug reaction					*Chlamydia* species	Other paraneoplastic conditions
Lupus erythematosus					Whipple's disease (rare)	Chronic granulomatous disease of childhood
Metastases					Schistosomiasis	
					Fungal infections	
					Viral infections (rare)	

CMV, cytomegalovirus; EBV, Epstein-Barr virus; *MAI, Mycobacterium avium-intracellulare.*

granulomas with associated neutrophils and lymphocytes. Giant cells and necrosis are rare.[93,94] In AIDS patients, the granulomas tend to be composed of aggregates of foamy macrophages in the parenchyma and portal tracts (see Fig. 34-26). Organisms are usually abundant on acid-fast stain in immunocompromised patients but rare in immunocompetent persons. Occasionally, particularly in AIDS patients, *MAI* forms pseudosarcomatous spindle-cell nodules that may mimic neoplasia (Fig. 34-27).[95] Culture and PCR may be useful diagnostic adjuncts. The differential diagnosis includes other causes of foamy macrophage aggregates, such as *Rhodococcus equi* and Whipple's disease. Other atypical mycobacteria, including *Mycobacterium kansasii* and bacilli Calmette-Guérin (BCG), occasionally cause liver disease.

Mycobacterium leprae

More than 60% of patients with lepromatous leprosy have hepatic involvement, along with about 20% of patients with tuberculoid leprosy.[96,97] Liver disease is often subclinical.[98] Histologically, findings vary with the type of leprosy. In lepromatous leprosy, aggregates of foamy histiocytes (lepra cells) containing numerous

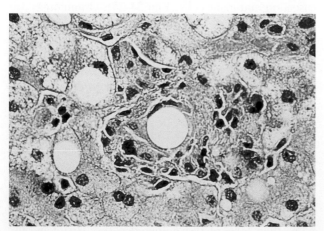

FIGURE 34–24. Fibrin-ring granulomas typically consist of an epithelioid granuloma with a central lipid vacuole surrounded by a fibrin ring (fibrin stain). (Photographs courtesy of Dr. Randall Lee.)

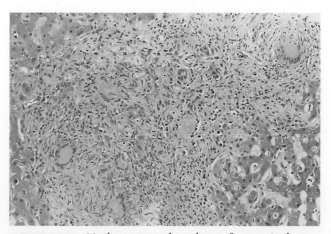

FIGURE 34–25. *Myobacterium tuberculosis* infection. Coalescent epithelioid granulomas with numerous giant cells are seen in portal tracts.

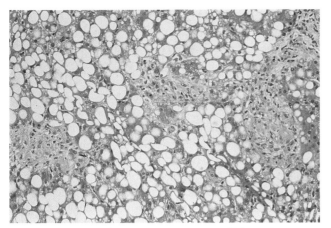

FIGURE 34–26. *Myobacterium avium-intracellulare.* Aggregates of foamy macrophages are present in the liver parenchyma of an HIV-positive patient.

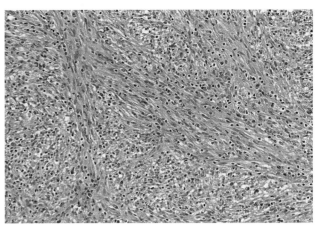

FIGURE 34–27. *Myobacterium avium-intracellulare.* Occasionally *MAI* induces pseudosarcomatous spindles cell nodules in the liver.

acid-fast bacilli are seen within portal tracts and lobules. Giant cells and discrete granulomas are rarely seen, and accompanying inflammation is minimal. In tuberculoid leprosy, discrete, tuberculoid granulomas are usually seen with associated giant cells. Bacilli are rare in this variant. Some patients manifest histologic features somewhere between lepromatous and tuberculoid granulomatous lesions.[98]

Bartonella Species

Bartonella henselae is the most common cause of cat-scratch disease (CSD).[99] Patients usually present with isolated lymphadenopathy in an area draining a cat-scratch inoculation, but a small percentage of patients (1% to 2%) develop disseminated infection. These patients usually lack the characteristic skin papule and superficial adenopathy but have generalized symptoms

such as weight loss, fever, and malaise. Liver lesions are usually multiple and associated with abdominal lymphadenopathy.[100] Hepatic CSD patients are often younger than 10 years of age and are usually not immunocompromised. Patients generally respond well to antibiotic therapy.

The characteristic histologic lesion of hepatic CSD consists of irregular, stellate microabscesses surrounded by an inner layer of palisading histiocytes, a surrounding rim of lymphocytes, and an outermost thick layer of fibrous tissue (Fig. 34-28). This outer fibrous zone is very pronounced in liver CSD. The lesions may vary widely within the same specimen, ranging from early microabscesses to older lesions consisting of fibrosis and granulation tissue.[100] The differential diagnosis primarily includes other infections. Diagnostic aids include patient history with specific questions pertaining to cat exposure, silver stains (Warthin-Starry or

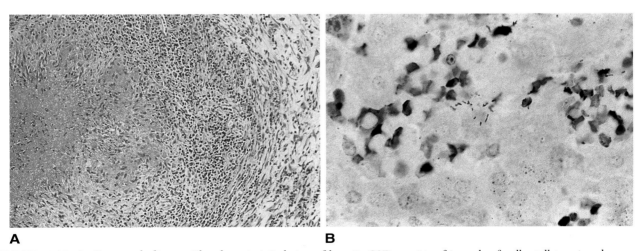

A   **B**

FIGURE 34–28. A, Cat-scratch disease. The characteristic lesion of hepatic CSD consists of irregular, focally stellate microabscesses surrounded by an inner layer of palisading histiocytes, an outer rim of lymphocytes, and a thick layer of fibrous tissue. **B,** Small pleomorphic bacilli are occasionally detectable in necrotic areas on silver impregnation stains (Warthin-Starry).

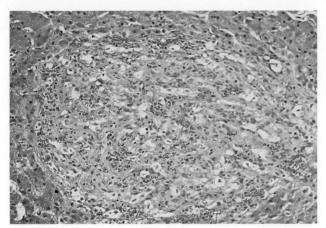

FIGURE 34–29. Hepatic bacillary angiomatosis consists of multiple slitlike vascular spaces within a fibromyxoid stroma with an associated mixed inflammatory infiltrate.

Steiner), molecular assays, and enzyme-linked immunosorbent assay (ELISA) at some centers.

Both *Bartonella* species (*B. henselae* and *B. quintana*) are associated with hepatic bacillary angiomatosis/peliosis.[101] These lesions consist of multiple slitlike or cystic vascular spaces within a fibromyxoid stroma, often with associated mixed inflammatory infiltrate and focal necrosis (Fig. 34-29).[102] Bacillary angiomatosis/peliosis is usually found in HIV-positive patients and may mimic Kaposi's sarcoma or other vascular tumors; well-formed vessels, a neutrophilic infiltrate, and organisms seen on silver precipitation stains help to distinguish bacillary angiomatosis.

Brucella Species

This disease occurs primarily in domestic and barnyard animals; humans contract infection through occupational exposure and by ingesting contaminated food. Patients generally present with fever, malaise, headache, and arthralgias; lymphadenopathy and hepatosplenomegaly may also occur. Hepatic involvement is seen in approximately half of cases.[103] Liver biopsy specimens often reveal noncaseating granulomatous inflammation, sometimes with accompanying giant cells.[103-105] Granulomas may be discrete and epithelioid or small and poorly formed. Some patients manifest only a nonspecific reactive hepatitis.[104,105] Organisms are difficult to culture and are rarely seen on special stains. Serologic studies and an appropriate exposure history are most helpful for clinicians in making the diagnosis.

Rickettsia and Similar Species

Most rickettsial illnesses affect the liver, although involvement may be subclinical. *Coxiella burnetii*

(causative agent of Q fever) is perhaps the most noteworthy of this group owing to its characteristic fibrin-ring granulomas. This lesion consists of an epithelioid granuloma with a central lipid vacuole surrounded by a fibrin ring (see Fig. 34-24); many Q fever granulomas are intermediate between epithelioid and fibrin ring types.[106,107] *Rickettsia conorii*, the causative agent of boutonneuse fever and South African tickbite fever, may cause either granulomas or a nongranulomatous reactive hepatitis.[108] *Rickettsia rickettsii* (Rocky Mountain spotted fever) causes a mixed portal inflammatory infiltrate, endotheliitis, cholestasis, and erythrophagocytosis.[109] *Rickettsia typhi* (murine typhus) may also involve the liver with similar histologic changes.[110] Organisms in the rickettsial illnesses are difficult to detect; thus, immunofluorescent stains and serologic studies may be helpful.

SPIROCHETE INFECTIONS

Syphilis

Both congenital and acquired syphilis (at any stage) may involve the liver. In congenital hepatic syphilis, neonates have hepatomegaly, jaundice, and elevated serum bilirubin and transaminases.[111] Histologic changes, which may be indistinguishable from those of neonatal hepatitis of other causes, include striking pericellular fibrosis with an associated mononuclear cell infiltrate, extramedullary hematopoiesis, and, rarely, small granulomas. Permanent liver damage rarely occurs if treatment is instituted.[111-113]

The reported prevalence of liver involvement in early acquired syphilis varies widely, ranging from 1% to 50%. Generally, hepatic involvement is reflected only by abnormal laboratory tests, but jaundice, hepatomegaly, abdominal pain, and markedly elevated alkaline phosphatase have been reported.[114-116] The histologic findings in both primary and secondary syphilis encompass a broad scope, ranging from unremarkable to nonspecific reactive changes to marked necroinflammatory changes.[114,115] Rarely, granulomas, cholestasis, vasculitis, and bile duct damage have been described.[116] Sinusoidal fibrosis may be present and may persist after treatment. Spirochetes may be identifiable in some cases, and serologic tests may be useful diagnostic aids.

The rarely seen but often discussed pathologic lesion of tertiary syphilis is the gumma, a nodular focus of caseous necrosis surrounded by a fibrous inflamed wall, scattered granulomas, and associated endarteritis.[117,118] Healing leads to the grossly distorted, scarred liver known as *hepar lobatum*. Clinically, nodular gummas may be confused with neoplasms or other infections.

Other spirochetal infections that may involve the liver include leptospirosis (Weil's disease) and those caused by *Borrelia* species (causative agents of Lyme disease and other relapsing febrile illnesses). These infections usually result in a nonspecific reactive hepatitis. Silver impregnation stains may reveal organisms; serologic studies and immunostains may also be of diagnostic value.

MISCELLANEOUS BACTERIAL INFECTIONS

Salmonella Species

Acute systemic *Salmonella* species infections, especially those associated with enteric fever, often involve the liver. The characteristic lesion is the typhoid nodule (even with nontyphoid *Salmonella* species)—an aggregate of Kupffer cells admixed with scattered lymphocytes.[119,120] Organisms are rarely detected.

Whipple's Disease *(Tropheryma whippelii)*

Rarely, Whipple's bacillus has been identified within the liver, occasionally even in the absence of small bowel involvement.[121,122] Histologically, these PAS-positive bacilli are present within Kupffer cells. Often, no significant inflammatory response is noted, but epithelioid granulomas in association with Whipple's disease are well documented.[122] Electron microscopy and PCR assays may be useful diagnostic aids. The differential diagnosis includes *MAI* infection and infection caused by other intracellular organisms such as *Histoplasma capsulatum* and *R. equi*.

Other infections that may affect the liver include those associated with the *Chlamydia* species, which can cause both perihepatitis (Fitz-Hugh–Curtis syndrome) and hepatitis; *R. equi*, which causes a granulomatous inflammatory pattern that mimics *MAI*; and *Pseudomonas pseudomallei* (melioidosis), which may cause either small neutrophilic microabscesses or granulomas.

Fungal Infections of the Liver

Hepatic fungal infections are generally part of a disseminated process that occurs in immunocompromised patients, although rare cases have been described in healthy persons. The clinical features are similar regardless of the fungus involved and include hepatomegaly, abdominal pain, and elevated transaminases and bilirubin.[123] Although fungi are often seen on routine hematoxylin and eosin sections in fulminant infection, GMS and PAS stains remain invaluable diagnostic aids. Fungi can sometimes be correctly classified in tissue sections according to morphology. It should be stressed, however, that culture should be relied on as

the gold standard of speciation; antifungal therapy may vary according to the type of fungus. A table of morphologic features of various fungal infections is provided in Chapter 3.

CANDIDA SPECIES

The *Candida* species is the most common cause of disseminated fungal infection in immunocompromised hosts, and liver involvement is frequent. Grossly, the liver contains multiple yellow-white nodules ranging in size from 1 to 2 cm.[124,125] The typical inflammatory reaction is granulomatous, often with a suppurative central area and variable necrosis. Giant cells are occasionally present. Surrounding palisading histiocytes and a fibrous scar may be seen, similar to hepatic CSD. Nonspecific findings such as cholestasis, portal inflammation, ductular proliferation, and sinusoidal dilatation near the inflammatory lesion are often present.[124-126] Organisms are generally seen in the center of the inflammatory lesion but may be few and only focally present. *Candida albicans* and *Candida tropicalis* produce budding yeast, hyphae, and pseudohyphae. *Candida (Torulopsis) glabrata* produces only tiny budding yeast, similar to the *Histoplasma* species.[126]

ASPERGILLUS SPECIES

Aspergillus infection generally begins in the lungs and occurs almost exclusively in immunocompromised patients. Grossly, affected livers show necrosis and the characteristic "target" lesion, consisting of a necrotic central zone with a hyperemic rim. The analogous histologic lesion is a nodular infarct centered on a blood vessel containing fungi. Inflammatory response ranges from minimal to marked neutrophilic infiltrates; granulomatous inflammation is sometimes seen.[123,126] The hyphae of *Aspergillus* are septate and branch dichotomously (equally) at acute angles. The pathology of mucormycosis and related Zygomycetes is similar to that of aspergillosis, but these organisms have broad, ribbon-like, pauciseptate hyphae that branch randomly at various angles.[126]

HISTOPLASMOSIS

H. capsulatum is endemic to the central United States. Hepatic involvement occurs in more than 90% of patients with disseminated infection. Patients occasionally present with signs of liver disease and do not always have concomitant pulmonary involvement. Discrete granulomas and giant cells are seen in only a minority of cases; most biopsy specimens reveal portal lymphohistiocytic inflammation and sinusoidal Kupffer cell hyperplasia (Fig. 34-30). Organisms are generally present within both portal macrophages and Kupffer

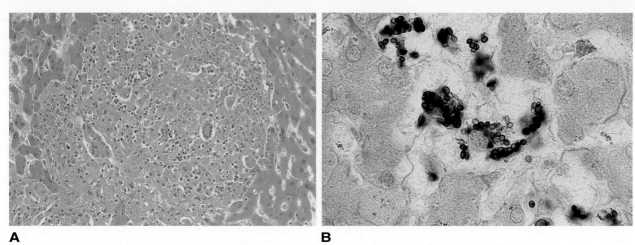

FIGURE 34–30. A, Histoplasmosis. Nodular portal lymphohistiocytic inflammation is typical of hepatic histoplasmosis. **B,** Sinusoidal Kupffer cells contain typical *Histoplasma* organisms (Gomori silver stain).

cells. In immunocompromised patients, large numbers of organisms may be seen with virtually no tissue reaction.[127] *Histoplasma* organisms are small, ovoid, usually intracellular yeast forms with small buds at the more pointed pole. *Penicillium marneffei*, a fungus endemic to Southeast Asia, resembles *H. capsulatum* but is more sausage shaped and has a central cross wall rather than a bud.

CRYPTOCOCCUS NEOFORMANS

Cryptococci are the most common cause of systemic mycosis in patients with AIDS.[128] The inflammatory reaction is variable and depends on the immune status of the host, ranging from a suppurative, necrotizing inflammatory reaction with granulomatous features to virtually no reaction at all in immunocompromised hosts.[126,129,130] Purely granulomatous responses are sometimes seen. The *Cryptococcus* organism is a round to oval yeast with narrow-based budding and often considerable variation in size. The mucopolysaccharide capsular material stains with Alcian blue, mucicarmine, and colloidal iron; Gomori silver stains (GMS) are positive. Cryptococcosis may also involve the biliary tree.

Other fungal infections that are occasionally seen in the liver include *Pneumocystis carinii*, *Blastomyces dermatitidis*, *Paracoccidioides brasiliensis* (South American blastomycosis), and *Coccidioides immitis.*

The differential diagnosis includes other suppurative and granulomatous processes, especially bacterial and mycobacterial infections. Noninfectious causes of hepatic granulomas should be considered, although these are less likely if suppuration and necrosis are prominent. Helpful diagnostic aids, in addition to culture, include serologic assays, antigen tests, and immunohistochemistry.

Parasitic Infections of the Liver

PROTOZOA

Malaria

Hepatic sequelae of malarial infection (e.g., jaundice, hepatomegaly, and elevated transaminase levels) are common, but hepatic failure does not ensue. Grossly, affected livers are enlarged and congested with a gray or dark brown appearance caused by malarial pigment deposition. Concomitantly, the most striking microscopic feature is hemozoin pigment within macrophages along sinusoids, in portal tracts, and in erythrocytes. The pigment forms dark brown clumps that do not react with iron stains. Nonspecific associated changes include mild portal lymphocytosis, erythrophagocytosis, lipofuscin pigment, and Kupffer cell hyperplasia.[131,132] Parasites may be visible within erythrocytes. Babesiosis is a tick-borne zoonotic illness that is clinicopathologically similar to malaria; serologic tests may be useful in distinguishing them.

Entamoeba histolytica

Hepatic amebiasis occurs when invasive colonic lesions seed the portal vein circulation, but many patients with hepatic lesions do not have a history of gastrointestinal complaints.[133] Clinically, patients present with fever, abdominal pain/tenderness, leukocytosis, and hepatomegaly; jaundice, weight loss, and malaise are variably present.[133] Patients may have elevated alkaline phosphatase and transaminase levels.

Grossly, abscesses may be solitary or multiple.[134] Lesions range from pale, necrotic nodules to irregularly shaped abscesses with fibrous capsules and contents reportedly resembling anchovy paste; size ranges

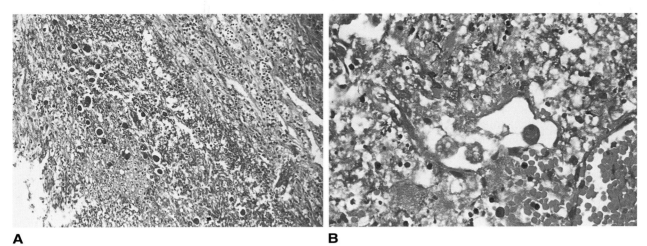

A   **B**

FIGURE 34–31. **A,** Amebic abscesses consist of necrotic material with prominent nuclear debris and relatively few inflammatory cells (PAS). **B,** Organisms may be present at the advancing edge. (Photographs courtesy of Dr. David Walker.)

from barely discernible to larger than 20 cm.[133,134] Occasionally, amebic abscesses rupture through the capsule into the peritoneum, or they may extend to involve surrounding organs and even the skin.[134] Histologically, the earliest lesion involves amebic trophozoites within sinusoids with focal necrosis and a neutrophilic infiltrate. In advanced disease, lesions consist predominantly of necrotic material containing nuclear debris and few inflammatory cells. Mononuclear cells and organisms may be present at the advancing edge; neutrophils are rare (Fig. 34-31). Eventually, peripheral granulation tissue and fibrosis develop. The amebae themselves resemble large macrophages (see Chapter 3) with foamy cytoplasm and a round eccentric nucleus; ingested red blood cells are pathognomonic of *E. histolytica*.

Radiographically, the abscesses may mimic neoplasms. Otherwise, the main item in the differential diagnosis is pyogenic liver abscess; aspiration and culture are invaluable in resolving this differential, and sometimes amebae are identifiable in the aspirate. The ciliate *Balantidium coli* can produce clinicopathologic changes similar to amebiasis.

FLAGELLATES

Visceral Leishmaniasis (Kala-Azar)

Visceral leishmaniasis is most often seen in AIDS patients. The typical hepatic pathologic finding is hyperplastic Kupffer cells (and, rarely, hepatocytes) containing amastigotes (tiny, round to oval organisms with the nucleus and kinetoplast in a "double-knot" configuration). The organism-laden macrophages may form small nodules or loosely formed granulomas. Fibrin-ring and epithelioid granulomas have been described.[135,136] *Leishmania* species organisms may be confused with similar organisms such as *Histoplasma*

species; *Leishmania* species organisms are GMS-negative, and *Histoplasma* species lack a kinetoplast.

Miscellaneous Flagellates

Rare reports of granulomatous hepatitis and cholangitis have been associated with *Giardia lamblia*.[137]

COCCIDIANS

Coccidians can produce infection in both immunocompromised and healthy patients. Many infections are subclinical; although the most common manifestation is diarrhea, these infections also cause hepatobiliary disease.

Toxoplasma gondii

Hepatic toxoplasmosis is primarily a disease of the immunocompromised. *Toxoplasma* species hepatitis features cholestasis, a mononuclear cell infiltrate, and focal hepatocyte necrosis; both crescent-shaped tachyzoites and tissue cysts containing bradyzoites may be seen within hepatocytes.[138,139] Granulomatous hepatitis has been described as well, and giant cell hepatitis may be present in neonates. Immunohistochemistry, PCR, and serologic tests provide useful diagnostic aids.

Cryptosporidium parvum and Microsporidia

These most common causes of AIDS-related cholangiopathy are discussed in detail in Chapter 28. They are only rarely seen in the liver.[140-142] Disseminated *Isospora belli* has been rarely reported in the liver[143] and mesenteric lymph nodes.

HELMINTHS (NEMATODES, TREMATODES, CESTODES)

Helminths are more often a cause of serious disease in nations with deficient sanitation systems, poor socio-economic status, and hot, humid climates. However, they are occasionally seen in developed countries.

Hepatic helminthic infections manifest a wide range of clinicopathologic findings. The differential diagnosis often involves differentiating between types of worms. Other entities to consider include additional causes of granulomatous inflammation and hepatic abscess.

Nematodes

ASCARIS LUMBRICOIDES

This roundworm causes the most common human helminth infection. Clinical findings are variable and include hepatomegaly, cholecystitis, cholangitis, and hepatic abscess. Cholangitic superinfection by enteric bacteria is common. These large worms (up to 20 cm) may be identified within the biliary tree with accompanying reactive epithelial changes. Abscesses may contain worm remnants or, rarely, eggs with associated inflammation (often prominent eosinophils) and necrosis.[144,145]

TOXOCARIASIS

Toxocara canis is the most common cause of visceral larvae migrans. Patients generally present with hepatomegaly, fever, leukocytosis, eosinophilia, and pulmonary and central nervous system disturbances. Histologically, central eosinophilic abscesses are seen with Charcot-Leyden crystals and associated granulomatous inflammation.[146] Larval remnants are occasionally identified. As lesions heal, fibrous scars develop. Many other helminths can cause visceral larvae migrans, including *Toxocara cati*, *Strongyloides stercoralis*, and *Capillaria* and *Ascaris* species.[146]

ENTEROBIUS VERMICULARIS (PINWORMS)

Pinworms are one of the most common human parasites. The rare pinworm granuloma is a hyalinized nodule with peripheral inflammation. Central necrosis with eggs and worm remnants may be present.[147,148]

STRONGYLOIDES STERCORALIS

Many patients with this infection are asymptomatic, but the worm's capability for autoinfection allows it to reside in the host and produce illness for upward of 30 years. Hepatic involvement is generally part of disseminated disease. Livers show larvae within portal vessels and sinusoids; associated inflammation ranges from none to a nonspecific mixed inflammatory infiltrate. Granulomas are sometimes seen.[149]

Trematodes

SCHISTOSOMIASIS

Schistosomiasis is the most common cause of portal hypertension in the world. Most hepatobiliary disease is caused by *Schistosoma mansoni*, *Schistosoma japonicum*, or *Schistosoma mekongi* because these organisms prefer mesenteric and portal veins. Once settled in their vein of choice, adult worms copulate and produce thousands of eggs in their lifetimes; approximately 50% of these eggs remain within the body.[150] Hypersensitivity to the eggs themselves is actually the underlying cause of disease, and resultant inflammation leads to fibrosis and obstructive hepatobiliary disease.[150] Symptomatic patients present with splenomegaly and signs of portal hypertension, particularly bleeding; hepatic function is usually preserved.

Grossly, livers are enlarged and nodular; on cut surface, the typical portal fibrosis, known as pipestem or Symmers' fibrosis, may be observed. Portal tracts are enlarged and stellate, but liver acinar architecture is essentially unremarkable. Histologic features vary with duration of disease. Early schistosomiasis features portal inflammation with numerous eosinophils, Kupffer cell hyperplasia, and focal hepatocyte necrosis, but ova are rarely seen. In chronic disease, a granulomatous reaction to the eggs typically occurs; the eggs are present in varying numbers within both granulomas and fibrotic areas (Fig. 34-32). Mixed portal inflammation and giant cells are noted. Ultimately, portal tracts become large and densely sclerotic, and fibrous septa link portal tracts together. Sinusoidal fibrosis may also develop. As fibrosis progresses, eggs may be difficult to find. Schistosomal pigment, similar to malarial pigment, is often present within Kupffer cells and macrophages.[92,150,151] Granulomas and fibrosis also affect portal vein branches, leading to phlebitis, sclerosis, and thrombosis. Eventually, portal veins are obstructed

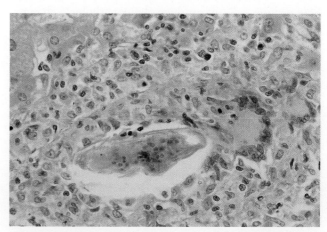

FIGURE 34–32. Portal granulomatous reaction to the schistosoma eggs. (Photograph courtesy of Dr. George F. Gray, Jr.)

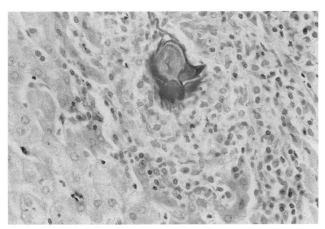

FIGURE 34–33. *Schistosoma mansoni* is acid-fast and has a prominent lateral spine (Fite stain). (Photograph courtesy of Dr. George F. Gray, Jr.)

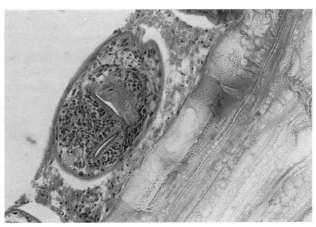

FIGURE 34–35. The inner lining of the cyst consists of epithelial cells giving rise to the brood capsules from which scoleces develop. The outer cyst layers comprise hyalinized, acellular, PAS-positive material. (Photograph courtesy of Dr. George F. Gray, Jr.)

and destroyed with subsequent proliferation of hepatic arterial branches.[92]

The eggs themselves are large. *S. mansoni* has an acid-fast shell (Fig. 34-33) and a prominent lateral spine, but exact speciation of schistosomes within the liver is difficult. The nematode of the *Capillaria* species should be considered in the differential diagnosis because the eggs are somewhat similar.

Other trematodes infecting the liver and biliary tree include flukes, *Opisthorchis sinensis*, and other *Opisthorchis* species (which are associated with the development of cholangiocarcinoma),[152,153] as well as *Fasciola hepatica*, which may cause calculi, cholangitis, obstructive jaundice, and a granulomatous hepatitis.[154]

Cestodes

ECHINOCOCCUS GRANULOSUS AND RELATED SPECIES

Hydatid disease is often subclinical, but some patients exhibit hepatomegaly, marked abdominal enlargement and distention, and ascites. Secondary

infection of the cysts may also develop. Ultimately, some patients manifest liver failure, portal hypertension, involvement of adjacent organs, and death.[155,156] Grossly, the cysts are large, unilocular, and rounded. The cyst fluid is strikingly antigenic and may lead to anaphylaxis if spilled into the abdominal cavity. The inner layer of the cysts consists of a thin lining of epithelial cells, giving rise to the brood capsules from which scoleces, or immature heads of adult worms, develop (Figs. 34-34 and 34-35). The outer cyst layers comprise hyalinized, PAS-positive material, surrounded by granulation tissue and fibrosis.[157] Daughter cysts may develop within the main cyst. The differential diagnosis includes other cystic lesions. The scolex of the worm distinguishes hydatid disease from amebic abscess, pyogenic abscess, and noninfectious processes such as fibropolycystic liver disease.

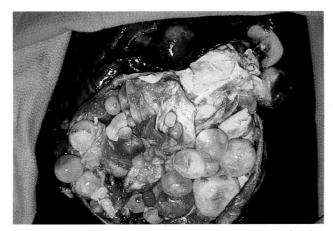

FIGURE 34–34. Grossly, echinococcal cysts are large, unilocular, and rounded. (Photograph courtesy of Dr. George F. Gray, Jr.)

References

1. Lee W: Acute liver failure. N Engl J Med 329:1862-1872, 1993.
2. Alter M, Gallagher M, Morris T, et al: Acute non A-E hepatitis in the US and the role of hepatitis G virus infection. Sentinel Counties Viral Hepatitis Study Team. N Engl J Med 336:741-746, 1997.
3. Centers for Disease Control and Prevention: Prevention of hepatitis A through active or passive immunization. Recommendations of the Advisory Committee on Immunization Practices (ACIP). MMWR 44:1-30, 1996.
4. Kemmer N, Miskovsky E: Hepatitis A. Infect Dis Clin North Am 14:605-615, 2000.
5. Befeler A, DiBisceglie A: Hepatitis B. Infect Dis Clin North Am 14:617-632, 2000.
6. Conry-Cantilena C, VanRaden M, Gibble J, et al: Routes of infection, viremia, and liver disease in blood donors found to have hepatitis C virus infection. N Engl J Med 334:1691-1696, 1996.
7. Centers for Disease Control and Prevention: Recommendations for prevention and control of hepatitis C (HCV) infection and HCV-related chronic disease. MMWR CDC Surveill Summ 47:1-39, 1998.

8. Alter M, Purcell R, Shih J, et al: Detection of antibody to hepatitis C virus in prospectively followed transfusion recipients with acute and chronic non-A, non-B hepatitis. N Engl J Med 321:1494-1500, 1989.

9. Cheney C, Chopra S, Graham C: Hepatitis C. Infect Dis Clin North Am 14:633-667, 2000.

10. Mendenhall C, Seeff L, Diehl A, et al: Antibodies to hepatitis B virus and hepatitis C virus in alcoholic hepatitis and cirrhosis: Their prevalence and clinical relevance. The VA Cooperative Study Group (No. 119). Hepatology 14:581-589, 1991.

11. Hoofnagle J: Hepatitis C: The clinical spectrum of disease. Hepatology 26:15S-20S, 1997.

12. Misiani R, Bellavita P, Fenili D, et al: Hepatitis C virus infection in patients with essential mixed cryoglobulinemia. Ann Intern Med 117:573-577, 1992.

13. Chuang T, Brashear R, Lewis C: Porphyria cutanea tarda and hepatitis C virus: A case-control study and meta-analysis of the literature. J Am Acad Dermatol 41:31-36, 1999.

14. Bulaj Z, Phillips J, Ajioka R, et al: Hemochromatosis genes and other factors contributing to the pathogenesis of porphyria cutanea tarda. Blood 95:1565-1571, 2000.

15. Hsu S-C, Syu W-J, Ting L-T, et al: Immunohistochemical differentiation of hepatitis D virus genotypes. Hepatology 32:1111-1116, 2000.

16. Buitrago B, Popper H, Hadler S, et al: Specific histologic features of Santa Marta hepatitis: A severe form of hepatitis delta-virus infection in northern South America. Hepatology 6:1285-1291, 1986.

17. Koonin E, Gorbalenya A, Purdy M, et al: Computer-assisted assignment of functional domains in the nonstructural polyprotein of hepatitis E virus: Delineation of an additional group of positive-strand RNA plant and animal viruses. Proc Natl Acad Sci U S A 89:8259-8263, 1992.

18. Krawczynski K, Aggarwal R, Kamili S: Hepatitis E. Infect Dis Clin North Am 3:669-687, 2000.

19. Gupta D, Smetana H: The histopathology of viral hepatitis as seen in the Delhi epidemic (1955-56). Indian J Med Res 45(Suppl): 101-113, 1957.

20. Alter H, Nakatsuji Y, Melpolder J, et al: The incidence of transfusion-associated hepatitis G virus infection and its relation to liver disease. N Engl J Med 336:747-754, 1997.

21. Takahashi K, Hoshino H, Ohta Y, et al: Very high prevalence of TT virus (TTV) infection in general population of Japan revealed by a new set of PCR primers. Hepatol Res 12:233-239, 1998.

22. Umemura T, Yeo AET, Sottini A, et al: SEN virus infection and its relationship to transfusion-associated hepatitis. Hepatology 33:1303-1311, 2001.

23. Hanau C, Munoz SJ, Rubin R: Histopathologic heterogeneity in fulminant hepatic failure. Hepatology 21:345-351, 1994.

24. Boyer J, Klatskin G: Pattern of necrosis in acute viral hepatitis: Prognostic value of bridging (subacute) hepatic necrosis. N Engl J Med 283:1063-1071, 1970.

25. Schmid M, Pirovino M, Altorfer J, et al: Acute viral hepatitis B with bridging necrosis: A follow-up study. Liver 1:222-229, 1981.

26. Wiener M, Enat R, Gellei B, et al: Bridging hepatic necrosis in acute viral hepatitis. Isr J Med Sci 20:33-36, 1984.

27. Reynoso-Paz S, Coppel R, MacKay I, et al: The immunobiology of bile and biliary epithelium. Hepatology 30:351-357, 1999.

28. International Working Party: Terminology of chronic hepatitis. World Congresses of Gastroenterology. Am J Gastroenterol 90:181-189, 1995.

29. Desmet VJ, Gerber M, Hoofnagle J, et al: Classification of chronic hepatitis: Diagnosis, grading and staging. Hepatology 19:1513-1520, 1994.

30. Knodell R, Ishak K, Black W, et al: Formulation and application of a numerical scoring system for assessing histological activity in asymptomatic chronic active hepatitis. Hepatology 1:431-435, 1981.

31. Payen J-L, Izopet J, Galindo-Migeot V, et al: Better efficacy of a 12-month interferon alfa-2b retreatment in patients with chronic hepatitis C relapsing after a 6-month treatment: A multicenter, controlled, randomized trial. Hepatology 28:1680-1686, 1998.

32. Lai C, Chien R, Leung N, et al: A one-year trial of lamivudine for chronic hepatitis B. Asia Hepatitis Lamivudine Study Group. N Engl J Med 339:61-68, 1998.

33. Ishak K, Baptista A, Bianchi L, et al: Histologic grading and staging of chronic hepatitis. J Hepatol 22:696-699, 1995.

34. Bedossa P, Poynard T: An algorithm for the grading of activity in chronic hepatitis C. Hepatology 24:289-293, 1996.

35. Hytiroglou P, Thung S, Gerber M: Histologic classification and quantitation of the severity of chronic hepatitis: Keep it simple! Semin Liver Dis 15:414-421, 1995.

36. Batts K, Ludwig J: Chronic hepatitis: An update on terminology and reporting. Am J Surg Pathol 19:1409-1417, 1995.

37. Scheuer PJ: Classification of chronic viral hepatitis: A need for reassessment. J Hepatol 13:372-374, 1991.

38. Tsui W: New classification of chronic hepatitis and more. Adv Anat Pathol 3:64-70, 1996.

39. Chisari FV, Ferrari C: Hepatitis B immunopathology. Semin Immunopathol 17:261-281, 1995.

40. Bianchi L, Desmet VJ, Popper H, et al: Histologic patterns of liver disease in hemophiliacs, with special reference to morphologic characteristics of non-A, non-B hepatitis. Semin Liver Dis 7:203-209, 1987.

41. Lefkowitch JH, Apfelbaum TF: Non-A, non-B hepatitis: Characterization of liver biopsy pathology. J Clin Gastroenterol 11:225-232, 1989.

42. Emile JF, Sebagh M, Feray C, et al: The presence of epithelioid granulomas in hepatitis C virus-related cirrhosis. Hum Pathol 24:1095-1097, 1993.

43. Lefkowitch JH, Schiff ER, Davis GL, et al: Pathological diagnosis of chronic hepatitis C: A multicenter comparative study with chronic hepatitis B. Gastroenterology 104:595-603, 1993.

44. Nayak N, Sathar S: Immunohistochemical detection of hepatitis C virus antigen in paraffin embedded liver biopsies from patients with chronic liver disease. Acta Histochem 101:409-419, 1999.

45. Liaw Y-F: Role of hepatitis C virus in dual and triple hepatitis infection. Hepatology 22:1101-1108, 1995.

46. Kobayashi M, Tanaka E, Sodeyama T, et al: The natural course of chronic hepatitis C: A comparison between patients with genotypes 1 and 2 hepatitis C viruses. Hepatology 23:695-699, 1996.

47. Poynard T, Bedossa P, Opolon P: Natural history of liver fibrosis progression in patients with chronic hepatitis C. Lancet 349:825-832, 1997.

48. Adinolfi L, Utili R, Andreana A, et al: Serum HCV RNA levels correlate with histological liver damage and concur with steatosis in the progression of chronic hepatitis C. Dig Dis Sci 46:1677-1683, 2001.

49. Yano M, Kumada H, Kage M, et al: The long term pathologic evolution of chronic hepatitis C. Hepatology 23:1334-1340, 1996.

50. Adinolfi LE, Gambardella M, Andreana A, et al: Steatosis accelerates the progression of liver damage of chronic hepatitis C patients and correlates with specific HCV genotype and visceral obesity. Hepatology 33:1358-1364, 2001.

51. Fontana R, Israel J, LeClair P, et al: Iron reduction before and during interferon therapy of chronic hepatitis C: Results of a multicenter, randomized controlled trial. Hepatology 31:730-736, 2000.

52. Kilpatrick ZM: Structural and functional abnormalities of liver in infectious mononucleosis. Arch Intern Med 117:47-53, 1966.

53. Purtilo DT, DeFlorio D, Hutt LM, et al: Variable phenotypic expression of an X-linked recessive lymphoproliferative syndrome. N Engl J Med 297:1077-1080, 1977.

54. Lucas SB: Other viral and infectious diseases and HIV-related liver disease. In MacSween RNM, Anthony PP, Scheuer PJ, et al (eds): Pathology of the Liver, 3rd ed. Hong Kong, Churchill Livingstone, 1994, pp 269-315.

55. Randhawa PS, Markin RS, Starzl TE, et al: Epstein-Barr virus associated syndromes in immunosuppressed liver transplant recipients: Clinical profile and recognition on routine allograft biopsy. Am J Surg Pathol 14:538-548, 1990.

56. Steeper TA, Horwitz CA, Ablashi DV, et al: The spectrum of clinical and laboratory findings resulting from human herpesvirus-6 (HHV-6) in patients with mononucleosis-like illnesses not resulting from Epstein-Barr virus or cytomegalovirus. Am J Clin Pathol 93:776-783, 1990.

57. Eddleston M, Peacock S, Juniper M, et al: Severe cytomegalovirus infection in immunocompetent patients. Clin Infect Dis 24:52-56, 1997.

58. Snover DC, Horwitz CA: Liver disease in cytomegalovirus mononucleosis: A light microscopical and immunoperoxidase study of six cases. Hepatology 4:408-412, 1984.

59. Kanj SS, Sharara AI, Clavien P-A, et al: Cytomegalovirus infection following liver transplantation: Review of the literature. Clin Infect Dis 22:537-549, 1996.

60. Snover DC, Hutton S, Balfour HH Jr, et al: Cytomegalovirus infection of the liver in transplant recipients. J Clin Gastroenterol 9:659-665, 1987.

61. Ten Napel CHH, Houthoff HJ, The TH: Cytomegalovirus hepatitis in normal and immune compromised hosts. Liver 4:184-194, 1984.

62. Clarke J, Craig RM, Saffro R, et al: Cytomegalovirus granulomatous hepatitis. Am J Med 66:264-269, 1979.

63. Lobdell DH: 'Ring' granulomas in cytomegalovirus hepatitis. Arch Pathol Lab Med 111:881-882, 1987.

64. Becroft DM: Prenatal cytomegalovirus infection: Epidemiology, pathology, and pathogenesis. Perspect Pediatr Pathol 6:203-241, 1981.

65. Chetty R, Roskell DE: Cytomegalovirus infection in the gastrointestinal tract. J Clin Pathol 47:968-972, 1994.

66. Lamps LW, Pinson CW, Shyr Y, et al: The significance of micro-abscesses in liver transplant biopsies: A clinicopathologic study. Hepatology 28:1532-1537, 1998.

67. Raga J, Chrystal V, Coovadia HM: Usefulness of clinical features and liver biopsy in diagnosis of disseminated herpes simplex infection. Arch Dis Child 59:820-824, 1984.

68. Goodman ZD, Ishak KG, Sessterhenn IA: Herpes simplex hepatitis in apparently immunocompetent adults. Am J Clin Pathol 85:694-699, 1986.

69. Krilov LR, Rubin LG, Frogel M, et al: Disseminated adenovirus infection with hepatic necrosis in patients with human immunodeficiency virus infection and other immunodeficiency states. Rev Infect Dis 12:303-307, 1990.

70. Koneru B, Jaffe R, Esquivel CO, et al: Adenoviral infections in pediatric liver transplant recipients. JAMA 258:489-492, 1987.

71. Ishak KG, Walker DH, Coetzer JAW, et al: Viral hemorrhagic fevers with hepatic involvement: Pathologic aspects with clinical correlations. Prog Liver Dis 7:495-515, 1982.

72. Walker DH, McCormick JB, Johnson KM, et al: Pathologic and virologic study of fatal Lassa fever in man. Am J Pathol 107:349-356, 1982.

73. Couvelard A, Marianneau P, Bedel C, et al: Report of a fatal case of dengue infection with hepatitis: Demonstration of dengue antigens in hepatocytes and liver apoptosis. Hum Pathol 30:1106-1110, 1999.

74. Molina JM, Welker Y, Ferchal F, et al: Hepatitis associated with primary HIV infection. Gastroenterology 102:739-746, 1992.

75. Risdall RJ, McKenna RW, Nesbit ME, et al: Virus associated hemophagocytic syndrome—a benign histiocytic proliferation distinct from malignant histiocytosis. Cancer 44:993-1002, 1979.

76. Okano M, Gross TG: Epstein-Barr virus-associated hemophagocytic syndrome and fatal infectious mononucleosis. Am J Hematol 53:111-115, 1996.

77. Tsui WMS, Wong KF, Tse CCH: Liver changes in reactive hemophagocytic syndrome. Liver 12:363-367, 1992.

78. Kandel G, Marcon NE: Pyogenic liver abscess: New concepts of an old disease. Am J Gastroenterol 79:65-71, 1984.

79. Miyamoto MI, Fang FC: Pyogenic liver abscess involving Actinomyces: Case report and review. Clin Infect Dis 16:303-309, 1993.

80. Robboy SJ, Vickery AL Jr: Tinctorial and morphologic properties distinguishing actinomycosis and nocardiosis. N Engl J Med 282:593-596, 1970.

81. Greenstein AJ, Lowenthal D, Hammer GS, et al: Continuing changing patterns of disease in pyogenic liver abscess: A study of 38 patients. Am J Gastroenterol 79:217-226, 1984.

82. Branum GD, Tyson G, Branum MA, et al: Hepatic abscess: Changes in etiology, diagnosis, and management. Ann Surg 212:655-662, 1990.

83. Ortega TJ, Hutchins LF, Rice J, et al: Tularemic hepatitis presenting as obstructive jaundice. Gastroenterology 91:461-463, 1986.

84. Gebauer K, Herrmann R, Hall JC, et al: Hepatic involvement in listeriosis. Aust N Z J Med 19:486-487, 1989.

85. Zimmerman HJ, Fang M, Utili R, et al: Jaundice due to bacterial infection. Gastroenterology 77:362-374, 1979.

86. Caruana JA Jr, Montes M, Camara DS, et al: Functional and histopathologic changes in the liver during sepsis. Surg Gynecol Obstet 154:653-656, 1982.

87. Lefkowitch JH: Bile ductular cholestasis: An ominous histopathologic sign related to sepsis and "cholangitis lenta." Hum Pathol 13:19-24, 1982.

88. Harrington PT, Gutierrez JJ, Ramirez-Ronda CH, et al: Granulomatous hepatitis. Rev Infect Dis 4:638-655, 1982.

89. Marazuela M, Moreno A, Yebra M, et al: Hepatic fibrin-ring granulomas: A clinicopathologic study of 23 patients. Hum Pathol 22:607-613, 1991.

90. Essop AR, Posen JA, Hodkinson JH, et al: Tuberculosis hepatitis: A clinical review of 96 cases. Q J Med 53:465-477, 1984.

91. Oliva A, Duarte B, Jonasson O, et al: The nodular form of local hepatic tuberculosis: A review. J Clin Gastroenterol 12:166-173, 1990.

92. Ishak KG. Granulomas of the liver. In Ioachim HL (ed): Pathology of Granulomas. New York, Raven Press, 1983, pp 314-319.

93. Farhi DC, Mason UG III, Horsburgh CR Jr: Pathologic findings in disseminated Mycobacterium avium-intracellulare infection. Am J Clin Pathol 85:67-72, 1986.

94. Klatt EC, Jensen DF, Meyer PR: Pathology of Mycobacterium avium-intracellulare infection in acquired immunodeficiency syndrome. Hum Pathol 18:709-714, 1987.

95. Kahn E, Greco MA, Daum F, et al: Hepatic pathology in pediatric acquired immunodeficiency syndrome. Hum Pathol 22:1111-1119, 1991.

96. Karat ABA, Job CK, Rao PSS: Liver in leprosy: Histological and biochemical findings. Br Med J 1:307-310, 1971.

97 Chen TSN, Drutz DJ, Whelan GE: Hepatic granulomas in leprosy: Their relation to bacteremia. Arch Pathol Lab Med 100:182-185, 1976.

98. Sehgal VN, Tyagi SP, Kumar S, et al: Microscopic pathology of the liver in leprosy patients. Int J Derm 11:168-172, 1972.

99. Scott MA, McCurley TL, Vnencak-Jones CL, et al: Cat scratch disease: Detection of B. henselae DNA in archival biopsies from patients with clinically, serologically, and histologically defined disease. Am J Pathol 149:2161-2167, 1996.

100. Lamps LW, Gray GF, Scott MA: The histologic spectrum of hepatic cat scratch disease. Am J Surg Pathol 20:1253-1259, 1996.

101. Koehler JE, Sanchez MA, Garrido CS, et al: Molecular epidemiology of Bartonella infections in patients with bacillary angiomatosis-peliosis. N Engl J Med 337:1876-1883, 1997.

102. Slater LN, Welch DF, Min KW: Rochalimaea henselae causes bacillary angiomatosis and peliosis hepatis. Arch Intern Med 152:602-606, 1992.

103. Williams RK, Crossley K: Acute and chronic hepatic involvement of brucellosis. Gastroenterology 83:455-458, 1982.

104. Ablin J, Mevorach D, Eliakim R: Brucellosis and the gastrointestinal tract: The odd couple. J Clin Gastroenterol 24:25-29, 1997.

105. Cervantes F, Carbonell J, Bruguera M, et al: Liver disease in brucellosis: A clinical and pathological study of 40 cases. Post Med J 58:346-350, 1982.

106. Srigley JR, Vellend H, Palmer N, et al: Q-fever: The liver and bone marrow pathology. Am J Surg Pathol 9:752-758, 1985.

107. Pellegrin M, Delsol G, Auvergnat JC, et al: Granulomatous hepatitis in Q fever. Hum Pathol 11:51-57, 1980.

108. Walker DH, Gear JHS: Correlation of the distribution of Rickettsia conorii, microscopic lesions, and clinical features in South African tick bite fever. Am J Trop Med Hyg 34:361-371, 1985.

109. Adams JS, Walker DH: The liver in Rocky Mountain spotted fever. Am J Clin Pathol 75:156-161, 1981.

110. Walker DH, Parks FM, Betz TG, et al: Histopathology and immunohistologic demonstration of the distribution of Rickettsia typhi in fatal murine typhus. Am J Clin Pathol 91:720-724, 1989.

111. Oppenheimer EH, Dahms BB: Congenital syphilis in the fetus and neonate. Perspect Pediatr Pathol 6:115-138, 1981.

112. Shah MC, Barton LL: Congenital syphilitic hepatitis. Pediatr Infect Dis J 8:891-892, 1989.

113. Wright DJM, Berry CL: Liver involvement in congenital syphilis. Br J Vener Dis 50:241, 1974.

114. Schlossberg D: Syphilitic hepatitis: A case report and review of the literature. Am J Gastroenterol 82:552-553, 1987.

115. Veeravahu M: Diagnosis of liver involvement by early syphilis: A critical review. Arch Intern Med 145:132-134, 1985.

116. Romeu J, Rybak B, Dave P, et al: Spirochetal vasculitis and bile ductular damage in early hepatic syphilis. Am J Gastroenterol 74:352-354, 1980.

117. Maincent G, Labadie H, Fabre M, et al: Tertiary hepatic syphilis: A treatable cause of multinodular liver. Dig Dis Sci 42:447-450, 1997.

118. Parnis R: Gumma of the liver. Br J Surg 62:236, 1975.

119. Scully RE, Mark EJ, McNeely WF, et al: Case records of the Massachusetts General Hospital. N Engl J Med 345:201-205, 2001.

120. Nasrallah SM, Nassar VH: Enteric fever: A cliniocopathologic study of 104 cases. Am J Gastroenterol 69:63-69, 1978.

121. Misra PS, Lebwohl P, Laufer H: Hepatic and appendiceal Whipple's disease with negative jejunal biopsies. Am J Gastroenterol 75:302-306, 1981.

122. Cho C, Linscheer WG, Hirschkorn MA, et al: Sarcoidlike granulomas as an early manifestation of Whipple's disease. Gastroenterology 87:941-947, 1984.

123. Park GR, Lamp BD, Milne LJR, et al: Disseminated aspergillosis occurring in patients with respiratory, renal, and hepatic failure. Lancet 2:179-183, 1982.

124. Johnson TL, Barnett JL, Appelman HD, et al: *Candida* hepatitis: Histopathologic diagnosis. Am J Surg Pathol 12:716-720, 1988.

125. Thaler M, Pastakia B, Shawker TH, et al: Hepatic candidiasis in cancer patients: The evolving picture of the syndrome. Ann Intern Med 108:88-100, 1988.

126. Chandler FW, Watts JC: Pathologic Diagnosis of Fungal Infections. Chicago, ASCP Press, 1987.

127. Lamps LW, Molina CP, Haggitt RC, et al: The pathologic spectrum of gastrointestinal and hepatic histoplasmosis. Am J Clin Pathol 113:64-72, 2000.

128. Bonacini M, Nussbaum J, Ahluwalia C: Gastrointestinal, hepatic, and pancreatic involvement with *Cryptococcus neoformans* in AIDS. J Clin Gastroenterol 12:295-297, 1990.

129. Wilkins MJ, Lindley R, Dourakis SP, et al: Surgical pathology of the liver in HIV infection. Histopathology 18:459-464, 1991.

130. Washington K, Gottfried MR, Wilson ML: Gastrointestinal cryptococcosis. Mod Pathol 4:707-711, 1991.

131. de Brito T, Barone AA, Faria RM: Human liver biopsy in *P. falciparum* and *P. vivax* malaria: A light and electron microscopy study. Virchows Arch A Pathol Pathol Anat 348:220-229, 1969.

132. Imes GD, Neafie RC: Babesiosis. In Binford CH, Connor DH, (eds): Pathology of Tropical and Extraordinary Diseases. Washington, DC, AFIP, 1976, pp 301-302.

133. Greenstein AJ, Barth J, Dicker A, et al: Amebic liver abscess: A study of 11 cases compared with a series of 38 patients with pyogenic liver abscess. Am J Gastroenterol 80:472-478, 1985.

134. Brandt H, Tamayo RP: Pathology of human amebiasis. Hum Pathol 1:351-385, 1970.

135. Daneshbod K: Visceral leishmaniasis (kala-azar) in Iran: A pathologic and electron microscopic study. Am J Clin Pathol 57:156-166, 1971.

136. Moreno A, Marazuela M, Yebra M, et al: Hepatic fibrin-ring granulomas in visceral leishmaniasis. Gastroenterology 95:1123-1126, 1988.

137. Roberts-Thomson IC, Anders RF, Bhathal PS: Granulomatous hepatitis and cholangitis associated with giardiasis. Gastroenterology 83:480-483, 1982.

138. Bonacini M, Kanel G, Alamy M: Duodenal and hepatic toxoplasmosis in a patient with HIV infection: Review of the literature. Am J Gastroenterol 91:1838-1840, 1996.

139. Bertoli F, Espino M, Arosemena JR, et al: A spectrum in the pathology of toxoplasmosis in patients with acquired immuno-deficiency syndrome. Arch Pathol Lab Med 119:214-224, 1995.

140. Glasgow BJ, Anders K, Layfield LJ, et al: Clinical and pathologic findings of the liver in the acquired immune deficiency syndrome (AIDS). Am J Clin Pathol 83:582-588, 1985.

141. Sheikh RA, Prindiville TP, Yenamandra S, et al: Microsporidial AIDS cholangiopathy due to *Encephalitozoon intestinalis*. Am J Gastroenterol 95:2364-2371, 2000.

142. Terada S, Redy KR, Jeffers LJ, et al: Microsporidian hepatitis in the acquired immunodeficiency syndrome. Ann Intern Med 107:61-62, 1987.

143. Michiels JF, Hofman P, Bernard E, et al: Intestinal and extraintestinal *Isospora belli* infection in an AIDS patient. Pathol Res Pract 190:1089-1094, 1994.

144. Javid G, Wani NA, Gulzar GM, et al: *Ascaris*-induced liver abscess. World J Surg 23:1191-1194, 1999.

145. Fogaca HS, Oliveira CS, Barbosa HT, et al: Liver pseudotumor: A rare manifestation of hepatic granulomata caused by *Ascaris lumbricoides* ova. Am J Gastroenterol 95:2099-2101, 2000.

146. Bhatia V, Sarin SK: Hepatic visceral larva migrans: Evolution of the lesion, diagnosis, and role of high-dose albendazole therapy. Am J Gastroenterol 89:624-627, 1994.

147. Daly JJ, Baker GF: Pinworm granuloma of the liver. Am J Trop Med Hyg 33:62-64, 1984.

148. Mondou EN, Gnepp DR: Hepatic granuloma resulting from *Enterobius vermicularis*. Am J Clin Pathol 91:97-100, 1989.

149. Poltera AA, Katsimbura N: Granulomatous hepatitis due to *Strongyloides stercoralis*. J Pathol 113:241-246, 1973.

150. Warren KS: The pathology, pathobiology, and pathogenesis of schistosomiasis. Nature 273:609-612, 1978.

151. Grimaud JA, Borojevic R: Chronic human *Schistosomiasis mansoni*. Lab Invest 36:268-273, 1977.

152. Ona FV, Dytoc JN: *Clonorchis*-associated cholangiocarcinoma: A report of two cases with unusual manifestations. Gastroenterology 101:831-839, 1991.

153. Riganti M, Pungpak S, Punpoowong B, et al: Human pathology of *Opisthorchis viverrini* infection: A comparison of adults and children. South Asia J Trop Med Pub Health 20:95-100, 1989.

154. Acosta-Ferreira W, Vercelli-Retta J, Falconi LM: *Fasciola hepatica* human infection. Virchows Arch A Pathol Anat Histol 383:319-327, 1979.

155. Akinoglu A, Demiryurek H, Guzel C: Alveolar hydatid disease of the liver: A report on thirty-nine surgical cases in Eastern Anatolia, Turkey. Am J Trop Med Hyg 45:182-189, 1991.

156. Honma K, Sasano N, Andoh N, et al: Hepatic alveolar echinococcosis invading pancreas, vertebrae, and spinal cord. Hum Pathol 13:944-946, 1982.

157. Sparks AK, Connor DH, Neafie RC: Echinococcosis. In Binford CH, Connor DH (eds): Pathology of Tropical and Extraordinary Diseases. Washington, DC, AFIP, 1976, pp 530-533.

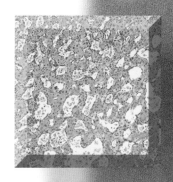

CHAPTER 35

Autoimmune and Cholestatic Disorders of the Liver

KENNETH P. BATTS

◼ Introduction

In this chapter, the focus is on three main syndromes of putative autoimmune etiology—autoimmune hepatitis (AIH), primary biliary cirrhosis (PBC), and primary sclerosing cholangitis (PSC). In addition, some uncommon noncongenital chronic biliary diseases that can mimic PBC and PSC are discussed.

◼ Autoimmune Hepatitis

Although it was referred to in the past as *autoimmune-type chronic active hepatitis*, it has been suggested that the preferred term is *autoimmune hepatitis (AIH)* because it is an a priori chronic disease.[1] Briefly, autoimmune hepatitis is a syndrome characterized by predominance in females, an association with polyclonal hypergammaglobulinemia, a variety of circulating autoantibodies, an immunogenetic predisposition (HLA-B8, -DR3, or -DR4), absence of viral infection, and a usually favorable response to immunosuppressive therapy.

The major symptoms and findings of AIH have been incorporated by the International Autoimmune Hepatitis Group into a scoring system, the sum of which describes the probability of the diagnosis of AIH.[1] Summarized in Table 35-1, the main principle of this scoring system is that a combination of clinical and laboratory features can, in aggregate, be useful in predicting the likelihood of a patient's having autoimmune hepatitis. Knowledge of these parameters during interpretation of a diagnostic liver sample can be extremely helpful. Briefly, factors that favor AIH are female sex, a hepatitic rather than a cholestatic liver enzyme profile (serum aminotransferases are elevated more prominently than alkaline phosphatase), hypergammaglobulinemia, presence of serum autoantibodies (see under Pathogenesis), and absence of evidence of virus-, drug-, or alcohol-related liver disease. A clinical and biochemical response to immunosuppressive therapy is also an important criterion.[1]

CLINICAL AND DEMOGRAPHIC DATA

There is a clear female predominance for AIH in the range of 8:1.[2,3] In addition, a subtype of AIH is characterized by high-titer anti–liver/kidney/microsomal antibody (anti-LKM), sometimes referred to as *AIH type IIa*,[4] that is more common among children, girls more frequently than boys.[5]

Individuals with certain HLA types are at increased risk for AIH, although testing for such phenotypes is not commonly necessary in daily practice. The HLA-A1, -B8, -DR3, and -DR4 phenotypes are associated with type I AIH.[1,4]

Serum biochemical test values vary considerably, reflecting grade and stage. During periods of inactive (quiescent) disease, serum alanine aminotransferase (ALT) and aspartate aminotransferase (AST) values may

TABLE 35-1. Scoring System for Diagnosis of Autoimmune Hepatitis: Minimum Required Parameters[1]

Parameters	Score
Sex	
Female	+2
Male	0
Serum ratio of elevation of alkaline phosphatase vs. aminotransferase	
>3.0	−2
<3.0	+2
Serum total globulin, gamma globulin, or IgG (times upper limit of normal)	
>2.0	+3
1.5–2.0	+2
1.0–1.5	+1
<1.0	0
Serum autoantibody titers: Adult—ANA, ASMA, or LKM-1	
>1:80	+3
1:80	+2
1:40	+1
<1:40	0
Serum autoantibody titers: Children—ANA or LKM-1	
>1:20 (ANA, LKM-1, or ASMA)	+3
1:10 or 1:20 (ANA, LKM-1) or 1:20 (ASMA)	+2
<1:10 (ANA, LKM-1) or <1:20 (ASMA)	0
Serum antimitochondrial antibody	
Positive	−2
Negative	0
Viral markers: Anti–hepatitis A IgM, HBsAb, or IgM anti-HBc	−3
Anti–hepatitis C positive	−2
Hepatitis C RNA positive in serum by PCR	−3
Positive test indicating active hepatitis from other virus	−3
Seronegative for all of the above	+3
History of hepatotoxic drug use or parenteral blood product exposure	
Yes	−2
No	+1
Alcohol average consumption	
Male <35 g/day or female <25 g/day	+2
Male 35–80 g/day or female 25–40 g/day	+2
Male 50–80 g/day or female 40–60 g/day	+2
Male <80 g/day or female <60 g/day	+2
Other autoimmune diseases in patient or first-degree relative	+1
Interpretation of aggregate scores	
Definite AIH: >15 before treatment, >17 after treatment	
Probable AIH: 10 to 15 before treatment, and 12 to 17 after treatment	

AIH, autoimmune hepatitis; ANA, antinuclear antibodies; ASMA, anti–smooth muscle antibody; IgG, immunoglobulin G; LKM, liver/kidney/microsomal antibody; PCR, polymerase chain reaction.

be normal. However, in "flares" of disease, the serum aminotransferase values range from the low hundreds to well in excess of 1000 IU/mL. Serum alkaline phosphatase values are generally normal to minimally elevated. Bilirubin values are often normal but may be elevated during severe flares. Hypergammaglobulinemia,

evident even in early-stage disease, is a hallmark and in part a defining feature of AIH.[1] As AIH progresses to cirrhosis, bilirubin levels rise and biochemical evidence of cirrhosis (such as thrombocytopenia, decreased serum albumin, and prolonged prothrombin time) becomes apparent.

PATHOGENESIS

Similar to other autoimmune diseases, AIH is a reflection of a defect in suppressor T cells that leads to disordered immunoregulation and production of a variety of autoantibodies, some of which appear to act against hepatocyte surface antigens. Although most of the autoantibodies seen in AIH are not specific for AIH and may not act directly in the pathogenesis of the disease, their identification may be helpful diagnostically.

Antinuclear antibodies (ANAs) are seen in approximately 80% of patients with AIH, typically in titers greater than 1:40. Anti–smooth muscle antibody (ASMA) is seen in about 70% of AIH patients, again typically in titers greater than 1:40. The presence of high-titer ANA and/or ASMA, in an overall context of AIH, defines type I AIH, which is the most common and the prototypical form of the disease. Both ANA and ASMA can be identified in serum in the absence of AIH or any other liver disease; however, it is not uncommon for low-titer ANA to be detected in patients with other chronic liver disease such as hepatitis C, alcoholic liver disease, or nonalcoholic steatohepatitis.[6] The presence of low-titer anti-LKM is a defining feature of type II AIH and is generally found in the absence of high-titer ANA or ASMA. High-titer anti-LKM in the absence of anti–hepatitis C antibody (anti-HCV) has been designated type IIa AIH,[4] or just type II.[7] This uncommon form of AIH is most often seen in children. Low-titer anti-LKM in the presence of anti-HCV has been designated type IIb AIH by some, although it is probably not an important pathologic entity. This form may more appropriately be viewed as a variant of hepatitis C that has autoimmune features. Antibodies against soluble liver antigen (SLA), liver pancreas (LP), and asialoglycoprotein receptor (ASGPR) can also be found but are less often diagnostically useful.[8]

Although the precise nature of the immune attack on liver remains incompletely defined, based on the histopathology it can be inferred that hepatocytes rather than biliary epithelial cells are the target of attack. Necrosis of hepatocytes is usually most prominent at the limiting plate (zone 1 or periportal hepatocytes), where the process has been traditionally designated "piecemeal necrosis," with more recent terms being *interface hepatitis*[9] and *troxis hepatitis*.[10] A predominant attack of hepatocytes in zone 3 (pericentral) also occurs in some cases,[11] conceptually representing centrilobular piecemeal necrosis. Last, necrosis of random hepatocytes

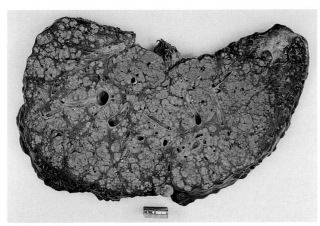

FIGURE 35–1. Cirrhosis secondary to autoimmune hepatitis. Although is the liver usually tan-brown, as shown here, occasionally it may have a greenish apperance. (Photo courtesy of Drs. Herschel Carpenter and Gerald Dayharsh, Mayo Clinic, Rochester, MN.)

TABLE 35-2. Comparative Histopathology of Necroinflammatory Features in Autoimmune Hepatitis, Primary Biliary Cirrhosis, and Primary Sclerosing Cholangitis

	Inflammation			Necrosis	
	Portal	Periportal	Lobular	Interface	Lobular
Autoimmune Hepatitis					
Grade 0	0–2+	0	0–1+	0	0
Grade 1	1–3+	1+	1–2+	≤1+	≤1+
Grade 2	2–4+	1–2+	1–2+	≤2+	≤2+
Grade 3	2–4+	2–3+	2–3+	≤3+	≤3+
Grade 4	2–4+	2–4+	3–4+	≤4+	≤4+
Primary Biliary Cirrhosis					
Stage I	2–4+	≤1+	1+	0	0
Stage II	2–4+	≤1+	1+	0	0
Stage III	2–4+	≤1+	1+	0	0
Stage IV	2–4+	≤1+	1+	0	0
Primary Sclerosing Cholangitis					
Stage 1	1–2+	≤1+	0	0	0
Stage 2	1–3+	≤1+	0	0	0
Stage 3	1–3+	≤1+	0	0	0
Stage 4	1–3+	≤1+	0	0	0

throughout the hepatic lobules is common and is recognizable as acidophil bodies.

PATHOLOGIC FEATURES

Gross Pathology

Gross examination of the liver in AIH plays little role diagnostically. In early-stage disease, the liver usually appears normal. In episodes of severe activity, if submassive or massive hepatocyte necrosis occurs, the external surface of the liver may appear grossly shriveled; cross sections show areas of confluent parenchymal collapse. As the disease progresses, cirrhosis may eventually occur, composed of variably sized tan to brown nodules (Fig. 35-1), similar to chronic viral hepatitis. Occasionally, a greenish discoloration may be noted, similar to that seen in chronic biliary disorders.

Microscopic Pathology

Although the histopathologic lesions in AIH vary considerably according to the grade and stage of the process (Table 35-2), chronic inflammation composed primarily of lymphocytes with a considerable number of plasma cells in portal tracts is a near-constant feature. During periods of quiescent disease ("remission"), however, portal inflammation may be the sole histologic abnormality; in some cases, negligible inflammation and an essentially normal liver are found (Fig. 35-2). A small number of intraepithelial lymphocytes may be seen within bile duct epithelium; however, bile duct destruction and loss are not features of AIH.

During flares of disease activity, lymphocytic piecemeal necrosis, the hallmark lesion of AIH, is observed. This lesion is characteristic of AIH but is not specific; lymphocytic piecemeal necrosis is also seen in viral and drug-associated chronic hepatitis,[12,13] as well as in primary biliary cirrhosis and other conditions. Lymphocytic piecemeal necrosis (interface hepatitis) is characterized by a prominent lymphohistiocytic infiltrate at mesenchymal/parenchymal junctions with accompanying evidence of local liver cell damage (Fig. 35-3**A**). This damage may appear in the form of overt necrosis of entire hepatocytes (acidophil bodies) or as slow destruction of hepatocytes caused by ingestion of small portions of cytoplasm by activated lymphocytes, described vividly by Wang and associates as *troxis*, the Greek word translated

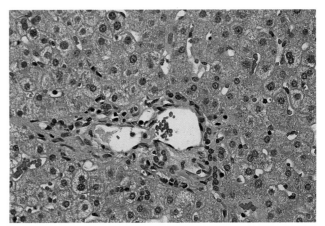

FIGURE 35–2. Autoimmune hepatitis in remission following immunosuppressive therapy. This portal tract is essentially normal. The patient has been treated with azathioprine for 6 years after onset of clinically and histologically typical autoimmune hepatitis, with normalization of serum liver tests.

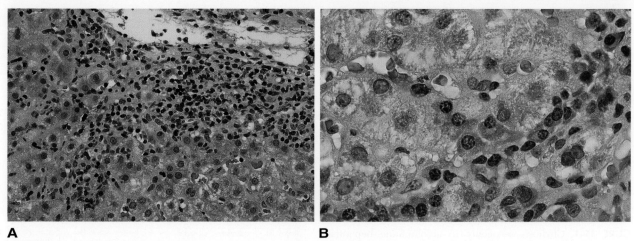

A   **B**

FIGURE 35–3. Interface hepatitis in autoimmune hepatitis. Also known traditionally as "piecemeal necrosis" and more recently as "troxis hepatitis," this is characterized by the presence of lymphocytes extending into zone 1 (periportal) hepatocytes with accompanying evidence of hepatocyte damage. **A,** At low to medium magnification, this causes a blurred limiting plate. **B,** In autoimmune hepatitis, plasma cells are often conspicuous, in contrast to hepatitis B or C.

as "to gnaw or chew."[10] In AIH, plasma cells are usually conspicuous, particularly in comparison with chronic viral hepatitis (Fig. 35-3**B**).

In addition to portal and periportal inflammatory infiltrates, lobular damage is commonly seen in AIH, manifested by variable degrees of anisonucleosis, ballooning degeneration, hepatocellular swelling, "neocholangiole" formation, bile (rarely), and acidophil bodies accompanied by variable lymphocytic and plasmacytic inflammation (Fig. 35-4). The degree of lobular damage contributes to the grade of disease. Although the hepatocellular damage is generally pan-lobular, in some cases, zone 3 (centrilobular) damage may be accentuated,[13] resembling periportal interface hepatitis (Fig. 35-5). Lobular hepatitis is often prominent during disease flares but may completely resolve, either spontaneously or as a result of immunosuppression. These features, similar to those in viral hepatitis, can be assessed semiquantitatively and used to assign a grade of activity. As compared with chronic hepatitis C, AIH is prone to a much broader range of disease activity, from completely inactive to submassive or massive necrosis with confluent necrosis (see Fig. 35-4).

Cholestasis is generally not present, but a mild degree of cholestasis may be seen in more severe examples of lobular hepatitis (Fig. 35-6). In contrast to hepatitis C, steatosis is not a usual feature of AIH.

Similar to chronic viral hepatitis, a progression in stage from portal to periportal to bridging fibrosis and cirrhosis is seen in AIH. Even after cirrhosis has occurred, piecemeal necrosis may persist along fibrous septa or regenerative nodules (active cirrhosis). Alternatively, the inflammation may subside, eventuating in a bland, inactive cirrhosis.

Although AIH is an a priori chronic disease, theoretically at some point the disease begins and could

be regarded as acute. Relatively little has been written about the histopathology of acute-onset AIH. Lefkowitch and colleagues reported hepatocyte swelling, acidophil bodies, fat, cholestasis, piecemeal necrosis, and portal plasma cells in the original liver biopsy specimens of two patients who clinically had AIH.[14] A study examining liver samples from patients with clinical disease of less than 6 months' duration found that with the exception of one case of lobular hepatitis with confluent necrosis (submassive hepatic necrosis), a vast majority (25 of 26) of patients already had histologic changes that suggested chronicity, either soft evidence (i.e., portal inflammation and fibrosis; 7 of 26 cases) or hard evidence (at least bridging fibrosis; 18 of 26 cases).[15] This suggested that most presentations of clinically acute AIH actually represent flares of previously occult chronic disease. It was further supported by observations in a related study that found that autoimmune hepatitis of less than 3 months' duration was indistinguishable by clinical and laboratory features from known disease of 12 months' duration or longer.[16] These findings support the view that AIH is an a priori chronic disease.[1]

DIFFERENTIAL DIAGNOSIS

Acute-Onset Autoimmune Hepatitis

The histologic differential diagnosis of autoimmune hepatitis is rather broad and depends somewhat on the clinical context. For cases presenting as severe, clinically acute hepatitis with prominent hepatocyte necrosis, the major differential considerations include a severe drug/toxic injury or a fulminant viral hepatitis related to hepatitis A or B or, rarely, Epstein-Barr virus (EBV) or another systemic virus (Table 35-3). Distinguishing between AIH and drug/toxin-associated hepatitis in this

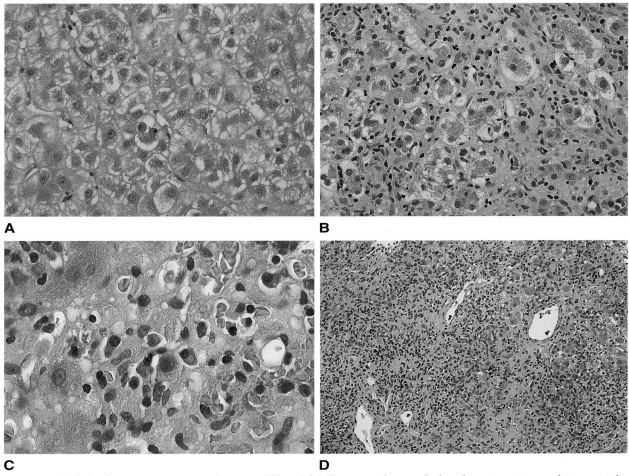

FIGURE 35–4. Lobular damage in autoimmune hepatitis. Although lobules are nearly normal when disease is quiescent, during periods of disease activity, lobules demonstrate acidophil bodies **(A),** hepatocellular swelling and disarray **(B),** and chronic inflammation with plasma cells **(C).** When disease is severe, confluent necrosis may be seen **(D).**

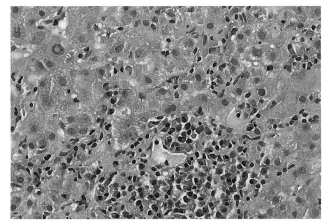

FIGURE 35–5. Zone 3 (centrilobular) damage in autoimmune hepatitis. Zone 3 necrosis and interface hepatitis–like inflammation can be seen in some cases of autoimmune hepatitis, in contrast to chronic viral hepatitis but similar to some examples of drug-associated hepatitis.

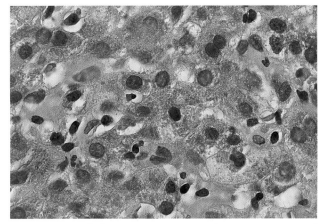

FIGURE 35–6. Cholestasis in autoimmune hepatitis. An unusual feature that is more typical of drug-associated hepatitis, bile can be seen in occasional examples of autoimmune hepatitis, as shown here.

TABLE 35-3. Major Differential Diagnosis of Autoimmune Hepatitis

Disease Pattern	Diagnosis
"Acute-onset" pattern of dominant lobular hepatitis	Acute viral hepatitis—HBV, HAV, EBV
"Chronic" pattern of predominant portal and periportal inflammation	Drug-associated hepatitis Primary sclerosing cholangitis Primary biliary cirrhosis Chronic hepatitis C Chronic hepatitis B Nonspecific reactive hepatitis

EBV, Epstein-Barr virus; HAV, hepatitis A; HBV, hepatitis B.

context can usually be accomplished by applying the principles of the scoring system of Johnson and coworkers[1] (see Table 35-1), which uses, among other items, autoantibody status and the presence of hypergammaglobulinemia. Careful history taking regarding the drug/toxins can often be helpful as well. In equivocal cases, a rapid response to immunosuppressive therapy can help support a diagnosis of AIH. Regarding the differential between AIH and acute viral hepatitis in this setting, viral serology testing for hepatitis A (HAV) and B (HBV) and EBV is generally quite reliable. Acute hepatitis C is rarely a diagnostic concern; however, assay for HCV RNA in serum by means of a sensitive qualitative test is the best tool to use in this setting because the development of anti-HCV may occur subsequent to the hepatitic episode.

Chronic Autoimmune Hepatitis

The histopathology associated with typical AIH—that is, the classic pattern of chronic active hepatitis—elicits a differential diagnosis with chronic HBV (with or without delta hepatitis), HCV, PBC, PSC, and, rarely, chronic drug-related hepatitis (see Table 35-3).

The differential with chronic viral hepatitis is most often readily resolved serologically; however, morphologic clues exist (Table 35-4). Examples of brisk (grade 3 or 4) active chronic hepatitis generally exclude HCV because HCV almost always exhibits minimal to mild disease with transaminases generally not exceeding 200 to 300 IU/mL. On occasion, chronic HCV may show fairly prominent plasma cells. This has been designated by Czaja and associates as chronic hepatitis C with autoimmune features[17]; it likely accounts for examples of AIH type IIa or III, as described earlier. Chronic hepatitis B may exhibit considerable disease activity that can mimic flares of AIH but usually in the context of superimposed delta hepatitis infection or emergence of a mutant strain of HBV. The presence of fairly prominent plasma cells helps to distinguish AIH from chronic HBV; however, the serologic profile is the most reliable means of identifying chronic hepatitis B.

TABLE 35-4. Differentiation of Autoimmune Hepatitis and Chronic Viral Hepatitis

Diseases	Helpful Hints
AIH vs. HCV	Apply clinical criteria (scoring system) for AIH[1] Plasma cells may also be seen in HCV; not very helpful HCV RNA in serum diagnostic of HCV; HCV serology less helpful Grade 3 or 4 disease seen in AIH but very rare in HCV Mild steatosis common in HCV; not a feature of AIH
AIH vs. HBV	Apply clinical criteria (scoring system) for AIH[1] Plasma cells typical of AIH; usually fairly few in HBV HBV DNA, HBsAg, and HBeAg in serum diagnostic of HBV Ground-glass hepatocytes = HBV Immunoperoxidase staining for HBsAg and/or HBcAg = HBV

AIH, autoimmune hepatitis; HBV hepatitis B; HCV, hepatitis C.

The differential between AIH and the two main chronic biliary diseases, PBC and PSC, is usually fairly straightforward histologically, serologically, and biochemically (cholestatic enzyme pattern in PBC and PSC vs. a hepatitic pattern in AIH) (Table 35-5; see also Table 35-2). However, overlap syndromes of AIH and PBC, as well as AIH and PSC, are well described and are discussed in the following section. Although both PBC and PSC may demonstrate some spillover of lymphocytes across the limiting plate into zone 1,

TABLE 35-5. Differentiation of Autoimmune Liver Diseases

Diseases	Helpful Hints
AIH vs. PBC	Apply clinical criteria (scoring system) for AIH[1] Plasma cells plus hepatocellular necrosis = AIH AMA plus cholestatic serum enzyme profile = PBC Florid duct lesion = PBC "Biliary" cirrhosis and/or duct loss = PBC Overlap syndrome is not uncommon
AIH vs. PBC	Apply clinical criteria (scoring system) for AIH[1] Plasma cells plus hepatocellular necrosis = AIH Abnormal cholangiogram = PSC Fibrous obliterative cholangitis = PSC "Biliary" cirrhosis and/or duct loss = PSC Overlap syndrome occasionally seen
PBC vs. PSC	Usually more extensive portal inflammation in PBC Greater number of plasma cells in PBC Florid duct lesions only in PBC Fibrous-obliterative cholangitis only in PSC Sinusoidal lymphocytosis in PBC Abnormal cholangiogram = PSC

AIH, autoimmune hepatitis; PBC, primary biliary cirrhosis; PSC primary sclerosing cholangitis.

neither PBC nor PSC should demonstrate overt hepatocyte necrosis to any significant degree. The number of portal plasma cells seen in PBC may be similar to the number seen in AIH; PSC generally demonstrates fewer. Although AIH, PBC, and PSC can all demonstrate lymphocytes within biliary epithelium (lymphocytic cholangitis), destruction of ducts and resultant ductopenia are much less common in AIH.[18] The florid duct lesions of PBC and the fibrous obliterative lesions of PSC should not be seen in pure examples of AIH.

OVERLAP SYNDROMES

Just as autoimmune diseases of other organs may coexist, there is evidence that autoimmune liver diseases may on occasion coexist or "overlap." Most commonly, this occurs as AIH and PBC or autoimmune cholangitis (AC), but associations of AIH and PSC have also been described.[19-22] The AIH/PSC overlap may be more common among children with autoimmune liver disease, as prospective performance of cholangiography in children with ANA, ASMA, and/or anti-LKM in serum found that half of patients had abnormal cholangiograms.[23] Because the therapy for AIH differs considerably from that for the chronic biliary diseases (i.e., PBC and PSC), these overlap syndromes may cause considerable therapeutic dilemmas.

In the evaluation of potential overlap syndromes, there should be compelling histologic and clinical evidence of both a hepatitic and a chronic biliary component. For example, the mere presence of lymphocytic cholangitis in tissue from an otherwise typical case of autoimmune hepatitis should not suggest coexistent PBC or PSC. Similarly, the presence of mild lymphocytic piecemeal necrosis in otherwise typical examples of PBC or PSC should not suggest an autoimmune hepatitis component. Consideration for true overlap syndromes should arise when there is significant lobular activity, manifested by hepatocellular swelling and acidophil bodies, as well as convincing florid duct lesions (in PBC) or fibrous obliterative lesions and/or typical cholangiographic findings (in PSC). Correlation with laboratory values is often helpful in these ambiguous cases; therapy should be tailored on a case-by-case basis.

REPORTING AIH—GRADING AND STAGING

In generating an interpretive biopsy report, it is advisable that an etiologic diagnosis be rendered (in this instance, autoimmune hepatitis) whenever possible following integration of clinical data with histologic findings. For AIH, grading the degree of inflammatory activity is also appropriate. The choice of grading system is best left to the discretion of the pathologist and constituent clinicians. The simplest system for grading

TABLE 35-6. Staging of Autoimmune Hepatitis and Chronic Hepatitis B and C*

Degree of Fibrosis	Score		
	Scheuer[24-26]	METAVIR[27]	Ishak[29]
No fibrosis	0	0	0
Portal fibrosis	1	1	1
Periportal fibrosis	2†	2†	2
Bridging fibrosis			
Rare	2	2	3
Considerable	3	3	4
Cirrhosis	4	4	
Rare nodules			5
Well developed			6

*See also Table 34-3.
†Rare septa may be seen.

activity is a none/minimal/mild/moderate/severe scale, corresponding to a numeric grade of 0 through 4, respectively.[24-26] This system is based on the degree of piecemeal necrosis and lobular necrosis, as indicated in Table 35-2; if there is a discrepancy between the two, the more severe of the two components prevails. The French METAVIR system is fairly similar but uses a 0 to 3 scale.[27] The Knodell scoring system has been popular since its publication in 1981[28] and provides a useful scoring system that is amenable to studies, but it has drawbacks in its original form of blurring the distinction between necroinflammatory activity (grade) and fibrosis (stage). This problem was rectified in an updated version published by Ishak and coworkers in 1995.[29]

It is also appropriate that an assessment of the degree of fibrosis (stage) be provided. A variety of schemes exist, and again, the choice of system is best left to the discretion of the pathologist based on input from constituent clinicians. The simplest system is a 0 to 4 scale that corresponds to none, portal, periportal, and bridging fibrosis, and cirrhosis, respectively (Table 35-6).[24-26] The French METAVIR system is fairly similar and uses a 0 to 4 scale[27]; the updated Knodell system by Ishak uses a 0 to 6 scheme.[29]

DISEASE COURSE AND TREATMENT

Most cases of AIH respond to immunosuppressive therapy. This is most commonly provided as corticosteroids, with or without azathioprine, initially. Eventually, many patients can be weaned from corticosteroids and maintained with azathioprine alone; approximately 20% can be weaned from all immunosuppression. For cases that progress to cirrhosis, liver transplantation is a satisfactory therapy for AIH; however, AIH can recur within the allograft. Recurrent disease is often asymptomatic and at 4 to 5 years of follow-up does not appear to be associated with significant fibrosis or morbidity.[30] Continued follow-up of these patients is necessary, however, so that the ultimate long-term outcomes can be determined.

Primary Biliary Cirrhosis

PBC is a chronic duct-destructive disease that results in progressive cholestasis and can progress to cirrhosis. Although the precise pathogenesis remains uncertain, considerable evidence indicates that it is an autoimmune disease. This disease is associated with a number of nonhepatic autoimmune diseases and several serum autoantibodies, and histologic changes indicate an autoimmune attack; these changes include lymphocytic and granulomatous destruction of intralobular and septal bile ducts with plasma cells in the background. The defining autoantibody in classic PBC is the antimitochondrial antibody (AMA) that is directed against the E2 component of pyruvate dehydrogenase.[31]

The traditional term *primary biliary cirrhosis* is commonly used, even though it is descriptive of only the last stage of disease. Thus, more appropriate terms would be *the syndrome of PBC* or the alternative term, *chronic nonsuppurative destructive cholangitis*.[32-34] Although this latter term is fitting, it would also apply to other conditions such as irreversible hepatic allograft rejection. It would appear that the term *primary biliary cirrhosis* is thoroughly entrenched in the literature at this point and is likely to remain the term of choice. The relationship of PBC with similar disease that lacks serum AMA (AC) is discussed in the following section.

CLINICAL AND DEMOGRAPHIC DATA

About 90% of patients with PBC are female, and presentation is typically between the ages of 40 and 60 years (with a range from 20 to 80 years).[35] There are reports of PBC occurring around the world, and all races appear to be susceptible. In a largely white population in Olmsted County, MN, the age-adjusted incidence of PBC has been estimated as 4.5 and 0.7 per 100,000 for women and men, respectively, with corresponding prevalences of 65.4 and 12.1 per 100,000.[36] Coexistence of PBC with a wide variety of other autoimmune diseases has been well described, with the strongest associations appearing to be with the connective tissue disorders (e.g., rheumatoid arthritis, CREST syndrome [calcinosis, Raynaud's disease, esophageal dysmotility, sclerodactyly, and telangiectasia], systemic lupus erythematosus, dermatomyositis, interstitial lung disease, and autoimmune thyroid disease).[37] An association between celiac disease and PBC has been described[38]; however, it most likely represents clustering of diseases in patients prone to autoimmune conditions rather than a direct pathogenetic link.

In early stages, PBC is usually asymptomatic and is detected only through identification of abnormal serum liver tests. In early disease, elevated serum levels of alkaline phosphatase and gamma-glutamyltransferase (GGT) are invariably present; serum cholesterol levels are usually elevated, and serum bilirubin levels are normal to minimally elevated (<2 mg/100 mL). Serum ALT and AST levels are generally normal or at most mildly elevated.

In more advanced disease, the same general biochemical patterns persist, but bilirubin levels progressively rise and biochemical stigmata of cirrhosis (i.e., decreased serum albumin, prolonged prothrombin time, thrombocytopenia) become apparent. In later stages of disease, the signs and symptoms of disease can be divided into those related to progressive cholestasis and those related to cirrhosis. Among the former are pruritus, xanthomas, jaundice, and osteoporosis. The signs and symptoms of cirrhosis in PBC are those common to all causes of cirrhosis—for example, esophagogastric varices, ascites, spider angiomas, and splenomegaly.

DISEASE COURSE

Survival in untreated patients with PBC depends on the phase of disease in which it was detected. Among asymptomatic individuals, the median predicted survival is 16 years, a time course that is shorter than that of a control population.[39] In contrast, patients who present with symptoms have a significantly shorter median survival of 7.5 years. Of asymptomatic individuals, 33% continue to be asymptomatic at a median of 12.1 years; however, once symptoms develop, their survival is similar to that quoted for symptomatic patients.[39] Patients with PBC are also at increased risk for developing hepatocellular carcinoma (HCC),[40] although the risk is probably not as high as that seen in cirrhosis due to viral hepatitis, hemochromatosis, or alcohol.

A mathematical model for predicting survival in PBC independent of biopsy, referred to as the *Mayo Model*, has been developed[41] and validated.[42] This model uses data (patient's age, serum bilirubin and albumin levels, prothrombin time, and presence or absence of edema) to estimate the likely survival time.

PATHOGENESIS

There is strong evidence that PBC represents an autoimmune attack directed at biliary epithelium. This is supported by the immunohistochemical demonstration on biliary epithelium of a protein that is cross-reactive with antibodies to the PDH-E2 complex (AMAs). This protein has similarly been demonstrated on the allograft biliary epithelium of patients with recurrent PBC after liver transplant.[43] Although it is characteristic of PBC, AMA is detected in only approximately 90% of patients with clinically and histologically typical PBC, and it can be seen in patients without typical clinical and histologic features of PBC.[44] The 10% of patients with AMA-negative PBC are discussed in greater detail in the following section.

The inflammatory cell milieu, the lymphocytic and granulomatous duct destruction, the associated autoimmune diseases of other organs, and the presence of overlap syndromes of PBC and AIH all provide strong evidence that PBC is an autoimmune process. The precise pathogenesis remains unknown; however, similar to other autoimmune processes, T-cell–mediated cytotoxicity and molecular mimicry[45,46] likely play a central role. An intriguing hypothesis regarding the potential role of a transmissible retrovirus has also been proposed.[47]

PATHOLOGIC FEATURES

Gross Pathology

In early-stage disease, the entire liver is often slightly enlarged and variably bile stained. In later stages, a typically macronodular cirrhosis evolves, generally with an intense green hue that reflects progressive cholestasis (Fig. 35-7). In contrast to PSC, cholangiectases and cholangitic abscesses are not seen.

Microscopic Pathology

The hallmark lesion of PBC is destructive cholangitis that affects interlobular and septal bile ducts and results in duct loss and subsequent biliary cirrhosis. The term *nonsuppurative destructive cholangitis* accurately describes these lesions, but the more succinct term *florid duct lesion* is more commonly used.[48] Because these lesions are focal, they may be missed by liver biopsy. The florid duct lesion is characterized by a portal lymphocytic infiltrate and epithelioid cells that are centered around septal and interlobular bile ducts with evidence of bile duct damage and destruction. Characteristic features include the disruption of the bile duct basement membrane, the presence of intraepithelial lymphocytes and plasma cells, evidence of epithelial cell damage manifested by cytoplasmic vacuolization and regenerative hyperplasia with occasional mitotic figures, and often but not always granuloma formation. Thus, florid duct lesions may reflect either granulomatous duct destruction (Fig. 35-8) or more severe examples of lymphocytic cholangitis (Fig. 35-9). The bile duct damage in florid duct lesions is segmental, not only in the longitudinal axis of the duct but often also in cross section, with only a portion of the duct being affected; granulomas often are poorly defined and tend to be associated with the bile duct in an eccentric fashion, although concentric involvement is also seen. Granulomas are also present within portal lymphocytic infiltrates without an obvious connection to a bile duct; less commonly, they are found in the hepatic lobule. Over time, interlobular and septal bile ducts vanish, and only small lymphohistiocytic aggregates remain, at least for some time.

The aforementioned bile duct changes are accompanied by a portal lymphoplasmacytic infiltrate (Fig. 35-10**A**) that is generally dense but may be patchy in early stages, may contain lymphoid aggregates and follicles, and typically has conspicuous plasma cells, as well as a mild eosinophil component.[49] The portal lymphoid infiltrate may, at times, spill over into the lobules and mimic lymphocytic piecemeal necrosis (Fig. 35-10**B**). True lymphocytic piecemeal necrosis also develops, albeit mildly.

The lobules in PBC are usually essentially normal, and the hepatocytes are regular in size without acidophil bodies. In some cases, a considerable number of lymphocytes may aggregate in hepatic sinusoids in a single-file fashion, potentially mimicking a lymphoproliferative disorder (Fig. 35-11**A**). Scattered, generally small, noncaseating lobular granulomas may be seen as well (Fig. 35-11**B**).

In early-stage disease, subtle nodular regenerative hyperplasia in nearly half of patients has been noted (see Chapter 38), perhaps reflecting portal venule damage by adjacent granulomas and potentially contributing to the early development of portal hypertension.[50]

The progression of early PBC to cirrhosis has been divided into four histologic stages.[51] Although florid duct lesions may be seen at any stage, they are most common in stages I and II (Table 35-7). Stage I is characterized by a strictly portal lymphocytic infiltrate (portal stage) with or without a florid duct lesion. In stage II, added features include piecemeal necrosis and delicate periportal fibrosis, often with ductular proliferation (periportal stage). The septal stage (stage III) is characterized by bridging necrosis or fibrous septa, and

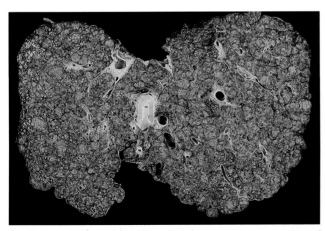

FIGURE 35–7. Primary biliary cirrhosis—gross appearance of stage IV disease. A mixture of tan and green regenerative nodules is typical. (Photo courtesy of Drs. Herschel Carpenter and Gerald Dayharsh, Mayo Clinic, Rochester, MN.)

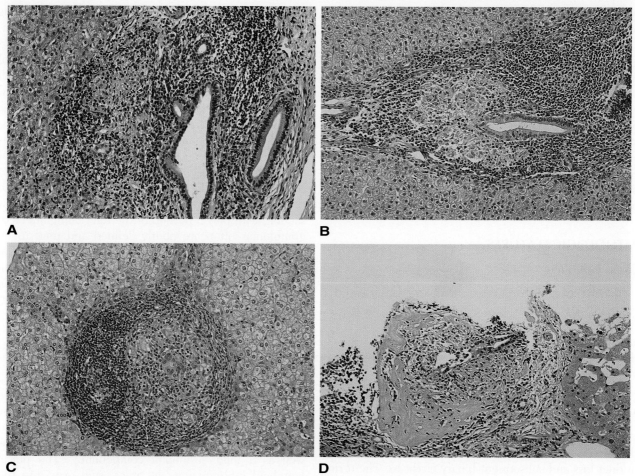

A

B

C

D

FIGURE 35–8. Granulomatous duct destruction in primary biliary cirrhosis. Also referred to as "florid duct lesion," these are characterized by granulomatous and lymphocytic cholangitis, which varies from ill-defined subtle lesions (**A**) to more obvious granulomas (**B** and **C**) to occasionally sclerotic granulomas (**D**). These can involve ducts eccentrically or concentrically and are associated with breakdown of the basement membrane and eventual duct loss. Granulomatous duct destruction is often patchy, as evidenced by the sparing of some portal tracts, some portions of one bile duct (**B**), and some bile ducts within one portal tract (**A**).

stage IV fibrosis is associated with nodular regeneration (cirrhotic stage). The regenerative nodules in PBC and in PSC are often not as regular and round as those seen in other forms of cirrhosis, often having "garland-shaped" irregular outlines, not unlike a jigsaw puzzle piece. A progressive loss of ducts can be noted early in the disease, with ductopenia usually being prominent in stage III and often nearly complete when stage IV is reached. Florid duct lesions become less common with advancing stage,[48] presumably reflecting loss of the target biliary epithelium.

Periportal hepatocyte degeneration, thought to reflect bile acid (cholate) stasis, helps to distinguish PBC and PSC from chronic hepatitis of autoimmune, viral, or drug etiology.[52] This feature becomes more prominent with advancing stage of disease and is extremely similar in PBC and PSC. The presence of proliferating ductules at the limiting plate (Fig. 35-12**A** and **B**) has been referred to as *biliary piecemeal necrosis*, in contrast to the lymphocytic piecemeal necrosis of AIH.[53] Biliary

piecemeal necrosis is often accompanied by feathery degeneration of periportal or paraseptal hepatocytes, Mallory bodies, and deposition of orcein-positive copper-protein complexes (Fig. 35-12**C** and **D**). The combined low-magnification effect of these is a characteristic edema of periportal connective tissue around regenerative nodules that can impart a halo-like effect (Fig. 35-12**E**).

DIFFERENTIAL DIAGNOSIS

Primary biliary cirrhosis shares many histologic features with PSC; in liver biopsy specimens, the two entities may be indistinguishable, particularly because the pathognomonic lesion of PBC (florid duct lesion) is less often seen in late-stage disease, and the pathognomonic lesion of PSC (fibrous obliterative cholangitis) may not have been sampled. In general, the portal inflammation is more intense in PBC than in PSC, and PBC commonly demonstrates mild sinusoidal lympho-

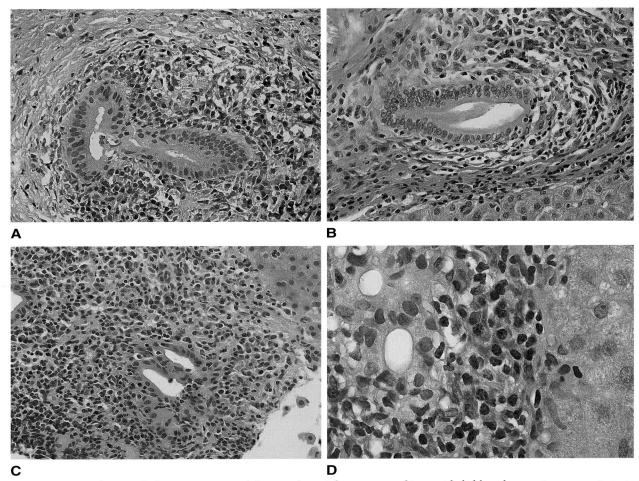

FIGURE 35–9. Lymphocytic cholangitis in primary biliary cirrhosis. The presence of intraepithelial lymphocytes is common in typical (AMA-positive) PBC (**A**), as well as in autoimmune cholangitis (AMA-negative PBC) (**B**). When associated with duct destruction, these have also been referred to as "florid duct lesions" in both typical PBC (**C**) and autoimmune cholangitis (**D**), but they can also be seen in PSC, AIH, and chronic viral and drug-associated hepatitis.

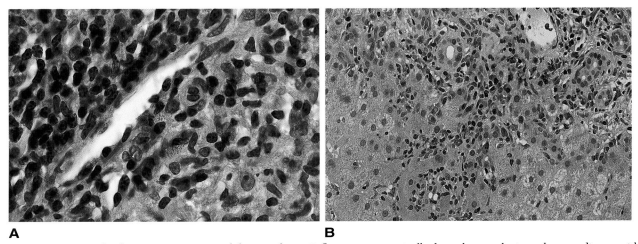

FIGURE 35–10. Portal inflammation in primary biliary cirrhosis. Inflammation is typically dense but patchy in early-stage disease with lymphocytes predominating but plasma cells also being conspicuous; eosinophils are also present in small numbers (**A**). Some spillover into periportal areas is also not uncommon, but overt hepatocyte necrosis is generally not seen (**B**).

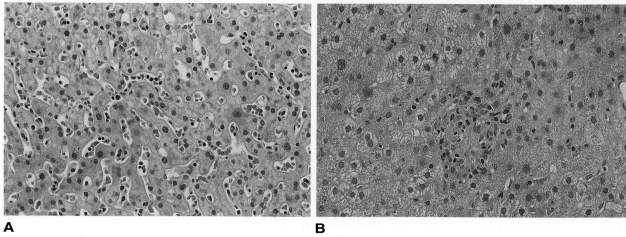

A

B

FIGURE 35–11. Hepatic lobule findings in primary biliary cirrhosis. Although the hepatocytes are generally quiescent, some degree of sinusoidal lymphocytosis is common in PBC (**A**), and occasional granulomas may be seen (**B**).

cytosis, a feature not seen in PSC (see Tables 35-2, 35-5, 35-7, and 35-8).

In their early stages, histologic manifestations of PBC and PSC may be indistinguishable from HCV, HBC, or AIH in that all can share the features of chronic active hepatitis, that is, portal and periportal inflammation (see Table 35-2). The presence of individual necrotic hepatocytes is not a feature of PBC or PSC; in contrast, these are present in active forms of chronic viral or autoimmune hepatitis. Although all of these features may demonstrate lymphocyte spillover into periportal areas (interface hepatitis), visibly necrotic hepatocytes associated with this are uncommon in both PBC and PSC.

Granulomatous duct destruction is fairly specific for PBC and AC, but there are a few mimics (Table 35-8). Florid duct lesions have rarely been described in

hepatitis C.[54] Uncommonly, drugs may cause lesions imitating the florid duct lesion of PBC; carbamazepine can cause both a granulomatous hepatitis and acute cholangitis.[55] Sarcoidosis can mimic PBC, particularly because duct loss, a cholestatic clinical picture, and rarely, cirrhosis may occur.[56] The granulomas in sarcoidosis are generally better developed and more numerous than those in PBC, and these granulomas are only randomly associated with bile ducts in sarcoidosis. In general, the background portal inflammation is more intense in PBC than in sarcoidosis.

TREATMENT

A variety of therapies were initially attempted for treatment of PBC with little success, including a variety of immunosuppressive drugs (azathioprine, D-penicillamine, corticosteroids, cyclosporin A, and methotrexate) and the antifibrotic agent colchicine.[37] Since the early 1990s, a number of trials using a synthetic bile acid called ursodeoxycholic acid (UDCA) have been undertaken. UDCA is believed to reverse the potential hepatotoxicity of bile acids and inhibit eosinophil degranulation[49]; it may also have some immunosuppressive effect but is not known to have significant adverse effects. Multiple trials at different institutions have shown that UDCA can improve serum biochemical tests of liver function.[57-60] UDCA appears to have little to no effect on hepatic inflammation[61] or the frequency of florid duct lesion development,[60] but long-term (>5 years) UDCA therapy appears to decrease the rate of progression to cirrhosis.[62] In UDCA-treated patients, the progression to cirrhosis is 4% and 17% at 5 and 10 years, respectively, for patients with stage I disease; 12% and 27%, respectively, for patients with initial stage II disease; and 59% and 76%, respectively, for patients with stage III disease.[63]

Survival benefits of UDCA in PBC remain somewhat controversial. A meta-analysis of multiple trials in 1997

TABLE 35-7. Comparative Intrahepatic Bile Duct Findings in Autoimmune Hepatitis, Primary Biliary Cirrhosis, and Primary Sclerosing Cholangitis

	Lymphocytic Cholangitis	Florid Duct Lesion	Fibrous Cholangitis	Duct Loss (Ductopenia)
Autoimmune Hepatitis				
Grade 0	0–1+	0	0	0
Grade 1	0–1+	0	0	0
Grade 2	1–2+	0	0	0
Grade 3	1–2+	0	0	0
Grade 4	1–2+	0	0	0
Primary Biliary Cirrhosis				
Stage I	2–4+	Common	0	0
Stage II	2–4+	Common	0	1+
Stage III	2–4+	Common	0	1–3+
Stage IV	0–2+	Few	0	3–4+
Primary Sclerosing Cholangitis				
Stage I	1–2+	0	Common	0
Stage II	2–3+	0	Common	1+
Stage III	2–3+	0	Common	2–3+
Stage IV	2–3+	0	Usual	3–4+

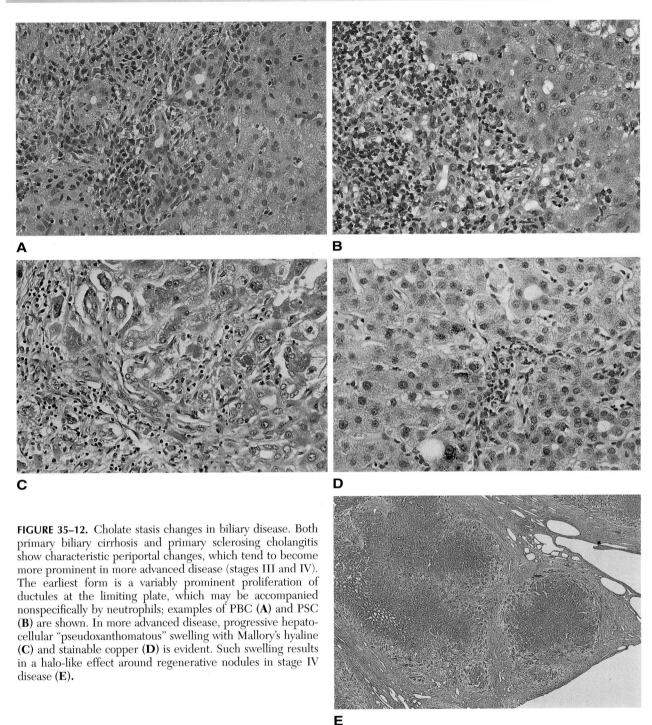

FIGURE 35–12. Cholate stasis changes in biliary disease. Both primary biliary cirrhosis and primary sclerosing cholangitis show characteristic periportal changes, which tend to become more prominent in more advanced disease (stages III and IV). The earliest form is a variably prominent proliferation of ductules at the limiting plate, which may be accompanied nonspecifically by neutrophils; examples of PBC (**A**) and PSC (**B**) are shown. In more advanced disease, progressive hepatocellular "pseudoxanthomatous" swelling with Mallory's hyaline (**C**) and stainable copper (**D**) is evident. Such swelling results in a halo-like effect around regenerative nodules in stage IV disease (**E**).

showed an improvement in survival free of transplantation in patients with moderate to severe disease.[64] A subsequent meta-analysis in 1999 concluded that UDCA had no effect on incidence of death, transplantation, or complications of liver disease,[65] although the methods of this analysis were questioned by some.[66]

For patients with decompensated cirrhosis, orthotopic liver transplantation (OLT) has emerged as an effective therapy. With the use of the Mayo model, predicted versus actual survival rates in patients undergoing liver transplantation were 55% and 79%, respectively, at 2 years after OLT, and 22% and 68%, respectively, at 7 years after OLT.[67] Although this was initially controversial, there now seems to be agreement that PBC can recur after OLT.[68] Most cases to date have been asymptomatic and of early stage, with the identification of recurrent disease depending on the identification of otherwise unexplained, definite granulomatous duct destruction.[69] Other less specific but typical features include dense but patchy portal inflammation, duc-

TABLE 35-8. Major Differential Diagnosis of Primary Biliary Cirrhosis/Autoimmune Cholangitis

Component	Diagnosis
Portal inflammation	Primary sclerosing cholangitis
	Autoimmune hepatitis
	Chronic hepatitis C
	Chronic hepatitis B
Bile duct loss	Nonspecific reactive hepatitis
	Primary sclerosing cholangitis
	Idiopathic adulthood ductopenia
	Ischemic cholangitis
	Childhood paucity of intrahepatic bile ducts (syndromic and nonsyndromic)
	Alpha-1-antitrypsin–associated duct loss
	Rare viral or drug-associated loss
Granulomatous duct destruction (florid duct lesion)	Sarcoidosis
	Drug (e.g., carbamazepine)
	Hepatitis C (rare)

topenia, copper in periportal hepatocytes, and ductular proliferation with rare cases of advanced fibrosis/cirrhosis.[70] The incidence of recurrent disease depends on the vigor of post-OLT liver sampling; however, in a cohort undergoing yearly biopsy, approximately 8% of patients at 2 to 6 years after OLT were noted to have recurrent PBC.[69] It is anticipated that with longer follow-up, a higher incidence of recurrent disease and cases with more advanced disease will be identified.

AUTOIMMUNE CHOLANGITIS

The term *autoimmune cholangitis* was first used in Germany in 1987[71] to describe cases that resembled PBC histologically and clinically but had an autoantibody pattern that appeared to reflect autoimmune hepatitis. In the mid-1990s, a number of publications addressed this issue,[72-75] focusing primarily on the question of whether AC should be considered AMA-negative PBC, an overlap syndrome with autoimmune hepatitis, or a separate entity. The relationship between PBC and AC remains undecided, but prevailing evidence suggests that AC is likely equivalent to AMA-negative PBC, and that UDCA rather than corticosteroids is an appropriate therapy. The response of AC to UDCA and the behavior of AC after OLT seem to be similar to the characteristics of AMA-positive PBC.[76]

OVERLAP SYNDROMES

Examples of coexistent PBC and AIH have been well described.[77-79] Ideally, coexistent histologic and clinical features of both PBC (elevations in cholestatic serum enzymes, positive AMA, presence of florid duct lesions) and AIH (elevations in serum transaminases, significant titers of serum ANA or ASMA, hepatocellular necrosis)

should be present. In many instances, however, identification of the two components is less than clear, and the frequency with which overlap syndromes are identified varies considerably, based on the stringency of criteria used. A modification of the International Autoimmune Hepatitis Group scoring system has been applied to overlap PBC-AIH; however, the applicability of this is questionable in that almost 20% of PBC cases are designated as probable AIH overlap.[79] Treatment of the PBC component with UDCA and the AIH component with corticosteroids and/or azathioprine seems reasonable.[77] Generally, clinicians treat the disease that seems to be predominant, using UDCA if there is greater cholestasis and corticosteroids if hepatitis is more pronounced. Because osteopenic bone disease is a common complication of biliary types of cirrhosis, caution should be used in administering corticosteroid therapy because of the associated risk of exacerbating the bone disease.

Primary Sclerosing Cholangitis

PSC is a biliary disorder characterized by potential involvement of (1) the extrahepatic biliary tree (large duct PSC), (2) both the extrahepatic and the intrahepatic biliary tree, including smaller bile ducts, and (3) in approximately 6% of cases, only the intrahepatic biliary tree (small duct PSC).[80,81] In addition, involvement of the gallbladder by PSC has been described,[82] and polypoid gallbladder lesions in PSC are not uncommonly malignant.[83] A fibroinflammatory process affecting the biliary tree that mimics PSC has been reported in patients with autoimmune pancreatitis[84]; however, in contrast to "true" PSC, these lesions appear to respond to corticosteroid therapy, suggesting that they might not be truly related.

CLINICAL AND DEMOGRAPHIC DATA

Patients with PSC are typically adults. Approximately 70% of patients with PSC also have chronic ulcerative colitis (UC), although only about 5% of patients with UC have PSC.[85] Patients with HLA haplotypes -A1, -B8, -DR3, -DR4, and -DRW52A are at increased risk.[86,87] In addition to its association with UC, other evidence of abnormal immune regulation includes the presence of perinuclear antinuclear cytoplasmic antibodies (p-ANCAs) in the majority and an association with other autoimmune diseases such as thyroiditis, diabetes, and autoimmune hepatitis.

Serum tests reflect a chronic cholestatic process. In early stages, elevations of alkaline phosphatase and GGT are universal, elevations in serum cholesterol are common, serum alanine and aspartate aminotransferases are nearly normal, and serum bilirubin level is minimally

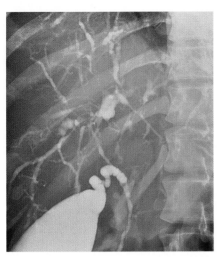

FIGURE 35–13. Abnormal cholangiogram in primary sclerosing cholangitis. The presence of multiple beaded areas with intervening stricture areas is typical of primary sclerosing cholangitis (*shown here*). Occasionally, infectious, eosinophilic, or ischemic cholangitis can show similar features. (Photo courtesy of Dr. John Poterucha, Mayo Clinic, Rochester, MN.)

elevated or normal. As the disease progresses, bilirubin levels rise and biochemical evidence of cirrhosis (such as thrombocytopenia and decreased serum albumin) becomes apparent.

The hallmark clinical lesion of PSC is an abnormal cholangiogram. With the exception of small duct PSC, cholangiography establishes the diagnosis of PSC by virtue of the characteristic, diffusely distributed, segmental, and multifocal strictures that lead to a "beaded" appearance of the cholangiogram (Fig. 35-13).[88,89] Rarely, other conditions reveal similar cholangiographic findings, however (see under Differential Diagnosis).

PATHOGENESIS

The precise pathogenesis of PSC remains uncertain. Similar to PBC, the combination of clinical, biochemical, and morphologic features clearly indicates that PSC is a reflection of an immune-mediated attack on biliary epithelium. However, in contrast to PBC, in which the direct immune target seems to be the biliary epithelium by virtue of prominent damage to the biliary epithelium proper, actual damage to biliary epithelium often is not apparent in early PSC, and concentric fibrosis is the dominant histologic feature. It has been speculated that progressive periductal fibrosis may interrupt fluid and nutrient exchange between the peribiliary capillary plexus and the bile duct epithelium[90]; this may then lead to epithelial necrosis and, eventually, obliteration of the lumen. The histologic changes seen in PSC certainly are compatible with an immunologic attack on components of the subepithelial mesenchyme, leading to secondary fibrosis and possible ischemic epithelial

damage.[90] Further evidence for a possible role for microvascular damage in PSC includes the striking morphologic similarities between PSC and ischemic cholangitis, particularly post liver transplantation,[91] and the observed displacement of peribiliary capillaries away from bile ducts by connective tissue in PSC.[92]

DISEASE COURSE

Survival among untreated patients with PSC depends on the stage of disease at diagnosis and the degree of cholangiographically evident bile duct abnormality. Typical survival from time of diagnosis to death or liver transplantation ranges from 12 to 18 years, and the degree of cholangiographic disease is inversely correlated with survival.[93,94] The time course of progression has been assessed through examination of paired biopsy samples.[95] In patients with stage II disease, progression was noted in 42%, 66%, and 93% of patients at 1, 2, and 5 years, respectively; in stage III disease, progression was noted in 14%, 25%, and 52%, respectively. Patients with PSC have an approximately 4% to 14% risk of developing cholangiocarcinoma,[96] which is associated with an extremely poor prognosis.[97] Patients with small duct PSC, which is associated with a more favorable course than classic PSC, are comparable with the general population and are likely to have a lesser risk of developing hepatobiliary malignancy.[98] Several mathematical models for predicting survival in PSC independent of biopsy have been developed, based on serum bilirubin, aspartate aminotransferase, and albumin levels plus variceal bleeding,[93] cholangiographic findings,[94] or serum bilirubin and albumin, as well as patient age at diagnosis.[99]

PATHOLOGIC FEATURES

Gross Pathology

In early-stage disease, the entire liver is often slightly enlarged and variably bile stained. In later stages, similar to PBC, a typically macronodular cirrhosis evolves, generally with an intense green hue, reflecting progressive cholestasis (Fig. 35-14**A**). In contrast to PBC, cholangiectases and cholangitic abscesses may be evident. Cholangiectases are recognizable as cystic collections of bilious and sometimes calculous dark green material that may be up to several centimeters in size and are generally seen in the hilar region of the liver (Fig. 35-14**B**). Cholangitic abscesses, which presumably reflect superinfection of the cholangiectases, often have a more yellow appearance than cholangiectases (Fig. 35-14**C**). The large intrahepatic ducts and the extrahepatic ducts may develop areas of gross stricture and concentric fibrosis as well. If cholangiocarcinomas or bile duct carcinomas occur, these are recognizable as typically firm, white, sclerotic masses.

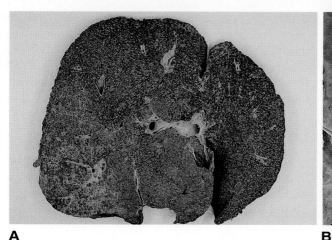

A

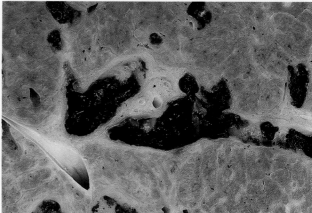

B

C

FIGURE 35–14. Gross pathology findings in primary sclerosing cholangitis (PSC). The liver in PSC typically has a green color, which becomes progressively dark with advancing stage; cirrhosis is illustrated here (**A**). Many cases at resection or autopsy demonstrate cholangiectases, which are evident grossly as aggregates of dark green bilious material along the large ducts (**B**). Less commonly, cholangitic abscesses may be seen, presumably representing superinfected cholangiectases. These tend to be more yellow than cholangiectases (**C**). (Photos courtesy of Drs. Herschel Carpenter and Gerald Dayharsh, Mayo Clinic, Rochester, MN.)

Microscopic Pathology

LARGE DUCTS

Biopsy from the extrahepatic bile ducts shows a thickened, fibrotic wall with a mixed inflammatory infiltrate. However, these alterations are nonspecific in that strictures unrelated to PSC (e.g., after bile duct surgery or the passage of gallstones with associated duct damage) can have similar features.[100] Alterations in large intrahepatic ducts mimic those in the extrahepatic ducts; both show segmental duct fibrosis with stricture. These areas of stricture frequently alternate with cholangiectases and occasionally cholangitic abscesses. Histologically, cholangiectases demonstrate duct dilatation, epithelial atrophy with focal denudation, and mixed bilious material, neutrophils, and granulation tissue at the sites of denudation (Fig. 35-15**A**). Cholangitic abscesses are similar but tend to have a more exuberant population of neutrophils (Fig. 35-15**B**). Although these lesions are strongly suggestive of PSC, they are rarely seen in liver biopsy samples.

LIVER

The hallmark lesion of PSC is fibrous cholangitis that may affect large ducts (perihilar intrahepatic or extra-

hepatic) and/or small ducts. When PSC affects small ducts but the large ducts appear unaffected, the term *small duct PSC* has been used.[80] Fibrous cholangitis is characterized by a mixed inflammatory infiltrate in or adjacent to the damaged duct with extensive concentric collagen deposition, presenting as a fibrous collar around the duct and epithelial atrophy (Fig. 35-16**A** and **B**). The lesions are frequently focal, similar to the florid duct lesions of PBC. The end stage of fibrous cholangitis, sometimes referred to as *fibrous-obliterative cholangitis*, is characterized by loss of epithelium and formation of fibrous scars, which serve as the only evidence of the obliterated duct (Fig. 35-16**C** and **D**). Unfortunately, this near-diagnostic fibrous-obliterative cholangitis is rare among biopsy specimens. Ductopenia without presence of ductal scars is the most common biopsy finding in advanced PSC.

Over time, PSC proceeds through various histologic stages, similar to PBC (see Tables 35-2 and 35-7).[100] Stage I is characterized by portal edema and inflammation and ductal proliferation. At this stage, changes may be indistinguishable from those of incomplete large duct obstruction of other etiology, or they may resemble stage I PBC. Stage II is characterized by periportal fibrosis and inflammation with or without ductular

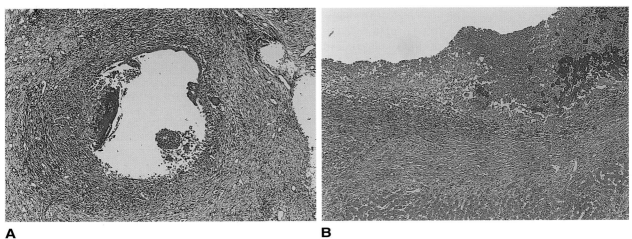

A   **B**

FIGURE 35–15. Histopathology of cholangiectases and cholangitic abscesses in primary sclerosing cholangitis. Both lesions affect large intrahepatic and extrahepatic bile ducts. Cholangiectases show duct dilatation, focal epithelial atrophy and loss, and a resulting mixture of bile, neutrophils, and granulation tissue along areas of denuded epithelium **(A).** Cholangitic abscesses likely reflect the same basic process with added bacterial superinfection, which results in a subjectively larger number of neutrophils **(B).** See Figures 35-14**B** and **C** for gross examples of these lesions.

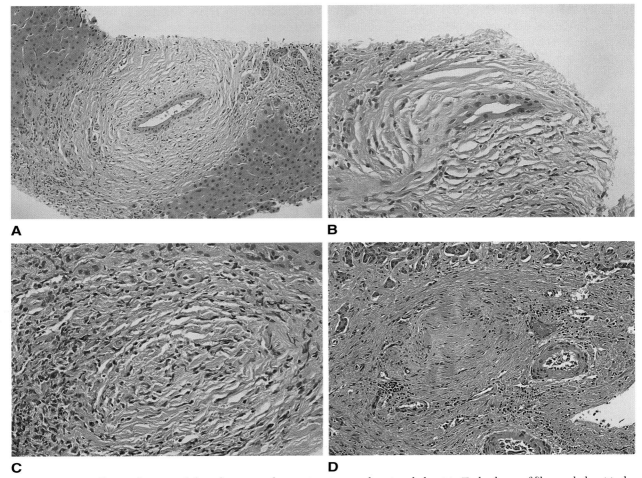

A   **B**

C   **D**

FIGURE 35–16. Small to medium-sized duct-destructive lesions in primary sclerosing cholangitis. Early phases of fibrous cholangitis show concentric periductal fibrosis with mild epithelial atrophy **(A).** Intermediate phases show a greater degree of fibrosis and epithelial atrophy **(B).** The end result, referred to as "fibrous obliterative cholangitis," is a fibrous nodule without epithelium, typically adjacent to a hepatic artery, reflecting the total obliteration of the duct **(C** and **D).**

proliferation; scant lymphocytic piecemeal necrosis may be present. In stage III disease, fibrous septa extend between adjacent portal tracts, and ductopenia becomes more prominent. Biliary piecemeal necrosis and cholate stasis changes identical to those described with PBC also may become apparent (see Figs. 35-12A through E). As in PBC, stage IV disease is the cirrhotic stage and is characterized by irregular garland-shaped regenerative nodules that usually are accompanied by ductular and biliary piecemeal necrosis, forming halos around their periphery. Tissue samples often show near-complete loss of the interlobular bile ducts at this stage.

DIFFERENTIAL DIAGNOSIS

The differential diagnosis of PSC falls into two main categories—histologic and cholangiographic—with some entities falling into both categories (Table 35-9; see also Table 35-5). Histologic mimics may arise based on similarities in pattern of inflammation or based on similar bile duct damage.

Inflammatory mimics include the major chronic hepatitides (AIH, chronic HCV, and chronic HBV) and PBC/AC. PSC lacks the necrotic hepatocytes commonly seen in AIH, HBV, and HCV in both lobules and periportal areas. The number of plasma cells in PSC generally is lower than that seen in AIH and PBC. The sinusoidal lymphocytosis seen in PBC is much less conspicuous in PSC as well. Lymphocytic cholangitis can be seen in PSC and in PBC, AIH, HCV, and HBV, although destructive cholangitis is seen only in PSC and PBC.

Bile duct destruction with concentric periductal fibrosis, superficial epithelial necrosis, cholangiectases,

TABLE 35-9. Major Differential Diagnosis of Primary Sclerosing Cholangitis

Component	Diagnosis
Portal inflammation	Primary biliary cirrhosis/autoimmune cholangitis
	Autoimmune hepatitis
	Chronic hepatitis C
	Chronic hepatitis B
	Nonspecific reactive hepatitis
Bile duct loss	Primary biliary cirrhosis/autoimmune cholangitis
	Idiopathic adulthood ductopenia
	Ischemic cholangitis
	Childhood paucity of intrahepatic bile ducts (syndromic and nonsyndromic)
	Alpha-1-antitrypsin–associated duct loss
	Rare viral or drug-associated loss
Abnormal cholangiogram	Ischemic cholangitis
	Eosinophilic cholangitis
	Sclerosing cholangitis associated with autoimmune pancreatitis
	Infective/AIDS-related cholangitis

and biliary strictures that are indistinguishable from PSC can be seen in ischemic cholangitis (Fig. 35-17).[101] In contrast to the hepatic parenchyma with a dual arterial/venous blood supply, the biliary tree is dependent on arterial supply, which is commonly derived from branches of the hepatic and gastroduodenal arteries. Damage to these vessels with subsequent ischemic cholangitis has been reported in the context of liver transplantation (related to both technical factors and ABO incompatibility), hepatic arterial chemotherapy (often floxuridine) infusion, vasculitis,[101] and surgical occlusion of the hepatic artery.[102]

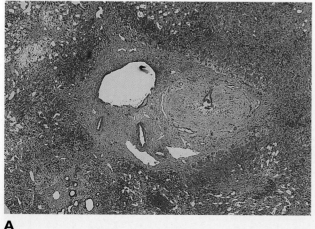

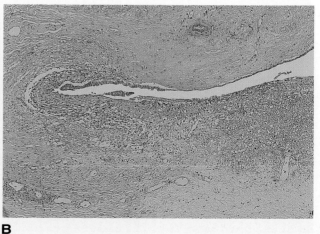

A   **B**

FIGURE 35–17. Bile duct damage in ischemic cholangitis, mimicking primary sclerosing cholangitis. **A,** In this case of ischemic biliary damage secondary to hepatic vein thrombosis (Budd-Chiari syndrome) and presumed venous stasis affecting the biliary tree, the biliary epithelium is attenuated, and concentric periductal fibrosis occurs, as in Figures 35-16A and **B. B,** Similar changes can be seen with disruption of arterial blood supply to the bile ducts, in this case secondary to hepatic artery infusion of chemotherapy (floxuridine) (Masson's trichrome).

A chronic bile-destructive syndrome that may result in a biliary-type cirrhosis has been associated with alpha-1-antitrypsin (A1AT) deficiency (see Chapter 41). This occurs more commonly in the pediatric age group and with homozygous disease and less commonly in adults and with heterozygous disease.[103]

Idiopathic adulthood ductopenia (IAD) is a syndrome characterized by progressive duct loss and its complications without apparent explanation (i.e., no morphologic or serologic features of PBC/AC, no abnormal cholangiogram or history of inflammatory bowel disease [IBD] to suggest PSC, and no other known bile-destructive condition). Patients with IAD appear to fall into two categories—those with progressive disease that may lead to liver transplantation and those with a benign course.[104] Rather than a distinct syndrome, IAD may represent a mixture of late-onset paucity of intrahepatic bile ducts, small duct PSC in the absence of IBD, autoimmune cholangitis in the absence of granulomas or typical serum autoantibodies, and postviral duct destruction.[104]

Cholangiographic mimics of PSC include eosinophilic cholangitis,[105] AIDS-related cholangiopathy (often referred to as cytomegalovirus or cryptosporidium),[106] cholangitis associated with autoimmune pancreatitis,[84] and ischemia.[101] Resolution with corticosteroid therapy is expected with eosinophilic cholangitis and autoimmune pancreatitis but not with PSC or ischemic or infectious cholangitis.

TREATMENT

To date, no effective medical therapy has been recommended[107]; however, UDCA does appear to improve results of serum biochemical tests (alkaline phosphatase, GGT).[108] Endoscopic therapy directed at relieving dominant biliary strictures can significantly improve survival and symptoms among patients with PSC.[109,110]

For patients with decompensated cirrhosis, OLT has emerged as an effective therapy. Disease recurrence in hepatic allografts occurs at an incidence of between 5% and 20% at 4.5 years, but to date, this has not been associated with a statistically significant decrease in patient survival.[111] Diagnosis of recurrent PSC is often difficult because biliary tract ischemia and bile duct anastomotic strictures can mimic PSC in individual cases, and most data supporting recurrence come from studies analyzing large series in a multivariate fashion.[111,112]

OVERLAP SYNDROMES

Overlap syndromes between PSC and AIH are well described (see under Overlap Syndromes in the Autoimmune Hepatitis section).

References

1. Johnson PJ, McFarlane IG: Meeting report: International autoimmune hepatitis group. Hepatology 18:998-1005, 1993.
2. Donaldson P, Doherty D, Underhill J, et al: The molecular genetics of autoimmune liver disease. Hepatology 20:225-239, 1994.
3. Manns MP, Kruger M: Immunogenetics of chronic liver diseases. Gastroenterology 106:1676-1697, 1994.
4. Sherlock S, Dooley J: Chronic hepatitis. In Sherlock S, Dooley J: Diseases of the Liver and Biliary System, 10th ed. Malden, MA, Blackwell Scientific, 1997, pp 303-335.
5. Homberg JC, Abuaf JC, Bernard O, et al: Chronic active hepatitis associated with anti-liver/kidney/microsome antibody type I: A second type of "autoimmune" hepatitis. Hepatology 7:1333-1339, 1987.
6. Hay JE, Czaja AJ, Rakela J, et al: The nature of chronic unexplained transaminase elevations of a mild to moderate degree in asymptomatic patients. Hepatology 9:193-197, 1989.
7. Desmet VJ, Gerber M, Hoofnagle JH, et al: Classification of chronic hepatitis: Diagnosis, grading, and staging. Hepatology 19:1513-1520, 1994.
8. Strassbourg CP, Manns MP: Autoimmune hepatitis vs. viral hepatitis C. Liver 15:225-232, 1995.
9. Baptista A, Bianchi L, DeGroote L, et al: The diagnostic significance of periportal hepatitic necrosis and inflammation. Histopathology 12:569-579, 1988.
10. Wang MX, Morgan T, Lungo W, et al: "Piecemeal" necrosis: Renamed troxis necrosis. Exp Mol Pathol 71:137-146, 2001.
11. Pratt DS, Fawaz KA, Rabson A, et al: A novel histological lesion in glucocorticoid-responsive chronic hepatitis. Gastroenterology 113:664-668, 1997.
12. Popper H, Geller SA: Pathogenetic considerations in the histologic diagnosis of drug-induced injury. In Fenoglio CM, Wolff M (eds): Progress in Surgical Pathology, vol III. New York, Masson, 1981, pp 233-246.
13. Wright R: Drug-induced chronic hepatitis. Springer Semin Immunopathol 3:331-338, 1980.
14. Lefkowitch JH, Apfelbaum TF, Weinberg L, et al: Acute liver biopsy lesions in early autoimmune ("lupoid") chronic active hepatitis. Liver 4:379-386, 1984.
15. Burgart LJ, Batts KP, Czaja AJ: Recent-onset autoimmune hepatitis: Biopsy findings and clinical correlations. Am J Surg Pathol 19:699-708, 1995.
16. Nikias GA, Batts KP, Czaja AJ: The nature and prognostic implications of autoimmune hepatitis with an acute presentation. J Hepatol 21:866-887, 1994.
17. Czaja AJ, Carpenter HA: Histological findings in chronic hepatitis C with autoimmune features. Hepatology 26:459-466, 1997.
18. Czaja AJ, Carpenter HA: Autoimmune hepatitis with incidental histologic features of bile duct injury. Hepatology 34:659-665, 2001.
19. Colombato LA, Alvarez F, Cote J, et al: Autoimmune cholangiopathy: The result of consecutive primary biliary cirrhosis and autoimmune hepatitis? Gastroenterology 107:1839-1843, 1994.
20. Rubel LR, Seeff LB, Patel V: Primary biliary cirrhosis—primary sclerosing cholangitis overlap syndrome. Arch Pathol Lab Med 108:360-361, 1984.
21. Wurbs D, Klein R, Terracciano LM, et al: A 28-year-old woman with a combined hepatitic/cholestatic syndrome (clinical conference). Hepatology 22:1598-1605, 1995.
22. Rabinovitz M, Demetris AJ, Bou-Abboud CF, et al: Simultaneous occurrence of primary sclerosing cholangitis and autoimmune chronic active hepatitis in a patient with ulcerative colitis. Dig Dis Sci 37:1606-1611, 1992.
23. Gregorio GV, Portmann B, Karani J, et al: Autoimmune hepatitis/sclerosing cholangitis overlap syndrome in childhood: A 16-year prospective study. Hepatology 33:544-554, 2001.
24. Batts KP, Ludwig JL: Chronic hepatitis. An update on terminology and reporting. Am J Surg Pathol 19:1409-1417, 1995.
25. Scheuer PJ: The nomenclature of chronic hepatitis: Time for a change. J Hepatol 22:112-114, 1995.
26. Desmet VJ, Gerber M, Hoofnagle JH, et al: Classification of chronic hepatitis: Diagnosis, grading and staging. Hepatology 19:1513-1520, 1994.
27. Poynard T, Bedossa P, Opolon P: Natural history of liver fibrosis progression in patients with chronic hepatitis C. The OBSVIRC,

METAVIR, CLINIVIR, and DOSVIRC groups. Lancet 349:825-832, 1979.

28. Knodell RG, Ishak KG, Black WC, et al: Formulation and application of numerical scoring system for assessing histological activity in asymptomatic chronic active hepatitis. Hepatology 1:431-435, 1981.

29. Ishak KG, Baptista A, Bianchi L, et al: Histological grading and staging of chronic hepatitis. J Hepatol 22:696-699, 1995.

30. Gonzalez-Koch A, Czaja AJ, Carpenter HA, et al: Recurrent autoimmune hepatitis after orthotopic liver transplantation. Liver Transpl 7:302-310, 2001.

31. Van de Water J, Gershwin ME, Leung P, et al: The auto-epitope of the 74-kD mitochondrial autoantigen of primary biliary cirrhosis corresponds to the functional site of dihydrolipoamide acetyltransferase. J Exp Med 167:1791-1799, 1988.

32. Ludwig J, Czaja AJ, Dickson ER, et al: Manifestations of non-suppurative cholangitis in chronic hepatobiliary diseases: Morphologic spectrum, clinical correlations, and terminology. Liver 4:105-116, 1984.

33. Ludwig J: New concepts in biliary cirrhosis. Semin Liver Dis 7:293-301, 1987.

34. Rubin E, Schaffner F, Popper H: Primary biliary cirrhosis: Chronic nonsuppurative destructive cholangitis. Am J Pathol 46:387-407, 1965.

35. Mistry P, Seymour CA: Primary biliary cirrhosis—from Thomas Addison to the 1990's. Q J Med 82:185-196, 1992.

36. Kim WR, Lindor KD, Locke GR, et al: Epidemiology and natural history of primary biliary cirrhosis in a US community. Gastroenterology 119:1631-1636, 2000.

37. Sherlock S, Dooley J: Primary biliary cirrhosis. In Sherlock S, Dooley J: Diseases of the Liver and Biliary System, 10th ed. Malden, MA, Blackwell Scientific, 1997, pp 239-252.

38. Floreani A, Betterle C, Baragiotta A, et al: Prevalence of celiac disease in primary biliary cirrhosis and of antimitochondrial antibodies in adult celiac disease patients in Italy. Dig Liver Dis 34:258-261, 2002.

39. Mahl TC, Shockcor W, Boyer JL: Primary biliary cirrhosis: Survival of a large cohort of symptomatic and asymptomatic patients followed for 24 years. J Hepatol 20:707-713, 1994.

40. Gores GJ: Yes, hepatocellular cancer does occur in primary biliary cirrhosis. Liver Transpl 8:570-571, 2002.

41. Dickson ER, Grambsch PM, Fleming TR, et al: Prognosis in primary biliary cirrhosis: Model for decision making. Hepatology 10:1-7, 1989.

42. Grambsch PM, Dickson ER, Kaplan M, et al: Extramural cross-validation of the Mayo primary biliary cirrhosis survival model establishes its generalizability. Hepatology 10:846-850, 1989.

43. Van de Water J, Gerson LB, Ferrell LD, et al: Immunohistochemical evidence of disease recurrence after liver transplantation for primary biliary cirrhosis. Hepatology 24:1079-1084, 1996.

44. Tanaka A, Miyakawa H, Luketic VA, et al: The diagnostic value of anti-mitochondrial antibodies, especially in primary biliary cirrhosis. Cell Mol Biol (Noisy-le-grand) 48:295-299, 2002.

45. Mackay IR: Hepatoimmunology: A perspective. Immunol Cell Biol 80:36-44, 2002.

46. Nishio A, Keeffe EB, Gershwin ME: Primary biliary cirrhosis: Lessons learned from an organ-specific disease. Clin Exp Med 1:165-178, 2001.

47. Mason A, Nair S: Primary biliary cirrhosis: New thoughts on pathophysiology and treatment. Curr Gastroenterol Rep 4:45-51, 2002.

48. Combes B, Markin RS, Wheeler DE, et al: The effect of ursodeoxycholic acid on the florid duct lesion of primary biliary cirrhosis. Hepatology 30:602-605, 1999.

49. Yamazaki K, Suzuki K, Nakamura A, et al: Ursodeoxycholic acid inhibits eosinophil degranulation in patients with primary biliary cirrhosis. Hepatology 30:71-78, 1999.

50. Colina F, Pinedo F, Solis JA, et al: Nodular regenerative hyperplasia of the liver in early histological stages of primary biliary cirrhosis. Gastroenterology 102:1319-1324, 1992.

51. Ludwig J, Dickson ER, McDonald GSA: Staging of nonsuppurative destructive cholangitis (syndrome of primary biliary cirrhosis). Virchows Arch A Pathol Anat Histol 379:103-112, 1978.

52. Ludwig J: New concepts in biliary cirrhosis. Semin Liver Dis 7:293-301, 1987.

53. Popper H: The problem of histologic evaluation of primary biliary cirrhosis. Virchows Arch A Pathol Anat Histol 379:99-102, 1978.

54. Harada K, Minato H, Hiramatsu K, et al: Epithelioid cell granulomas in chronic hepatitis C: Immunohistochemical character and histological marker of favorable response to interferon-alpha therapy. Histopathology 33:216-221, 1998.

55. Larrey D, Hadengue A, Pessayre D, et al: Carbamazepine-induced acute cholangitis. Dig Dis Sci 32:554-557, 1987.

56. Ishak KG: Sarcoidosis of the liver and bile ducts. Mayo Clin Proc 73:467-472, 1998.

57. Poupon RE, Poupon R, Balkau B: Ursodiol for the long-term treatment of primary biliary cirrhosis. The UDCA-PBC study group. N Engl J Med 330:1342-1347, 1994.

58. Heathcote EJ, Cauch-Dudek K, Walker V, et al: The Canadian Multicenter Double-blind Randomized Controlled Trial of ursodeoxycholic acid in primary biliary cirrhosis. Hepatology 19:1149-1156, 1994.

59. Combes B, Carithers RL, Maddrey WC, et al: A randomized, double-blind, placebo-controlled trial of ursodeoxycholic acid in primary biliary cirrhosis. Hepatology 22:759-766, 1995.

60. Lindor KD, Dickson ER, Jorgenson RA, et al: The combination of ursodeoxycholic acid and methotrexate for patients with primary biliary cirrhosis: The results of a pilot study. Hepatology 22:1158-1162, 1995.

61. Batts KP, Jorgenson RA, Dickson ER, et al: Effects of ursodeoxycholic acid on hepatic inflammation and histological stage in patients with primary biliary cirrhosis. Am J Gastroenterol 91:2314-2317, 1996.

62. Angulo P, Batts KP, Therneau TM, et al: Long-term ursodeoxycholic acid delays histological progression in primary biliary cirrhosis. Hepatology 29:644-647, 1999.

63. Corpechot C, Carrat F, Poupon R, et al: Primary biliary cirrhosis: Incidence and predictive factors of cirrhosis development in ursodiol-treated patients. Gastroenterology 122:652-658, 2002.

64. Poupon RE, Lindor KD, Cauch-Dudek K, et al: Combined analysis of randomized controlled trials of ursodeoxycholic acid in primary biliary cirrhosis. Gastroenterology 113:884-890, 1997.

65. Goulis J, Leandro G, Burroughs AK: Randomised controlled trials of ursodeoxycholic-acid therapy for primary biliary cirrhosis: A meta-analysis. Lancet 354:1053-1060, 1999.

66. Lindor KD, Poupon R, Poupon R, et al: Ursodeoxycholic acid for primary biliary cirrhosis. Lancet 355:657-658, 2000.

67. Tinmouth J, Tomlinson G, Heathcote EJ, et al: Benefit of transplantation in primary biliary cirrhosis between 1985-1997. Transplantation 73:224-227, 2002.

68. Faust TW: Recurrent primary biliary cirrhosis, primary sclerosing cholangitis, and autoimmune hepatitis after transplantation. Liver Transpl 7(Suppl 1):S99-S108, 2001.

69. Balan V, Batts KP, Porayko MK, et al: Histological evidence for recurrence of primary biliary cirrhosis after liver transplantation. Hepatology 18:1392-1398, 1993.

70. Hubscher SG, Elias E, Buckels JA, et al: Primary biliary cirrhosis. Histological evidence of disease recurrence after liver transplantation. J Hepatol 18:173-184, 1993.

71. Brunner G, Klinge O: Ein der chronisch-destruierenden nicht-eitrigen Cholangitis ähnliches Krankheitsbild mit antinukleären Antikörpern (Immunocholangitis). Dtsch Med Wochenschr 112:1454-1458, 1987.

72. Taylor S, Dean P, Riely C: Primary autoimmune cholangitis: An alternative to antibody-negative primary biliary cirrhosis. Am J Surg Pathol 18:91-99, 1994.

73. Michieletti P, Bassendine M, Heathcote E, et al: Antimitochondrial antibody negative primary biliary cirrhosis: A distinct syndrome of autoimmune cholangitis. Gut 35:260-265, 1994.

74. Goodman ZD, McNally PR, Davis DR, et al: Autoimmune cholangitis: A variant of primary biliary cirrhosis. Clinicopathologic and serologic correlations in 200 cases. Dig Dis Sci 40:1232-1242, 1995.

75. Ben-Ari Z, Dhillon A, Sherlock S: Autoimmune cholangiopathy: Part of the spectrum of autoimmune chronic active hepatitis. Hepatology 18:10-15, 1993.

76. Kim WR, Poterucha JJ, Jorgenson RA, et al: Does antimitochondrial antibody status affect response to treatment in patients with primary biliary cirrhosis? Outcomes of ursodeoxycholic acid therapy and liver transplantation. Hepatology 26:22-26, 1997.

77. Chazoullieres O, Wendum D, Serfaty L, et al: Primary biliary cirrhosis—autoimmune hepatitis overlap syndrome: Clinical features and response to therapy. Hepatology 28:296-301, 1998.

78. Lohse AW, zum Buschenfelde KH, Franz B, et al: Characterization of the overlap syndrome of primary biliary cirrhosis (PBC) and autoimmune hepatitis: Evidence for it being a hepatitic form of PBC in genetically susceptible individuals. Hepatology 29:1078-1084, 1999.

79. Talwalker JA, Keach JC, Angulo P, et al: Overlap of autoimmune hepatitis and primary biliary cirrhosis: An evaluation of a modified scoring system. Am J Gastroenterol 97:1191-1197, 2002.

80. Wee A, Ludwig J: Pericholangitis in chronic ulcerative colitis: Primary sclerosing cholangitis of the small bile ducts. Ann Intern Med 102:581-587, 1985.

81. Angulo P, Larson DR, Therneau T, et al: Time course of histological progession in primary sclerosing cholangitis. Am J Gastroenterol 94:3310-3313, 1999.

82. Jessurun J, Bolio-Solis A, Manivel JC: Diffuse lymphoplasmacytic acalculous cholecystitis: A distinctive form of chronic cholecystitis associated with primary sclerosing cholangitis. Hum Pathol 29:512-517, 1998.

83. Buckles DC, Lindor KD, Larusso NF, et al: In primary sclerosing cholangitis, gallbladder polyps are frequently malignant. Am J Gastroenterol 97:1138-1142, 2002.

84. Kazumori H, Ashizawa N, Moriyama N, et al: Primary sclerosing pancreatitis and cholangitis. Int J Pancreatol 24:123-127, 1998.

85. Olsson R, Danielsson A, Jarnerot G, et al: Prevalence of primary sclerosing cholangitis in patients with chronic ulcerative colitis. Gastroenterology 100:1319-1323, 1991.

86. Chapman RWG, Varghese Z, Gaul R, et al: Association of primary sclerosing cholangitis with HLA B-8. Gut 24:38-41, 1983.

87. Donaldson PT, Farrant JM, Wilkinson ML, et al: Dual association of HLA DR2 and DR3 with primary sclerosing cholangitis. Hepatology 13:129-133, 1991.

88. Lefkowitch JH, Martin EC: Primary sclerosing cholangitis. Prog Liver Dis 8:557-580, 1986.

89. MacCarty RL, LaRusso NF, Wiesner RH, et al: Primary sclerosing cholangitis: Findings on cholangiography and pancreatography. Radiology 149:39-44, 1983.

90. Nakanuma Y, Hirai N, Kono N, et al: Histological and ultrastructural examination of the intrahepatic biliary tree in primary sclerosing cholangitis. Liver 6:317-325, 1986.

91. Ludwig J, Batts KP, MacCarty RL: Ischemic cholangitis in hepatic allografts. Mayo Clin Proc 67:519-526, 1992.

92. Washington K, Clavien PA, Killenberg P: Peribiliary vascular plexus in primary sclerosing cholangitis and primary biliary cirrhosis. Hum Pathol 28:791-795, 1997.

93. Kim WR, Therneau TM, Wiesner RH, et al: A revised natural history model for primary sclerosing cholangitis. Mayo Clin Proc 75:688-694, 2000.

94. Ponsioen Cy, Vrouenraets SM, Prawirodirdjo W, et al: Natural history of primary sclerosing cholangitis and prognostic value of cholangiography in a Dutch population. Gut 51:562-566, 2002.

95. Angulo P, Larson DR, Therneau TM, et al: Time course of histological progression in primary sclerosing cholangitis. Am J Gastroenterol 94:3310-3313, 1999.

96. Kaya M, de Groen PC, Angulo P, et al: Treatment of cholangio-carcinoma complicating primary sclerosing cholangitis: The Mayo Clinic experience. Am J Gastroenterol 96:1164-1169, 2001.

97. Bergquist A, Ekbom A, Olsson R, et al: Hepatic and extrahepatic malignancies in primary sclerosing cholangitis. J Hepatol 36:321-327, 2002.

98. Angulo P, Maor-Kendler Y, Lindor KD: Small-duct primary sclerosing cholangitis: A long-term follow-up study. Hepatology 35:1494-1500, 2002.

99. Boberg KM, Rocca G, Egeland T, et al: Time-dependent Cox regression model is superior in prediction of prognosis in primary sclerosing cholangitis. Hepatology 35:652-657, 2002.

100. Ludwig J, Barham SS, LaRusso NF, et al: Morphologic features of chronic hepatitis associated with primary sclerosing cholangitis and chronic ulcerative colitis. Hepatology 1:632-640, 1981.

101. Batts KP: Ischemic cholangitis. Mayo Clin Proc 73:380-385, 1998.

102. Gomez M, Scotto B, Roger R, et al: Ischemic cholangitis after ligation of the hepatic artery: A case report. J Radiol 83:736-738, 2002.

103. Graziadei IW, Joseph JJ, Wiesner RH, et al: Increased risk of chronic liver failure in adults with heterozygous alpha-1-antitryspin deficiency. Hepatology 28:1058-1063, 1998.

104. Ludwig J: Idiopathic adulthood ductopenia: An update. Mayo Clin Proc 73:285-291, 1998.

105. Grauer L, Padilla VM, Bouza L, et al: Eosinophilic sclerosing cholangitis associated with hypereosinophilic syndrome. Am J Gastroenterol 88:1764-1769, 1993.

106. Benhamou Y, Caumes E, Gerosa Y, et al: AIDS-related cholangiopathy. Critical analysis of a prospective series of 26 patients. Dig Dis Sci 38:1113-1118, 1993.

107. Meier PN, Manns MP: Medical and endoscopic treatment in primary sclerosing cholangitis. Best Pract Res Clin Gastroenterol 15:657-666, 2001.

108. van Hoogstraten HJ, Wolfhagen FH, van de Meeberg PC, et al: Ursodeoxycholic acid therapy for primary sclerosing cholangitis. Results of a 2-year randomized controlled trial to evaluate single versus multiple daily doses. J Hepatol 29:417-423, 1998.

109. Baluyut AR, Sherman S, Lehman GA, et al: Impact of endoscopic therapy on the survival of patients with primary sclerosing cholangitis. Gastrointest Endosc 53:308-312, 2001.

110. Stiehl A, Rudolph G, Kloters-plachky P, et al: Development of dominant bile duct stenoses in patients with primary sclerosing cholangitis treated with ursodeoxycholic acid: Outcome after endoscopic treatment. J Hepatol 36:151-156, 2002.

111. Graziadei IW: Recurrence of primary sclerosing cholangitis after liver transplantation. Liver Transpl 8:575-581, 2002.

112. Graziadei IW, Wiesner RH, Batts KP, et al: Recurrence of primary sclerosing cholangitis following liver transplantation. Hepatology 29:1050-1056, 1999.

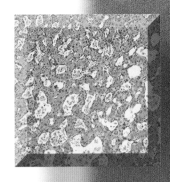

CHAPTER 36

Toxic and Drug-Induced Disorders of the Liver

PAULETTE BIOULAC-SAGE • CHARLES BALABAUD

Introduction

Because the liver is the major site of drug metabolism, it is often the target of drug-induced injury. Despite improvements in preclinical and clinical toxicologic studies and in the safety analysis of clinical trials, the frequency of drug hepatotoxicity has remained unchanged over the past 10 years. Adverse chemical reactions are not confined to pharmaceutical drugs (i.e., the drug itself and excipients [vehicles]) used for classic therapeutic purposes. Vitamins and herbal medicines also represent potential hepatotoxins. Furthermore, various toxins can give rise to hepatotoxicity, beginning with alcohol and also including illicit drugs (e.g., cocaine, heroin, ecstasy), criminal poisons, and environmental and industrial toxins (e.g., natural toxicants, mushrooms, industrial chemicals, pesticides). Circumstances of exposure to all forms of liver toxicants are listed in Table 36-1.[1]

All drugs and toxins can be potentially hepatotoxic, and essentially all forms of hepatic lesions can be encountered. Particular lesions that are more likely to be drug induced are discussed in detail in this chapter. Hepatotoxicity also gives rise to an extensive variety of clinical expressions, acute or chronic, that lead in extreme cases to fulminant hepatitis or cirrhosis, respectively. In this area of hepatology, as in others, clinicopathologic correlations are essential. Even with such correlations, the diagnosis of drug-induced hepatotoxicity remains difficult.

Drug-induced hepatotoxicity is a significant clinical problem and should be included in the differential diagnosis of any patient with hepatic laboratory abnormalities or with hepatic dysfunction. Although hepatocytes are the cells of obvious concern, the primary target of some drugs may be endothelial cells, Kupffer cells, hepatic stellate cells, or cholangiocytes. Current preclinical test systems for hepatotoxicity are inadequate, reflecting our limited understanding of the mechanisms of drug toxicity, particularly the "hypersensitivity" and "idiosyncratic" types of reactions. Hence, hepatotoxicity

TABLE 36-1. Circumstances of Exposure to Liver Toxicants
Drugs
Treatment: prescription medication, over-the-counter drug abuse
Self-poisoning, especially suicide attempts
Natural Toxicants
Food
Food contaminants
Alcohol abuse
Folk and herbal medicine
Bacterial infection
Fungal, insect, and scorpion toxins
Industrial Chemicals and Pesticides
Industrial accidents
Household accidents with chemical products
Self-poisoning with chemical products
Low-level chronic exposure at the workplace
Environmental pollution

From Kahl R: Toxic liver injury. In Bircher J, Benhamou JP, McIntyre N, et al (eds): Oxford Textbook of Clinical Hepatology, 2nd ed. New York, Oxford University Press, 1999, pp 1319-1334.

is a problem with major economic impact in that it is the most frequent cause of postmarketing withdrawal of new medications. For the pathologist, keeping the potential of toxin- or drug-induced hepatic damage in mind is the important first step in recognizing hepatotoxicity.

We consider here the main pathologic lesions attributed to drugs and toxins, as well as some recent pathogenic data. General readings concerning this topic and/or detailed descriptions of hepatotoxicity produced by individual drugs may be found in specialized books,[2] chapters,[3-5] and recent detailed papers.[6-10]

◼ Pertinent Clinical Features

DEMOGRAPHIC DATA

Drug-induced liver injury accounts for about 10% of cases of acute hepatitis in adult patients and for more than 40% in those over 50 years of age[7]; it accounts for 10% to 20% of fulminant and subfulminant hepatitis[11] and for 2% to 5% of patients hospitalized for jaundice. The risk of a fulminant course is much greater for drug-induced (20%) than for viral (1%) acute hepatitis. However, drugs are much less often incriminated in chronic hepatitis and cirrhosis (less than 1% of cases).

The overall number of drugs liable to be toxic to the liver exceeds 1100, and this long list must be frequently updated.[12] The highest frequency of hepatotoxicity for marketed drugs is around 1% (i.e., for tacrine), but for the majority of drugs, the risk is low (1/10,000 to 1/100,000) or extremely low (1/100,000 to 1/1,000,000 [antihistaminic compounds, penicillin]).

In addition, overdoses of certain drugs are well known to be extremely toxic, not only in the context of a therapeutic misadventure (or with repeated doses, particularly in cases of excessive alcohol ingestion) but also as a method of suicide. In the latter instance, acetaminophen (paracetamol) is the most frequent suicidal overdose encountered among adolescents and young adult women in Great Britain and the United States.

The potential hepatotoxicity of herbal remedies commonly used for self-medication (i.e., alternative or "natural" treatments) and of other botanicals (e.g., well-known mushroom poisoning from *Amanita phalloides*) must also be remembered. The list of ascertained or suspected hepatotoxic herbal components (e.g., Chinese herbs, Germander[13]) is long, but the extent of their responsibility remains unclear.[14]

An increased consumption of illicit drugs such as heroin, cocaine, and ecstasy ("Rave" parties) is a major preoccupation among adolescents today, whatever the route of administration, that is, intranasally, intravenously, or by smoking.[15] In many cases, hepatotoxicity is potentiated by other drugs or by alcohol.

DIFFERENTIAL DIAGNOSIS AND DIAGNOSTIC CRITERIA

Hepatic lesions attributed to drugs and toxins are numerous and various. Their recognition is important because they may mimic all forms of acute or chronic hepatitis, as well as different types of cholestatic or vascular hepatopathy. In addition, some liver tumors, in particular, hepatocellular adenoma and angiosarcoma, may be attributed to drugs and toxins. Thus, the pathologist must consider possible hepatotoxicity in the differential diagnosis of virtually all morphologic lesions. Critical chronologic and clinical diagnostic criteria are provided in Table 36-2. Chronologic criteria, although essential, require precise history taking, which is not always possible. Clinical criteria[16] and laboratory data may eliminate other causes of hepatopathy. Nevertheless, for different reasons, major difficulties remain in the definitive diagnosis of drug-induced liver disease (Table 36-3),

---

TABLE 36-2. Diagnostic Criteria

Chronologic Criteria
- Interval between the beginning of treatment and the onset of liver injury: 1 week–3 months (shorter after readministration)
- Regression of liver laboratory abnormalities after withdrawal of the treatment (decrease of more than 50% in a week)
- Relapse of liver laboratory abnormalities after accidental or intentional readministration of the offending drug

Clinical Criteria
Elimination of Other Causes
- Previous hepatic or biliary disease
- Alcohol abuse
- Viral hepatitis (HAV, HBV, HCV, HDV, CMV, Epstein-Barr virus, herpesvirus, etc.)
- Biliary obstruction (ultrasonography, MRI)
- Autoimmune hepatitis/cholangitis
- Liver ischemia
- Wilson's disease
- Bacterial infection (*Listeria*, *Campylobacter*, *Salmonella*)

Positive Clinical Criteria
- Age >50 yr
- Intake of many drugs
- Intake of a known hepatotoxic agent
- Specific serum autoantibodies: anti-M6, anti-LKM2, anti–CYP 1A2, anti–CYP 2E1
- Drug analysis in blood: acetaminophen (paracetamol), vitamin A
- Hypersensitivity manifestations (fever, chills, skin rash, hypereosinophilia)

Liver Biopsy (not necessarily required but indicated for the following purposes)
- Eliminate other causes of liver injury
- Show lesions suggestive of drug-induced hepatotoxicity
- Define lesions for new drugs

HAV, hepatitis A virus; HBV, hepatitis B virus; HCV, hepatitis C virus; HDV, hepatitis D virus; CMV, cytomegalovirus; MRI, magnetic resonance imaging.

Adapted from Larrey D: Drug-induced liver diseases. J Hepatol 32:77-88, 2000.

TABLE 36-3. Major Difficulties in the Diagnosis of Drug-Induced Liver Disease

Nonspecific clinical features
Treated disease itself may lead to liver abnormalities (bacterial infection)
Intake of several hepatotoxic drugs (i.e., combined antituberculosis agents)
Compounds considered safe (herbal remedies)
Drug prescription difficult to analyze
- Inaccurate history
- Automedication
- Masked information
  - Illegal compounds
  - Offending agent not considered a "drug" by the patient
- Forgotten information (elderly)
Fulminant hepatitis with comatose patient

Adapted from Larrey D: Drug-induced liver diseases. J Hepatol 32:77-88, 2000.

even though liver biopsy may reveal features suggestive of drug toxicity.

PREDICTION OF HEPATOTOXICITY

Because of variability in both drug exposure and patient susceptibility, anticipating hepatotoxicity depends on both the type of drug and the particular patient being treated (Table 36-4). On one hand, some acquired factors may enhance the susceptibility of one particular drug. On the other hand, various genetic factors such as deficiency in different types of cytochromes P-450 or in other enzymatic and metabolic pathways may contribute to drug hepatotoxicity (Table 36-5).[7] Unfortunately, idiosyncratic reactions that eventually can be severe and even fatal cannot be predicted. For example, troglitazone,

TABLE 36-4. Assessing the Likelihood of Hepatotoxicity

Drug Factors
- Drug is massively absorbed in the digestive tract
- Drug is metabolized by cytochrome P-450
- Drug belongs to a family with well-documented hepatotoxicity
- Drug exhibits a molecular structure predisposing to the formation of reactive metabolites

Patient Factors

Constitutional and Acquired Risk Factors		Examples of Increased Probability
Age	>60 yr	Isoniazid, nitrofurantoin
	Children	Valproic acid, salicylates
Sex	Women	Methyldopa, nitrofurantoin
	Men	Azathioprine
Nutrition	Obesity	Halothane
	Fasting/malnutrition	Acetaminophen (paracetamol)
Pregnancy		Acetaminophen (paracetamol), tetracycline
Chronic alcohol abuse		Acetaminophen (paracetamol)
Intake of other drugs	Enzyme induction	Rifampicin, isioniazid
	Enzyme inhibition	Troleandomycin, estrogens
Disease	HIV infection	Cotrimoxazole/sulfonamides

Genetic Factors (see Table 36-5)

which was an approved drug on the market for the treatment of diabetes mellitus, is a recent example of idiosyncratic, direct hepatocyte toxicity that led to an unacceptable rate of acute hepatic failure; it has been removed from the market.[17-19]

TABLE 36-5. Genetic Factors Contributing to Drug Hepatotoxicity

Genetic Deficiency	Drugs	Comments
CYP2D6	Perhexiline	Enzyme deficiency: 6% of white population. Perhexiline toxicity: 75% of patients are CYP2D6 deficient.
CYP2C19	Atrium*	Enzyme deficiency: 3% to 5% of white population. Atrium toxicity: all patients have a complete or partial deficiency.
NAT2	Sulfonamides, dihydralazine	Transmitted as an autosomal recessive trait. High frequency of the slow acetylation phenotype. The deficiency contributes to but is not sufficient for the toxicity.
Sulfoxidation	Chlorpromazine	Not proven.
Glutathione synthetase	Acetaminophen (paracetamol)	Uncommon condition; deficient subjects are more susceptible to paracetamol hepatotoxicity.
Glutathione S-transferase type T	Tacrine	Needs to be confirmed.
Hepatic detoxification capacity for reactive metabolites	Halothane, phenytoin, carbamazepine, amineptine, sulfonamides	Deficiencies are observed in patients and some members of their family. Precise defects are not identified.
Genetic variations in the immune system	Halothane, tricyclic antidepressants, chlorpromazine, etc.	Association between several HLA haplotypes and some hepatotoxic drugs.

*Febarbamate, difebarbamate, phenobarbital.
HLA; human leukocyte antigen; NAT2, *N*-acetyltransferase 2.

TABLE 36-6. Causality Assessment

- *Very likely* (rare): Drug overdose; relapse after accidental readministration; specific features of drug hepatitis
- *Compatible* (many cases): No specific criteria; suggestive chronology; absence of other causes
- *Doubtful* (frequent): Missing information (chronology, clinical data); no specific criteria; frequent in fulminant hepatitis
- *Incompatible:* Demonstration of another cause; incompatible chronology; be aware that hepatitis can occur after discontinuation of treatment (i.e., halothane, clavulanic acid–amoxicillin)

Causality can be assessed with more or less certainty if a clear chronologic linkage and correlation between drug type and hepatotoxic event can be established (Table 36-6). However, it is difficult to provide definitive proof of responsibility for an offending drug because its readministration is ill advised. Withdrawal of the drug, usually followed by a return to normality, is good supporting evidence.

PREVENTION OF DRUG HEPATOTOXICITY

Assessment of host toxicity is performed before and after marketing of all drugs. After marketing, simple rules can be applied to prevent drug hepatotoxicity (Table 36-7).

TABLE 36-7. Prevention of Drug Hepatotoxicity

Before Marketing
Detection of toxicity in animals or cellular models
Safety analysis in healthy volunteers and patients
After Marketing
Avoid readministration of the offending drug
Avoid readministration of drugs belonging to the same biochemical family
Avoid simultaneous administration of several drugs:
- Cytochrome P-450 inhibitors: Cimetidine, ketoconazole, methoxsalen, oleandomycin may be nonselective (cimetidine) or selective for a given cytochrome P-450 isoform
- Cytochrome P-450 inducers: Rifampicine, barbiturates, phenytoin; more selectively, omeprazole for CYP1A1 and CYP1A2
Control administration of drugs to patients with malnutrition (lack of defense against reactive metabolites) and to alcoholic patients
Be aware that elderly patients are more susceptible to drug hepatotoxicity
Be careful when administering drugs to HIV patients:
- Coadministration of many drugs
- Decreased ability to detoxify drugs (malnutrition)
- Higher susceptibility to some drugs (sulfonamides)
Genetic factors: genotyping and phenotyping tests are not widely available
Follow-up of aminotransferase levels is useful for detecting hepatotoxicity

TREATMENT AND PROGNOSIS

The only example of well-established treatment for drug-induced hepatotoxicity is the prevention of hepatitis in patients with acetaminophen (paracetamol) overdose by administration of *N*-acetylcysteine within the first 10 hours to detoxify formed reactive metabolites.[20] In other cases, no specific treatment is given for drug-induced liver injury; the main measure instead is to stop administration of the offending agent. The usefulness of corticosteroids in immunoallergic hepatitis has not been demonstrated. The administration of ursodeoxycholic acid has been proposed for long-lasting chronic cholestasis and as symptomatic treatment for the relief of pruritus or as compensation for vitamin malabsorption.[7] In the worst case—drug- or toxin-induced fulminant hepatic failure—liver transplantation may be required.

The prognosis of drug-induced hepatotoxicity is excellent when the injury is acute, the cause is recognized, and the offending agent withdrawn before severe acute injury or chronic injury occurs. In the setting of chronic hepatitis (as with amiodarone, alpha-methyldopa, or methotrexate), progression to fibrosis and eventual cirrhosis may occur over an extended period. Withdrawal of the drug at a late date minimizes the risk of continued progression, but reversal of fibrosis is rare. An important caveat is the risk of alcohol-induced synergistic injury. Intake of alcohol in the setting of drug-induced chronic hepatitis may exacerbate the severity of injury and cause continued progression toward cirrhosis even after the drug has been withdrawn.

▇ Categories of Toxic Liver Injury

Drug hepatotoxicity is classified as intrinsic or idiosyncratic. Intrinsic hepatotoxicity is predictable, dose dependent, and often characteristic of a particular agent taken in large quantities (e.g., acetaminophen). The mechanism of injury can be direct—by damaging cells and organelles—or indirect—by conversion of a xenobiotic into an active toxin or through an immune-mediated mechanism. Idiosyncratic hepatotoxicity, the most frequent form of hepatotoxicity, corresponds to unpredictable reactions according to the host, individual genetic variations in the metabolism of drugs, and environmental factors. The formation of reactive metabolites is a frequent mechanism for idiosyncratic reactions and hence is highly dependent on the metabolic capacity of the host. The different categories of hepatic damage can be etiologically pure, but most of the time, a mixture of lesions in the same liver is produced by the same or different mechanisms. Furthermore, a single drug may give rise to different aspects of hepatotoxicity in different patients (e.g., hepatitis, cholestasis, or granulomas arising from the same drug).

TABLE 36-8. Main Functions of Sinusoidal Liver Cells

Kupffer Cells
Endocytosis (viruses, bacteria, protozoa)
Presenting antigen to lymphocytes
Secretion of cytokines (inflammation: TNF-α; IL-1, -6, -12, -18; IFN-α and -γ fibrosis: TGF-β)
Secretion of prostaglandins (PGI$_2$, PGE$_2$) and reactive oxygen species

Sinusoidal Endothelial Cells
Receptor-mediated endocytosis (scavenger, Ag-presenting cell)
Synthesis of extracellular matrix components (collagens III and IV, fibronectin)
Secretion of cytokines (IL-1, -6) and eicosanoids (PGE$_2$)
Secretion of NO
Recruitment of leukocytes (adhesion, extravasation)

Hepatic Stellate Cells
Storage of vitamin A
Synthesis of extracellular matrix components, mainly after activation into myofibroblasts (collagens, glycoproteins, proteoglycans)
Degradation of the extracellular matrix (degrading enzymes; metalloproteinases and their inhibitors; TIMPS)
Vasomotor regulation: secretion of endothelin-1 (vasoconstriction) and NO (vasodilatation)

Liver-Associated Natural Killer Cells (NK, T, NT/T)
Antiviral, antitumor, and pathogenic inflammatory responses

IL, interleukins; IFN, interferon; NO, nitric oxide; PG, prostaglandin; TIMPS, tissue inhibitors of metalloproteinases; TGF, transforming growth factor; TNF, tumor necrosis factor.

Adverse drug reactions affect mainly hepatocytes and bile duct epithelial cells but may also damage sinusoidal cells. Although the functions of hepatocytes and bile duct epithelial cells are well appreciated, it is worth noting the physiologic functions of sinusoidal cells as given in Table 36-8. The spatial organization of vessels, lobules, and sinusoids is illustrated in Figure 36-1. The different types of morphologic changes are given for each, and some examples of damaging drugs are listed in Table 36-9. For simplicity, these are classified according to the main histologic target.

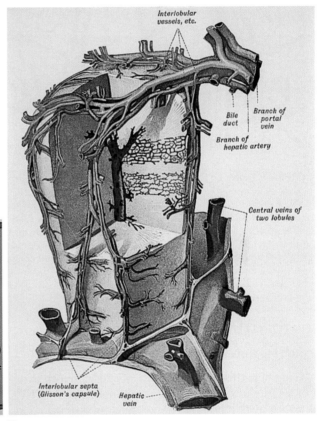

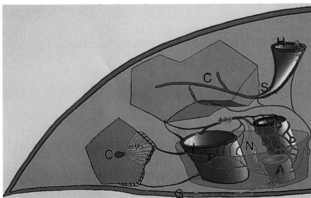

A   **B**

FIGURE 36–1. Schematic representation of liver architecture. A, Diagrammatic representation of hepatic artery compartmentalization in mammalian livers shows two systems of the artery (A) within and outside of the portal tract. In the portal tract (*lower right*), the artery feeds the bile duct (B) as the peribiliary vascular plexus, the portal tract interstitium, including nerve (N), and the wall of the portal vein (P). Drainage of these vascular beds is collected as a hepatic artery–derived portal system (APS), which joins the portal vein (1) in the tract or at the inlet venule on entering the lobule. The hepatic artery therefore supplements the portal blood flow via the APS. Outside the portal tract, the artery dissociates itself (*asterisks*) to supply Glisson's capsule (G), which drains into subcapsular lobules, and the walls of the hepatic venous system, including the central (C), sublobular (S), and hepatic (H) veins. The latter are the pathways by which arterial blood can bypass the hepatic parenchyma into the hepatic vein (2). Note that in the lobule, inlet venules perfuse the lobular bed as conical sectors, the hepatic microcirculatory subunits (HMS). (From Ekataksin W, Kaneda K: Liver microvascular architecture: An insight into the pathophysiology of portal hypertension. Semin Liver Dis 19:359-382, 1999.) **B,** Wax reconstruction (by A. Vierling) of a lobule of the liver of a pig. A portion of the lobule has been cut away to show the bile capillaries and sinusoids. (After Braus.) (From Bloom W, Fawcett DW: Liver and gallbladder. In Bloom W, Fawcett DW: A Textbook of Histology, 10th ed. Philadelphia, WB Saunders, 1975, p 689.)

Continued

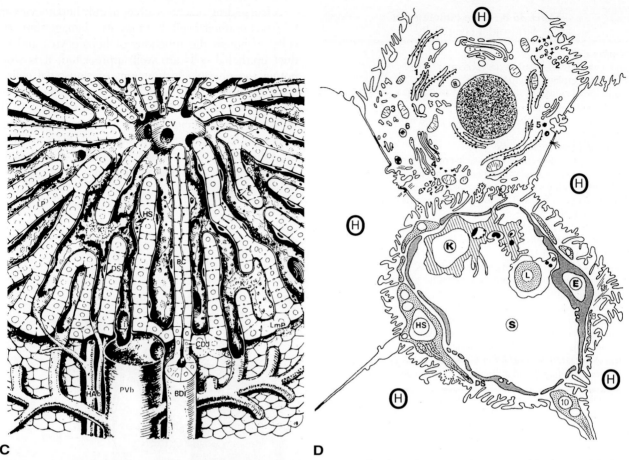

C

D

FIGURE 36–1, cont'd C, Diagram of a lobule. This schematic figure summarizes the three-dimensional structure of the hepatic lobule as revealed by scanning electron microscopy. CV, central vein; K, Kupffer cell; HS, hepatic stellate cell; BC, bile canaliculus; SEC, sinusoidal endothelial cell; S, sinusoid populated with large and small fenestrations (these latter mainly arranged in clusters); DS, Disse space; HAb, hepatic artery branch; PVb, portal vein branch; CDJ, canaliculoductular junction; BDI, bile ductule; LmP, limiting plate; LP, liver plates. (Modified from Muto M: A scanning electron microscopic study on endothelial cells and Kupffer cells in rat liver sinusoids. Arch Histol Jpn 37:369-386, 1975. **D,** Schematic representation of the hepatic parenchyma and sinusoids. H, hepatocyte; HS, hepatic stellate cell; K, Kupffer cell: HS, hepatic stellate cell containing lipid droplets (vitamin A) with their process in the Disse space; E, sinusoidal endothelial cell with fenestrae; DS, Disse space—between the sinusoidal membrane of hepatocyte and the sinusoidal endothelial cell—contains the extracellular matrix; L, liver-associated lymphocyte; 1, rough endoplasmic reticulum; 2, smooth endoplasmic reticulum; 3, mitochondria; 4, Golgi apparatus; 5, lysosomes; 6, peroxisomes.

HEPATOCELLULAR INJURY

Acute Hepatocellular Injury

Acute hepatitis represents 90% of drug-induced liver diseases, defined by alanine aminotransferase (ALT) elevations two times the upper limit of normal as a marker of hepatocyte cytolysis. Elevations in alkaline phosphatase (AP) are an enzymatic marker of cholestasis in that this enzyme is present on the apical membranes of both hepatocytes and bile duct epithelial cells.[21] Acute hepatocellular injury may be predominantly cytolytic (ratio ALT/AP ≥ 5) or cholestatic (ALT/AP ≤ 2), or it may occur in a combined form (ALT/AP between 2 and 5).

PREDOMINANT CYTOLYSIS

This form of drug-induced acute hepatitis resembles acute viral hepatitis with no specific features; numerous drugs can be incriminated (see Table 36-9). It ranges from mild hepatitis with rapid improvement after removal of the offending drug to severe, even fatal liver failure.

Spotty Necrosis. When predominantly cytolytic, necrosis can affect isolated hepatocytes in the lobule (spotty necrosis), either resembling viral hepatitis or taking on a "mononucleosis-like" form. In the former type, ballooning and/or apoptotic hepatocytes, often in small foci, are distributed at random in the lobule, with no or few inflammatory cells. Often, neutrophils and eosinophils are present in the lobule and in some portal tracts. Kupffer cells are often hypertrophied and contain pigments (lipofuscin, hemosiderin). Their prominent activation, associated with sinusoidal lymphocytosis, characterizes the variant form of mononucleosis hepatitis–like injury, as is seen with phenytoin.

Submassive Necrosis. Liver necrosis (whether it appears as ballooning degeneration, apoptotic bodies,

TABLE 36-9. Pathologic Effects of Drugs and Toxicity on the Liver

Type of Injury	Main Drugs
Hepatocellular	
Acute hepatocellular injury	
• *Predominantly cytolytic*	*Conventional drugs*
	Without hypersensitivity: paracetamol, isoniazid, ketoconazole, valproic acid
	With hypersensitivity: NSAIDs (almost all drugs), sulfonamides, almost all antidepressants (tricyclic, iproniazid), halothane, and derivatives
	New causative drugs
	Psychotropic and neurotropic drugs (e.g., tacrine), anti-HIV (e.g., didanosine, zidovudine), antimycotics (terbinafine), cytokines and growth factors (interleukins, G-CSF), antidiabetic agents (troglitazone)
	Herbal medicines
	Pyrrolizidine alkaloids (crotaloria, *Senecio*)
	Germander, Chinese herbal preparations
	Illegal compounds
	Cocaine, ecstasy
	Excipients
	Sodium saccharinate, polysorbate, propylene glycol
	Chemical agents
	Carbon tetrachloride, trichloroethylene, tetrachloroethylene, toluene, dimethylformamide, vinyl chloride
• *Predominantly cholestatic*	
Pure cholestasis	Oral contraceptives, estrogens, estrogens + troleandomycin or erythromycin, androgens, tamoxifen, azathioprine, cytarabine
Cholestasis + mild cytolysis ("cholestatic hepatitis")	*Conventional drugs*
	Phenothiazines, NSAIDs, macrolides, sulfonamides, beta-lactam antibiotics, tricyclic antidepressants, carbamazepine, amoxicillin/clavulanic acid, gold salts, propoxyphene
	New drugs
	Anti-HIV: didanosine, zidovudine, stavudine, ritonavir
	Interleukins: IL-2, IL-6, IL-12
• *Mixed-pattern acute hepatitis*	
Chronic hepatocellular injury	
• *Chronic hepatitis (with risk of cirrhosis)*	Valproic acid, amiodarone, aspirin, benzarone, halothane, iproniazid, isoniazide, methotrexate, methyldopa, nitrofurantoin, papaverine, herbal medicines (Germander)
Steatosis/steatohepatitis/phospholipidosis	
• *Microvesicular*	Aspirin, tetracycline, valproic acid, alcohol, NSAIDs, anti-HIV drugs, fialuridine
• *Macrovesicular steatosis*	Alcohol, methotrexate, corticosteroids
• *NASH (from steatosis to cirrhosis)*	DEAEH, amiodarone, perhexiline maleate, anti-HIV, corticosteroids, tamoxifen
• *Phospholipidosis*	DEAEH, amiodarone, perhexiline maleate, TPN
Miscellaneous	
• *Pigment accumulation*	
Lipofuscin	Phenothiazines, aminopyrine
Hemosiderin	Excess dietary iron, alcoholism, TPN
• *Ground-glass changes*	Phenobarbital, phenytoin, cyanamide
• *Anisonucleosis*	Methotrexate
• *Increased mitoses*	Colchicine, arsenic
Bile Duct	
Acute cholangitis	
• *Cholestasis + bile duct degeneration without/ with inflammation*	Phenothiazines, ajmaline, carbamazepine, tricyclic antidepressants, macrolides, amoxycillin/clavulanic acid, dextropropoxyphene
Chronic cholangitis ± ductopenia	
• *Primary biliary cirrhosis–like*	Phenothiazines, ajmaline, arsenical derivatives, tricyclic antidepressants
	Macrolides, thiobendazole, tetracycline, fenofibrate
	Herbal medicines (Germander)
• *Primary sclerosing cholangitis–like*	Arterial infusion with floxuridine, formol, and hypertonic saline injection into hydatid cyst, hepatic artery embolization
Vascular	
Sinusoids	
• *Sinusoidal dilatation/ peliosis*	Oral contraceptives, estrogens, anabolic steroids, azathioprine, vitamin A, tamoxifen, danazol, heroin

Continued

TABLE 36-9. Pathologic Effects of Drugs and Toxicity on the Liver—cont'd

Type of Injury—cont'd	Main Drugs—cont'd
Hepatic vein lesions	
• *Large HV thrombosis: Budd-Chiari*	Oral contraceptives, dacarbazine, irradiation, total parenteral nutrition
• *Sublobular/small centrilobular vein: veno-occlusive disease*	Pyrrolizidine alkaloids, azathioprine, antineoplastic agents, alcohol, heroin
Portal vein lesions	
• *Hepatoportal sclerosis*	Arsenic, azathioprine, Thorotrast
• *Nodular regenerative hyperplasia*	Spanish toxic oil, oral contraceptives, azathioprine
Hepatic artery lesions	
• *Intimal hyperplasia*	Oral contraceptives
Sinusoidal Cells	
Hepatic stellate cells	
• *Hypertrophy (lipid storage) without/with perisinusoidal fibrosis*	Vitamin A, methotrexate, azathioprine, 6-mercaptopurine
Kupffer cells/macrophages	
• *Storage*	Talc, polyvinyl pyrrolidone, silicone, barium
• *Phospholipidosis*	Amiodarone
• *Granulomatous reactions*	
Epithelioid granulomas	Quinidine, hydralazine, phenytoin
Fibrin-ring granulomas	Allopurinol
Granulomatous hepatitis (cytolytic without/with cholestasis)	Phenylbutazone
Lipogranulomas	Mineral oil ingestion
Lipogranulomas with black pigments	Gold salts
Foreign body granulomas	Talc, suture surgical material
Sinusoidal endothelial cells	(See Hepatic vein lesions)
Tumors	
Benign: hepatocellular adenoma (± intratumoral hemorrhage, subcapsular hematoma, rupture)	Oral contraceptives, anabolic/androgenic steroids, estrogens
Malignant	
• *Angiosarcoma*	Vinyl chloride, Thorotrast
• *Hepatocellular carcinoma*	Oral contraceptives, anabolic/androgenic steroids, Thorotrast
• *Intrahepatic cholangiocarcinoma*	Thorotrast

DEAEH, diethylaminoethoxyhexestrol; G-CSF, granulocyte cell-stimulating factor; HIV, human immunodeficiency virus; NASH, nonalcoholic steatohepatitis; NSAIDs, nonsteroidal anti-inflammatory drugs; TPN, total parenteral nutrition.

or coagulative necrosis) occurs mainly in centrilobular zones, leading to dropout of individual hepatocytes. Extension of hepatocyte death to the midzonal areas leads to formation of well-demarcated, more or less confluent necrotic areas that contrast with surviving parenchymal zones, leading to an aspect of "maplike" hepatitis (Fig. 36-2). In collapsed zones, reticulin framework and endothelial cells are still preserved, mixed with a variable number of inflammatory cells and numerous hypertrophied Kupffer cells/macrophages that contain brown ceroid pigment. Several drugs may be responsible (see Table 36-9). Predominantly periportal necrosis can occur, but more rarely than the centrilobular type, with illicit drugs such as cocaine (Fig. 36-3) or with other toxins (e.g., halogenated hydrocarbons).

Massive Necrosis. This type of injury involves nearly all of the lobule, leads to features of fulminant hepatitis requiring liver transplantation, and can occur with most drugs that cause centrilobular necrosis. The most common example is suicidal or accidental overdose of acetaminophen (paracetamol[22]) (Fig. 36-4) or halothane (Fig. 36-5), but other drugs can be causative as well (see Table 36-9). The same pattern of injury can be seen after mushroom poisoning with *A. phalloides* (Fig. 36-6), with other environmental or illicit drugs such as ecstasy, and with other toxins that may cause this kind of confluent necrosis.[23-28] Such severe injury can leave only a few spared periportal hepatocytes, which often exhibit microvesicular or macrovesicular steatosis (see Fig. 36-6B). Collapsed stroma is intermingled with

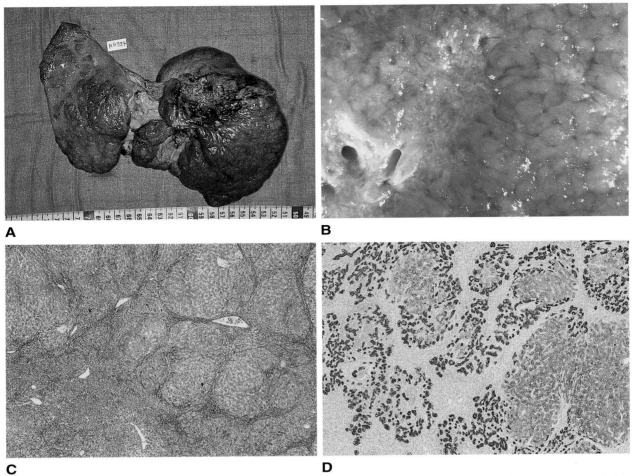

FIGURE 36–2. Subfulminant hepatitis in a 47-year-old woman related to alpidem (Ananxyl), taken for 6 months (150 mg/day). **A,** Dysmorphic explanted liver with large atrophic areas between nodular parenchymal areas of regeneration. **B,** Section of explanted liver showing areas of collapse (*on the left*) contrasting with areas of persisting yellow-tan parenchyma (*on the right*) (fresh tissue seen under a lens). **C,** "Maplike" hepatitis. Large areas of collapse (*on the left*) with loose connective tissue contrasting with surviving parenchymal areas (*on the right*) (Masson's trichrome). **D,** In collapsed areas, there is a prominent ductular proliferation mixed with some inflammatory cells (pancytokeratin [KL-1] immunostain).

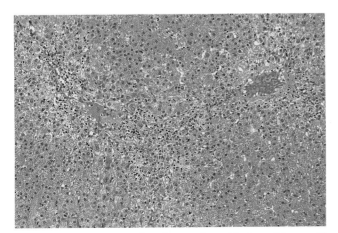

FIGURE 36–3. Cocaine-induced acute hepatitis in a 20-year-old man: perivenular and bridging necrosis, mixed with inflammatory reaction. (Case provided by Dr. M. Chevallier, Lyon, France.)

prominent bile ductular proliferation and a few inflammatory cells and Kupffer cells. The contrast between the severity of parenchymal necrosis and a poorly developed inflammatory portal reaction increases the likelihood that hepatotoxicity (as opposed to viral infection) is the cause of the massive necrosis.

PREDOMINANT CHOLESTASIS

This pattern of damage is characteristic of anabolic or contraceptive steroids. It is characterized by prominent intrahepatic cholestasis ("bland cholestasis"), predominantly in centrilobular hepatocytes, with formation of canalicular plugs; sometimes, an aspect of feathery degeneration of hepatocytes and liver cell rosettes is seen in cases of prolonged cholestasis. Discontinuation

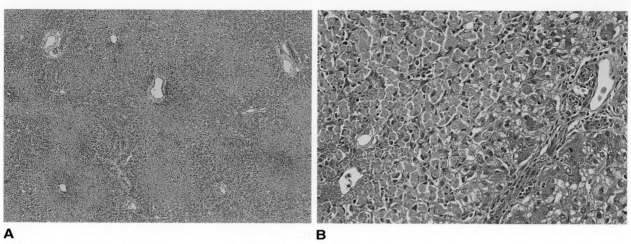

A   **B**

FIGURE 36–4. Fulminant liver failure in a 1-year-old baby with a history of acetaminophen (paracetamol) overdose (therapeutic misadventure: fourfold therapeutic doses for 4 days); section from liver explant. **A,** Submassive confluent centrilobular and midlobular necrosis with congestion around terminal hepatic veins. **B,** Centrilobular and midlobular necrosis of coagulative type (shrunken, eosinophilic hepatocytes, without nuclei), sparing only a rim of periportal hepatocytes, sometimes steatotic. (Case provided by Linda D. Ferrell, University of California, San Francisco.)

of the offending drug is usually followed by complete recovery.

Mild hepatocyte ballooning/necrosis or apoptotic bodies are often associated. This latter damage can be more pronounced, leading to a combined cytolytic and cholestatic hepatitis (Fig. 36-7) that is frequently associated with immunoallergic manifestations.[29] Many drugs may cause cholestatic or the mixed pattern type of acute hepatitis (see Table 36-9). In both forms, the prognosis is better than that in pure acute hepatocellular hepatitis, as described earlier.

Whatever the form and intensity of hepatocellular damage, a centrilobular predominance of lesions and the presence of scattered eosinophils argue for drug hepatotoxicity.

PATHOGENESIS

Mechanisms of drug-induced acute hepatitis are complex.[3] They are rarely direct (e.g., lovastatin); only massive doses of foreign substances and/or extensive metabolism of a particular xenobiotic may lead to such direct toxicity. Drug-induced acute hepatitis is mainly the result of the formation of hepatotoxic reactive metabolites, often involving the cytochrome P-450 system. The role of cytochrome P-450 in the formation of reactive metabolites and the protective mechanisms involving, for example, glutathione are schematically summarized in Table 36-10. The end result of this in situ reaction of reactive metabolites may be either apoptosis or cytolytic necrosis. However, for many drugs, the

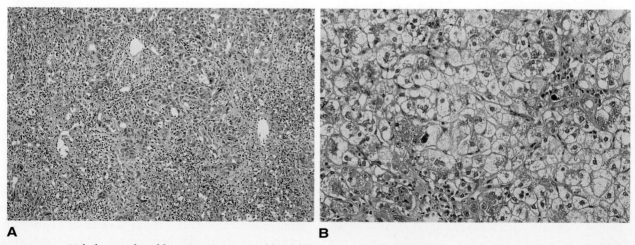

A   **B**

FIGURE 36–5. Halothane-induced hepatitis in a 6-year-old girl following a second anesthesia 1 year after initial exposure; section from liver explant. **A,** Bridging, extensive collapse with severe centrilobular hemorrhagic necrosis, prominent ductular proliferation, mixed inflammation of portal tracts and parenchyma with neutrophilic component. **B,** Foamy degeneration of hepatocytes and canalicular cholestasis. (Case provided by Bernard Portmann, King's College Hospital, London.)

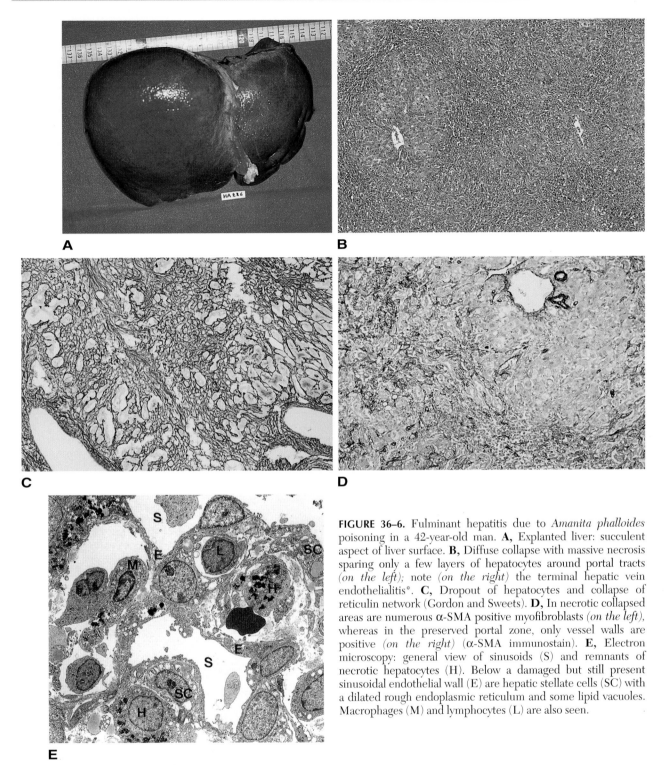

FIGURE 36–6. Fulminant hepatitis due to *Amanita phalloides* poisoning in a 42-year-old man. **A,** Explanted liver: succulent aspect of liver surface. **B,** Diffuse collapse with massive necrosis sparing only a few layers of hepatocytes around portal tracts *(on the left);* note *(on the right)* the terminal hepatic vein endothelialitis°. **C,** Dropout of hepatocytes and collapse of reticulin network (Gordon and Sweets). **D,** In necrotic collapsed areas are numerous α-SMA positive myofibroblasts *(on the left)*, whereas in the preserved portal zone, only vessel walls are positive *(on the right)* (α-SMA immunostain). **E,** Electron microscopy: general view of sinusoids (S) and remnants of necrotic hepatocytes (H). Below a damaged but still present sinusoidal endothelial wall (E) are hepatic stellate cells (SC) with a dilated rough endoplasmic reticulum and some lipid vacuoles. Macrophages (M) and lymphocytes (L) are also seen.

formation of reactive metabolites may be minimal, so that at most mild elevation of serum aminotransferases is seen.

The covalent binding of reactive metabolites to intra-cellular or circulating proteins modifies the "self" of the individual (see Table 36-10). In some subjects, this modification may "mislead" the immune system into mounting an immune attack against hepatocytes. The immune attack may be directed against either the modified self (Fig. 36-8) or the self itself when autoimmunity is directed, in part, against unmodified epitopes of proteins. Some of these autoantigens are themselves cytochrome P-450. Mechanisms leading to anti–cytochrome P-450 autoantibodies remain unknown. Cytochrome P-450 present on the plasma membrane of hepatocytes probably plays a role. As an example, halothane hepatitis is a paradigm for immune-mediated

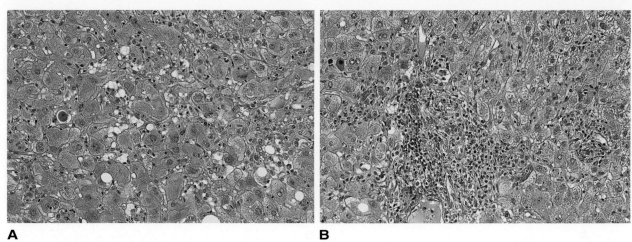

A   **B**

FIGURE 36–7. Mixed cytolytic and cholestatic hepatitis in a 64-year-old man taking several hepatotoxic drugs (oral hypoglycemic, hypolipemic drugs and omeprazole). **A,** Prominent centrilobular cholestasis with ballooning of hepatocytes *(on the right)*, associated with spotty necrosis *(apoptotic body on the left)*. **B,** There is also a moderate polymorphous portal infiltrate with ductular proliferation and interface hepatitis.

TABLE 36-10. Mechanisms of Drug-induced Acute Hepatitis

The cytochrome P-450 system, located mainly in the liver (hepatocytes), predominantly in the centrilobular zone:
Able to metabolize and eliminate essentially all liposoluble xenobiotics of the environment, as well as most drugs used at present.
The various cytochrome P-450s share the same oxidizing center (the heme moiety) and a similar architecture but differ in their protein
   moieties. Each cytochrome P-450 metabolizes partially overlapping, but largely different, sets of xenobiotics.
Several xenobiotics are transformed by cytochrome P-450s into stable metabolites; many others are oxidized into unstable, chemically
   reactive intermediates. The reactive metabolites can attack hepatic constituents (e.g., DNA, unsaturated lipids, proteins, glutathione).
Reactive metabolites are formed mainly through oxidative reactions.
The cytochrome P-450 isoenzymes are under genetic control, and the hepatic level of a given isoenzyme varies considerably among
   different people.
Microsomal enzyme induction by drugs administrated concurrently may promote the formation of reactive metabolites.
Chronic ethanol ingestion increases a particular isoenzyme of cytochrome P-450 (P-450 2E1) that activates acetaminophen
   (paracetamol).
Protective mechanisms:
 • Inactivation of cytochrome P-450 by some reactive intermediates
 • Glutathione
   • Glutathione serves as a molecular sink for electrophilic metabolites; the reaction is accelerated by several cytosolic and
      microsomal glutathione S-transferases
   • Fasting decreases glutathione content
   • Pregnancy decreases the capacity for the liver to resynthesize glutathione
 • Other protective mechanisms:
   • Several other enzymes may catalyze the rearrangement of reactive metabolites into stable metabolites
In situ reaction of reactive metabolites: molecular lesions
 • First type of molecular lesion: lipid peroxidation (may extend from one lipid to the other)
 • Second type of molecular lesion:
   • Electrophilic metabolites (react with and covalently bind to several nucleophilic groups of proteins)
   • Reaction with the SH group of glutathione, resulting in its depletion together with
     • Direct covalent binding to protein thiols
     • And/or direct oxidation of protein thiols
   • Depletion of protein thiols: several toxicologic consequences:
     • Destruction of the microfilament network
     • Increase in cellular Ca^{2+}, activation of calcium-dependent proteases, cell damage
     • Permeabilization of the mitochondrial inner membrane
The immune system: immune attack against:
 • The modified self: formation of alkylated proteins degraded into alkylated peptides, different from the self of the individual
 • The self: formation of anti–cytochrome P-450 antibodies (drug-induced autoimmune hepatitis) (e.g., tienilic acid [cytochrome P-450 2C9], dihydralazine [cytochrome P-450 1A2])

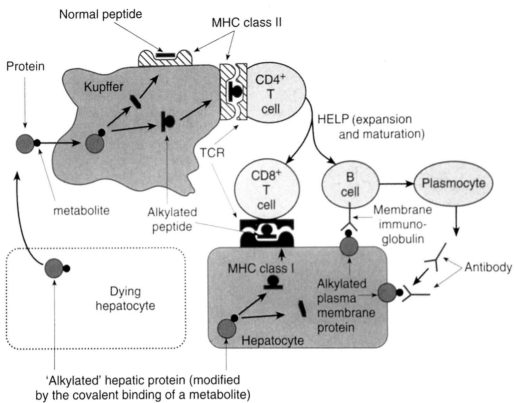

FIGURE 36–8. Hypothetical mechanisms of immunization by, and against, the modified self. (From Pessayre D, Larrey D, Biour M: Drug-induced liver injury. In Bircher J, Benhamou JP, McIntyre N, et al [eds]: Oxford Textbook of Clinical Hepatology, 2nd ed. New York, Oxford University Press, 1999, pp 1261-1315.)

drug hepatotoxicity,[30,31] with the presence of antibodies in the serum of patients. Genetic factors affecting hepatic drug metabolism and the polymorphism of major histocompatibility complex molecules may explain the particular susceptibility of some subjects. Toxic hepatitis due only to activation of the host immune system (autoimmunity), without a contribution from direct hepatic metabolism of an exogenous drug, is quite infrequent. It is usually associated with hypersensitivity manifestations such as fever, rash, and blood eosinophilia.

Chronic Hepatocellular Injury

Chronic drug-induced hepatitis has the same morphologic features as other causes of chronic hepatitis with variable degrees of activity (mild, moderate, or severe) and fibrosis (Fig. 36-9). Complete serologic tests are necessary for eliminating a viral or autoimmune hepatitis and affirming the responsibility of a hepatotoxic agent (see Table 36-9) such as certain drugs[32] or herbs.[33,34] Diagnosis can be very difficult, however, because on the one hand, chronic drug-induced hepatitis can resemble autoimmune hepatitis, and on the other hand, the drug can also be a trigger of autoimmunity. Chronic drug-induced hepatitis can progress to fibrosis and even cirrhosis; this has been suspected after long-term methotrexate treatment (with frequently additional risk

factors) or exposure to toxins such as arsenic or vinyl chloride or in cases of hypervitaminosis A.[35]

Steatosis and Steatohepatitis

Steatosis (fatty liver) and steatohepatitis (fatty liver with inflammation) represent two of the most frequent

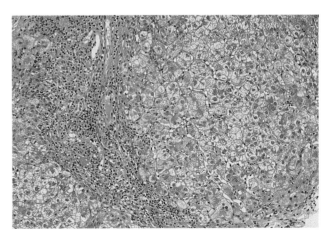

FIGURE 36–9. Diclofenac-induced hepatitis in a 74-year-old woman with rheumatoid arthritis. Shown are features of chronic hepatitis with portal fibrosis and moderate neutrophilic portal infiltrate with spillover associated with ballooned hepatocytes. (Case provided by Wilson Tsui, Caritas Medical Center, Kowloon, Hong Kong.)

pathologic manifestations of hepatotoxicity. Steatosis and steatohepatitis may be due to alcohol ingestion or may be a manifestation of central obesity, diabetes, or hypertriglyceridemia with insulin resistance. However, drugs must always be considered as a potential cause of steatosis and steatohepatitis as well. In patients who are not alcohol abusers, these two conditions are designated as nonalcoholic fatty liver disease (NAFLD). Although the term *nonalcoholic fatty liver disease* encompasses both steatosis and steatohepatitis, the term *nonalcoholic steatohepatitis* (NASH) refers specifically to the presence of an inflamed steatotic liver in a nonalcoholic patient.

ALCOHOLIC LIVER DISEASE

Excessive alcohol (ethanol) consumption is the leading cause of liver disease in most Western countries. Currently 67% of Americans older than age 18 years consume alcohol. More than 14 million Americans meet the criteria for alcohol abuse and/or dependence, which corresponds to a prevalence of 7.4% among adults over age 18. The incidence of alcoholism is higher in men (11%) than in women (4%).[36]

CLINICAL FEATURES

Acute ingestion of up to 80 g of alcohol (eight beers or 7 ounces of 80-proof liquor) generally produces mild, reversible hepatic changes, such as fatty liver. Daily intake of at least 80 g of alcohol generates a significant risk for severe hepatic injury, and daily ingestion of at least 160 g for 10 to 20 years is often associated with severe chronic hepatic injury. However, only 10% to 15% of alcoholics develop cirrhosis. In fact, cirrhosis may develop without any antecedent evidence of steatosis or alcoholic hepatitis.

Acute alcohol exposure may induce microvesicular steatosis, regardless of the individual's general pattern of alcohol consumption. In contrast, chronic alcohol consumption has a variety of adverse effects and induces three distinctive, albeit overlapping, forms of liver disease: (1) steatosis, (2) hepatitis, and (3) cirrhosis. These three forms of liver pathology are collectively referred to as alcoholic liver disease.[37] Because the first two conditions may develop independently of each other, this pattern of disease does not necessarily represent a continuum of changes.

Patients with alcohol-induced steatosis may present with hepatomegaly and a mild elevation of serum bilirubin and alkaline phosphatase levels. Alternatively, there may be no clinical or biochemical evidence of liver disease. Severe hepatic compromise is unusual. Alcohol withdrawal and the provision of an adequate diet is usually sufficient treatment for alcohol-induced steatosis.

In contrast, alcoholic hepatitis is an acute disease that usually follows a bout of heavy alcohol consumption. Symptoms and laboratory abnormalities may range from minimal to severe (fulminant hepatic failure). Between these two extremes, patients may present with nonspecific symptoms such as malaise, anorexia, weight loss, upper abdominal discomfort, and tender hepatomegaly, and laboratory findings of hyperbilirubinemia, elevated alkaline phosphatase levels, and neutrophilic leukocytosis. Rarely, an acute cholestatic syndrome that resembles large bile duct obstruction may develop. The prognosis is unpredictable; each bout of hepatitis incurs about a 10% to 20% risk of death. With repeated bouts, cirrhosis develops in about one third of patients within a few years. Alcoholic hepatitis may also be superimposed on established cirrhosis. With proper nutrition and total cessation of alcohol consumption, alcoholic hepatitis may resolve slowly. However, in some patients, hepatitis persists despite abstinence and eventually progresses to cirrhosis.

The manifestations of alcoholic cirrhosis are similar to other forms of cirrhosis, as discussed in Chapter 37. The first signs of alcohol-related cirrhosis are often due to complications of portal hypertension, including life-threatening variceal hemorrhage. Alternatively, malaise, weakness, weight loss, and loss of appetite may precede the appearance of jaundice, ascites, and peripheral edema, the latter due to impaired synthesis of albumin. The stigmata of cirrhosis (e.g., grossly distended abdomen, wasted extremities, caput medusae) may also be dramatically evident. Laboratory findings reflect the presence of evolving hepatic injury, with elevated serum aminotransaminase levels, hyperbilirubinemia, a variable elevation of serum alkaline phosphatase, hypoproteinemia (globulins, albumin, and clotting factors), and anemia. In some instances, a liver biopsy may be indicated, because in about 10% to 20% of cases of presumed alcoholic cirrhosis, another unrelated disease process may be inadvertently discovered on biopsy. Finally, cirrhosis may also be clinically silent, discovered only at autopsy or when other conditions such as infection or trauma tip the scale toward hepatic insufficiency.

Although an alcoholic patient with cirrhosis may die of unrelated causes, the 5-year survival rate is only 50% to 60% in those who continue to consume alcohol. In such patients, the immediate causes of death include hepatic coma, massive gastrointestinal hemorrhage from esophageal varices, intercurrent infection, hepatorenal syndrome, and hepatocellular carcinoma (in 3% to 6% of cases).

PATHOGENESIS

Alcohol causes hepatocellular injury via a variety of mechanisms. Pure hepatocellular steatosis results from shunting of normal substrates away from catabolism and toward lipid biosynthesis, impaired assembly and secretion of lipoproteins, and increased peripheral catabolism of fat.[38] Alcohol also impairs hepatic metabolism of methionine, which leads to decreased intrahepatic glutathione (GSH) levels, thereby sensitizing the liver to oxidative injury. Furthermore, induction of cytochromes P-450, especially CYP2E1, increases catabolism of alcohol in the endoplasmic reticulum, but it produces reactive oxygen species in the process. These molecules react with membranes and proteins detrimental to hepatocellular function. The induction of cytochromes P-450 also augments bioconversion of other drugs to toxic metabolites. Alcohol also directly affects microtubular and mitochondrial function and membrane fluidity. Acetaldehyde (the major intermediate metabolite of alcohol en route to acetate production) induces lipid peroxidation and acetaldehyde-protein adduct formation, further disrupting cytoskeletal and membrane function. Finally, alcohol intake induces an immunologic attack on hepatic neoantigens, possibly the result of alcohol-induced or acetaldehyde-induced alteration in hepatic proteins.

Alcohol is often a major caloric source in alcoholics, displacing other nutrients and leading to malnutrition and vitamin deficiencies (such as vitamin B_{12}). This effect is compounded by impaired digestive function, primarily related to chronic gastric and intestinal mucosal damage, and pancreatitis.

Alcohol-induced hepatic inflammation and activation of perisinusoidal stellate cells to become myofibroblasts and to deposit extracellular connective tissue matrix is a response to many converging events, such as activation of hepatic macrophages (both Kupffer cells and infiltrating macrophages), with release of proinflammatory cytokines (tumor necrosis factor α, interleukins-1 and -6, transforming growth factor β); amplification of cytokine stimuli by platelet-activating factor (PAF), a lecithin-related lipid released by endothelial cells and Kupffer cells; and influx of neutrophils into the parenchyma with release of their noxious substances. These various events are set in motion by the local toxic effects of alcohol and by alcohol-induced release of bacterial endotoxin into the portal circulation. Alcohol also induces release of endothelins from sinusoidal endothelial cells. Endothelins are potent vasoconstrictors and induce myofibroblast-like perisinusoidal stellate cells to contract, decreasing sinusoidal perfusion and causing regional hypoxia of the parenchyma. This then promotes parenchymal extinction, as discussed in Chapter 37.

The net effect is a chronic disorder featuring steatosis, hepatitis, progressive fibrosis, and marked derangement of vascular perfusion. In essence, alcoholic liver disease may be regarded as a maladaptive state in which the liver responds in an increasingly harmful manner to a stimulus (alcohol) that originally was only marginally harmful.

PATHOLOGIC FEATURES

Steatosis (Fatty Liver). Following intake of alcohol, microvesicular steatosis occurs in hepatocytes. With

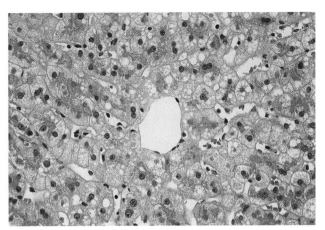

FIGURE 36–10. Alcoholic foamy degeneration: microvesicular steatosis of centrilobular hepatocytes.

chronic intake of alcohol, large clear macrovesicular steatotic globules develop, compressing and displacing the cell nucleus to the periphery of the hepatocyte. This transformation is initially centrilobular in location (Fig. 36-10), but in severe cases, it may involve the entire lobule. Macroscopically, fatty liver of chronic alcoholism induces a large (up to 4 to 6 kg), soft organ that is yellow, greasy, and readily fractured with handling. Although there is little or no fibrosis at the outset of alcoholic steatosis, with continued alcohol intake, fibrous tissue develops around the terminal hepatic veins and extends into adjacent sinusoids (Fig. 36-11).

Alcoholic Hepatitis. This is characterized by four features (Fig. 36-12):

1. Hepatocyte swelling and necrosis, evident as single or scattered foci of cells undergoing swelling (ballooning) and necrosis.

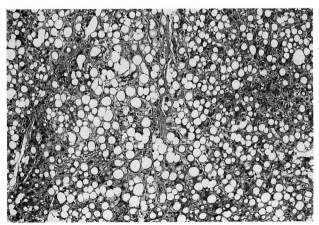

FIGURE 36–11. Recurrent alcoholic steatosis in a 50-year-old woman who underwent liver transplantation 1 year ago for alcoholic cirrhosis. Massive macrovesicular steatosis is associated with zone 3 perisinusoidal and terminal hepatic vein fibrosis (Masson's trichome).

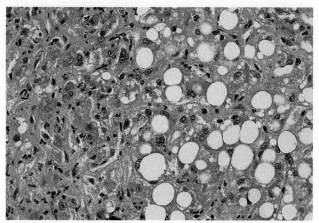

FIGURE 36–12. Acute alcoholic hepatitis superimposed on cirrhosis in a 52-year-old man. Macrovesicular steatosis is associated with prominent Mallory bodies (*on the left*) intermingled with neutrophils.

2. Mallory bodies, which are tangled skeins of cytokeratin intermediate filaments and other proteins, and are visible as eosinophilic cytoplasmic inclusions in degenerating hepatocytes. These inclusions are a characteristic but nonspecific feature of alcoholic liver disease, because they also are seen in other disorders such as primary biliary cirrhosis, Wilson's disease, chronic cholestatic syndromes, and hepatocellular tumors.
3. Neutrophilic inflammation, which involves the lobules and accumulates around degenerating hepatocytes, particularly those with Mallory bodies. Lymphocytes and macrophages also enter portal tracts and may spill into the parenchyma.
4. Fibrosis, sinusoidal and perivenular, but occasionally periportal as well, particularly with repeated bouts of heavy alcohol intake.

In addition to these features, some cases show cholestasis and a mild deposition of hemosiderin (iron) in hepatocytes and Kupffer cells. Macroscopically, the liver is usually mottled red with bile-stained areas. Although the liver may be of normal or even increased size, it often contains visible nodules and fibrosis indicative of evolution to cirrhosis.

Alcoholic Cirrhosis. The final and irreversible form of alcoholic liver disease usually evolves slowly and insidiously. At first, the cirrhotic liver is yellow-tan, fatty, and enlarged, usually weighing over 2 kg. Over the span of years it is transformed into a brown, shrunken, nonfatty organ, sometimes less than 1 kg in weight. Arguably, cirrhosis may develop more rapidly in the setting of alcoholic hepatitis, within 1 to 2 years. Initially, the developing fibrous septa are delicate and extend through sinusoids from central to portal regions as well as from portal tract to portal tract. Regenerative activity of entrapped parenchymal hepatocytes generates fairly uniformly sized "micronodules." With time,

nodularity becomes more prominent, and a mixed micronodular-macronodular pattern may develop (discussed in Chapter 37). As fibrous septa dissect and surround nodules, the liver becomes more fibrotic, loses fat, and shrinks progressively. Parenchymal islands become engulfed by wide bands of fibrous tissue. Ischemic necrosis and fibrous obliteration of nodules eventually create a broad expanse of tough, pale scar tissue ("Laënnec's cirrhosis"). Bile stasis often develops as well. However, Mallory bodies are only rarely evident at this stage. Thus, end-stage alcoholic cirrhosis resembles, both macroscopically and microscopically, cirrhosis that develops from viral hepatitis, as well as other causes.

NONALCOHOLIC FATTY LIVER DISEASE

CLINICAL FEATURES

Nonalcoholic fatty liver disease (NAFLD) is defined pathologically as a condition that resembles alcohol-induced liver disease but occurs in patients who are not heavy drinkers.[39] Men and women of many races are affected, with the following strong associations: obesity, dyslipidemia, hyperinsulinemia and insulin resistance, overt type 2 diabetes, and a variety of drugs (discussed separately below). Although NAFLD is ultimately a diagnosis of exclusion, it is the most likely explanation for the elevated serum aminotransferase and/or gamma-glutamyltranspeptidase values documented in 24% of the general population. It is estimated that 31% of American men and 16% of American women have NAFLD, which represents approximately 31 million Americans.

Patients with NAFLD are largely asymptomatic, showing abnormalities often only in their laboratory parameters. Hence, there is debate as to whether NAFLD actually represents a disease versus an aberrant "physiologic" condition. However, with increasing recognition of NAFLD since the 1990s, it is now thought to account for up to 70% of cases of chronic hepatitis of unknown etiology. Indeed, up to 10% to 30% of patients with NAFLD eventually develop cirrhosis. Hence, NAFLD is now considered to be the most common cause of "cryptogenic" cirrhosis, with its attendant morbidity and mortality. In fact, the epidemic of obesity in the United States heightens concern that NAFLD will further increase in prevalence. There is also growing evidence that NAFLD contributes to the progression of other liver diseases such as hepatitis C viral infection. The incidence of hepatocellular carcinoma in NAFLD is, essentially, unknown.

PATHOGENESIS

A "multiple-hit" hypothesis is proposed for the pathogenesis of NAFLD, which suggests that fatty livers are unusually vulnerable to oxidants and may develop steatohepatitis when secondary insults generate sufficient oxidants to cause liver cell death and inflammation.[40] Patients with NAFLD have high hepatic free fatty acid levels and high mitochondrial β-oxidation rates, thus increasing the delivery of electrons to the mitochondrial respiratory chain.[41] This leads to the "first hit," namely generation of a fatty liver through diversion of excess electrons to triglyceride biosynthesis. However, the imbalance between high mitochondrial electron input and restricted electron outflow may cause over-reduction of respiratory chain components, which increasingly react with oxygen to form reactive oxygen species (ROS), in particular the superoxide anion radical. This is the "second hit." ROS then oxidize unsaturated lipids to release lipid peroxidation products, such as malondialdehyde, that react with mitochondrial DNA and proteins. Hepatocellular antioxidants such as glutathione are depleted, rendering the cells more susceptible to additional ROS-induced injury. Ongoing mitochondrial injury further blocks the flow of electrons in the respiratory chain and exacerbates hepatocellular injury through the generation of more ROS. In essence, a steatotic hepatocyte is unable to tolerate oxidative or apoptotic stress.

It has been hypothesized that lipid peroxidation and general ROS-mediated hepatocellular injury then may induce formation of hepatic tumor necrosis factor α (TNF-α), which represents the "third hit." Perisinusoidal stellate cells are thereby stimulated to convert to myofibroblasts and deposit extracellular connective tissue. TNF-α also induces Fas ligand expression on hepatocytes, thereby triggering hepatocellular apoptosis. A progressive "multi-hit" cycle of hepatocellular destruction, cytokine-induced parenchymal inflammation, and stellate cell fibrogenesis is thus set in motion.

Particular attention is given to the role of an intracellular enzyme, termed *inhibitor of kappa beta kinase* (IKKβ), based on animal studies.[42] IKKβ activates nuclear factor kappa beta (NF-κβ), a nuclear transcription factor, which induces the synthesis of TNF-α. Genetic susceptibility to IKKβ activation and/or chronic environmental activation of IKKβ activity and TNF-α expression may underlie the progression of NAFLD to NASH.

PATHOLOGIC FEATURES

The characteristic feature of NAFLD is steatosis that consists of both large and small vesicles of fat, predominantly triglycerides, within hepatocytes.[43] At the benign end of the spectrum, there is usually no appreciable inflammation, hepatocyte death, or scarring (despite persistent elevation of serum liver enzymes).

In contrast, nonalcoholic steatohepatitis (NASH) is an intermediate form of liver damage. Liver biopsies show hepatocellular steatosis, scattered Mallory bodies, and occasional hepatocytes undergoing apoptosis or ballooning degeneration. Multiple foci of parenchymal

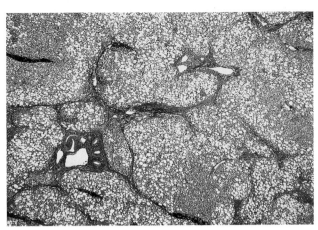

FIGURE 36–13. Nonalcoholic steatohepatitis with progressive fibrosis. This low-power photomicrograph from a morbidly obese patient demonstrates extensive macrovesicular steatosis throughout the liver parenchyma. This trichrome-stained tissue section exhibits fibrous septa that bridge between centrilobular regions and portal tracts; cirrhosis has not yet developed.

inflammation are present. In particular, neutrophils may be scattered throughout the parenchyma, particularly in the immediate vicinity of hepatocytes that contain Mallory bodies or degenerating hepatocytes.

Unlike the severe degree of parenchymal inflammation and damage characteristic of alcoholic hepatitis, NASH generally shows a milder appearance, often containing only scattered foci of parenchymal inflammation and hepatocellular degeneration, in an otherwise steatotic liver. Nevertheless, sinusoidal fibrosis may develop over a period of many years, initially in a centrilobular location but eventually leading to portal-to-central bridging (Fig. 36-13). Cirrhosis develops as a result of years of subclinical progression of the inflammatory and fibrotic processes.

DRUG-INDUCED STEATOSIS AND STEATOHEPATITIS

Drugs may induce either microvesicular or macrovesicular steatosis, steatohepatitis, or a combination thereof. Microvesicular steatosis is the more serious form. It appears as numerous small fat droplets that fill the cytoplasm of enlarged hepatocytes without peripheral displacement of the cell nucleus. Special stains for lipid, such as Oil Red O or Sudan black, are sometimes necessary for differentiating microvesicular steatosis from clear cell degeneration. A large number of drugs have been incriminated in the pathogenesis of steatosis (see Table 36-9). These include aspirin (acetylsalicylic acid) and valproic acid, which are more toxic in children and may lead to a Reye's-like syndrome (Fig. 36-14); tetracycline, particularly in pregnant women; several antiviral nucleoside analogues, such as fialuridine in hepatitis B virus hepatitis[44]; and a variety of new drugs such as didanosine, zidovudine,[45,46] and stavudine.

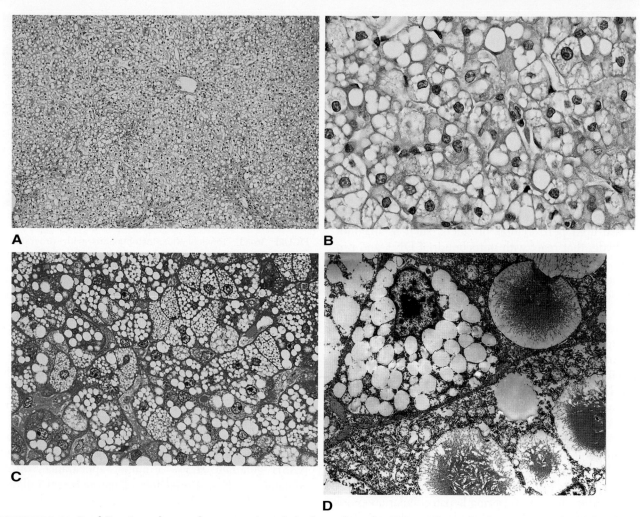

A

B

C

D

FIGURE 36–14. Fatal Reye's syndrome after aspirin (acetylsalicylic acid) intake (600 mg/day, 3 days) in a 15-month-old female. **A,** Panlobular, microvesicular steatosis. **B,** A few steatotic macrovacuoles are intermingled with microvesicular steatosis. **C,** Swollen hepatocytes are filled with lipidic microvacuoles surrounding the central nucleus—1-μm-thick epon section (toluidine blue). **D,** In this hepatocyte *(top)*, lipidic microvacuoles fill the whole cytoplasm, indenting the nucleus, whereas a portion of another hepatocyte contains macrovacuoles of lipids (electron microscopy).

In some severe cases, microvesicular steatosis may be associated with centrilobular cholestasis and/or necrosis, such as with valproic acid or anti-HIV drug-induced hepatotoxicity (Fig. 36-15).

Because the underlying pathogenesis of drug-induced microvesicular steatosis is related to damage to the intracellular mitochondrial oxidative pathways, acute liver failure or chronic liver injury may ensue. Thus, drug-induced microvesicular steatosis may develop into a severe form of hepatic injury. This condition may resemble inherited metabolic diseases, such as the congenital enzymatic errors and mitochondrial cytopathic disorders of oxidative phosphorylation.[47] In patients with drug-induced hepatic microvesicular steatosis, in vitro and/or in vivo diagnostic studies can be conducted to assess the level of mitochondrial injury.[48] These studies include investigation of abnormal mitochondrial

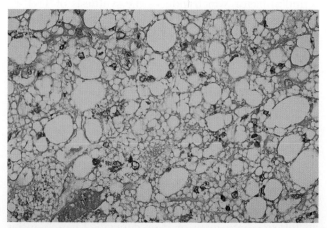

FIGURE 36–15. Fatal acute liver failure in an HIV patient, a 49-year-old treated with didanosine and zidovudine for 8 weeks: mixed, massive steatosis, predominantly microvesicular with hepatocanalicular cholestasis.

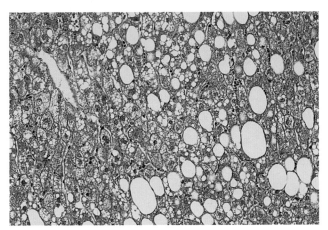

FIGURE 36–16. Macrovesicular steatosis associated with slight perisinusoidal and centrilobular vein fibrosis in a 54-year-old psoriatic patient treated with methotrexate for a long time (Masson's trichrome).

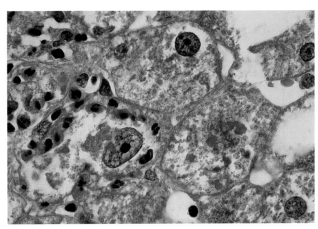

FIGURE 36–17. Nonalcoholic steatohepatitis induced by amiodarone in a 60-year-old patient. Mallory bodies are surrounded by neutrophils ("satellitosis"). (Case provided by P. Callard, Tenon Hospital, Paris.)

morphology, depletion of mitochondrial DNA, anomalies of respiratory chain enzymes and lactate production, and accumulation of drug (i.e. fialuridine) in both mitochondrial and chromosomal DNA.[49]

Macrovesicular steatosis is a more indolent form of steatosis. This is characterized by the presence of one or more large intracytoplasmic fat droplets that displace the hepatocellular nucleus to the periphery of the cell, often indenting the nucleus. Glucocorticoids and methotrexate are pharmaceutical agents that cause macrovesicular steatosis as the predominant histologic lesion. This occurs mainly in the centrilobular zone, often surrounding a thickened terminal hepatic vein and often associated with perisinusoidal fibrosis (Fig. 36-16). Drug-induced macrovesicular steatosis may either be the only histologic abnormality or may be associated with various degrees of microvesicular steatosis, thereby resembling alcohol-induced steatosis.

As discussed above for NASH, steatohepatitis refers to the combination of steatosis and hepatocyte degeneration (especially ballooning degeneration and Mallory body formation) combined with an inflammatory infiltrate (polymorphonuclear cells mixed with lymphocytes). Most cases are accompanied by some degree of pericellular fibrosis, which can progress to bridging fibrosis and cirrhosis.[50] Some types of drugs that are known to cause steatohepatitis include diethylaminoethoxyhexestrol (DEAEH), perhexiline maleate, amiodarone, and tamoxifen (Fig. 36-17; see Table 36-9).[51-54] These four cationic amphophilic compounds have a lipophilic moiety and an amine function that can become protonated. A high intramitochondrial concentration of protonated forms inhibits β-oxidation, which causes steatosis and leads to the mitochondrial formation of reactive oxygen species (ROS). ROS can trigger steatohepatitis by lipid peroxidation, cytokine release, and Fas ligand induction. All of these mechanisms can

lead to hepatocyte death, fibrosis, and chemotaxis of neutrophils (Fig. 36-18).[55] Drug-induced steatohepatitis (NASH) may coexist with other factors such as obesity and diabetes.

PHOSPHOLIPIDOSIS

In humans, phospholipidosis has been mainly observed in association with three antianginal drugs: DEAEH, perhexiline maleate,[3] and amiodarone,[56] and rarely with some types of antibiotics.[57] It can also be induced by parenteral nutrition.[58] In this particular type of injury (Fig. 36-19), hepatocytes and Kupffer cells are enlarged and appear foamy by light microscopy. By electron microscopy, the cytoplasm of affected cells is filled with characteristic lamellated and membrane-bound bodies, which correspond to phospholipids and/or gangliosides, and resembles the morphology observed in Niemann-Pick disease. In contrast to NASH, phospholipidosis is a dose-related change.[52]

The pathogenesis of injury is related to the fact that, uncharged, lipophilic drugs can easily cross the lysosomal membrane of cells. In this acidic intralysosomal milieu, the drug is protonated, becomes more water soluble, and accumulates inside lysosomes. Protonated forms of the drug bind with phospholipids, hampering the action of intralysosomal phospholipases. The accumulation of drug-phospholipid complexes generates large lysosomes filled with pseudomyelinic figures. Because of the very slow dissociation of the drug-phospholipid complexes, the drug may be detectable in plasma several months after discontinuation of treatment.

DIFFERENTIAL DIAGNOSIS OF STEATOSIS AND STEATOHEPATITIS

The most important factor to aid in the differential diagnosis of steatotic liver disease is the clinical history of the patient. Exclusion of drugs known to cause

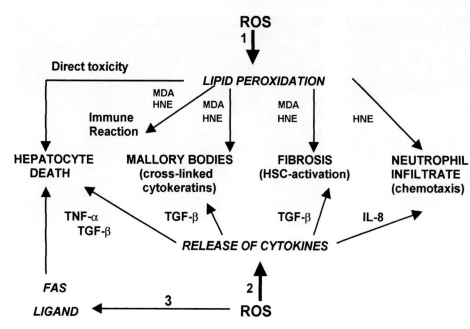

FIGURE 36–18. Mechanisms of induction of steatohepatitis from reactive oxygen species (ROS) through lipid peroxidation (1), release of cytokines (2), and Fas ligand induction (3). MDA, malondialdehyde; HNE, 4-hydroxynonenal; HSC, hepatic stellate cell; TGF, transforming growth factor; TNF, tumor necrosis factor. (From Pessayre D, Berson A, Fromenty B, et al: Mitochondria in steatohepatitis. Semin Liver Dis 21:57-69, 2001.

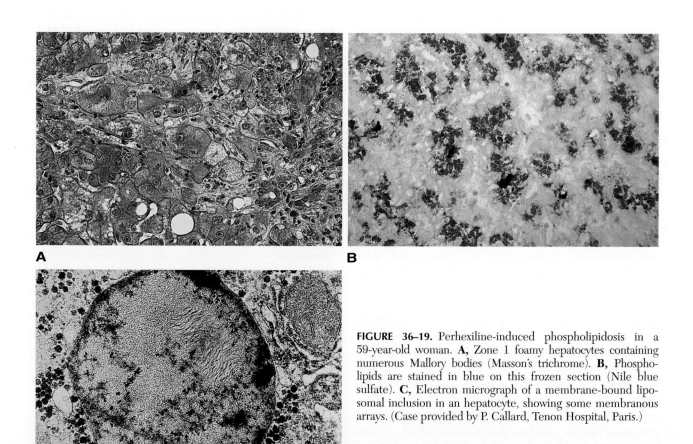

FIGURE 36–19. Perhexiline-induced phospholipidosis in a 59-year-old woman. **A,** Zone 1 foamy hepatocytes containing numerous Mallory bodies (Masson's trichrome). **B,** Phospholipids are stained in blue on this frozen section (Nile blue sulfate). **C,** Electron micrograph of a membrane-bound liposomal inclusion in an hepatocyte, showing some membranous arrays. (Case provided by P. Callard, Tenon Hospital, Paris.)

hepatic steatosis and/or steatohepatitis, and a thorough appreciation of the patient's alcohol intake is crucial. Morphologically, differentiating drug-induced from alcoholic steatohepatitis is often very difficult. Similar to alcoholic-induced damage, drug-induced steatohepatitis shows Mallory bodies mainly located in ballooned hepatocytes in zone 3, or randomly distributed in the lobule. However, some drugs, such as amiodarone, may induce involvement of zone 1 hepatocytes.[43]

Differentiation of alcohol-induced steatosis/hepatitis from NAFLD/NASH also depends heavily on the appropriate clinical history. However, it is now known that a minimal intake of alcohol does not necessary exclude a diagnosis of NAFLD. Morphologically, it is not possible to reliably distinguish alcohol-induced steatosis from nonalcoholic steatosis. However, in the case of NASH, parenchymal inflammation and hepatocellular degeneration (Mallory body formation, apoptosis, ballooning) usually coexists with moderate to severe hepatocellular steatosis. This is in contrast to alcoholic hepatitis and to severe drug-induced steatohepatitis, in which fat droplets within hepatocytes usually diminish in the presence of a severe onslaught of inflammation, fibrosis, and hepatocellular destruction.

Miscellaneous Hepatocellular Injury

PIGMENT ACCUMULATION

Lipofuscins accumulate in hepatocytes, particularly in the centrilobular zone, during various types of drug-induced damage such as that caused by phenothiazine or aminopyrine. In cases of excess dietary iron, alcoholism, parenteral nutrition, or transfusion, hemosiderin can be found in hepatocytes, but it is predominantly noted in sinusoidal lining cells (e.g., Kupffer cells).

GROUND-GLASS/ADAPTIVE CHANGES

Ground-glass inclusions (periodic acid–Schiff [PAS]-positive) correspond to complex material (e.g., glycogen, fragments of lysosomes, and other organelles) accumulated in periportal hepatocytes of patients taking cyanamide, which is used in alcohol aversion therapy. Such hepatocytes resemble ground-glass cells of chronic hepatitis B virus (HBV) infection or Lafora's inclusions.

Some other adaptive changes of hepatocytes are represented by an abundant and pale cytoplasm (Fig. 36-20), due to enhanced smooth endoplasmic reticulum induced by long-term treatment with anticonvulsant drugs such as phenobarbital or phenytoin.

ANISONUCLEOSIS AND INCREASED MITOSES

Anisonucleosis (marked variability in hepatocyte nuclear size) is a consistent finding in the biopsy specimens of patients taking methotrexate. Mitoses are strikingly increased in cases of colchicine therapy and in acute arsenic intoxication.[59]

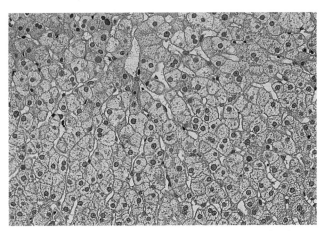

FIGURE 36–20. Adaptative changes of hepatocytes in this biopsy from a 39-year-old patient taking phenobarbital. Hepatocytes have an enlarged and pale-staining cytoplasm.

BILE DUCT INJURY

Acute Cholangitis

Acute cholestasis may be accompanied by bile duct degeneration with or without obvious inflammation. Some hepatotoxins such as Spanish toxic oil, the herbicide paraquat, or transcatheter hepatic artery embolization can lead to a nearly pure bile duct necrosis, whereas acute cholangitis has been reported with several drugs[7,9,60] such as amoxicillin/clavulanic acid (Augmentin). It corresponds to a focal destructive cholangiopathy surrounded by a polymorphous infiltrate (Fig. 36-21). Acute cholangitis may be followed by prolonged cholestasis and ductopenia, directly related to the severity of the early acute damage to bile ducts.[61]

Chronic Cholangitis

Most cases of drug-induced bile duct injury improve rapidly after withdrawal of the medication. About 10% of patients, however, experience a chronic cholestatic disease. This delayed cholestatic syndrome is defined as persistence of jaundice for longer than 6 months, or as biologic abnormalities (increase of alkaline phosphatase and gamma-glutamyltranspeptidase) apparent longer than 1 year after interruption of the drug.

At this chronic phase, lesions predominate in portal tracts with a moderate polymorphonuclear infiltrate and ductular proliferation, associated with ductopenia of small biliary channels and resembling a primary biliary cirrhosis (PBC). Numerous drugs can lead to these PBC-like features (see Table 36-9) with cholestasis, more or less portal fibrosis, inflammation, and bile duct damage (Fig. 36-22), culminating in marked ductopenia (called *vanishing bile duct syndrome*); this has been reported to occur, for example, with chlorpromazine, various antimicrobial agents, and injections of the

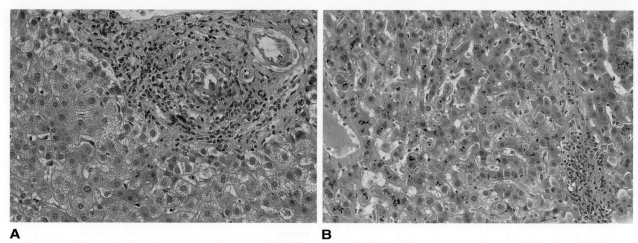

A   **B**

FIGURE 36–21. Amoxicillin-induced focal destructive cholangiopathy in a 65-year-old man (6 days). **A,** Mixed portal inflammatory infiltrate with cells involving a damaged bile duct. **B,** Centrilobular cholestasis with bile plugs within canaliculi and cytoplasm of hepatocytes. (Case provided by Dr. M. Chevallier, Lyon, France.)

hepatic artery with chemotherapeutic agents for the treatment of metastatic colon cancer (Fig. 36-23).[62-64] Parenteral nutrition may also be associated with cholestasis and ductular proliferation, along with hepatocellular damage, fibrosis, and even cirrhosis (Fig. 36-24).[65,66]

Mechanisms of drug-induced lesions of *small bile ducts* remain largely unknown. However, it is thought that the initial destruction of bile ducts may be immunologically mediated. The causative drug or one of its metabolites may trigger an immune response directed against the normal biliary epithelium.

When large bile ducts are involved (as with 5-fluorouracil), it has been suggested that damage may occur primarily to arteries; bile duct ischemia and loss may follow, with ensuing fibrosis. Histologically, the damage resembles primary sclerosing cholangitis. In a few cases, chronic cholangitis does not regress after withdrawal of the offending drug, leading to end-stage biliary cirrhosis.

Cellular mechanisms of cholestasis with some corresponding examples of drugs are summarized in Table 36-11.[67]

VASCULAR INJURY

Drugs and chemicals can cause lesions at all levels of the vascular system (i.e., portal vein and branches,

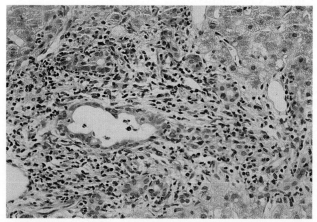

FIGURE 36–22. Flucloxacillin-induced chronic cholangitis in a 72-year-old woman. Shown is a dilated interlobular bile duct with damaged epithelium penetrated by some inflammatory cells in an enlarged portal tract containing moderate neutrophilic inflammation with eosinophils and ductular proliferation: aspect of primary biliary cirrhosis-like chronic cholangitis. (Case provided by Jurgen Rode, Royal Darwin Hospital, Darwin, Australia.)

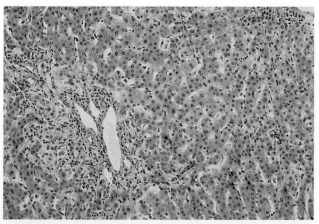

FIGURE 36–23. Thiabendazole toxicity in a 27-year-old man who developed cholestatic liver disease following treatment of a presumed parasitic diarrheal infection: aspect of vanishing bile duct syndrome, with mild portal inflammation. (Case provided by Dr. Dale Snover, Fairview Southdale Hospital, Edina, MN.)

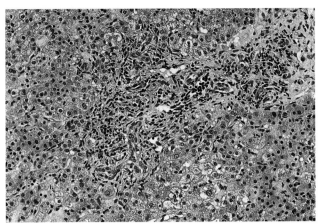

FIGURE 36–24. Total parenteral nutrition in a 43-year-old woman who had serious burns. These are enlarged fibrotic portal tracts with ductular proliferation and mixed inflammatory infiltrate; hepatocytes appear ballooned and clarified with moderate cholestasis.

hepatic artery, sinusoids, central veins, hepatic veins). Often, the same drug can cause several of these vascular lesions, suggesting a basic, common mechanism such as toxicity to endothelial cells.[68] The molecular or cellular mechanisms remain essentially unknown; impair-

ment of sinusoidal endothelial cell glutathione and nitric oxide metabolic pathways appears to play an important role.[69]

Sinusoids

SINUSOIDAL DILATATION

Sinusoidal dilatation is a frequent incidental finding in patients taking oral contraceptives for a long time; it predominates in the periportal zone and is usually of no clinical consequence (Fig. 36-25).[70] On the contrary, sinusoidal dilatation induced by azathioprine may lead to fibrosis and even cirrhosis after several years; nodular regenerative hyperplasia may also be associated (Fig. 36-26). Microvascular alterations (e.g., sinusoidal dilatation, perisinusoidal fibrosis), mainly in the centrilobular zone, have been described in abusers of heroin. This agent is thought to have direct vascular toxic effects that are potentially reversible when the drug is stopped.[71]

PELIOSIS

This is rarer, is reported with various drugs (see Table 36-9), and is characterized by more or less blood-

TABLE 36–11. Cellular Mechanisms of Cholestasis

Mechanism		Agent
Altered plasma membrane lipid composition		Estrogens, chlorpromazine, monohydroxy bile acids
↓		
Decreased membrane fluidity		
↓		
Decreased transport function	Na⁺/K⁺ ATPase Na⁺/H⁺ exchange Bile acid update Bile acid excretion	Endotoxin, inflammatory cytokines, estrogens
+		
Microtubular dysfunction		Colchicine
↓		
Impaired transcellular transport (vesicles)		Chlorpromazine, phorbol esters
+		
Microfilament dysfunction		Phalloidin, cytochalasin B, chlorpromazine, norethandrolone
↓		
Increased biliary permeability (tight junction or canalicular membrane)		Estrogens Monohydroxy bile acids
↑		
Biliary obstruction		
↑		
Precipitation in bile ductules		Monohydroxy bile acids, chlorpromazine
Portal vasoconstriction		Chlorpromazine, phorbol esters

Adapted from Gleeson D, Boyer JL: Intrahepatic cholestasis. In Bircher J, Benhamou JP (eds): Oxford Textbook of Clinical Hepatology, 2nd ed. New York, Oxford University Press, 1999, pp 1591-1620.

In the decreased transport function row, the "+" and "Microtubular dysfunction" relationship and the biological equations use Na^+/K^+ ATPase, Na^+/H^+ exchange notation.

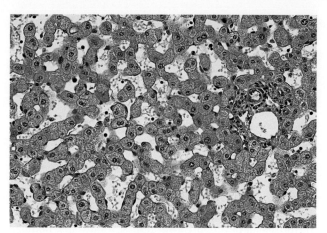

FIGURE 36–25. Sinusoidal dilatation in a 45-year-old woman with long-term use of oral contraceptives.

filled spaces haphazardly distributed within the lobule that lack an endothelial lining. Most cases are asymptomatic; long-standing peliosis (Fig. 36-27) may, however, lead to perisinusoidal fibrosis or to nodular regenerative hyperplasia (discussed further in Chapter 38).

Hepatic Vein

Lesions of veno-occlusive disease (VOD) correspond to nonthrombotic obstruction of small terminal hepatic veins, which appear narrowed or occluded with loose subintimal mesenchyme and fibrosis (Fig. 36-28). VOD may complicate treatment with different anticancerous drugs and may also result from intake of toxins such as alcohol, heroin, or some herbal remedies containing pyrrolizidine alkaloids. The irradiation and chemotherapy

used before bone marrow transplantation are also a major cause of VOD; in this context, it is frequently severe with a high mortality rate.[72] VOD occurs frequently in renal transplant patients treated with immunosuppressive agents and corticoids; it is often associated with peliosis and may be followed by nodular regenerative hyperplasia. VOD may be acute or chronic. In either instance, if severe enough, it may lead to massive parenchymal collapse (Fig. 36-29) and hepatic failure. The liver of a patient treated with radiation may also exhibit aspects of chronic VOD (Fig. 36-30) or Budd-Chiari syndrome.

Alkylating agents such as cyclophosphamide, busulfan, and melphalan are the main inducers of VOD, which is directly related to the formation of highly toxic metabolites. The unpredictable occurrence of VOD may be due to genetic polymorphisms in exporters that remove toxic metabolites.

Budd-Chiari syndrome (see Chapter 38) corresponds to obstruction by the thrombosis of large hepatic veins, leading to hepatic congestion and necrosis of the ischemic centrilobular hepatocytes, followed by an acute or chronic course. When it appears in women taking oral contraceptives, Budd-Chiari syndrome is nearly always associated with coagulative abnormalities or a latent myeloproliferative disease.[73]

Portal Vein

Lesions of hepatoportal sclerosis have been reported with some immunosuppressive agents and in arsenic intoxication. This lesion is characterized by sclerosis of small portal venules, followed by periportal fibrosis without development of cirrhosis, yet leading to noncirrhotic portal hypertension.

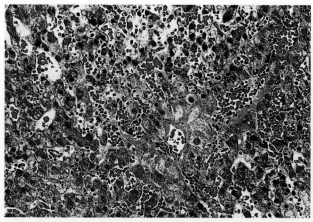
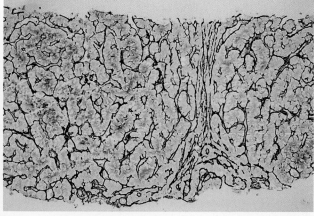

A **B**

FIGURE 36–26. Renal transplant patient taking azathioprine. **A,** Prominent sinusoidal dilatation associated with perisinusoidal and central vein fibrosis (Masson's trichrome). **B,** Typical aspect of nodular regenerative hyperplasia; atrophic hepatocytic plates between enhanced reticulin network separate nodular areas (Gordon and Sweets).

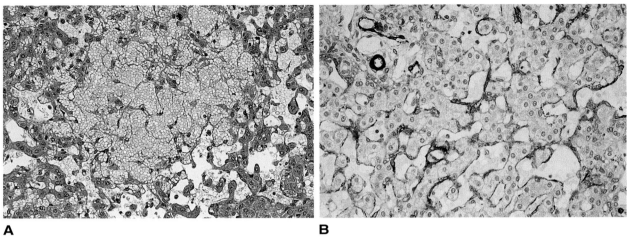

A   **B**

FIGURE 36–27. Anticancerous chemotherapy in a 4-year-old boy before surgery for hepatoblastoma, nontumoral liver. **A,** Areas of peliosis and sinusoidal dilatation. **B,** Alpha–smooth muscle antibody (α-SMA)–positive hepatic stellate cells underlying dilated sinusoids (α-SMA immunostain).

Nodular regenerative hyperplasia may be associated with or may be the consequence of sinusoidal dilatation and peliosis, as has been described (see Fig. 36-26**B**).

Hepatic Artery

Intimal hyperplasia of the hepatic artery has been reported in association with oral contraceptive exposure. It usually remains asymptomatic but rarely may lead to necrohemorrhagic lesions of the liver. Sclerosing lesions of hepatic artery branches caused by intra-arterial drug infusions and leading to bile duct injury have been discussed under Chronic Cholangitis.

SINUSOIDAL CELLS

Hepatic Stellate Cells

In hypervitaminosis A (Fig. 36-31), hypertrophied hepatic stellate cells (HSCs) containing abundant lipid droplets between the sinusoidal endothelial lining and the hepatocyte plates are visible on light microscopy. This HSC hypertrophy is often accompanied by sinusoidal dilatation and prominent perisinusoidal fibrosis. Lipid loading is better visualized on epon 1-μm thick sections and, of course, on electron microscopy. Extracellular matrix is deposited in the space of Disse, often with a more or less complete basement membrane and underlying the sinusoidal endothelial cells. This

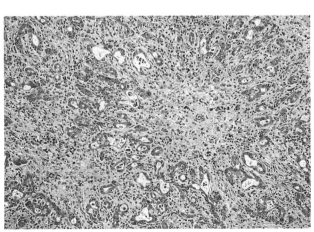

FIGURE 36–28. Subacute veno-occlusive disease in a 19-year-old male patient treated by anticancerous chemotherapy (actinomycin-Oncovin) for a Ewing's sarcoma. The wall of this hepatic vein is thickened and the lumen narrowed by a subintimal deposition of loose connective tissue. In the lobule, the reticulin network is enhance (Gordon and Sweets).

FIGURE 36–29. Fatal subfulminant hepatitis attributable to herbal remedies in a 28-year-old man: aspect of chronic veno-occlusive disease with massive collapse, confluent necrosis, cholangitis, and prominent ductural cholestasis. (Case provided by James M. Crawford, University of Florida, Gainesville, FL.)

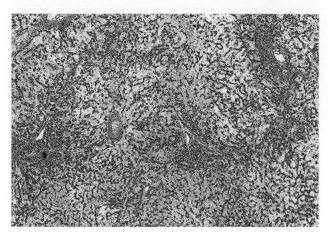

FIGURE 36–30. Liver in a 50-year-old man, 1 year after radiotherapy for a retroperitoneal sarcoma, showing chronic venoocclusive disease with marked sinusoidal congestive dilatation and atrophy of disorganized hepatocytic plates.

condition usually remains asymptomatic for a long time[74] until large cumulative doses lead to more or less severe fibrosis and even cirrhosis with portal hypertension. Deposition of perisinusoidal fibrosis is the result of myofibroblastic transformation of HSCs (their "activated" phenotype); expression of alpha–smooth muscle actin is a characteristic feature of activated HSC.

Some lesser degrees of HSC lipid storage, with or without an obvious perisinusoidal fibrosis (Fig. 36-32), exist with drugs such as methotrexate or other immunosuppressive drugs. Methotrexate hepatotoxicity is probably enhanced by several intrinsic factors (e.g., psoriasis, diabetes, obesity) and by concomitant alcohol exposure. Methotrexate-induced fibrosis develops insidiously but may lead to severe fibrosis and cirrhosis.

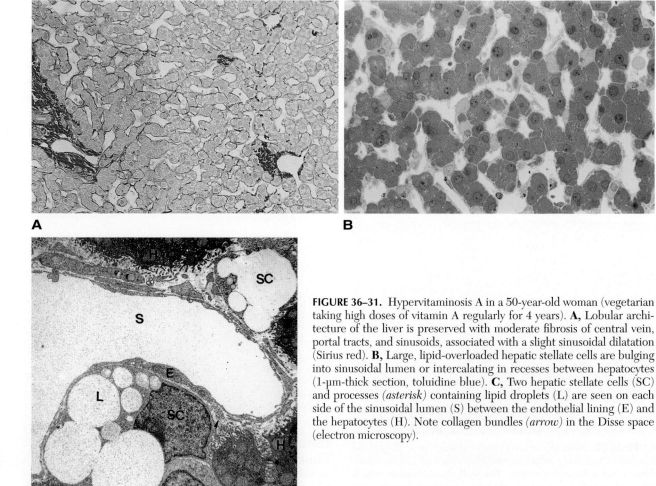

FIGURE 36–31. Hypervitaminosis A in a 50-year-old woman (vegetarian taking high doses of vitamin A regularly for 4 years). **A,** Lobular architecture of the liver is preserved with moderate fibrosis of central vein, portal tracts, and sinusoids, associated with a slight sinusoidal dilatation (Sirius red). **B,** Large, lipid-overloaded hepatic stellate cells are bulging into sinusoidal lumen or intercalating in recesses between hepatocytes (1-μm-thick section, toluidine blue). **C,** Two hepatic stellate cells (SC) and processes (asterisk) containing lipid droplets (L) are seen on each side of the sinusoidal lumen (S) between the endothelial lining (E) and the hepatocytes (H). Note collagen bundles (arrow) in the Disse space (electron microscopy).

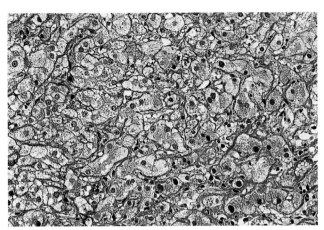

FIGURE 36–32. Polyarthritis treated by immunosuppressive agents in a 62-year-old woman. Prominent perisinusoidal fibrosis and hypertrophy of hepatic stellate cells *(in the middle)* is associated with nodular regenerative hyperplasia *(not seen)* (Masson's trichrome).

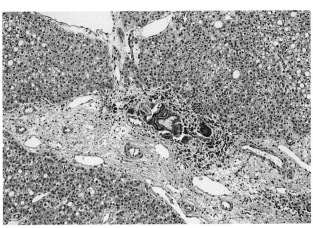

FIGURE 36–34. Foreign body granuloma around a branch of hepatic artery embolized with particles of polyvinyl alcohol for stopping hemorrhage of a ruptured hepatocellular adenoma in a 27-year-old man.

Kupffer Cells and Macrophages

Some drugs, toxins, or foreign materials are phagocytosed by Kupffer cells and other liver macrophages. Some of them, such as polyvinylpyrrolidone (stained with Congo red), talc, silicone (seen with phase contrast), gold, and Thorotrast, exhibit characteristic features that are visible with the use of standard or special techniques. Phospholipidosis, as described for hepatocytes, can involve Kupffer cells as well.

GRANULOMATOUS REACTIONS

Numerous drugs (see Table 36-9) lead to different forms of granulomatous reaction that can be isolated or can form part of a cytolytic or cholestatic hepatitis.

The most frequent drugs cause noncaseating epithelioid granulomas of variable size, located in portal tracts and/or in the lobule (Fig. 36-33). Some drugs such as phenylbutazone can lead to granulomatous hepatitis with granulomas, accompanied by some degree of hepatocytic degeneration and/or intrahepatic cholestasis. Granulomas with a fibrin ring resembling those seen in Q fever are rare but can be seen with allopurinol. Lipogranulomas can be induced by mineral oil ingestion or by gold salts[75]; macrophages contain fine black or brown pigmented granules. Foreign body granulomas can appear around talc, surgical suture material, or embolization material. Therapeutic embolization is performed either through a branch of the hepatic artery (i.e., for embolization of a tumor or for stopping hemorrhage of a ruptured liver tumor [Fig. 36-34]) or through a portal vein branch (i.e., for generating

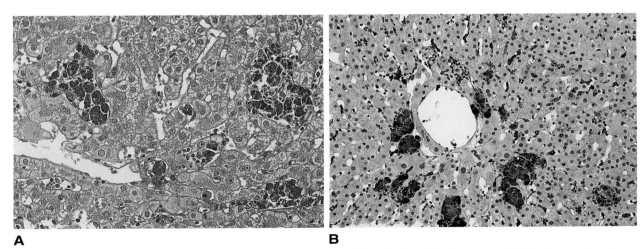

A   **B**

FIGURE 36–33. Granulomatous hepatitis related to Atrium (association of phenobarbital, febarbamate, and difebarbamate) in a 72-year-old man. **A,** Small epithelioid granulomas predominate in centrilobular zone. Macrophages contain PAS-positive material, diastase resistant. **B,** Macrophages in granuloma, as well as Kupffer cells in sinusoids, are well identified by KP-1 (anti-CD68) immunostaining.

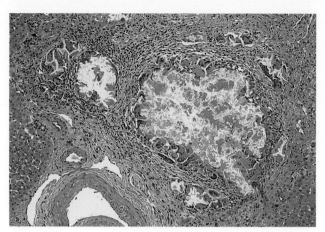

FIGURE 36–35. Foreign body granuloma around a branch of portal vein occluded by embolized material (mixture of histoacryl and lipiodol), before resection of the atrophic lobe containing colon carcinoma metastasis.

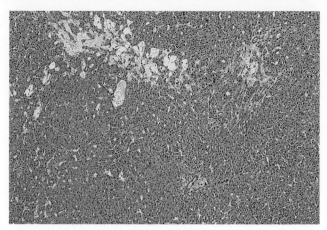

FIGURE 36–36. Hepatocellular adenoma with areas of peliosis in a 23-year-old man treated with androgens for an anaplastic anemia.

compensatory hypertrophy of a well-vascularized lobe before surgical resection of the other embolized atrophic lobe containing tumor [Fig. 36-35]).

Activated Kupffer cells and macrophages as well as neutrophils in the vicinity of granulomas are implicated as mediators of hepatotoxicity through the secretion of various cytokines and cytotoxic soluble factors[76] and the production of reactive metabolites. Secreted inflammatory mediators can play both protective and pathologic roles in hepatotoxicity, depending on the nature of the toxin and on individual susceptibility.

HEPATIC TUMORS

A limited set of drug-induced hepatic tumors may be diagnosed (see Chapter 42). Hepatocellular adenoma is most often associated with exposure to oral contra-

ceptives (OCs) or anabolic/androgenic steroids (Fig. 36-36).[77] Adenomas are classically complicated by intratumoral hemorrhage, rupture, and formation of subcapsular hematoma. Their transformation or the de novo occurrence of hepatocellular carcinoma is much rarer but has been well documented (Fig. 36-37).[78] A role for OCs in the development and increased size of focal nodular hyperplasia is still debated but not confirmed.

The occurrence of angiosarcoma, cholangiocarcinoma, and hepatocellular carcinoma has been demonstrated after Thorotrast administration, following latency periods of several decades. With discontinuance of Thorotrast usage in 1955, this risk is now of historic interest only. The contrast agent is recognizable inside Kupffer cells in liver tissue surrounding the tumor (Fig. 36-38). As an occupational exposure, vinyl chloride also is associated with the occurrence of angiosarcoma.

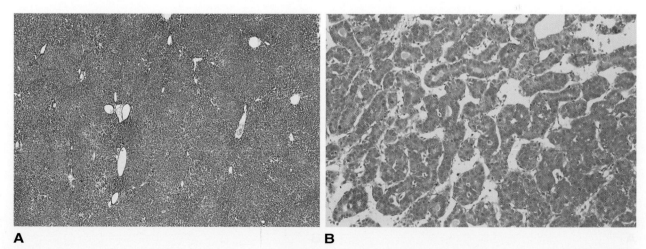

A　　　　　　　　　　　**B**

FIGURE 36–37. A, Large hepatocellular adenoma in a 24-year-old woman taking oral contraceptives for 4 years, incomplete resection. **B,** Twelve years later (two pregnancies, then oral contraceptive intake): large and multifocal trabecular and pseudoglandular hepatocellular carcinoma.

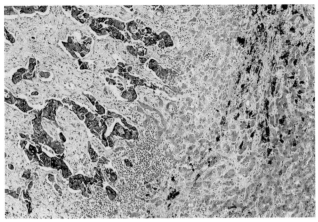 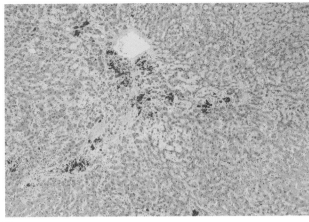

A   **B**

FIGURE 36–38. Cholangiocarcinoma developed in a Thorotrast-induced liver injury. **A,** Thorotrast granules are deposited in macrophages (*on the right*) at the border of the cholangiocarcinoma (*on the left*) (cytokeratin 7 immunostain). **B,** In zones of Thorotrast deposits (nontumoral liver), sinusoidal dilatation, peliosis, and atrophy of hepatocytic plates, related to Thorotrast injury, are also seen. (Case provided by A. Paul Dhillon, Royal Free Hospital, London.)

References

1. Kahl R: Toxic liver injury. In Bircher J, Benhamou JP, McIntyre N, et al (eds): Oxford Textbook of Clinical Hepatology, 2nd ed. New York, Oxford University Press, 1999, pp 1319-1334.
2. Zimmerman HJ: Hepatotoxicity. The Adverse Effects of Drugs and Other Chemicals on the Liver, 2nd ed. Philadelphia, Lippincott Williams & Wilkins, 1999.
3. Pessayre D, Larrey D, Biour M: Drug-induced liver injury. In Bircher J, Benhamou JP, McIntyre N, et al (eds): Oxford Textbook of Clinical Hepatology, 2nd ed. New York, Oxford University Press, 1999, pp 1261-1315.
4. Scheuer PJ, Lefkowitch JH: Drugs and toxins. In Scheuer PJ, Lefkowitch JH (eds): Liver Biopsy Interpretation, 6th ed. Philadelphia, WB Saunders, 2000, pp 134-150.
5. Zimmerman HJ, Ishak KG: Hepatic injury due to drugs and toxins. In MacSween RNM, Anthony PP, Scheuer PJ, et al (eds): Pathology of the Liver, 4th ed. Edinburgh, Churchill Livingstone, 2001.
6. Aithal PG, Day CP: The natural history of histologically proved drug induced liver disease. Gut 44:731-735, 1999.
7. Larrey D: Drug-induced liver disease. J Hepatol 32:77-88, 2000.
8. Pirmohamed M, Breckenridge AM, Kitteringham NR, et al: Adverse drug reactions. BMJ 316:1295-1298, 1998.
9. Vial T, Biour M, Descotes J, et al: Antibiotic-associated hepatitis: Update from 1990. Ann Pharmacother 31:204-220, 1997.
10. Lewis JH: Drug-induced liver disease. Med Clin North Am 84:1275-1311, 2000.
11. Bernuau J, Benhamou JP: Fulminant and subfulminant liver failure. In Bircher J, Benhamou JP, McIntyre N, et al (eds): Oxford Textbooks of Clinical Hepatology, 2nd ed, vol 2. Oxford, Oxford University Press, 1999, pp 1341-1372.
12. Biour M, Poupon R, Grange JD, et al: Hépatotoxicité des médicaments. 13ème mise à jour du fichier bibliographique des atteintes hépatiques et des médicaments responsables. Gastroenterol Clin Biol 24:1052-1091, 2000.
13. Larrey D: Hepatotoxicity of herbal remedies. J Hepatol 26:47-51, 1997.
14. Stickel F, Egerer G, Seitz HK: Hepatotoxicity of botanicals. Publ Health Nutr 3:113-124, 2000.
15. Mallat A, Dhumeaux D: Cocaine and the liver. J Hepatol 12:275-278, 1991.
16. Maria VAJ, Victorino RMM: Development and validation of a clinical scale for the diagnosis of drug-induced hepatitis. Hepatology 26:664-669, 1997.
17. Fukano M, Amano S, Sato J, et al: Subacute hepatic failure associated with a new antidiabetic agent, troglitazone: A case report with autopsy examination. Hum Pathol 31:250-253, 2000.
18. Kohlroser J, Mathai J, Reichheld J, et al: Hepatotoxicity due to troglitazone: Report of two cases and review of adverse events reported to the United States Food and Drug Administration. Am J Gastroenterol 95:272-276, 2000.
19. Murphy EJ, Davern TJ, Shakil AO, et al: Troglitazone-induced fulminant hepatic failure. Acute Liver Failure Study Group. Dig Dis Sci 45:549-553, 2000.
20. O'Grady JG: Paracetamol-induced acute liver failure: Prevention and management. J Hepatol 26:41-46, 1997.
21. Benichou C: Criteria of drug-induced liver disorders. Report of an International Consensus Meeting. J Hepatol 11:272-276, 1990.
22. Andrade RJ, Lucena MI, Garcia-Escano MD, et al: Severe idiosyncratic acute hepatic injury caused by paracetamol. J Hepatol 28:1078, 1998.
23. Andreu V, Mas A, Bruguera M, et al: Ecstasy: A common cause of severe acute hepatotoxicity. J Hepatol 29:394-397, 1998.
24. Ellis AJ, Wendon JA, Portmann B, et al: Acute liver damage and ecstasy ingestion. Gut 38:454-458, 1996.
25. Fidler H, Dhillon A, Gertner D, et al: Chronic ecstasy (3,4-methylenedioxymetamphetamine) abuse: A recurrent and unpredictable cause of severe acute hepatitis. J Hepatol 25:563-566, 1996.
26. Milroy CM, Clark JC, Forrest ARW: Pathology of deaths associated with "ecstasy" and "eve" misuse. J Clin Pathol 49:149-153, 1996.
27. Silva MO, Roth D, Reddy KR, et al: Hepatic dysfunction accompanying acute cocaine intoxication. J Hepatol 12:312-315, 1991.
28. Wanless IR, Dore S, Gopinath N, et al: Histopathology of cocaine hepatotoxicity. Report of four patients. Gastroenterology 98:497-501, 1990.
29. Erlinger S: Drug-induced cholestasis. J Hepatol 26:1-4, 1997.
30. Neuberger J: Halothane hepatitis. Eur J Gastroenterol Hepatol 10:631-633, 1998.
31. Kenna JG: Immunoallergic drug-induced hepatitis: Lessons from halothane. J Hepatol 26:5-12, 1997.
32. Banks AT, Zimmerman HJ, Ishak KG, et al: Diclofenac-associated hepatotoxicity: Analysis of 180 cases reported to the Food and Drug Administration as adverse reactions. Hepatology 22:820-827, 1995.
33. Kamiyama T, Nouchi T, Kojima S, et al: Autoimmune hepatitis triggered by administration of an herbal medicine. Am J Gastroenterol 92:703-704, 1997.
34. Picciotto A, Campo N, Brizzolara R, et al: Chronic hepatitis induced by Jin Bu Huan. J Hepatol 28:165-167, 1998.
35. Jorens PG, Michielsen PP, Pelckmans PA, et al: Vitamin A abuse: Development of cirrhosis despite cessation of vitamin A. A six-year clinical and histopathological follow-up. Liver 12:381-386, 1992.
36. Kim WR, Brown RS, Terrault NA, El-Serag: Burden of liver disease in the United States: Summary of a workshop. Hepatology 36:227-242, 2002.

37. Crawford JM: The liver and biliary tree. In Kumar V, Fausto N, Abbas A (eds): Robbins Pathologic Basis of Disease, 7th ed. Philadelphia, WB Saunders, 2004 (in press).

38. Tsukamoto H, Lu SC: Current concepts in the pathogenesis of alcoholic liver injury. FASEB J 15:1335-1349,2001.

39. Clark JM, Brancati FL, Diehl AM: Nonalcoholic fatty liver disease. Gastroenterology 122:1649-1657,2002.

40. Koteish A, Diehl AM: Animal models of steatosis. Semin Liver Dis 21:89-104, 2001.

41. Pessayre D, Berson A, Fromenty B, Mansouri A: Mitochondria in steatohepatitis. Semin Liver Dis 21:57-69, 2001.

42. Yuan M, Konstantopoulos N, Lee J, et al: Reversal of obesity and diet-induced insulin resistance with salicylates or targeted disruption of IKKbeta. Science 293:1673-1677, 2001.

43. Burt AD, Mutton A, Day C: Diagnosis and interpretation of steatosis and steatohepatitis. Semin Diagn Pathol 15:246-258, 1998.

44. McKenzie R, Fried MW, Sallie R, et al: Hepatic failure and lactic acidosis due to fialuridine (FIAU), an investigational nucleoside analogue for chronic hepatitis B. N Engl J Med 333:1099-1105, 1995.

45. Bissuel F, Bruneel F, Habersetzer F, et al: Fulminant hepatitis with severe lactate acidosis in HIV-infected patients on didanosine therapy. J Intern Med 235:367-371, 1994.

46. Chariot P, Drogou I, de Lacroix-Szmania I, et al: Zidovudine-induced mitochondrial disorder with massive liver steatosis, myopathy, lactic acidosis, and mitochondrial DNA depletion. J Hepatol 30:156-160, 1999.

47. Fromenty B, Berson A, Pessayre D: Microvesicular steatosis and steatohepatitis: Role of mitochondrial dysfunction and lipid peroxidation. J Hepatol 26:13-22, 1997.

48. Bissel DM, Gores GJ, Laskin DL, et al: Drug-induced liver injury: Mechanisms and test systems. Hepatology 33:1009-1013, 2001.

49. Tennant BC, Baldwin BH, Graham LA, et al: Antiviral activity and toxicity of fialuridine in the woodchuck model of hepatitis B virus infection. Hepatology 38:179-191, 1998.

50. Brunt EM: Nonalcoholic steatohepatitis: Definition and pathology. Semin Liver Dis 21:3-16, 2001.

51. Barbany G, Uzzan F, Larrey D, et al: Alcoholic-like liver lesions induced by nifedipine. J Hepatol 9:252-255, 1989.

52. Chitturi S, Farrell GC: Etiopathogenesis of nonalcoholic steatohepatitis. Semin Liver Dis 21:27-41, 2001.

53. Cotrim HP, Andrade ZA, Parana R, et al: Nonalcoholic steatohepatitis. A toxic liver disease in industrial workers. Liver 19:299-304, 1999.

54. Pinto HC, Baptista A, Camilo ME, et al: Tamoxifen-associated steatohepatitis: Report of three cases. J Hepatol 23:95-97, 1995.

55. Pessayre D, Berson A, Fromenty B, et al: Mitochondria in steatohepatitis. Semin Liver Dis 21:57-69, 2001.

56. Lewis JH, Mullick F, Ishak KG, et al: Histopathological analysis of suspected amiodarone hepatotoxicity. Hum Pathol 21:59-67, 1990.

57. Munoz SJ, Martinez-Hernandez A, Maddrey WC: Intrahepatic cholestasis and phospholipidosis associated with the use of trimethoprim-sulfamethoxazole. Hepatology 12:342-347, 1990.

58. Degott C, Messing B, Moreau D, et al: Liver phospholipidosis induced by parenteral nutrition: Histologic, histochemical, and ultrastructural investigations. Gastroenterology 95:183-191, 1988.

59. Brenard R, Laterre PF, Reynaert M, et al: Increased hepatocytic mitotic activity as a diagnostic marker of acute arsenic intoxication. A report of two cases. J Hepatol 25:218-220, 1996.

60. Ryley NG, Fleming KA, Chapman RWG: Focal destructive cholangiopathy associated with amoxycillin/clavulanic acid (Augmentin). J Hepatol 23:278-282, 1995.

61. Degott C, Feldmann G, Larrey D, et al: Drug-induced prolonged cholestasis in adults: A histological semi-quantitative study demonstrating progressive ductopenia. Hepatology 15:244-251, 1992.

62. Davies MH, Harrisson RF, Elias E, et al: Antibiotic-associated acute vanishing bile duct syndrome: A pattern associated with severe, prolonged, intrahepatic cholestasis. J Hepatol 20:112-116, 1994.

63. Desmet VJ: Vanishing bile duct syndrome in drug-induced liver disease. J Hepatol 26:31-35, 1997.

64. Eckstein RP, Dowsett JF, Lunzer MR: Flucloxacillin induced liver disease: Histopathological findings at biopsy and autopsy. Pathology 25:223-228, 1993.

65. Body JJ, Bleiberg H, Bron D, et al: Total parenteral nutrition-induced cholestasis mimicking large bile duct obstruction. Histopathology 6:787-792, 1982.

66. Quigley EM, Marsh MN, Shaffer JL, et al: Hepatobiliary complications of total parenteral nutrition. Gastroenterology 104:286-301, 1993.

67. Gleeson D, Boyer JL: Intrahepatic cholestasis. In Bircher J, Benhamou JP, McIntyre N, et al (eds): Oxford Textbook of Clinical Hepatology, 2nd ed. New York, Oxford University Press, 1999, pp 1591-1620.

68. Zafrani ES, Pinaudeau Y, Dhumeaux D: Drug-induced vascular lesions of the liver. Arch Intern Med 143:495-502, 1983.

69. DeLeve LD: Glutathione defense in non-parenchymal cells. Semin Liver Dis 18:403-413, 1998.

70. Valla D, Benhamou JP: Liver diseases related to oral contraceptives. Dig Dis 6:76-86, 1988.

71. Trigueiro de Araujo MS, Gerard F, Chossegros P, et al: Vascular hepatotoxicity related to heroin addiction. Virchows Arch 417:497-503, 1990.

72. McDonald GB, Shulman HM, Wolford JL, et al: Liver disease after human marrow transplantation. Semin Liver 7:210-229, 1987.

73. Valla D, Le MG, Poynard T, et al: Risk of hepatic vein thrombosis in relation to recent use of oral contraceptives. A case-control study. Gastroenterology 90:807-811, 1986.

74. Bioulac-Sage P, Quinton A, Saric J, et al: Chance discovery of hepatic fibrosis in patient with asymptomatic hypervitaminosis A. Arch Pathol Lab Med 112:505-509, 1988.

75. Landas SK, Mitros FA, Furst DE, et al: Lipogranulomas and gold in the liver in rheumatoid arthritis. Am J Surg Pathol 16:171-174, 1992.

76. Laskin DL, Pendino KJ: Macrophages and inflammatory mediators in tissue injury. Ann Rev Pharmacol Toxicol 35:655-677, 1995.

77. Ishak KG: Hepatic lesions caused by anabolic and contraceptive steroids. Semin Liver Dis 1:116-128, 1981.

78. Neuberger J, Forman D, Doll R, et al: Oral contraceptives and hepatocellular carcinoma. BMJ 291:1355-1357, 1986.

CHAPTER 37

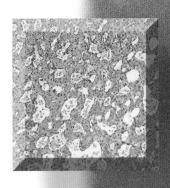

Cirrhosis

IAN R. WANLESS • JAMES M. CRAWFORD

Introduction

Cirrhosis is among the top ten causes of death in the Western world. In the United States, cirrhosis is the ninth leading cause of death. Cirrhosis is also an important cause of morbidity. It is listed as a diagnosis on approximately 1% of discharges from non-Federal hospitals for patients aged 15 years and older. *Cirrhosis* is a term that implies consequences that are unrelated to the primary etiology. These consequences are both mechanical—involving intrahepatic and extrahepatic shunting of blood with risk of bleeding from esophageal varices—and functional—leading to failure of the liver to perform the physiologic roles of the organ. Likewise, most forms of cirrhosis carry a risk of hepatocellular carcinoma. Cirrhosis results largely from alcohol abuse, chronic hepatitis, biliary disease, iron overload, and inherited metabolic defects. Although each insult may cause progressive injury to the liver, the enormous functional reserve of the liver masks to some extent the clinical impact of early liver damage. However, with progression of disease or strategic disruption of bile flow over months to years, impaired hepatic function may become life threatening.

Definition

Cirrhosis is defined anatomically by the presence throughout the liver of fibrous septa that subdivide the parenchyma into nodules,[1] as shown in Figure 37-1. Each of the required elements of fibrous septa and architectural disturbance occurs in a spectrum from minimal to severe.

Several features are critical to the definition. First, the parenchymal architecture of the entire liver is disrupted by interconnecting fibrous scars. Localized hepatic scarring does not constitute cirrhosis. Second, fibrous scars may be present in the form of delicate bands connecting portal tracts and centrilobular terminal hepatic veins in a portal-to-portal, portal-to-central, and/or central-to-central pattern, or they may occur as broad fibrous tracts obliterating multiple adjacent lobules. Third, parenchymal nodules are created by fibrotic isolation of islands of hepatic parenchyma. These nodules may vary from micronodules (smaller than 3 mm in diameter) to macronodules (3 mm to several centimeters in diameter).

Some qualifying comments are in order. First, fibrous subdivision of the liver parenchyma into isolated islands is requisite for the diagnosis; regeneration of these islands is not. Hence, fibrosis that evolves rapidly over several months may still produce a cirrhotic organ, even if insufficient time has passed for substantive expansion of the islands into spherical nodules by regeneration. Second, the distance from portal tract to terminal hepatic vein is on the order of 0.8 to 1.5 mm, so scarring at the lobular level may produce nodularity on a millimeter scale. However, the hepatic capacity for regeneration is enormous, and parenchymal regeneration in the face of more slowly developing fibrosis may produce nodules of several centimeters in diameter. Third, parenchymal islands do not have to be simple polygons or spheres. Portal tract–based fibrosis may produce a much more coarsely subdivided and irregular cirrhotic liver.

Because of the qualitative nature of the definition of cirrhosis, its diagnosis depends on arbitrary limits.

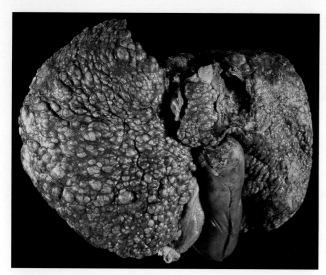

FIGURE 37–1. Cirrhosis caused by hepatitis B virus. This dorsal view shows a coarsely nodular capsular surface, shrinkage of the right lobe, and compensatory hypertrophy of the left lobe.

Specifically, the point at which a liver with chronic hepatitis and fibrous scarring truly becomes cirrhotic is arbitrary and cannot easily be established on the basis of percutaneous needle biopsy tissue (which represents less than 1/10,000 of the liver mass). Moreover, cirrhotic livers exhibit a spectrum of severity, with fibrous septa that are few or numerous and thin or broad, and liver parenchyma that has nodules of uniform or variable size and contour. Fortunately, clinical data provide valuable guidance as to whether abnormal findings observed in percutaneous liver biopsy tissue are representative of the whole liver. Supporting clinical data include physical examination findings (e.g., ascites, caput medusa, spider angiomata, gynecomastia) and impressions gained from imaging studies or intraoperative visualization of the organ. Laboratory data may not reveal abnormalities. Serum levels for albumin, clotting factors, urea, alkaline phosphatase, aminotransferases, and bilirubin may be normal in a patient who has quiescent cirrhosis with minimal ongoing damage, and who has not yet developed hepatic failure. Conversely, a patient with massive hepatic necrosis and hepatic failure may not have cirrhosis, despite profound abnormalities in these serum parameters. Hence, laboratory data per se do not establish a diagnosis of cirrhosis.

Occasionally, a severe focal injury to the liver results in focal changes that are histologically indistinguishable from cirrhosis on percutaneous needle biopsy specimens. This focal change is not considered true cirrhosis, as the remainder of the liver may be undamaged. When the question of focal damage arises, definitive information derived from clinical evaluation and from imaging studies on the general status of the liver, or a biopsy sample from elsewhere in the liver, is critical in determining whether a fibrotic process is actually focal or diffuse.

◼ Pathogenesis

Liver cirrhosis is not strictly the end result of hepatic scarring. Rather, it is a dynamic, biphasic process dominated on one hand by progressive parenchymal fibrosis, and on the other by severe disruption of vascular architecture and distortion of normal lobular architecture. Detailed consideration is given to the pathogenesis of cirrhosis in this chapter because it provides insight into histopathologic interpretation of the cirrhotic liver.

The three major mechanisms that combine to create cirrhosis are cell death, deposition of aberrant extracellular matrix (fibrosis), and vascular reorganization. The cirrhotic process is usually initiated by hepatocellular death (discussion of which is beyond the scope of this chapter), but only after cell death has occurred consistently and persistently over a long period of time. Cell death can occur in any form of liver injury and does not define cirrhosis. For example, an acute overdose of acetaminophen causes severe hepatic necrosis and may kill the patient, but it will not produce chronic liver injury in those who survive. In contrast, small doses of alcohol that alone are insufficient to cause more than a small degree of hepatic parenchymal injury are quite capable of producing cirrhosis when ingested on a daily basis for a number of years.

Two additional processes critical to the pathophysiology of cirrhosis are regeneration and changes in metabolic zonation. These will be discussed in turn.

FIBROSIS

In the normal liver, interstitial collagens (types I and III) are concentrated in portal tracts and around central veins, with occasional bundles in the space of Disse. Delicate strands of type IV collagen (reticulin) course alongside hepatocytes in the space of Disse. In cirrhosis, excessive collagen of types I and III is laid down in portal tracts, and aberrant deposition of this collagen is noted along sinusoids in the lobule, creating delicate or broad septal tracts. Concomitantly, the sinusoidal vascular channel is converted into a capillary channel with a basement membrane (to be discussed), such that blood/hepatocyte solute exchange is impaired despite maintenance of absolute hepatocyte volume.[2]

Activation of Stellate Cells

Extracellular matrix in the normal liver may be produced by hepatocytes, perisinusoidal stellate cells, and sinusoidal endothelial cells. The major source of excess collagen in cirrhosis appears to be stellate cells (Ito cells).[3] Normally, stellate cells are quiescent and reside within the subendothelial space of Disse and sometimes in the perisinusoidal recess between hepatocytes. Although normally functioning as vitamin A and fat-storing cells, during the development of cirrhosis they proliferate, lose their retinyl ester stores, and transform into myofibroblast-like cells that are positive immunohistochemically for alpha-smooth muscle actin.[4] Stellate cells are activated by inflammatory mediators to commence collagen synthesis.[5] Simultaneously, activation of tissue metalloproteinases occurs.[6] The greatest activation of stellate cells occurs in areas of severe hepatocellular necrosis and inflammation.[7] Stellate cell activation and sinusoidal fibrosis are readily reversible within weeks of cessation of injury.[8]

Chronic disease leads to sustained activation of stellate cells. When stellate cells are activated in low-grade disease, the collagen deposition is local and delicate with sinusoidal pericellular fibrosis. This is most easily appreciated in the perivenular regions (centrilobular, Rappaport zone 3). Over years, the liver is subdivided by fibrous septa, with ample opportunity for regeneration of hepatocytes to form nodules. Alternatively, widespread injury to hepatocytes, as occurs in alcoholic hepatitis and some forms of drug injury (e.g., amiodarone), may activate stellate cells throughout the liver, leading to extensive deposition of sinusoidal collagen over a period of months and development of a cirrhotic liver without substantive opportunity for formation of spheroid parenchymal nodules.

Activation of Portal Tract Myofibroblasts

During biliary-type fibrogenesis, sinusoidal stellate cells proliferate and migrate toward the portal tracts, but it is not yet clear whether they migrate into portal tracts.[9] Instead, injury within portal tracts, particularly of biliary origin, leads to activation of portal tract myofibroblasts. These cells become prominent around bile ducts and bile ductules upon obstruction to bile flow downstream or primary damage to local bile ducts.[10,11] It is unclear whether these cells represent previously quiescent resident myofibroblasts or are the product of an epithelial-to-mesenchymal transition by bile duct epithelial cells themselves.[12] Peribiliary myofibroblasts are capable of rapid proliferation and deposition of collagen. As a result, fibrosis arising from biliary tract disease can run an aggressive course, as occurs in complete biliary obstruction seen in extrahepatic biliary atresia, in which the liver becomes cirrhotic by 9 weeks of age (see Chapter 41). At the opposite end of the spectrum is the exceedingly indolent progression of portal tract fibrosis to cirrhosis over 20 or more years in primary biliary cirrhosis (see Chapter 35). A curious feature of biliary-type fibrosis is that the lobular parenchyma is not induced to regenerate substantively until the liver is substantively fibrotic. Hence, biliary-type fibrosis subdivides the liver in a jigsaw-like pattern during its progression, and cirrhosis may be a late feature.

Parenchymal Extinction

Parenchymal extinction is defined as a focal loss of contiguous hepatocytes (Fig. 37-2).[13] Extinction lesions may involve a small portion of an acinus or larger units of one or more adjacent acini or even a whole lobe. The contiguous cell loss is the result of focal ischemia caused by obstruction of veins or sinusoids. The size of extinction lesions depends on the size of the obstructed vessels. Small regions of extinction are most easily recognized by the close approximation of hepatic veins and portal tracts, a lesion called an *adhesion* (Figs. 37-3 and 37-4). The concept of parenchymal extinction is important because it indicates that (1) parenchymal extinction is not directly caused by the initial hepatocellular injury but is an epiphenomenon caused by innocent bystander injury of local vessels, (2) each parenchymal extinction lesion has its own natural history and may be in an early or late stage of healing, (3) cirrhosis occurs when numerous independent and discrete parenchymal extinction lesions accumulate throughout the liver, and (4) the form of cirrhosis is largely determined by the distribution of the vascular injury. It must be noted that parenchymal extinction can continue to occur long after cirrhosis is established, leading to slow conversion of a marginally functional liver into an organ incapable of sustaining life.

Vascular obstruction may affect portal veins, hepatic arteries, and hepatic veins. The distribution of parenchymal extinction is dependent on the distribution of vascular obstruction. Importantly, localized combined obstruction of inflow vessels (especially portal vein radicles) and outflow hepatic veins guarantees obliteration of the intervening parenchyma.

The pathogenesis of vascular obstruction depends on the size of the vessels. Most small vessel obliteration occurs secondary to local inflammation.[14,15] Although thrombosis may be important in veins of all sizes, it is the exclusive mechanism for blocking of medium-sized and large veins. Most parenchymal injury is produced by obstruction of veins larger than 100 μm because obstruction at this site cannot be easily circumvented by collateral flow in sinusoids. Obstruction of several adjacent sinusoids is also difficult to circumvent.

Outcome of Fibrosis

In cirrhosis, all types of collagens, glycoproteins, and proteoglycans can increase to twice the normal level normally found in the liver.[16] Aberrant deposition of extracellular matrix within the hepatic parenchyma leads to deposition of fibrillar proteins within the space of Disse, creating a major barrier for solute exchange between hepatocytes and sinusoidal blood.[17] On a percent area basis, total extracellular matrix components can increase from 5% in normal liver to 25% to 40% in cirrhosis.[18] The total matrix in the space of Disse

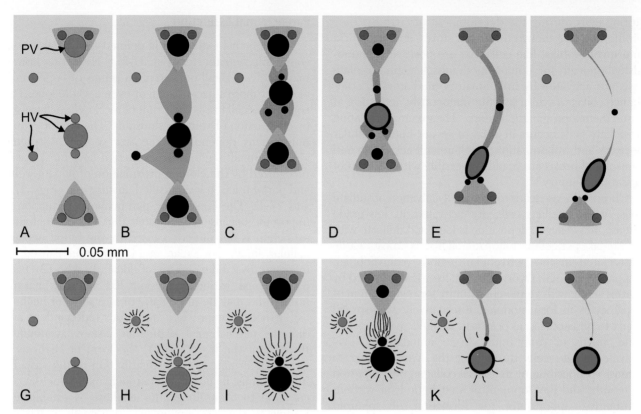

0.05 mm

FIGURE 37–2. Diagrammatic depiction of tissue remodeling in chronic hepatitis **(A-F)** and in alcoholic liver disease **(G-L)** during the development and regression of cirrhosis. Normal acini are shown in **A** and **G** with the sequence of events leading to small regions of parenchymal extinction in the following panels. Obstructed veins are shown as black circles. **B,** Obliteration of small portal and hepatic veins occurs early in the development of cirrhosis in response to local inflammatory damage. The supplied parenchyma becomes ischemic. **C** and **D,** Ischemic parenchyma shrinks and is replaced by fibrosis (process of extinction). The shrinkage is accompanied by close approximation of adjacent vascular structures. **E,** Septa are deformed and stretched by asymmetrical expansion of regenerating hepatocytes. **F,** Fibrous septa are resorbed. They become progressively thinner and then perforate before disappearing. Small residual tags may extend from portal tracts. Trapped portal structures and hepatic veins are released from the septa and are recognizable as deformed remnants that are irregularly distributed. Residual hepatic veins are often described as *ectopic*. Note the absence of portal veins. In alcoholic disease **(G-L),** the sequence of events may differ from that of other forms of chronic liver disease. **H,** Sinusoidal fibrosis is often prominent before the development of parenchymal collapse, leading to a pericellular pattern of fibrosis. **I** and **J,** Inflammation and fibrosis lead to hepatic and portal vein obliteration with secondary condensation of preformed sinusoidal collagen fibers into a septum. **K** and **L,** After prolonged periods of inactivity, sinusoidal fibrosis and septa are resorbed. (Modified from Wanless IR, Nakashima E, Sherman M: Regression of human cirrhosis. Morphologic features and the genesis of incomplete septal cirrhosis. Arch Pathol Lab Med 124:1599-1607, 2000; Wanless IR: Physioanatomic considerations. In Schiff ER, Sorrell MF, Maddrey WC [eds]: Schiff's Diseases of the Liver, 9th ed. Philadelphia, Lippincott-Raven, 2003, p 43.)

can increase and change its character to the extent that it can be identified on routine light microscopy. In particular, the change in the contents of the space of Disse from delicate interspersed strands of fibrillar collagen (types III and IV) to a dense matrix of basement membrane–type matrix proteins closes the space of Disse to protein exchange between hepatocytes and plasma. In general, abnormal matrix deposition within the space of Disse occurs in those parts of the parenchyma where cell injury and inflammation are greatest.

Reversal of Cirrhosis

Cirrhosis is viewed as the end stage in the evolution of many different types of chronic liver disease. How-

ever, clinical reports indicate that with cessation of the injurious process, cirrhosis may reverse.[13,19-21] These reports describe patients whose full-blown cirrhosis has subsided to a form of incomplete septal cirrhosis or apparent absence of fibrosis following successful treatment of hereditary hemochromatosis,[22,23] autoimmune hepatitis,[24] and Wilson's disease.[25] A reduction in fibrosis has been noted also in primary biliary cirrhosis,[26] schistosomiasis,[27] and extrahepatic biliary obstruction.[28] Clearly, reduction in fibrosis is a goal of antiviral therapy in viral hepatitis (see Chapter 34).

However, even with substantial resorption of fibrous tissue septa, restoration of the hepatic architecture to a normal state never occurs. Rather, depending on how much extracellular matrix resorbs and where, the possibility of incomplete septal cirrhosis, in which

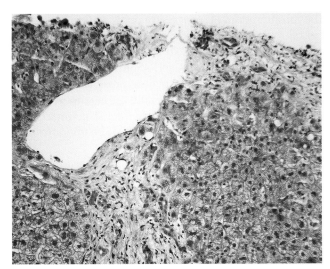

FIGURE 37–3. Photomicrograph of chronic hepatitis C showing fibrous adhesions between two portal tracts *(top right and bottom left)* and a hepatic vein. The structures are closely approximated, indicating substantial loss of tissue volume. Note the fibrous intimal thickening of the hepatic vein *(top right)* (Masson's trichrome).

incomplete resorption of fibrous tissue occurs in both the parenchyma and the portal tracts, may remain. Alternatively, complete resorption of fibrous tissue from the parenchyma with continuing prominent portal tract fibrosis engenders hepatoportal sclerosis. Resorption of all fibrous tissue with continuation of irregular vascular supply to the parenchyma engenders nodular regenerative hyperplasia because the well-vascularized regions of parenchyma hypertrophy. These latter two conditions are perhaps erroneously viewed as

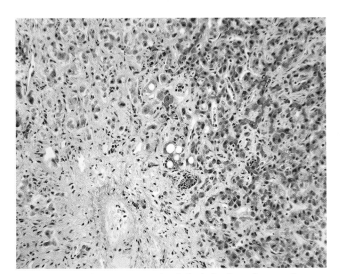

FIGURE 37–4. Photomicrograph of alcoholic liver disease showing diffuse pericellular fibrosis delimited by intact hepatocytes in single-cell plates. Adjacent to the obstructed hepatic vein *(left),* the hepatocytes have dropped out, apparently allowing the pericellular fibrosis to collapse into a dense mass that will form a septum. This is analogous to **J** in Figure 37-2.

"vascular" abnormalities; as such, they are discussed in Chapter 38.

Nonuniformity of vascular supply to the liver parenchyma is also proposed as an underlying cause for de novo development of incomplete septal cirrhosis.[29] The pathogenesis is thought to be the result of recurrent emboli, composed of platelet aggregates and formed within the portal venous system or spleen.[29,30]

Collectively, incomplete septal cirrhosis, nodular regenerative hyperplasia, partial nodular transformation, and focal nodular hyperplasia are thought to be interrelated disorders with a common pathogenesis related to abnormalities in the vascular supply.[31] Obliterative portal venopathy is postulated to produce nodular hyperplastic lesions by inducing nonuniformity of the blood supply to the parenchyma.[30,32,33] The hypothesis is attractive in that it unites several entities with similar morphologic features, but the underlying causes of vascular obliteration are not fully understood. Regardless, the hypothesis does, however, (1) explain the considerable overlap and diagnostic confusion associated with these entities, (2) provide a mechanism for focality of disease in some instances and diffuse disease in others, and (3) offer a rational explanation for the lack of any clinically overt disease or of any inflammatory component.

VASCULAR REORGANIZATION

Vascular modifications during the development of cirrhosis are central to the development of the cirrhotic state.[34] In normal liver, sinusoidal endothelial cells lack a basement membrane and exhibit fenestrations approximately 100 nm in diameter, occupying between 2% and 3% of the area of the endothelial cell. Deposition of extracellular matrix in the space of Disse is accompanied by the loss of fenestrations in the sinusoidal endothelial cells.[35] With the development of cirrhosis, the diameter of the fenestrations slightly decreases, but the area occupancy ("porosity") drops to below 0.5%.[36] Because of this, in combination with the deposition of aberrant extracellular matrix in the space of Disse by stellate cells, the sinusoidal space comes to resemble a capillary rather than a channel for exchange of solutes between hepatocytes and plasma.[35] In particular, hepatocellular secretion of proteins (e.g., albumin, clotting factors, lipoproteins) is greatly impaired.

The changes in fluid dynamics are dramatic.[37] First, sclerosis of the portal tracts and their vascular branches increases presinusoidal vascular resistance. Second, acquisition of myofibers by perisinusoidal stellate cells increases sinusoidal vascular resistance because tonic contraction of these "myofibroblasts" constricts the sinusoidal vascular channels. Third, fibrosis in the perivenular region of the lobule may partially obstruct vascular outflow, creating postsinusoidal vascular resistance.

With the formation of bona fide bridging fibrous septa between portal tracts and terminal hepatic veins, portovenous and arteriovenous shunting occurs, effectively bypassing the parenchymal nodules. As fibrosis progresses to cirrhosis, shunted blood flow through the "fast" vascular channels leaves the remainder of the hepatic parenchyma almost bereft of meaningful blood flow.[38] This explains the increased blood flow observed in sinusoids of the cirrhotic liver in the midst of relative underperfusion of the liver parenchyma as a whole. A remarkable fraction of nutritive blood flow may therefore pass through these intrahepatic functional shunts, contributing to ongoing hepatocellular necrosis and parenchymal extinction. In fact, in advanced cirrhosis, most of the hepatic blood supply seems to cross the liver via these channels.[38] Unfortunately, an increased transhepatic vascular resistance is maintained through further compression of the shunt channels by regenerating nodules.

The final insult is vascular thrombosis, as noted earlier. In angiographic and ultrasonographic studies, portal vein thrombosis has been found in 0.6% to 16.6% of cirrhotic patients,[39] and grossly visible portal vein fibrosis or thrombosis has been noted in 39% of cirrhotic livers at autopsy.[40] Veno-occlusive lesions of hepatic veins smaller than 0.2 mm in diameter have been seen in up to 74% of cirrhotic livers examined at autopsy.[41-43] Obliterative lesions in 36% of portal veins and 70% of hepatic veins have been detected in cirrhotic livers removed at liver transplantation.[44] The distribution of portal vein obliterative lesions is more uniform than that in hepatic veins, each consistent with the concept of propagation of multifocal thrombi downstream from their site of origin. Portal vein lesions have been associated with prominent regional variation in the size of cirrhotic nodules. Hepatic vein lesions have been associated with regions of confluent fibrosis and parenchymal extinction. The compelling conclusion is that thrombosis of medium-sized and large portal veins and of hepatic veins is a common occurrence in cirrhosis, and that these events are important in causing the progression of parenchymal extinction to full-blown cirrhosis.

REGENERATION

Hepatocytes, bile duct epithelial cells, and resident hepatic progenitor cells maintain the ability to multiply throughout adult life.[45] Depending on the type of injurious agent, the nature of the liver disease, and the extent of hepatic destruction, liver regeneration may occur by at least two mechanisms.[46-48] First, adult differentiated hepatocytes may undergo division and replication, responding quickly to liver damage associated with mild to moderate hepatocellular loss. Second, more extensive or massive hepatic necrosis stimulates the proliferation of progenitor cells within the periportal region. Proliferation of these cells gives rise first to ductular hepatocytes, in which ductular structures containing cuboidal cells and slightly larger cells with mitochondria-rich cytoplasm are present. Over time, these cells mature into definitive hepatocytes and possibly repopulate damaged bile duct structures. Each of these regenerative mechanisms may be operative as a liver evolves toward cirrhosis.

In addition to the presence of scattered mitotic figures, hepatocellular regeneration is recognized by the twinning of liver cell plates. This is evident as a double line of hepatocytes with nuclei seemingly running in parallel. Twinning of cell plates may remain for some months after regeneration before new sinusoidal channels develop and nuclear alignments dissipate.[49] Second, if regeneration is recent, the hepatocytes lack lipofuscin because this pigment accumulates over time in the normal liver. Third, increased numbers of binucleate or multinucleate hepatocytes are noted, reflecting the replication of nuclear material. Hepatocyte nuclei may be more uniform in size in that anisonucleosis increases with age in the normal liver and hence may not be as evident in the regenerating liver.

To the extent that fibrosis and cell death precede hepatocellular regeneration, a parenchymal island may simply be carved out of the preexisting parenchyma. It is not until hepatocellular regeneration occurs that the characteristic nodular transformation of cirrhosis becomes manifest. With thickening of liver cell plates, the parenchyma expands against the constraining fibrous septa and acquires a spherical shape. Hepatocyte plates abutting the fibrous septa become compressed and are bent outward by the less-constrained plates toward the interior of the nodule.

The ultimate size of the nodule is determined in part by the anatomic location of the antecedent fibrous septa. If matrix deposition is occurring at the acinar level, then the ensuing nodules will grow out of monoacinar units and will be small. If matrix deposition encompasses many acinar units (multiacinar), the growing nodules may be much larger and will retain components of the preexisting acini, including intact portal tracts.

In some cases of cirrhosis, vast expanses of bile ductules within fibrous septa coexist with interspersed hepatocellular nodules. These may occur in cirrhosis of almost any cause and are not necessarily the result of biliary obstruction.[50] Hyperplasia of ductules is associated with lengthening and increased tortuosity of existing channels and with extensive sprouting of new channels. This change is reminiscent of the massive proliferation of ductular structures within the hepatic parenchyma or at the interface between parenchyma and portal tracts that occurs in massive hepatic necrosis, and it implicates the proliferation of periportal progenitor cells.[45,51,52] Over time, these ductular structures may mature into hepatocellular parenchyma or bile ductules. Thus, expanses of bile ductules in occasional cirrhotic livers point toward occasions in the recent past where extensive parenchymal destruction occurred; these ductules represent the intermediate stage of a massive regenerative response.[53]

ZONATION

In the previous discussion, fibrosis is simply viewed as parenchymal (i.e., uniform along the sinusoid) or portal-tract based. The most dramatic example of a zonal pattern of fibrosis is the initial perivenular fibrosis that occurs during chronic exposure to alcohol and results from the hepatocellular injury that typically occurs in this region of the lobule.[54,55] Subsequent to the perivenular fibrosis, septal fibrosis develops, connecting portal tracts to terminal hepatic veins (portal/central) and following the principles of fibrogenesis and microvascular transformation discussed earlier.

A separate question regards the zonal distribution of hepatocellular metabolism and whether it changes in cirrhosis.[56] In the normal liver, heterogeneity in hepatocellular metabolism is observed, with hepatocytes in the periportal region exhibiting different patterns of enzyme complements than those seen in the perivenular region.[57] Immunohistochemical study of hepatocellular enzymes normally exhibiting zonal distributions can serve as a guide to alterations in disease states. In cirrhosis arising from perivenular hepatic damage and sublobular fibrosis (e.g., as caused by alcohol), the afferent vascular channels appear to penetrate to the center of parenchymal nodules with efferent vascular flow at the periphery.[56] The zonation of the liver parenchyma is lost[58] or even reversed with a periportal hepatocellular phenotype toward the center of cirrhotic nodules and a pericentral hepatocellular phenotype at the periphery.[56] This disruption of normal metabolic architecture may contribute to the metabolic disorders associated with alcoholic cirrhosis.[59] In contrast, in biliary-type cirrhosis, the periportal hepatocellular phenotype is retained along fibrous septa,[60-62] lending credence to the observation that metabolic derangement occurs late in biliary-type fibrosis (e.g., primary biliary cirrhosis).

Glutamine synthetase is an enzyme with a distribution that normally is almost exclusively perivenular and restricted to a layer of two to four hepatocytes around the terminal hepatic vein. Glutamine synthetase is undetectable in cirrhotic nodules and hepatocyte clusters isolated in fibrous septa, regardless of the cause of cirrhosis.[62] Given that glutamine synthesis is a critical step in the fixing of free ammonia for elimination via the urea cycle, loss of glutamine synthetase expression may lead to the increased ammonia concentrations found in blood and hence may indirectly contribute to the pathogenesis of hepatic encephalopathy.

These findings also suggest that the center of nodules is not necessarily an efferent zone, despite the prominence of venous vascular channels at nodule centers. Conversely, the periphery of cirrhotic nodules cannot be considered as homologous to the periportal zone of the hepatic lobule. Thus, profound alterations in the metabolic zonation of parenchymal nodules are seen in the cirrhotic liver, with substantive differences between nodules arising in the setting of toxic/metabolic damage brought about by alcohol versus those caused by biliary damage resulting from biliary obstruction.

■ Morphology

MACROSCOPIC FEATURES

Several patterns of cirrhosis are recognized whose variations depend on the severity of the underlying liver disease, the degree of microcirculatory damage leading to parenchymal extinction, and the duration of inactivity before histologic examination (Table 37-1).[63] The main macroscopic types of cirrhosis are micronodular and macronodular; the diameter of most nodules is smaller than or equal to 3 mm in the former and greater than 3 mm in the latter.[64,65] The basis for the 3-mm cutoff is empirical and is not grounded in anatomy because the normal hepatic acinus is on the order of 0.8 to 1.6 mm in diameter.[66]

Micronodular Cirrhosis

The overall shape and external appearance of the liver in early micronodular cirrhosis may not be greatly altered. The nodules on the cut surface are small and uniform in appearance but may be difficult to define. Fibrosis is diffusely distributed as fine, indistinct bands between nodules; occasionally, these may be broader and may define more clearly the nodules on both the cut and the capsular surfaces. In the early stages, before the fibrous subdivision of the liver is complete, the liver

---

TABLE 37–1. Anatomic Classification of Cirrhosis and Related Forms of Chronic Liver Disease

Micronodular cirrhosis
Macronodular cirrhosis
Mixed micronodular/macronodular cirrhosis
Postnecrotic cirrhosis following subacute massive necrosis
Noncirrhotic portal hypertension
    Incomplete septal cirrhosis
    Hepatoportal sclerosis (see Chapter 38)
    Nodular regenerative hyperplasia (see Chapter 38)
Cirrhosis with regional parenchymal extinction

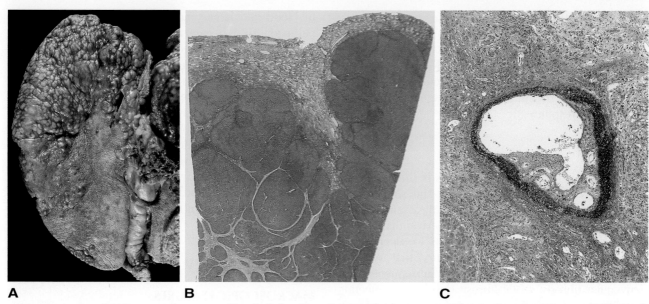

A   **B**   **C**

FIGURE 37–5. A and **B,** Severe cirrhosis caused by alcohol and hepatitis C with a large region of parenchymal extinction noted beneath the capsule of the left lobe. **C,** Such large regions of fibrosis are invariably associated with intimal thickening of medium-sized hepatic veins.

may become enlarged. In the case of fatty alcoholic liver disease, it may actually be softer than the normal liver. However, with advancing disease, the liver shrinks and becomes progressively harder, until at the end stage, more fibrous tissue than parenchyma is evident on cut section. The liver surface becomes studded with a myriad of small protruding nodules. Severe regional extinction in micronodular cirrhosis may continue, generating large contiguous regions of collapse and fibrosis in the interior of the liver (Fig. 37-5).[67] This end-stage, micronodular form of cirrhosis best fits the description of Laënnec's cirrhosis.

Alcohol is most frequently associated with micronodular cirrhosis in Europe and North America. Less common causes for this pattern include hemochromatosis, biliary obstruction, chronic hepatic venous outflow obstruction (cardiac cirrhosis, see Chapter 38), and many of the metabolic diseases of infancy and childhood that affect the liver. Alcoholic liver disease may show a diffuse tan or yellow color caused by severe fatty change; in the setting dominated by alcoholic hepatitis, red may be a more typical color. In hemochromatosis, heavy iron deposition imparts a dark reddish-brown color to the liver. Destructive biliary diseases such as primary biliary cirrhosis or primary sclerosing cholangitis render the liver a deep yellow or green color; they also impart to the liver capsule a progressive fine septal scarring pattern resembling "pigskin." Distinguishing macroscopic features are rarely noted in micronodular cirrhosis caused by drug toxicity.

Macronodular Cirrhosis

Liver size and shape in macronodular cirrhosis are much more variable. The liver is frequently enlarged, but in association with clinical liver failure, it is more typically small and may weigh less than 1000 g. The parenchyma exhibits large, bulging nodules separated by fibrous bands that vary considerably in width, but the liver retains its overall anatomic shape. Early stages of macronodular cirrhosis may reveal slender fibrous bands, but as liver injury and parenchymal damage progress, these fibrous bands become broader and denser, producing marked grooving and retraction that are evident on the capsular surface in particular. Diseases that tend to produce a de novo macronodular cirrhosis include chronic viral hepatitis and autoimmune hepatitis.

Supplementary Considerations

Incomplete Septal Cirrhosis. Incomplete septal cirrhosis is a highly regressed form of cirrhosis that is often associated with portal hypertension but normal hepatocellular function.[68-70] Macroscopically, the liver may exhibit only delicate fibrous septa on cut sections (Fig. 37-6). The liver may reveal no significant distortion, or it may exhibit residual bulging nodules. Because portal vein thrombosis is often the complication that leads to portal hypertension in these cases, gross examination should include inspection of the portal vein system.

Mixed Micronodular/Macronodular Cirrhosis. The World Health Organization (WHO) classification

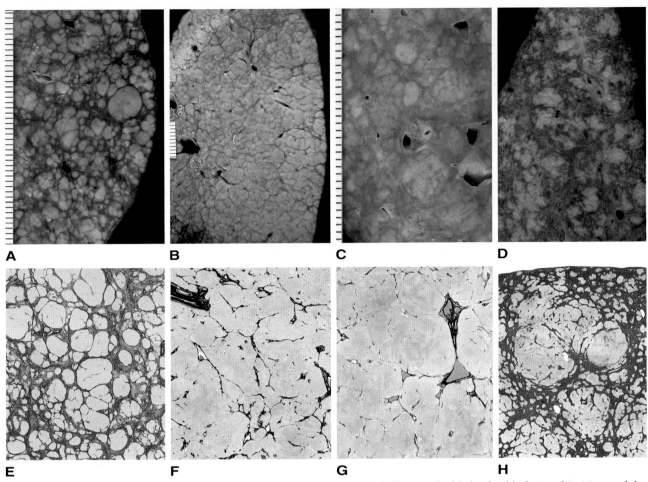

FIGURE 37–6. Examples of cirrhosis showing a cut surface. Trichrome stain with fibrosis is highlighted in black. **A** and **B,** Micronodular cirrhosis caused by hepatitis C virus. Most nodules are smaller than 3 mm in diameter, and septa are fairly broad. **C** and **D,** Regressed incomplete cirrhosis caused by hepatitis B virus. The septa are delicate and often incomplete. **E** and **F,** Incomplete septal cirrhosis caused by hepatitis B virus. The nodules are more apparent grossly than histologically. Most septa are delicate and incomplete. **G** and **H,** Primary biliary cirrhosis. The largest nodules are pale against a green cholestatic background with small cirrhotic nodules.

defines a mixed category of cirrhosis wherein nodules larger and smaller than 3 mm coexist. Mixed cirrhosis is often found in primary biliary cirrhosis and primary sclerosing cholangitis (Fig. 37-6**G** and **H**). The ebb and flow of hepatic fibrogenesis and the regenerative activity are sufficiently variable to limit the reliability of any classification scheme based on morphology alone. In any liver, the tendency is for small nodules to increase in size over time; this is counterbalanced by constraints imposed by fibrous scarring and parenchymal extinction.[71] Hence, liver cirrhosis resulting from any cause may evolve into a mixed micronodular/macronodular pattern.

Postnecrotic Cirrhosis Following Submassive Hepatic Necrosis. A severe bout of acute hepatitis with large contiguous regions of extinction and lesser regions of regenerative tissue gives rise to this form of cirrhosis, which has earned the name postnecrotic cirrhosis (Fig. 37-7).[72] The coarse scarring of postnecrotic cirrhosis, also called *posthepatitic cirrhosis* by Gall,[73] leads to a grossly misshapen liver with large regenerative regions of liver parenchyma separated by dense fibrous scars. Because many patients suffer subacute hepatic failure, these livers are usually severely cholestatic even though the original hepatitis may have resolved.

Macronodules. Unusually large regenerating nodules may occur in a cirrhotic liver. Preferably called *macroregenerative nodules*,[74] these nodules are evident as 0.5-cm-diameter nodules on a background of nodules smaller than 0.3 cm in diameter, or they may stand out as gigantic nodules that reach up to 10 cm in diameter. They may bulge from the liver surface or may be embedded deep within the hepatic substance. Any nodule substantially larger than its neighbors merits sampling for histopathologic examination. Macroscopic

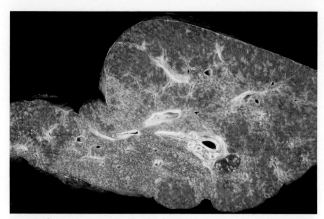

FIGURE 37–7. Fulminant hepatitis, idiopathic. The green regions contain regenerating hepatocytes. The brown regions are totally collapsed without residual hepatocytes. Fibrosis in such livers is usually minimal, but patients who survive several months may have sufficient fibrosis to be considered to have a form of cirrhosis.

features characteristic of a regenerative, nonmalignant nodule include a color similar to that of other cirrhotic nodules and minimal bulging of the cut surface.

Hepatocellular Carcinoma. Gross evaluation of any cirrhotic liver must include examination for the presence of hepatocellular carcinoma. In contrast to macroregenerative nodules, hepatocellular carcinomas arising in cirrhotic livers may exhibit altered coloration (including a more pale appearance resulting from absent bile formation, or a more red appearance caused by enhanced blood flow) and bulging of the cut surface. Necrosis or hemorrhage is likely to be seen only in large malignant nodules; these two macroscopic features are not requisite correlates of histologic malignancy. Any large cirrhotic nodule with an interior alteration in coloration, either concentric or eccentric, is called a *nodule-in-nodule*. These foci may simply be regenerative but merit histologic sampling in the event that malignant transformation has occurred within an otherwise enlarged cirrhotic nodule. The pathologist must also be alert to the presence of multiple malignant nodules. Given that malignant transformation may occur in nodules smaller than 0.5 cm in diameter, sectioning the liver at 0.3- to 0.5-cm intervals is required for adequate gross examination of the cirrhotic liver.

Portal Vein Thrombosis. Portal vein thrombosis is a common complication of portal hypertension and is particularly common when hepatocellular carcinoma invades the vascular tree. Hence, thrombi within the portal vascular system must be traced back to their intrahepatic terminus, enabling potential confirmation of the presence of a fleshy, nonthrombotic tumor mass.

Ischemic Extinction of Nodules. Necrosis of cirrhotic nodules may occur in association with systemic hypotension that accompanies a variceal bleed. Affected nodules show the classic changes of infarction, becoming bright yellow with a peripheral zone of congestion and new vessel formation.

Hepar Lobatum. An extraordinary aberration of hepatic architecture may arise from the deep scarring that occurs in syphilis acquired in adulthood. The process of chronic spirochetal infection with gumma formation leads to the deposition of broad septal scars within the hepatic parenchyma. The severe contraction of these scars, accompanied by a robust regenerative response of the unaffected liver, leads to deep clefting of the liver surface, so-called hepar lobatum. Although hepar lobatum may be confused macroscopically with cirrhosis, it is not a true form of cirrhosis. The regenerating liver is not nodular but is made up of deranged remnants of liver lobes.

MICROSCOPIC FEATURES

The microscopic features of cirrhosis are more easily generalized than the macroscopic features. As expected, fibrous subdivision of the liver parenchyma with isolation of parenchymal islands is the sine qua non for a diagnosis of cirrhosis. Application of these criteria, however, brings its challenges, particularly on liver biopsy specimens.

Natural History of Cirrhosis

The histologic appearance of cirrhosis varies according to the age of the accumulated extinction lesions (Figs. 37-8 and 37-9). If the causative injury continues, new parenchymal extinction lesions coexist with old ones. Parenchymal extinction, which is usually accompanied by inflammation, constitutes activity; an active cirrhosis is a cirrhotic liver that shows persistent destruction of residual tissue. Conversely, if the causative injury is no longer present, the liver will contain only lesions in the late stages of repair, and the cirrhosis can be considered quiescent (see Fig. 37-6). These overall concepts are presented in Figure 37-10.

New extinction lesions represent areas of bridging necrosis or focal intense congestion with atrophy and clusters of apoptotic cells. Moreover, careful examination of the vascular channels—both septal and intraparenchymal—may reveal organized thrombi that result from chaotic and sluggish blood flow, loss of anticoagulant function, and the prothrombotic effects of sepsis and cholestasis. Thrombosis of medium-sized or large hepatic veins produces large regions of extinction, which lead to marked irregularity of the cirrhotic liver (see Fig. 37-5).[67] By definition, ongoing parenchymal extinction is seen only in livers with moderate to severe activity.

Old lesions of parenchymal extinction predominate in livers in which the primary disease has remitted,

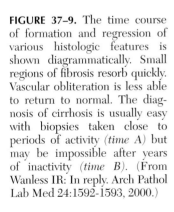

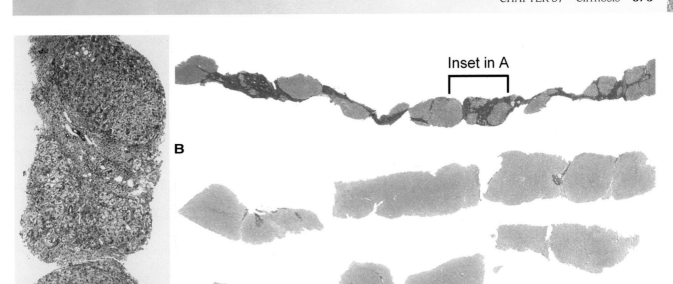

A C

FIGURE 37–8. Fibrous septa regress and disappear with time, as illustrated by this patient with chronic hepatitis B and cirrhosis (**A** and **B**). After successful treatment with lamivudine, a biopsy 2.5 years later (**C**) showed marked reduction in fibrous septation. (From Wanless IR, Nakashima E, Sherman M: Regression of human cirrhosis. Morphologic features and the genesis of incomplete septal cirrhosis. Arch Pathol Lab Med 124:1599-1607, 2000.)

FIGURE 37–9. The time course of formation and regression of various histologic features is shown diagrammatically. Small regions of fibrosis resorb quickly. Vascular obliteration is less able to return to normal. The diagnosis of cirrhosis is usually easy with biopsies taken close to periods of activity (*time A*) but may be impossible after years of inactivity (*time B*). (From Wanless IR: In reply. Arch Pathol Lab Med 24:1592-1593, 2000.)

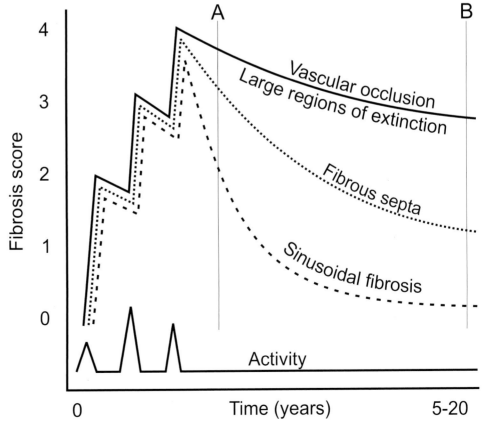

Natural History of Chronic Liver Disease

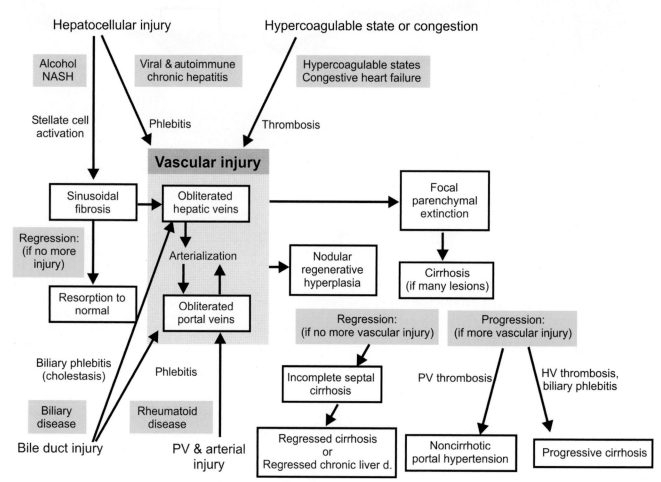

FIGURE 37–10. Diagram summarizing the factors that determine the natural history of chronic liver disease. There are five principal classes of disease that lead to chronic liver disease *(blue boxes)*. Most patients with chronic liver disease have hepatocellular injury. This may lead to local activation of stellate cells and sinusoidal fibrosis that is largely reversible. Patients who develop obliteration of vessels, especially small hepatic veins, develop parenchymal collapse (extinction) that heals as fibrous septa. When septa are numerous, the histologic features of cirrhosis are present. Biliary disease and rheumatoid disease are associated with predominant portal tract disease. Rheumatoid disease usually affects the portal vessels, leading to multifocal atrophy of parenchyma with minimal fibrous septation, a condition recognized as nodular regenerative hyperplasia. In biliary disease, portal inflammation is an early event leading to portal tract expansion and sometimes presinusoidal portal hypertension; zone 3 cholestasis occurs later, leading to bile salt injury of small hepatic veins. Thus, the order of vascular events is different, but accumulation of extinction lesions eventually leads to cirrhosis. The outcome depends on the time course of disease activity *(green boxes)*. If injury ceases, regression occurs as all extant lesions heal and new lesions do not appear. If injury continues, new lesions develop, progressive collapse and fibrosis occur, as a result of the continuing primary injury, secondary thrombotic events, or secondary bile salt injury to hepatic veins.

either spontaneously or after successful treatment.[13] Fibrosis may be progressively removed from extinction lesions so that broad septa become delicate in appearance, and delicate septa become incomplete or disappear. Thus, micronodular cirrhosis may remodel to macronodular cirrhosis or incomplete septal cirrhosis, or it may eventually be near normal in appearance. Arteriovenous shunts are recognized as focal regions of sinusoidal congestion and hepatocellular atrophy; their presence can be confirmed by the presence of CD34-positive sinusoidal endothelial cells.[13]

Micronodular Cirrhosis

Normal liver acini are approximately 1 mm in diameter. Because micronodular cirrhosis arises from subdivisions of parenchymal acini, cirrhotic nodules may be smaller then 1 mm in diameter. Tiny nodules may enlarge as they regenerate but are severely confined by the surrounding fibrous tissue. Virtually every acinus is affected in this form of cirrhosis; usually no anatomically intact acini are detected. Fibrous septa connect portal tracts to their adjacent terminal hepatic venules. Thus, zones 1, 2, and 3 of the acinus are transected by fibrovascular septa. Depending on the cause, fibrosis may be dominant in one zone (e.g., around the portal tracts [zone 1] in hemochromatosis or around the terminal hepatic venules [zone 3] in alcoholic liver disease), but cirrhosis should not be considered fully developed if fibrosis is restricted only to these zones.

The characteristic feature of micronodular cirrhosis is deposition of fibrous septa along the sinusoidal channels that connect portal tracts to terminal hepatic veins. Frequently, multiple adjacent sinusoids exhibit fibrosis; this is a particularly characteristic feature of the evolving cirrhosis of alcohol- and drug-induced micronodular cirrhosis. In three dimensions, the fibrous bands are plates of fibrous tissue rich in newly formed blood vessels.[34]

Micronodular cirrhosis seems to be most commonly associated with diseases in which the uniform and generalized effect of a hepatotoxic agent or metabolic derangement is seen on the smallest parenchymal units in the liver. For example, in alcoholic liver disease, every acinus has been regularly exposed to high levels of alcohol. In cirrhosis arising in the setting of severe alcoholic hepatitis, the rate of fibrous tissue deposition may be so rapid (over weeks to months) as to render nodular regeneration almost impossible. In this setting, extensive hepatocellular degeneration with steatosis, ballooning, and Mallory body formation is accompanied by a mixed neutrophilic and mononuclear pattern of inflammation. Nodule formation may be minimal, yet the liver is transformed into a densely fibrotic organ with fibrous septa that seem to traverse almost every sinusoid. This extreme degree of micronodular cirrhosis raises the question of at what point the definition of cirrhosis is fulfilled, yet few will argue that such a fibrotic liver is not cirrhotic. Alternatively, a smoldering form of alcoholic hepatitis may proceed to a more mixed micronodular/macronodular pattern of cirrhosis, possibly caused by a more portally based pattern of fibrous deposition.

Macronodular Cirrhosis

The histology of macronodular cirrhosis is highly variable, particularly when it is evaluated by percutaneous liver biopsy (see under Liver Biopsy Procedures). This pattern typically exhibits large nodules delimited by abnormal septa, in which multiple hepatic acini are incorporated into single nodules. During the early to intermediate stages of evolution, residual portal tracts and portal tract/hepatic vein acinar units may be evident. Cell plates within the multiacinar nodules are often single with little evidence of twinning, but they do not show the regular radial orientation present between the portal tracts and hepatic veins of a normal acinus. Abnormal cell plate patterns probably reflect altered blood flow through the parenchyma, as

has been discussed earlier. One outcome of an abnormal vascular flow through the parenchyma is an increase in the number of venous channels within the parenchymal nodules. As has been noted under the heading Pathogenesis, whether these represent afferent or efferent vascular channels is open to debate. Although this finding cannot be regarded as diagnostic on its own, the possibility of macronodular cirrhosis must be considered whenever abnormal hepatocellular plate patterns and excess veins are noted in a needle liver biopsy specimen that does not contain identifiable portal tracts.

Incomplete Septal Cirrhosis

In this pattern, slender fibrovascular septa extend from portal tracts into the parenchyma but do not connect with other portal tracts or hepatic veins. These septa demarcate large, rather inconspicuous nodules.[75] Intrasinusoidal collagen distant from the septa is not obviously increased, and little evidence of hepatocellular damage or inflammation is noted. Portal tracts are variably attenuated, and an increased number of parenchymal venous channels is noted. This abnormal architecture is present throughout the liver in a variable mixture of thickened hepatocellular plates, dilated sinusoids, and compression of sinusoids between hyperplastic plates.[76] The plate pattern is disorganized with irregular orientation of plates to portal tracts and terminal hepatic veins. Histologic indicators of the original causative agent are usually absent.

In a patient with portal hypertension, diagnosing incomplete septal cirrhosis on liver biopsy specimens is exceedingly difficult, as is distinguishing it from hepatoportal sclerosis and nodular regenerative hyperplasia (see Chapter 38). When large expanses of liver are available for examination, both the fibrous septa extending out from portal tracts and the disorganized plate architecture of incomplete septal cirrhosis are absent in hepatoportal sclerosis. The chief distinction between incomplete septal cirrhosis and nodular regenerative hyperplasia is the absence of parenchymal fibrous tissue and the presence of clear spherical nodules in the latter. In every instance, a reticulin stain is often helpful in assessing parenchymal architecture; a trichrome stain is needed for collagen assessment.

Histologic Features of Specific Etiologic Subtypes

CHRONIC HEPATITIS

The most frequent forms of chronic hepatitis are hepatitis B, hepatitis C, and autoimmune hepatitis. These diseases are usually diagnosed on clinical grounds, especially with serologic tests. On histologic examination of the cirrhotic liver, hepatitis B infection may be diagnosed by the presence of cytoplasmic inclusions (ground-glass cells) or by immunohistochemical staining for hepatitis B surface and core antigens. With current techniques, hepatitis C may be detected in tissue only with difficulty. Chronic hepatitis C infection is suggested by the presence of portal tract lymphoid aggregates and scattered foci of parenchymal macrovesicular steatosis. These are not reliable histologic findings in the cirrhotic liver because virtually any form of chronic hepatitis can leave behind residual foci of lymphocytic inflammation. The possibility of coinfection with hepatitis B and hepatitis C must also be kept in mind. Finally, the cirrhosis associated with autoimmune hepatitis may be quite active, or it may simply be a quiescent cirrhosis resulting from injury incurred years earlier. Indeed, many cases of cryptogenic cirrhosis may represent end-stage autoimmune hepatitis. Hence, it is unrealistic for the clinician to expect that histopathologic examination of a cirrhotic liver will readily establish an etiologic diagnosis of autoimmune hepatitis.

The pattern of cirrhosis varies with the history of underlying disease activity. As a low-grade necroinflammatory disease, hepatitis C usually causes only small regions of liver cell extinction that, over time and when numerous, may lead to micronodular or mixed micronodular/macronodular cirrhosis. Hepatitis B and autoimmune hepatitis produce larger regions of extinction, eventually leading to the formation of large regenerative nodules and macronodular cirrhosis.

FATTY LIVER DISEASE

Fatty liver disease may be caused by alcohol abuse or other toxic/metabolic states. Insulin excess, as is seen in obesity or type 2 diabetes mellitus, is a common cause as well. The non–alcohol-associated cases are collectively known as *nonalcoholic steatohepatitis* or *nonalcoholic fatty liver disease*.[77] The latter term is preferred because it allows the inclusion of cases without definite evidence of steatohepatitis.

Fatty liver disease is characterized by macrovesicular steatosis with or without evidence of activity (steatohepatitis). Steatohepatitis is defined by the presence of ballooning necrosis and pigmented macrophages scattered in zone 3. Mallory bodies and neutrophils are noted in most active cases.

Simple steatosis typically does not progress to cirrhosis.[78] Rather, fibrosis develops in steatohepatitis with deposition of delicate fibers in the walls of zone 3 sinusoids. When small hepatic veins are obliterated during this process, focal parenchymal collapse is noted, along with approximation of portal tracts and adjacent hepatic veins with minimal deposition of collagen.[15] Broad fibrous septa occur when larger regions of

parenchyma collapse. Sinusoidal fibrosis, occasionally called *chicken-wire fibrosis*, may occur after local activation of sinusoidal stellate cells or after the splitting and repopulation of broad fibrous septa. A similar sequence of events can occur with chronic viral disease and other etiologic types of cirrhosis; thus, pericellular fibrosis is characteristic but not pathognomonic of fatty liver disease.

Alcoholic and nonalcoholic liver diseases are often identical in histologic appearance.[79] However, severe activity with numerous Mallory bodies and neutrophils is seen more often in alcoholic disease. Minimal steatohepatitis often occurs in patients with chronic hepatitis C, so that the cause of elevated aminotransferases may be difficult to determine except by a trial of dietary restraint. In end-stage cirrhosis caused by fatty liver disease, steatosis and steatohepatitis may be focal or absent; biopsies may not be able to confirm the diagnosis.

CHRONIC BILIARY DISEASE

Liver disease exhibiting chronic retention of biliary products is usually caused by duct obstruction and rarely by chronic hepatocellular dysfunction due to cholestatic drug reactions or inherited transport protein defects. In adults, duct obstruction is most commonly seen in primary biliary cirrhosis and primary sclerosing cholangitis.[80] By the time cirrhosis develops, inflammatory bile duct destruction in these disorders is usually complete; thus, diagnostic lesions are not usually present. Instead, only nonspecific features of biliary obstruction are typically seen—septal edema and neutrophilic inflammation, bile ductular proliferation (although these, too, may be few in number), ductular and hepatocellular cholestasis, degenerative swelling of periseptal hepatocytes (cholate stasis), Mallory body formation and copper retention in periseptal hepatocytes, liver cell rosettes, and clusters of bile-stained foamy macrophages within parenchymal nodules. Some suggest that a jigsaw pattern of nodules with molding of nodules to each other indicates chronic biliary-type cirrhosis.

Biliary fibrosis is topographically variable. Fibrosis in primary sclerosing cholangitis and cystic fibrosis is particularly variable. Whole liver segments may undergo liver cell extinction or may be spared, depending on the distribution of duct obstruction.

Occasionally, primary sclerosing cholangitis may be suggested by identification of hepatic arteries with a clearly identifiable companion fibrous cord (Fig. 37-11). As has been discussed, the bile duct–obstructed liver is subdivided extensively by fibrous septa before the parenchyma undergoes nodular transformation. Hence, preexisting portal tract relationships may be retained. Identification of a portal vein/hepatic artery pair associated with a sclerotic cord of similar diameter as the

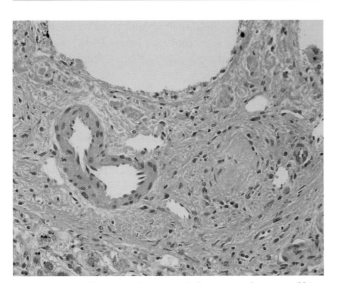

FIGURE 37–11. Primary sclerosing cholangitis at the time of liver transplantation. A clearly identifiable hepatic artery is accompanied only by a fibrous cord; there is no visible bile duct.

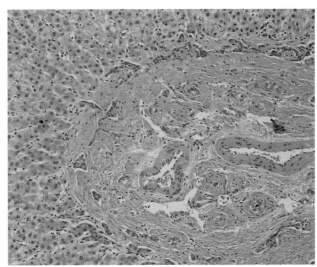

FIGURE 37–12. Biliary atresia, early to severe. A broad fibrous tract contains a central cluster of hypertrophied hepatic arteries and an irregular circumferential array of bile ductular elements around the periphery.

hepatic artery allows suggestion of primary sclerosing cholangitis as the cause.

Biliary Atresia. Chapter 41 describes the histologic features of extrahepatic biliary atresia (EHBA) on percutaneous liver biopsy specimens in comparison with the histologic features of neonatal hepatitis. This chapter discusses cirrhosis arising from EHBA, which is usually assessed in an explanted liver. The progressive findings that occur with increasing age (from birth to 2 years of life) include progressive portal and periportal fibrosis, ballooning degeneration of hepatocytes at the portal tract/parenchymal interface, and, at the extreme, copper accumulation and Mallory body formation in periportal hepatocytes and bile lakes in the parenchyma. Although the inciting injury is obliteration of the extrahepatic biliary tree, paucity of intrahepatic bile ducts develops within 4 to 5 months, with progression to virtual absence of intrahepatic bile ducts and full-blown biliary cirrhosis within 8 to 9 months.

The exception to this sequence is early severe biliary atresia, in which an intrinsic malformation of the intrahepatic biliary tree may be noted.[81,82] In this form, the biliary tree does not form normally from the embryonic ductal plate.[83] This results in portal tracts that do not contain interlobular bile ducts but rather include residual ductal plate remnants concentrically placed around the periphery of portal tracts.[84,85] Accompanying this ductal plate malformation is hypertrophy of hepatic arterial elements toward the center of the portal tracts, as well as a robust fibrous mesenchyme. Rapidly evolving cirrhosis over the following weeks to months retains circumferential ductal plate remnants embedded in broad fibrous septa and closely approximated hypertrophied arteries toward the center of these septa (Fig. 37-12). Identification of these features in a liver explant

favors a diagnosis of early severe biliary cirrhosis over the more conventional form of EHBA.

Cystic Fibrosis. In cystic fibrosis, thick mucus–laden bile focally blocks bile flow, leading to focal or regional biliary fibrosis. With long-term survival of cystic fibrosis patients, a greater portion of the liver may become involved, leading to a form of multilobular cirrhosis with broad fibrous bands and coarse nodularity. Notably, cirrhosis develops in less than 10% of patients with cystic fibrosis.[86] Dilated major bile ducts with inspissated mucinous contents and upstream dense biliary fibrosis are characteristic histologic features.

METAL OVERLOAD STATES

Iron and copper are deposited in the liver in hemochromatosis and Wilson's disease (*ATP7B* disease; see Chapter 41), respectively. Iron overload is usually genetically determined (*HFE* disease; see Chapter 41) but may be acquired secondarily through ingestion or by transfusion.[87] As with so many other forms of cirrhosis, definitive diagnosis through histologic examination of a cirrhotic liver is difficult. Metals in the cirrhotic liver may suggest but are not intrinsically diagnostic of hereditary hemochromatosis or Wilson's disease. Rather, definitive diagnosis usually rests on molecular analysis of the genome.[88]

Iron. Although iron and copper may be detected in the liver by histochemistry, low to moderate levels of both metals may accumulate in severe cirrhosis of other causes. In particular, iron overload is a well-documented phenomenon in alcoholic cirrhosis,[89] attributable to redistribution of iron stores from other sites in the body.[90] In general, hemosiderosis is common in nonbiliary forms of cirrhosis but is uncommon in the biliary forms.[91] Large amounts of stored iron cause slow progression of fibrosis; this progression is often enhanced by cofactors such as steatohepatitis or viral infection.[92] Hence, the pattern of fibrosis is not diagnostically useful.

An interesting phenomenon is heterogeneous accumulation of iron in cirrhotic livers. On the one hand, regenerative nodules arising in the livers of patients with hereditary hemochromatosis may be free of iron staining. This is presumably due to rapid growth of nodular parenchyma, such that iron accumulation has not yet occurred. On the other hand, large regenerative nodules that selectively accumulate stainable iron in otherwise iron-free cirrhotic livers have been reported.[93-95] These nodules exhibit a higher incidence of hyperplastic hepatocellular foci, suggesting that iron-accumulating large regenerative nodules are preneoplastic.

Copper. In Wilson's disease, excess copper deposition occurs throughout the hepatic parenchyma. The cirrhotic liver is marked by distribution of copper throughout parenchymal nodules. This is in contrast to the copper accumulation that occurs predominantly in periseptal hepatocytes in biliary cirrhosis, because copper is eliminated from the body principally via biliary secretion.[96] The hepatocellular degenerative features of Wilson's disease (i.e., steatosis, Mallory bodies, ballooning degeneration, glycogenated hepatocellular nuclei) often persist during fibrosis. However, because these histologic features are present in many toxic conditions, once again care must be taken to avoid overinterpretation of these findings.

Indian Childhood Cirrhosis. First reported by Sen in 1887,[97] this entity was thought to be peculiar to the Indian subcontinent. However, an increasing number of cases have now been reported in whites and Native Americans.[98-101] Morbidity and mortality from the disease are high, the age range of affected children is from 6 months to 5 years, and a family predilection is often noted. Clinically, the disease is characterized by hepatosplenomegaly and hepatocellular failure that eventually progresses to death. The earliest histologic change is steatosis. With progression of disease, ballooning hepatocytes, focal necrosis, prominent Mallory body formation, marked pericellular fibrosis, and an interstitial mixed acute and chronic inflammatory infiltrate develop. A prominent feature is a marked accumulation of copper, as detected by copper stain or by quantitative measures. Progression to micronodular cirrhosis eventually occurs.

CONGESTIVE CIRRHOSIS

A congestive element occurs in the genesis of all types of cirrhosis and is caused by increased vascular resistance of the hepatic vascular bed. The distinct category of congestive cirrhosis refers to the condition in which the initiating lesion is obstruction of medium-sized to large hepatic veins, as is seen in congestive heart failure and hepatic vein thrombosis (Budd-Chiari syndrome).

Congestive heart failure by itself causes only sinusoidal dilatation and mild hepatocellular atrophy. Livers in this condition develop fibrosis only when additional obliteration of hepatic and portal veins occurs.[63] Because the venous lesions form after thrombosis, congestive fibrosis is variable from one region to another and may occur quickly. Complete cirrhosis is seldom attributed to congestive failure alone.

In Budd-Chiari syndrome, hepatic vein obstruction is dominant, leading to a pattern of venocentric fibrosis, also known as *reversed-nodularity cirrhosis*.[102] Subsequent portal vein thrombosis frequently occurs and may explain the transition to a venoportal pattern of fibrosis wherein portal tracts become incorporated into the fibrous septa.

Evaluating the Cirrhotic Liver

Cirrhotic liver specimens are obtained as a result of liver transplantation or partial hepatectomy. The clinical indication for liver transplantation is almost always hepatic failure. Besides documenting the presence of cirrhosis, the pathologist should also note features that may point toward a specific underlying causative process. Resection specimens should be examined for weight, color, capsule thickness, relative size of the lobes, regional parenchymal collapse, and the patency of ducts, vessels, and any prosthetic stents. Uncomplicated cirrhosis is usually uniform in appearance. Heterogeneity in the macroscopic pattern of cirrhosis should prompt extra sampling of vessels and ducts to help the pathologist to identify occlusions of these structures.

A critical role of the pathologist is to identify or exclude hepatocellular carcinoma. In an extensive 6-year series of 422 hepatocellular carcinomas identified in explanted livers, 60% were known at the time of transplantation, and 40% were identified only upon examination of the explanted liver.[103] Almost half (47%) of the 190 patient deaths that occurred during the follow-up period were due to recurrent hepatocellular carcinoma. Key prognostic features for recurrence and death included poorly differentiated histologic grade, vascular invasion, positive hilar lymph nodes, and tumor size greater than 5.0 cm in maximal diameter. On gross examination, therefore, the liver should be sectioned at no more than 0.5-cm intervals so that suspicious nodules of 0.5 cm or greater in diameter can be identified.

Nodules of variable size, color, or texture may be an indication of neoplasia.

Preoperative ablative therapy of a known hepatic mass lesion is increasingly performed before liver transplantation or partial hepatectomy. The pathologist should document the presence of necrotic lesions on both gross and histologic examination and should take sections to determine whether any viable rim of tumor remains and whether vascular invasion or lymphatic metastasis may be present.

LIVER BIOPSY PROCEDURES

Liver biopsy specimen assessment helps in establishing the severity of necroinflammatory and fibrotic liver injury (grade and stage, respectively) and may provide insight into cause. However, clinically cirrhotic patients are not without comorbidity, and the risks of percutaneous liver biopsy (especially for hematoma and intra-abdominal hemorrhage) are potentially increased owing to coagulopathy and ascites. If need is sufficiently great in spite of clinical contraindications, transjugular hepatic biopsy may be required.

Because the definition of cirrhosis requires involvement of the entire liver, the liver biopsy specimen should be representative of the whole, even though it includes only a minute portion of the liver. However, fibrosis in evolving chronic liver disease may be concentrated into fibrous septa that are not necessarily distributed uniformly throughout the liver; therefore, sampling errors may occur. False-negative diagnoses are possible in cases of macronodular cirrhosis in which the nodules are 0.5 cm or greater in diameter.[104-106] Diagnosis of cirrhosis is more easily made in cases of micronodular cirrhosis because entire nodules may be encompassed by the 0.6- to 1.4-mm diameter of the tissue fragment.[76] In all instances, reticulin stain may provide evidence of spherical nodule formation that may not be revealed on the trichrome stain.

Choice of Technique

The four main liver biopsy procedures are open wedge biopsy, cutting liver biopsy, fine-needle aspiration biopsy, and transjugular biopsy.

Open Wedge Biopsy. Open wedge biopsy specimens of the liver are obtained from the convexity of the liver surface or by resection of a small portion of the most inferior edge of the right lobe. In the former, Glisson's capsule is present on one of the three faces of the triangular specimen. In the latter, Glisson's capsule is present on two of the three faces.

The great risk of histologic evaluation of such specimens is misinterpretation of normal anatomy. A normal array of fibrous septa penetrate from Glisson's capsule to a depth of approximately 0.5 cm in the liver parenchyma, partially ensheathing subcapsular portal tracts in more than half of individuals[107] and extending between subcapsular portal tracts to terminal hepatic veins in one quarter of the population.[108] Hence, fibrous tissue may be excessively represented in the subcapsular area such that cirrhosis may be erroneously diagnosed. The observant pathologist will recognize a rapid decrement in the amount of fibrous tissue that is 0.2 to 0.5 cm deep to the capsule; thus, misinterpretation should be avoided. However, if this is the only tissue available, staging of liver fibrosis cannot be performed accurately. Surgeons are strongly encouraged to obtain cutting needle biopsy specimens as well. In our experience, the needle biopsy specimen, despite its smaller size, is almost always more informative than other types of specimens.

Cutting Needle Biopsy. Percutaneous cutting needle biopsies are usually performed percutaneously with a 16-, 18-, or 20-gauge needle, and rarely with a 14-gauge needle.[109] Percutaneous needle biopsy specimens can usually provide a diagnosis of cirrhosis on the first attempt; multiple needle passes are needed only if tissue is not obtained on the first pass.[110] However, cirrhotic livers yield tissue more reluctantly than do nonfibrotic livers, and the end result of needle biopsies may be only fragments of misshapen liver parenchyma, rather than a cylindrical core of tissue. Moreover, biopsy needles tend to reflect off hard fibrous tissue and to selectively sample softer areas of parenchyma[110-113]; thus, needle biopsy may be inadequate for assessing the severity of fibrosis or cirrhosis.

Ideally, the needle cuts through fibrous tissue and parenchyma alike, enabling identification of fibrous septa that encompass parenchymal nodules. To the extent that a cutting needle harvests only parenchymal nodules, the liver tissue is substantially fragmented upon ejection from the cutting needle. The degree of fragmentation alone cannot be used as a criterion for cirrhosis because even normal liver may be substantially fragmented by the time the final histologic sections are prepared.[114] Rather, a critical feature of cirrhotic liver tissue fragments, best observed by connective tissue stains, is the rounded fragments of parenchyma that show concentrically oriented compressed liver cell plates at the periphery, along with curvilinear rims of connective tissue (Fig. 37-13).

Fine-Needle Aspiration Biopsy and Transjugular Biopsy. Fine-needle aspiration biopsy, which is most often performed with a 21-gauge needle, yields an array of isolated fragments of hepatic parenchyma. Transjugular biopsy also yields fragments of hepatic parenchyma, along with segments of the hepatic vein wall. Although transjugular biopsy specimens are often small, in experienced hands diagnostic tissue can be obtained in more than 90% of cases.[115]

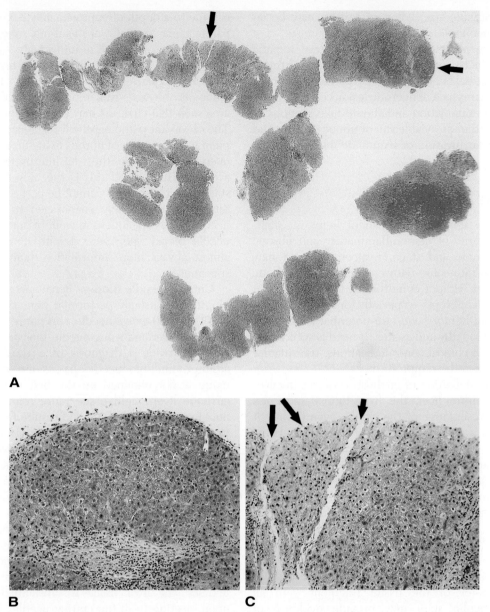

A

B   **C**

FIGURE 37–13. A, Percutaneous needle biopsy of cirrhotic liver shows fragmentation into a dozen pieces. Most of the fragments have curved edges, suggesting the fracture planes are at the margins of cirrhotic nodules. Regions at the arrow are enlarged in lower panels. **B,** Rounded edge with a circumferential rim of connective tissue. **C,** Connective tissue is often absent at the edge, but rounded shapes *(long arrows)* are suggestive of fracture at sites of fibrous septa. Fracture lines not occurring at fibrous septa are usually not curved but straight or irregular *(short arrow)* (Masson's trichrome).

Histologic Examination of the Liver Biopsy Specimen

Regardless of how a sample is obtained, biopsy specimens from patients with chronic liver disease are examined for lobular architecture (including the relationship between portal tracts and terminal hepatic veins), the degree of hepatocyte damage, and the degree of fibrosis, inflammatory infiltration, and parenchymal regeneration and nodule formation. To the extent that fibrous septa encompass regenerative nodules in the tissue sample, a definitive diagnosis of cirrhosis can be made. The pathologist must always be alert to the presence of hepatocellular carcinoma and its antecedent lesions.

Staging of Fibrosis

Many publications describe methods for semiquantitative estimation of fibrosis, as reviewed by Brunt.[116] Two staging systems are widely used for chronic hepatitis (METAVIR[117] and Ishak[118]), as are two different systems for chronic biliary disease (Scheuer[119] and Ludwig[120]). These systems vary in the number of

TABLE 37–2. Laënnec Scoring System for Grading Fibrosis in Liver Biopsy Specimens

Grade	Name	Criteria: Septa (thickness and number)	Descriptive Examples
0	No definite fibrosis		
1	Minimal fibrosis	+/−	No septa or rare thin septum; possible portal expansion or mild sinusoidal fibrosis
2	Mild fibrosis	+	Occasional thin septa; possible portal expansion or mild sinusoidal fibrosis
3	Moderate fibrosis	++	Moderate thin septa, up to incomplete cirrhosis
4A	Cirrhosis—mild, definite, or probable	+++	Market septation with rounded contours or visible nodules. Most septa are thin (one broad septum allowed)
4B	Moderate cirrhosis	++++	At least two broad septa, but no very broad septa; less than half of biopsy length composed of minute nodules
4C	Severe cirrhosis	+++++	At least one very broad septum; more than half of biopsy length composed of minute nodules (micronodular cirrhosis)

categories (0 to 4, 0 to 6, and 1 to 4) and in the definitions of the categories. These definitions include several qualitative histologic parameters, thereby introducing an opportunity for variation in interpretation. None of these systems acknowledges that cirrhosis may be mild or severe, although the Ishak system allows for evolving cirrhosis in its 0 to 6 scale for fibrosis.[118] All staging systems are empirically defined categories and are not necessarily linear with respect to rate of progression or clinical dysfunction.

The Laënnec system, presented in Table 37-2, offers a number of advantages.[121,122] This system is designed to be applied to all types of chronic liver disease. Thus, chronic hepatitis, fatty liver disease, hemochromatosis, and chronic biliary disease are all graded on a scale of 0 to 4, with cirrhosis assigned a grade of 4. In recognition of the variable degree of severity noted among cirrhotic livers, cirrhosis is divided into subgrades 4A, 4B, and 4C. The definitions of each grade are simplified to allow concentration on a single histologic parameter, that of the fibrous septum. Fibrous septa are graded according to their width and number. As a minor variation of the METAVIR system, the Laënnec system can easily be compared with historical data. The expanded scale allows detection of changes over time in patients with cirrhosis. Although it is not discussed here in detail, the Laënnec system also reports grade of activity on a scale of 0 to 4 and notes specific causative features.

Stage should be estimated with a connective tissue stain such as Masson's trichrome. The reticulin stain is useful for detecting delicate, highly resorbed septa. Curved contours help to confirm the presence of a septum when the lesion is otherwise indefinite. Biopsy reports should include comments on the size of the biopsy specimen and the degree of fragmentation noted.

Obliteration of portal and hepatic veins is an important element in chronic liver disease. When regressed cirrhosis occurs with no visible septa, detection of obliterated veins may help the clinician to distinguish it from normal liver tissue. Immunostain for CD34 may help in the detection of arterialized sinusoids that would otherwise appear normal. Fibrosis in the vicinity of neoplasms should be evaluated with caution because this may be a local reaction to the tumor.

DIFFERENTIAL DIAGNOSIS IN LIVER BIOPSY EVALUATION OF CIRRHOSIS

Three key clinical indications are required for biopsy of a presumed cirrhotic liver.

Establish or Exclude the Diagnosis of Cirrhosis. The first indication is to establish or exclude the diagnosis of cirrhosis. This requires consideration of the architecture of the liver, as has been discussed. The differential diagnosis for a patient with possible cirrhosis includes a lesser degree of fibrosis in a chronically diseased liver, and causes of noncirrhotic portal hypertension that include incomplete septal cirrhosis, hepatoportal sclerosis, and nodular regenerative hyperplasia. Criteria needed for establishing a diagnosis of cirrhosis, to the extent that it is possible to do so on the basis of a liver biopsy specimen, are discussed under Microscopic Features. A false-positive diagnosis is most likely to occur when a wedge liver biopsy is interpreted; a false-negative diagnosis is most likely to occur during interpretation of a biopsy specimen from a liver with macronodular cirrhosis. Nevertheless, a correct diagnosis can be achieved in more than 90% of cases.

Compared with cirrhosis, incomplete septal cirrhosis can be suggested when delicate fibrous septa link portal-to-portal and/or portal-to-central regions with evidence of some spherical deformation of the liver parenchyma on reticulin stain. In particular, portal tracts and terminal hepatic veins in close approximation and linked by fibrous septa are seen in incomplete septal cirrhosis. Hepatoportal sclerosis is suggested by the presence of essentially normal parenchymal architecture with portal tracts that are expanded by dense sclerotic tissue and in which portal veins are difficult to identify. Nodular regenerative hyperplasia is suggested by essentially normal portal tracts, but with definitive nodular transformation of the parenchyma without fibrosis. On hematoxylin and eosin stain, this is evident as alternating areas of hypertrophied and atrophic hepatocytes; on reticulin stain, curvilinear atrophic liver cell plates appear to surround disorganized hypertrophied plates.

Seek a Cause. The second reason for liver biopsy of a cirrhotic liver is to seek a cause; this is a difficult exercise. When a cause has not been established on clinical grounds before biopsy, the pathologist has only a limited ability to determine cause on the basis of the end-stage cirrhotic liver tissue. In adults, obvious opportunity arises for diagnosing hereditary hemochromatosis (*HFE* disease) and alpha-1-antitrypsin deficiency. More difficult is the identification of viral hepatitis, autoimmune hepatitis, drug toxicity, alcoholic liver disease, nonalcoholic fatty liver disease, Wilson's disease, and other forms of biliary disease as an underlying cause. The characteristic histologic features, which are often obliterated by the time cirrhosis develops, are nonspecific. An approach to liver biopsy in childhood liver disease is presented in Chapter 41.

Evaluate a Mass Lesion. The third reason for liver biopsy of a cirrhotic liver is evaluation of a mass lesion. Chapter 42 discusses the differential assessment of benign cirrhotic nodules, dysplastic foci and nodules, and hepatocellular carcinoma in the cirrhotic liver.

References

1. Crawford JM: Cirrhosis. In MacSween RNM, Anthony PP, Scheuer PJ, et al (eds): Pathology of the Liver, 4th ed. New York, Churchill Livingstone, 2002, pp 575-619.
2. Ohara N, Schaffner T, Reichen J: Structure-function relationship in secondary biliary cirrhosis in the rat. Stereologic and hemodynamic characterization of a model. J Hepatol 17:155-162, 1993.
3. Friedman SL: Seminars in medicine of the Beth Israel Hospital, Boston: The cellular basis of hepatic fibrosis—mechanisms and treatment strategies. N Engl J Med 328:1828-1835, 1993.
4. Mathew J, Geerts A, Burt AD: Pathobiology of hepatic stellate cells. Hepatogastroenterology 43:72-91, 1996.
5. Friedman SL, Maher JJ, Bissell DM: Mechanisms and therapy of hepatic fibrosis: Report of the AASLD Single Topic Basic Research Conference. Hepatology 32:1403-1408, 2000.
6. Arthur MJ, Iredale JP, Mann DA: Tissue inhibitors of metalloproteinases: Role in liver fibrosis and alcoholic liver disease. Alcohol Clin Exp Res 23:940-943, 1999.
7. Enzan H, Himeno H, Iwamura S, et al: Sequential changes in human Ito cells and their relation to postnecrotic liver fibrosis in massive and submassive hepatic necrosis. Virchows Arch Int J Pathol 426:95-101, 1995.
8. Iredale JP: Hepatic stellate cell behavior during resolution of liver injury. Semin Liver Dis 21:427-436, 2001.
9. Kinnman N, Francoz C, Barbu V, et al: The myofibroblastic conversion of peribiliary fibrogenic cells distinct from hepatic stellate cells is stimulated by platelet-derived growth factor during liver fibrogenesis. Lab Invest 83:163-173, 2003.
10. Tuchweber B, Desmoulière A, Costa AM, et al: Myofibroblastic differentiation and extracellular matrix deposition in early stages of cholestatic fibrosis in rat liver. Curr Top Pathol 93:103-109, 1999.
11. Tuchweber B, Desmoulière A, Bochaton-Piallat ML, et al: Proliferation and phenotypic modulation of portal fibroblasts in the early stages of cholestatic fibrosis in the rat. Lab Invest 74:265-278, 1996.
12. Tang L, Tanaka Y, Marumo F, Sato C: Phenotypic change in portal fibroblasts in biliary fibrosis. Liver 14:76-82, 1994.
13. Wanless IR, Nakashima E, Sherman M: Regression of human cirrhosis: Morphologic features and the genesis of incomplete septal cirrhosis. Arch Pathol Lab Med 124:1599-1607, 2000.
14. Wanless IR, Shimamatsu K: Phlebitis in viral and autoimmune chronic hepatitis and primary biliary cirrhosis. Possible role in the histogenesis of cirrhosis. Mod Pathol 10:147A, 1997.
15. Wanless IR, Shiota K, Heathcote EJ: Role of hepatic vein obliteration in the progression of non-alcoholic steatohepatitis (NASH) to cirrhosis. Hepatology 36:730A, 2002.
16. Murata K, Ochiai Y, Akaashio K: Polydispersity of acidic glycosaminoglycan components in human liver and the changes at different stages in liver cirrhosis. Gastroenterology 89:1249-1257, 1985.
17. Martinez-Hernandez A, Martinez J: The role of capillarization in hepatic failure: Studies in carbon tetrachloride–induced cirrhosis. Hepatology 14:864-874, 1991.
18. James J, Bosch KS, Zuyderhoudt FM, et al: Histophotometric estimation of volume density of collagen as an indication of fibrosis in rat liver. Histochemistry 85:129-133, 1986.
19. Williams R, Smith P, Spicer E, et al: Venesection therapy in idiopathic haemochromatosis. Q J Med 38:1-16, 1969.
20. Bunton GL, Cameron GR: Regeneration of liver after biliary cirrhosis. Ann N Y Acad Sci 111:412-421, 1963.
21. Yeong ML, Nicholson GI, Lee SP: Regression of biliary cirrhosis following choledochal cyst drainage. Gastroenterology 82:332-335, 1982.
22. Powell LW, Kerr JF: Reversal of "cirrhosis" in idiopathic haemochromatosis following long-term intensive venesection therapy. Aust Ann Med 19:54-57, 1970.
23. Blumberg RS, Chopra S, Ibrahim R, et al: Primary hepatocellular carcinoma in idiopathic hemochromatosis after reversal of cirrhosis. Gastroenterology 95:1399-1402, 1988.
24. Dufour JF, DeLellis R, Kaplan MM: Reversibility of hepatic fibrosis in autoimmune hepatitis. Ann Intern Med 127:981-985, 1997.
25. Falkmer S, Samuelson G, Sjolin S: Penicillamine-induced normalization of clinical signs, and liver morphology and histochemistry in a case of Wilson's disease. Pediatrics 45:260-268, 1970.
26. Kaplan MM, DeLellis RA, Wolfe HJ: Sustained biochemical and histologic remission of primary biliary cirrhosis in response to medical treatment. Ann Intern Med 126:682-688, 1997.
27. Dunn MA, Cheever AW, Paglia LM, et al: Reversal of advanced liver fibrosis in rabbits with Schistosomiasis japonica. Am J Trop Med Hyg 50:499-505, 1994.
28. Greenwel P, Geerts A, Ogata I, et al: Liver fibrosis. In Arias I, Boyer J, Fausto N, et al (eds): The Liver: Biology and Pathobiology, 3rd ed. New York, Raven, 1994, pp 1367-1381.
29. Wanless IR, Godwin TA, Allen F, et al: Nodular regenerative hyperplasia of the liver in hematologic disorders: A possible response to obliterative venopathy. Medicine 59:367-379, 1980.
30. Barnett JL, Appelman HD, Moseley RH: A familial form of incomplete septal cirrhosis. Gastroenterology 102:674-678, 1992.
31. Sciot R, Staessen D, Van Damme B, et al: Incomplete septal cirrhosis: Histopathological aspects. Histopathology 13:593-603, 1988.
32. Wanless IR, Lentz JS, Roberts EA: Partial nodular transformation of liver in an adult with persistent ductus venosus. Arch Pathol Lab Med 109:427-432, 1985.
33. Wanless IR, Mawdsley C, Adams R: On the pathogenesis of focal nodular hyperplasia of the liver. Hepatology 5:1194-1200, 1985.
34. Rappaport AM, MacPhee PJ, Fisher MM, et al: The scarring of the liver acini (cirrhosis). Tridimensional and microcirculatory considerations. Virchows Arch A 402:107-137, 1983.

35. Arias IM: The biology of hepatic endothelial cell fenestrae. Prog Liver Dis 9:11-26, 1990.
36. Mori T, Okanoue T, Sawa Y, et al: Defenestration of the sinusoidal endothelial cell in a rat model of cirrhosis. Hepatology 17:891-897, 1993.
37. Picchiotti R, Mingazzini PL, Scucchi L, et al: Correlations between sinusoidal pressure and liver morphology in cirrhosis. J Hepatol 20:364-369, 1994.
38. Sherman IA, Pappas SC, Fisher MM: Hepatic microvascular changes associated with development of liver fibrosis and cirrhosis. Am J Physiol 258:H460-H465, 1990.
39. Gaiani S, Bolondi L, Li Bassi S, et al: Prevalence of spontaneous hepatofugal portal flow in liver cirrhosis. Clinical and endoscopic correlation in 228 patients. Gastroenterology 100:160-167, 1991.
40. Hou PC, McFadzean AJS: Thrombosis and intimal thickening in the portal system in cirrhosis of the liver. J Pathol Bact 89:473-480, 1965.
41. Goodman ZD, Ishak KG: Occlusive venous lesions in alcoholic liver disease. A study of 200 cases. Gastroenterology 83:786-796, 1982.
42. Nakanuma Y, Ohta G, Doishita K: Quantitation and serial section observations of focal venocclusive lesions of hepatic veins in liver cirrhosis. Virchows Arch A 405:429-438, 1985.
43. Burt AD, MacSween RN: Hepatic vein lesions in alcoholic liver disease: Retrospective biopsy and necropsy study. J Clin Pathol 39:63-67, 1986.
44. Wanless IR, Wong F, Blendis LM, et al: Hepatic and portal vein thrombosis in cirrhosis: Possible role in development of parenchymal extinction and portal hypertension. Hepatology 21:1238-1247, 1995.
45. Rubin EM, Martin AA, Thung SN, et al: Morphometric and immunohistochemical characterization of human liver regeneration. Am J Pathol 147:397-404, 1995.
46. Gerber MA, Thung SN: Liver stem cells and development. Lab Invest 68:253-254, 1993.
47. Gerber MA, Thung SN, Sirica AE (eds): The role of cell types in hepatocarcinogenesis. In Cell Lineages in Human Liver Development, Regeneration, and Transformation. Boca Raton, CRC Press, 1992, pp 209-226.
48. Grisham JW: Migration of hepatocytes along hepatic plates and stem cell-fed hepatocyte lineages. Am J Pathol 144:849-854, 1994.
49. Ross MA, Sander CM, Kleeb TB, et al: Spatiotemporal expression of angiogenesis growth factor receptors during the revascularization of regenerating rat liver. Hepatology 34:1135-1148, 2001.
50. Masuko K, Rubin E, Popper H: Proliferation of bile ducts in cirrhosis. Arch Pathol Lab Med 78:421-431, 1964.
51. Crosby HA, Hubscher S, Fabris L, et al: Immunolocalization of putative human liver progenitor cells in livers from patients with end-stage primary biliary cirrhosis and sclerosing cholangitis using the monoclonal antibody OV-6. Am J Pathol 152:771-779, 1998.
52. Theise ND, Saxena R, Portmann BC, et al: The canals of Hering and hepatic stem cells in humans. Hepatology 30:1425-1433, 1999.
53. Kossor DC, Meunier PC, Dulik DM, et al: Bile duct obstruction is not a prerequisite for type 1 biliary epithelial cell hyperplasia. Toxicol Appl Pharmacol 152:327-338, 1998.
54. Nakano M, Lieber CS: Ultrastructure of initial stages of perivenular fibrosis in alcohol-fed baboons. Am J Pathol 106:145-155, 1982.
55. Nakano M, Worner TM, Lieber CS: Perivenular fibrosis in alcoholic liver injury: Ultrastructure and histologic progression. Gastroenterology 83:777-785, 1982.
56. Sokal EM, Trivedi P, Portmann B, et al: Adaptive changes of metabolic zonation during the development of cirrhosis in growing rats. Gastroenterology 99:785-792, 1990.
57. Gumucio JJ, Chianale J: Liver cell heterogeneity and liver function. In Arias IM, Jakoby WB, Popper H, et al (eds): The Liver: Biology and Pathobiology, 2nd ed. New York, Raven Press, 1988, pp 931-947.
58. Racine-Samson L, Scoazec JY, D'Errico A, et al: The metabolic organization of the adult human liver: A comparative study of normal, fibrotic, and cirrhotic liver tissue. Hepatology 24:104-113, 1996.
59. Gebhardt R, Reichen J: Changes in distribution and activity of glutamine synthetase in carbon tetrachloride-induced cirrhosis in the rat: Potential role in hyperammonemia. Hepatology 20:684-691, 1994.
60. Reference deleted.
61. Sokal EM, Collette E, Buts JP: Persistence of a liver metabolic zonation in extra-hepatic biliary atresia cirrhotic livers. Pediatr Res 30:286-289, 1991.
62. Racine-Samson L, Scoazec JY, D'Errico A, et al: The metabolic organization of the adult human liver: A comparative study of normal, fibrotic, and cirrhotic liver tissue. Hepatology 24:104-113, 1996.
63. Wanless IR, Liu JJ, Butany J: Role of thrombosis in the pathogenesis of congestive hepatic fibrosis (cardiac cirrhosis). Hepatology 21:1232-1237, 1995.
64. Popper H: Pathologic aspects of cirrhosis. Am J Pathol 87:228-264, 1977.
65. Anthony PP, Ishak KG, Nayak NC, et al: The morphology of cirrhosis. Recommendations on definition, nomenclature, and classification by a working group sponsored by the World Health Organization. J Clin Pathol 31:395-414, 1978.
66. Moragas A, Allende H, Sans M, et al: Mathematical morphologic analysis of liver cirrhosis: Correlation with etiology, clinical score and hepatocellular carcinoma. Anal Quant Cytol Histol 14:483-490, 1992.
67. Wanless IR, Wong F, Blendis LM, et al: Hepatic and portal vein thrombosis in cirrhosis: Possible role in development of parenchymal extinction and portal hypertension. Hepatology 21:1238-1247, 1995.
68. Sciot R, Staessen D, Van Damme B, et al: Incomplete septal cirrhosis: Histopathological aspects. Histopathology 13:593-603, 1988.
69. Nevens F, Staessen D, Sciot R, et al: Clinical aspects of incomplete septal cirrhosis in comparison with macronodular cirrhosis. Gastroenterology 106:459-463, 1994.
70. Nakashima E, Kage M, Wanless IR: Idiopathic portal hypertension: Histologic evidence that some cases may be regressed cirrhosis with portal vein thrombosis. Hepatology 30:218A, 1999.
71. Fauerholdt L, Schlichting P, Christensen E, et al: Conversion of micronodular cirrhosis into macronodular cirrhosis. Hepatology 3:928-931, 1983.
72. Popper H, Rubin E, Krus S, et al: Postnecrotic cirrhosis in alcoholics. Gastroenterology 39:669, 1960.
73. Gall EA: Posthepatitic, postnecrotic, and nutritional cirrhosis. A pathologic analysis. Am J Pathol 36:241-258, 1960.
74. Wanless IR, International Working Party, Crawford JM: Terminology of nodular hepatocellular lesions. Hepatology 22:983-993, 1995.
75. Popper H, Ingelfinger F, Relman A, et al (eds): What Are the Major Types of Hepatic Cirrhosis? Controversies in Internal Medicine. Philadelphia, WB Saunders, 1966, p 233.
76. Sciot R, Staessen D, Van Damme B, et al: Incomplete septal cirrhosis: Histopathological aspects. Histopathology 13:593-603, 1988.
77. Brunt EM: Alcoholic and nonalcoholic steatohepatitis. Clin Liver Dis 6:399-420, 2002.
78. Teli MR, James OF, Burt AD, et al: The natural history of non-alcoholic fatty liver: A follow-up study. Hepatology 22:1714-1719, 1995.
79. Diehl AM, Goodman Z, Ishak KG: Alcohol-like liver disease in nonalcoholics. A clinical and histologic comparison with alcohol-induced liver injury. Gastroenterology 95:1056-1062, 1988.
80. Ludwig J: The pathology of primary biliary cirrhosis and autoimmune cholangitis. Baillieres Best Pract Res Clin Gastroenterol 14:601-613, 2000.
81. Raweily EA, Gibson AA, Burt AD: Abnormalities of intrahepatic bile ducts in extrahepatic biliary atresia. Histopathology 17:521-527, 1990.
82. Desmet VJ: Ludwig symposium on biliary disorders—part I. Pathogenesis of ductal plate abnormalities. Mayo Clin Proc 73:80-89, 1998.
83. Crawford JM: Development of the intrahepatic biliary tree. Semin Liver Dis 22:213-226, 2002.
84. Tan CE, Davenport M, Driver M, et al: Does the morphology of the extrahepatic biliary remnants in biliary atresia influence survival? A review of 205 cases. J Pediatr Surg 29:1459-1464, 1994.
85. Low Y, Vijayhan V, Tan CEL: The prognostic value of ductal plate malformation and other histologic parameters in biliary atresia: An immunohistochemical study. J Pediatr 139:320-322, 2001.
86. Feigelson J, Anagnostopoulos C, Poquet M, et al: Liver cirrhosis in cystic fibrosis—therapeutic implications and long term follow up. Arch Dis Child 68:653-657, 1993.

87. Britton RS, Fleming RE, Parkkila S, et al: Pathogenesis of hereditary hemochromatosis: Genetics and beyond. Semin Gastrointest Dis 13:68-79, 2002.
88. Andrews NC: Metal transporters and disease. Curr Opin Chem Biol 6:181-186, 2002.
89. Loréal O, Deugnier Y, Moirand R, et al: Liver fibrosis in genetic hemochromatosis. Respective roles of iron and non-iron-related factors in 127 homozygous patients. J Hepatol 16:122-127, 1992.
90. LeSage GD, Baldus WP, Fairbanks VF, et al: Hemochromatosis: Genetic or alcohol-induced? Gastroenterology 84:1471-1477, 1983.
91. Elzouki AN, Hulterantz R, Stal P, et al: Increased PiZ gene frequency for alpha 1 antitrypsin in patients with genetic haemochromatosis. Gut 36:922-926, 1995.
92. Angelucci E, Muretto P, Nicolucci A, et al: Effects of iron overload and hepatitis C virus positivity in determining progression of liver fibrosis in thalassemia following bone marrow transplantation. Blood 100:17-21, 2002.
93. Terada T, Nakanuma Y: Survey of iron-accumulative macroregenerative nodules in cirrhotic livers. Hepatology 10:851-854, 1989.
94. Terada T, Kadoya M, Nakanuma Y, et al: Iron-accumulating adenomatous hyperplastic nodule with malignant foci in the cirrhotic liver: Histopathologic, quantitative iron, and magnetic resonance imaging in vitro studies. Cancer 65:1994-2000, 1990.
95. Murakami T, Nakamura H, Hori S, et al: CT and MRI of siderotic regenerating nodules in hepatic cirrhosis. J Comput Assist Tomogr 16:578-582, 1992.
96. Elmes ME, Clarkson JP, Mahy NJ, et al: Metallothionein and copper in liver disease with copper retention—a histopathological study. J Pathol 158:131-137, 1989.
97. Sen BC: Enlargement of the liver in children. Indian Med Gaz 22:343, 1887.
98. Muller-Hocker J, Meyer U, Wiebecke B, et al: Copper storage disease of the liver and chronic dietary copper intoxication in two further German infants mimicking Indian childhood cirrhosis. Pathol Res Pract 183:39-45, 1987.
99. Lefkowitch J, Honig C, King M, et al: Hepatic copper overload and features of Indian childhood cirrhosis in an American sibship. N Engl J Med 307:271-277, 1982.
100. Maggiore G, De Giacomo C, Sessa F, et al: Idiopathic copper toxicosis in a child. J Pediatr Gastroenterol Nutr 6:980-983, 1987.
101. Adamson M, Reiner B, Olson JL, et al: Indian childhood cirrhosis in an American child. Gastroenterology 102:1771-1777, 1992.
102. Tanaka M, Wanless IR: Pathology of the liver in Budd-Chiari syndrome: Portal vein thrombosis and the histogenesis of venocentric cirrhosis, veno-portal cirrhosis, and large regenerative nodules. Hepatology 27:488-496, 1998.
103. Klintmalm GB: Liver transplantation for hepatocellular carcinoma: A registry report of the impact of tumor characteristics on outcome. Ann Surg 228:479-490, 1998.
104. Scheuer PJ: Liver biopsy in the diagnosis of cirrhosis. Gut 11:275-278, 1970.
105. Sherlock S: Diseases of the Liver and Biliary System, 8th ed. London, Blackwell Scientific Publications, 1989, p 36.
106. Soloway RD, Baggenstoss AH, Schoenfield LJ, et al: Observer error and sampling variability tested in evaluation of hepatitis and cirrhosis by liver biopsy. Am J Dig Dis 16:1082-1086, 1971.
107. Petrelli M, Scheuer PJ: Variation in subcapsular liver structure and its significance in the interpretation of wedge biopsies. J Clin Pathol 20:743-748, 1967.
108. Ansell ID: The uses of liver biopsy. Postgrad Med J 45:202-207, 1969.
109. Hopper KD, Baird DE, Reddy VV, et al: Efficacy of automated biopsy guns versus conventional biopsy needles in the pygmy pig. Radiology 176:671-676, 1990.
110. Abdi W, Millan JC, Mezey E: Sampling variability on percutaneous liver biopsy. Arch Intern Med 139:667-669, 1979.
111. Nakamura T, Nakamura S, Aikawa T, et al: Morphological classification of liver cirrhosis based upon measurement of per cent of interstitial tissue in liver biopsy specimens. Tohoku J Exp Med 87:110-122, 1965.
112. Buschmann RJ, Ryoo JW: Hepatic structural correlates of liver fibrosis: A morphometric analysis. Exp Mol Pathol 50:114-124, 1989.
113. Ryoo JW, Buschmann RJ: Comparison of intralobar non-parenchyma, subcapsular non-parenchyma, and liver capsule thickness. J Clin Pathol 42:740-744, 1978.
114. Crawford AR, Lin XZ, Crawford JM: The normal adult human liver biopsy: A quantitative reference standard. Hepatology 28:323-331, 1998.
115. Sawyerr AM, McCormick PA, Tennyson GS, et al: A comparison of transjugular and plugged-percutaneous liver biopsy in patients with impaired coagulation. J Hepatol 17:81-85, 1993.
116. Brunt EM: Grading and staging the histopathological lesions of chronic hepatitis: The Knodell histology activity index and beyond. Hepatology 31:241-246, 2000.
117. Poynard T, Bedossa P, Opolon P: Natural history of liver fibrosis progression in patients with chronic hepatitis C. The OBSVIRC, METAVIR, CLINIVIR, and DOSVIRC groups. Lancet 349:825-832, 1997.
118. Ishak K, Baptista A, Bianchi L, et al: Histological grading and staging of chronic hepatitis. J Hepatol 22:696-699, 1995.
119. Scheuer P: Primary biliary cirrhosis. Proc R Soc Med 60:1257-1260, 1967.
120. Ludwig J: Etiology of biliary cirrhosis: Diagnostic features and a new classification. Zentralbl Allg Pathol 134:132-141, 1988.
121. Kutami R, Girgrah N, Wanless IR, et al: The Laennec grading system for assessment of hepatic fibrosis: Validation by correlation with wedged hepatic vein pressure and clinical features. Hepatology 32:407A.
122. Wanless IR, Sweeney G, Dhillon AP, et al: Lack of progressive hepatic fibrosis during long-term therapy with deferiprone in subjects with transfusion-dependent beta-thalassemia. Blood 100:1566-1569, 2002.

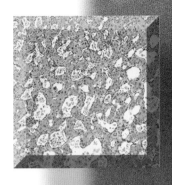

CHAPTER 38

Vascular Disorders of the Liver

IAN R. WANLESS

◼ Introduction

The vasculature of the liver is unique in that it has two afferent supplies—arterial and splanchnic. This arrangement is responsible for the great variety of histologic patterns produced by vascular compromise. The pattern is a reflection of the number and size of vessels involved and whether obstruction is rapidly or slowly progressive. These parameters are determined by the primary disease process. In most liver diseases, the primary injury affects hepatocytes or duct cells, and the vascular damage is secondary. However, there are many primary disorders of the hepatic vasculature, and these are the focus of this chapter.

The clinical presentation of hepatic vascular obstruction varies with the location of the block. Obstruction of portal veins is usually silent initially, but if severe it leads to varices, generally without ascites or liver failure. Obstruction of hepatic arteries is usually silent but may produce necrosis of hepatocytes or bile ducts if combined with hypotension or another vascular lesion or if it occurs in the post-transplant state. Obstruction of hepatic veins tends to cause increased formation of hepatic lymph, leading to ascites and, if severe, to splanchnic varices and hepatic failure. Diseases involving hepatic vein obstruction usually result in cirrhosis (see Chapter 37).

Hepatocytes can manifest two levels of ischemic injury. Atrophy is a reduction in cell size that occurs in response to mild ischemia; it is typically seen with pure portal vein obstruction or mild outflow obstruction. If additional obstruction involves the hepatic vein or

artery in the same region, cell death occurs. Primary obstruction of the hepatic veins also leads to hepatocellular death. After hepatocytes die, local collapse of the tissue usually occurs with secondary fibrosis, a lesion called *extinction*. When extinction is widespread, the accumulated lesions are recognized as cirrhosis (see Chapter 37 for greater detail). If widespread atrophy is noted without fibrosis, regenerative changes of better-vascularized areas lead to hepatocellular nodules that are separated by regions of atrophy, yielding two major patterns—nodular regenerative hyperplasia when the nodules are small and diffuse, and large regenerative nodules when the pattern is more heterogeneous.

Vascular disease also has a direct effect on bile duct epithelial cells. Arterial compromise is particularly important in that bile ducts derive their vascular supply exclusively from arteries. The most dramatic example is occlusion of the hepatic artery following liver transplantation, which leads to necrosis of the major bile ducts. Discerning the causative role of ischemia in bile duct disease in the native liver has been more difficult.

The position of the liver between the capillary bed of the intestines and the heart accounts for the important clinical effects of portal hypertension caused by obstruction of blood vessels in the liver. Portal hypertension is commonly classified as cirrhotic or noncirrhotic according to the histology of the liver parenchyma. Before 1945, approximately 40% of patients with portal hypertension were thought to have noncirrhotic portal hypertension.[1] In recent years, that percentage has dropped to less than 1%. The decline in noncirrhotic portal hypertension is largely due to improved diagnosis of cirrhosis. This explanation was recognized after the discovery that cirrhosis is largely reversible after successful treatment of primary liver disease, as can be provided by antiviral agents or abstinence from alcohol.[2-5] Thus, formerly cirrhotic patients may have subsequent biopsy specimens that lack the histologic criteria for diagnosis of cirrhosis. These patients often continue to have portal hypertension because regeneration of portal and hepatic veins lags behind the resorption of bridging fibrous septa. These patients with regressed cirrhosis then fall into the category of hepatic vascular disease; thus, they merit discussion in this chapter.

Vascular disease is often classified according to the size and type of the vessels involved. This is useful because various etiologic types of liver disease target different portions of the vasculature. However, thrombi can propagate and hepatic vein obstruction can lead to secondary portal vein thrombosis, so histologic classification is often mixed.

Although hepatic vessels have some unique properties, they respond to stress in ways that are similar to those of other organs. Thus, the cause of hepatic vascular disease can usefully be considered in terms of the elements of Virchow's triad—vascular injury, obstruction, and hypercoagulable states. This formulation is used in the discussion of hepatic vascular disease that follows.

▋ Portal Vein Disease (Portal Vein Obstruction)

CLINICAL FEATURES

Most adult patients with large portal vein obstruction have symptomatic cirrhosis, and the portal vein lesion is discovered during imaging studies. In the absence of cirrhosis, large portal vein obstruction is asymptomatic until the onset of bleeding varices; ascites is usually absent. During the asymptomatic period, evidence of portal hypertension, especially splenomegaly or thrombocytopenia, often leads to diagnosis through imaging studies. The portal vein may appear to be absent, or multiple local collaterals may provide an appearance called *cavernous transformation*. Large collaterals develop in the round ligament in 5% of patients; rarely, this presents with a bruit or an umbilical caput medusa. Round ligament collaterals represent dilated paraumbilical veins that communicate with the left portal vein. Large collaterals between the extrahepatic portal vein and the renal or adrenal veins are frequent. Numerous smaller collaterals are seen during imaging or abdominal surgery. Secondary aneurysmal dilatation of the portal vein may occur.

In contrast to this indolent natural history, acute portal vein obstruction accompanied by thrombosis of

the mesenteric veins may be catastrophic, leading to infarction of the intestines. This sequence often occurs in a setting of abdominal sepsis, trauma with vascular injury, cirrhosis, or growth of hepatocellular carcinoma into the main portal vein.

The portal vein branches are hypoplastic in patients with persistent ductus venosus or in those with other congenital anomalies of the major vessels. Hepatic encephalopathy with hyperammonemia may be a presenting feature when portosystemic shunting is prominent.

Obstruction confined to the small portal veins is a rare cause of portal hypertension that tends to be milder than that seen with large portal vein block. Features of the causative disease usually dominate the clinical appearance.

PATHOGENESIS

Thrombosis is the most frequent mechanism of large portal vein obstruction. Following from Virchow's triad, thrombosis is usually secondary to obstruction, venous inflammation, or a hypercoagulable state (Tables 38-1 through 38-3). Obstruction usually occurs secondary to cirrhosis but may be related to tumor in the hepatic hilum or pancreas, or to small portal vein disease in

TABLE 38–1. Hypercoagulable States Associated With Large Venous Obstruction in the Liver

	References	
Hypercoagulable State	Portal Vein Thrombosis	Hepatic Vein Thrombosis
Myeloproliferative Disease		
Latent myeloproliferative disease	99–101	100–102
Polycythemia vera	99, 103, 104	105
Agnogenic myeloid metaplasia	99, 104	104
Paroxysmal nocturnal hemoglobinuria	99, 106	107–109
Idiopathic thrombocytosis	99, 110, 111	
Chronic myeloid leukemia	112	113
Promyelocytic leukemia		114, 115
Multiple myeloma		116
Genetic Anomalies		
Protein C deficiency	117–119	101, 120
Protein S deficiency	119, 121–123	101
Antithrombin III deficiency	124	125, 126
Factor II G20201A	127	128, 129
Factor V Leiden	101, 130	101, 131
Heparin cofactor II deficiency	132	
Plasminogen deficiency		133
Dysfibrinogenemia		134
Other Hypercoagulable States		
Pregnancy	135	136
Oral contraceptive therapy	137	105, 138–140
Lupus anticoagulant or antiphospholipid antibodies	141	74, 101, 142–149
Idiopathic thrombocytopenic purpura		105

TABLE 38–2. Tumors and Other Stasis Lesions Associated With Large Venous Obstruction in the Liver

Tumor/Lesion	References Portal Vein Thrombosis or Obstruction	References Hepatic Vein Thrombosis
Tumors		
Hepatocellular carcinoma	106, 150	151, 152
Carcinoma of pancreas	153, 154	
Renal cell carcinoma		155
Adrenal carcinoma		156
Hodgkin's disease		157
Epithelioid hemangioendothelioma		158
Wilms' tumor		159
Leiomyosarcoma or leiomyoma		152, 160–162
Metastatic neoplasm		152
Other Stasis Lesions		
Cirrhosis	150, 163–165	166
Primary biliary cirrhosis	167	
Primary sclerosing cholangitis		
Splenectomy	168, 169	
Retroperitoneal fibrosis	170	
Congestive heart failure		166
Constrictive pericarditis		171, 172
Membranous obstruction of inferior vena cava		173, 174
Obstruction of superior vena cava		175
Other congenital anomalies		176, 177
Umbilical cord redundancy or placental thrombosis		178
Portal vein atresia or absence		
Atrial myxoma		179
Sickle cell disease		180
Hydatid cyst		181
Hepatic abscess		182, 183
Hematoma		184

TABLE 38–3. Vascular Injury and Inflammatory Conditions Associated With Large Venous Obstruction in the Liver

Condition	References Portal Vein Thrombosis	References Hepatic Vein Thrombosis
Behçet's disease	185	185–187
Trauma	1, 188	189–193
Catheterization	194	195
Sarcoidosis	196, 197	198, 199
Umbilical sepsis	112	
Pylephlebitis	103, 200–202	
Congenital hepatic fibrosis	185, 203, 204	
Cytomegalovirus infection	205	
Hematopoietic cell transplantation	206	
Esophageal sclerotherapy	207, 208	
Schistosomiasis	209	
Inflammatory bowel disease	210–212	
Ventriculoatrial shunt		213
Sclerotherapy		207
Amyloidosis		214
Vasculitis or tissue inflammation		176
Tuberculosis		215
Fungal vasculitis		216, 217
Idiopathic granulomatous venulitis		218
Filariasis		219
Inflammatory bowel disease		166, 220, 221
Mixed connective tissue disease		222
Protein-losing enteropathy		223, 224
Celiac disease		225
5q–syndrome and hypereosinophilia		226

early primary biliary cirrhosis. Vascular injury may be caused by hilar bile leak in primary sclerosing cholangitis or post-transplant biliary necrosis, splanchnic sepsis, variceal sclerotherapy, or trauma. Trauma may be blunt abdominal injury or surgical intervention, as occurs with splenectomy, umbilical vein catheterization, portacaval shunt, transjugular intrahepatic portosystemic shunt (TIPS) insertion, or the Kasai procedure. Hypercoagulable states may be inherited abnormalities of the clotting cascade or acquired abnormalities of the platelets, as in polycythemia vera and other myeloproliferative diseases (see Table 38-1). Coincidental hypercoagulable states have been documented to contribute to thrombosis when underlying cirrhosis is noted.[6]

Agenesis of the portal vein and large spontaneous shunts may be associated with other congenital anomalies.[7] In patients with cirrhosis, large-caliber shunts are usually placed secondary to portal hypertension. Arterial shunts are considered with arterial diseases.

Obliteration of small portal veins (obliterative portal venopathy) may develop after thrombus propagates from larger veins, or it may occur secondary to local inflammation in the portal tracts in any chronic disease, including primary biliary cirrhosis, primary sclerosing cholangitis, sarcoidosis, polyarteritis nodosa, and congenital hepatic fibrosis. A variety of vasculotoxins, including azathioprine, cyclophosphamide, methotrexate, and arsenic, may be responsible. In some geographic regions, schistosomiasis is the most frequent cause of portal vein disease and portal hypertension.

PATHOLOGIC FEATURES

Portal vein thrombus is usually seen in the healed state after recanalization and fibrosis have occurred. The healing process may be nearly complete such that no residual changes or only slight pearly thickening of the intima may be seen grossly. In other instances, residual high-grade obstruction may cause marked intraluminal fibrosis involving numerous racemose channels (Fig. 38-1). Thrombi in large and medium-sized portal veins may recanalize almost completely,

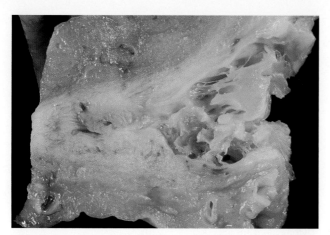

FIGURE 38–1. Organized portal vein thrombosis near the bifurcation with numerous recanalized channels and subtotal obstruction of the lumen. This appearance has been called *cavernous transformation.*

leaving a layer of residual intimal fibrosis (Fig. 38-2), or they may remain largely occluded (Fig. 38-3). Multiple layers of collagen indicate recurrent thrombosis. As thrombi heal with a granulation tissue response, small arteries are often seen within the neointima. When thrombosis or inflammatory injury involves small portal veins, the vein walls usually disappear completely within a few weeks of the event. An elastic and connective tissue stain, such as the elastic trichrome, is useful for identifying the residua of vein walls. (Masson's trichrome stain alone is also informative.) Muscle bundles may mark the location of the vein (see Fig. 38-3), especially if muscular hyperplasia is present.

After organization of a thrombotic or inflammatory event, obliterated small portal veins have a nonspecific appearance, but several clues may indicate the origin of the lesions. Portal granulomas may be seen in sarcoidosis and primary biliary cirrhosis; duct paucity favors the latter (Fig. 38-4). Granulomas in sarcoidosis are usually numerous, but in burned-out disease, they may resorb, making diagnosis difficult. Eggs of *Schistosoma* species may occur with or without granulomatous inflammation (Fig. 38-5). These eggs are few with *Schistosoma mansoni* and numerous with *Schistosoma japonicum.* Active or healed arteritis may suggest polyarteritis nodosa or another rheumatologic condition. Irregular and dilated ducts are found in most portal tracts in congenital hepatic fibrosis and in occasional portal tracts in polycystic disease of the liver and/or kidney. Thorotrast deposits in portal macrophages may be associated with obliteration of small portal veins and noncirrhotic portal hypertension (Fig. 38-6). If marked parenchymal congestion and/or obstruction of hepatic veins is noted, the portal vein block is likely secondary to stasis with thrombosis.

Patients with noncirrhotic portal hypertension usually have portal vein intimal fibrosis and delicate septa, suggesting regressed cirrhosis and superimposed portal vein thrombosis.[8] The patients with noncirrhotic portal hypertension reported under the term *hepatoportal sclerosis*[9] probably had portal vein thrombosis (see further discussion in Chapter 37). After portal vein obliteration, the parenchyma becomes atrophic with crowding of portal tracts. There may be a localized region of sinusoidal dilatation called an infarct of Zahn (see under Sinusoidal Dilatation). Atrophy may be uniform or mixed with small regenerative nodules in a pattern called *nodular regenerative hyperplasia* (see later).

DIFFERENTIAL DIAGNOSIS

The diagnosis of portal vein disease does not rest on histologic appearance alone but requires consideration of clinical and imaging information. The most useful task in a patient with portal hypertension is to confirm the presence or absence of cirrhosis, including regressed cirrhosis. This allows investigation to be directed at likely causative agents. Biopsy specimen size is important in giving the pathologist the confidence to exclude cirrhosis. Cirrhosis, particularly when highly regressed, is frequently missed when biopsy specimens are shorter than 2 cm. Regressed cirrhosis is suggested by reduction in both portal and hepatic veins, delicate remnants of fibrous septa, and irregular arrangements of portal structures and hepatic veins, typically with hepatic veins in close approximation to portal tracts. If small portal veins are obliterated, the acinar arrangement is normal, and hepatic veins are patent, the disease likely involves only the portal veins or portal tracts. Irregularity of parenchyma with atrophy and hyperplasia (i.e., nodular regenerative hyperplasia) suggests small vessel disease, even if this is not indicated in the biopsy specimen. Similar changes may occur adjacent to mass lesions, including neoplasms and abscesses.

Biopsy is seldom indicated for the identification of large portal vein disease because peripheral biopsy specimens do not sample these vessels. Recanalization of large portal vein thrombi makes these lesions elusive from a clinical point of view. Past thrombosis is indicated by prominent intimal fibrosis of portal veins, especially those larger than 200 µm in diameter. No specific histologic features can be used to diagnose hypercoagulable states. However, hepatomegaly, marked splenomegaly, and extramedullary hematopoiesis in the liver are often found in myeloproliferative disease, even without hepatic vascular disease.

Obliteration of small portal veins is nonspecific. Lesions associated with inflammatory obliteration of small portal veins should be sought, including duct lesions of primary biliary cirrhosis, granulomas of sarcoidosis and schistosomiasis, and arteritis. Obliteration of sub-

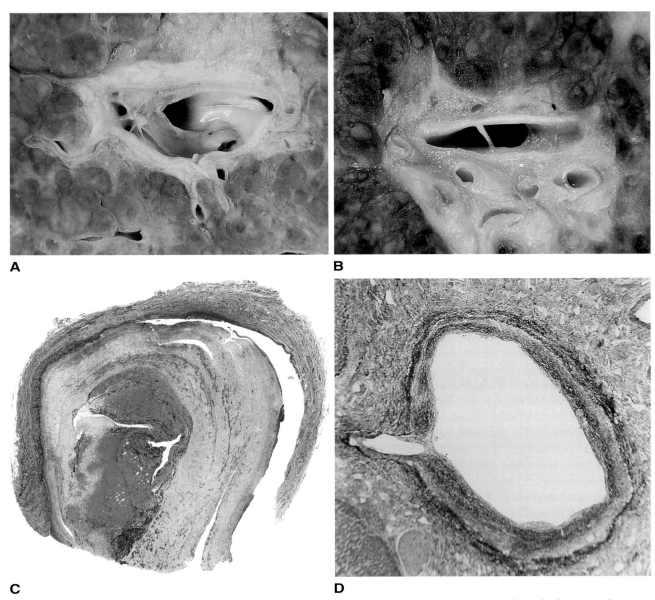

FIGURE 38–2. Portal vein thrombosis. **A,** Lobar portal vein with moderate stenosis from organized thrombus. The liver is cirrhotic. **B,** Lobar portal vein with delicate web as reflection of organized thrombus. **C,** Transverse section of the main portal vein showing several layers of organized thrombus, including a central region of recent thrombus (elastic trichrome). **D,** Medium-sized portal vein with concentric intimal fibrous thickening (Masson's trichrome).

capsular small portal veins is a common event among aged individuals.[10] However, if a majority of small portal veins are missing, this is likely to be a significant finding.

Hepatic Vein Disease (Hepatic Vein Outflow Obstruction)

CLINICAL FEATURES

Hepatic vein outflow obstruction occurs in all types of chronic liver disease. The principal conditions discussed here are those in which vascular disease is prominent or cirrhosis is not a constant feature.

Thrombosis of Large Hepatic Veins. Symptomatic obstruction of all three hepatic veins—Budd-Chiari syndrome—typically presents with painful hepatomegaly, ascites, and liver failure. Increasingly, patients are being discovered with minimal symptoms and with imaging studies that show involvement of only one or two of the main hepatic veins.[11] Thrombi in large hepatic veins often recanalize early in the course of Budd-Chiari syndrome so that some patients present with cryptogenic cirrhosis and patent large hepatic veins on imaging studies. Obstruction of the vena cava is associated with dilated veins on the abdominal wall and chest and edema of the legs.[12] Disease course is generally chronic, with less severe hepatic dysfunction

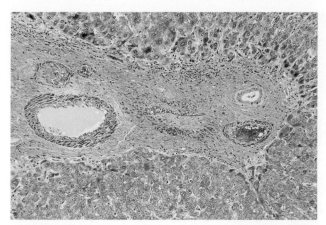

FIGURE 38–3. Portal vein obliteration in a noncirrhotic liver. The portal vein wall is severely sclerosed. The original wall is identified by a row of muscle bundles (Masson's trichrome).

compared with patients with isolated hepatic vein disease.[13] Thrombosis typically recurs, leading to episodic worsening of disease. As a result of sluggish or reversed flow in the portal veins, thrombosis of the large portal veins occurs in 10% to 20% of patients with hepatic vein obstruction. Blood from the caudate lobe drains directly into the inferior vena cava via the inferior right hepatic vein. If this vein is spared from the thrombotic process, the caudate lobe may undergo segmental hyperplasia.[14] This caudate hyperplasia or large regenerative nodules elsewhere in the liver may resemble neoplasms.[15] Long-standing Budd-Chiari syndrome is a recognized cause of hepatocellular carcinoma, especially among patients with thrombotic involvement of the vena cava.[13]

Veno-occlusive Disease or Sinusoidal Obstruction Syndrome. Small hepatic vein obstruction occurs gradually in chronic diseases that lead to cirrhosis, and it is essential to the evolution of cirrhosis (see Chapter 37).

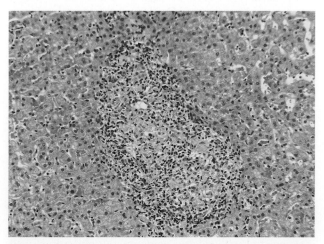

FIGURE 38–4. Obliterated small portal vein in early-stage primary biliary cirrhosis. The vein is replaced by granulomatous inflammation, and the duct is absent.

When lesions develop acutely, the condition is called *veno-occlusive disease* or *sinusoidal obstruction syndrome*. Presenting features include weight gain, ascites, hepatomegaly, and jaundice. Veno-occlusive disease occurs most frequently following bone marrow transplantation (see Chapter 39), but it may also occur in the setting of herbal medicine overdose or radiation injury (see Chapter 36).

PATHOGENESIS

Budd-Chiari Syndrome. As in portal vein disease, Virchow's triad is useful with contributions from hypercoagulable states, obstructing mass lesions, and local vascular injury (see Tables 38-1 through 38-3). Thrombosis is the most common cause of large hepatic vein obstruction. This may occur in otherwise normal livers or in livers with an obstructing lesion such as a neoplasm or cirrhosis. Amebic abscess is an important cause of hepatic vein disease in developing countries. Sarcoidosis may involve medium-sized and large hepatic veins. As is evident from Table 38-1, hypercoagulable states are often associated with hepatic vein thrombosis. Oral contraceptives and pregnancy are important stimuli of the coagulation cascade. Other predisposing factors include paroxysmal nocturnal hemoglobinuria, factor V Leiden, prothrombin G20210A, and protein C deficiency, among others (see Table 38-1). Frequently, patients have more than one risk factor, typically an underlying hypercoagulable state followed by an acute initiating event such as commencement of oral contraceptives, pregnancy, trauma, or infection.[16]

Membranous obstruction of the vena cava is a short or long segmental narrowing that is believed to be an organized thrombus that has undergone partial resorption.[17] This is not to be confused with the Eustachian valve, which is a normal vein valve encountered in some individuals in the inferior vena cava just above the effluence of the hepatic veins and below the diaphragm. Although membranous obstruction of the vena cava is rare in Western countries, a majority of patients with Budd-Chiari syndrome in developing countries have such membranous obstruction, known as *obliterative hepatocavopathy*.[18] These patients do not usually have a recognized hypercoagulable state. Recurrent infections or other environmental factors appear to initiate caval injury, and hepatic outflow occurs only after thrombosis extends to the ostia of the hepatic veins.[18] Hepatocellular carcinoma may occur in Budd-Chiari syndrome, usually decades after onset of symptoms of liver disease. This complication is more frequent among patients with obliterative hepatocavopathy.

Veno-occlusive Disease. Obliteration of small hepatic veins is noted in diseases leading to cirrhosis (as discussed in Chapter 37). Vessel lesions are usually caused by adjacent parenchymal inflammation (Fig. 38-7). In

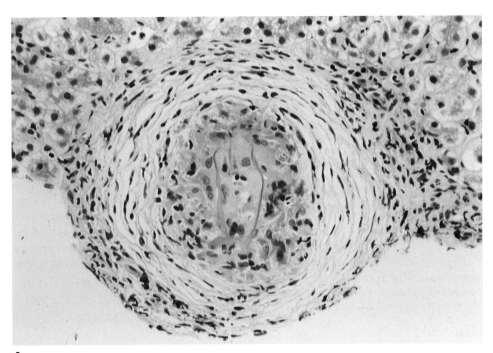

FIGURE 38–5. Schistosomiasis. **A,** *S. mansoni* egg surrounded by a fibrous granuloma. The large lateral spine is not visible in this section. The portal vein is not seen and is presumably obliterated. **B,** *S. japonicum* is characterized by numerous small eggs with a small lateral spine that is rarely visible in histologic sections. **C,** *Schistosoma* pigment in portal macrophages.

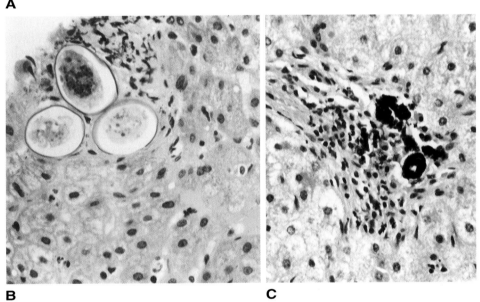

veno-occlusive disease, obstructive lesions occur after administration of toxic doses of various radiomimetic drugs, which are typically given in preparation for bone marrow transplantation. The earliest anatomic event is necrosis of sinusoidal endothelial cells. Because of this pathogenic consideration, veno-occlusive disease is discussed more fully later under Veno-occlusive Disease and Sinusoidal Obstruction Syndrome (and see Chapter 39).

PATHOLOGIC FEATURES

Budd-Chiari Syndrome. Acute obstruction of all three hepatic veins causes marked congestion of the obstructed parenchyma, producing a massively engorged liver. Subacute thrombotic occlusion, as occurs in most instances, leads to hepatomegaly with congestion and fibrosis (Fig. 38-8). Given the sluggish blood flow through the liver, secondary thrombosis of small and large portal veins may be observed. Liver biopsy specimens reveal perivenular necrosis, intra-parenchymal hemorrhage, and fibrosis. Large and medium-sized hepatic veins show intimal fibrosis, usually with multiple layers, suggesting recurrent thrombosis. Multiple luminal channels or delicate webs may indicate previous thrombosis. Pure hepatic vein thrombosis causes a venocentric pattern of septation (so-called reversed nodularity) whereby portal tracts are

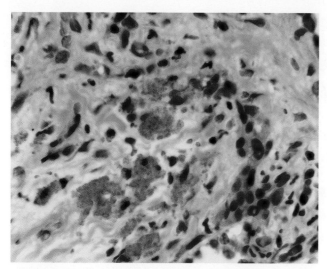

FIGURE 38–6. Thorotrast accumulates in macrophages as coarse granules in portal tracts and other organs (Masson's trichrome). This patient presented with angiosarcoma 42 years after exposure to Thorotrast. Thorotrast was visible on x-ray within liver, spleen, and abdominal lymph nodes.

seldom incorporated into the septa. Venoportal septa and venoportal cirrhosis are seen when secondary portal vein thrombosis has occurred; these septa involve portal tracts. Venoportal cirrhosis is the form seen with most causes of cirrhosis. Lesser degrees of parenchymal disease with atrophy and hyperplasia may reveal a pattern of nodular regenerative hyperplasia. A small number of large regenerative nodules are found in the majority of livers with hepatic vein thrombosis; these are easily misdiagnosed on imaging and histologic examination as neoplasms or focal nodular hyperplasia.

Cardiac Cirrhosis. Long-standing obstruction to hepatic venous outflow, as occurs in right-sided heart failure or constrictive pericarditis, causes mild atrophy

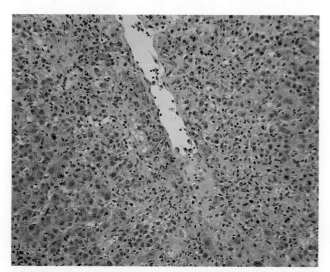

FIGURE 38–7. Active phlebitis of a small hepatic vein in autoimmune hepatitis.

of zone 3 hepatocytes with sinusoidal dilatation. In regions showing evidence of hepatic vein thrombosis, a venocentric pattern of fibrous septation is noted.[19] Nodules completely surrounded by collagen are rarely seen, so in most cases, the term *cardiac sclerosis* is preferable to *cardiac cirrhosis*.

Hepar Lobatum. This is a condition wherein deep furrows in the capsule cause a lobe to be segmented. This gross anatomic finding is usually accompanied by nearly normal parenchyma. Hepar lobatum may be caused by any disease with focal obstruction of large adjacent portal and hepatic veins; it is most often seen in Hodgkin's disease, metastatic breast carcinoma, and syphilitic gummata (Fig. 38-9). The typical appearance of hepar lobatum is expected when the primary lesion causes obstruction of vessels but tumor growth is muted or in remission.

DIAGNOSIS

Biopsy is very useful for diagnosing hepatic vein outflow obstruction, especially when clinical features are not definitive. Once the diagnosis has been established, however, biopsy is not helpful in most instances. Anatomic variation can produce significant sampling problems, such that serum alanine transaminase (ALT) elevation is a better predictor of ongoing necrosis and progressive decline of function. Biopsy specimens obtained by the transvenous route may sample thrombotic material from the lumen of a large vein; in this instance, the biopsy is useful, even if liver parenchyma is not obtained. The cause of hepatic vein disease may be visible histologically. Lesions that might be found include vasculitis, thrombus, neoplasm, granulomas of sarcoidosis (Fig. 38-10), sickled red cells (Fig. 38-11), an abscess wall, and specific infectious agents such as amebae and fungi. Extramedullary hematopoiesis suggests polycythemia vera or another myeloproliferative disease.

Hypercoagulable states require laboratory investigation. Myeloproliferative diseases may be evident from abnormal blood counts. Culture of bone marrow can reveal subclinical myeloproliferative disease if red cell colonies form in vitro without exogenous erythropoietin stimulation. Protein S and C deficiencies are difficult to diagnose because hepatic failure depresses plasma levels of these molecules. Genetic mutations involving coagulation factors are easily detected because the defect does not vary with the plasma level of the gene product.

DIFFERENTIAL DIAGNOSIS

Severe congestion or hemorrhage into the liver cell plates is suggestive of hepatic vein disease, but severe congestive heart failure and constrictive pericarditis

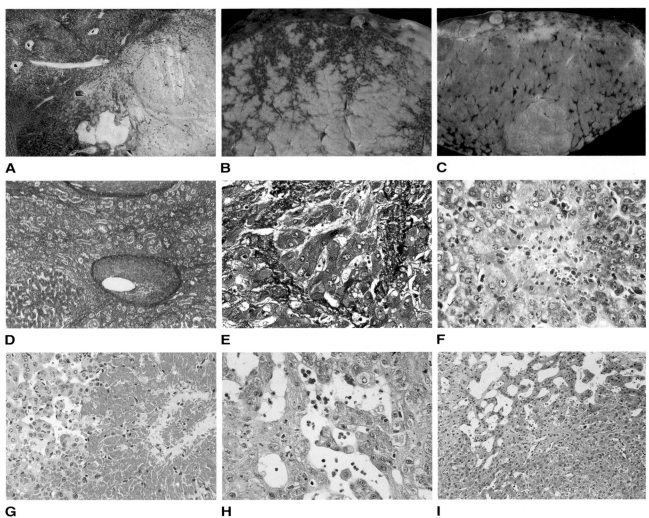

FIGURE 38–8. Budd-Chiari syndrome. **A,** Cut liver surface. Marked variation in severity from mild on right to severe on left. There is a recent infarct at bottom center. The patient had chronic disease with an episode of marked serum aminotransferase elevation shortly before transplantation. **B,** Moderately severe but heterogeneous disease with nodular regeneration in regions near patent hepatic veins. **C,** Moderate disease with large regenerative nodule. **D,** Elastic trichrome stain demonstrates the original vein wall and highlights the intimal fibrosis. **E,** This liver with hepatic vein thrombosis was resected more than 20 years after onset of clinical liver disease. Many medium hepatic veins are remodeled with hepatocytes residing in the former lumen (elastic trichrome). **F,** Small hepatic vein showing a lumen replaced by fibroinflammatory tissue. This lesion is nearly identical to the lesion in veno-occlusive disease in Figure 38-13 (Masson's trichrome). **G,** Recent venous obstruction with marked zone 3 dropout, hemorrhage into the plates, atrophy of surviving hepatocytes, and early organization of the hepatic vein. **H,** Chronic Budd-Chiari syndrome with marked sinusoidal dilatation and sinusoidal fibrosis and atrophy of the few surviving hepatocytes (Masson's trichrome). **I,** Chronic Budd-Chiari syndrome with region showing sinusoidal dilatation and hepatocellular atrophy but no fibrosis.

may cause similar changes. Local congestion and ischemic necrosis are occasionally seen in cirrhosis of any cause, so risk factors for the usual types of cirrhosis should be excluded before it is assumed that hepatic vein thrombosis is the causative lesion.

Differentiation of cirrhosis of long-standing Budd-Chiari syndrome from other types of cirrhosis may be difficult even with large samples of tissue. After regeneration in Budd-Chiari syndrome, the liver may reveal surprisingly little congestion. Differentiation requires an assessment of post-thrombotic changes in medium-sized to large hepatic veins, which is minimal in most posthepatitic cirrhotic livers.

Hepatocellular carcinoma or another neoplasm should be considered if any mass effect is seen on imaging. Large regenerative nodules are frequent in Budd-Chiari syndrome; diagnosis should be supported by surveillance to exclude malignant behavior.

Fibrous obliteration of small hepatic veins is found in any chronic liver disease, but involvement of veins larger than 100 μm, prominent intimal fibrosis, or parenchymal congestion suggests hepatic vein thrombosis. Budd-Chiari syndrome and veno-occlusive disease may be identical histologically. They may be differentiated by history or by examination of medium-sized or large hepatic veins.

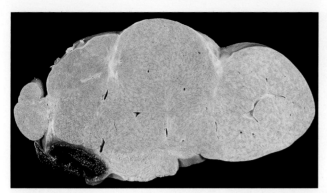

FIGURE 38–9. Hepar lobatum from patient with Hodgkin's disease in remission. The liver is subdivided by thin fibrous septa, causing deep clefts in the capsule. The left lobe is hypertrophied, and the right lobe is atrophic, as witnessed by the marked displacement of the gallbladder.

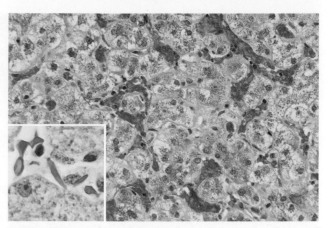

FIGURE 38–11. Sickle cell disease shows characteristic clumps of densely packed red blood cells blocking sinusoids. *Inset* shows a sickled red cell (Masson's trichrome).

Sinusoidal and Microvascular Disease

The sinusoids have a critical role as conduits that bring blood and nutrients to hepatocytes. The normal sinusoidal wall is composed of highly fenestrated endothelial cells and delicate fibrillar matrix with no defined basement membrane or occlusive pericytes.[20] Stellate cells reside in the subendothelial space of Disse. These cells contain droplets of retinyl esters and produce collagen in response to inflammation. They also have contractile properties activated by endothelin-1 and inhibited by nitric oxide.[21,22] The sinusoids must adapt to physiologic and pathologic alterations in arterial and venous blood flow. Thus, many diseases involve histologic changes in sinusoids and in the small veins.

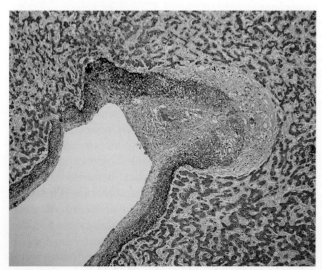

FIGURE 38–10. Sarcoidosis. This 1.5-mm-diameter hepatic vein has granulomas involving intima, media, and adventitia (elastic trichrome).

SINUSOIDAL DILATATION

In the normal liver, sinusoid diameter and hepatocyte size are uniform across the liver. This uniformity is lost when local obstruction of small portal or hepatic veins occurs, along with local compensatory increase in arterial flow. Regional portal vein obstruction leads to localized sinusoidal dilatation and hepatocellular atrophy. The resulting localized increase in the blood space is seen as a darkened region known as an *infarct of Zahn*.[23] When many adjacent obstructive portal vein lesions occur, atrophy causes the portal tracts to become crowded together. Typically, these lesions are seen adjacent to neoplasms or with focal portal vein thrombosis. In chronic congestive heart failure and constrictive pericarditis, a diffuse increase in sinusoidal pressure is noted that leads to mild zone 3 hepatocellular atrophy and sinusoidal dilatation. Sinusoidal dilatation is also seen in patients with chronic wasting illnesses,[24] such as tuberculosis, acquired immunodeficiency syndrome,[24,25] and malignancies, notably Hodgkin's disease[26] and renal cell carcinoma,[27,28] and within nodules of severe cirrhosis. Dilatation of zone 1 and 2 sinusoids occurs during pregnancy and in women taking oral contraceptives.[29,30] The mechanism of this effect may be related to mild diffuse angiogenesis and increased arterial blood flow. Sickle cell disease characteristically has small clumps of sickled red blood cells within sinusoids (see Fig. 38-11). In this disease, sinusoidal fibrosis is often seen; cirrhosis is rarely found but is usually related to coincidental viral or other liver disease.

Differential Diagnosis

History should be sought for cardiac disease, chronic wasting diseases, oral contraceptive use, sickle cell disease, and imaging evidence of mass lesions. Chronic passive congestion generally has zone 3 dilatation; that resulting from contraceptive use is usually found in zone 1. Hemorrhage into the liver cell plates or hepatic vein intimal thickening or obliteration suggests some form of hepatic vein outflow obstruction.

PELIOSIS HEPATIS

Peliosis hepatis is the presence of blood-filled spaces in the liver, resulting from focal rupture of sinusoidal walls.[31] Peliosis varies from minimal lesions that are asymptomatic and grossly inapparent to massive lesions that may present with cholestasis, liver failure, portal hypertension, a vascular mass lesion, or spontaneous rupture. Calcifications have been seen radiologically.[32] Peliosis has been associated with anabolic steroids, tamoxifen, corticosteroids, azathioprine, methotrexate, 6-thioguanine, 6-mercaptopurine, vinyl chloride, arsenic, Thorotrast, and hairy cell leukemia.[7,33,34] *Bartonella* infection causes bacillary peliosis, generally in immunosuppressed patients.

Pathologic Features

Peliosis hepatis results from focal rupture of sinusoidal walls. The endothelial lining may be lost during lesion development but is regained in chronic lesions (Fig. 38-12).[35] Severe peliosis is characterized by defoliation of sinusoids off portal tracts so that the latter extend into the cystic blood-filled cavity. In *Bartonella* infection, the organisms may be seen as a haze on hematoxylin and eosin stain but are well seen with the Warthin-Starry stain.[36] Peliosis may be associated with sinusoidal dilatation, but plate structure is intact.

Differential Diagnosis

Peliosis hepatis should be distinguished from collapse of the liver cell plates from hepatocellular dropout (evacuation). Peliosis may occur within hepatocellular adenoma and hepatocellular carcinoma. The endothelial cells of peliosis hepatis should also be examined carefully because angiosarcoma may contain areas of peliosis lined by malignant cells.

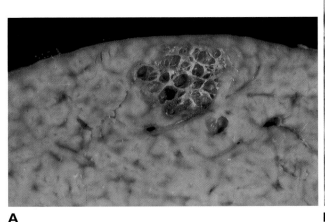

A

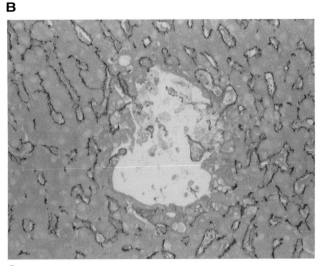

B

C

FIGURE 38–12. Peliosis hepatis. **A,** Cut section of a 1-cm-diameter lesion. The portal tract connective tissue denuded of hepatocyte cords forms a network within the lesion. The same liver had larger lesions with cavities 8 cm in diameter. **B,** This small (1 mm) lesion contains macrophages. They were not visible grossly. **C,** The same lesion on reticulin stain shows lysis of the reticulin at the site of peliosis.

SINUSOIDAL INJURY AND FIBROSIS

Because of their close proximity to hepatocytes, sinusoids are injured in all forms of acute and chronic hepatitis. This injury is most often appreciated when many contiguous hepatocytes drop out. If the dropout spans all acinar zones, the outcome is bridging necrosis. If contiguous dropout involves only zone 3, there may be no collapse of the reticulin framework, yielding a lesion called *evacuation of the liver cell plates*.[37] This is most commonly seen in allograft rejection, acetaminophen toxicity, and chronic hepatitis. Bridging necrosis heals as lesions of parenchymal extinction—the building blocks of cirrhosis.

Sinusoidal obstruction is seldom significant unless it is acute and massive (see under Veno-occlusive Disease and Sinusoidal Obstruction Syndrome) because, given time, sinusoids are easily bypassed and regenerated. It was hypothesized many years ago that chronic sinusoidal obstruction might be a cause of noncirrhotic portal hypertension. However, the absence of clinical portal hypertension in most patients with diffuse sinusoidal amyloid deposits suggests that this mechanism is rarely important.

Sinusoids are normally lined by CD34- endothelial cells. In chronic liver disease, the endothelium becomes CD34+, at first near the portal tracts. In severe cirrhosis, the entire sinusoidal bed may be involved.[5] This capillarization is likely a chronic response of sinusoids to arterialization. Other features of capillarization include decreased fenestration of the endothelial cells, increased collagen and other matrix proteins in the space of Disse, and loss of microvilli on the hepatocellular surface.[38,39] Sinusoidal endothelial cells in hepatocellular carcinoma are also CD34+.

Differential Diagnosis

Sinusoidal fibrosis may be seen in any chronic liver disease, although it is most prominent in alcoholic disease, nonalcoholic steatohepatitis,[40] hepatic vein thrombosis, vitamin A toxicity,[41] congenital syphilis, sickle cell disease, and Gaucher's disease. Because sinusoidal fibrosis is resorbed or compacted into septa, it is usually an indicator of recently active sinusoidal injury.[5]

VENO-OCCLUSIVE DISEASE AND SINUSOIDAL OBSTRUCTION SYNDROME

Many drugs and toxins can cause injury to the endothelial cells of sinusoids and small veins.[42] When the toxicity is acute and severe, widespread simultaneous necrosis of sinusoidal endothelial cells is noted, resulting in rapid weight gain, ascites, and hepatic failure. This acute phenomenon is called the sinusoidal obstruction syndrome (SOS).[43] Among survivors, the sinusoidal lesions become less apparent over time, and

the major residual lesion is fibrous obliteration of small hepatic veins. This pattern of disease was called veno-occlusive disease (VOD)[44] because the acute sinusoidal lesions were not appreciated until they were demonstrated experimentally many years later.[43,45]

Initial observations of VOD involved subjects exposed to pyrrolizidine alkaloids. These compounds are found in plants of the genera *Senecio*, *Heliotropium*, *Crotalaria*, and others. Epidemics of pyrrolizidine alkaloid toxicity occur in arid regions when toxin-containing plants overgrow fields during periods of drought. Livestock are affected when they graze in these fields, and humans are affected when they eat bread grown on affected fields. Herbal medicines made from toxic plants, commonly called bush tea, may cause severe disease, especially in young children.

In recent years, VOD (or SOS) has usually occurred in patients prepared for transplantation of bone marrow or stem cells using myeloablative doses of radiomimetic drugs and irradiation (see Chapter 39).[43,46] The drugs most often implicated are cyclophosphamide, busulfan, and recently, gemtuzumab ozogamicin (Mylotarg).[47] Occasionally, VOD develops in patients given lower doses of drugs and toxins, including azathioprine, cysteamine, dacarbazine, dactinomycin, BCNU, 6-mercaptopurine, 6-thioguanine, busulfan, dimethylbusulfan, cytosine arabinoside, cyclophosphamide, indicine-N-oxide, mustine-HCl, doxorubicin (Adriamycin), urethane, vincristine, mitomycin-C, etoposide, arsenic, Thorotrast, and intra-arterial fluorodeoxyuridine.[48-50] Patients who survive the acute SOS usually recover completely, generally with some asymptomatic VOD lesions; residual portal hypertension or cirrhosis is rare and is usually related to intercurrent disease, especially hepatitis C.[51] Cirrhosis appears to be more frequent among survivors of pyrrolizidine alkaloid–induced VOD.[52]

Pathologic Features

During the first 2 weeks of disease, marked diffuse hemorrhage occurs into the liver cell plates.[53] Hepatic veins are difficult to find because of the suffusion of blood. When Masson's trichrome fails to demonstrate hepatic veins, examination under polarized light may reveal the collagen bundles of the hepatic veins. After several weeks, congestion or dropout in zone 3 sinusoids, sinusoidal fibrosis, and eccentric intimal fibrosis are seen in small hepatic veins smaller than 200 μm in diameter (Fig. 38-13). The cirrhosis seen in survivors of pyrrolizidine toxicity may be indistinguishable from other types of cirrhosis.[52]

Differential Diagnosis

Biopsy is seldom performed because the clinical features, including timing after bone marrow transplanta-

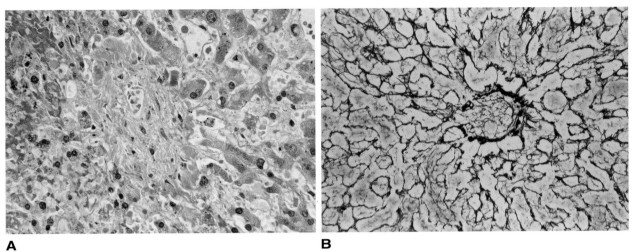

A   **B**

FIGURE 38–13. Veno-occlusive disease following bone marrow transplantation (**A**) and after chemotheraphy for a solid tumor (**B**) (Masson's trichrome and reticulin).

tion, weight gain, and ascites, are usually sufficient for the diagnosis. Atypical features such as prominent cholestasis or liver failure may lead to a biopsy with a differential of sepsis, graft-versus-host disease, drug reaction, recurrent tumor, intercurrent viral disease, or decompensation of preexisting cirrhosis.

SINUSOIDAL CELLULAR INFILTRATION

Extramedullary hematopoiesis, characterized by megakaryocytes, normoblasts, and other hematopoietic cells, is seen in normal infants, after cardiac bypass surgery and other stresses, and in myeloproliferative states. Malignant cells of many types, especially those of lymphoma and hairy cell leukemia, may cause ischemic features and hepatic failure.[34,54-56]

AMYLOIDOSIS AND LIGHT CHAIN DEPOSITION DISEASE

Clinical Features

Amyloidosis may present with hepatomegaly, cholestasis, hepatic failure, ascites, or portal hypertension.[57,58] Other features include renal failure, nephrotic syndrome, and cardiomyopathy. Light chain deposition disease may also present with hepatomegaly, cholestasis, or hepatic failure.[59,60]

Pathologic Features

Great variation is noted in the severity and distribution of hepatic amyloid deposits (Fig. 38-14). Although arterial and sinusoidal deposits are most commonly encountered, small globular deposits may occur in portal or parenchymal regions,[61,62] and large and small bile ducts and peribiliary glands may have subepithelial deposits.[63,64] The pattern of distribution does not distinguish between AA and AL amyloidosis.[65] Apolipoprotein A1 amyloidosis involves interstitial deposits in portal tracts.[66] In transthyretin amyloidosis, hepatic deposition is largely confined to the nerves, and clinical liver disease is absent.

Severe sinusoidal involvement impedes hepatocellular nutrition, leading to atrophy and dropout of hepatocytes, especially in zone 1. Venous involvement may lead to regional worsening of hepatocyte loss and condensation of the amyloid matrix into a confluent mass (amyloidoma). Nodular regenerative hyperplasia may occur with amyloidosis.[67]

Marked amyloid deposits can be easily recognized on routine stains. Amyloid deposits stain weakly with eosin and d-PAS (periodic acid–Schiff with diastase) stains and are usually positive with the Congo red stain. Minimal involvement may be demonstrated with Congo red staining followed by examination under polarized light to detect apple-green birefringence. The thioflavin-T stain and immunostain for P component are more sensitive than Congo red. Congophilia of AA amyloid is abolished by permanganate treatment. Light chain deposition disease may involve sinusoidal deposits that resemble amyloid on hematoxylin and eosin and d-PAS stains.[59] These deposits have a granular ultrastructure; amyloid deposits are fibrillar.

Diagnosis

Diagnosis of amyloidosis may be made with biopsy specimens of the rectum, abdominal fat pad, labial salivary glands, or liver. Injection of radiolabeled serum amyloid P component followed by scintigraphy is a sensitive and specific method for making a diagnosis of both AA and AL amyloidosis. This method avoids the need for biopsy and demonstrates body distribution of the deposits.[68]

PART THREE Liver

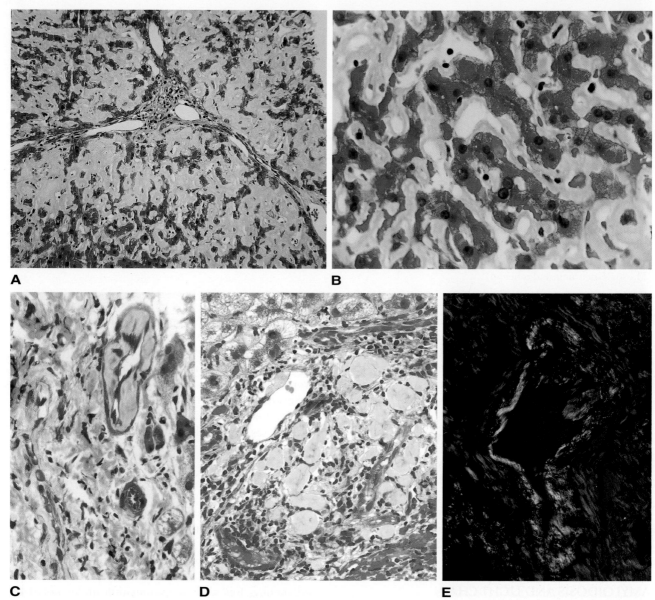

FIGURE 38–14. Amyloidosis. **A,** Marked zone 1 perisinusoidal deposition is seen with atrophy of hepatocytes (Masson's trichrome). **B,** Same biopsy shows marked expansion of the space of Disse with amorphous gray-blue amyloid (Masson's trichrome). **C,** Amyloid deposition in artery *(top right)* and portal vein wall *(lower left)* (Masson's trichrome). **D,** Globular amyloid in portal tract (Masson's trichrome). **E,** Arterial amyloid is viewed under polarized light. The amyloid is apple-green or orange (Congo red stain).

Arterial Disease

The arterial tree of the liver is frequently involved in systemic disease but is seldom symptomatic because of compensation from portal vein flow. The hepatic arterial tree reflects lesions likely to be found in many organs. For example, hyaline arteriosclerosis is often prominent in aged individuals. Systemic amyloidosis may involve the hepatic arteries, as well as portal and hepatic veins, interstitial tissue, and sinusoids (as was discussed under Amyloidosis and Light Chain Deposition Disease).

Showers of atheromatous emboli may lead to a decline in function or the development of infarcts, especially if hypotension or congestive heart failure is present.[69,70]

Arteritis of large and medium-sized vessels may be seen in polyarteritis or rheumatoid arthritis. This is usually silent, although hepatic rupture has been reported.[71,72] Small vessel arteritis, with lupus or rheumatoid arthritis, is usually silent but may result in significant obliteration of adjacent portal veins, causing nodular regenerative hyperplasia revealed on biopsy specimens and portal hypertension.[73-75]

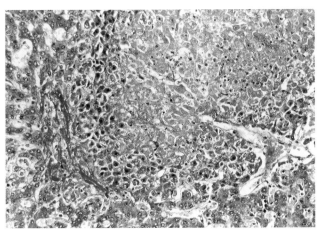

FIGURE 38–15. Infarct in a child with hypotension and sepsis. Recent thrombus can be seen in the adjacent hepatic vein. The infarct is presumably a result of hypotension and superimposed local thrombosis.

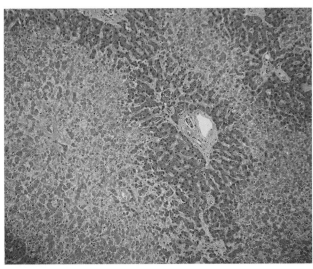

FIGURE 38–16. Ischemic necrosis. Postmortem liver shows preserved periportal parenchyma and necrosis of the entire region near the terminal hepatic veins.

ISCHEMIC LIVER INJURY AND CIRCULATORY COLLAPSE

Patients with circulatory collapse have low arterial pressure as well as reduced oxygen tension in the portal vein blood. Typically, such patients develop a sharp rise in serum aminotransferases with or without liver failure. These enzymes also fall rapidly in those who survive. Histologically, diffuse zone 3 coagulative necrosis or focal necrosis may occur. Infarction in the liver is defined as ischemic necrosis involving two or more contiguous complete acini (including zones 1 and 2). Infarcts occur when any two of portal vein, hepatic vein, and hepatic artery are involved in the same unit of tissue (Fig. 38-15). In the presence of hypotension, less vascular obstruction is needed. Often, no vascular obstruction can be identified.[69]

Hepatic infarction has been associated with Budd-Chiari syndrome, hepatic trauma, hepatic transplantation,[76] hepatic catheterization,[77] laparoscopic cholecystectomy,[78] TIPS insertion,[79] and alcohol injection.[80] A variety of hypercoagulable states and vascular injury syndromes have been reported, such as disseminated intravascular coagulation, sepsis, toxemia of pregnancy or HELLP syndrome (i.e., hemolysis, elevated liver enzymes, and low platelet count), arteritis,[81] sickle cell disease,[82] and oral contraceptive use.[83]

Pathologic Features

Right-sided cardiac decompensation leads to passive congestion of the liver (see under Hepatic Vein Outflow Obstruction). Left-sided cardiac failure or shock may lead to zonal coagulative necrosis (Fig. 38-16). With chronic passive congestion or zonal necrosis, a uniform accentuation of the acinar patterns occurs, giving a pattern known as *nutmeg liver* (Fig. 38-17). Although

zone 3 is usually most sensitive to ischemia, isolated zone 2 necrosis may be seen after shock.[84] Single cell calcification may occur. Apoptotic bodies generally are found at the interface between healthy and coagulated hepatocytes. Zone 1 necrosis is typical of diseases producing intravascular fibrin deposition such as toxemia of pregnancy and disseminated intravascular coagulation. The fibrin in these conditions may be in arterioles, portal venules, and zone 1 sinusoids.

Differential Diagnosis

Diagnosis is usually made on the basis of history. The differential diagnosis of zone 3 necrosis includes drug-induced necrosis, especially with acetaminophen or cocaine. Obtaining a history of exposure to these agents may require special effort. Vasculitis, fibrin, venous thrombi, and sickled red cells should be sought. Herpesvirus typically produces focal necrosis that resembles infarcts, except that the margins of necrosis do not follow acinar landmarks, and viral inclusions are usually seen. Atrophy and sinusoidal dilatation suggest underlying chronic cardiac disease.[85]

HEPATIC ARTERY THROMBOSIS

Hepatic artery obstruction, as seen with thrombosis or after post-traumatic ligation, is usually well tolerated unless there is hypotension or disseminated intravascular coagulation, with which infarction may occur. After transplantation, the ducts of the implanted liver do not have the rich, anastomosing arterial bed of the native liver and are therefore totally dependent on the intact flow in the hepatic artery. Thrombosis of this vessel leads to ischemic necrosis and leak of bile that

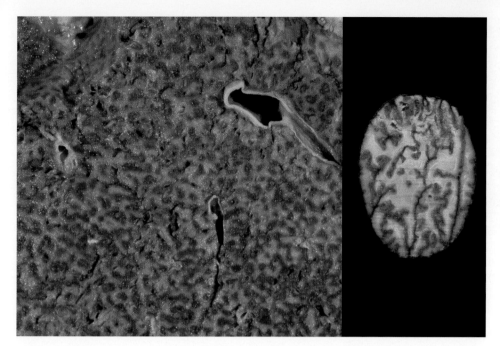

FIGURE 38–17. Ischemic necrosis. Cut section of formalin-fixed postmortem liver shows variegated pattern of hemorrhagic necrotic zone 3 parenchyma and preserved periportal parenchyma. This pattern is similar to that seen in a sliced nutmeg *(right)*.

causes necrosis of the perihilar parenchyma (Fig. 38-18).[86] The resulting necrotic debris often harbors *Candida* species or other microorganisms. Partial biliary obstruction eventually leads to liver failure, necessitating replacement of the organ. Hepatic artery cannulation and infusion with floxuridine or other agents often lead to a similar biliary ischemia and eventual stenosis of large ducts.[87,88]

ARTERIOPORTAL AND ARTERIOVENOUS SHUNTS

Large shunts between a splanchnic artery and a portal or hepatic vein most commonly develop months or years after the occurrence of penetrating trauma

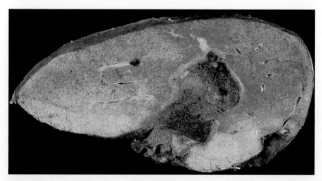

FIGURE 38–18. Liver that failed several months after transplantation. Hepatic artery thrombosis was noted early after transplantation, before the onset of progressive cholestasis. The hilar region is necrotic and bile-stained because of necrosis of the large bile ducts. A medium-sized duct is also necrotic *(left of center)*.

such as a gunshot wound or liver biopsy.[89,90] Occasionally, these anomalies of development are found early in life or are a result of abnormal vascular remodeling, such as that seen in hereditary hemorrhagic telangiectasia. Increased arterial flow in the liver may be inapparent but can present with a bruit, high-output congestive heart failure, ascites, diarrhea, weight loss, protein-losing enteropathy, or hemobilia.[91] When the shunt involves the portal vein, portal hypertension is the most important effect. Diagnosis depends on the finding of a dilated high-flow channel on Doppler ultrasonography or other imaging studies. One may see double vasculature on an arteriogram with the arterial tree and early retrograde filling of the parallel portal venous tree. The portal vein may be thrombosed. Histologically, numerous congested capillaries and arterioles are found in or adjacent to portal tracts.[92] Large regenerative nodules similar to focal nodular hyperplasia may also be noted.

■ Nodular Hyperplasia

Nodular hyperplasia is a family of conditions in which benign and apparently regenerative hepatocytes form nodules. The conditions are classified according to the size, distribution, and histologic appearance of the nodules.[93,94]

LARGE REGENERATIVE NODULES

Large regenerative nodules (LRNs) are masses of parenchyma that measure up to many centimeters and arise in response to parenchymal injury or vascular abnormality. They are to be distinguished from the neoplastic liver nodules discussed in Chapter 42. They occur in cirrhosis, organizing massive hepatic necrosis, Budd-Chiari syndrome (see Fig. 38-8), Rendu-Osler-Weber disease, and portal vein absence or thrombosis; they also appear adjacent to mass lesions such as hepatocellular carcinoma.[93] *Partial nodular transformation* is an obsolete term applied to noncirrhotic livers that have a large perihilar nodule in patients with portal hypertension; too few lesions have been published to provide a full understanding of their character, but they were likely LRNs.

Pathologic Features

LRNs have a fairly constant appearance histologically, being supplied by portal tracts that contain arteries and ducts with or without portal veins. Ductular proliferation usually accompanies cholestasis. Hepatocytes range from normal to moderately reactive. Livers in Budd-Chiari syndrome commonly have LRNs, but hepatocellular carcinoma also occurs in long-standing disease. Reactive nodules occurring in portal vein absence or portal vein hypoplasia have usually been classified as focal nodular hyperplasia.

Differential Diagnosis

The differential diagnosis includes hepatocellular carcinoma and other malignant lesions, lobar hyperplasia in Budd-Chiari syndrome, primary sclerosing cholangitis, and biliary atresia.

FOCAL NODULAR HYPERPLASIA

Focal nodular hyperplasia (FNH) is a large, regenerative nodule with characteristic clinical and histologic features (see Chapter 42). FNH is the most frequent type of LRN and the most frequent benign solid liver lesion, occurring in approximately 3% of the adult population. Ninety percent of patients are women of childbearing age, two thirds of whom are using oral contraceptives. FNH also occurs in children and the elderly. Although they usually present as an incidental finding, the lesions may cause pain and, rarely, hemorrhage. Hepatic hemangioma coexists in 20% of patients. A variety of systemic vascular anomalies have been found, including absence of portal vein, dysplasia and spontaneous rupture of systemic arteries, hereditary hemorrhagic telangiectasia, and vascular anomalies in the brain.[95] Astrocytoma and meningioma have also been reported. Hepatic imaging studies characteristically show increased arterial flow with a large artery, centripetal flow, and prolonged opacification.

Pathologic Features

Lesions of FNH may be a few millimeters or up to 10 or more centimeters in diameter. The cut surface shows a central fibrous region with radiating branches and a well-demarcated, multinodular, pale parenchyma (Fig. 38-19). The central region reveals large vessels, fibrosis, and proliferating ductules but usually no ducts or portal veins. The liver plate structure is relatively normal or slightly widened. Hepatocytes display alternating areas of hyperplasia and atrophy, creating many small nodules

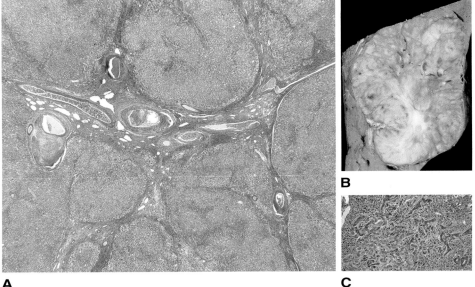

FIGURE 38–19. Focal nodular hyperplasia (FNH). **A,** The central scar contains large vessels and fibrous septa resembling cirrhosis. **B,** Cut section shows typical central stellate scar. The FNH is paler than the adjacent noncirrhotic parenchyma. **C,** Foci of ductular proliferation are present; this is a useful feature for distinguishing the lesion from adenoma.

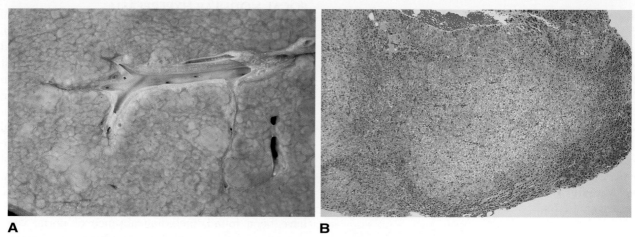

A   **B**

FIGURE 38–20. Nodular regenerative hyperplasia. **A,** Cut section of a liver with early-stage primary biliary cirrhosis. **B,** Alternating regions of atrophy and nonatrophic parenchyma and minimal parenchymal fibrosis are seen (Masson's trichrome).

within the entire FNH lesion. Sinusoids are mostly compressed in the usual solid type and are dilated in the telangiectatic type of FNH.[95,96] FNH-like nodules that contain portal veins or ducts may be considered to be LRNs that are FNH precursor lesions.[97]

Differential Diagnosis

Focal nodular hyperplasia is most often confused with hepatic adenoma. The latter has no ductules and less periarterial collagen than FNH. Adenoma is also more uniform without alternating areas of hyperplasia and atrophy. Focal areas within FNH may resemble adenoma. A zone of hyperplasia may occur adjacent to the fibrolamellar type of hepatocellular carcinoma. This lesion usually does not have all the features of FNH. The key tissue features suggestive of FNH on percutaneous biopsy (either cutting needle or fine needle) include strands of fibrous tissue containing mononuclear inflammatory cells and bile duct elements. These are not present in adenoma. Adenoma is suggested by biopsy tissue that consists only of benign hepatocellular parenchyma; the presence of hepatic arteries unaccompanied by other portal vein structures (portal vein, bile duct, or ductules) strongly suggests adenoma.

NODULAR REGENERATIVE HYPERPLASIA

Nodular regenerative hyperplasia (NRH) arises when intrahepatic circulation is heterogeneous, particularly in the portal veins and arteries. Mild outflow obstruction, as is seen with congestive failure or focal small hepatic vein obliteration, may contribute to the findings, but major outflow obstruction causes more severe hepatocyte loss, leading to cirrhosis rather than NRH.

Any portal tract inflammatory disease, especially primary biliary cirrhosis, polyarteritis nodosa, systemic

sclerosis, systemic lupus erythematosus, and rheumatoid arteritis, can cause predominant afferent block and NRH.[98]

Pathologic Features

NRH is defined as a diffuse nodularity in the parenchyma without fibrosis (Fig. 38-20). The 1- to 2-mm nodules are separated by regions of atrophy. This condition may be asymptomatic or associated with portal hypertension, usually without ascites. The capsular surface reveals minimal irregularities that may be mistaken for cirrhosis.

Differential Diagnosis

Unlike in cirrhosis, the nodules are separated by atrophic parenchyma only. Occasionally, a liver with NRH contains large regenerative nodules that might suggest hepatocellular or metastatic carcinoma clinically. Alternatively, in some patients, metastatic carcinoma can obstruct sufficient numbers of small portal and hepatic veins to cause NRH as a mass effect.

References

1. Whipple AO: The problem of portal hypertension in relation to the hepatosplenopathies. Ann Surg 122:449-475, 1945.
2. Powell LW, Kerr JF: Reversal of "cirrhosis" in idiopathic haemochromatosis following long-term intensive venesection therapy. Australas Ann Med 19:54-57, 1970.
3. Iredale JP, Benyon RC, Pickering J, et al: Mechanisms of spontaneous resolution of rat liver fibrosis. Hepatic stellate cell apoptosis and reduced hepatic expression of metalloproteinase inhibitors. J Clin Invest 102:538-549, 1998.
4. Dufour JF, DeLellis R, Kaplan MM: Regression of hepatic fibrosis in hepatitis C with long-term interferon treatment. Dig Dis Sci 43:2573-2576, 1998.
5. Wanless IR, Nakashima E, Sherman M: Regression of human cirrhosis: Morphologic features and the genesis of incomplete septal cirrhosis. Arch Pathol Lab Med 124:1599-1607, 2000.

6. Amitrano L, Guardascione MA, Brancaccio V, et al: Portal and mesenteric venous thrombosis in cirrhotic patients. Gastroenterology 123:1409-1410, 2002.

7. Wanless IR: Vascular disorders. In MacSween RNM, Burt AD, Portmann BC, et al (eds): Pathology of the Liver, 4th ed. Edinburgh, Churchill Livingstone, 2002, pp 539-574.

8. Nakashima E, Kage M, Wanless IR: Idiopathic portal hypertension: Histologic evidence that some cases may be regressed cirrhosis with portal vein thrombosis. Hepatology 30:218A, 1999.

9. Mikkelsen WP, Edmondson HA, Peters RL, et al: Extra- and intrahepatic portal hypertension without cirrhosis (hepatoportal sclerosis). Ann Surg 162:602-618, 1965.

10. Wanless IR, Bernier V, Seger M: Intrahepatic portal sclerosis in patients without history of liver disease: An autopsy study. Am J Pathol 106:63-70, 1982.

11. Valla D, Hadengue A, el Younsi M, et al: Hepatic venous outflow block caused by short-length hepatic vein stenoses. Hepatology 25:814-819, 1997.

12. Okuda H, Yamagata H, Obata H, et al: Epidemiological and clinical features of Budd-Chiari syndrome in Japan. J Hepatol 22:1-9, 1995.

13. Rector WG Jr, Xu YH, Goldstein L, et al: Membranous obstruction of the inferior vena cava in the United States. Medicine (Baltimore) 64:134-143, 1985.

14. Meindok H, Langer B: Liver scan in Budd-Chiari syndrome. J Nucl Med 17:365-368, 1976.

15. Tanaka M, Wanless IR: Pathology of the liver in Budd-Chiari syndrome: Portal vein thrombosis and the histogenesis of veno-centric cirrhosis, veno-portal cirrhosis, and large regenerative nodules. Hepatology 27:488-496, 1998.

16. Valla D, Denninger MH, Casadevall N, et al: Thrombose de la veine porte et des veines hepatiques: Combinaisons d'affections thrombogenes multiples et de facteurs locaux (abstract). Gastroenterol Clin Biol 21:731, 1997.

17. Kage M, Arakawa M, Kojiro M, et al: Histopathology of membranous obstruction of the inferior vena cava in the Budd-Chiari syndrome. Gastroenterology 102:2081-2090, 1992.

18. Okuda K, Kage M, Shrestha SM: Proposal of a new nomenclature for Budd-Chiari syndrome: Hepatic vein thrombosis versus thrombosis of the inferior vena cava at its hepatic portion. Hepatology 28:1191-1198, 1998.

19. Wanless IR, Liu JJ, Butany J: Role of thrombosis in the pathogenesis of congestive hepatic fibrosis (cardiac cirrhosis). Hepatology 21:1232-1237, 1995.

20. Wisse E, Braet F, Luo D, et al: Structure and function of sinusoidal lining cells in the liver. Toxicol Pathol 24:100-111, 1996.

21. Rockey DC: Hepatic blood flow regulation by stellate cells in normal and injured liver. Semin Liver Dis 21:337-349, 2001.

22. Shah V: Cellular and molecular basis of portal hypertension. Clin Liver Dis 5:629-644, 2001.

23. Shimamatsu K, Wanless IR: Role of ischemia in causing apoptosis, atrophy, and nodular hyperplasia in human liver. Hepatology 26:343-350, 1997.

24. Bruguera M, Aranguibel F, Ros E Jr: Incidence and clinical significance of sinusoidal dilatation in liver biopsies. Gastroenterology 75:474-478, 1978.

25. Welch K, Finkbeiner W, Alpers CE, et al: Autopsy findings in the acquired immune deficiency syndrome. JAMA 252:1152-1159, 1984.

26. Bain BJ, Coghlan SJ, Chong KC, et al: Hepatic sinusoidal ectasia in association with Hodgkin's disease. Postgrad Med J 58:182-184, 1982.

27. Delpre G, Ilie B, Papo J, et al: Hypernephroma with nonmetastatic liver dysfunction (Stauffer syndrome) and hypercalcemia. Am J Gastroenterol 72:239-247, 1979.

28. Aoyagi T, Mori I, Ueyama Y, et al: Sinusoidal dilatation of the liver as a paraneoplastic manifestation of renal cell carcinoma. Hum Pathol 20:1193-1197, 1989.

29. Winckler K, Poulsen H: Liver disease with periportal sinusoidal dilatation. A possible complication to contraceptive steroids. Scand J Gastroenterol 10:699-704, 1975.

30. Spellberg MA, Mirro J, Chowdhury L: Hepatic sinusoidal dilatation related to oral contraceptives. Am J Gastroenterol 72:248-252, 1979.

31. Zak FG: Peliosis hepatis. Am J Pathol 26:1-15, 1950.

32. Muradali D, Wilson SR, Wanless IR, et al: Peliosis hepatis with intrahepatic calcifications. J Ultrasound Med 15:257-260, 1996.

33. Degott C, Rueff B, Kreis H, et al: Peliosis hepatis in recipients of renal transplants. Gut 19:748-753, 1978.

34. Zafrani ES, Degos F, Guigui B, et al: The hepatic sinusoid in hairy cell leukemia. An ultrastructural study of 12 cases. Hum Pathol 18:801-807, 1987.

35. Wold LE, Ludwig J: Peliosis hepatis: Two morphologic variants? Hum Pathol 12:388-389, 1981.

36. Perkocha LA, Geaghan SM, Yen TSB, et al: Clinical and pathological features of bacillary peliosis hepatis in association with human immunodeficiency virus infection. N Engl J Med 323:1581-1586, 1990.

37. Wanless IR: Vascular disorders. In MacSween RNM, Burt AD, Portmann BC, et al (eds): Pathology of the Liver, 4th ed. Edinburgh, Churchill Livingstone, 2002, p 553.

38. Schaffner F, Popper H: Capillarization of hepatic sinusoids in man. Gastroenterology 44:239-242, 1963.

39. Babbs C, Haboubi NY, Mellor JM, et al: Endothelial cell transformation in primary biliary cirrhosis: A morphological and biochemical study. Hepatology 11:723-729, 1990.

40. Latry P, Bioulac-Sage P, Echinard E, et al: Perisinusoidal fibrosis and basement membrane-like material in the livers of diabetic patients. Hum Pathol 18:775-780, 1987.

41. Zafrani ES, Bernuau D, Feldmann G: Peliosis-like ultrastructural changes of the hepatic sinusoids in human chronic hypervitaminosis A: Report of 3 cases. Hum Pathol 15:1166-1170, 1984.

42. McDonald G, Hinds MS, Fisher LD, et al: Veno-occlusive disease of the liver and multiorgan failure after bone marrow transplantation: A cohort study of 355 patients. Ann Intern Med 118:255-267, 1993.

43. DeLeve LD, Ito Y, Bethea NW, et al: Embolization by sinusoidal lining cells obstructs the microcirculation in rat sinusoidal obstruction syndrome (hepatic venooclusive disease). Am J Physiol Gastrointest Liver Physiol (in press).

44. Bras G, Jelliffe DB, Stuart KL: Veno-occlusive disease of the liver with non-portal type of cirrhosis, occurring in Jamaica. Arch Pathol 57:285-300, 1954.

45. Rappaport AM, Knoblauch M, Zelin S, et al: Experimental hepatic veno-occlusive disease: In vivo microcirculatory study. Adv Microcirc 2:69-79, 1969.

46. McDonald GB, Slattery JT, Bouvier ME, et al: Cyclophosphamide metabolism, liver toxicity, and mortality following hematopoietic stem cell transplantation. Blood 101:2043-2048, 2003.

47. Rajvanshi P, Shulman HM, Sievers EL, et al: Hepatic sinusoidal obstruction after gemtuzumab ozogamicin (Mylotarg) therapy. Blood 99:2310-2314, 2002.

48. Ortega JA, Donaldson SS, Ivy SP, et al: Venoocclusive disease of the liver after chemotherapy with vincristine, actinomycin D, and cyclophosphamide for the treatment of rhabdomyosarcoma. A report of the Intergroup Rhabdomyosarcoma Study Group. Children's Cancer Group, the Pediatric Oncology Group, and the Pediatric Intergroup Statistical Center. Cancer 79:2435-2439, 1997.

49. Czauderna P, Chyczewski L, Lech K, et al: Experimental model of hepatic venoocclusive disease (VOD) caused by dactinomycin—preliminary report about hepatoprotective effect of amifostine. Med Sci Monit 6:446-453, 2000.

50. Czauderna P, Katski K, Kowalczyk J, et al: Venoocclusive liver disease (VOD) as a complication of Wilms' tumour management in the series of consecutive 206 patients. Eur J Pediatr Surg 10:300-303, 2000.

51. Strasser SI, Sullivan KM, Myerson D, et al: Cirrhosis of the liver in long-term marrow transplant survivors. Blood 93:3259-3266, 1999.

52. Tandon BN, Joshi YK, Sud R, et al: Follow-up of survivors of epidemic veno-occlusive disease in India (letter). Lancet 1:730, 1984.

53. Shulman HM, Fisher LB, Schoch HG, et al: Veno-occlusive disease of the liver after marrow transplantation: Histological correlates of clinical signs and symptoms. Hepatology 19:1171-1181, 1994.

54. Trudel M, Aramendi T, Caplan S: Large-cell lymphoma presenting with hepatic sinusoidal infiltration. Arch Pathol Lab Med 115:821-824, 1991.

55. Evans MA, Gastineau DA, Ludwig J: Relapsing hairy cell leukemia presenting as fulminant hepatitis. Am J Med 92:209-212, 1992.

56. Costa F, Choy CG, Seiter K, et al: Hepatic outflow obstruction and liver failure due to leukemic cell infiltration in chronic lymphocytic leukemia. Leuk Lymphoma 30:403-410, 1998.

57. Iwai M, Ishii Y, Mori T, et al: Cholestatic jaundice in two patients with primary amyloidosis: Ultrastructural findings of the liver. J Clin Gastroenterol 28:162-166, 1999.

58. Mohr A, Miehlke S, Klauck S, et al: Hepatomegaly and cholestasis as primary clinical manifestations of an AL-kappa amyloidosis. Eur J Gastroenterol Hepatol 11:921-925, 1999.

59. Faa G, Van Eyken P, De Vos R, et al: Light chain deposition disease of the liver associated with AL-type amyloidosis and severe cholestasis. J Hepatol 12:75-82, 1991.

60. Michopoulos S, Petraki K, Petraki C, et al: Light chain deposition disease of the liver without renal involvement in a patient with multiple myeloma related to liver failure and rapid fatal outcome. Dig Dis Sci 47:730-734, 2002.

61. Kanel GC, Uchida T, Peters RL: Globular hepatic amyloid-an unusual morphologic presentation. Hepatology 1:647-652, 1981.

62. French SW, Schloss GT, Stillwan AE: Unusual amyloid bodies in human liver. Am J Clin Pathol 75:400-402, 1981.

63. Sasaki M, Nakanuma Y, Terada T, et al: Amyloid deposition in intrahepatic large bile ducts and peribiliary glands in systemic amyloidosis. Hepatology 12:743-746, 1990.

64. Terada T, Hirata K, Hisada Y, et al: Obstructive jaundice caused by the deposition of amyloid-like substances in the extrahepatic and large intrahepatic bile ducts in a patient with multiple myeloma. Histopathology 24:485-487, 1994.

65. Buck FS, Koss MN: Hepatic amyloidosis: Morphologic differences between systemic AL and AA types. Hum Pathol 22:904-907, 1991.

66. Shaz BH, Lewis WD, Skinner M, et al: Livers from patients with apolipoprotein A-I amyloidosis are not suitable as "domino" donors. Mod Pathol 14:577-580, 2001.

67. Kitazono M, Saito Y, Kinoshita M, et al: Nodular regenerative hyperplasia of the liver in a patient with multiple myeloma and systemic amyloidosis. Acta Pathol Jpn 35:961-967, 1985.

68. Lovat LB, Persey MR, Madhoo S, et al: The liver in systemic amyloidosis: Insights from 123I serum amyloid P component scintigraphy in 484 patients. Gut 42:727-734, 1998.

69. Chen V, Hamilton J, Qizilbash A: Hepatic infarction. Arch Pathol Lab Med 100:32-36, 1976.

70. Ueda T, Mizushige K, Izumi Y, et al: Hepatic infarction caused by an embolus from an atherosclerotic lesion—a case report. Angiology 49:165-168, 1998.

71. Hocking WG, Lasser K, Ungerer R, et al: Spontaneous hepatic rupture in rheumatoid arthritis. Arch Intern Med 141:792-794, 1981.

72. Parangi S, Oz MC, Blume RS, et al: Hepatobiliary complications of polyarteritis nodosa. Arch Surg 126:909-912, 1991.

73. Reynolds WJ, Wanless IR: Nodular regenerative hyperplasia of the liver in a patient with rheumatoid vasculitis: A morphometric study suggesting a role for hepatic arteritis in the pathogenesis. J Rheumatol 11:838-842, 1984.

74. Nakamura H, Uehara H, Okada T, et al: Occlusion of small hepatic veins associated with systemic lupus erythematosus with the lupus anticoagulant and anti-cardiolipin antibody. Hepatogastroenterology 36:393-397, 1989.

75. Kuramochi S, Tashiro Y, Torikata C, et al: Systemic lupus erythematosus associated with multiple nodular hyperplasia of the liver. Acta Pathol Jpn 32:547-560, 1982.

76. Hung CF, Tseng JH, Jeng LB, et al: Isolated caudate lobe infarct after orthoptic liver transplantation. Transplant Proc 32:2223-2224, 2000.

77. Abe S, Yamasaki T, Nakano K, et al: Multiple hepatic infarction after transcatheter arterial infusion with SMANCS. J Gastroenterol 36:415-421, 2001.

78. Wong MD, Lucas CE: Liver infarction after laparoscopic cholecystectomy injury to the right hepatic artery and portal vein. Am Surg 67:410-411, 2001.

79. Mayan H, Kantor R, Rimon U, et al: Fatal liver infarction after transjugular intrahepatic portosystemic shunt procedure. Liver 21:361-364, 2001.

80. Seki T, Wakabayashi M, Nakagawa T, et al: Hepatic infarction following percutaneous ethanol injection therapy for hepatocellular carcinoma. Eur J Gastroenterol Hepatol 10:915-918, 1998.

81. Iuliano L, Gurgo A, Gualdi G, et al: Succeeding onset of hepatic, splenic, and renal infarction in polyarteritis nodosa. Am J Gastroenterol 95:1837-1838, 2000.

82. Gauthier N, Cornud F, Vissuzaine C: Liver infarction in sickle cell disease. AJR Am J Roentgenol 144:1089-1090, 1985.

83. Jacobs MB: Hepatic infarction related to oral contraceptive use. Arch Intern Med 144:642-643, 1984.

84. Bynum TE, Boitnott JK, Maddrey WC: Ischemic hepatitis. Dig Dis Sci 24:129-135, 1979.

85. Arcidi JM Jr, Moore GW, Hutchins GM: Hepatic morphology in cardiac dysfunction. A clinicopathologic study of 1000 subjects at autopsy. Am J Pathol 104:159-166, 1981.

86. Ludwig J, Batts KP, MacCarty RL: Ischemic cholangitis in hepatic allografts. Mayo Clin Proc 67:519-526, 1992.

87. Ludwig J, Kim CH, Wiesner RH, et al: Floxuridine-induced sclerosing cholangitis: An ischemic cholangiopathy? Hepatology 9:215-218, 1989.

88. Shrikhande S, Friess H, Kleeff J, et al: Bile duct infarction following intraarterial hepatic chemotherapy mimicking multiple liver metastasis: Report of a case and review of the literature. Dig Dis Sci 47:338-344, 2002.

89. Okuda K, Musha H, Nakajima Y, et al: Frequency of intrahepatic arteriovenous fistula as a sequela to percutaneous needle puncture of the liver. Gastroenterology 74:1204-1207, 1978.

90. Strodel WE, Eckhauser FE, Lemmer JH, et al: Presentation and perioperative management of arterioportal fistulas. Arch Surg 122:563-571, 1987.

91. Van Way CW, Crane JM, Riddell DH, et al: Arteriovenous fistula in the portal circulation. Surgery 70:876-890, 1971.

92. Donovan AJ, Reynolds TB, Mikkelsen WP, et al: Systemic-portal arteriovenous fistulas: Pathologic and hemodynamic observations in two patients. Surgery 66:474-482, 1969.

93. International Working Party: Terminology of nodular hepatocellular lesions. Hepatology 22:983-993, 1995.

94. Wanless IR: Benign liver tumors. Clin Liver Dis 6:513-526, 2002.

95. Wanless IR, Albrecht S, Bilbao J, et al: Multiple focal nodular hyperplasia of the liver associated with vascular malformations of various organs and neoplasia of the brain: A new syndrome. Mod Pathol 2:456-462, 1989.

96. Nguyen BN, Flejou JF, Terris B, et al: Focal nodular hyperplasia of the liver: A comprehensive pathologic study of 305 lesions and recognition of new histologic forms. Am J Surg Pathol 23:1441-1454, 1999.

97. Wanless IR: Focal nodular hyperplasia of the liver: Comments on the pathogenesis. Arch Pathol Lab Med 124:1105-1107, 2000.

98. Wanless IR: Micronodular transformation (nodular regenerative hyperplasia) of the liver: A report of 64 cases among 2500 autopsies and a new classification of benign hepatocellular nodules. Hepatology 11:787-797, 1990.

99. Valla D, Casadevall N, Huisse MG, et al: Etiology of portal vein thrombosis in adults: A prospective evaluation of primary myeloproliferative disorders. Gastroenterology 94:1063-1069, 1988.

100. Pagliuca A, Mufti GJ, Janossa-Tahernia M, et al: In vitro colony culture and chromosomal studies in hepatic and portal vein thrombosis—possible evidence of an occult myeloproliferative state. Q J Med 76:981-989, 1990.

101. Denninger MH, Helley D, Valla D, et al: Prospective evaluation of the prevalence of factor V Leiden mutation in portal or hepatic vein thrombosis. Thromb Haemost 78:1297-1298, 1997.

102. Valla D, Casadevall N, Lacombe N, et al: Primary myeloproliferative disorders and hepatic vein thrombosis: A prospective study of erythroid colony formation in vitro in 20 patients with Budd-Chiari syndrome. Ann Intern Med 103:329-334, 1985.

103. Simonds JP: Chronic occlusion of the portal vein. Arch Surg 33:397-424, 1936.

104. Wanless IR, Peterson P, Das A, et al: Hepatic vascular disease and portal hypertension in polycythemia vera and agnogenic myeloid metaplasia: A clinicopathological study of 145 patients examined at autopsy. Hepatology 12:1166-1174, 1990.

105. Klein AS, Sitzmann JV, Coleman J, et al: Current management of the Budd-Chiari syndrome. Ann Surg 212:144-149, 1990.

106. McDermott WV, Bothe A, Clouse ME, et al: Noncirrhotic portal hypertension in adults. Am J Surg 141:514-518, 1981.

107. Ludwig J, Hashimoto E, McGill DB, et al: Classification of hepatic venous outflow obstruction: Ambiguous terminology of the Budd-Chiari syndrome. Mayo Clin Proc 65:51-55, 1990.

108. Valla D, Dhumeaux D, Babany G, et al: Hepatic vein thrombosis in paroxysmal nocturnal hemoglobinuria: A spectrum from asymptomatic occlusion of hepatic venules to fatal Budd-Chiari syndrome. Gastroenterology 93:569-575, 1987.

109. Leibowitz AI, Hartmann RC: The Budd-Chiari syndrome and paroxysmal nocturnal hemoglobinuria. Br J Hematol 48:1-6, 1981.

110. Klemperer P: Cavernous transformation of the portal vein Its relation to Banti's disease. Arch Pathol Lab Med 6:353-377, 1928.

111. Shaldon S, Sherlock S: Portal hypertension in the myeloproliferative syndrome and the reticuloses. Am J Med 32:758-764, 1962.

112. Thompson EN, Sherlock S: The aetiology of portal vein thrombosis with particular reference to the role of infection and exchange transfusion. Q J Med 33:465-480, 1964.

113. Wang Z, Zhu Y, Wang S, et al: Recognition and management of Budd-Chiari syndrome. A report of 100 cases. J Vasc Surg 10:149-156, 1989.

114. Riccio JA, Colley AT, Cera PJ: Hepatic vein thrombosis (Budd-Chiari syndrome) in the microgranular variant of acute promyelocytic leukemia. Am J Clin Pathol 92:366-371, 1989.

115. Chillar RK, Paladugu RR: Hepatic vein thrombosis (acute Budd-Chiari syndrome) in acute leukemia. Am J Med Sci 282:153-156, 1981.

116. Tsuji H, Murai K, Kobayashi K, et al: Multiple myeloma associated with Budd-Chiari syndrome. Hepatogastroenterology 37(suppl 2):97-99, 1990.

117. Orozco H, Guraieb E, Takahashi T, et al: Deficiency of protein C in patients with portal vein thrombosis. Hepatology 8:1110-1111, 1988.

118. Valla D, Denninger MH, Delvigne JM, et al: Portal vein thrombosis with ruptured oesophageal varices as presenting manifestation of hereditary protein C deficiency. Gut 29:856-859, 1988.

119. Harward TR, Green D, Bergan JJ, et al: Mesenteric venous thrombosis. J Vasc Surg 9:328-333, 1989.

120. Couffinhal T, Bonnet J, Benchimol D, et al: A case of the Budd-Chiari syndrome attributed to a deficit in protein C. Eur Heart J 12:266-269, 1991.

121. Klar E, Buhr H, Zimmermann R: Protein C deficiency with recurrent infarct of the small intestine. Chirurg 61:59-62, 1990.

122. Seifert M, Fleck U, Vogel G, et al: Partial portal vein and mesenteric vein thrombosis in familial protein S deficiency. Chirurg 65:1143-1147, 1994.

123. Zigrossi P, Campanini M, Bordin G, et al: Portal and mesenteric thrombosis in protein S (pS) deficiency. Am J Gastroenterol 91:163-165, 1996.

124. Odegard QR, Abildgaard U: Antifactor Xa activity in thrombophilia. Studies in a family with AT-III deficiency. Scand J Hematol 18:86-90, 1977.

125. Das M, Carroll S: Antithrombin III deficiency: An etiology of Budd-Chiari syndrome. Surgery 97:242-245, 1985.

126. McClure S, Dincsoy HP, Glueck H: Budd-Chiari syndrome and antithrombin III deficiency. Am J Clin Pathol 78:236-241, 1982.

127. Chamouard P, Pencreach E, Maloisel F, et al: Frequent factor II G20210A mutation in idiopathic portal vein thrombosis. Gastroenterology 116:144-148, 1999.

128. De Stefano V, Chiusolo P, Paciaroni K, et al: Hepatic vein thrombosis in a patient with mutant prothrombin 20210A allele (letter). Thromb Haemost 80:519, 1998.

129. Bucciarelli P, Franchi F, Alatri A, et al: Budd-Chiari syndrome in a patient heterozygous for the G20210A mutation of the prothrombin gene (letter). Thromb Haemost 79:445-446, 1998.

130. Heresbach D, Pagenault M, Gueret P, et al: Leiden factor V mutation in four patients with small bowel infarctions. Gastroenterology 113:322-325, 1997.

131. Mahmoud AE, Elias E, Beauchamp N, et al: Prevalence of the factor V Leiden mutation in hepatic and portal vein thrombosis. Gut 40:798-800, 1997.

132. Schved JF, Gris JC, Aguilar-Martinez P, et al: Recurrent venous thromboembolism caused by heparin cofactor II deficiency. A case. Presse Med 20:1211-1214, 1991.

133. Balian A, Valla D, Naveau S, et al: Post-traumatic membranous obstruction of the inferior vena cava associated with a hypercoagulable state. J Hepatol 28:723-726, 1998.

134. Min AD, Atillasoy EO, Schwartz ME, et al: Reassessing the role of medical therapy in the management of hepatic vein thrombosis (see comments). Liver Transpl Surg 3:423-429, 1997.

135. Webb LJ, Sherlock S: The aetiology, presentation and natural history of extra-hepatic portal venous obstruction. Q J Med 48:627-639, 1979.

136. Khuroo M, Datta DV: Budd-Chiari syndrome following pregnancy. Report of 16 cases, with roentgenologic, hemodynamic and histo-

logic studies of the hepatic outflow tract. Am J Med 68:113-121, 1980.

137. Capron JP, Lemay JL, Muir JF, et al: Portal vein thrombosis and fatal pulmonary thromboembolism associated with oral contraceptive treatment. J Clin Gastroenterol 3:295-298, 1981.

138. Lewis JH, Tice HL, Zimmerman HJ: Budd-Chiari syndrome associated with oral contraceptive steroids. Review of treatment of 47 cases. Dig Dis Sci 28:673-683, 1983.

139. Maddrey WC: Hepatic vein thrombosis (Budd-Chiari syndrome): Possible association with the use of oral contraceptives. Semin Liver Dis 7:32-39, 1987.

140. Valla D, Le GM, Poynard T, et al: Risk of hepatic vein thrombosis in relation to recent use of oral contraceptive: A case-control study. Gastroenterology 90:807-811, 1986.

141. Collier JD, Sale J, Friend PJ, et al: Graft loss and the antiphospholipid syndrome following liver transplantation. J Hepatol 29:999-1003, 1998.

142. Pomeroy C, Knodell RG, Swaim WR, et al: Budd-Chiari syndrome in a patient with the lupus anticoagulant. Gastroenterology 86:158-161, 1984.

143. Farrant JM, Judge M, Thompson RP: Thrombotic cutaneous nodules and hepatic vein thrombosis in the anticardiolipin syndrome. Clin Exp Dermatol 14:306-308, 1989.

144. Terabayashi H, Okuda K, Nomura F, et al: Transformation of inferior vena caval thrombosis to membranous obstruction in a patient with the lupus anticoagulant. Gastroenterology 91:219-224, 1986.

145. Van Steenbergen W, Beyls J, Vermylen J, et al: Lupus anticoagulant and thrombosis of the hepatic veins (Budd-Chiari syndrome). Report of three patients and review of the literature. J Hepatol 3:87-94, 1986.

146. Asherson RA, Thompson RP, MacLachlan N, et al: Budd Chiari syndrome, visceral arterial occlusions, recurrent fetal loss and the "lupus anticoagulant" in systemic lupus erythematosus. J Rheumatol 16:219-224, 1989.

147. Asherson RA, Khamashta MA, Hughes GR: The hepatic complications of the antiphospholipid antibodies (editorial). Clin Exp Rheumatol 9:341-344, 1991.

148. Pelletier S, Landi B, Piette JC, et al: Antiphospholipid syndrome as the second cause of non-tumorous Budd-Chiari syndrome. J Hepatol 21:76-80, 1994.

149. Kim JH, Ha HK, Yoon KH, et al: CT features of abdominal manifestations of primary antiphospholipid syndrome. J Comput Assist Tomogr 23:678-683, 1999.

150. Albacete RA, Matthews MJ, Saini N: Portal vein thromboses in malignant hepatoma. Ann Intern Med 67:337-348, 1967.

151. Reynolds TB: Budd-Chiari syndrome. In Schiff L, Schiff ER (eds): Diseases of the Liver, 6th ed. Philadelphia, JB Lippincott, 1987, pp 1466-1473.

152. Fortner JG, Kallum BO, Kim DK: Surgical management of hepatic vein occlusion by tumor. Arch Surg 112:727-728, 1977.

153. Die Goyanes A, Pack GT, Bowden L: Cancer of the body and tail of the pancreas. Rev Surg 28:153-175, 1971.

154. McDermott WV Jr: Portal hypertension secondary to pancreatic disease. Ann Surg 152:147-150, 1960.

155. Spapen HD, Volckaert A, Bourgain C, et al: Acute Budd-Chiari syndrome with portosystemic encephalopathy as first sign of renal carcinoma. Br J Urol 62:274-275, 1988.

156. Carbonnel F, Valla D, Menu Y, et al: Acute Budd-Chiari syndrome as first manifestation of adrenocortical carcinoma. J Clin Gastroenterol 10:441-444, 1988.

157. Bhaskar KVS, Joshi K, Banerjee CK, et al: Peliosis hepatis in Hodgkin's disease: An infrequent association (letter). Am J Gastroenterol 85:628-629, 1990.

158. Walsh MM, Hytiroglou P, Thung SN, et al: Epithelioid hemangioendothelioma of the liver mimicking Budd-Chiari syndrome. Arch Pathol Lab Med 122:846-848, 1998.

159. Jose B, Narayan PI, Pietsch JB, et al: Budd-Chiari syndrome secondary to hepatic vein thrombus from Wilm's tumor. Case report and literature review. J Kentucky Med Assoc 87:174-176, 1989.

160. Imakita M, Yutani C, Ishibashi-Ueda H, et al: Primary leiomyosarcoma of the inferior vena cava with Budd-Chiari syndrome. Acta Pathol Japan 39:73-77, 1989.

161. Lee PK, Teixeira OH, Simons JA, et al: Atypical hepatic vein leiomyoma extending into the right atrium: An unusual cause of the Budd-Chiari syndrome. Can J Cardiol 6:107-110, 1990.

162. Pollanen M, Butany J, Chiasson D: Leiomyocarcoma of the inferior vena cava. Arch Pathol Lab Med 111:1085-1087, 1987.

163. Hunt AH, Whittard BR: Thrombosis of the portal vein in cirrhosis hepatis. Lancet 1:281-284, 1954.

164. Chang HP, McFadzean AJS: Thrombosis and intimal thickening in the portal system in cirrhosis of the liver. J Pathol Bacteriol 89:473-480, 1965.

165. Wanless IR, Wong F, Blendis LM, et al: Hepatic and portal vein thrombosis in cirrhosis: Possible role in development of parenchymal extinction and portal hypertension. Hepatology 21:1238-1247, 1995.

166. Averbuch M, Aderka D, Winer Z, et al: Budd-Chiari syndrome in Israel: Predisposing factors, prognosis, and early identification of high-risk patients. J Clin Gastroenterol 13:321-324, 1991.

167. Wenzel JS, Donohoe A, Ford KL 3rd, et al: Primary biliary cirrhosis: MR imaging findings and description of MR imaging periportal halo sign. AJR Am J Roentgenol 176:885-889, 2001.

168. Bilbao JI, Rodriguez-Cabello J, Longo J, et al: Portal thrombosis: Percutaneous transhepatic treatment with urokinase—a case report. Gastrointest Radiol 14:326-328, 1989.

169. Perel Y, Dhermy D, Carrere A, et al: Portal vein thrombosis after splenectomy for hereditary stomatocytosis in childhood. Eur J Pediatr 158:628-630, 1999.

170. Mosimann F, Mange B: Portal hypertension as a complication of idiopathic retroperitoneal fibrosis. Br J Surg 67:804, 1980.

171. Lorenzo MJ, Gual Corts M, Morato Griera J: The syndrome of Budd-Chiari associated with constrictive pericarditis and complete thrombosis of the inferior vena cava. Rev Clin Esp 152:407-410, 1979.

172. Paul O, Castleman B, White PD: Chronic constrictive pericarditis: A study of 53 cases. Am J Med Sci 216:361-377, 1948.

173. Hirooka M, Kimura C: Membranous obstruction of the hepatic portion of the inferior vena cava. Surgical correction and etiological study. Arch Surg 100:656-663, 1970.

174. Okuda K, Ostrow JD: Clinical conference: Membranous type of Budd-Chiari syndrome. J Clin Gastroenterol 6:81-88, 1984.

175. Fonkalsrud EW, Linde LM, Longmire WPJ: Portal hypertension from idiopathic superior vena caval obstruction. JAMA 196:115-118, 1966.

176. Gentil-Kocher S, Bernard O, Brunelle F, et al: Budd-Chiari syndrome in children: Report of 22 cases. J Pediatr 113:30-38, 1988.

177. Correa de Araujo R, Bestetti RB, Oliveira JSM: An unusual case of Budd-Chiari syndrome—a case report. Angiology 39:193-198, 1988.

178. Dahms BB, Boyd T, Redline RW: Severe perinatal liver disease associated with fetal thrombotic vasculopathy. Pediatr Dev Pathol 5:80-85, 2002.

179. Feingold ML, Litwak RL, Geller SS, et al: Budd-Chiari syndrome caused by a right atrial tumor. Arch Intern Med 127:292-295, 1971.

180. Sty JR: Ultrasonography: Hepatic vein thrombosis in sickle cell anemia. Am J Pediatr Hematol-Oncol 4:213-215, 1982.

181. Koshy A, Bhusnurmath SR, Mitra SK, et al: Hydatid disease associated with hepatic outflow tract obstruction. Am J Gastroenterol 74:274-278, 1980.

182. Parker RGF: Occlusion of the hepatic veins in man. Medicine 38:369-402, 1959.

183. Aikat BK, Bhusnurmath SR, Chhuttani PN, et al: Hepatic vein obstruction—a retrospective analysis of 72 autopsies and biopsies. Indian J Med Res 67:128-144, 1978.

184. Nicoloff DM, Fortuny IE, Pewall RA: Acute Budd-Chiari syndrome secondary to intrahepatic hematoma following blunt abdominal trauma: Treatment by open intracardiac surgery. J Thorac Cardiovasc Surg 47:225-229, 1964.

185. Bayraktar Y, Balkanci F, Kayhan B, et al: Congenital hepatic fibrosis associated with cavernous transformation of the portal vein. Hepatogastroenterology 44:1588-1594, 1997.

186. al-Dalaan A, al-Balaa S, Ali MA, et al: Budd-Chiari syndrome in association with Behçet's disease. J Rheumatol 18:622-626, 1991.

187. Bismuth E, Hadengue A, Hammel P, et al: Hepatic vein thrombosis in Behçet's disease. Hepatology 11:969-974, 1990.

188. Maddrey WC, Sen Gupta KP, Basu Mallik KC, et al: Extrahepatic obstruction of the portal venous system. Surg Gynecol Obstet 127:989-998, 1968.

189. Klein MD, Philippart AI: Posttraumatic Budd-Chiari syndrome with late reversibility of hepatic venous obstruction. J Pediatr Surg 14:661-663, 1979.

190. Millikan WJ Jr, Henderson JM, Sewell CW, et al: Approach to the spectrum of Budd-Chiari syndrome: Which patients require portal decompression? Am J Surg 149:167-176, 1985.

191. Hales MR, Scatliff JH: Thrombosis of the inferior vena cava and hepatic veins (Budd-Chiari syndrome). Ann Intern Med 65:768-781, 1966.

192. Chamberlain DW, Walter JB: The relationship of Budd-Chiari syndrome to oral contraceptives and trauma. Can Med Assoc J 101:618, 1969.

193. Campbell DA, Rolles K, Jameson N, et al: Hepatic transplantation with perioperative and long term anticoagulation as treatment for Budd-Chiari syndrome. Surg Gynecol Obstet 166:511-518, 1988.

194. Lauridsen UB, Enk B, Gammeltoft A: Oesophageal varices as a late complication to neonatal umbilical vein catheterization. Acta Pediatr Scand 67:633-636, 1978.

195. Estrada V, Gutierrez FM, Cortes M, et al: Budd-Chiari syndrome as a complication of the catheterization of the subclavian vein (letter). Am J Gastroenterol 86:250-251, 1991.

196. Valla D, Pessegueiro-Miranda H, Degott C, et al: Hepatic sarcoidosis with portal hypertension. A report of seven cases with a review of the literature. Q J Med 63:531-544, 1987.

197. Moreno-Merlo F, Wanless IR, Shimamatsu K, et al: The role of granulomatous phlebitis and thrombosis in the pathogenesis of cirrhosis and portal hypertension in sarcoidosis. Hepatology 26:554-560, 1997.

198. Natalino MR, Goyette RE, Owensby LC, et al: The Budd-Chiari syndrome in sarcoidosis. JAMA 239:2657-2658, 1978.

199. Russi EW, Bansky G, Pfaltz M, et al: Budd-Chiari syndrome in sarcoidosis. Am J Gastroenterol 81:71-75, 1986.

200. Lin CS: Suppurative pylephlebitis and liver abscess complicating colonic diverticulitis: Report of two cases and review of literature. Mt Sinai J Med 40:48-55, 1973.

201. Wanless IR: The pathophysiology of non-cirrhotic portal hypertension: A pathologist's perspective. In Boyer JL, Bianchi L (eds): Falk Symposium 44: Liver Cirrhosis. Proceedings of the VIIth International Congress of Liver Diseases. Lancaster, Pa, MTP Press, 1987, pp 293-311.

202. Slovis TL, Haller JO, Cohen HL, et al: Complicated appendiceal inflammatory disease in children: Pylephlebitis and liver abscess. Radiology 171:823-825, 1989.

203. Delamarre J, Fabre V, Remond A, et al: [Portal venous system calcifications. Study of 3 cases and review of the literature.] Gastroenterol Clin Biol 15:254-260, 1991.

204. Besnard M, Pariente D, Hadchouel M, et al: Portal cavernoma in congenital hepatic fibrosis. Angiographic reports of 10 pediatric cases. Pediatr Radiol 24:61-65, 1994.

205. Inacio C, Hillaire S, Valla D, et al: Case report: Cytomegalovirus infection as a cause of acute portal vein thrombosis. J Gastroenterol Hepatol 12:287-288, 1997.

206. Kikuchi K, Rudolph R, Murakami C, et al: Portal vein thrombosis after hematopoietic cell transplantation: Frequency, treatment and outcome. Bone Marrow Transplant 29:329-333, 2002.

207. Hunter GC, Steinkirchner T, Burbige EJ, et al: Venous complications of sclerotherapy for esophageal varices. Am J Surg 156:497-501, 1988.

208. Thatcher BS, Sivak MV, Ferguson DR, et al: Mesenteric venous thrombosis as a possible complication of endoscopic sclerotherapy. Am J Gastroenterol 81:126-129, 1986.

209. Andrade ZA, Peixoto E, Guerret S, et al: Hepatic connective tissue changes in hepatosplenic schistosomiasis. Hum Pathol 23:566-573, 1992.

210. Talbot RW, Heppell J, Dozois RR, et al: Vascular complications of inflammatory bowel disease. Mayo Clin Proc 61:140-145, 1986.

211. Capron JP, Remond A, Lebrec D, et al: Gastrointestinal bleeding due to chronic portal vein thrombosis in ulcerative colitis. Dig Dis Sci 24:232-235, 1979.

212. Aronson AR, Steinheber FU: Portal vein thrombosis in ulcerative colitis. NY State J Med 71:2310-2311, 1971.

213. O'Shea PA: Inferior vena cava and hepatic vein thrombosis as a rare complication of ventriculoatrial shunt. J Neurosurg 48:143-145, 1978.

214. Paliard P, Bretagnolle M, Collet P, et al: Inferior vena cava thrombosis with Budd-Chiari syndrome during the course of hepatic and digestive amyloidosis. Gastroenterol Clin Biol 7:919-922, 1983.

215. Victor S, Jayanthi V, Madanagopalan N: Budd-Chiari syndrome in a child with hepatic tuberculosis. Indian Heart J 41:279, 1989.
216. Vallaeys JH, Praet MM, Roels HJ, et al: The Budd-Chiari syndrome caused by a zygomycete. A new pathogenesis of hepatic vein thrombosis. Arch Pathol Lab Med 113:1171-1174, 1989.
217. Young RC: The Budd-Chiari syndrome caused by *Aspergillus*. Two patients with vascular invasion of the hepatic veins. Arch Intern Med 124:754-757, 1969.
218. Young ID, Clark RN, Manley PN, et al: Response to steroids in Budd-Chiari syndrome caused by idiopathic granulomatous venulitis. Gastroenterology 94:503-507, 1988.
219. Victor S: In Okuda K (ed): 2nd International Symposium on Budd-Chiari Syndrome, 1991. Kyoto, Japan, 1991.
220. Maccini DM, Berg JC, Bell GA: Budd-Chiari syndrome and Crohn's disease. An unreported association. Dig Dis Sci 34:1933-1936, 1989.
221. Brinson RR, Curtis WD, Schuman BM, et al: Recovery from hepatic vein thrombosis (Budd-Chiari syndrome) complicating ulcerative colitis. Dig Dis Sci 33:1615-1620, 1988.
222. Cosnes J, Robert A, Levy VG, et al: Budd-Chiari syndrome in a patient with mixed connective-tissue disease. Dig Dis Sci 25:467-469, 1980.
223. Shani M, Theodor E, Frand M, et al: A family with protein-losing enteropathy. Gastroenterology 66:433-445, 1974.
224. Tsuchiya M, Oshio C, Asakura H, et al: Budd-Chiari syndrome associated with protein-losing enteropathy. Gastroenterology 75:114-117, 1978.
225. Marteau P, Cadranel JF, Messing B, et al: Association of hepatic vein obstruction and coeliac disease in North African subjects. J Hepatol 20:650-653, 1994.
226. Zylberberg H, Valla D, Viguie F, et al: Budd-Chiari syndrome associated with 5q deletion and hypereosinophilia. J Clin Gastroenterol 23:66-68, 1996.

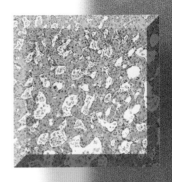

CHAPTER 39

Transplantation Pathology of the Liver

ANTHONY J. DEMETRIS • JAMES M. CRAWFORD
MIKE NALESNIK • PARMJEET RANDHAWA
TONG WU • MARIDA MINERVINI

◼ Introduction

The pathology of liver transplantation is a broad topic. It covers the entire gamut of native liver pathology, as well as a variety of new diseases that occur as a result of situations unique to allografts. Examples include "preservation" injury, rejection, mechanical problems related to unique aspects of the operative procedure(s), and infections and neoplasms occurring in immunosuppressed hosts. This chapter provides practical information needed by any practicing pathologist who wishes to effectively participate in a liver transplant program. Descriptions of the allograft syndromes include a brief introduction and overview of pathophysiologic concepts, followed by clinical presentation and correlations, microscopic pathology, and differential diagnosis. This approach reflects the reliance of transplant pathology on pathophysiologic concepts and clinicopathologic correlations. Reliance strictly on morphologic findings is discouraged because new variables that can influence the microscopic pathology are frequently introduced into patient management.

◼ Information Helpful in Specimen Evaluation

Interpretation of post-transplant specimens requires knowledge of the original disease, of the time since transplantation, and of the operative approach used. These variables greatly influence patient susceptibility to certain complications and consequently affect the histopathologic differential diagnosis. The list of disease indications for liver transplantation for cadaveric donors in the United States during the calendar year 2001 is given in Table 39-1.

The standard operation is an orthotopic liver transplant procedure[1] during which the recipient portal vein, hepatic artery, bile duct, and vena cava are connected to the corresponding donor structures by end-to-end anastomoses performed after donor cholecystectomy.[1] The donor and recipient are matched for size and ABO blood group. Refer to a standard text for explanations of numerous surgical variations.[2] In general, the more technically demanding operative approaches and those that deviate from reconstruction of the normal anatomy are associated with an increased risk of complications. For example, the risk of hepatic artery thrombosis is increased in small-caliber vessels from pediatric donors and recipients.[1] Any operative manipulation of the donor liver before transplantation, such as the use of "split" livers, reduced-size livers, and living donors, generally increases the risk of vascular and biliary tract complications. In addition, split livers and those from living donors undergo compensatory hyperplasia after transplantation. Consequently, these grafts frequently show changes representing growth and adaptive responses to the operation and physiologic demands of the recipient that can be mistaken for pathology.

TABLE 39-1. Indications for Liver Transplantation for Cadaveric Donors in the United States During the Calendar Year 2001

Diagnosis	Number	%
Fulminant hepatic failure	417	9
Other	455	10
Alcohol	784	17
Metabolic disease	171	4
Primary liver malignancy	157	3
Primary biliary cirrhosis	194	4
Primary sclerosing cholangitis	233	5
Biliary atresia	174	4
Cirrhosis: Cryptogenic, idiopathic, and other	419	9
Hepatitis B virus cirrhosis	211	5
Hepatitis C virus cirrhosis	1302	28
Autoimmune cirrhosis	150	3
Total	**4667**	**100**

Data obtained from the United Network for Organ Sharing (UNOS) Web site at http:/www.OPTN.org.

When signing off on cases, we primarily rely on electronic medical records and our in-house information portal software Electronic Data Interface for Transplantation (EDIT[3]) for pertinent clinical and laboratory information. Any relevant previous biopsy specimens should be reviewed together with the current one. This not only establishes a baseline for each allograft but also facilitates interpretation of the effects of therapy and/or disease progression. Conducting the initial histologic review without clinical information minimizes bias, but the final interpretation must be based on complete clinicopathologic correlation.

Special Considerations for Specific Specimens

PRETRANSPLANT BIOPSIES

Needle biopsies taken early in the pretransplant recipient course can help diagnose the underlying disease when morphologic clues of etiology may be masked under end-stage cirrhosis at the time of transplantation. In addition, patients with fulminant hepatic failure may be referred for transplantation without a firm diagnosis or thorough workup. In such cases, pathologists may be requested to evaluate frozen sections and/or "rapidly processed" slides of the native liver obtained via a transjugular biopsy. The etiologic and prognostic significance of microscopic findings may be helpful in assessment of the potential outcome for a specific treatment and the reversibility of the process. In turn, these findings influence the need for and the timing of transplantation.

Removal or control of a specific and potentially treatable or reversible acute insult can lead to regener-

ation of the native liver. This outcome is preferable to transplantation. Examples include herpes simplex hepatitis, ischemic injury, and acetaminophen toxicity. It must be emphasized, however, that the histopathology is only one laboratory result that should be combined with other clinical and laboratory data. The recipient surgeon is ultimately responsible for the final decision of whether to proceed with or delay transplantation.

NATIVE HEPATECTOMY SPECIMENS

Every attempt should be made to correctly diagnose the disease that led to the need for transplantation because disease recurrence is a major problem in long-term survivors. It is not uncommon for pathologists to revisit native liver slides to determine whether unexplained findings in biopsies obtained after transplantation resemble those seen in the native hepatectomy specimen.

Gross examination of native hepatectomy specimens should be done according to a predefined protocol. First, the liver is weighed and the external surface examined. The gallbladder, if present, is opened longitudinally, starting at the fundus. The incision is extended up through the common bile duct and right and left hepatic ducts into the hepatic parenchyma. Then, the hepatic artery and the portal vein are identified in the hilum and opened longitudinally, starting at the resection line and extending up into the parenchyma. Any abnormalities are noted. Next, the hepatic vein(s) or vena cava, if present, is identified and dissected back into the hepatic parenchyma.

It is extremely important that the native liver be sliced thinly and serially in a horizontal plane at 0.5- to 1.0-cm intervals; slices produced are then similar to those observed on a computed axial tomography (CAT) scan. Any regenerative nodule that by virtue of size or color distinguishes itself from the surrounding cirrhotic parenchyma should be sampled (Fig. 39-1). The location of any other intrahepatic defect is recorded, and the lesion is sampled. In our experience, small, clinically undetected hepatocellular carcinomas are the most common unexpected gross finding. Microscopic sections other than those from suspicious nodules or obvious anatomic defects are taken according to a protocol. Routine sections should include right and left hepatic lobes; resection margins of the hepatic artery; portal and hepatic veins and bile duct; and a deep hilar section. Bulk frozen sections, embedded and frozen in optimum cold temperature (OCT) compound, and bulk formalin-fixed tissue from each patient are saved in an "in-house" tissue bank.

FAILED ALLOGRAFTS

Causes of liver allograft failure vary with the time that has passed since transplantation. Most failures

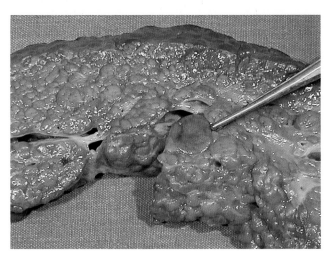

FIGURE 39–1. This gross image of a cirrhotic native liver shows well-developed mixed cirrhosis. A large grossly atypical and suspicious nodule is located at the tip of the forceps and is easily distinguished from the surrounding regenerative nodules. Any nodule that distinguishes itself from the surrounding nodules by size or color should be sampled for microscopic examination.

within the first several weeks after transplantation are related to "preservation" injury or primary nonfunction, vascular thrombosis, and patient death.[4,5] Acute cellular rejection is relatively uncommon as a cause of early graft failure unless immunosuppressive therapy was deliberately withdrawn; humoral rejection is also uncommon.[4,6] Late graft failures (>1 year) are usually attributable to delayed manifestations of technical complications such as vascular thrombosis or biliary sludge syndrome, recurrent disease, and patient death.[4,7] In contrast to other solid organ allografts, chronic rejection of a transplanted liver is a relatively uncommon cause of graft failure, and the incidence is decreasing.[4,8]

Determination of the precise cause of allograft failure often requires review of previous biopsies and correlation with the clinical course. The gross examination is the same as that used for native hepatectomy specimens,[9] as has been described above. Special attention is paid to the inspection and dissection of hilar structures, including the anastomoses. This may require the assistance of the operative surgeon. Necrosis of hilar structures, especially the bile duct wall, with bile leakage into the hilar connective tissue and superimposed bacterial and fungal infection are common in allografts with arterial thrombosis. Microscopic sections are taken according to the same protocol used in native livers.

POST-TRANSPLANT ALLOGRAFT NEEDLE BIOPSIES

Post-transplant allograft needle biopsies are obtained to determine the cause of graft dysfunction or to examine the immunologic and/or architectural status of the allograft. Proper triage of the tissue specimen depends on the clinical differential diagnosis, which in turn depends on the time that has passed since transplantation. Most diagnostically important histopathologic studies can be completed on routinely processed, formalin-fixed, paraffin-embedded sections. Immunofluorescence staining to exclude humoral rejection requires fresh frozen tissue. We routinely prepare only two hematoxylin and eosin (H&E)-stained slides from each biopsy, each of which contains a ribbon of sections. Trichrome, iron, periodic acid–Schiff with diastase (d-PAS), and any other special histochemical or immunohistochemical stains are ordered on indication only after the H&E findings are reviewed. Our signout table is equipped with a multiheaded microscope and a computer for use in accessing electronic medical records and laboratory results. Various allograft syndromes tend to occur at characteristic time intervals since transplantation (Table 39-2).

Evaluation of the Donor Liver

FROZEN SECTIONS OF CADAVERIC DONORS

The macroscopic appearance of the donor organ, preexisting donor disease, or the clinical history or circumstances surrounding donor death or the harvesting procedure can raise doubts about the suitability of a donor organ for transplantation. This uncertainty frequently prompts requests for frozen section evaluation of a donor liver. The following guidelines were developed over the past two decades at University of Pittsburgh Medical Center; use of this approach avoids a number of pitfalls (Table 39-3).

The biopsy specimen should be freshly obtained, preferably in the presence of the pathologist. The pathologist should grossly inspect the donor liver and should assist in choosing the biopsy site (Fig. 39-2). A 1.0-cm^2 wedge or a 2.0-cm-long needle core from the anterior inferior edge of the liver is adequate in most cases when anticipated changes are diffuse. If there is any question about the heterogeneity of a particular gross finding, several biopsy specimens are obtained from different areas of the liver.

The liver tissue should be transported to the frozen section area on a paper towel moistened with preservation fluid (e.g., University of Wisconsin solution). Immersion in saline or preservation fluid for longer than a few minutes should be avoided because this can lead to artifactual changes within the section. Instead, the sample should be immediately frozen and examined. Finally, microscopic pathology should be correlated with the complete donor history and laboratory values before a diagnosis or opinion is given.

TABLE 39-2. Approximate Timing of Common Allograft Syndromes

Syndrome	Clinical Associations/Observations	Peak Time Period
"Preservation" injury	Older, hemodynamically unstable and hypernatremic donors Long cold (>14 hr) or warm (>120 minutes) ischemic time Reconstruction of vascular anastomoses Poor bile production	Can be recognized in postreperfusion biopsies and might persist for several months depending on the severity of the injury
Rejection		
Humoral rejection	ABO-incompatible donor; high-titer (>1:32) lymphocytotoxic crossmatch	Immediately after reperfusion, persisting for several weeks
Acute cellular rejection	Younger, "healthier" female and inadequately immunosuppressed recipients; those with autoimmune disorders	Three days to 6 weeks; later onset is usually associated with inadequate immunosuppression or coexistent viral infection
Chronic rejection	Moderate or severe or persistent episodes of acute rejection; noncompliant and inadequately immunosuppressed patients (e.g., infections, tumors, PTLD)	Bimodal distribution; early peak during first year and later increase in noncompliant and inadequately immunosuppressed patients
Mechanical Problems		
Hepatic artery thrombosis	Pediatric (small-caliber) vessels; donor and/or recipient atherosclerosis; suboptimal or difficult arterial anastomosis; large difference in vessel caliber across anastomosis (see text)	Bimodal distribution; early peak between 0 and 4 weeks, and later peak between 18 and 36 months (see text)
Biliary tract infarction, obstruction, or stricturing	Arterial insufficiency or thrombosis; difficult biliary anastomosis; original disease of primary sclerosing cholangitis	Variable
Venous outflow obstruction	Difficult "piggyback" hepatic vein reconstruction; cardiac failure	Usually during the first several weeks
Infections		
"Opportunistic" viral and fungal infections (e.g., CMV, HSV, VZ, EBV, *Candida* species, *Aspergillus* species)	Seropositive donors to seronegative recipients (often pediatric); overimmunosuppressed recipients	0 to 8 weeks, much less common thereafter except for EBV-related PTLDs and other EBV-related tumors (see text)
Recurrent Diseases		
Recurrent or new onset of viral or autoimmune hepatitis (e.g., HBV, HCV)	Original disease of HBV, HCV, or autoimmune hepatitis	Usually first becomes apparent 4 to 6 weeks after transplantation and persists thereafter, but earlier onset (within 2 weeks) in aggressive cases
PBC and PSC	Original disease of PBC or PSC; donor-recipient MHC-DR matching for PBC patients, weaning of immunosuppression	Usually longer than 6 months after transplantation; incidence of PSC increases over time after transplantation
Alcohol abuse	High per-day alcohol intake before transplantation; noncompliance with treatment protocols; γ-GTP: ALP ratio > 1.4	Usually >6 months
Nonalcoholic steatohepatitis	Original disease of nonalcoholic steatohepatitis or cryptogenic cirrhosis; persistent risk factors for NASH after transplantation	Usually >3 to 4 weeks

ALP, alkaline phosphatase; CMV, cytomegalovirus; DR, donor-recipient; EBV, Epstein-Barr virus; γ-GTP, gamma-glutamyltranspeptidase; HSV, herpes simplex virus; HBV, hepatitis B virus; HCV, hepatitis C virus; MHC, major histocompatibility complex; NASH, nonalcoholic steatohepatitis; PBC, primary biliary cirrhosis; PSC, primary sclerosing cholangitis; PTLD, post-transplant lymphoproliferative disease; VZ, varicella-zoster virus.

Clinical history and biopsy findings that absolutely disqualify donor organs for transplantation include (1) a number of serologically diagnosed infections (e.g., human immunodeficiency virus [HIV]); (2) certain central nervous system (CNS) and most extra-CNS malignancies; (3) sepsis (e.g., in association with a biopsy, operation, or shunt); and (4) a liver donor biopsy specimen that shows widespread necrosis/apoptosis, as well as severe macrovesicular steatosis involving 50% or more of the hepatocyte volume.[10-13]

Several clinical parameters and microscopic pathology are relative contraindications and render a donor "marginal." Such donor organs are generally considered suboptimal but are not disqualified because many show excellent postoperative function. Unfortunately, our ability to predict the postoperative function of an

TABLE 39-3. Pitfalls to Avoid in Preparation and Interpretation of Frozen Sections of Cadaveric Donor Livers

Pitfall	Artifact/Consequence	Method to Avoid Pitfall
Storage of fatty liver tissue in preservative solution or placement of fatty liver tissue on dry paper towel	Fat leaches out of tissue, and severity of steatosis is underestimated, resulting in inappropriate use of donor organ that should be discarded	Grossly inspect donor liver, obtain fresh biopsy specimen, and immediately freeze; avoid immersion of biopsy specimen in preservation solution altogether. Instead, transport tissue from operating room to frozen section room on *paper towel moistened with preservation solution,* and cut deep into block before taking a section for staining. Place needle biopsy specimens at 45-degree angle with cryostat blade.
Storage of biopsy specimen in "physiologic" saline	Hepatocyte cytology can be significantly distorted; hepatocytes can assume a crenated/necrotic appearance; hepatocyte injury can be overestimated	Use University of Wisconsin solution or other preservation fluid, if needed. Preferred method is to avoid immersion of biopsy in preservation solution altogether. Instead, follow above procedure.
Difficulty cutting frozen section	Suspect fatty or necrotic liver; misinterpretation of findings and inappropriate use or disqualification of donor organ on basis of biopsy findings	Follow above procedure.
Difficulty estimating early subtle ischemic hepatocyte injury because of tissue storage (see above), preparation, or staining	Ischemic injury may be overestimated or missed altogether; misinterpretation of findings and inappropriate use of disqualification of donor organ on basis of biopsy findings	Cut six to eight serial sections, and stain each for increasing length of time in eosin. One or two of the sections will optimize recognition of the difference between ischemically damaged and healthy hepatocytes; then, correlate with serial liver injury tests.

individual marginal donor is sorely in need of improvement. Factors that render donors marginal include older age (>65 years), long cold ischemic time (>13 to 15 hours), donor hemodynamic instability, use of vasopressors, hypernatremia, obesity, hepatitis B virus (HBV) or hepatitis C virus (HCV) infection or anti-hepatitis B core (HBc) antibody positivity, grossly fatty liver, and presence of a liver mass, fibrosis, or other focal lesion or history of cancer (Table 39-4).[13-15]

The greater the number of factors that render a donor marginal, the more likely it is that graft dysfunction or failure will occur after transplantation.[13-15] For example, the combination of a 68-year-old donor liver with a long cold ischemic time (>15 hours) and hepatic artery atherosclerosis with 30% macrovesicular steatosis is likely to disqualify the donor liver. In the absence of microscopic pathology that might impact organ function or recovery, the pathologist is unable to predict the

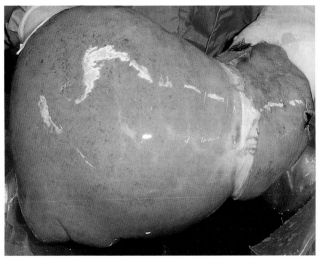
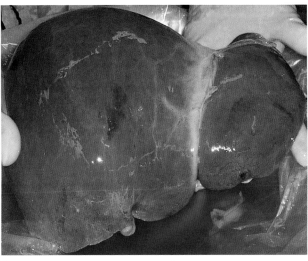

A **B**

FIGURE 39-2. Comparison of the gross appearance of **(A)** a fatty donor liver from **(B)** a normal-appearing donor liver. Needle biopsy sampling of the liver in **A** revealed more than 50% macrovesicular steatosis (see Figure 39-3).

TABLE 39-4. Clinicopathologic Analysis of Marginal Cadaveric Donors

Clinical History/Circumstances	Histopathologic Findings	Comments
Biopsy Findings May Not Be Helpful		
Older donor age (>65 years)	Centrilobular lipofuscin, centrilobular sinusoidal widening/hepatocyte atrophy, and hepatocyte anisonucleosis	In general, older donor livers do not function as well as younger donors and take longer to recover from injury; but individual cases vary and dysfunction/recovery potential cannot be predicted from biopsy findings.
Nonheartbeating donor	Harvesting usually occurs shortly after cessation of heartbeat and often there are no histopathologic changes. When changes are present, they vary widely from nonspecific findings (most common) to widespread coagulative necrosis (organ should be discarded).	Depending on circumstances of harvesting, pathology may or may not be helpful. However, nonheartbeating donors generally show higher rates of complications and failure than do traditional donors.
Prolonged donor ICU stay (>3 to 4 days)	Reactive hepatitis with mononuclear portal inflammation and mild ductular reaction simulating chronic hepatitis	Biopsy findings cannot predict dysfunction
History of extra-CNS malignancy	Not applicable, unless a liver mass is detected; donor liver biopsy should not be used as a screening tool.	Generally disqualifies organ donor depending on circumstances including type of malignancy
CNS malignancy	Not applicable unless a liver mass is detected; donor liver biopsy should not be used as a screening tool.	Depends on histologic subtype of tumor and whether CNS lesion was manipulated (biopsy, operation) and blood-brain barrier was breached
Donor hypernatremia	No consistent histopathologic findings	Biopsy generally not helpful
Biopsy Findings Usually Helpful		
Donor obesity or liver is grossly fatty	>50% macrovesicular steatosis disqualifies organ; 10% to 50% macrovesicular steatosis is usually associated with suboptimal post-transplant function; microvesicular steatosis is often associated with a period of warm ischemia but does not reliably predict post-transplant dysfunction.	Biopsy should be freshly obtained and immediately frozen to prevent artifacts that can underestimate the severity of the steatosis (see Table 39-2).
Masses, focal fibrosis, and other focal lesions	Benign and malignant tumors, granulomas, and areas of fibrosis	Malignant tumors and hepatic adenomas disqualify the donor. Focal nodular hyperplasia and bile duct adenomas can be resected and livers used; liver with old infectious granulomas can generally be used, but infection workup is needed after transplant (see text).
Chronic viral hepatitis type B or C, or anti-HBc–positive donors	Low-grade chronic hepatitis (mHAI ≤ 4) and low fibrous stage (≤1) most common; more severe inflammation and fibrosis generally eliminated on gross examination. Anti-HBc-positive donors may not show any significant pathology (see text). Subcapsular biopsy can overestimate the severity of fibrosis.	HBV-positive or HCV-positive donors with low-grade chronic hepatitis and minimal fibrosis are triaged to HBV-positive and HCV-positive recipients, respectively, after informed consent. Anti-HBc–positive donors can transmit HBV infection to naïve recipients (see text).
Donor hemodynamic instability, hypotensive episodes, use of vasopressors	Varying degrees of ischemic hepatocellular injury ranging from cytoaggregation to microvesicular steatosis, apoptosis, and zonal coagulative necrosis	Changes can be subtle (see Table 39-2); correlation with serial liver injury tests in donor before harvesting is helpful.
Severe donor atherosclerosis	Variable but moderate (>50%) narrowing of intrahepatic branches of the hepatic artery by fibrointimal hyperplasia should render liver highly suspect.	Significant sampling problem exists; severity of atherosclerosis in donor aorta and other organs useful for comparison in borderline cases

adequacy of post-transplant organ function on the basis of frozen section light microscopic evaluation before the operation.

Microscopic pathology may or may not be helpful in the evaluation of a marginal donor (see Table 39-3).[11,12,16] Biopsy findings represent just one laboratory result used by the recipient surgeon, who is ultimately responsible for the decision of whether to use or dispose of the donor organ.

Donor macrovesicular steatosis is one of the most common reasons for obtaining a frozen section. This is not surprising given the prevalence of obesity in the United States. At UPMC, the severity of steatosis is roughly estimated on H&E-stained slides alone; in our experience, fat stains are not necessary. Our cutoff for donor disqualification is macrovesicular steatosis involving roughly 50% or more of the hepatocyte volume seen on low-power microscopic examination (Fig. 39-3). More precise measurement of steatosis is generally not required. Post-transplant dysfunction associated with donor macrovesicular steatosis is proportionate to severity. Even livers with less than 50% macrovesicular steatosis are at increased risk for dysfunction early after transplantation, but graft failure is not common.[10-13,16] Microvesicular steatosis, on the other hand, is often found after a short period of warm ischemia or other insults, and in our experience it usually does not adversely affect the clinical course after transplantation.

Because recurrent HCV infection is universal after liver transplantation, and because, in general, HCV is an indolent disease, many centers use HCV-positive

donors. At UPMC, we routinely screen such donors by frozen section histology at the time of harvesting. Those donor livers that show mild inflammation and fibrosis are used only after informed consent is obtained from the recipient. Formal evaluation of the policy to use HCV-positive donors shows that the rates of recurrent hepatitis and serious disease after transplantation are not affected by the HCV status of the donor.[17] Thus, minimally diseased, HCV-positive donor organs that otherwise would have been discarded can be used to prolong the life of a recipient with end-stage HCV-induced liver failure; graft and patient survival rates are similar to those of HCV-negative donors.[18]

Livers from anti-HBc positive donors might be considered marginal because they can transmit HBV to recipients, especially those with no previous exposure to HBV.[19] However, biopsy evaluation of such livers usually does not provide any useful information because a majority do not show any specific features of HBV-induced liver disease.

BIOPSY EVALUATION OF THE LIVING DONOR

Living donors are being used increasingly to supplement the significant shortage of cadaveric donors. A maximum mass of about 70% to 80% of liver volume can be safely removed from healthy donors. A hyperdynamic portal circulation also limits the minimal mass of liver tissue to about 1% of body mass or about 30% of expected liver volume that can be safely transplanted into cirrhotic recipients.[20,21] Exceeding either limitation usually leads to an increased rate of complications, the most feared being catastrophic liver failure.[20,21] Therefore, the left lobe can often be used for adult-to-pediatric transplants, but adult-to-adult living donor transplantation usually requires right lobe donation[22,23]; this is a major operation with mortality roughly estimated at about 2 in 700.[24]

A conservative approach to donor evaluation is used at most centers in an effort to minimize the risks of donation. A thorough step-wise medical and surgical evaluation includes screening for any major medical diseases, obesity, previous major abdominal surgery, infectious diseases that could be transmitted to the recipient, psychosocial instability, and any liver function abnormality or disease that might put the donor at risk.[24] Abnormalities detected during the workup can disqualify a potential donor or may signal the need for a liver biopsy.

We routinely biopsy all living donors, although this practice is not mandatory. Ryan and associates[25] subjected 100 consecutive living donors to liver biopsy and found that body mass index was not as accurate as liver biopsy in determining the severity of hepatic steatosis. In addition, three patients were disqualified

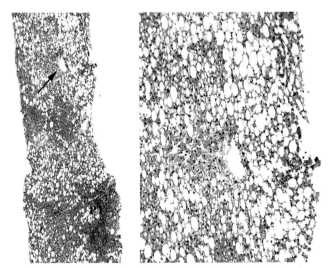

FIGURE 39–3. Microscopic examination of the grossly fatty liver shown in Figure 39-2 shows macrovesicular steatosis involving more than 50% of the hepatocyte volume in the lobules. The *arrow* shown on the left side of the photomicrograph points toward a central vein shown at higher magnification on the right side of the photomicrograph. PT, portal tract.

because of occult liver disease, such as low-grade chronic hepatitis, portal fibrosis, and unclassified vascular abnormalities. Our results have been similar: We have detected unsuspected macrovesicular steatosis and have disqualified livers with greater than 30% steatosis; another prospective donor with steatohepatitis and bridging fibrosis was detected during protocol biopsy specimen evaluation.

■ Determination of Causes of Graft Dysfunction After Transplantation

"PRESERVATION" OR ISCHEMIC INJURY AND PRIMARY DYSFUNCTION

"Preservation," or harvesting, injury refers to damage that causes dysfunction immediately after transplantation but is not readily explainable on the basis of a technical or a vascular insult, arterial or venous thrombosis, alloimmunologic or adverse drug reaction, toxin exposure, or infection. Insults that contribute to preservation injury include donor and recipient hypotension and other causes of warm ischemia, metabolic abnormalities, cold ischemia during organ preservation, and reperfusion injury.

Pathophysiology

Warm ischemia occurs when the organ is kept at body temperature but is inadequately perfused with blood before or during harvesting and during rewarming after implantation. Warm ischemia is thought to preferentially damage hepatocytes and is not usually a clinical problem if it is kept to under 120 minutes.[26,27] Cold ischemia occurs during storage in preservation fluid and ice bath immersion; it preferentially damages sinusoidal endothelial cells.[12,28] General guidelines suggest that cold ischemic time should be kept to less than 15 hours, if possible. Although longer cold ischemic times can be tolerated, patient outcome is jeopardized; increased rates of dysfunction, post-transplant complications, and allograft failure may be noted.[14,29]

Even though hypothermia reduces the metabolic rate and prolongs the time that anoxic cells can retain essential metabolic function,[28] ischemic injury causes loss of mitochondrial respiration and, consequently, adenosine triphosphate (ATP) depletion. This is followed by deterioration in energy-dependent metabolic pathways and transport processes[28] and activation of proteinases and metalloproteinases, which in turn causes lifting of the sinusoidal endothelial cells from the underlying matrix. Loss of sinusoidal microvascular integrity and function and subsequent interference with hepatic blood flow after revascularization are thought to be the major determinants of loss of graft viability.[12,28,30]

However, damage to hepatocytes and biliary epithelial cells and the interaction between parenchymal and nonparenchymal cells are receiving increased attention as important determinants of graft viability.[31] Donor livers with preexisting steatosis show an increased susceptibility to both warm and cold ischemic injury.[31,32]

Complete revascularization and reperfusion with blood cause Kupffer cell activation mediated by priming with tumor necrosis factor-α from the intestines.[28,30] The hypoxia and subsequent reoxygenation lead to activation of complement factors. Activated Kupffer cells release reactive oxygen species that induce a network of cytokines, which in turn contribute granulocyte accumulation within the sinusoids.[28,30] All of these processes lead to an imbalance of vasoconstrictors over vasodilators—an additional important factor contributing to microcirculatory failure. Agents that favor vasodilatation, such as endothelin antagonists, can lessen reperfusion injury, whereas those that favor vasoconstriction can worsen it.[28] Neutrophils secondarily contribute to the damage by releasing reactive oxygen species and proteases.

Bile duct cells are directly susceptible to preservation and reperfusion injury, as well as to the toxic actions of hydrophobic bile salts.[31] The biliary tree is flushed during preservation, but residual bile remains and long cold ischemic times increase the number of biliary epithelial cells shed into the bile after transplantation.[33] This might explain the increased incidence of biliary sludge syndrome seen in marginal grafts and in those with long donor cold ischemic times.[34] In addition, biliary epithelial damage likely contributes to the prolonged cholestatic phase of the preservation-reperfusion syndrome.

Clinical Features

Poor bile production and persistent elevation of serum lactate after complete revascularization are the most reliable early signs of significant preservation injury.[35-37] Marked elevation of serum alanine transaminase (ALT) and aspartate transaminase (AST) to levels greater than 2500 IU/mL during the first few days after transplantation usually signals relatively severe damage.[12] In such cases, if the graft survives the initial insult, the transaminases rapidly normalize after the first few days.[30,31] This is followed by a prolonged cholestatic phase with elevations in total serum bilirubin and gamma-glutamyltranspeptidase (γ-GTP).[9,12,30,31] The general trend is toward gradual improvement, but resolution of abnormal bilirubin values and restoration of normal architecture may require several months.[9,12]

Reperfusion of a donor liver with preexisting macrovesicular steatosis results in a characteristic intraoperative syndrome manifest as fibrinolysis and wound site bleeding. Oozing from disrupted vessels makes it difficult for hemostasis to be achieved.[10,38]

The recovery of recipients who were critically ill before transplantation becomes even more complicated and protracted when they receive a fatty or marginal donor liver.

Microscopic Pathology

Even though cold ischemic injury preferentially damages sinusoidal endothelial cells, routine light microscopic examination on either frozen or permanent section cannot be used before implantation to accurately assess the damage or to predict post-transplant allograft function; electron microscopy is required.[12] Light microscopic examination of biopsy specimens obtained after reperfusion is more informative.

Biopsy specimens obtained within hours of complete revascularization (so-called reperfusion biopsies) show the damage and, with reasonable accuracy, can predict poor allograft function during the first few post-operative weeks.[12] Indicators of severe preservation injury in reperfusion biopsy specimens include zonal or confluent coagulative necrosis, particularly if periportal or bridging, and severe neutrophilic exudation. The subcapsular parenchyma is especially susceptible to damage.[39] A needle biopsy specimen taken from this area may show more severe pathology than is seen in the deeper parenchyma. Neutrophilia without necrosis (so-called surgical hepatitis) can be seen to result from operative manipulation of the liver alone and is not a sign of severe injury.

Histopathologic evidence of a repair response usually begins within 2 to 3 days after transplantation and is proportionate to the severity of the insult. Mild hepatocellular injury such as microvesicular steatosis, hepatocellular cytoaggregation (i.e., rounding up of hepatocyte cytoplasm with detachment from adjacent hepatocytes), and hepatocellular swelling[9,12] is rapidly reversible. Reparative responses in such cases are usually limited to hepatocellular mitosis, twinning of the plates, and nuclear enlargement (Fig. 39-4). Mild centrilobular hepatocellular swelling and hepatocanalicular cholestasis may persist for several weeks.

Response to more severe injury varies with the location of the hepatocyte necrosis. Centrilobular hepatocyte dropout usually triggers mitosis in neighboring viable zone 2 hepatocytes that rapidly proliferate to restore the normal architecture. Periportal and bridging necrosis with architectural collapse triggers cholangiolar proliferation[9,12] that can link adjacent portal tracts and distort the architecture. More severe injury is also usually accompanied by centrilobular hepatocellular swelling and hepatocanalicular and cholangiolar cholestasis (Fig. 39-5)[9,12]—changes that can persist for 1 or 2 months or longer. If the graft recovers, the normal lobular architecture will eventually be restored if the patient does not develop biliary strictures.

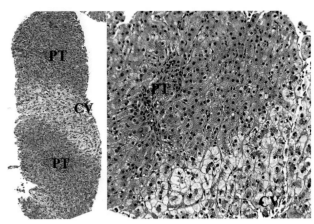

FIGURE 39–4. Mild preservation/reperfusion injury is characterized by centrilobular hepatocyte swelling and mild hepatocanalicular cholestasis. Note the absence of portal inflammation and cholangiolar proliferation at the interface zone. PT, portal tract; CV, central vein.

Reperfusion of a donor liver with preexisting macrovesicular steatosis results in lysis of some fat-containing hepatocytes and release of the lipid droplets into the sinusoids (Fig. 39-6). Extracellular lipid droplets coalesce into large fat globules, which clog sinusoidal blood flow. This triggers local fibrin deposition, neutrophilia, and red blood cell congestion.[10] If the liver recovers, the large fat globules eventually resolve over a period of several weeks.

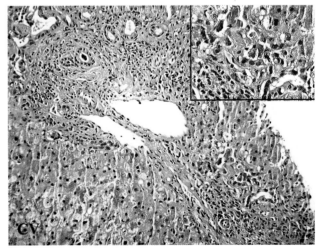

FIGURE 39–5. Severe preservation/reperfusion injury is characterized by centrilobular hepatocyte swelling, hepatocanalicular cholestasis, and portal tract expansion because of cholongiolar proliferation at the interface zone, which is often accompanied by mild nonspecific inflammation and cholangiolar bile plugs *(inset)*. These changes can persist for up to several months or longer after transplantation; such patients are at risk for developing biliary sludge. CV, central vein.

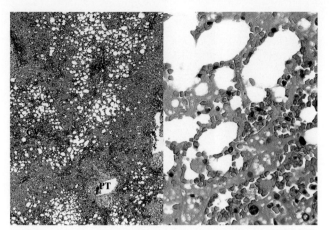

FIGURE 39–6. Reperfusion of a donor liver with severe macrovesicular steatosis results in release of the fat globules into the sinusoids because of hepatocyte injury during preservation and reperfusion. These fat globules coalesce with other fat globules, leading to large open spaces in the sinusoids shown on the left side of this diagram. These large intrasinusoidal fat globules shown at higher magnification on the right side of the image cause focal fibrin deposition, congestion, and mild neutrophilia. PT, portal tract; CV, central vein.

Differential Diagnosis

The histopathologic differential diagnosis includes sepsis, biliary obstruction, humoral rejection, and cholestatic hepatitis. The pathophysiologic mechanisms of injury are similar in sepsis, preservation injury, and humoral rejection and include sinusoidal endothelial cell injury with poor microvascular flow and coagulative necrosis. In such cases, considerable reliance is placed on the clinical history for guidance in further analysis and interpretation. Donor age, cold and warm ischemic times, operative difficulties, clinical profile, and blood culture and crossmatch results often help the pathologist to determine what type of additional testing (e.g., immunofluorescent staining) might distinguish among these possibilities. In most instances, however, preservation injury and technical problems prove to be the culprits early after transplantation.

The histopathologic distinction between preservation injury and obstruction/cholangitis can be accomplished by close examination of the "true" bile ducts contained within the portal tract connective tissue and comparison with the "cholangioles" located at the interface zone. In obstruction or cholangitis, the usual findings are periductal lamellar edema surrounding the true bile ducts, accompanied by neutrophils within the lumen or infiltrating between biliary epithelial cells. These changes are not seen in preservation injury. Instead, acute pericholangiolitis is noted in preservation injury. Both disorders can show marked centrilobular hepatocanalicular cholangiolar cholestasis and intralobular neutrophil clusters. Fortunately, a T-tube stent, the long limb of which is brought to the skin surface, is usually kept in

place for the first several months after transplantation, when this difficulty most frequently arises. This helps to prevent biliary obstruction and provides ready access for monitoring of bile flow and biliary tract patency.

The distinction between preservation injury and cholestatic hepatitis is based on the clinical history and time since transplantation. Cholestatic hepatitis has been reported only in patients infected with HBV or HCV; it is unusual before 2 to 3 weeks after transplantation and generally worsens with time unless the patient is specifically treated with decreased immunosuppression and/or antiviral therapy. In contrast, preservation injury begins immediately after transplantation and generally improves over time after transplantation.

An additional problem is recognition of acute rejection superimposed on preservation injury. Acute rejection superimposed on preservation injury is recognized by the appearance of mild to moderate mixed portal inflammation containing blastic lymphocytes, especially eosinophils combined with infiltration and damage to true bile ducts. Mononuclear inflammation of portal and central veins provides additional support for the diagnosis of acute rejection.

Finally, apoptotic bodies or coagulative necrosis in a biopsy specimen obtained more than several days after transplantation should not be attributed to preservation injury.[31] Only 4 to 6 hours are required for a normal hepatocyte to undergo the entire apoptotic cycle; therefore, the presence of apoptotic bodies usually signifies an additional, usually ischemic, insult.

VASCULAR COMPLICATIONS IN TRANSPLANTATION

Vascular complications are the most common major technical problem leading to serious allograft damage and failure. Most manifest during the first several months after transplantation and, one way or another, are related to the anastomosis, manipulation of the vascular tree, preexisting vascular disease, metabolic or physiologic abnormalities that predispose to thrombosis, or a combination of these factors. Examples include anastomotic narrowing and other irregularities such as intimal flaps, intimal and/or medial tears, dramatic reductions in caliber across a suture line, or the creation of "kinks" or abnormal tortuosity.[35-37,40] Potential problems are compounded by preexisting atherosclerotic disease and any factors that increase the technical difficulty of completing the vascular anastomosis, such as small-caliber vessels in pediatric recipients or abnormal anatomy (e.g., piggyback vena caval anastomosis). Finally, physiologic or metabolic abnormalities that decrease hepatic blood flow or predispose to thrombosis, such as clotting abnormalities, rejection, infection, and cardiac failure, also increase the risk of complications, especially at sites of abnormal anatomy.

Vascular interposition grafts or small arterial (most often iliac) or venous segments used to link the donor and recipient arteries or veins, respectively, are a convenient "plumbing" solution but also a source of problems. They increase the number of anastomoses required for vascular reconstruction.[1] Vascular grafts cryopreserved or stored in preservation fluid for one to several days before implantation may be marginally viable at the time of placement and may serve as a thrombogenic or atherogenic stimulus or nidus of infection.

Hepatic Artery Thrombosis

OVERVIEW AND PATHOPHYSIOLOGY

The hepatic arterial tree is the most frequent source of vascular complications after liver transplantation and a major cause of allograft dysfunction and failure.[35-37,40] Unlike native livers, an allograft is devoid of collateral arterial circulation, at least early after transplantation. This increases susceptibility to ischemic injury.

The pathophysiologic consequences of inadequate arterial flow are related primarily to ischemia of structures supplied predominantly or exclusively by the hepatic artery. These include the extrahepatic and intrahepatic bile ducts, hilar and portal tract connective tissue, and lymph nodes. This in turn eventually leads to biliary tract strictures, cholangitic abscesses, and the biliary sludge syndrome. All of these complications have been lumped together under the phrase *ischemic cholangitis*.[9,41]

Most arterial complications occur within the first 2 months after transplantation. A second wave of technically related arterial thromboses occurs between 1 and 3 years after transplantation.[42] A less than perfect anastomosis causes turbulent arterial flow immediately downstream from the suture line. This eventually leads to arterial narrowing and thrombosis. In addition, arterial interposition vascular grafts frequently develop fibrointimal hyperplasia more quickly than is seen in the native or allograft arterial vasculature, predisposing to thrombosis and its subsequent complications.

CLINICAL FEATURES

Symptoms, when present, are usually related to hepatic infarcts, abscesses, and/or impaired bile flow. Included are right upper abdominal pain/discomfort, intermittent fever, bacteremia/fungemia, bile peritonitis, and jaundice. Occasionally, fulminant hepatic failure may be seen if large areas of the liver are infarcted. If sufficient collaterals have developed, the patient may be asymptomatic.

MICROSCOPIC PATHOLOGY

Needle biopsy specimen evaluation is an unreliable method for establishing the diagnosis of hepatic artery thrombosis.[9,43] The histologic changes are varied, and

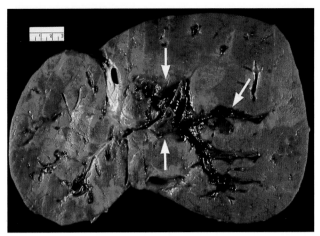

FIGURE 39–7. This is the typical gross appearance of a liver allograft that failed because of hepatic artery thrombosis. The *arrows* outline necrosis of the hepatic hilar structures, including the large bile ducts. This causes leakage of bile into the surrounding connective tissue and parenchyma. Note also the mottled appearance of the subcapsular hepatic parenchyma. A peripheral core needle biopsy could be misleading if it sampled a more viable area.

the structures that are most commonly affected—the hilum and large bile ducts—are not routinely sampled. Thus, peripheral core needle biopsy specimens are subject to greater sampling error than usual. They may show a completely normal appearance, frank coagulative necrosis or marked centrilobular hepatocyte swelling, cholangiolar proliferation with or without bile plugs, and acute cholangiolitis. In some cases, spotty acidophilic necrosis of hepatocytes, or so-called ischemic hepatitis, can mimic acute viral hepatitis. These sampling problems should be remembered when attempts are made to salvage an allograft through arterial thrombectomy. The surgeon may be encouraged by a grossly and microscopically viable appearance at the capsular surface, only to be disappointed later by allograft failure resulting from necrosis of the bile ducts (Fig. 39-7). Hepatic artery thrombosis may also present as biliary tract obstruction.

Examination of failed allografts with hepatic artery thrombosis often reveals transmural necrosis of hilar bile ducts with leakage of bile into the surrounding connective tissue (Fig. 39-8). The necrotic tissue is not infrequently colonized by bacterial and fungal colonies; special staining for microorganisms should be carried out routinely.

DIFFERENTIAL DIAGNOSIS

Hepatic artery narrowing or thrombosis can mimic almost every histopathologic syndrome associated with graft dysfunction, including biliary tract obstruction and cholangitis, acute and chronic rejection, and acute and chronic viral hepatitis. The biopsy specimen may even

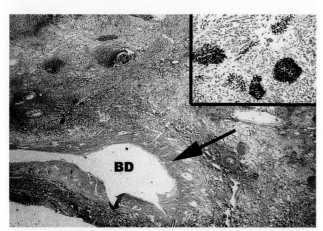

FIGURE 39–8. This is the typical microscopic appearance of a hilar section of a liver allograft that failed from hepatic artery thrombosis. Note the epithelial denudation and mural necrosis of the large bile duct (BD) and leakage of the bile into the surrounding connective tissue. The *arrow* points to the area shown in the *inset*. Necrotic tissue should be routinely subjected to Gram and Grocott staining to detect microorganisms, which are frequently present. In this case, *Candida* colonies were detected (*inset*, Grocott stain).

be unremarkable, either because the patient has developed vascular collaterals and the thrombosis is inconsequential or because necrosis of hilar bile ducts has occurred but changes secondary to biliary sludging have not yet developed in the periphery. More frequent findings include biliary tract obstruction or stricturing. The association of arterial thrombosis with biliary tract complications is so common that examination for hepatic arterial patency is standard practice when biliary tract complications are encountered.[41]

Portal Vein Thrombosis

OVERVIEW AND PATHOPHYSIOLOGY

Portal vein complications such as thrombosis, stricture, and poor flow resulting from persistent collateral circulation or hypotension are uncommon early after transplantation.[35-37,40,44] However, the portal vein is a major source of blood flow, and suboptimal flow or complete occlusion is usually clinically significant. The incidence of complications is increased when cryopreserved venous interposition grafts are used.[45] Long-surviving cirrhotic allografts are more susceptible to portal vein thrombosis than are noncirrhotic allografts.

CLINICAL FEATURES

Complete portal vein thrombosis of a noncirrhotic allograft can result in massive hepatic failure, or the patient can present with signs and symptoms of portal hypertension with massive ascites and edema. If the thrombus is partial or if only narrowing is present, relapsing fever and miliary seeding of the liver with

bacteria may be encountered. Symptoms of portal vein thrombosis in a cirrhotic allograft are the same as those in a native liver with cirrhosis—variceal hemorrhage, splenomegaly, and ascites.

MICROSCOPIC PATHOLOGY

As with hepatic artery thrombosis, the microscopic pathology can be varied and depend on the severity of portal vein flow compromise and the time after transplantation. Complete obstruction early after transplantation is often associated with massive coagulative necrosis. Suboptimal portal flow because of strictures, kinks, or persistent collateral circulation may cause zonal (often periportal or midzonal) coagulative necrosis, hepatocyte atrophy (small size), unexplained zonal or panlobular steatosis, apoptosis, or nodular regenerative hyperplasia–like changes. Bacterial or fungal infection of a partial portal vein thrombus can lead to miliary seeding of the liver with small abscesses.

DIFFERENTIAL DIAGNOSIS

Unexplained zonal ischemic or hepatocellular changes, similar to those described previously, should raise the possibility of compromised portal vein blood flow, which can be evaluated by ultrasound or angiography. Portal vein complications uncommonly show inflammation, and particular attention should be paid to the size and shape of the portal vein branches and their relationship to the parenchyma.

Hepatic Vein and Vena Caval Complications

OVERVIEW AND PATHOPHYSIOLOGY

Hepatic vein and vena caval complications are relatively uncommon but not rare. When they do occur, the clinical history usually includes descriptions of difficulties with reconstruction of the venous outflow tract or alternative anastomoses such as the piggyback approach.[1] Significant stenosis or thrombosis is mostly always associated with either clinical or histopathologic consequences.

CLINICAL FEATURES

The clinical manifestations of severe stenosis or thrombosis resemble the Budd-Chiari syndrome and include hepatic enlargement, tenderness, and ascites and edema. Less severe stenosis might initially result only in histopathologic manifestations, or an increase in the portal vein/vena cava pressure gradient may be noted.

MICROSCOPIC PATHOLOGY

Typical acute findings include congestion and hemorrhage involving the hepatic venules and surrounding perivenular sinusoids. This is often associated with hepatocyte necrosis and dropout. Red blood cell stasis can usually be observed within the lumina of at least some of the hepatic venules. Other findings include changes in nodular regenerative hyperplasia. Perivenular fibrosis also frequently develops, particularly if outflow obstruction is severe or of long duration.

DIFFERENTIAL DIAGNOSIS

Centrilobular or perivenular congestion, hemorrhage, and hepatocyte necrosis can be caused by mechanical outflow obstruction and immune-mediated injury such as acute and chronic rejection, adverse drug reaction, and viral and autoimmune hepatitis. The major difference between mechanical and immune-mediated causes is the presence of perivenular mononuclear inflammation in the latter. Involvement of most central veins suggests a global insult, such as a mechanical problem, an adverse drug reaction, or rejection, whereas patchy involvement is more common with viral or autoimmune hepatitis. However, the inflammation can be transient in some cases of immune-mediated injury and may present at a later stage when it is indistinguishable from mechanical causes of venous outflow obstruction.[46] The focus of any coexistent portal necroinflammatory activity can provide additional information useful in distinguishing between these possibilities—inflammatory damage to bile ducts and portal veins suggests coexistent rejection, whereas prominent interface activity indicates coexistent viral or autoimmune hepatitis. Review of the original disease, operative anatomy, previous rejection history, and results of venous flow and pressure studies is needed in many cases if the underlying cause is to be determined.

BILE DUCT COMPLICATIONS

Overview and Physiology

The biliary tract is usually reconstructed by means of either a duct-to-duct or a choledochojejunal anastomosis. The two most common factors underlying biliary tract complications are ischemic injury and iatrogenically introduced abnormal anatomy, both of which predispose to mucosal damage and inadequate drainage or inordinate reflux. Mucosal or mural damage can lead to anastomotic dehiscence, transmural necrosis and bile leakage, cholangitic abscesses, ascending cholangitis, anastomotic or intrahepatic stricturing, bile casts, obstruction, or biliary-vascular fistulas.[43,47,48]

Several causes of biliary tract ischemia other than frank arterial thrombosis or narrowing are known. These include prolonged cold ischemia[34] and preformed anti-donor antibodies (anti-major histocompatibility complex [MHC] or ABO blood group).[6] The latter can cause arterial vasospasm and immunologic damage to the artery and peribiliary arterial plexus.[6] Biliary tract complications are more common after living donor[49,50]

and split liver transplant operations.[51] Once all other causes of biliary tract complications have been reasonably excluded, the possibility of recurrent disease should be entertained in primary sclerosing cholangitis (PSC) patients.

Clinical Features

Minor biliary tract problems such as strictures and stones are the most common and are usually first suspected when selective elevation of g-GTP and alkaline phosphatase is noted on routine liver injury testing. Actual clinical symptoms are less frequently seen. Biliary imaging studies are used to confirm the diagnosis.[43,47,48] When the T tube is still in place early after transplantation, cholangiograms are routinely performed before clamping (1 week), at the time of T-tube removal (3 months), and when indicated in patients with clinical or biochemical evidence suggestive of biliary obstruction.

Major biliary tract complications such as complete obstruction, cholangitic abscesses, and ascending cholangitis often present with fever, jaundice, upper right quadrant pain, and intermittent bacteremia. These usually require surgical correction, if possible.

Microscopic Pathology

The histopathologic changes associated with biliary tract complications in allografts are the same as those encountered in native livers. Most of these complications are recognized by predominantly neutrophilic portal inflammation, periductal edema, and intraepithelial and intraluminal neutrophils within the true bile ducts. Mild ductular proliferation, centrilobular hepatocanalicular cholestasis, and small clusters of neutrophils throughout the lobules are also commonly seen. Chronic biliary tract strictures may be associated with chronic portal inflammation, biliary epithelial cell senescence, and patchy small bile duct loss. This constellation of findings can closely mimic chronic rejection, which is discussed later.

Red blood cells in bile duct lumina or, conversely, bile concretions surrounded by foreign body giant cells in blood vessels are abnormal and signal the presence of a biliary-vascular fistula. Prompt surgical intervention is often needed when either finding is encountered. Periductal hemorrhage surrounding small interlobular bile ducts is not an uncommon finding when a biopsy specimen is obtained within a day after transhepatic cholangiography.[52] Such patients are usually asymptomatic, and the findings generally resolve without intervention.

Differential Diagnosis

The histopathologic differential diagnosis depends on the time that has passed since transplantation.

Within the first several weeks, biliary obstruction/cholangitis can be difficult to distinguish from preservation injury and acute rejection, particularly if the patient was treated with increased immunosuppression before the biopsy specimen was taken. The distinction between preservation injury and biliary obstruction was discussed under Preservation Injury.

The most important features for distinguishing between acute rejection and biliary obstruction/cholangitis are the composition of the portal inflammation, the presence of a ductular reaction, the cytologic appearance of the biliary epithelial cells, and the presence of perivenular mononuclear inflammation. In biliary obstruction/cholangitis, neutrophils usually predominate, the biliary epithelial cells retain a relatively normal nucleus-to-cytoplasm ratio, and perivenular mononuclear inflammation is absent. In acute rejection, the portal inflammation comprises lymphocytes, plasma cells, and eosinophils, the last of which may be striking or may actually predominate when patients are treated with steroid-sparing immunosuppressive regimens.[53] In addition, the biliary epithelial cells show distinct reactive changes in rejection such as an increased nucleus-to-cytoplasm ratio. Perivenular inflammation is a feature that further distinguishes acute rejection from acute cholangitis/obstruction.

More than 6 months after transplantation, biliary obstruction or stricturing can mimic acute and chronic rejection, viral hepatitis, and recurrent autoimmune disorders. Chronic intermittent biliary obstruction or cholangitis, as seen in patients with the biliary sludge syndrome, may be associated with a mixed or even a predominantly mononuclear portal infiltrate and biliary epithelial cell senescent changes.[54] Portal fibrosis with mild duct proliferation, mild portal neutrophilic or eosinophilic inflammation, and mild centrilobular cholestasis are features that should suggest obstructive cholangiopathy. A clinical and laboratory clue that biliary tract pathology is masquerading as acute rejection is that the patient is more than 6 months post transplant and has adequate immunosuppressive drug levels with preferential elevation of gamma-glutamyltranspeptidase (γ-GTP) and alkaline phosphatase.[55] Late-onset acute rejection is unusual in this circumstance.

Chronic obstructive cholangiopathy may also mimic chronic viral hepatitis. Cholangitis, rather than acute cholangiolitis, and lobular disarray, which is seen in viral hepatitis but not in cholangiopathy, are useful distinguishing features. The profile of liver injury test elevations is also usually helpful. Exclusion of viral pathogens through adjuvant testing procedures can be used to rule out viral infection. It should be remembered, however, that biliary tract problems might be first suspected on biopsy, but cholangiography (magnetic resonance cholangiopancreatography [MRCP], endoscopic retrograde cholangiopancreatography [ERCP, duct-to-duct] or percutaneous transhepatic cholangiography [PTC]) is needed to confirm the diagnosis.

REJECTION

All patients are potentially at risk for the development of rejection, but the incidence and severity of rejection are greater in certain patient populations and under certain circumstances. In general, younger, healthier (e.g., Child's A, lack of renal failure, good muscle mass), black, and female recipients and patients with disorders of immune regulation (e.g., primary biliary cirrhosis [PBC], PSC, autoimmune hepatitis) before transplantation show higher incidences and severity of acute and chronic rejection.[56] Responsiveness to the allograft is enhanced by previous exposure to the same or similar alloantigens via blood transfusions or previous transplants or pregnancies. Inadequate immunosuppression is also a major risk factor.

Rejection in liver allografts is categorized as humoral, acute (cellular), and chronic.[57] Humoral rejection usually occurs within the first several weeks after transplantation and is mediated primarily by antibodies. The acute (cellular) type can occur at any time after transplantation but is most common during the first month and is mediated primarily by cell-mediated immune mechanisms. Chronic rejection usually develops as a direct result of severe or persistent and unresolved acute rejection and is probably mediated by a combination of both antibodies and cell-mediated mechanisms. Each is discussed in greater detail in the following sections.

Humoral Rejection

Liver allografts are much less susceptible to humoral rejection because of preformed lymphocytotoxic antibodies than are other solid organ allografts.[6] Therefore, crossmatch results do not routinely influence the decision to proceed with transplantation. However, crossing ABO blood group barriers is still generally avoided because doing so leads to a high incidence (~60%) of humoral rejection in unconditioned recipients.[6] Nevertheless, some groups still employ ABO-incompatible liver transplantation with reasonable results in candidates with fulminant hepatic failure or in pediatric recipients, in whom the need can be more urgent because the donor pool is limited. If ABO-incompatible recipients are preconditioned with splenectomy, cytoreductive therapy, and/or plasmapheresis,[58] graft failure from acute humoral rejection can generally be avoided. However, such patients are still at risk for late complications of humoral rejection, such as infarcts, and for ischemic cholangitis.[41,59,60]

Living donor liver allografts seem to be more susceptible to humoral rejection than are whole liver cadaveric donors.[61] This is likely related to the further strain on already precarious blood flow that is seen in living donors early after transplantation.

PATHOPHYSIOLOGY

The isoagglutinins and anti-MHC lymphocytotoxic antibodies can cause accelerated liver allograft injury and failure but rarely in a hyperacute fashion.[6] The consequences of antidonor antibodies vary with the class, the titer, the timing of the antibody response, and the density and distribution of target antigens in the organ.[6,62] Preformed antibodies directed at antigens expressed on endothelial cells, such as the isoagglutinins and the lymphocytotoxic (anti-MHC class I) antibodies, are the most dangerous. Binding of antibodies to the graft vasculature causes complement fixation, endothelial damage, deposition of platelet-fibrin thrombi, and initiation of the clotting and fibrinolytic cascades. Subsequent microvascular thrombosis, arterial vasospasm, and coagulopathy act in concert to impair blood flow and cause hemorrhagic necrosis.

Relatively high-titer antibodies are needed to overcome the natural resistance of liver allografts to humoral rejection. This resistance is attributable to (1) secretion by the donor liver of soluble MHC class I antigens that bind to and neutralize the antibodies, (2) Kupffer cell phagocytosis of subsequent immune complexes and activated platelet aggregates, (3) the dual afferent hepatic blood supply, (4) the unique hepatic sinusoidal microvasculature, which is devoid of a conventional basement membrane,[6,63] and (5) possibly a homologous source of complement.[64]

In general, isoagglutinins cause significantly more injury than do lymphocytotoxic antibodies, which do not routinely cause damage unless they are present in high titer (>1:32) and are of the immunoglobulin G (IgG) class.[6,65] The relative risk of damage from lymphocytotoxic antibodies should be kept in perspective. Positive crossmatch results are encountered in 8% to 12% of recipients, and only 30% have relatively high titers. Thus, the patient population at risk for severe humoral rejection is fairly small. Consequently, it may be overlooked as a cause of dysfunction or failure if it occurs only once or twice per year in programs that carry out fewer than 100 procedures per year.

CLINICAL FEATURES

Allograft dysfunction from humoral rejection usually manifests over a period of hours to days rather than minutes to hours.[6] The first signs of serious injury can develop in the operating room after complete revascularization. The liver might reperfuse uniformly and produce bile initially, but then it becomes hard and swollen before bile flow slows or stops altogether. Difficulty in achieving hemostasis and an inordinate need for platelets and blood component replacement

therapy signal the initiation of an intrahepatic consumptive coagulopathy.

Intraoperative events are rarely serious enough to warrant abortion of the procedure or performance of immediate retransplantation. Instead, a relentless rise in serum levels of liver enzymes during the first several post-transplant days and other signs of impending hepatic failure signal the onset of severe humoral rejection.

In cases of suspected humoral rejection, hepatic angiograms are often used to exclude an arterial thrombosis. Segmental narrowing or a sausage-link appearance[6] and diffuse luminal narrowing with poor peripheral changes are suggestive of immunologically mediated arterial vasospasm. In severe cases, these changes are accompanied by marked increases in serum transaminases and other systemic signs of synthetic and functional hepatic failure. Frequent presentation includes a persistent rise in serum bilirubin during the first week after transplantation accompanied by refractory thrombocytopenia, low complement activity, and a biopsy showing changes similar to those described for preservation injury or biliary obstruction.[65] Ischemic biliary necrosis later manifests as biliary sludge; obstructive cholangiopathy and small bile duct loss are other late manifestations of early humorally mediated arterial injury, vasospasm, and thrombosis.

PATHOLOGIC FEATURES

The microscopic features vary with the timing of the biopsy and the presensitized state.[6] Biopsy specimens of ABO-incompatible organs obtained within 2 to 6 hours after reperfusion show prominent red blood cell and focal neutrophil sludging in the sinusoids, focal platelet-fibrin thrombi in portal and central veins, and acidophilic hepatocyte necrosis. These changes can progress within 1 to 2 days to large areas of confluent coagulative hepatocyte necrosis, prominent sinusoidal and venous congestion, and hemorrhage into the portal tract connective tissue. Portal veins often show circumferential fibrin deposition. Arteries occasionally show neutrophilic and/or necrotizing arteritis, but more common findings include endothelial cell hypertrophy and evidence of arterial vasospasm, such as mural myocyte vacuolization, wrinkling of the elastic lamina, and thickening of the wall with narrowing of the lumen.

Mild portal neutrophilia usually appears at 2 to 3 days, along with focal cholangiolar proliferation. The histologic features up to this point are difficult to separate from preservation injury, unless convincing immune deposits are detected. Thereafter, progressive hemorrhagic infarction of the organ can occur in ABO-incompatible organs.

Antibody-mediated injury in patients harboring preformed lymphocytotoxic antibodies is generally less florid, but rare cases mimic ABO-incompatible allografts. Reperfusion biopsies contain platelet aggregates in the portal or central veins more often than do crossmatch-negative controls, but red blood cell congestion is usually not a significant finding. Spotty acidophilic necrosis of hepatocytes and centrilobular hepatocellular swelling, accompanied by cholangiolar proliferation and hepatocanalicular cholestasis, often appear during the first week after transplantation. Inflammatory or necrotizing arteritis is rare.

The gross appearance of failed ABO-incompatible grafts at the time of retransplantation is similar to that of other organ allografts undergoing hyperacute rejection: They are enlarged, cyanotic, and mottled with areas of necrosis. Rupture of the capsule is occasionally seen. Hepatic artery or portal vein thrombosis is not uncommon. Hilar changes include congestion of the peribiliary vascular plexus, partially organized thrombi in arterial branches, and focal mural necrosis of large septal bile ducts. Long-term sequelae of an early humoral insult can include biliary sludge and stricturing with obstructive cholangiopathy, obliterative arteriopathy and loss of small bile ducts, or chronic rejection.

Immune deposits are ephemeral in humoral rejection. Even in allografts that are known to be affected, deposits are usually detectable only in postreperfusion biopsies and for a few days after transplantation. Thereafter, immune deposits become patchy in distribution and may be difficult to distinguish from background staining. IgM and C1q alone frequently become lodged in necrotic arterial walls, regardless of the cause of damage; therefore, they should not be interpreted as evidence of humoral rejection. C4d staining, which is a reliable marker of humoral rejection in kidney allografts, has not been systematically studied in liver allografts. In florid cases of humoral rejection, selective deposits of IgG and/or immunoglobulin M (IgM), along with C3 and C4 in perihilar arteries, portal veins, and the peribiliary plexus, can be seen with diffuse sinusoidal staining.

DIFFERENTIAL DIAGNOSIS

Severe humoral rejection in an ABO-incompatible organ is difficult to distinguish from hemorrhagic liver necrosis caused by severe hypotension, sepsis, or vascular thrombosis. The distinction is often based on the results of clinicopathologic correlation and immunofluorescence analyses rather than on routine microscopic pathology, unless clear-cut inflammatory arteritis is detected. Knowing that the allograft is ABO blood group incompatible, recognizing the injury described earlier, and correlating findings with the clinical course often provide enough information for the pathologist to confidently distinguish between these entities.

In ABO-compatible organs, humoral rejection is difficult to distinguish from preservation injury, although the presensitization state and the post-transplant clinical profile can provide useful information (see under Clinical Presentation). A patient with a short cold ischemic time and a positive crossmatch at high titer that persists after transplantation, and who develops refractory and otherwise unexplained thrombocytopenia and low complement levels, should be suspected of experiencing humoral rejection.[65]

Acute Rejection

Acute (cellular) rejection has been defined as "inflammation of the allograft, elicited by a genetic disparity between the donor and the recipient, primarily affecting interlobular bile ducts and vascular endothelia, including portal and hepatic veins and occasionally the hepatic artery and its branches."[57] Most episodes occur within 30 days after transplantation and are precipitated by the mass migration of donor cells into recipient lymphoid tissues.[66,67] Early acute rejection episodes are usually controlled easily by increased immunosuppression and rarely lead to allograft failure.[3]

Risk factors for the development of acute rejection within the first several months depend on the immunosuppressive regimen but usually include younger recipient age; healthier recipients (e.g., normal serum creatinine, Child's classification); donor-recipient MHC-DR mismatch; patients with immune-dysregulated syndromes such as PSC, autoimmune hepatitis, and PBC; long cold ischemic time; and increased donor age.[56] Late-onset acute rejection occurring more than 1 year after transplantation is often associated with inadequate immunosuppression, is more difficult to control, and more frequently leads to allograft failure.[56]

PATHOPHYSIOLOGY

Recognition of the allograft as foreign through central and peripheral sensitization triggers a cascade of events that change the microenvironment of the allograft. Local secretion of cytokines and chemokines alters the expression of various MHC, adhesion, and co-stimulatory molecules on various cell populations within the liver (Tables 39-5 and 39-6). This results in the retention of a greater number of inflammatory cells within the graft, especially in the portal tracts and perivenular tissues. The biliary epithelia of small bile ducts, the endothelia of portal and central veins, and the hepatic artery branches (in severe rejection) are preferentially targeted for injury.

Various immunologic effector mechanisms contribute to graft injury during acute rejection. Antibody- and complement-mediated injury, cytolytic T-cell lympholysis (Fas-FasL interactions), and effector molecules and cytokines released from various inflammatory cells (e.g., tumor necrosis factor [TNF], eosinophil cationic protein, reactive oxygen species) can directly injure bile ducts[68] and endothelial cells. Endothelial cell damage may in turn interfere with blood flow, indirectly leading to ischemic injury.[69] The exuberance of inflammation and

TABLE 39-5. Hepatic Expression of Major Histocompatibility Complex Molecules, Adhesion Molecules, and Tissue-Specific Antigens in Normal and Rejecting Livers

	Class I MHC	Class II MHC	CD58 (LFA-3)	CD54 & CD102 (ICAM-1, -2)	CD62E ELAM-1	CD62	CD106 VCAM-1	Tissue-Specific Antigens
Normal liver								
Hepatocytes	+	–	–	–/–	–	–	–	Yes
BEC	+	–	–	–/–	–	–	–	Yes
Kupffer	+	+	+	+/–	–	–	–	Unlikely
Artery	+	–	–	–/++	–	–	–	Unlikely
Sinusoid	+	–	–	+/+	–	–	–	Possible
Portal vein	+	–	+	–/–	±	±	–	Unlikely
Acute cellular rejection								
Hepatocytes	++	+	+	+/–	–	–	–	Yes
BEC	++	+++	+	+/–	–	–	–	Yes
Kupffer	++	++	+	+/–	–	–	+	Unlikely
Artery	+	±	+	±/++	±	+	+	Unlikely
Sinusoid	+	+	+	++/+	–	–	–	Possible
Portal vein	+	±	+	+/+	+	+	+	Unlikely
Ductopenic rejection								
Hepatocytes	++	+	+	+/–	–	–	–	Yes
BEC	++	+++	+	+/–	–	–	–	Yes
Kupffer	++	++	+	+/–	–	–	+	Unlikely
Artery	+	±	+	+/++	+	++	+	Unlikely
Sinusoid	+	+	+	+++/+	–	–	±	Possible
Portal vein	+	±	++	+/+	++	++	++	Unlikely

BEC, biliary epithelial cell.
From Vierling JM: Immunology of acute and chronic hepatic allograft rejection. Liver Transpl Surg 5:S1-S20, 1999.

the severity of damage are used to histologically grade acute rejection. The most feared consequence of acute rejection is rapid allograft failure, which usually occurs because of immunologically mediated microcirculatory failure and poor arterial flow or thrombosis. The second most feared (but relatively uncommon) complication of acute rejection is the development of chronic rejection.[70]

TABLE 39-6. Banff Grading of Acute Liver Allograft Rejection[75]

Global Assessment*	Criteria
Indeterminate	Portal inflammatory infiltrate that fails to meet the criteria for the diagnosis of acute rejection (see text)
Mild	Rejection infiltrate in a minority of the triads, that is, generally mild and confined to within the portal spaces
Moderate	Rejection infiltrate expanding most or all of the triads
Severe	As above for moderate, with spillover into periportal areas and moderate to severe perivenular inflammation that extends into the hepatic parenchyma and is associated with perivenular hepatocyte necrosis

Note: Global assessment of rejection grade mode on a review of the biopsy and after the diagnosis of rejection has been established.

*Verbal description of mild, moderate, or severe acute rejection could also be labeled as grade I, II, and III, respectively.

CLINICAL FEATURES

Acute rejection usually first occurs between 5 and 30 days after transplantation. Earlier or later presentations may be seen in presensitized patients or in those who receive less than optimal baseline immunosuppression. Clinical findings are often absent in early or mild acute rejection. In late or severe cases, fever, as well as enlargement, cyanosis, and tenderness of the allograft, frequently occurs. Bile drainage from a T tube often becomes thin and pale, and the flow is decreased. Occasionally, ascites develops because of increased intrahepatic pressure, liver swelling, and increased production of lymphatic fluid.[71]

Liver dysfunction usually manifests as concomitant nonselective elevation of some or all of the standard liver injury tests, including total bilirubin, ALT, aspartate aminotransferase, γ-GTP, and alkaline phosphatase (ALP).[71] Peripheral blood leukocytosis and eosinophilia are also frequently noted. Biochemical tests of the peripheral blood often reveal elevation of various interleukin levels or their receptors—neopterin, amyloid A protein, and antidonor class I MHC antibodies. Unfortunately, all clinical and laboratory findings lack sensitivity or specificity. The diagnosis is suspected on clinical grounds and is confirmed by examination of a core needle biopsy specimen, which has become the gold standard method of establishing the diagnosis.

The decision to increase immunosuppressive therapy is usually based on a combination of clinical and histopathologic parameters. In general, patients with indeterminate and mild acute rejection without significant liver function abnormalities are not treated with increased immunosuppression, and this approach does not usually lead to long-term sequelae.[3,72,73] Patients with mild acute rejection who show significant liver function abnormalities and those with moderate and severe acute rejection are generally given enhanced immunosuppressive treatment because of a small but definitely increased risk of graft loss and the possible development of chronic rejection.[3,74]

MICROSCOPIC PATHOLOGY AND GRADING

Because little controversy has been expressed regarding the histopathology of acute rejection, and because most groups report similar if not identical findings, specific bibliographic references to particular features are not included here.[3,71,75] Acute rejection is characterized by (1) predominantly mononuclear but mixed portal inflammation comprising blastic or activated lymphocytes, neutrophils, and eosinophils, (2) subendothelial inflammation of portal and/or terminal hepatic venules, and (3) bile duct inflammation and damage.[71,75] Minimal diagnostic criteria needed to establish the diagnosis of acute rejection are two of the previously mentioned histologic features. The diagnosis is strengthened if more than 50% of the ducts or central veins are damaged, or if unequivocal endotheliitis of portal or terminal hepatic vein branches can be identified. Microscopic pathology associated with severe injury (and used for histopathologic grading) includes perivenular inflammation, centrilobular necrosis, arteritis, and inflammatory bridging.[3,71,75]

The composition and location of inflammation are important features in the recognition of acute rejection and are dependent on the immunosuppressive protocol. Blastic and smaller mononuclear cells usually constitute the majority population, but eosinophils are often conspicuous and can predominate in patients treated with steroid-sparing immunosuppressive regimens (Fig. 39-9). Mononuclear cells tunnel underneath the portal and central vein endothelium, a process referred to as *endotheliitis*, or *endothelialitis*. This much-publicized feature of acute rejection can be seen with other causes of allograft dysfunction and should not be relied on too heavily, particularly if it is only a focal finding.

Immunophenotypic analysis of acute rejection infiltrates shows a predominance of T lymphocytes, dominated by the CD8+ subset in the portal tracts, particularly in damaged bile ducts.[76,77] Minority populations of B cells, macrophages, and other leukocytes are also present,[76-78] including occasional donor and recipient dendritic cells. In general, immunohistochemical analysis of the portal infiltrate is not clinically useful, except when distinction is drawn between acute rejection (T-cell predominant) and a post-transplant lymphoproliferative

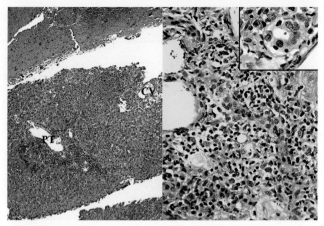

FIGURE 39–9. The typical low-power appearance of mild acute rejection *(left).* Note the mild portal inflammation. *Right,* At higher magnification, the typical appearance of the "acute rejection infiltrate." It consists of blastic and smaller lymphocytes, eosinophils, and occasional neutrophils and macrophages. The *inset* at the upper right shows bile duct damage in greater detail. Note the lymphocytes inside the basement membrane of the duct, the perinuclear vacuolization, and the mitotic figure at 6 to 7 o'clock. PT, portal tract; CV, central vein.

disorder (B-cell predominant; also see under Differential Diagnosis).

Inflammatory damage to small bile ducts manifests as lymphocytes inside the basement membrane associated with biliary epithelial cell alterations such as paranuclear vacuolization, increased nucleus-to-cytoplasm ratio, mitoses, nucleoli, occasional apoptotic bodies, and cytoplasmic eosinophilia. Luminal disruption with breaks in the basement membrane signifies severe bile duct damage. Peribiliary granulomas are not a feature of either acute or chronic rejection; in our experience, their presence is indicative of a non–rejection-related cause of duct injury (e.g., recurrent PBC) or infection.

Inflammatory or necrotizing arteritis is an important feature that is used in the recognition and grading of severe acute rejection; however, the vessels most commonly affected are located in the hilum and are not usually accessible by needle biopsy. In addition, histopathologic recognition of arteritis in peripheral needle biopsies is poorly reproducible.[79] Therefore, arteritis is not generally included in the grading schema unless it has been unequivocally identified in an artery branch containing an internal elastic lamina.

Occasionally, acute rejection can manifest as predominantly or exclusively perivenular inflammation.[80,81] This form of acute rejection is usually associated with perivenular hepatocyte necrosis, dropout, hemorrhage, and pigmented macrophages (Fig. 39-10); in severe cases, it can lead to perivenular fibrosis and a Budd-Chiari or veno-occlusive–like clinical syndrome.[46]

Lobular findings include mild Kupffer cell hypertrophy and a slight increase in inflammatory cells in the

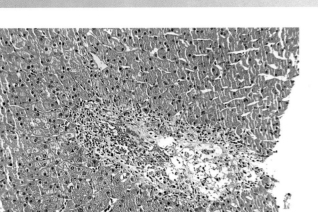

FIGURE 39–10. Acute rejection can present as predominantly perivenular inflammation with little or no portal inflammation or bile duct damage, as shown here. However, to make the diagnosis of acute rejection with this finding, a majority of the central veins should be involved, and other causes of perivenular inflammation and congestion should be excluded (see text).

sinusoids. Infiltration of the sinusoids and the connective tissue surrounding the central vein by cells similar to the portal tract infiltrate, or so-called central venulitis, can be seen in up to 30% of acute rejection episodes. In severe acute rejection, zonal centrilobular congestion, hemorrhage, hepatocyte necrosis, and dropout accompany the perivenular inflammation (Fig. 39-11).

Several well-known systems are used for grading acute rejection,[3,71,75] but the Banff schema represents the consensus opinion of a group of recognized expert liver transplant pathologists, hepatologists, and surgeons from many of the major hepatic transplant centers in North America, Europe, and Asia.[75] It incorporates concepts from these earlier systems that satisfied requirements for simplicity, reproducibility, scientific correctness, and clinical utility.

The Banff schema (see Table 39-6; Table 39-7) includes a descriptive grade of indeterminate, mild, moderate, and severe, along with a semiquantitative rejection activity index (RAI).[75] The latter component, adopted from the European grading system,[74] is the conceptual equivalent of the hepatitis activity index. The RAI scores the prevalence and severity of three separate features—portal inflammation, bile duct damage, and subendothelial inflammation—on a scale of 0 to 3. These components are then added together for a total RAI score.

The higher the total RAI score, the more severe the rejection episode will be, and the more likely it is that the allograft will fail from acute rejection or will develop chronic rejection.[3,75] The total RAI score for indeterminate or acute rejection usually ranges between 1 and 2. Mild acute rejection biopsy specimens usually score between 3 and 4, moderate between 5 and 6; biopsies with severe acute rejection usually attain a total RAI score of greater than 6. Although the maximum possible total is 9, biopsies rarely achieve this score.[3] Instead, most episodes of acute rejection are mild, have a total RAI less than 6, respond to increased immunosuppression, and do not lead to significant fibrosis, bile duct loss, or arteriopathy in subsequent or follow-up biopsies.[3]

Additional immunosuppression should not be given before a biopsy specimen is obtained because histopathologic interpretation is made more difficult. Treatment with increased immunosuppression may cause some of the infiltrate to subside within 24 hours; subendothelial infiltration of veins is one of the first findings affected. In addition, centrilobular hepatocyte swelling and hepatocanalicular cholestasis may appear after treatment. It usually takes 7 to 10 days after treatment for the changes to completely resolve.

DIFFERENTIAL DIAGNOSIS

The differential diagnosis for acute rejection depends on the time that has passed since transplantation. During the first several months, acute rejection can be distinguished from preservation injury and acute cholangitis by several key features, discussed under Preservation or Ischemic Injury and Primary Dysfunction.

At between 3 and 10 weeks after liver transplantation, acute rejection can be particularly difficult to distinguish from recurrent or viral hepatitis B or C. Rejection and recurrent hepatitis show predominantly mononuclear portal inflammation, bile duct damage, and Kupffer cell hypertrophy with variable acidophilic necrosis of

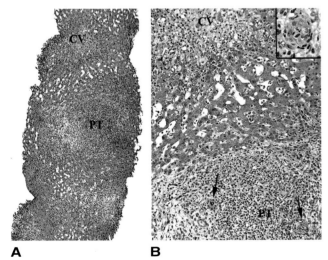

A   **B**

FIGURE 39–11. Severe acute rejection is characterized by marked portal expansion because of inflammation, along with perivenular inflammation and hepatocyte dropout as shown in **A**. **B** shows at higher magnification the prominent portal inflammation, bile duct damage *(arrows and inset),* and perivenular inflammation with hepatocyte dropout. PT, portal tract, CV, central vein.

TABLE 39-7. Acute Rejection Activity Index (RAI)[75]

Category	Criteria	Score
Portal inflammation	Mostly lymphocytic inflammation involving, but not noticeably expanding, a minority of the triads	1
	Expansion of most or all of the triads by a mixed infiltrate containing lymphocytes with occasional blasts, neutrophils, and eosinophils	2
	Marked expansion of most or all of the triads by a mixed infiltrate containing numerous blasts and eosinophils with inflammatory spillover into the periportal parenchyma	3
Bile duct inflammation damage	A minority of the ducts are cuffed and infiltrated by inflammatory cells and show only mild reactive changes such as increased nucleus-to-cytoplasm ratio of the epithelial cells	1
	Most or all of the ducts infiltrated by inflammatory cells. More than an occasional duct shows degenerative changes such as nuclear pleomorphism, disordered polarity, and cytoplasmic vacuolization of the epithelium	2
	As above for a score of 2, with most or all of the ducts showing degenerative changes or focal luminal disruption	3
Venous endothelial inflammation	Subendothelial lymphocytic infiltration involving some, but not a majority, of the portal and/or hepatic venules	1
	Subendothelial infiltration involving most or all of the portal and/or hepatic venules	2
	As above for a score of 2, with moderate or severe perivenular inflammation that extends into the perivenular parenchyma and is associated with perivenular hepatocyte necrosis	3

Note: Total Score = Sum of Components. Criteria that can be used to score liver allograft biopsies with acute rejection, as defined by the World Gastroenterology Consensus Document.

hepatocytes. The distinction is made through close examination of the severity and prevalence of bile duct damage, interface activity, lobular changes, and perivenular inflammation and hepatocyte dropout. In acute rejection, inflammatory bile duct damage and perivenular inflammation, if present, usually involve a majority of the ducts and central veins, respectively. In contrast, only occasional bile ducts are damaged in recurrent viral hepatitis; perivenular inflammation, if present, involves a minority of central veins. Conversely, interface activity involves most of the portal tracts; lobular changes are more severe and are conspicuous in recurrent hepatitis. More than 10 weeks after transplantation, distinguishing between chronic viral or autoimmune hepatitis and rejection is usually not a problem and is based on these same features.

More than 6 months after transplantation, acute rejection must also be distinguished from chronic biliary tract strictures, post-transplant lymphoproliferative disorders, and recurrent viral or autoimmune hepatitis. Chronic biliary tract strictures can produce microscopic pathology in peripheral core needle biopsy specimens that are virtually indistinguishable from those of acute rejection. In these cases, it is helpful for the pathologist to remember that acute rejection occurring longer than 6 months after transplantation is unusual in adequately immunosuppressed patients. Therefore, simply checking the blood levels of baseline immunosuppressive drugs and the liver injury test profile often provides sufficient data to suggest a cholangiogram before immunosuppressive therapy is increased. Subtle histopathologic clues that favor chronic biliary strictures over acute rejection include sinusoidal clusters of neutrophils, periportal deposition of elemental copper, centrilobular hepatocanalicular cholestasis, and lamellar periductal

edema involving any of the sampled bile ducts. Distinguishing viral or autoimmune hepatitis from rejection in biopsies obtained more than 6 months after transplantation is based on the same guidelines proposed at earlier time points.

Chronic Rejection

Chronic rejection has been defined as an immunologic injury to the liver allograft that usually evolves from severe or persistent acute rejection and results in potentially irreversible damage to the bile ducts, arteries, and veins.[70] It currently affects about 3% to 5% of liver allograft recipients by 5 years after transplantation, which is a dramatic decrease since the 1980s, when the incidence was 15% to 20%.[70] The decline is probably attributable to improved recognition and control of acute and early phases of chronic rejection, combined with the unique immunologic properties of liver allografts and the remarkable ability of the liver to regenerate without fibrosis. Nevertheless, chronic rejection has not been entirely eliminated and is still an important cause of late liver allograft dysfunction and failure.

The term *chronic* technically implies a time parameter, but none is intended[71] because chronic rejection often occurs within several months after transplantation, and allograft failure typically occurs within the first year after transplantation.[70] In contrast to other vascularized allografts, the incidence of chronic rejection in the liver does not appear to increase with time after transplantation. However, a small group of patients is known to develop late-onset chronic rejection. These patients usually suffer from complications of overimmunosuppression; the baseline drugs are often decreased or discontinued altogether because of immunosuppression-related complications.[82] Older terms for chronic rejection, such as *vanishing bile duct syndrome* or *ductopenic rejection*, are fading from use because bile duct loss is now recognized as just one of several histopathologic features of chronic rejection.[70,71]

Risk factors have generally been divided into two general categories. The first and most important comprises alloantigen-dependent, immunologic, or rejection-related factors. Among these, the number and severity of acute rejection episodes are the most significant,[56,70] regardless of the immunosuppressive regimen. In cyclosporine-treated cohorts, late-onset acute rejection episodes; younger recipient age; male-to-female sex mismatch; a primary diagnosis of autoimmune hepatitis or biliary disease; baseline immunosuppression; interactions between MHC-DR3, TNF-2 status, and cytomegalovirus (CMV) infection[83]; and nonwhite recipient race have all been associated with an increased risk of chronic rejection.[70] The role of histocompatibility differences is still controversial, as is the effect of CMV infection.

In a large tacrolimus-treated cohort, many of the matching factors described earlier for the cyclosporine-treated patients were not a significant risk factor for chronic rejection, but the influence of the number and severity of acute rejection episodes remained.[82] Non–alloantigen-dependent or nonimmunologic risk factors that contribute to the development of chronic rejection include donor age greater than 40 years.[82]

PATHOPHYSIOLOGY

Because chronic rejection primarily evolves from severe or multiple recurrent and uncontrolled acute rejection episodes,[3,82,84,85] many of the immunologic mechanisms of injury discussed for acute rejection are likely to be relevant to chronic rejection.[70,86] Bile duct damage and loss in chronic rejection are due to a combination of direct immunologic damage by the effector mechanisms of acute rejection and indirect ischemic damage because of obliterative arteriopathy, small artery/arteriolar loss, and destruction of the peribiliary capillary plexus.[87,88] Cumulative damage results in enhanced biliary epithelial cell senescence,[54] which manifests as distinct cytologic changes recognizable on routine light microscopy and enhanced expression of nuclear p21 without Ki67 labeling.[54] These changes precede bile duct loss.[70,84]

CLINICAL FEATURES

A clinical diagnosis of chronic rejection is usually suspected in a patient with a history of acute rejection who develops progressive cholestasis and an increase in canalicular enzymes and is unresponsive to antirejection treatment.[71] Three clinical settings are typical, including the following: (1) the end stage of unresolved acute

rejection; (2) after multiple episodes of acute rejection; and (3) indolent evolution without preceding clinically recognized episodes of acute rejection. The first two scenarios are by far the most common and usually occur within the first year after transplantation. The last situation is relatively uncommon and may simply reflect inadequate monitoring. Late-onset chronic rejection occurring longer than 1 year after transplantation is typically seen in inadequately immunosuppressed patients, either as a result of noncompliance or because immunosuppression has had to be lowered because of infectious, neoplastic, or toxic complications of overimmunosuppression.[82]

Unresolved or indolent rejection may become apparent only because of a persistent elevation in liver injury tests. Standard liver injury tests usually reveal a progressive cholestatic pattern that manifests as preferential elevation of γ-GTP and ALP.[55,71,89] Transition from acute to chronic rejection may be marked by a persistent elevation of alanine aminotransferase and total bilirubin that presages allograft failure.[80,82,84] Clinical symptoms, when present, usually resemble those of acute rejection until allograft dysfunction becomes severe enough to cause jaundice. Biliary sludging or the appearance of biliary strictures, appearance of hepatic infarcts, and finally, loss of hepatic synthetic function (which can manifest as coagulopathy and malnutrition) are other late findings presaging allograft failure.[71] Selective hepatic angiography that shows pruning of the intrahepatic arteries with poor peripheral filling and segmental narrowing can also be used to support the diagnosis of chronic rejection.[71,90]

MICROSCOPIC PATHOLOGY AND STAGING

The portal tracts and perivenular regions are primarily affected by chronic rejection, and changes in these areas are divided into early and late stages (Table 39-8). Portal tract changes in early chronic rejection include mild lymphocytic cholangitis (Fig. 39-12), which leads to biliary epithelial cell senescence changes (Fig. 39-13), eventually followed by loss of small bile ducts in the later stages (Fig. 39-14). Compared with portal inflammation in acute rejection, the portal inflammation in chronic rejection is usually less severe and contains primarily lymphocytes and plasma cells; mast cells[91] and eosinophils are much less common.

Distinct histopathologic changes of biliary epithelial cell senescence[54] presage bile duct loss. These include eosinophilic transformation of the biliary epithelial cytoplasm, uneven nuclear spacing, syncytia formation, nuclear enlargement and hyperchromasia resembling cytologic dysplasia (see Fig. 39-13), and ducts only partially lined by biliary epithelial cells. The nucleus of senescent biliary epithelial cells stains positive for p21$^{WAF1/Cip1}$ (but not for Ki67), an inhibitor of cell cycle progression that becomes upregulated in cells under severe stress or that show replicative senescence.[54]

TABLE 39-8. Features of Early and Late Chronic Liver Allograft Rejection[70]

Structure	Early Chronic Rejection	Late Chronic Rejection
Small bile ducts (<60 μm)	Bile duct loss in <50% of portal tracts. Degenerative change involving a majority of ducts—eosinophilic transformation of the cytoplasm; nuclear hyperchromasia; uneven nuclear spacing; ducts only partially lined by biliary epithelial cells	Loss in ≥50% of portal tracts; degenerative changes in remaining bile ducts
Terminal hepatic venules and zone 3 hepatocytes	Intimal/luminal inflammation Lytic zone 3 necrosis and inflammation Mild perivenular fibrosis	Focal obliteration Variable inflammation Severe perivenular fibrosis, defined as central-to-central bridging fibrosis
Portal tract hepatic arterioles	Occasional loss involving <25% of portal tracts	Loss involving >25% of portal tracts
Other	So-called transition hepatitis with spotty necrosis of hepatocytes	Sinusoidal foam cell accumulation; marked cholestasis
Large perihilar hepatic artery branches	Intimal inflammation, focal foam cell deposition without luminal compromise	Luminal narrowing by subintimal foam cells, fibrointimal proliferation
Large perihilar bile ducts	Inflammation damage and focal foam cell deposition	Mural fibrosis

From Demetris A, Adams D, Bellamy C, et al: Update of the International Banff Schema for Liver Allograft Rejection: Working recommendations for the histopathologic staging and reporting of chronic rejection. An international panel. Hepatology 31:792-799, 2000.

Late-stage chronic rejection manifests as bile duct and arteriolar loss, the severity of which is based on quantitative morphometry.

Crawford and colleagues[92] defined a portal tract as "a focus within the parenchyma containing connective tissue (by Masson's trichrome stain) and at least two luminal structures embedded in the connective tissue mesenchyme, each with a continuous connective tissue circumference." According to this definition, in a normal liver, 93 ± 6% and 91 ± 7% of portal tracts contain bile ducts and hepatic artery branches, respectively.[92] Somewhat lower figures were cited by others using larger tissue samples.[87] With the use of two standard deviations from the normal as a cutoff, bile duct loss is considered present when less than 80% of the portal tracts contain bile ducts; arterial loss is considered present when less than 77% of the portal tracts contain hepatic artery branches.

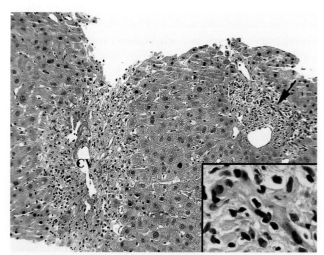

FIGURE 39–12. This photomicrograph shows a case in transition between acute and chronic rejection. Note the mild portal inflammation, duct damage *(arrow)*, and early biliary epithelial senescence changes. The *arrow* points toward the damaged bile duct shown at higher magnification in the *inset*. Note also the perivenular inflammation, hepatocyte dropout, and early fibrosis. CV, central vein.

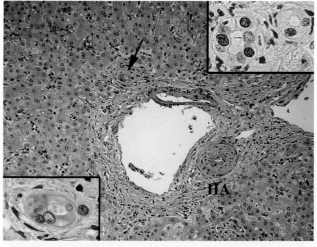

FIGURE 39–13. Early chronic rejection is characterized by biliary epithelial cell senescence changes *(arrow and lower left inset)* such as cytoplasmic eosinophilia, syncytia formation, ducts only partially lined by biliary epithelial cells, and expression of *p21* *(upper right inset)* without simultaneous expression of Ki67. Note also the fibrointimal hyperplasia and luminal narrowing of the hepatic artery branch (HA).

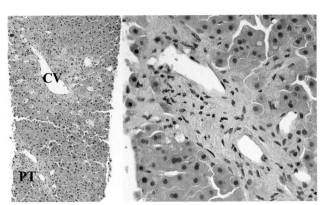

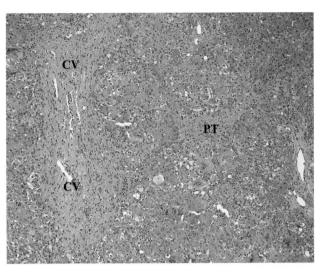

FIGURE 39–14. The late stage of chronic rejection in the portal tracts is characterized by loss of the bile ducts and small hepatic artery branches, as shown in this panel. The portal tract from the left side of the panel is shown at higher magnification on the right side of the panel. PT, portal tract; CV, central vein.

FIGURE 39–15. The late stage of chronic rejection in the lobule is characterized by severe perivenular fibrosis with focal central vein obliteration and at least focal central-to-central bridging fibrosis as shown in this photomicrograph. PT, portal tract; CV, central vein.

When both bile duct and arterial losses are seen,[87,88] recognition and counting of the portal tracts can be problematic. In such cases, recognition of portal tracts should be based primarily on the location (cholestasis in chronic rejection is centrilobular), shape, and internal structure of the connective tissue mesenchyme. Determination of bile duct and arterial loss in these cases should be based on a count of the total number of portal tracts with and without bile ducts and arteries and on a comparison with expected values from normal livers. A ductular reaction at the interface zone is unusual in chronic rejection unless the liver is recovering from chronic rejection, in which case a ductular reaction can precede the regrowth of bile ducts.[84,93,94]

The early phase of chronic rejection in the terminal hepatic venules and surrounding perivenular parenchyma is characterized by subendothelial and perivenular mononuclear inflammation.[70,85] This is accompanied by perivenular hepatocyte dropout and an accumulation of pigment-laden macrophages and mild perivenular fibrosis.[70] Spotty acidophilic necrosis of hepatocytes, or so-called transitional hepatitis, may occur during evolution from early to late stages of chronic rejection.[95]

Late chronic rejection is characterized by severe (bridging) perivenular fibrosis with at least focal central-to-central bridging and occasional obliteration of terminal hepatic venules (Fig. 39-15).[70] A well-developed cirrhosis from chronic rejection is unusual until the late stages, when venous obliteration leads to areas of parenchymal extinction.[86] True regenerative nodules are uncommon, perhaps because the combination of venous and arterial obliteration blunts any regenerative response.[96]

Other common findings in late chronic rejection include perivenular hepatocyte ballooning and dropout, along with centrilobular hepatocanalicular cholestasis, nodular regenerative hyperplasia–like changes, and intrasinusoidal foam cell clusters. The clusters of foamy macrophages likely represent a nonspecific response to

cholestasis and therefore, alone, are not diagnostic of chronic rejection.

The final diagnosis of chronic rejection should be based on various combinations of clinical, radiologic, laboratory, and microscopic pathology. In a biopsy specimen, the minimum diagnostic criteria for chronic rejection comprise (1) senescent changes, affecting a majority of the bile ducts, with or without bile duct loss; or (2) convincing foam cell obliterative arteriopathy; or (3) bile duct loss affecting greater than 50% of the portal tracts.[70]

The diagnosis of chronic rejection is easier to establish in an explanted failed allograft, and characteristic sequential changes that develop in the branches of the hepatic arterial tree can be appreciated. Arteriopathy is usually seen in at least some of the muscular arteries in the hilum, except in cases characterized by bile duct loss and/or perivenular fibrosis alone.

Sequential changes in the hepatic arterial tree include a progressive accumulation of the foamy macrophages triggering proliferation of donor-derived subintimal myofibroblasts (Fig. 39-16). In severely affected arteries, the entire wall may be completely replaced by foam cells or may be completely obliterated, leading to arterial thrombosis and subsequent necrosis of the large bile ducts. This is followed by thinning of media as the arteries attempt to dilate and compensate for the reduced arterial flow. Eventually, the foam cells are replaced by intimal myofibroblasts.

Other changes in the major hilar bile ducts include focal sloughing of the epithelium, papillary intraluminal hyperplasia, mural fibrosis, and acute and chronic inflammation. Foamy macrophages may also be seen around bile ducts and veins in the connective tissue.

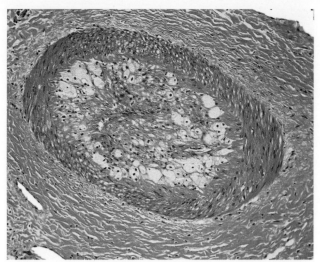

FIGURE 39–16. The obliterative arteriopathy of chronic rejection is usually restricted to the first- and second-order branches of the hepatic artery in the liver hilum, although occasionally it can be seen in the periphery, as is shown in Figure 39-13. This figure shows the typical appearance of obliterative arteriopathy in a hilar artery from a failed allograft. It is characterized by luminal narrowing because of intimal thickening. The intimal thickening is related to deposition of foamy macrophages and proliferation of myofibroblasts. The media often become thinned as the vessels try to dilate to compensate for the luminal narrowing. However, the compensation mechanisms eventually fail, resulting in ischemic damage to the organ.

The staging of chronic rejection (see Table 39-8) assumes that the diagnosis has already been correctly established.[70] Early chronic rejection implies that a significant potential for recovery exists if the insult can be controlled or removed. Late chronic rejection suggests that the potential for recovery is limited, and perhaps retransplantation should be considered. However, more study is needed in this area because it is not well established that all patients sequentially proceed in an orderly fashion from the early to the late stages of chronic rejection. Some patients appear to persist in the acute/early stage for months or years; others rapidly develop severe fibrosis and late changes. In addition, some cases show either bile duct loss or foam cell arteriopathy alone, but usually both features are found together.[70]

The decision to proceed with retransplantation should be based on both clinical and histopathologic parameters such as progressive decline in synthetic function, superimposed hepatic artery thrombosis, and bile duct necrosis or biliary sludging. The important practical implication of chronic rejection staging is that the biopsy findings do not absolutely define a point of no return; they provide information about the likelihood of reversal.

DIFFERENTIAL DIAGNOSIS

Because arteries with pathognomonic changes are rarely present in needle biopsy specimens, considerable significance is placed on damage to and loss of small bile ducts and perivenular fibrosis.[70] However, a similar pattern of ductal injury and ductopenia can occur as a result of nonrejection-related complications such as obstructive cholangiopathy (including recurrent PSC), hepatic artery stricturing or thrombosis, adverse drug reactions, and CMV infection. In cases of chronic rejection identified by biliary epithelial senescence or loss or perivenular fibrosis alone, other, nonrejection-related causes of ductal injury and loss or perivenular fibrosis, which histopathologically appear similar to chronic rejection, should be reasonably excluded. Bile duct loss in some portal tracts accompanied by a ductular reaction in other portal tracts should raise the suspicion of a biliary tract stricture. Cholangiography and/or angiography may be required in some cases to distinguish between chronic rejection and biliary obstruction. In other cases, isolated ductopenia involving less than 50% of the portal tracts can be seen without significant elevation of liver injury tests. Whether these uncommon cases are an early phase of chronic rejection is uncertain.

Isolated perivenular fibrosis may be caused by mechanical outflow obstruction, adverse drug reactions, or all of the nonrejection causes of veno-occlusive disease and Budd-Chiari syndrome in native livers.[97]

The safest approach to the diagnosis of chronic rejection in any setting is to review previous biopsies and to closely correlate the microscopic pathology with the clinical course. The usual scenario is a history of severe or unresolved acute rejection preceding the development of histologic findings interpreted as chronic rejection.

BACTERIAL AND FUNGAL INFECTIONS

The most serious opportunistic fungal and viral infections generally occur within the first 2 months after transplantation. Late-onset infections occurring after 6 months tend to be bacterial in origin. Early after transplantation, the more serious opportunistic infections are related to the high levels of immunosuppression used to prevent rejection and stress from the operation. Although a high index of suspicion should always be maintained, clinical histories that should arouse the suspicion of an infection include fever, anastomotic or wound dehiscence, retransplantation, persistent abdominal pain, and vascular thrombosis. Bacterial and fungal infections most commonly arise in nonviable tissue. Such tissue should be routinely subjected to special stains for bacteria and fungi. Although inflammation and granulomas are always good markers of potential infection, they may or may not be present because of immunosuppression. Histopathologic changes associated with common bacterial or fungal infections are well known to most surgical pathologists and are not discussed here.

VIRAL INFECTIONS

Viral hepatitis types B and C are leading indications for liver transplantation worldwide. Because reinfection of the allograft is nearly universal in those with active viral replication before transplantation and because blood products are screened, HBV and HCV infections are largely restricted to those who had these viruses before transplantation. However, new cases that develop after transplantation are not rare.[98] The manifestations and evolution of HBV and HCV in liver allografts are similar to those in the general population, except that viral replication is enhanced and subsequent disease is usually more aggressive after transplantation. Markedly enhanced levels of viral replication can lead to atypical clinical and histopathologic presentations, as described in the following section.

Opportunistic Hepatitis Viruses

The immunosuppression needed to prevent rejection also renders liver allograft recipients vulnerable to hepatitis caused by opportunistic hepatitis viruses such as CMV, Epstein-Barr virus (EBV), herpes simplex (HSV) or varicella-zoster (VZ), and adenovirus. These viruses do not usually cause acute hepatitis in the general population, and none causes chronic hepatitis in either the general population or liver allograft recipients.

Most adult liver allograft recipients have been infected and latently carry these opportunistic viruses, whereas pediatric recipients and a minority of adults may not have been previously exposed. These naïve allograft recipients usually develop more severe CMV, EBV, HSV, and VZ disease after transplantation. The onset of clinical disease is usually associated with enhanced viral replication; therefore, peripheral blood monitoring for viral antigens or nucleic acids is used to guide preemptive lowering of immunosuppression or treatment with specific antiviral agents.[99]

CYTOMEGALOVIRUS HEPATITIS

OVERVIEW AND PATHOPHYSIOLOGY

CMV is the most commonly encountered opportunistic viral infection in liver allograft recipients, but effective prophylactic and preemptive therapies have greatly lessened the incidence and impact of symptomatic disease.[100-102] When symptomatic infection or disease does develop, it usually does so between 3 and 8 weeks after transplantation, toward the end of or shortly after a cycle of increased immunosuppressive therapy used to treat acute rejection. Disease may be the result of recrudescence in a carrier, or it may occur as an acquired disease in naïve recipients via transmission through blood products or the donor organ. Seronegative recipients who receive seropositive donor organs are at the greatest risk of developing symptomatic disease.[103-106] Viral infection

and latency in granulocytes or endothelial cells[107] and monocytes may explain the early appearance of viral antigens in the sinusoidal cells.[103] CMV infection is thought to be a risk factor for hepatic artery thrombosis, especially in pediatric patients,[108,109] and for chronic rejection.[56]

CLINICAL FEATURES

Signs and symptoms of active CMV infection include fever, diarrhea, gastrointestinal ulcers, leukopenia, and low-grade hepatitis with modestly elevated liver injury tests results.[110] Any organ system may be involved, depending on the extent of viral dissemination. Respiratory insufficiency and retinitis occur when the disease is severe. Occasionally, CMV can cause a syndrome that mimics EBV-associated post-transplant lymphoproliferative disorders and that includes mild liver function abnormalities, lymphadenopathy, fever, and atypical lymphocytosis.[110]

MICROSCOPIC PATHOLOGY

The histopathologic manifestations of active CMV infection depend, in part, on the immune status of the host. In heavily immunosuppressed and untreated naïve recipients, any cell type of the liver may be infected. The CMV-infected cells develop large eosinophilic intranuclear inclusions surrounded by a clear halo and occasionally small basophilic or amphophilic cytoplasmic inclusions. Despite widespread CMV infestation of the liver allograft, submassive or massive necrosis from CMV alone has never been seen.[110]

In the occasional patient who develops active disease, CMV hepatitis is usually characterized by spotty lobular necrosis, Kupffer cell hypertrophy, and mild lobular disarray. Hepatocytes near the necrotic cells may contain nuclear and/or cytoplasmic inclusions (Fig. 39-17) and are often surrounded by neutrophils (microabscess) or clusters of macrophages and lymphocytes (microgranulomas). Mild plasmacytic and lymphocytic portal inflammation, associated with bile duct cell infiltration and damage, may also be seen, mimicking or actually associated with acute or chronic rejection. Bile duct loss has been associated with persistent CMV infection of the allograft.[111,112]

On occasion, the characteristic parenchymal alterations described earlier may be seen, without clear evidence of cytomegaly or nuclear or cytoplasmic CMV inclusions. In such cases, immunoperoxidase staining for early viral antigens or in situ hybridization can be used to detect infected cells. In addition, "activated" or rapidly dividing tissues such as young granulation tissue, proliferating cholangioles seen in ischemically damaged livers, edges of infarcts, abscesses, or other intra-parenchymal defects provide fertile soil for CMV growth.[9] When such tissue is encountered, a more careful search for CMV is warranted.

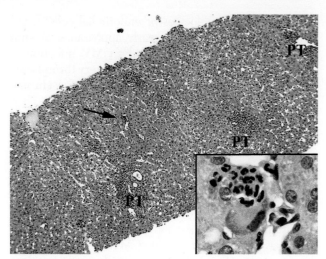

FIGURE 39–17. CMV hepatitis often shows mononuclear or mixed portal inflammation and focal bile duct damage accompanied by small clusters of neutrophils (microabscesses; *arrow and lower right inset*) or macrophages (microgranulomas) scattered randomly throughout the lobules. Examination of the microabscess at the tip of the *arrow* at higher magnification *(lower right inset)* shows the characteristic cytomegaly, eosinophilic intranuclear inclusion, and small basophilic cytoplasmic inclusions. PT, portal tract.

DIFFERENTIAL DIAGNOSIS

When no viral inclusions are detected, CMV hepatitis may be difficult to distinguish from early HBV or HCV recurrence and, on occasion, EBV hepatitis. When inclusions are seen, CMV may still be difficult to distinguish from HSV infection because both can cause multinucleation and intranuclear eosinophilic inclusions. However, CMV-infected cells may also show small basophilic or amphophilic cytoplasmic inclusions that are not seen in HSV. Also, the circumscribed zones of coagulative necrosis characteristic of HSV generally are not encountered with CMV.

In the absence of inclusions, subtle clues that can be used to distinguish between CMV and early acute HBV or HCV include less lobular disarray and hepatocyte swelling in CMV. Conversely, microabscesses or microgranulomas are not generally seen in HBV or HCV. The final diagnosis, however, often relies on adjuvant techniques such as immunoperoxidase staining for viral antigens (CMV, HBV) or in situ hybridization for viral nucleic acids (EBV) and correlation with the clinical profile.

Cases of CMV hepatitis resembling EBV hepatitis reveal mild lymphoplasmacytic portal and lobular inflammation. Blastic and atypical lymphocytes may or may not be present. Microgranulomas are usually seen in the lobules, although characteristic CMV inclusions are absent. Deeper cuts into the block, immunoperoxidase stains for EBV and CMV viral antigens, and in situ hybridization for EBV nucleic acids are usually required to establish the final diagnosis.

A difficult challenge involves determining whether the liver injury occurred because of residual CMV hepatitis or because of onset of acute or chronic rejection resulting from the low immunosuppression levels used to treat the viral infection. This occurs because CMV hepatitis most commonly develops in patients who have recently completed an augmented immunosuppressive regimen for rejection and are therefore at risk for rejection and CMV. Further complicating the issue is the report by O'Grady and others showing an association between CMV infection and chronic rejection.[111,112] Others have not seen this association.[113] In our experience, CMV inclusions or antigens in the biopsy are generally given priority, the immunosuppressive therapy dosage is reduced, and ganciclovir is given. Follow-up biopsy after 1 to 2 weeks, if liver function abnormalities persist, is used to monitor therapy.

HERPES SIMPLEX AND VARICELLA-ZOSTER VIRAL HEPATITIS

Both subtypes of HSV (types I and II) and VZ have been identified as causes of liver allograft hepatitis.[110] These have been seen as early as 3 days post transplant and can occur any time thereafter. The clinical presentation includes fever, vesicular skin rashes, fatigue, and body pain, combined with serologic evidence of hepatic injury. If HSV hepatitis goes unrecognized, it can rapidly lead to submassive or massive hepatic necrosis, hypotension, disseminated intravascular coagulation, and metabolic acidosis.[114] Fulminant cases occur more often in patients without evidence of previous immunity. Early recognition achieved by needle biopsy sampling is particularly crucial because effective pharmacologic therapy is available.

MICROSCOPIC PATHOLOGY

Two histopathologic patterns of HSV hepatitis have been identified[114]—localized and diffuse. Separation of the two may be related to swiftness in establishing the diagnosis, level of immune competence, and evidence of previous immunity. Common to both are circumscribed areas of coagulative-type necrosis that show no respect for the lobular architecture.[110,114] Ghosts of hepatocytes, intermixed with neutrophils and nuclear debris, are seen in the center of the lesions. More viable hepatocytes at the periphery may be slightly enlarged and may contain "smudgy," ground-glass nuclei or characteristic Cowdry type A eosinophilic inclusions (Fig. 39-18).

We have not been able to reliably separate HSV from VZ on the basis of H&E slides alone. Multinucleate cells are occasionally present, but, not infrequently, changes diagnostic of HSV or VZ are absent on H&E slides. In such cases, immunoperoxidase stains for HSV antigens may be confirmatory. Some antibody preparations used to detect HSV subtypes show considerable cross-reactivity, making it difficult for HSV I to be

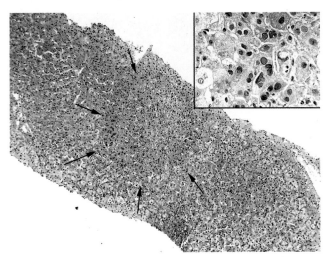

FIGURE 39–18. Herpes simplex and varicella-zoster virus hepatitis are characterized by "maplike" areas of necrosis that do not show any respect for the underlying liver architecture *(outlined by arrows)*. Examination of the cells at the edge of the area of necrosis at higher magnification *(inset)* shows the characteristic eosinophilic intranuclear inclusions of the herpes simplex and varicella-zoster virus; immunoperoxidase staining is needed to distinguish these two viruses.

separated from HSV II by means of immunohistochemistry. Cross-reactivity between VZ and HSV with the use of monoclonal antibodies has not been a problem in our experience.

DIFFERENTIAL DIAGNOSIS

If a histopathologic diagnosis of HSV or VZ viral hepatitis is even considered, regardless of whether the diagnosis is confirmed, clinical physicians should be immediately notified. Necrotic herpes hepatitis lesions can be difficult to distinguish from the edge of an infarct or an area of ischemic necrosis. The most reliable finding is an inclusion body, but unequivocal HSV inclusions may not be present. Frequently, only cells with a smudged nuclear chromatin are seen. In such cases, it is our policy to overdiagnose HSV hepatitis because without the highly effective acyclovir treatment, HSV and VZ viral hepatitis can rapidly cause liver failure and death.

It can also be difficult to distinguish HSV/VZ from CMV hepatitis. HSV is associated with large areas of coagulative-type necrosis, whereas CMV alone rarely causes significant hepatocyte necrosis. In addition, CMV hepatitis may reveal both nuclear and cytoplasmic inclusions, whereas HSV inclusions are exclusively nuclear.

EPSTEIN-BARR VIRUS

OVERVIEW AND PATHOPHYSIOLOGY

EBV lies dormant in B lymphocytes and some epithelial cells after the immune system effectively controls viral replication following a primary infection. In vitro, EBV infection immortalizes B lymphocytes. In vivo, control of the virus is maintained by T-cell immune surveillance that keeps viral replication and B-cell proliferation in check.[115,116] However, potent immunosuppressive therapy depresses immune surveillance, which leads to enhanced viral replication and the various disease manifestations discussed under Clinical Presentation below. For a more detailed discussion of the pathophysiology of the interactions of EBV, the reader is referred elsewhere.[115,116]

CLINICAL FEATURES

Many clinicopathologic manifestations of active EBV infection can occur after transplantation. In adults with preexisting immunity, up to 1% to 2% develop persistent and/or recurrent disease (EBV) after transplantation that can manifest as hepatitis, gastroenteritis, post-transplant lymphoproliferative disease (PTLD; including the B-cell type),[117-120] Hodgkin's disease,[121] T-cell lesions,[122] and smooth muscle stromal tumors.[123] The incidence of disease is higher and the severity is worse among pediatric patients and adults who were seronegative before transplantation and received a seropositive donor organ.[115-119]

Other risk factors for serious EBV-associated disease such as PTLDs include heavy immunosuppression, underlying Langerhans' cell histiocytosis,[124] and CMV disease.[125] In contrast, the risk of developing PTLD late in the post-transplant course appears to be influenced not by the type of immunosuppressive agents employed but rather by the duration of any immunosuppression.[126]

The systemic viral syndrome associated with EBV often resembles that seen with classic infectious mononucleosis. Fever, lymphadenitis, pharyngitis, and jaundice[115-119] are typical findings. Atypical signs and symptoms include jaw pain, arthralgia, joint space effusions, diarrhea, encephalitis, pneumonitis, mediastinal lymphadenopathy, and ascites.[115-119] Laboratory investigation usually reveals elevation of the hepatocellular liver enzymes; circulating atypical lymphocytes and pancytopenia are noted on occasion.[115-119] Monitoring of the peripheral blood for EBV nucleic acids is used to guide preemptive reductions in immunosuppression before more serious manifestations occur.[127]

Unresolved and/or recurrent EBV syndromes most often culminate in the development of a PTLD.[115,116] Although PTLDs may involve any site in the body, they most commonly affect the lymph nodes, hepatic allografts, and the gastrointestinal tract. Signs and symptoms attributable to a mass lesion at the site of involvement are common. Withdrawal or dramatic reduction in immunosuppression with the addition of antiviral agents such as acyclovir is the first line of therapy, regardless of the clinical or histopathologic manifestations or the clonality of the lesion.[115,116] This maneuver attempts to restore immune regulation or surveillance. If this is unsuccessful, supplemental treatment with anti-CD20 antibodies or conventional chemotherapy should be considered.[115,116]

MICROSCOPIC PATHOLOGY

Histopathologic manifestations of EBV-associated disorders in the allograft range from nonspecific portal and sinusoidal lymphocytosis (classic EBV hepatitis) to malignant-appearing PTLDs.[117-119,128] Occasional EBV-containing cells can also be detected in rejection and other disorders in patients with increased levels of viral replication.[128]

Reactive or nonspecific EBV hepatitis usually shows mild portal and sinusoidal mononuclear infiltrates composed of small or mildly atypical lymphocytes. Conspicuous lining up of lymphocytes in the sinusoids should suggest an EBV-related disorder, which can be confirmed by in situ hybridization for EBV RNA (EBER). Lobular changes include focal hepatocellular swelling, mild acidophilic necrosis of hepatocytes, and mild lobular disarray.[117-119] Regenerative activity, including double-layered plates, pseudoacinar formation, and mitotic figures, is common.

Patients with less effective control of viral replication evolve toward a PTLD. The key to recognition of liver allograft involvement is the presence of atypical cells in the portal inflammation. In early cases, these atypical cells are intermixed with small and blastic lymphocytes, plasmacytoid lymphocytes, and plasma cells.[117-119] In late or well-developed lesions, the atypical cells predominate. Subendothelial localization of lymphocytes can be seen in the portal or central veins, similar to acute rejection.

Allograft involvement by frank PTLD manifests as maplike enlargement of portal tracts caused by sheets of monomorphic atypical immunoblastic cells (Fig. 39-19), which obscure the normal architectural landmarks.[117-119] Smaller aggregates composed of similar cells can be seen in the sinusoids, and on occasion, focal areas of necrosis are present. Cytologically, the infiltrate resembles an immunoblastic lymphoma, and usually many more cells with atypical cytologic features are seen, including occasional Reed-Sternberg–like cells. The diagnosis is confirmed by in situ hybridization for the EBER sequence. The reader is referred elsewhere for a detailed discussion of the extrahepatic manifestation of PTLD in lymph nodes and other tissues.[115,116]

In cases of suspected PTLD, our routine workup includes immunohistochemical stains for kappa and lambda light chains, CD20 (to determine possible responsiveness to anti-CD20 antibodies),[115] and EBV antigens, as well as in situ hybridization for EBER RNA. If enough fresh tissue is available, a portion is also submitted for flow cytometry and molecular analyses for more detailed phenotypic characterization and immunoglobulin gene rearrangements, respectively.

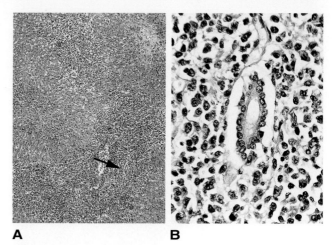

A   **B**

FIGURE 39–19. Liver allograft involvement by a post-transplant lymphoproliferative disorder often takes the form of maplike enlargement of the portal tracts (**A**) by a population of atypical mononuclear cells comprising atypical blastic lymphocytes, some of which usually show evidence of plasmacytoid differentiation. Note that there is little bile duct damage in this case (*arrow* in **A,** highlighted in **B**), despite the presence of a marked portal infiltrate. Compare the composition of this infiltrate typical of PTLD with that of acute rejection shown in Figure 39-11.

DIFFERENTIAL DIAGNOSIS

EBV hepatitis is most often confused with acute rejection, nonspecific "reactive hepatitis," and acute hepatitis due to HCV or CMV.[117-119] Both hepatitis C and EBV hepatitis can reveal sinusoidal lymphocytosis. However, biopsy specimens with EBV hepatitis usually contain at least some cytologically atypical cells, whereas HCV usually evokes a response of small, round, inactive-appearing lymphocytes in the sinusoids and portal tracts.[117-119] Compared with acute rejection, eosinophils and neutrophils are much less common in EBV-related disorders. The portal infiltrate in EBV-related disorders is less pleomorphic, consisting primarily of activated and immunoblastic mononuclear cells, many of which show features of plasmacytic differentiation. Bile duct damage can be seen with EBV, but the severity and prevalence of duct damage are less than would be expected for acute rejection, based on the severity of the portal infiltrate.[117-119] We have also observed several cases of EBV-associated disorders that developed bile duct loss. As with CMV, it is uncertain whether the duct loss is a result of the EBV infection or of rejection that developed because of decreased immunosuppression.

Availability of EBER probe technology is a necessity for interpretation of allograft biopsies and has led to a greater appreciation of the extent of EBV infection in this population.[117-119] However, EBER probe results must be interpreted with caution.[129] Rare cells containing the EBER sequence are not uncommon in the general population and are found with increased frequency in allograft recipients. The significance of rare EBER-positive cells in biopsy specimens is open to debate,[129] but clustering of such cells into aggregates or the presence of EBER-positive cells in tissues showing other histopathologic features of EBV-associated disease is indicative of enhanced EBV replication. In our experience, such patients are at increased risk of developing a PTLD; more frequent peripheral blood monitoring is recommended, and cautious immunosuppression management is warranted. It should also be emphasized that some histologically typical PTLDs may fail to show evidence of EBV infection. This phenomenon is becoming increasingly recognized, accounting for up to 31% of PTLDs in some series.[130]

ADENOVIRAL HEPATITIS

OVERVIEW AND PATHOPHYSIOLOGY

Adenoviral infection and disease after liver transplantation are largely limited to the pediatric population,[131,132] although occasional cases have been seen in adults.[133] Presumably most adults already have protective immunity and thus are less susceptible. Viral subtypes 1, 2, and 5 have been isolated from the lung, gastrointestinal tract, and liver in patients with fever, respiratory distress, diarrhea, and liver dysfunction.[131,132,134] The onset of disease usually occurs between 1 and 10 weeks after transplantation, and biopsy histopathology is used to ascertain the diagnosis. Hepatitis is most often caused by viral subtype 5, but subtypes 2, 11, and 16 have been associated with hepatitis in the general population and could be expected to infect and cause hepatitis in liver allograft recipients.[131,132]

MICROSCOPIC PATHOLOGY

Adenoviral hepatitis is histopathologically distinctive, but some experience is required if the diagnosis is to be established with certainty. The most characteristic findings are "poxlike" granulomas, consisting almost entirely of macrophages, often accompanied by small maplike areas of necrosis, which are spread randomly throughout the parenchyma; the latter characteristic resembles HSV hepatitis.[131-133] Adenoviral inclusions are often found in the nuclei of hepatocytes near the edges of necrotic zones and/or granulomas (Fig. 39-20). Diagnostic inclusions are characterized by a central granular inclusion. Other virus-containing nuclei assume a smudgy appearance. Crowding of chromatin toward the nuclear membrane often imparts a muffin-shape appearance to the nucleus. Immunohistochemical staining is confirmatory.

DIFFERENTIAL DIAGNOSIS

Adenoviral hepatitis can be confused with other causes of focal hepatic necrosis and hepatic granulomas such as infarcts and deep fungal or mycobacterial infections, which can be excluded by microbiologic cultures of the biopsy and negative special stains for granuloma-causing organisms. CMV and HSV-VZ should also be distinguished from adenovirus. The granulomas associated with adenovirus consist almost entirely of macrophages and are much larger than the microgranulomas of CMV; multinucleated giant cells are rare. In contrast, CMV causes cytomegaly and produces eosinophilic intranuclear inclusions surrounded by a clear halo and basophilic or amphophilic small cytoplasmic inclusions. Adenovirus does not cause cytomegaly, the nucleus is often "smudgy-appearing," and no cytoplasmic inclusions are seen. The hepatocyte necrosis associated with adenovirus is generally less than that seen with HSV or VZ hepatitis, although isolated cases can appear similar. In such cases, reliance on immunoperoxidase stains for specific viral antigens is needed.

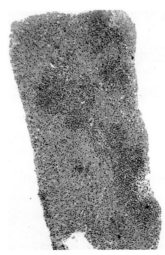
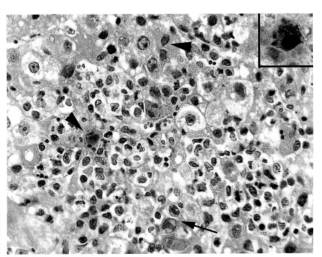

FIGURE 39–20. Adenovirus hepatitis often shows granulomatoid aggregates of macrophages and fewer lymphocytes associated with hepatocellular necrosis (**A**). Other cases can present with large "maplike" areas of necrosis, similar to herpes simplex or varicella-zoster. **B,** The key to establishing the diagnosis of adenovirus hepatitis is the recognition of the characteristic "smudge cells" *(arrowheads)* and intranuclear inclusions *(arrow),* which can be confirmed by immunoperoxidase staining *(inset).*

A   **B**

Hepatitis Virus Infections (A, B, C, and D)

HEPATITIS A

We have not as yet identified hepatitis A (HAV) as a cause of allograft dysfunction. However, Fagan and coworkers[135] showed hepatic persistence (or reinfection) of a liver allograft in a recipient who required transplantation for HAV-induced fulminant hepatic failure. Extrahepatic reservoirs of the virus were thought to account for reinfection of the allografted liver.

HEPATITIS B AND DELTA

Hepatitis B virus (HBV) infection, with or without delta coinfection, is largely restricted to patients whose original liver disease was caused by this virus. Livers from anti-HBc positive donors can transmit HBV to recipients, especially those with no previous exposure to HBV.[19,136]

Virtually all patients who show evidence of viral replication before transplantation (i.e., hepatitis Be antigen (*HBeAg*-seropositive or HBV DNA–positive) will reinfect their allograft. Reinfection and recurrent disease are less predictable in patients who had HBV-induced fulminant liver failure or in those with chronic liver disease who had become anti-HBe–positive and serum HBV DNA– and HBeAg-negative before transplantation[137-143]: Approximately 10% to 25% of these patients will not reinfect the allograft, nor will they develop HBV disease. Despite donor and blood product screening, a small number of patients without previous HBV disease will acquire HBV infection during or after transplantation.[98,144]

Various treatment modalities such as hepatitis B immune globulin (polyclonal and monoclonal), active vaccination with hepatitis B surface antigen (HBsAg), α-interferon, and antiviral drugs such as foscarnet, ganciclovir, famciclovir, and lamivudine[145] are used in an attempt to prevent recurrent infection of the allograft and progressive HBV liver disease after transplantation. Unfortunately, the cycle of reinfection cannot be broken because of the high infectivity of HBV, the extrahepatic reservoirs of HBV, and the ability of HBV to integrate into the genome. However, these treatments keep viral replication in check and thus effectively control recurrent disease and enable long-term survival.[145] Major drawbacks, however, include the high cost of indefinite drug therapy and the emergence of viral mutants that escape pharmacologic control.

PATHOPHYSIOLOGY

Under normal circumstances in nonimmunosuppressed hosts, HBV is generally considered to be noncytopathic, and liver damage is mediated primarily by immunologic mechanisms. A recent study of allograft recipients by Marinos and associates[146] suggests that the same concepts apply to the majority of liver allograft recipients. They propose that HBV peptides are presented to recirculating recipient T-helper cells in association with MHC class II molecules by the host antigen presenting cells that repopulate the allograft after transplantation.[147,148] Recognition of viral antigens by the preexposed T-helper cells leads to expansion and activation of antigen-specific TH1-type CD4+ lymphocytes, which release IFN-γ, the most potent activator of monocytes/macrophages. This activation results in the production of proinflammatory cytokines, especially TNF-α. These two cytokines (IFN-γ and TNF-α) cause damage by (1) recruiting and activating nonspecific inflammatory cells; (2) upregulating tumor necrosis factor receptor expression, making the hepatocytes more vulnerable to the cytolytic and apoptotic actions of TNF-α; (3) exerting a direct cytotoxic effect on the HBsAg-expressing hepatocytes; and (4) inducing local mediators of tissue injury such as nitric oxide. All these mechanisms can operate independent of MHC matching between the host and donor and the immunosuppression.[146]

In a minority of patients, most of whom are over-immunosuppressed, massive viral replication can lead directly to liver injury with little or no hepatic inflammation, suggesting that under these special circumstances, the virus may be directly cytopathic.[138-140]

CLINICAL FEATURES

Recurrent HBV hepatitis usually first manifests at about 6 to 8 weeks after transplantation. The most common presentation involves mild elevations of liver injury test results. Nausea, vomiting, jaundice, and hepatic failure signal more severe recurrent disease. The clinical syndrome, therefore, is not significantly different from the viral hepatitis seen in other immunosuppressed or even nonimmunosuppressed patients in the general population.[137-140] Needle biopsy evaluation confirms the diagnosis.

MICROSCOPIC FEATURES

The histopathologic presentation of hepatitis B infection in hepatic allografts is similar to that seen in nonallograft livers, although local treatment policies can influence the microscopic pathology.[137,138,149,150] In particular, antiviral therapy can effectively control viral replication and limit the tissue pathology. However, untreated or inadequately treated patients and those harboring resistant viral mutants often eventually develop chronic disease, and a typical progression from an acute to a chronic hepatitis occurs. Cirrhosis can develop with striking rapidity.[137-142] Occasional patients show histopathologic resolution of disease activity after a bout of acute hepatitis. Rare patients actually "clear" or immunologically control the virus after transplantation.

In most patients who develop disease, the acute phase presents within 4 to 6 weeks after transplantation, coincident with expression of hepatitis core antigen in the cytoplasm of occasional hepatocytes.[137,138] This is followed by spread of the core antigen, appearance of the surface antigen in a large number of hepatocytes,[137,138] appearance of lobular necroinflammatory activity, Kupffer cell hypertrophy, lobular disarray, and varying amounts of portal inflammation. Even though patients are immunosuppressed, a small percentage can develop bridging or even submassive necrosis, particularly if immunosuppression is lowered or withdrawn.[137]

The most common scenario in those with active viral replication is evolution into chronic hepatitis, characterized by lymphoplasmacytic portal inflammation with relative sparing of the bile ducts and portal veins. This is associated with interface activity of varying severity characterized by extension of lymphocytes and macrophages into the edge of the lobule combined with cholangiolar proliferation. Lobular findings at this time include hepatocytes with a ground-glass cytoplasm or sanded nuclei that stain positively for hepatitis B surface antigen and core antigen, respectively, accompanied by lobular disarray, Kupffer cell hypertrophy, and lobular necroinflammatory activity.

A pattern of liver injury associated with HBV is not commonly encountered in the general population; it is related to massive viral replication because of the effects of overimmunosuppression and MHC nonidentity between the liver and the recipient.[138,140,149,150] It can also occur with the emergence of viral mutants. Usual findings in this presentation include marked hepatocyte swelling, lobular disarray, and cholestasis combined with cholangiolar proliferation but little or no portal or lobular inflammation. These cases usually reveal massive hepatocellular expression of the hepatitis B core (Fig. 39-21) and/or surface antigen (Fig. 39-22) in the degenerating hepatocytes that show swelling, steatosis, or necrosis. Such cases often progress to portal and periportal sinusoidal fibrosis and lobular collapse without a significant inflammatory component.[138-141,149,150] High levels of viral replication and antigen expression have led several groups to suggest that HBV is directly cytopathic under these special circumstances.[138-141,149,150]

The Cambridge group has suggested the term *fibrosing cholestatic hepatitis*[140] to describe this peculiar form of hepatitis; Benner and colleagues[150] preferred *fibrosing cytolytic hepatitis* to describe a similar, if not the same, set of findings. Phillips and coworkers[149] emphasized the heavy viral burden in liver allograft recipients, which caused swelling of the endoplasmic reticulum and hepatocellular degenerative changes. They drew particular attention to the presence of hepatocellular steatosis and coined the terms *steatoviral* and *fibroviral* hepatitis B to accentuate the features of fat and fibrosis.[149] The exact relationship between the terms proposed by Phillips[149] and those proposed by Benner[150] and Davies[140] is uncertain, but in general they

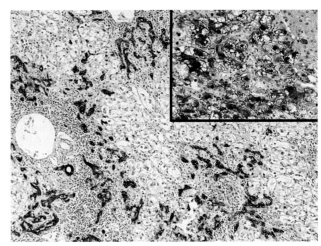

FIGURE 39–21. This photomicrograph shows a case of fibrosing cholestatic hepatitis stained with CK19 to illustrate a basic feature of this disorder—the marked cholangiolar proliferation, which is accompanied by hepatocyte swelling. The swollen and degenerating hepatocytes in the lobules often show marked overproduction of hepatitis B core antigen, which is usually nuclear, except in the presence of massive viral replication, when it spills over into the cytoplasm, as is shown in the *inset.* A similar case with overproduction of surface antigen is shown in Figure 39-22.

appear to describe a similar set of findings associated with massive viral replication. Finally, overproduction of the surface antigen can be seen in the vast majority of hepatocytes containing a ground-glass cytoplasm, similar to HBsAg transgenic mice.[151]

As in the general population, delta agent coinfection may complicate reinfection of the allograft by HBV. Follow-up of such patients has yielded somewhat conflicting results, with reports of both more and less severe disease after transplantation.[143,152,153] In addition,

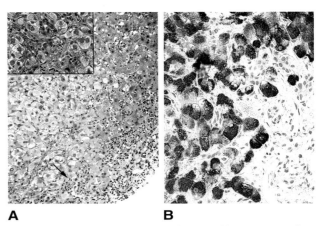

A   **B**

FIGURE 39–22. A, Marked overproduction of hepatitis B surface antigen can lead to degeneration of hepatocytes and cholangiolar proliferation, very similar to the case shown in Figure 39-21. Note the cholangiolar proliferation (*arrow* and *inset*) often associated with pericholangiolar fibrosis. **B,** Stained for hepatitis B surface antigen.

reports conflict about the cytopathic effect of hepatitis D virus (HDV) after transplantation and its relationship to HBV replication. David and associates[154] have noted that HDV hepatitis associated with nonreplicative HBV infection resulted in hepatitic lesions similar to those described earlier as fibrosing cholestatic, fibrosing cytolytic, or steatoviral hepatitis, but without hepatitis B core antigen (HBcAg) expression in the liver. In contrast, when active HBV replication was present, the HBV + HDV hepatitis in the allograft produced necroinflammatory activity similar to that seen in B and D viral hepatitis in patients from the general population.[154]

DIFFERENTIAL DIAGNOSIS

Acute hepatitis B is most often confused with acute hepatitis caused by other viruses. Distinction is usually achieved with the aid of special studies to detect viral antigens and/or nucleic acids in the blood or tissues, or antibody reactions to the virus. Acute rejection and acute or chronic hepatitis can also be confused with each other.[137,138] This differential was discussed earlier under Acute Reaction.

Finally, infection of the allograft by HBV does not equate with HBV disease or, for that matter, exclude rejection.[138] Detection of either core antigen or surface antigen by immunohistochemistry may occur in allografts that otherwise have all the features of acute or chronic rejection.[138]

HEPATITIS C VIRUS

Chronic hepatitis C virus (HCV)-induced cirrhosis is one of the most common indications for liver transplantation throughout the world.[155] At most large centers, it accounts for about 30% of all patients undergoing hepatic replacement.[156-159] Reinfection of the liver allograft with HCV after transplantation and subsequent systemic viremia are practically a universal event that likely occurs within hours after transplantation.[160,161] Fortunately, the screening of blood products for HCV has led to a low incidence of de novo infection, which is on the order of 0.84% in some studies[162,163] but as high as 10% to 20% in others.[98,164]

In most recipients, recurrent infection leads to recurrent hepatitis and recapitulation of the same sequence of events that originally led to liver transplantation. Similar to the original infection, recurrent disease in the majority of allograft recipients evolves slowly; thus, hepatic replacement can significantly prolong survival.[157] However, a smaller percentage of allograft recipients develop very aggressive disease after transplantation.[165] The development of new and more effective antiviral drugs offers the potential of breaking this disheartening cycle of infection, hepatitis, fibrosis, and eventually cirrhosis.

Even if newer antiviral agents can effectively cure HCV infection before transplantation, HCV-induced cirrhosis requiring liver transplantation will continue to be a major problem for the foreseeable future. The incidence of infection in the general population ranges from 1% to 3% in low-incidence areas to 25% to 30% in high-risk countries or regions. Thus, understanding of important issues related to recurrence of HCV infection/disease in the liver allograft is essential for optimal patient management.

Because most HCV infections in liver allograft recipients represent recurrent or persistent disease, the distribution of HCV genotypes after transplantation generally reflects that seen in the recipient population of that particular center before the operation. In several European centers[166,167] and in a North American site,[168] type 1b is the most prevalent, accounting for 25% to 60% of patients. In another large American study, type 1a is the predominant genotype.[168]

PATHOPHYSIOLOGY

The pathogenesis of HCV infection in the allograft is similar to that in native livers, except that a greater viral burden is noted in allograft recipients because of the baseline immunosuppression needed to control rejection.[169-171] Consequently, a greater percentage of allograft recipients experience aggressive disease.[155,165] The already enhanced viral burden in allograft recipients plateaus at 1 month after transplantation and peaks at the time of onset of acute hepatitis (between 1 and 4 months after transplantation). This peak is associated with T-cell infiltration and Fas-mediated hepatocyte apoptosis,[172] manifest as lobular hepatitis and described below under Microscopic Pathology. Chronic HCV seems to be associated with activation of TH1-type inflammatory, profibrotic, and proapoptotic pathways.[171]

Various factors appear to influence the outcomes of HCV infection after transplantation. These include the year of transplantation (worse in recent years),[173] patient race (worse in blacks),[173] the degree of pretransplantation viremia (worse with high levels),[173,174] MHC compatibility, the presence of HCV genotypes that are more pathogenic (worse in genotype 1), the integrity of the cellular immune response, quasi-species homogeneity (worse with viral diversity),[175] and the type and amount of immunosuppression (greater immunosuppression, worse outcome).[173,176-178]

Increased immunosuppression to control episodes of acute rejection has been associated with an increased incidence and earlier onset of more severe recurrent acute and/or chronic HCV-induced disease in the liver allograft. Immunosuppressive agents associated with a higher incidence of HCV include interleukin-2 (IL-2) receptor antibodies,[179] corticosteroids,[176,177,180] azathioprine, OKT3, and total immunosuppression.[176,180]

Studies examining the influence of the primary immunosuppressant on the post-transplant course of

HCV have yielded mixed results. Some show that the baseline immunosuppressive agent did not significantly influence recurrent HCV disease activity,[169,174,177,181] whereas others suggest that more powerful baseline drugs, such as tacrolimus, foster the development of more aggressive disease after transplantation.[182] Mueller and coworkers[183] suggested that tacrolimus use in HCV-positive recipients was associated with a higher incidence of acute rejection, which in turn might influence the hepatitic activity in that additional treatment with corticosteroids might be required. In a small series of HCV-positive renal transplant recipients in whom the confounding influence of rejection could be avoided, the baseline immunosuppressive agent did not affect the hepatitis C disease activity in the native liver.[184] Post-transplant viral titers are similar in patients with recurrent and acquired infection. Although continued study is needed, it is safe to conclude that heavy treatment for rejection increases viral titers and the risk of aggressive disease such as fibrosing cholestatic hepatitis (see later under Microscopic Pathology).

Some studies show that various HCV genotypes are not associated with specific clinical courses of recurrent HCV infection,[162,174,185] but many of them report an earlier onset and/or an increased incidence of disease, higher viremia, and/or greater severity of hepatitis in patients infected with type 1 viruses.[166,168,169,186-188] Even in studies in which the disease appears to be more severe in those with type 1b virus, no significant differences are noted in patient or graft survival by genotype. In addition, no specific qualitative histopathologic features can be used to distinguish between the several different viral genotypes on the basis of routine histopathology alone. However, continued long-term studies are needed to evaluate the effects of viral genotype on HCV disease after transplantation.

When an HCV-positive donor liver is implanted into an HCV-positive recipient, Laskus and associates[189] showed that within a few months after transplantation, either the donor (57%) or the recipient (43%) strain predominated. Subtype 1b and type 1 (1a + 1b) appeared to have a replicative advantage because they became the predominant strains in all recipient/donor pairs in which they were present. This is consistent with several studies that show a more aggressive course associated with genotype 1b and higher levels of viremia.[190,191] It is interesting to note that patients retaining their own strain were found to have significantly more active liver disease than those infected by the donor strain.[189] This may be related to the existence of primed lymphocytes within HCV-positive recipients.

Cholestatic HCV seems to be a disease of direct HCV cytopathic injury related to extreme virus levels, an intrahepatic T-helper subtype 2 cell (TH2)-like response, and lack of a specific HCV-directed response.[192]

CLINICAL FEATURES

The clinical presentation of HCV hepatitis is virtually identical to that seen in the general population. The early phase of the disease is often asymptomatic and is detectable only by an elevation in liver injury test results. Hepatitis develops in a majority of patients after transplantation and manifests primarily by persistent elevation in liver injury tests (especially ALT and AST) to 4 to 8 times normal levels. Liver injury test results may further increase when the first histologic signs of hepatitis appear, usually at between 3 and 6 weeks after transplantation, but an earlier onset within 10 to 14 days has also been observed. Fatigue, nausea, jaundice, and other typical signs of acute hepatitis are less frequent, and fulminant liver failure is uncommon. When it occurs, massive viral replication is usually seen.[160,163,193-195] Needle biopsy evaluation is used to confirm the diagnosis.

Severe recurrent HCV can manifest as fibrosing cholestatic hepatitis, characterized clinically by malaise, jaundice, and a marked increase in cholestatic liver injury tests, such as bilirubin, alkaline phosphatase, and gamma-glutamyl transpeptidase. The disease often evolves subacutely over a period of weeks to months with the development of functional liver failure with encephalopathy and/or cirrhosis. The key to early recognition relies on suspicion by both the clinical physician and the pathologist.

By 5 years after transplantation, approximately 5% to 20% of patients have cirrhosis caused by recurrent hepatitis.[165,175,196,197]

MICROSCOPIC PATHOLOGY

The histopathologic appearance of HCV in the liver allograft is similar to that seen in the general population. The virus likely infects the allograft within minutes after transplantation, and the first reliable histopathologic features that can be used to detect disease activity usually appear within 3 to 6 weeks, although in some cases, histopathologic signs of recurrence can be detected in as little as 10 to 14 days. Once infection occurs, development of the disease usually follows a predictable evolution through several well-recognized clinical and histopathologic phases,[43,157,198,199] although atypical presentations can occur.

The acute or initial phase is usually characterized by lobular hepatitis. Typical features include lobular disarray, Kupffer cell hypertrophy, spotty acidophilic hepatocyte necrosis, mild sinusoidal lymphocytosis, and variable degrees of mononuclear portal inflammation. Macrovesicular steatosis of periportal and midzonal hepatocytes is also often seen. Portal inflammation is usually mild. Lymphocytes invading the basement membrane and reactive changes of the biliary epithelium can be focally seen, but these changes are neither severe nor widespread. Typically, they involve less than 50% of the bile ducts. Some studies show that acute lobular hepatitis on biopsy is accompanied by a steep increase in HCV RNA levels and the appearance of core and NS4 antigens in the graft[190]; others show no strong relationship between level of viremia and degree of hepatic damage.[170]

During the transition from acute to chronic hepatitis, lobular changes usually start to wane and portal inflammation increases. This is accompanied by the appearance of interface activity, including an accompanying ductular reaction that begins to distort the architecture.

The chronic phase usually begins between 4 and 12 months after transplantation, and the predominant features are portal inflammation and periportal hepatitis with varying degrees of interface activity, lobular disarray, and necroinflammatory activity. Again, inflammatory bile duct damage can be seen, but it is usually not severe or widespread, and there is no bile duct loss. Inflammation beneath the endothelium and/or around the connective tissue sheath of the central vein, known in the liver as *central venulitis*, can also be seen in an occasional vessel. But, similar to the duct damage, it is neither severe nor widespread and typically involves less than 50% of terminal hepatic venules.

One notable atypical HCV presentation is fibrosing cholestatic hepatitis (Fig. 39-23). It is characterized by extensive centrilobular hepatocyte swelling and degeneration, cholestasis, spotty acidophilic hepatocyte necrosis, and Kupffer cell hypertrophy, combined with portal tract expansion because of ductular proliferation, fibrosis, and a mild mixed or even neutrophilic predominant portal infiltrate.[198,200]

Several studies have specifically examined the effects of viral genotype and titers on quantitative and qualitative aspects of the histopathology of recurrent HCV. Some studies showed no correlation between viral titers and the severity of liver damage[201]; others showed that HCV RNA was higher during the lobular phase of the infection and that progression to the chronic phase with interface activity was associated with a highly significant decrease in liver HCV RNA. Other studies have shown that ballooning degeneration and cholestasis at initial presentation[202,203] are associated with the subsequent development of allograft cirrhosis.[202,203] In one study, no significant difference was noted in the histopathology of recurrent versus de novo disease, whereas in another, de novo infection more often led to significant disease.[198]

DIFFERENTIAL DIAGNOSIS

The differential diagnosis includes acute and chronic rejection, recurrent non-HCV viral hepatitis (e.g., HBV, CMV, EBV), recurrent autoimmune hepatitis, recurrent PBC, recurrent PSC, and bile duct obstruction.[55,194,198] Definitive exclusion of chronic HCV liver disease is based on negative reverse transcription polymerase chain reaction (RT-PCR) results for HCV on liver tissue. HBV is identified on the basis of viral antigens, which are present and detected in the serum or with immunoperoxidase staining of tissue specimens.

Cholestatic hepatitis can be difficult to distinguish from bile duct obstruction and hepatic artery thrombosis. Portal edema and portal (rather than periportal) neutrophilia are common in duct obstruction and/or acute cholangitis. In contrast, cholangiolar proliferation and acute cholangiolitis without portal edema are more characteristic of cholestatic hepatitis. In addition, lobular disarray and marked hepatocellular swelling are more usual for viral hepatitis in contrast to duct obstruction.

Acute rejection may be extremely difficult to distinguish from chronic viral hepatitis C mostly because both can show portal inflammation and bile duct damage. In addition, acute and/or chronic rejection and recurrent HCV can occur together, making it difficult in some cases to determine the more important cause of allograft injury. In such cases, the pathologist should first determine whether acute rejection is present. The key features used to identify acute rejection include (1) the prevalence and severity of mononuclear inflammatory bile duct damage and biliary epithelial senescence changes (Fig. 39-24), and (2) the prevalence and severity of central vein inflammation and fibrosis. If either of these features involves a majority of bile ducts or central veins, then acute or chronic rejection, respectively, is present. Conversely, key features used to identify HCV include the prevalence and severity of (1) spotty lobular necrosis,[204] (2) interface activity, and (3) ductular reaction, all of which are usually inconspicuous in rejection. In addition, prevalent and prominent type I and II ductular reactions[205] provide strong evidence of

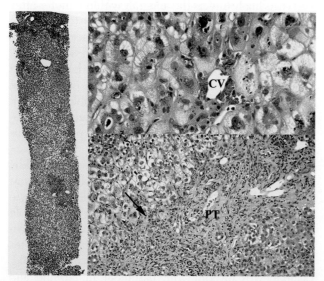

FIGURE 39–23. Fibrosing cholestatic hepatitis can also be seen with HCV infection, as is shown in this composite image. In our experience, this presentation of HCV is also associated with marked viral replication, as measured by virus nucleic acids in the serum. CV, central vein; PT, portal tract.

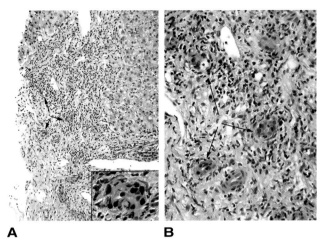

A   **B**

FIGURE 39–24. The diagnosis of acute rejection can be established in a liver allograft with chronic hepatitis C. The biopsy illustrated in this composite was obtained 9 months after transplantation. A biopsy obtained two months before this sample showed changes typical of chronic hepatitis C. In the interval, the patient was treated with dramatic lowering of the immunosuppression and a combination of interferon and ribavirin, which led to nearly nondetectable viral nucleic acids in the peripheral blood but a new onset of jaundice and marked elevation of the GGTP. Note the mononuclear portal inflammation with only mild interface activity (**A**). However, prominent lymphocytic bile duct damage involved a majority of the bile ducts (*arrows*). **B,** Higher magnification of the region highlighted with the *arrows* in **A.**

a nonrejection-related cause of allograft dysfunction. Taking the risk of treating acute rejection with increased immunosuppression in the context of recurrent HCV should be based on thorough clinicopathologic correlations that take into consideration the severity of findings (mild rejection may not require treatment), the level of viral titers (avoid treatment with high titers), and the liver injury test profile.

The time after transplantation is useful in distinguishing acute rejection from recurrent HCV. During the first several weeks after transplantation, HCV is an uncommon cause of allograft dysfunction, although in isolated cases, the typical sequence of changes described earlier can begin in only 10 to 14 days. Most cases of recurrent hepatitis C begin at between 3 and 8 weeks after transplantation. In contrast, most acute rejection episodes occur within the first 30 days, with a median of 8 days.[206]

Distinguishing HCV from HBV, autoimmune hepatitis, drug-induced hepatitis, PBC, and obstructive cholangiopathy is based on a complete clinical, biochemical, serologic, and histopathologic profile. For example, the distinction between recurrent and new-onset autoimmune hepatitis and HCV is largely based on the clinical profile and the results of laboratory tests other than the liver biopsy, such as autoantibodies (e.g., anti-nuclear antibody [ANA], anti-smooth muscle antibody [ASMA], and liver kidney microsomal [LKM] antibody). No specific histopathologic features can reliably distinguish between autoimmune and HCV-induced hepatitis in an individual case. However, similar to native livers, it has been our experience that autoimmune disease reveals more plasma-cell rich inflammation, less steatosis, and fewer portal lymphoid nodules than does recurrent HCV.

Several groups have reported a higher incidence of chronic rejection in HCV-positive recipients.[159,207,208] Several possible nonexclusionary explanations can be offered for this association. First, it is well known that viral infections can cause an inflammatory microenvironment within an allograft, which in turn can upregulate adhesion, co-stimulatory, and MHC antigens. All of these factors acting in concert can precipitate a rejection response. Partial MHC class I compatibility between the donor and the recipient might permit MHC-restricted T cell–mediated response to viral infection simultaneously with an allogeneic response.[209] These scenarios are made even more likely if immunosuppression is concomitantly reduced or an immune stimulator like α-interferon is added[210,211]; both of these approaches are used to treat the viral infection.

▌ Recurrent Diseases and Diseases Induced by Transplantation

For the purpose of this discussion, recurrent native liver diseases can be categorized as follows: (1) infectious (e.g., viral hepatitis A, B, C, D), (2) dysregulated immunity (autoimmune hepatitis, PBC, PSC, and overlap syndromes), (3) primary hepatic malignancies (hepatocellular and cholangiocarcinomas), (4) toxic conditions (e.g., alcohol, adverse drug reactions, drug overdoses), and (5) hepatically based (e.g., alpha-1-antitrypsin deficiency, Wilson's disease) and extrahepatically based metabolic disorders (e.g., hemochromatosis, Gaucher's disease, cystic fibrosis).

Recurrence of infectious disorders is common.[35-37] Virtually all patients with active HBV or HCV infection before transplantation will reinfect the new liver and develop at least some degree of chronic hepatitis; in general, the post-transplant disease is generally more virulent than the one that occurred before transplantation because of the immunosuppression and the enhanced viral replication. Details as to the incidence and severity of recurrent viral hepatitis and its clinical and histopathologic presentations are given in the respective sections on those disorders.

Disorders of immune regulation such as PBC, autoimmune hepatitis, and sclerosing cholangitis also commonly recur after liver transplantation, but the incidence of recurrence is lower than for viral hepatitis. In addition, recurrent disease is often less severe than the same disease before transplantation.[212]

Within 5 years after transplantation, roughly 25% to 50% of patients with PBC, PSC, or autoimmune disease develop some evidence of recurrent disease. For this particular category of diseases, however, it is not uncommon to be confronted with clinical and microscopic pathology that are suggestive but not diagnostic of disease recurrence. This problem arises because the diagnosis is based on variable combinations of clinical, serologic, histopathologic, and radiographic findings, and a similar constellation of findings can occur outside of the setting of recurrent disease. For example, many causes of intrahepatic biliary strictures are known besides recurrent PSC. In addition, autoantibodies present before transplantation and used to establish the diagnosis often persist afterward, albeit at lower titers, even in the absence of clinical or histopathologic evidence of recurrent disease. Consequently, we divide recurrent disease after liver transplantation into definite, probable, and possible categories. Each is discussed more fully in the following respective sections on specific diseases.

Liver transplantation for primary hepatic malignancies (mostly hepatocellular carcinoma and bile duct or cholangiocarcinoma) is chosen according to the stage of the disease at the time of transplantation.[213-215] In general, early-stage hepatocellular carcinomas without vascular invasion are cured by liver transplantation. Microscopic vascular invasion is a powerful predictor of hepatocellular carcinoma recurrence, as are multiple liver tumors and larger overall tumor burden (Table 39-9). Bile duct adenocarcinomas and cholangiocarcinomas have a poor prognosis after liver transplantation because most cases are discovered only after significant invasion into the surrounding liver has occurred.

Toxic insults and adverse drug reactions also do not recur after transplantation unless the patient is again exposed to the same agent, which is obviously a problem with alcoholics.

Jaffe[216] separated liver transplantation for metabolic diseases into three categories: (1) The liver is the prime site of the defect, and involvement leads to end-stage liver disease (Table 39-10); (2) the liver is the site of the defect, but the predominant effects are systemic and not hepatotoxic (Table 39-11); and (3) the defect lies somewhere outside of the liver, and the effects on the liver are largely secondary (Table 39-12). The first group of patients are prime candidates for liver replacement because the cirrhotic liver is replaced by a genetically and structurally normal one that cures the disease. Examples include type 1 tyrosinemia, alpha-1-antitrypsin deficiency, Wilson's disease, neonatal hemochromatosis, and types 1, 3, and 4 glycogen storage disease.[216] In the second group, the liver may be structurally normal or near normal, and the goal is to alleviate the systemic disease burden of abnormal liver physiology. Examples include familial amyloid polyneuropathy, type 1 oxalosis, urea cycle defects and hyperammonemia syndromes,

familial hypercholesterolemia, and hepatic clotting factor disorders.[216] In the third group, the liver is vulnerable to recurrent disease because the metabolic disorder persists, but a survival advantage and/or improved quality of life is the primary driving factor behind liver replacement.[216] Examples include storage diseases and lysosomal storage diseases such as Niemann-Pick, Gaucher's, cystinosis, and erythropoietic protoporphyria.

Other diseases of uncertain origin also can recur after liver transplantation. These include sarcoidosis,[217] idiopathic granulomatous hepatitis,[55] postinfantile giant cell hepatitis,[218] and the Budd-Chiari syndrome.[35-37]

SPECIAL CONSIDERATIONS—COMMON RECURRENT DISEASES

Primary Biliary Cirrhosis

OVERVIEW AND PATHOPHYSIOLOGY

PBC is a relatively common indication for liver transplantation at some large centers. It has been reported to recur in 0% to 90% of patients after 1 to 19 years following liver transplantation, but an average incidence of 20% at 5 years is typical[212] (see Table 39-9). New-onset PBC is rare, although the senior author has observed at least one convincing but unreported case in a patient with coexistent HCV infection. There are many reasons for the broad range of incidences in the various studies, including the certainty of the pretransplant and post-transplant diagnosis, immunosuppressive agents used and management policies followed, the use of protocol biopsies, the length of post-transplant follow-up, operative techniques, and other factors that would influence biliary tract physiology during or after transplantation.[212]

For example, one study showed that 28 of 38 (74%) PBC patients developed immunohistochemical evidence of altered expression of the immunodominant mitochondrial autoantigen of PBC (pyruvate dehydrogenase complex-E2), sometimes within days after transplantation.[219] However, only 8 of these patients developed routine histopathologic and clinical evidence of recurrent PBC. Another study was unable to confirm this finding.[220] Centers that conduct protocol biopsies tend to report a higher incidence of recurrent disease compared with centers that biopsy only upon indication. Nevertheless, there is widespread agreement that PBC does indeed recur in the liver allograft; closely studying this patient population provides an opportunity to gain insight into the underlying cause.

Although PBC is often classified as an autoimmune disease, evidence supporting this contention can be challenged because PBC in native livers does not respond favorably to increased immunosuppression, and there is no universal association with MHC types, as with autoimmune hepatitis. In fact, patients treated with one of

TABLE 39-9. Recurrence of the Original Disease After Liver Transplantation

Original Disease	Incidence of Recurrence (at ~5 years)	Comments	References
Viral Hepatitis			
HAV	<5%	Preexisting anti-HAV titers decline following OLTx, but recurrent or new-onset HAV is rare after OLTx	135, 310, 311
HBV/HDV	Variable	Rate of recurrence depends on viral status at time of OLTx: especially high (100%) in HBV/DNA- or HBeAg-positive recipients. Natural course of recurrent disease is dismal without therapy but is significantly improved by treatment with various antiviral reagents (see text). Good long-term survival with minimal disease activity if viral replication kept in check. Long-term problems include cost of therapy and emergence of viral mutants	138, 142, 145, 312–315
HCV	Nearly 100%*	Reinfection nearly universal and high incidence of recurrent chronic hepatitis. Risk factors for rapidly progressive recurrent disease include transplantation in recent years, advanced donor age, high immunosuppression, high viral load (before or early after transplant), early recurrence within several weeks or months after transplantation, and ballooning and cholestasis in liver biopsies early after transplantation. Five percent to 30% of patients with recurrence develop cirrhosis within 5 years	197, 316–323
Disorders of Immune Regulation			
Autoimmune hepatitis	25%–42%*	Risk factors for recurrence in some studies include MHC-DR3-negative and -DR4-positive recipients, patients with high-grade inflammation in native liver, steroid withdrawal and weaning from other immunosuppressives, and young recipient age; children may also develop a more aggressive form of recurrent disease	Reviewed in 212
PBC	20%–90%*	Recurrence risk increased by immunosuppression regimen (tacrolimus > CyA), steroid withdrawal, and weaning from other immunosuppressives, as well as MHC-DR matching (Dvorchik, unpublished observation)	Reviewed in 212
PSC	~30%*	Incidence appears to increase with time after transplantation, but specific risk factors for recurrence are difficult to identify. Recurrent disease has little impact on patient or graft survival up to 5 to 7 years after transplantation	Reviewed in 212
Toxic Diseases			
Alcoholic	13%–50%	Rate of recidivism difficult to precisely document, and coexisting diseases (e.g., HCV, hemochromatosis, alpha-1-antitrypsin heterozygotes, head and neck cancers) are frequently present. Severe relapse can lead to graft loss or patient death, but recurrent alcoholic liver disease is not a significant problem for the majority of alcoholics up to 6 years after transplantation	248, 249, 252, 257
NASH	25%–100%*	Incidence depends on whether NASH or cryptogenic cirrhosis was the original diagnosis	324–326
Malignancies			
HCC	See comments	Recurrence depends on size (less likely with single tumor <5 cm or three tumors each <3 cm), stage ≤T2, and histologic grade (well differentiated), as well as absence of vascular invasion and lymph node metastasis. Multiparameter modeling systems used to predict recurrence after OLTx and, thus, eligibility for OLTx	215, 327–333
Bile duct/CC	See comments	Prognosis is generally poor, but patients with peripheral cholangiocarcinomas and those early-stage hilar tumors (stages 0–II) without lymph node metastasis and negative resection margins can show reasonable (~40%) 5-year survival	334–337

*Incidence depends on definition and whether protocol biopsies were obtained.

CC, cholangiocarcinoma; CyA, cyclosporin A; HAV, hepatitis A virus; HBV, hepatitis B virus; HCC, hepatocellular carcinoma; HCV, hepatitis C virus; HDV, hepatitis D virus; MHC, major histocompatibility complex; NASH, nonalcoholic steatohepatitis; OLTx, orthotopic liver transplant; PBC, primary biliary cirrhosis; PSC, primary sclerosing cholangitis.

TABLE 39-10. Metabolic Disease Treated by Liver Transplantation Where the Primary Defect Lies Within the Liver and Is Associated With Liver Disease

Disease	Explanation of Disease and Alternative Treatment	Associated Liver Disease	Correction of Metabolic Defect	References
Alpha-1-antitrypsin deficiency	Mutations in protease inhibitor synthesized in liver lead to defective transport from endoplasmic reticulum because of protein misfolding. No alternative treatments	Cirrhosis	Partial; patients are biochemically chimeric because protease inhibitor is produced by other cells, but no evidence of recurrent liver disease	338, 339
Wilson's disease	Autosomal recessive gene mapped to chromosome 13q14-q21.1, which codes for abnormal copper-transporting ATPase and leads to increased biliary copper excretion, decreased copper binding to ceruloplasmin, and copper accumulation in tissues. Alternative therapy: Pharmacologic therapy available to reduce copper absorption and stimulate endogenous proteins that block copper toxicity (zinc) or chelating agents to remove copper from the body	Fulminant hepatic failure and/or cirrhosis	Yes, but usually indicated now in patients presenting with liver failure	340–342
Tyrosinemia	Fumaroylacetoacetate hydrolase deficiency leads to accumulation of toxic intermediates that cause hepatocyte and DNA damage, leading to cirrhosis and liver tumors. Alternative therapy: Pharmacologic—2-(2-nitro-4-trifluoromethylbenzoyl) cyclohexane-1-3-dione (NTBC), which lessens the need for liver replacement	Cirrhosis, hepatoma	Nearly complete	343, 344
Types I and Ib glycogen storage disease	Glucose-6-phosphatase deficiency leads to storage products in liver that cause fibrosis. Alternative therapy: Nocturnal nasogastric infusion of glucose or orally administered cornstarch	Glycogen storage, fibrosis, tumors	Yes, but may not cure associated renal disease	345, 346
Type III glycogen storage disease	Autosomal recessive deficiency of amylo-1,6-glucosidase, 4-alpha-glucanotransferase enzyme (AGL, or glycogen debranching enzyme) leads to storage products in liver that cause fibrosis	Liver fibrosis and adenomas	Incomplete; extrahepatic manifestations may progress	346
Type IV glycogen storage disease	Amylo-1:4,1:6-transglucosidase (branching enzyme) defect. Amylopectin accumulation leads to liver fibrosis/cirrhosis	Cirrhosis	Incomplete; extrahepatic manifestations may or may not improve, depending on variant of disease	342, 346
Inborn errors of bile acid synthesis	Defective synthesis of bile acid synthesis (see ref 347 for listing of specific enzyme defects) leads to cholestasis and liver injury. Alternative treatment with bile acids (cholic acid)	Cholestasis and liver failure	Yes	347

TABLE 39-11. Metabolic Disease Treated by Liver Transplantation Where the Primary Defect Lies Inside of the Liver, But Liver Is Often Normal or Near Normal

Disease	Explanation of Disease and Alternative Treatment	Associated Liver Disease	Correction of Metabolic Defect	References
Familial amyloid polyneuropathy (FAP)	Defective transthyretin (prealbumin) molecule accumulates as amyloid in extrahepatic (endoneurial, gastrointestinal and intracardiac) organs No alternative therapy	Mild liver abnormalities with amyloid deposits in portal tracts and nerve trunks; use of FAP-affected liver is controversial (see refs 348 to 350)	Nearly complete; extrahepatic amyloid deposits may not resolve, but natural history of disease is improved	351, 352
Crigler-Najjar syndrome	Glucuronyltransferase deficiency leads to unconjugated hyperbilirubinemia and neuronal injury. Alternative therapy: Pharmacologic and phototherapy	None	Yes	353, 354
Type I hyperoxaluria	Peroxisomal alanine:gloxylate aminotransferase deficiency leads to deposition of calcium oxalate crystals in the tissue, especially kidneys. Alternative therapy: Pharmacologic (pyridoxine, crystalline inhibitors) and high fluid intake	None	Yes, but may or may not prevent or reverse kidney disease, which is major limiting factor	216, 347, 355
Urea cycle enzyme deficiencies	X-linked recessive disorders; biosynthesis of urea dependent on six enzymes, all of which are located in liver. Alternative therapy: Pharmacologic	None	Yes	216, 347
Protein C deficiency	Defective C protein synthesis, resulting in predisposition to thrombosis. Alternative therapy: Oral anticoagulation and blood component therapy; replacement gene therapy anticipated	None	Yes	356
Familial hypercholesterolemia	Low-density lipoprotein receptor deficiency, low-density lipoprotein overproduction lead to accelerated atherosclerosis. Alternative therapy: Pharmacologic	None	Incomplete	216, 357
Hemophilia A	Factor VIII deficiency leads to bleeding tendency. Alternative therapy: Recombinant protein or gene therapy	None; cirrhosis occurs as a complication of blood component therapy	Yes	358, 359
Hemophilia B	Factor IX deficiency leads to bleeding tendency. Alternative therapy: Recombinant protein or gene therapy	None; cirrhosis occurs as complication of blood component therapy	Yes	216, 360

the more potent immunosuppressive agents such as tacrolimus show a higher incidence and an earlier onset of recurrent PBC than do patients maintained on cyclosporine[221,222] (unpublished observation). Recurrent PBC is also common after living-related liver transplantation[223] and after steroid withdrawal.[224,225] An association with MHC-DR matching (Dvorchick, unpublished observation), suggests that antigen presenting cells might play a pivotal role in this disease.[226]

CLINICAL FEATURES

In the vast majority of patients, the first signs of recurrent PBC usually occur more than 6 months after transplantation. Most patients are diagnosed with early-stage disease and are asymptomatic, coming to clinical attention because of a preferential increase in routinely monitored ALP and gamma-glutamyltranspeptidase. However, we have observed rare patients who develop an acute febrile onset with increased liver injury test results,

TABLE 39-12. Metabolic Disease Treated by Liver Transplantation Where the Primary Defect Lies Outside the Liver

Disease	Explanation of Disease and Alternative Treatment	Associated Liver Disease	Correction of Metabolic Defect	References
Hemochromatosis (or inadvertent transplantation of donor with hemochromatosis)	Autosomal recessive disorder associated with point mutation C282Y in *HFE* gene, which results in increased iron absorption from intestine and possibly defective storage in hepatocytes, which causes liver injury and fibrosis, although all patients with iron overload may not have same metabolic defect; disease development not fully understood. Alternative therapy: Chelating agents and phlebotomy	Cirrhosis	Uncertain because of limited follow-up, relatively low frequency of *HFE* mutations in native livers with iron overload, and treatment to avoid exposure to iron. Little impact up to 5 years after transplantation	Reviewed in 361, 362
Niemann-Pick disease	Defect in *NPC1* gene; sphingomyelinase deficiency leads to dysregulation of cholesterol trafficking	None	Not known	216, 363
Sea-blue histiocyte syndrome	Unknown, neurovisceral lipochrome storage	Cirrhosis	No	364
Erythropoietic protoporphyria	Hepatic ferrochelatase deficiency, overproduction of protoporphyrin by erythropoietic tissues. Alternative therapy: Heme-albumin preparations and supportive	Cirrhosis	Incomplete; OLTx considered palliative	365–367
Cystinosis	Lysosomal storage disorder mapped to chromosome 17p defect apparently lies in impaired ATPase cystine transport across lysosomal membranes and accumulation of cystine crystals in lysosomes. Alternative therapy: Pharmacologic	Does not generally cause liver disease; one patient developed intrahepatic crystal deposits in liver with perivenular fibrosis and recurrent disease in the allograft (see ref 216)	No	216
Cystic fibrosis	Autosomal recessive mutations in chloride channel gene; cystic fibrosis transmembrane conductance regulator (CFTR) results in inspissated secretions in lung and liver. Alternative therapy: Supportive, nutritional, and antibiotic	Biliary fibrosis/cirrhosis	Cures liver disease, and if liver transplant is done early, lung function can improve	368–370

combined with a mixed biliary and hepatitic histology within 2 months after transplantation (unpublished observation).

As the disease progresses, patients can develop cholestatic symptoms similar to those seen before transplantation such as jaundice, itching, hepatosplenomegaly, and portal hypertension. Antimitochondrial antibodies are of little additional benefit in the diagnosis of recurrent PBC because they remain elevated in the majority of patients after transplantation.[212] The diagnosis is established on needle biopsies of the allograft. The effect of treatment with ursodeoxycholic acid on recurrent disease has not been systematically investigated, but the expectation is that the results will be similar to those seen in native livers.

MICROSCOPIC PATHOLOGY

The routine histopathologic manifestations of recurrent PBC are identical to those seen in the native liver. Noninfectious granulomatous duct damage producing breaks in the ductal basement membranes or "florid duct" lesions are diagnostic of disease recurrence in the proper setting (Fig. 39-25). Portal granulomas have been identified in patients with HCV infection,[227] although this observation is not common in our experience, and these granulomas are rarely associated with significant ductal damage.

Unfortunately, diagnostic florid duct lesions are not always present. Prominent but patchy lymphocytic cholangitis accompanied by portal lymphoid nodules

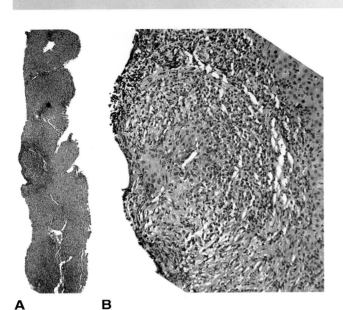

A B

FIGURE 39–25. The histopathologic manifestations of recurrent primary biliary cirrhosis are identical to those in native livers. Note the patchy portal mononuclear portal inflammation shown in **A. B** shows a florid duct lesion at higher magnification. This finding is diagnostic of recurrent PBC in the proper setting (see text).

containing germinal centers and an interface ductular reaction are findings strongly suggestive of recurrent disease. In the proper setting, such cases are best classified as probable recurrent PBC.

Lobular findings in recurrent PBC are nonspecific and usually include mild spotty necrosis, Kupffer cell hypertrophy, a slight increase in sinusoidal lymphocytes, mild nodular regenerative hyperplastic changes, and Kupffer cell granulomas. As the disease progresses, development of biliary fibrosis and cholatestasis and deposition of copper and copper-associated proteins at the edge of the lobules provide strongly supportive evidence of recurrent PBC if other causes for biliary tract pathology have been excluded.

In the absence of pathognomonic or strongly suggestive findings, the histopathologic diagnosis of recurrent PBC is less certain. For example, possible recurrent PBC might first manifest as an unexplained chronic hepatitis,[55,228] either because the duct damage was missed on biopsy or because the recurrent disease manifested as autoimmune hepatitis.[229] In addition, findings of recurrent PBC can overlap with recurrent autoimmune hepatitis,[228] and plasma cell–rich periportal hepatitis early after transplantation has been suggested as an early marker, predictive of PBC recurrence.[230]

DIFFERENTIAL DIAGNOSIS

Recurrent PBC can be confused with acute and chronic rejection; chronic biliary tract obstruction and structuring; chronic viral, autoimmune, or idiopathic hepatitis; and adverse drug reactions. The key to establishing the diagnosis of recurrent PBC with certainty is identification of granulomatous duct destruction or florid duct lesions in the proper context, which excludes other causes (e.g., fungal or acid-fast bacterial infections and HCV). Prominent focal lymphocytic cholangitis accompanied by portal lymphoid nodules containing germinal centers and an interface ductular reaction are findings strongly suggestive but not absolutely diagnostic of recurrent disease.

In cases without diagnostic findings, development of a "biliary gestalt" eventually points toward recurrent PBC and distinguishes such cases from other nonbiliary causes of chronic allograft dysfunction. The most helpful findings in this context include a ductular reaction at the interface zone, periportal clearing or edema, cholatestasis, and accumulation of copper or copper-associated pigment in periportal hepatocytes, as well as patchy small bile duct loss. It is assumed that these findings are occurring in the absence of evidence of large bile duct obstruction or stricturing or other causes of chronic cholangiopathy.

Neither acute nor chronic rejection shows a ductular reaction or leads to biliary fibrosis or biliary cirrhosis. In addition, the portal inflammation and rejection–associated lymphocytic cholangitis usually involves a majority of portal tracts and preferentially involves small bile ducts (<20 µm in smallest diameter), whereas PBC-associated portal inflammation and lymphocytic cholangitis are typically patchy and preferentially involve medium-sized bile ducts (>40 µm in shortest diameter). Chronic hepatitis does not lead to chronic progressive biliary pathology.

Some PBC patients have developed autoimmune hepatitis after liver transplantation.[229] It is uncertain whether this represents a switching of autoimmune disease from PBC to autoimmune hepatitis, new-onset autoimmune hepatitis, or an alternative form of rejection.[231] Such patients may not develop a biliary gestalt and need to be distinguished from those with other causes of chronic hepatitis, such as HBV or HCV infection and adverse drug reactions.

Recurrent and New-Onset Autoimmune Hepatitis

OVERVIEW AND PATHOPHYSIOLOGY

The diagnosis of autoimmune hepatitis in a native liver is based on a combination of clinical, pathologic, and serologic findings, together with the exclusion of other causes of chronic liver injury.[232] The diagnosis of autoimmune hepatitis after transplantation is even more problematic because of a conceptual and pathophysiologic overlap with rejection and other late post-transplant complications.[231,233] Further complicating the issue is the observation that autoantibodies present before transplantation often persist after transplantation, albeit usually at lower titers,[234,235] even in those with histopathologic evidence of recurrent hepatitis. Therefore, we advocate using relatively strict criteria, such as those proposed by the International Scoring System,[232] to establish with certainty the diagnosis of recurrent or new-onset autoimmune hepatitis.

At a minimum, the diagnosis of autoimmune hepatitis in an allograft should be based on chronic hepatitis histopathology on liver biopsy, accompanied by persistent elevation of liver injury test results, a negative RT-PCR for HBV and HCV infection, and no other evidence of a cause for chronic hepatitis.[231] An unequivocal diagnosis of autoimmune hepatitis before transplantation is needed to diagnose recurrent disease. Regardless of these difficulties, strong evidence from a number of centers indicates that recurrent autoimmune hepatitis develops in roughly 30% of recipients by 5 years, usually first manifest longer than 1 year after transplantation.[212]

Risk factors for the development of recurrent autoimmune hepatitis include suboptimal immunosuppression, MHC-DR3–negative and -DR4–positive recipients, the type of autoimmune disease (greater recurrence incidence with type I versus type II), severe inflammation in the native liver before transplantation, and the duration of follow-up since transplantation.[212] Children are at increased risk for new-onset autoimmune hepatitis after transplantation.[212] This observation is probably attributable to the immaturity of the pediatric immune system, including an active thymus susceptible to damage from calcineurin-inhibiting immunosuppressive drugs and subsequent premature release of autoreactive clones into the periphery.[236]

Rejection reactions, especially chronic rejection, also trigger autoimmune effector pathways.[237,238] This most likely accounts for the conceptual and histopathologic overlap between rejection and autoimmune hepatitis long after transplantation.[231,233]

DIFFERENTIAL DIAGNOSIS

Once chronic hepatitis is recognized on histopathology, complete clinicopathologic and serologic correlation is needed to establish with certainty a diagnosis of recurrent or new-onset autoimmune hepatitis. Most importantly, there must be persistent liver injury test result elevations, and other causes of chronic hepatitis such as hepatitis B and C virus infection, recurrent PBC or PSC, chronic obstructive cholangiopathy, adverse drug reactions, and acute rejection must be reasonably excluded. Distinguishing autoimmune hepatitis from acute and chronic rejection is done according to the same guidelines as those used to distinguish rejection from viral hepatitis (see under Hepatitis C Virus).

Recurrent Primary Sclerosing Cholangitis

OVERVIEW AND PATHOPHYSIOLOGY

PSC is a disease of unknown origin that often arises in patients with coexistent ulcerative colitis. It recurs in about 30% of patients within 5 years after transplantation.[212] The presence of hilar bile duct cancer before transplantation significantly degrades survival after transplantation.[239,240] Coexistent ulcerative colitis generally worsens after transplantation,[241,242] and the risk of developing and dying from colon cancer is substantial.[243] Patients with PSC are also at greater risk for acute and chronic and steroid-resistant rejection.[240,244]

Establishing the diagnosis of recurrent PSC can be difficult because many other insults, such as ischemic injury from prolonged preservation or nonheartbeating donors, imperfect biliary anastomoses, inadequate hepatic arterial flow, and humoral rejection, can also cause nonanastomotic intrahepatic biliary strictures that mimic recurrent PSC. Graziadei and associates[245] restrictively defined recurrent PSC using both positive and negative criteria. The definition included a confirmed diagnosis of PSC before transplantation and cholangiographically confirmed biliary strictures occurring more than 90 days after transplantation, or biopsy findings showing fibrous cholangitis and/or fibro-obliterative lesions with or without ductopenia, biliary fibrosis, or biliary cirrhosis—all in the absence of hepatic artery thrombosis/stenosis, established chronic (ductopenic) rejection, anastomotic strictures alone, nonanastomotic strictures occurring before post-transplantation day 90, and ABO incompatibility between donor and recipient. Nevertheless, otherwise unexplained nonanastomotic intrahepatic biliary strictures occur with greater frequency after transplantation in patients who had PSC before liver replacement.[212]

CLINICAL FEATURES

Recurrent PSC usually first manifests longer than 6 months after transplantation and, in our experience, appears to increase over time after transplantation.[212] Nonanastomotic intrahepatic strictures developing before 90 days after transplantation are usually not attributable to recurrent disease. The early stage of recurrent disease usually first comes to clinical attention because of selective elevation of ALP and gamma-glutamyltranspeptidase. Recurrent disease usually progresses over a period of years. Symptoms of ascending cholangitis and biliary cirrhosis can develop, but up to 5 years after transplantation, patient and allograft survival are not adversely influenced.[212] Cholangiographic findings helpful in distinguishing recurrent disease from other causes of biliary strictures include mural irregularity, diverticulum-like outpouchings, and an overall appearance resembling PSC in the native liver.[246]

MICROSCOPIC PATHOLOGY

Microscopic pathology is identical to that described for native livers with sclerosing cholangitis and other causes of biliary tract obstruction or stricturing. Early stages are characterized by mild nonspecific acute and chronic pericholangitis, often accompanied by a mild type I ductular reaction involving a variable percentage of portal tracts (Fig. 39-26). As the disease progresses, a biliary gestalt develops that includes irregular fibrous expansion of most portal tracts accompanied by variable portal edema and a ductular reaction. In established cases, periductal lamellar edema (or fibrous cholangitis), intraepithelial or intraluminal neutrophils, pigmented macrophages in the portal connective tissue, and periportal deposition of golden pigment and copper and copper-associated protein signal chronically impaired bile flow. Focal small bile duct loss can also be seen. Superimposed acute cholangitis can lead to marked portal periductal and intraductal neutrophilia. As in other biliary diseases, the spatial relationship between the expanded portal tracts and the central veins remains intact until late.

Lobular findings early in recurrent disease include Kupffer cell hypertrophy, lobular neutrophil clusters, and mild nodular regenerative hyperplasia changes with thickening of the periportal plates and slight displacement of the central veins. Later stages are characterized by the development of biliary cirrhosis, cholestasis, intralobular foam cell clusters, marked deposition of copper and copper-associated protein, and Mallory's hyaline at the edge of the nodules.

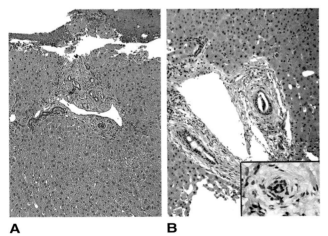

A   **B**

FIGURE 39–26. In our experience, recurrent PSC cannot be reliably distinguished from other causes of biliary tract obstruction or stricturing on the basis of a peripheral core needle biopsy alone. Clinicopathologic and radiologic correlation are needed to establish the diagnosis of recurrent PSC with certainty (see text). Typical early findings shown in this biopsy specimen include mild portal expansion because of a ductular reaction and mild portal fibrosis (**A**), periductal lamellar edema (**B**), and fibrous cholangitis (*inset*).

DIFFERENTIAL DIAGNOSIS

An important first step in recognizing recurrent PSC and distinguishing it from other causes of chronic allograft dysfunction is recognition of the early stages of a biliary gestalt, described earlier. This impression can be reinforced by preferential elevation of gamma-glutamyltranspeptidase and ALP. Clinicopathologic correlation is needed to determine whether the changes can be attributed to recurrent PSC or to other causes of biliary tract obstruction or stricturing. Harrison and colleagues[247] suggested that the presence of classic fibro-obliterative duct lesions might be restricted to liver allograft recipients who had PSC before transplantation. However, we have seen similar lesions in patients with ischemic cholangitis and in those with chronic reflux cholangiopathy. In our experience, a diagnosis of recurrent PSC is most reliable when based on a combination of clinical, histopathologic, and radiographic findings.

TOXIC AND METABOLIC DISEASES

Recurrent Alcoholic and Nonalcoholic Steatohepatitis

OVERVIEW AND PATHOPHYSIOLOGY

End-stage alcoholic liver disease is a leading indication for liver transplantation at many large centers (see Table 39-1), although nonalcoholic steatohepatitis (NASH) affects a minority of recipients before transplantation. Despite rigorous pretransplant screening programs that attempt to identify patients who are likely to relapse after transplantation, recurrent alcohol abuse can be a direct cause of allograft dysfunction, or it can indirectly contribute to allograft dysfunction because of rejection related to noncompliance with immunosuppression.[248,249]

The exact incidence of recurrent alcohol use/abuse after transplantation is difficult to determine with certainty, but reported values range from 15% to 50% by 5 years after transplantation.[250-252] Most patients who develop cirrhosis because of NASH maintain risk factors for recurrent disease after transplantation. Many patients also newly develop risk factors for NASH after transplantation because of the immunosuppressive drugs.

Although a minority of patients experience a rapid downhill course after transplantation because of recidivism and recurrent alcoholic steatohepatitis or NASH,[253-255] most alcoholics do not, and recurrent disease has a relatively small impact on long-term patient and allograft survival.[248,252,256] The discussion of the pathophysiologic mechanisms of liver injury associated with nonalcoholic or alcohol-related steatohepatitis is beyond the scope of this chapter.

CLINICAL FEATURES

Problems with alcohol recidivism are usually detected because of elevation of liver injury test results that are routinely obtained in liver transplant populations,[248] missed medical appointments,[257] inappropriate social behavior,[55] and noncompliance with immunosuppression.[248,249] We have found that a high gamma-glutamyltranspeptidase–to–ALP ratio identifies potential alcohol recurrence.[55,248] NASH is usually first detected on protocol or on indicated allograft biopsies.

MICROSCOPIC PATHOLOGY

The microscopic pathology of alcohol abuse in a liver allograft is virtually identical to that seen in the general population and will not be covered here in any significant detail. The most common finding in liver allograft recipients with documented relapse is mixed but predominantly microvesicular steatosis involving primarily the centrilobular hepatocytes (Fig. 39-27). The zonal pattern is usually distinctive.[55,248,252,253] In more severe cases, so-called foamy degeneration of centrilobular hepatocytes can occur,[55] and these changes can progress to fully developed alcoholic hepatitis with Mallory's hyaline, ballooning degeneration of hepatocytes, and associated lobular inflammation. Persistent or recurrent alcoholic hepatitis leads to perivenular and subsinusoidal fibrosis. Occasional patients with relapse show only increased iron deposition in the reticular endothelial cells and hepatocytes sometimes without steatosis.[55] Not infrequently, changes in coexistent viral hepatitis (especially HCV) or biliary obstruction will be identified. In cases with coexistent disorders, rapid progression of liver fibrosis and architectural distortion can be seen as a result of the combination of alcoholic liver disease and hepatitis.[248,253]

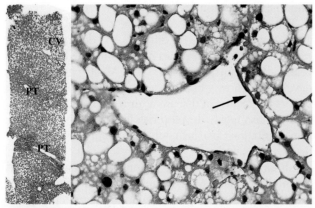

FIGURE 39–27. Recurrent alcohol abuse is most often characterized by centrilobular-predominant mixed macrovesicular and microvesicular steatosis (*arrow, right side of panel*). More severe recidivism can lead to frank alcoholic hepatitis with Malloy's hyaline, foamy degeneration of hepatocytes, and perivenular fibrosis, identical to the findings in native livers. PT, portal tract; CV, central vein.

DIFFERENTIAL DIAGNOSIS

The differential diagnosis for recurrent alcoholism and NASH includes all of the disorders known to cause steatohepatitis in the general population, and then some. Included are obesity, poorly controlled diabetes, insulin resistance, intestinal bypass surgery, malabsorption, hyperlipidemia, and toxicities of several drugs.[258] In the allograft recipient, we have also seen steatohepatitis develop in association with portal vein steal syndrome, whereby the nutrient-rich portal blood bypasses the liver and elicits centrilobular steatosis. Nausea-induced rapid weight loss because of adverse reaction to medications has caused similar changes in our experience. A thorough clinicopathologic correlation is needed to substantiate a suspicion of alcohol relapse or metabolic abnormalities leading to NASH. Awareness of the original disease(s) and a detailed clinical history, including current alcohol use, blood alcohol levels, and the ratio of gamma-glutamyltranspeptidase to ALP, can be used to distinguish between these possibilities.

Idiopathic Post-transplant Hepatitis

Idiopathic post-transplant hepatitis is a diagnosis coined by Hubscher[231] to describe a group of patients who have no clinical or serologic evidence of viral hepatitis infection, autoimmunity, or adverse drug reaction but show mononuclear portal inflammation with variable interface activity on liver allograft biopsy. By definition, bile duct damage and venous endothelial inflammation are not conspicuous. Hubscher also included in this category cases with inflammatory changes in zone 3, sometimes with foci of confluent necrosis.[231] However, we might characterize such patients as having acute rejection.[80,81] Regardless, the diagnosis of idiopathic post-transplant hepatitis is a valid one. Most programs that monitor long-term causes of allograft dysfunction and conduct protocol biopsies encounter cases with unexplained chronic hepatitis, as defined earlier.

Most cases of idiopathic post-transplant hepatitis are identified longer than 6 months after transplantation. Most patients so identified are asymptomatic, although minor elevation in liver injury test results is not uncommon. One subgroup of these patients represents recurrent autoimmune hepatitis.[231] Another subgroup likely represents acute rejection and will respond to increased immunosuppression.[80,81,231] Approximately 5% of patients followed for a minimum of 10 years develop progressive fibrosis resulting in established cirrhosis.[231]

The differential diagnosis for idiopathic post-transplant hepatitis is the same as that for hepatitis B or C virus infection or autoimmune hepatitis, all of which have been previously described.

LONG-TERM CHANGES NOT READILY EXPLAINED BY RECURRENT DISEASE

Several studies[55] examining the structural integrity of the allograft and causes of dysfunction in recipients who have survived for from 1 to 19 years after liver transplantation were remarkably similar, although the recipient pool, immunosuppressive management policies, and study designs differed. Most remarkable of all was the relatively low incidence of acute and chronic rejection, which varied from 4% to 38%. Recurrence of the original disease, especially viral hepatitis, was a leading cause of dysfunction, and obstructive cholangiopathy also was surprisingly common. Pappo and coworkers[55] drew particular attention to the point that awareness of the original disease, recent changes in immunosuppressive management policies, a review of previous biopsies, the clinical profile, and the result of any therapeutic or diagnostic tests or interventions should be incorporated with the biopsy findings to facilitate correct identification of the causes of late allograft dysfunction.

Several histopathologic changes in long-surviving allografts cannot be attributed to recurrence of a specific disease. These include mild lymphocytic portal inflammation without significant duct damage or venulitis or interface activity; portal arterial and arteriolar thickening and hyalinization; and a spectrum of nodular regenerative hyperplastic changes, characterized on one end by thickening of the plates and pseudorosette formation and on the other end by frank nodular regenerative hyperplasia with portal hypertension.[55]

Adverse Drug Reactions and Toxic Injury

As a general rule, the morphologic manifestations induced by a particular agent in an allograft are the same as those described for nonallografted livers and are not discussed here. The exception may be drugs that induce an immunologic response or altered self-antigens that may precipitate or drive the reaction. The use of azathioprine as an immunosuppressant in liver allograft recipients has been associated with the development of centrilobular necrosis and central vein and sinusoidal fibrosis in the short term[259]; nodular regenerative hyperplasia has been seen with long-term usage.[260]

◼ Bone Marrow Transplantation: The Hepatic Perspective

Liver disease, ranging from mild and reversible elevation of serum aminotransferases to fatal hepatic failure, occurs in up to 80% of patients following liver transplantation.[261] Patterns of damage fall into the broad categories of toxic injury due to medication, recurrence of the primary disease, and immunologically mediated injury (Table 39-13).[262] Liver toxicity generally is attributed to the cytoreductive therapy used during induction for bone marrow transplantation and may take the form of a generalized impairment of liver function in the immediate post-transplantation period, veno-occlusive disease in the weeks following transplantation, or nodular regenerative hyperplasia months later.[263] Systemic infection involving the liver or infection by hepatotrophic viruses is an ever-present threat. Emerging from this morass of potential problems is the clinical syndrome of graft-versus-host disease (GVHD), featuring to varying degrees skin rashes, diarrhea, and weight loss, as well as predominantly cholestatic liver dysfunction.[264]

TABLE 39-13. Differential Diagnosis of Hepatic Dysfunction in Bone Marrow Transplantation Patients

Timing	Common Causes	Less Common Causes
Pretransplant	Viral hepatitis Malignancy	Drug toxicity Veno-occlusive disease Opportunistic infections Biliary tract disease
Days 0–25	Veno-occlusive disease Drug toxicity	Graft-versus-host disease Opportunistic infections Nodular regenerative hyperplasia Total parenteral nutrition toxicity Cholestasis of sepsis
Days 25–100	Acute graft-versus-host disease Veno-occlusive disease Opportunistic infections Drug toxicity	Acalculous cholecystitis Total parenteral nutrition toxicity Nodular regenerative hyperplasia
Days >100	Chronic graft-versus-host disease Viral hepatitis (hepatotropic)	Opportunistic infections Drug toxicity Epstein-Barr virus–induced lymphoma

DRUG TOXICITY

Liver toxicity describes the general syndrome that occurs after cytoreductive therapy and before bone marrow transplantation; it affects up to one half of all such patients.[261] Sudden weight gain and the development of hepatomegaly and tenderness are the initial signs of liver toxicity; these typically occur on day 0 or 1, or 8 to 10 days after initiation of cytoreductive therapy. With severe liver toxicity, in which serum bilirubin values exceed 15 mg/dL and weight gains approach 10 to 15 kg, mortality exceeds 90%.[265] Although persistent severe liver dysfunction is a harbinger of a fatal outcome, liver disease per se is not usually the direct cause of death; most patients die from septicemia, pneumonia, bleeding, and/or multiorgan failure. Patients who undergo bone marrow transplantation for nonmalignant conditions are less likely to develop liver toxicity because the doses of cytoreductive therapy are generally lower than those given for malignancy.[266] Pretransplant hepatitis (caused by elevation of serum aminotransferases) is a risk factor for liver toxicity after transplantation.

Given the risks of percutaneous, transjugular, and operative liver biopsy in the immediate post-transplant period, liver tissue is not usually available for examination unless fungal liver disease is a serious consideration. With the passage of time after transplantation, liver biopsy may be increasingly necessary to sort out the diagnostic possibilities in these patients.

VENO-OCCLUSIVE DISEASE

Veno-occlusive disease (VOD) is a singular form of liver toxicity that occurs as a result of the cytotoxicity of induction therapy (discussed also in Chapters 36 and 38). This entity first achieved notoriety in 1954, when obliteration of hepatic vein radicals was described in Jamaican drinkers of bush tea[267]; this was subsequently attributed to the ingestion of plant pyrrolizidine alkaloids.[268] Currently, VOD is most often encountered in the bone marrow transplantation population. Apparent risk factors include transplantation for malignancy (as opposed to conditions such as aplastic anemia, which do not require such intense conditioning); patient age older than 15 years; and, in particular, abnormal pretransplant serum levels of liver enzymes.[266] The incidence of VOD after bone marrow transplantation has varied from 21% to 25% in allogeneic graft recipients to 5% in recipients of autologous bone marrow.[262] Criteria for a clinical diagnosis of VOD include the occurrence of at least two of the three following symptoms during the first month after bone marrow transplantation: jaundice, development of tender hepatomegaly and right upper quadrant pain, ascites, and/or unexplained weight gain. Serum aminotransferase levels may also rise substantially but do not differentiate between potential causes of liver injury.

Microscopic Pathology

VOD may exhibit acute, subacute, and chronic features, depending on when liver material is obtained. Unfortunately, because this disease is focal, diagnostic features may not be evident on liver biopsy.

In acute disease, striking centrilobular congestion is seen, with centrilobular hepatocellular necrosis and accumulation of hemosiderin-laden macrophages. The terminal hepatic venules exhibit intimal edema without obvious fibrin deposition or thrombosis. VOD presumably arises from toxic injury to the sinusoidal endothelium.[269] Sinusoidal endothelial cells are more susceptible than hepatocytes to toxic injury resulting from the conditions that cause this disease. The cells round up and slough off the sinusoidal wall, embolizing downstream and obstructing sinusoidal blood flow. This is accompanied by dissection of erythrocytes into the space of Disse and downstream accumulation of cellular debris in the terminal hepatic vein. Proliferation of perisinusoidal stellate cells and subendothelial fibroblasts in the terminal hepatic vein follows, with deposition of extracellular matrix. Obliterative changes in the terminal hepatic vein are secondary to sinusoidal damage, hence the recommended alternative name of *sinusoidal obstruction syndrome*.[269] Liver biopsy specimens are almost never obtained during the acute stage.

Over days to weeks (subacute), collagen deposition occurs in and around the affected terminal hepatic venule. This leads to progressive obliteration of the venule, which is easily identified with special stains for either collagen or reticulin (see Fig. 38-13).[261] Obvious centrilobular congestion without readily identifiable terminal hepatic veins on H&E stain should prompt the use of connective tissue stains to exclude VOD.

With persistence of the VOD lesion into weeks to months (chronic), dense perivenular fibrosis radiating out into the parenchyma develops. The scar tissue contains hemosiderin-laden macrophages, and terminal hepatic vein lumina cannot be identified. Notably, congestion is minimal at this stage. Severe destruction of lobular parenchyma may be seen and, rarely, evolution to cirrhosis.

Differential Diagnosis

Diagnoses to be excluded, if possible, include GVHD (see under Graft-Versus-Host Disease); other causes of venous outflow obstruction such as Budd-Chiari syndrome and congestive heart failure; drug reactions, including the toxic effects of hyperalimentation; and infections such as viral hepatitis, fungi, and sepsis. The pathology of Budd-Chiari syndrome features centrilobular congestion and potentially parenchymal destruction but without the occlusion of terminal hepatic veins seen in VOD. Drug reactions exhibit parenchymal damage with hepatocellular apoptosis, cholestasis, and parenchymal inflammation. Although severe VOD may cause similar histology in its more severe stages, identification of terminal hepatic vein lesions is readily made in such cases. The clinical features of post-transplantation drug toxicity and the specific condition of VOD are similar; no specific management is recommended for either condition other than supportive care. Hence, there is less need for a specific diagnosis of VOD to be made by liver biopsy in these unstable patients than there is need to exclude other potential causes of hepatic dysfunction.

GRAFT-VERSUS-HOST DISEASE

Bone marrow transplantation involves the grafting of donor bone marrow cells into an immunosuppressed patient whose marrow has been abrogated by cytoreductive therapy. This disease has been separated into acute and chronic forms, with acute GVHD usually developing within 7 to 50 days after marrow transplantation and chronic GVHD evolving 100 or more days after transplantation.

Three conditions are necessary for the development of GVHD against host tissues: (1) infusion of immunocompetent cells; (2) histocompatibility differences between donor and recipient; and (3) inability of the recipient to destroy donor cells. Thus, GVHD usually arises in the setting of allogeneic bone marrow transplantation, with the likelihood that GVHD will develop increasing with the degree of histoincompatibility between donor and recipient. However, this disease also has been reported following autologous and syngeneic bone marrow transplants and, rarely, following solid organ transplantation other than transplantation of the liver (owing to the resident lymphocytes transplanted with the solid organ).

Clinical symptoms of GVHD consist of skin changes, diarrhea, and weight loss, reflecting involvement of the epithelium of the skin, alimentary tract, liver, and other tissues (such as mucous membranes, bronchial epithelium, and muscles).

Although acute and chronic GVHD appear to be related, sufficient differences are noted both clinically and histologically to indicate that they represent distinct processes.[270] In general, acute GVHD is dominated by necrosis of the undifferentiated proliferating epithelial cells of the skin, gastrointestinal tract, and liver. Chronic GVHD tends to affect more differentiated cells and eventually leads to fibrosis.[271,272] In both cases, it is the disruption of the protective mucosal epithelial barriers that may have the most dire clinical consequences.

Acute Graft-Versus-Host Disease

CLINICAL FEATURES

In acute GVHD, liver dysfunction may develop within days but more commonly manifests within 2 to 4 weeks after transplantation as a gradual rise in serum levels of both direct and indirect bilirubin and in ALP and aminotransferases. Hepatomegaly may occur, usually without pain. The syndrome of acute GVHD includes the appearance of a red, maculopapular rash on the trunk, soles, palms, and ears, which may progress to total body involvement with bullae formation and desquamation in severe cases. Intestinal symptoms include crampy abdominal pain, anorexia, nausea, vomiting, watery or bloody diarrhea, and paralytic ileus. With progression to severe disease, coagulopathy and bleeding diathesis may develop, along with hepatic failure with ascites and encephalopathy. Full-scale destruction of the epithelium of the alimentary tract in the most advanced cases leads to fatal sepsis. The incidence of acute GVHD ranges from 10% to more than 80% of bone marrow recipients, depending on the degree of histoincompatibility, the number of T cells in the graft, the patient's age (incidence increases with age), and the immunoprophylactic regimen.

MICROSCOPIC PATHOLOGY

The nonspecific features of acute GVHD are a hepatitis-like picture with cholestatic and ballooning hepatocytes, frequent apoptotic hepatocytes, and lymphocytic infiltration of the lobule, resembling drug- or virally induced hepatitis. More useful for the diagnosis of acute GVHD is mild portal tract inflammation with infiltration of lymphocytes into the biliary epithelium, causing vacuolation and necrosis of interlobular bile ducts and their ultimate destruction (Fig. 39-28). Endothelial attack, manifest as endotheliitis and similar to that observed in allograft rejection of the transplanted liver, is an uncommon finding in hepatic GVHD.[273] It is important to note that the characteristic morphologic changes due to GVHD may not be obvious in the early stage of the diseases. For example, bile duct damage can be identified only rarely in the first 35 days after bone marrow transplantation in patients.[274] In addition, clinical improvements in grafting regimens, widespread use of prophylaxis, and improved clinical management have not only reduced the incidence and severity of hepatic GVHD but at the same time rendered the histologic diagnosis of GVHD more difficult.

The sine qua non of acute GVHD of the liver is direct attack of donor lymphocytes on bile duct epithelial cells.[262,270,274,275] The bile ducts most frequently involved are of small caliber.[276] Lymphocytic infiltrates are seen surrounding, invading, and disrupting the walls of interlobular bile ducts. Lymphocytic attachment is accompanied by necrosis of bile duct epithelial cells, evidenced as cytoplasmic vacuolization, nuclear pleomorphism or loss of nuclei, and sloughing of epithelial cells into the bile duct lumina. Residual duct epithelial cells may become attenuated to the point of appearing squamous around a portion of the duct circumference. The withered

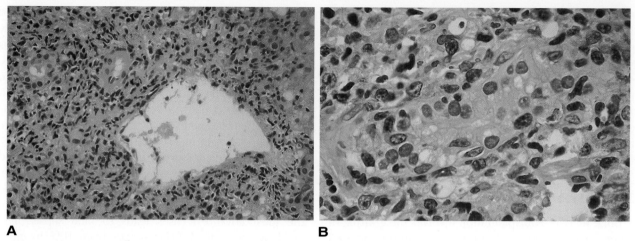

A   **B**

FIGURE 39–28. Acute graft-versus-host disease. **A,** Medium-power image of a portal tract, containing an activated mixed inflammatory infiltrate, portal vein endothelitis, and a difficult-to-discern interlobular bile duct *(left)*. **B,** High-power image of a bile duct, surrounded and infiltrated by mononuclear inflammatory cells.

appearance of the ductal epithelium is to be distinguished from the heaped-up, reactive duct epithelial cells commonly encountered in viral hepatitis, particularly with infection of hepatitis C virus.[277] Because patients with acute GVHD are usually pancytopenic, the degree of bile duct and portal tract inflammation may be minimal, despite obvious damage to the bile ducts.

DIFFERENTIAL DIAGNOSIS

Certainty of diagnosis of acute GVHD is based on the extent of clinical findings and the exclusion of drug toxicity and infection. Unlike in VOD, weight gain and right upper quadrant pain are rare. The sine qua non of histopathologic diagnosis of acute GVHD in liver biopsy is selective epithelial damage of the bile ducts. Rigorous adherence to the diagnostic criteria is essential if overdiagnosis of GVHD and potentially disastrous immunosuppression are to be avoided.

Chronic Graft-Versus-Host Disease

Chronic GVHD is conventionally defined as a syndrome arising after day 100. It may arise as an inexorable extension of acute GVHD after a disease-free interval or de novo, without previous episodes of acute GVHD. Because the syndrome of chronic GVHD may develop as early as 40 to 50 days after transplantation, the time frames for acute and chronic GVHD can overlap. However, unlike acute GVHD, chronic GVHD is a heterogeneous disease that involves a much wider range of organ systems, including skin, gastrointestinal tract, liver, minor salivary glands, lymph nodes, mouth, eyes, lungs, and musculoskeletal system, thereby constituting a blend of autoimmune syndromes.[270,278]

CLINICAL FEATURES

Limited chronic GVHD consists of localized skin disease and/or mild liver dysfunction. The designation of severe chronic GVHD is reserved for patients with generalized skin involvement or localized skin involvement or liver dysfunction with one of the following: severe chronic liver damage by histology; eye, mucosalivary, or mucosal involvement; or disease involvement of other target organs.[279] Chronic GVHD can significantly affect the quality of life of long-term survivors and can also lead to mortality.[280] The incidence of chronic GVHD in bone marrow transplant recipients ranges from 30% to 60%, with acute GVHD increasing the likelihood of chronic GVHD in allogeneic bone marrow recipients.

MICROSCOPIC PATHOLOGY

Chronic GVHD is characterized chiefly by portal infiltration by lymphocytes without or with plasma cells or eosinophils and damage to interlobular bile ducts.[263] These bile ducts are generally of small size[281] (<45 mm in diameter). Although bile duct epithelial degeneration resembling that of acute GVHD may be observed, more commonly damaged bile duct epithelial cells appear eosinophilic and coagulated when compared with healthy neighboring cells (Fig. 39-29). As with acute GVHD, lymphocytes are seen in close point contact with bile duct epithelial cells. Loss of bile ducts is a relatively late phenomenon in chronic GVHD, although it has been observed as early as 1 month after bone marrow transplantation.[282,283] Regardless of the time frame, bile duct loss may lead to a vanishing bile duct syndrome or to outright cirrhosis.[284-287] Unlike in acute GVHD, hepatocellular damage is minimal in most cases of chronic GVHD, except for the fact that the loss of interlobular bile ducts gives rise to progressive hepatocellular cholestasis. In the more advanced stages of

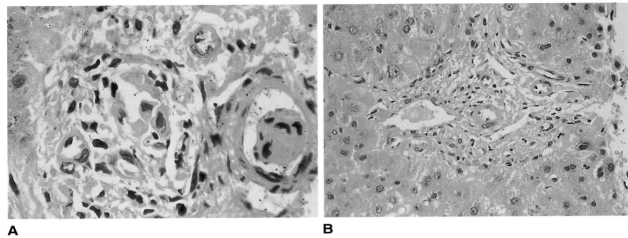

A   **B**

FIGURE 39–29. Chronic graft-versus-host disease. **A,** High-power image of a portal tract, showing one circular structure with degenerated cellular material within *(right)* and a second cluster of degenerating cells *(center);* these represent degenerating interlobular bile ducts. Only minimal mononuclear inflammation in seen. **B,** Medium-power image of a portal tract, showing portal vein and hepatic artery elements but no evident interlobular bile duct, which indicates bile duct paucity.

chronic GVHD, hepatocellular cholestasis may be so severe as to lead to actual degeneration of hepatocytes, particularly along the portal tract margins. Venous endotheliitis is not a prominent feature of chronic GVHD. Noncaseating granulomas in the portal tract are encountered only rarely.

An unusual form of hepatic GVHD has been recently reported. Patients with chronic GVHD of the liver exhibited significantly elevated transaminases and significant parenchymal damage on liver biopsy, resembling acute viral hepatitis.[288-291] However, the characteristic bile duct destructive features of chronic GVHD were still present. Therefore, liver biopsy plays an important role in the accurate diagnosis of long-term survivors of bone marrow transplantation with a hepatitic syndrome as well.

Features of acute and chronic GVHD vary greatly in severity from one portal tract to another, and the damage to interlobular and septal bile ducts is segmental.[270,274,292] This variability can make difficult the interpretation of liver biopsy specimens. The diagnosis of GVHD is reinforced by demonstration using molecular techniques that the inflammatory cells in the liver are of donor origin,[293] although this is not part of the usual diagnostic armamentarium. Nevertheless, the biopsy diagnosis of hepatic GVHD has a sensitivity of 66%, a specificity of 91%, and a predictive value of 86%[274]; little alteration has been seen in the histologic diagnosis of hepatic GVHD over the past 20 years except for recognition of the severe hepatitic form.

DIFFERENTIAL DIAGNOSIS

Chronic GVHD is the most common cause of cholestatic liver disease in long-term survivors of bone marrow transplantation and may occur in other transplantation settings. However, elevations of liver indices

(i.e., serum bilirubin, ALP, aminotransferases) are nonspecific in that they can result from cholestatic drug injury, sepsis, hepatic infection with hepatotropic viruses or opportunistic microorganisms, recurrence of malignancy, or development of post-transplant lymphoproliferative disorder (PTLD). These elevations can also occur with extrahepatic biliary disease (e.g., stones, infection). Moreover, because chronic GVHD and viral hepatitis may coexist in the same patient, elevations of serum aminotransferases cannot distinguish between these etiologies. Hence, as with acute GVHD, rigorous adherence to the criteria required for diagnosing chronic GVHD on liver biopsy examination is critical in the clinical management of these complex patients.

The Role of Liver Biopsy in Graft-Versus-Host Disease

Liver biopsy in the setting of acute GVHD is not usually required because skin or gastrointestinal tract biopsies are generally sufficient to establish the diagnosis, and the risk of liver biopsy may be unacceptably high. However, because abnormal serum liver enzyme values can persist after improvement in other organs following treatment, liver biopsy may be needed to exclude coexistent disease such as viral infection. In the acute situation (<100 days after transplantation), liver biopsy can play an important role in the exclusion of causes of hepatic damage, but diagnosis of hepatic GVHD itself may be difficult. Biopsy specimens from the earliest stages of hepatic GVHD (<35 days after transplantation) show hepatocyte apoptosis and portal tract inflammatory infiltrates that are nonspecific. In addition, hemodynamic instability of more severely affected patients often precludes the use of liver needle biopsy. Fine-needle aspiration biopsy, which carries a much lower risk of bleeding complications, has been used to evaluate the degree of inflammatory reaction in acute GVHD,[294] but the procedure provides only minimal histologic information. Transvenous biopsy via the jugular vein is an alternative, and in experienced hands it may provide satisfactory amounts of hepatic tissue. Laparoscopic biopsy also has been of value in obtaining liver tissue from these fragile patients.[295] For these various reasons, liver biopsies in the early weeks after transplantation are not widely used for the diagnosis of GVHD, but they may play a role if other conditions are suspected.

In contrast, liver needle biopsies are an important diagnostic test for establishing a diagnosis of chronic GVHD following bone marrow transplantation. Although there is considerable overlap among the histologic changes caused by different diseases, the bile duct injury of hepatic GVHD serves as an important discriminator. Specifically, the finding of extensive bile duct damage involving more than 50% of bile ducts with minimal inflammatory changes, or evidence of bile duct paucity (<80% of portal tracts containing bile ducts[92]) is highly suggestive of GVHD. Although it is observed infrequently, the presence of endotheliitis of portal or terminal veins is even more predictive of GVHD. Parenchymal inflammation and hepatocyte necrosis, cholestasis, and secondary bile ductular proliferation are not satisfactory discriminators between GVHD and other etiologies such as drug toxicity, hepatotropic and nonhepatotropic viral infection, and bile duct obstruction. Of great importance is the need to avoid misdiagnosis of the infiltrate of PTLD as GVHD because therapy for GVHD is diametrically opposite that for EBV-induced PTLD.

Avoidance of false-positive diagnosis requires both careful correlation with clinical data and appropriate caution in invoking GVHD as the solitary diagnosis. Given the common occurrence of bile duct damage or loss in hepatic GVHD, false-negative diagnoses are less of a problem than is false positivity. However, patchy distribution of the bile duct lesion may lead to its absence in needle biopsy specimens from patients with milder forms of the disease. Finally, pretransplant biopsies on all patients with evidence of preexisting liver disease help to reduce the likelihood of misinterpretation of previous liver disease as newly evolving GVHD.

NODULAR REGENERATIVE HYPERPLASIA

Nodular regenerative hyperplasia (NRH) is discussed elsewhere (see Chapter 38), but several comments here are in order. This condition has been reported following solid organ (primarily renal) and bone marrow transplantation.[296-298] NRH also has occurred one to two decades after liver transplantation.[297] The presumed common event is smoldering vascular injury that results from abnormal activation of the immune system, similar to the rheumatologic conditions normally associated with NRH.

The clinical syndrome of NRH, hepatomegaly, and ascites may be confused with the symptoms of VOD. In fact, in a retrospective study of 103 liver specimens (biopsy or autopsy) from bone marrow transplant patients at the University of Minnesota, VOD was found to be less frequent (9%) than NRH (23%), with overlapping time frames.[297] Thus, this entity must be considered in patients exhibiting liver dysfunction after bone marrow transplantation; diagnosis can be established only by histologic examination of liver tissue. Diagnosis can be extremely difficult because of the small samples of tissue obtained. The key to diagnosis, or at least implication, of NRH as the cause of hepatomegaly and portal hypertension is the performance of a reticulin stain to discern the nodularity of the liver parenchyma while excluding the presence of fibrous septa.[299] NRH is of minimal clinical impact, unlike other hepatic complications of bone marrow transplantation. Hence, consideration of this possibility in a patient with unexplained portal hypertension may provide immense assurance to an otherwise stable long-term survivor of transplantation.

INFECTION

Systemic infection with hepatic involvement is an ever-present possibility in the bone marrow transplant patient, and liver biopsy may assist in the assessment of fungal or opportunistic viral infection. Hepatotropic viral infection definitely occurs in patients with hematopoietic disorders and may recur in the post-transplant period. Finally, even in the absence of direct hepatic infection, endotoxemia or sepsis may induce severe hepatic cholestasis.[300] Hence, one must always be alert for the possibility of infection.

Liver Pathology After Transplantation of Other Solid Organs

Chronic viral hepatitis and opportunistic infections such as cytomegalovirus occur in recipients of other solid organs, such as kidney, heart, lung, small intestine, or pancreas. Fatal cases of adenovirus and herpesvirus infection have been reported.[301,302] The histologic severity of HBV-related liver disease increases following renal transplantation and may progress more rapidly to cirrhosis.[303,304] A high prevalence of HCV infection also occurs among recipients of renal transplants, usually as the result of long-term hemodialysis.[305] In some cases, HCV infection may be aggressive with rapid progression to cirrhosis.[306] A severe cholestatic form of HCV infection also has been described in cardiac and renal allograft recipients.[307,308] Severe fibrosing cholestatic hepatitis also may occur in patients serologically negative for HBV and HCV; this is attributed to the combined effects of cytomegalovirus infection and azathioprine toxicity.[309] As has been noted, GVHD affecting the liver may also occur following solid organ transplantation caused by the donor lymphoid tissue transplanted with such organs. Finally, the occurrence of nodular regenerative hyperplasia following solid organ transplantation has been mentioned.

Acknowledgments

The editorial assistance and patience of Mrs. Linda Askren are gratefully acknowledged. We are also grateful to our surgical colleagues and mentors who have provided the specimens and the environment in which to study them. Because of space limitations, we have had to limit the number of primary literature citations and have relied on review articles.

References

1. Starzl TE: History of liver and other splanchnic organ transplantation. In Busuttil R, Klintmalm G (eds): Transplantation of the Liver. Philadelphia, WB Saunders, 1996, pp 3-22.
2. Klintmalm G, Busuttil R: Transplantation of the Liver. Philadelphia, WB Saunders, 1996.
3. Demetris AJ, Ruppert K, Dvorchik I, et al: Real-time monitoring of acute liver-allograft rejection using the Banff schema. Transplantation 74:1290-1296, 2002.
4. Jain A, Reyes J, Kashyap R, et al: Long-term survival after liver transplantation in 4,000 consecutive patients at a single center. Ann Surg 232:490-500, 2000.
5. Sieders E, Peeters PM, TenVergert EM, et al: Graft loss after pediatric liver transplantation. Ann Surg 235:125-132, 2002.
6. Demetris AJ, Murase N, Nakamura K, et al: Immunopathology of antibodies as effectors of orthotopic liver allograft rejection. Semin Liver Dis 12:51-59, 1992.
7. Rabkin JM, de La Melena V, Orloff SL, et al: Late mortality after orthotopic liver transplantation. Am J Surg 181:475-479, 2001.
8. Jain A, Demetris AJ, Kashyap R, et al: Does tacrolimus offer virtual freedom from chronic rejection after primary liver transplantation? Risk and prognostic factors in 1,048 liver transplantations with a mean follow-up of 6 years. Liver Transpl Surg 7:623-630, 2001.
9. Demetris AJ, Jaffe R, Starzl TE: A review of adult and pediatric post-transplant liver pathology. Pathol Annu 22:347-386, 1987.
10. Todo S, Demetris AJ, Makowka L, et al: Primary nonfunction of hepatic allografts with preexisting fatty infiltration. Transplantation 47:903-905, 1989.
11. Kakizoe S, Yanaga K, Starzl TE, et al: Frozen section of liver biopsy for the evaluation of liver allografts. Transplant Proc 22:416-417, 1990.
12. Kakizoe S, Yanaga K, Starzl TE, et al: Evaluation of protocol before transplantation and after reperfusion biopsies from human orthotopic liver allografts: Considerations of preservation and early immunological injury. Hepatology 11:932-941, 1990.
13. Zamboni F, Franchello A, David E, et al: Effect of macrovescicular steatosis and other donor and recipient characteristics on the outcome of liver transplantation. Clin Transplant 15:53-57, 2001.
14. Briceno J, Solorzano G, Pera C: A proposal for scoring marginal liver grafts. Transpl Int 13(suppl 1):S249-S252, 2000.
15. Loinaz C, Gonzalez EM: Marginal donors in liver transplantation. Hepatogastroenterology 47:256-263, 2000.
16. Markin RS, Wisecarver JL, Radio SJ, et al: Frozen section evaluation of donor livers before transplantation. Transplantation 56:1403-1409, 1993.
17. Testa G, Goldstein RM, Netto G, et al: Long-term outcome of patients transplanted with livers from hepatitis C-positive donors. Transplantation 65:925-929, 1998.
18. Velidedeoglu E, Desai NM, Campos L, et al: The outcome of liver grafts procured from hepatitis C-positive donors. Transplantation 73:582-587, 2002.
19. Dodson SF, Issa S, Araya V, et al: Infectivity of hepatic allografts with antibodies to hepatitis B virus. Transplantation 64:1582-1584, 1997.
20. Ben-Haim M, Emre S, Fishbein TM, et al: Critical graft size in adult-to-adult living donor liver transplantation: Impact of the recipient's disease. Liver Transpl 7:948-953, 2001.
21. Nishizaki T, Ikegami T, Hiroshige S, et al: Small graft for living donor liver transplantation. Ann Surg 233:575-580, 2001.
22. Marcos A, Fisher RA, Ham JM, et al: Selection and outcome of living donors for adult to adult right lobe transplantation. Transplantation 69:2410-2415, 2000.
23. Shimada M, Shiotani S, Ninomiya M, et al: Characteristics of liver grafts in living-donor adult liver transplantation: Comparison between right- and left-lobe grafts. Arch Surg 137:1174-1179, 2002.
24. Trotter JF, Wachs M, Everson GT, et al: Adult-to-adult transplantation of the right hepatic lobe from a living donor. N Engl J Med 346:1074-1082, 2002.
25. Ryan CK, Johnson LA, Germin BI, et al: One hundred consecutive hepatic biopsies in the workup of living donors for right lobe liver transplantation. Liver Transpl 8:1114-1122, 2002.
26. Takada Y, Taniguchi H, Fukunaga K, et al: Prolonged hepatic warm ischemia in non-heart-beating donors: Protective effects of FK506 and a platelet activating factor antagonist in porcine liver transplantation. Surgery 123:692-698, 1998.
27. Kootstra G, Kievit J, Nederstigt A: Organ donors: Heartbeating and non-heartbeating. World J Surg 26:181-184, 2002.
28. Bilzer M, Gerbes AL: Preservation injury of the liver: Mechanisms and novel therapeutic strategies. J Hepatol 32:508-515, 2000.
29. Porte RJ, Ploeg RJ, Hansen B, et al: Long-term graft survival after liver transplantation in the UW era: Late effects of cold ischemia and primary dysfunction. European Multicentre Study Group. Transpl Int 11(suppl 1):S164-S167, 1998.
30. Lichtman SN, Lemasters JJ: Role of cytokines and cytokine-producing cells in reperfusion injury to the liver. Semin Liver Dis 19:171-187, 1999.
31. Kukan M, Haddad PS: Role of hepatocytes and bile duct cells in preservation-reperfusion injury of liver grafts. Liver Transpl 7:381-400, 2001.
32. Hayashi M, Tokunaga Y, Fujita T, et al: The effects of cold preservation on steatotic graft viability in rat liver transplantation. Transplantation 56:282-287, 1993.
33. Carrasco L, Sanchez-Bueno F, Sola J, et al: Effects of cold ischemia time on the graft after orthotopic liver transplantation. A bile cytological study. Transplantation 61:393-396, 1996.
34. McDonald V, Matalon TA, Patel SK, et al: Biliary strictures in hepatic transplantation. J Vasc Interv Radiol 2:533-538, 1991.
35. Starzl TE, Demetris AJ: Liver transplantation: A 31-year perspective. Part I. Curr Probl Surg 27:55-116, 1990.
36. Starzl TE, Demetris AJ: Liver transplantation: A 31-year perspective. Part II. Curr Probl Surg 27:123-178, 1990.
37. Starzl TE, Demetris AJ: Liver transplantation: A 31-year perspective. Part III. Curr Probl Surg 27:187-240, 1990.
38. D'Alessandro AM, Kalayoglu M, Sollinger HW, et al: The predictive value of donor liver biopsies on the development of primary nonfunction after orthotopic liver transplantation. Transplant Proc 23:1536-1537, 1991.
39. Russo PA, Yunis EJ: Subcapsular hepatic necrosis in orthotopic liver allografts. Hepatology 6:708-713, 1986.
40. Lerut JP, Gordon RD, Tzakis AG, et al: The hepatic artery in orthotopic liver transplantation. Helv Chir Acta 55:367-378, 1988.
41. Ludwig J, Batts KP, MacCarty RL: Ischemic cholangitis in hepatic allografts. Mayo Clin Proc 67:519-526, 1992.
42. Backman L, Gibbs J, Levy M, et al: Causes of late graft loss after liver transplantation. Transplantation 55:1078-1082, 1993.
43. Demetris A, Kakizoe S: Pathology of liver transplantation. In Williams JW (ed): Hepatic Transplantation. Philadelphia, WB Saunders, 1990, pp 61-111.
44. Lerut J, Tzakis AG, Bron K, et al: Complications of venous reconstruction in human orthotopic liver transplantation. Ann Surg 205:404-414, 1987.

45. Kuang AA, Renz JF, Ferrell LD, et al: Failure patterns of cryopreserved vein grafts in liver transplantation. Transplantation 62:742-747, 1996.

46. Sebagh M, Debette M, Samuel D, et al: "Silent" presentation of veno-occlusive disease after liver transplantation as part of the process of cellular rejection with endothelial predilection. Hepatology 30:1144-1150, 1999.

47. Sanchez-Urdazpal L, Gores GJ, Ward EM, et al: Diagnostic features and clinical outcome of ischemic-type biliary complications after liver transplantation. Hepatology 17:605-609, 1993.

48. Lerut J, Gordon RD, Iwatsuki S, et al: Biliary tract complications in human orthotopic liver transplantation. Transplantation 43:47-51, 1987.

49. Testa G, Malago M, Broelseh CE: Complications of biliary tract in liver transplantation. World J Surg 25:1296-1299, 2001.

50. Cheng YF, Chen YS, Huang TL, et al: Biliary complications in living related liver transplantation. Chang Gung Med J 24:174-180, 2001.

51. Amersi F, Farmer DG, Busuttil RW: Fifteen-year experience with adult and pediatric liver transplantation at the University of California, Los Angeles. Clin Transpl 255-261, 1998.

52. Hartshorne N, Hartman G, Markin RS, et al: Bile duct hemorrhage: A biopsy finding after cholangiography or biliary tree manipulation. Liver 12:137-139, 1992.

53. Nagral A, Ben-Ari Z, Dhillon AP, et al: Eosinophils in acute cellular rejection in liver allografts. Liver Transpl Surg 4:355-362, 1998.

54. Lunz JG 3rd, Contrucci S, Ruppert K, et al: Replicative senescence of biliary epithelial cells precedes bile duct loss in chronic liver allograft rejection: Increased expression of p21(WAF1/Cip1) as a disease marker and the influence of immunosuppressive drugs. Am J Pathol 158:1379-1390, 2001.

55. Pappo O, Ramos H, Starzl TE, et al: Structural integrity and identification of causes of liver allograft dysfunction occurring more than 5 years after transplantation. Am J Surg Pathol 19:192-206, 1995.

56. Neuberger J: Incidence, timing, and risk factors for acute and chronic rejection. Liver Transpl Surg 5:S30-S36, 1999.

57. Terminology of chronic hepatitis, hepatic allograft rejection, and nodular lesions of the liver: Summary of recommendations developed by an international working party, supported by the World Congresses of Gastroenterology, Los Angeles, 1994. Am J Gastroenterol 89:S177-S181, 1994.

58. Fischel RJ, Ascher NL, Payne WD, et al: Pediatric liver transplantation across ABO blood group barriers. Transplant Proc 21:2221-2222, 1989.

59. Demetris AJ: Ischemic cholangitis. Mayo Clin Proc 67:601-602, 1992.

60. Batts KP: Ischemic cholangitis. Mayo Clin Proc 73:380-385, 1998.

61. Takakura K, Kiuchi T, Kasahara M, et al: Clinical implications of flow cytometry crossmatch with T or B cells in living donor liver transplantation. Clin Transpl 15:309-316, 2001.

62. Furuya T, Murase N, Nakamura K, et al: Preformed lymphocytotoxic antibodies: The effects of class, titer and specificity on liver vs. heart allografts. Hepatology 16:1415-1422, 1992.

63. Demetris AJ, Markus BH: Immunopathology of liver transplantation. Crit Rev Immunol 9:67-92, 1989.

64. Valdivia LA, Fung JJ, Demetris AJ, et al: Donor species complement after liver xenotransplantation. The mechanism of protection from hyperacute rejection. Transplantation 57:918-922, 1994.

65. Manez R, Kelly RH, Kobayashi M, et al: Immunoglobulin G lymphocytotoxic antibodies in clinical liver transplantation: Studies toward further defining their significance. Hepatology 21:1345-1352, 1995.

66. Demetris AJ, Qian S, Sun H, et al: Early events in liver allograft rejection. Delineation of sites of simultaneous intragraft and recipient lymphoid tissue sensitization. Am J Pathol 138:609-618, 1991.

67. Demetris AJ, Murase N, Fujisaki S, et al: Hematolymphoid cell trafficking, microchimerism, and GVH reactions after liver, bone marrow, and heart transplantation. Transplant Proc 25:3337-3344, 1993.

68. Nawaz S, Fennell RH: Apoptosis of bile duct epithelial cells in hepatic allograft rejection. Histopathology 25:137-142, 1994.

69. Vierling JM: Immunology of acute and chronic hepatic allograft rejection. Liver Transpl Surg 5:S1-S20, 1999.

70. Demetris A, Adams D, Bellamy C, et al: Update of the International Banff Schema for Liver Allograft Rejection: Working recommendations for the histopathologic staging and reporting of chronic rejection. An international panel. Hepatology 31:792-799, 2000.

71. Terminology for hepatic allograft rejection. International Working Party. Hepatology 22:648-654, 1995.

72. Seiler CA, Renner EL, Czerniak A, et al: Early acute cellular rejection: No effect on late hepatic allograft function in man. Transpl Int 12:195-201, 1999.

73. Dousset B, Conti F, Cherruau B, et al: Is acute rejection deleterious to long-term liver allograft function? J Hepatol 29:660-668, 1998.

74. Hubscher S: Diagnosis and grading of liver allograft rejection: A European perspective. Transplant Proc 28:504-507, 1996.

75. Banff schema for grading liver allograft rejection: An international consensus document. Hepatology 25:658-663, 1997.

76. Demetris AJ, Lasky S, Van Thiel DH, et al: Induction of DR/IA antigens in human liver allografts. An immunocytochemical and clinicopathologic analysis of twenty failed grafts. Transplantation 40:504-509, 1985.

77. McCaughan GW, Davies JS, Waugh JA, et al: A quantitative analysis of T lymphocyte populations in human liver allografts undergoing rejection: The use of monoclonal antibodies and double immunolabeling. Hepatology 12:1305-1313, 1990.

78. Steinhoff G, Behrend M, Wonigeit K: Expression of adhesion molecules on lymphocytes/monocytes and hepatocytes in human liver grafts. Hum Immunol 28:123-127, 1990.

79. Demetris AJ, Belle SH, Hart J, et al: Intraobserver and interobserver variation in the histopathological assessment of liver allograft rejection. The Liver Transplantation Database (LTD) Investigators. Hepatology 14:751-755, 1991.

80. Demetris AJ, Fung JJ, Todo S, et al: Conversion of liver allograft recipients from cyclosporine to FK506 immunosuppressive therapy—a clinicopathologic study of 96 patients. Transplantation 53:1056-1062, 1992.

81. Tsamandas AC, Jain AB, Felekouras ES, et al: Central venulitis in the allograft liver: A clinicopathologic study. Transplantation 64:252-257, 1997.

82. Blakolmer K, Jain A, Ruppert K, et al: Chronic liver allograft rejection in a population treated primarily with tacrolimus as baseline immunosuppression: Long-term follow-up and evaluation of features for histopathological staging. Transplantation 69:2330-2336, 2000.

83. Evans PC, Smith S, Hirschfield G, et al: Recipient HLA-DR3, tumour necrosis factor-alpha promoter allele-2 (tumour necrosis factor-2) and cytomegalovirus infection are interrelated risk factors for chronic rejection of liver grafts. J Hepatol 34:711-715, 2001.

84. Blakolmer K, Seaberg EC, Batts K, et al: Analysis of the reversibility of chronic liver allograft rejection implications for a staging schema. Am J Surg Pathol 23:1328-1339, 1999.

85. Neil DA, Hubscher SG: Histologic and biochemical changes during the evolution of chronic rejection of liver allografts. Hepatology 35:639-651, 2002.

86. Nakazawa Y, Jonsson JR, Walker NI, et al: Fibrous obliterative lesions of veins contribute to progressive fibrosis in chronic liver allograft rejection. Hepatology 32:1240-1247, 2000.

87. Oguma S, Belle S, Starzl TE, et al: A histometric analysis of chronically rejected human liver allografts: Insights into the mechanisms of bile duct loss: Direct immunologic and ischemic factors. Hepatology 9:204-209, 1989.

88. Matsumoto Y, McCaughan GW, Painter DM, et al: Evidence that portal tract microvascular destruction precedes bile duct loss in human liver allograft rejection. Transplantation 56:69-75, 1993.

89. Demetris AJ, Seaberg EC, Batts KP, et al: Chronic liver allograft rejection: A National Institute of Diabetes and Digestive and Kidney Diseases interinstitutional study analyzing the reliability of current criteria and proposal of an expanded definition. National Institute of Diabetes and Digestive and Kidney Diseases Liver Transplantation Database. Am J Surg Pathol 22:28-39, 1998.

90. White RM, Zajko AB, Demetris AJ, et al: Liver transplant rejection: Angiographic findings in 35 patients. AJR Am J Roentgenol 148:1095-1098, 1987.

91. O'Keeffe C, Baird AW, Nolan N, et al: Mast cell hyperplasia in chronic rejection after liver transplantation. Liver Transpl 8:50-57, 2002.

92. Crawford AR, Lin XZ, Crawford JM: The normal adult human liver biopsy: A quantitative reference standard. Hepatology 28:323-331, 1998.

93. Freese DK, Snover DC, Sharp HL, et al: Chronic rejection after liver transplantation: A study of clinical, histopathological and immunological features. Hepatology 13:882-891, 1991.

94. Hubscher SG, Buckels JA, Elias E, et al: Vanishing bile-duct syndrome following liver transplantation—is it reversible? Transplantation 51:1004-1010, 1991.

95. Quaglia AF, Del Vecchio Blanco G, Greaves R, et al: Development of ductopaenic liver allograft rejection includes a "hepatitic" phase prior to duct loss. J Hepatol 33:773-780, 2000.

96. Wanless I: Physioanatomic considerations. In Schiff ER, Sorrell MF, Maddrey WC (eds): Diseases of the Liver, 8th ed. Philadelphia, Lippincott Williams & Wilkins, 1999, pp 3-37.

97. MacSween RN, Burt AD, Portmann B, et al (eds): Pathology of the Liver, 4th ed. Philadelphia, Churchill Livingstone, 2002, p 982.

98. Cavallari A, De Raffele E, Bellusci R, et al: De novo hepatitis B and C viral infection after liver transplantation. World J Surg 21:78-84, 1997.

99. Bai X, Rogers BB, Harkins PC, et al: Predictive value of quantitative PCR-based viral burden analysis for eight human herpesviruses in pediatric solid organ transplant patients. J Mol Diagn 2:191-201, 2000.

100. Badley AD, Seaberg EC, Porayko MK, et al: Prophylaxis of cytomegalovirus infection in liver transplantation: A randomized trial comparing a combination of ganciclovir and acyclovir to acyclovir. NIDDK Liver Transplantation Database. Transplantation 64:66-73, 1997.

101. Barkholt L, Lewensohn-Fuchs I, Ericzon BG, et al: High-dose acyclovir prophylaxis reduces cytomegalovirus disease in liver transplant patients. Transpl Infect Dis 1:89-97, 1999.

102. McGavin JK, Goa KL: Ganciclovir: An update of its use in the prevention of cytomegalovirus infection and disease in transplant recipients. Drugs 61:1153-1183, 2001.

103. Theise ND, Conn M, Thung SN: Localization of cytomegalovirus antigens in liver allografts over time. Hum Pathol 24:103-108, 1993.

104. Bronsther O, Makowka L, Jaffe R, et al: Occurrence of cytomegalovirus hepatitis in liver transplant patients. J Med Virol 24:423-434, 1988.

105. Snover DC, Hutton S, Balfour HH Jr, et al: Cytomegalovirus infection of the liver in transplant recipients. J Clin Gastroenterol 9:659-665, 1987.

106. Wiesner RH, Marin E, Porayko MK, et al: Advances in the diagnosis, treatment, and prevention of cytomegalovirus infections after liver transplantation. Gastroenterol Clin North Am 22:351-366, 1993.

107. Toorkey CB, Carrigan DR: Immunohistochemical detection of an immediate early antigen of human cytomegalovirus in normal tissues. J Infect Dis 160:741-751, 1989.

108. Oh CK, Pelletier SJ, Sawyer RG, et al: Uni- and multi-variate analysis of risk factors for early and late hepatic artery thrombosis after liver transplantation. Transplantation 71:767-772, 2001.

109. Pastacaldi S, Teixeira R, Montalto P, et al: Hepatic artery thrombosis after orthotopic liver transplantation: A review of nonsurgical causes. Liver Transpl 7:75-81, 2001.

110. Demetris A, Tsamandas A, Delaney CP, et al: Pathology of liver transplantation. In Busuttil R, Klintmalm G (eds): Transplantation of the Liver. Philadelphia, WB Saunders, 1996, pp 681-723.

111. O'Grady JG, Alexander GJ, Sutherland S, et al: Cytomegalovirus infection and donor/recipient HLA antigens: Interdependent co-factors in pathogenesis of vanishing bile-duct syndrome after liver transplantation. Lancet 2:302-305, 1988.

112. Lautenschlager I, Hockerstedt K, Jalanko H, et al: Persistent cytomegalovirus in liver allografts with chronic rejection. Hepatology 25:190-194, 1997.

113. Paya CV, Wiesner RH, Hermans PE, et al: Lack of association between cytomegalovirus infection, HLA matching and the vanishing bile duct syndrome after liver transplantation. Hepatology 16:66-70, 1992.

114. Kusne S, Schwartz M, Breinig MK, et al: Herpes simplex virus hepatitis after solid organ transplantation in adults. J Infect Dis 163:1001-1007, 1991.

115. Nalesnik MA: Clinicopathologic characteristics of post-transplant lymphoproliferative disorders. Recent Results Cancer Res 159:9-18, 2002.

116. Nalesnik MA: The diverse pathology of post-transplant lymphoproliferative disorders: The importance of a standardized approach. Transpl Infect Dis 3:88-96, 2001.

117. Randhawa PS, Markin RS, Starzl TE, et al: Epstein-Barr virus-associated syndromes in immunosuppressed liver transplant recipients. Clinical profile and recognition on routine allograft biopsy. Am J Surg Pathol 14:538-547, 1990.

118. Randhawa PS, Jaffe R, Demetris AJ, et al: The systemic distribution of Epstein-Barr virus genomes in fatal post-transplantation lymphoproliferative disorders. An in situ hybridization study. Am J Pathol 138:1027-1033, 1991.

119. Randhawa PS, Jaffe R, Demetris AJ, et al: Expression of Epstein-Barr virus-encoded small RNA (by the EBER-1 gene) in liver specimens from transplant recipients with post-transplantation lymphoproliferative disease. N Engl J Med 327:1710-1714, 1992.

120. Nalesnik MA, Jaffe R, Starzl TE, et al: The pathology of posttransplant lymphoproliferative disorders occurring in the setting of cyclosporine A-prednisone immunosuppression. Am J Pathol 133:173-192, 1988.

121. Bierman PJ, Vose JM, Langnas AN, et al: Hodgkin's disease following solid organ transplantation. Ann Oncol 7:265-270, 1996.

122. Sivaraman P, Lye WC: Epstein-Barr virus-associated T-cell lymphoma in solid organ transplant recipients. Biomed Pharmacother 55:366-368, 2001.

123. Lee ES, Locker J, Nalesnik M, et al: The association of Epstein-Barr virus with smooth-muscle tumors occurring after organ transplantation. N Engl J Med 332:19-25, 1995.

124. Newell KA, Alonso EM, Whitington PF, et al: Posttransplant lymphoproliferative disease in pediatric liver transplantation. Interplay between primary Epstein-Barr virus infection and immunosuppression. Transplantation 62:370-375, 1996.

125. Manez R, Breinig MC, Linden P, et al: Posttransplant lymphoproliferative disease in primary Epstein-Barr virus infection after liver transplantation: The role of cytomegalovirus disease. J Infect Dis 176:1462-1467, 1997.

126. Cockfield SM: Identifying the patient at risk for post-transplant lymphoproliferative disorder. Transpl Infect Dis 3:70-78, 2001.

127. Matsukura T, Yokoi A, Egawa H, et al: Significance of serial real-time PCR monitoring of EBV genome load in living donor liver transplantation. Clin Transpl 16:107-112, 2002.

128. Randhawa P, Blakolmer K, Kashyap R, et al: Allograft liver biopsy in patients with Epstein-Barr virus-associated posttransplant lymphoproliferative disease. Am J Surg Pathol 25:324-330, 2001.

129. Hubscher SG, Williams A, Davison SM, et al: Epstein-Barr virus in inflammatory diseases of the liver and liver allografts: An in situ hybridization study. Hepatology 20:899-907, 1994.

130. Muti G, Cantoni S, Oreste P, et al: Post-transplant lymphoproliferative disorders: Improved outcome after clinico-pathologically tailored treatment. Haematologica 87:67-77, 2002.

131. Koneru B, Jaffe R, Esquivel CO, et al: Adenoviral infections in pediatric liver transplant recipients. JAMA 258:489-492, 1987.

132. Michaels MG, Green M, Wald ER, et al: Adenovirus infection in pediatric liver transplant recipients. J Infect Dis 165:170-174, 1992.

133. Saad RS, Demetris AJ, Lee RG, et al: Adenovirus hepatitis in the adult allograft liver. Transplantation 64:1483-1485, 1997.

134. McGrath D, Falagas ME, Freeman R, et al: Adenovirus infection in adult orthotopic liver transplant recipients: Incidence and clinical significance. J Infect Dis 177:459-462, 1998.

135. Fagan E, Yousef G, Brahm J, et al: Persistence of hepatitis A virus in fulminant hepatitis and after liver transplantation. J Med Virol 30:131-136, 1990.

136. Uemoto S, Sugiyama K, Marusawa H, et al: Transmission of hepatitis B virus from hepatitis B core antibody-positive donors in living related liver transplants. Transplantation 65:494-499, 1998.

137. Demetris AJ, Jaffe R, Sheahan DG, et al: Recurrent hepatitis B in liver allograft recipients. Differentiation between viral hepatitis B and rejection. Am J Pathol 125:161-172, 1986.

138. Demetris AJ, Todo S, Van Thiel DH, et al: Evolution of hepatitis B virus liver disease after hepatic replacement. Practical and theoretical considerations. Am J Pathol 137:667-676, 1990.

139. O'Grady JG, Smith HM, Davies SE, et al: Hepatitis B virus reinfection after orthotopic liver transplantation. Serological and clinical implications. J Hepatol 14:104-111, 1992.

140. Davies SE, Portmann BC, O'Grady JG, et al: Hepatic histological findings after transplantation for chronic hepatitis B virus infection, including a unique pattern of fibrosing cholestatic hepatitis. Hepatology 13:150-157, 1991.

141. Mason AL, Wick M, White HM, et al: Increased hepatocyte expression of hepatitis B virus transcription in patients with features of fibrosing cholestatic hepatitis. Gastroenterology 105:237-244, 1993.

142. Todo S, Demetris AJ, Van Thiel D, et al: Orthotopic liver transplantation for patients with hepatitis B virus-related liver disease. Hepatology 13:619-626, 1991.

143. Samuel D, Bismuth H: Liver transplantation for hepatitis B. Gastroenterol Clin North Am 22:271-283, 1993.

144. Prieto M, Gomez MD, Berenguer M, et al: De novo hepatitis B after liver transplantation from hepatitis B core antibody-positive donors in an area with high prevalence of anti-HBc positivity in the donor population. Liver Transpl 7:51-58, 2001.

145. Vargas HE, Dodson FS, Rakela J: A concise update on the status of liver transplantation for hepatitis B virus: The challenges in 2002. Liver Transpl 8:2-9, 2002.

146. Marinos G, Rossol S, Carucci P, et al: Immunopathogenesis of hepatitis B virus recurrence after liver transplantation. Transplantation 69:559-568, 2000.

147. Porter KA: Pathology of liver transplantation. Transplant Rev 2:129-170, 1969.

148. Gouw AS, Houthoff HJ, Huitema S, et al: Expression of major histocompatibility complex antigens and replacement of donor cells by recipient ones in human liver grafts. Transplantation 43:291-296, 1987.

149. Phillips MJ, Cameron R, Flowers MA, et al: Post-transplant recurrent hepatitis B viral liver disease. Viral-burden, steatoviral, and fibroviral hepatitis B. Am J Pathol 140:1295-1308, 1992.

150. Benner KG, Lee RG, Keeffe EB, et al: Fibrosing cytolytic liver failure secondary to recurrent hepatitis B after liver transplantation. Gastroenterology 103:1307-1312, 1992.

151. Chisari FV, Filippi P, Buras J, et al: Structural and pathological effects of synthesis of hepatitis B virus large envelope polypeptide in transgenic mice. Proc Natl Acad Sci U S A 84:6909-6913, 1987.

152. Rizzetto M, Macagno S, Chiaberge E, et al: Liver transplantation in hepatitis delta virus disease. Lancet 2:469-471, 1987.

153. Reynes M, Zignego L, Samuel D, et al: Graft hepatitis delta virus reinfection after orthotopic liver transplantation in HDV cirrhosis. Transplant Proc 21:2424-2425, 1989.

154. David E, Rahier J, Pucci A, et al: Recurrence of hepatitis D (delta) in liver transplants: Histopathological aspects. Gastroenterology 104:1122-1128, 1993.

155. Bernard PH, Le Bail B, Rullier A, et al: Recurrence and accelerated progression of hepatitis C following liver transplantation. Semin Liver Dis 20:533-538, 2000.

156. Ascher NL, Lake JR, Emond J, et al: Liver transplantation for hepatitis C virus-related cirrhosis. Hepatology 20:24S-27S, 1994.

157. Randhawa PS, Demetris AJ: Hepatitis C virus infection in liver allografts. Pathol Annu 30:203-226, 1995.

158. Fishman JA, Rubin RH, Koziel MJ, et al: Hepatitis C virus and organ transplantation. Transplantation 62:147-154, 1996.

159. Lumbreras C, Colina F, Loinaz C, et al: Clinical, virological, and histologic evolution of hepatitis C virus infection in liver transplant recipients. Clin Infect Dis 26:48-55, 1998.

160. Feray C, Samuel D, Thiers V, et al: Reinfection of liver graft by hepatitis C virus after liver transplantation. J Clin Invest 89:1361-1365, 1992.

161. Weinstein JS, Poterucha JJ, Zein N, et al: Epidemiology and natural history of hepatitis C infections in liver transplant recipients. J Hepatol 22:154-159, 1995.

162. Arnold JC, Kraus T, Otto G, et al: Recurrent hepatitis C virus infection after liver transplantation. Transplant Proc 24:2646-2647, 1992.

163. Mateo R, Demetris A, Sico E, et al: Early detection of de novo hepatitis C infection in patients after liver transplantation by reverse transcriptase polymerase chain reaction. Surgery 114:442-448, 1993.

164. Marzano A, Smedile A, Abate M, et al: Hepatitis type C after orthotopic liver transplantation: Reinfection and disease recurrence. J Hepatol 21:961-965, 1994.

165. Sanchez-Fueyo A, Restrepo JC, Quinto L, et al: Impact of the recurrence of hepatitis C virus infection after liver transplantation on the long-term viability of the graft. Transplantation 73:56-63, 2002.

166. Belli LS, Silini E, Alberti A, et al: Hepatitis C virus genotypes, hepatitis, and hepatitis C virus recurrence after liver transplantation. Liver Transpl Surg 2:200-205, 1996.

167. Feray C, Gigou M, Samuel D, et al: Influence of the genotypes of hepatitis C virus on the severity of recurrent liver disease after liver transplantation. Gastroenterology 108:1088-1096, 1995.

168. Gayowski T, Singh N, Marino IR, et al: Hepatitis C virus genotypes in liver transplant recipients: Impact on posttransplant recurrence, infections, response to interferon-alpha therapy and outcome. Transplantation 64:422-426, 1997.

169. Gane EJ, Portmann BC, Naoumov NV, et al: Long-term outcome of hepatitis C infection after liver transplantation. N Engl J Med 334:815-820, 1996.

170. Chazouilleres O, Kim M, Combs C, et al: Quantitation of hepatitis C virus RNA in liver transplant recipients. Gastroenterology 106:994-999, 1994.

171. McCaughan GW, Zekry A: Pathogenesis of hepatitis C virus recurrence in the liver allograft. Liver Transpl 8:S7-S13, 2002.

172. Crespo J, Rivero M, Mayorga M, et al: Involvement of the fas system in hepatitis C virus recurrence after liver transplantation. Liver Transpl 6:562-569, 2000.

173. Berenguer M, Ferrell L, Watson J, et al: HCV-related fibrosis progression following liver transplantation: Iincrease in recent years. J Hepatol 32:673-684, 2000.

174. Charlton M, Seaberg E, Wiesner R, et al: Predictors of patient and graft survival following liver transplantation for hepatitis C. Hepatology 28:823-830, 1998.

175. Burroughs AK: Posttransplantation prevention and treatment of recurrent hepatitis C. Liver Transpl 6:S35-S40, 2000.

176. Sheiner PA, Schwartz ME, Mor E, et al: Severe or multiple rejection episodes are associated with early recurrence of hepatitis C after orthotopic liver transplantation. Hepatology 21:30-34, 1995.

177. Berenguer M, Prieto M, Cordoba J, et al: Early development of chronic active hepatitis in recurrent hepatitis C virus infection after liver transplantation: Association with treatment of rejection. J Hepatol 28:756-763, 1998.

178. Ahmed A, Keeffe EB: Hepatitis C virus and liver transplantation. Clin Liver Dis 5:1073-1090, 2001.

179. Boker KH, Dalley G, Bahr MJ, et al: Long-term outcome of hepatitis C virus infection after liver transplantation. Hepatology 25:203-210, 1997.

180. Singh N, Gayowski T, Ndimbie OK, et al: Recurrent hepatitis C virus hepatitis in liver transplant recipients receiving tacrolimus: Association with rejection and increased immunosuppression after transplantation. Surgery 119:452-456, 1996.

181. Zervos XA, Weppler D, Fragulidis GP, et al: Comparison of tacrolimus with microemulsion cyclosporine as primary immunosuppression in hepatitis C patients after liver transplantation. Transplantation 65:1044-1046, 1998.

182. Johnson MW, Washburn WK, Freeman RB, et al: Hepatitis C viral infection in liver transplantation. Arch Surg 131:284-291, 1996.

183. Mueller AR, Platz KP, Blumhardt G, et al: The optimal immunosuppressant after liver transplantation according to diagnosis: Cyclosporine A or FK506? Clin Transplant 9:176-184, 1995.

184. Roth D, Zucker K, Cirocco R, et al: A prospective study of hepatitis C virus infection in renal allograft recipients. Transplantation 61:886-889, 1996.

185. Zhou S, Terrault NA, Ferrell L, et al: Severity of liver disease in liver transplantation recipients with hepatitis C virus infection: Relationship to genotype and level of viremia. Hepatology 24:1041-1046, 1996.

186. Caccamo L, Gridelli B, Sampietro M, et al: Hepatitis C virus genotypes and reinfection of the graft during long-term follow-up in 35 liver transplant recipients. Transpl Int 9:S204-S209, 1996.

187. Gordon FD, Poterucha JJ, Germer J, et al: Relationship between hepatitis C genotype and severity of recurrent hepatitis C after liver transplantation. Transplantation 63:1419-1423, 1997.

188. Gigou M, Roque-Afonso AM, Falissard B, et al: Genetic clustering of hepatitis C virus strains and severity of recurrent hepatitis after liver transplantation. J Virol 75:11292-11297, 2001.

189. Laskus T, Wang LF, Rakela J, et al: Dynamic behavior of hepatitis C virus in chronically infected patients receiving liver graft from infected donors. Virology 220:171-176, 1996.

190. Gane EJ, Naoumov NV, Qian KP, et al: A longitudinal analysis of hepatitis C virus replication following liver transplantation. Gastroenterology 110:167-177, 1996.

191. Di Martino V, Saurini F, Samuel D, et al: Long-term longitudinal study of intrahepatic hepatitis C virus replication after liver transplantation. Hepatology 26:1343-1350, 1997.

192. Zekry A, Bishop GA, Bowen DG, et al: Intrahepatic cytokine profiles associated with posttransplantation hepatitis C virus-related liver injury. Liver Transpl 8:292-301, 2002.

193. Wright TL, Donegan E, Hsu HH, et al: Recurrent and acquired hepatitis C viral infection in liver transplant recipients. Gastroenterology 103:317-322, 1992.

194. Thung SN, Shim KS, Shieh YS, et al: Hepatitis C in liver allografts. Arch Pathol Lab Med 117:145-149, 1993.

195. Wright TL: Liver transplantation for chronic hepatitis C viral infection. Gastroenterol Clin North Am 22:231-242, 1993.

196. Paik SW, Tan HP, Klein AS, et al: Outcome of orthotopic liver transplantation in patients with hepatitis C. Dig Dis Sci 47:450-455, 2002.

197. Berenguer M: Natural history of recurrent hepatitis C. Liver Transpl 8:S14-S18, 2002.

198. Ferrell LD, Wright TL, Roberts J, et al: Hepatitis C viral infection in liver transplant recipients. Hepatology 16:865-876, 1992.

199. Greenson JK, Svoboda-Newman SM, Merion RM, et al: Histologic progression of recurrent hepatitis C in liver transplant allografts. Am J Surg Pathol 20:731-738, 1996.

200. Tsamandas AC, Furukawa H, Abu-Elmagd K, et al: Liver allograft pathology in liver/small bowel or multivisceral recipients. Mod Pathol 9:767-773, 1996.

201. Asanza CG, Garcia-Monzon C, Clemente G, et al: Immunohistochemical evidence of immunopathogenetic mechanisms in chronic hepatitis C recurrence after liver transplantation. Hepatology 26:755-763, 1997.

202. Rosen HR, Gretch DR, Oehlke M, et al: Timing and severity of initial hepatitis C recurrence as predictors of long-term liver allograft injury. Transplantation 65:1178-1182, 1998.

203. Rosen HR, Martin P: Hepatitis C infection in patients undergoing liver retransplantation. Transplantation 66:1612-1616, 1998.

204. Saxena R, Crawford JM, Navarro VJ, et al: Utilization of acidophil bodies in the diagnosis of recurrent hepatitis C infection after orthotopic liver transplantation. Mod Pathol 15:897-903, 2002.

205. Demetris AJ: Immunopathology of the human biliary tree. In Sirica AE, Longnecker DS (eds): Biliary and Pancreatic Ductal Epithelia. Pathobiology and Pathophysiology. New York, Marcel Dekker, 1997, pp 127-180.

206. Wiesner RH, Demetris AJ, Belle SH, et al: Acute hepatic allograft rejection: Incidence, risk factors, and impact on outcome. Hepatology 28:638-645, 1998.

207. Charco R, Vargas V, Allende H, et al: Is hepatitis C virus recurrence a risk factor for chronic liver allograft rejection? Transpl Int 9:S195-S197, 1996.

208. Hoffmann RM, Gunther C, Diepolder HM, et al: Hepatitis C virus infection as a possible risk factor for ductopenic rejection (vanishing bile duct syndrome) after liver transplantation. Transpl Int 8:353-359, 1995.

209. Ontanon J, Muro M, Garcia-Alonso AM, et al: Effect of partial HLA class I match on acute rejection in viral pre-infected human liver allograft recipients. Transplantation 65:1047-1053, 1998.

210. Jain A, Demetris AJ, Manez R, et al: Incidence and severity of acute allograft rejection in liver transplant recipients treated with alfa interferon. Liver Transpl Surg 4:197-203, 1998.

211. Dousset B, Conti F, Houssin D, et al: Acute vanishing bile duct syndrome after interferon therapy for recurrent HCV infection in liver-transplant recipients. N Engl J Med 330:1160-1161, 1994.

212. Faust TW: Recurrent primary biliary cirrhosis, primary sclerosing cholangitis, and autoimmune hepatitis after transplantation. Liver Transpl 7:S99-S108, 2001.

213. Iwatsuki S, Gordon RD, Shaw BW Jr, et al: Role of liver transplantation in cancer therapy. Ann Surg 202:401-407, 1985.

214. Iwatsuki S, Starzl TE, Sheahan DG, et al: Hepatic resection versus transplantation for hepatocellular carcinoma. Ann Surg 214:221-228, 1991.

215. Iwatsuki S, Starzl TE: Role of liver transplantation in the treatment of hepatocellular carcinoma. Semin Surg Oncol 9:337-340, 1993.

216. Jaffe R: Liver transplant pathology in pediatric metabolic disorders. Pediatr Dev Pathol 1:102-117, 1998.

217. Hunt J, Gordon FD, Jenkins RL, et al: Sarcoidosis with selective involvement of a second liver allograft: Report of a case and review of the literature. Mod Pathol 12:325-328, 1999.

218. Pappo O, Yunis E, Jordan JA, et al: Recurrent and de novo giant cell hepatitis after orthotopic liver transplantation. Am J Surg Pathol 18:804-813, 1994.

219. Van de Water J, Gerson LB, Ferrell LD, et al: Immunohistochemical evidence of disease recurrence after liver transplantation for primary biliary cirrhosis. Hepatology 24:1079-1084, 1996.

220. Neuberger J, Wallace L, Joplin R, et al: Hepatic distribution of E2 component of pyruvate dehydrogenase complex after transplantation. Hepatology 22:798-801, 1995.

221. Dmitrewski J, Hubscher SG, Mayer AD, et al: Recurrence of primary biliary cirrhosis in the liver allograft: The effect of immuno-suppression. J Hepatol 24:253-257, 1996.

222. Liermann Garcia RF, Evangelista Garcia C, McMaster P, et al: Transplantation for primary biliary cirrhosis: Retrospective analysis of 400 patients in a single center. Hepatology 33:22-27, 2001.

223. Hashimoto E, Shimada M, Noguchi S, et al: Disease recurrence after living liver transplantation for primary biliary cirrhosis: A clinical and histological follow-up study. Liver Transpl 7:588-595, 2001.

224. Mazariegos GV, Reyes J, Marino IR, et al: Weaning of immuno-suppression in liver transplant recipients. Transplantation 63:243-249, 1997.

225. Ramos HC, Reyes J, Abu-Elmagd K, et al: Weaning of immuno-suppression in long-term liver transplant recipients. Transplantation 59:212-217, 1995.

226. Demetris AJ, Sever C, Kakizoe S, et al: S100 protein positive dendritic cells in primary biliary cirrhosis and other chronic inflammatory liver diseases. Relevance to pathogenesis? Am J Pathol 134:741-747, 1989.

227. Farges O, Bismuth H, Sebagh M, et al: Granulomatous destruction of bile ducts after liver transplantation: Primary biliary cirrhosis recurrence or hepatitis C virus infection? Hepatology 21:1765-1767, 1995.

228. Hubscher SG, Elias E, Buckels JA, et al: Primary biliary cirrhosis. Histological evidence of disease recurrence after liver transplantation. J Hepatol 18:173-184, 1993.

229. Jones DE, James OF, Portmann B, et al: Development of auto-immune hepatitis following liver transplantation for primary biliary cirrhosis. Hepatology 30:53-57, 1999.

230. Sebagh M, Farges O, Dubel L, et al: Histological features predictive of recurrence of primary biliary cirrhosis after liver transplantation. Transplantation 65:1328-1333, 1998.

231. Hubscher SG: Recurrent autoimmune hepatitis after liver trans-plantation: Diagnostic criteria, risk factors, and outcome. Liver Transpl 7:285-291, 2001.

232. Alvarez F, Berg PA, Bianchi FB, et al: International Autoimmune Hepatitis Group Report: Review of criteria for diagnosis of autoimmune hepatitis. J Hepatol 31:929-938, 1999.

233. Demetris AJ, Murase N, Delaney CP: Overlap between allo- and autoimmunity in the rat and human evidence for important contribtuions for dendritic and regulatory cells. Graft 6:21-32, 2003.

234. Ratziu V, Samuel D, Sebagh M, et al: Long-term follow-up after liver transplantation for autoimmune hepatitis: Evidence of recurrence of primary disease. J Hepatol 30:131-141, 1999.

235. Reich DJ, Fiel I, Guarrera JV, et al: Liver transplantation for autoimmune hepatitis. Hepatology 32:693-700, 2000.

236. Czaja AJ: Autoimmune hepatitis after liver transplantation and other lessons of self-intolerance. Liver Transpl 8:505-513, 2002.

237. Duclos-Vallee JC, Johanet C, Bach JF, et al: Autoantibodies associated with acute rejection after liver transplantation for type-2 autoimmune hepatitis. J Hepatol 33:163-166, 2000.

238. Graze PR, Gale RP: Chronic graft versus host disease: A syndrome of disordered immunity. Am J Med 66:611-620, 1979.

239. Goss JA, Shackleton CR, Farmer DG, et al: Orthotopic liver trans-plantation for primary sclerosing cholangitis. A 12-year single center experience. Ann Surg 225:472-481, 1997.

240. Graziadei IW, Wiesner RH, Marotta PJ, et al: Long-term results of patients undergoing liver transplantation for primary sclerosing cholangitis. Hepatology 30:1121-1127, 1999.

241. Gow PJ, Chapman RW: Liver transplantation for primary sclerosing cholangitis. Liver 20:97-103, 2000.

242. Dvorchik I, Subotin M, Demetris AJ, et al: Effect of liver trans-plantation on inflammatory bowel disease in patients with primary sclerosing cholangitis. Hepatology 35:380-384, 2002.

243. Narumi S, Roberts JP, Emond JC, et al: Liver transplantation for sclerosing cholangitis. Hepatology 22:451-457, 1995.

244. Jeyarajah DR, Netto GJ, Lee SP, et al: Recurrent primary sclerosing cholangitis after orthotopic liver transplantation: Is chronic rejection part of the disease process? Transplantation 66:1300-1306, 1998.

245. Graziadei IW, Wiesner RH, Batts KP, et al: Recurrence of primary sclerosing cholangitis following liver transplantation. Hepatology 29:1050-1056, 1999.

246. Sheng R, Campbell WL, Zajko AB, et al: Cholangiographic features of biliary strictures after liver transplantation for primary sclerosing cholangitis: Evidence of recurrent disease. AJR Am J Roentgenol 166:1109-1113, 1996.

247. Harrison RF, Davies MH, Neuberger JM, et al: Fibrous and obliterative cholangitis in liver allografts: Evidence of recurrent primary sclerosing cholangitis? Hepatology 20:356-361, 1994.

248. Bellamy CO, DiMartini AM, Ruppert K, et al: Liver transplantation for alcoholic cirrhosis: Long term follow-up and impact of disease recurrence. Transplantation 72:619-626, 2001.

249. Lucey MR, Carr K, Beresford TP, et al: Alcohol use after liver transplantation in alcoholics: A clinical cohort follow-up study. Hepatology 25:1223-1227, 1997.

250. Osorio RW, Ascher NL, Avery M, et al: Predicting recidivism after orthotopic liver transplantation for alcoholic liver disease. Hepatology 20:105-110, 1994.

251. Berlakovich GA, Steininger R, Herbst F, et al: Efficacy of liver transplantation for alcoholic cirrhosis with respect to recidivism and compliance. Transplantation 58:560-565, 1994.

252. Burra P, Mioni D, Cecchetto A, et al: Histological features after liver transplantation in alcoholic cirrhotics. J Hepatol 34:716-722, 2001.

253. Conjeevaram HS, Hart J, Lissoos TW, et al: Rapidly progressive liver injury and fatal alcoholic hepatitis occurring after liver transplantation in alcoholic patients. Transplantation 67:1562-1568, 1999.

254. Molloy RM, Komorowski R, Varma RR: Recurrent nonalcoholic steatohepatitis and cirrhosis after liver transplantation. Liver Transpl Surg 3:177-178, 1997.

255. Tang H, Boulton R, Gunson B, et al: Patterns of alcohol consumption after liver transplantation. Gut 43:140-145, 1998.

256. Yusoff IF, House AK, De Boer WB, et al: Disease recurrence after liver transplantation in Western Australia. J Gastroenterol Hepatol 17:203-207, 2002.

257. Abosh D, Rosser B, Kaita K, et al: Outcomes following liver transplantation for patients with alcohol- versus nonalcohol-induced liver disease. Can J Gastroenterol 14:851-855, 2000.

258. Lee R: Acute hepatitis. In Diagnostic Liver Pathology. St. Louis, Mosby-Year Book, 1994, pp 23-66.

259. Sterneck M, Wiesner R, Ascher N, et al: Azathioprine hepatotoxicity after liver transplantation. Hepatology 14:806-810, 1991.

260. Gane E, Portmann B, Saxena R, et al: Nodular regenerative hyperplasia of the liver graft after liver transplantation. Hepatology 20:88-94, 1994.

261. McDonald GB, Shulman HM, Wolford JL, et al: Liver disease after human marrow transplantation. Semin Liver Dis 7:210-229, 1987.

262. Crawford J, Ferrell L: The Liver in transplantation. In Rustgi V, Van Thiel D (eds): The Liver in Systemic Diseases. New York, Raven Press, 1993, pp 337-364.

263. Shulman HM, Fisher LB, Schoch HG, et al: Veno-occlusive disease of the liver after marrow transplantation: Histological correlates of clinical signs and symptoms. Hepatology 19:1171-1181, 1994.

264. Crawford J: Graft versus host disease of the liver. In Ferrara J, Deeg J, Burakoff S (eds): Graft vs. Host Disease, 2nd ed. New York, Marcel Dekker, 1996, pp 315-336.

265. McDonald GB, Sharma P, Matthews DE, et al: The clinical course of 53 patients with veno-occlusive disease of the liver after marrow transplantation. Transplantation 39:603-608, 1985.

266. McDonald GB, Sharma P, Matthews DE, et al: Veno-occlusive disease of the liver after bone marrow transplantation: Diagnosis, incidence, and predisposing factors. Hepatology 4:116-122, 1984.

267. Bras G, Jelliffe D, Stuart K: Veno-occlusive disease of liver with nonportal type of cirrhosis, occurring in Jamaica. Arch Pathol Lab Med 57:285-300, 1954.

268. McLean EK: The toxic actions of pyrrolizidine (senecio) alkaloids. Pharmacol Rev 22:429-483, 1970.

269. Bearman SI: Avoiding hepatic veno-occlusive disease: What do we know and where are we going? Bone Marrow Transplant 27:1113-1120, 2001.

270. Snover DC: Acute and chronic graft versus host disease: Histopathological evidence for two distinct pathogenetic mechanisms. Hum Pathol 15:202-205, 1984.

271. Snover D: Acute and chronic graft-versus host disease. In Burakoff S, Geeg H, Ferrar J et al (eds): Graft-Versus-Host Disease: Immunology, Pathophysiology, and Treatment. New York, Marcel Dekker, 1990, pp 337-353.

272. Shulman HM: Pathology of chronic graft-vs.-host disease. In Burakoff S, Geeg H, Ferrar J (eds): Graft-Versus-Host Disease: Immunology, Pathophysiology, and Treatment. New York, Marcel Dekker, 1990, pp 587-614.

273. Snover DC, Weisdorf SA, Ramsay NK, et al: Hepatic graft versus host disease: A study of the predictive value of liver biopsy in diagnosis. Hepatology 4:123-130, 1984.

274. Shulman HM, Sharma P, Amos D, et al: A coded histologic study of hepatic graft-versus-host disease after human bone marrow transplantation. Hepatology 8:463-470, 1988.

275. Shulman HM, Gooley T, Dudley MD, et al: Utility of transvenous liver biopsies and wedged hepatic venous pressure measurements in sixty marrow transplant recipients. Transplantation 59:1015-1022, 1995.

276. Tanaka M, Umihara J, Shimmoto K, et al: The pathogenesis of graft-versus-host reaction in the intrahepatic bile duct. An immunohistochemical study. Acta Pathol Jpn 39:648-655, 1989.

277. Bach N, Thung SN, Schaffner F: The histological features of chronic hepatitis C and autoimmune chronic hepatitis: A comparative analysis. Hepatology 15:572-577, 1992.

278. Teshima T, Ferrara JL: Understanding the alloresponse: New approaches to graft-versus-host disease prevention. Semin Hematol 39:15-22, 2002.

279. Shulman HM, Sullivan KM, Weiden PL, et al: Chronic graft-versus-host syndrome in man. A long-term clinicopathologic study of 20 Seattle patients. Am J Med 69:204-217, 1980.

280. Socie G, Stone JV, Wingard JR, et al: Long-term survival and late deaths after allogeneic bone marrow transplantation. Late Effects Working Committee of the International Bone Marrow Transplant Registry. N Engl J Med 341:14-21, 1999.

281. Vierling JM: Immune disorders of the liver and bile duct. Gastroenterol Clin North Am 21:427-449, 1992.

282. Andersen CB, Horn T, Sehested M, et al: Graft-versus-host disease: Liver morphology and pheno/genotypes of inflammatory cells and target cells in sex-mismatched allogeneic bone marrow transplant patients. Transplant Proc 25:1250-1254, 1993.

283. Yeh KH, Hsieh HC, Tang JL, et al: Severe isolated acute hepatic graft-versus-host disease with vanishing bile duct syndrome. Bone Marrow Transplant 14:319-321, 1994.

284. Yau JC, Zander AR, Srigley JR, et al: Chronic graft-versus-host disease complicated by micronodular cirrhosis and esophageal varices. Transplantation 41:129-130, 1986.

285. Knapp AB, Crawford JM, Rappeport JM, et al: Cirrhosis as a consequence of graft-versus-host disease. Gastroenterology 92:513-519, 1987.

286. Stechschulte DJ Jr, Fishback JL, Emami A, et al: Secondary biliary cirrhosis as a consequence of graft-versus-host disease. Gastroenterology 98:223-225, 1990.

287. Urban CH, Deutschmann A, Kerbl R, et al: Organ tolerance following cadaveric liver transplantation for chronic graft-versus-host disease after allogeneic bone marrow transplantation. Bone Marrow Transplant 30:535-537, 2002.

288. Strasser SI, Shulman HM, Flowers ME, et al: Chronic graft-versus-host disease of the liver: Presentation as an acute hepatitis. Hepatology 32:1265-1271, 2000.

289. Fujii N, Takenaka K, Shinagawa K, et al: Hepatic graft-versus-host disease presenting as an acute hepatitis after allogeneic peripheral blood stem cell transplantation. Bone Marrow Transplant 27:1007-1010, 2001.

290. Akpek G, Boitnott JK, Lee LA, et al: Hepatitic variant of graft-versus-host disease after donor lymphocyte infusion. Blood 100:3903-3907, 2002.

291. Malik AH, Collins RH Jr, Saboorian MH, et al: Chronic graft-versus-host disease after hematopoietic cell transplantation presenting as an acute hepatitis. Am J Gastroenterol 96:588-590, 2001.

292. Williams FH, Thiele DL: The role of major histocompatibility complex and non-major histocompatibility complex encoded antigens in generation of bile duct lesions during hepatic graft-vs.-host

responses mediated by helper or cytotoxic T cells. Hepatology 19:980-988, 1994.

293. Au WY, Ma SK, Kwong YL, et al: Graft-versus-host disease after liver transplantation: Documentation by fluorescent in situ hybridisation and human leucocyte antigen typing. Clin Transplant 14:174-177, 2000.

294. Picardi M, De Rosa G, Muretto P, et al: Ultrasound-guided fine needle cutting biopsy for the characterization of diffuse liver diseases in bone marrow transplant patients. Bone Marrow Transplant 22:571-573, 1998.

295. Iqbal M, Creger RJ, Fox RM, et al: Laparoscopic liver biopsy to evaluate hepatic dysfunction in patients with hematologic malignancies: A useful tool to effect changes in management. Bone Marrow Transplant 17:655-662, 1996.

296. Naber AH, Van Haelst U, Yap SH: Nodular regenerative hyperplasia of the liver: An important cause of portal hypertension in noncirrhotic patients. J Hepatol 12:94-99, 1991.

297. Snover DC, Weisdorf S, Bloomer J, et al: Nodular regenerative hyperplasia of the liver following bone marrow transplantation. Hepatology 9:443-448, 1989.

298. Morales JM, Prieto C, Colina F, et al: Nodular regenerative hyperplasia of the liver in renal transplantation. Transplant Proc 19:3694-3696, 1987.

299. Stromeyer FW, Ishak KG: Nodular transformation (nodular "regenerative" hyperplasia) of the liver. A clinicopathologic study of 30 cases. Hum Pathol 12:60-71, 1981.

300. Crawford JM, Boyer JL: Clinicopathology conferences: Inflammation-induced cholestasis. Hepatology 28:253-260, 1998.

301. Norris SH, Butler TC, Glass N, et al: Fatal hepatic necrosis caused by disseminated type 5 adenovirus infection in a renal transplant recipient. Am J Nephrol 9:101-105, 1989.

302. Ludwig J, Batts K: Transplantation pathology. In MacSween R, Anthony P, Scheuer P, et al (eds): Pathology of the Liver, 3rd ed. Edinburgh, Churchill Livingstone, 1994, pp 766-786.

303. Fairley CK, Mijch A, Gust ID, et al: The increased risk of fatal liver disease in renal transplant patients who are hepatitis Be antigen and/or HBV DNA positive. Transplantation 52:497-500, 1991.

304. Fornairon S, Pol S, Legendre C, et al: The long-term virologic and pathologic impact of renal transplantation on chronic hepatitis B virus infection. Transplantation 62:297-299, 1996.

305. Roth D: Hepatitis C virus infection and the renal allograft recipient. Nephron 71:249-253, 1995.

306. Brunson ME, Lau JY, Davis GL, et al: Non-A, non-B hepatitis and elevated serum aminotransferases in renal transplant patients. Correlation with hepatitis C infection. Transplantation 56:1364-1367, 1993.

307. Lim HL, Lau GK, Davis GL, et al: Cholestatic hepatitis leading to hepatic failure in a patient with organ-transmitted hepatitis C virus infection. Gastroenterology 106:248-251, 1994.

308. Delladetsima JK, Boletis JN, Makris F, et al: Fibrosing cholestatic hepatitis in renal transplant recipients with hepatitis C virus infection. Liver Transpl Surg 5:294-300, 1999.

309. Munoz de Bustillo E, Benito A, Colina F, et al: Fibrosing cholestatic hepatitis-like syndrome in hepatitis B virus-negative and hepatitis C virus-negative renal transplant recipients. Am J Kidney Dis 38:640-645, 2001.

310. Gane E, Sallie R, Saleh M, et al: Clinical recurrence of hepatitis A following liver transplantation for acute liver failure. J Med Virol 45:35-39, 1995.

311. McCaughan GW, Torzillo PJ: Hepatitis A, liver transplants and indigenous communities. Med J Aust 172:6-7, 2000.

312. Steinmuller T, Seehofer D, Rayes N, et al: Increasing applicability of liver transplantation for patients with hepatitis B-related liver disease. Hepatology 35:1528-1535, 2002.

313. Neumann UP, Langrehr JM, Naumann U, et al: Impact of HLA-compatibilities in patients undergoing liver transplantation for HBV-cirrhosis. Clin Transplant 16:122-129, 2002.

314. Hasegawa K, Hashimoto E, Kanai N, et al: Living-related partial liver transplantation for decompensated hepatitis B without reactivation of hepatitis B in the following 30 months. J Gastroenterol 36:637-642, 2001.

315. Samuel D, Zignego AL, Reynes M, et al: Long-term clinical and virological outcome after liver transplantation for cirrhosis caused by chronic delta hepatitis. Hepatology 21:333-339, 1995.

316. Willems M, Metselaar HJ, Tilanus HW, et al: Liver transplantation and hepatitis C. Transpl Int 15:61-72, 2002.

317. Pruthi J, Medkiff KA, Esrason KT, et al: Analysis of causes of death in liver transplant recipients who survived more than 3 years. Liver Transpl 7:811-815, 2001.

318. Teixeira R, Papatheodoridis GV, Burroughs AK: Management of recurrent hepatitis C after liver transplantation. J Viral Hepat 8:159-168, 2001.

319. Rosen HR, Martin P: Hepatitis B and C in the liver transplant recipient. Semin Liver Dis 20:465-480, 2000.

320. Rosen HR: Retransplantation for hepatitis C: Implications of different policies. Liver Transpl 6:S41-S46, 2000.

321. Teixeira R, Pastacaldi S, Papatheodoridis GV, et al: Recurrent hepatitis C after liver transplantation. J Med Virol 61:443-454, 2000.

322. Terrault NA: Hepatitis C virus and liver transplantation. Semin Gastrointest Dis 11:96-114, 2000.

323. Vargas HE, Laskus T, Wang LF, et al: Outcome of liver transplantation in hepatitis C virus-infected patients who received hepatitis C virus-infected grafts. Gastroenterology 117:149-153, 1999.

324. Kim WR, Poterucha JJ, Porayko MK, et al: Recurrence of nonalcoholic steatohepatitis following liver transplantation. Transplantation 62:1802-1805, 1996.

325. Contos MJ, Cales W, Sterling RK, et al: Development of nonalcoholic fatty liver disease after orthotopic liver transplantation for cryptogenic cirrhosis. Liver Transpl 7:363-373, 2001.

326. Charlton M, Kasparova P, Weston S, et al: Frequency of nonalcoholic steatohepatitis as a cause of advanced liver disease. Liver Transpl 7:608-614, 2001.

327. Wong LL: Current status of liver transplantation for hepatocellular cancer. Am J Surg 183:309-316, 2002.

328. Figueras J, Ibanez L, Ramos E, et al: Selection criteria for liver transplantation in early-stage hepatocellular carcinoma with cirrhosis: Results of a multicenter study. Liver Transpl 7:877-883, 2001.

329. Frilling A, Malago M, Broelsch CE: Current status of liver transplantation for treatment of hepatocellular carcinoma. Dig Dis 19:333-337, 2001.

330. Iwatsuki S, Dvorchik I, Marsh JW, et al: Liver transplantation for hepatocellular carcinoma: A proposal of a prognostic scoring system. J Am Coll Surg 191:389-394, 2000.

331. Klintmalm GB: Liver transplantation for hepatocellular carcinoma: A registry report of the impact of tumor characteristics on outcome. Ann Surg 228:479-490, 1998.

332. Marsh JW, Casavilla A, Iwatsuki S, et al: Predicting the risk of tumor recurrence following transplantation for hepatocellular carcinoma. Hepatology 26:1689-1691, 1997.

333. Tamura S, Kato T, Berho M, et al: Impact of histological grade of hepatocellular carcinoma on the outcome of liver transplantation. Arch Surg 136:25-30, 2001.

334. Casavilla FA, Marsh JW, Iwatsuki S, et al: Hepatic resection and transplantation for peripheral cholangiocarcinoma. J Am Coll Surg 185:429-436, 1997.

335. Iwatsuki S, Todo S, Marsh JW, et al: Treatment of hilar cholangiocarcinoma (Klatskin tumors) with hepatic resection or transplantation. J Am Coll Surg 187:358-364, 1998.

336. Meyer CG, Penn I, James L: Liver transplantation for cholangiocarcinoma: Results in 207 patients. Transplantation 69:1633-1637, 2000.

337. Weimann A, Varnholt H, Schlitt HJ, et al: Retrospective analysis of prognostic factors after liver resection and transplantation for cholangiocellular carcinoma. Br J Surg 87:1182-1187, 2000.

338. Starzl T: Surgery for metabolic liver disease. In McDermott WV (ed): Surgery of the Liver. Boston, Blackwell Scientific Publications, 1986, pp 127-136.

339. Putnam CW, Porter KA, Peters RL, et al: Liver replacement for alpha1-antitrypsin deficiency. Surgery 81:258-261, 1977.

340. DuBois RS, Rodgerson DO, Martineau G, et al: Orthotopic liver transplantation for Wilson's disease. Lancet 1:505-508, 1971.

341. Groth CG, Dubois RS, Corman J, et al: Metabolic effects of hepatic replacement in Wilson's disease. Transplant Proc 5:829-833, 1973.

342. Zitelli BJ, Malatack JJ, Gartner JC, et al: Orthotopic liver transplantation in children with hepatic-based metabolic disease. Transplant Proc 15:1284-1287, 1983.

343. Fisch RO, McCabe ER, Doeden D, et al: Homotransplantation of the liver in a patient with hepatoma and hereditary tyrosinemia. J Pediatr 93:592-596, 1978.
344. Starzl TE, Zitelli BJ, Shaw BW Jr, et al: Changing concepts: Liver replacement for hereditary tyrosinemia and hepatoma. J Pediatr 106:604-606, 1985.
345. Malatack JJ, Finegold DN, Iwatsuki S, et al: Liver transplantation for type I glycogen storage disease. Lancet 1:1073-1075, 1983.
346. Matern D, Starzl TE, Arnaout W, et al: Liver transplantation for glycogen storage disease types I, III, and IV. Eur J Pediatr 158:S43-S48, 1999.
347. Kayler LK, Merion RM, Lee S, et al: Long-term survival after liver transplantation in children with metabolic disorders. Pediatr Transplant 6:295-300, 2002.
348. Figueras J, Pares D, Munar-Ques M, et al: Experience with domino or sequential liver transplantation in familial patients with amyloid polyneuropathy. Transplant Proc 34:307-308, 2002.
349. Shaz BH, Lewis WD, Skinner M, et al: Livers from patients with apolipoprotein A-I amyloidosis are not suitable as "domino" donors. Mod Pathol 14:577-580, 2001.
350. Nishizaki T, Kishikawa K, Yoshizumi T, et al: Domino liver transplantation from a living related donor. Transplantation 70:1236-1239, 2000.
351. de Carvalho M, Conceicao I, Bentes C, et al: Long-term quantitative evaluation of liver transplantation in familial amyloid polyneuropathy (Portuguese V30M). Amyloid 9:126-133, 2002.
352. Suhr OB, Ericzon BG, Friman S: Long-term follow-up of survival of liver transplant recipients with familial amyloid polyneuropathy (Portuguese type). Liver Transpl 8:787-794, 2002.
353. Wolff H, Otto G, Giest H: Liver transplantation in Crigler-Najjar syndrome. A case report. Transplantation 42:84, 1986.
354. Kaufman SS, Wood RP, Shaw BW Jr, et al: Orthotopic liver transplantation for type I Crigler-Najjar syndrome. Hepatology 6:1259-1262, 1986.
355. Shneider BL: Pediatric liver transplantation in metabolic disease: Clinical decision making. Pediatr Transplant 6:25-29, 2002.
356. Casella JF, Lewis JH, Bontempo FA, et al: Successful treatment of homozygous protein C deficiency by hepatic transplantation. Lancet 1:435-438, 1988.
357. Starzl TE, Bilheimer DW, Bahnson HT, et al: Heart-liver transplantation in a patient with familial hypercholesterolaemia. Lancet 1:1382-1383, 1984.
358. Lewis JH, Bontempo FA, Spero JA, et al: Liver transplantation in a hemophiliac. N Engl J Med 312:1189-1190, 1985.
359. Bontempo FA, Lewis JH, Gorenc TJ, et al: Liver transplantation in hemophilia A. Blood 69:1721-1724, 1987.
360. Merion RM, Delius RE, Campbell DA Jr, et al: Orthotopic liver transplantation totally corrects factor IX deficiency in hemophilia B. Surgery 104:929-931, 1988.
361. Brandhagen DJ: Liver transplantation for hereditary hemochromatosis. Liver Transpl 7:663-672, 2001.
362. Brandhagen DJ, Alvarez W, Therneau TM, et al: Iron overload in cirrhosis-HFE genotypes and outcome after liver transplantation. Hepatology 31:456-460, 2000.
363. Daloze P, Delvin EE, Glorieux FH, et al: Replacement therapy for inherited enzyme deficiency: Liver orthotopic transplantation in Niemann-Pick disease type A. Am J Med Genet 1:229-239, 1977.
364. Gartner JC Jr, Bergman I, Malatack JJ, et al: Progression of neurovisceral storage disease with supranuclear ophthalmoplegia following orthotopic liver transplantation. Pediatrics 77:104-106, 1986.
365. Samuel D, Boboc B, Bernuau J, et al: Liver transplantation for protoporphyria. Evidence for the predominant role of the erythropoietic tissue in protoporphyrin overproduction. Gastroenterology 95:816-819, 1988.
366. de Torres I, Demetris AJ, Randhawa PS: Recurrent hepatic allograft injury in erythropoietic protoporphyria. Transplantation 61:1412-1413, 1996.
367. Dellon ES, Szczepiorkowski ZM, Dzik WH, et al: Treatment of recurrent allograft dysfunction with intravenous hematin after liver transplantation for erythropoietic protoporphyria. Transplantation 73:911-915, 2002.
368. Cox KL, Ward RE, Furgiuele TL, et al: Orthotopic liver transplantation in patients with cystic fibrosis. Pediatrics 80:571-574, 1987.
369. Mieles LA, Orenstein D, Teperman L, et al: Liver transplantation in cystic fibrosis. Lancet 1:1073, 1989.
370. Milkiewicz P, Skiba G, Kelly D, et al: Transplantation for cystic fibrosis: Outcome following early liver transplantation. J Gastroenterol Hepatol 17:208-213, 2002.

CHAPTER 40

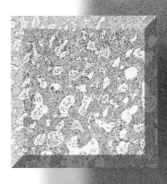

Liver Pathology in Pregnancy

KAMRAN BADIZADEGAN • JACQUELINE L. WOLF

■ Introduction

Pregnancy, an altered physiologic state designed to support a developing fetus, may be associated with specific pathophysiologic and pathologic complications. Although gastrointestinal complaints are common in pregnancy, symptoms due to de novo abnormalities of the liver are relatively uncommon. When present, however, their prompt diagnosis and treatment is of utmost importance because of the potentially high maternal and fetal morbidity and mortality associated with them. This chapter focuses on the diagnosis of liver diseases unique to pregnancy. In practice, however, the differential diagnoses must be broadened to include the full spectrum of liver and biliary abnormalities. In fact, the most common abnormalities of the liver and the biliary tree during pregnancy result from common diseases such as viral hepatitis and gallstone disease. The subject of this chapter has also been the topic of several excellent clinical and clinicopathologic reviews, to which the reader is referred for additional reading.[1-7] Unlike other chapters in this book, differential diagnosis per se is not featured because the panoply of hepatic diseases constitute the differential diagnosis of hepatic disease in pregnancy. Among those diseases specific to pregnancy discussed here, there is little room for confusion.

■ Clinical and Laboratory Aids in Assessment

Hepatic histopathology in pregnancy is often nonspecific. A basic knowledge of clinical history and physical signs and symptoms is therefore essential for adequate evaluation of liver pathology during pregnancy. The time of symptom onset in relation to the weeks of gestation and the signs and symptoms themselves are helpful in limiting the differential diagnosis of hepatic pathology in pregnancy. For instance, severe nausea and vomiting during the first trimester are key features for the diagnosis of hyperemesis gravidarum. Nausea and vomiting of later onset, however, are suggestive of preeclampsia when accompanied by headache and peripheral edema, and of hepatic rupture when accompanied by abdominal pain with or without systemic hypotension. Pruritus, particularly of the palms and soles, is characteristic of intrahepatic cholestasis of pregnancy and typically precedes the clinical onset of jaundice. Right upper quadrant and midabdominal pain may indicate acute fatty liver of pregnancy or hepatic rupture, both of which require immediate clinical intervention. Signs and symptoms of acute and chronic viral hepatitis and extrahepatic biliary disease are the same in pregnancy as they are in nonpregnant women. Clinical signs and symptoms are discussed in greater detail under each heading, and an overall summary is presented in Table 40-1.

TABLE 40–1. Clinical and Laboratory Aids in the Diagnosis of Common Liver Diseases in Pregnancy

Condition	Trimester	Signs and Symptoms	Laboratory Findings (Serum or Blood)
Intrahepatic cholestasis of pregnancy	Late 1st–3rd	Pruritus ± Jaundice	↑ Bile acids (30x–100x) ↑ Aminotransferases (1x–4x) ↑ Bilirubin (<5–6 mg/dL) ± ↑ Cholesterol and triglycerides
Acute fatty liver of pregnancy	Late 2nd–3rd	Nausea and vomiting Abdominal pain ± Jaundice	↑ Aminotransferases (1x–5x) ↑ Bilirubin (<10 mg/dL) ↑ Uric acid DIC Hypoglycemia
Preeclampsia/eclampsia	Late 2nd–3rd	Abdominal pain Hypertension Edema Mental status changes	↑ Aminotransferases (1x–100x) ↑ Uric acid ↑ Bilirubin (<5 mg/dL) DIC
HELLP syndrome	3rd	Systemic symptoms Abdominal pain ± Hypertension	Similar to preeclampsia/eclampsia Hemolysis Thrombocytopenia (<100,000/mm³)
Hepatic rupture	3rd	Acute abdominal pain ± Nausea and vomiting ± Hypotension	Similar to preeclampsia/eclampsia
Hyperemesis gravidarum	1st–early 2nd	Nausea and vomiting	↑ Aminotransferases (1x–2x) ↑ Bilirubin (<4–5 mg/dL)
Viral hepatitis	1st–3rd	Nausea and vomiting ± Fever	↑ Aminotransferases (10x–100x) ↑ Bilirubin Positive hepatitis serology

DIC, disseminated intravascular coagulation; HELLP, hemolysis, elevated liver enzymes, and low platelets.

Evaluation of liver disease in pregnancy is also complicated by physiologic changes in liver function test parameters as a function of gestational age. In spite of these well-known but poorly characterized alterations, almost all clinical laboratories use a normal adult population for reference ranges for liver function tests, thus leaving the evaluation of liver function abnormalities to the subjective judgment of clinicians and surgical pathologists. A summary of the most important changes is presented in the following sections, but the reader is referred to the original literature for a detailed discussion of the facts and controversies regarding changes in liver test parameters in normal pregnancy.[8-12]

Compared with that of age-matched nonpregnant women, the serum albumin level is significantly lower during all three trimesters and can decrease by as much as 60% during the second trimester, most likely because of hemodilution. Serum alkaline phosphatase activity rises during pregnancy and is significantly higher (by as much as a factor of 4) during the third trimester compared with that of nonpregnant women, although most of the activity originates from the placenta.

Serum levels of alanine aminotransferase (ALT), aspartate aminotransferase (AST), gamma-glutamyltranspeptidase (GGT), 5′-nucleotidase (5′-NT), bilirubin, total bile acids, and prothrombin time (PT) remain within reference range during normal pregnancy. Within the reference range, serum ALT levels may be on average slightly higher during the second trimester; serum GGT levels appear to be on average lower during the second and third trimesters compared with nonpregnant controls. Serum 5′-NT levels are higher during the second and third trimesters compared with the first trimester and compared with nonpregnant controls, but average increases are small (10% to 25%), and all values are well within the normal reference range. Total, free, and conjugated bilirubin levels may be lower than nonpregnant controls in all trimesters, with the most significant changes (up to 50%) noted in total and free bilirubin levels in the second and third trimesters. Serum triglycerides are higher in pregnancy, and cholesterol levels may increase by as much as 200% during the third trimester. Coagulation factors VII to X have been reported to be higher during pregnancy, and fibrinogen levels may increase by up to 50%. Alpha- and beta-globulins are also higher, although gamma-globulin levels decrease.

The microscopic appearance of the liver in uncomplicated pregnancy is thought to be "normal." Minor nonspecific changes that have been described include nuclear pleomorphism, increased glycogen, mild steatosis, mild portal inflammation, and reactive Kupffer cells.[13-17]

Intrahepatic Cholestasis of Pregnancy

As the name implies, intrahepatic cholestasis of pregnancy (IHCP) is a disease characterized by cholestasis within the liver without biliary duct obstruction.

Although the overall incidence of IHCP is estimated to be 0.5% to 1%,[2] wide geographic variations have been noted, with reported rates of up to 22% in parts of Chile, 9% in Bolivia, 2% to 3% in Sweden, less than 1% in Australia, and less than 0.2% in France, China, and Canada.[1,2] Furthermore, the prevalence of IHCP in high-incidence regions such as Chile has been decreasing over the past few decades for unknown reasons. IHCP is reported to be genetically transmitted as a sex-linked dominant trait, and genetic linkages to human leukocyte histocompatibility antigens (HLA) have been established.[18-20] There is an increased risk of IHCP with progesterone use in pregnancy and among women with a family history of oral contraceptive– or pregnancy-induced cholestasis and in women with a personal history of oral contraceptive–induced cholestasis.[21,22] The recurrence rate of IHCP in subsequent pregnancies is estimated at 40% to 60%, and a dietary link to selenium has been recently suggested.[23]

CLINICAL FEATURES

IHCP occurs most commonly in the third trimester but can occur in any trimester. Pruritus, which is the presenting symptom in almost all affected women, tends to be more severe at night and most often affects the palms, the soles, and the trunk. Jaundice occurs in 10% to 25% of cases, making IHCP the second leading cause of jaundice in pregnancy (after viral hepatitis). When jaundice occurs, it typically follows the onset of pruritus by 2 to 4 weeks. Other symptoms such as dark urine, light stools or steatorrhea, nausea, vomiting, and abdominal discomfort may also be present.[1,2,22] Symptoms of IHCP typically persist for the duration of pregnancy but resolve within 1 to 2 weeks after delivery. The maternal outcome in IHCP is generally favorable, and there is no permanent liver damage.[2,21,24] In contrast, the fetal complications of IHCP are more serious and consist of prematurity (19% to 60%), fetal distress (22% to 33%), meconium staining (increased by a factor of 1.5), and perinatal death (1% to 2%).[21,25]

Laboratory findings in IHCP include a mildly elevated serum bilirubin (mostly direct), mildly elevated serum transaminases, and markedly elevated serum bile acids (see Table 40-1).[2,26]

PATHOLOGIC FEATURES

Because the diagnosis of IHCP is typically made according to clinical criteria, liver histopathology in IHCP has not been extensively reported. Findings are thought to be subtle and consist primarily of hepatocellular bile and canalicular bile plugs, predominantly in a pericentral distribution with minimal to no hepatocellular necrosis and minimal portal inflammation (Fig. 40-1).[3,27,28] The histologic differential diagnosis of

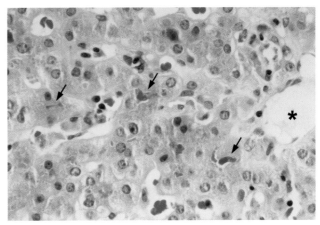

FIGURE 40–1. Liver biopsy specimen of a 19-year-old woman with benign recurrent intrahepatic cholestasis who presented with jaundice early in the second trimester. High-power view of hepatic parenchyma in the vicinity of a central vein (*asterisk*) shows moderate cholestasis with prominent canalicular bile plugs (*arrows*). A minimal mononuclear infiltrate is noted in the portal tracts, and occasional acidophilic bodies are present (not shown).

intrahepatic cholestasis is broad and includes such common entities as drug-induced hepatocellular injury and early extrahepatic biliary obstruction.

PATHOGENESIS

The pathogenesis of IHCP is not clearly delineated. Current evidence points to altered metabolism of steroid hormones and bile acids, and a mechanistic role for estrogen or a related compound has been suggested.[22,29] At the same time, genetic studies have shown IHCP to be an inherited disease with linkage to HLA antigens.[18-20] The most direct data about one possible etiology of IHCP, however, have recently come from genetic studies of a specific subset of patients in whom IHCP is associated with elevated serum GGT activity. Two pedigrees have been reported with IHCP in the mothers of children with autosomal recessive progressive familial intrahepatic cholestasis (PFIC) *and* elevated serum GGT activity (also known as type 3 PFIC).[30,31] Affected children have homozygous mutations in the *MDR3* gene, and heterozygous mothers have IHCP. Human MDR3 is a class III multidrug resistance (MDR) P-glycoprotein (homologous to mdr2 in mice) that mediates the translocation of phosphatidylcholine across the bile canalicular membrane of the hepatocyte.

Dixon and associates investigated eight women with IHCP and raised serum GGT activity with no family history of PFIC, to specifically determine the role of MDR3 in this patient population.[32] DNA sequence analysis revealed a heterozygous missense mutation in the MDR3 gene, resulting in the expression of a nonfunctional protein at the cell surface in one of eight patients. Two more recent reports on the association between MDR3 and IHCP provide further evidence for a defect in protein trafficking in the pathogenesis of some forms of IHCP.[33,34] In addition to these compelling data regarding the role of MDR3 in the pathogenesis of this disease, IHCP has been reported in association with benign recurrent intrahepatic cholestasis (BRIC; see Fig. 40-1). BRIC is associated with a mutation in the same region of chromosome 18 as type 1 PFIC, in which the affected patients have normal serum GGT activity,[35] suggesting the presence of other mechanistic pathways for yet another subset of women with IHCP. It is not surprising that different defects in transport across the hepatocyte canalicular membrane can lead to similar clinical phenotypes, which we collectively recognize as IHCP.

Acute Fatty Liver of Pregnancy

Acute fatty liver of pregnancy (AFLP) is a potentially fatal complication for the mother and the fetus. Although AFLP used to be considered an extremely rare disease, it is now believed to occur in as many as 1 in 13,000 to 16,000 pregnancies.[36,37] AFLP is classically associated with first pregnancies, twin gestations, and male fetuses. It generally occurs late in the third trimester or in the immediate postpartum period.[36-41] In a rare case, AFLP was reported to occur in a 35-year-old multipara at 22 weeks' gestation.[42]

CLINICAL FEATURES

The most common clinical presentation of AFLP is the triad of abdominal pain, nausea, and vomiting. Other associated symptoms include headache, fatigue, malaise, and anorexia. These prodromal symptoms are typically followed by jaundice as the disease progresses. In later stages or in severe cases, progressive hepatic failure may occur, accompanied by coagulopathy, encephalopathy, and renal failure. AFLP may be associated with preeclampsia in a significant number of patients (20% to 40%).[38,43,44] In such cases, the presenting signs and symptoms also include those of pregnancy-induced hypertensive disorders. A rare association between AFLP and IHCP has also been reported,[45] in which the patient initially presented with pruritus, which is a more typical presentation for a primary cholestatic disease than for AFLP.

Because early diagnosis and prompt treatment of AFLP are essential to maternal and fetal well-being, liver function tests must be measured immediately in any pregnant woman past 22 to 24 weeks' gestation who presents with any of the previously mentioned symptoms. The liver function tests in AFLP are typically suggestive of mild to moderate hepatocellular damage

and cholestasis (see Table 40-1). Serum aminotransferase levels are almost always elevated in AFLP but rarely to the extent observed in acute viral hepatitis. The bilirubin level is normal early in the course, but it rises if pregnancy is not terminated. Alkaline phosphatase levels are also elevated, but distinguishing hepatic from placental isoenzymes may not be practical. The peripheral blood may show leukocytosis and evidence of disseminated intravascular coagulation. Blood urea nitrogen and serum creatinine levels may be elevated, but uric acid levels are disproportionately high, making them diagnostically valuable. Blood glucose levels are typically low, to the extent that clinically significant hypoglycemia may occur.

Regardless of cause or type of presentation, the mainstay of therapy for AFLP is early delivery and supportive care.

PATHOLOGIC FEATURES

The diagnosis of AFLP is commonly made without the need for a liver biopsy. Nevertheless, the microscopic hallmark of AFLP is hepatocellular microvesicular steatosis. Classically, steatosis involves the pericentral zone and spares the periportal hepatocytes, but periportal involvement has also been described.[41,46] In most cases, the fat droplets are large enough and their location well enough preserved to produce a readily recognizable vacuolar change on routine hematoxylin and eosin (H&E) sections (Fig. 40-2**A**). Occasionally, however, the individual fat droplets may be too small or too poorly preserved to result in a classic vacuolar pattern on routine H&E sections (Figs. 40-2**B** and **C**). Under these circumstances, hepatocytes may look essentially normal, be somewhat dilated, or exhibit diffuse cytoplasmic ballooning not readily distinguishable from "ballooning degeneration" of other forms of acute hepatocellular damage. It is therefore paramount that at least a small portion of a liver biopsy specimen obtained for the clinical suspicion of AFLP should be processed as a frozen section for Oil Red O or Sudan black staining, or it should be submitted for electron microscopy.

The histopathologic differential diagnosis of AFLP is broad and includes essentially all toxic, metabolic, and drug-induced conditions that lead to microvesicular steatosis. Definitive diagnosis of AFLP can therefore be made only in conjunction with clinical findings.

Although fatty change is considered to be the diagnostic histologic hallmark of AFLP, a host of other significant abnormalities were also reported in a detailed study of 35 cases by Rolfes and Ishak.[41] Hypertrophied Kupffer cells containing lipid or lipofuscin were prominent in the areas of fatty change in the majority of cases. Evidence of intrahepatic cholestasis, including bile canalicular plugs and acute cholangiolitis, was seen

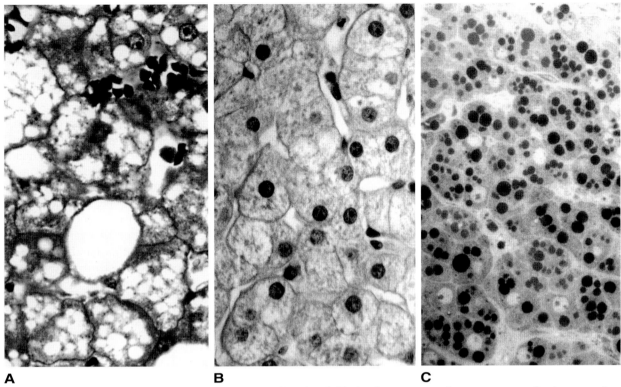

A   **B**   **C**

FIGURE 40–2. Classic microvesicular steatosis is often readily identifiable by the presence of numerous optically clear vacuoles on routine hematoxylin and eosin (H&E) stains, as shown in **A.** This liver biopsy specimen, which was obtained from a 32-year-old female who presented at 34 weeks' gestation with mildly increased transaminases and a "giant fatty liver" on ultrasound, also contained scattered hepatocytes with macrovesicular steatosis, as shown here. Special studies for fat are required in evaluation of liver biopsies suspected of fatty change because microvesicular steatosis may not be apparent on routine H&E stains, as shown in this biopsy specimen of a patient with suspected metabolic disease unrelated to pregnancy **(B).** In contrast, toluidine blue–stained plastic sections of an adjacent piece of the same biopsy specimen shown in **B** clearly demonstrated the presence of numerous hepatocellular fat droplets **(C).**

in two thirds of cases. Significant mononuclear lobular inflammation (comparable to acute viral hepatitis) and inflammation of the central veins were present in 25% of cases. In addition, 75% showed evidence of extramedullary hematopoiesis with prominent megakaryocytes and cells of erythroid lineage. Most notable in its absence in this large series of cases was sinusoidal fibrin deposition. In spite of the frequent presence of clinical signs and symptoms of pregnancy-induced hypertensive disorders in patients with AFLP,[38,43,44] the absence of fibrin deposition was taken as evidence at the time for no histologic overlap between these two entities.[41]

PATHOGENESIS

The pathogenesis of AFLP is unknown, but a strong association between fetal long-chain 3-hydroxyacyl-CoA dehydrogenase (LCHAD) deficiency and maternal AFLP has been established.[47-51] LCHAD catalyzes the third step in β oxidation of long-chain fatty acids, and its

activity is present on the C-terminal portion of the alpha subunit of the mitochondrial trifunctional protein, which also contains the active site of long-chain 2,3-enoyl-CoA hydratase and long-chain 3-ketoacyl-CoA thiolase. It is interesting that so far only one specific mutation in the alpha subunit of the mitochondrial trifunctional protein (glutamic acid to glutamine at residue 474) has been shown to be associated with maternal liver disease during pregnancy[50,51]; other mutations in fetuses with LCHAD deficiency do not appear to have an association with maternal liver disease.[51] A second fatty acid oxidation defect, hepatic carnitine palmitoyltransferase (CPT I) deficiency, has also been recently associated with maternal AFLP.[52] This finding further strengthens the arguments for a mechanistic association between deficiencies in mitochondrial fatty acid metabolism and AFLP, with the unique feature of a metabolic deficiency in the fetus placing the mother at risk for liver disease (usually it is the other way around).

Pregnancy-Induced Hypertensive Disorders (Preeclampsia and Eclampsia)

Preeclampsia is a systemic disorder characterized by hypertension, proteinuria, peripheral edema, and coagulation abnormalities with variable degrees of disseminated intravascular coagulation (DIC).[52-56] When neurologic abnormalities such as hyperreflexia and seizures are present, the condition is referred to as eclampsia. Preeclampsia occurs in 5% to 10% of all pregnancies, and it is classically a disease of primigravidas. Progression to eclampsia is rare, occurring in only 0.1% to 0.2% of all pregnancies, but when it happens, it is associated with significant maternal and fetal morbidity and mortality. Clinical risk factors and associated clinical conditions include diabetes, extremes of maternal age, family history of preeclampsia or eclampsia, multiple gestations, molar pregnancies, hydrops fetalis, polyhydramnios, and renal disease. Preeclampsia and eclampsia usually become clinically manifest after 20 weeks of gestation, and they are most common near term.

CLINICAL FEATURES

Liver is a nonspecific target organ for preeclampsia and eclampsia. Liver function abnormalities often include variably increased aminotransferases, which may be accompanied by a mild increase in serum bilirubin, alkaline phosphatase, and uric acid levels (see Table 40-1). Additional clinical laboratory findings include thrombocytopenia and evidence of DIC with microangiopathic hemolysis.

The systemic manifestations of preeclampsia/eclampsia seem to be associated with endothelial dysfunction.[57] Markers of endothelial activation can be demonstrated in women with preeclampsia. Furthermore, the appearance of some serologic markers of endothelial activation precedes clinically evident disease; their disappearance accompanies resolution of the disease.[57] This systemic disease appears to be a consequence of interactions between a hypoperfused placenta and maternal factors, leading to endothelial activation and systemic vascular injury. There also appears to be a genetic component to this abnormal maternal-fetal interaction,[53] but the precise components of maternal or fetal genotypes that contribute to the disease are not yet identified.

PATHOLOGIC FEATURES

Hepatic involvement in preeclampsia and eclampsia is morphologically suspected by the presence of patchy parenchymal and subcapsular hemorrhagic foci. Micro-scopically, the periportal zone is preferentially affected and may reveal a combination of fibrin deposition, hemorrhage, and hepatocellular necrosis (Fig. 40-3A).[3,14,58,59] Thrombi and evidence of endothelial damage may also be seen in the branches of the hepatic arteries and, less commonly, in the portal veins. In practice, the diagnosis is made clinically, and the classic pathologic changes discussed previously are seen only in rare instances of maternal death due to severe disease. Liver biopsies may be done—but rarely are—in patients with mild or clinically indeterminate liver disease, in whom the finding may be limited to mild and focal portal or periportal disease. Because of the focal nature of the hepatic involvement, the absence of specific findings on a liver biopsy should not be used as definitive evidence against preeclampsia. On the other hand, the presence of these findings is not specific to hypertensive disorders, and a nearly identical morphology may be seen in association with other conditions of altered hemostasis such as hypercoagulable status (Fig. 40-3B).

HELLP Syndrome

The triad of *h*emolysis, *e*levated *l*iver enzymes, and *l*ow *p*latelets, or HELLP syndrome, often occurs in the third trimester in association with preeclampsia/eclampsia. In a large study of approximately 12,000 pregnancies complicated by hypertensive disorders, HELLP syndrome was diagnosed in 20% of patients with severe preeclampsia and 10% of patients with eclampsia.[60] This paradoxically inverse relationship between HELLP syndrome and preeclampsia/eclampsia, however, was not seen in another large study that found a stronger association with eclampsia (35%) than with preeclampsia (12%).[61] Lack of standard quantitative diagnostic criteria for preeclampsia, eclampsia, and HELLP syndrome confounds these and other studies and may be partly responsible for the observed discrepancies.

CLINICAL FEATURES

The peak period of clinical onset appears to be between 27 and 36 weeks' gestation, and a significant number of cases are clinically diagnosed in the immediate postpartum period.[60] The most common presenting symptoms are abdominal pain (65% of cases), nausea or vomiting (36%), and headache (31%).[60] The risk of recurrence of HELLP syndrome in subsequent pregnancies has been reported from 3% to 27% in different studies.[62,63] HELLP syndrome is associated with significant maternal and fetal complications.[60,64,65] Maternal mortality is currently 1% or less, and the most serious maternal morbidity appears to be related to DIC, abruptio placentae, acute renal

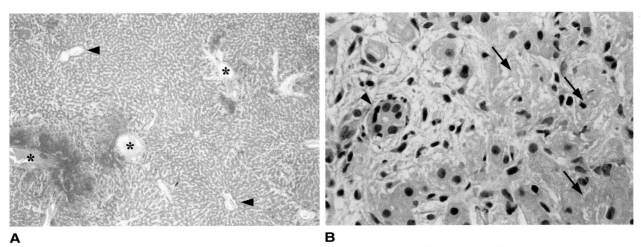

A   **B**

FIGURE 40–3. A, Classic histopathology of eclampsia is characterized by patchy areas of hemorrhage, fibrin deposition, and hepato-cellular necrosis in the vicinity of the portal tracts (asterisks). The pericentral areas *(arrowheads)* are virtually free of disease, and no significant inflammatory infiltrate is seen. **B,** The liver biopsy specimen also shows fibrin in the vicinity of a portal tract *(arrowhead points to the bile duct)* with obliteration of sinusoids and damaged periportal hepatocytes *(arrows).* This biopsy specimen, which came from a 30-year-old pregnant woman with abnormal liver function tests, could be distinguished from a pregnancy-induced hypertensive disorder only on the basis of clinical data (first-trimester pregnancy and a hypercoagulable state with antiphospholipid antibodies).

failure, and pulmonary edema.[60,61] Infants born to mothers with HELLP syndrome are at significantly increased risk for low birth weight and prematurity.[64,65] The mortality rate and the rate of other neonatal complications do not appear to be significantly different compared with matched neonates born to mothers without HELLP syndrome who were treated in a neonatal intensive care unit.[65]

PATHOLOGIC FEATURES AND PATHOGENESIS

In the classic form of HELLP syndrome (associated with preeclampsia/eclampsia), the pathogenesis and the laboratory findings, including liver histopathology, are not significantly different from those of preeclampsia and eclampsia (see Table 40-1). One of the most intriguing features of HELLP syndrome, however, is its proposed association with AFLP and LCHAD deficiency, as reported in a number of recent studies.[47,48,51,58] Although such an association would remarkably link two divergent pathologic mechanisms (one of presumed endothelial activation and one of mitochondrial fatty acid oxidation), its validity must await further confirmation. Significant overlap has been noted between the criteria that are commonly used to diagnose AFLP[39,41] and those used to diagnose HELLP syndrome in the previous studies.[47,48,51,66] Potentially because of such overlap, three of the six patients originally diagnosed with HELLP syndrome in the study by Ibdah and colleagues were reclassified as having AFLP during the course of their illness.[51] Furthermore, in a recent genetic study of the Dutch

population prompted by the reported associations between LCHAD deficiency and HELLP syndrome, no statistically significant difference was identified in a common LCHAD deficiency mutation between 113 women with HELLP syndrome and the general population.[67]

Hepatic Rupture

Hepatic rupture is a potentially catastrophic complication of pregnancy, with a reported incidence of 0.4 to 2.2 in 100,000 deliveries.[68,69] Although a vast majority of reported cases have occurred in the setting of hypertensive disorders (e.g., preeclampsia, eclampsia, and HELLP syndrome), more than 80% of these cases have been reported to occur in relatively older multigravidas.[70-72] This patient population is somewhat different from the average population with preeclampsia, eclampsia, or HELLP syndrome, which consists primarily of younger primigravidas. Large subcapsular hematomas, the setting in which most cases of hepatic rupture occur, have been reported in 0.9% of pregnant women with HELLP syndrome who appear to have a high risk for this complication.[60] Spontaneous hepatic rupture in pregnancy has also been reported in uncomplicated pregnancies[73] and in patients with AFLP,[74] connective tissue disorders,[75] hepatic abscesses,[76] liver masses,[77,78] history of cocaine use,[79] and abdominal trauma.[80] Regardless of the underlying cause, hepatic rupture typically presents with acute abdominal pain associated with nausea and vomiting, followed by abdominal distention and hypovolemic shock; emergent

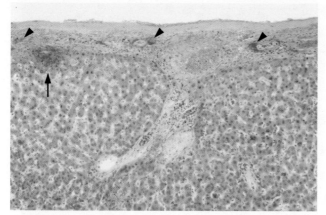

FIGURE 40–4. Multiple subcapsular hematomas *(arrow)* and multifocal intracapsular hemorrhages *(arrowheads)* were present in this fatal case of eclampsia. As is demonstrated in this photomicrograph, vascular branches of the portal tracts are in direct continuity with Glisson's capsules, and periportal hemorrhages often extend into and beneath the capsule, providing the background for large hematomas that may eventually stretch the capsule enough to cause a rupture.

surgical and medical treatment is required. Recurrence of rupture in subsequent pregnancies is rare.

PATHOGENESIS

The pathologic processes that lead to hepatic rupture are not well understood, and they are most likely as varied as the underlying causes of rupture. In hypertensive disorders, the most likely sequence of events is intrahepatic or intracapsular hemorrhage with tissue disruption leading to hematoma formation followed by distention and rupture of the capsule (Fig. 40-4). The events initiating intrahepatic hemorrhage in hypertensive disorders are unknown, but they are most likely related to parenchymal ischemia that occurs as a result of either fibrin thrombi or reduced blood flow due to endothelial dysfunction. Hepatic rupture is most commonly associated with hematomas that occur on the superior and anterior aspects of the right lobe of the liver. The gross and microscopic pathology is essentially that of the underlying condition with associated hematoma and rupture.

■ Hyperemesis Gravidarum

Nausea and vomiting are common during pregnancy, occurring in more than half of all pregnant women.[81] Nausea and vomiting most commonly begin between the fourth and seventh weeks of gestation, and they typically regress by the 16th week. Hyperemesis gravidarum, in contrast, is a severe and intractable form of nausea and vomiting that causes secondary abnor-

malities such as dehydration and electrolyte imbalance. Hyperemesis gravidarum is diagnosed in less than 2% of all pregnancies and may be associated with mildly elevated bilirubin and transaminases (see Table 40-1).[81,82]

Maternal abnormalities promptly return to normal with supportive treatment. Perinatal outcome in patients with hyperemesis gravidarum has been the subject of debate. Although older studies reported growth retardation and anomalies in infants of women with severe hyperemesis gravidarum,[83] these findings have not been confirmed in subsequent studies of perinatal outcomes.[84,85]

Liver histology in hyperemesis gravidarum is typically normal but may include mild steatosis, mild cholestasis, or occasional necrotic hepatocytes.[86,87] No specific mechanisms of liver damage have been described, and the mild hepatic abnormalities are thought to be secondary to dehydration and other systemic disturbances associated with hyperemesis.

■ Hepatitis E Infection

Viral hepatitis may present at any time during pregnancy, and its clinical and histopathologic diagnosis is the same as in nongravid patients. With the exception of hepatitis E virus (HEV) infection, the clinical course of viral hepatitis does not seem to be affected by pregnancy. HEV is a nonenveloped RNA virus that is uncommon in the United States but is responsible for large epidemics of acute hepatitis in southeast and central Asia, the Middle East, parts of Africa, and Mexico.[88] Hepatitis E is enterically transmitted and presents after an incubation period of 8 to 10 weeks with a clinical illness resembling other forms of acute viral hepatitis. The attack rate is the highest in young adults, with a population-based average mortality of less than 0.6% (compared with up to 4% in hospitalized patients).[88] In pregnant women, however, the illness can be particularly severe, with mortality rates reaching as high as 25%.[88] Anti-HEV immunoglobulin M (IgM) antibody appears early during clinical illness but disappears rapidly over a few months. Anti-HEV immunoglobulin G (IgG) antibody appears later and persists for at least a few years. Because no vaccines and no specific treatments are currently available, pregnant women should avoid contact with individuals suspected of HEV infection.

PATHOLOGIC FEATURES

Histopathology of confirmed HEV infection in pregnant women or others has been described only rarely. In general, the histopathology is that of an acute cholestatic hepatitis with some resemblance to acute hepatitis A infection.[89-91] Findings include a dense portal inflammatory infiltrate with canalicular bile stasis and occasional cholestatic hepatocellular rosettes. Varying degrees of hepatocellular damage may be noted with ballooned hepatocytes, acidophilic bodies, and focal or confluent hepatocellular necrosis. The main histologic differential diagnosis in pregnancy is seen with IHCP, in which case markedly elevated transaminases may be helpful in distinguishing viral hepatitis from IHCP, in which transaminases are typically only mildly elevated (see Table 40-1).

PATHOGENESIS

The pathobiology of HEV infection is not well known. In experimental HEV infection, it has been shown that hepatocellular injury is initially linked to hepatic viral replication but is later continued in spite of the appearance of anti-HEV antibodies and the disappearance of HEV antigen, suggesting an indirect mechanism of damage.[92]

Herpesvirus Infections

Clinically significant liver disease due to nonhepatitic viral infection is uncommon, but it can be devastating in pregnancy. With the exception of herpesviruses, such viral infections are generally neither more common nor more severe in pregnancy. Among the different serotypes, herpes simplex virus (HSV) infections are the most common, with a seropositivity rate of up to 30% for HSV-2 in a large cohort of pregnant women.[93] Dissemination of HSV from the primary site of infection is often associated with primary or secondary immunodeficiency states, but in rare occasions it may occur in otherwise healthy individuals. A disproportionate number of disseminated infections in otherwise healthy individuals appear to be associated with pregnancy, particularly during the third trimester.[94,95] Suspicion of the disease and prompt diagnosis with liver biopsy, culture, and serologic tests are important because treatment with antiviral agents may be successful in controlling a disease that otherwise would have extremely high maternal and fetal mortality rates. Tissue diagnosis in clinically suspected cases is particularly important because classic mucocutaneous vesicular lesions may be absent in a significant number of pregnancy-associated cases.[94,95] Other members of the herpesvirus family, including the cytomegalovirus and the varicella-zoster virus, can also result in fulminant hepatic disease in pregnancy.

PATHOLOGIC FEATURES

Liver pathology in affected individuals is characterized by irregular areas of hemorrhage and necrosis without significant inflammation but with classic viral inclusions in the surrounding hepatocytes. The underlying factors predisposing some pregnant women to more severe herpesvirus infections are not known, but altered immunity during the course of pregnancy is likely to play a role.

Budd-Chiari Syndrome

Budd-Chiari syndrome is the clinical manifestation of hepatic venous outflow obstruction; it is classically caused by thrombotic occlusion of hepatic vein branches or the inferior vena cava. Pregnancy, including the early postpartum period, accounts for approximately 5% to 15% of all documented cases.[96,97] Classic presentation with abdominal pain, hepatomegaly, and ascites is often insidious, although a disproportionate number of pregnancy-related cases appear to have acute onset and to be associated with massive ischemic damage.[96,97] Recent studies suggest that factor V Leiden deficiency may be responsible for this atypical presentation during pregnancy.

In a study of 63 cases by Deltenre and coworkers, Budd-Chiari syndrome with massive ischemic necrosis was encountered only in carriers of factor V Leiden mutation, three of whom (75%) were pregnant; the fourth was on oral contraceptives.[97] Another rare case of severe acute Budd-Chiari syndrome with factor V Leiden mutation in pregnancy has also been separately reported.[98] The liver histopathology and the pathogenesis of Budd-Chiari syndrome in pregnancy are the same as those in nonpregnant patients.

Conclusions

The liver is affected by many of the pathophysiologic and hormonal effects of pregnancy. Although many of the hepatic disorders encountered during pregnancy are similar to those affecting the nonpregnant population, liver diseases specific to pregnancy can have a profound impact on the maternal and fetal outcome. Liver pathology in pregnancy-related disorders may be subtle and nonspecific, and clinicopathologic correlation can be confounded by physiologic changes in liver function. The primary role of the pathologist in the diagnosis of liver disease in pregnancy is either to provide confirmatory evidence for a clinically suspected diagnosis or to guide the clinical team toward an alternative diagnosis. For these goals to be accomplished, a clear dialogue must take place between clinicians and pathologists to convey clinically relevant data and to ensure proper handling and triage of the biopsy material.

References

1. Wolf JL: Liver disease in pregnancy. Med Clin North Am 80:1167, 1996.
2. Schorr-Lesnick B, Lebovics E, Dworkin B, et al: Liver diseases unique to pregnancy. Am J Gastroenterol 86:659, 1991.
3. Rolfes DB, Ishak KG: Liver disease in pregnancy. Histopathology 10:555, 1986.
4. Riely CA: Liver disease in the pregnant patient. American College of Gastroenterology. Am J Gastroenterol 94:1728, 1999.
5. Knox TA, Olans LB: Liver disease in pregnancy. N Engl J Med 335:569, 1996.
6. Sandu BS, Sanyal AJ: Pregnancy and liver disease. Gastroenterol Clin North Am 32:407, 2003.
7. Maroo S, Wolf JL: The liver in pregnancy. In Friedman LS, Keeffe EB (eds): Handbook of Liver Diseases, 2nd ed. Philadelphia, Elsevier Science, 2003.
8. Jarnfelt-Samsioe A, Eriksson B, Waldenstrom J, et al: Serum bile acids, gamma-glutamyltransferase and routine liver function tests in emetic and nonemetic pregnancies. Gynecol Obstet Invest 21:169, 1986.
9. Girling JC, Dow E, Smith JH: Liver function tests in pre-eclampsia: Importance of comparison with a reference range derived for normal pregnancy. Br J Obstet Gynaecol 104:246, 1997.
10. Carter J: Liver function in normal pregnancy. Aust N Z J Obstet Gynaecol 30:296, 1990.
11. Higgins JR, Walshe JJ, Darling MR: Liver function tests in pre-eclampsia: Importance of comparison with a reference range derived for normal pregnancy. Br J Obstet Gynaecol 104:1215, 1997.
12. Bacq Y, Zarka O, Brechot JF, et al: Liver function tests in normal pregnancy: A prospective study of 103 pregnant women and 103 matched controls. Hepatology 23:1030, 1996.
13. Ishak KG: Hepatic lesions caused by anabolic and contraceptive steroids. Semin Liver Dis 1:116, 1981.
14. Gonzalez-Angulo A, Aznar-Ramos R, Marquez-Monter H, et al: The ultrastructure of liver cells in women under steroid therapy. I. Normal pregnancy and trophoblastic growths. Acta Endocrinol (Copenh) 65:193, 1970.
15. Perez V, Gorodisch S, Casavilla F, et al: Ultrastructure of human liver at the end of normal pregnancy. Am J Obstet Gynecol 110:428, 1971.
16. Antia FP, Bharadwaj TP, Watsa MC, et al: Liver in normal pregnancy, pre-eclampsia, and eclampsia. Lancet ii:776, 1958.
17. Steven MM: Pregnancy and liver disease. Gut 22:592, 1981.
18. Holzbach RT, Sivak DA, Braun WE: Familial recurrent intrahepatic cholestasis of pregnancy: A genetic study providing evidence for transmission of a sex-limited, dominant trait. Gastroenterology 85:175, 1983.
19. Mella JG, Roschmann E, Glasinovic JC, et al: Exploring the genetic role of the HLA-DPB1 locus in Chileans with intrahepatic cholestasis of pregnancy. J Hepatol 24:320, 1996.
20. Reyes H, Wegmann ME, Segovia N, et al: HLA in Chileans with intrahepatic cholestasis of pregnancy. Hepatology 2:463, 1982.
21. Reyes H: Review: Intrahepatic cholestasis. A puzzling disorder of pregnancy. J Gastroenterol Hepatol 12:211, 1997.
22. Davidson KM: Intrahepatic cholestasis of pregnancy. Semin Perinatol 22:104, 1998.
23. Reyes H, Baez ME, Gonzalez MC, et al: Selenium, zinc and copper plasma levels in intrahepatic cholestasis of pregnancy, in normal pregnancies and in healthy individuals, in Chile. J Hepatol 32:542, 2000.
24. Fisk NM, Bye WB, Storey GN: Maternal features of obstetric cholestasis: 20 years experience at King George V Hospital. Aust N Z J Obstet Gynaecol 28:172, 1988.
25. Fisk NM, Storey GN: Fetal outcome in obstetric cholestasis. Br J Obstet Gynaecol 95:1137, 1988.
26. Lunzer M, Barnes P, Byth K, et al: Serum bile acid concentrations during pregnancy and their relationship to obstetric cholestasis. Gastroenterology 91:825, 1986.
27. Wilson JA: Intrahepatic cholestasis of pregnancy with marked elevation of transaminases in a black American. Dig Dis Sci 32:665, 1987.
28. Haemmerli UP, Wyss HI: Recurrent intrahepatic cholestasis of pregnancy. Report of six cases, and review of the literature. Medicine (Baltimore) 46:299, 1967.
29. Mullally BA, Housen WF: Intrahepatic cholestasis of frequency: Review of the literature. Obstet Gynaecol Surv 57:47, 2002.
30. de Vree JM, Jacquemin E, Sturm E, et al: Mutations in the MDR3 gene cause progressive familial intrahepatic cholestasis. Proc Natl Acad Sci U S A 95:282, 1998.
31. Jacquemin E, Cresteil D, Manouvrier S, et al: Heterozygous non-sense mutation of the MDR3 gene in familial intrahepatic cholestasis of pregnancy. Lancet 353:210, 1999.
32. Dixon PH, Weerasekera N, Linton KJ, et al: Heterozygous MDR3 missense mutation associated with intrahepatic cholestasis of pregnancy: Evidence for a defect in protein trafficking. Hum Mol Genet 9:1209, 2000.
33. Gendrot C, Bacq Y, Brechot MC, et al: A second heterozygous MDR3 nonsense mutation associated with intrahepatic cholestasis of pregnancy. J Med Genet 40:e32, 2003.
34. Lucena JF, Herrero JI, Quiroga JB, et al: A multidrug resistance 3 gene mutation causing cholelithiasis, cholestasis of pregnancy, and adulthood biliary cirrhosis. Gastroenterology 124:1037, 2003.
35. Bull LN, van Eijk MJ, Pawlikowska L, et al: A gene encoding a P-type ATPase mutated in two forms of hereditary cholestasis. Nat Genet 18:219, 1998.
36. Pockros PJ, Peters RL, Reynolds TB: Idiopathic fatty liver of pregnancy: Findings in ten cases. Medicine (Baltimore) 63:1, 1984.
37. Reyes H, Sandoval L, Wainstein A, et al: Acute fatty liver of pregnancy: A clinical study of 12 episodes in 11 patients. Gut 35:101, 1994.
38. Cejudo Carranza E, Helguera Martinez A, Garcia Caceres E: Acute fatty liver in pregnancy. Experience of 7 years. Ginecol Obstet Mex 68:191, 2000.
39. Kaplan MM: Acute fatty liver of pregnancy. N Engl J Med 313:367, 1985.
40. Riely CA: Acute fatty liver of pregnancy. Semin Liver Dis 7:47, 1987.
41. Rolfes DB, Ishak KG: Acute fatty liver of pregnancy: A clinico-pathologic study of 35 cases. Hepatology 5:1149, 1985.
42. Monga M, Katz AR: Acute fatty liver in the second trimester. Obstet Gynecol 93:811, 1999.
43. Riely CA, Latham PS, Romero R, et al: Acute fatty liver of pregnancy. A reassessment based on observations in nine patients. Ann Intern Med 106:703, 1987.
44. Brown MA, Passaris G, Carlton MA: Pregnancy-induced hyper-tension and acute fatty liver of pregnancy: Atypical presentations. Am J Obstet Gynecol 163:1154, 1990.
45. Vanjak D, Moreau R, Roche-Sicot J, et al: Intrahepatic cholestasis of pregnancy and acute fatty liver of pregnancy. An unusual but favorable association? Gastroenterology 100:1123, 1991.
46. Burroughs AK, Seong NH, Dojcinov DM, et al: Idiopathic acute fatty liver of pregnancy in 12 patients. Q J Med 51:481, 1982.
47. Tyni T, Ekholm E, Pihko H: Pregnancy complications are frequent in long-chain 3-hydroxyacyl-coenzyme A dehydrogenase deficiency. Am J Obstet Gynecol 178:603, 1998.
48. Wilcken B, Leung KC, Hammond J, et al: Pregnancy and fetal long-chain 3-hydroxyacyl coenzyme A dehydrogenase deficiency. Lancet 341:407, 1993.
49. Ibdah JA, Dasouki MJ, Strauss AW: Long-chain 3-hydroxyacyl-CoA dehydrogenase deficiency: Variable expressivity of maternal illness during pregnancy and unusual presentation with infantile cholestasis and hypocalcaemia. J Inherit Metab Dis 22:811, 1999.
50. Sims HF, Brackett JC, Powell CK, et al: The molecular basis of pediatric long chain 3-hydroxyacyl-CoA dehydrogenase deficiency associated with maternal acute fatty liver of pregnancy. Proc Natl Acad Sci U S A 92:841, 1995.
51. Ibdah JA, Bennett MJ, Rinaldo P, et al: A fetal fatty-acid oxidation disorder as a cause of liver disease in pregnant women. N Engl J Med 340:1723, 1999.
52. Innes AM, Seargeant LE, Balachandra K, et al: Hepatic carnitine palmitoyltransferase I deficiency presenting as maternal illness in pregnancy. Pediatr Res 47:43, 2000.
53. Roberts JM, Cooper DW: Pathogenesis and genetics of pre-eclampsia. Lancet 357:53, 2001.
54. Dietl J: The pathogenesis of pre-eclampsia: New aspects. J Perinat Med 28:464, 2000.
55. Kenny L, Baker PN: Maternal pathophysiology in pre-eclampsia. Baillieres Best Pract Res Clin Obstet Gynaecol 13:59, 1999.
56. Mattar F, Sibai BM: Eclampsia. VIII. Risk factors for maternal morbidity. Am J Obstet Gynecol 182:307, 2000.
57. Roberts JM: Endothelial dysfunction in preeclampsia. Semin Reprod Endocrinol 16:5, 1998.

58. Arias F, Mancilla-Jimenez R: Hepatic fibrinogen deposits in pre-eclampsia. Immunofluorescent evidence. N Engl J Med 295:578, 1976.
59. McKay DG: Clinical significance of the pathology of toxemia of pregnancy. Circulation 30(suppl 2):66, 1964.
60. Sibai BM, Ramadan MK, Usta I, et al: Maternal morbidity and mortality in 442 pregnancies with hemolysis, elevated liver enzymes, and low platelets (HELLP syndrome). Am J Obstet Gynecol 169:1000, 1993.
61. Vigil-De Gracia P: Pregnancy complicated by pre-eclampsia-eclampsia with HELLP syndrome. Int J Gynaecol Obstet 72:17, 2001.
62. Sibai BM, Ramadan MK, Chari RS, et al: Pregnancies complicated by HELLP syndrome (hemolysis, elevated liver enzymes, and low platelets): Subsequent pregnancy outcome and long-term prognosis. Am J Obstet Gynecol 172:125, 1995.
63. Sullivan CA, Magann EF, Perry KG Jr, et al: The recurrence risk of the syndrome of hemolysis, elevated liver enzymes, and low platelets (HELLP) in subsequent gestations. Am J Obstet Gynecol 171:940, 1994.
64. Harms K, Rath W, Herting E, et al: Maternal hemolysis, elevated liver enzymes, low platelet count, and neonatal outcome. Am J Perinatol 12:1, 1995.
65. Kandler C, Kevekordes B, Zenker M, et al: Prognosis of children born to mothers with HELLP-syndrome. J Perinat Med 26:486, 1998.
66. Treem WR, Shoup ME, Hale DE, et al: Acute fatty liver of pregnancy, hemolysis, elevated liver enzymes, and low platelets syndrome, and long chain 3-hydroxyacyl-coenzyme A dehydrogenase deficiency. Am J Gastroenterol 91:2293, 1996.
67. den Boer ME, Ijlst L, Wijburg FA, et al: Heterozygosity for the common LCHAD mutation (1528g>C) is not a major cause of HELLP syndrome and the prevalence of the mutation in the Dutch population is low. Pediatr Res 48:151, 2000.
68. Smith LG Jr, Moise KJ Jr, Dildy GA 3rd, et al: Spontaneous rupture of liver during pregnancy: Current therapy. Obstet Gynecol 77:171, 1991.
69. Hibbard LT: Spontaneous rupture of the liver in pregnancy: A report of eight cases. Am J Obstet Gynecol 126:334, 1976.
70. Aziz S, Merrell RC, Collins JA: Spontaneous hepatic hemorrhage during pregnancy. Am J Surg 146:680, 1983.
71. Henny CP, Lim AE, Brummelkamp WH, et al: A review of the importance of acute multidisciplinary treatment following spontaneous rupture of the liver capsule during pregnancy. Surg Gynecol Obstet 156:593, 1983.
72. Sheikh RA, Yasmeen S, Pauly MP, et al: Spontaneous intrahepatic hemorrhage and hepatic rupture in the HELLP syndrome: Four cases and a review. J Clin Gastroenterol 28:323, 1999.
73. Matsuda Y, Maeda T, Hatae M: Spontaneous rupture of the liver in an uncomplicated pregnancy. J Obstet Gynaecol Res 23:449, 1997.
74. Minuk GY, Lui RC, Kelly JK: Rupture of the liver associated with acute fatty liver of pregnancy. Am J Gastroenterol 82:457, 1987.
75. Gelbmann CM, Kollinger M, Gmeinwieser J, et al: Spontaneous rupture of liver in a patient with Ehlers-Danlos disease type IV. Dig Dis Sci 42:1724, 1997.
76. Cowan DB, Houlton MC: Rupture of an amoebic liver abscess in pregnancy. A case report. S Afr Med J 53:460, 1978.
77. Monks PL, Fryar BG, Biggs WW: Spontaneous rupture of an hepatic adenoma in pregnancy with survival of mother and fetus. Aust N Z J Obstet Gynaecol 26:155, 1986.
78. Hsu KL, Ko SF, Cheng YF, et al: Spontaneous rupture of hepatocellular carcinoma during pregnancy. Obstet Gynecol 98:913, 2001.
79. Moen MD, Caliendo MJ, Marshall W, et al: Hepatic rupture in pregnancy associated with cocaine use. Obstet Gynecol 82:687, 1993.
80. Icely S, Chez RA: Traumatic liver rupture in pregnancy. Am J Obstet Gynecol 180:1030, 1999.
81. Eliakim R, Abulafia O, Sherer DM: Hyperemesis gravidarum: A current review. Am J Perinatol 17:207, 2000.
82. Morali GA, Braverman DZ: Abnormal liver enzymes and ketonuria in hyperemesis gravidarum. A retrospective review of 80 patients. J Clin Gastroenterol 12:303, 1990.
83. Gross S, Librach C, Cecutti A: Maternal weight loss associated with hyperemesis gravidarum: A predictor of fetal outcome. Am J Obstet Gynecol 160:906, 1989.
84. Hallak M, Tsalamandris K, Dombrowski MP, et al: Hyperemesis gravidarum. Effects on fetal outcome. J Reprod Med 41:871, 1996.
85. Tsang IS, Katz VL, Wells SD: Maternal and fetal outcomes in hyperemesis gravidarum. Int J Gynaecol Obstet 55:231, 1996.
86. Larrey D, Rueff B, Feldmann G, et al: Recurrent jaundice caused by recurrent hyperemesis gravidarum. Gut 25:1414, 1984.
87. Adams RH, Gordon J, Combes B: Hyperemesis gravidarum. I. Evidence of hepatic dysfunction. Obstet Gynecol 31:659, 1968.
88. Aggarwal R, Krawczynski K: Hepatitis E: An overview and recent advances in clinical and laboratory research. J Gastroenterol Hepatol 15:9, 2000.
89. De Cock KM, Bradley DW, Sandford NL, et al: Epidemic non-A, non-B hepatitis in patients from Pakistan. Ann Intern Med 106:227, 1987.
90. Asher LV, Innis BL, Shrestha MP, et al: Virus-like particles in the liver of a patient with fulminant hepatitis and antibody to hepatitis E virus. J Med Virol 31:229, 1990.
91. Dienes HP, Hutteroth T, Bianchi L, et al: Hepatitis A-like non-A, non-B hepatitis: Light and electron microscopic observations of three cases. Virchows Arch A Pathol Anat Histopathol 409:657, 1986.
92. Longer CF, Denny SL, Caudill JD, et al: Experimental hepatitis E: Pathogenesis in cynomolgus macaques (Macaca fascicularis). J Infect Dis 168:602, 1993.
93. Frenkel LM, Garratty EM, Shen JP, et al: Clinical reactivation of herpes simplex virus type 2 infection in seropositive pregnant women with no history of genital herpes. Ann Intern Med 118:414, 1993.
94. Young EJ, Chafizadeh E, Oliveira VL, et al: Disseminated herpesvirus infection during pregnancy. Clin Infect Dis 22:51, 1996.
95. Kang AH, Graves CR: Herpes simplex hepatitis in pregnancy: A case report and review of the literature. Obstet Gynecol Surv 54:463, 1999.
96. Khuroo MS, Datta DV: Budd-Chiari syndrome following pregnancy. Report of 16 cases, with roentgenologic, hemodynamic and histologic studies of the hepatic outflow tract. Am J Med 68:113, 1980.
97. Deltenre P, Denninger MH, Hillaire S, et al: Factor V Leiden related Budd-Chiari syndrome. Gut 48:264, 2001.
98. Fickert P, Ramschak H, Kenner L, et al: Acute Budd-Chiari syndrome with fulminant hepatic failure in a pregnant woman with factor V Leiden mutation. Gastroenterology 111:1670, 1996.

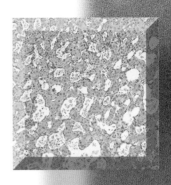

CHAPTER 41

Inherited and Developmental Disorders of the Liver

A. S. KNISELY • JAMES M. CRAWFORD

◼ Introduction

Diagnostic assessment of inherited and metabolic disorders of the liver falls into two general categories: (1) assessment of liver disease in the infant or young child and (2) assessment of liver disease in the adolescent or adult. In the former instance, presentation of the full compendium for diagnostic evaluation of the pediatric liver biopsy is beyond the scope of this chapter, and so the primary focus is on specimen processing and triage. In the latter instance, three major diseases are considered—HFE disease (hereditary hemochromatosis), ATP7B disease (Wilson's disease), and alpha-1-antitrypsin storage disorder (A1ATSD). In addition, a striking set of developmental abnormalities of the biliary tree merits comment.

◼ The Pediatric Liver Biopsy

BIOPSY SPECIMENS IN GENERAL PATHOLOGY PRACTICE

Pathologists in general practice do not often interpret pediatric liver biopsy specimens. The numbers and availability of pediatric hospitals have increased in recent years, and infants, children, and adolescents with liver disease may likely be attended in a specialized regional facility. Pediatric liver biopsy specimens are generally seen by subspecialty pathologists. However, the numbers of community-based pediatric gastro-enterologists also have increased in recent years. These individuals may offer pediatric specialty services, including liver biopsy, at general or community hospitals.

General pathologists at institutions where pediatric gastroenterologists practice must decide if they wish to attempt full diagnostic evaluation of pediatric liver biopsy specimens. If they do, an excellent compendium is available to guide them[1] (this chapter makes no attempt to recapitulate it). If they do not, another option exists.

That option is triage. Some pathologists may prefer to conduct preliminary evaluation of a pediatric liver biopsy specimen while reserving material for study in consultation. To do so facilitates a provisional diagnosis, adequate for revealing appropriate early steps in directing patient care and later to be integrated with other findings. This course often is taken with lymph node or kidney biopsy specimens. To adopt it with pediatric liver biopsy specimens may be prudent. This section is written specifically for the purpose of discussing initial pediatric liver biopsy specimen evaluation and triage.

SPECIMEN HANDLING AT THE BEDSIDE AND THEREAFTER

Whichever route is followed (triage or full evaluation), the first step is the same. For information not to be lost, the biopsy specimen must be correctly handled. Studies useful in the evaluation of pediatric liver biopsy specimens include not only light microscopy but also enzymologic work, transmission electron microscopy, and, to an ever-increasing degree, molecular genetics analysis. How can material best be preserved for all these purposes, so that liver biopsy does not have to be repeated?

Harvesting pediatric liver biopsy tissue properly is the responsibility of the person who undertakes the biopsy, whether gastroenterologist, hepatologist, or radiologist, and not that of the pathologist. Fortunately, processing of pediatric liver biopsy tissue to specialty care standards is not difficult, but arrangements should be in place before elective liver biopsy is conducted in pediatric patients.

- Liquid nitrogen at the bedside and storage at –80°C are required. Cores of tissue aggregating optimally to 2 cm in length should be snap-frozen immediately for preservation of mRNA. Tissue fragments should then be placed in a specimen vial in an air-excluded fashion to prevent desiccation. Portions can be retrieved for any of the molecular genetic analyses required.
- A small portion (0.3 cm) should be placed in electron microscopy fixative and held for potential further processing.
- A 1-cm portion should be fixed directly in formalin. Saline or transport media should not be used because liver tissue in such solutions becomes distorted and suboptimal. The core for light microscopy should be placed in a mesh cassette. Biopsy sponges, which distort the tissue, are unnecessary after the specimen has spent an hour in formalin.

The formalin-fixed specimen should then be processed routinely for light microscopy. Serial sections should be obtained. At the Institute of Liver Studies at King's College Hospital, a ribbon of 20 sections is cut and picked up on ten slides, two sections per slide. The sections on two slides (the first and last pairs of sections in the ribbon) are stained with hematoxylin and eosin (H&E). Periodic acid–Schiff with diastase (d-PAS), orcein, Perls', and modified Gordon and Sweets (gold toning omitted) reticulin techniques are used to stain four pairs of intervening sections. The others in the ribbon are held as "blanks." Abundant tissue remains in the block.

This approach, which enables evaluation of 12 stained sections on six slides, generally yields enough information for short-term clinical management. Following that, should the patient's care be transferred to another institution or should an opinion in consultation be sought, one of the H&E-stained sections and the block can readily be supplied. Snap-frozen and electron microscopy–fixed tissue can be held until questions of histologic diagnosis are resolved. It then can be discarded or placed in formalin and processed into paraffin.

CLINICAL INDICATIONS AND BIOPSY INTERPRETATION

Other than liver biopsy after liver or bone marrow transplantation (see Chapter 39), pediatric liver biopsies generally are done to evaluate a small number of conditions, including the following:

- Conjugated hyperbilirubinemia in the young infant, several weeks after birth
- Tumor (see Chapter 42)
- Liver injury, inflammation, and fibrosis in older children

The most common indication for pediatric liver biopsy at the Institute of Liver Studies is conjugated hyperbilirubinemia in the infant several weeks after birth. At this age, extrahepatic biliary atresia (EHBA) is effectively the one condition underlying conjugated hyperbilirubinemia that is potentially amenable to surgical palliation. Choledochal cysts that produce jaundice shortly after birth are exceptionally rare and are diagnosed by imaging studies, not by liver biopsy. EHBA must be recognized quickly if hepatic portoenterostomy is to succeed in reestablishing biliary drainage.[2] Biopsy specimens from such patients sometimes are obtained before results are available from noninvasive studies, such as protease inhibitor typing to assess the possibility of A1ATSD.

A smaller but substantial portion of our workload relates to primary diagnosis of tumor and assessments of liver injury, inflammation, and fibrosis in older children. When liver disease is manifest after the neonatal period, clinical studies generally identify a cause for liver disease before biopsy is completed. Usual causes include hepatitis B virus or hepatitis C virus infection, inherited storage disorders, steatosis, ATP7B disease (Wilson's disease), drug- or autoimmunity-associated disease, and cholangiopathy, although, on occasion, we are asked to evaluate liver tissue from a child with portal hypertension in whom none of these conditions is strongly suspected.

As a result, and if practice at King's College Hospital can be taken as a guide, pediatric liver biopsy usually is performed not to answer the question "What is it?" but to find the answer to the question "How bad is it?" Even when EHBA is suspected, the primary question to be answered is "Are the findings more compatible with EHBA than with another disorder?" Data to which clinical colleagues have access will likely help narrow the list of potential diagnoses. For best results, accordingly, pediatric liver biopsy specimens should be interpreted only after review with the treating physician of clinical, imaging, and laboratory studies. Similarly, although findings in pediatric liver biopsy specimens may contribute to management decisions, they are unlikely to be the only factors considered when such decisions are made.

NORMAL AND POTENTIALLY MISLEADING FEATURES OF THE LIVER IN INFANTS AND CHILDREN

Although many features of the livers of infants and children are the same as those of the livers of adolescents and adults, some differ. These differences can lead to misinterpretation. They fall into several categories, among them architecture, cellular populations, hepatocyte contents, and responses to injury.

Architecture

The liver grows with the child. From birth at term to age 1 month, the liver doubles in weight; it doubles again by age 12 months.[3] The dimensions of the hepatic lobule remain constant as an infant grows, but hepatocyte cords may be two cells thick into the fourth postnatal year. This "hyperplasia" is physiologic. It is to be distinguished from regenerative hyperplasia in settings of fibrosis, inflammation, and abnormal vascular supply.

Cellular Populations

Hematopoietic elements are commonly seen in liver biopsy specimens taken during the first postnatal months. Granulopoiesis tends to predominate in portal tracts, erythropoiesis in the lobule. These elements are to be distinguished from inflammatory infiltrates.

Hepatocyte Contents

First, the term infant liver normally may contain copper-binding protein and copper (demonstrable by either the orcein or the rhodanine technique, respectively) and granules of hemosiderin in periportal hepatocytes, especially until a postnatal age of approximately 3 months. These are dispersed as the infant grows. These deposits are physiologic. Not until well past the neonatal period can they be adduced as evidence for iron storage disease or cholangiopathy. Second, hepatocyte alterations in various storage disorders may be inconspicuous in early infancy by comparison with those in later infancy or childhood (as in A1ATSD, discussed later).

The one exception to this statement about physiologic iron deposition occurs in the newborn child presenting with liver failure attributable to severe liver injury in utero. Marked iron deposits may be present in hepatocytes, giving rise to the term *neonatal iron storage disease*, or *neonatal hemochromatosis*.[4] Severe fibrosis also is invariably present in this condition. Extrahepatic iron accumulation spares the reticuloendothelial system.[5] The finding of perinatal siderosis is nonspecific and only points to the development of severe liver injury during gestation. Notably, when

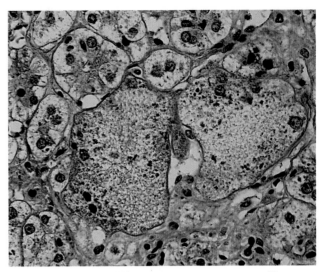

FIGURE 41–1. Giant cell hepatocyte, present in neonatal hepatitis. Masson's trichrome stain.

measured by quantitative chemical analysis, the amount of iron present in the liver is not increased.[6]

Responses to Injury

"Giant cell" hepatocytes containing bile pigment are commonly found in infants with liver disease of various causes and are by themselves not specific for cause. They are formed by breakdown of cell/cell borders, generally with partial preservation of canalicular aspects (Fig. 41-1).[7] This finding can persist well into childhood when liver disease of neonatal onset does not resolve. Although unusual in adults, giant cell change of hepatocytes is associated with autoimmune disease.[8] This association is not present in early infancy but can manifest in early childhood.[9]

Observation of a few scattered hepatocytes with three or four nuclei does not warrant assigning the diagnosis of giant cell hepatitis (GCH) in a young child with a clinical diagnosis of neonatal hepatitis (NH). Rather, the histologic findings in the spectrum of disorders known as NH/GCH includes giant cell change of hepatocytes, intralobular cholestasis, necrosis of hepatocytes, and intrahepatic hematopoiesis. NH/GCH is a nonspecific change in infancy that can be found in EHBA, A1ATSD, and many other conditions. An underlying cause should be carefully excluded before the nonspecific pathologic designation NH/GCH is given.

PRINCIPLES OF DIAGNOSIS

Liver disease in infancy often (but not always) manifests as cholestasis with conjugated hyperbilirubinemia. This tendency, even in disorders that in later life are hepatitic rather than cholestatic, is generally ascribed to the immaturity in early life of hepatic secretory and excretory functions. Lists of disorders that present with infantile conjugated hyperbilirubinemia, when comprehensive, are long indeed and are available elsewhere.[1,10] These include infections, mitochondriopathies, metabolic disorders primarily affecting either intrahepatic or extrahepatic functions, toxic hepatopathies, and syndromes with mechanisms not yet classified.[11,12] Most important clinically is to distinguish obstructive (extrahepatic) cholestasis, which often can be palliated to good long-term effect, from cholestasis of other causes. In practice, this means recognizing EHBA.

EXTRAHEPATIC BILIARY ATRESIA

EHBA accounts for more than 30% of all neonates presenting with cholestasis. Its incidence is 1 in 10,000 live births; it usually occurs on a sporadic basis without a family history. Infants with EHBA are of normal gestational age and birth weight and look well except for cholestatic jaundice, which brings them for medical attention in the first few weeks of life. Clinical biochemistry indices of hepatobiliary injury fit no specific pattern. Serum concentrations of gamma-glutamyl-transpeptidase activity are an exception; if these are not elevated, obstructive cholestasis is not a consideration. Ultrasonography must be performed to exclude biliary tract anomalies such as choledochal cyst. Percutaneous liver biopsy is then justified to determine whether histologic features of large bile duct obstruction are present.

Pathology

The usual pattern of findings in EHBA in the infantile liver is well described.[13] Nonspecific changes include parenchymal cholestasis, with giant cell trans-

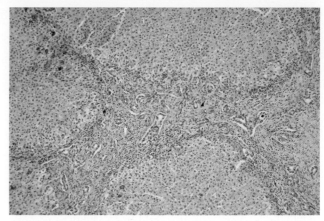

FIGURE 41–2. The portal tract in extrahepatic biliary atresia, demonstrating increased numbers of bile duct profiles and severe cholestasis in the periportal parenchyma.

formation in 15% of cases. Diagnostic findings include bile plugs within bile duct lumina (as distinct from the lumina of neocholangioles at the margins of portal tracts) and increased numbers of bile duct profiles (Fig. 41-2).[14] Although these features may strongly suggest EHBA, they are not pathognomonic because portal tracts in A1ATSD (and, more rarely, in neonatal sclerosing cholangitis) can appear similar. Edema and sparse acute inflammation in portal tracts are to be expected, as is relatively slight lobular disarray.

Extensive lobular disease, more characteristic of NH without or with giant cells (GCH), can be seen in EHBA (Fig 41-3). Indeed, EHBA and NH/GCH have been thought to represent points on a continuum of manifestations of the same disorder.[15] Lobular changes should not be allowed to distract attention from portal tract features. Moreover, nonclassic features of EHBA, in

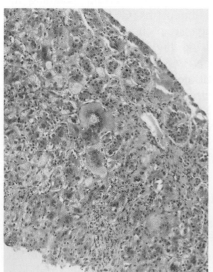

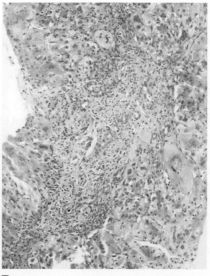

FIGURE 41–3. A, Lobular changes of "neonatal hepatitis" in EHBA. Marked lobular disarray with giant cell transformation is present. **B,** Portal tract of same patient, with bile plug *(lower left of center),* edema, and proliferated ductules. Periportal hepatocytes are not steatotic.

A   **B**

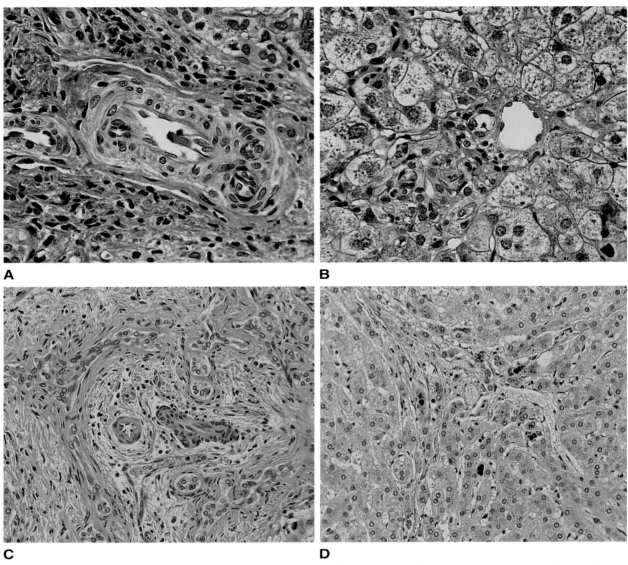

FIGURE 41–4. Nonclassic features of portal tracts in EHBA. **A,** Arterial hypertrophy, without an accompanying interlobular bile duct. **B,** Portal tract with no interlobular bile duct, but otherwise unremarkable (Masson's trichome). **C,** Ductal plate malformation with fibrosed portal tract, centrally located hepatic arteries, and a peripheral rim of ductular structures. **D,** Lack of bile plugs and lack of proliferated ducts (*second* biopsy specimen; obtained at age 8 weeks because findings on initial biopsy [at age 6½ weeks] suggested neonatal hepatitis); exploratory laparotomy and cholangiography were required for definitive diagnosis.

which loss of intrahepatic bile ducts is seen rather than proliferation, may be noted on initial percutaneous liver biopsy, confusing the histologic picture (Fig. 41-4).[14,16,17]

The accuracy of percutaneous liver biopsy in the diagnosis of EHBA is reported as 60% to 95%, "depending on the skill of the pathologist."[17] This skill appears to be a matter not only of slide interpretation but also of liaison with clinical colleagues in that the classic obstructive findings of bile duct proliferation and inspissated bile plugs are encountered in only 65% of biopsies[13,17]; the other 35% have features more suggestive of NH/GCH. EHBA can be exceedingly difficult to diagnose, even for the most experienced pediatric hepatopathologist. Each author of this chapter can cite recent personal cases in which diagnosis (and treat-

ment) of EHBA was delayed because of the absence of clearly diagnostic features in percutaneous liver biopsy material.

The decision to proceed to biliary tract exploration in a young infant for possible hepatic portoenterostomy does not rest only on histopathologic findings in a liver biopsy specimen. Acholic stools, irregular contours of the gallbladder on sonographic study, and findings on endoscopic choledochography all may indicate that EHBA is present. Even the argument that liver biopsy is superfluous to diagnosis can be made. The opinion that "it is preferable to err on the side of overdiagnosis of the surgical disorders"[18]—the disorders in which conjugated hyperbilirubinemia of infancy can be palliated by surgery—perhaps overestimates the role of the pathologist and may no longer be tenable. "Features compatible with distal biliary tract obstruction" is a diagnostic formulation often used at the Institute of Liver Studies.

Differential Diagnosis

If EHBA can be reasonably excluded on the basis of clinical findings and percutaneous liver biopsy, further evaluation of the specimen and of the patient is best conducted in referral because the list of conditions to be considered is overwhelmingly long. Review of several other conditions is in order, however, for the non-specialist pathologist who reviews pediatric liver biopsy materials in conducting triage.

ALPHA-1-ANTITRYPSIN STORAGE DISORDER (A1ATSD) AT PRESENTATION IN INFANCY

This disorder is discussed more thoroughly under Alpha-1-Antitrypsin Storage Disease. Two aspects of liver biopsy specimens from infants with A1ATSD and conjugated hyperbilirubinemia can be particularly misleading. The globules of d-PAS–staining material in periportal hepatocytes that characterize livers from children and adults with A1ATSD are not recognizable in early infancy. Bile pigment, hemosiderin, and copper-binding protein all can be found in periportal hepatocytes. On d-PAS staining, all mark as fine granules. Scanty accumulations of alpha-1-antitrypsin (A1AT) cannot be distinguished against this background,[19] so that A1ATSD must be excluded definitively by protease inhibitor typing. At the Institute of Liver Studies, immunohistochemical demonstration of A1AT, using

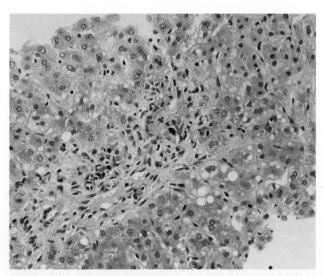

FIGURE 41–5. Portal tract in alpha-1-antitrypsin storage disorder. Macrovesicular steatosis of periportal hepatocytes is present. A bile plug suggests distal obstruction.

antibodies against usual A1AT or against the Z variant, has not been of value in early infancy.

A1ATSD also can mimic EHBA convincingly with portal tract changes that include edema, scant acute inflammation, proliferated bile ductules, and bile plugs within bile duct lumina (Fig 41-5). Periportal macro-vesicular steatosis in the infant with neonatal hepatitis is a tip-off that A1ATSD may be present,[20] although this association does not permit firm distinctions when phenotypes otherwise largely overlap.

PAUCITY OF INTRAHEPATIC (INTERLOBULAR) BILE DUCTS

Some instances of conjugated hyperbilirubinemia of infancy (and later childhood) are associated with a complex of cardiac, vertebral, and ocular malformations. Interlobular bile ducts may be present early in the course of the disorder but may not be demonstrable on follow-up biopsy.[21] This combination of extrahepatic abnormalities and deficiency of interlobular bile ducts is known as Alagille syndrome.

Although no significant portal tract inflammation is typically seen, the findings in liver biopsy specimens from patients with Alagille syndrome otherwise cannot be distinguished from those in liver biopsy specimens from patients who lack bile ducts for other reasons. Various infective, metabolic, and endocrine disorders are associated with conjugated hyperbilirubinemia and deficiency of interlobular bile ducts. An example is A1ATSD, as shown in Figure 41-6. The normal ratio of bile ducts to interlobular portal tracts is 9:10,[22-24] so that a finding of only four bile ducts among five portal tracts may point toward the possibility of paucity of interlobular bile ducts. In Alagille syndrome, bile duct loss may worsen over time, and rebiopsy may demonstrate that disease has progressed.[25] When sections are assessed, large portal tracts and their bile ducts should not be considered, nor should incomplete portal tracts whose margins were transected by the biopsy trocar.

It is important to note that initial criteria for bile duct enumeration were established before immunohisto-chemical staining for bile duct cytokeratins became widely available.[23] A subsequent morphologic study specifically used routine stains to ensure relevance to examination of routine sections.[22] The reported ratio of nine bile ducts to ten portal tracts therefore does not take into account hypoplastic interlobular ducts that often can be detected as threadlike or single-cell structures in sections immunostained for cytokeratins,[26] although they are not apparent in routinely stained parallel sections. Distinctions between *paucity* and *hypoplasia* of interlobular bile ducts also are not clearly drawn; paucity may be present in H&E-stained sections, and cytokeratin immunostaining demonstrates hypoplasia. Caution and precision are recommended in

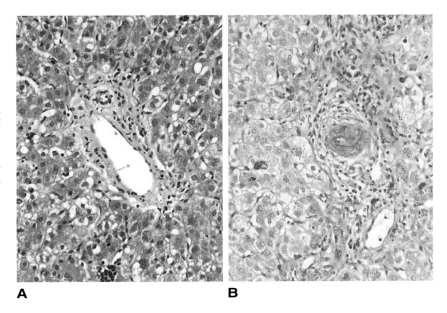

FIGURE 41–6. Portal tracts in alpha-1-antitrypsin storage disorder, showing paucity of interlobular bile ducts in evolution. **A,** Cross section of portal space lacking bile duct. **B,** Cross section of portal space in which bile duct obliteration by fibrous reaction is apparent (diastase–periodic acid–Schiff [d-PAS]).

the use of these terms; any report should stipulate how bile ducts and portal tracts were counted.

Paucity of interlobular bile ducts, like NH/GCH, is not a diagnosis so much as an observation. As with NH/GCH, the observation should prompt careful evaluation for potential underlying disorders.

SUMMARY

Diagnosis in pediatric liver biopsy specimens depends on close communication with clinical staff. This is necessary to ensure both that biopsy specimens are handled without precluding certain approaches to diagnosis and that interpretations issued take into account clinical information of significance. The pathologist should be acquainted with usual features of the normal liver in infancy and childhood and with specifically pediatric patterns of reaction to injury. Biopsy materials should readily be referred for consultation.

▮ Inherited Metabolic Disease in the Adolescent and Adult

Three inherited metabolic disorders known to present in adolescence or adulthood must be understood by every pathologist who examines liver biopsy specimens. These are HFE disease (hereditary hemochromatosis, type 1), ATP7B disease (Wilson's disease), and A1ATSD. The approaches to sampling at liver biopsy and to specimen processing that are described earlier for pediatric specimens enable the most complete analysis of these three disorders; however, specimen procurement for adolescents and adults rarely involves detailed

bedside processing of the specimen. Hence, the pathologist may need to alert the performing physician of necessary special processing, preferably in advance of performance of the liver biopsy. Specific points for attention and possible sources of diagnostic error are presented in the following section.

HFE DISEASE (HEREDITARY HEMOCHROMATOSIS, TYPE 1)

The total body iron pool ranges from 2 to 6 g in normal adults; about 0.5 g is stored in the liver, 98% of which is found in hepatocytes. *Hemochromatosis* is defined as excessive accumulation of body iron, most of which is deposited in parenchymal organs such as the liver and pancreas. Because humans do not have a major excretory pathway for iron, hemochromatosis either results from a genetic defect causing excessive iron absorption or is acquired as a consequence of parenteral administration of iron (usually in the form of transfusions). *Hereditary hemochromatosis*, also now called HFE disease, is a homozygous recessive inherited disorder, in which total body iron accumulation may exceed 50 g. Dysregulation of enteric iron absorption in hereditary hemochromatosis leads to accumulation of iron over decades, first in liver and then in extrahepatic sites. Symptoms do not usually occur until the fifth or sixth decade of life, when they manifest with the severe consequences of cardiomyopathy, diabetes mellitus, cirrhosis, and, potentially, hepatocellular carcinoma.

In Western European populations, specific mutations in the *HFE* gene underlie the inherited dysregulation of enteric iron uptake, in which iron is absorbed in excess of body needs. HFE, a major histocompatibility complex (MHC)-like protein encoded by the *HFE* gene, and β_2-microglobulin form a complex in the basolateral membrane of the duodenal crypt precursor of the absorptive enterocyte. In the presence of several specific mutations in *HFE*, through mechanisms not yet well understood, this regulatory complex fails to appropriately program the absorption of iron from the gut lumen for throughput into portal venous plasma. Absorption of iron is not downregulated when systemic iron stores are adequate or high, leading to progressive body iron loading. The most common protein mutation identified in HFE disease is C282Y (tyrosine for cytosine, amino acid 282), caused by the nucleotide substitution G845A (adenine for guanine, nucleotide 845); it is found in more than 70% of patients with clinically diagnosed nontransfusional iron overload. The mutation is common in Northern European populations, in which the prevalence of homozygosity is approximately 1 of 220, and that of heterozygosity is approximately 1 of 9. Analyses to detect this mutation are commercially available.

Iron toxicity causes fibrosis and dysfunction; in the pituitary, this manifests as hypogonadism; in the synovium, as arthritis; in the heart, as cardiomyopathy; in the pancreas, as diabetes; in the skin, as pigmentation; and in the liver, as a micronodular cirrhosis with an attendant risk of hepatocellular carcinoma. Screening for iron overload, which begins with assessment of serum indices of iron-binding capacity and content, can be supplemented by magnetic resonance imaging studies of parenchymal organs. Although general population screening for molecular mutations is feasible and is worth considering given the prevalence of the C282Y mutation, penetrance of iron overloading reportedly occurs in only 20% of homozygotes.[27] Hence, liver biopsy remains the single most important diagnostic test for HFE disease. Liver biopsy may be prompted by elevations in serum indices of iron content or in serum aminotransferases that are found during routine examination or during the evaluation of general malaise. Alternatively, more specific symptomatology, as from frank portal hypertension, may prompt liver biopsy.

Pathologic Features

In the liver, iron becomes evident first as golden-yellow hemosiderin granules in the cytoplasm of periportal hepatocytes (Fig. 41-7**A**) because they are the first exposed to excessive iron in portal blood. These hepatocytes take up iron and store it first as dispersed hemosiderin within the cytoplasm and ultimately as hemosiderin granules within lysosomes. Because lysosomes are distributed predominantly in the subapical region of hepatocytes, a pericanalicular localization of the lysosomal hemosiderin granules occurs; these granules stain blue with the Prussian blue stain. Hence, a chickenwire-like distribution of Prussian blue–positive granules within periportal hepatocytes is the first histologic indication of HFE disease (Fig. 41-7**B**).

With increasing iron load, progressive involvement of the rest of the lobule is noted, along with accumulation of hemosiderin granules in bile duct epithelium and in Kupffer cells. This occurs in contradistinction to transfusional iron overload, in which Kupffer cells are the first to accumulate iron, followed by hepatocytes. Assuming that the observed Prussian blue–reactive iron is predominantly hepatocellular, a five-point semi-quantitative scale can be used to grade the intensity of stainable iron deposits from 0 (none) through 4 (extending throughout the lobule, visible as clumps, and dispersed within hepatocytes[28]). Siderosis should be mentioned in the biopsy report, as should suggested evaluation for systemic iron overloading (quantitation of

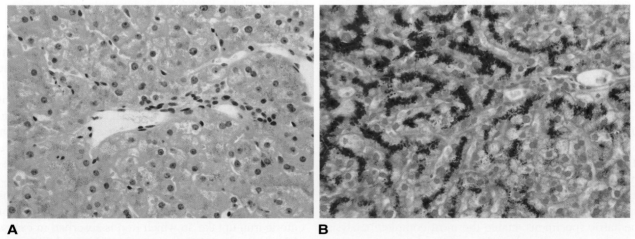

A   **B**

FIGURE 41–7. HFE disease (hereditary hemochromatosis). **A,** Pericanalicular brown granules in periportal hepatocytes. **B,** Same specimen stained with Prussian blue stain, demonstrating strong blue color of the pericanalicular hemosiderin granules.

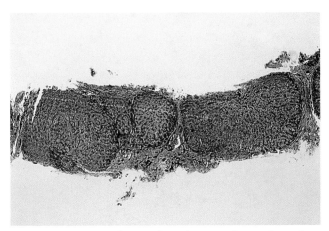

FIGURE 41–8. HFE disease, liver biopsy. This cirrhotic liver demonstrates extensive iron deposition by Prussian blue stain.

serum transferrin saturation and serum ferritin concentrations, if not already performed) and *HFE* analysis in the patient and in his or her near relatives.

Iron is a direct hepatotoxin, and inflammation is characteristically absent. Fibrous septa develop slowly, leading ultimately to a micronodular pattern of cirrhosis in an intensely pigmented liver (Fig. 41-8). Notably, the presence of inflammation of any sort, such as mononuclear infiltrates in portal tracts, should prompt consideration of coexistent causes of chronic liver disease.

Biochemical determination of hepatic iron concentration in unfixed tissue is the standard for quantitating hepatic iron content. In normal individuals, the iron content of unfixed liver tissue is less than 1000 µg per 1 g dry weight of liver. Adult patients with HFE disease exhibit more than 10,000 µg iron/1 g dry weight; hepatic iron concentrations in excess of 22,000 µg/g dry weight are associated with the development of fibrosis and cirrhosis. Because iron accumulation is lifelong, an *iron index* is also employed, in which quantitative iron content is divided by the patient's age as a guide to the probability of HFE disease.[29] Although liver tissue may be excavated from a paraffin block for quantitative iron analysis (a not uncommon request after the biopsy tissue has been processed), leaching of iron from the liver tissue during processing may introduce error into the quantitative iron measurement. Moreover, molecular analysis of tissue retrieved from the paraffin block may well become the new standard for diagnosis of HFE disease.[30,31]

The most common causes of *secondary hemochromatosis* are the hemolytic anemias associated with ineffective erythropoiesis. In these disorders, excess iron accumulation results not only from transfusions but also from increased intestinal iron absorption. Transfusions alone as a cause of systemic siderosis, as in aplastic anemias, lead to parenchymal organ injury only in extreme cases. *Alcoholic cirrhosis* is often associated

with a modest increase in stainable iron within liver cells and should not be misinterpreted as HFE disease. However, this iron accumulation represents alcohol-induced redistribution of iron because total body iron is not significantly increased. A rather unusual form of iron overload resembling HFE disease occurs in sub-Saharan Africa; it results from ingestion of large quantities of alcoholic beverages fermented in iron utensils (Bantu siderosis). Home brewing in steel drums continues to this day, and a genetic susceptibility in this population has been identified.[32] Neonatal iron storage disorder has been discussed earlier.

Heterozygotes for *HFE* mutations are not generally thought to cause liver disease, although their hepatic iron levels approach levels intermediate between normal and those of homozygotes over the lifetime of the individual. However, about a third of heterozygotes develop some degree of liver fibrosis.[33] Increased iron may also exacerbate liver injury from coexistent hepatitis C infection or alcoholic liver disease, but it does not appear to worsen the severity of nonalcoholic steatohepatitis.[34]

Differential Diagnosis

Identification of granular brown pigment in the hepatocytes of an uninflamed liver generates a small differential diagnosis—iron versus lipofuscin, bile pigment, or Dubin-Johnson pigment.

First, exclusion of bile pigment is readily achieved by lowering the condenser of the microscope to determine whether the pigment is refractile; bile is not, whereas lipofuscin and hemosiderin are refractile. Bile pigment in a cholestatic hepatocyte is also distributed in a floccular fashion throughout the cytoplasm and is not localized to the pericanalicular region. Bile accumulates in the canalicular space, even in nonobstructive cholestasis. Bile does not stain blue on Prussian blue stain. It does stain green on Hall's stain.

Second, lipofuscin accumulates predominantly in pericentral hepatocytes unlike iron, which accumulates first in periportal hepatocytes (Fig. 41-9). Therefore, the presence of pericentral granular brown pigment in hepatocytes without evident granular pigment in periportal hepatocytes essentially excludes iron. Of course, lipofuscin does not stain blue on Prussian blue stain.

Third, in Dubin-Johnson syndrome, a benign autosomal recessive condition in which biliary secretion of bilirubin pigments is defective, hepatocytes contain multiple large, nonrefractile globular inclusions containing dark brown pigment (Fig. 41-10). It is curious that this pigment appears to comprise polymers of epinephrine, rather than bilirubin pigment.[35] Usually, no clinical difficulty is associated with identification in jaundiced individuals with Dubin-Johnson syndrome.

The key differential diagnosis depends on distinguishing HFE disease from secondary iron overload. As

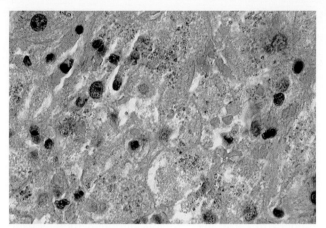

FIGURE 41–9. Brown granules of lipofuscin in pericentral hepatocytes.

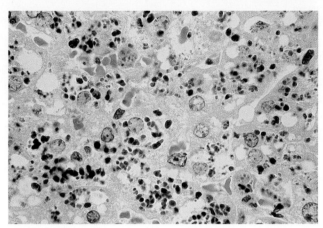

FIGURE 41–10. Dubin Johnson syndrome, showing large non-refractile globular inclusions within hepatocytes.

has been noted, the latter features accumulation of hemosiderin in Kupffer cells with later spillover into hepatocytes; HFE disease exhibits only a minor component of Kupffer cell siderosis, even in the end-stage cirrhotic liver. The non-HFE disease reticuloendothelial pattern reliably predicts the absence of homozygosity for the C282Y mutation (Fig. 41-11).[36] Finally, inflammation seen in the hemochromatotic liver points to an additional cause of liver injury.

Clinical Features

HFE disease is autosomal recessive and hence has no sex predominance; however, clinical and histologic evidence of tissue injury is more common at any given age among men than among women. This reflects physiologic iron losses in women through the menses and transfer of iron to the conceptus during gestation. The clinical manifestations of HFE disease generally are first apparent in the fifth decade—with the sex proviso as described—and these manifestations result from end-stage parenchymal disease. Death in HFE disease may result from cirrhosis or cardiac disease. A significant cause of death is hepatocellular carcinoma; the risk is 200-fold greater than in the general population, and treatment for iron overload does not remove the risk for this aggressive neoplasm. Hepatocellular carcinoma can occur in patients who have been successfully treated by phlebotomy with normalization of their systemic iron levels, and even in those whose cirrhosis has been reversed.[37]

Given these severe outcomes of HFE disease and the ease of treatment with phlebotomy, earlier liver biopsy offers the opportunity to diagnose abnormal iron loading and to intervene, with phlebotomy, in the natural course of the disease. Siblings of a proband should be genetically evaluated. Given the high incidence of the C282Y mutation in Northern European populations,

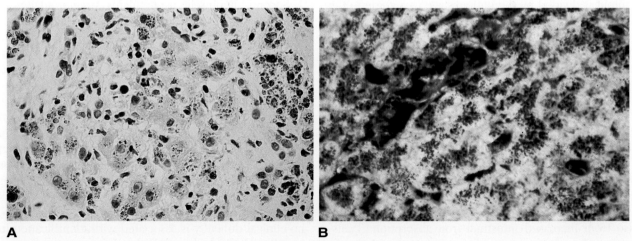

A   **B**

FIGURE 41–11. Liver in secondary iron overload. **A,** Large, dense brown granules of hemosiderin are present in Kupffer cells; smaller granules are present in hepatocytes. **B,** Dense Kupffer cell iron deposition is seen along with hepatocellular deposition; this is the "reticuloendothelial" pattern of iron deposition (Prussian blue stain).

such evaluation may be appropriate for parents and children of a proband as well. Whether liver biopsy is appropriate in persons known to be homozygous for the C282Y mutation who have clinical biochemistry evidence of iron overload (i.e., high serum concentrations of ferritin, high serum transferrin saturation) for the assessment of fibrosis and siderosis remains a matter for debate.

ATP7B DISEASE (WILSON'S DISEASE)

This autosomal recessive disorder is marked by the accumulation of toxic levels of copper in many tissues and organs, principally the liver, brain, and eye. The gene for Wilson's disease, designated *ATP7B*, is found on chromosome 13 and encodes a 7.5-kB transcript for a transmembrane copper-transporting ATPase, located on the hepatocyte canalicular membrane.[38] More than 30 mutations in this gene have been identified, effectively excluding currently available screening approaches for identifying the disorder. *An overwhelming majority of patients are compound heterozygotes containing different mutations of the Wilson's disease gene on each allele.* Other than inbred "carrier populations," the frequency of mutated alleles is 1 in 200, engendering a prevalence of the disease of approximately 1 in 30,000 to 1 in 50,000. Clinically significant mutations disable the canalicular membrane copper-exporting ATPase that *ATP7B* encodes, thereby leading to accumulation of copper in hepatocyte cytoplasm. This copper is segregated in lysosomal complexes with metallothioneins. These sulfhydryl-rich proteins (copper-binding proteins) can be identified as black-brown flecks in orcein-stained sections; the copper bound to them appears as red-orange flecks in rhodanine-stained sections. Both the copper-binding proteins and copper appear earliest in periportal hepatocytes and ultimately throughout the lobule. When the capacity to segregate copper within the liver is exceeded, spillover from the liver and damage at extrahepatic sites begin. Parkinsonism or behavioral changes that can amount to psychosis, which can be caused by accumulations of copper in the brain, are the first sign of disease in some patients. Liver dysfunction in ATP7B disease is most commonly identified as an increase in serum concentrations of transaminase activity, which in our experience is noted at the time of an intercurrent illness. This then prompts liver biopsy.

Pathologic Features

The liver often bears the brunt of injury in Wilson's disease; hepatic changes range from relatively minor to massive damage. Fatty changes may be mild to moderate with vacuolated nuclei (glycogen or water) and occasional hepatocyte focal necrosis. An acute hepatitis can exhibit features mimicking acute viral hepatitis, save possibly for the accompanying fatty change. The chronic hepatitis of Wilson's disease exhibits moderate to severe inflammation and hepatocyte necrosis, with the particular features of macrovesicular steatosis, vacuolated hepatocellular nuclei, and Mallory bodies (Fig. 41-12). With progression of chronic hepatitis, cirrhosis develops. Massive liver necrosis is a rare manifestation that is indistinguishable from that caused by viruses or drugs. Excessive copper deposition can often be demonstrated by special stains (rhodanine stain for copper, orcein stain for copper-associated

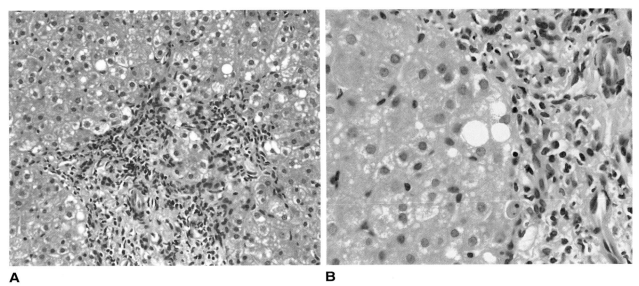

A   **B**

FIGURE 41–12. Wilson's disease, showing the characteristic (but not specific) chronic hepatitis. **A,** Portal tract, with mild inflammation and mild interface hepatitis. Hepatocytes exhibit focal macrovesicular steatosis. **B,** Portal tract interface, showing an apoptotic hepatocyte.

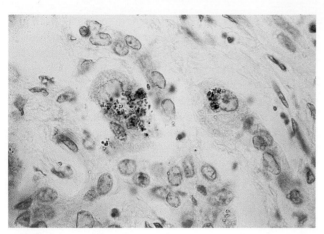

FIGURE 41–13. Wilson disease, showing retained copper within hepatocytes (rhodanine stain).

protein). Because copper also accumulates in chronic obstructive cholestasis, and because histology cannot reliably distinguish Wilson's disease from virus- and drug-induced hepatitis, demonstration of hepatic copper content in excess of 250 µg/1 g dry weight is most helpful in diagnosis. It is important to note that assessment of hepatic copper content can be performed only on fresh liver tissue obtained with a needle that has been rinsed with chelating solution before use to remove trace copper levels.

The finding of chronic hepatitis with fibrosis and steatosis on liver biopsy, particularly in children 5 years of age through adolescence, requires action. First, these findings in a child require specific histochemical evaluation for copper (rhodanine stain, Fig. 41-13) and metallothioneins (orcein stain). Second, because copper and metallothionein are not always histochemically demonstrable, these findings must also prompt an attempt to identify copper overload clinically (e.g., urinary excretion before and after administration of chelators); a comment to this effect in the biopsy report is appropriate.

Differential Diagnosis

ATP7B disease can present clinically in the second decade of life with moderate to severe chronic hepatitis or fully developed cirrhosis. By the third decade of life, severe fibrosis and/or cirrhosis is the most common. Hence, ATP7B disease must be included in the differential diagnosis of virtually every case of chronic hepatitis presenting in the second to fourth decades of life. Identification of steatosis, Mallory bodies, and hepatitis with chronic inflammation and fibrosis, although attributable to other causes such as alcohol, should especially prompt consideration of ATP7B disease. Presentation and diagnosis of ATP7B disease beyond the fourth decade are rare; therefore, this disease falls off the list of differential diagnoses.

Clinical Features

The age at onset and the clinical presentation of Wilson's disease are extremely variable, but the disorder rarely manifests before 6 years of age. The most common presentation is acute or chronic liver disease. Neuropsychiatric manifestations, including mild behavioral changes, frank psychosis, or a Parkinson's disease–like syndrome, are the initial features in most remaining cases.

Diagnosis of ATP7B disease is important because chelation of copper by drugs excreted in the urine can halt or reverse damage in probands. Siblings of persons in whom the diagnosis is made also should be evaluated. Ceruloplasmin concentrations in serum often are low in ATP7B disease for reasons that are not known. However, because inflammation may elevate serum concentrations of acute phase reactants, including ceruloplasmin, normal serum concentrations of ceruloplasmin do not exclude ATP7B disease from consideration. Quantitation of copper excretion in urine and, if possible, of copper in liver tissue is the approach that is considered definitive. The advantage of systematically snap-freezing aliquots of liver biopsy specimens again is apparent in that this may permit tissue copper studies even if ATP7B disease was not considered before biopsy—chelation of environmental copper notwithstanding.

ALPHA-1-ANTITRYPSIN STORAGE DISEASE (A1ATSD)

Alpha-1-antitrypsin deficiency is an autosomal recessive disorder marked by abnormally low serum levels of this major protease inhibitor. The major function of this protein is the inhibition of proteases, particularly the normal process of neutrophil release of elastase, cathepsin G, and proteinase 3 at sites of inflammation. Alpha-1-antitrypsin deficiency leads to the development of pulmonary emphysema because a relative lack of this protein permits tissue-destructive enzymes to run amok.

A1AT is a small, 394–amino acid plasma glycoprotein synthesized predominantly by hepatocytes. The encoding gene, *SERPINA1*, is located on human chromosome 14 and is polymorphic. At least 75 A1AT forms have been identified, denoted alphabetically by their relative migration on an isoelectric gel. The general notation is *Pi* for *protease inhibitor* and an alphabetic letter for the migration position on the gel; two letters denote the genotype of the two alleles. The most common genotype is PiMM, occurring in 90% of individuals (in the traditional sense, this would be the wild-type genotype). Most allelic variants exhibit conservative substitutions in the polypeptide chain and produce normally functioning levels of A1AT. Some deficiency variants, including the PiS variant, result in a reduction in serum concentrations of A1AT without clinical manifestations. Rare variants called *Pi-null* have no detectable serum

A1AT. The most common clinically relevant genetic mutation is PiZ; homozygotes for the PiZ protein (designated PiZZ homozygotes) have circulating A1AT levels that are only 10% of normal levels. Affected individuals are at high risk for developing pulmonary disease.

Expression of alleles is autosomal codominant; consequently, PiMZ heterozygotes have intermediate plasma levels of A1AT. The gene frequency of PiZ is 0.0122 in the North American white population, yielding a PiZZ genotype frequency of approximately 1 in 7000. However, because of the frequency of earlier presentation when compared with HFE disease, A1ATSD is the most commonly diagnosed genetic liver disease in infants and children.

The liver synthesizes A1AT for secretion into plasma, but it does not require A1AT for its own function. However, the gene defects that lead to defective secretion of A1AT may be accompanied by excessive accumulation of abnormal A1AT peptides in hepatocytes. Specifically, patients with mutated A1AT exhibit a selective defect in movement of this secretory protein from the endoplasmic reticulum (ER) to the Golgi apparatus; this event is most marked for the PiZ polypeptide, attributable to a single amino acid substitution of Glu_{342} to Lys_{342}. The mutant polypeptide is abnormally folded, blocking its movement along the remainder of the secretory pathway. All individuals with the PiZZ genotype accumulate A1AT in the ER of hepatocytes, but not all manifest liver disease. Those who have additional defects in the degradation of retained proteins in the ER are at risk for development of liver disease.[39] Hence, the hepatic disease is better referred to as *alpha-1-antitrypsin storage disease (A1ATSD)* and will be so named for the remainder of this discussion.

Pathologic Features

Accumulated A1AT within endoplasmic reticulum of hepatocytes can cause hepatocellular injury; such disease is most frequent with homozygosity for the *SERPINA1* Z (PiZ) mutation. In about 10% to 20% of affected infants,[40] this takes the form of a cholestatic hepatitis of infancy resembling neonatal hepatitis or biliary atresia, with bile ductular proliferation, hepatocellular and canalicular cholestasis, and occasionally giant cell transformation of hepatocytes and hepatocyte rosetting.[41] Up to 10% of these young patients may demonstrate paucity of intrahepatic bile ducts and a patent but narrow extrahepatic biliary tree by cholangiogram. The diagnostic globules of A1AT may not be prominent in the young child, leading to potential misdiagnosis of this disorder. As noted in the discussion under Alpha-1-Antitrypsin Storage Disorder (A1ATSD) at Presentation in Infancy, periportal macrovesicular steatosis in the infant with neonatal hepatitis should prompt serologic or genotypic consideration of A1ATSD.[20]

Many persons with the PiZZ serotype, however, do not become ill as infants and may instead present with cirrhosis in their fourth decade or even later. Moreover, after early infancy, globules of A1AT retained within cytoplasm are easily found in periportal hepatocytes on histologic sections digested with diastase and stained with periodic acid–Schiff technique (d-PAS–stained sections; Fig. 41-14). These magenta globules increase in size with advancing patient age. Their nature can be confirmed on immunostaining for A1AT. To demonstrate A1AT within such globules in a patient with cirrhosis, however, does not permit the inference that the patient has the PiZZ serotype. Liver disease of other causes can predispose to globule formation in persons who are heterozygous for the PiZ mutation (the PiMZ genotype).[42] Genotyping, therefore, is required for

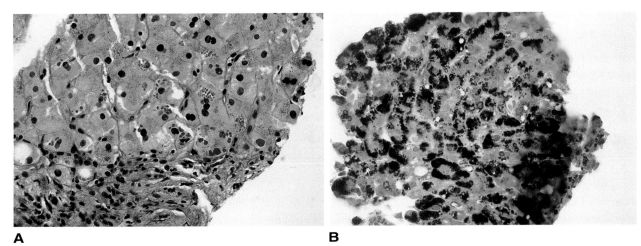

A   **B**

FIGURE 41–14. Alpha-1-antitrypsin storage disorder. **A,** Fibrotic liver, demonstrating periseptal hepatocellular globular inclusions. **B,** Same liver, with globular inclusions highlighted by immunohistochemistry for alpha-1-antitrypsin.

definitive diagnosis of Pi status and, along with sero-typing, should be suggested in the surgical pathology report when d-PAS–stained sections of liver contain characteristic globules. Congestion globules within hepatocytes, ascribed to nonspecific imbibition of plasma proteins, must be considered as possible confounders; however, they tend to occur in centrilobular regions. The rare storage disorders that mimic A1ATSD are beyond the scope of this text.

A1AT-deficient individuals who escape severe liver disease in childhood generally remain free of symptomatic liver disease until late in life,[43] although the adolescent may present with symptoms related to hepatitis or cirrhosis. By 50 years of age, an additional 20% of PiZZ individuals develop cirrhosis. The cirrhosis of the adult A1ATSD patient exhibits mixed nodule size, with variable portal inflammation containing lymphocytes and mild fat accumulation, usually in periportal hepatocytes. Necrosis of hepatocytes is not a prominent feature. Other than the A1AT globules, the features of A1ATSD are not specific.

Clinical Features

Several relevant clinical considerations have been noted in A1ATSD. First, although A1ATSD is primarily a morphologic diagnosis, A1AT deficiency is a serologic diagnosis. The two often are coupled, but they need not be; null alleles of *SERPIN1A* can lead to failure to synthesize any A1AT. A1AT then is demonstrable neither in the serum nor in hepatocytes, and no liver injury is noted (i.e., A1AT deficiency without A1ATSD). Second, regardless of the status of liver injury (because some livers may be free of significant injury), the finding of hepatocellular globular inclusions, particularly periportal ones, raises the possibility of A1AT deficiency. Deficiency of circulating A1AT carries the implied consequence of increased susceptibility to emphysema and to aneurysmal vascular disease, both of which are consequences of unchecked proteolytic activity. Hence, alerting caregivers to the possibility of A1AT deficiency is clinically important, regardless of liver status. Finally, hepatocellular carcinoma develops in 2% to 3% of PiZZ adults, usually but not always in the setting of cirrhosis. The modality for treatment and cure of severe hepatic disease at any age is orthotopic liver transplantation.

SUMMARY

That we discuss here only three inherited metabolic disorders in the adolescent and adult population is no grounds for complacency. The level of expectation that general pathologists will correctly diagnose inherited and metabolic disease involving the adolescent or adult liver is modest at present; however, we think that practitioners are likely to be held responsible soon, if

not for definitive diagnosis, then for preservation of tissue in ways that ensure that definitive diagnosis is not precluded. The standards that apply for pediatric diagnosis may well come to hold for adolescent and adult diagnosis as well. This development is due especially to recent rapid progress in human genetics. Mutations in the same gene may lead to variation in the clinical severity of a particular disorder. The more severe variants often manifest in infancy or childhood; the less severe variants in adolescence or adulthood.

Genes that underlie specific disorders that are apparent in the pediatric liver are being identified in increasing numbers, and the adult liver may soon be the beneficiary of expanded genetic insights as well. With gene identification come, in parallel, development of antibodies against gene products and reevaluation of morphologic findings in biopsy specimens with molecular/biologic correlation. These tools permit revision of diagnostic categories for greater precision. Molecular analysis is becoming the standard of practice in pediatric liver disease. It is not unreasonable to anticipate extension of such a standard to evaluation of the adolescent and adult liver.

Carrying this idea further, the diagnostic category of *cholestasis due to drug reaction*, for example, is likely to be replaced by a declaration of molecular defects in the cholestatic liver, which serve as molecular sentinels in the adult. Assigning such precise diagnostic insight will have a major impact on intervention strategies. Hence, we anticipate that evidence for abnormal distribution or regulation of various canalicular transporters[44] or for nucleotide polymorphisms associated with disease must be sought at the proteomic or genetic level. Investigational work of this sort will require forethought at the time specimens are obtained.

We believe that recent brisk advances in genomics and proteomics mean that the standard of care in histopathology practice and the quantities of resources devoted to specimen handling are certain to rise. We predict that good practice in the handling of liver biopsy specimens from adolescents and adults may well require adoption across the board of (1) snap-freezing and banking aliquots of tissue with (2) triage to specialty practitioners after preliminary evaluation, as has been recommended for pediatric specimens.

Abnormal Development of the Biliary Tract

In addition to Alagille syndrome (discussed under Paucity of Intrahepatic [Intralobar] Bile Ducts), a striking set of developmental abnormalities can affect the intrahepatic biliary tract. These are collectively referred to as *ductal plate malformations* (DPMs), based on the concept that embryologic arrest of ductal plate development is the underlying cause.[45] Distinctions between these conditions are not sharp. A spectrum of histologic abnormalities may be encountered in one patient's liver or in the livers of different family members of a proband, suggesting that the molecular origins of these conditions play a role in similar developmental pathways. The confusing and overlapping histology of these lesions may lead to misdiagnosis of cirrhosis in children and adults. It is important to note that there is a variably increased incidence of primary hepatic malignancies among patients with these conditions.[46]

VON MEYENBURG COMPLEX

A von Meyenburg complex comprises a variable number of bile ducts embedded in a fibrous, sometimes hyalinized, stroma (Fig. 41-15).[45] Each lumen may contain inspissated bile concrements, and the lumina may interconnect. These complexes, which have been described as bile duct microhamartomas,[47] are incidental findings upon examination of liver tissue. They are usually small and multiple, located in the subcapsular region and throughout both lobes of the liver.[48] It is interesting to note that they are found in the interlobular region, either in continuity with or merged into portal tracts (as seen in Fig. 41-15). Desmet[45] hypothesizes that they arise as a result of arrest or perturbation of remodeling of the ductal plates in the later phases of embryologic development of the intrahepatic biliary tract. Von Meyenburg complexes are often seen as incidental lesions in the liver of patients with congenital hepatic fibrosis or polycystic liver disease (described next), supporting Desmet's hypothesis. Neoplastic transformation of von Meyenburg complexes occurs rarely.[46]

CONGENITAL HEPATIC FIBROSIS

Splenomegaly and portal hypertension can prompt liver biopsy in otherwise clinically well children or ado-

lescents without clinical/laboratory evidence of cholestasis or hepatocellular injury. In addition to previously unrecognized liver disease from other causes, ending in a "burnt-out" or cryptogenic cirrhosis, the possibility of congenital hepatic fibrosis (CHF) must be considered as a cause of portal hypertension. CHF occurs typically as an autosomal recessive disease and is usually associated with autosomal recessive polycystic kidney disease (ARPKD).[45] Among children undergoing kidney transplantation for ARPKD, complications of CHF develop in 79%.[49] CHF has been reported to occur in families with autosomal dominant polycystic kidney disease.[50-52]

Pathologic Features

The liver is of normal size but exhibits irregular whitish areas of fibrosis (Fig. 41-16**A**). On microscopy, portal tracts are expanded by connective tissue that forms portal–portal bridging septa and by increased numbers of bile duct profiles (Fig. 41-16**B**). The most striking feature reveals persistent ductal plate remnants along the margins of portal tracts. Two clues to the diagnosis of CHF should be sought specifically (Fig. 41-17). The first is that portal vein branches may be hypoplastic or absent in CHF,[53] which is not the case in usual cirrhosis. The second is that bile duct lumina may be ectatic or may mouth directly into the lobule in CHF. Again, this is not the case in usual cirrhosis. Both these features of CHF reflect the ductal plate malformation complex.[45] CHF can be associated with renal cystic disease that is clinically silent at the time of liver biopsy.

In light of the occasional findings of von Meyenburg complex and cystic lesions in the liver of patients with CHF, considerable variability is seen in the morphology of CHF. Variability also occurs because of the gradual disappearance of bile duct profiles with increasing periportal fibrosis, superimposed bouts of cholangitis with bile duct destruction, and the variable evolution of coexisting cystic lesions.[45] Primary hepatic malignancies are reported to occur in 1% of patients with CHF.[54]

Clinical Features

The interesting association of CHF with ARPKD has been noted. The latter typically presents with severe renal impairment in neonates or infants, and it may be lethal at birth from pulmonary insufficiency. ARPKD arises from a genetic mutation at chromosome 6p21.[55] The hepatic lesions in ARPKD are fairly uniform and seldom give rise to macroscopically visible liver cysts.[45] Rather, portal tracts may be enlarged by connective tissue and contain numerous, somewhat dilated bile duct profiles. Normal tubular interlobular bile ducts in the center of portal tracts are often missing. This histology corresponds to incompletely remodeled ductal plates. In keeping with the normal development of the

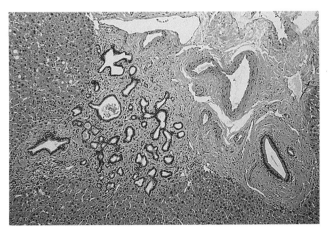

FIGURE 41–15. Von Meyenburg complex.

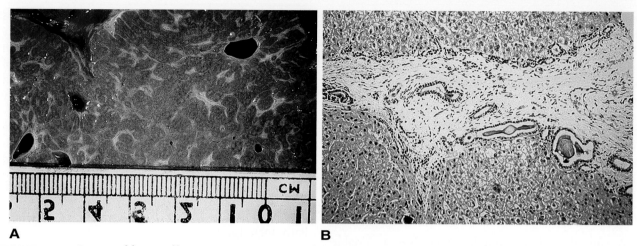

FIGURE 41–16. Congenital hepatic fibrosis. **A,** Gross specimen, showing dense fibrous bands subdividing the liver without definitive formation of nodules. **B,** Low-power photomicrograph, showing diagnostic dense fibrosis of portal tracts with numerous marginal dilated bile ductular profiles.

biliary tract, these malformed bile ducts are found to be in continuity with the rest of the biliary system. For those children with a less severe renal lesion, CHF arises in older childhood and adolescence.[56] With advancing age, the number of bile duct profiles decreases, and an increase is noted in fibrosis of portal tracts. Similarly, renal cysts become less numerous and are associated with increasing interstitial fibrosis.[57] CHF may be accompanied by isolated anomalies of the gallbladder or common bile duct[58,59] or may be associated with dilatation of the large intrahepatic bile ducts of Caroli's disease.[45,60] A CHF-like histologic lesion is also a major feature of the rare autosomal recessive Meckel's syndrome.[61]

POLYCYSTIC LIVER DISEASE

Polycystic diseases of the liver represent a variable group of clinical conditions, almost always associated with autosomal dominant polycystic kidney disease (ADPKD) but with marked variability in expression. An age-dependent increase in hepatic cyst prevalence (from 20% of patients in their third decade of life to 75% by the seventh decade) is noted in ADPKD. At any stage, women are more likely than men to have more and larger cysts, and nulliparous women who have never used estrogens are less likely to have cysts than those who have been pregnant and/or used hormones.[62] Autosomal dominant polycystic liver disease (ADPLD) can occur independently of ADPKD, as has been docu-

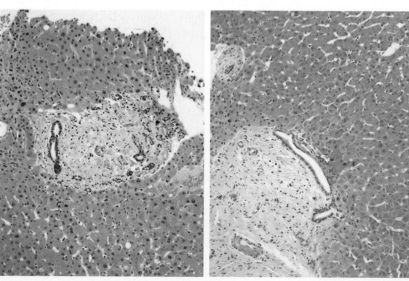

FIGURE 41–17. Typical changes in congenital hepatic fibrosis. **A,** No portal vein radicle is seen. **B,** A dilated bile duct lies at the margin of a portal tract, its lumen in continuity with a presumed canal of Hering.

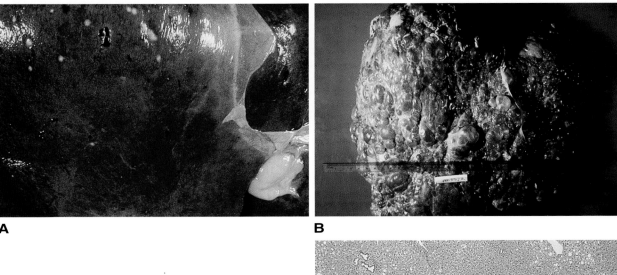

A   B

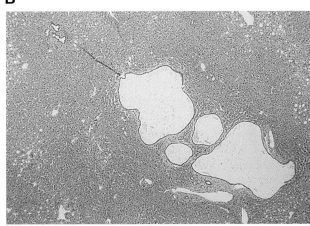

C

FIGURE 41-18. Polycystic liver disease. **A,** Incidental liver cyst *(upper left)* in a postmortem liver with small metastatic tumor deposits. **B,** Massive involvement of the liver by polycystic liver disease. **C,** Photomicrograph showing liver cyst lined by simple biliary epithelium.

mented in a large retrospective study of medicolegal autopsies in Finland.[63] A locus for ADPLD has been identified on chromosome 19p13.2-13.1, but this 12.5-cm locus precludes ready speculation about candidate genes.[64] ADPKD is one of the more common hereditary diseases, occurring in 1 in 1000 individuals. It is characterized by the progressive development and enlargement of multiple fluid-filled cysts in the kidneys, which may ultimately lead to end-stage renal disease.

Pathologic Features

Hepatic involvement in polycystic liver disease can be completely incidental, as illustrated in Figure 41-18**A.** Alternatively, the liver itself may reveal massive involvement (Fig. 41-18**B**) that is not unlike that seen in renal disease. The cysts are lined by a simple biliary epithelium (Fig. 41-18**C**). Careful histomorphometric analysis demonstrates a strong positive correlation between the density of biliary microhamartomas (in essence, von Meyenburg complexes) and the severity of polycystic liver disease.[65] This finding supports the view that hepatic cysts in ADPKD result from cystic dilatation of biliary microhamartomas, along with separation

over time of cysts from the biliary ducts from which they have been derived.

Clinical Features

Polycystic liver disease usually presents as an asymptomatic enlarged liver. However, significant symptoms, including abdominal pain, orthopnea, dyspnea, early satiety, abdominal pain, and abdominal distention, can occur in up to 20% of cases. These are mechanical symptoms that result from the massive liver enlargement. Fatal hepatic failure with venous compression and ascites is distinctly uncommon.[66]

CAROLI'S DISEASE AND CAROLI'S SYNDROME

Caroli's disease is defined as congenital dilatation of the large intrahepatic bile ducts—left and right hepatic ducts, segmental ducts, and area branches. A pure type characterized by ectasia of the intrahepatic bile ducts without further histologic abnormalities is referred to as *Caroli's disease.* A combined type in which Caroli's disease is associated with lesions of CHF is referred to as *Caroli's syndrome.*[45] The mode of inheritance of these conditions is controversial. Caroli's disease per se is not associated with the renal malformations (ARPKD) that accompany CHF, and the bile duct abnormalities may be confined to only part of the organ. Caroli's disease may be associated with a choledochal cyst.[67] In contrast, Caroli's syndrome (with its accompanying CHF) affects the whole liver and is transmitted as an inherited trait—autosomal recessive in some reports[68] and autosomal dominant in others without[69] or with[70] association with ADPKD.

Pathologic Features

In the simplest form of Caroli's disease, abnormalities consist of focal dilatation of the large intrahepatic bile ducts with predominant involvement of the segmental ducts.[71] These dilated cystic ducts are in continuity with the rest of the biliary system. In Caroli's syndrome, the major ducts of the intrahepatic biliary tree are extensively dilated, and histologic CHF is seen in the liver corpus. Large duct ectasias predispose to repeated attacks of cholangitis, and there is risk of portal hypertension (from the CHF), intrahepatic lithiasis, amyloidosis, and cholangiocarcinoma.[45] Recurrent cholangitis may be difficult to control and may lead to death of the patient from uncontrolled biliary infection within 5 to 10 years after onset of the recurrent cholangitis. Malignancy (cholangiocarcinoma) occurs in up to 7% of patients with Caroli's syndrome.[72,73] The pathogenesis of Caroli's disease involves putatively total or partial arrest of remodeling of the ductal plate of the large intrahepatic bile ducts.[45] This hypothesis is supported by the persistence of vascular bridges across the cystically dilated bile duct lumina, readily identifiable on imaging.[74,75]

■ Conclusion

Performance of any liver biopsy in the infant or child requires rigorous attention to proper bedside processing of the liver specimen so that maximum information can be obtained and the need for subsequent liver biopsy can be avoided. Critical distinctions between findings suggestive of biliary obstruction, and hence extrahepatic biliary atresia, versus findings of absence of obstruction (and the large differential diagnosis generated) may be difficult in some cases. Cases should be referred readily for consultation to subspecialist pediatric hepatopathologists. Regardless of which pathologist is rendering the final opinion, histopathologic findings must always be considered in concert with other clinical findings, including laboratory data, radiographic findings, and, obviously, history and physical examination findings.

Liver disease in the adolescent and young adult may result from the most common causes of hepatic injury such as viral hepatitis, or it may be attributable to the specific inherited conditions of HFE disease (hereditary hemochromatosis, type 1), ATP7B disease (Wilson's disease), and A1ATSD. These conditions must be considered in the differential diagnosis for every liver biopsy examined in this age group, and all liver pathologists examining such liver biopsy specimens should be able to recognize the features of these conditions. We anticipate that the same rigorous specimen processing guidelines used for liver biopsy specimens from infants and children will be required for the adolescent and young adult age group.

Finally, pathologists should be able to recognize the incidental von Meyenburg complex and, when suggestive histologic features are present, should raise the possibility of a hepatic DPM with its considerations for congenital hepatic fibrosis, polycystic liver disease, Caroli's disease, and Caroli's syndrome.

Through application of the diagnostic principles presented in this chapter, inherited and developmental disorders of the liver will be successfully recognized.

References

1. Ishak KG, Sharp HL, Schwarzenberg SJ: Metabolic errors and liver disease. In MacSween RMN, Burt AD, Portmann BC, et al (eds): Pathology of the Liver, 4th ed. London, Churchill Livingstone, 2002, pp 155-255.
2. McKiernan PJ, Baker AJ, Kelly DA: The frequency and outcome of biliary atresia in the UK and Ireland. Lancet 355:25-29, 2000.
3. Stocker JT, Dehner LP: Pediatric Pathology, 1st ed. Philadelphia, JB Lippincott, 1992.
4. Vobra P, Haller C, Emre S, et al: Neonatal hemochromatosis: The importance of early recognition of liver failure. J Pediatr 136:537-541, 2000.
5. Knisely AS: Neonatal hemochromatosis. Adv Pediatr 39:383-403, 1992.
6. Silver MM, Valberg LS, Cutz E, et al: Hepatic morphology and iron quantitation in perinatal hemochromatosis: Comparison with a large perinatal control population, including cases with chronic liver disease. Am J Pathol 143:1312-1325, 1993.
7. Koukoulis G, Mieli-Vergani G, Portmann B: Infantile liver giant cells: Immunohistological study of their proliferative state and possible mechanisms of formation. Pediatr Dev Pathol 2:353-359, 1999.
8. Labowitz J, Finklestein S, Rabinovitz M: Postinfantile giant cell hepatitis complicating ulcerative colitis: A case report and review of the literature. Am J Gastroenterol 96:1274-1277, 2001.
9. Perez-Atayde AR, Sirlin SM, Jonas M: Coombs-positive autoimmune hemolytic anemia and postinfantile giant cell hepatitis in children. Pediatr Pathol 14:69-77, 1994.
10. Jonas MM, Perez-Atayde AR: Liver disease in infancy and childhood. In Schiff ER, Sorrell MF, Maddrey WC (eds): Diseases of the Liver, 9th ed. Philadelphia, Lippincott Williams & Wilkins, 2003, pp 1459-1496.
11. Jevon GP, Dimmick JE: Histopathologic approach to metabolic liver disease: Part 1. Pediatr Dev Pathol 1:179-199, 1998.
12. Jevon GP, Dimmick JE: Histopathologic approach to metabolic liver disease: Part 2. Pediatr Dev Pathol 1:261-269, 1998.
13. Desmet VJ: Embryology of the liver and intrahepatic biliary tract, and overview of malformations of the bile duct. In McIntyre N, Benhamou J-P, Bircher J, et al (eds): The Oxford Textbooks of Clinical Hepatology, vol 1. Oxford, Oxford University Press, 1991, pp 497-519.

14. Cocjin J, Rosenthal P, Buslon V, et al: Bile ductule formation in fetal, neonatal, and infant livers compared with extrahepatic biliary atresia. Hepatology 24:568-574, 1996.

15. Landing BH: Considerations of the pathogenesis of neonatal hepatitis, biliary atresia and choledochal cyst—the concept of infantile obstructive cholangiopathy. Prog Pediatr Surg 6:113-139, 1974.

16. Low Y, Vijayhan V, Tan CEL: The prognostic value of ductal plate malformation and other histologic parameters in biliary atresia: An immunohistochemical study. J Pediatr 139:320-322, 2001.

17. Raweily EA, Gibson AA, Burt AD: Abnormalities of intrahepatic bile ducts in extrahepatic biliary atresia. Histopathology 17:521-527, 1990.

18. Snover DC: Biopsy Diagnosis of Liver Disease. Baltimore, Williams & Wilkins, 1992.

19. Talbot IC, Mowat AP: Liver disease in infancy: Histological features and relationship to alpha-antitrypsin phenotype. J Clin Pathol 28:559-563, 1975.

20. Amarapurkar A, Somers S, Knisely AS, et al: Steatosis of periportal hepatocytes is associated with alpha-1-antitrypsin storage disorder at presentation in infancy (abstract). Lab Invest 82:309A-310A, 2002.

21. Deutsch GH, Sokol RJ, Stathos TH, et al: Proliferation to paucity: Evolution of bile duct abnormalities in a case of Alagille syndrome. Pediatr Dev Pathol 4:559-563, 2001.

22. Crawford AR, Lin XZ, Crawford JM: The normal adult human liver biopsy: A quantitative reference standard. Hepatology 28:323-331, 1998.

23. Alagille D: Intrahepatic biliary atresia (hepatic ductular hypoplasia). In Berenberg SR (ed): Liver Diseases in Infancy and Childhood. Dordrecht, The Netherlands, Martinez Nijhoff, 1976, pp 129-142.

24. Crawford JM: Development of the intrahepatic biliary tree. Semin Liver Dis 22:213-226, 2002.

25. Kahn E: Paucity of interlobular bile ducts: Arteriohepatic dysplasia and nonsyndromic duct paucity. Perspect Pediatr Pathol 14:168-215, 1991.

26. Theise ND, Saxena R, Portmann BC, et al: Canals of Hering and hepatic stem cells in humans. Hepatology 30:1425-1433, 1999.

27. Bacon BR, Olynyk JK, Brunt EM, et al: HFE genotype in patients with hemochromatosis and other liver diseases. Ann Intern Med 130:953-962, 1999.

28. Ludwig J, Batts K, Moyer T, et al: Liver biopsy diagnosis of homozygous hemochromatosis: A diagnostic algorithm. Mayo Clin Proc 68:263-267, 1993.

29. Deugnier YM, Turlin B, Powell LW, et al: Differentiation between heterozygotes and homozygotes in genetic hemochromatosis by means of a histological hepatic iron-index. A study of 192 cases. Hepatology 17:30-34, 1993.

30. Bartolo C, McAndrew PE, Sosolik RC, et al: Differential diagnosis of hereditary hemochromatosis from other liver disorders by genetic analysis. Gene mutation analysis of patients previously diagnosed with hemochromatosis by liver biopsy. Arch Pathol Lab Med 122:633-637, 1998.

31. Nash S, Marconi S, Sikorska K, et al: Role of liver biopsy in the diagnosis of hepatic iron overload in the era of genetic testing. Am J Clin Pathol 118:73-81, 2002.

32. Moyo VM, Mandishona E, Hasstedt SJ, et al: Evidence of genetic transmission in African iron overload. Blood 91:1076-1082, 1998.

33. Schöniger-Hekele M, Müller C, Polli C, et al: Liver pathology in compound heterozygous patients for hemochromatosis. Liver 22:295-301, 2002.

34. Chittur S, Weltman M, Farrell GC, et al: HFE mutations, hepatic iron, and fibrosis: Ethnic-specific association of NASH with C282Y but not with fibrotic severity. Hepatology 36:142-149, 2002.

35. Kitamura T, Alroy J, Gatmaitan Z, et al: Defective biliary excretion of epinephrine metabolites in mutant (TR-) rats: Relation to the pathogenesis of black liver in the Dubin-Johnson syndrome and Corriedale sheep with an analogous excretory defect. Hepatology 15:1154-1159, 1992.

36. Brunt EM, Olynyk JK, Britton RS, et al: Histological evaluation of iron in liver biopsies: Relationship to HFE mutations. Am J Gastroenterol 95:1788-1793, 2000.

37. Britte MRC, Thomas LA, Balaratnam N, et al: Hepatocellular carcinoma arising in non-cirrhotic liver in genetic haemochromatosis. Scand J Gastroenterol 35:889-893, 2000.

38. Llanos RM, Mercer JF: The molecular basis of copper homeostasis copper-related disorders. DNA Cell Biol 21:259-270, 2002.

39. Perlmutter DH: Liver injury in alpha-1-antitrypsin deficiency: An aggravated protein induces mitochondrial injury. J Clin Invest 110:1579-1583, 2002.

40. Sveger T: Prospective study of children with a-1-antitrypsin deficiency: Eight-year-old follow-up. J Pediatr 104:91-94, 1989.

41. Deutsch J, Becker H, Aubock L: Histopathological features of liver disease in alpha-1-antitrypsin deficiency. Acta Paediatr Suppl 393:8-12, 1994.

42. Pittschieler K: Liver involvement in alpha1-antitrypsin-deficient phenotypes PiSZ and PiMZ. Acta Paediatr 91:239-240, 2002.

43. Larsson C: Natural history and life expectancy in severe alpha 1-antitrypsin deficiency, Pi Z. Acta Med Scand 204:345-351, 1978.

44. Milkiewicz P, Chilton AP, Hubscher SG, et al: Antidepressant induced cholestasis: Hepatocellular redistribution of multidrug resistant protein (MRP2). Gut 52:300-303, 2003.

45. Desmet VJ: Ludwig symposium on biliary disorders—Part I. Pathogenesis of ductal plate abnormalities. Mayo Clin Proc 73:80-89, 1998.

46. Jain D, Sarode VR, Abdul-Karim FW, et al: Evidence for the neoplastic transformation of von-Meyenburg complexes. Am J Surg Pathol 24:1131-1139, 2000.

47. Thommesen N: Biliary hamartomas (von Meyenburg complexes) in liver needle biopsies. Acta Pathol Microbiol Scand A 86:93-99, 1978.

48. Chung EB: Multiple bile-duct hamartomas. Cancer 26:287-296, 1970.

49. Khan K, Schwarzenberg SJ, Sharp HL, et al: Morbidity from congenital hepatic fibrosis after renal transplantation for autosomal recessive polycystic kidney disease. Am J Transplant 2:360-365, 2002.

50. Cobben JM, Breuning MH, Schoots C, et al: Congenital hepatic fibrosis in autosomal-dominant polycystic kidney disease. Kidney Int 38:880-885, 1990.

51. Matsuda O, Ideura T, Shinoda T, et al: Polycystic kidney of autosomal dominant inheritance, polycystic liver and congenital hepatic fibrosis in a single kindred. Am J Nephrol 10:237-241, 1990.

52. Kaczorowski JM, Halterman JS, Spitalnik P, et al: Congenital hepatic fibrosis and autosomal dominant polycystic kidney disease. Pediatr Pathol Mol Med 20:245-248, 2001.

53. Desmet VJ: What is congenital hepatic fibrosis? Histopathology 20:465-477, 1992.

54. Scott J, Scousha S, Thomas HC, et al: Bile duct carcinoma: A late complication of congenital hepatic fibrosis. Am J Gastroenterol 73:113-119, 1980.

55. Zerres K, Mucher G, Bachner L, et al: Mapping of the gene for autosomal recessive polycystic kidney disease (ARPKD) to chromosome 6p21cen. Nat Genet 7:429-432, 1994.

56. Kaplan BS, Fay J, Shah V, et al: Autosomal recessive polycystic kidney disease. Pediatr Nephrol 3:43-49, 1989.

57. Premkumar A, Berdon WE, Levy J, et al: The emergence of hepatic fibrosis and portal hypertension in infants and children with autosomal recessive polycystic kidney disease: Initial and follow-up sonographic and radiographic findings. Pediatr Radiol 18:123-129, 1988.

58. Alvarez F, Bernard O, Brunelle F, et al: Congenital hepatic fibrosis in children. J Pediatr 99:370-375, 1981.

59. Kerr DNS, Okonkwo S, Choa RG: Congenital hepatic fibrosis: The long-term prognosis. Gut 19:514-520, 1978.

60. D'Agata IDA, Jonas JA, Perez-Atayde AR, et al: Combined cystic disease of the liver and kidney. Semin Liver Dis 14:215-228, 1994.

61. Sergi C, Adam S, Kahl P, et al: Study of the malformation of ductal plate of the liver in Meckel syndrome and review of other syndromes presenting with this anomaly. Pediatr Dev Pathol 3:568-583, 2000.

62. Gabow PA, Johnson AM, Kaehny WD, et al: Risk factors for the development of hepatic cysts in autosomal dominant polycystic kidney disease. Hepatology 11:1033-1037, 1990.

63. Karhunen PJ, Tenhu M: Adult polycystic liver and kidney diseases are separate entities. Clin Genet 30:29-37, 1986.

64. Reynolds DM, Falk CT, Li A, et al: Identification of a locus for autosomal dominant polycystic liver disease, on chromosome 19p13.2-13.1. Am J Hum Genet 67:1598-1604, 2000.

65. Ramos A, Torres VE, Holley KE, et al: The liver in autosomal dominant polycystic kidney disease. Arch Pathol Lab Med 114:180-184, 1992.

66. Vauthey J-N, Maddern GJ, Kolbinger P, et al: Clinical experience with adult polycystic liver disease. Br J Surg 79:562-565, 1992.

67. Henry X, Marrasse E, Stoppa R, et al: Association maladie de Caroli-kyste du cholédoque-fibrose hépatique congénitale-polykystose rénale. Chirurgie 113:834-843, 1987.

68. Benhamou J-P: Syndrome de Caroli. Med Ther 1:253-256, 1995.

69. Tsuchida Y, Sato T, Sanjo K, et al: Evaluation of long-term results of Caroli's disease: 21 years' observation of a family with autosomal "dominant" inheritance, and review of the literature. Hepatogastro-enterology 42:175-181, 1995.

70. Jordon D, Harpaz N, Thung SN: Caroli's disease and adult polycystic kidney disease: A rarely recognized association. Liver 9:30-35, 1989.

71. Caroli J, Corcos V: Maladies des voies biliares intrahepatiques segmentaires. Paris, Masson, 1964.

72. Bloustein PA: Association of carcinoma with congenital cystic conditions of the liver and bile ducts. Am J Gastroenterol 67:40-46, 1977.

73. Taylor AC, Palmer KR: Caroli's disease. Eur J Gastroenterol Hepatol 10:105-108, 1998.

74. Marchal GJ, Desmet VJ, Proesmans WC, et al: Caroli disease: High-frequency US and pathologic findings. Radiology 158:507-511, 1986.

75. Choi BI, Yeon KM, Kim SH, et al: Caroli disease: Central dot sign in CT. Radiology 174:161-163, 1990.

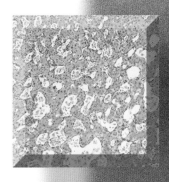

CHAPTER 42

Benign and Malignant Tumors of the Liver

LINDA D. FERRELL

◼ Introduction

Primary tumors of the liver are divided into benign and malignant epithelial and nonepithelial neoplasms. Epithelial neoplasms are the most common and fall predominantly into the hepatocellular and bile ductular types. Other non-neoplastic tumor-like lesions of various types may be of significance as well. The World Health Organization's classification scheme, which includes both neoplasms and tumor-like lesions, is provided in Table 42-1.

◼ Tumor Resection Specimens: Reporting

Verification of tumor type and status as a primary or metastatic neoplasm or a non-neoplastic tumor is the most important consideration in diagnosis. Descriptive comments should focus on information important for tumor staging, such as tumor size (smaller or larger than 2 cm), number of lesions (single or multiple), specific lobes (or segments) involved, local extension of lesion outside of the liver, and presence or absence of gross vascular invasion, especially notation of which of the major vessels (portal or hepatic vein) is involved. Microscopic evaluation of a mass should involve adequate numbers of sections relative to tumor size for evaluation of vascular invasion or extension outside of Glisson's capsule.[1,2] Sections near the edge of the tumor are generally recommended for detection of vascular invasion if gross invasion is not noted. Any gross observation of possible large vessel invasion should be documented microscopically. A section of non-neoplastic liver should also be included for identification of any significant pathology.

Generally, it is recommended that surgical margins of the resection should be inked before the tumor is sectioned for more definitive evaluation of the distance from the margin to the tumor; the status of the resection margins should be included in the report. Some studies have suggested that a tumor-free margin of at least 1 cm may be directly related to a better prognosis for some malignant tumor types.[3] Other studies have shown that extensive resection of hepatocellular carcinoma (HCC) is preferable to limited excision when the lesion is small.[1] Thus, the distance from the tumor to the closest margin of resection should be documented.

BIOPSY SAMPLES—SPECIAL CONSIDERATIONS

Both small core and fine-needle aspiration biopsies (FNABs) are often used successfully for the diagnosis of specific tumor types (see Chapter 33). However, the clinician must remember that the accuracy of the FNAB may be enhanced by the use of extra tissue preparations such as cell buttons for evaluation of the microhistology of paraffin-embedded sections of the sample collected

TABLE 42–1. World Health Organization Classification of Primary Liver Tumors and Tumor-like Lesions

Epithelial Tumors or Tumor-like Lesions	Nonepithelial Tumors or Tumor-like Lesions
Benign	Benign
Large regenerative nodule	Hemangioma
Low-grade dysplastic nodule	Angiomyolipoma
High-grade (borderline) dysplastic nodule	Infantile hemangioendothelioma
Hepatocellular adenoma	Mesenchymal hamartoma
Focal nodular hyperplasia	Localized fibrous tumor
Bile duct adenoma	Solitary necrotic nodule
Bile duct hamartoma	Inflammatory pseudotumor
Biliary cystadenoma	Infectious cyst
Intraductal biliary papillomatosis	Other rare benign tumors
Congenital biliary cyst	Malignant
Focal fatty change	Epithelioid hemangioendothelioma
Malignant	Angiosarcoma
Hepatocellular carcinoma, including fibrolamellar variant	Undifferentiated sarcoma (embryonal sarcoma)
Combined hepatocellular and cholangiolar carcinoma	Lymphoma and other hematopoietic tumors
Cholangiocarcinoma—peripheral, hilar, and extrahepatic types	Kaposi's sarcoma
Biliary cystadenocarcinoma	Other malignant tumors
Intraductal papillary adenocarcinoma	

from the FNAB material.[4] Use of such methodology is especially helpful in the evaluation of well-differentiated lesions of hepatocellular type, in which subtle cytologic features such as cell size, crowding of nuclei, and increased nucleus-to-cytoplasm ratio or architectural features such as formation of trabeculae or width of cell plates may be difficult to assess on the basis of smears alone. In these instances, the use of histologic sections in combination with well-prepared smears is highly successful in differentiating the well-differentiated HCC from other lesions such as adenoma, focal nodular hyperplasia, a large regenerative nodule, or dysplastic nodules. In addition, preparation of the cell button in cases of poorly differentiated neoplasm or in tumors with unusual morphology may result in more accurate diagnoses through the application of immunoperoxidase techniques to these samples.

Because the biopsy material is often limited in amount, it is recommended that slides of unstained material also be cut when the block is initially sectioned to ensure that sufficient material will be available if it becomes necessary to evaluate additional level sections or other stains. It is also advised that the usual panel of stains (which often includes trichrome, reticulin, diastase/periodic acid–Schiff [d-PAS], and iron stains) should not be ordered automatically at the time of gross examination because this excess sectioning (before examination of the hematoxylin and eosin [H&E] morphology) often depletes the block of diagnostic material such that sufficient tissue may not be available for other more diagnostic stains.

◼ Hepatocellular Tumors*

BENIGN LESIONS IN THE NONCIRRHOTIC LIVER

Hepatic Adenoma

CLINICAL FEATURES

Hepatic adenomas (HAs) are rare tumors that are seen almost exclusively in young women during their reproductive years and only rarely occur in men[6,7] or children.[8] HA may be single or multifocal; the latter condition is known as *multiple hepatocellular adenomatosis*. These tumors occur in a liver that is histologically normal or nearly normal.[5] The clinical presentation is generally that of an abdominal mass, but some patients also have complaints of abdominal pain, discomfort, or nausea, and a significant number present with hemoperitoneum.[9] Serum alkaline phosphatase may be elevated, but serum alpha-fetoprotein (AFP) levels are generally normal or minimally elevated. Radiographically, the lesions show an enhanced vascular pattern.

PATHOGENESIS

Many HAs are thought to result from the use of oral contraceptives[10] or anabolic steroids. However, with the

---

*The International Working Party of 1994 attempted to better define the diagnostic criteria of benign and malignant hepatocellular nodules of the liver, which resulted in the nomenclature that has been incorporated into this chapter.[5]

low-dose pills now widely used, their incidence may be decreasing. Some HAs associated with oral contraceptives appear to regress after cessation of the drugs, but others do not. Other risk factors for the development of adenomas include metabolic disorders (especially the carbohydrate metabolic disorders such as the glycogen storage diseases I and IV), galactosemia, and familial diabetes mellitus, as well as tyrosinemia.[11] The consensus of the International Working Party is that the diagnosis of adenoma should not be assigned for a lesion arising in a cirrhotic liver unless regression is evident when the stimulus is removed, or unless one of the risk factors described here is present.[5] Rarely, HCCs have been found arising within HAs.[10,12]

PATHOLOGIC FEATURES

GROSS PATHOLOGY

HAs are round tumors that tend to bulge on cut section; they are soft and are typically somewhat lighter in color than the surrounding liver, but their appearance may vary if necrosis or hemorrhage is present. HA generally lacks significant evidence of fibrosis or nodularity, but rarely, such features may be present.[12] Usually, a capsule is not present. Rarely, adenoma may have a slate-gray to black color caused by large amounts of lipofuscin pigment, the so-called black adenoma.[11]

MICROSCOPIC PATHOLOGY

HAs are composed of a relatively uniform population of hepatocytes arranged in cell plates that are one to three cells thick (Fig. 42-1). These cell plates are usually more irregular and nonlinear than those in the normal liver. A key feature is that the reticulin framework of the cell plates is intact or only focally decreased. The tumor

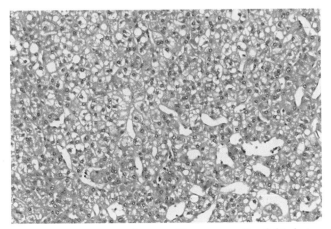

FIGURE 42–1. Hepatic adenoma. The tumor cells of this lesion have nuclear cytologic features similar to those of normal liver. The cytoplasm of the tumor cells is very pale in this case, consistent with increased glycogen in the cytoplasm. The cell plate architecture is preserved, and cell plates are often two cells thick as seen here. Focal mild dilation of sinusoids is also present.

cells are usually about the same size as those in the normal liver, but they may also be slightly smaller or larger compared with normal hepatocytes. Even if the size of the cells varies, however, the nucleus-to-cytoplasm ratio remains about the same as that in normal liver. The cytoplasm of the tumor cells may be eosinophilic or clear, or it may contain fat droplets; bile stasis, lipofuscin pigment, or Mallory's hyaline stain may be noted. Other variations in cellular morphology such as multinucleated hepatocytic tumor cells and focally atypical or pleomorphic hepatocytes may also be present. Regardless of the cellular morphology, mitotic figures are absent or extremely rare.

Variations in architecture such as formation of acini (i.e., pseudoglands or glandlike structures composed of hepatocytes) are relatively common findings; such acinar structures may contain bile. Alterations in the sinusoids may also be noted; these may appear compressed, resulting in a somewhat uniform, solid appearance to the tumor, or alternatively, sinusoidal dilation and peliosis hepatis may be present. Large arterial vessels are often prominent. Kupffer cells may be seen but tend to be fewer in number than in the normal liver. HAs may or may not be encapsulated, and, if a capsule is present, it is often only partially complete with foci of tumor cells merging with the adjacent parenchyma at sites where the capsule is absent. Adenomas associated with anabolic steroids are more likely to show nuclear atypia, peliosis hepatis, or a prominent acinar (pseudoglandular) pattern.[5,11] No portal zones are seen. Areas of infarction and hemorrhage are relatively frequent findings.

SPECIAL STUDIES

HA stains positively for the usual hepatocellular markers, including the cytokeratin marker CAM 5.2 and the canalicular marker polyclonal carcinoembryonic antigen (CEA). HAs often show CD34 positivity on the endothelial cells lining the cell plates, similar to that seen in HCC, so this marker cannot be used to distinguish the two lesions.[13] AFP is negative in these lesions.

DIFFERENTIAL DIAGNOSIS

The key issue is the differentiation of HA from focal nodular hyperplasia (Table 42-2) or from well-differentiated HCC. For HA, the relatively uniform cell population resembling normal liver and lacking mitotic activity, the lack of cell plates greater than three cells thick, and an intact reticulin framework lining the cell plates help to distinguish the lesion from well-differentiated HCC. For differentiation from focal nodular hyperplasia, the presence of isolated arteries and the lack of nodularity, fibrous bands, a central fibrous zone, or proliferating bile ductules are the most helpful features. However, one must be careful not to

TABLE 42–2. Comparison of Hepatic Adenoma and Focal Nodular Hyperplasia

Morphology	Hepatic Adenoma	Focal Nodular Hyperplasia
Hepatocytes	Similar in size, slightly larger or smaller than in normal liver; more cellular pleomorphism may occur. Cytoplasmic glycogen or fat may be present.	Usually normal in size; no significant cytologic abnormalities; rare foci of cellular pleomorphism may be seen. Cytoplasmic glycogen or fat may be present.
Bile ductules	None present	Present in fibrovascular zone, edges of hepatocytic nodules
Vessels or other blood-filled spaces	Large vessels often seen but without significant connective tissue zone around vessels; small to medium isolated hepatic arteries are typical; peliosis hepatis and sinusoidal dilatation may be seen	Abnormal large muscular vessels generally surrounded by a zone of connective tissue stroma
Connective tissue component	Occasional fibrous septa; encapsulation can be seen but tends to be discontinuous	Fibrovascular central zone; can vary from myxoid to more dense collagen; not encapsulated. Chronic inflammatory infiltrates may be present.
Cell plate architecture	1 to 3 cells wide; often appears regenerative	1 to 3 cells wide; plates can be compressed to give impression of solid growth. Wider cell plates may be prominent.
Reticulin stain	Normal or slightly decreased staining along the cell plates	Normal pattern with staining along the cell plates
Other features	Age >10 yr; almost always female; normal serum alpha-fetoprotein (AFP); possible increased alkaline phosphatase	Young adults; female > male; normal AFP

confuse acinar formation seen in HA for bile ductules. The distinction among these lesions may be difficult, especially on small samples. At this time, immunohistochemistry does not appear to be helpful in distinguishing HA from either of these two lesions.

Focal Nodular Hyperplasia

CLINICAL FEATURES

Focal nodular hyperplasia (FNH) is a benign, non-neoplastic lesion that is most commonly seen in young women.[7,9] However, a significant number of these lesions may be seen in men. Similar to HAs, FNHs are usually solitary lesions but may be multifocal in 20% to 30% of cases.[5,14] Classic FNH often is noted as an incidental finding, but it may also present with complications caused by large lesion size (only rarely resulting from hemorrhage[14]) or with complaints of upper abdominal pain. Nodules similar to FNH have been described adjacent to hemangiomas. Some patients with the so-called multiple FNH syndrome have at least two FNH lesions associated with one or more lesions such as hepatic hemangioma, an arterial structural defect, vascular malformation, meningioma, and astrocytoma.[5] A rare variant of FNH, the telangiectatic type, is commonly associated with the multiple FNH syndrome.[11] Some patients may have abnormal liver function tests, most with gamma-glutamyltranspeptidase activity.[14]

PATHOGENESIS

Unlike HA, FNH is not thought to develop because of the use of oral contraceptives, but many speculate that this lesion may increase in size with their use or regress with their cessation. The currently favored hypothesis for the development of FNH is that it represents a hyperplastic and altered growth response to changes in blood flow in the parenchyma surrounding a preexisting arterial malformation.[15] The presence of numerous abnormal muscular vessels within the lesion and the fact that some of these lesions or similar hyperplastic foci have been noted in association with hemangiomas and the Budd-Chiari syndrome lend support to this theory. (The International Working Party has recommended that FNH-like lesions associated with the Budd-Chiari syndrome and Rendu-Osler-Weber disease should not be designated as FNH, but rather should be referred to as *regenerative nodules*). FNH has no known malignant potential, and in spite of its rare association with fibrolamellar HCC, most feel that the lesion itself does not progress to carcinoma. Instead, it is speculated that the association of FNH with fibrolamellar HCC may represent a hyperplastic response in the adjacent parenchyma to the increased vascularity of the carcinoma. Some have proposed that nodules in FNH may have clonal features, but at this time this is still controversial.

PATHOLOGIC FEATURES

GROSS PATHOLOGY

FNH has a nodular appearance (which may suggest the appearance of macronodular cirrhosis) and tends to be lighter brown than the adjacent liver. These lesions are often located near the capsule of the liver, which may cause the surface of the liver to have a localized nodular appearance mimicking cirrhosis; occasionally, the lesions may be pedunculated. The edges of FNH appear demarcated from the adjacent normal parenchyma because of the nodularity, but no fibrous capsule is present. The lesions may vary considerably in size. Most have a central fibrous scar, which consists of fibrovascular tissue (usually not dense scar tissue), but this central focus of connective tissue may be absent. A rare variant of this lesion, the telangiectatic type, does not have the central fibrous zone but rather has a gross appearance of either HA or a vascular lesion such as hemangioma or peliosis hepatis.

MICROSCOPIC PATHOLOGY

The classic type of FNH is composed of mostly normal-appearing hepatocytes arranged in incomplete nodules that are partially separated by fibrous tissue; these tend to extend from the central fibrous zone when it is present. An important feature is the variable number of bile ductular structures present within the fibrous stroma and at the edge of the nodules. The cell plate architecture with an intact reticulin framework is similar to that in normal liver, but the cell plates are usually wider (two to three cells thick), as in a regenerative nodule. The hepatocytes in this lesion may demonstrate increased glycogen in the cytoplasm, as well as other findings such as focal fatty change, bile stasis, lipofuscin, iron pigment, copper-associated protein, and Mallory bodies.[5] Some foci of atypical hepatocytes with larger nuclei and mild hyperchromasia, with or without conspicuous nucleoli, may be present.

Another important diagnostic feature is the presence of medium-sized to large, thick-walled muscular vessels, which often exhibit myointimal myxoid or fibromuscular hyperplastic changes (Fig. 42-2). These vessels are not components of a portal tract in that no large duct of similar caliber or portal vein is associated with them. In fact, usually no normal portal tracts are present within the lesion, although a bile duct of intermediate or large caliber may be found in the central fibrous zone in rare cases.[14] Sinusoids may be somewhat dilated, and Kupffer cells may be seen. Inflammatory cell infiltrates are relatively common and generally consist of lymphocytes, although neutrophils and eosinophils may be found, especially around bile ductular structures. Rarely, granulomas may be seen.

The telangiectatic variant contains dilated, blood-filled vascular spaces instead of a central fibrous zone, so the gross appearance may be more typical of adenoma, hemangioma, or peliosis hepatis. The arteries in this variant are smaller and more numerous than those in typical FNH, and the fibrous septa are less prominent.[5,14]

Other, relatively rare, nonclassic forms may occur, including forms that lack the central fibrous zone, with macroscopic and microscopic appearances mimicking adenoma and the telangiectatic form. Thick-walled vessels are present, at least in part of these lesions, and bile ductular proliferation is always noted; this latter feature may be focal and subtle.[14]

SPECIAL STUDIES

Similar to HA, FNH stains positively for the usual hepatocellular markers, including the cytokeratin marker CAM 5.2 and the canalicular marker polyclonal CEA. In addition, CD34 is often positive on the endothelial cells lining the cell plates, so again, this marker cannot be used to distinguish this lesion from adenoma or HCC.[13] AFP is also negative in these lesions.

DIFFERENTIAL DIAGNOSIS

FNH resembles HA or normal liver on small biopsy samples. One of the most important distinguishing features of FNH is the bile ductular structures (see Table 42-2). Because of the relative paucity of bile ductular findings, a large sample of core needle biopsy or a wedge biopsy is likely to be necessary for this diagnosis to be confirmed. The finding of large vessels with abnormal hyperplastic features surrounded by connective tissue may also be helpful because larger vessels in adenoma tend to have a more normal configuration and lack significant perivascular connective tissue stroma.

BENIGN LESIONS IN THE CIRRHOTIC LIVER

A brief overview of the currently recommended terminology used for cytologic changes is necessary as a prelude to the discussion of nodules within the cirrhotic liver. The cirrhotic nodule frequently contains scattered enlarged hepatocytes with abundant cytoplasm and atypical, enlarged nuclei, but the nucleus-to-cytoplasm ratio is relatively normal (Fig. 42-3). This cytologic feature was designated *large cell dysplasia* in the past,

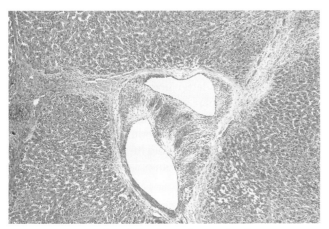

FIGURE 42–2. Focal nodular hyperplasia. This lesion contains abnormal muscular vessels that lack associated bile ducts of similar size.

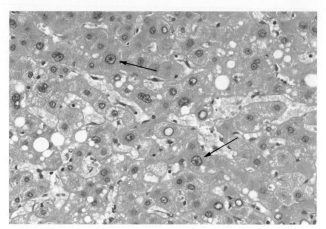

FIGURE 42–3. Large cell change. Focal hepatocytes have a markedly enlarged nucleus as well as more abundant cytoplasm (*arrows*). These large nuclei are scattered rather than clustered in one site.

but now the International Working Party has recommended the term *large cell change*[5] for this finding because the consensus is that this lesion is not likely to be truly dysplastic, and this cellular change is too frequently seen for a premalignant process to be assumed.[16]

Similarly, cirrhotic nodules may contain hepatocytes smaller than normal with normal, slightly smaller, or slightly larger nuclei and scant cytoplasm, which results in an overall increase in the nucleus-to-cytoplasm ratio (Fig. 42-4). This cytologic feature was previously designated *small cell dysplasia*, but the International Working Party has recommended the term *small cell change* for this process.[5] Again, the current consensus is that small cell features in cirrhotic livers could be regenerative rather than dysplastic, and they may be preneoplastic only in certain instances when the cells are arranged in clusters within a cirrhotic nodule. These clusters of small cells may be present in any nodule in the cirrhotic

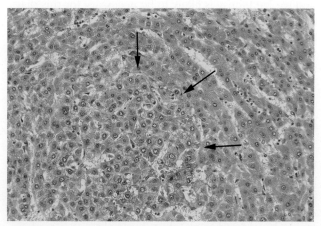

FIGURE 42–4. High-grade dysplastic focus with small cell change. Note the "nodule" of smaller cells with higher ratios associated with some thickening of the cell plates (*arrows*).

liver, may be a focus of no more than 1 to 2 mm in diameter, and may appear like a nodule within a nodule (see Fig. 42-4). This type of change has been designated by the International Working Party *dysplastic focus*, without further grading into low or high grade[5]; it has been noted to have a high prevalence in diseases such as chronic hepatitis B virus (HBV) and hepatitis C virus (HCV), alpha-1-antitrypsin deficiency, and tyrosinemia.[5] Dysplastic foci may also contain cells with enlarged nuclei with hyperchromasia, with the spectrum of nuclear atypia varying from minimal to severe. Cytoplasmic fat or glycogen may differ in content from the surrounding liver. The same International Working Party recommended that the term *dysplasia* be used only in the previously described dysplastic foci or for bona fide dysplastic nodules, and not for scattered cytologic changes within the cirrhotic liver.

Large Regenerative Nodule (Macroregenerative Nodule) and Low-Grade Dysplastic Nodule

NOMENCLATURE

In the cirrhotic liver, benign nodules that are larger than the typical cirrhotic nodule have been referred to by various names, including *large regenerative nodule*,[5] *macroregenerative nodule*, and *adenomatous hyperplasia*. In contrast, the low-grade dysplastic nodule in the cirrhotic liver is thought to represent a clonal proliferation of hepatocytes. However, gross and standard microscopic features of large regenerative nodules and of low-grade dysplastic nodules are often indistinguishable. For this reason, the descriptions in this section apply to both lesions. In practice, many do not try to distinguish large regenerative nodules from low-grade dysplastic nodules because clonality studies may be the only mechanism by which to do so. Rather, in practice, the terms are almost used interchangeably to represent a nodule that is distinct from the surrounding cirrhotic liver but lacks the cytologic or architectural abnormalities seen in the high-grade dysplastic nodule.

For similar nodules in the noncirrhotic liver, the International Working Party has recommended the designation *multiacinar regenerative nodules* or *adenomatous hyperplasia*.[5] These latter nodules tend to occur in the setting of Budd-Chiari syndrome or portal vein thrombosis, or as sequelae of necrosis with regeneration. These large regenerative nodules and multiacinar regenerative nodules are thought to be a reactive process rather than a clonal preneoplastic lesion.

CLINICAL FEATURES

Large regenerative nodules/low-grade dysplastic nodules occur in the setting of cirrhosis, with a few exceptions when they are noted in the setting of chronic liver disease without fully developed cirrhosis.[17] They are often found as incidental findings at autopsy or at the time of transplantation, but they may also be noted on radiographic studies. Serum AFP is normal or within the low abnormal range expected for the underlying chronic liver disease/cirrhosis.

PATHOGENESIS

These nodules are generally considered benign lesions and may represent either regenerative foci or presumed clonal proliferations in a liver with chronic disease. Nodules with this benign histologic pattern have been associated with an increased incidence of HCC, and in some instances, they may be predisposed to the development of HCC.[18] However, it is important to point out that almost all past studies of these nodules have not attempted to define the lesions as regenerative or clonal but rather have defined them as lacking features of high-grade dysplastic nodules or HCC on routine histologic examination. Hence, the literature may be somewhat contradictory, and one cannot definitively state at this time whether the regenerative nodules and the clonal nodules have similar risks for association with HCC. Regardless, these distinctive nodules are more typically seen in cirrhosis due to HBV, HCV, alcohol, and hemochromatosis, but they are unlikely to be seen in primary biliary cirrhosis. Risk factors for these nodules thus tend to be the same as those for HCC.

PATHOLOGIC FEATURES

GROSS PATHOLOGY

Large regenerative nodules/low-grade dysplastic nodules are larger than other cirrhotic nodules. The lower limit for size is generally accepted as between 0.8 and 1 cm in diameter, and these lesions are almost always smaller than 3 cm in greatest diameter. These nodules tend to bulge on cut section; the edges of the nodules are rounded and sharply circumscribed, and they may be more deeply bile stained or paler yellow to tan than other cirrhotic nodules.

MICROSCOPIC PATHOLOGY

These nodules histologically resemble cirrhotic nodules. They have an intact reticulin framework similar to normal liver, and the cell plates are one or two cells in thickness (Fig. 42-5). The hepatocytes typically have unremarkable cytology, although some focal variations in cell size, especially scattered large cell changes similar to those seen in the other cirrhotic nodules, may be present in the large regenerative nodule. The low-grade dysplastic nodule would probably be expected to have a more uniform population of hepatocytes owing to its clonal nature, but many specific features of this type of clonal nodule have not been definitively established. Findings such as Mallory bodies,

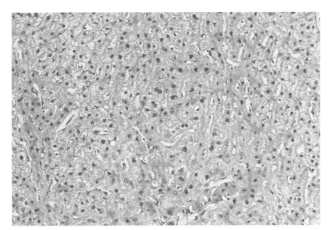

FIGURE 42–5. Macroregenerative or low-grade dysplastic nodule. The cytology of the cells is similar to that seen in normal liver, and the cell plate architecture is preserved.

bile stasis, clear cell cytoplasmic changes, iron or copper deposits, a slight decrease in cell size,[19] and focal or diffuse fatty change may be present. Portal tracts are usually present within the nodule, and bile ductular proliferation may be prominent, but fibrous septa extending into the nodule without the complete triad of duct, vein, and artery may be noted as well.[20]

SPECIAL STUDIES

Studies of the vascularity of these lesions have shown that they tend to have a greater number of arteries that lack the other components of a portal zone, the so-called unpaired artery. However, staining for CD34 or CD31 as a marker for sinusoidal capillarization is essentially the same as that seen in cirrhotic nodules; some peripheral staining is present at the edges of the nodule.[21,22] The nodules are negative for AFP[23] and otherwise show staining patterns similar to those expected in normal liver for cytokeratin and polyclonal CEA.

DIFFERENTIAL DIAGNOSIS

The size of this nodule differentiates it from other cirrhotic nodules. Rarely, a nodule with this pattern of histology may lack portal zones, but this does not warrant a diagnosis of adenoma in the cirrhotic liver unless one of the risk factors discussed earlier for adenoma is present. The features differentiating these nodules from high-grade dysplastic nodules and from small, well-differentiated HCCs are outlined in Table 42-3.

High-Grade Dysplastic (Borderline) Nodules

CLINICAL FEATURES

The high-grade dysplastic nodule,[5,20] which is also known as *borderline nodule*,[19] *type II macroregenerative nodule, atypical adenomatous hyperplasia,*

TABLE 42–3. Diagnostic Features: Large Regenerative and Dysplastic Nodules, Well-Differentiated Hepatocellular Carcinoma

Morphology	Large Regenerative (Macroregenerative) Nodule	Low-Grade Dysplastic Nodule	High-Grade Dysplastic (Borderline) Nodule	Well-Differentiated Hepatocellular Carcinoma
Overall hepatocyte size	Similar to cirrhotic nodules	A uniform population of hepatocytes with essentially normal cytologic features, suggesting a clonal proliferation	Variable, usually close to normal size or slightly smaller	Smaller or larger cells; diffuse-type changes most common
Small cell change, or nuclear density >2× normal	Absent or only scattered cells	Absent or only scattered cells	Occasional small foci, but nuclear density >2× normal; can be diffuse or prominent; dysplastic focus may have appearance of a nodule within a larger nodule	Small foci to large zones commonly present
Large cell change	Scattered cells may be present	Absent	Scattered cells may be present; zones of cells unlikely unless in dysplastic focus	May be present instead of, or in addition to, small cell change
Cell plates ≥3 cells thick, and presence of trabeculae	Absent	Absent	May see some plates >3 cells thick, but no zones of trabeculae present	Trabeculae commonly seen
Reticulin framework	Intact as in cirrhotic nodule, no foci of increased or absent reticulin	Intact	Focal loss or decreased reticulin	Usually, reticulin is extensively lost; occasionally, reticulin staining is more prominent with thickened bands separating tumor cell plates
Increased iron deposits	Sometimes present	Unknown	Sometimes present	Almost always absent, even in the setting of a siderotic liver
Periphery of nodule	Well circumscribed	Well circumscribed	Some with irregular edges	Common to see infiltrative or irregular edges
Portal zones or fibrous tissue zones	Almost always present; focal bile ductular proliferation may be present; normal portal structures usually seen	Probably present	Normal portal zones often seen within larger dysplastic nodules	No intact portal zones present unless entrapped near edge of tumor; fibrous zones or bands may be present, separating cell plates

and *atypical macroregenerative nodule*, almost always occurs in a cirrhotic liver. Serum AFP is normal or in the range seen with underlying chronic liver disease/cirrhosis. Most recommend that these lesions should be excised or ablated because they are believed to represent the beginning stages of a premalignant process.

PATHOGENESIS

This type of nodule, which typically occurs in the setting of cirrhosis, is considered to be a premalignant change on the pathway to the development of HCC.

PATHOLOGIC FEATURES

GROSS PATHOLOGY

These nodules have essentially the same gross features as large regenerative/low-grade dysplastic nodules with the exception that some of them may appear to be less well circumscribed or to have irregular edges.

MICROSCOPIC PATHOLOGY

When dysplastic changes are noted uniformly throughout the nodule, then the nodule is designated a *high-grade dysplastic nodule*. (A nodule containing one or more dysplastic foci is designated a *dysplastic nodule* [see Fig. 42-4].) The atypical features seen are not overtly diagnostic for HCC but are more atypical than expected in the usual cirrhotic nodule. The nodule is often recognized by zones of small cell change (see Fig. 42-4) with increased nucleus-to-cytoplasm ratio, also designated *increased nuclear density*, which is defined as the estimated number of hepatocyte nuclei per microscopic field compared with that in the normal liver.[19] Large cell change is rarely a feature of high-grade dysplastic nodules, but if it is, the focus must be a discrete zone of atypical cells rather than enlarged nuclei scattered singly throughout a nodule.

Other common features include the focal zones of cell plates up to three cells thick, a focal decrease in the reticulin framework, and mild dilatation of sinusoids. These nodules may also contain foci of Mallory bodies, fat, clear cell changes, cytoplasmic basophilia, bile, and portal tracts. Iron deposits may be present, but high-grade dysplastic lesions tend to lack iron deposits in contrast to low-grade nodules, in which iron deposits are more common. The edges of the nodule may be irregular, and focal acini (pseudoglands) may be present.

DIFFERENTIAL DIAGNOSIS

This lesion is differentiated from overt HCC by features such as those described in Table 42-3. Features that are probably most helpful for the diagnosis of HCC include the presence of mitotic figures in moderate numbers, trabeculae, cell plates greater than three cells thick, nuclear density greater than two times normal, marked reduction in reticulin framework, numerous unpaired arteries, and absence of portal zones.

MALIGNANT LESIONS

Hepatocellular Carcinoma and Variants

CLINICAL FEATURES

HCC, the most common malignant primary tumor in the liver, is usually seen in the setting of cirrhosis (noted in approximately 85% of cases[24]). Lesions smaller than 1.5 cm generally do not enhance on radiographic angiography, and HCC may be more or less echogenic than the adjacent liver. A high serum AFP level (>1000 ng/mL) is seen in almost two thirds of cases of large tumors[24]; tumors smaller than 2 to 3 cm are unlikely to have an elevated serum AFP.[23] Elevations of serum AFP of less than 500 ng/mL may be seen in many liver disorders, and elevations from 500 to 1000 ng/mL are suggestive of HCC but are not as reliably specific. Prognosis is typically correlated with staging for lymph node and distant metastases and with histologic features that may be evaluated routinely on resection samples, such as vascular invasion, adequacy of surgical resection margins (with at least 1 cm typically recommended),

number and location of lesions, and size of tumor. The relationship of histologic tumor grade or subtype of HCC to prognosis is considered by most to be not as important as these factors,[6] except when the histology is that of fibrolamellar HCC (see under Fibrolamellar Variant of Hepatocellular Carcinoma). Liver transplantation has been shown to be an effective form of therapy for HCCs smaller than 5 cm in greatest diameter and without evidence of large vessel invasion. Alternative therapies such as cryoablation, percutaneous ethanol injection, and transarterial chemoembolization have also been used, predominantly in inoperable cases, to improve length of survival.

PATHOGENESIS

The major etiologic association for HCC is cirrhosis, but HBV or HCV infection also is a predisposing factor. Patients with cirrhosis due to hemochromatosis and alpha-1-antitrypsin disease may also have an increased risk of HCC compared with patients with cirrhosis due to other causes (excluding HBV and HCV). Other risk factors include exposure to Thorotrast (thorium dioxide), aflatoxins, and estrogenic steroids.[10]

PATHOLOGIC FEATURES

GROSS PATHOLOGY

Most HCCs arise in the cirrhotic liver. HCC may be more bile stained or paler than the adjacent liver, and it may have irregular borders or even satellite nodules. Large vein invasion and a fibrous capsule may be noted in association with large tumors. Small HCC is generally defined as HCC measuring less than 2 cm in diameter; these small tumors usually lack gross vascular invasion, necrosis, and hemorrhagic zones.

MICROSCOPIC PATHOLOGY

Several typical histologic patterns of HCC[6] have been described by the World Health Organization.

1. *Trabecular pattern.* The most common is the trabecular pattern, also known as the *sinusoidal pattern* (Fig. 42-6). In this variant, tumor morphology mimics the cell plate architecture of normal liver but with important differences. First, the cell plates in trabecular HCC are three cells thick or greater, compared with the plates of normal or regenerative liver, which are only one or two cells thick. As in normal liver, tumor cell plates are lined with endothelial cells. However, on reticulin stain, the reticulin framework is often absent or may be markedly decreased or distorted with irregular or absent staining of the edges of the trabeculae (Fig. 42-7). Tumor cells often have features of small cell change (see Figs. 42-6 and 42-7). Large cell change may also be noted but is

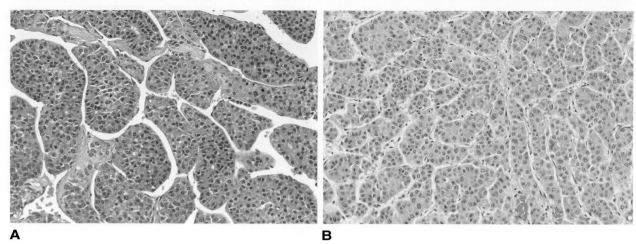

A **B**

FIGURE 42–6. A, Hepatocellular carcinoma, trabecular type. The cell plate architecture shows wide plates forming trabeculae and somewhat dilated sinusoids. The trabeculae are lined by endothelial cells. Bile stasis and small cell change are also present. **B,** Hepatocellular carcinoma, trabecular type. The cell plates are equal to or wider than 3 cells thick in most of this area of tumor. Small cell change is also present.

probably less frequently seen except in higher-grade tumors. Often, foci of small or large cell change are admixed. Kupffer cells are typically absent.

2. *Acinar pattern.* The acinar pattern of HCC, also called *pseudoglandular* or *adenoid*, is less common than the trabecular type. The defining feature in this variant is the glandlike spaces, or acini, lined by hepatocytic tumor cells (Fig. 42-8). These acinar structures are formed by the dilatation or expansion of bile canaliculi, and they often contain bile or proteinaceous material. Less frequently, the spaces are a result of central necrosis of the trabeculae and so may instead contain protein, cellular debris, or macrophages. Because of the formation of these glandlike

spaces, one must not mistake this lesion for adenocarcinoma. The acinar pattern is frequently admixed as a minor component with the trabecular pattern (see Fig. 42-7).

3. *Solid pattern.* The solid or *compact* pattern of HCC is a relatively uncommon variant characterized by dense aggregates of tumor cells that may seem to lack endothelial cell–lined trabeculae or cell plates (Fig. 42-9); however, careful examination with endothelial cell markers often reveals the presence of compressed trabeculae. Loss of the reticulin framework is typically seen as well in solid, crowded zones.

4. *Scirrhous pattern.* The final pattern is the scirrhous pattern, which contains focal to diffuse, prominent areas of fibrosis that may be associated

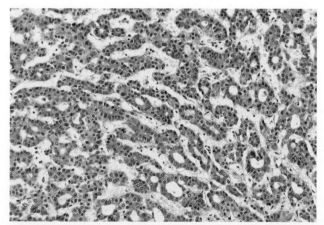

FIGURE 42–7. Hepatocellular carcinoma, trabecular type. Reticulin stain shows complete loss of the reticulin framework (which would be visible as black strands of subendothelial connective tissue). The cell plates are relatively thin, and pseudoglands (acinar structures) are also present (reticulin stain).

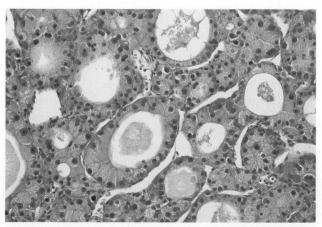

FIGURE 42–8. Hepatocellular carcinoma, pseudoglandular (acinar) type. The hepatocytes form glandlike structures that contain proteinaceous debris but also contain bile (not shown here).

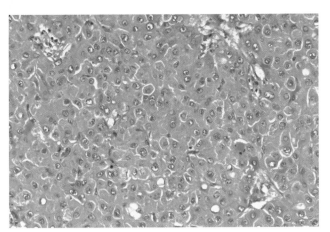

FIGURE 42–9. Hepatocellular carcinoma, solid type. The tumor cells are arranged in sheets without definable cell plate or trabecular architecture.

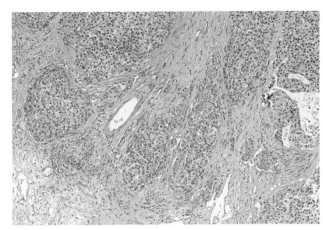

FIGURE 42–10. Hepatocellular carcinoma, scirrhous type. The tumor nests are separated by fibrous connective tissue.

with any of the patterns described here (Fig. 42-10). Occasionally, the tumor cell plates (or trabeculae) may be separated by increased amounts of connective tissue instead of by endothelial cell–lined sinusoidal spaces. In these instances, reticulin staining is usually increased in the bands of connective tissue rather than decreased, as has been described for the trabecular pattern of HCC. The thickened cell plates, which are separated by this prominent reticulin framework, often have a linear or ribbon-like arrangement. This pattern could be subclassified as a form of scirrhous HCC as well, although the overall amount of fibrous tissue may not be as great as has typically been described (Fig. 42-11). Differentiation of scirrhous HCC from fibrolamellar HCC (discussed under Fibrolamellar Hepatocellular Carcinoma) is based on identification of

the particular cytologic features of the latter, as well as on the different clinical settings in which these two tumors occur.

The cytologic features of HCC within any of these patterns tend to resemble those of normal hepatocytes, with variable degrees of nuclear atypia ranging from essentially normal to abnormal angular nuclei with clumped chromatin. Tumor cells often maintain a polygonal shape and have round vesicular nuclei and prominent nucleoli—typical features of hepatocytic differentiation. Intranuclear vacuoles (composed of cytoplasmic invaginations) and glycogenation of nuclei (another feature seen in normal liver) are fairly common findings (Fig. 42-12). Small cell change (as described earlier) is probably the most common atypical cytologic change, but large cell change and giant and/or pleomorphic cells may be present as either a diffuse or a focal finding (see Fig. 42-12). The amount of cytoplasm

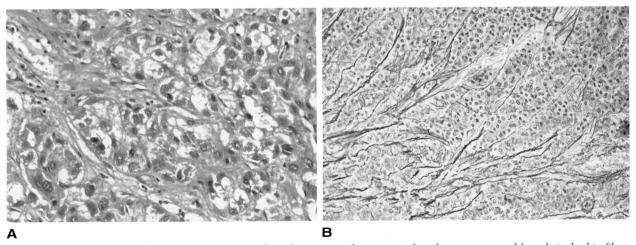

A   **B**

FIGURE 42–11. A, Hepatocellular carcinoma, variant of scirrhous type. The tumor trabeculae are separated by relatively thin fibrous bands. Extensive Mallory's hyaline is present within many of the tumor cells. **B,** Hepatocellular carcinoma, variant of scirrhous type. Reticulin stain shows increased staining for reticulin fibers along the thin fibrous septa that separate the tumor trabeculae. The tumor plates tend to line up in a side-by-side (ribbon-like) pattern.

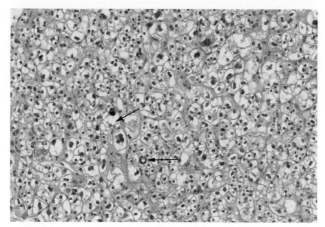

FIGURE 42–12. Hepatocellular carcinoma, clear cell variant. This tumor shows prominent cytoplasmic clear cell change. In addition, an occasional intranuclear vacuole, focally enlarged pleomorphic nuclei, and some eosinophilic cytoplasmic globules are present *(arrows)*.

may vary, and it is often slightly more basophilic than that seen in normal hepatocytes. The cytoplasm may also have a granular appearance or may be exceptionally oxyphilic owing to the presence of large numbers of mitochondria. Cytoplasmic inclusions such as Mallory bodies or globular acidophilic bodies composed of proteins, including albumin, fibrinogen, alpha-1-antitrypsin, or ferritin, may be present (see Fig. 42-12).

Fat (Fig. 42-13), glycogen, or even water may be prominent as well, giving the cells a clear cell appearance (see Fig. 42-12), which has been described as the clear cell variant of HCC. If the entire tumor shows this type of clear cell change and if it occurs in the noncirrhotic liver, it may be difficult to differentiate HCC from other clear cell tumors such as metastatic renal cell carcinoma. Other cytoplasmic changes that are seen much less frequently include pale bodies

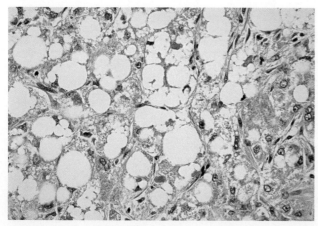

FIGURE 42–13. Hepatocellular carcinoma with prominent fatty change. This portion of the tumor shows prominent fat droplets within the tumor cell cytoplasm.

(which are round to oval, lightly eosinophilic or clear cytoplasmic structures most frequently seen in the fibrolamellar variant of HCC; see under Fibrolamellar Hepatocellular Carcinoma), ground-glass cells containing hepatitis B surface antigen (HBsAg) (present in some patients with HBV infection),[25] and dark-brown to black pigment like that seen in the Dubin-Johnson syndrome. Rare forms of HCC with a prominent spindle cell component and a small cell type have been described.

HISTOLOGIC GRADING OF HCC

The grading of HCC has traditionally been based on three or four grades, according to the system developed by Edmondson and Steiner in 1954.[26] These investigators originally defined four grades that were distinguished by proportional increases in the nucleus-to-cytoplasm ratio, variability in nuclear shape, hyperchromasia, and loss of cell plate architecture from low- to high-grade tumors. These grades are still used[6] with some modifications.

Some of Edmondson/Steiner's grade I tumors with minimal cytologic atypia and architectural distortion were recognized as malignant only by their association with admixtures of higher grades of HCC or by the presence of metastatic lesions.[24,26] With the current criteria now available as established by the International Working Party,[5] stricter definition for "grade I" lesions may possibly differentiate some of these as simply dysplastic nodules. Ideally, a true grade I HCC still exhibits definitive architectural features of malignancy (as per Table 42-3), even though it shows little to no cytologic atypia.

Grade II tumors are still well differentiated and still have a typical trabecular pattern but with increased nuclear size as compared with grade I tumors. Grade II lesions may also contain acinar structures and bile.

Grade III tumors are moderately differentiated and have greater cytologic and architectural variability than do grade II lesions. Multinucleated and giant cells are often seen focally, and, in contrast to grade II lesions, bile is often not present. When trabeculae are present, they are typically wider and/or more variable in structure than those in grade II tumors.

Grade IV consists of poorly differentiated tumors or anaplastic lesions for which classification as HCC is difficult without the appropriate clinical setting, such as cirrhosis or significantly elevated serum AFP. Grade IV lesions may include spindle cell and small cell components as well.

An alternative three-grade system is often used, with grade I representing well-differentiated lesions (grades I and II from the previously described system combined); grade II, moderately differentiated lesions; and grade III, poorly differentiated and anaplastic lesions.

Regardless of which grading system is used, vascular invasion and poor differentiation are independent findings indicative of a poorer prognosis.

SPECIAL STUDIES

AFP is a reasonably specific marker for HCC; however, the staining tends to be patchy and completely absent in up to half of HCCs; it has been noted to be absent in small, well-differentiated HCCs.[27] Polyclonal CEA, which highlights the bile canaliculi, is another highly specific marker for hepatocellular differentiation,[27] but it tends to stain only the well- to moderately differentiated lesions. This stain also delineates outer cellular membranes in adenocarcinomas, which may potentially mimic a canalicular pattern on tangential sectioning. A relatively new hepatocyte antibody (DAKO clone OCH1E5.2.10) may also prove to be relatively specific for hepatocellular differentiation. This antibody stains in a granular pattern within the cytoplasm to varying degrees within tumors with hepatocytic differentiation, but as with polyclonal CEA, it tends to be less sensitive for poorly differentiated HCCs.[27,28]

Cytokeratins 8 and 18 (present in the CAM 5.2 stain) are generally seen in tumors with hepatocellular differentiation; AE1/AE3, which contains most other keratin types but not 8 and 18, is often negative. However, both of these cytokeratins stain most adenocarcinomas, so the CAM 5.2 cannot be used in isolation. In addition, cytokeratin 7 tends to be negative in the majority of HCCs but, in our experience, focally stains smaller ductular-like hepatocytes or some acinar structures within HCC; cytokeratin 20 is essentially always negative. CD10 stains the cytoplasmic surface of the hepatocyte, and CD34 typically stains the endothelium-lined trabeculae in HCC and highlights their increased vascularity.

DIFFERENTIAL DIAGNOSIS

Immunoperoxidase studies are not helpful in differentiating benign from malignant hepatocellular tumors; however, they may help to distinguish HCC from other tumors in the liver. Most diagnostic problems arise in differentiating benign hepatocellular tumors such as adenoma or focal nodular hyperplasia from well-differentiated HCC, or poorly differentiated HCC from other primary or metastatic neoplasms. Well-differentiated HCC may be differentiated from large regenerative/low-grade dysplastic nodules and high-grade dysplastic nodules by features noted in Table 42-3.

DISTINCTION FROM ADENOCARCINOMA

Monoclonal CEA is often diffusely positive in some types of adenocarcinoma and usually does not stain hepatocellular tumors. LeuM1, B72.3, and Lewis blood group[x] (Le[x]) tend to be positive in adenocarcinomas and negative in HCC[29] and, when used in combination with

the monoclonal CEA and perhaps the hepatocyte antibody (see earlier under Special Studies), may be helpful in distinguishing poorly differentiated adenocarcinoma from HCC. Routine histochemical stains for the epithelial mucins such as mucicarmine or d-PAS are often helpful because mucins should not be present in HCC except in combined HCC/cholangiocarcinoma and in some cases of fibrolamellar variant of HCC (FLHCC). One must take some care in the interpretation of the d-PAS stain, however, because this method also reacts with many cytoplasmic glycoproteins produced by hepatocytes, resulting in a possible false-positive interpretation. A combination of the profiles of cytokeratins 7, 19, and 20 may be helpful because these tend to be positive in cholangiocarcinoma (cytokeratin 19 is essentially always positive in cholangiocarcinoma) or metastatic carcinoma[30-32] and negative in HCC.[31,33]

DISTINCTION FROM NEUROENDOCRINE TUMORS

HCC may also be difficult to distinguish from a neuroendocrine neoplasm because both may form acinar or trabecular-like structures, and both may be composed of relatively large tumor cells with abundant eosinophilic cytoplasm and round nuclei. Features that favor a neuroendocrine tumor in such cases include a prominent vascular or capillary network and/or stromal hyalinization. These neuroendocrine tumors may rarely arise as a primary lesion in the liver; otherwise, they are almost always metastatic.[24] Focal neuroendocrine differentiation, including the fibrolamellar variant, has been noted in HCC, as well as in hepatoblastoma, with the use of various markers such as neuron-specific enolase (NSE), protein gene product 9.5 (PGP 9.5), vasoactive intestinal peptide (VIP), calcitonin, and S100,[34-36] but diffuse staining with a marker such as chromogranin or synaptophysin would strongly support the diagnosis of a neuroendocrine tumor.

DISTINCTION FROM OTHER TUMOR TYPES

Clear cell carcinomas in the liver may pose a diagnostic challenge in distinguishing the clear cell variant of HCC from clear cell renal cell carcinoma that is metastatic to the liver.[28] In a cirrhotic liver, the diagnosis of clear cell variant of HCC may be made with enough certainty that stains are not necessary. However, for lesions in a noncirrhotic liver without significant AFP elevation, the likelihood of a metastatic lesion makes differentiation more critical. Keratin profiles are not helpful because both of these tumors typically show similar staining (positive for CAM 5.2, negative for cytokeratins 7 and 20). However, HCC of these clear cell types often demonstrates polyclonal CEA canalicular staining; renal cell carcinomas show no canalicular pattern. Other useful markers are epithelial membrane antigen (EMA), which tends to be positive in renal cell carcinoma and negative in HCC, and the hepatocyte antibody (see earlier under Special Studies) that does not stain renal cell carcinoma.

Melanomas may also mimic HCCs, but S100 and HMB-45 are usually but not always negative in hepatocellular tumors. Rarely, an adrenocortical tumor may need to be distinguished from a primary hepatocellular tumor. In these instances, positive staining for inhibin A,[37] which has a high percentage of positivity in adrenal tumors but not in hepatocytic lesions, may be helpful, in addition to the hepatocyte markers previously discussed such as polyclonal CEA and hepatocyte antibody. The use of immunohistochemistry in the differentiation of HCC from primary mesenchymal tumors is described later under Mesenchymal Tumors.

Fibrolamellar Variant of Hepatocellular Carcinoma

FLHCC occurs in the noncirrhotic liver in young adults (mean age, 26 years; females > males) and, with this strict definition (as is generally accepted), has a better prognosis than does typical HCC of similar size. Lesions with similar morphology have been noted in the cirrhotic liver,[38-40] but these HCCs should not be diagnosed as FLHCC by convention owing to their much more variable outcome.

CLINICAL FEATURES

Presentation may be accompanied by complaints such as abdominal pain or swelling, anorexia, weight loss, jaundice, and, rarely, hemoperitoneum. No definitive risk factors have been identified. Nodular hyperplastic changes have been noted adjacent to FLHCC,[41,42] but most researchers concur that this is a secondary affect caused by vascular changes within the liver adjacent to the tumor rather than a suggestion that FLHCC arises in association with FNH. Serum AFP levels are usually normal; only rarely have high levels been reported.[38,39] Complete excision of the involved lobe is the current therapy of choice. When tumor location precludes resection, liver transplantation has been done, but the outcome is not as favorable.

PATHOLOGIC FEATURES

GROSS PATHOLOGY

FLHCC is a well-circumscribed, nodular, yellow to brown tumor with fibrosis. Rarely, a prominent central, fibrous zone similar to that of FNH[38] may be present. Larger tumors may show foci of hemorrhage and necrosis; satellite lesions are rare.

MICROSCOPIC PATHOLOGY

The cellular component of FLHCC consists of small to large clusters or sheets of tumor cells separated by dense bands of lamellar fibrous tissue (Fig. 42-14).

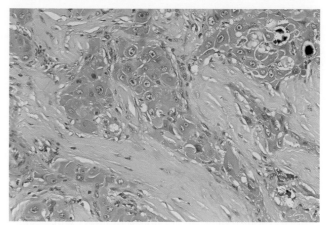

FIGURE 42–14. Fibrolamellar variant of hepatocellular carcinoma. The tumor cells have a distinctive eosinophilic and granular cytoplasm, polygonal shape, and relatively large round nuclei with prominent nucleoli. The tumor cells are arranged in small groups and are separated by dense lamellar collagen.

These tumor cells tend to have a polygonal shape, and they routinely comprise eosinophilic and granular cytoplasm. Nuclei are large, with prominent nucleoli easily identified. Other cytoplasmic features include the "pale body," which may contain fibrinogen and/or albumin, and d-PAS–positive bodies, which probably represent various glycoprotein secretions. Other focal features that may be noted include acinar structures, bile, multinucleated tumor cells, copper, fat, epithelioid granulomas, and peliosis hepatis. Neuroendocrine markers (see earlier under Distinction From Neuroendocrine Tumors) have been reported to be focally positive but have no known clinical significance.[36] Glandular differentiation with mucin secretion and zones of trabecular HCC have also been noted[43]; it is not clear whether these variations result in a poorer prognosis.

Combined Hepatocellular/Cholangiolar Carcinoma

Combined (or mixed) hepatocellular/cholangiolar carcinoma (HCC/CC) may account for up to 5% of all primary carcinomas of the liver.[43] The risk factors are essentially the same as those for HCC alone.

DIAGNOSTIC FEATURES

Combined HCC/CC includes a mixture of hepatocellular and ductular elements scattered throughout the tumor (Fig. 42-15).[6] Collision tumors, in which each element is separated or appears side by side, are not considered to fall into this combined category, according to the World Health Organization classification.[6] Findings on percutaneous needle biopsies of combined HCC/CC may be confusing because a glandular or ductular malignancy is sampled in a patient with risk

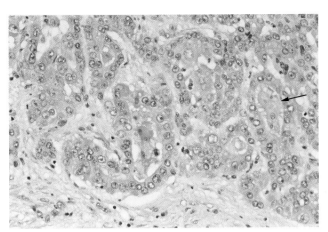

FIGURE 42–15. Combined hepatocellular cholangiocarcinoma. This example shows bile present in a glandlike structure as well as faint blue mucin *(arrow)*. More prominent mucin was noted in other areas of the tumor.

conditions for HCC. Thus, combined HCC/CC tumor should be kept in the differential diagnosis for primary liver malignancies sampled by needle biopsy.

SPECIAL STUDIES

Cytoplasmic mucin and/or immunoperoxidase stain for keratin types such as AE1/AE3 and cytokeratins 19 or 20 (as seen in ductular tumors) may be used to identify the cholangiocarcinoma component. Cytokeratin 7 also identifies ductular components, but this may stain cells within HCC as well, so caution should be used in interpretation of cytokeratin 7 alone. Bile production by tumor cells or immunoperoxidase positivity for markers specific for hepatocytes such as AFP, polyclonal CEA, and hepatocyte antibody may help to reveal the hepatocellular component.

Sclerosing Hepatic Carcinoma

This term has been used to refer to a mixture of hepatocellular, cholangiolar, and combined HCC/CCs with tubular neoplastic structures embedded in a fibrous stroma that are typically associated with hypercalcemia.[44]

Hepatoblastoma

Hepatoblastoma (HB) is the most common malignant liver tumor in children; about 66% occur in children younger than 2 years of age, and 90% occur before the age of 5. This tumor may occasionally arise in older children[45,46] and rarely in adults.[47] The lesion has a surprising male preponderance of almost 2 to 1. Associations with other congenital conditions such as Beckwith-Wiedemann syndrome,[46] cleft palate, diaphragmatic hernia,[48] Down syndrome, familial polyposis coli,[49] hemihypertrophy, renal malformation, and other chromosomal abnormalities[50] may be noted in as many as one third of reported cases.

Presenting symptoms such as an abdominal mass, failure to thrive, and loss of weight are relatively common. Less common are features such as vomiting, diarrhea, and jaundice. A patient may rarely present with signs of precocious puberty such as virilization, which is associated with production of human chorionic gonadotropin (HCG) by the tumor.[51] Serum AFP is nearly always elevated and has proved to be a useful marker for tumor recurrence or metastasis after therapy. Prognosis is directly related to complete surgical excision and tumor stage.[52] The treatment of choice is thus complete surgical resection, but chemotherapy is often used preoperatively to reduce tumor size, as well as for treatment of residual tumor and nonresectable tumors. Some histologic subtypes (see under Microscopic Pathology, below), such as the pure fetal types, are thought by some to have a better prognosis after complete resection[45] than do fetal/embryonal or mixed patterns. Other subtypes, such as small cell and macrotrabecular types, may worsen the prognosis.[52] Tumor-free margins are thought to be important for prognosis, but vascular invasion probably does not have a significant effect on outcome.[45] Other factors thought to be associated with a more adverse outcome include age of presentation younger than 1 year, large tumor size, and involvement of vital structures.

PATHOLOGIC FEATURES

GROSS PATHOLOGY

HB occurs in the noncirrhotic liver, typically as a large, single mass. Gross appearance may be variable, but the tumor is often multinodular with foci of hemorrhage and necrosis. Because grossly different nodules or zones within the tumor may represent different histologic components, which in turn may correlate with prognosis, adequate sections of these various areas must be taken. After chemotherapy, tumors may be necrotic, and their mesenchymal components, especially the osteoid, often remain prominent.[53]

MICROSCOPIC PATHOLOGY

The two subtypes of differentiation most commonly seen in HB are the epithelial and mixed epithelial/mesenchymal types. The epithelial type presents typically as a combination of two histologic forms—the embryonal and fetal patterns; rarely, a pure fetal subtype may occur. The mixed epithelial/mesenchymal subtype is usually composed of two epithelial patterns admixed with a spindle cell mesenchyme; osteoid is also a common finding.

Within the epithelial subtype, the embryonal pattern is the more "immature" form; it consists of small tumor

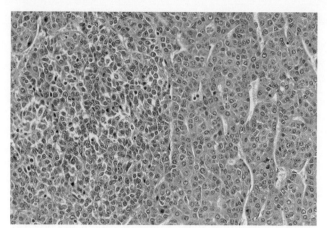

FIGURE 42–16. Hepatoblastoma. The embryonal component *(left)* shows small, rather undifferentiated tumor cells arranged in a somewhat ribbon-like pattern. The fetal component *(right)* shows better-differentiated tumor cells with pink cytoplasm and round nuclei, arranged in thickened trabeculae.

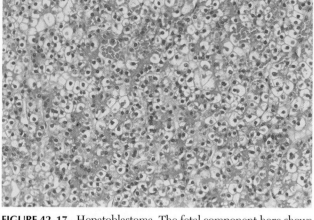

FIGURE 42–17. Hepatoblastoma. The fetal component here shows an alternating white and pink pattern of staining of the cytoplasm of the tumor cells.

cells with fairly round to oval nuclei and scant basophilic cytoplasm, which tend to form tubular, acinar, or ribbon-like arrangements (Fig. 42-16). The fetal pattern is the other, more "mature" form that more closely resembles fetal liver and includes tumor cell arrangement in plates or cords (see Fig. 42-16). The tumor cells in the fetal pattern are typically smaller than normal hepatocytes but are slightly larger than the tumor cells in the embryonal pattern; they show cytoplasmic changes of hepatocellular differentiation. The tumor cells in the fetal pattern also have moderate amounts of eosinophilic and/or clear cytoplasm, with clear cell changes caused by the presence of lipids and/or glycogen. Both eosinophilic and clear cytoplasmic features often occur in the same tumor and result in a distinctive, alternating pink and white appearance (Fig. 42-17). Nuclei in the fetal pattern are typically small and round, similar to normal fetal liver cells. In both patterns, mitotic figures are rare. Extramedullary hematopoiesis is often present and is usually associated with the fetal component.

Less commonly seen subtypes of HB include the small cell undifferentiated type, the macrotrabecular type, and the mixed type with teratoid features. The small cell type consists of sheets of tumor cells without evidence of hepatocellular differentiation. These cells have scant cytoplasm that is similar to that of neuroblastoma; therefore, one of the other typical patterns of HB must be present for this possibility to be excluded. The macrotrabecular type forms wide trabeculae that must be greater than 10 cells thick. Fetal and/or embryonal types of tumor cells typically make up these trabeculae, but a less common pattern of larger cells with more cytoplasm may rarely be seen, which may histologically mimic HCC. Again, the presence of other patterns of HB and their occurrence in a noncirrhotic liver may help to distinguish this variant of macro-

trabecular HB from HCC arising in a child. A tumor with a limited macrotrabecular component should probably be classified according to the other predominant patterns.[52] Mixed-type HB with teratoid features contains both epithelial and mesenchymal components, as well as foci of other tissue types such as intestinal-type glandular elements, squamous epithelium, melanin pigment, other mesenchymal elements such as cartilage or skeletal muscle, or neural tissue.

SPECIAL STUDIES

HB stains positively for AFP in the embryonal component,[35] and both hepatocyte antibody (see above under Hepatocellular Carcinoma and Variants, Special Studies) and polyclonal CEA stain the epithelial component, especially the fetal component, of this tumor.[28] Focal neuroendocrine staining with chromogranin A has been reported in the embryonal, fetal, and osteoid components.[35,54]

DIFFERENTIAL DIAGNOSIS

Pure fetal HB may be histologically similar to hepatic adenoma; tumor cells tend to be smaller in HB than in adenoma, and the alternating pink and white cytoplasmic staining pattern of HB is typically not seen in adenoma. However, the lesions are conventionally separated by clinical parameters as well. For example, hepatic adenoma essentially does not occur before age 5, except in association with a metabolic disorder such as glycogen storage disease, and serum AFP is not elevated in adenoma. Clinical parameters also play an important role in distinguishing the macrotrabecular variant of HB from HCC in that the latter essentially occurs only in this young age group in the presence of preexisting liver disease or metabolic disorder (usually in the setting of cirrhosis).

▮ Ductular Lesions

BENIGN DUCTULAR LESIONS

Biliary Hamartoma

CLINICAL FEATURES

Biliary hamartoma (BH), or the von Meyenburg complex, is thought to represent a ductal plate malformation; therefore, these lesions are often seen as part of the spectrum of polycystic disease in the liver and other organs.

PATHOLOGIC FEATURES

GROSS PATHOLOGY

BH is a small (usually smaller than 0.5 cm), gray to white, irregularly shaped lesion; multifocality is common.

MICROSCOPIC PATHOLOGY

BH consists of numerous small to medium-sized ductules, which are typically more dilated than normal ducts and are separated by dense collagen (Fig. 42-18). These typically are located within and at the edges of a portal zone. The ductules are lined by small, cuboidal to flattened epithelium with round to oval nuclei; they are also more irregularly shaped than normal ducts and may contain eosinophilic debris or inspissated bile.

Bile Duct Adenoma

CLINICAL FEATURES

Bile duct adenoma (BDA) is a less common lesion than BH. The designation *adenoma* may be a misnomer in that most feel this lesion does not represent a true neoplasm but rather a localized ductular proliferation at a site of previous injury[55] or a form of peribiliary gland hamartoma.[56] Lesions are usually discovered as incidental findings and may be biopsied at the time of surgery (often for frozen section) to exclude metastatic disease.

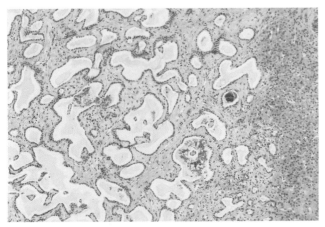

FIGURE 42–18. Bile duct hamartoma. The lesion shows dilated ductular structures lined by cuboidal to flattened bile duct epithelium. Some of these structures contain bile.

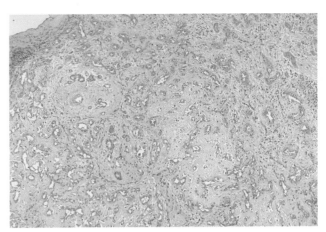

FIGURE 42–19. Bile duct adenoma. In this case, the lesion is located immediately beneath the capsule of the liver. The ductules are relatively evenly spaced and form small curvilinear glandular structures separated by fibrous tissue. Inflammation is scant, and the cytology of the ductules is unremarkable.

PATHOLOGIC FEATURES

GROSS PATHOLOGY

BDAs are small lesions (usually less than 2 cm in diameter); they are firm, white to gray-tan, and well circumscribed. Typically, they are noted in a subcapsular location, but they may be found deep in the parenchyma. BDAs may be single or multifocal.

MICROSCROPIC PATHOLOGY

The ductules in BDA are more uniform in size without the appearance of dilatation and with less intervening fibrous stroma than is found in the ductules of hamartomas (Fig. 42-19). Although the fibrous stroma is typically not as pronounced as that in hamartoma, the amount of collagenization may vary considerably, and focal zones of dense collagen may be present. The ductules tend to have a tubular or curvilinear shape and are lined by cuboidal epithelium with bland, round to oval nuclei without mitotic activity. Mucinous metaplasia of the epithelium, alpha-1-antitrypsin droplets, and neuroendocrine differentiation may be noted in the tubular lining cells. Typically, residual portal tracts are often preserved within or near the edge of the lesion, and small aggregates of lymphocytes are present at the periphery.

Hepatobiliary (Biliary) Cystadenoma (and Cystadenocarcinoma)

CLINICAL FEATURES

Hepatobiliary, or biliary, cystadenomas are rare lesions, with a higher incidence among women and histologic counterparts in the pancreas and ovary. These cystic tumors are typically associated with an ovarian type of stroma when they occur in women, but not in men.

Lesions may also be associated with the development of cystadenocarcinoma, which tends to be a low-grade adenocarcinoma in women but has greater malignant potential in men.

PATHOLOGIC FEATURES

GROSS PATHOLOGY

Hepatobiliary cystadenomas are almost always multi-locular with a smooth or somewhat trabeculated inner surface to the cyst walls. The cysts contain fluid of variable appearance, including serous, mucinous, gelatinous, occasionally hemorrhagic, or even purulent. No communication occurs between the cysts and the biliary tree. Large polypoid projections from or dense masses in the wall of a cyst often indicate zones of malignant transformation.

MICROSCOPIC PATHOLOGY

Cysts are lined by a single layer of epithelial cells, usually of a mucinous type. The cells may vary from flattened to cuboidal to columnar, and small papillary tufts may be present along the surface. Epithelial nuclei are bland and basally located without mitotic activity. The underlying stroma often has an appearance similar to that of ovarian stroma (when the lesion occurs in a woman), but this stroma may not be uniformly present. A more densely hyalinized stroma often separates the ovarian-like stroma from the adjacent liver. Cyst walls may also be lined focally by macrophages, calcifications, or scarlike tissue.

Cystadenocarcinomas arising in this lesion often have a tubulopapillary type of histology.[57] Features such as marked nuclear pleomorphism, loss of polarity, mitotic figures, and multilayering of the epithelium all could suggest the possibility of transformation to malignancy and may be designated *in situ cystadenocarcinoma*,[57] but invasion of tumor into the stroma is the best evidence for the presence of carcinoma.

Simple Cyst

CLINICAL FEATURES

Simple biliary cysts are generally an incidental finding. When multiple cysts are noted, they often represent a component of polycystic disease and are accompanied by von Meyenburg complexes (biliary hamartomas). Simple cysts have no or only slight premalignant potential.

PATHOLOGIC FEATURES

GROSS PATHOLOGY

Simple cysts are usually found in a subcapsular location, but some may occur deeper in the parenchyma. They typically contain a clear, light-yellow fluid.

MICROSCOPIC PATHOLOGY

Simple cysts are lined by a cuboidal to low columnar epithelium with a fibrous wall. This epithelium may be disrupted or flattened, and the wall may be thickened. Evidence for reactive changes such as recent or remote hemorrhage in the cyst wall may be present.

Other Rare Benign Biliary Tumors or Lesions

Biliary adenofibroma is a recently described, extremely rare entity that is considered benign.[58] The lesion consists of ductular and stromal elements with solid and microcystic regions. The ductular components may be similar to those in bile duct adenoma, and they often have tortuous or branching configurations. Others are dilated to form microcysts. The epithelium lining the ducts is cuboidal to low columnar, but it is often more flattened along the dilated microcysts. The cytoplasm of the ductal cells is amphophilic, and foci of apocrine change may be seen. Occasional epithelial tufts and mitotic figures may also be detected. No mucin is produced, but some cysts may contain an eosinophilic fluid. The stroma, which is composed of spindly fibroblasts and a patchy, moderate inflammatory infiltrate, forms well-defined septa between the glands.

Serous cystadenoma, which is similar grossly and microscopically to microcystic adenoma (serous cyst-adenoma) of the pancreas, has only rarely been described to occur in the liver.[57] Similar to its pancreatic counterpart, this tumor consists of multiple microcysts lined by cuboidal epithelium that contains glycogen (and so is PAS-positive).

Biloma is a term used for a large, encapsulated collection of bile located outside of the bile ducts and often found in perihepatic tissues around the gall-bladder. These collections of bile usually occur secondary to trauma or iatrogenic injury, and treatment is often surgical excision. The lesion consists of bilious debris admixed with and surrounded by inflammatory cells and macrophages, the latter of which may often have a xanthomatous appearance. Often, an exuberant fibrous connective tissue reaction occurs at the periphery of the bile, which accounts for the encapsulated appearance of the lesion.

MALIGNANT DUCTULAR LESIONS

Cholangiocarcinoma

CLINICAL FEATURES

Cholangiocarcinoma typically occurs in the elderly, with both sexes affected equally. In general, no association with cirrhosis has been noted, although patients with primary sclerosing cholangitis do have a significantly increased risk of developing this tumor.[59,60]

The tumor is most prevalent in Southeast Asia, where liver fluke infestation with *Clonorchis* species and *Opisthorchis* species is high. Other possible risk factors include congenital anomalies of the biliary tree such as von Meyenburg complex,[61] choledochal cyst,[62] Caroli's disease,[63] anomalous arrangements of the pancreatic and common bile ducts,[64] hepatolithiasis,[65] and use of Thorotrast.[66] Presenting systems vary with location of the tumor; four locations are often designated separately as peripheral (intrahepatic), hilar,[67] extrahepatic, and intraductal. Extrahepatic lesions are discussed in greater detail in Chapter 29. The peripheral type usually remains asymptomatic until the tumor is in a late stage; the hilar, extrahepatic, and intraductal types present with signs of obstruction. Prognosis for the peripheral, hilar, and extrahepatic types is dismal, usually because the disease has reached an advanced stage by the time it is diagnosed, rendering surgical removal difficult if not impossible; however, the length of survival may be increased when tumor-free surgical margins may be attained.[3]

The intraductal papillary type, also known as *intraductal papillomatosis*,[6] *biliary papillomatosis*, or *intraductal papillary tumor*, generally involves extensive areas of intrahepatic and/or extrahepatic bile ducts, with preference for the latter. Men are more greatly affected than women at a ratio of about 2.4:1, and patients are usually middle-aged and older (mean age, 60). Although histologically benign in most cases, the lesion is generally regarded in the clinical setting as a borderline or low-grade malignant tumor because of its tendency to recur, its multicentricity, its ability to undergo malignant transformation and metastasize (although only rarely),[24] and its significant morbidity and mortality, which are caused by its intraductal growth pattern and subsequent complications such as recurrent bouts of cholangitis and obstructive jaundice and episodes of sepsis and hemobilia. Even when invasion occurs, the incidence of metastasis is still much less than in other forms of cholangiocarcinoma. In spite of the fact that most of these intraductal papillary tumors may not become invasive or metastasize, because of the multi-centric nature of the lesions, the possibility of a cure without liver transplantation is unlikely. Even then, the lesion may possibly recur in the extrahepatic ducts.

PATHOLOGIC FEATURES

GROSS PATHOLOGY

The peripheral, hilar, and extrahepatic variants of cholangiocarcinoma are usually firm, white-tan lesions caused by dense fibrous stroma within the lesions. In contrast, the intraductal papillomatous variants are soft, polypoid, or cauliflower-like lesions that protrude into the large ducts and cause ductal dilatation; these lesions are typically multifocal.

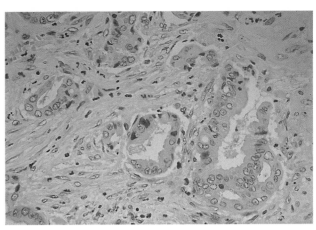

FIGURE 42–20. Cholangiocarcinoma, ductal type. Malignant ductular structures are embedded in an inflamed fibrous stroma. The epithelium is cuboidal and shows considerable variability in cytologic features.

MICROSCROPIC PATHOLOGY

Peripheral, hilar, and extrahepatic variants are adeno-carcinomas that typically have a significant component of dense fibrous stroma. These tumors often are well differentiated, with tubular gland formation and minimal cytologic changes; however, foci of atypia with increased nucleus-to-cytoplasm ratios, prominent nucleoli, variations in nuclear size, and loss of polarity are often seen (Fig. 42-20). Features that have been noted to support the diagnosis of carcinoma over that of a benign hyperplastic or reactive process include the formation of intracytoplasmic lumina and a focal cribriform pattern. In addition, multilayering of nuclei and intraluminal cellular debris may be helpful features that suggest the possibility of malignancy.

Intraductal papillomatosis,[6] or biliary papillomatosis (along with its invasive form, papillary adeno-carcinoma), grows into the duct lumina as a multifocal, papillary lesion. The architecture consists of papillae lined by columnar epithelial cells supported by a delicate fibrovascular stroma (Fig. 42-21). The nuclei are round to oval and basally located, without significant multilayering. The cytoplasm is generally abundant and mucinous, but clear or oncocytic differentiation, as well as intestinal metaplasia with goblet cell change, may also be seen. Mitotic figures are infrequent. Frank invasion of the stalk and underlying periductular tissues must occur if adenocarcinoma is to be diagnosed.

SPECIAL STUDIES

Immunoperoxidase and mucin staining may be used to differentiate cholangiocarcinoma from HCC, as has been described (see above under Hepatocellular Carcinoma and Variants, Distinction From Adenocarcinoma). However, differentiation from metastatic adenocarcinoma may be problematic if no primary is known to be

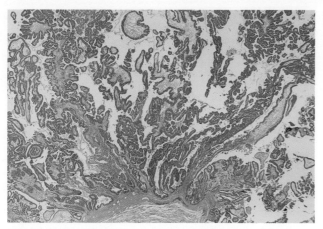

FIGURE 42–21. Cholangiocarcinoma, papillary type. The tumor grows in thin, delicate fronds. This focus does not show invasion, but this was present in other parts of the tumor.

present at another site. An adenocarcinoma composed of tall columnar cells with an adenomatous pattern, a focal cribriform pattern, lack of intraepithelial mucin, and the presence of luminal necrotic debris is more suggestive of metastatic colonic carcinoma than of primary cholangiocarcinoma. The latter usually shows greater intraepithelial mucinous differentiation or is composed of glands lined by low columnar to cuboidal cells. Cytokeratin profiles for types 7, 19, and 20 have also proved to be helpful in differentiating primary from metastatic lesions. The cholangiocarcinoma is generally cytokeratin 7– and cytokeratin 19–positive and cytokeratin 20–negative; metastatic colorectal adenocarcinoma is cytokeratin 7–negative in about 90% of cases but is usually positive for either cytokeratin 19 or 20.[30,31] Another marker that could be helpful is Le^x, which often shows cytoplasmic and membranous reactivity in cholangiocarcinoma but only cytoplasmic reactivity in metastatic carcinoma. In contrast, LeuM1 and B72.3 are likely to reveal the opposite pattern, with cytoplasmic staining in cholangiocarcinoma and cytoplasmic and membranous staining in metastatic adenocarcinoma.[29]

■ Mesenchymal Tumors

BENIGN MESENCHYMAL LESIONS

Mesenchymal Hamartoma

CLINICAL FEATURES

Mesenchymal hamartoma (MH) is a benign tumor that occurs primarily in young children, predominantly presenting at younger than 2 years of age. It is the third most common tumor of the liver in this age group[68] (following hepatoblastoma and infantile hemangio-

endothelioma). The patient often presents with such clinical symptoms as a palpable liver mass, abdominal enlargement, or respiratory distress caused by compression by the tumor. No risk for malignant transformation has been noted.

PATHOLOGIC FEATURES

GROSS PATHOLOGY

The tumor may be solid or cystic; solid areas of this tumor are typically tan. When cysts are present, they contain a translucent fluid or a gelatinous material.[46,68] These cysts may form from the degeneration of loose mesenchymal tissue of the tumor; it is thought that the tumor probably enlarges through continued accumulation of fluid within these cysts.

MICROSCOPIC PATHOLOGY

MH has both epithelial and stromal components. The former consist of relatively normal-appearing hepatocytes and bile ducts, both of which are surrounded by varying amounts of myxoid to fibrous stroma (Fig. 42-22). The hepatocytes are cytologically unremarkable and are arranged for the most part either in small clusters or in larger groups with retention of the cell plate architecture as occurs in normal liver. Bile duct structures are typically arranged in a branching pattern and often are associated with an acute inflammatory infiltrate in the duct walls or adjacent to it. Cystic spaces, when present, may be lined by flattened to cuboidal epithelial cells surrounded by loose to dense fibrous tissue (see Fig. 42-22). Cysts may lack lining cells as well. The stroma generally contains increased numbers of small vascular structures (but the cysts are not lined by endothelial cells), spindle cells, and

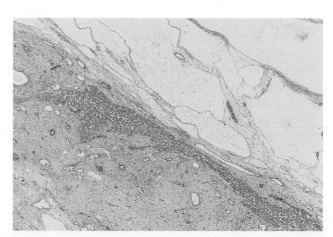

FIGURE 42–22. Mesenchymal hamartoma. Multiple thin-walled cysts (*upper right*) are present. The solid component of this lesion consists of cytologically unremarkable hepatocytes arranged in clusters that have a preserved cell plate architecture. The hepatocyte clusters are separated by a myxoid stroma that contains ductular elements.

inflammatory cells. No normal portal zones are present. Extramedullary hematopoiesis is often noted.

Hemangioma

PATHOLOGIC FEATURES

Hemangioma is the most common primary tumor of the liver. This benign vascular neoplasm is usually noted as an incidental finding at surgery or autopsy, but it may require surgical excision because of the possibility of hemorrhage or because of its large size.[69] It has been suggested that estrogen therapy may lead to enlargement of the tumor.[69] Rarely, thrombotic events within a large hemangioma may be associated with thrombocytopenia.[70] These tumors are occasionally multiple in the liver and may be associated with hemangiomas at other sites as part of von Hippel-Lindau disease or skeletal/systemic hemangiomatosis syndrome.[71]

GROSS PATHOLOGY

Hemangiomas are well-circumscribed, red to red-brown tumors. They almost always have a spongy texture or honeycombed surface that represents the cavernous vascular component; many also have undergone thrombosis and sclerosis, resulting in a firm, white to white-tan appearance.

MICROSCOPIC PATHOLOGY

The hallmark of this tumor is its cavernous vascular channels. The walls of these channels consist of fibrous stromal bands lined by a single layer of flattened endothelial cells without cytologic atypia or mitotic activity (Fig. 42-23). Sclerotic zones may be present and extensive. Thrombosed channels may also be seen. Extensively sclerotic hemangiomas may have only a few remaining vascular channels and so may mimic a localized scar.

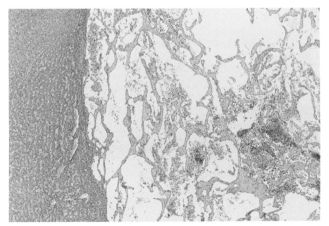

FIGURE 42–23. Cavernous hemangioma. The tumor is composed of large vascular channels that are lined by flattened endothelial cells lining a fibrous stroma.

Infantile Hemangioendothelioma

CLINICAL FEATURES

Infantile hemangioendothelioma (IHE) is the second most common tumor in children younger than 3 years of age, second only to hepatoblastoma; almost all reported cases have occurred in infants younger than 6 months of age. The tumor is almost twice as common in girls as in boys.[72,73] It is often multifocal within the liver, and in about 10% of patients, hemangiomas are found in other organs as well.[6] The tumors may be associated with other congenital anomalies, such as bilateral renal agenesis, Beckwith-Wiedemann syndrome, hemihypertrophy, and meningomyelocele.[6,72] Clinical presentation may occur as an abdominal mass or distention (with hepatomegaly), jaundice, diarrhea, constipation, vomiting,[72] congestive heart failure, or failure to thrive. Other, less common findings include thrombocytopenia due to sequestration of platelets within the tumor(s) and rupture with hemoperitoneum.[9]

These tumors are generally benign histologically, but because of their multifocality and/or large size, patients have a high mortality rate resulting from cardiac or hepatic failure.[72] These tumors may regress, but therapy such as resection, embolization, hepatic arterial ligation, or chemotherapy/radiation is often necessary for patient survival.[73] Angiosarcoma may rarely arise in this lesion.[74]

PATHOLOGIC FINDINGS

GROSS PATHOLOGY

IHE is often a poorly circumscribed lesion that may be solid and cystic with variable hemorrhagic foci. These foci typically alternate with fibrotic (solid) zones. The tumors are multifocal.

MICROSCOPIC PATHOLOGY

Two histologic subtypes have been described for this lesion, although practically speaking, distinguishing the two may be difficult. Type I is defined by a mixture of large numbers of small vascular channels and fewer large, irregularly shaped spaces with a cavernous appearance (Fig. 42-24); both types of vascular channels are lined by a single layer of endothelial cells. Vascular spaces are separated by a poorly developed stroma with only scattered collagen or reticulin fibers. Small bile ducts and hepatocytes may be seen in the stroma as well, often near the periphery of the tumor (see Fig. 42-24). Focal necrosis, hemorrhage, fibrosis, and calcification are often present. Type II lesions contain endothelial cells with more atypical cytologic features, with mitotic activity and hyperchromasia, and arranged in a more complex budding or branching pattern[70] than that noted in type I lesions.

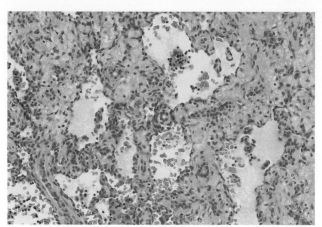

FIGURE 42–24. Infantile hemangioendothelioma. Vascular tumor channels are lined by endothelial cells. Occasional residual bile duct elements are present in the fibrous stroma.

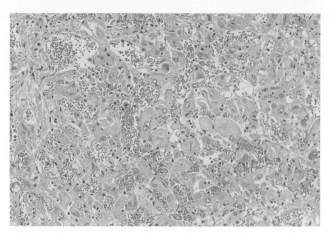

FIGURE 42–25. Angiomyolipoma. The tumor consists of epithelioid cells with abundant eosinophilic cytoplasm and nuclei with prominent nucleoli, with dilated vascular channels.

SPECIAL STUDIES

Endothelial cells of the tumor stain with CD34, CD31, and factor VIII. Stromal cells underlying the basement membrane of capillary structures are positive for alpha–smooth muscle actin HHF35 and negative for desmin, a profile consistent with pericytes.[75]

Angiomyolipoma

CLINICAL FEATURES

Angiomyolipomas (AMLs) are only rarely noted in the liver. The tumor often presents in the 30- to 40-year-old age group in both men and women.[76,77] Some tumors occur in the setting of tuberous sclerosis, but many do not.[76,77] The tumor is thought to arise from the perivascular epithelioid cell (PEC); related lesions in other organs include the clear cell "sugar" tumor and lymphangioleiomyomatosis of the lung.[78]

PATHOLOGIC FEATURES

GROSS PATHOLOGY

AML may present as a large, variably colored tumor caused by fat, necrosis, and hemorrhage.[76,77]

MICROSCOPIC PATHOLOGY

This lesion usually is composed of various elements, including smooth muscle–like cells, blood vessels, fat, and hematopoietic tissue. The smooth muscle–like differentiation is often the most prominent in liver AML and consists of either epithelioid or spindled cells, often surrounding the vessels. Epithelioid cells have a rounded or polygonal shape with abundant eosinophilic cytoplasm (Fig. 42-25). Nuclei are typically large and round with prominent nucleoli, but their appearance

may vary. The cytoplasmic contents may be oncocytic and may be condensed around the nucleus with a clear zone near the cell membrane, giving the appearance of a spider's web (Fig. 42-26).[77] Spindled cells include eosinophilic cytoplasm and small oval nuclei. Trabeculae, usually composed mostly of epithelioid types of cells, have also been noted. Either the epithelioid or the spindle cell component may predominate to the exclusion of the other. The vascular component is typically made up of thick-walled arterial or venous-like channels admixed with thin-walled, venous-like spaces. The fatty tissue consists of mature fat cells scattered throughout the tumor singly or as clusters or sheets of cells; however, in liver variants of this lesion, the fat component may be scant or absent. Foam cells containing fine droplets of lipid may also often be seen. Peliotic spaces closely associated with areas of hemorrhage are noted.

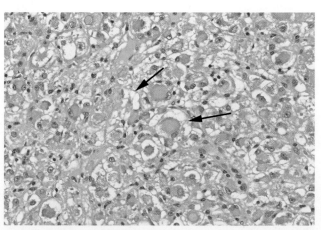

FIGURE 42–26. Angiomyolipoma. Epithelioid cells with abundant cytoplasm. Some tumor cells show a concentration of the cytoplasm in the center of the cell with peripheral clearing near the cell membrane, the so-called spider-web appearance (*arrows*).

These spaces mostly lack an endothelial lining. Prominent dense lymphoid aggregates composed of a mixture of T and B cells may be noted as well. Rarely, inflammatory cells may be associated with the stromal spindle cell component of the tumor, mimicking inflammatory pseudotumor. Rarely, hemosiderin and melanin pigments are noted. Variable numbers of hematopoietic elements, including megakaryocytes and erythroid and myeloid precursors, are often present.

SPECIAL STUDIES

Most diagnostic problems arise when (1) epithelioid smooth muscle–like cells predominate within the tumor as large, round nuclei with prominent nucleoli and (2) abundant eosinophilic cytoplasm mimics HCC or hepatic adenoma. In addition, any formation of trabeculae containing epithelioid cells closely mimics HCC. Therefore, immunohistochemistry may be helpful in identifying the tumor as AML rather than HCC or adenoma by demonstrating positivity for HMB-45 and smooth muscle actin in the smooth muscle–like cells. Spindle cells often stain more strongly for smooth muscle actin, and epithelioid cells stain for HMB-45.[77] Desmin positivity has been noted in spindle cells as well.[77] Stains for keratin are negative. S100 has been noted to be focally positive in AML as well, generally staining both epithelioid and fat cells.[77] A combination of spindled and epithelioid cells may also mimic metastatic melanoma, so HMB-45 positivity for AML may add to the confusion.

Inflammatory Pseudotumor

CLINICAL FEATURES

Inflammatory pseudotumor (IPT) is a rare, inflammatory, fibrosing lesion that may be found in other organs besides the liver.[79-81] Patients may present with abdominal pain, fever, chills, jaundice, vomiting, and weight loss. Lesions have also been reported in association with chronic cholangitis.[79] The lesion may be mistaken clinically for cholangiocarcinoma if it is in the hilar region. Evidence for Epstein-Barr virus has been noted in tumors from various sites, including the liver.[82] Some have also suggested the possibility of an association with proliferation of follicular dendritic reticulum cells.[82]

PATHOLOGIC FEATURES

GROSS PATHOLOGY

The appearance may vary considerably, especially in the larger lesions, and foci of fibrosis, hemorrhage, and necrosis are present.[81] The tumor may also vary considerably in size, may be solitary or multiple, and may arise in the porta hepatis or elsewhere in the liver parenchyma.[81]

MICROSCOPIC PATHOLOGY

IPT consists of a mixture of inflammatory and fibrous tissue, but the relative degrees of these components may be variable. The inflammatory component of the lesion usually contains a polyclonal population of plasma cells,[79,80] but neutrophils, eosinophils, lymphocytes (predominantly T cells), and macrophages (often xanthomatous) are also often present to some degree. The spindle cell component is made up of fibroblasts, and sclerotic foci are common. Mitotic figures may be seen but should not be numerous,[81] and abnormal mitotic figures should not be seen. Occasionally, granulomas or phlebitis (or varying degrees of venous obstruction) may be noted.[79,80]

SPECIAL STUDIES

IPTs should be differentiated from other sarcomas such as angiosarcoma or metastatic gastrointestinal stromal tumor. In these latter sarcomas, cellular atypia and frequent mitotic figures should be noted; also, sarcomas typically lack numerous inflammatory cells. Immunohistochemistry may be helpful as well in that angiosarcomas stain positively for factor VIII and other vascular endothelial markers (including CD34), and metastatic gastrointestinal tumors react with CD117 as well as CD34. The differentiation from follicular dendritic cell (FDC) tumor may be more difficult; however, the absence of plasma cells and the presence of pleomorphic tumor cells in FDC, as well as specific markers for FDC such as CD21, CD35, and R4/23, should help distinguish the two lesions.[83]

MALIGNANT MESENCHYMAL LESIONS

Angiosarcoma

CLINICAL FEATURES

Angiosarcoma is a rare primary malignant tumor that usually occurs in middle-aged adults but has also been noted rarely in children, sometimes in the setting of infantile hemangioendothelioma.[74] Other definitive associations include Thorotrast and vinyl chloride exposure,[84] but many of these tumors have no apparent etiologic factor. Presenting signs include hepatomegaly, ascites, jaundice, thrombocytopenia, hemoperitoneum, and liver failure. The mean survival after diagnosis is 6 months.

PATHOLOGIC FEATURES

GROSS PATHOLOGY

Angiosarcomas are often large hemorrhagic tumors with indistinct borders and variable solid or cystic areas, the latter usually containing blood. Satellite nodules may be present.

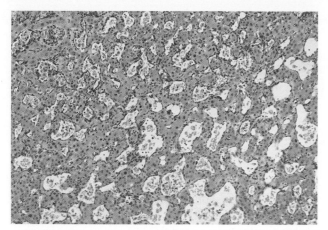

FIGURE 42–27. Angiosarcoma. The malignant cells show atypical cytologic features and line the hepatocyte cell plates in a scaffold-like arrangement. Sinusoids are dilated.

MICROSCOPIC PATHOLOGY

The tumor typically has a mixed pattern of histology, with sinusoidal, solid, papillary, and cavernous types of growth. The sinusoidal pattern is the most distinctive growth pattern in the liver. In this pattern, endothelial cells line both sides of the hepatic cell plates in a scaffold-like arrangement that dissects the plates, often resulting in sinusoidal dilatation (Fig. 42-27). The tumor cells lining the cell plates are more numerous, more hyperchromatic, and larger than normal endothelial cells. This sinusoidal pattern is more likely to be noted at the periphery of the tumor and so may represent an early outgrowth of the tumor, which then later transforms into the solid or papillary form. The solid pattern may have a fascicular or whorled appearance, or it may resemble fibrosarcoma. The papillary pattern consists of nodules of stroma lined by tumor cells that protrude into a lumen (Fig. 42-28). This cavernous pattern consists of large, blood-filled spaces and is commonly seen with any of the other patterns.

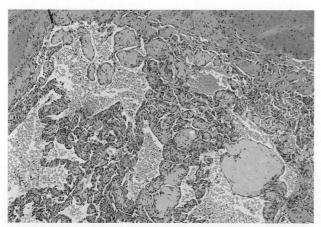

FIGURE 42–28. Angiosarcoma. Some vascular spaces are cavernous, and a focal papillary pattern is seen where nodules of stroma lined by the tumor cells protrude into a lumen.

SPECIAL STUDIES

Endothelial markers such as factor VIII, CD31, and CD34 are typically positive on tumor cells, but not all tumor cells may stain. Factor VIII is the most sensitive and specific marker for the tumor.

Epithelioid Hemangioendothelioma

CLINICAL FEATURES

Epithelioid hemangioendothelioma (EHE) is a rare, low-grade malignancy that occurs in adults of any age but tends to be more common among women.[85] Many lesions are discovered as an incidental finding, but presenting symptoms may include upper abdominal mass or discomfort. Serum alkaline phosphatase levels may be elevated. Liver transplantation may be a reasonable means of treatment in unresectable cases,[86] showing a survival similar to that of HCC of the same stage. Overall, the prognosis is better than that of angiosarcoma, even if excision is incomplete or extrahepatic metastases are present.

PATHOLOGIC FEATURES

GROSS PATHOLOGY

EHE is a firm, white to yellow tumor that often has an ill-defined border. The tumor is often multifocal with involvement of both right and left liver lobes. Focal calcification may be present and causes a somewhat gritty consistency.

MICROSCOPIC PATHOLOGY

The cells constituting this tumor may be dendritic or epithelioid in appearance. The former are irregularly shaped, elongated, or stellate cells with branching processes. The cell cytoplasm may contain a vacuole that represents an intracellular "capillary" luminal space. The epithelioid tumor cells are rounder with more abundant cytoplasm than is found in the dendritic cells. These cells often form small papillations or tufts within thin-walled vascular spaces (Fig. 42-29). Both cell types are surrounded by a myxoid to fibrous stroma. Calcification of the more dense type of stroma may be seen. The tumor tends to grow around and leave intact preexisting structures such as portal zones and residual hepatocytes, or bile ducts may be present within the tumor, especially near the periphery of the lesion. The tumor also has a marked predilection for invading larger vascular structures such as portal and central veins, thereby mimicking the histologic appearance of vascular thrombosis. Scattered inflammatory cells such as lymphocytes and neutrophils are often seen.

SPECIAL STUDIES

Histologic differentiation of this lesion from adenocarcinoma (including cholangiocarcinoma) or HCC may

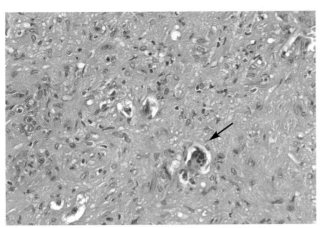

FIGURE 42–29. Epithelioid hemangioendothelioma. The tumor cells can be dendritic or epithelioid and are separated by a myxoid to fibrous stroma. Some tumor cells form small tufts within capillary lumina *(arrow)*, and cells with a single vacuolated lumen can be present.

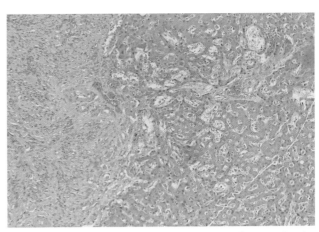

FIGURE 42–30. Kaposi's sarcoma. The tumor tends to involve the portal zones in a solid pattern of spindle cell proliferation *(left)*, but when the tumor cells extend into the lobule, they grow along the sinusoidal space, resulting in sinusoidal dilation and peliosis *(right)*.

be problematic on routine staining. However, immunohistochemical staining for endothelial markers on the tumor cells, such as CD34, CD31, and/or factor VIII, confirms the diagnosis of EHE. Care must be taken, however, not to mistake focal keratin positivity in this tumor (a result of either entrapped hepatocytes or ducts) for carcinoma; keratin can also stain some tumor cells.[87] Another diagnostic problem may be the differentiation of EHE from venous thrombosis/veno-occlusive disease because tumor growth within large vessels may mimic an organizing thrombus.

Kaposi's Sarcoma

CLINICAL FEATURES

Kaposi's sarcoma (KS) most often occurs in the liver in the setting of acquired immunodeficiency syndrome (AIDS), usually only after the tumor is known to be present at other sites.

PATHOLOGIC FEATURES

GROSS PATHOLOGY

Most findings of KS in the liver are similar to those seen at other sites. The tumor may have a fibrous to hemorrhagic, multifocal appearance, often centering around portal triads.

MICROSCOPIC PATHOLOGY

The tumor consists of spindle cell proliferations that form slitlike spaces or, in larger lesions, a more solid, fibrosarcomatous-type pattern (Fig. 42-30). As at other sites, cellular pleomorphism and mitotic activity are minimal, and extravasation of erythrocytes, hemosiderin deposits, and small eosinophilic globules is typically present. One pattern that is typically seen only in the

liver is the growth of spindled tumor cells into and along the sinusoidal spaces, usually at the periphery of tumor nodules. This pattern of growth results in dilated channels that contain erythrocytes that replace the normal sinusoids—findings that have a peliotic appearance (see Fig. 42-30). The tumor also tends to surround or infiltrate the portal zone, often leaving the hepatic artery and interlobular bile duct intact.

SPECIAL STUDIES

Tumor cells are positive for endothelial markers, including CD31 and CD34, that may be useful in helping to differentiate KS from fibroblastic proliferations. Tumor positivity for herpes virus 8 is pathognomonic.

Undifferentiated (Embryonal) Sarcoma

CLINICAL FEATURES

Embryonal sarcoma is a rare tumor that typically occurs in children between the ages of 6 and 10, with some occurring in a slightly older age group (younger than age 20).[88] The presenting features are often those of a mass or of abdominal pain.[88,89] Complete surgical excision generally offers the best outcome.[89]

PATHOLOGIC FEATURES

GROSS PATHOLOGY

Embryonal sarcomas are usually large, soft tumors with variably cystic and solid areas and a white, shiny or gelatinous or mucoid surface. Additional areas of necrosis and hemorrhage are often noted.

MICROSCOPIC PATHOLOGY

These tumors contain a mixture of spindled and stellate cells embedded in a myxoid stroma. The tumor

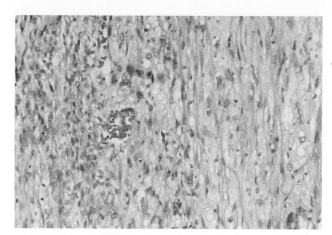

FIGURE 42–31. Undifferentiated (embryonal) sarcoma. The tumor cells are spindled to stellate. The stroma is typically myxoid, as seen here.

cells have a granular to bubbly, light pink cytoplasm, and many contain cytoplasmic globules of various sizes that are d-PAS–positive (Fig. 42-31). These globules may also be noted in the stroma. Other cellular features include the presence of other large atypical tumor cells with hyperchromatic nuclei, as well as multinucleated tumor cells. The surrounding stroma is usually myxoid, but some dense collagen deposits may be seen. Mitotic figures are usually numerous. Hematopoiesis is often noted, and entrapped hepatocytes and/or ductules may be observed at the tumor's periphery.

SPECIAL STUDIES

Tumor cells of the lesion have been shown to stain immunohistochemically for vimentin, alpha-1-antitrypsin, and alpha-1-antichymotrypsin.[89]

Hematopoietic Malignancies

All types of leukemias and lymphomas (e.g., Hodgkin's and non-Hodgkin's) may secondarily involve the liver.[90] The leukemias typically exhibit a diffuse pattern of infiltration of the sinusoids by leukemic cells, with the exception that chronic lymphocytic and acute lymphoblastic leukemia often involve the portal zones, which are more typical of the lymphoma pattern of infiltrate. Hairy cell leukemia may also be associated with the formation of a peliosis hepatis–like lesion consisting of dilated sinusoids lined by tumor cells.

In Hodgkin's disease (HD), the tumor typically involves the liver as nodular masses within the portal zones. Reed-Sternberg cells should be noted for a definitive diagnosis, but the presence of an infiltrate composed of lymphocytes and admixed with plasma cells, eosinophils, and some atypical cells is consistent with HD if the diagnosis is already well established at

another site. Occasionally, epithelioid granulomas may be found in either the parenchyma or the portal zones, but these granulomas alone without the other features noted here would not be sufficient to confirm a diagnosis of liver involvement by HD. Rarely, intrahepatic cholestasis, occasionally associated with a paucity of bile ducts, may be seen in HD as well.[91]

Non-Hodgkin's lymphomas usually involve the liver as a metastatic lesion by forming nodular masses in the portal tracts. Some lymphomas may show sinusoidal infiltration by the tumor cells, similar to that seen in leukemia.[90] Liver involvement is especially common among peripheral T-cell lymphomas, occurring in as many as 50% of patients.[92] Intrahepatic cholestasis and epithelioid granulomas similar to those seen in HD have also been noted. Non-Hodgkin's lymphoma as a primary lesion only rarely occurs in the liver in children or adults; many of these lymphomas have been reported in association with AIDS. These tumors are primarily solitary or multiple masses, and they are usually morphologically high-grade lesions.

Other Benign Lesions or Neoplasms

Benign neoplasms that have also been noted in the liver include chondroma,[93] fibroma, leiomyoma, lipoma, lymphangioma, myxoma,[70] schwannoma,[94] solitary fibrous tumor,[95] and adrenal and pancreatic rests.[96] Granular cell tumors may involve the biliary tract.[97]

Focal fatty change (FFC) is a localized zone of hepatocytes that contain abundant fat. This lesion is often subcapsular and may be confused grossly or radiographically with a neoplasm. FFC may be associated with diabetes or alcoholic hepatitis.[98]

Solitary necrotic nodules are rare non-neoplastic lesions that consist of a central zone of amorphous, eosinophilic debris rimmed by a hyalinized fibrotic capsule that contains prominent elastic fibers. These lesions may be clinically mistaken for metastatic disease and rarely have been noted in association with parasitic infection.[99]

Other Malignant Tumors

Carcinoid, fibrosarcoma, malignant fibrous histiocytoma, follicular dendritic cell tumor, leiomyosarcoma, liposarcoma, malignant mesenchymoma, malignant mixed tumor, osteosarcoma, pheochromocytoma, plasmacytoma, malignant rhabdoid tumor, rhabdomyosarcoma, malignant schwannoma, squamous carcinoma, malignant trophoblastic tumor, teratoma, and yolk sac tumor have all been described as primary malignancies in the liver.[83,84,96,100-108]

References

1. Torii A, Harada A, Nonami T, et al: Tumor localization as a prognostic factor in hepatocellular carcinoma. Hepatogastroenterology 41:16-19, 1994.

2. Hamazaki K, Mimura H, Orita K, et al: Surgical treatment for hepatocellular carcinoma (HCC) 3 cm or less than 3 cm in diameter. Hepatogastroenterology 6:485-588, 1992.

3. Schoenthaler R, Phillips T, Castro J, et al: Carcinoma of the extrahepatic bile ducts: The University of California at San Francisco experience. Ann Surg 219:267-274, 1994.

4. Ljung B, Ferrell L: Fine needle aspiration biopsy of the liver: Diagnostic problems. In Ferrell L (ed): Diagnostic Problems in Liver Pathology. Pathology: State of the Art Reviews. Philadelphia, Hanley & Belfus, 1994, pp 161-184.

5. Wanless I, Callea F, Craig J, et al: Terminology of nodular lesions of the liver. Hepatology 25:983-993, 1995.

6. Ishak KG, Anthony PP, Sobin LH, et al: Histological Typing of Tumours of the Liver, 2nd ed. Berlin, Springer-Verlag, 1994.

7. Craig J, Peters R, Edmondson H: Benign tumors and tumor-like conditions. In Hartmann W, Sobin L (eds): Tumors of the Liver and Intrahepatic Bile Ducts. Washington, DC, Armed Forces Institute of Pathology, 1989, pp 8-98.

8. Wheeler D, Edmondson H, Reynolds T: Spontaneous liver cell adenoma in children. Am J Clin Pathol 85:6-12, 1986.

9. Ishak K, Rabin L: Benign tumors of the liver. Med Clin North Am 59:995-1013, 1975.

10. Tao L: Oral contraceptive-associated liver cell adenoma and hepatocellular carcinoma: Cytomorphology and mechanism of malignant transformation. Cancer 68:341-347, 1991.

11. Hytiroglou P, Theise N: Differential diagnosis of hepatocellular nodular lesions. Semin Diagn Pathol 15:285-299, 1998.

12. Ferrell L: Hepatocellular carcinoma arising in a focus of multilobular adenoma. Am J Surg Pathol 17:525-529, 1993.

13. Kong C, Appenzeller M, Ferrell L: Utility of CD34 reactivity in evaluating focal nodular hepatocellular lesions sampled by fine needle aspiration biopsy. Acta Cytol 44:218-222, 2000.

14. Nguyen B, Flejou J, Terris B, et al: Focal nodular hyperplasia of the liver: A comprehensive pathologic study of 305 lesions and recognition of new histologic forms. Am J Surg Pathol 23:1441-1454, 1999.

15. Wanless I, Mawdsley C, Adams R: On the pathogenesis of focal nodular hyperplasia of the liver. Hepatology 5:1194-1200, 1985.

16. Crawford JM: Pathologic assessment of liver cell dysplasia and benign liver tumors: Differentiation from malignant tumors. Semin Diagn Pathol 7:115-128, 1990.

17. Theise N, Lopook J, Thung S: A macroregenerative nodule containing multiple foci of hepatocellular carcinoma in a noncirrhotic liver. Hepatology 17:993-996, 1993.

18. Nakanuma Y, Terada T, Ueda K, et al: Adenomatous hyperplasia of the liver as a precancerous lesion. Liver 13:1-9, 1993.

19. Ferrell L, Crawford JM, Dhillon A, et al: Proposal for standardized criteria for the diagnosis of benign, borderline, and malignant hepatocellular lesions arising in chronic advanced liver disease. Am J Surg Pathol 17:1113-1123, 1993.

20. Ferrell L: Hepatocellular nodules in the cirrhotic liver: Diagnostic features and proposed nomenclature. In Ferrell L (ed): Diagnostic Problems in Liver Pathology. Pathology: State of the Art Reviews. Philadelphia, Hanley & Belfus, 1994, pp 105-117.

21. Park Y, Yang C-T, Fernandez G, et al: Neoangiogenesis and sinusoidal "capillarization" in dysplastic nodules of the liver. Am J Surg Pathol 22:656-662, 1998.

22. Roncalli M, Roz E, Goggi G, et al: The vascular profile of regenerative and dysplastic nodules of the cirrhotic liver: Implications for diagnosis and classification. Hepatology 30:1174-1178, 1999.

23. Theise N, Fiel I, Hytiroglou P, et al: Macroregenerative nodules in cirrhosis are not associated with elevated serum or stainable tissue alpha-fetoprotein. Liver 15:30-34, 1995.

24. Craig J, Peters R, Edmondson H: Primary malignant epithelial tumors. In Hartmann W, Sobin L (eds): Tumors of the Liver and Intrahepatic Bile Ducts. Washington, DC, Armed Forces Institute of Pathology, 1989, pp 123-214.

25. Stromeyer F, Ishak K, Gerber M, et al: Ground-glass cells in hepatocellular carcinoma. Am J Clin Pathol 74:254-258, 1980.

26. Edmondson H, Steiner P: Primary carcinoma of the liver: A study of 100 cases among 48,900 necropsies. Cancer 1:462-503, 1954.

27. Minervini M, Demetris A, Lee R, et al: Utilization of hepatocyte-specific antibody in the immunocytochemical evaluation of liver tumors. Mod Pathol 10:686-692, 1997.

28. Murakata L, Ishak K, Nzeako U: Clear cell carcinoma of the liver: A comparative immunohistochemical study with renal clear cell carcinoma. Mod Pathol 13:874-881, 2000.

29. Fucich L, Cheles M, Thung S, et al: Primary versus metastatic hepatic carcinoma: An immunohistochemical study of 34 cases. Arch Pathol Lab Med 118:927-930, 1994.

30. Maeda T, Kajiyama K, Adachi E, et al: The expression of cytokeratins 7, 19, 20 in primary and metastatic carcinomas of the liver. Mod Pathol 9:901-909, 1996.

31. Wang N, Zee S, Zarbo R, et al: Coordinate expression of cytokeratins 7 and 20 defines unique subsets of carcinomas. Appl Immunohistochem 3:99-107, 1995.

32. Rullier A, Le Bail B, Fawaz R, et al: Cytokeratin 7 and 20 expression in cholangiocarcinomas varies along the biliary tract but still differs from that in colorectal carcinoma metastases. Am J Surg Pathol 24:870-876, 2000.

33. Chu P, Wu E, Weiss L: Cytokeratin 7 and cytokeratin 20 expression in epithelial neoplasms: A survey of 435 cases. Mod Pathol 13:962-972, 2000.

34. Garcia de Davila M, Gonzalez-Crussi F, Mangkornkanok M: Fibrolamellar carcinoma of the liver in a child: Ultrastructural and immunohistologic aspects. Pediatr Pathol 7:319-331, 1987.

35. Ruck P, Harms D, Kaiserling E: Neuroendocrine differentiation in hepatoblastoma: An immunohistochemical investigation. Am J Surg Pathol 14:847-855, 1990.

36. Wang J, Dhillon A, Sankey E, et al: Neuroendocrine differentiation in primary neoplasms of the liver. J Pathol 163:61-67, 1991.

37. Renshaw A, Granter S: A comparison of A103 and inhibin reactivity in adrenal cortical tumors: Distinction from hepatocellular carcinoma and renal tumors. Mod Pathol 11:1160-1164, 1998.

38. Craig J, Peters R, Edmondson H, et al: Fibrolamellar carcinoma of the liver: A tumor of adolescents and young adults with distinctive clinico-pathologic features. Cancer 46:372-379, 1980.

39. Berman M, Libbey N, Foster J: Hepatocellular carcinoma: Polygonal cell type with fibrous stroma—an atypical variant with a favorable prognosis. Cancer 46:1448-1455, 1980.

40. Berman M, Sheahan D: Fibrolamellar carcinoma of the liver: An immunohistochemical study of nineteen cases and a review of the literature. Hum Pathol 19:784-794, 1988.

41. Saxena R, Humphreys S, Williams R, et al: Nodular hyperplasia surrounding fibrolamellar carcinoma: A zone of arterialized liver parenchyma. Histopathology 25:275-278, 1994.

42. Saul S, Titelbaum D, Gansler T, et al: The fibrolamellar variant of hepatocellular carcinoma: Its association with focal nodular hyperplasia. Cancer 60:3049-3055, 1987.

43. Goodman Z, Ishak K, Langloss J, et al: Combined hepatocellular-cholangiocarcinoma: A histologic and immunohistochemical study. Cancer 55:124-135, 1985.

44. Omata M, Peters R, Tatters D: Sclerosing hepatic carcinoma: Relationship to hypercalcemia. Liver 1:33-49, 1981.

45. Haas J, Muczynski K, Krailo M, et al: Histopathology and prognosis in childhood hepatoblastoma and hepatocarcinoma. Cancer 64:1082-1095, 1989.

46. Weinberg A, Finegold M: Primary hepatic tumors of childhood. Hum Pathol 14:512-537, 1983.

47. Altmann H: Epithelial and mixed hepatoblastoma in the adult. Pathol Res Pract 188:16-26, 1992.

48. Anthony P: Tumours and tumour-like lesions of the liver and biliary tract. In MacSween R, Anthony P, Scheuer P, et al (eds): Pathology of the Liver, 3rd ed. Edinburgh, Churchill Livingstone, 1994, pp 635-711.

49. Haggitt R, Reid B: Hereditary gastrointestinal polyposis syndromes. Am J Surg Pathol 10:871-887, 1986.

50. Stocker J: Hepatoblastoma. Semin Diagn Pathol 11:136-143, 1994.

51. Abbassi V, Hoy G, Weintraub B: HCG production by hepatoblastoma causing isosexual precocious puberty. Pediatr Res 13:375-381, 1979.

52. Conran R, Hitchcock C, Waclawiw M, et al: Hepatoblastoma: The prognostic significance of histologic type. Pediatr Pathol 12:167-183, 1992.

53. Saxena R, Leake J, Shafford E, et al: Chemotherapy effects on hepatoblastoma: A histological study. Am J Surg Pathol 17:1266-1271, 1993.

54. Ruck P, Kaiserling E: Melanin-containing hepatoblastoma with endocrine differentiation: An immunohistochemical and ultrastructural study. Cancer 72:361-368, 1993.

55. Allaire G, Rabin L, Ishak K, et al: Bile duct adenoma: A study of 152 cases. Am J Surg Pathol 12:708-715, 1988.

56. Bhathal P, Hughes N, Goodman Z: The so-called bile duct adenoma is a peribiliary gland hamartoma. Am J Surg Pathol 20:858-864, 1996.

57. Devaney K, Goodman Z, Ishak K: Hepatobiliary cystadenoma and cystadenocarcinoma: A light microscopic and immunohistochemical study of 70 patients. Am J Surg Pathol 18:1078-1091, 1994.

58. Tsui W, Loo K, Chow L, et al: Biliary adenofibroma. Am J Surg Pathol 17:186-192, 1993.

59. Wee A, Ludwig J, Coffey R, et al: Hepatobiliary carcinoma associated with primary sclerosing cholangitis and chronic ulcerative colitis. Hum Pathol 16:719-726, 1985.

60. Chalasani N, Baluyut A, Ismail A, et al: Cholangiocarcinoma in patients with primary sclerosing cholangitis: A multicenter case-control study. Hepatology 31:7-11, 2000.

61. Honda N, Cobb C, Lechago J: Bile duct carcinoma associated with multiple von Meyenberg complexes in the liver. Hum Pathol 17:1287-1290, 1986.

62. Todani T, Watanabe Y, Toki A, et al: Carcinomas related to choledochal cysts with internal drainage operations. Surg Gynecol Obstet 164:61-64, 1987.

63. Chauduri P, Chauduri B, Schuler J, et al: Carcinoma associated with congenital cystic dilatation of bile ducts. Arch Surg 117:1349-1351, 1982.

64. Sameshima Y, Uchimura M, Muto Y, et al: Coexistent carcinoma in congenital dilatation of the bile duct and anomalous arrangement of the pancreatico-bile duct: Carcinogenesis of coexistent gall bladder carcinoma. Cancer 60:1883-1890, 1987.

65. Koga A, Ichimiya H, Yamaguchi K, et al: Hepatolithiasis associated with cholangiocarcinoma. Cancer 55:2826-2829, 1985.

66. Rubel L, Ishak K: Thorotrast-associated cholangiocarcinoma. Cancer 50:1408-1415, 1982.

67. Klatskin G: Adenocarcinoma of the hepatic duct at its bifurcation within the porta hepatis: An unusual tumor with distinctive clinical and pathological features. Am J Med 38:241-256, 1965.

68. Stocker J, Ishak K: Mesenchymal hamartoma of the liver: Report of 30 cases and review of the literature. Pediatr Pathol 1:245-267, 1983.

69. Hobbs K: Hepatic hemangiomas. World J Surg 14:468-471, 1990.

70. Craig J, Peters R, Edmondson H: Benign mesenchymal tumors and tumor-like conditions. In Hartmann W, Sobin L (eds): Tumors of the Liver and Intrahepatic Bile Ducts. Washington, DC, Armed Forces Institute of Pathology, 1989, pp 63-101.

71. Kane R, Newman A: Diffuse skeletal and hepatic hemangiomatosis. California Med 118:41-44, 1973.

72. Dehner L, Ishak K: Vascular tumors of the liver in infants and children: A study of 30 cases and review of the literature. Arch Pathol 92:101-111, 1971.

73. Stanley P, Geer G, Miller J, et al: Infantile hepatic hemangiomas: Clinical features, radiologic investigations, and treatment of 20 patients. Cancer 64:936-949, 1989.

74. Selby D, Stocker J, Ishak K: Angiosarcoma of the liver in childhood: A clinicopathologic and follow-up study of 10 cases. Pediatr Pathol 12:485-498, 1992.

75. Cerar A, Dolenc-Strazar Z, Bartenjev D: Infantile hemangioendothelioma of the liver in a neonate: Immunohistochemical observations. Am J Surg Pathol 20:871-876, 1996.

76. Goodman Z, Ishak K: Angiomyolipomas of the liver. Am J Surg Pathol 8:745-750, 1984.

77. Tsui W, Colombari R, Bonetti F, et al: Hepatic angiomyolipoma: Delineation of unusual morphological variants. Am J Surg Pathol 23:34-48, 1999.

78. Bonetti F, Pea M, Martignoni G, et al: The perivascular epithelioid cell and related lesions. Adv Anat Pathol 4:343-358, 1997.

79. Nakanuma Y, Tsuneyama K, Masuda S, et al: Hepatic inflammatory pseudotumor associated with chronic cholangitis: Report of three cases. Hum Pathol 25:86-91, 1994.

80. Anthony P, Telesinghe P: Inflammatory pseudotumor of the liver. J Clin Pathol 39:761-768, 1986.

81. Shek T, Ng I, Chan K: Inflammatory pseudotumor of the liver: Report of four cases and review of the literature. Am J Surg Pathol 17:231-238, 1993.

82. Selves J, Meggetto F, Brousset P, et al: Inflammatory pseudotumor of the liver: Evidence for follicular dendritic reticulum cell proliferation associated with clonal Epstein-Barr virus. Am J Surg Pathol 20:747-753, 1996.

83. Shek T, Ho F, Ng I, et al: Follicular dendritic cell tumor of the liver: Evidence for an Epstein-Barr virus-related clonal proliferation of follicular dencritic cells. Am J Surg Pathol 20:313-324, 1996.

84. Craig J, Peters R, Edmondson H: Primary malignant mesenchymal tumors. In Hartmann W, Sobin L (eds): Tumors of the Liver and Intrahepatic Bile Ducts. Washington, DC, Armed Forces Institute of Pathology, 1989, pp 223-255.

85. Ishak K, Sesterhenn I, Goodman Z, et al: Epithelioid hemangioendothelioma of the liver: A clinicopathologic and follow-up study of 32 cases. Hum Pathol 15:839-852, 1984.

86. Madariaga J, Marino I, Karavias D, et al: Long-term results after liver transplantation for primary hepatic epithelioid hemangioendothelioma. Ann Surg Oncol 2:483-487, 1995.

87. Gray M, Rosenberg A, Dickersin G, et al: Cytokeratin expression in epithelioid vascular neoplasms. Hum Pathol 21:212-217, 1990.

88. Stocker J, Ishak K: Undifferentiated (embryonal) sarcoma of the liver: Report of 31 cases. Cancer 42:336-348, 1978.

89. Lack E, Schloo B, Azumi N, et al: Undifferentiated (embryonal) sarcoma of the liver: Clinical and pathologic study of 16 cases with emphasis on immunohistochemical features. Am J Surg Pathol 15:1-16, 1991.

90. Scheimberg I, Pollock D, Collins P, et al: Pathology of the liver in leukaemia and lymphoma. Histopathology 26:311-321, 1995.

91. Hubscher S, Lumley M, Elias E: Vanishing bile duct syndrome: A possible mechanism for intrahepatic cholestasis in Hodgkin's lymphoma. Hepatology 17:70-77, 1993.

92. Jaffe E: Malignant lymphomas: Pathology of liver involvement. Semin Liver Dis 7:257-268, 1987.

93. Fried R, Wardzala A, Willson R, et al: Benign cartilaginous tumor (chondroma) of the liver. Gastroenterology 103:678-680, 1992.

94. Hytiroglou P, Linton P, Klion F, et al: Benign schwannoma of the liver. Arch Pathol Lab Med 117:216-218, 1993.

95. Kottke-Marchant K, Hart W, Broughan T: Localized fibrous tumor (localized fibrous mesothelioma) of the liver. Cancer 64:1096-1102, 1989.

96. Craig J, Peters R, Edmondson H: Tumors of heterotopic tissue and uncertain origin. In Hartmann W, Sobin L (eds): Tumors of the Liver and Intrahepatic Bile Ducts. Washington, DC, Armed Forces Institute of Pathology, 1989, pp 102-122.

97. Eisen R, Kirby W, O'Quinn J: Granular cell tumor of the biliary tree: A report of two cases and a review of the literature. Am J Surg Pathol 15:460-465, 1991.

98. Kudo M, Ikekubo K, Yamamoto K, et al: Focal fatty infiltration of the liver in acute alcoholic liver injury: Hot spots with radiocolloid SPECT scan. Am J Gastroenterol 84:948-952, 1989.

99. Tsui W, Yuen R, Chow L, et al: Solitary necrotic nodule of the liver: Parasitic origin? J Clin Pathol 45:975-978, 1992.

100. Demirhan B, Sokmensuer C, Karakayali H, et al: Primary extramedullary plasmacytoma of the liver. J Clin Pathol 50:74-76, 1997.

101. Weichhold W, Labouyrie E, Merlio J, et al: Primary extramedullary plasmacytoma of the liver. Am J Surg Pathol 19:1197-1202, 1995.

102. Cozzutto C, Bernardi B, Comelli A, et al: Malignant mesenchymoma of the liver in children: A clinicopathologic and ultrastructural study. Hum Pathol 12:481-485, 1981.

103. Kawarada Y, Uehara S, Noda M, et al: Nonhepatocytic malignant mixed tumor primary in the liver: Report of two cases. Cancer 55:1790-1798, 1985.

104. Parham D, Peiper S, Robicheaux G, et al: Malignant rhabdoid tumor of the liver: Evidence for epithelial differentiation. Arch Pathol Lab Med 112:61-64, 1988.

105. Parham D, Weeks D, Beckwith J: The clinicopathologic spectrum of putative extrarenal rhabdoid tumors: An analysis of 42 cases studied with immunohistochemistry or electron microscopy. Am J Surg Pathol 18:1010-1029, 1994.

106. Heaton G, Matthews T, Christopherson W: Malignant trophoblastic tumors with massive hemorrhage presenting as liver primary: A report of two cases. Am J Surg Pathol 10:342-347, 1986.

107. Gresham G, Rue L: Squamous cell carcinoma of the liver. Hum Pathol 16:413-416, 1985.

108. Nelson V, Fernandes NF, Woolf GM, et al: Primary liposarcoma of the liver: A case report and review of literature. Arch Pathol Lab Med 125:410-412, 2001.

Index

Note: Page numbers followed by f indicate figures; those followed by t indicate tables; those followed by b indicate boxed material.